a

Pediatric Primary Care

A Handbook for Nurse Practitioners

Pediatric Primary Care

A Handbook for Nurse Practitioners

3rd Edition

Catherine E. Burns, PhD, RN, CPNP, FAAN
Professor Emeritus
Primary Health Care Nurse Practitioner Specialty
Oregon Health Science University School of Nursing
Portland, Oregon

Ardys M. Dunn, PhD, RN, PNP
Associate Professor, Retired
University of Portland School of Nursing
Portland, Oregon

Margaret A. Brady, PhD, RN, CPNP
Professor
California State University Long Beach
Department of Nursing
Pediatric Nurse Practitioner
Miller Children's Hospital
Long Beach, California

Nancy Barber Starr, MS, RN, CPNP
Pediatric Nurse Practitioner
Aurora Pediatric Associates
Aurora, Colorado

Catherine G. Blosser, MPA:HA, RN, CPNP
Pediatric Nurse Practitioner
Multnomah County Health Department
Portland, Oregon

SAUNDERS
An Imprint of Elsevier

SAUNDERS
An Imprint of Elsevier

11830 Westline Industrial Drive
St. Louis, Missouri 63146

Pediatric Primary Care: A Handbook for Nurse Practitioners
ISBN 0-7216-0185-5

NOTICE

Nursing is an ever-changing field. Standard safety precautions must be followed, but as new research and clinical experience broaden our knowledge, changes in treatment and drug therapy may become necessary or appropriate. Readers are advised to check the most current product information provided by the manufacturer of each drug to be administered to verify the recommended dose, the method and duration of administration, and contraindications. It is the responsibility of the licensed prescriber, relying on experience and knowledge of the patient, to determine dosages and the best treatment for each individual patient. Neither the publisher nor the author assumes any liability for any injury and/or damage to persons or property arising from this publication.

Previous editions copyrighted 2000, 1996

International Standard Book Number 0-7216-0185-5

Vice President, Nursing and Health Professions: Sally Schrefer
Executive Publisher, Nursing: Barbara Nelson Cullen
Acquisitions Editor: Sandra Clark Brown
Senior Developmental Editor: Cindi Anderson
Publishing Services Manager: Catherine Jackson
Senior Project Manager: Jeff Patterson
Designer: Kathi Gosche

Printed in the United States of America

Last digit is the print number: 9 8 7 6 5 4 3 2 1

The Child's Name is Today

We are guilty of many errors and faults,
but our worst crime is abandoning the children,
neglecting the fountain of life.
Many of the things we need can wait.
The child cannot.
Right now is the time his bones are being formed,
his blood is being made,
and his senses are being developed.
To him we cannot answer, "Tomorrow".
His name is "Today".

Gabriela Mistral (1889-1957) 1945
Nobel Laureate in Literature, Chile

This book is dedicated to the infants, children, and adolescents
and their families about whom the book was written,
wishing them health, loving support,
and happiness,
the real goals of this book.

Contributors

Constance Blair Brehm, PhD, RN, CFNP
Associate Professor
School of Nursing
Azusa Pacific University
Azusa, California
Chapter 40: Common Injuries

Barbara Jones Deloian, PhD, RN, CPNP
Pediatric Nurse Practitioner
Professor, Adjunct, UCHSC, School of Nursing
Clinical Instructor, UCHSC, School of Medicine, Department of Pediatrics
The Children's Hospital, Child Development Unit
University of Colorado Health Sciences Center, JFK Partners
Denver, Colorado
Chapter 5: Developmental Management in Pediatric Primary Care
Chapter 6: Developmental Management of Infants
Chapter 8: Developmental Management of School-Age Children (with Bonnie Gance-Cleveland)

Judith W. Fisher, RN, MHS, FNP
Lead Nurse Practitioner for Adolescent Health
School-Based Health Care Program
Multnomah County Health Department
Portland, Oregon
Chapter 9: Developmental Management of Adolescents

Bonnie Gance-Cleveland, PhD, RNC, PNP
Associate Professor
University of Arkansas for Medical Sciences
Director of Nursing Research
Arkansas Children's Hospital
Little Rock, Arkansas
Chapter 8: Developmental Management of School-Age Children (with Barbara Jones Deloian)

Nan M. Gaylord, PhD, RN, CPNP
Assistant Professor
Coordinator, Nursing of Women and Children Graduate Track
College of Nursing
University of Tennessee
Knoxville, Tennessee
Chapter 35: Genitourinary Disorders

Catherine J. Goodhue, NM, RN, CPNP
Clinical Instructor, Graduate Nursing
School of Nursing
Azusa Pacific University
Azusa, California;
Pediatric Nurse Practitioner
Division of Clinical Immunology and Allergy
Childrens Hospital of Los Angeles
Los Angeles, California
Chapter 25: Atopic Disorders and Rheumatic Diseases
Chapter 32: Respiratory Disorders

Steven Goodstein, MS, MT, (ASCP)
Assistant Professor
Department of Pathology
Oregon Health and Science University
Portland, Oregon
Appendix C: Normal Laboratory Values

Kevin J. Hale, DDS
Adjunct Clinical Assistant Professor
Department of Pediatric Dentistry
University of Michigan
Ann Arbor, Michigan;
Private Practice, Pediatric Dentistry
Brighton, Michigan
Chapter 34: Dental and Oral Diseases (with Charles Poland)

Denise A. Hall, BS, ACMPE (Nominee)
Practice Administrator
Aurora Pediatric Associates
Aurora, Colorado
Chapter 44: Practice Management Strategies for a Health Care Practice

Pamela J. Hellings, RN, PhD, CPNP
Professor Emerita
Oregon Health & Science University School of Nursing
Portland, Oregon
Chapter 13: Breastfeeding
Chapter 41: Genetic Disorders

Gail M. Houck, RN, PhD, PMHNP
Professor and Program Director
Academic Graduate & Interdisciplinary Programs
Oregon Health & Science University
Portland, Oregon
Chapter 21: Coping and Stress Tolerance

Janie Huff-Slankard, MSN, RN, CPNP
Pediatric Nurse Practitioner
Calcagno Pediatrics
Gresham, Oregon
Chapter 1: Child Health Status in the United States

Sheila M. Kodadek, PhD, RN
Professor, Child, Adolescent, and Family Nursing
School of Nursing
Oregon Health & Science University
Portland, Oregon,
Chapter 3: Family Assessment in Pediatric Primary Care

Linda M. Kollar, RN, MSN
Director of Clinical Services
Division of Adolescent Medicine
Cincinnati Children's Hospital Medical Center
Cincinnati, Ohio
Chapter 36: Gynecologic Conditions

Mary A. Murphy, PhD, CPNP
Senior Instructor
Department of Pediatrics
University of Colorado School of Medicine
Development Management of Infants, Toddlers, Preschoolers, and School Age Children
Denver, Colorado
Chapter 7: Developmental Management of Toddlers and Preschoolers
Chapter 5: Developmental Management in Pediatric Primary Care

Deborah K. Parks, RN, DSN, PNP
Boston & Hughes, P.C.
Houston, Texas
Chapter 39: Perinatal Conditions (with Robert Yetman)

Ann Marie Petersen-Smith, MS, RN, CPNP
Pediatric Nurse Practitioner
Emergency Department
The Children's Hospital
Denver, Colorado
Chapter 30: Ear Disorders
Chapter 33: Gastrointestinal Disorders

Charles Poland III, DDS
Associate Professor, Pediatric Dentistry
Indiana University School of Dentistry
Private Practice, Pediatric Dentistry
Indianapolis, Indiana
Chapter 34: Dental and Oral Diseases (with Kevin Hale)

Jean Betschart Roemer, MN, MSN, CPNP, CDE
Pediatric Nurse Practitioner
University of Pittsburgh
Children's Hospital of Pittsburgh
Pittsburgh, Pennsylvania
Chapter 26: Endocrine and Metabolic Diseases

Kathleen Shelton, PNP, PhD
Training Director, LEND Project
Child Development & Rehabilitation Center
Portland, Oregon
Chapter 17: Cognitive-Perceptual Patterns

Martha K. Swartz, PhD (c), APRN, BC, PNP
Associate Professor and Director, PNP Specialty
Yale University School of Nursing
New Haven, Connecticut
Chapter 27: Hematologic Diseases

Peggy Vernon, RN, MA, CPNP
Nurse Practitioner
Aurora/Parker Skin Care Center
Instructor
Regis University
University of Colorado
Denver, Colorado
Chapter 37: Dermatologic Diseases

Teri Moser Woo, RN, MS, CPNP
Instructor
School of Nursing
University of Portland
Portland, Oregon
Appendix A: Medications

Robert J. Yetman, MD
Professor of Pediatrics: Director, Division of Community and General Pediatrics
Department of Pediatrics
University of Texas-Houston Medical School
Houston, Texas
Chapter 39: Perinatal Conditions (with Deborah Parks)

Preface

We are delighted to introduce the third edition of *Pediatric Primary Care: A Handbook for Nurse Practitioners.* As with the first and second editions, this book is designed for advanced practice nurses serving the primary health care needs of infants, children, and adolescents. Pediatric nurse practitioners (PNPs) and family nurse practitioners are anticipated to be our primary audience, but pediatricians, family physicians, pediatric clinical nurse specialists, community health nurses, pediatric ambulatory care nurses, school nurses, and other primary care providers should also find the book to be a valuable resource. Our goal has been to provide a textbook for nurse practitioner students as well as a handbook for clinicians. Feedback from our readers over the past several years indicates that we achieved our goal: both students and experienced clinicians find *Pediatric Primary Care* to be a key resource for their work and study.

Each of the authors brings a special perspective to the subject of pediatric primary health care: nurse practitioner educators, practicing PNPs, and a PNP with long experience working in and teaching community health. Each author has unique areas of expertise—development, nursing theory, cultural competence, and extensive experience with a variety of health care problems. Several other specialists have been invited to contribute to the work. Some have continued from the previous two editions, whereas other contributing authors are new.

ORGANIZATION OF THE BOOK

After four introductory chapters that discuss child health issues and assessment of children in the context of their families and cultures, the book is organized into four major sections—Introduction to Primary Care, Development, Functional Health Patterns, and Diseases. Some features of the third edition that we are excited about include the following:

- Color figures of some important ear, skin, and dental pathologies to help with diagnosis
- A new chapter on practice management, an area of increasing concern and interest for clinicians
- An updated chapter on infectious diseases that addresses helminthic zoonoses, new viruses, and agents of bioterrorism, including clinical features for diagnosis and management
- An extensive table of current medications used in pediatric primary care
- More tables to facilitate differential diagnosis of related conditions or conditions that have some common elements
- More tables to summarize management strategies for common conditions
- Resource boxes at the end of chapters that include websites to access organizations and printed materials that may be useful for clinicians and their clients
- Improved formatting of the text to make it even easier to read

Every chapter has been updated to bring the most current information available to the reader.

We have maintained key features that have made the first two editions so successful:

- An assessment chapter that emphasizes a holistic approach, including identification of both medical and nursing problems
- Attention to family and cultural factors
- Emphasis on prevention and management of problems from the PNP's point of view and scope of practice
- Explicit reference to *Healthy People 2010* guidelines (U.S. Department of Health and Human Services [USDHHS], 2000), *Bright Futures, Guidelines for Adolescent Preventive Services (GAPS)* (Elster and Kuznets, 1994), nurse practitioner competencies, and practice guidelines from the U.S. Preventive Services Task Force, the American Academy of Pediatrics, and others
- Introduction of key concepts and foundations for care in a narrative format followed by identification and management of diagnoses discussed using an outline format
- Organization of information into tables and appendices for quick access and efficient use by working nurse practitioners and nurses
- Selection of an expanded list of common medical and nursing diagnoses that are managed by primary care providers in practice

The authors assume that the reader has a baccalaureate degree in nursing and advanced course work in physiology, child development, health assessment, pharmacology, and family systems. Thus this book guides clinical application of concepts important to the nursing specialty, primary health care of children and their families.

Introductory Section

Chapter 1 begins with a review of the major morbidity and mortality statistics highlighting the health problems of children in the United States. The chapter then identifies the important goals for health care of children and describes several sets of current guidelines and standards designed to safeguard primary care of the nation's children. Working with managed care organizations is discussed. Chapter 2 presents the health assessment of the child, including both history and physical examination data. The chapter uses a model that supports identification and management of development, functional health patterns, and disease problems. Chapters 3 and 4 highlight important family and cultural components of care to be incorporated into the assessment and management plans for all clients.

Development Section

The development section includes five chapters—an introduction to development for primary care and chapters on infants, toddlers and preschoolers, school-age children, and adolescents. Each chapter begins with a review of the major developmental theories used to understand children in the particular age group. The assessment of developmental needs of children in primary care is then reviewed. Topics for discussion with parents are outlined. Several important developmental issues for each age group are discussed from a problem-oriented perspective. Application of principles of child development to primary care is the key feature for these chapters. Red flags are described to alert the NP about key developmental problem indicators.

Functional Health Patterns Section

Functional health patterns (Gordon, 1987) serve as the organizational framework of this section. Eleven patterns are common to people of all cultures and ages. The first seven chapters provide a platform for discussing health promotion through the various components of healthy living—health maintenance, nutrition, breast-feeding, elimination, sleep, and activity and sports participation. The remaining functional health pattern chapters are more psychosocial in nature—self-perception; role relationships where issues of child abuse are addressed; coping and stress tolerance to explore mental health problems of children; cognitive/perceptual patterns to discuss attention deficit/hyperactivity disorder and problems of blindness, deafness, and autism; sexuality; and values and beliefs. In all of these chapters, foundations of psychology and the basic sciences are first introduced and then applied to common problems of children. North American Nursing Diagnosis Association (NANDA) nursing diagnoses related to the respective health pattern are identified in boxes near the end of each chapter. Normative behaviors are discussed, and the assessment process is reviewed. Current guidelines or standards for care and management strategies with which the clinician should be familiar are identified. Common problems of each pattern are presented with the aid of a problem-oriented framework.

Diseases Section

The section of the book related to diseases is organized with a chapter for each of the main components of the *International Classification of Diseases*, 22 chapters in all. This section begins with an introductory chapter that outlines approaches to diseases and their management. The infectious diseases chapter then reviews key communicable diseases and includes a comprehensive subsection on immunizations. A major set of chapters focuses on principal body systems, with additional chapters devoted to neonatology, genetics, and uncomplicated trauma. An environmental health chapter discusses these emerging important issues. A chapter on complementary therapies promotes PNPs' knowledge about many of the less traditional health care strategies that families may be using.

Each chapter follows the same format throughout, standards and guidelines for care are highlighted, the physiologic and assessment parameters are discussed, management strategies are identified, and management of common problems is presented in a problem-oriented format. Each disease or condition is explained as follows:

- Description
- Etiology and incidence
- Clinical findings (history, physical examination, laboratory and other studies)
- Differential diagnosis
- Management
- Complications
- Preventive and patient education measures

Tables highlight and summarize differential diagnoses, management, and other pertinent information. The scope of practice of the nurse practitioner is always kept in mind with appropriate referral and consultation points identified. At the end of many chapters, useful resources are listed, such as national organizations for various disorders.

Practice Management Section

A new chapter on practice management has been included in this edition. In the current health care marketplace, it is increasingly important that the nurse practitioner be aware of issues of productivity, compliance with state and federal laws, quality-of-care indicators, and successful business practices that will ensure viability.

Appendices

The appendices include sections on common drugs used in pediatric primary care settings, growth parameters, laboratory data, and *Healthy People 2010* standards related to children. The appendices are designed for easy access to reference data.

Summary

This book is written by and for nurse practitioners interested in the primary health care of children. It provides a comprehensive resource for students and serves as a reference for practicing clinicians. The book is conceptually organized around domains of interest to PNPs—development; functional health patterns related to health maintenance and psychosocial well-being of children and their families; and diseases of children that require intervention, monitoring, and/or referral. The book uses a problem-oriented focus consistent with the education of PNPs and has been written using the latest standards and guidelines available. Content is consistent with the major recommendations for primary care of children in the United States. We are delighted to bring forward a third edition of this much-needed resource for nurse practitioners who work with and for children.

Catherine E. Burns, PhD, RN, CPNP, FAAN

Ardys M. Dunn, PhD, RN, PNP

Margaret A. Brady, PhD, RN, CPNP

Nancy Barber Starr, MS, RN, CPNP

Catherine G. Blosser, MPA:HA, RN, CPNP

REFERENCES

Elster A, Kuznets N: *AMA Guidelines for Adolescent Preventive Services (GAPS)*, Baltimore, 1994, Williams & Wilkins.

Gordon M: *Nursing diagnosis: process and application*, New York, 1987, McGraw-Hill.

US Department of Health and Human Services: *Healthy People 2010: understanding and improving health*, ed 2, Washington, DC, 2000, US Government Printing Office.

Acknowledgments

A book of this size and complexity could never have been completed without considerable help—the work of the contributors who researched, wrote, and revised content; the consultation and review of experts in various specialties who critiqued drafts and provided important perspectives and guidance; and the essential technical support from those who managed the production of the manuscript and the final product. Another kind of help came from family and friends who offered unending support and encouragement for the duration of the project. We are indebted to so many people and want to say thanks to them all. The following are some of the many people we want to acknowledge.

CONTRIBUTORS TO THE SECOND EDITION

These people were instrumental in helping us develop the second edition of the book. Although they are not authors in this edition, their ideas and work have contributed greatly to our work, and we are deeply indebted to them:
Patricia Billings, CPNP
Melanie Canady, CPNP
Natalie Cheffer, PNP
Jeffrey Dean, DDS
Connie Evers, RD
Diane Montgomery, CPNP
Linda Wildey

Technical Support

Janie Huff-Slankard, PNP, Portland, Oregon

Family And Friends

Jerry and Jennifer Burns; Jill, Cory, and Alyssa Nordstrom; and in memory of my parents, Leslie and Frances Meyer. *Catherine E. Burns*

Marvin, Malcolm, and Philip Dunn; Liz Flynn; and other family and friends. *Ardys M. Dunn*

Mary, Martha, Greg, and Katie, and other family and friends. *Margaret A. Brady*

Jon and Jonah and AnnaMei Starr, my APA colleagues, and in memory of Janet Barber. *Nancy Barber Starr*

Terry Dolan, family, and in memory of my father, John A. Blosser. *Catherine G. Blosser*

Contents

UNIT 1

Pediatric Primary Care Foundations

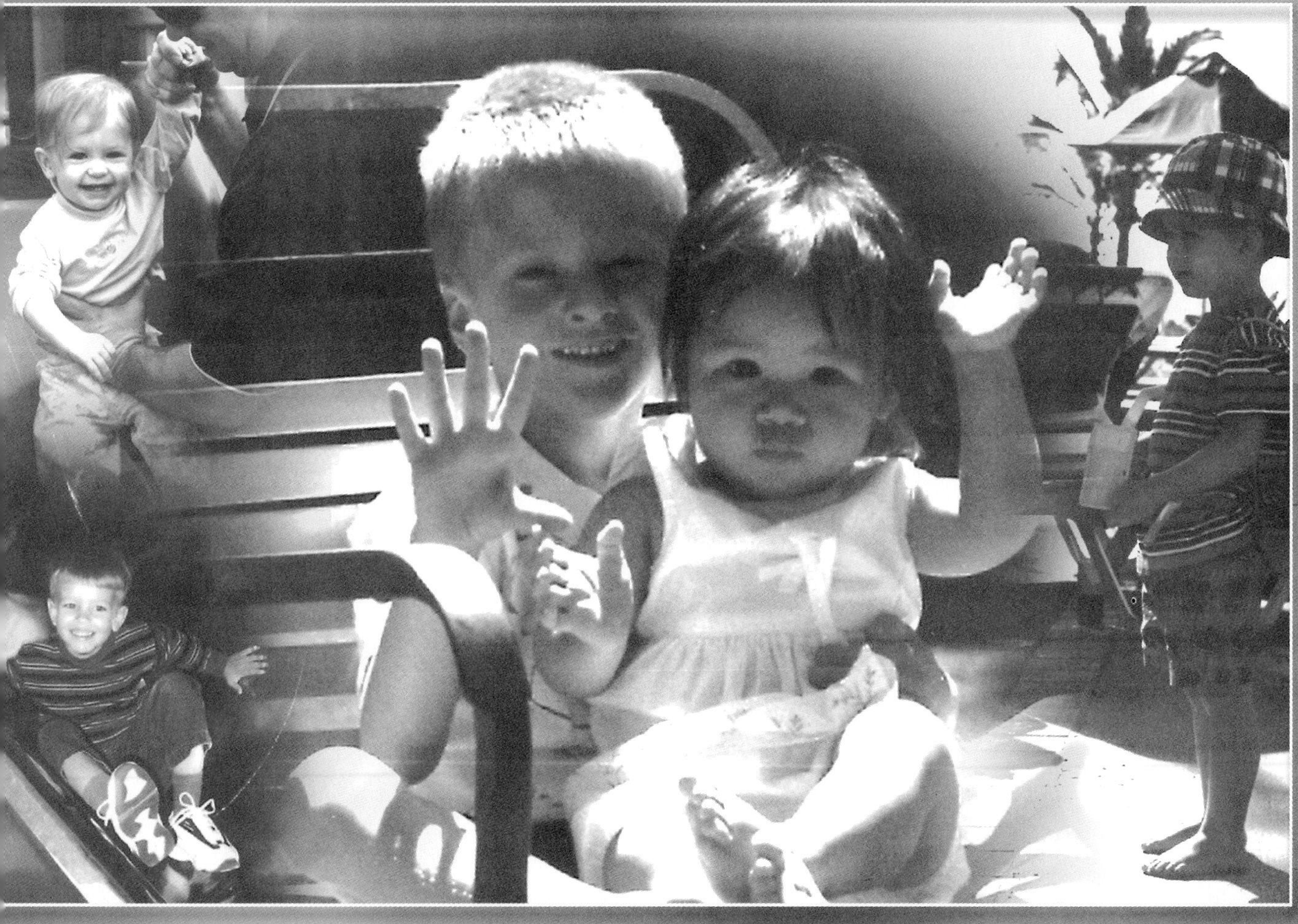

1 Child Health Status in the United States

Catherine E. Burns, Janie Huff-Slankard

America's children represent the future of the country. Society has given the families of those children responsibility for raising them in loving and stable homes in the belief that nurtured, healthy children will be productive citizens and leaders for coming generations. Far too many children, however, are growing up without the benefits of families with adequate resources. Millions of children grow up hungry, neglected, abused, living in unsafe environments, and receiving inadequate education. The nation's commitment to children should involve providing for them directly, as well as ensuring opportunities for families to be successful in their child-rearing efforts. Primary health care providers have unique opportunities to be involved with families and children as they work to solve the problems of living to achieve and maintain hopeful, fulfilled lives.

This book describes the health of children and their families, their development, their health problems, and their health care. This chapter presents the status of children's health in America. Standards and guidelines for health care of children are identified because they represent the goals to be achieved. The role of the nurse practitioner (NP) in the delivery of health care is defined. Children need to be healthy if they are to achieve their maximum potential as productive, happy people.

CHILD HEALTH STATUS IN AMERICA

Morbidity and Mortality Data on Children

In 2000, 86 million children through age 21 represented 31.2% of the total population. Adolescents currently make up almost 40 million of these youth (U.S. Department of Health and Human Services [USDHHS], 2001). Many indicators are used to measure the health status of children in the United States: low-birth-weight rate, infant mortality rate, child death rate, teen death rate, and teen birth rate. Other indicators include the violent crime arrest rate, the percentage of teens who are high school dropouts, and the percentage of children who live in poverty or single-parent households. A variety of these indicators are discussed in this book. If health care providers are to substantially influence the health of children, they need to understand child health risks and primary sources of disease and death among children. Furthermore, the government and major professional organizations have established goals for health care and guidelines to provide preventive care efficiently and effectively. Providers need to adopt these goals for their own practices.

Infant Mortality Rate (0 to 12 months)

The 2000 infant death rate in the United States fell to an all-time low of 6.9 per 1000 live births (Hoyert et al, 2001). In Healthy *People 2010: National Health Promotion and Disease Prevention Objectives for the Year 2010*, the infant death rate goal for the year 2010 is 4.5 per 1000 live births (USDHHS, 2000). Despite the good news of 2000 and a downward trend over many years, some striking disparities can be noted. Infant mortality rates continue to be different for blacks and whites. Based on preliminary data of 1998-1999, infants of black mothers were 2.5 times more likely to die than were infants of white mothers (USDHHS, 2001). Although the child poverty rate in 1999 was the lowest since 1979, infants born into poor families are 50% more likely to die than children born into families with incomes above the poverty line (Annie E. Casey Foundation, 2001). See Fig. 1-1 for infant mortality rates.

In 1997 the United States ranked twenty-seventh in infant mortality rate, behind such places as the Czech Republic, Portugal, Greece, and Cuba (USDHHS, 2001). Congenital malformations, shorter gestation and its consequent disorders, sudden infant death syndrome (SIDS), and

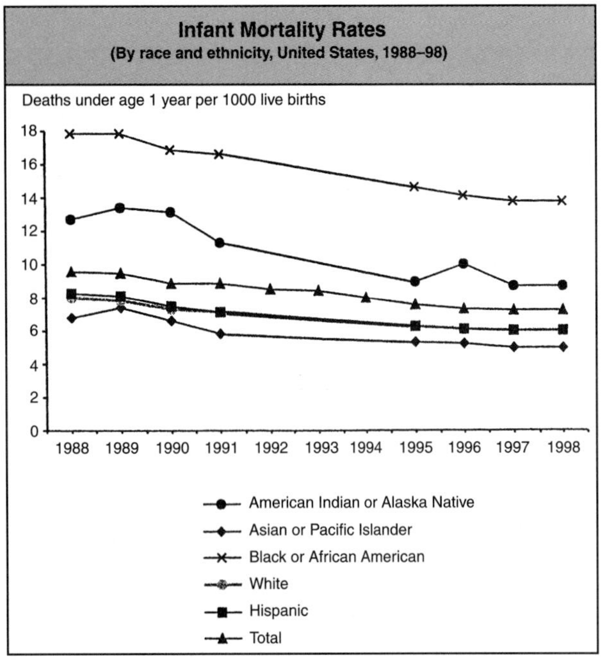

FIGURE 1-1 Infant mortality rates. Data for 1998 are preliminary; 1992-1994 linked live birth–infant death files are not available. *Note*: Data for white and Hispanic overlap from 1991 to 1998. (Data from US Department of Health and Human Services: *Healthy people 2010: understanding and improving health*, ed 2, Washington, DC, 2000, US Government Printing Office.)

maternal complications are the leading causes of infant mortality. Even though SIDS continues to rank high in infant mortality, deaths from SIDS have decreased by 21% since the "back to sleep" recommendation from the American Academy of Pediatrics in 1992. Although unintentional injury still ranks seventh in cause of death in infants, deaths have decreased by 4.7% from 1999 (Hoyert et al, 2001).

Infant Health and Morbidity

Of all live births in 2000, 7.6% had low birth weight (1500 to 2499 g). The proportion of low-birth-weight babies has not changed significantly since the 1970s, due partially to an increased rate of multiple births. Low birth weight continues to be one of the four leading causes of infant death. Infants in the low-birth-weight category have a 6 times higher risk of death before their first birthday. Of these, infants weighing less than 1500 g have a 96 times higher risk of death than do babies having a normal birth weight (Hoyert et al, 2001). Black infants are twice as likely to be low birth weight as white infants (Children's Defense Fund, 2002).

Teen birth rates are important to assess because teen childbearing diminishes the life opportunities of both child and mother, significantly more so if the teenager has two or more children. Four of five teen births are to first-time young mothers. In 2000 the birth rate for teenagers age 15 to 19 years declined to a record low of 48.7 per 1000, and the overall rates for teenagers, regardless of age, have declined from 1999 to 2000. The live birth rate for teens age 10 to 14 was 0.9 per 1000; 27.5 per 1000 for those age 15 to 17 years, a historic low rate for this age-group; and 79.5 per 1000 for those 18 to 19 years old.

Race and ethnic origin continue to be factors in the teen birth rate. In 2000, the rate for black teen mothers 15 to 19 years old was high (79.2 per 1000). However, here again, there was a dramatic fall in teen birth rates in black teens age 15 to 17 (50.2 per 1000). On the other hand, the rate for Hispanic teens has not decreased significantly for any age-group since 1991. Birth rates for teens by age, race, and Hispanic origin can be seen in Fig. 1-2 (Hoyert et al, 2001).

Child Mortality Rate (1 to 12 years)

Injuries are important to assess in pediatric populations because they account for so much of the total mortality and morbidity statistics for children. Injuries are classified as unintentional (such as burns and falls) or intentional (homicides and suicides). Unintentional injuries to young infants are most often due to burns, drowning, and falls. Poisonings are added to the list when infants gain mobility.

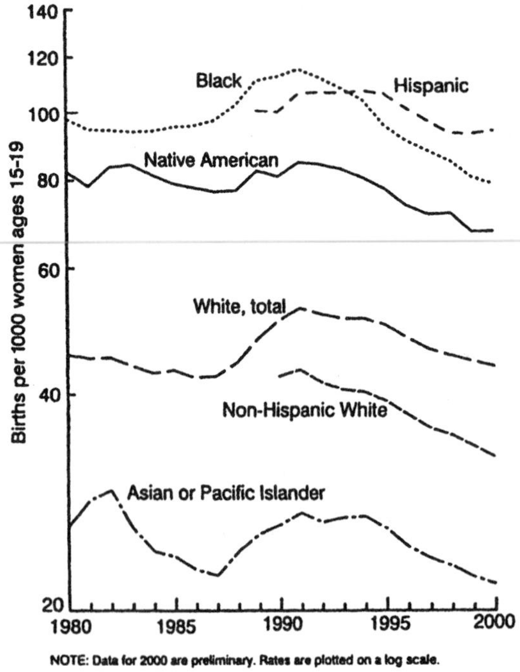

FIGURE 1-2 Teen birth rates by race. (From Hoyert D et al: Annual summary of vital statistics: 2000, *Pediatrics* 108:1241, 2001.)

In 2000 the overall death rates decreased 6% for 1- to 4-year-olds, 5% for 5- to 9-year-olds, and 3% for 10- to 19-year-olds. Depending on the age-group, from 36% to 48.8% of child deaths resulted from unintentional injuries. Of all age-groups, the highest death rate from unintentional injuries was for 15- to 19-year-olds and is believed to be a result of increased motor vehicle accidents. Homicides have decreased in all age-groups, as have the numbers of deaths from diseases of the heart. One of the more disturbing statistics is a 25% increase in intentional self-harm among 10- to 14-year-olds (Hoyert et al, 2001). See Table 1-1 for leading causes of death in children and adolescents.

Child Health and Morbidity

Morbidity and health of children can be measured by chronic health conditions and children with special health care needs. Unfortunately, no recent statistics have been gathered for these children, but beginning in 2002, national surveys were initiated to collect data for this population in an effort to determine need for services and status of these children (USDHHS, 2001).

General health status of children is measured in many ways. Morbidity and mortality rates are relatively easy to figure statistically, as are immunization rates. The measurement of parents' perception of their child's health is another indicator of child health. In 2000 parents reported that 82% of children were in very good or excellent health. Unfortunately, living below the poverty level also is shown to affect health status. Only 70% of parents living in poverty reported their child's health to be very good or excellent. Race also has shown a difference with fewer black and Hispanic parents reporting very good or excellent health of their children.

In 2000 chronic health conditions limited children's activities in 7% of children 5 to 17 years of age. In children less than 5 years of age, that number was only 3%, but the disparity between statistics may be related to the fact that children are less likely to have been diagnosed with a chronic condition until they are of school age (America's Children, 2002).

Childhood morbidity is also measured by injury statistics, which include bicycle injuries, motor vehicle accidents, playground accidents, and poisonings. Motor vehicle accident injuries rise in relation to age with 35% among 1- to 4-year-olds, 56% among 5- to 9-year-olds, and 63% among 10- to 14-year-olds (Centers for Disease Control and Prevention [CDC], 2002). Serious head injuries and brain injuries from not wearing bicycle helmets contribute significantly to the morbidity of children. Recent estimates indicate that only 25% of children 5 to 14 years old wear a helmet, and the percentage drops to 15% when looking at teenagers in high school (Youth Risk Behavior Surveillance, 2002). The *Healthy People 2010* goal is to increase this number to 50% in teenagers in grades 9 to 12 (USDHHS, 2000). Poison exposures and poisonings numbered 2 million, 52.7% of which were among children younger than 6 years old (Litovitz et al, 2001). Playground injuries account for 200,000 emergency department visits annually with an estimated cost of $1.2 billion; 35% of these injuries are considered serious (fractures, dislocations, concussions, amputations) (CDC, *www.cdc.gov/ncipc/factsheets/playgr.htm*, 2002).

Adolescent Mortality Rate (13 to 19 Years)

Adolescent (13 to 19 years old) death rates have continued to decline since 1990. In 1999, 69.8 deaths per 100,000 were reported. Of these, over 50% were related to injuries. Seventy percent of mortality is related to seven risk-taking behaviors (Brindes et al, 2002):

- Drug and alcohol use
- Unsafe sexual behaviors
- Violence
- Injury-related behaviors
- Tobacco use
- Decreased physical activity
- Poor dietary habits

TABLE 1-1 ***Leading Causes of Death in Children and Adolescents***

Rank	Ages 1-4	Ages 5-9	Ages 10-14	Ages 15-19
1	Unintentional injury, 36%	Unintentional injury, 41%	Unintentional injury, 37.7%	Unintentional injury, 48.8%
2	Congenital malformation, 9.5%	Malignant neoplasm, 15.4%	Malignant neoplasm, 12.6%	Homicide, 13.8%
3	Malignant neoplasm, 8%	Congenital anomaly, 6.1%	Suicide, 7.2%	Suicide, 11.7%
4	Homicide, 6.4%	Homicide, 4.4%	Homicide, 5.4%	Malignant neoplasm, 5.4%
5	Heart disease, 3.4%	Heart disease, 3.1%	Congenital anomaly, 4.6%	Heart disease, 2.8%

From US Department of Health and Human Services: *Healthy people 2010: understanding and improving health,* ed 2, Washington, DC, 2000, US Government Printing Office.

Motor vehicle traffic injuries increased to 53%, whereas firearm-related homicides (8.6%) and firearm-related suicides (4.9%) decreased. Disparities continue when the data are analyzed by race and ethnicity. Firearm-related homicide was highest in the black population, at 57% of these homicides, and lowest for whites, at 2.9%. Firearm-related suicide was highest in Alaska Native/American Indian youth, at 18.7%, and lowest in Hispanic youth, at 5.6%. Cancer, heart disease, and birth defects account for the remainder of adolescent mortality (America's Children, 2002).

Adolescent Health and Morbidity

Education has always been a key predictor for health and life outcomes. Despite the importance of education, 1.5 million teens (age 16 to 19 years) were not in school or had not graduated from high school in 1999. Although the 10% dropout rate was unchanged from 1990 to 1999, the rate fell in 24 states, rose in 15 states and was unchanged in 11 states (Annie E. Casey Foundation, 2002). In 1999 the percentage of adolescents in the United States not in school, working, in the military, or defining themselves as homemakers ranged from 4% in Iowa, Minnesota, and Nebraska to 15% in the District of Columbia (Annie E. Casey Foundation, 2002). The juvenile violent crime arrest rates increased 70% from 1986 to 1991 but declined 12% in 1995 and 1996. Youths arrested in 1999 numbered 1.7 million. Of those incarcerated in prisons, 20% ($n = 236$) were held in adult facilities. Although victimization of children is highest in the younger population, 5.9 per 1000 among 16- to 17-year-olds still represents significant morbidity in this age-group (USDHHS, 2001).

Some adolescents face additional health risks. Brindes and associates (2002) have identified some key factors that contribute to teen morbidity: chronic physical or mental conditions; foster or group home care; undocumented, migrant, or new immigrant status; homelessness; incarceration; pregnancy; parenting; and poverty.

The Youth Risk Behavior Survey, which monitors six major health risk behaviors in the U.S. population that are related to the *Healthy People 2010* goals, queries students in grades 9 to 12 annually. Results from 2001 provide a picture of the health issues of these adolescents. Because the survey is administered annually, trends can be identified. Between 1991 and 2001, here are some of the key findings (Youth Risk Behavior Surveillance, 2002):

- Significant *decreases* occurred in teens who
  - Never or rarely wore a seatbelt (25% to 14%)
  - Participated in a physical fight (42% to 33%)
  - Seriously considered suicide (29% to 19%)
  - Planned and attempted suicide (19% to 15%)
  - Carried a weapon (26% to 17%)
  - Had sexual intercourse with more than four partners (54% to 46% males and 19% to 14% females)
  - Reported current cigarette smoking (decreases from 1997 to 2001, from 36.4% in males and 16.7% in females to 29% in males and 14% in females)
  - Reported enrollment in daily physical education classes (42% to 32%)
- Significant *increases* occurred in teens who
  - Reported lifetime and current marijuana use (increases from 1991 to 1997 and decreases from 1997 to 2001 with overall changes of 31% to 42% in males and 15% to 24% in females)
  - Reported lifetime and current cocaine use (6% to 9% in males and 2% to 4% in females)
  - Used a condom at last sexual intercourse (46% to 58%)

In 1999 chlamydia was the most common sexually transmitted infection (STI) in adolescents, while gonorrhea and syphilis rates declined. Although antibiotics are effective in treating STIs, significant morbidity from pelvic inflammatory disease and infertility continue to affect the untreated victims (USDHHS, 2001).

Three hundred twelve new cases of acquired immunodeficiency syndrome (AIDS) were reported in 1999 among 13- to 19-year-olds (USDHHS, 2001). The number of AIDS cases reported among adolescents (13- to 19-year-olds) and young adults has risen steadily since 1981(Leslie, Sarah, & Palfrey, 1998). Although the number of newly diagnosed young adults with AIDS decreased by 10% from 1999 to 2000, 46% of those patients were in the 13- to 19-year-old adolescent population (USDHHS, 2001).

Fifty-eight percent of the total population with AIDS are men and 42% are women. White adolescents represent 29% of those cases, 57% of whom were exposed through blood transfusions or clotting factor for hemophilia and 19% through male-to-male sexual contact. However, only 6.4% of the newly reported cases among adolescents in 1999 identified acquisition of the virus through clotting factor and hemophilia. Thus, this source of infection now seems controlled. Forty-nine percent of adolescent AIDS cases were among black non-Hispanics; 35% were infected through heterosexual contact and 24% through male-to-male sexual contact. Forty-two percent of adolescent AIDS cases were among females, with 40% of them infected through heterosexual contact and 15% through injecting drugs (USDHHS, 2001).

Immunizations

The U.S. government monitors immunization levels across the country through the National Immunization Survey. Data on the 2001 immunization rates for completion of the combined 4:3:1:3 series (4 diptheria/tetanus/pertussis [DTaP/DT/DTP] vaccine, 3 polio vaccine, 1 of any measles/mumps/rubella [MMR] vaccine, 3 *Haemophilus influenzae* B [HIB] vaccine) revealed a 71% vaccination level, up from 1997. The highest level of compliance was reported in Massachusetts at 80.1% and the lowest in New Mexico at 58.9% (CDC, *www.cdc.gov/nip/coverage/NIS/01/TAB9-24months_iap.xls*, 2001). Race and ethnicity continue to affect rates of immunization, with white non-Hispanics at 79%, Hispanics at 73%, and blacks at 71%. Poverty level rates remained stable. Varicella coverage increased from 58% in 1999 to 68% in 2000, with gains in all ethnic and racial groups (USDHHS, 2001).

Social Factors Influencing Child Health

Child well-being is directly linked to the poverty status of the family. The United States currently ranks seventeenth of 17 developed countries in the proportion of children living in poverty. Among industrialized nations, only Russia ranks lower than the United States in the child poverty rate. The U.S. child poverty rate in 2001 was 16.1% (Annie E. Casey Foundation, 2002). Children in poverty have higher mortality rates, poorer health at birth, poorer growth, and more physical morbidity from respiratory infections, gastrointestinal infections, wheezing, failure to thrive, anemia, asthma, dental caries, otitis media, and visual loss. They also have higher accident rates and more psychologic and developmental disorders.

Fifty-seven per cent of the 11.5 million children living in poverty live in homes of single mothers (USDHHS, 2001). The percentage of births to single mothers seems to have stabilized over the past 5 years. Interestingly, stepchildren living in married-couple families have the same negative child outcomes as children in single-parent families (Annie E. Casey Foundation, 2002). A record number of children were in foster care in 1999, although the number adopted from foster care increased (Children's Defense Fund, 2002).

Access to Health Care

Measurement of health status includes access to health care. Twelve percent, or 8.4 million children, in 2000 had no health care insurance at any time during the year as compared with 13% in 1999. By race, 75% of Hispanic children, 87% of black children, and 93% of white children were covered by health insurance at one time or another in 2000 (America's Children, 2002). Almost 25% of children living in poverty have no health insurance (USDHHS, 2001).

The health status of black and low-income children is worse than that of other children, and they receive the fewest health services of all children. There are 5.8 million children eligible for Medicaid or the Children's Health Insurance Plan (CHIP) (Children's Defense Fund, 2002). The welfare reform legislation enacted federally in 1996 has resulted in significantly fewer children receiving public benefits, a decrease of 28% in the first 2 years. There have also been significant declines in the number of children with Medicaid health insurance, food stamps, and supplemental security income (SSI) coverage if handicapped. The significant increase in uninsured children limits their access to care (Smith et al, 2000).

Access to care is a function of insurance coverage, as well as a function of the area in which one lives. Nearly 43 million people, almost half of them women of childbearing age and children, lived in underserved areas. These settings included both rural and inner-city areas with shortages of physicians and clinics. The recommended number of visits to a health care provider in the first year of life is eight; three visits are recommended in the second year and then yearly visits are recommended until age 6. In 1998, 12% of 5- to 9-year-olds and 6% of 2- to 4-year-olds had not seen a provider in the past year. Hispanic children were twice as likely as white children to have lacked a provider (USDHHS, 2001).

In summary, although the incidence and prevalence rates for many health problems of children have improved over the past several years, there are significant disparities by race, economic status, age of parents, and other factors. Many children lack access to the benefits of the health care available in the United States.

Managed Care Effects on Child Health

The health of U.S. children is significantly affected by the health care delivery system in the communities in which they live. Managed care has become a dominant health care system in most states, although it is less successful economically than first thought. This system was developed in response to excessive, uncontrolled costs of health care. Employers and the government have supported the development of managed care through cost-conscious insurance plans. The main features of managed health care plans are

- Strong incentives for members to obtain care only from selected providers and hospitals that are part of the plan
- Control of access to specialty care, diagnostic tests, and hospitalization
- Shared financial risk among doctors, the health plan, and other health professionals through capitated payments or bonuses and penalties

Whereas the main problem of fee-for-service care was excessive charges, the main problem of managed care may be lack of provision of needed services.

These plans were designed to meet the health needs of working adults. However, in many states, Medicaid clients are also enrolled in managed care plans. Because the health care needs of children are unique, managed care plans need to create benefits packages that meet children's needs. These benefits packages include preventive health care, immunizations, anticipatory guidance, psychosocial counseling, and access to prompt care for acute illnesses. Pediatric specialists need to receive fair reimbursement rates to provide care for children with chronic or disabling conditions and be available providers to children enrolled in managed care plans. Care needs to be coordinated among the home, managed care organization, school, day care, and other service providers. Parents need to be involved in decisions made about their child's health care. Managed care organizations should be accountable for the health care of enrollees and rewarded for improving the health of their pediatric population (David and Lucile Packard Foundation, 1998).

Health care outcomes are difficult to measure. Evidence-based care offering guidance to clinicians for many common conditions and health maintenance has been shown to improve care. Individual clinicians and consumer groups need to be involved with regular quality-of-care reviews and contribute to the criteria by which care is evaluated. The Health Plan Employer Data and Information Set (HEDIS) developed by the National Committee for Quality Assurance is most frequently used as a measure of access and quality services. Most Medicaid and CHIP programs require HEDIS data from participating health care systems to evaluate services to children. HEDIS data include the following:

- Child and adolescent immunization rates
- Treatment for childhood ear infections
- Low-birth-weight babies
- Children's access to primary care providers and dentists
- Annual dental visits
- Availability of language interpretation services
- Well child visits for children and teens

Use of published report cards on these data from all health care systems for children can inform communities about the quality of the services available to their children and families. Patient and family satisfaction is also important to assess regularly; they must be viewed as partners in the health care plan. A variety of evidence-based guidelines for the health care of children are identified later in this chapter.

HEALTH, HEALTH PROMOTION, DISEASE PREVENTION, AND PRIMARY CARE DEFINITIONS

Health, Health Promotion, and Disease Prevention

The American Nurses' Association defines *health* as "a dynamic state of being in which the developmental and behavioral potential of an individual is realized to the fullest extent possible. . . . The presence of illness does not preclude health nor does optimal health preclude illness" (American Nurses' Association, 1995). The process of achieving one's optimal potential is influenced by systems both within and outside the individual, including biologic, cognitive, and emotional systems within the person, as well as the social, economic, and political systems of family, community, race, culture, and country.

Health promotion focuses on moving individuals to actualize their full potential, whereas disease prevention focuses on stabilizing the human organism to resist disease. Health promotion depends on active participation by the client to develop and maintain a lifestyle that maximizes well-being. It cannot be achieved solely by the activities of the primary health care provider, although that person is essential to identify risks, help the individual develop a health promotion plan, offer support and motivation for changing health behavior, and evaluate progress over time. Health promotion activities must also occur at the family, community, and society levels and be guided by primary care providers and health experts who design interventions helpful to groups of people. Fluoride supplementation in water supplies, laws requiring seat belt use, community health fairs, and regulations related to the content of school lunches and clean air standards are examples of broader efforts to promote health and prevent disease.

Primary Care

Primary care includes the following elements: first-contact care, comprehensive care, coordinated or integrated care, and care that is longitudinal rather than episodic. First-contact care is the extent to which a patient contacts the source of care whenever that person perceives a new need for care. Comprehensive means that it includes all the health problems of the individual. Coordination of care entails a health care provider's ability to provide for continuity of information within that provider's practice setting, as well as coordinating specialists' care on behalf of the child and family. Providing longitudinal care refers to the extent to which a provider serves as a source of care over time regardless of the presence of a particular type of problem (U.S. Congress, Office of Technology Assessment, 1991).

A somewhat more recent definition that is widely cited reads as follows:

> Primary care is the provision of integrated, accessible health care services by clinicians who are accountable for addressing a large majority of personal health care needs, developing a sustained partnership with patients, and practicing in the context of family and community (Institute of Medicine, Committee on the Future of Primary Care, 1994).

Primary care must be incorporated into the health care delivery system as a basic tenet; availability of primary care services for all children and families is essential. Primary health care, including minor acute and chronic illness and well-child care, may be provided in traditional offices and clinics but may also be found in settings such as the workplace, schools, churches, child care centers, and mobile units. Primary care should also be incorporated into the work of tertiary care centers—that is, children with serious illnesses also need primary care. Primary care providers include some physicians (internal medicine, family practice, pediatrics, and sometimes obstetrics/gynecology), NPs, and physician assistants.

IMPLEMENTING HEALTH PROMOTION AND DISEASE PREVENTION IN PRACTICE

National Health Goals

In 1990, under the leadership of Dr. Louis Sullivan, then Secretary of Health and Human Services, national health promotion and disease prevention objectives were released in a report called *Healthy People 2000: National Health Promotion and Disease Prevention Objectives for the Year 2000* (USDHHS, 1990). Objectives have now been extended to 2010, including 28 focus areas and 467 objectives within the focus areas (USDHHS, 2000). The major health indicators used to measure goals are found in Box 1-1. The goals are listed in Box 1-2. It is important for primary care providers to understand these goals because they influence practice guidelines and allocation of federal and state resources. They should guide health

BOX 1-1 ***Healthy People 2010 Major Health Indicators***

- Physical activity
- Overweight/obesity
- Tobacco use
- Substance abuse
- Responsible sexual behavior
- Mental health
- Injury and violence
- Environmental quality
- Immunizations
- Access to health care

From US Department of Health and Human Services: *Healthy people 2010: understanding and improving health*, ed 2, Washington, DC, 2000, US Government Printing Office.

BOX 1-2 ***Healthy People 2010: Understanding and Improving Health Goals****

Access to Quality Health Services

Goal: Improve access to comprehensive, high-quality health care across a continuum of care.

Cancer

Goal: Reduce the number of new cancer cases, as well as the illness, disability, and death caused by cancer.

Chronic Kidney Disease

Goal: Reduce new cases of chronic kidney disease and its complications, disability, death, and economic costs.

Diabetes

Goal: Through prevention programs, reduce the disease and economic burden of diabetes, and improve the quality of life for all persons who have or are at risk for diabetes.

Disability and Secondary Conditions

Goal: Promote the health of people with disabilities, prevent secondary conditions, and eliminate disparities between people with and without disabilities in the U.S. population.

Education and Community-Based Programs

Goal: Increase the quality, availability, and effectiveness of educational and community-based programs designed to prevent disease and improve the health and quality of life.

Environmental Health

Goal: Promote health for all through a healthy environment.

Family Planning

Goal: Improve pregnancy planning and spacing and prevent unintended pregnancy.

Continued

BOX 1-2 *Healthy People 2010: Understanding and Improving Health Goals**—cont'd*

Food Safety

Goal: Reduce the number of food-borne illnesses.

Human Immunodeficiency Virus Infection

Goal: Prevent HIV transmission and associated morbidity and mortality by (1) ensuring that all persons at risk for HIV infection know their serostatus, (2) ensuring that persons not infected with HIV remain uninfected, (3) ensuring that persons infected with HIV do not transmit HIV to others, and (4) ensuring that those infected with HIV are accessing the most effective therapies possible.

Immunization and Infectious Diseases

Goal: Prevent disease, disability, and death from infectious diseases, including vaccine-preventable diseases.

Injury/Violence Prevention

Goal: Reduce injuries, disabilities, and deaths caused by unintentional injuries and violence.

Maternal, Infant, and Child Care

Goal: Improve the health and well-being of women, infants, children, and families.

Mental Health and Mental Disorders

Goal: Improve mental health and ensure access to appropriate, quality mental health services.

Nutrition and Overweight

Goal: Promote health and reduce chronic disease associated with diet and weight.

Occupational Safety and Health

Goal: Promote the health and safety of people at work through prevention and early intervention.

Oral Health

Goal: Prevent and control oral and craniofacial diseases, conditions, and injuries and improve access to related services.

Physical Activity and Fitness

Goal: Improve health, fitness, and quality of life through daily physical activity.

Public Health Infrastructure

Goal: Ensure that federal, tribal, state, and local health agencies have the infrastructure to provide essential public health services effectively.

Respiratory Diseases

Goal: Promote respiratory health through better prevention, detection, treatment, and education efforts.

Sexually Transmitted Diseases

Goal: Promote responsible sexual behaviors, strengthen community capacity, and increase access to quality services to prevent sexually transmitted diseases (STDs) and their complications.

Substance Abuse

Goal: Reduce substance abuse to protect the health, safety, and quality of life of all, especially children.

Tobacco Use

Goal: Reduce illness, disability, and death related to tobacco use and exposure to secondhand smoke.

Vision and Hearing

Goal: Improve the visual and hearing health of the nation through prevention, early detection, treatment, and rehabilitation.

From US Department of Health and Human Services: *Healthy people 2010: understanding and improving health*, ed 2, Washington, DC, 2000, US Government Printing Office.

*Objectives for each goal can be found in Appendix D.

care decisions and patient education for all patients. If the statistical trends are to be modified to reduce morbidity and mortality rates, health supervision must become ever more efficient and effective. The traditional health care of the past is insufficient given the current needs and changes needed to be achieved through community-wide efforts, as well as individual case progress. National goals are intended to provide direction for changes in the health care delivery system, most of which must occur in the primary health care arena.

Clinical Preventive Services: Health Supervision

Clinical preventive services can be viewed as evidence-based care guidelines. These services include screening tests, immunizations, and preventive counseling—all areas of expertise for NPs. They are designed as cost-effective means to achieve the national goals. NPs should be familiar with several sets of guidelines for providing clinical preventive services. The American Academy of Pediatrics (AAP) guidelines for health supervision are found in the book *Guidelines for Health Supervision III, revised* (AAP, 2002). The AAP's recommendations for preventive health care (AAP, 2000) provide a summary of health promotion assessments and interventions for each age-group. This guideline is presented in Table 1-2. The AAP's recommendations are also incorporated throughout this text. *Bright Futures: Guidelines for Health Supervision of Infants, Children, and Adolescents is a book* of guidelines that supports *Healthy People 2010* goals. It was developed by the Bureau of Maternal and Child Health and the Health Care Financing Administration (HCFA) (Green & Palfrey, 2002). These guidelines provide information for conducting health promotion visits from infancy through adolescence.

AMA Guidelines for Adolescent Preventive Services (GAPS) (Elster & Kuznets, 1994) provides another set of guidelines developed by experts on adolescence under the sponsorship of the American Medical Association (AMA). Their 24 recommendations are summarized in Box 1-3. The rationale and suggested interventions found in GAPS are also incorporated into this text. It is recommended that primary care providers be familiar with both the *Bright Futures* and *GAPS* guidelines. They were developed because teens have been one of the most at-risk groups across the life span and because many adult health conditions begin in adolescence. Further, teens access preventive health care less than other age-groups do (Brindes et al, 2002).

Another widely accepted publication is the *Clinician's Handbook of Preventive Services*, second edition (U.S. Public Health Service, 1998), prepared by the U.S. Preventive Services Task Force. This book rigorously reviews evidence for 169 interventions to prevent 60 different illnesses and conditions across the life span. It is made clinically accessible through the Putting Prevention into Practice (PPIP) program.

The PPIP program is designed to assist clinicians to implement the *Clinician's Handbook of Preventive Services* recommendations. Like the *Bright Futures* project, the PPIP program offers strategies for patients, providers, and office systems to increase the likelihood that the recommendations will indeed be followed. PPIP's *Child Health Guide* and *Personal Health Guide* (for adults) are passport-size, patient-held records that also provide information about the recommended services. The *Clinician's Handbook of Preventive Services* (U.S. Public Health Service, 1998) is a manual of 62 chapters, each including steps to delivery of a service, recommendations from major authorities, and provider resources. Finally, the office materials include chart flow sheets to track the clinical preventive services status of clients, prevention prescription pads to contract with patients for behavioral changes, reminder postcards, chart stickers and Post-It notes to remind providers of needed services, and posters for waiting and examining rooms with age-specific timelines for delivery of services.

Bright Futures offers similar resources to promote use of the guidelines in primary care practice. The *Bright Futures* program is called the *Healthy Steps Initiative.* It was initiated by the Commonwealth Fund in New York and implemented by the Boston University School of Medicine (Lawrence, Magee, & Bernard, 2001).

Clinical preventive services guidelines need to be part of the practice of every primary health care provider. Whether the clinician chooses the PPIP program, the *Bright Futures* guidelines, the *GAPS* recommendations, or all three, one should select and define the standard of care for practice. The clinical setting is designed to support delivery of those services by incorporating the guidelines into the plan of care for every patient, whether sick or well. One goal of sick care should always be to move the patient back into the health promotion arena, thereby providing appropriate health promotion services even to sick patients. For example, recommendations for providing immunizations are much more flexible than they were several years ago. In many cases, immunizations should be given to patients coming for illness visits.

Numerous guidelines can be found for the diagnosis and management of most common pediatric health problems, as well as preventive care of children with special needs and newborn care. Some guidelines include management of acute and chronic asthma, fever in young children, gastroenteritis, hearing screening, infectious diseases, otitis media with effusion, pain, sickle cell disease, attention deficit/hyperactivity disorder, diabetes, and many others. They are referred to in this book within the appropriate chapters. The Agency for Health Care Policy and Research spearheaded the development of guidelines to decrease the variability of practice and improve the adequacy of outcome measures. Managed care organizations have also supported the guidelines movement to promote uniformity of clinical outcomes and to measure clinician performance, set policy, and drive management decisions about the best use of resources for groups of patients (Callender, 1999). Although development of quality guidelines is a rigorous process, the dissemination and implementation of guidelines in practice is probably more difficult. Habits and practice patterns of clinicians are difficult to change.

Barriers to the Use of Preventive Services

Many health care needs of children are unmet. More than 4.7 million children annually between 1993 and 1996 had

TABLE 1-2 *Recommendations for Preventive Health Care (RE9939). Committee of Practice and Ambulatory Medicine*

Each child and family is unique; therefore, these **Recommendations for Preventive Pediatric Health Care** are designed for the care of children who are receiving competent parenting, have no manifestations of any important health problems, and are growing and developing in satisfactory fashion. **Additional visits may become necessary** if circumstances suggest variations from normal.

These guidelines represent a consensus by the Committee on Practice and Ambulatory Medicine in consultation with national committees and sections of the American Academy of Pediatrics. The Committee emphasizes the great importance of continuity of care in comprehensive health supervision and the need to avoid **fragmentation of care**.

		Infancy[4]								Early Childhood[4]				
Age[5]	**Prenatal[1]**	**Newborn[2]**	**2-4 d[3]**	**By 1 mo**	**2 mo**	**4 mo**	**6 mo**	**9 mo**	**12 mo**	**15 mo**	**18 mo**	**24 mo**	**3 y**	**4 y**
History														
Initial/Interval	•	•	•	•	•	•	•	•	•	•	•	•	•	•
Measurements														
Height and weight		•	•	•	•	•	•	•	•	•	•	•	•	•
Head circumference		•	•	•	•	•	•	•	•	•	•	•		
Blood pressure													•	•
Sensory Screening														
Vision		S	S	S	S	S	S	S	S	S	S	S	O[6]	O
Hearing		O[7]	S	S	S	S	S	S	S	S	S	S	S	O
Developmental/ Behavioral Assessment[8]		•	•	•	•	•	•	•	•	•	•	•	•	•
Physical Examination[9]		•	•	•	•	•	•	•	•	•	•	•	•	•
Procedures—General[10]														
Hereditary/metabolic screening[11]		← (arrow, Newborn to By 1 mo)	•	→										
Immunization[12]		•	•	•	•	•	•	•	•	•	•	•	•	•
Hematocrit or hemoglobin[13]								• (arrow, 9 mo to 12 mo)	→	*	*	*	*	
Urinalysis														
Procedures—Patients at Risk														
Lead screening[16]								* (arrow, 9 mo to 12 mo)	→			*		
Tuberculin test[17]									*	*	*	*	*	*
Cholesterol screening[18]												*	*	*
STD screening[19]														
Pelvic exam[20]														
Anticipatory Guidance[21]	•	•	•	•	•	•	•	•	•	•	•	•	•	•
Injury prevention[22]	•	•	•	•	•	•	•	•	•	•	•	•	•	•
Violence protection[23]	•	•	•	•	•	•	•	•	•	•	•	•	•	•
Sleep positioning counseling[24]	•	•	•	•	•	•	•							
Nutrition counseling[25]	•	•	•	•	•	•	•	•	•	•	•	•	•	•
Dental Referral[26]									← (arrow, 3 y back to 12 mo)				•	

	Middle Childhood[4]				Adolescence[4]										
Age[5]	**5 y**	**6 y**	**8 y**	**10 y**	**11 y**	**12 y**	**13 y**	**14 y**	**15 y**	**16 y**	**17 y**	**18 y**	**19 y**	**20 y**	**21 y**
History															
Initial/interval	•	•	•	•	•	•	•	•	•	•	•	•	•	•	•
Measurements															
Height and weight	•	•	•	•	•	•	•	•	•	•	•	•	•	•	•
Head circumference															
Blood pressure	•	•	•	•	•	•	•	•	•	•	•	•	•	•	•
Sensory Screening															
Vision	O	O	O	O	S	O	S	S	O	S	S	O	S	S	S
Hearing	O	O	O	O	S	O	S	S	O	S	S	O	S	S	S
Developmental/ Behavioral Assessment[8]	•	•	•	•	•	•	•	•	•	•	•	•	•	•	•
Physical Examination[9]	•	•	•	•	•	•	•	•	•	•	•	•	•	•	•
Procedures—General[10]															
Hereditary/metabolic screening[11]															
Immunization[12]	•	•	•	•	•	•	•	•	•	•	•	•	•	•	•
Hematocrit or hemoglobin[13]	★				←		•[14]								→
Urinalysis	•				←					•[15]					→
Procedures—Patients at Risk															
Lead screening[16]															
Tuberculin test[17]	★	★	★	★	★	★	★	★	★	★	★	★	★	★	★
Cholesterol screening[18]	★	★	★	★	★	★	★	★	★	★	★	★	★	★	★
STD screening[19]					★	★	★	★	★	★	★	★	★	★	★
Pelvic exam[20]					★	★	★	★	★	★	★	★ ←	★[20]	★	★ →
Anticipatory Guidance[21]	•	•	•	•	•	•	•	•	•	•	•	•	•	•	•
Injury prevention[22]	•	•	•	•	•	•	•	•	•	•	•	•	•	•	•
Violence protection[23]	•	•	•	•	•	•	•	•	•	•	•	•	•	•	•
Sleep positioning counseling[24]															
Nutrition counseling[25]	•	•	•	•	•	•	•	•	•	•	•	•	•	•	•
Dental Referral[26]															

From American Academy of Pediatrics: Recommendations for preventive pediatric health care. Committee on Practice and Ambulatory Medicine, *Pediatrics* 105:645, 2000.

1. A prenatal visit is recommended for parents who are at high risk, for first-time parents, and for those who request a conference. The prenatal visit should include anticipatory guidance, pertinent medical history, and a discussion of benefits of breastfeeding and planned method of feeding per the AAP statement, "The Prenatal Visit" (1996).
2. Every infant should have a newborn evaluation after birth. Breastfeeding should be encouraged and instruction and support offered. Every breastfeeding infant should have an evaluation 48 to 72 hours after discharge from the hospital to include weight, formal breastfeeding evaluation, encouragement, and instruction as recommended in the AAP statement, "Breastfeeding and the Use of Human Milk" (1997).
3. For newborns discharged less than 48 hours after delivery per the AAP statement, "Hospital Stay for Healthy Term Newborns" (1995).
4. Developmental, psychosocial, and chronic disease issues for children and adolescents may require frequent counseling and treatment visits separate from preventive care visits.
5. If a child comes under care for the first time at any point on the schedule, or if any items are not accomplished at the suggested age, the schedule should be brought up to date at the earliest possible time.
6. If the patient is uncooperative, rescreen within 6 months.

Continued

TABLE 1-2 ***Recommendations for Preventive Health Care (RE9939). Committee of Practice and Ambulatory Medicine—cont'd***

7. All newborns should be screened per the AAP Task Force on Newborn and Infant Hearing statement, "Newborn and Infant Hearing Loss: Detection and Intervention" (1999).
8. By history and appropriate physical examination: if suspicious, by specific objective developmental testing. Parenting skills should be fostered at every visit.
9. At each visit, a complete physical examination is essential, with infant totally unclothed, older child undressed and suitably draped.
10. These may be modified, depending on entry point into schedule and individual need.
11. Metabolic screening (e.g., thyroid, hemoglobinopathies, phenylketonuria, galactosemia) should be done according to state law.
12. Schedule(s) per the Committee on Infectious Diseases, published annually in the January edition of *Pediatrics*. Every visit should be an opportunity to update and complete a child's immunizations.
13. See AAP *Pediatric Nutrition Handbook* (1998) for a discussion of universal and selective screening options. Consider earlier screening for high-risk infants (e.g., premature infants and low-birth-weight infants). See also Recommendations to prevent and control iron deficiency in the United States, *MMWR* 47(RR-3):1-29, 1998.
14. All menstruating adolescents should be screened annually.
15. Conduct dipstick urinalysis for leukocytes annually for sexually active male and female adolescents.
16. For children at risk of lead exposure consult the AAP statement, "Screening for Elevated Blood Levels" (1998). Additionally, screening should be done in accordance with state law where applicable.
17. TB testing per recommendations of the Committee on Infectious Diseases, published in the current edition of *Red Book: Report of the Committee on Infectious Diseases*. Testing should be done on recognition of high-risk factors.
18. Cholesterol screening for high-risk patients per the AAP statement, "Cholesterol in Childhood" (1998). If family history cannot be ascertained and other risk factors are present, screening should be at the discretion of the physician.
19. All sexually active patients should be screened for sexually transmitted diseases (STDs).
20. All sexually active females should have a pelvic examination. A pelvic examination and routine Pap smear should be offered as part of preventive health maintenance between ages 18 and 21 years.
21. Age-appropriate discussion and counseling should be an integral part of each visit for care per the AAP *Guidelines for Health Supervision III* (1998).
22. From birth to age 12, refer to the AAP injury prevention program (TIPP9r) as described in *A Guide to Safety Counseling in Office Practice* (1994).
23. Violence prevention and management for all patients per the AAP statement, "The Role of the Pediatrician in Youth Violence Prevention in Clinical Practice and at the Community Level" (1999).
24. Parents and caregivers should be advised to place healthy infants on their backs when putting them to sleep. Side positioning is a reasonable alternative but carries a slightly higher risk of SIDS. Consult the AAP statement, "Changing Concepts of Sudden Infant Death Syndrome: Implications for Infant Sleeping Environment and Sleep Position" (2000).
25. Age-appropriate nutrition counseling should be an integral part of each visit per the AAP *Handbook of Nutrition* (1998).
26. Earlier initial dental examinations may be appropriate for some children. Subsequent examinations as prescribed by dentist.

Key:
• = to be performed
⋆ = to be performed for patients at risk
S = subjective, by history
O = objective, by a standard testing method
◄—•—► = the range during which a service may be provided, with the dot indicating the preferred age

Note:
Special chemical, immunologic, and endocrine testing is usually carried out on specific indications. Testing other than newborn (e.g., inborn errors of metabolism, sickle cell disease) is discretionary with the physician.
The recommendations in this statement do not indicate an exclusive course of treatment or serve as a standard of medical care. Variations, taking into account individual circumstances, may be appropriate.

BOX 1-3 *American Medical Association Guidelines for Adolescent Preventive Services*

I. Recommendations for Delivery of Health Services

Recommendation 1: From ages 11 to 21, all adolescents should have an annual routine health visit. Visits should address biomedical and psychosocial aspects of health with a preventive focus. A complete physical examination should be performed during three of these visits—11-14 years, 15-17 years, and 18-21 years—unless more frequent examinations are warranted by clinical signs or symptoms.

Recommendation 2: Preventive services should be age and developmentally appropriate and sensitive to individual and sociocultural differences.

Recommendation 3: Physicians should establish office policies regarding confidential care for adolescents and how parents will be involved in that care. These policies should be made clear to adolescents and their parents.

II. Recommendations for Health Guidance

Recommendation 4: Parents or other adult caregivers of adolescents should receive health guidance at least once during early adolescence, middle adolescence, and late adolescence.

Normative adolescent development (physical, sexual, and emotional), signs and symptoms of disease and emotional stress, parenting behavior that promotes healthy adolescent adjustment, benefits of discussing health-related behavior with their adolescents, planning family activities, and acting as a role model should be discussed with parents or caregivers.

Caregivers or parents should be advised of methods for helping their adolescents avoid potentially harmful behavior such as monitoring and managing the use of motor vehicles, avoiding weapons in the home, removing weapons and potentially lethal medications from homes of adolescents with suicidal intent, and monitoring social and recreational activities to restrict sexual behavior and tobacco, alcohol, and other drug use.

Recommendation 5: All adolescents should receive health guidance annually to promote a better understanding of their physical growth, their psychosocial and psychosexual development, and the importance of becoming actively involved in decisions about health care.

Recommendation 6: All adolescents should receive health guidance annually to promote the reduction of injuries, including avoidance of the use of alcohol or drugs while operating motor vehicles or where impaired judgment may lead to injury, and the use of safety devices, including safety belts, helmets, and appropriate sports protective devices.

Recommendation 7: All adolescents should receive health guidance annually about dietary habits, including the benefits of a healthy diet and ways to achieve a healthy diet and safe weight management.

Recommendation 8: All adolescents should receive health guidance annually about the benefits of exercise and should be encouraged to engage in safe exercise regularly.

Recommendation 9: All adolescents should receive health guidance annually regarding responsible sexual behavior, including abstinence. Latex condoms to prevent STDs and appropriate methods of birth control should be made available with instructions on how to use them effectively. Counseling should include effectiveness of abstinence; HIV transmission, dangers, and prevention by latex condoms; and sensible sexual behavior for those who are not sexually active, as well as for those who are using condoms and birth control appropriately.

Recommendation 10: All adolescents should receive health guidance to promote avoidance of tobacco, alcohol, abusable substances, and anabolic steroids.

III. Recommendations for Screening

Recommendation 11: All adolescents should be screened annually for hypertension according to the National Heart, Lung, and Blood Institute Second Task Force on Blood Pressure Control in Children.

Recommendation 12: Selected adolescents should be screened to determine their risk for hyperlipidemia and adult coronary disease, as per the protocol developed by the Expert Panel on Blood Cholesterol Levels in Children and Adolescents. High-risk adolescents include those with serum cholesterol levels greater than 240 mg/dl who are older than 19 years and those with an unknown family history of parents or grandparents with coronary artery disease.

Recommendation 13: All adolescents should be screened annually for eating disorders and obesity by determining weight and stature and asking about body image and dieting patterns.

Recommendation 14: All adolescents should be asked annually about their use of tobacco products, including cigarettes and smokeless tobacco.

Recommendation 15: All adolescents should be asked annually about the use of alcohol and other abusable substances and their use of over-the-counter or prescription drugs for nonmedical purposes, including anabolic steroids.

Continued

BOX 1-3 *American Medical Association Guidelines for Adolescent Preventive Services—cont'd*

Recommendation 16: All adolescents should be asked annually about their involvement in sexual behavior that may result in unintended pregnancy and STDs, including HIV infection.

Recommendation 17: Sexually active adolescents should be screened for STDs.

Recommendation 18: Adolescents at risk for HIV infection should be offered confidential HIV screening with the ELISA and confirmatory tests.

Risk factors include intravenous drug use, STD infection, residence in a high-prevalence area, more than one sexual partner in the past 6 months, exchange of sex for drugs or money, male gender and engaging in sex with another male, or a sexual partner at risk for HIV infection.

Recommendation 19: Female adolescents who are sexually active or any female 18 years or older should be screened annually for cervical cancer by use of a Papanicolaou test.

Recommendation 20: All adolescents should be asked annually about behavior or emotions that indicate recurrent or severe depression or a risk of suicide.

Recommendation 21: All adolescents should be asked annually about a history of emotional, physical, or sexual abuse.

Recommendation 22: All adolescents should be asked annually about learning or school problems.

Recommendation 23: Adolescents should receive a tuberculin skin test if they have been exposed to active tuberculosis, have lived in a homeless shelter, have been incarcerated, have lived in or come from an area with a high prevalence of tuberculosis, or are currently working in a health care setting.

IV. Recommendations for Immunizations

Recommendation 24: All adolescents should receive prophylactic immunizations according to the guidelines established by the federally convened Advisory Committee on Immunization Practices.

From Elster A, Kuznets N: *AMA guidelines for adolescent preventive services (GAPS)*, Baltimore, 1994, Williams & Wilkins.
ELISA, Enzyme-linked immunosorbent assay; *HIV*, human immunodeficiency virus; *STD*, sexually transmitted disease.

at least one unmet need, the most common being dental care (Newacheck et al, 2000).

A variety of barriers to the provision of clinical preventive services by all primary care providers exist: uncertainty about the guidelines, lack of reimbursement, lack of time, limited patient education efforts associated with lack of commitment to facilitate behavior changes, lack of office system organization, clinician attitudes more focused on acute care than prevention, and less feedback from patients and the agency about the effects of preventive care. In other words, primary care providers cannot blame low immunization rates only on access-to-care issues on the patient side of the equation!

It is hoped that health care initiatives will reduce the financial barriers to child health care. Recommended clinical preventive services should be included in the essential benefits packages of all insurance plans. They are designed to decrease costs either through decreasing unnecessary services or through prevention of unnecessary morbidity and mortality. The barriers related to clinician attitudes, motivation, and office systems are harder to eliminate, but if the health of America's children and adults is to improve, they must be addressed.

Health promotion work with patients and families needs to be individualized. Cultural diversity, family values and lifestyles, and economics are all important factors to consider in helping families plan for their health. Health promotion care also needs to be viewed as a longitudinal process. Planning must be done across visits. Families need to understand the plan over time and whether they are on target with their health promotion activities (e.g., the status of immunization series completion, the next immunizations required, and the time at which they should be given). Continuity of care should be viewed over time. Continuity should also be viewed across health and human services centers. In other words, care provided by a variety of professionals (including social workers, therapists, teachers, physicians, nurses, and others) across agencies and time should be integrated and "seamless."

NURSE PRACTITIONERS AND MANAGED CARE

Child health care has changed considerably over the past 20 years. Financing and organization of services have changed to a system of managed care. The number of child visits to primary care providers increased 22% between 1979 and 1998, and the average patient age decreased from 6.7 to 5.7 years. The ethnic diversity of clients has increased, with a greater proportion of visits by Hispanics and Asians. Shifts in the frequencies with which some common conditions are diagnosed and treated have also been observed. Counseling has apparently increased in primary care visits (Ferris et al, 1998). Another study of this type is merited to document changes in the twenty-first century.

NPs as well as physicians are expected to be efficient, effective providers. Unlike physicians, NPs are expected to provide more health teaching and bring a more holistic perspective to their analysis of patient and family problems. NPs manage health as well as illness. They are first and foremost nurses. As advanced practice nurses, they must be expert nurses using practical wisdom and knowledge and pattern recognition skills, as well as possessing theoretical knowledge from graduate studies. They must be able to apply all the knowledge and skills they have to specific patient care situations, considering a variety of options with families. It is a complex role (Oberle & Allen, 2001).

The problem-oriented and health promotion models for care, which are themes of this book, are discussed in Chapter 2. Comprehensive care of children includes assessment and management of diseases, daily living problems (functional health problems), and developmental problems. Community-based care is another theme for NP practice that is less emphasized in this book but is nonetheless important.

Despite the pleasures of working with children, the problems NPs face, such as juggling the expectations of employers and managed care payers versus the needs and expectations of their patients and families, make providing care stressful for many. Unfortunately, much of their work becomes invisible when billed under physician names. With the current system of 85% reimbursement to NPs as direct providers under Medicaid and Medicare, many are reluctant to take the penalty of loss of revenue for their practice to be acknowledged as providers in their own right. Nurse practitioners, as an important provider group, need to be well versed in reimbursement strategies but must also shift their practices based on the dynamics of the health care system. Some of these issues are discussed further in the last chapter of this book.

Utilization of clinical preventive services guidelines, working with auxiliary personnel to eliminate the nonprofessional tasks of the day, and working toward management of paperwork by clerical personnel for reimbursement and referrals will increase efficiency. Nurse practitioners should promote full utilization of registered nurses in ambulatory care, a frequently underestimated and underused workforce.

Generation of data about the effectiveness of NP services, as well as NPs' economic value to a practice, will continue to be important to NP viability as providers of the future. Patient and family satisfaction with NPs can have

RESOURCE BOX

Agency for Healthcare Research and Quality
www.ahcpr.gov

National Guideline Clearinghouse
www.guidelines.gov

American Academy of Pediatrics
www.aap.org

Annie E. Casey Foundation
Kids Count Data Book
www.acef.org

Bright Futures
www.brightfutures.org

Centers for Disease Control and Prevention
www.cdc.gov.nchs

Child health statistics
www.childstats.gov

Department of Health and Human Services statistics
www.hrsa.gov

Guidelines for Adolescent Preventive Services
www.ama-assn.org/ama/upload/mm/39/gapsmono.pdf

Healthy People 2010
www.health.gov/healthypeople/

MD Choice—practice guidelines
www.mdchoice.com

PPIP 2001: a step-by-step guide to delivering clinical preventive services—a systems approach
www.ahrq.gov/ppip/manual/manual.pdf

To Leave No Child Behind
www.childrensdefense.org

Youth Risk Behavior Surveillance System
www.cdc.gov/necdphp/dash/yrbs/

important effects on the system as it shifts to meet consumer demands; one must remember that employers as well as employees are current consumers of health care insurance plans.

SUMMARY

It must be understood that much of the work of NPs and other primary health care providers is in the realm of common illness management and coordination of care for children with serious and chronic illnesses. However, the real long-term positive impact of primary health care occurs when health-promoting activities are provided to patients and their families in such a way that they are participants in, not recipients of, their health care. Health for children as they grow is essential because it helps them cope in an increasingly complex world and achieve their dreams.

REFERENCES

American Academy of Pediatrics: Recommendations for preventive pediatric health care. Committee on Practice and Ambulatory Medicine, *Pediatrics* 105:645, 2000.

American Academy of Pediatrics, Committee on Practice and Ambulatory Medicine: *Guidelines for health supervision III, revised*, Elk Grove, IL, 2002, American Academy of Pediatrics.

American Nurses' Association: *Nursing's social policy statement*, Kansas City, MO, 1995, American Nurses' Association.

America's Children: Key national indicators of well-being. Available at *www.childstats.gov*, 2002.

Annie E. Casey Foundation Center for the Study of Social Policy: *Kids count data book*, Washington, DC, 2002, Annie E. Casey Foundation.

Brindes C et al: Adolescent access to health care services and clinical preventive health care: crossing the great divide, *Pediatr Ann* 31:575-581, 2002.

Callender D: Pediatric practice guidelines: Implications for nurse practitioners, *J Pediatr Prim Care* 13:105-111, 1999.

Centers for Disease Control and Prevention: Available at *www.childstats.gov*, 2002.

Centers for Disease Control and Prevention, National Center for Injury Prevention and Control: Factsheet: playground injuries. Available at *www.cdc.gov/ncipc/factsheets/playgr.htm*, 2002.

Centers for Disease Control and Prevention, National Immunization Program: National Immunization Survey: estimated coverage with individual vaccines and selected vaccination series by 24 months of age by state and immunization plan area. Available at *www.cdc.gov/nip/coverage/NIS/01/TAB9-24months_iap.xls*, 2001.

Children's Defense Fund: *The state of America's children*, Washington, DC, 2002, Children's Defense Fund.

David and Lucile Packard Foundation: Children and managed health care, *Future of Children* 8(2), 1998.

Elster A, Kuznets N: *AMA guidelines for adolescent preventive services (GAPS)*, Baltimore, 1994, Williams & Wilkins.

Ferris T et al: Changes in the daily practice of primary care for children, *Arch Pediatr Adolesc Med* 152:227-233, 1998.

Green M, Palfrey J: *Bright futures: guidelines for health supervision of infants, children, and adolescents*, ed 2, revised, Arlington, VA, 2002, National Center for Education in Maternal and Child Health.

Hoyert D et al: Annual summary of vital statistics: 2000, *Pediatrics* 108:1241-1255, Dec 2001.

Institute of Medicine, Committee on the Future of Primary Care: *Defining primary care: an interim report*, Washington, DC, 1994, Division of Health Care Services.

Lawrence P, Magee T, Bernard A: Reshaping primary care: the Healthy Steps Initiative, *J Pediatr Health Care* 15:58-62, 2001.

Leslie L, Sarah R, Palfrey J: Child health care in changing times, *Pediatrics* 101:746-752, 1998.

Litovitz TL et al: 2000 annual report of American Association of Poison Control Centers Toxic Exposure Surveillance System, *Am J Emerg Med* 19:337-396, 2001.

Newacheck P et al: The unmet health needs of America's children, *Pediatrics* 105:989-997, 2000.

Oberle K, Allen M: The nature of advanced practice nursing, *Nurs Outlook* 49:148-153, 2001.

Smith L et al: Implications of welfare reform for child health: emerging challenges for clinical practice and policy, *Pediatrics* 105:1117-1125, 2000.

US Congress, Office of Technology Assessment: *Adolescent health*, vol 1, *Summary and policy options*, OTA-H-468, Washington, DC, 1991, Office of Technology Assessment.

US Department of Health and Human Services: *Healthy people 2000: national health promotion and disease prevention objectives for the year 2000*, pub no (PHS) 91-50212, Washington, DC, 1990, US Government Printing Office.

US Department of Health and Human Services: *Healthy people 2010: understanding and improving health*, ed 2, Washington, DC, 2000, US Government Printing Office.

US Department of Health and Human Services, Maternal and Child Health Bureau: *Child health USA*, Washington, DC, 2001, US Government Printing Office.

US Public Health Service: *Clinician's handbook of preventive services*, ed 2, McLean, VA, 1998, International Medical Publishers.

Youth Risk Behavior Surveillance—United States, 2001, *MMWR CDC Surveill Summ* 5/ss-4, June 28, 2002.

2

Child Assessment in Pediatric Primary Care

Catherine E. Burns

A careful, complete, and thoughtful assessment of the child's health status is absolutely essential to provide excellent primary health care. This assessment is based on knowledge of child development, family structure and functions, culture, anatomy and physiology, pathophysiology, pharmacology, health care delivery systems, communities, and standards of primary health care for children. The assessment must also be viewed through the lens of the provider's experience to allow the provider to modify perceptions and validate data on the basis of previous work. When providers analyze patient care situations, they are engaged in critical thinking. This chapter cannot teach critical thinking, nor does it teach physical assessment. Rather, it provides frameworks for gathering data to facilitate expert decision making. It is assumed that the reader already knows how to do a complete physical examination and has some experience working with children and families in health care settings. It is also assumed that nurse practitioners (NPs) have the requisite knowledge in the areas just listed.

An important corollary to health assessment is the skill to communicate information obtained in both oral and written forms. A record of the care given must always be written to communicate the provider's logical thinking based on data obtained. This record is important because it provides information for later care, serves as a communication link with other providers, documents the quality of care provided, may be used for research purposes, and serves as a legal and billing document. Verbal communication of health care information is also essential. The words must paint a picture of the child and family for the reader (e.g., a consultant). Knowledge of the classic format used by other health care providers is important. Using that same format or one that is closely related facilitates efficient communication about patient problems.

This chapter provides the basic framework for health assessment of children. In-depth assessments related to specific topics are included in later chapters. The outline for assessment of children in this chapter is consistent with the organization for the entire text. Development, daily living problems, and diseases are the three domains for pediatric nurse practitioner (PNP) practice and are the major units of this book. Each chapter provides comprehensive information about topics that are categorized within one of those domains.

PEDIATRIC NURSE PRACTITIONER ASSESSMENT COMPETENCIES

In 2002 the U.S. Department of Health and Human Services (USDHHS), Division of Nursing, published a document of NP primary care competencies (USDHHS, 2002). The competencies were developed by representatives of all major NP organizations and include competencies expected both for all NPs and for specialty practices, such as PNPs. Those competencies serve as standards for practice, which can be used to develop curricula, test graduates for board certification, and educate the public and health care industry about the care that an NP will deliver to his or her clients. Competencies related to assessment and decision making for NPs in general and PNPs in particular are found in Box 2-1. (There are other competencies not included here.)

BOX 2-1 *Assessment and Management Competencies for Nurse Practitioners*

Items selected for this box reflect the content of this chapter—collection of the health history, completion of the physical examination, diagnostic reasoning, communication via charting and verbal reports, and communication with the patient and family to promote the caregiving role of the nurse practitioner. Many other competencies that relate to other aspects of the nurse practitioner's work are found in the original competencies document (USDHHS, 2002)

COMPETENCIES: ALL NURSE PRACTITIONERS

Domain 1: Management of Patient Health/Illness Status

1. Demonstrates critical thinking and diagnostic reasoning skills in clinical decision making.
2. Obtains a comprehensive and problem-focused health history from the patient.
3. Performs a comprehensive and problem-focused physical examination.
4. Analyzes the data collected to determine health status.
5. Formulates a problem list.
6. Assesses, diagnoses, monitors, coordinates, and manages the health/illness status of patients over time and supports the patient through the dying process.
7. Demonstrates knowledge of pathophysiology of acute and chronic diseases or conditions commonly seen in practice.
8. Communicates the patient's health status using appropriate terminology, format, and technology.
9. Applies principles of epidemiology and demography in clinical practice by recognizing populations at risk, patterns of disease, and effectiveness of prevention and intervention.
10. Uses community/public health assessment information in evaluating patient needs, initiating referrals, coordinating care, and program planning.
11. Applies theories to guide practice.
12. Applies, conducts research studies pertinent to areas of practice.

[...]

19. Orders, may perform, and interprets common screening and diagnostic tests.
20. Evaluates results of interventions using accepted outcome criteria, revises the plan accordingly, and consults/refers when needed.
21. Schedules follow-up visits to appropriately monitor patients and evaluate health/illness care.

Domain 2: The Nurse Practitioner–Patient Relationship

1. Creates a climate of mutual trust and establishes partnerships with patients.
2. Validates and verifies findings with patients.
3. Creates a relationship with patients that acknowledges their strengths and assists patients in addressing their needs.
4. Communicates a sense of "being present" with the patient and provides comfort and emotional support.
5. Evaluates the impact of life transitions on the health/ illness status of patients and the impact of health and illness on patients (individuals, families, and communities).
6. Applies principles of self-efficacy/empowerment in promoting behavior change.
7. Preserves the patient's control over decision making; assesses the patient's commitment to the jointly determined, mutually acceptable plan of care; and fosters the patient's personal responsibility for health.
8. Maintains confidentiality while communicating data, plans, and results in a manner that preserves the dignity and privacy of the patient and provides a legal record of care.

[...]

12. Evaluates patient's and caregiver's support systems.

PEDIATRIC NURSE PRACTITIONER COMPETENCIES

I. Health Promotion, Health Protection, Disease Prevention, and Treatment.

A. Assessment of Health Status

1. Obtains and documents a relevant health history for children.
2. Performs age-appropriate screening for developmental and behavioral concerns, such as speech/language development, learning disabilities, and behavioral and mental health concerns.
3. Assesses the child's developmental status based on developmental theories recognizing the individual differences in temperament, reactions to selected developmental tasks and situational crises, and coping styles and strategies.
4. Identifies and analyzes factors that affect the child's growth and development, such as the following:
   - Genetic background
   - Prenatal factors
   - Temperament
   - Family and cultural influences
   - Parenting style
   - Environmental milieu (e.g., day care, school, neighborhood, community)
   - Health status
   - Significant life events (trauma, loss, violence, etc.)
5. Adapts and performs the history and screening procedures according to the child's developmental age, behavior, and reason for contact.

BOX 2-1 *Assessment and Management Competencies for Nurse Practitioners—cont'd*

6. Performs and records a complete, accurate, and systematic pediatric physical assessment.
7. Recognizes variations of normal including genetic, ethnic, physiologic, and anatomic differences.
8. Assesses for evidence of child abuse and neglect and the effects of violence on the child.
9. Analyzes the family system to identify factors that influence the health of the child and adolescent, including, but not limited to, the following:
   - Parental occupation/education/developmental level
   - Family support system
   - Family dynamics
   - Family values and beliefs
   - Family management style
   - Family stresses
   - Social morbidities, including poverty and illiteracy
   - Management of and coping with chronic illness
10. Assesses patient's health risks, including, but not limited to, the following:
   - Developmental level
   - Genetic/family history
   - Immunization status
   - Nutritional status
   - Risk-taking behavior
   - Environmental factors
   - Family issues
   - Social support
11. Assesses patient's and family's knowledge and behavior regarding leading health indicators, including, but not limited to, the following:
   - Physical activity
   - Eating disorders
   - Tobacco use
   - Substance abuse
   - Responsible sexual behavior
   - Mental health
   - Injury/violence
   - Environmental quality
   - Immunizations
   - Access to health care

B. Diagnosis of Health Status

The pediatric nurse practitioner (PNP) is engaged in the diagnosis of health status. This diagnostic process includes critical thinking, differential diagnosis, and the integration and interpretation of various forms of data. These competencies describe this role of the PNP.

1. Differentiates between normal and abnormal development in relation to anatomic findings, physiologic findings, motor findings, cognitive findings, psychologic findings, and social behavior of the child.
2. Identifies etiology, natural history, developmental considerations, pathogenesis, and clinical manifestations of common disease processes in children.
3. Identifies nutritional conditions and behavioral feeding issues.
4. Orders and interprets age- and situation-appropriate screening, laboratory tests, and other diagnostic tests, including, but not limited to, hematocrit, lead level, tuberculosis testing, ova, and parasites.
5. Collaborates in the diagnosis of children with special health needs and disabilities.

C. Plan of Care and Implementation of Treatment

The objectives of planning and implementing therapeutic interventions are to return the patient to a stable state and to optimize the patient's health. These competencies describe the pediatric nurse practitioner's role in stabilizing the patient, minimizing physical and psychologic complications, and maximizing the patient's health potential.

1. Promotes healthy nutritional practices, including promotion and management of breastfeeding, national nutritional programs, and nutritional intake considering food preferences and avoidance of food sensitivities.
2. Provides interventions to modify behavior associated with health risks such as tobacco and substance use, lack of physical activity, nutritional patterns, sexual activity, and violence.
3. Refers children with developmental disabilities and chronic illnesses to appropriate community agencies and for family support and specialty care as needed.
4. Incorporates health objectives into individual educational plans (IEPs) for children with special needs.
5. Assists the parent/child in coping with developmental behaviors and in facilitating the child's developmental potential.
6. Manages common pediatric illnesses/conditions and behavioral problems of children.
7. Performs common primary care procedures, including, but not limited to, suturing, splinting, Papanicolaou (Pap) tests, and microscopy.
8. Develops, implements, and evaluates health maintenance and health promotion services for the child/family by including teaching, counseling, advising, and anticipatory guidance.
9. Activates child protective services and other resources on behalf of children at risk.
10. Prescribes drugs and other therapies, recognizing the pharmacodynamic and pharmacokinetic processes and the effects of drug selection and dosing regimens on children.
11. Collaborates in planning for transition to adult health care.

Continued

BOX 2-1 *Assessment and Management Competencies for Nurse Practitioners—cont'd*

12. Applies child-centered research that contributes to positive change in the health of or the health care delivered to children.

II. Pediatric Nurse Practitioner–Patient Relationship

Competencies in this area demonstrate the personal, collegial, and collaborative approach, which enhances the pediatric nurse practitioner's effectiveness in patient care. The competencies speak to the critical importance of interpersonal transactions as they relate to therapeutic patient outcomes.

1. Adapts the pediatric nurse practitioner–patient relationship to the changing nature of the child's cognitive and psychosocial environment.
2. Communicates effectively with children of all developmental levels.
3. Communicates effectively with family members, including multigenerational family members.

Note: Competencies continue within the teaching-coaching, professional role, managing and negotiating health care delivery systems, monitoring and ensuring the quality of health care practice, and cultural competence domains.

From US Department of Health and Human Services: *Nurse practitioner competencies in specialty areas: adult, family, gerontological, pediatric, and women's health*, Rockville, MD, 2002, US Department of Health and Human Services.

THE ASSESSMENT MODEL

When analyzing patient problems, most NPs are comfortable with classification of diseases using the following categories of the *International Classification of Diseases*, ninth revised edition, *Clinical Modification* (ICD-9-CM) (USDHHS, 1981): infectious, endocrine, nutritional, metabolic, immunologic, respiratory, cardiovascular, and so on. NPs consistently record the disease diagnoses they make for problems in these body systems. One reason that NPs use this classification system so easily is that the classic health history format used drives decision making into these categories. This classic health history format is listed in Box 2-2.

The classic medical history is written to expand on the chief complaint, which is generally a physical problem. Issues such as nutrition, development, and activities of daily living are included, primarily as they relate to various diseases. This classification system works well and has generally been taught to physicians and NPs. The system fails, however, to provide a framework for integrating nursing aspects of NP work into the problem list and management plan. Without that framework, NPs may fail to clearly identify and document the unique contributions they make as nurses providing primary health care. Without that identification, the special aspects of their work with patients remain invisible.

An alternative model is offered in this chapter that integrates the nursing and medical aspects of NP work conceptually and clinically. This assessment model (Burns, 1991a, 1992a, 1992b) is based on the assumption that patient problems can be grouped into three distinct domains: developmental problems, functional health problems, and diseases.

The pediatric problems that NPs manage in primary care are organized into an integrated taxonomy or classification

BOX 2-2 *The Classic Health History*

I. Patient identifying information: Name, birth date, sex, address, record number, and name of historian, along with relationship to the patient stated
II. Chief complaint (C/C)
III. History of present illness (HPI)
IV. Past medical history (PMH)
   A. Prenatal, natal, postnatal
   B. Past illnesses
   C. Allergies
   D. Accidents
   E. Hospitalizations
   F. Immunization history
   G. Nutrition history
   H. Growth
   I. Development
V. Review of systems (RDS): As found in Disease Domain Database described previously with the following added:
   A. Psychologic—colic, breath holding, thumb sucking, head banging, fears, tics, behavior disorders, temper tantrums, nail biting, hair pulling, masturbation. Adjustment to home, school, neighborhood. Temperament—activity level, predictability, moods, intensity of reactions, adaptability, initial responses, distractibility. Sleep—amount, habits, problems
VI. Family history (FH)
VII. Socioeconomic (SE)
   A. Occupations of father and mother
   B. Time spent with child by parents, activities together
   C. Finances—adequacy
   D. Persons in the home
   E. House or apartment living arrangements
   F. General relationship of family members
   G. Community support systems—friends, church, agencies involved with family

list of medical and nursing diagnoses sorted by the three domains, which form a framework for analysis of the problems (Box 2-3).

Developmental Problems

This domain includes the long-term issues of development and maturation over the life span. In pediatrics, developmental issues are prominent. Missing a developmental problem or failing to plan for its management is as serious as missing diabetes mellitus or a dislocated hip. Both physical and developmental problems can affect the child's entire future if not remedied or managed to minimize their effects. NPs assess for developmental problems in the areas of gross motor, fine motor, speech and language, cognitive, and social and adaptive behaviors.

BOX 2-3 *Integrated Classification System of Diagnoses for Use by Nurse Practitioners*

Domain I: Development Diagnoses

- Cognitive development
  - Cognitive delay
  - Learning disorder
- Language development
  - Language delay
  - Speech delay
- Motor development
  - Gross motor delay
  - Fine motor delay
- Social development
  - Social development delay
  - Attachment failure

Domain II: Functional Health Diagnoses

- Health perception/health management pattern
  - Adjustment impaired
  - Health maintenance alteration
  - Health-seeking behavior
  - Home maintenance management impaired
  - Home care resources inadequate
  - Knowledge deficits
  - Noncompliance
  - Risk of injury—suffocation/poisoning/trauma/aspiration
  - Self-care deficits, dressing/toileting/hygiene
  - Skill deficit
  - Therapeutic regimen management ineffective—individual/family
  - Decisional conflict
- Nutritional-metabolic pattern
  - Anorexia
  - Anorexia nervosa
  - Breastfeeding ineffective/interrupted/effective
  - Bulimia
  - Colic
  - Infant feeding pattern ineffective
  - Nausea
  - Nutrition alterations less than/greater than body requirements
  - Swallowing impaired
- Elimination pattern
  - Constipation
  - Encopresis
  - Enuresis
  - Incontinence, bowel/urinary
- Activity/exercise pattern
  - Activity intolerance
  - Diversional activities deficit
  - Fatigue
  - Physical mobility impaired
- Sleep pattern
  - Sleep pattern disturbance
- Cognitive/perceptual pattern
  - Attention deficit disorder
  - Disorganized infant behavior
  - Memory impaired
  - Potential for enhanced organized infant behavior
  - Sensory-perceptual alteration
  - Blind
  - Deaf
- Self-perception/self-concept pattern
  - Depression
  - Body image disturbance
  - Self-esteem disturbance, chronic/situational
  - Personal identity disturbance
- Role relationships pattern
  - Abuse
  - Caregiver role strain
  - Communication impaired—verbal
  - Family coping ineffective, disabling/compromised/potential for growth
  - Family process alteration
  - Family process alteration: alcoholism
  - Loneliness, risk for
  - Parenting alteration
  - Parental role conflict
  - Risk of alteration in parent/infant/child attachment
  - Role performance alteration

Continued

BOX 2-3 *Integrated Classification System of Diagnoses for Use by Nurse Practitioners—cont'd*

- Social interaction impaired
- Social isolation

Sexuality pattern
- Pregnancy
- Sexual dysfunction
- Sexual pattern alteration

Coping/stress tolerance pattern
- Anxiety
- Comfort alteration
- Coping, individual, ineffective/defensive
- Fear
- Pain/chronic pain
- Posttrauma response
- Rape-trauma response
- Self-mutilation risk
- Grieving, anticipatory/dysfunctional
- Hopelessness
- Ineffective denial
- Powerlessness
- Substance misuse
- Violence potential, self/others

Values/beliefs pattern
- Potential for enhanced spiritual well-being
- Spiritual distress

Domain III: Pediatric Disease Diagnoses

Infectious diseases
- Candidiasis
- Chickenpox
- Diarrhea
- Giardiasis
- Gonorrhea
- Herpes simplex
- Infection, potential for
- Influenza
- Parasites
- Roseola
- Scabies
- Tuberculosis
- Viral hepatitis
- Viral warts

Endocrine, nutritional, metabolic, and immune diseases
- Fluid volume excess
- Fluid volume deficit
- Food allergy
- Thyroid disorders
- Diabetes mellitus
- Immune deficiency disease

Diseases of blood and blood-forming organs
- Anemias
- Jaundice
- Leukemia

Neurologic/sense organ diseases
- Central nervous system—epilepsy/seizures, cerebral palsy
- Eye—amblyopia, conjunctivitis, dacryocystitis, myopia, strabismus
- Ear—otitis externa, otitis media, serous otitis

Circulatory system diseases
- Cardiac output decreased
- Congenital heart disease

Respiratory system disease
- Acute nasopharyngitis
- Airway clearance ineffective
- Allergic rhinitis
- Asthma
- Bronchiolitis
- Croup
- Pharyngitis
- Pneumonia
- Tonsillitis

Digestive system diseases
- Acute abdomen
- Constipation (not encopresis)
- Diarrhea
- Hernia
- Swallowing impaired
- Vomiting

Dental disorders
- Caries
- Dentition impairment
- Malocclusion
- Oral mucous membrane alteration

Genitourinary system disorders
- Adhesions
- Cryptorchidism
- Hydrocele
- Hypospadias
- Incontinence
- Urinary tract infection
- Urinary elimination alteration
- Urinary retention
- Menstrual disorder
- Vaginitis

Skin diseases
- Acne
- Atopic dermatitis
- Cellulitis
- Contact dermatitis
- Folliculitis
- Impetigo
- Nevus
- Seborrhea
- Urticaria

BOX 2-3 ***Integrated Classification System of Diagnoses for Use by Nurse Practitioners—cont'd***

Musculoskeletal diseases
- Developmental dislocated hip
- Genu varum/valgum
- Internal tibial torsion
- Lordosis
- Metatarsus adductus
- Osgood-Schlatter disease
- Scoliosis

Symptoms/signs/ill-defined conditions
- Hypotonia
- Jaundice
- Lack of physiologic maturity
- Temperature alteration—hypothermia, hyperthermia

Injury and poisoning
- Abrasion
- Bee sting
- Burn
- Contusion
- Corneal abrasion
- Fracture
- Insect bite
- Sprain/strain
- Injury, high risk for

Data from Burns C: Development and content validity testing of a comprehensive classification of diagnoses for use by pediatric nurse practitioners, *Nurs Diagn* 2:93-104, 1991.

Functional Health Problems

Functional health problems are derived from Gordon's functional health patterns (Gordon, 1987). These patterns provide a way of thinking about the problems that nurses have always managed independently. They represent the universal health behavior patterns of all humans, no matter what their culture, sex, age, or economic status. Gordon's 11 patterns include health beliefs and behavior, nutrition, elimination, activity, sleep, role relationships, coping, self-perception, cognitive/perceptual, sexuality, and values/beliefs. Nursing's primary mission is management of these problems to maximize a person's health. In hospital settings, nurses help patients eat or receive nutrition, facilitate sleep, promote coping with illness, and maximize activity (even if only rolling a comatose patient from side to side). In primary care, NPs are also concerned about these issues, although their management strategies differ with the nature and complexity of the problems.

Labels for the problems from this domain are derived primarily from the North American Nursing Diagnosis Association (NANDA) taxonomy terms (NANDA, 2003). The NANDA taxonomy is expanded and updated every 2 years. It was first developed in the 1980s and thus represents a taxonomy of phenomena important to nursing in its early stages, as compared, for instance, with the taxonomy for disease diagnoses. Diagnoses can be statements of health, risks, or existing difficulties.

Diseases

Diseases are conditions assessed and managed at the tissue or organ level of analysis. The diagnoses found in this domain generally come from the ICD-9-CM, as well as some physiologic diagnoses from NANDA. Otitis media, streptococcal pharyngitis, and appendicitis are examples of disease diagnoses. It is not expected that NPs use nursing diagnosis language for traditional disease diagnoses. For example, "seborrheic dermatitis" would not be called "alteration in skin integrity."

The *International Classification of Diseases* has been under development for more than 100 years and is designed to represent the phenomena of concern to physicians. It is broad and mature in scope. It represents physiologic problems of patients extremely well but does not include labels, or rubrics, for the behavioral, social, and developmental problems that NPs also manage. The ICD-9-CM listings are recognized by many insurance carriers for billing purposes and, as such, have become the "currency" for much health care delivery in the United States, whereas the NANDA nursing diagnoses have not yet achieved that recognition. Fortunately, many diagnoses similar to those in the NANDA classification can be found in the medical listings, thus facilitating reimbursement for nursing aspects of NP work.

Problem Interactions

The concept of interactions of problems across domains is important to understand. For instance, iron deficiency anemia can be considered a disease if looked at from the effects of lack of iron on heme production, red blood cells, oxygen transport, and cellular metabolism. The NP can diagnose this disease and prescribe an iron supplement to manage the problem at this physiologic level. However, if the problem is found to be related to a lack of iron in the diet, the NP can choose to intervene at the daily living–nutrition level, call the problem "nutrition: less than body requirements for iron," and teach the family how to increase the selection of iron-rich foods for the table. Iron deficiency has also been shown to cause developmental delays. If a goal for the visit is to provide additional support in the school setting, a developmental problem would be diagnosed.

A particular domain can also serve as the context for the problem in another area. For instance, Down syndrome, a chromosomal disorder, can be the etiology or context for a cognitive development problem. If the intervention is for cognition, a developmental problem of cognitive delay is listed. Content issues for which the NP is planning interventions are the diagnoses. The contextual issues are not the diagnoses.

The most important point to remember is that interventions must be based on or derived from diagnoses. A situation should never arise in which the NP intervenes without explicit reasons for doing so. The reasons are stated as diagnoses, either actual or potential, and enumerated in the problem list. The preventive work (i.e., to avoid potential problems) done by NPs also needs to be identified. Diagnoses, as well as interventions, need to be recorded.

THE DATABASE

The Child Health History

It is said that 80% of diagnoses are made on the basis of the history. The physical examination only provides a view of the situation as it is at the moment. It is often a cloudy picture because the body frequently responds similarly to different assaults. It is the history of the problem—its onset, duration, progress, associated symptoms, meaning, and effects on daily living—that brings the health care provider to an understanding in sufficient depth to choose appropriate management. Functional health and developmental problems present the same issues for the provider. A thorough, thoughtful history is essential.

The pediatric health history has several unique aspects. First, the participants in the conversation include more than just the patient and provider. Second, the topics emphasized will vary significantly depending on the child's developmental stage. Third, the process of communication with the child will vary with his or her age.

The Environment for Data Collection

Primary health care is delivered in many settings, not just examination rooms in outpatient clinics. Wherever the patient and the family are to be cared for, privacy must be ensured. People should have places to sit down, and the room in which the examination is conducted should be well lighted and allow the patient to lie down comfortably. The examiner must be able to work comfortably, too. The environment must be safe, given the developmental ages of the children to be cared for, and should present an atmosphere of warmth and welcome.

The health care provider should sit down during the history to make data collection a conversation, to equalize the status of clients and examiner, and to help clients feel that they have time to talk. Sitting also helps the provider conserve energy for a busy day.

For young children, the conversation time gives them the opportunity to become familiar with the examiner and setting, which is essential for cooperation when needed. Remember that young children are learning the "script" for health care visits. The visit should help them learn a script that is understandable and not too stressful. When the script is to be varied (e.g., no immunizations this visit), alert them of the change with cues and explanations for the new experiences of this visit and the likelihood that the new script will be repeated at future visits. All those in the room need to be addressed at one time or another. Health care is a family event in pediatrics.

The NP is also observing parent-child interactions during the visit. For example, are the parents responding to their baby? Can the parent set limits on a preschooler's behavior? Do the parents contribute to the school-age child's self-esteem? Cues to mental health problems in any family member or the child should be addressed (Green & Palfrey, 2002).

For adolescents, the history can be started with the parents and teen together; however, they need to then separate, with the NP getting information from the parents and the teen independently.

The well child visit should begin with open-ended questions to allow child and family to voice their concerns. Development, feeding and diet, accident prevention, growth, family and social relationships, and anticipatory guidance should all be addressed during the visit.

The Initial (Complete) Health History

Data can be collected verbally, through record review, via written forms completed by the family, or through a combination of these methods. It might not be practical for data to be fully collected on the first visit; rather, the collection can be staged according to the visit priorities. When time with patients is limited, it is common to ask new families to come early for their first appointment to complete a written history before meeting the NP. Notation of any missing data should be made so that further baseline data can be collected at the next visit.

The model used in this book integrates the classic medical history with a functional health patterns approach that leads to identification of problems specific to the three domains (Box 2-4). It uses a basic problem-oriented format that begins with subjective data (the history), moves to objective data (the physical examination, laboratory, and test data), then lists the problems by domain (identified through the subjective and objective data), and finally, plans care, problem by problem. The items listed under each topic are meant to serve as suggestions; they are not required data to obtain from every patient. As children age, the emphasis will change (e.g., less time spent on birth and infancy histories). The history needs to be individualized, considering family, culture, health status, and environment. The complete format should be *mastered* so that it becomes core to the provider's approach to all patient situations. If data are

BOX 2-4 *Problem-oriented Health Record for NPs with Consideration of Disease, Daily Living, and Development Domains*

I. Preliminary Information
- Date:
- Name:
- Birth date:
- Record no.:
- Corrected age for preterm infant younger than 2 yr:
- Caregiver's name:
- Address:
- Phone:
- Informant, relationship to patient, reliability as historian:
- Referral source:

II. Database: Subjective Information

A. Contextual information
1. Family/household profile
   - People in the home:
   - Home environment description:
   - Family care issues (time, energy, needs of other family members, emotional stresses):
2. School/employment:
3. Agencies involved with family:

B. Chief complaints (CC)
1. Concern #1:
   - History of Present Illness (HPI):
2. Concern #2:
   - HPI:

C. Disease history database
1. Past medical history
   a. Prenatal:
   b. Perinatal—birth weight, length, head circumference, delivery, and postpartum course
   c. Past disease profile:
   d. Current health problems (put in table below):

Diagnosis	Date	Provider	Current Status
1.			
2.			
3.			

   - Operations/hospitalizations
   - Injuries:
   - Allergies—food, environmental, medications:
   - Growth:
   - Immunizations:
   - Medications:
2. Review of systems
   - General:
   - Skin:
   - Head:
   - EENT:
   - Respiratory:
   - Cardiovascular:
   - GU:
   - GI:
   - Musculoskeletal:
   - Neurologic:
   - Endocrine:
   - Hematologic:
   - Dental:
3. Family history of diseases
   - Mother, father (age, health):
   - Mother's pregnancy history:
   - Familial diseases:
   - Genogram (pedigree for single disease genetics history) if appropriate to explain genetic transmission in family or health of various family members:
4. Environmental history
   - Air quality/tobacco smoke
   - Water quality
   - Exposures to soils with toxins/pesticides/heavy metals
   - Food-borne exposures
   - Noise exposure

Continued

BOX 2-4 *Problem-oriented Health Record for NPs with Consideration of Disease, Daily Living, and Development Domains—cont'd*

D. Daily living problems database
1. Health maintenance/health perceptions
   Primary care provider:
      Last visit:
   Dentist:
      Last visit:
   Knowledge and skills for caregiving/self-care:
   Safety measures:
      Car:
      Smoke alarms:
      Occupational:
      Guns locked:
      Sports equipment:
   Home and health management/resource issues:
2. Nutrition
   Diet—breakfast, lunch, dinner:
   Supplements:
   Feeding strategies/patterns:
   Restricitions—calories, other:
3. Activities
   Amount and type of activities:
   Play:
   Limitations/equipment:
4. Sleep
   Number of hours—night, naps:
   Disturbances:
5. Elimination
   Urinary:
   Bowel:
6. Role relationships
   Family patterns:
   Parenting patterns:
   Peers/social support:
   Communication—verbal, nonverbal:
7. Coping/temperament and discipline
   Substance use/abuse—alcohol, drugs, tobacco:
   Indicators of depression, anxiety, mental health disorders:
8. Cognitive/perceptual problems
   Cognitive disturbances/school performance:
   Hearing deficit:
   Vision deficit:
   Kinesthetic disturbance:
   Attention deficits/hyperactivity:
9. Self-perception/self-concept
   Role identity:
   Self-concept/self-esteem, body image:
10. Sexual and menstrual patterns
11. Values/beliefs/religious patterns

E. Developmental issues—past milestones and current skills
1. Motor development:
   Gross motor development:
   Fine motor development:
2. Language development:
3. Cognitive development:
4. Social development:
5. Development test scores:

III. Database: Objective Information

A. Physical examination

Age:	Sex:	Height:	Weight:
HC:	BP:	TPR:	BMI:

1. General appearance:
2. Skin:
3. Head:
4. Eyes:
5. Ears:
6. Nose:
7. Mouth:
8. Neck:
9. Chest/breasts:
10. Lungs:
11. Heart:
12. Abdomen;
13. Genitalia:
14. Anus/rectum:
15. Musculoskeletal:
16. Neurologic
    Motor—tone, strength:
    Reflexes:
    Primitive reflexes:
    Cranial nerves:
    Responsiveness:
    Extraneous movements:
    Gait/position:
    Cerebellar, including coordination, balance, nystagmus:
    Sensory function:

B. Screening/laboratory data
1. Hct/Hgb:
2. Hearing:
3. Vision:
4. TB:
5. Metabolic/newborn screens:
6. Other:

C. Data from other disciplines
   Physical therapy, occupational therapy, speech therapy, audiology, social work, psychology, medicine, home health, education:

BOX 2-4 *Problem-oriented Health Record for NPs with Consideration of Disease, Daily Living, and Development Domains—cont'd*

IV. Problem List (Use Classification of Diagnoses List)
Include all chief complaints and problems identified during the assessment. Categorize diagnoses by the following:
1. Diseases:
2. Daily living problems:
3. Developmental problems:

V. Plan
For each problem, describe plans, including diagnostic, therapeutic, and educational activities:
A. Disease problems:
B. Daily living problems:
C. Developmental problems:
D. Disposition/return appointments and purpose:

Adapted from Burns C: A new assessment model and tool for nurse practitioners, *Pediatri Health Care* 6:76-79, 1992.
BP, blood pressure; *EENT*, eyes, ears, nose, throat; *GI*, gastrointestinal; *GU*, genitourinary; *HC*, head circumference; *Hct*, hematocrit; *Hgb*, hemoglobin; *TB*, tuberculosis; *TPR*, temperature, pulse, respirations; *BMI*, body mass index.

omitted, the omissions should be by choice, not by an error committed through haste, distraction, ignorance, or habit.

The adolescent history needs special modification because adolescents' health care needs, risks, and developmental characteristics are so different from those of infants and young children, and because they are interviewed directly. See Box 2-5 for a modification of the initial health history for adolescents.

Patient Identifying Information. Data here are standard to medical records: date, name, medical record number, birth date, sex, address, phone number, and names of other family members. The information about the informant is designed

BOX 2-5 *Problem-oriented History for Adolescents*

I. Database—Subjective Information
- A. Contextual information
  1. With whom do you live?
  2. In the past year, have there been any changes in your immediate family such as
     - Marriage, separation, divorce
     - Serious illness or injury
     - Loss of job
     - Move/change of address
     - Change of school
     - Births, deaths
     - Other
  3. What languages are spoken in your home?
- B. Chief complaint
- C. Past medical history
  1. In the past year, have you had any injury or illness that made you miss school or cut down on activities, or that required medical care?
  2. Have you been hospitalized in the past year?
  3. Do you have any illnesses or medical conditions?
  4. Are you taking any medications?
  5. Have you been exposed to tuberculosis in the past year?
  6. Have you stayed overnight in a homeless shelter, jail, or detention center in the past year?
  7. Girls only: Have you had a period? Date of last one
- D. Review of systems
  1. Do you have any questions or concerns about
     - Height/weight
     - Blood pressure
     - Headaches/migraines
     - Eyes/vision
     - Hearing/ears/earaches
     - Nose
     - Frequent colds
     - Mouth/teeth (frequency of tooth brushing, flossing)
     - Neck/back
     - Chest pain
     - Coughing/wheezing
     - Breasts
     - Heart
     - Stomach
     - Nausea/vomiting
     - Diarrhea/constipation

Continued

BOX 2-5 *Problem-oriented History for Adolescents—cont'd*

Skin (rash, acne, sore, use of sunscreen)
Muscle or joint pain
Frequent or painful urination
Sexual organs/genitals
Menstruation/periods
Sexual activity
Future plans/job
Physical or sexual abuse
Masturation
Cancer or dying
Other (explain)

II. Functional Health Database

A. Health maintenance/health perception
1. Do you usually wear a helmet for rollerblade, bicycle, skateboard, motorcycle, or all-terrain vehicle use?
2. Do you usually wear a seat belt when riding in a car, truck, or van?
3. In the past year, have you been in a car when the driver has been drinking or using drugs?
4. Do you use electric tools or heavy equipment at work or home?
5. Do you have questions or concerns about avoiding accidents or injuries?

B. Nutrition
1. Do you eat from the four food groups almost every day?
2. Do you have any diet/food/appetite concerns?
3. Are you eating in secret?
4. Are you satisfied with your eating patterns?
5. Do you prefer a change in your current weight?
6. Have you tried to lose weight or control weight by vomiting, taking diet pills or laxatives, or starving yourself?
7. Do you have concerns about your weight?

C. Activities
1. Do you watch television or play video games more than 2 hours per day?
2. Are you involved with exercises that make you sweat and breathe hard at least three times per week?
3. What do you do after school?
4. Do you have physical problems that limit your exercise?
5. Do you have questions or concerns about exercise or physical activity?

D. Sleep
1. Do you have trouble sleeping?
2. Do you have trouble with tiredness?

E. Elimination habits
1. Do you sometimes wet the bed?

F. Role relationships
1. Do you have at least one friend you really like and feel you can talk to?
2. Do parents or guardian usually listen to you and take your feelings seriously?
3. Do you and your parents or guardian do things together on a regular basis such as eating meals, attending religious activities, performing chores or errands, playing sports, or watching television?
4. Is there a lot of tension or conflict in your home?
5. Do you have questions or concerns about family or friends?

G. Coping/temperament and discipline
1. Alcohol
   In the past year, did you or friends get drunk or very high on alcoholic beverages?
   Have you ever consumed alcohol and then done any of the following: driven a vehicle, gone swimming or boating, gotten in a fight, used tools or equipment, done something you later regretted?
   Have you been criticized or gotten in trouble because of drinking?
   Do you have any questions or concerns about alcohol?
2. Drugs
   Do you or your friends ever use marijuana or street drugs?
   Some drugs can be bought at a store without a doctor's prescription. Do you ever use nonprescription drugs to get to sleep, stay awake, calm down, get high, or enhance your sports performance?
   Have you ever used steroids without a doctor telling you to do so?
   Do you have any questions or concerns about drugs or drug use?
3. Tobacco
   Do you or your friends ever smoke cigarettes or use smokeless tobacco?
   Does anyone you live with smoke cigarettes or use smokeless tobacco?
   Do you have any questions or concerns about cigarettes or other tobacco products?
4. Emotions
   Have you had fun during the past 2 weeks?
   In general, are you happy with the way things are going for you these days?
   During the past few weeks, have you often felt sad or down with nothing to look forward to?

BOX 2-5 *Problem-oriented History for Adolescents—cont'd*

Have you ever seriously thought about killing yourself, made a plan to kill yourself, or actually tried to kill yourself?
Do you think counseling would help you or someone in your family?
Do you have any questions or concerns about physical, sexual, or emotional abuse?

5. Weapons/violence
   Do you or does anyone you live with have a gun, rifle, shotgun, or other firearm in your home?
   In the past year, have you ever carried a gun, knife, razorblade, club, or other weapon?
   Have you been in a physical fight during the past 3 months?
   Are guns or violence a problem in your neighborhood?
   Have you ever witnessed a violent act?
   When you are angry, do you ever get violent?
   Do you have any questions or concerns about violence or your safety?

H. Cognitive/perceptual problems
   In general, do you like school? Why?
   Are your grades this year better on worse than the year before? What are your usual grades?
   Have you ever had to repeat a grade in school?
   Do you cut classes or skip school?
   How many days of school have you missed this year?
   Have you ever been suspended or dropped out of school?
   Do you have any questions or concerns about school or your learning?

I. Self-perception/self-concept
   1. Do you have any concerns about the size or shape of your body or your physical appearance?
   2. What do you like about yourself?
   3. What do you do best?
   4. If you could, what would you change about your life or yourself?

J. Sexual and menstrual
   1. Do you date?
   2. Do you or your friends have sexual intercourse?
   3. Do you think you might be gay, lesbian, or bisexual?
   4. Have you ever been told that you have a sexually transmitted disease such as gonorrhea, genital herpes, chlamydia, trichomonas, syphilis, hepatitis, genital warts, AIDS, or HIV infection?
   5. Do you have any questions or concerns about sex or relationships?
   6. Are you worried about getting pregnant (girls) or do you worry about getting someone pregnant (boys)?
   7. Have you ever been forced to do something sexual that you didn't want to do?
   8. Do you practice abstinence?
   9. Do you use a birth control method? If so, which one(s)?
   10. Do you want information or supplies to prevent pregnancy or sexually transmitted diseases, including HIV?

K. Values and beliefs/religious
   1. Are you involved with any religious groups or activities on a regular basis?

III. Development Database

Throughout the history, listen for data that allow you to assess the following areas (see Developmental Management of Adolescents, Chapter 9):

A. Motor development
   1. All teens should be active and skilled in a variety of physical activities and sports.
   2. Fine motor development should also be mature. Special arts/crafts or occupational activities may be learned.

B. Cognitive development
   1. Early adolescents are still concrete and generally present rather than future oriented. Questions can be answered quite literally.
   2. Middle adolescents can use and understand if-then statements. They are able to understand long-term consequences and think of the future. They might challenge many ideas and rules with their newfound skills in logic and reasoning.
   3. Late adolescents are able to consider options before making decisions, engage in sophisticated moral reasoning, and use principles to guide their decisions.

C. Social development
   1. Early adolescents are egocentric in thinking. They can vacillate between childish and mature behavior, especially around their parents. Their peers are usually of the same sex. Group activities are the norm.
   2. Middle adolescents are concerned with their identity within society and less concerned with their sexual identity unless they are struggling with recognizing their homosexuality. They tend to distance themselves from parents, spend less time at home, and increasingly challenge parental control. Cliques or friends prevail, with only a few close friends. Physical intimacy can occur during this stage, and romantic partners are common.

Continued

BOX 2-5 *Problem-oriented History for Adolescents—cont'd*

3. Late adolescents have distanced themselves from parents and then reestablished relationships with family on a new basis of independence. Romantic, emotional intimacy appears.

D. School/vocational development
1. Early adolescents are usually adjusting to the expectations of middle school. Setting priorities and completing homework independently can be a challenge. Future goals are often unrealistic and change frequently.
2. Middle adolescents are entering high school and beginning to develop an awareness that their performance in school will affect their future options for work or college. They do not usually have specific ideas about future vocations in mind.
3. Late adolescents are making decisions about vocations, college, working, or entering the military.

Adapted from American Medical Association, Department of Adolescent Health: *Guidelines for adolescent preventive services (GAPS) user's manual,* Chicago, 1994, American Medical Association.

to give the reader a sense of the probability that the history is accurate and complete and from a knowledgeable source.

The Database—Subjective Information

Contextual Information. The intent of this section is to identify family, day care, school, work, or community agency factors that form the context of the child's life and need to be considered in planning care.

- People in the home
- Home environment description: Apartment, home, or farm? Fenced yard or unsafe neighborhood?
- Family care issues: Primary caregiver? Who helps? What stresses are faced by the caregiver? Do other family members require more attention than the patient? Is the caregiver well both physically and emotionally?
- Family structure issues: Is this a two-parent family, a single-parent family, or a foster home? Are divorced parents dividing caregiving, and what is the meaning of the family structure for the child? How much time do parents and the child spend in the home together, given job, school, and other obligations? Is this a latchkey child?
- Family financial issues: Health insurance? Money for basic necessities? Does the child have an allowance or access to money? What are the sources of money—jobs or welfare? Are financial issues causing family stress?
- School/employment: Where does the child go for day care, school, or work (if an adolescent)? What is the quality of the setting?
- Agencies involved: What other community agencies know this child or family?
- What resources and family support systems are being used and with what success?

Chief Complaint and History of Present Problem

- Concerns: What brings the child to the clinic today? The chief complaint is a brief statement of the problem and its duration. Remember that new concerns can arise at any point during the visit. Agendas can be hidden or unconscious. The chief complaint or complaints can involve disease, the functional health pattern, or development.
- Present problem history: For each concern, a chronologic description should be made that includes onset, duration, characteristics or symptoms, exposure to illnesses or other causative factors, similar problems in other family members or neighbors, previous episodes of similar illnesses or symptoms, previous diagnostic measures, pertinent negative data, things that have been tried in attempts to manage the concern and their success, and the meaning of the concern for the family and child.

Disease Domain Database

1. Medical history:
   - Prenatal: Planned pregnancy? When did prenatal care begin? What was the mother's health during pregnancy? Drug, alcohol, and tobacco use? Illnesses and medications? Weight gain? Accidents? (With age and history of a healthy baby, these sections may become less significant.)
   - Perinatal: Where was the baby born and who delivered the infant? Duration and process of labor? Vaginal or cesarean delivery and process? Anesthesia? Infant response to labor and delivery (breathing, crying)? Resuscitation needed? Apgar scores? Birth weight, length, and head circumference? Gestational age? Neonatal course: Infections or other health problems, physiologic stabilization, feeding, responsiveness? Jaundice? Weight at discharge? Hospital duration? Neonatal follow-up over the first few weeks? (Again, with age and health, this section is given less attention.)

- Past diseases profile: What health problems has the child experienced, and what have the outcomes been? Who has provided care? Infectious diseases?
- Other current health problems (not related to the chief complaint): What problems does the child have now? What was the date of onset? Who is the principal care provider for each problem, and what is the current status (e.g., medications, awaiting surgery, problem in remission)?
- Operations/hospitalizations/emergency department visits: Has the child been hospitalized for any reason? Why, when, where, outcomes? Response to hospitalization? Problems resolved? Emergency department visits? Why, when, and outcomes?
- Injuries: What significant injuries has the child experienced? What care was needed, was care sought at emergency department(s), and does the child currently have any sequelae?
- Allergies: Allergies to foods, medications, or environmental factors? How are the allergies manifested? What care is given?
- Growth: What has the child's growth pattern been? (Always plot growth data on a growth grid to assess progress.) Is the child similar in size to peers? Are clothing sizes changing? Has growth been a worry for the child or family?
- Immunizations and laboratory tests: Obtain a record with dates for all immunizations received in the past. Reactions? Blood tests and screening tests?
- Medications: Is the child taking any medications (prescription drugs, over-the-counter agents, and folk remedies)? What? Why? How much? Responses to the medication?

2. Review of systems: Remember that this section documents the history of body systems, not the physical assessment findings.
   - General: Is the child considered to be well, happy, and developing normally?
   - Skin: History of birthmarks, lesions, or skin conditions?
   - Head: Head trauma? Head growth—microcephaly, macrocephaly? Headaches?
   - Eyes, ears, nose, throat: Vision and eye problems? Hearing and ear problems? Nose—discharge or bleeding episodes, breathing interference? Throat problems or infections?
   - Respiratory: Breathing problems? Respiratory infections? Blue spells? Cough? Snoring at night or obstructive sleep apnea?
   - Cardiovascular: Heart murmur history? Cyanosis? Blood pressure problems? Activity intolerance? Syncope?
   - Gastrointestinal: Infections, diarrhea, constipation, vomiting, or reflux? Structural problems? Anal itching or fissures? Stomachaches?
   - Genitourinary: Infections, discharges? Structural problems? Stream appearance? Frequency or burning?
   - Gynecologic: Menarche and menstrual history including length of menses, frequency of cycle, cramps, and clots? Vaginal discharge or bleeding? Itching?
   - Musculoskeletal: Movement or structural problems? Broken bones or joint sprains? Joint inflammation?
   - Neurologic: Seizures? Movement disorders? Tremors? Tics? Loss-of-consciousness episodes?
   - Endocrine: Problems with growth or pubescence?
   - Hematologic: Anemia history or symptoms? Blood transfusions? Bleeding disorders?
   - Dentition: Number of teeth and eruption pattern? Dental trauma? Dental care? Use of fluoride? Teeth brushing? Toothaches?
3. Family history of diseases:
   - Mother and father: Ages and health history.
   - Mother's pregnancy history: Number of pregnancies, births, status of offspring.
   - Familial diseases: Age, sex, and health status of each family member. Familial and communicable diseases such as diabetes, epilepsy, tuberculosis, hypertension or heart disease, cancer, sickle cell anemia, birth defects, known genetic disorders?
   - Genogram: Draw out a genogram of the family members, including sex, age, and health status of each member. (See Chapters 3 and 41 for genogram and pedigree notations.)
4. Environmental history: This section is used to consider toxic exposures. What foods does the child eat and how are they prepared? What is the quality of the child's living environment(s)—water and air quality? Pesticides used? Chemicals/heavy metals near or in the home? Tobacco smoke and lead exposure?

Functional Health Domain Database. The questions in this section are organized by functional health patterns and relate to the nursing diagnoses for each pattern.

1. Health maintenance/health perceptions: All people take steps to influence and protect their health. These choices include selection of health care providers, use of safety devices, learning how to take care of oneself, and daily care of the body. Nursing diagnoses can include health-seeking behavior, altered health maintenance, or noncompliance to a preventive or adaptive health care regimen. Usual data include the following:
   - Usual primary care provider—last visit?
   - Dentist—last visit?

- Child's self-care or caregiver needs for more knowledge of caregiving?
- Health care recommendations that the family chooses not to follow?
- Safety measures used: Car seats or seat belts? Smoke and carbon monoxide alarms? Window screens? Home safety measures? Pools? Firearms in the home?
- Routine health promotion regimens?
- Home and health management resource issues for the chronically ill or handicapped child? Home nursing? Equipment needs? Transportation needs?

2. Nutrition: Quality and quantity of the daily diet and the processes of feeding and swallowing. Data to support diagnoses such as nutrition, less than or greater than body requirements; anorexia; bulimia; impaired swallowing; and breastfeeding issues would be found in this section.
   - Daily diet—breakfast, lunch, snacks, and dinner?
   - Supplements/vitamins?
   - Feeding patterns—meal times and snack times? Feeding strategies? Self-feeding skills? Breastfeeding and bottle-feeding issues?
   - Nutritional restrictions—calories, other?
   - Satisfaction with weight?
   - Difficulties chewing or swallowing?
3. Activities: Physical mobility as well as the diversional and occupational activities of daily life should be described here.
   - Amount, timing, and types of physical activities?
   - Television and computer/electronic games time?
   - Reading time?
   - Play opportunities and activities in which the child engages?
   - Sports, organized activities, and hobbies of older children and adolescents?
   - Activity limitations caused by health problems?
   - Special equipment used or needed to support mobility?
4. Sleep: Sleep and rest patterns are described here. Hours? Disturbances for the child or family? Sleep aids? Sleep position for infants.
5. Elimination: Problems of elimination can be analyzed at the physiologic level of the genitourinary or gastrointestinal systems or in terms of daily living patterns. Enuresis and encopresis are daily living problems (bowel and bladder habits) that fall in this area. Physiologically, the child is well but the elimination habits are problematic.
   - Urinary patterns: Bed wetting? Toilet training? Voiding schedule?
   - Bowel patterns: Constipation or soiling? Stooling patterns? Toilet training?
6. Role relationships: Role relationships include family relationships and relationships with peers and friends in the community. Both family and individual diagnoses need to be considered here. Family coping, family process alteration, parenting alteration, abuse, and social interaction or isolation can be addressed.
   - Family interactions: Between parents? Parents and children? With other family members?
   - Parenting style and activities?
   - Peers/social supports for the child and family? Special adults in the child's life?
   - Communication with and by the child: Verbal? Nonverbal?
   - School performance for school-age children and teens.
7. Coping/temperament and discipline used: People select and use a variety of coping strategies in their daily lives. Temperament is also important to understand child behavior and likely responses to the environment. Discipline strategies used in families are important to identify. Anxiety, fear, hopelessness, grief, powerlessness, substance abuse, pain, and potential for violence might be identified nursing diagnoses.
   - Stressors for the child and family? Losses?
   - Coping strategies of the child and caregivers?
   - Use of alcohol or drugs?
   - Temperament characteristics of the child and the "fit" with other family members?
   - Problem behavior, discipline strategies used and their outcomes?
8. Cognitive/perceptual: Cognitive or perceptual problems are identified here. Attention deficit disorder is an example.
   - Hearing or vision problems?
   - Learning disorders?
   - Attention problems?
   - Adaptations made at home and school to assist the child, especially for problems of comprehension.
9. Self-perception/self-concept: Personal role identity, body image, and self-esteem are issues identified in this functional health domain.
   - Satisfaction with self?
   - Feelings of depression?
10. Sexual: All people have sexuality issues that affect their lives. Within their sexual preferences and habits, problems are identified when these patterns are interrupted or viewed as problematic by the client or family. Pregnancy, viewed from the psychosocial perspective, is also a sexual issue that should be explored.
    - Sexual habits?
    - Sexual relationships?
    - Development of sexual identity?

11. Values and beliefs: In this last section, the NP explores spiritual patterns and personal values and beliefs that affect the child's health.
    - Involvement with church?
    - Religious rituals?
    - Sense of alienation?
    - Sense of spiritual meaning in one's life
    - Values the family wants to impart to their children?

Development Domain Database. The levels of motor, language, cognitive, and social development are assessed and documented in this area. Both past milestones and current functioning are important. Sometimes, developmental tests are administered to provide data in this area.

- Motor landmarks—sitting, standing, walking, and so on
- Language landmarks—words, sentences, intelligibility, comprehension
- Personal and social—play, attachment, self-care, peer relationships
- Scholastic grade and progress

The Interval History

The complete history should need to be completed only once for new patients. After that, for routine scheduled health maintenance visits, the history is updated only from the last contact to the present. The format remains the same as for the complete history; however, questions are modified to verify that the situations are as they were in the past or to add new information. All areas of the history should be assessed.

The Episodic History

Many times, patients come for help with specific problems. The history includes the chief complaint and history of present illness sections of the complete history. The framework for dealing with these problems is as follows, with each symptom analyzed in chronologic sequence.

Symptom Analysis

1. Onset—initial and episodic; date and time, sudden or gradual, setting
2. Location of pain—local, radiation, generalized, superficial, or deep
3. Duration—how long, has it eased, gotten worse?
4. Characteristics and course:
   Symptom quality: Nature of symptoms
   Symptom quantity: Severity, frequency, volume, number, size or extent, degree of functional impairment
   Course: Continuous or intermittent, pattern of variation
5. Activating (precipitating) and aggravating factors
6. Relieving factors and patient's reactions to symptoms
7. Tests and treatment: What, when, where, who, and results, including complications and sequelae

Even though the patient comes in for a specific problem, always ask some screening questions that tap into the other domains of the history—disease, daily living, and developmental. At visits for minor illnesses, health promotion and disease prevention issues should be considered, as well as the problem at hand. An immunization history and vaccinations, if appropriate, should be completed at every visit.

The Psychosocial Problem History

Psychosocial or behavioral problems also must be assessed (Green, Sullivan, & Eichberg, 2002). Some considerations are summarized in Box 2-6. Much of the data related to psychosocial concerns will be collected in the functional health pattern domain database.

BOX 2-6 *Suggestions for the Psychosocial Complaint History*

1. Use good communication skills—*listen.* Nonjudgmental approach. Seek a balanced give and take of information.
2. Interview the child or adolescent alone as well as with parents. Time alone with the preschooler may be used for play or drawing.
3. Have questionnaires or checklists from parents, teachers, child care workers available. Use the information in the interview.
4. Be alert to emotional tone and interactions among family members.
5. Review the context for the concern:
   - Information about parents and family members: illnesses, mental health problems, poverty, employment, violence, social isolation
   - Information about the child: school, peer relationships, temperament, neglect or abuse history, foster home placements, losses
   - Information about child-parent relationships: attachment disorder, unrealistic expectations, poor family communication, lack of knowledge of child development and appropriate parenting
6. The history of present illness becomes an amalgam of information from the multiple sources—child, parents, others. Do not assume that both parents have the same views of the issues.
7. Remember that the interview itself may be therapeutic.

From Green M, Sullivan P, Eichberg C: Avoid a "Swiss cheese" history when psychosocial complaints are on the menu, *Contemp Pediatr* 19:115, 2002.

The Physical Examination and Laboratory and Other Studies

The Physical Examination

The physical examination is conducted following the history, although younger children might do better with developmental testing preceding the physical examination. Height, weight, head circumference, body mass index (BMI), and vital signs are recorded. Principal findings that the NP is expected to identify are presented in the following list. Screening tests for hearing and vision, as well as laboratory data and data from other disciplines, are included as other types of objective information. More experienced NPs collect some of the history while conducting the physical examination.

1. General appearance: Ill or well, distressed, alert, cooperative, body build. Reaction to parents. Characteristic position, movements, nutrition, developmental appearance as contrasted with the stated age.
2. Skin: Color—pigmentation, cyanosis, jaundice, carotenemia, erythema, pallor. Vascular—visible veins, arteries. Eruptions, petechiae, ecchymosis, hives, rashes, nevi. Nodules. Texture, scaling, striae, scars. Sweat, edema, turgor. Subcutaneous tissue. Distribution and color of hair. Nail appearance.
3. Lymph nodes: Occipital, postauricular, preauricular, cervical, parotid, submaxillary, sublingual, axillary, epitrochlear, inguinal. Size, mobility, tenderness, heat.
4. Head: Position, shape, sutures, fontanels. Size—circumference, microcephaly, macrocephaly, hydrocephaly. Facial paralysis, twitching.
5. Eyes: Vision, visual fields, cover test. Blinking. Position: exophthalmos, enophthalmos, hypertelorism, hypotelorism. Movements: strabismus, extraocular movements, nystagmus. Ptosis, eyelids, sclera, conjunctivae. Lesions—styes, chalazion. Corneas, corneal reflex. Discharge. Pupils, accommodation, iris. Retina, red reflex, fundus.
6. Ears: Anomalies. Position. Discharge. Tenderness. Canals. Tympanic membranes: redness, light reflex, landmarks, bulging or retraction, perforation, mobility. Mastoid. Hearing. Vestibular function.
7. Nose: Shape. Alae nasi, flaring. Mucosa, secretions, bleeding, airway. Septum. Polyps, tumors.
8. Mouth: Odor. Teeth—number, edges, occlusion, caries, formation, color. Gums—discoloration, bleeding. Buccal mucosa, tongue—coating, protrusion, color, tremor. Palate—cleft, arch. Tonsils—size, color, exudate. Pharynx—appearance, color, lesions.
9. Neck: Size. Anomalies—webbing, edema, nodes, masses. Sternocleidomastoids. Trachea. Thyroid. Vessels. Motion—head drop, tilting, nodding, range of motion.
10. Chest: Shape—circumference, symmetry, Harrison groove. Movement—flaring, expansion, abdominal/thoracic breathing, intercostal retractions.
11. Breasts: Tanner stage of development, symmetry, redness, heat, tenderness, lumps. Gynecomastia.
12. Lungs: Respiration—type, rate, dyspnea. Exercise tolerance. Cough, hemoptysis, sputum. Palpation—masses, tenderness, fremitus. Percussion—dullness, hyperresonance, diaphragm. Auscultation—breath sounds, crackles (rales), rubs, rhonchi, wheezes, vocal resonance.
13. Cardiovascular/heart: Blood pressure and pulse rate.
    - Inspection: Vascularity, bulging, impulse. Distress, cyanosis, edema, clubbing, pulsations, venous distention.
    - Palpation: Femoral pulses, point of maximal impulse, thrill.
    - Auscultation: First and second heart sounds, rhythm, split, third heart sound, gallop, friction rub, venous hum, murmurs.
14. Abdomen:
    - Inspection: Shape, distention, transillumination. Umbilicus, diastasis rectus, veins. Peristaltic, gastric waves.
    - Auscultation: Bowel sounds, bruits.
    - Palpation: Superficial or deep tenderness, rebound. Spleen, liver, masses, kidneys, bladder, uterus.
    - Percussion: Masses, fluid, flatus.
15. Genitalia: Discharge, foreign body. Tags. Labia, adhesions, vagina, clitoris. Penis—hypospadias, epispadias, phimosis. Meatus, scrotum, testes, hydrocele, hernia. Cremasteric reflex. Tanner staging. Vaginal, bimanual examination for teenage girls. (Pelvic examination observations are discussed further in Chapter 36.)
16. Anus and rectum: Buttocks, fistula, fissure, prolapse, polyps, hemorrhoids, rashes. Rectal—rectum, fistula, megacolon, masses, prostate, uterus, tenderness. Sensation.
17. Musculoskeletal: Anomalies, length, clubbing, pain, tenderness, temperature, swelling, shape, symmetry.
    - Gait: Stance, balance, limp. Foot position.
    - Spine: Tufts of hair, dimples, masses, spina bifida, tenderness, mobility, scoliosis.
    - Posture: Lordosis, kyphosis.
    - Joints: Heat, tenderness, mobility, swelling, effusion.
    - Muscles: Development, pain, tone, spasm, paralysis, rigidity, contractures, atrophy.
18. Nervous system:
    - General impression, abilities, responsiveness, position, spontaneous movements, play activity.

Development—consistent with age or current level.
State of consciousness, irritability, seizure activity.
Gait, stance, limp, ataxia. Coordination, Romberg sign.
Tremors, twitching, choreiform movements, athetosis, spasticity, paralysis, flaccidity.
Reflexes: Superficial, deep tendon, clonus, Chvostek sign.
Primitive reflexes: Moro, tonic neck, Babinski, grasp, suck. Thumb position.
Sensation: Hyperesthesia, paresthesia, temperature, touch. Stereognosis.
Cranial nerves I to XII.
Hearing and vision.

Other Data

Laboratory and Radiographic Data. Record hearing, vision, hematocrit or other blood tests, lead, urinalysis, newborn screening tests, tuberculosis screening.

Developmental and Psychologic Test Scores. Scores need to be recorded and considered when problems are being identified.

Data from Other Disciplines. Summarize social work, nutrition, physical therapy, occupational therapy, medical specialist, speech pathology, education, and other reports.

Creating the Problem List

The problem list is derived from analysis of the subjective and objective data collected. Differential diagnosis is the clinical decision-making process used to derive the problems listed (Fig. 2-1). To use this process, the clinician considers all the possible diagnoses for the problems presented by the patient. Then the factors that support or rule out each of the various options considered are analyzed. Identification of the best fit of the patient's subjective and objective data with the possible diagnoses is the goal. If further data are needed to confirm a diagnosis, collection of these data is incorporated into the plan. For example, the differential diagnoses for coryza (a runny nose) include, among others, allergic rhinitis, upper respiratory infection, and a foreign body in the nose. The NP uses data about related symptoms (e.g., itchy eyes, a sore throat, systemic symptoms, or bilateral or unilateral drainage from the nostrils) to choose which diagnosis best fits the child's picture. That analysis for fit is the diagnostic reasoning process.

Functional health problems and developmental problems are also subject to the notion of differential diagnosis. For example, a child who is not sleeping well might be fearful, a trained night feeder, or experiencing episodes of obstructive sleep apnea. The interventions for each problem are different. Thus the NP must use the differential

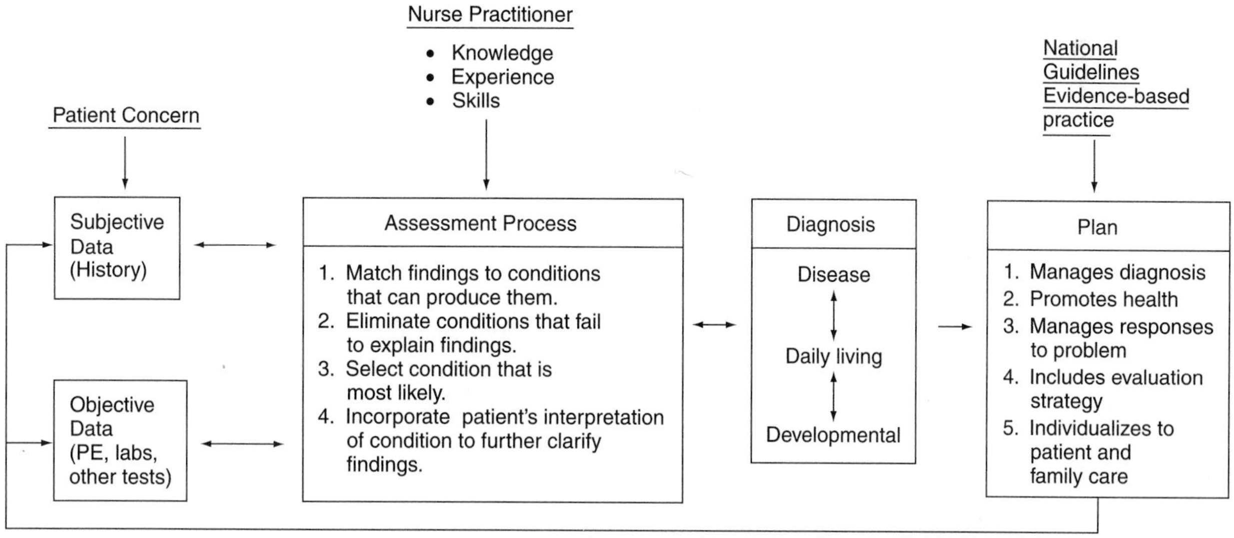

FIGURE 2-1 Model for clinical decision-making. The NP will take the patient's concern and clarify it with subjective and objective data. As the NP works, he or she will use past experience and skills to facilitate the assessment process. The process, which happens both during and after data collection, involves decision-making to find the best match between standardized diagnoses and the patient's findings. Once the diagnosis is made, a plan is then developed, using national evidence-based guidelines where appropriate, to achieve the five goals listed. Sometimes the development of the plan requires further data collection. Data from Burns C: Development and content validity testing of a comprehensive classification of diagnoses for use by pediatric nurse practitioners, *Nurs Diagn* 2:93-104, 1991.

diagnosis process to identify the problem or problems at hand. A problem should never be included on the problem list that is not supported by subjective and objective data found and recorded in the database. "Rule out" should not be listed as a diagnosis. The diagnosis would be the unexplained symptom, for example, "dysuria" or "dysuria, rule out urinary tract infection."

Creating the Management Plan

A plan must be developed for every identified problem. It is helpful to consider diagnostic, therapeutic, and educational interventions for every problem listed. Of course, not every problem requires work in all three areas, but they should be considered. The management activities are listed in the record. The plan should always include a recommendation for the next visit and what is to be done at that visit in an attempt to move the patient into a health maintenance pattern rather than being seen only episodically. Just as the problem list must be consistent with the data at hand, plans must address diagnoses that are included in the problem list. In other words, the plan is internally consistent with the data and diagnoses.

VALIDATING DATA COLLECTION

Data collection for clinical practice, just as for research, must be as reliable and valid as possible. To assist with reliability, consider the following techniques (Burns, 1991b): test-retest, interrater reliability, and internal consistency.

Test-Retest

Ask the question again later. Take a blood pressure reading twice. Look for the physical finding a second time a bit later.

Interrater Reliability

Ask someone else to listen, palpate, and so on for the same finding. Does someone else get the same answer to the same question you asked?

Internal Consistency

Look for a logical consistency to the findings you are getting. If something is "out of sync," question it. For example, do the height points on the graph line up, or is one significantly off the trajectory? If there is significant variation, consider a measuring error before looking for a health problem that has altered growth. Does the history support the physical findings? Does the story keep changing?

Algorithms, protocols, and flow sheets can improve the consistency and reliability of the data collected, especially when several staff members are involved with the data for a given patient.

To assess the validity, or meaning, of data collected, the provider should consider sources of error:

- Do the cumulative data fit and support a given diagnosis? If not, perhaps the diagnosis was inadequate or an error in data collection, sequencing, or interpretation occurred.
- Was the diagnosis made on the basis of one isolated finding or a cluster? For instance, diagnosing pneumonia after hearing a cough and diagnosing failure to thrive with one growth measurement are mono-operation bias errors.
- Sometimes two problems occur with overlapping findings. One problem might be missed while the other is pursued.
- The patient might change the data provided because of stress or worry about the outcomes of the assessment visit. Both findings and their meaning to patients need to be explored with the patient and family.
- Provider expectations can also threaten accurate diagnosing.
- Were cues missed or questions unasked?
- Data are often compared with specific criteria (e.g., heights and weights for age are known, developmental milestones are established, laboratory norms are set for children of different ages). Which test has been used? What is its specificity and sensitivity? Is the right criterion being used?
- Clinicians constantly need to attend to age, sex, race, culture, and other issues when they consider data. Is it likely for a white child to have sickle cell disease? What diagnoses should one consider when a teenage girl has abdominal pain, as opposed to the diagnoses possible for a boy of the same age?

SUMMARY

The assessment of a child and family is the basis for all the primary care work that NPs do. The knowledge and skills needed for accurate, comprehensive, individualized care are considerable and will expand over time. Data collection begins with collection of a health history. A physical examination and laboratory and developmental testing data are added to the historical findings. From the total database, the clinician develops a list of diagnoses and a plan of care for each. Errors either in data collection or in analysis can result in diagnostic errors, which always need to be minimized.

REFERENCES

Burns C: Development and content validity testing of a comprehensive classification of diagnoses for use by pediatric nurse practitioners, *Nurs Diagn* 2:93-104, 1991a.

Burns C: Parallels between research and diagnosis: the reliability and validity issues of clinical practice, *Nurs Pract* 16:42-50, 1991b.

Burns C: A new assessment model and tool for nurse practitioners, *J Pediatr Health Care* 6:73-81, 1992a.

Burns C: Using a comprehensive taxonomy of diagnoses to describe the practice of pediatric nurse practitioners: findings of a field study, *J Pediatr Health Care* 7:115-121, 1992b.

Gordon M: *Nursing diagnosis: process and application*, New York, 1987, McGraw-Hill.

Green M, Palfrey J: *Bright futures: guidelines for health supervision of infants, children, and adolescents*, ed 2, revised, Arlington, VA, 2002, National Center for Education in Maternal and Child Health.

Green M, Sullivan P, Eichberg C: Avoid a "Swiss cheese" history when psychosocial complaints are on the menu, *Contemp Pediatr* 19:115-125, 2002.

North American Nursing Diagnosis Association: *NANDA nursing diagnoses: definitions and classification 2003-2004*, Philadelphia, 2003, North American Nursing Diagnosis Association.

US Department of Health and Human Services, National Center for Health Statistics: *International classification of diseases*, rev ed 9, *Clinical modification*, DHHS pub no PHS 80-1260, Washington, DC, 1981, US Government Printing Office.

US Department of Health and Human Services: *Nurse practitioner primary care competencies in specialty areas: adult, family, gerontological, pediatric, and women's health*, Washington, DC, 2002, US Government Printing Office.

3

Family Assessment in Pediatric Primary Care

Sheila M. Kodadek

Family-centered, community-based primary care for children is recognized as the best possible practice model for providing health care services to children and their families. Nurse practitioners (NPs) perhaps understand this point better than any other group of primary care providers, but they, like their colleagues, face significant challenges in implementing family-centered care. At minimum, family-centered care is perceived as time consuming. In addition, families are still too often viewed from a pathology-based model borrowed from psychiatry and psychology, and primary care providers often report feeling inadequate to the task of working with the complex and often stressed families they meet in their practices (Wells & Stein, 1999).

However daunting the perceived barriers to family-centered care, investing in family assessment and management is essential in contemporary pediatric primary care practice. Duffy (1988) wrote over a decade ago that understanding family health promotion begins with understanding family dynamics. Research has repeatedly demonstrated that a mother's level of education, her beliefs and attitudes about health, and her own health practices have a significant influence on the health status of her children. As fathers have increasingly become involved in their children's health care, questions about relationships between characteristics of fathers and family health behavior are being raised. It is not surprising that parents who believe that they can improve their health status by practicing health promotion behavior tend to raise children who share similar beliefs.

Research has provided us with definitive evidence that children, from birth through adolescence, need nurturing time and attention from the significant adults in their lives (Gross et al, 2001; Gunnar, 1998; Resnick et al, 1997). These significant adults most often are the child's birth or adoptive parents, but they may also be grandparents, extended family members, or foster parents. Evidence is strong that when children are raised without this consistent, affectionate attention and without sensitive interactions with a caring adult, the results can be devastating for both the child and society (Belsky et al, 2001; Gunnar et al, 1996; Nachmias et al, 1996; Perry & Pollard, 1998). In contrast, when a parent or another significant adult responds consistently and sensitively to a child's needs, such as a need to play, to eat, to sleep, to be comforted, or to be left alone, the child is likely to grow up competent to initiate and build strong, nurturing relationships (Gunnar, 1998; Resnick et al, 1997).

Histories of physical or emotional neglect alone have increasingly been associated with children and adolescents who are withdrawn, anxious, and socially isolated (Ogawa et al, 1997; Perry & Pollard, 1998). Although inadequate or poor parenting is linked in the literature to factors such as poverty, substance abuse, and minimal education, contemporary research suggests that a poor "fit" between a child and a significant adult can occur in any family, including those in which the adults are well educated, socially competent, and economically successful (Perry & Pollard, 1998). For example, parents who value competition and athletic success may be a good parenting fit for their daughter, who is star of her soccer team. However, they may not be able to connect with their younger son, who prefers reading to sports and who avoids competition in all forms.

This chapter begins with the assumption that families are central to and inseparable from the health of children. It is based on a family health promotion framework that assumes that the vast majority of family members are competent, want to do what is best for their children, and desire to be active participants in their children's health care. It describes characteristics of expert nursing practice with families. Finally, this chapter presents an approach to family assessment that can be incorporated with relative ease into a busy primary care practice.

BACKGROUND

It is said that three families are present in every primary care encounter: the family of the patient, the family of the NP, and the "family" of the practice, agency, or unit. The health- and illness-related beliefs, values, and behavior of each of these families have a significant potential to influence the outcome of the encounter.

Research evidence links expert nursing practice in a variety of settings and specialties with knowledge and skills in family nursing, particularly because such nursing practice reflects an appreciation of the complex interactions linking the health status of individuals with their families (Chesla, 1996; Kitzman et al, 1997; Olds et al, 1997). Family nursing practice is based on the assumption that families are influential in how an individual defines health. Families also teach behaviors used to promote health, prevent disease, and manage illnesses and healing. These assumptions go far beyond the biologic contribution made through blood ties within families and equally far beyond the limited view of families as convenient (or unavoidable) caregivers.

The importance of family can be seen more readily in delivery of primary care to children than to adults. In general, pediatric NPs encounter far more family members in the course of their practice than do adult primary care providers. A child is usually accompanied by a family member who, at minimum, is legally responsible for the child's welfare. As stated earlier, children are dependent on their families "to create a nurturing environment to assure physical survival and personal development" (Terkelsen, 1980). In turn, NPs are dependent on families, primarily on parents, to accomplish health-related goals for children. Entering into a true partnership with parents, with NPs as expert consultants, sets the stage for optimal pediatric health care (Dokken & Sydnor-Greenberg, 2001; Schuster et al, 2000).

Expert nursing practice that honors the family's critical roles in a child's health outcomes is characterized by the following: recognition and validation of the family's primary position in a child's world; provision of perspective, knowledge, and skills to families; facilitation of access of family members to ill or suffering members; assistance for family members who need to emotionally reconnect with ill or suffering members; and assistance for families to mobilize their healing capacities when needed (Chesla, 1996). This level of expert care is possible when NPs have knowledge of normal family development and family systems, are aware of their own participation in systems, and incorporate systematic family assessment in their practice.

THE ASSESSMENT MODEL

Family assessment in primary care practice with children requires attention to family structure, family life cycle stage, family functioning, and social network. In other words, a basic family assessment addresses characteristics of the family, transitions that the family is experiencing, how family members interact and get things done, what they believe and value, and how they interact with the community.

It is important to recognize that NPs' own definitions of family and healthy family functioning are culturally and temporally bound, determine who is and who is not family, and can profoundly affect assessment, treatment, and outcomes. NPs might find it useful to periodically examine their own assumptions and beliefs regarding families and use the knowledge gained to foster increased sensitivity and openness to the rich diversity that their clients present.

Legal definitions of *family* usually address bonds of blood, marriage, and adoption. A significant number of contemporary families do not fit such restrictive definitions. To address this reality, Whall (1986) defined *family* as "a self-identified group of two or more individuals whose association is characterized by special terms, who may or may not be related by bloodlines or law, but who function in such a way that they consider themselves to be a family." Wherever NPs' personal definitions might fall on a continuum of inclusiveness, it is imperative that they know and understand the implications of that definition in practice.

Many family assessment models and tools can be used in primary care practice. The following is a baseline assessment model that provides NPs with essential data on which to build a management plan. It is tailored for a relatively busy practice, can be done in stages across visits, and invites additional data entries to update the family database over time.

Family Structure and Roles

Assessment of a family's structure and roles includes the composition of the family or household, demographic data, intergenerational data, and information about family roles. Implicit in the data is the way the family defines itself (i.e., who the family says is "family") and how the family gets its work done.

Families come in many forms today, including two-parent families, single-parent families, families headed by grandparents or other family members, blended families or stepfamilies, and foster families. Specific issues are addressed for these and other forms in the section on targeted assessments later in this chapter.

Family Life Cycle

Family life cycle assessment includes data on the present family life cycle stage (such as a family with young children), family life cycle transitions or developmental crises (such as serious illness of a frail, elderly grandparent), and family life cycle events that are untimely or "out of sync" (such as the terminal illness of a young wife and mother).

Family Functioning

Healthy family functioning should result in what Terkelsen, in his classic paper, called the "good-enough family" (1980). Families have both strengths and limitations, but the majority of families are able to meet most of their members' needs most of the time. This is a hopeful stance, one that allows for the less than perfect family to feel successful and empowered.

Characteristics of healthy family functioning have been identified by a number of researchers, and lists of characteristics differ. For example, deChesnay (1986) used an extensive research literature review to identify healthy families as those characterized by open communication, mutual respect and support, differentiation, shared problem solving, shared decision making, flexibility, and enhancement of personal growth of members. Additions to that list might include a sense of play and humor (Curran, 1983), a shared spiritual value system (Curran, 1983; Lewis et al, 1976; Stinnett, Chesser, & DeFrain, 1979), and a shared value of service to others (Curran, 1983).

Family Social Network

The family's social network includes those persons, activities, agencies, and institutions that have the potential to support, harm, or drain energy from the family. Assessing the family's relationships with extended family, friends, and the community provides information on which to base recommendations and further assessment.

FAMILY DATABASE

Genograms and Ecomaps

The construction of genograms and ecomaps, two approaches to developing a family database, is described in the following sections. Neither requires the purchase of standardized assessment tools, and both can be updated over time, a characteristic making them valuable to NPs in understanding patterns in children and families. Together, the genogram and ecomap assist NPs in assessing family structure and roles, life cycle transitions, family functioning, and social networks in a relatively quick and efficient manner. Both have the advantage of providing a means for interacting with children and their family members in a focused, nonthreatening way around potentially complex and difficult issues. Both also are inherently appealing to families. They help families see themselves in new ways and provide ways for families to be partners in their own diagnosis and management.

Clinicians who use genograms and ecomaps in their practice frequently come to the conclusion that the tools are as useful for intervention as they are for assessment. In addition, nurse clinicians working with children find that including the children in the construction and updating of genograms and ecomaps helps children be active in their own care and provides data on family interactions (Visscher & Clore, 1992).

Genograms

Genograms are sociometric, paper-and-pencil tools used to depict a family's composition and history across generations (Fig. 3-1). Although not essential, computer programs to facilitate genogram data management have become available in recent years and can be easily included in computerized patient records. These programs have made updating genogram data easy and efficient. Genograms are appealing to clinicians because they provide graphic representations of complex family data; they allow clinicians to map family structure clearly and to update the picture as it emerges; they are an efficient clinical summary; they make it easier for clinicians to keep in mind family members, patterns, and events that may have recurring significance in a family's ongoing care; they help clinicians think systematically about how events and relationships in their clients' lives are related to patterns of health and illness; and they are a subjective, interpretive tool with which the clinician can generate tentative hypotheses for further systematic evaluation (Like, Rogers, & McGoldrick, 1988; McGoldrick, 1999; McGoldrick & Gerson, 1985; Rogers & Cohn, 1987; Visscher & Clore, 1992).

Priorities for organizing genogram data for clinical use rely less on formal blood and legal links and more on

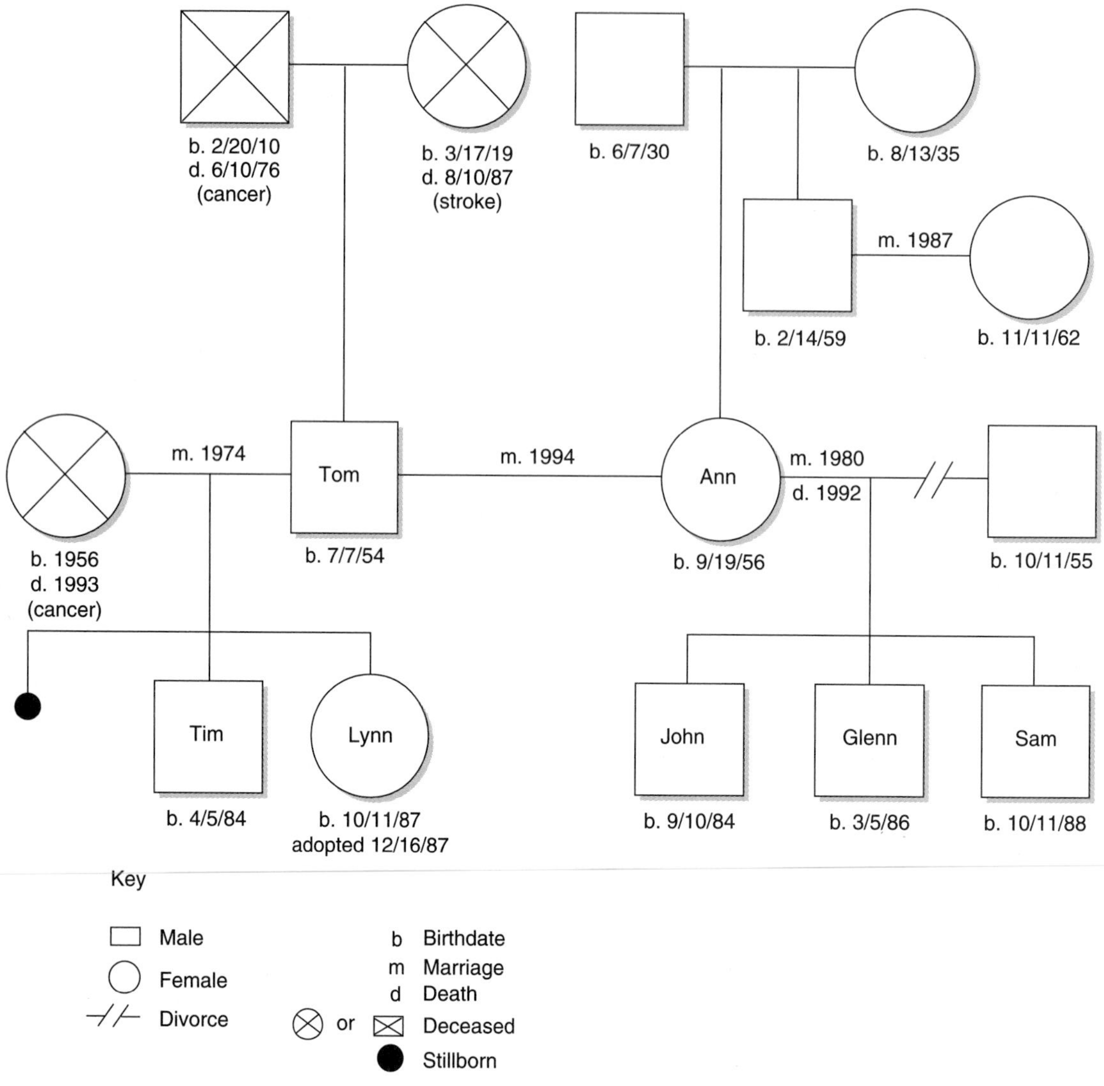

FIGURE 3-1 A three-generational genogram.

repetitive symptoms and relationships or functioning patterns seen across the family or over generations. Genograms highlight coincidences of dates, such as deaths and symptoms, and the impact of change and untimely life cycle transitions (McGoldrick & Gerson, 1985).

Genograms are meant to be a part of a general health assessment. They are most effective when constructed during an initial visit with children and their families and then revised as new information becomes available.

The NP begins by drawing a basic family tree, with the family members present guiding identification of family members. Because the primary purpose of using a genogram in primary care is not to trace genetic lines, the use of symbols to indicate relationships can be less rigorous. In fact, it can be more informative and useful to learn who is living in a household than who is related by blood or birth.

Conventional symbols used in genograms can be seen in Fig. 3-1. Again, the purpose of the family genogram is primarily psychosocial, and symbols that speak eloquently to legal and blood lines may be perceived as offensive to both parents and children. For example, use of solid lines to connect birth children to parents and broken lines to connect adopted children to parents may be precise but may also suggest parent-child relationship differences that do not exist. In practice, it is more informative and respectful to let the family decide how to indicate relationships.

As mentioned earlier, it is clinically useful to identify members of the current household in which children live.

This objective can be met by drawing a circle around the members of the genogram who currently live together; for example, the circle may include parents and three children, or it may include one of two parents, two of three children, and a grandparent. It is also useful to include at least three generations of the family.

Health history information, including serious medical, behavioral, and emotional problems, can be noted on the genogram; examples include drug or alcohol problems, serious problems with the law, and causes of death. Likewise, family information that is significant to the health of the child can be included, such as ethnic background, language spoken in the home, education of parents, occupations, religious affiliation, major family moves, and current location of family members. Significant others who live with or are important to the family should be included, including family friends, foster children, and baby-sitters. In some cases, the significant other is a family pet.

Practical pointers include using pencil instead of pen, unless there are legal or institutional requirements to use a pen; leaving space at the bottom of the page for notes; and including a key to notations or unusual symbols. It also is useful to provide child patients with their own paper and pencils or crayons to use while conducting the interview; they might even draw a picture of their family for you.

The genogram interview can begin with an open question, such as "Tell me about your family." It can be addressed to children, to parents, or to both. As the genogram is being constructed, questions can be used to elicit information about family functioning. McGoldrick and Gerson (1985) suggest the following order of questions; the specific questions are suggestions only and are not exhaustive.

Chief Problem and the Immediate Family

Family Composition and Structure

- Who is in your family?
- Who currently lives with you and your child?
- If the relationships are not clear: How are you related to the members of your household?
- If divorce or separation is involved: Where does the child's other parent live? What are the custody and visitation agreements? How often does the child see or hear from the other parent?
- Who in your family was involved in the decision to come here today?
- If a health-related problem is involved:
- How do other members of your family see this problem?
- With whom will you discuss today's visit when you go home?

Current Family Situation. An understanding of the current family situation is helpful, especially if a significant time period has elapsed since the child and family were last seen. Understanding changes that the family is facing and where they are in the family life cycle is also important:

- Have there been any major stresses in your family since your last visit?
- Have there been any changes in your family since your last visit?
- What, if any, changes do you anticipate in the near future?

Extended Family Context. The following questions suggest a way to begin to collect data about extended family members. This information may not seem relevant to parents or children, but patterns that can have an impact on children's health often do not become evident until this kind of intergenerational mapping is done. This more extensive mapping of a family may be used when the clinical picture includes conflicting information or when the effectiveness of a prevention activity is a concern. For example, knowing that both the mother and grandmother of the young adolescent in your office became pregnant at 14 and dropped out of high school may be helpful in deciding how to best use a brief visit.

It would help me to help your child if I knew more about your child's grandparents, aunts, uncles, and other relatives. Let's begin with your mother's family.

- When was your mother born? Where? Who were her parents?
- Who was in her family while she was growing up?
- Is she living? (If yes) Where does she live now? How often do you have contact with her? (If no) When did she die? What was the cause of death?
- How did she meet your father? When were they married (if applicable)? (And so on.)

Demographic Data. Demographic data include dates of birth, death, adoption, marriage, separation, divorce, significant illness, and major family events; culture/ethnicity; religion; education; and occupations. The NP can probe for more information about specific data as they appear to be significant in a given situation. For example, faith and strength of adherence to a specific religion may have an unexpected impact on care decisions for a child. Disagreement about adherence within a family may result in mixed messages and uneven follow-through with a treatment plan.

Historical Perspective. Knowledge of the timing and repetition of significant family events or behavior may be helpful. For example, adolescent pregnancy, alcohol abuse, dropping out of high school, and suicide may be patterns of behavior in a family's intergenerational history.

If gaps in data become evident, they need to be explored. It is also helpful to keep in mind events external to the family that may have influenced family choices. For example, the years of conflict in Vietnam interrupted many life plans, with effects seen in the present generation. Immigration, voluntary or forced, can have an impact on family health status. Natural disasters such as floods, hurricanes, and droughts have changed family histories and the health status of family members.

Family Relationships and Roles. In developing the database, NPs can begin to probe for family relationships and roles. For example, understanding how parents make decisions and solve problems can be useful in helping parents improve health promotion practices. Examples of questions that can lead to an increased appreciation for a specific family include the following:

- How would you describe your parenting style? How does it compare with your partner's?
- Who in your family is responsible for monitoring your children's health?
- What does your family enjoy most about this child?
- What are some of the things you do together as a family? How often?
- How do you generally make important decisions in your family?
- To whom does your child tend to tell problems and concerns?
- How do family members show their support for one another?
- How well do you think your family adapts to change?
- How does your family nurture the interests and talents of each individual family member?
- To whom do you go for advice about being a good parent? Why do you go to that person?
- How do you deal with unwanted advice from family members about raising your child(ren)?

In summary, genograms provide clinicians with data about family structure, life cycle fit, patterns repeating across generations, life experiences, and relational patterns (Like, Rogers, & McGoldrick, 1988; McGoldrick, 1999; McGoldrick & Gerson, 1985).

Targeted Assessments. Families come with a variety of issues, some related to the composition and structure of the family, others related to variables such as socioeconomic and health status. Family-related issues have the potential to influence the health and well-being of children and adolescents in significant ways. Although much about family assessment remains constant across families, it is useful to pay attention to some of the unique potential family variations.

Two-Parent Families. Two-parent families include married couples with children, unmarried couples with children, remarried couples with blended families (or stepfamilies), and gay or lesbian couples. Two-parent families experience the same stressors as do single-parent families, but children in two-parent families tend to have social, economic, and health advantages. Parent educational levels, economic status, and health status are generally higher in two-parent families than in single-parent families (Annie E. Casey Foundation, 2002; Ford-Gilboe, 2000). There is also the fact, seldom researched but often cited by parents, that even when the division of labor is uneven, it is still a relief to have another adult with whom to share the work of raising children (Ford-Gilboe, 2000).

The following questions may help two-parent families explore how they share their parenting and the impact on their child:

- How do you decide who does what at home?
- Who has primary responsibility for daily child care? How is that working?
- Who has primary responsibility for health care and appointments? How is that working?

Working Parents and Child Care. When a single parent works outside the home or both parents in a two-parent family work outside the home, specific considerations involve all members of the family. Carter (1999, p. 252) identified three "unresolved problems" related to work and families: men's unequal contributions to housework, workplace inflexibility, and the increasing number of hours both men and women are spending outside the home, all of which can affect parenting. A large number of studies have explored the impact of maternal employment on children's maternal attachment, with mixed results. Whereas some researchers have found weakened attachment bonds, others have found no effect (Broom, 1998). Researchers have identified protective factors that are in the socioeconomic realm, including educated parents, financial security, and parents' psychologic well-being (Broom, 1998; Kneipp, 2002). The following are examples of questions to help parents explore the interface between work and home:

- How many hours do you work outside the home in a typical week? How does that affect your family life?
- What tensions do you anticipate (or are you experiencing) to be associated with balancing work and home?
- What child care arrangements have you made? How satisfactory are they? What would you change if you could?
- How do you manage care for a child who is ill on a workday?

Multiple Births. A family faced with caring for newborn twins, triplets, or more, even while delighted, can be quickly overwhelmed by the responsibility and amount of work involved. Assessing parents' level of fatigue, ability to seek and accept support, and plans for ongoing care is useful to both the NP and the parents.

- Have things gone as you expected with the babies?
- When you have questions about their care, whom do you ask?
- Have you had help from your partner? Family members? Friends?
- How are your babies similar? How do they differ from one another?
- How have you managed those times that happen to all new parents when you feel overwhelmed?
- How have the babies' sibling(s) responded to them?

Families with a Premature Infant. Low-birth-weight and premature infants present special issues for new parents. There may be an extended time between the birth of the child and being able to bring the child home. Concerns about the child's physiologic vulnerability may arise. Almost certainly, costs and time commitments around the care of the infant will be increased. Parents may have similar concerns to those of parents of a full-term newborn, but their fears and anxieties about being responsible for a seemingly fragile newborn may be close to overwhelming.

Similar to the situation of a multiple birth, exploring who is caring for the child and who is helping the parents is a priority.

Families Raising a Child with a Chronic Illness. Parents caring for a child with a significant medical or developmental challenge, whether it be a chronic illness, a disabling condition, or a developmental disability, are responsible for their child's daily medical care, monitoring, and management (O'Brien, 2001). The care can be minimal or consume hours of every day and night. The monitoring can be casual or meticulous; the management, routine or complex. Survival may be a realistic concern.

The impact of a chronic illness or disabling condition on a family, including the child, parents, siblings, and extended family, is influenced not only by the diagnosis and its sequelae, but also by the meaning it has for the family and individual members. Time may or may not help; for example, the overall stress of living with the aftermath of a diagnosis may not lessen, but specific concerns may.

While all developmental levels present challenges and opportunities for these families, the interface between families and schools around developmental and health issues can be particularly difficult. Parents generally want their child to be placed in a situation in which he or she has the maximum opportunity to be successful. Parents also want their child to be as "normal" as possible. Both of these goals may require a great deal of planning and negotiation with school teachers and staff. Sydnor-Greenberg and Dokken (2000) identified five recommendations to help parents and children cope with schools, camps, and other settings:

- Communicate details about the child's needs.
- Recognize that education and knowledge about chronic illness vary widely among individuals.
- Be flexibile around rules surrounding treatment.
- Advocate for parents' needs.
- Promote self-care and self-advocacy for the children themselves.

Knafl and Deatrick have described the process of normalization in these families (Deatrick, Knafl, & Murphy-Moore, 1999; Knafl et al, 1996; Knafl, Deatrick, & Kirby, 2001). Parents acknowledge the condition and potential impact, redefine (or adapt) their definition of normal to fit their family, engage in behaviors that fit the definition of normal, develop a treatment regimen that also fits, and interact with others based on the view that the child and family are normal (Knafl et al, 2001). Normalization promotion as a nursing intervention can be a powerful tool.

Often parents become both medical experts in their child's diagnosis and management and experts in their child's idiosyncratic responses. They expect to be treated seriously and with respect, and they set high standards for their child's health care providers.

Health care providers can find it a challenge to work with parents raising a child with a significant health problem. Providers can feel tested and challenged; they may be taken by surprise by angry responses from parents, responses that do not appear to be justified. In a classic paper, Thorne and Robinson (1988) described three phases of this relationship between health care providers and health care recipients or family caregivers. Naïve trusting was the first stage, a time when the family assumed that its perspective was shared by the professionals who cared for their family members, and that the family members' involvement as caregivers would be respected and acknowledged. Family members also assumed that all professionals would be highly knowledgeable and skilled, and would be honest and direct in communications. As ongoing interactions with health care professionals taught families that these assumptions were not valid, a second phase, characterized by disenchantment, occurred. Anger was often the primary expression of this disenchantment, reflecting the loss of trust in health care providers, and family members moved toward trying to protect their family member. Finally, but not inevitably, family members moved to a phase called *guarded alliance.* The no longer naïve family members were able to reconstruct trust on a more sophisticated level. Trust was now shared with individual professionals, and it had to be earned.

The following questions may help demonstrate a provider's appreciation for the family's perspective and concerns:

- How are things going on a day-to-day basis with your child's care?

- How is the management affecting your child's relationships with other children?
- How is school going?
- How is the management affecting family life?
- What are your hopes for the future? Your concerns?
- What do you need most right now to better care for your whole family?

Blended Families. A *blended family* is one in which two adults create a reorganized family by joining together with their children from previous relationships. Although this term usually refers to families created by remarriage after divorce, it is also used to describe families created by remarriage after the death of spouses. Assessing how the children are coping with the significant changes in their lives can help both the NP and the parents direct their attention.

- Have things gone as you expected they would in your new family?
- How is each child coping with the new family?
- How do their responses vary with their ages and developmental levels?
- How has their child care or school situation changed and how have they responded?
- What do the parents identify as the most significant loss for each child in the blended family? The most significant benefit?
- How are the relationships between parents (including stepparent) and children?
- How are the relationships among the stepsiblings?
- How are the parents handling discipline issues?

Single-Parent Families. The number of children living in single-parent households rose from 12.8 million in 1990 to 16.8 million in 2000 (Annie E. Casey Foundation, 2002). Although the vast majority of single parents are women, increasingly fathers are raising their children in single-parent homes. Today, single parents may be adolescents enrolled in welfare programs or company executives with live-in nannies. Clearly, understanding the family context is fundamental to assessing these families.

Single-parent households may be headed by a divorced parent or by a parent who has never been married. In general, children living with a divorced parent have an advantage; divorced parents tend to be older, with more years of schooling completed and with higher levels of income than do parents who have never been married. Children in single-parent families benefit when both parents are involved in their lives, regardless of marital or living arrangements.

Single parents across socioeconomic parameters all experience the demands and burdens of raising a child alone. Even with help, the weight of responsibility is felt and exacerbated by lack of time and role strain (Kneipp, 2002; Lipman et al, 2002; Lutenbacher, 2002). Single parents sometimes have difficulty accessing health care. Research suggests that affordability is a more significant issue than time pressures or workplace demands (Kneipp, 2002). The relatively large proportion of single parents who are classified as "working poor" puts them above the income level for subsidized care and below the level where they could realistically afford health insurance.

Questions probing how the parent is managing as a single parent can be useful. Examples include the following:

- What is the best thing about being your child's only parent?
- What is most challenging for you about being a single parent?
- How do you get the support you need as a parent?
- What would most help you raise your child at this point in time?

Adolescent Parents. Adolescents who become parents generally face the problems inherent when a major role is assumed before the adolescent is developmentally ready. Adolescent parents have developmental needs of their own, and not infrequently their needs are in conflict with those of their children. In addition, children of adolescent mothers are more likely than children of older mothers to have a low birth weight, to have ongoing health problems during childhood, to grow up in homes without fathers, and to be raised in poverty or near poverty. Questions that can help formulate an idea about the environment in which a child will be raised include exploring the adolescent parent's own support system, attitudes toward parenting, and source of parenting advice. In addition, it is helpful to understand the adolescent's school status, child care arrangements, financial situation, and plans for the future.

Gay/Lesbian Parent Families. Gay and lesbian parents face the problems of all parents, with an added concern about societal attitudes and behavior that add stress to their lives and the lives of their children. These parents generally need support in raising their children to deal with beliefs and attitudes that may include isolation and teasing. Assessing the ability of these families to find and use community support is important, as is exploring their ideas about how they will prepare their children to handle curiosity, possible negative responses, and the experience of "being different."

Adoptive Parent Families. Adoptive parents come in every variety—married couples, single parents, gay and lesbian parents, grandparents or other extended family members, and so on. Assessment of these families includes asking about the legal status of the adoption, the timing of the adoption in the child's life, arrangements regarding involvement of the birth parents or other family members, decisions about how and when to tell the child about being adopted, and potential health concerns related to the birth parents or family, if known.

Grandparents Raising Grandchildren. According to the 2000 U.S. census, 6.3% of U.S. children under 18 live in grandparent-headed households, a 29.7% increase since the 1990 census; these percentages include all socioeconomic and ethnic groups (U.S. Census Bureau, 2003). The reasons why grandparents assume parenting responsibility for their grandchildren vary, but they rarely do so unless the parent is unable or unwilling to parent. In the United States, substance abuse, parental illness, and parental maturity are primary reasons (Kelley, 1993; Monsen, 2001). Death of a parent, child abuse and neglect, and incarceration also are reasons for placement with grandparents.

Grandparents face significant legal issues around custody, adoption, guardianship, and foster care (Caliandro & Hughes, 1998). Trying to enroll a grandchild in school can lead to a minefield of legal issues. In addition, although some states provide financial assistance to grandparents, others do not. Grandparents may have difficulty accessing and paying for health care (Casper & Bryson, 2000). For example, some insurance carriers do not allow grandchildren as dependents. Grandparents may be in their thirties or their eighties, and may have boundless or flagging energy. They may be still active in a job they love, or they may have looked forward to enjoying their retirement and new challenges. They may be thrilled to be parenting again, or they may be clinically depressed. There is no "one size fits all" template.

Compounding the practical and economic issues are the psychologic and emotional responses of all involved. Grief, anger, confusion, resentment, and depression all can describe reactions of both grandparents and their grandchildren (Caliandro & Hughes, 1998; Kelley, 1993). At the same time, relief that the grandchildren are safe, loved, and nurtured also can be present. Sensitivity and openness to grandparents can allow them to express their ambivalence and concerns. Expressed respect and appreciation can help form a working partnership.

Knowledge of resources can be especially helpful (Monsen, 2001). The American Association of Retired Persons (AARP) has a website for grandparents that includes excellent resources, including information for grandparents parenting grandchildren. The site includes information about financial assistance, including the Temporary Assistance to Needy Families (TANF) program, online and community-based support groups, books and other literature, and a wide range of other resources (see Resource Box: Grandparents Raising Grandchildren).

Foster Parent Families. Children are placed in foster care for a variety of reasons. Substance abuse by biologic family members is the leading cause; the effects of family substance abuse on children are many and profound (Barton, 1999). Children may be placed in foster care because they need specialized medical, psychiatric/mental health, and developmental assistance beyond the ability of their biologic parents to provide. The children may need to be removed from a chaotic and unsafe family environment. They may have been abandoned or orphaned. These children, first and foremost, are at risk for deep-seated feelings of insecurity, loss, and anger. Assessment of these families includes exploration of the child's history that resulted in foster family placement, identification of health issues that precipitated or resulted from separation from the birth parents, and evaluation of the foster parent.

Foster parents have a difficult role in society. They want to be treated with respect and to have their care and knowledge of the foster child acknowledged. They want to have the assistance they need to provide the best care possible to the children in their care. However, they report that their concerns and needs often are not recognized by health care professionals (Barton, 1999). Exploring concerns the foster parent has with his or her parenting, with attention not only to the child's needs, but also to the foster family's needs, may help establish a working relationship that can work for the benefit of all (Barton, 1999; Gottesman, 2001). Again, providing resources can be helpful. The Child Welfare League of America's website has excellent information and resources about and for family foster care providers. In addition, the National Foster Parent Association provides support and caregiving information for foster families (see Resource Box: Foster Families).

Displaced or Homeless Families. The number of homeless children in the United States is growing, with substance abuse and poverty as prime reasons for the growth. Homeless children and their families have difficulty with the most basic needs of food, shelter, and clothing. Accessing education and health care may be difficult to impossible. The health care visit may be in response to a crisis that could not be denied, but assessment should include well child care, including immunizations, on the operating principle that any visit is better than no visit.

Poverty and Families. Families are facing poverty in increasing numbers, and children are the most at risk. Two-parent families, with both working, may be struggling to meet basic needs. For example, in some states welfare reform has resulted in the working poor, who make too much to qualify for subsidized health care, having to choose between keeping a job that helps feed their family or meeting their children's health needs (Heymann & Earle, 1999).

Ecomaps

Ecomaps are similar to genograms in their inherent and deceptive simplicity (Fig. 3-2). Ecomaps depict, in a clear and dynamic way, "the major systems that are a part of the family's life and the nature of the family's relationship with the various systems" (Hartman, 1995). Mapping of family relationships within and outside family boundaries highlights the nature of those relationships, their potential for support, conflicts in the relationships, and areas of current or potential strain and stress.

As with genograms, all that is needed is a piece of paper and a pencil. A large circle representing the family boundary is drawn in the center of the paper; smaller circles representing different parts of the environment (individuals, organizations and institutions, hobbies, work, and so on) are drawn around the large circle. Inside the large circle, a genogram depiction of the family members in the household is drawn. Family members are then asked to label the smaller circles with those people, places, and activities, whether enjoyable, stressful, or both, that make up their world. Examples of labels include extended family members, friends, work, school, band practice, church or synagogue, camping, exercise, and health care. Connections between individual family members or the family as a whole and the smaller circles are then drawn. Coded lines and brief descriptions are used to indicate the strength and quality of the relationships. Common codes for the lines are found in the key for Fig. 3-2:

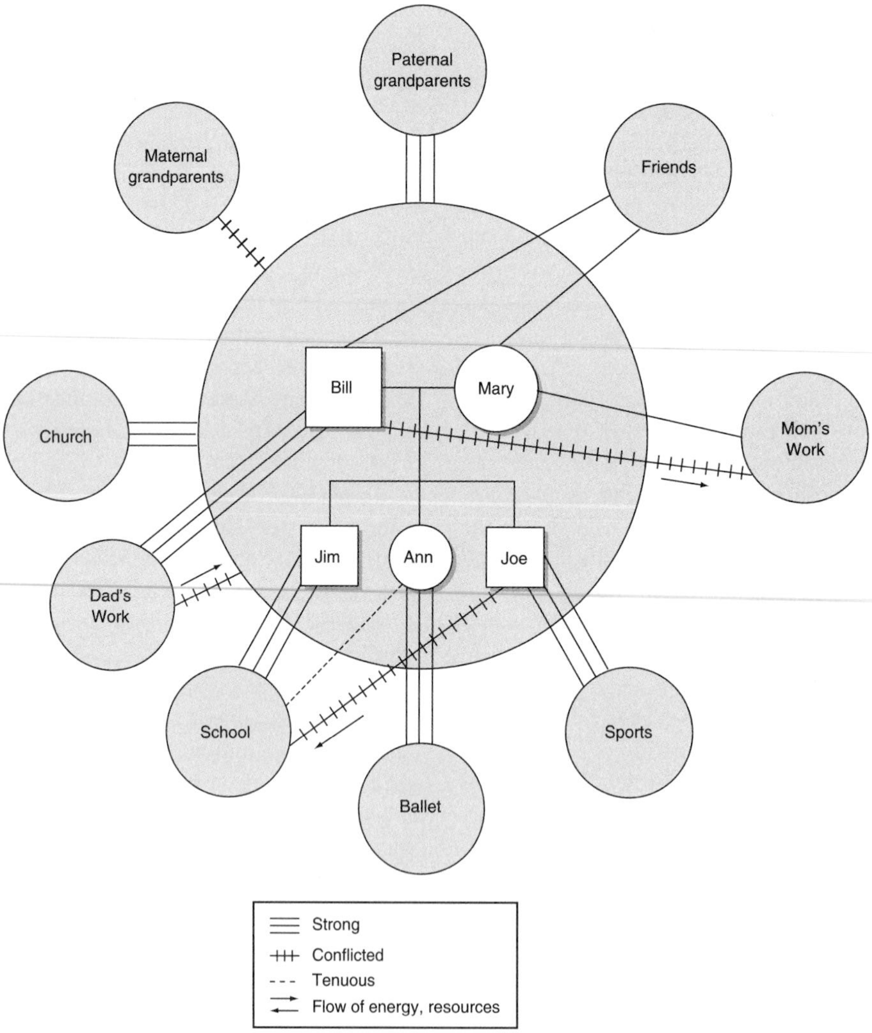

FIGURE 3-2 Ecomap showing family with three children. Ecomaps can provide additional data.

Direction of the flow of energy, resources, or interest can be indicated by drawing arrows along the connecting lines. An example is a family with three children, one of whom loves school and does well (three solid lines with arrows pointing from school to the child), one of whom is an indifferent student but likes the social aspect of school (a dotted line with no arrows), and one who has serious academic problems and dreads going to school each morning (a solid line with hatch marks and arrows pointing from the child to school) (see Fig. 3-2).

Sometimes the whole family is connected to an activity, and the energy flow is similar for all members. For example, a family might identify a particular family friend as supportive. In other cases, the experience differs across family members. For example, family vacations may be positive for all members of the family except adolescents, who would prefer to stay home near their friends. A scarcity of connections outside the household suggests isolation and may be a problem if the family needs significant support during a crisis. A sheet full of circles may indicate a family overcommitted and overwhelmed by activities and responsibilities.

In summary, ecomaps provide both additional data about a family's social network and potential for social support. They also provide a way of validating information from the genogram interview, especially around family relationships and roles.

Selected Family Assessment Tools

The process of constructing a genogram and ecomap results in a fairly complete picture of the family's composition, social network, and family functioning. However, at times additional information is needed. The following assessment models and tools offer NPs other resources that are clinically relevant and reasonably efficient. In addition, the tools have research evidence of reliability and validity supporting their use in practice (Box 3-1).

BOX 3-1 *Family Assessment Tools*

Comprehensive Family Assessment Models

These models provide ways to organize family assessment material. They can provide NPs with a database characterized by both breadth and depth.

- Calgary Family Assessment Model (CFAM) (Wright & Leahey, 1994)
- Family Health Assessment Form (Friedman, 1986)

Family Assessment Screening Tool

This screening tool is quick to administer (5 minutes) and provides an overview assessment of family functioning.

- Family Apgar (Smilkstein, 1978)

Family Functioning Tools

These tools vary in length and complexity, but all are easy to score and provide NPs with in-depth data about family functioning.

- Family Adaptability and Cohesion Evaluation Scale (FACES III) (Olson, Portner, & Lavee, 1985) (Source: Family Social Sciences, University of Minnesota, 290 McNeal Hall, St Paul, MN 55108)
- Family Environment Scale (FES) (Moos, 1974)
- Feetham Family Functioning Survey (FFFS) (Feetham & Humerick, 1982)

Family Stress and Coping Tools

These tools provide NPs with information about how families define and manage stress. They can be used to help families self-diagnose their strengths and identify areas needing modification.

- Assessing Adolescent Stress: Adolescent-Family Inventory of Life Events and Changes (A-FILE) (Olson et al, 1982) (Source: Family Social Sciences, University of Minnesota, 290 McNeal Hall, St Paul, MN 55108)
- Family Inventory of Life Events (FILE) (McCubbin & Patterson, 1983) (Source: McCubbin HI, Thompson AI: Family assessment inventories for research and practice. In Family Stress and Coping Project. Madison, WI, University of Wisconsin, 1987)
- Family Coping Strategies (F-COPES) (Olson, Sprenkle, & Russell, 1979) (Source: McCubbin HI, Thompson AI: Family assessment inventories for research and practice. In Family Stress and Coping Project. Madison, WI, University of Wisconsin, 1987)

Creating the Problem List

The problem list is derived from data collected during the family assessment. Similar to the child health assessment process, NPs working with family members identify possible family issues and problems and weigh them against what they know is occurring within the family at that time. If further data are needed, time should be designated to explore the area of concern in more detail.

Creating the Management Plan

Again, similar to the child health assessment, a plan should be developed in collaboration with family members for every identified problem or issue. Management plans should be written in the record and evaluated at the next visit.

Research suggests that few, if any, adequately functioning families seek professional help for normal transitions in the life cycle (Olson et al, 1989). Requests for assistance with parenting, routine family caregiving, or other normative stressors can be met in the context of primary care practice. Education and supportive counseling can be done with a variety of strategies, including listening with empathy; normalizing when appropriate; providing individualized anticipatory guidance; offering suggestions of books, videos, and audiotapes; and referring to community support groups when appropriate and available.

Family conferences are a useful strategy for NPs when a pattern of recurring problems can be observed or when the family would clearly benefit from a group educational session. Family conferences are also essential at times of significant family stress or transition, including the onset of chronic illness, serious acute illness, significant psychosocial issues, lifestyle problems, terminal illness, and death.

Long-term management of significant family problems, problems that exceed a family's ability to adapt, or problems that exceed an NP's skills, time, or resources require referral for family therapy or counseling. Findings of family violence, chemical dependency, chronic depression or anxiety, or child neglect or maltreatment require a referral and, in some cases, a report to appropriate authorities. A list of family therapists and counselors is useful to have available for families in or near crisis. Families that are not functioning optimally but whose members are not endangered may need time to recognize their need for assistance.

RESOURCE BOX

Grandparents Raising Grandchildren

American Association of Retired Persons (AARP) Grandparent Information Center:
www.aarp.org/confacts/health/grandsupport.html

Support Groups for Grandparents Raising Grandchildren:
www.aarp.org/confacts/health/grandsupport.html

Today's Grandparent Magazine:
www.todaysgrandparent.com/

GrandsPlace—website for grandparents raising grandchildren:
www.grandsplace.com/

Grand Parent Again:
www.grandsplace.com/

NPs who use a family perspective in their practice do not need every possible bit of information about a family, nor do they need to interact with all family members. Incorporating a sensitivity to family issues in health care recommendations can be a major contribution to a family's well-being, even if the only person with whom NPs communicate is a worried parent.

RESOURCE BOX

Foster Families

Child Welfare League of America, Family Foster Care
www.cwla.org/programs/fostercare/

Casey Family Programs National Center for Resource Family Support
www.fostercaremonth.org

Children's Bureau Express
www.calib.com/cbexpress

The National Foster Parent Association
www.nfpainc.org

Rowell Foster Children's Positive Plan
www.rowellfosterchildren.org

Connect for Kids
www.connectforkids.org/content1552/content.htm

NURSING DIAGNOSES RELATED TO FAMILIES

- Ineffective role performance
- Impaired parenting and risk for impaired parenting
- Risk for impaired parent/infant/child attachment
- Interrupted family processes
- Caregiver role strain and risk for caregiver role strain
- Dysfunctional family processes: alcoholism
- Parental role conflict
- Disabled family coping, compromised family coping, readiness for enhanced family coping
- Ineffective family therapeutic regimen management
- Impaired social interaction
- Relocation stress syndrome
- Impaired home maintenance

From North American Nursing Diagnosis Association (NANDA): *NANDA nursing diagnoses: definitions and classification 2001-2002*, Philadelphia, 2001, The Association.

REFERENCES

Annie E. Casey Foundation: Kids count data book online summary and findings, 2002. Available at *www.aecf.org/kidscount/kc2002/summary/summary12.htm* (accessed Jan 20, 2003).

Barton SJ: Family matters: promoting family-centered care with foster families, *Pediatr Nurs* 25(1):57-59, 1999.

Belsky J et al: Child-rearing antecedents of intergenerational relations in young adulthood: a prospective study, *Dev Psychol* 37(6):801-813, 2001.

Broom BL: Parental sensitivity to infants and toddlers in dual-earner and single-earner families, *Nurs Res* 47(3):162-170, 1998.

Caliandro G, Hughes C: The experience of being a grandmother who is the primary caregiver for her HIV-positive grandchild, *Nurs Res* 47(2):107-113, 1998.

Carter B: Becoming parents: the family with young children. In Carter C, McGoldrick M, editors: *The expanded family life cycle: individual, family, and social perspectives*, ed 3, Boston, 1999, Allyn & Bacon.

Casper LM, Bryson KR: *Co-resident grandparents and their grandchildren: grandparent maintained families*, Population Division, Fertility and Family Statistics Branch, working paper no 26, Washington, DC, 2000, US Census Bureau.

Chesla C: Reconciling technological and family care in critical-care nursing, *Image* 28:199-203, 1996.

Curran D: *Traits of a healthy family*, New York, 1983, Ballantine.

Deatrick JA, Knafl KA, Murphy-Moore C: Clarifying the concept of normalization, *Image* 31:209-214, 1999.

deChesnay M: Promoting healthy family functioning in acute care units, *J Pediatr Nurs* 1:96-101, 1986.

Dokken DL, Sydnor-Greenberg N: Communication in health-care: the parents' perspective, *J Child Fam Nurs* 4(1):71-75, 2001.

Duffy ME: Health promotion in the family: current findings and directives for nursing research, *J Adv Nurs* 13:109-117, 1988.

Feetham SL, Humerick SS: The Feetham Family Functioning Survey. In Humerick SS, editor: *Analysis of current assessment strategies in the health care of young children and childbearing families*, East Norwalk, CT, 1982, Appleton-Century-Crofts.

Ford-Gilboe M: Dispelling myths and creating opportunity: a comparison of strengths of single-parent and two-parent families, *ANS Adv Nurs Sci* 23(1):41-58, 2000.

Friedman MM: *Family nursing: theory and assessment*, ed 2, East Norwalk, CT, 1986, Appleton-Century-Crofts.

Gottesman MM: Children in foster care: a nursing perspective on research, policy, and child health issues, *J Soc Pediatr Nurses* 6(2):55-64, 2001.

Gross SJ et al: Impact of family structure and stability on academic outcome in preterm children at 10 years of age, *J Pediatr* 138:169-174, 2001.

Gunnar MR: Quality of early care and buffering of neuro-endocrine stress reactions: potential effects on the developing human brain, *Prev Med* 27:209-211, 1998.

Gunnar MR et al: Stress reactivity and attachment security, *Dev Psychobiol* 29:191-204, 1996.

Hartman A: Diagrammatic assessment of family relationships, *Families in Society* 76(2):11-122, 1995.

Heymann SJ, Earle A: The impact of welfare reform on parents' ability to care for their children's health, *Am J Public Health* 89(4):502-505, 1999.

Kelley SJ: Caregiver stress in grandparents raising grandchildren, *Image* 25(4):331-337, 1993.

Kitzman H et al: Effect of prenatal and infancy home visitation by nurses on pregnancy outcomes, childhood injuries, and repeated childbearing, *JAMA* 278:644-652, 1997.

Knafl KA et al: Family response to childhood chronic illness: description of management styles, *J Pediatr Nurs* 11:315-326, 1996.

Knafl KA, Deatrick JA, Kirby A: Normalization promotion. In Craft-Rosenberg M, Denehy J, editors: *Nursing interventions for infants, children, and families*, Thousand Oaks, CA, 2001, Sage.

Kneipp SM: The relationships among employment, paid sick leave, and difficulty obtaining health care of single mothers with young children, *Policy Polit Nurs Pract* 3(1):20-30, 2002.

Lewis JM et al: *No single thread: psychological health in family systems*, New York, 1976, Brunner/Mazel.

Like RC, Rogers J, McGoldrick M: Reading and interpreting genograms: a systematic approach, *J Fam Pract* 28:407-412, 1988.

Lipman EL et al: Child well-being in single-mother families, *J Am Acad Child Adolesc Psychiatry* 41(1):75-82, 2002.

Lutenbacher M: Relationships between psychosocial factors and abusive parenting attitudes in low-income single mothers, *Nurs Res* 51(3):158-167, 2002.

McCubbin HI, Patterson JM: Stress: the family inventory of life events. In Fillsinger EE, editor: *Marriage and family assessment: a sourcebook for family therapy*, Beverly Hills, CA, 1983, Sage.

McGoldrick M: History, genograms, and the family life cycle. In Carter C, McGoldrick M, editors: *The expanded family life cycle: individual, family, and social perspectives*, ed 3, Boston, 1999, Allyn & Bacon.

McGoldrick M, Gerson R: *Genograms in family assessment*, New York, 1985, Norton.

Monsen RB: Raising kids, grandparents bear a burden, *J Pediatr Nurs* 16(2):130-131, 2001.

Moos R: *Family environment scales*, Palo Alto, CA, 1974, Consulting Psychologists Press.

Nachmias M et al: Behavioral inhibition and stress reactivity: the moderating role of attachment security, *Child Dev* 67:508-522, 1996.

O'Brien ME: Living in a house of cards: family experiences with long-term childhood technology dependence, *J Pediatr Nurs* 16(1):13-22, 2001.

Ogawa JR et al: Development and the fragmented self: longitudinal study of dissociative symptomatology in a nonclinical sample, *Dev Psychopathol* 9:855-879, 1997.

Olds DL et al: Long term effects of home visitation on maternal life course and child abuse and neglect: fifteen year follow-up of a randomized trial, *JAMA* 278:637-643, 1997.

Olson D et al: *Family inventories*, St Paul, MN, 1982, University of Minnesota.

Olson DH et al: *Families: what makes them work*, Beverly Hills, CA, 1989, Sage.

Olson DH, Portner J, Lavee Y: *FACES III*, St Paul, MN, 1985, Family Social Sciences, University of Minnesota.

Olson DH, Sprenkle DH, Russell CS: Circumplex model of marital and family systems. I. Cohesion and adaptability dimensions, family types, and clinical applications, *Fam Process* 18:3-28, 1979.

Perry BD, Pollard R: Homeostasis, stress, trauma, and adaptation: a neurodevelopmental view of childhood trauma, *Child Adolesc Psychiatr Clin North Am* 7:33-51, 1998.

Resnick MD et al: Protecting adolescents from harm: findings from the National Longitudinal Study on Adolescent Health, *JAMA* 278:823-832, 1997.

Rogers JC, Cohn P: Impact of a screening family genogram on first encounters in primary care, *Fam Pract* 4:291-301, 1987.

Schuster MA et al: Anticipatory guidance: what information do parents receive? What information do they want? *Arch Pediatr Adolesc Med* 154(12):1191-1198, 2000.

Smilkstein G: The family APGAR: A proposal for a family function test and its use by physicians, *J Fam Pract* 6:1231-1239, 1978.

Stinnett N, Chesser B, DeFrain J, editors: *Building family strengths: blueprints for action*, Lincoln, NE, 1979, University of Nebraska.

Sydnor-Greenberg N, Dokken D: Helping parents and children cope with chronic conditions in school, *J Child Fam Nurs* 3(6): 447-451, 2000.

Terkelsen KG: Toward a theory of the family life cycle. In Carter EA, McGoldrick M, editors: *The family life cycle: a framework for family theory*, New York, 1980, Gardner.

Thorne SE, Robinson CA: Health care relationships: the chronic illness perspective, *Res Nurs Health* 11:293-300, 1988.

US Census Bureau: QT-02. Profile of selected social characteristics, 2000. Available at *http://factfinder.census.gov/servlet/QTTable?ds_name = D&geo_id = D&qr_name = ACS_C2SS_EST_G00_QT02&_lang = en* (accessed Feb 23, 2003).

Visscher EM, Clore ER: The genogram: a strategy for assessment, *J Pediatr Health Care* 6:361-367, 1992.

Wells RD, Stein MT: Special families. In Dixon SD, Stein MT, editors: *Encounters with children: pediatric behavior and development*, ed 3, St Louis, 1999, Mosby.

Whall AL: The family as the unit of care in nursing: a historical review, *Public Health Nurs* 3:240-249, 1986.

Wright LM, Leahey M: *Nurses and families: a guide to family assessment and intervention*, ed 2, Philadelphia, 1994, FA Davis.

4 Cultural Perspectives for Primary Health Care

Ardys M. Dunn

CULTURE

The definition of *culture*, articulated years ago by noted anthropologist Alfred Kroeber, and synthesized from some 164 anthropologic sources, still applies today. Culture is a set of "patterns, explicit and implicit, of and for behavior." It is "acquired and transmitted by symbols" and is based on "traditional (i.e., historically derived and selected) ideas and . . . their attached values; culture systems may, on the one hand, be considered as products of action, on the other as conditioning elements of further action" (Kroeber, 1952). In an anthropologic and sociologic sense, culture is a social construction of the relationships within and among groups of human beings. It is based on ethnicity, race, religion, class, and geography. The term *ethnicity* is used to identify groups of people within society, each of which shares distinctive traits and customs. Race, in contrast, classifies humans according to specific physical characteristics (e.g., pigmentation, facial features). Humans also differ by religion, social class, and the physical place in which they experience life. All of these qualities contribute to shaping the culture of the social group. No one quality is definitive of culture, and within cultural groups, individuals show great variation in behavior and beliefs.

Characteristics of Culture

Although each cultural group possesses a unique identity, all cultures have certain common characteristics. These universal characteristics of culture represent the framework by which cultures function (Table 4-1).

Culture Is Dynamic and Shared

As both a product and function of human interaction, culture is constantly evolving. The concept of self (identity) and the roles played in society are culturally dependent (Berger & Luckmann, 1966), created through the ongoing interaction of individuals with others and with their environment. In most societies, a dominant group is clearly evident. The culture of this dominant group shapes the lifestyle and collective consciousness of the community, functions as the guardian and sustainer of the controlling value system, and is the prime allocator of rewards. Generally, individuals in a society learn to identify with the dominant cultural framework and incorporate its traditions and customs into their daily life and decision making. The extent to which this sharing of culture occurs is termed *cultural embeddedness*. Many factors influence the degree of cultural embeddedness, including level of education, socioeconomic status, social class, country of origin of individuals or their ancestors, exposure to other cultures, lifestyle (e.g., urban vs. rural), length of stay in the host country, and the exact region of the host country in which individuals grow up, reside, or both.

Individuals may also identify with a minority group (i.e., a group that shares racial or ethnic characteristics that differ from those of the dominant group) or have one or more subcultural affiliations based on social class, religion, occupation, or socioeconomic status. In diverse societies, especially where minority groups are large or their members are vocal proponents of retaining their cultural integrity, assimilation into the dominant culture may not

TABLE 4-1 ***Universal Characteristics of Culture***

Characteristic	Significance
Culture is dynamic.	Beliefs and practices of groups are created through interactions among people and between people and their physical and social environments. Beliefs, customs, and values change over time as new interactions occur and to meet the needs of the social group. Although cultures evolve, there is a tendency for stability and cultural continuity.
Culture is shared.	Members of a cultural group share group ways of thinking, doing, and interacting.
Culture is learned.	Cultural groups teach members the "rules" or expectations of that culture.
Culture is based on symbols.	Language is the primary mechanism for transmitting and interpreting culture. Humans use artifacts (e.g., clothing, food, music, religious icons) and rituals to communicate within and among cultures.
Culture is integrated.	Cultural norms, beliefs, customs, and values span all areas of social life (e.g., the lessons learned in the family extend into the school setting), providing coherence to the social group. There may be significant variation from one arena of social life to another (e.g., language used in the home may differ from that used in school or workplace).

be easy or automatic, and cultural confusion or conflict may occur. Characteristics (e.g., skin color, religion) that set a minority group apart from the dominant group may result in collective discrimination within the society. Ethnocentrism and racism create and perpetuate the distinctions of dominant and minority groups. Ethnocentrism is the belief that one's own ethnic culture or subculture is superior to all others. Racism is the assumption of inherent racial superiority or inferiority with consequent discrimination (Buck, 2001).

An individual or group that straddles two or more cultures and embraces more than one set of values is termed *bicultural*, but efforts to achieve this status can be a source of considerable stress. Tremendous intraethnic diversity may exist in life perspective, values, problem-solving strategies, and customs among individual members of dominant and minority groups. Thus one can expect to see variations within as well as between cultures. In diverse societies, both the dominant and minority groups will change as a result of their interactions.

Culture Is Learned

The elements of culture are transmitted from one generation to another through a complicated process of social interaction. This socialization process shapes a child's reality; through it, children learn how to perceive the world, the values, ideologies, and rules that motivate and define behavior. This learning is facilitated by the long period of dependency that humans have before reaching physical and social maturity (Erikson, 1964), and depends on the child's temperament (Carey & McDevitt, 1995) and biologic capabilities.

A number of social institutions influence and support cultural socialization, including the family, school, peer groups, and the media.

Family. The family is the first socializing force an individual encounters. A powerful primary group, the family exposes the child to a set of values in the context of intensely personal relationships, as well as material and psychologic support. It is here that children first learn patterns of socially appropriate behavior. Each culture possesses its own values, attitudes, and practices with regard to families and child rearing, providing care and guidance in culturally prescribed ways. Family dynamics can facilitate conformity to the prevailing standards and codes of behavior. As active family members, children develop their personalities and a sense of self; they are given the opportunity to identify feelings and emotions, express ideas and thoughts, and practice interactional skills that they will use throughout their lives.

School. The school functions to expand the child's socialization beyond the boundaries of the family. Schools serve as models for much of the adult social world, providing the groundwork for developing methods of negotiating one's way within the institutions of adult society (e.g., workplace, politics, or organized recreation). For many children, schools may provide stability, opportunities for creative expression, and learning. A sense of collective identity and responsibility to the group may grow as children engage in school activities.

Peer Group. Peer groups also play a powerful role in socializing children to their culture. Peer groups can place children in a position of social equality unlike the socially inferior position that they may experience at home or in their school role. Through peer interactions, children explore their identities, give and receive validation of appropriate behavior, and further consolidate a sense of self.

Media. Television, radio, magazines, newspapers, films, and electronic media (e.g., Internet, chat rooms) have an enormous influence on the cultural socialization of children, especially in contemporary America. As an audience, Americans are conditioned to receive mass culture passively via these vehicles. Through the media, the child is exposed to a wide array of values, many of which may conflict with those of the family or the school. A number of authorities have expressed concern about the negative effect this exposure has on children's health (Kennedy, 2000).

Culture Is Symbolic

Communication takes place between humans using cultural symbols such as language (verbal and nonverbal), dress, food, music, dance, sports, and other activities. The extent to which individuals understand and master these cultural symbols will shape their self-concept, how others perceive them, and their ability to function within and contribute to their culture.

Culture Is Integrated

Culture is reflected in and influences every aspect of an individual's life. The cultural values, beliefs, and behaviors taught are embedded in the fabric of one's life and can be generalized from one social arena to another. Ideas about the appropriate behavior of children may extend from the family to the school to the community (e.g., "Children should be respectful to adults"). On the other hand, a cultural group may have different expectations in different roles; for example, language used among peers in the street may be very different from that used in the school or at home. Attitudes and behaviors regarding health, wellness, disease, and disability are an intricate part of this cultural framework.

PROVIDING CULTURALLY COMPETENT CARE

According to the U.S. Census Bureau (2000), by 2020 approximately 45% of individuals 20 years of age and younger will be from minority groups. Change in immigration patterns in the last decade alone has created a remarkable diversity of cultures in America. As national economies become more global, and as transportation and communication systems become more sophisticated, interdependence between countries and their peoples will continue to increase. Nurse practitioners (NPs) will see more clients from cultures different than their own, and they will need to become more culturally competent in the care they provide. This effort by health care providers to develop cultural competency in order to provide high-quality care is an excellent example of the dynamic nature of culture—health care in America will change because of the intercultural exchange among clients and providers.

Developing Cultural Competence

Cultural competence is the ability to communicate among cultures and demonstrate cultural skill outside one's culture of origin (Dunn, 2002). It is based on empathy, respect, and knowledge (Campinha-Bacote, 2002) and requires a fundamental recognition and valuing of culture as a distinctive way of life. The culturally competent provider's focus is not on how to interact with clients so that they will comply with a medical regimen. Instead, culturally competent providers work with clients to increase mutual understanding, strengthen clients' control of their health, and construct more healthful decisions.

To achieve cultural competence, providers must work to understand and, if necessary, change their worldview; become familiar with core cultural issues; increase their knowledge about core cultural issues related to health and illness; and become knowledgeable about the cultural groups with whom they work, in general and in terms of health and illness (Carrillo, Green, & Betancourt, 1999).

Worldview

A worldview is a conceptual framework that allows members of a social group or culture to answer fundamental questions such as "How does the world function?" "Why does it operate that way?" "Where is it going?" "What does it mean? What values, ethics, and moral standards is it working from?" "How should we act?" and "What is true—or false? What is knowledge?" In the United States, the dominant worldview tends to reflect an activistic, rational-mastery, future-oriented approach to life. It is based on a sense of independence and autonomy, and it values acquisition and power. Diversity of ideas, race, ethnicity, and lifestyle may be given little value unless they are useful to those in power; incidents of discrimination based on race, gender, age, or sexual orientation can be outcomes of this perception.

Various aspects of worldviews have been identified and are frequently presented as dichotomies for purposes of comparison: for example, individualism versus collectivism; masculinity versus femininity; power distance; and uncertainty avoidance (Hofstede, 1983). An example related to health care would be the U.S. culture of "individualism," in which clients make their own decisions about treatment, as opposed to a Southeast Asian culture (e.g., Hmong), in which the family is actively involved in deciding what treatment will be done. The dualistic thinking reflected in these taxonomies has come under criticism as being too simplistic, however, because it does not help explain the subtle nuances of cultures or the complexities of behaviors of members of social groups (Voronov & Singer, 2002). Critics assert that in order to understand human behavior, one must look at interaction within the larger socioecologic context. Not all Hmong clients rely on family members to help them make decisions about health treatments, for example; nor do all Americans make their decisions independently. Though culture is a vital element in why people make the choices they do, those choices depend on many other factors as well.

For health care providers working with clients from a cultural group other than their own, this means two things: First, NPs need to examine their own worldview, look at what social and cultural dynamics affect their thinking and behavior, and determine how this influences their practice and interaction with clients. A relevant example might be NPs who work with adolescents. NPs are a part of our "adult culture." To effectively work with adolescents, NPs need to reflect on what their "adult" perceptions are regarding teenagers and how those perceptions structure their approach to the client. There are additional dynamics to consider: NPs have experienced their own adolescence and have had their worldview shaped by that experience. They bring those perceptions to the interaction with their adolescent client (some providers have said, "Two people walk into the exam room when I see an adolescent—me as an adult NP, and me when I was 16 years old"). How does the NP's worldview affect her or his thinking about this client? How does it influence the way the NP interacts with the client? Additionally, the current "socioecologic" dynamics of the NP may be important to consider; perhaps he or she is struggling with a rebellious teenager at home. This personal concern could change the NP's ability to provide high-quality care to adolescents.

Second, NPs must be open to understanding the worldview of their clients and be willing to adapt their own in order to find the most effective way of providing health care. For example, problem-solving approaches vary among cultures. Not everyone solves problems in the linear, cause-and-effect way characteristic of the dominant culture in the United States. If NPs present a health problem and its solution in a linear fashion and insist that their patients and families use the same perspective, they should not be surprised if the patient is sometimes "noncompliant." An example might be a child who has a fever. Based on their worldview, NPs begin a diagnostic process of examination and laboratory testing to rule out causes, with some idea of an infectious agent in the back of their mind that may need to be treated with an antibiotic. The family, however, may have a more reflective, circuitous problem-solving style, part of which is a wait-and-see attitude, letting the child's body do what it will in response to the fever; and part of which means providing support in traditional cultural ways that involve preparation and time (e.g., sweats, prayer, chicken soup). If NPs do not listen to the family's understanding of the problem, and simply instruct the family to do what they say, the family may not follow through.

Core Cultural Issues

Core cultural issues are those qualities that are "universal (i.e., every culture has them) but specific (i.e., every culture expresses them differently)" (Dunn, 2002, p. 107). One cannot know all there is to know about all cultural groups, but knowledge will be enhanced if core cultural issues are used to learn about and understand different cultural groups. Table 4-2 outlines these issues and provides several examples of each. NPs can work with their clients from specific cultural groups to identify how that culture expresses these core issues.

Specific Cultural Groups

Becoming knowledgeable about the specific cultural groups with whom NPs work is essential in order to provide sensitive, relevant care. In addition to examining general cultural characteristics of clients (see Table 4-2), one needs to look at how culture influences clients' understanding and management of health and illness. Questions that allow clients and families to explain the cultural context of their illness, what they believe about its causes and what they think might be a way to treat it, can give NPs significant insight into how to best work with clients (Kleinman, Eisenberg, & Good, 1978) (Box 4-1).

When developing the plan of care, incorporate culture-related practices whenever possible and appropriate. Delivering care in a nonjudgmental manner does not call for NPs to abdicate their own standards. Rather, NPs should think in terms of the context within which those standards exist. It is helpful to ask the following questions: Is the culture-related practice efficacious? Is it safe? If it is beneficial, the NP should encourage it. The NP may determine that it is safe but has no therapeutic benefit; the client, however, may believe in it, and this belief can have a powerful placebo effect. If the treatment is not safe, further negotiation must happen as the NP explains why he or she does

TABLE 4-2 *Core Cultural Issues*

Cultural Characteristics	Example
Physical and biologic characteristics	Bone structure, hair, skin
Self-orientation and worldview	Individualistic (centered on self and one's needs) vs. collectivistic (person is part of larger whole, functions within context of community and history)
Concepts of time, space, and physical distance	What is the comfortable distance between individuals during conversation; when and how is it appropriate to touch a client?
Style and pattern of communication	Who speaks for the family, and, when do they do so, what language is used; are introductory comments or questions expected; is language formal?
Physical and social activities expected of group members	Muslim women are expected to cover their faces when in public; young Latino women may be expected to have a male family member escort when they go out
Relationships with others, often based on gender, age, or social class	Father in family may make decisions for other family members; grandmother may be first person consulted for health problems
Systems of social organization	Older children in Southeast Asian family may live at home with parents, contribute to family income; attendance at religious services and participation in church activities may be focus of social life
Relationships with nature	Belief in animism (inanimate natural objects [e.g., wind, earth, rocks] have spiritual quality); sense of responsibility and stewardship toward environment; view that environment is unsafe (e.g., "cleanliness is next to godliness")

not recommend it and what options would be better. An example might be treatments for gastrointestinal distress in children used by some Mexican families: One treatment involves rubbing the child's abdomen and body with an uncooked egg in the shell, a technique that is not likely to affect the biologic cause of the gastritis. The egg treatment is not harmful, however, and may comfort both parent (being able to do something) and child (because of the massage and attention). If the family wishes to use it, it should be encouraged. Another treatment for gastritis, however, is *greta*, a lead-based powder that is mixed with water and given to the child orally. *Greta* does not affect the cause of the gastritis and is a serious health risk to the child; it is the NP's responsibility to explain why it should not be given and explore with the family what alternatives are possible.

When doing cultural assessments, the NP must view cultural characteristics as being on a continuum, recognizing that not all individuals from the same social group have the same characteristics. Intraethnic variations must be anticipated and incorporated into the plan of care for a truly individualized approach. Attempting to fit a family or individual into any preconceived cultural framework is not cultural sensitivity—it is stereotyping. The distinction between individualizing care based on cultural characteristics and stereotyping is a fine one. Stereotyping and cross-cultural comparisons are to be avoided because they interfere with the development of basic trust and threaten the success of the therapeutic relationship and the plan of care.

BOX 4-1 *Identifying Cultural Meaning of Illness for Families*

- What is the problem called?
- What does the family believe is happening?
- What do you think caused the problem?
- Why do you think it started when it did?
- How has this illness affected you and the family?
- What are the chief problems this sickness has caused?
- How severe is the sickness?
- Will it have a short or long course?
- What kind of treatment should the patient receive?
- What are the most important results you hope to have happen from this treatment?
- What treatments have you already tried?
- What helped in the past?
- What do you fear most about your sickness?
- Are you afraid to tell your relatives or friends? What are you fearful might happen?

Communication Strategies

Culturally competent NPs work to develop a relationship of trust with clients and create a welcoming atmosphere in the health care setting. A relationship built on trust allows NP and client to actively negotiate for mutually acceptable interventions of care.

Communication strategies that NPs use in their interactions with clients can facilitate the message that they recognize and respect clients' beliefs and approaches to health and illness, and provide the basis for effective negotiation. Clearly, it is important to be able to speak the client's language, to be linguistically appropriate. But that ability alone is not sufficient and may not always be possible. Other concepts to consider when providing linguistically and culturally appropriate care include the following (Health Resources and Services Administration, 2001):

- Recognizing the linguistic variations within a cultural group
- Recognizing the cultural variations within a language group
- Recognizing the variations in literacy levels in all language groups

Context

Context is a characteristic of culture that influences how verbal and nonverbal communications are constructed and delivered, as well as the recipient's perception and response. Context lends structure to communication, influencing not just how individuals interpret messages but how they respond to them. Awareness of context is invaluable in communicating with individuals and families. According to Hall (1977), cultural groups tend to vary from "high context" to "low context."

A cultural group in which members send and receive verbal and nonverbal messages according to well-defined rules is referred to as high context. Among these groups, the context of the message (e.g., the situation in which the communication takes place, the status of the speaker, and the nonverbal aspects of the message) is more significant than what is actually said. As a result of the emphasis on context, individuals from high-context cultures tend to be less direct in their verbal statements and extremely sensitive to nonverbal and situational cues. In encounters with clients who engage in highly contextual communication, the client may speak very little and be extremely sensitive to the NP's body language and situational cues. Reliance on validation and clarification techniques, as well as less explicit or direct verbal messages, promotes a therapeutic relationship with these clients (Porter & Samovar, 1997).

In low-context cultures, the emphasis is on the content of the verbal message. Few rules are observed in communicating, and the status of the speaker is of little significance. Verbal communication is direct and explicit, and nonverbal and situational cues are not as significant as in high-context cultures. The NP should be very clear in verbal communication with clients from low-context cultures, recognizing that they may not pick up on situational and nonverbal cues.

Time and Spatial Perspectives as Forms of Nonverbal Communication

Time. Some cultures view time as steady, predictable, and mobile. It is always moving forward, and the impressions of past, present, and future are distinct—it is "monochronic," one thing at a time (Hall, 1990). For others, the reality of time exists only in relation to events occurring. "Polychronic" time is characterized by "the simultaneous occurrence of many things and by a great involvement with people" (Hall, 1990, p. 14). From this perspective, there is no such thing as early or late. The future is less important than the present, and problems of daily survival take priority over far-reaching goals. An understanding of these differences can aid providers in looking at their clients' actions, especially failed treatment plans, from a different and less judgmental perspective.

Space. Human beings seek to maintain a certain spatial distance from others. This desire for control over a certain amount of personal space is known as *territoriality*, and although it varies from one individual to another, Watson (1980) found a correlation between personal space requirements and culture. Three dimensions or zones of spatial distancing are recognized: The *intimate zone* allows close proximity and is reserved for family members and those in the roles of caregiver, comforter, and protector; the *personal zone* provides more spatial distance between individuals and is reserved for friends and close acquaintances; and the *public zone* is the spatial distance expected between co-workers and individuals in business encounters. This sense of personal space can be perceived not only visually, but through sound, smell, and touch (Hall, 1990).

The degree of territoriality and the amount of space considered appropriate in each zone varies from one individual to another and is influenced by gender, age, and situation, as well as culture. Most people are not consciously aware of their personal space requirements and the variables that influence spatial distance. Unconsciously, they may give nonverbal cues, such as turning to avoid direct face-to-face contact or stepping back, to indicate that they need more personal space (Giger & Davidhizar, 1995). A tendency to move closer, lean forward, and maintain direct eye contact for sustained periods indicates the need for less spatial distance.

Failure to recognize and respect an individual's personal space needs may be interpreted as a threatening invasion of personal space or a lack of caring and compassion, depending on the situation. An awareness of territoriality and appropriate responses to cues received with regard to the spatial needs of an individual client or family enhance the development of a satisfactory client-provider relationship.

Talking with the Family

The initial approach to talking with the family sets the tone for ongoing interactions. In general, a good way to begin a visit is to use the family's surname when addressing the parent or parents, or ask what they prefer to be called. Regardless of the culture, it is best not to assume that it is acceptable to call an adult (particularly one who is older than the provider) by his or her first name. All family members who accompany the child should be acknowledged. For some cultural groups, the presence of numerous family members represents an expression of respect and caring for children and their parents. When family elders are present, they should be included in all conversations and decision making that take place regarding the child.

Some clients may view an interrogative approach (asking questions) as intrusive, thus interfering with the development of a trusting relationship. The NP should be sensitive to signs of discomfort, such as evasive answers or visible uneasiness, and switch from asking questions to making gentle declarative statements based on observations and information already acquired.

Extensive note taking in the family's presence can also cause uneasiness. If this occurs, the NP should stop the note taking and listen more intently. Follow the parent's lead with regard to eye contact. Among some cultures and in different regions across the United States, consistent eye contact can be perceived as threatening or rude. In others, breaking eye contact frequently may be interpreted as a sign of disrespect or boredom.

In general, a low tone of voice helps calm anxious patients and parents. The provider should also resist the temptation to talk fast. Focus on the parent first, and ask permission before touching the infant or young child. This shows respect for the parent and can also have a calming effect on the child.

Out of respect for the authority of the practitioner, the parent or patient may not wish to ask questions or request clarification, so the NP should encourage questions and check frequently for understanding.

Culturally Sensitive Patient Education

It is incorrect to assume that all clients and their families value and benefit from patient education material. Although members of low-context cultures may seek and appreciate written educational material, it may be overwhelming for members of high-context cultures who are trying to interpret a myriad of nonverbal and situational cues as well as the verbal message associated with the visit. The best approach is to make clients aware of the written educational material that is available and let them know they may take it if they wish.

Any instructions for home management should be written in simple terms in the client's native language or in the language in which parents or caregivers are literate (this may not be the same as the native language), and educational efforts should be directed toward any elder family members present, fathers as well as mothers. Abbreviations should be avoided, and all written material should be reviewed with the patient, parent, or both, with the help of an interpreter when necessary. Do not assume that all parents can read English or their own native language. However, assessing literacy must be done with sensitivity, because illiteracy is a source of shame among some peoples.

Using an Interpreter

The importance of using a qualified interpreter cannot be overemphasized. Interpreters who are familiar with the culture as well as the language are especially helpful, because they are likely to be more sensitive to the nonverbal cues inherent in a patient's presentation of the complaint. The term *cultural broker* is used to describe an individual who bridges two or more cultures and can translate both linguistic and cultural meaning.

In some immigrant communities, especially those that are small, there may be few qualified interpreters. Also, as members of a small, closely knit community, both interpreter and client may find it awkward to discuss sensitive personal information in the NP's office and then return to their culturally prescribed social roles in the community. In larger immigrant communities, several languages or dialects may be spoken; and language barriers may arise even among people who speak the same language, because communication patterns differ among classes, subcultures, and regions of the country of origin. Contracting with a commercial telephone interpreter service may be a possibility in cases such as these.

Qualified interpreters must be well-trained professionals who are able to communicate to the client that they can be trusted to keep information confidential. When family members or unqualified persons are relied on to translate, patient confidentiality, as well as provider and family understanding, can be jeopardized.

The qualified interpreter stands or sits behind the provider so as not to interfere with eye contact between the patient, the parent, and the provider. In some instances, the interpreter can even stand or sit behind a screen if privacy is an issue. If topics related to sexuality are to be discussed, interpreters should be of the same sex as the patient.

The interpreter should make an effort to translate the dialogue as closely and accurately as possible for both parties. When a provider's yes-or-no question results in a lengthy response, the interpreter must ensure that the provider is apprised of the whole statement, including any seemingly unrelated data. It is especially difficult to convey emotion through verbal translation, and this component of communication may be lost or diminished when interpreters are used. This should not be perceived as lack of concern on the part of the patient or family, and the NP should be alert for nonverbal cues. Nonverbal cues may have their own cultural connotative meaning, however, so clarification may be necessary (e.g., "You seem very upset; I noticed your face change when we talked about ______. Are you worried about _____?"). Regarding instructions for home management, it may be helpful if the interpreter can write instructions for the family in the family's language and review them again before the family leaves.

Interpreters should work toward the following goals:

- Making the clients' description and understanding of the problem clear to the provider
- Communicating accurately the provider's interpretation and explanation of a health problem (e.g., pathophysiology) to the client
- Facilitating the discussion to develop a management plan
- Assessing patient and parents' level of knowledge and understanding of what is being said.

Recognizing Culture Shock

The process of emigrating—leaving one's homeland to settle in a different country—presents the individual and the family with many challenges. Changes in diet, exposure to unfamiliar environmental hazards, and lack of appropriate immunity may threaten physical health. In addition, considerable energy is required to interpret and respond to the unfamiliar behavior and symbols individuals encounter on a daily basis as they attempt to meet basic and complex needs in the absence of familiar resources. The feelings of helplessness and exhaustion that may ensue are part of the phenomenon known as *culture shock*, first identified by anthropologists in the 1950s (Oberg, 1960).

Culture shock affects the physical, emotional, and psychologic well-being of every member of the family and may take many months to overcome. Generally, individuals progress through stages of culture shock: Initially, they may be fascinated with the novelty of the new culture, then become hostile or highly critical, before moving on to adjustment and acceptance. The degree of culture shock that is experienced depends on many variables, including social status, personality characteristics, age, occupation, available support systems, familiarity with the dominant language, general state of health, and the extent of cultural differences between the home and host countries. For immigrants from areas of the world where they have experienced displacement, trauma, abuse, and fear, culture shock may be complicated by delayed responses to stress.

In the presence of health care providers, patients and perhaps their family members as well may appear inappropriately complacent or overreactive. Rather than being noncompliant or uncooperative, they may, in reality, be experiencing culture shock. NPs can facilitate clients' successful management of culture shock by clearly and patiently explaining what is happening with the client; providing clear, relevant information about how the health system works; acknowledging the client's sense of confusion as normal; and giving positive feedback for the client's efforts.

NPs who care for clients and families from culturally diverse backgrounds frequently experience culture shock, too. Lack of knowledge of differences in cultural practices, beliefs, and values can result in feelings of helplessness, frustration, and inadequacy for everyone involved in the helping relationship. NPs can reduce their own culture shock and that of their clients by learning about the different cultural groups they work with and recognizing the signs of culture shock in their clients and themselves.

CULTURES IN AMERICAN SOCIETY

The population of the United States consists of numerous ethnic groups, races, and subcultures and is becoming increasingly diverse. It is often broken down into the dominant white middle class and a number of minority groups, including African Americans, Hispanic Americans, Asian Americans, Native Americans, Russian Americans, and Arab Americans. Within each of these categories, there are many subgroups. For example, most providers would include families from Iran, Syria, Eritrea, Somalia, Egypt, and Iraq in the category of "Arab Americans," yet the cultural differences between each are immeasurable, and, though they may share some common characteristics, each is unique. To present accurate descriptions of each cultural group with whom NPs will work is beyond the scope of this text. Instead, Table 4-3 lists some of the more common health issues found in some cultural groups. The Resource Box lists a number of resources that providers can use to access information that best suits their particular practice.

Providing culturally competent care is increasingly required of health care providers. It is a challenge that requires personal reflection, as well as significant change in beliefs, attitudes, and practices. Fortunately, NPs are not alone in the process. By working sensitively with clients of

TABLE 4-3 *Health Issues More Common in a Particular Cultural Group*

Cultural Group	Health Issue
African American	High infant mortality rate
	Sickle cell trait and disease
	Hypertension
	Obesity
	Type 2 diabetes mellitus
	Type 1 diabetes mellitus with beta-cell destruction
	Slipped capital femoral epiphysis
	Blount disease
	Lead poisoning due to environmental exposure in urban areas
	Violence
Asian American	Lactose intolerance
	Tuberculosis, dental caries, malnutrition among some recent immigrants
	Cleft lip and palate
Caucasian	Rett syndrome (girls)
	Tay-Sachs disease (Ashkenazi Jewish; French Canadian)
	Tyrosinemia (French Canadian; Scandinavian)
	Celiac disease
	Cystic fibrosis
	Phenylketonuria (Northern European)
	Pyloric stenosis (Northern European)
	Blount disease (Northern European)
	Lactose intolerance
	Type 1 diabetes mellitus
	Glutaric aciduria type 1 (Amish and Hutterites; Canadian)
Latino	Dental caries
	Obesity
	Type 2 diabetes mellitus
	Blount disease
	Asthma
	Teenage pregnancy
Native American (American Indian)	Otitis media
	Poor prenatal care, low-birth-weight babies, high infant mortality rate
	Alcoholism
	Unintentional injury
Samoan/Polynesian	Dermatologic conditions
	Obesity
	Slipped capital femoral epiphysis
Russian American	Obesity
	Alcoholism

RESOURCE BOX

Cultural Perspectives

Centers for Medicare and Medicaid Services (CMS)
www.cms.gov/healthplans/quality/project03.asp
Guidelines for medical practices to develop and implement culturally and linguistically appropriate services:
Providing Oral Linguistic Services: A Guide for Managed Care Plans
Planning Culturally and Linguistically Appropriate Services: A Guide for Managed Care Plans

Cross Cultural Health Care Program
www.xculture.org
1-206-860-0329
Cultural competence training, interpreter training, research, and educational materials; links to community profiles for range of diverse populations

Diversity, Health and Health Care
www.gasi.org/diversity.htm

EthnoMed
www.ethnomed.org
Detailed information regarding cultural characteristics of diverse populations

Montana Area Health Education Center
1-406-994-6001
ahec.msu.montana.edu/students/culture.html
Designed for students, but excellent links for all providers to cultural resources

National Center for Cultural Competence
www.georgetown.edu/research/gucdc/nccc/
1-800-788-2066
Training opportunities; links to national resources for health care to diver.se populations

Continued

RESOURCE BOX

Cultural Perspectives—cont'd

Northwest Center for Physician-Patient Communication
www.tfme.org/nwppc.htm
1-503-36-2234
Information and training program of the Foundation for Medical Excellence

Office of Minority Health Information Center
U.S. Public Health Service
U.S. Department of Health and Human Services
www.omhrc.gov/clas
Guidelines for culturally and linguistically appropriate services in health care

Resource for Cross-Cultural Health Care
www.diversityrx.org
Sponsored by the National Conference of State Legislatures (NCSL); Resources for Cross Cultural Health Care (RCCHC); and the Henry J. Kaiser Family Foundation of Menlo Park, CA

Educational opportunities for professionals; legislative, policy, and advocacy information about cultural groups

Society of Medical Interpreters
www.sominet.org/
Professional association with educational offers, networking; list of interpreters for wide range of languages in Pacific Northwest/Seattle area

State University of New York Institute of Technology
www.sunyit.edu/library/html/culturedmed/bib/medical/
Extensive bibliographies, information, and links on a wide range of cultural groups, refugees and immigrants, standards, interpreters, dictionaries, etc.

diversity, sharing ideas and information, and learning from and about each other, both clients and NPs can become full participants in creating a new cultural context for the health and illness experience.

REFERENCES

Berger P, Luckmann T: *The social construction of reality*, New York, 1966, Doubleday.

Buck PD: *Worked to the bone: race, class, power, and privilege in Kentucky*, New York, 2001, Monthly Review Press.

Campinha-Bacote J: The process of cultural competence in the delivery of health care services: a model of care, *J Transcult Nurs* 13:181-184, 2002.

Carey WB, McDevitt SC: *Coping with children's temperament: a guide for professionals*, New York, 1995, Basic Books.

Carrillo JE, Green AR, Betancourt JR: Cross-cultural primary care: a patient-based approach, *Ann Intern Med* 130:829-834, 1999.

Dunn AM: Culture competence and the primary care provider, *J Pediatr Health Care* 16:105-111, 2002.

Erikson E: *Childhood and society*, New York, 1964, Norton.

Giger JN, Davidhizar RE: *Transcultural nursing: assessment and intervention*, St Louis, 1995, Mosby.

Hall ET: *Beyond culture*, Garden City, NY, 1977, Anchor Press/Doubleday.

Hall ET: *Understanding cultural differences*, Yarmouth, ME, 1990, Intercultural Press.

Health Resources and Services Administration: *Cultural competence works: using cultural competence to improve the quality of health care for diverse populations and add value to managed care arrangements*, Washington, DC, 2001, US Department of Health and Human Services.

Hofstede G: Dimensions of national cultures in fifty countries and three regions. In Deregowski JB, Dziurawiec S, Annis RC, editors: *Expiscations in cross-cultural psychology: selected papers from the Sixth International Conference of the International Association for Cross-Cultural Psychology held at Aberdeen, July 20-23, 1982*, Lisse, Netherlands, 1983, Swets & Zeitlinger.

Kennedy C: Examining television as an influence on children's health behaviors, *J Pediatr Nurs* 15:272-281, 2000.

Kleinman A, Eisenberg L, Good B: Culture, illness and care: clinical lessons from anthropologic and cross-cultural research, *Ann Intern Med* 88:251-258, 1978.

Kroeber AL: *The nature of culture*, Chicago, 1952, University of Chicago Press.

Oberg K: Culture shock: adjustment to new cultural environment, *Practical Anthropology* 7:177-182, 1960.

Porter RE, Samovar LA: *Intercultural communication: a reader*, ed 8, Belmont, CA, 1997, Wadsworth.

US Census Bureau, Population Division: *Population projections program*, Washington, DC, 2000, US Census Bureau.

Voronov M, Singer JA: The myth of individualism-collectivism: a critical review, *J Soc Psychol* 142:461-480, 2002.

Watson OM: *Proxemic behavior: a cross-cultural study*, The Hague, Netherlands, 1980, Mouton.

UNIT 2

Management of Development

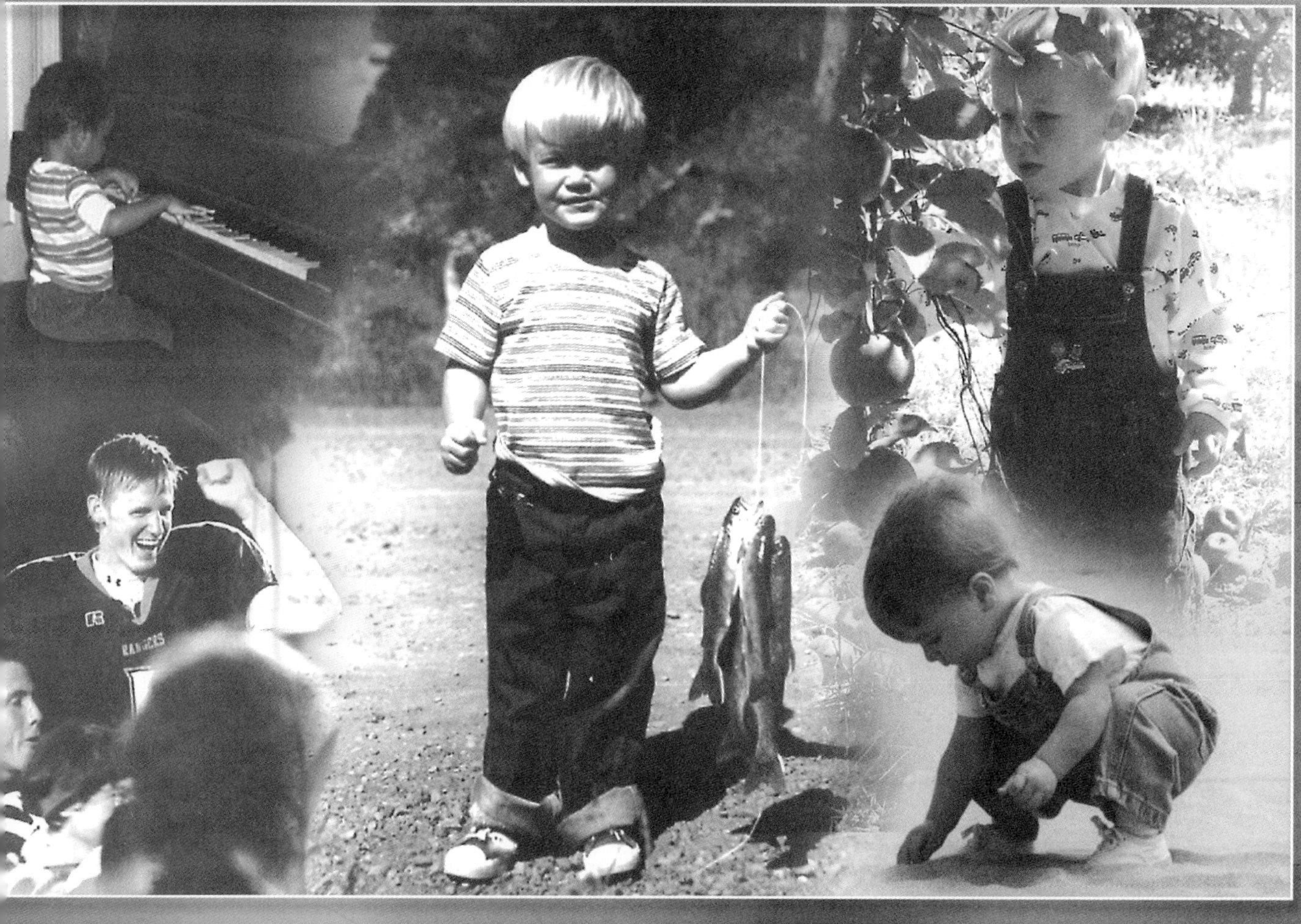

5 Developmental Management in Pediatric Primary Care

Barbara Jones Deloian, Mary A. Murphy

Primary care providers have a responsibility to monitor children's overall physical and psychosocial development and to provide anticipatory guidance to families as children grow. This requires a strong background in child development and knowledge of clinical strategies that will help parents better understand their child's development. Nurse practitioners (NPs) who work with parents and their children share in the parents' pride as their child accomplishes a new developmental task. NPs assist parents to understand the challenges that new accomplishments create and how parents may best handle these challenges. Modern approaches to managing children's well-being today differ dramatically from those that prevailed at the turn of the last century, when health supervision consisted of a brief examination to detect communicable or contagious diseases. As the twenty-first century begins, significant social, economic, and demographic changes continue to influence the American family and affect children's health. Children's health supervision must take a broader approach than would be necessary only for detection of disease.

The Classification of Child and Adolescent Mental Health Diagnoses in Primary Care: Diagnostic and Statistical Manual for Primary Care (DSM-PC), Child and Adolescent Version (Wolraich, Felice, & Drotar, 1996) establishes a comprehensive description of the physical and psychosocial developmental concerns of childhood and adolescence. The pediatric primary care provider must have a sound knowledge of these developmental issues (Dixon & Stein, 2000). This chapter presents an introduction to principles of development, developmental theories, methods of developmental assessment, and identification and management of developmental problems. Chapters 6 through 9 review developmental theories, describe normal patterns of development, identify "red flags" related to development, and recommend anticipatory guidance for families of infants, toddlers and preschoolers, school-age children, and adolescents.

DEVELOPMENTAL PRINCIPLES

Development is a lifelong, dynamic process. Achievement of changes in one phase sets the stage for the next phase. Development is also a dynamic and reciprocal process that occurs between the child's internal and external environment. Key principles are often used to understand concepts of development. Exactly how these principles are manifested in a particular child depends on the child's genetic background, personality, and intrauterine and extrauterine environmental factors.

Principle 1. Growth and development are orderly and sequential. Although children differ in rates and timing of developmental changes, they generally follow certain predictable stages or phases. Specific examples include the rapid growth during the first year of life, progress toward independence throughout childhood, and the unfolding of secondary sex characteristics during adolescence.

Principle 2. The pace of growth and development is specific for each child. Developmental changes vary considerably for each child. Some children demonstrate early skill in motor coordination, others in language acquisition. These changes represent the uniqueness of each child.

Principle 3. Development occurs in a cephalocaudal and proximodistal direction. An example of this principle is seen as infants develop increasing motor coordination, gaining head control before sitting and walking. Similarly, developmental progress is seen in controlled movements that occur near the midline of the body first, such as rolling over. Eventually, distal coordination of the hands, such as mastery of the pincer grasp, occurs.

Principle 4. Growth and development become increasingly integrated. Behavior that is often taken for granted, such as self-feeding, occurs as a result of numerous small changes and skills acquired by the child. Simple skills and behaviors are integrated into more complex behaviors as the child grows and develops.

Principle 5. Developmental abilities become increasingly organized and differentiated. As a result of increasing maturation and experience, children's behaviors and responses to internal and external cues become more regulated, organized, and differentiated. The infant's crying and body movements in response to hunger cues are different from the toddler's walking to the refrigerator in response to the same cues.

Principle 6. Growth and development are affected by the child's internal and external environment. Opportunities for play, societal norms, cultural values, family traditions, and family beliefs all influence the development of children. Similarly, children influence their environment to achieve desired experiences and opportunities.

Principle 7. Certain periods are critical during growth and development. Critical periods are defined as points of time when developmental advances occur more readily than they do at other times. The occurrence of congenital anomalies when the fetus is exposed to certain viruses during fetal growth is one example.

Principle 8. Growth and development is a dynamic process influenced by many factors. Development is a continual process, often without smooth transitions. Phases of development are marked by periods of change, growth, and plateaus of stability. Efforts to predict and control the developmental process often emphasize the individual nature of development and the numerous individual factors that influence developmental outcomes (Cech & Martin, 2002).

DEVELOPMENTAL THEORIES

The study of developmental theories reveals a fascinating array of ideas about how children progress from infancy through adolescence, providing many perspectives on children's growth and development. NPs need to continue to stay abreast of changing ideas of child development and appreciate new developmental theories relating to children. Developmental theories are based on various cultures, personalities, environmental issues, philosophic beliefs, and investigative methods. Thus, when using a developmental perspective in practice, the NP should understand how the theory was developed and how it may relate to a particular family and child.

Developmental theories provide guidelines for understanding the unfolding of the child's behavior, personality, and physical abilities. Therefore it is necessary to combine several theories to understand the child as a whole person.

Ethology: Animal Studies

The study of animal behavior has led to some theoretic assumptions that assist in the study of child development. These include four major propositions on the concepts of bonding, altruism, social intelligence, and dominant and submissive behavior. Bowlby (1969) first generalized theories developed about animal behavior to bonding for humans. This was followed by Klaus and Kennel's work (1976), which emphasized the importance of early mother-infant contact that later became the basis for changes in hospital rooming-in care. Ainsworth, Bell, & Stayton (1971) continued to examine the elements of early attachment and separation in child development and personality.

Maturational Theories: Developmental Milestones

Early theories about human behavior set the stage for studies in child development. The religious and cultural beliefs based on the sinful and obstinate child that derive from Puritan beliefs can be seen currently in strict child-rearing practices. Rousseau's descriptions in 1762 of the natural, innately good growth of the child, if not misled by a "corrupt social environment," provided the foundation for maturational theories. Gesell (1940) is credited with the term *maturation* in reference to the orderly, sequential developmental changes that occur over time. He also described cycles of behavior that correspond to certain chronologic ages. His work resulted in the chronologic growth and development norms for motor, affective, linguistic, and social domains that are now used to assess developmental progress.

Lewin's work (1936) provided the identification of growth principles and the currently acknowledged stages, including infancy, early childhood, and adolescence. He also provided an understanding of the play and decision-making phases through which children progress.

Havighurst's work (1953), a summation of ideas from many theorists, popularized the concept of developmental tasks described as "successful achievement which leads to . . . happiness and to success with later tasks, while failure leads to unhappiness in the individual, disapproval by society, and difficulty with later tasks."

Cognitive-Structural Theories: Language and Thought

Cognitive-structural theories examine the ways in which children think, reason, and use language. They are based on assumptions of maturation of the central nervous system and children's interactions with their environment. Individual differences are ascribed to genetic endowment and environmental influences.

Jean Piaget's observations, many of which were of his own children, provide an understanding of children's cognitive development and their perception and use of the world around them. Piaget (1969) described how children actively use their life experiences, incorporating them into their own mental and physical being over time. He emphasized how children modify themselves depending on their environmental experiences and their stage-related level of competencies. Piaget described four stages of cognitive development (Table 5-1).

Sensorimotor Stage (Birth to 2 Years)

At this stage, children learn about the world through their actions and sensory and motor movements. Key concepts that are assimilated during this period include perception of object permanence, spatial relationships, causality, use of instruments, and combination of objects. The child's framework for learning is the self, and there is little cognitive connection to objects outside the self.

Preoperational Stage (2 to 7 Years)

Children next attempt to make sense of the world and reality. However, this is based on an egocentric perspective and is accomplished through certain mental operations that are linked to concrete objects. Children at this stage are not able to understand cause and effect. Therefore their reasoning is often flawed. Children are able to begin to use semiotic functioning, or the use of one thing to represent another. Intuitive reasoning emerges toward the end of this stage, but reasoning continues to be connected to the concrete reality of the here and now.

Concrete Operational Stage (7 to 12 Years)

Children are able to use symbols to represent concrete objects (here and now) and perform mental operations in their head. This process involves cognitive skills required to organize experiences and classify increasingly complex information. Most schoolwork requires functioning at this level with flexibility of thought, declining egocentrism, logical reasoning, and greater social cognition.

Formal Operational Stage (13 Years through Adulthood)

At this stage, children begin to think abstractly and to imagine different solutions to problems and different outcomes. During this stage, adolescents begin to develop increased awareness of degrees of illness, as well as personal control of one's health. Renewed egocentrism may be noted early in this stage as a result of lack of differentiation between what others are thinking and one's own thoughts. This egocentric thinking eventually gives way to appreciation of differences in judgment between the adolescent and other individuals, societies, and cultures, and becomes the basis of an adolescent's ability to think about politics, law, and society in terms of abstract principles and benefits rather than focusing only on the punitive aspects of societal laws.

Piaget's work was expanded by theorists such as Flavell (1977) and Siegler, Liebert, & Liebert (1973), who looked at specific intellectual capabilities via the information processing model, which included concepts of attention, perception, memory, and inferencing. The information processing model provides initial understanding of how mental activity leads progressively to more sophisticated ways of handling information.

Kohlberg (1969) provided a theoretic focus on moral development and socialization, emphasizing the process by which children learn the expectations and norms of their society and culture (see Table 5-1). Kohlberg's work primarily involved male participants. Gilligan (1982) suggested that female thoughts and actions involve significantly different objectives and goals.

Fowler's theory (1981) described the spiritual dimension of human life, or the development of faith. This theory addressed the process by which humans develop meaning for daily life. Faith is described as the structure that people use to build their lives. Fowler emphasized that achieving the stages is not due to intelligence but, rather, occurs through valuing, thinking, and interacting with others.

Criticism has been expressed that early theorists' work lacked experimental support, especially related to different cultural and socioeconomic settings. More research is being conducted to validate and test developmental theories, especially to gain a better understanding of the learning mechanisms of children who have visual or motor compromises and need special interventions.

TABLE 5-1 ***Comparison of Early Developmental Theorists***

		Kohlberg		Piaget		Erikson	
Age	**Freud**	**Stages**		**Stages/Substages**	**Characteristics**	**Psychologic Crisis**	**Themes**
0-12 mo	Oral stage	"Amoral" preconventional level	1: Punishment and obedience	Sensorimotor stage		Trust vs. mistrust	To get; to give in return
				1. Reflexive stage; 0-1 mo	Innate infant reflexes		
				2. Primary circular stage: 1-4 mo	Repetitive responses		
				3. Secondary circular stage: 4-8 mo	Outward-directed behaviors		
				4. Coordination of secondary circular stage: 8-12 mo	Object permanence and goal-directed behaviors		
12-18 mo				5. Tertiary circular reactions stage: 2-18 mo	Causality and object permanence through several steps	Autonomy vs. shame	To hold on; to let go
18-36 mo	Anal stage	Stages 1-2 conventional level	2: Instrumental realistic orientation	6. Mental combinations stage 18-24 mo	Memory used for problem solving		
3-6 yr	Oedipal stage	Stages 1-3	3: Interpersonal acceptance of "nice" girl and "good" boy social concept	Preoperational stage: 1. Preconceptual stage: 2-4 yr	Increased use of symbols, especially language; representational thought, egocentrism, assimilation, and symbolic play	Initiative vs. guilt	To make things; to play
				2. Intuitive stage: 4-7 yr	Increased symbolic functioning, language, decreasing egocentricity, imitation of reality		

6-11 yr	Latency stage	Stages 2-5	4: The "law and order" orientation 5: Social contract, and utilitarian orientation	Concrete operational stage	Flexible thought: understands rules of reversibility and deconcentration, conservation, and identity Declining egocentrism: ability to understand another's perspective Local reasoning: understands concepts of relation, ordering, conservation; able to classify objects Social cognition: improved sense of equality and justice	Industry vs. inferiority	To make things; to complete
12-17 yr	Adolescence (Oedipus complex)	Stages 4-6	6: Universal ethical principle orientation	Formal operational stage	Development of logical thinking, the ability to work with abstract ideas; able to synthesize and integrate concepts into larger schemes	Identity vs. role confusion	To be oneself; to share being oneself or not being oneself
17-30 yr	Young adult	Stages 4-6		Formal operational stage		Intimacy vs. isolation	To lose and find oneself in another

Psychoanalytic Theories
Personality and Emotions

Psychodynamic theorists have studied factors that influence the emotional and psychologic behavior of individuals. Personality includes the characteristics of temperament and motivation, as well as concepts related to self-esteem and self-concept. Sigmund Freud (1938) was one of the most influential theorists in this area. Freud sought to find links between the conscious mind and the body through the unconscious mind (see Table 5-1). Some of his most significant contributions were his descriptions of the interactions of id, ego, and superego (Thomas, 1985).

Anna Freud continued the work of her father, focusing particularly on children. It was through her studies that the implications of psychoanalysis for raising normal children were developed. She believed that psychoanalytic theory could help parents gain "insight into the potential harm done to young children during the critical years of their development by the manner in which their needs, drives, wishes, and emotional dependencies are met" (Freud, 1974).

Erikson (1964) also expanded Freud's theories, describing the stages of the individual through the life span (see Table 5-1). Each stage presents problems that the individual seeks to master. Erikson believed that if problems were not resolved, they would be revisited again at future stages.

Sullivan (1964) emphasized the importance of self-concept and the environmental influences that modulate it. He defined the most crucial cultural environment as the home and the parent. Sullivan posited that progression toward mature relationships is based on communication skills and the integration of social experiences inhibited or enhanced by the parents' relationship between themselves.

Mahler, Pine, & Bergman (1975) analyzed the development of an infant's evolving independence through study of the mother-infant dyad. Three phases of development were proposed: autism, symbiosis, and separation-individuation. These phases account for the gradually increasing awareness of the infant's sense of self and others. In the autistic phase (3 to 5 weeks of age), the infant has no concept of self but is working, physiologically, to achieve homeostasis in the extrauterine world. The second phase, symbiosis, refers to a period of undifferentiation or fusion with the mother in which infant and mother form a dual unity. Separation-individuation (from about 4 to 5 months of age onward) is characterized by a steady increase in awareness of the separateness of the self and the other. One indication of this is a specific, preferential smile in response to the mother. During differentiation, a subphase of separation-individuation (6 to 7 months of age), the infant uses visual and tactile exploration of the mother or caregiver. Practicing, a second subphase of separation-individuation, occurs as the infant explores movement toward more autonomous functions. Transitional objects, such as blankets or toys, make separation from the mother easier and help the infant establish familiarity with a broader segment of the world. The infant may move back and forth from the mother for emotional "refueling." During this practice period, weaning may be easier because the natural tendency for exploration and separation is occurring. Rapprochement, a third subphase of the separation-individuation phase (14 to 24 months), accounts for the child's use of the mother as an extension of self. Shyness with strangers and adverse reactions to separations may be due to a growing sense of vulnerability. A final subphase, consolidation (24 to 36 months), is demonstrated as the infant is able to separate from the mother without extreme anxiety. Symbolic play emerges, and the child is better able to delay gratification of needs.

Infant attachment within the context of separation and connectedness has been explored by Stern (1985), Emde and Buchsbaum (1990), and Rogoff (1990). They propose that infants develop a sense of self through the experience of the infant-caregiver relationship. The quality and consistency of relationships help the infant develop an affective, or emotional, sense of self. The early beginnings of the sense of self are based on three biologic principles: self-regulation, social fittedness, and affective monitoring (Emde, 1988). Infants with attachment security and a sense of connectedness are more likely to explore and be autonomous. This is called an *internal working model*, guiding the individual in later attachments. Rogoff's work (1990) defines the idea of intersubjectivity, that is, shared meaning or shared purpose between individuals. The parent guides the infant in connecting with others and experiencing mutuality. According to these theories, the major influences on infant development are social interactions and engagement of infants with their parents and objects in their world.

Behavioral Theories: Human
Actions and Interactions

Behaviorism is the study of the general laws of human behavior. Behaviorism focuses on the present and the ways that the environment influences human behavior. Skinner's view of child development focused on learning that was controlled through classic operant conditioning (1953). Behavior modification therapy is largely based on this theory. Bandura's social learning theory looked at imitation and modeling as a means of learning, emphasizing the social variables involved (Mott, 1990; Thomas, 1985). Bijou and Baer (1965) responded to critics of behaviorism's view of the child as a passive object. They expressed the notion that children's responses to environmental stimuli are dependent on their genetic structure and personal history (Thomas, 1985).

Humanistic Theories

Innermost Self

Maslow (1971), Buhler and Allen (1972), and Mahrer (1978) are the best known humanistic theorists. They focus on development throughout the life span. Maslow's hierarchy of needs included physiologic, safety, belongingness and love, esteem, and self-actualization needs (1971). He differentiated deficiency needs from growth or self-actualization needs. Rather than proposing stages through which children or adults mature, the humanists believe that individuals and those around them are responsible for any movement they make from one needs plateau to another; intrinsic forces do not move them along.

Ecologic Theories

Human ecology theory (Bronfenbrenner, 1979) emphasizes environmental influences more than most other developmental theories do. The key concepts of this perspective emphasize the interdependence of the settings (roles, interpersonal relations, and activities) that influence the developing child, both directly and indirectly. Children are viewed as dynamic entities who are increasingly able to restructure the settings in which they live. Environments also are seen as influencing children, leading to mutual accommodation and reciprocity. Children are influenced by the home and family, child care settings, schools, entertainment and recreational activities, their parents' work, and broad economic opportunities in society. Individuals' perceptions of the environment influence their behavior and development more than the objective reality does. Development is described as the growing capacity to discover, sustain, or alter the self or the environment. Finally, recognition is given to ecologic transitions or changes in an individual's role or setting, such as the birth of a sibling or changes in family structure. Routine and ritual within the family system can be powerful mediators of children's development (Fiese, 2002; Kubicek, 2002). The parent-child interaction also may be inhibited or enhanced by the parents' relationships. When the parent experiences positive mutual feelings, the parent-child relationship can be strengthened. Alternatively, when the parent experiences mutual antagonism or interference, the parent-child relationship may be impaired (Kelly & Barnard, 2000). These theories are especially useful to better understand the impact of domestic violence on a child's development and future.

Temperament

Chess and Thomas (1995) have provided much of the understanding about the effect of temperament on a child's behavior. Their work seeks to explain the role that temperament plays in children's behavior. During a child's infancy, the NP can explain to parents the individual variations in temperament and help parents understand how temperament may affect the child's behavior (Carey, 1998). The intent is to alleviate guilt and frustration about the child's behavior and to assist parents in developing strategies that enhance rather than exaggerate difficult temperamental characteristics. Chess and Thomas (1995) also introduced the concept of "goodness of fit" to describe the degree to which the child's environment and parents' characteristics, including the parents' temperament, are congruous with the child's natural temperamental characteristics. Scales that can be used to assess an individual child's temperament are listed in the Chapter 6 Resource Box. Table 5-2 further defines characteristics of temperamental differences.

CULTURAL FACTORS INFLUENCING DEVELOPMENT

Cultural and ethnic traditions are important considerations in the development of infants, children, adolescents, parents, and families. Differences have been identified in achievement of childhood developmental milestones for some cultural groups. This information, however, is insufficient when providing individualized care for a particular child and family. More accurate assessments of families and children come from understanding the specific culture of a family and community. To gain this knowledge about a family, additional assessment is needed beyond the traditional health history and physical examination. The NP's ongoing relationship with a particular family and the families within a community may be most helpful in this regard. A nonjudgmental attitude must be used with families to gain insight into their beliefs and values.

Tools, such as the genogram, ecomap, and family functioning model (Minuchin, 1974), can be particularly helpful in identifying family structure, strengths, and resources, as well as individual family health responses, beliefs, and practices. The Childhood Health Assessment Questionnaire (CHAQ) and Child Health Questionnaire (CHQ) have also been adapted to a number of cultural groups (Ruperto et al, 2001). The interview process is valuable for clarifying

TABLE 5-2 *Characteristics of Temperament*

Temperament Characteristic	Description
Activity	What is the child's activity level? Is the child moving all the time he or she is awake, some of the time, or rarely?
Rhythmicity	How predictable is the child's sleep/wake pattern, feeding schedule, and elimination pattern?
Approach/withdrawal	What is the child's response when presented with something new such as a new toy, a new experience, or a new person? Does he or she immediately approach or turn away?
Adaptability	How quickly does the child get used to new things? Quickly or not at all?
Threshold of response	How much stimulation does the child require for calming? A quiet voice and touch or more intense, loud voice or firm grasp?
Intensity of reaction	Are the child's responses (crying or laughing) very subtle or extremely intense?
Quality of mood	Is the child's mood usually outgoing, happy, joyful, pleasant or unfriendly, withdrawn, or quiet?
Distractibility	How easily is the child distracted by outside disturbance such as a phone ringing, TV, siblings?
Attention span and persistence	How long will the child continue to play with a particular toy or engage in a certain activity? Does this continue even when there are distractions?

families' unique qualities and resources and serving as an avenue for communicating interest in, and understanding of, individual families and their ethnic or cultural values, differences, and commonalities (see Chapters 3 and 4).

Nugent (1994) discusses three invaluable outcomes that can be achieved through cross-cultural studies of child development. First, these studies add an understanding of the diversity of parenting styles and belief systems, and, as such, they allow practitioners to move beyond their own worldview. Second, cross-cultural research provides a better understanding of the dynamic aspects of child-environment relationships and development. Third, practitioners become sensitive to carefully examine conventional programs and assessment tools for their appropriateness with different populations.

DEVELOPMENTAL ASSESSMENT

Significance for the Nurse Practitioner

Monitoring children's developmental progress brings the pleasure of watching their mastery of expected developmental milestones. With time, many practitioners develop an intuitive sense about the ages at which particular milestones should occur. Experience also brings an appreciation of individual differences in infants, families, and ethnic groups. It is difficult, however, for any practitioner to appreciate intuitively all the various developmental skills of a particular child. For example, a premature infant at or below the 5th percentile for height and weight may physically appear much younger. The discrepancy between size and age can result in an inaccurate estimate of the child's abilities. Consider an infant who is 15 months chronologically, 12 months adjusted age, but physically and developmentally at the 9 month level. If the NP evaluated this infant developmentally based on physical size, the development level might appear appropriate (size and development at 9 months). Consideration for age adjustment because of the infant's prematurity (adjustment to 12 months) still might not signal the need for intervention and referral. With the use of screening and assessment tools, it is more readily apparent that, despite the history of prematurity, the infant requires referral and intervention services. Despite the practitioner's intuitive knowledge of child development, using developmental screening and assessment tools is a necessary aspect of the NP's practice.

Developmental Surveillance

The concept of developmental surveillance as described by Dworkin (1989) provides the framework for this discussion. Surveillance encompasses all primary care activities related to the monitoring of the development of children, including the following (Dworkin, 1989):

- Obtaining a relevant developmental history
- Making accurate and informative observations of children
- Eliciting and attending to parental concerns
- Sharing opinions and concerns with other relevant professionals

Developmental surveillance involves more than simply asking developmental questions, completing a developmental screening checklist, asking how a child is doing in school, or completing a school physical examination. Emphasis is placed on monitoring development within the context of the child's overall well-being rather than viewing development during an isolated testing session.

Developmental surveillance is essential for early detection and treatment of, or intervention for, developmental delays, and can be conducted using a variety of screening tools (American Academy of Pediatrics [AAP], 2001a). Several assumptions underlie developmental surveillance. These include the following:

- Development is a self-fueling, ongoing process that requires physical and emotional energy.
- Development occurs in stages and is dynamic and interactional.
- Development is influenced by the child and his or her environment.
- Development occurs in "spurts and lulls." Periods of disorganization, disharmony, and turbulence are usually followed by periods of harmony, balance, and organization as new skills are integrated.
- All areas of development are interrelated.

Providing supportive care for children through developmental surveillance also is based on certain assumptions. These include the following:

- Children are generally healthy and have adaptive capabilities. Therefore the goal of the NP is to maintain health rather than solely to resolve problems.
- Individual differences among children are reflected in developmental variations. These arise, in part, from the unique characteristics of families, cultures, and social circumstances. Individual developmental variations and positive adaptations should be appreciated and facilitated.
- Children and families have the capacity to learn from and grow beyond their limitations when interventions are based on their abilities.
- Preventive health care for children includes developmentally supportive mental health care.

Definitions

Developmental Screening

Screening is considered a first-level contact with an individual to identify potential and actual developmental concerns. Developmental screening provides a quick, inexpensive method of describing the child's progress and enables the practitioner to document that progress over time, as well as identify developmental strengths objectively. It also serves as a tool for stimulating parent questions about development and facilitating parent education (Perrin & Stancin, 2002).

Screening techniques are generally viewed as appropriate for all children, although culture and life experiences may affect some outcomes and need to be taken into consideration. Screening is conducted on all children with the assumption that some will be identified as outside the normal limits. Variation from the norm on a screening tool requires closer, more in-depth examination. Referrals are based on scores outside the defined normal limits of the tool.

Developmental Assessment

In contrast to screening, an assessment is done when a more individualized approach is required to decide whether a developmental concern exists and how best to guide the plan of care and management of that concern. Assessment is considered to be at a second level of analysis, focusing on a more narrow, often complicated problem. Generally, assessments are conducted to fulfill three functions (Teti & Gibbs, 1990):

1. Confirm a developmental problem
2. Describe an infant's level of functioning in one or more developmental domains
3. Identify the type of problem

Areas of Developmental Screening and Assessment

Typical areas of developmental screening and assessment include language, motor, social, and cognitive skills. Screening and assessment should also examine the regulatory and sensory systems as a part of the child's overall development and functioning. Regulation refers to infants' daily patterns of sleep/wake cycles that include sleeping, eating, moving, responding, and reacting to their internal as well as external environment. Examination of sensory systems includes evaluation of the child's ability to receive and respond to both internal and external stimuli. Finally, although it is conceptually a part of the child's social skill set, review of parent-child interactions and the family and environmental context in which the child is living is important. A comprehensive approach to developmental screening and assessment that includes the areas of regulation and adaptive skills in daily routines will be presented for each age-group in the following chapters. Table 5-3 provides examples of information to gather within each of these areas.

Strategies for Developmental Screening and Assessment

Several key strategies are involved in both screening and assessment:

- Parent interview
- Child interview

TABLE 5-3 *Areas of Child Development*

Developmental Area	Definition
1. Physical development	Physical stability, growth, sexuality, temperament
2. Regulatory skills	State control and modulation, ability to manage sensory (e.g., light, noise, touch, movement) input from the external as well as internal environment; self-regulation and control
3. Adaptive skills/fine motor skills	Self-care skills that are involved in daily routines (e.g., feeding, bathing, dressing, play)
4. Motor skills	Skills that facilitate overall movement and locomotion
5. Communication/language	Verbal and nonverbal communication skills including behaviors, gestures, signs
6. Social-emotional development/parent-child interaction	Ability to interact with others and the environment and overall affect; the reciprocal relationship between the child and his or her caregivers
7. Cognitive/intellectual development	Cognitive and intellectual skills, including problem solving, decision making, and goal setting

- Observation of child's behavior
- Observation of child-parent interaction
- Parent questionnaire

Success using these strategies begins when the NP builds rapport and a trusting relationship with both parent and child. The parent interview is one in which the NP supports parents to share sensitive information, ask questions, and express concerns about their child's development. The interview of the child requires an understanding of child development and ages; the NP must know when approaching the child may be most difficult and be skilled in the use of age-appropriate strategies to engage the child. NPs also need to have the ability to relate to the child verbally and physically. One example would be to move to the same level as the child to establish eye contact. Gaining the parent's and child's trust and engagement in the interview process is critical to obtaining accurate and reliable information. Targeted questions around daily routines often provide insight into a child's daily activities, as well as parents' areas of concern. Examples of these questions are provided in Box 5-1.

BOX 5-1 *Interview Guide for Daily Routines*

- Tell me about your child's typical day.
- What aspects of your child's day are easy? What aspects are more challenging?
- How does your child communicate what he or she wants?
- Does your child show an ability to understand the feelings of others?
- How does your child act around others?
- To what extent has your child developed independence in eating, dressing, and toileting? Responsibilities at home, school, and community?
- How does your child get from one place to another (e.g., running, walking, transportation)?

A trusting relationship also enhances the NP's ability to accurately observe the child's behaviors. Observation of the child and the child's attention, activities, verbalization, connection with the parent, processing of information, quality of movements, cooperation, and ability to follow requests are all components of developmental screening and assessment. Box 5-2 lists specific observations that may be made during a feeding in a clinic or home visit, and Box 5-3 lists observations that can be made during a play or teaching activity with the parent.

BOX 5-2 *Observations during a Feeding*

- Positioning of the infant/child and the caregiver
  - Eye contact
  - Infant holding
  - Environmental distractions
- Suck, swallow, breathing coordination, and physiologic stability
- Infant/child comfort with eating
- Oral motor functioning
  - Lip closure, tongue, jaw movements, swallowing
- Endurance for feeding
- Sustained attention to feeding
- Stability of head and trunk control
- Ability to reach, grasp, hold, transfer objects
- Self-feeding skills and utensil use
- Coordination and quality of movements during feeding
- Infant's/child's anticipation of feeding
- Clarity of behavioral cues and use of vocalizations
- Responsiveness to caregivers' actions and verbalizations

BOX 5-3 *Observations during Spontaneous Play or a Teaching Activity*

- Positioning of the infant/child and the caregiver
  - Eye contact
  - Placement of toys within reach
  - Environmental distractions
- Success of gaining child's attention and sustained attention to play or teaching activity
- Tracking or following both visually or with verbal instructions and modeling
- Initiation of play activity
- Anticipation of songs or games
- Ability to reach, grasp, hold, transfer objects
- Coordination and quality of movements
- Clarity of behavioral cues and use of vocalizations
- Responsiveness to caregivers' actions and verbalizations

Often parent questionnaires are used in both developmental screening and assessment. Screening questionnaires are usually developed to meet the demands of a busy office and may have not been tested for reliability or validity. These may include such items as the Family History Questionnaire, Well Child Visit Update, 3-Day Diet History, Daily Routines Check, Weekly or Daily Diary, Denver Prescreening Developmental Questionnaire (PDQ), or Infant Irritability Scale. Questionnaires used for assessment often have been tested on large populations and have established reliability and validity so that they can be used to substantiate or rule out a particular diagnosis. These assessment tools are usually specific for a particular age-group or population.

Each of the following chapters will provide suggested tools that are age appropriate for purposes of developmental screening or assessment.

Strategies Specific to Developmental Screening

Because the purpose of developmental screening is the identification of children with developmental delays, NPs should consider doing developmental screening themselves. The completion of developmental screening also provides opportunities to answer specific parent questions and address parenting issues. When developmental screening is omitted or delegated to medical assistants or volunteers, parenting issues and anticipatory guidance might not be addressed within the context of a child's development, and important teaching opportunities may be missed. One focus of developmental surveillance is to build parental competence and confidence, which, in turn, enhances the child's overall well-being. Learning about their own child's unique developmental strengths and skills allows parents to increase their knowledge of development and create their own parenting style. When parents feel success in their current parenting role, they do a better job meeting their child's future needs.

NPs can use a variety of screening tools in their practices that will enhance both the efficiency and quality of their practice. Such tools also provide a consistent, reliable, and efficient method of documentation of the care provided. These tools generally require minimal training, have set standards for referral, and can be administered easily in a clinic setting (e.g., pure-tone audiometry; Denver Developmental Screening Tool II).

Strategies Specific to Developmental Assessment

Assessment tools or diagnostic tests are significantly different from screening tools and are appropriate when concerns require more in-depth evaluation. Assessment tools for developmental and behavioral diagnosis, home assessment, family assessment, parent-child interaction assessment, parent stress, and parental competency are most frequently used in research but may also be of value in the clinical setting. These tools can be used for a thorough assessment of the child within the family context, looking at the parent-child interaction as well as developing a substantiated diagnosis for the child. The information also improves the practitioner's ability to structure individualized interventions for both the child and the parents, and it can be used to evaluate the effectiveness of recommended interventions.

Because of the complexity of issues that might need evaluation, developmental assessment tools require more knowledge, practice, and skill to perform reliably, interpret the findings, and plan appropriate interventions. These tools generally require special training or credentials to administer accurately. The Bayley Scales of Infant Development and the Nursing Child Assessment Satellite Training (NCAST) Feeding and Teaching Scales that assess parent-child interaction are examples of assessment tools (Barnard, 1976, 1979; Bayley, 1993).

MANAGEMENT STRATEGIES IN CHILD DEVELOPMENT

Promoting Parent Development and Parent-Child Interaction: Anticipatory Guidance

Parental role development is described by authors using the ecologic model (Barnard, 1999; Bronfenbrenner, 1979; Sameroff & Chandler, 1975). This model stresses the fluid nature of early parent-child relationships and the importance of understanding the interactive and reciprocal relationships among parent, infant, and environment. Based on this model, the parental role develops in concert with the child's development, within the context of a unique environment. Barnard (1979) described two major nursing interventions that can be used to promote parental role development:

- Provide information and anticipatory guidance to parents and caregivers in order to assist them to facilitate the child's growth.
- Support parents so that they are able to center their energy and motivation on caring for their child.

The goal of anticipatory guidance is to help parents plan for and cope with anticipated changes, and to increase parenting skills, confidence, and competence in problem solving. It is intended to assist parents to adapt their parenting styles and strategies to their child's temperament, growth, and development and includes the following:

- Assess the child's developmental status.
- Determine the parents' knowledge of child development.
- Determine the parents' knowledge of and experience with the parent role.
- Assess the parents' problem-solving and coping skills.
- Instruct parents about normal child development and variations of that development as indicated. Provide educational information and materials as appropriate.
- Assist parents to develop realistic expectations of their child's development.
- Instruct parents about parenting strategies and concepts.
- Guide parents to appropriate community resources and support networks.
- Reassess and obtain feedback; reinforce healthy parental role development.

The NP's responsibility to promote parent development through anticipatory guidance has often been more of a challenge than providing physical care, especially in practices where time spent with patients is limited. The standard of care in pediatric practices should include opportunities for providers to address parenting issues or concerns. Quick, pat answers to complex parenting issues do not facilitate parental growth. Creative strategies can be used to structure prenatal visits, hospital discharge rounds, early discharge newborn follow-up, breastfeeding consultations, well-child visits, and referrals to achieve this standard. An organized parent support program in practice settings, for example, can help NPs to listen, hear, and act on parent concerns. Without an organized plan that connects the child's developmental needs, parents' concerns and educational needs, providers' abilities and resources, and community resources, it is easy to overlook, delay, or deny important parenting issues.

The interview and counseling conducted during anticipatory guidance should be guided by a consistent framework. Programs such as Touch Points (Brazelton, 1992), Bright Futures (Green, 2000), and the Parenting Pyramid (Webster-Stratton, 1994) (Fig. 5-1) can be used by the NP. Specific questions are suggested to elicit responses from parents and guide the visit, as well as provide anticipatory guidance and counseling. Stein (1998) emphasized the need for such an organized framework when approaching developmental and behavioral issues. He suggested focusing on four basic areas: developmental themes, temperament, family support, and resiliency (the ability to withstand stressors). He also emphasized the use of the teachable moment and role modeling during the office visit.

There is a wealth of popular literature available for parents to guide them as they raise their children. The NP can be an invaluable resource for parents by eliciting their questions, encouraging problem solving and decision making, providing suggestions and new strategies, engaging the parent during the visit, and reinforcing positive parent behaviors or actions. Providing parents with positive feedback builds parent confidence and establishes comfort for bringing forth more difficult concerns if such discussion is necessary. A trusting relationship between NPs and parents can be built by reinforcing those things a parent is doing well and by being open to teaching and listening to parent concerns. The practitioner-family relationship can be a powerful tool to guide family members' management of their child's temperament, behavior, and development. The benefit of establishing a long-term, continuous relationship with a child and family cannot be overestimated. (See Chapter 18 for a more in-depth discussion of parenting strategies.)

Certain "red flags" related to parent-child interactions indicate that assessment of the home environment, parent-child interaction, and child's development is indicated. Box 5-4 identifies some of these parental red flags.

When There Are Concerns about Delayed Development

Developmental Red Flags

Development among children is exceptionally varied. A 2-year-old girl may use full, complex sentences while her 3-year-old neighbor relies on three-word directives (e.g., "want milk, peeze") to get what he desires. Both can be normal, but the differences may be striking and parents may express concern that their child is "delayed." NPs should keep in mind certain red flags related to normal child development when seeing infants and children for well-child care or minor acute illnesses. These red

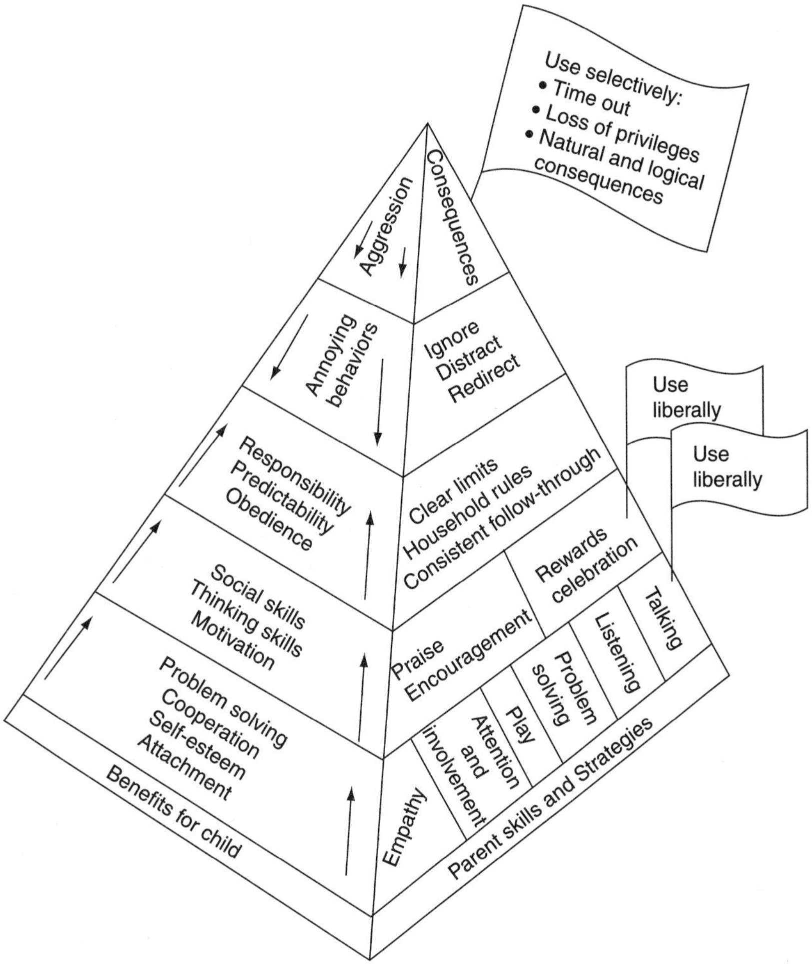

FIGURE 5-1 Parenting pyramid. (From Webster-Stratton C: *The incredible years: a trouble shooting guide for parents of children aged 3-8,* Toronto, Ontario, 1992, Umbrella Press.)

flags are highlighted in each of the following chapters in this unit.

If the NP notes a concern, a focused screening is necessary, followed by an in-depth assessment as appropriate. Subsequently, a decision must be made as to whether the child is progressing appropriately or whether intervention is indicated. Information from the history, physical examination, developmental screening and assessment, hearing and vision screening, and other tests that are indicated is essential in making this decision. It is also important to consider the etiology of developmental delays when making a judgment to intervene or refer (Box 5-5).

Understanding the possible etiology helps the NP to plan appropriate developmental care, including parent counseling, educational programs, and referral choices (e.g., which developmental specialist is most appropriate to further assess the child? Or which treatment modality, such as speech or physical therapy, would be most effective?). The discussion in Chapter 28 of the management of cerebral palsy illustrates the decision-making process the NP uses in cases of developmental delay. One cannot assume that waiting will remedy a problem, because even though developmental progress may occur, the rate and quality can be abnormal. Neither can one assume that all developmental problems can be fixed with home remedies (e.g., changing parenting or environmental factors). Sometimes, developmental problems are indicators of serious systemic, particularly neurologic, dysfunctions. Any child who fails to move ahead as expected or, worse yet, begins to deteriorate developmentally requires immediate and in-depth evaluation.

BOX 5-4 *Parenting Red Flags*

Moderate Concern

Disinclination to separate from child, or prematurely hastening separation
Signs of despondency, apathy, or hostility
Fearful, dependent, apprehensive
Disinterested in or rejecting of infant or child
Overly critical, mocking, and censuring of child; tendency to undermine child's confidence
Inconsistent in discipline or control; erratic in behavior
Highly restrictive and overly moralistic environment

Extreme Concern

Extreme depression and withdrawal; rejection of child
Intense hostility; aggression toward child
Uncontrollable fears, anxieties, guilt
Complete inability to function in family role
Severe moralistic prohibition of child's independent strivings
Domestic abuse or violence in the home
Self-destructive behaviors: alcohol or drug abuse

Talking with Parents about Developmental Delays

Talking with parents about specific developmental problems is always a challenge. For this reason, it is particularly helpful to have an opportunity to complete developmental assessments on an ongoing basis. Each infant and child has areas in which development is progressing, even if the progress is not consistent with usual development. Discussing these areas first provides parents with a framework to understand their child's unique strengths along with any developmental challenges. Typically, parents notice differences in the child first and seek reassurance or confirmation of problems from their health care provider. It is always important to discuss the child's strengths and limitations, as well as the parents' concerns.

Above all, it is important to be honest, positive, and realistic. Most often, the long-term prognosis for developmental delays is unknown because of continuing brain development. Parents want to know what they can do and, specifically, how they can assist their child. They also need support and time to cope with their own feelings (Harnel & Feldman, 1998). Different families have different expectations for their children, so a child with mild delay may be more devastating to one family than a child with severe developmental delays may be to another. Often, parents report that they have expressed their concerns to their health care provider only to be reassured. Later on, as problems become more obvious and a referral is finally made, they are frustrated that they were not listened to initially and that services to their child have been delayed.

BOX 5-5 *Etiologies of Developmental Delays*

- Central nervous system dysfunction
- Mental health problem
- Chronic disease affecting either functional abilities or activity tolerance (e.g., cardiovascular, visual, auditory)
- Child abuse and neglect
- Maternal or paternal stress
- Developmentally inappropriate animate or inanimate environment, or both
- Lack of parental knowledge of development
- Genetic syndromes
- Depression
- Attention-deficit hyperactivity disorder
- Autism spectrum
- Regulatory or sensory dysfunctions
- Unknown causes

Implementing Individualized Interventions

Early Intervention Programs. Children with developmental delays should receive appropriate referral or more frequent visits, or both, particularly during the first year of life (see Chapter 23 for a discussion of issues related to children with chronic illnesses) (Batshaw, 2002). Many later learning problems, difficulties with parent-child interaction, behavioral problems, and attachment problems can be managed effectively during the first year of life simply by offering parental counseling or referral to appropriate community services. The longer the problem lasts, the more difficult it is to resolve. Most communities have early infant education programs for infants and young children (birth to 3 years of age) provided for under Public Law 99-457, enacted at the federal level in 1986. This legislation requires developmental screening and early intervention programs for infants and young children at risk for developmental delay. The Individualized Family Service Plan (IFSP) is a process that includes the family in planning services for children. As primary care providers, NPs may be asked to participate in the meetings in which the IFSP is developed with the family. These programs can be established through school systems, health departments, or developmental programs and vary significantly in quality and comprehensiveness from one community to another. The importance of structured programs that stimulate growth of all children cannot be overestimated (Emde, Mann, & Bertacchi, 2001). NPs need to be familiar with community resources and educate community leaders and legislators about the developmental and health needs of children and families.

Areas that require special attention to guide nursing interventions include assessment of feeding, sleep, elimination, activity, temperament, and behavior. Nursing interventions, such as referrals to parent groups and recommendations regarding organization of the child's health records, are greatly appreciated by the family.

School Intervention Resources. Public Law 94-142, enacted in 1975, addresses the needs of children older than 3 years of age. Under this legislation, schools are mandated to provide appropriate education to all children with developmental delays, including opportunities for mainstreaming children with developmental delays or handicaps into regular classrooms. Special education services assist in this process through the development of an Individualized Education Plan (IEP).

Planning sessions for IFSPs or IEPs determine the school services that will be offered during a designated period of time for a particular child. If a child's or family's needs are not identified, services are not made available. Often, health care services are omitted when the overall health history of the child is not addressed. As the primary care provider for children, the NP should be available to be an advocate for families and children. In this role, the NP can help clarify children's needs and ensure that parental concerns, health care services, and educational services are appropriately coordinated (Jackson Allen & Vessey, 2004).

Family-Centered Care. Public Law 99-457 emphasizes family-centered care. This legislation also establishes a process in which families become active participants in determining the care of their children. The uniqueness of each family is to be respected, and families are considered to be active team participants. Nurses have stressed this focus with varying success. The American Academy of Pediatrics' Committee on Children with Disabilities has addressed the role of the pediatrician in developing IFSPs and IEPs and in providing family-centered care (AAP, 1998, 1999, 2001b). Educators are embracing the concept as well. The shift from child-centered to family-centered care is represented in Table 5-4.

Care and Service Coordination. As a coordinator of primary care, NPs identify and, when necessary, help develop community resources to serve families. NPs also help families to access these resources. It is important for the NP to become "community wise" through professional networks, parent groups, and educational connections. These resources are invaluable in assisting families locally. However, it is not enough simply to give a family a name and phone number of a referring agency. All too often, parents' calls lead to busy signals, disconnected numbers, or the wrong agency for their needs. These deterrents can discourage even the most willing family from pursuing needed resources for their child. Parents can also hesitate to seek resources because of apprehension about the outcome of the referral, costs, time constraints, or lack of understanding about the need for timely follow-up. When the NP intervenes to guide families through the referral process and coordinate services, parents have greater

TABLE 5-4 ***Comparison of Child-Centered and Family-Centered Care***

Child-Centered Care	Family-Centered Care
Goal: To take care of the child for the short term.	*Goal*: Parental empowerment and child advocacy for life of child.
• Child's needs are primary focus	• Family needs to assist the child are the focus
• Professionals decide on the plan of care	• Family and professionals decide on the plan of care
• Parents' opinions are not consistently requested	• Parents' ideas are requested and valued
• Families are considered part of a particular group	• Families are all considered to be unique
• Parents participate as observers	• Parents are considered to be equal members of the team at whatever level they are comfortable
• Parental differences are judged as not being in the best interest of the child	• Family culture, language, ethnicity, and structure are respected
• Test results of the child are the most important factor used to plan care	• Focus is on addressing parental concerns, issues, questions, and their need for assistance in problem solving
• One-way communication, professional to parent	• Two-way communication, with parents encouraged to have input into the child's care plan

RESOURCE BOX

Pediatric Primary Care Developmental Management

Bright Futures in Practice
www.brightfutures.org
Guidelines for assessment, anticipatory guidance, and health promotion for infants, children, and adolescents

Facts for Families
www.aacap.org/info_families/
American Academy of Pediatrics facts for families and other resources

Growth charts
www.cdc.gov/nchs/about/major/nhanes/growthcharts/charts.htm
New National Center for Health Statistics growth charts

Growth charts for Down syndrome
www.growthcharts.com

Measurement standards
www.odc.com/anthro/deskref/desktoc.html
Standards for anthropometry

NCAST
www.ncast.org
NCAST programs for nursing child assessment

Touch Points
www.touchpoints.org
Training based on the work of Dr. T. Berry Brazelton; incorporates relationship building and child development into professionals' practice.

Zero to Three
www.zerotothree.org
Multidisciplinary focus on care, research, and education for the first years of life

confidence in the new health care or educational resource and are more likely to achieve appropriate follow-up for their child.

SUMMARY

Effective management strategies in primary care maximize the strengths of children, parents, and families and lead to optimal health outcomes. The role of NPs in this process is complex. Focusing on social and psychologic needs of the child, NPs move beyond the standard well-child visit to comprehensive assessment of growth and development. NPs address parenting issues, examine the impact of environmental factors on health, facilitate access to community resources, and manage, coordinate, and collaborate in interdisciplinary care. This holistic approach is essential to ensure that children have every opportunity to achieve healthful, responsible, and happy adulthoods.

NURSING DIAGNOSES RELATED TO DEVELOPMENT

- Risk for disproportionate growth
- Delayed growth and development
- Risk for delayed development

REFERENCES

Ainsworth M, Bell S, Stayton D: Individual differences in strange-situation behavior of one year olds. In Schaffer HR, editor: *The origins of human social relations*, London, 1971, Academic Press.

American Academy of Pediatrics, Committee on Children with Disabilities: Managed care and children with special health care needs: a subject review, *Pediatrics* 102:657-659, 1998.

American Academy of Pediatrics, Committee on Children with Disabilities: The pediatrician's role in development and implementation of an Individual Education Plan (IEP) and/or an Individual Family Service Plan (IFSP), *Pediatrics* 104:124-126, 1999.

American Academy of Pediatrics, Committee on Children with Disabilities: Developmental surveillance and screening of infants and young children, *Pediatrics* 108:192-196, 2001a.

American Academy of Pediatrics, Committee on Children with Disabilities: Role of the pediatrician in family-centered early intervention services, *Pediatrics* 107:1155-1157, 2001b.

Barnard K: *Beginning rhythms: the emerging process of sleep wake behavior and self-regulation*, Seattle, 1999, NCAST Publications.

Barnard K: *NCAST instructors' manual*, Seattle, 1979, NCAST Publications.

Barnard K: *NCAST II learners' resource manual*, Seattle, 1976, NCAST, University of Washington.

Batshaw ML, editor: *Children with disabilities*, ed 5, Washington, DC, 2002, Paul H Brookes Publishing Company.

Bayley N: *Manual for the Bayley Scales of Infant Development*, ed 2, San Antonio, TX, 1993, The Psychological Corporation.

Bijou S, Baer D: *Child development II: universal stages of infancy*, New York, 1965, Appleton-Century-Crofts.

Bowlby J: *Attachment and loss*, vol 1, *Attachment*, New York, 1969, Basic Books.

Brazelton B: *Touchpoints: your child's emotional and behavioral development,* New York, 1992, Addison-Wesley.

Bronfenbrenner U: *The ecology of human development: experiments by nature and design,* Cambridge, MA, 1979, Harvard University Press.

Buhler C, Allen M: *Introduction to humanistic psychology,* Monterey, CA, 1972, Brooks/Cole.

Carey WB: Let's give temperament its due, *Contemp Pediatr* 15:91-113, 1998.

Cech DJ, Martin S: *Functional movement development across the life span,* Philadelphia, 2002, WB Saunders.

Chess T, Thomas A: *Temperament in clinical practice,* New York, 1995, Guilford Press.

Dixon S, Stein M, editors: *Encounters with children: pediatric behavior and development,* St Louis, 2000, Mosby.

Dworkin PH: British and American recommendations for developmental monitoring: the role of surveillance, *Pediatrics* 83:619-622, 1989.

Emde R: Development terminable and interminable. I. Innate and motivational factors from infancy, *Int J Psychoanalysis* 69:23-42, 1988.

Emde R, Buchsbaum H: "Didn't you hear my mommy?" Autonomy with connectedness in moral self emergence. In Cicchetti D, Beeghly M, editors: *The self in transition: infancy to childhood,* Chicago, 1990, University of Chicago Press.

Emde RN, Mann TL, Bertacchi J: Organizational environments that support mental health, *Zero to Three* 22:67-69, 2001.

Erikson E: *Insight and responsibility,* New York, 1964, Norton.

Fiese BH: Routines of daily living and rituals in family life: a glimpse at stability and change during the early child-raising years, *Zero to Three* 22:10-13, 2002.

Flavell J: *Cognitive development,* Englewood Cliffs, NJ, 1977, Prentice-Hall.

Fowler J: *Stages of faith: the psychology of human development and the quest for meaning,* New York, 1981, Harper & Row.

Freud A: *The writings of Anna Freud,* vol V, New York, 1974, International Universities Press.

Freud S: *An outline of psychoanalysis,* London, 1938, Hogarth.

Gesell A: *The first five years of life,* New York, 1940, Harper.

Gilligan C: *In a different voice: psychological theory and women's development,* Cambridge, MA, 1982, Harvard University Press.

Green M, editor: *Bright futures: guidelines for health supervision of infants, children, and adolescents,* ed 2, Arlington, VA, 2000, National Center for Education in Maternal and Child Health.

Harnel SC, Feldman HM: Focus on families: caring for children with special needs, *Contemp Pediatr* 15:141-155, 1998.

Havighurst R: *Human development and education,* New York, 1953, Longmans, Green.

Jackson Allen P, Vessey J: *Primary care of the child with a chronic condition,* ed 4, St Louis, 2004, Mosby.

Kelly JL, Barnard KE: Assessment of parent-child interaction: implications for early intervention. In Shonkoff JP, Meisels SJ, editors: *Handbook of early childhood education,* New York, 2000, Cambridge University Press.

Klaus M, Kennel J: *Maternal-infant bonding,* St Louis, 1976, Mosby.

Kohlberg L: Stage and sequence: the cognitive-development approach to socialization. In Gastin D, editor: *Handbook of socialization: theory and research,* New York, 1969, Rand McNally.

Kubicek L: Fresh perspectives on young children and family routines, *Zero to Three* 22:4-9, 2002.

Lewin K: *Principles of topological psychology,* New York, 1936, McGraw-Hill.

Mahler M, Pine F, Bergman A: *The psychological birth of the human infant,* New York, 1975, Basic Books.

Mahrer A: *Experiencing: a humanistic theory of psychology and psychiatry,* New York, 1978, Brunner/Mazel.

Maslow A: *The farther reaches of human nature,* New York, 1971, Viking.

Minuchin S: *Families and family therapy,* Cambridge, MA, 1974, Harvard University Press.

Mott S: Developmental theories: how the child grows. In Mott S, James SR, Sperhac A, editors: *Nursing care of children and families,* New York, 1990, Addison-Wesley.

Nugent JK: Cross-cultural studies of child development: implications for clinicians, *Zero to Three* 15:1-8, 1994.

Perrin E, Stancin T: A continuing dilemma: whether and how to screen for concerns about children's behavior, *Pediatr Rev* 23:264-275, 2002.

Piaget J: *The theory of stages in cognitive development,* New York, 1969, McGraw-Hill.

Rogoff B: *Apprenticeship in thinking: cognitive development in social context,* New York, 1990, Oxford University Press.

Ruperto N et al: Cross-cultural adaptation and psychometric evaluation of the Childhood Health Assessment Questionnaire (CHAQ) and the Child Health Questionnaire (CHQ) in 32 countries. Review of the general methodology, *Clin Exp Rheumatol* 19(4 suppl 23):S1-S9, 2001.

Sameroff A, Chandler M: Reproductive risks and the continuum of caretaking casualty. In Horowitz FD, editor: *Review of child development research,* Chicago, 1975, University of Chicago Press.

Siegler R, Liebert D, Liebert R: Inhelder and Piaget's pendulum problem, *Dev Psychol* 9:97-101, 1973.

Skinner BF: *Science and human behavior,* New York, 1953, The Macmillan Free Press.

Stein M: Preparing families for the toddler and preschool years, *Contemp Pediatr* 15:88-110, 1998.

Stern D: *The interpersonal world of the infant: a view from psychoanalysis and developmental psychology,* New York, 1985, Basic Books.

Sullivan H: *The fusion of psychiatry and social sciences,* New York, 1964, Norton.

Teti D, Gibbs E: *Interdisciplinary assessment of infants: a guide for early intervention professionals,* Baltimore, 1990, Paul H Brookes.

Thomas RM: *Comparing theories of child development,* Belmont, CA, 1985, Wadsworth.

Webster-Stratton C: *The incredible years: a trouble shooting guide for parents of children aged 3-8,* Toronto, Ontario, 1994, Umbrella Press.

Wolraich ML, Felice ME, Drotar D, editors: *The classification of child and adolescent mental health diagnoses in primary care: Diagnostic and Statistical Manual for Primary Care (DSM-PC), child and adolescent version,* Elk Grove Village, IL, 1996, American Academy of Pediatrics.

6 Developmental Management of Infants

Barbara Jones Deloian

Infancy is an exciting time for everyone involved—the infant, his or her immediate family, extended family members, and others in the infant's community. Nurse practitioners (NPs) are privileged to be able to work with families during this period of rapid, predictable (yet unique), and challenging change. When providing care to infants and their families, NPs have a responsibility to assess and monitor growth and development; educate parents about child development; offer guidance about ways to foster healthy growth and development; identify and manage health problems; guide, counsel, and support parents when dealing with their infant's health or illness; and collaborate with other providers as necessary.

Recent research on brain development has validated the notion that the child's experiences during the first years of life are critical to healthy physical, emotional, and intellectual development (Shonkoff & Phillips, 2000). During pregnancy and early life, the infant is affected by both internal physiologic and neurologic factors and external factors such as light, sound, touch, positioning, taste, and movement. An infant's ability to develop consistent and predictable responses to these internal and external stimuli during the first year of life is influenced by physical growth, brain development, the surrounding environment, and particularly the actions of the infant's caregivers. The infant's mastery of self-regulating behaviors depends on healthy biorhythms and sensitive, contingent caregivers (Anders, Goodlin-Jones, & Zelenko, 1998; Barnard, 1999). Nurturing relationships between infants and their adult caregivers strengthen all aspects of an infant's development (Dixon & Stein, 2000). NPs can give parents the information, support, and encouragement they need to be successful in their new role and ensure that their infant achieves optimal growth and development.

BIRTH RATES AND INFANT MORTALITY

Birth rates in the United States decreased slightly from 2000 to 2001, from 14.7 to 14.5 births per 1000 population. Between 1990 and 2001, the teen (15- to 19-year-olds) birth rate declined dramatically, from 59.5 to 45.3 births per 1000 population. Twin, triplet, and other multiple births, however, rose 3% from 2000 to 2001 (Martin et al, 2001). Infant mortality rate decreased from 7.1 deaths per 1000 births in 1999 to 6.9 deaths per 1000 births in 2000. The leading causes of infant mortality are congenital malformations and chromosomal abnormalities (20.7% of all infant deaths); low birth weight and prematurity (deaths due to this cause decreased by 4.6% to 15.4% from 1999 to 2000); and sudden infant death syndrome (SIDS) (20.9% of infant deaths). SIDS continues a decline that began in 1988 and may reflect the success of the Back-to-Sleep campaign, as well as the way SIDS is diagnosed in each community. Despite these declines, the United States ranks poorly in comparison with international infant mortality rates, and the infant mortality rate among black Americans continues to be more than twice the national average (14.0% in 2000) (Minino & Smith, 2001). Unintentional injuries also remain high, and almost 25% of infants and toddlers in the United States live in poverty.

DEVELOPMENT DURING THE FIRST YEAR OF LIFE

Birth to 1 Month of Age

Physical Development

The assessment of the neonate must begin with a determination of gestational age using the Dubowitz or similar gestational age scale (see Chapter 39). It is important to be aware of significant prematurity, intrauterine growth retardation (IUGR), and size for gestational age (i.e., either large for gestational age [LGA] or small for gestational age [SGA]). The reported gestational age, birth weight and length, and head circumference data are compared with the infant's gestational age as assessed by observation.

The infant may initially lose up to 5% to 10% of birth weight but should regain birth weight within 10 to 14 days. Weight gain after the initial loss will average 0.5 to 1 oz per day, or about 2 lb per month. Nutritional needs to promote growth are about 110 kcal/kg per day (see Chapter 12).

The stability of the infant's autonomic nervous system can be evaluated through heart rate, respiratory rate, temperature control, and color changes. The infant should demonstrate some degree of regulation of state and ease of transitions from deep sleep through crying. With the use of a variety of techniques, the newborn can be aroused to an alert state for feedings. The newborn infant sleeps about 16 hours a day and breastfeeds every 2 to 3 hours. Assessment for a normally pitched cry is important, because problems such as hypothyroidism and genetic disorders (e.g., cri du chat syndrome) can cause voice alterations.

Motor Skills Development

The newborn's flexed posture provides the infant with the ability to self-console when positioned so that the hands reach the face and mouth. Primary reflexes, such as sucking, rooting, asymmetric tonic neck, Moro, and grasp, should be present and symmetric. Passive muscle tone is evaluated within gestational age scales through observation of shoulder (scarf sign) and knee flexibility (popliteal angle). Arm and leg recoil provides information about the infant's active movements, particularly symmetry and coordination. Jerkiness and tremors may be noted. The neonatal period begins a remarkable series of fine and gross motor skill milestones for the infant (Table 6-1).

Communication and Language Development

The newborn infant is able to give clear signals of distress, such as crying, arching, or gagging. These help the caregiver respond to the infant's needs. The newborn also should be able to habituate to sound and light. Newborns use self-consoling or self-calming behaviors, such as sucking, moving hand to mouth, or grasping clothing, to keep organized or maintain their state.

Articulation, or the way that the structures of the nose and mouth mold the sounds emitted by the larynx, begins at birth with the infant's first cry. In the first few weeks of life, infants will make sounds of comfort and discomfort.

Social and Emotional Development

Social skills are evident as the newborn quiets readily to the parent's voice and demonstrates a brief smile. Using a soft voice, touching, and picking up the baby are ways the caregiver can console the newborn, because the infant is able to calm when listening to a quiet voice or sounds.

Cognitive Development

Vision is limited, but the newborn does have the ability to focus briefly on a face or bright object when it is brought into visual range. The infant is also able to visually track an object to midline. The sense of smell is most acute in newborns. Hearing is also fairly well developed.

Age 1 through 3 Months

Physical Development

From 1 through 3 months of life, the infant experiences many physical and developmental changes. The infant will continue to gain 0.5 to 1 oz per day with six to eight feedings daily, each lasting 30 to 40 minutes. Length increases about 3.5 cm per month and head circumference about 2 cm per month, with growth more rapid for the younger infant. Sleep cycles become more regular, about 15 to 16 hours per day, with defined sleep/wake patterns. The infant may need more organized play periods as sleep periods become consolidated with consistent naps. Many infants may have fussy periods in the late evening that may last 1 to 3 hours. If no regular nap schedule is established, fussiness may increase. At about 6 to 8 weeks the infant may experience a growth spurt and fuss to eat more frequently. This fussiness usually lasts for a short period. Mothers who are breastfeeding need extra encouragement during this time, because they may believe that they do not have enough milk for their babies. NPs should instruct mothers to follow their infant's cues for feeding, pointing out that the extra suckling will increase the milk supply sufficiently to meet their growing infant's needs. Elimination patterns become more regular, with several stools a day and wet diapers after each feeding.

Motor Skills Development

Fine motor skills begin to emerge as primitive reflexes become integrated. Infants attempt to grasp rattles, fingers, and clothing. They also are able to demonstrate visible head control, lifting the head off the bed about 45 degrees when in the prone position and showing little head droop when held in suspension. All their body movements should be symmetric (see Table 6-1).

TABLE 6-1 ***Fine Motor and Gross Motor Development Milestones for Infants and Preschoolers***

Age	Fine Motor Movement	Oral Movement	Gross Motor Movement
Birth	Flexion	Suckling tongue movements, extension-retraction of tongue, up and down jaw movements, low approximation of lips	Momentary head control when held sitting
1 mo	Extension, nondirected swipes	Rooting	Turns head when prone
4 mo	Directed swipes, corralling, reaching		Sits with support, rolls over, head steady in sitting
4-5 mo	Ulnar-palmar grasp		"Swims" in prone position, no head lag
6-7 mo	Radial-palmar grasp, raking	Sucking with negative oral cavity pressure, rhythmic jaw movements, firm approximation of lips	Sits independently, rocks on hands and knees, free head lift in supine
7-8 mo	Radial digital grasp	Phasic bite reflex, rhythmic bite and release pattern	Supports weight standing, bounces when held
7-9 mo	Scissors grasp	Munching, early chewing	Sits alone well, may crawl
9-10 mo	Voluntary release		Cruises, pivots while seated, pulls to stand
12 mo	Picks up pellet with pincer grasp	Chewing with spreading/rolling tongue movements, tongue lateralization, rotary jaw movements, controlled sustained bite	Walks with one hand held, stands alone momentarily
18 mo	Makes tower of four cubes, imitates scribbling, dumps pellet, puts blocks in large holes, drinks from cup with little spilling, can take off socks		Directed throwing, walks well independently, climbs into adult chair
24 mo	Makes tower of seven cubes, does circular scribbling, folds paper once imitatively, turns doorknobs, turns pages one at a time, unbuttons or unzips large fasteners, puts on coat with assistance		Throws overhand, runs well, kicks ball, up and down stairs placing both feet on each step
30 mo	Makes tower of nine cubes, makes vertical and horizontal strokes, imitates circle, buttons large button, uses fork in fist, twists jar lids		Jumps off ground with both feet
36 mo	Makes tower of 10 cubes, imitates bridge of three cubes, copies circle, snips with scissors, can brush teeth but not well, puts shoes on feet		Broad jumps, walks up stairs alternating feet, may pedal tricycle, balance one foot 2-3 sec
48 mo	Copies bridge from model, copies cross and square, cuts curved line with scissors, dresses self, strings small beads		Pedals tricycle, runs smoothly, hops on one foot, catches large ball
60 mo	Some can print name; copies triangle, opens lock with key, bathes self, cuts out simple shapes, pours from small pitcher		Walks downstairs alternating feet, catches bounced ball, skips, stands on one foot 7-8 sec

Data from many developmental tests.

Communication and Language Development

Parents should be encouraged to talk to their infants, cooing, smiling, and actively interacting. Infants will start to make cooing and babbling sounds, much to the delight of their parents (Table 6-2). However, body movements (e.g., snuggling, turning the head, arching the body) continue to be the primary form of communication, and NPs can help parents identify and become more skilled at interpreting their infant's cues.

Social and Emotional Development

The infant begins to become highly social, imitating the parent's expressions and visually following the parent. Infants are more responsive to sounds in their environment, attending to sounds by quieting body movements or demonstrating visual responses. The older infant may smile in response to parents. As infants become more active, alert, and responsive, parents may mistakenly assume that they can handle more activity and irregular

TABLE 6-2 ***Speech and Language Milestones: Areas for Assessment***

Age	Receptive Language	Expressive Language
0-3 mo	Attends to voice, turns head or eyes Startles to loud sounds Quiets in response to voice Smiles, coos, gurgles to voice	Undifferentiated but strong cry Coos and gurgles Single-syllable repetition /G/, /K/, /H/, and /NG/ appear
3-6 mo	Actively seeks sound source May look in response to name Responses may vary to angry or happy voice	Increased babbling, vocal play Laughs Increased repetitive babbling (gaga) Vocalizes to toys Spontaneous smile to verbal play Increased intensity and nasal tone Vocalizes to removal of toy Experiments with own voice
6-9 mo	May look at family member when named Inhibits to "no" Begins interest in pictures when named Individual words begin to take on meaning	Babbles tunefully Increased sound combinations Uses /M/, /N/, /B/, /D/, /T/ Initiates sounds such as click or kiss Uses nonspecific "mama" and "dada"
9-12 mo	Will give toy on request Understands simple commands Turns head to own name Understands "hot," "where's ...?" Responds with gestures to "bye-bye"	Increased imitating efforts Has one word with specific reference Accompanies vocalizations with gestures Jargon increases Imitates animal sounds
12-18 mo	Follows simple one-step commands Understands new words weekly Increased interest in named pictures Differentiates environmental sounds Points to familiar objects and body parts when named Understands simple questions Begins to distinguish "you" from "me"	All vowels, many consonants present Increased use of true words Jargon is sentence-like Shows "no" behavior Names a few pictures 10 words Can imitate nonspeech sounds (cough, tongue click)
18-24 mo	Follows two-step commands Vocabulary increases rapidly Enjoys simple stories Recognizes pronouns	Names some body parts Imitates two-word combinations Dramatic increase in vocabulary Speech combines jargon and words Names self Answers some questions Begins to combine words

TABLE 6-2 ***Speech and Language Milestones: Areas for Assessment—cont'd***

Age	Receptive Language	Expressive Language
24-30 mo	Understands prepositions *in* and *on* Seems to understand most of what is said Understands more reasoning ("when you are done, then . . .") Identifies object when given function (wear on feet, cook on)	Jargon reduced Two- to three-word sentences Repeats two digits Increased use of pronouns Asks simple questions Joins in songs and nursery rhymes
30-36 mo	Listens to adult conversations Understands preposition *under* Can categorize items by function Begins to recognize colors Begins to take turns Understands "big/little," "boy/girl"	Can repeat simple phrases and sentences Answers questions (wear on feet, to bed) Repeats three digits Uses regular plurals Can help tell simple story
36-42 mo	Understands *fast* Understands prepositions *behind* and *in front* Responds to simple three-part commands Increasing understanding of adjectives and plurals Understands "just one"	Understands and answers (cold, tired, hungry) Mostly three- to four-word sentences Gives full name Begins rote counting Begins to relate events Lots of questions, some beginning prepositions (on, in)
42-48 mo	Recognizes coins Begins to understand future and past tenses Understands number concepts—more than one	Uses prepositions Tells stories Can give function of objects Repeats larger than six-word sentences Repeats four digits Gives age Good intelligibility
48-60 mo	Responds to three-action commands	Asks "how" questions Answers verbally to questions such as "How are you?" Uses past and future tenses Can use conjunctions to string words and phrases together

Data from D. Anderson, Ph.D., Speech Pathologist, Portland, OR, using items from a variety of developmental tests.

stimulation than they are truly capable of. Developing sensitivity to infant cues for the need to rest or to have decreased stimulation is important.

Cognitive Development

By 4 to 8 weeks, infants readily begin to take in more of their environment, and when a face or toy is brought into visual range, the infant begins to visually track past midline, vertically, and horizontally. The infant may also begin to show variety in facial expressions, respond to sounds, and attempt to imitate mouthing movements. By 3 months, infants begin to enjoy toys and may wave their arms when a toy is brought into sight.

Age 4 through 5 Months

Physical Development

Infants 4 through 5 months of age usually begin to settle into regular patterns of eating, sleeping, and playing. Babies sleep 12 to 15 hours a day with five to six feedings a day. Somewhere between 4 and 6 months, infants will double their birth weight, gaining about 5 oz a week during this time. Their length increases about 2 cm per month, and head circumference increases about 1 cm per month. Growth may appear in spurts, rather than along an even curve. Weight gain can also be influenced by the amount of play activity and the sleep schedule. Although the infant's primary source of nutrition comes from breast milk or formula, parents may ask about when to begin feeding the infant solid foods. Rice cereal can be started in small amounts between 4 and 6 months. As other food is added, changes in stool consistency will be noted.

Motor Skills Development

Fine motor skills are demonstrated as infants play with their hands and begin to reach for and pull at clothing or other objects that are close. Eventually, they grasp toys and begin to grab at other objects, such as the parents' hair, earrings, or eyeglasses. They also start to place their hands on the breast or on the bottle in an attempt to hold or pat it.

Motor skills progress (see Table 6-1) as the Moro and asymmetric tonic neck reflexes are integrated, and there is no longer the obligation of arm extension with head turning. The Landau reflex emerges. Infants begin to roll, first from front to back and then from back to front, and can roll from one place to another. Head control becomes stronger and more sustained, and there should be no head lag when the baby is pulled to sit. When in the prone position, infants hold the head up at 45 degrees, gradually progressing to 90 degrees for sustained periods of time. The infant learns to sit, first in the tripod stance, then unassisted with the head held erect. Infants are able to lift their legs and bring their feet to their mouth. They bear full weight when standing and enjoy bouncing up and down in their parent's lap. All their body movements should be symmetric.

Communication and Language Development

Infants' social skills are increasing and verbal skills are becoming more evident (see Table 6-2). They begin babbling, using vowel sounds, cooing, and laughing quietly. They experiment with variations in tone and pitch, such as low-pitched chuckles and deeper laughs. Eventually, they begin to laugh out loud, much to the enjoyment of those around them. Their responses to sounds gradually become more localized, and they search for the sound of a bell or rattle.

Oral-motor development is a prerequisite for speech. Throughout infancy, oral development progresses from sucking and rooting to rhythmic biting and chewing. Beginning at about 6 months and continuing through 2 years of age, the child learns to chew by moving the jaw up and down while flattening and spreading the tongue, and to control biting by using rotary jaw movements with lateralization of tongue placement. These motor skills, essential for the production of speech, are among the most complex movements that the young child must master.

Social and Emotional Development

During this time, infants' social skills become more evident. Smiling spontaneously at parents and others while visually following the caregiver around the environment and turning the head a full 180 degrees is usual behavior. Babies at this age should promptly look at an object when it is placed in front of them; they notice things. The infant's increasing awareness of the environment facilitates more complex social interactions. Infants begin to recognize that their parents are responding to their needs. The infant will notice, for example, as the parent prepares to offer the breast or get a bottle ready for feeding. Because infants notice other things as well, parents can often distract them from demanding immediate gratification by talking, playing, or using other social interaction. As a result, infants learn that their hunger needs will be met, but that there are other satisfying interactions they can have with their parents. Infants at this age begin to more actively reciprocate their parents' attention and enjoy playing with their parents. Crying may reflect a need for social interaction, not just hunger. Parents are able to acknowledge their child's unique personality, and this reciprocal recognition is an important aspect of infant-parent attachment.

Cognitive Development

Visual exploration increases during this age, as infants look at mobiles, mirrors, their hands, and the toys that they are holding. Chewing and mouthing are other means of exploration that infants use to differentiate textures, tastes, and shapes. As their muscle control improves they are able to bring a toy to their mouth first when lying on their back and then when sitting.

Age 6 through 8 Months

Physical Development

As infants reduce their breast milk or formula intake and add solids to their diet, growth curves can change. Weight gain slows to 3 to 4 oz a week, or about 1 lb a month; length gains are about 1.2 to 1.5 cm per month; and head circumference increases about 0.5 cm per month. If concerns about a large head circumference exist, note each parent's hat size and continue to monitor the infant carefully. Teething for central incisors can begin at about 6 months and lateral incisors appear at about 8 months. The first childhood illness might occur at this time, if it has not already done so, and either of these events can disrupt the infant's previous sleep routine.

Motor Skills Development

Motor skills at this age need little encouragement for development. Infants sit erect for longer periods of time, and may scoot while in a sitting position. Crawling begins with the infant pushing up to hands and knees and rocking in place, then eventually mastering the rhythm of hands and knees working together. Infants may stand, fully supporting their weight, when their hands are held at shoulder height.

Infants' fine motor skills continue to be refined, and they are more adept at using their palm and all of their fingers to pick up objects. Initially, they rake at small objects and are able to hold a small cube, lifting it off the table. Gradually, they use fingers and thumb to pick up objects. They reach for and grasp toys, can hold a toy in each hand at the same time, and can transfer objects from one hand to another.

Communication and Language Development

Vocalizations continue to show increasing variety in pitch and tone, and imitation of specific speech sounds begins. Infants articulate single-sound units that may be vowels, consonants, or blends such as "ah," "ba," "da," "ga," "ch," and "bl." Gradually they progress to double-consonant sounds (e.g., "da-da") and occasionally will vocalize using three or more different syllables. They use "ma-ma" and "da-da" but not specifically for their parents. Infants can delight their parents as they respond to verbal cues, as well as play at making sounds and noises when alone. They enjoy imitating oral sounds such as raspberries and coughing.

Although infants' expressive language skills are limited, their receptive language can clearly be seen as they listen and respond to their parents' talking. Infants are able to distinguish facial expressions and gestures, may stop or quiet when their parent uses "no" or a different tone of voice, and will turn toward their parents' voices and other sounds, localizing directly to the sound.

Social and Emotional Development

The infant's individual personality and temperament continues to be expressed. At times, infants' increased ability to do things for themselves puts them at odds with their parents, and even if parents have learned to understand their infant's cues and allow reciprocity between themselves and the infant, control issues can arise. Infants use gestures such as pointing, reaching with outstretched arms, tugging, and throwing things to get their parent's attention and communicate their needs. As infants' abilities and desires become more complex and they expand their repertoire of communication cues, parents need to learn new parenting skills (e.g., how to handle a determined child) in order to meet their infant's social development needs.

Stranger anxiety may appear at this time, depending on the variety of caregivers infants have had and their individual temperament.

Cognitive Development

From 6 through 8 months, infant cognitive development demonstrates significant growth. The infant is able to see cause-and-effect relationships in activities such as ringing a bell; pulling on a string to retrieve a ring, train, or phone; and dropping a toy from the crib or highchair. They can follow a toy if it falls and remains within their visual field. For some older infants, beginning object permanence is evident. The infant is increasingly aware of surroundings and begins to express individual preferences more clearly. This is often a time when resistance to bedtime, feeding, and parental separation occurs.

Age 9 through 12 Months

Physical Development

At 9 to 10 months, the infant's growth may have begun to follow a different growth curve than the one established early in infancy. Growth spurts become more apparent to parents as the infant outgrows clothes "overnight." At the same time, illnesses, decreased solid food intake caused by teething, and the infant's increased activity level can slow the rate of growth. It becomes important to estimate the infant's total caloric intake if there is a significant decrease in the infant's growth or if feeding problems are present. Early intervention in feeding problems at this time can result in a much easier resolution (see Chapter 12).

Infants begin to show regular patterns in bowel and bladder elimination. Some parents interpret their ability to predict their infant's bowel movements as toilet training (see Chapter 14). Sleep problems, if managed with consistency, begin to resolve. Otherwise, there might still be struggles with bedtime.

Between 11 and 12 months, infants gain about 1 lb per month. Growth in length continues to occur in spurts. Eleven- to 12-month-olds usually eat solids well, want to feed themselves, and are able to recognize their own hunger or satiation needs. They usually do not eat the same amount at each meal and demonstrate specific food preferences. Some infants may still not have their central or lateral incisors, and food choices should be limited to foods that need not be chewed until the infant has these teeth. Feedings begin to follow a routine of breakfast, lunch, and dinner, with midmorning, afternoon, and bedtime snacks.

Motor Skills Development

Fine motor development allows older infants to entertain themselves for extended times. They are able to hold objects of different sizes and pick up small objects using the sides of the fingers and eventually a fine pincer grasp, most often transferring the object directly to their mouth. Infants at this age enjoy putting objects into containers and taking them out again, and, by 11 or 12 months, can stack blocks one on top of the other. They often begin to hold a cup with two hands but may still have difficulty sealing their lips around the edge of the cup to take sips.

At 9 to 10 months, most infants sit for long periods and crawl on hands and knees. They begin to "cruise," walking around furniture holding on with both hands, and are able to pull themselves off the floor to a standing position. They may begin to let themselves down from furniture with fairly good control. They also take steps if someone holds two hands and then one hand. Eventually they take a few steps from one object or person to another. They may momentarily stand alone, and some infants walk independently.

Communication and Language Development

Receptive language skills improve, and infants participate in games such as pat-a-cake and peek-a-boo. Babies at this age momentarily stop activity when they hear "no," but they do not truly understand what "no" means. They are still very focused on observing activities in their environment and, when given names of things, attend well to the new information. They enjoy songs and rhymes and may participate by "singing" along.

By 12 months, infants' expressive language has expanded to a total of three or four words. Words such as "da-da," "ma-ma," or "ba-ba" (for bottle) can be recognized. They are able to name a picture in a book, visually look for an object when named, and follow simple one-step requests.

Social and Emotional Development

Infants at this age demonstrate stranger wariness, and some demonstrate fear of new situations or experiences. Emotions such as affection, anger, jealousy, and anxiety become more evident in late infancy. However, once familiar with new people, particularly if introduced by their parents, babies enjoy initiating games and social interchanges. Overall, 11- to 12-month-olds appear to be in love with the world, love to explore, and have little understanding of those things that can cause them harm. They enjoy playing interactive games. They assist in dressing by extending an arm or leg and are able to retrieve the bottle if it is dropped. They take great pride in mastering new skills or overcoming their fears, and they look to others around them to take notice as well.

Cognitive Development

Cognitively, older infants are completing more complicated tasks, such as stacking and container play. They master object permanence and easily locate a toy placed out of sight or under a cloth. This skill allows them to take a more active role in playing hide-and-seek or peek-a-boo. They hold a crayon or pencil with their whole hand and will make dots on a piece of paper imitating a drawn line.

Their curiosity blossoms. Infants begin to explore not only visually and with mouthing and chewing, but also by grasping, poking, shaking, pushing, pulling, and stacking. They often develop their own games or explore different ways of playing with familiar toys or objects. Play and other activities become more spontaneous and self-directed, and the parent begins to take a more passive role. It is still important for parents to play with their infant, but, as cognitive skills increase, the play increasingly becomes child directed.

ASSESSMENT OF INFANTS

Monitoring the overall growth and development of the infant is critical, because change is rapid and if a problem is detected early, treatment can be started and outcomes are likely to be more positive. Each area of development is important to assess and discuss with parents, because behaviors seen in each vary greatly by age of the infant. Good assessment is facilitated through consistent visits with the same provider. Seeing the same provider on a regular basis strengthens the relationship between the parents and the NP and makes it easier to pursue follow-up questions and concerns, validate the efforts of parents, and reinforce their successes.

As noted in Chapter 5, there is a distinction between screening and assessment for diagnosis. The NP uses both strategies when working with infants. One of the most informative questions that can be asked of the parent is, "Tell me about your child's day." This will provide information about daily routines of feeding, bathing, naps and sleep, elimination, and play activities. It will also provide information about what areas may be most difficult for the parents and areas where suggestions may be most helpful. NPs can find that listening carefully to parents' responses to this question from visit to visit helps them truly understand the life of the infant and how best to assist an individual family.

Screening Strategies for Infants

The Prenatal Visit

Meeting with parents prenatally allows the NP to assess parents' knowledge and receptiveness to anticipatory guidance. The prenatal visit should include a discussion of the partnership between the primary care provider and the parent. NPs can reach parents prenatally in a variety of ways, such as participation in Lamaze classes or parent preparation classes. Teenage mothers-to-be can be contacted through their local school or social service programs. These meetings provide a foundation for later visits and establish the NP as a resource for the parents.

The Neonatal Visit

The hospital visit may be the least opportune time to discuss infant care because of the short stay and the mother's physiologic state, which reduces her ability to absorb new information. Ideally, a 48- to 72-hour postpartum home or office visit can be arranged to assess the infant's physiologic and neurologic status, especially as related to feeding and state regulation, and to do important infant care teaching. Owing to the short length of hospital stay, a visit at 1 to 2 weeks after birth is also needed to assess the infant's weight gain, elimination pattern, sleep/wake cycle, breastfeeding success, and parent-child interaction. Screening for metabolic conditions takes place at this visit as well.

The mutual regulatory patterns that are established during this period significantly influence later infant self-regulation and parental responses. Developmental screening tools are rarely sensitive enough to discern problems at this time. The NP's interviewing, observations, and clinical experience are the most useful factors for uncovering infant or parenting problems.

The 2 through 12 Months of Age Visits

After the first month of life, more common screening tools include the Ages and Stages Questionnaires, the Denver screening tools (Denver II or Denver PDQ Parent Questionnaire), Child Development Inventories, and the Parents' Evaluation of Developmental Status (PEDS). Parent-completed tools, such as the Ages and Stages Questionnaires, can be given to parents while waiting for the visit or mailed with a reminder notice for the well-child visits. Other tools may be used for specific areas of concern, such as the Infant-Toddler and Family Instrument (ITFI), the Temperament and Atypical Behavior Scale (TABS), and the Receptive-Expressive Emergent Language Scale (REEL) (see the Resource Box at the end of this chapter for more information about these tools).

It is recommended that a standardized developmental screening test be completed and documented on all children during the first year of life. A simple checklist of developmental milestones does not provide adequate developmental screening for a child. A visit at 8 months is an optimal time to implement a standardized developmental screening because of the significant developmental changes occurring at this time, the changes in parental control, the infant's developing autonomy, and the numerous questions parents have.

Diagnostic Developmental Assessment Strategies for Infants

Developmental assessment tools include the Brazelton Neonatal Behavioral Assessment Scale, the HOME Scale, the Bayley Scales of Infant Development, and the Nursing Child Assessment Satellite Training (NCAST) Scales (Feeding Scale, Teaching Scale, Sleep Activity Record, and Personal Environment Assessments). These tools require special training to use and take longer to administer than screening tools. Use of developmental assessment tools can ensure more timely, appropriate referrals and help establish individualized intervention strategies for clients.

It is beyond the scope of this chapter to provide a complete review of the screening and assessment tools available in the areas of infant development, parent-child interaction, and family assessment. The Resource Box at the end of this chapter lists additional information about commonly used assessment tools.

ANTICIPATORY GUIDANCE FOR INFANTS

Many of the issues of infancy can be addressed through education and anticipatory guidance of parents. New parents, in particular, can be bombarded with more information and opinions than they can manage—from their own parents, neighbors, friends, the popular media, and others. The NP can help them sort through the information, understand what it means, and decide what is best for their family. Acknowledging specific positive aspects of the parents' skills before offering anticipatory guidance will help ensure that parents are more receptive to new ideas or suggestions.

Approaches to Parent Education for Infants

Developmentally supportive care engages infants in activities that are tailored to their unique developmental capabilities. These "developmentally appropriate" activities are integrated into all aspects of the infant's daily routines. Through parent education, NPs can help parents learn about infant development, what activities will promote healthy development, and what the parent can do to provide secure, safe relationships in an environment that supports their child's development.

Steward and Steward (1973) first introduced the concept of a teaching loop, in which teaching interactions between the parent and child consist of four specific teaching behaviors (Table 6-3). These behaviors provide the infant with verbal instruction, modeling, and positive feedback. Parents are often observed using the teaching loop as infants learn to walk; but they are unaware they are using a formal teaching strategy. NPs can instruct parents about the teaching loop and encourage them to use it earlier and in other areas of development.

This teaching loop model also can be used by NPs to teach parents. When offering anticipatory guidance, NPs must be sensitive to parents' interest in and tolerance of the information presented. Too much information, or information that the parent feels is irrelevant, can be overwhelming. If parents come to the NP with a concern, listening carefully to their perception of the problem is important. Information can then be structured to more directly address those parental concerns.

Frequently, time limitations in a clinic or office setting lead to use of a "laundry list" of topics for anticipatory guidance rather than information individualized to the infant and family being seen. Alternative approaches can be effectively used to provide parent education. For example, groups of parents can be scheduled for classes during well-child care visits or in the evening. These classes work well because they bring parents together to problem solve commonly shared issues.

In addition to giving verbal instruction, NPs can model developmentally appropriate activities during the well-child examination, showing parents ways to interact with their infant that stimulate, comfort, or soothe the baby. During these demonstrations, parents can be asked to give examples of things they have done at home as they care for their infant. If a problem was discussed at a previous well-child care visit and a plan made to try certain activities (e.g., creating a nighttime ritual to manage a 10-month-old who refuses to go to sleep in her own bed), the NP reviews the outcome with the parent, and gives positive feedback and encouragement for the efforts made and successful results. NPs should also be alert for developmentally appropriate parent-child interactions in the office and reinforce the parents' behavior with positive feedback.

The goal for parent education in the early years is to provide tools for parents that will be used in the many challenging years to come. It is also intended to give parents the skills to become their child's advocates, capable and knowledgeable about their child's individual needs.

Birth to 1 Month of Age

By understanding the capabilities of the newborn, such as hearing, vision, states and state transition, and self-calming and self-consoling techniques, parents are better able to read infant cues and provide timely and appropriate care. In turn, the infant's responsive behaviors assist in building the parents' confidence and aid in their receptiveness to future anticipatory guidance. NPs can use the following interventions to help parents promote infant development during daily activities and routines.

TABLE 6-3 ***The Teaching Loop***

Behavior	Description of Behavior
Alerting	The parent gets the infant's attention and makes sure that the child is paying attention. This may occur by calling the infant's name, making a noise, or directing the child to the toy.
Instruction	The parent gives a specific instruction to the infant or child about the toy or task and what is to be done. This instruction should be short and may be either verbal or a demonstration, or both.
Performance	The parent then gives the infant or child time to explore the material, to attempt to practice the task or play with the toy as shown, or just to explore the toy, depending on the child's age. Many parents have trouble allowing the child the time just to explore the task; others may offer excessive time without offering any assistance.
Feedback	The parent makes some comment that may be positive or negative, such as "Good job," "Good try," or "No, that's not quite right; try it this way."

Data from Steward D, Steward M: The observation of Anglo-Mexican and Chinese-American mothers teaching their young sons, *Child Dev* 44:329-337, 1973.

Regulation and Sleep/Wake Patterns

- Discuss the need for infants to develop day/night cycles, because infants' days and nights are often mixed up. Suggest that parents use consistent daily routines to help the infant establish a good sleep/wake cycle.
- Encourage parents to place the infant in a bassinet or crib during the day to allow an easier transition from the parent to bed at night.
- Describe the infant's need for variety of movement, voice, or touch to awaken or move up in sleep/wake states, and describe the infant's need for rhythmicity of voice, movement, or touch to calm or reduce state level. Explain that some infants benefit from external stimuli, such as music, voice, or movement to calm down and develop self-regulation. Gentle massage or swaddling can help some infants adjust to state changes.
- Explain the infant's startle or Moro reflex and encourage parents to use slow, easy movements in their caregiving activities.

Strength and Motor Coordination

Infants' gradually increasing strength makes it possible for them to lift their heads. Parents should be instructed to place their infants in the supine position for sleep, but to give their babies "tummy time" when awake and alert, placing them in a prone position. Parents can be encouraged to interact with their infants during these "prone to play" periods, at least once or twice every day.

Feeding and Self-Care

- Explain that a primary developmental activity of the newborn is organizing feeding responses. Bringing the infant slowly to an awake state for feeding is the first step. Emphasize that if the infant becomes overstimulated or disorganized, it might be necessary to reduce external stimuli (e.g., lights and noise), increase the infant's flexion of arms and legs, or bundle the infant to assist with central nervous system control and improve feeding responses.
- Help parents understand the infant's need to set the suck-swallow pace for feeding. If milk flows through the breast or bottle too rapidly or too slowly, adjustments to help the baby manage the feeding pace are needed. Feedings that are more than 45 minutes long or feedings that are shorter than 20 minutes with follow-up feedings within an hour should be evaluated further.
- Discuss how the face-to-face feeding position encourages eye contact, social smiles, and parent-child communication and interaction.
- Describe how the infant's reach for breast or bottle represents beginning exploratory learning and should be encouraged. Parents also can encourage the grasp reflex while the baby is feeding through finger play or finger holding.
- Discuss how much infants should be expected to ingest in a feeding, and the importance of burping.
- Explain that urinary output is an indicator of adequate intake, and discuss how many wet diapers to expect.
- Discuss how to avoid nipple confusion, stimulate milk production, and return to work while breastfeeding (see Chapter 13).

Communication and Language

- Discuss the communication skills of babies that are seen during state changes, periods of alertness, feeding, and sleep routines. Parents must be alert to nonverbal infant communication (e.g., fussiness, turning the head away) in order to understand their infant's needs.
- Encourage parents to attend promptly to infant crying. When parents respond to the infant's cries, the infant develops a sense of trust in them.
- Have parents reinforce their infant's comfort sounds through verbal responses.

Social and Emotional Growth

- Describe the infant's ability to tolerate brief periods of social interaction; when in the alert state, the infant can orient to visual stimuli (e.g., a parent's smiling face) to maintain stability. It is helpful to demonstrate for parents how the infant achieves this alert state.
- Encourage parents to hold their infant. Many parents believe that holding spoils their child and do not understand the infant's need for emotional support and tactile contact.
- Discuss the role of sibling involvement with the new infant. Facilitating overall family development and emotional growth is important.
- Help parents feel successful to promote their development as parents. Parents' concerns should be followed up closely with support, guidance, and reassurance. Early success while caring for the new infant is essential for parents to enjoy their new role.

Cognitive and Environmental Stimulation

Encourage opportunities for the infant to look at things in the environment, such as mobiles. Avoid having the same objects in the environment on the same side of the crib day after day. Variety encourages infants to move their heads from side to side. It is also helpful to place infants at different ends of the bed periodically.

Age 1 through 3 Months

Regulation and Sleep/Wake Patterns

- Continue structuring the infant's day because of the infant's ongoing need for external routines to facilitate state organization.
- Reemphasize the use of repetitive stimulation (e.g., rocking or a soothing voice) for quieting, and stimulus variation (e.g., undressing, stroking, or voice intonations) for awakening.
- Discuss the still immature nervous system, especially while the infant continues to show the Moro or asymmetric tonic neck reflex.
- Explore sleeping arrangements and begin discussing the importance of establishing a nighttime ritual.

Strength and Motor Coordination

- Encourage parents to place the infant in different positions for play time. Supine position stimulates movement of hands, feet, and legs; prone position strengthens upper torso, neck, and arms.
- Encourage parents to hold their infant.

Feeding and Self-Care

- Greater feeding control occurs at this time, and the infant begins to demonstrate a stronger need for sucking.
- Drooling may appear, as salivary glands mature, but the infant is still developing the ability to swallow excessive saliva.
- Discuss the infant's need for nonnutritive sucking, such as sucking on fingers and toys as a way of learning about the environment.
- Discuss the purpose and use of a pacifier.
- Discuss the importance of social and developmental, as well as nutritional, aspects of feeding.
- Discuss the infant's individual cues for readiness to eat, as well as satiation.
- Give positive reinforcement for continued breastfeeding. Offer problem-solving suggestions if the mother is returning to work (see Chapter 13).
- Remind parents to encourage infants to look at their hands as they begin to use their hands for self-consoling and hand-to-mouth exploration.

Communication and Language

- Continue discussing parents' observations and intuitions about their infant. Reinforce parents' understanding and sensitivity to their infant's cues and sleep/wake states. Recommendations associated with the parents' own observations are the most supportive. Parents' confidence and competence will grow as their increasing skills are validated.
- Encourage parents to sing to, talk to, and rock their infants.

Social and Emotional Growth

- Discuss the benefits of responding to infant cries as soon as possible. Prompt, consistent responses assist infants to trust that their needs will be met and decrease the chances of crying later on.
- Discuss the emerging temperament of the infant and the parents' perceptions of the infant's behaviors (Carey, 1998).
- Advise parents of the increasing social needs of the infant and the infant's desire to play with the caregiver.
- Encourage social games and eye contact for longer periods of time but with sensitivity to the infant's level of tolerance.
- Support the parents' need to find time for their own relationships. Assist in identifying possible child care resources and criteria for selection.

Cognitive and Environmental Stimulation

- Explain that the infant's visual awareness is increasing. The baby requires more visual diversity, such as changes in position and location, and changes in stimulating objects such as a mobile or mirror.
- Discuss the importance of equipment and toys that are semirigid, are not painted, and have varying textures. Toys that rattle and make sounds are appropriate. These encourage waving arms and kicking legs.

Age 4 through 5 Months

Parents' confidence strengthens as they become more skilled at communicating with their infant and as the infant begins to reciprocate their attentions. The NP should emphasize to parents the benefits of consistency in daily activities. Consistency helps infants to have internal control of their overall development. It is also important to help parents see the uniqueness of their infant and develop an individualized approach in their caregiving.

Regulation and Sleep/Wake Patterns

- Explore ways to help infants resume sleep independently when they awaken at night. This assists parents to prepare for future changes in the infant's sleep/wake pattern. Have parents put infants to sleep in the crib while drowsy but not yet asleep. If they awaken at night, they are more likely to resume sleep without comforting from the parent.

- Discuss the importance of nighttime rituals.
- Discuss parents' perception of their infant's temperament. Note the parents' description of their infant as an easy, average, or challenging baby. Parents often compare their infant with other babies and need to understand the uniqueness of their infant, individualizing their activities to their baby's style of responsiveness.
- Discuss varied parenting approaches to infants of different temperaments, including patterns of eating and sleeping.
- Remind parents that crying still needs to be addressed in a consistent and timely manner.
- Demonstrate the use of gradually increasing caregiver facilitation (e.g., presence, face, voice, touch, holding) for quieting the infant.

Strength and Motor Coordination

- Discuss safety precautions as the child becomes more mobile.
- Emphasize that parental supervision is essential for child safety.
- Discuss the need for childproofing the home from the infant's eye level (e.g., locks on cabinets and gates for stairs). Encourage childproofing at relatives' homes, as well as child care or day care settings.
- Remind parents about the benefits of playpens.
- Discourage use of walkers.
- Encourage parental holding and supervised floor play.

Feeding and Self-Care

- Remind parents about salivary gland maturation, drooling, and the infant's developing ability to swallow excessive saliva.
- Discuss the infant's individual cues for readiness to eat, as well as satiation. Discuss the importance of allowing the infant to self-regulate the amount of feedings.
- Explain that the infant will be ready for solids as the gastrointestinal tract matures. Listen closely to parents' questions and beliefs and the influence of others on the introduction of solids (see Chapters 12 and 13).
- When solids are appropriate, discuss the importance of using a spoon instead of placing cereal in the bottle. This helps the infant develop new oral-motor skills; skills needed to suck and swallow milk from a bottle or breast differ from those needed to take cereal from a spoon.
- Explain the need to engage infants socially, interacting with the child during feeding. Encourage parents to make feeding a social and fun time.
- Encourage parents to allow their infants to pat the breast or bottle and place their hands on the bottle in anticipation of self-feeding at a later date. Discourage propping the bottle, however.
- Advise parents that infants gradually become less dependent on external calming. Encourage parents to note other methods of self-calming through play, vocalization, and visual stimuli.

Communication and Language

- Reinforce parents' "back and forth talking" with their infant, especially using changes in voice inflection and intonation.
- Encourage parents to talk to their infant during caregiving activities. This holds the infant's attention, especially when fussy and makes it easier to change diapers, prepare meals, and attend to the infant's needs in other ways. It also stimulates the infant's language skills.
- Discuss the benefits of looking at picture books and reading to infants even at this early age. Emphasize the importance of developing habits of quiet time, reading time, and parent-child together time. The NP may want to participate in the national early literacy program for children 6 months through 5 years of age, Reach Out and Read (ROAR; see Resource Box).

Social and Emotional Growth

- Reassure parents that responding to their baby's cries promotes the infant's sense of trust and will not cause the baby to be spoiled.
- Discuss the infant's continued need for nonnutritive sucking as a means of self-regulation. Sucking on fingers or toys requires different oral-motor movements from those needed to suck on a pacifier.
- Explore ongoing communication between parents about their roles and responsibilities. Fathers may be more comfortable handling their infant at this age, as the infant becomes responsive. Try to have both parents included in the routine well-child care visits in order to discuss parenting issues.
- Discuss parenting and discipline (see Chapters 5 and 18).
- Clarify each parent's expectations (e.g., to allow an infant to cry at bedtime or not).
- Discuss how parents plan to resolve differences in expectations.
- Differentiate discipline and teaching from punishment. Help parents understand their role as the infant's first teachers. Offer examples of healthy ways to handle infant behavior as the infant exerts his or her own personality.
- Provide information to parents related to child development and what parents can expect their child to be able to do. Recommend parenting classes that provide information on developmental milestones and anticipated changes.

- Discuss mothers' feelings regarding their time to themselves, return to work, and particular life stresses. Mothers' feelings are often reflected in infants' behaviors.
- Discuss parents' need to spend time together. The parents' emotional well-being is an important aspect of the infant's overall care.
- Discuss selection of good day care settings that are developmentally and environmentally appropriate.

Cognitive and Environmental Stimulation

- Discuss the infant's increasing activity and awake time. Counsel parents that infants need increased adult attention and will make efforts to draw attention by smiling, making sounds, or crying.
- Encourage parents to use a variety of types of stimulation, such as soft stuffed toys, rattles, a crib gym or busy box, and toys of different sizes, weights, shapes, materials, and colors.
- Provide examples of home objects that infants see every day that can be used as "toys" for stacking, shaking, and rolling.
- Explain that infants enjoy looking at themselves in a mirror. Putting a mirror by the changing table is a good diversion.
- Reinforce parents' efforts to provide new experiences for their infant, such as walks to the park, visiting neighbors, or trips to the grocery store.
- Remind parents that infants of all ages enjoy being talked to and played with affectionately.

Age 6 through 8 Months

This period can be one of enjoyment and pleasure for parents as they watch their infant accomplish new skills on a daily basis. It is also one of the most challenging times for parents, because previously successful parenting strategies and techniques may no longer be effective. Infants at this age demonstrate a wide range of developmental differences, with a few older infants beginning to walk, for example, while others are not yet crawling. Temperamental differences are also striking among 6- through 8-month-olds. In addition, parents may be confronted with comparisons and suggestions from relatives, friends, or neighbors that undermine their confidence. For these reasons, anticipatory guidance is particularly important to sustain parental confidence and increase parents' knowledge about their infant's unique development.

Regulation and Sleep/Wake Patterns

- Discuss infants' needs for assistance to resume sleep/wake patterns after teething or illness.
- Discuss the increased need to provide consistency and maintain a nighttime ritual that transitions from play time to sleep time (e.g., bath time and a story).
- Stress the importance of teaching infants to go to sleep in their own beds so that when they awaken at night they are able to return to sleep. Advise parents that nighttime awakenings are best handled with the least amount of caregiver intrusion (e.g., use face, voice, touch, and then holding).
- Remind parents that infants are more capable of waiting for gratification. Parents can use talking and tone of voice to distract, calm, and reassure the infant.

Strength and Motor Coordination

- Discuss opportunities for crawling and walking. Discourage use of walkers.
- Discuss safety needs related to the child's increasing mobility and poor understanding of dangers.
- Review aspects of childproofing the home, such as checking gates on stairs, padding sharp corners, covering electrical outlets, and keeping the cord on an iron safely out of the way. Ensure that parents have the telephone number for a poison control center handy.

Feeding and Self-Care

- Encourage infant self-feeding. Encourage handling of utensils, holding the bottle, and taking solids from a spoon. Advise parents that using two spoons, giving one to the infant to hold, may make mealtimes more satisfying for all.
- Encourage structured mealtimes, especially if there are feeding problems. Advise parents to use an infant seat or highchair and avoid opportunities for "grazing" (i.e., allowing small snacks).
- Discuss parents' feelings about messiness of feeding, finding ways to minimize the mess (e.g., sheet on the floor, small-sized portions of food).
- Describe the benefits of offering finger foods, using a spoon, and drinking from a cup.
- Discuss eventual weaning from breast or bottle to cup by encouraging cup feeding now.
- Discuss need to clean teeth and provide fluoride supplements if water supply is not fluoridated (see Chapter 34).

Communication and Language

- Encourage parents to talk to their infant in their everyday activities and respond to their infant's vocalizations.
- Have the parents show the infant pictures in books, on the wall, or in magazines; read to the infant.
- Demonstrate naming body parts while examining the infant in order to show the parents the infant's responsiveness.

Social and Emotional Growth

- Discuss parents' feelings regarding limit setting and consistency of care; parental consensus benefits the child.
- Discuss the infant's need for positive parental responsiveness and attention.

Cognitive and Environmental Stimulation

- Encourage toys that demonstrate cause and effect, stacking, and container play.
- Allow infants to initiate games and social activities on their own.
- Identify common favorite toys, such as wooden spoons, plastic bowls, pull toys, or telephone.

Age 9 through 12 Months

Depending on the transitions accomplished from 6 through 8 months, the 9- to 12-month period may be a leveling out of previous changes or the beginning of new developmental changes that require further parental adjustments. Frequent discrepancies between infant development and family readiness are common, and each child and family has its unique temperamental qualities. As a result, it becomes increasingly important to individualize counseling to the infant and family at hand. Each of the developmental areas should be addressed, and NPs can reinforce parents' positive child management strategies, as well as offer information and guidance to assist infant development in areas that are more challenging.

Regulation and Sleep/Wake Patterns

- Discuss the infant's need to rely on a favorite toy or blanket in new situations to maintain a sense of comfort or familiarity.
- Reinforce efforts to establish and maintain routine nighttime rituals, regular mealtimes, and consistency of caregivers. Discuss the child's need for predictability in the daily schedule in order to gain mastery over new situations.
- Discuss the child's temperament, which is becoming more evident in activity level, level of curiosity, and ease of adjusting to new situations. A child's temperament is not always consistent with that of other family members. This discrepancy can become an area of conflict and turmoil. Discussion of positive parenting strategies can generate creative solutions.

Strength and Motor Coordination

- Encourage the parents' natural tendency to "cheer" their children on as they refine old and achieve new motor skills. This parenting behavior can be used as an example of positive reinforcement for the child in other areas of development.
- Discuss the importance of childproofing the environment. Parents need help in anticipating their infant's next major developmental achievement and preparing for the child's natural curiosity. Babies at this age are often able to get into trouble but not get themselves out (e.g., falling into a bucket of water).
- Discuss the continuing need to check bath water temperature and avoid leaving the infant alone for even a few seconds in the tub. At this age, infants can sit well but are unable to right themselves if they fall over in a slippery tub.
- Provide the 24-hour poison control telephone number.
- Discuss the value of outings for both parents and child. Stress the need to supervise the child closely as the child becomes more mobile and is apt to wander away.
- Reinforce the need for placing medicine, cleaning agents, matches, and firearms in locked cabinets, not just out of reach. These safety precautions are a must for mobile older infants with increased fine motor skills and curiosity.

Feeding and Self-Care

- Counsel on dental hygiene and caries prevention (e.g., use a soft toothbrush or wrap a washcloth around the finger to cleanse teeth and gums).
- Encourage finger foods, self-feeding, and letting the child practice using utensils.
- Encourage giving the infant meals in a highchair and having the infant eat or snack with the rest of the family.
- Discuss control issues that can arise as the infant increases self-feeding activities.
- Assist parents to recognize satiation cues.
- Help keep the infant focused on meals by removing distracters (e.g., no toys or television), using verbal reinforcement, and talking about the meal.

Communication and Language

- Discuss the continuing need to encourage the infant's verbalizations and to use a teaching style to help the infant learn about the environment.
- Encourage use of words in all interactions with the child (e.g., ear, nose, cup, shoe).
- Demonstrate teaching of body parts (e.g., eyes, nose, mouth).
- Continue to encourage the infant's interest in picture books and willingness to pat and point to pictures on each page.
- Encourage "reading" stories several times a week for as long as the child tolerates (see Resource Box for reading program information).

Social and Emotional Growth

- Discuss the development of each child's will, desire for autonomy, need for control, and initiative. Explain the infant's ego growth and need to distinguish parent from self.
- Review the parent's "teaching role" and discipline vs. punishment.
- Introduce the teaching loop: attention, instruction, demonstration, practice, reinforcement (see Table 6-3).
- Emphasize distraction and use of infant curiosity to deal with difficult situations.
- Discuss parents' feelings about the infant's stranger anxiety and how parents handle this. Help parents establish a separation ritual that communicates to the child that the parent is leaving but will return.
- Discuss the energy parents need to deal with busy, mobile infants and ways to cope when exhaustion occurs.
- Discuss negotiation of parental roles and responsibilities.
- Provide positive reinforcement for parenting skills.

Cognitive and Environmental Stimulation

- Explore parents' expectations for later toilet training. Discuss the physiologic and cognitive development that is necessary for learning this skill.
- Discuss toys that demonstrate cause and effect. Advise parents that they might need to put some toys away and then bring them out at a later date to maintain curiosity and interest.
- Reinforce that the parents should allow the child to take the lead in play activities.
- Encourage books, music, blocks, stacking toys, container toys, pull toys, and toys that allow self-initiated activities.
- Encourage interactive games, such as peek-a-boo and pat-a-cake. Encourage parents to play ball with the infant, rolling or throwing the ball back and forth interactively. Interaction with the caregiver is still the most important activity for the child.
- Explore parental feelings when infants enjoy time away from the parent.
- Discuss infants' enjoyment of messy play (e.g., water, sand, and different textures).

COMMON DEVELOPMENTAL ISSUES FOR INFANTS

Parents' concerns during the infant's first year of life are often related to inexperience or lack of knowledge about what to expect as infants grow and develop. A minority of infants have a true developmental delay. The fact that their baby is "normal," however, does not make the parents' concern any less compelling, and the NP has a responsibility to answer parents' questions; provide essential information about development; make accurate assessments to rule out problems; and, should a problem be found, treat or refer appropriately and provide follow-up care and support. Some of the more common developmental issues that trouble parents are discussed in this section. When parents understand the complexity of infant growth and development, they are better able to make healthy decisions for their infants and family.

Sleep

Should babies sleep in the same bed with their parents? How much sleep does an infant need? How can an 8-month-old be convinced that it is all right to sleep through the night? These are just a few of the questions parents have about their infant's sleep. Although the answers to these, and other, questions will differ for each family and infant, and a fuller discussion of children's sleep and rest patterns is found in Chapter 16, there are some general principles that can help guide parents, including the following:

- The first month of life is one of transition from the warm, dark uterine environment in which the fetus lived with the rhythm of the mother's body, heartbeat, and respirations. Being in a similar environment, close to those rhythms, helps many infants relax and sleep.
- Parents must provide for the safety of infants during sleep; supine sleep position on a firm surface from which the infant cannot fall is recommended. If parents are exposed to alcohol, drugs, or medications that would cause either parent to sleep more soundly than usual, they should not have their infant sleep in the same bed with them.
- Infants require assistance to transition from an awake state into sleep.
- Feeding facilitates transition to sleep, especially for young infants.
- As the infant matures neurologically, ease of state transition increases and skills of self-regulation develop.
- Self-regulation of state is an important skill for infants to learn; learning to put themselves to sleep and to sleep as long as they need is an important developmental task.
- A consistent and predictable sleep routine, in a consistent and predictable location (for both naps and nighttime sleep) provides the infant with a foundation to establish self-regulation.

Feeding

Breastfeeding is recommended for the first 12 months of life. Feeding concerns or problems in infancy, in particular a less than expected weight gain or decrease in weight, should be addressed by a detailed feeding history, a minimum of a 3-day diet history and calorie analysis, and an observation of an infant feeding either in the clinic or at home. The infant's oral motor skills and general development should be assessed. A standardized feeding assessment using a tool such as the NCAST Feeding Scale provides information about the parent-child relationship and assists in the development of individualized recommendations for the parents (see Chapters 12 and 13).

Crying

Infant crying and irritability cause parents great concern as they worry that something is wrong. It also can become a great disruption to the family and create a strained parent-child relationship. Labeling the crying as "colic" when it occurs more than 3 hours a day, three times a week, and between 3 weeks and 3 months does little to console stressed parents. It is advisable to evaluate the crying duration and intensity, as well as what factors contribute to it and what factors offer relief. Assessment of the infant's sleep/wake activity and amount of direct holding also provides insight into how to assist the family. Parents can use a tool such as the NCAST Sleep Activity Record to evaluate the infant's daily feeding, sleep routine, and fussiness.

Teaching parents to understand their infant's behavioral cues and communication is an important first step in resolving frequent crying. Most often, infant irritability is reduced as the infant establishes a consistent sleep/wake cycle, especially daily naps. The sleep-deprived infant is likely to become irritable and demonstrate poor feeding routines. Parents can be instructed to be alert to the infant's cues of tiredness and assist their infant to transition more easily from the wake to sleep state.

Spitting Up

Helping parents differentiate between normal infant "spit-up," regurgitation, reflux, and vomiting is often critical in providing appropriate parent support. In addition to describing the differences to parents, it can be valuable to have them complete a 3-day diary with the frequency and events surrounding these episodes. Spitting up may be influenced by the infant's daily routine and schedule, including feedings; lack of sleep routines, incomplete feedings resulting in grazing, or overfeeding may be precursors. Reflux management and vomiting are discussed in Chapters 12 and 33.

CLASSIFICATION OF DEVELOPMENTAL DISORDERS IN INFANTS

When evaluating any developmental delay in an infant it is important to distinguish disorders that manifest as motor problems (e.g., cerebral palsy) and disorders that manifest as cognitive problems (e.g., mental retardation, specific deficits in processing, and seizures). Processing disorders include peripheral problems such as deafness and blindness; central processing disorders reflected in motor, language, and perceptual dysfunction; and behavioral problems.

Usually, the history provides the best clues to the diagnosis of developmental delay, although there are some limits to the history. Some problems, such as fetal alcohol syndrome, autism, or fragile X syndrome, may not have clear symptoms in infancy. In some cases, parents may not be able to recall exactly when their child achieved a particular milestone, or how long the infant has been demonstrating a particular behavior.

It is important to determine whether the problems are the result of neurodegeneration as opposed to a static encephalopathy. Developmental delays that appear during infancy are usually connected to dysfunctions of major organs, physiologic abnormalities, and physiologic imbalances. Later presentations may manifest as feeding problems and poor interaction with caregivers or the environment; these can indicate motor coordination problems or hearing and vision problems. Gross motor problems are most often identified after 9 months of age, although parents may report concerns earlier. The Diagnostic Classification Task Force (1995) has developed a systematic approach for organizing, describing, and managing developmental and mental health issues. The Bright Futures program also provides practical tools for clinicians (Green & Palfrey, 2002; Jellinek, Patel, & Froehle, 2002a, 2002b).

RED FLAGS FOR INFANTS

Although developmental problems are not typical in infants, they do appear, and the NP must be alert to "red flags" that indicate a possible problem. As the well-child history is taken, specific risk factors that contribute to development delays can be identified, including the following:

- Prenatal exposure to street drugs or alcohol
- Prematurity
- Low birth weight
- Anoxia or birth trauma
- Neonatal intensive care and long-term hospitalization
- Cardiovascular illnesses
- Endocrine and metabolic problems
- Genetic syndromes
- Failure to thrive
- Cerebral palsy
- Sensory problems
- Autism

Table 6-4 outlines developmental findings that are indications for referral to a child development center, the state's early child development identification program, or a child development specialist.

TABLE 6-4 *Developmental Red Flags: Newborns and Infants*

Age	Physical Development (Autonomic Stability/Regulation/Sleep/Temperament)	Gross Motor (Strength Coordination)	Fine Motor (Feeding/Self-Care)	Language/Hearing	Psychosocial/Emotional Skills	Cognitive and Visual Abilities
Newborn-1 mo	Lack of return to birth weight by 2 wk examination Poor coordination of suck/swallow Tachypnea/bradycardia with feedings Poor habituation to external stimuli	Asymmetric movements Hypertonia or hypotonia Asymmetric primitive reflexes	Hands held fisted Absent or asymmetric palmar grasp	No startle to sound or sudden noises No quieting to voice High-pitched cry	Diffuse nonverbal cues Poor state transitions Irritable	Doll's eyes No red light reflex Poor alert state
3 mo	Poor weight gain; less than 1 lb weight gain in 1 mo Head circumference increasing greater than 2 standard deviations on growth curve or showing no increase in size Continuing problems with poor suck/swallow Difficulty with regulation of sleep/wake cycle Fussy baby	Asymmetric movements Hypertonia or hypotonia No attempt to raise head on stomach	Hands fisted with oppositional thumb No hand-to-mouth activity Feedings taking longer than 45 minutes Consistently awakening hourly for feeding	Does not turn to voice, rattle, or bell No sounds, coos, squeals	Lack of social smile Withdrawn or depressed Lack of consistent, safe child care	No visual tracking Not able to fix on face or object
6 mo	Less than double birth weight Head circumference shows no increase Continuation of poor feeding or sleep regulation Difficulty with self-calming	Persistent primitive reflexes Does not attempt to sit with support Head lag with pull to sit Scissoring	Does not reach for objects, hold rattle, hold hands together Does not grasp at clothes	No babbling Does not respond to voice, bell, rattle, or loud noises even with startle	No smiles No response to play Solemn appearance	Not visually alert Does not reach for objects Does not look at caregiver

9 mo	Parent control issues with feeding or sleep Night awakening that persists Offered bottle in bed for sleep Difficulty with self-calming/ regulation	Does not sit even in tripod position No lateral prop reflex Asymmetric crawl, handedness, or other movements	No self-feeding No high chair sitting No solids Does not pick up toy with one hand	Lack of single or double consonant sounds Lack of response to name or voice Does not respond to any words	Intense stranger anxiety or absent stranger anxiety Does not seek comfort from caregiver with stress	Lack of visual awareness Lack of reaching out for toys Lack of toy exploration visually or orally
12 mo	Less than triple birth weight Losing more than 2 standard deviations on growth curve for weight, length, or head circumference Poor sleep/wake cycle Extreme inability to separate from parent	Not pulling self to stand Not moving around the environment to explore	Persistent mouthing Not attempting to feed self or hold cup Not able to hold toy in each hand or transfer objects	Inability to localize to sound Not imitating speech sounds Not using 2-3 words Does not point	No response to game playing No response to reading or interactive activities Withdrawn or solemn	Not visually following activities in the environment

RESOURCE BOX

Developmental Management of Infants

SCREENING TOOLS

Ages and Stages Questionnaire (ASQ)
Birth through 5 years
Paul H. Brookes Publishers
www.pbrookes.com/catalog/books/asq.htm
www.brookespublishing.com
1-800-638-3775

Batelle Developmental Inventory Screening Test
Riverside Publishing Company
www.riversidepublishing.com
1-800-323-9540

Child Development Inventories
Age 3 months through 6 years
www.dbpeds.org/articles/dbtesting/cdi.html
Behavioral Science Systems
Box 580274
Minneapolis, MN 55458
1-612-929-6220

Communication and Symbolic Behavior Scales Developmental Profile (CSBS DP)
Paul H. Brookes Publishers
www.pbrookes.com/catalog/books/asq.htm
www.brookespublishing.com
1-800-638-3775

Denver Screening Scales (Denver II)
Developmental Materials (DDM)
www.denverii.com/related.html
1-800-419-4729
1-303-355-4729

Early Start Online Library
Resource library of developmental and educational materials for assessment and teaching
www.edgateway.net

Infant-Toddler and Family Instrument (ITFI)
Age 6 through 36 months
Paul H. Brookes Publishers
www.pbrookes.com/catalog/books/asq.htm
www.brookespublishing.com
1-800-638-3775

Milani-Comparetti Motor Development
Meyer Rehabilitation Institute
www.unmc.edu/mmi
1-800-656-3937

Parents' Evaluation of Developmental Status (PEDS)
Birth through 8 years
Ellsworth & Vandermeer Press, Ltd.
www.pedstest.com
1-888-729-1697
1-615-226-4060

PDQ-II
Prescreening Developmental Questionnaire
Developmental Materials (DDM)
www.denverii.com/related.html
1-800-419-4729
1-303-355-4729

Receptive-Expressive Emergent Language Scale, second edition
Pro-Ed, Inc.
www.proedinc.com/store/index.php
1-800-879-3202

Temperament and Atypical Behavior Scale (TABS)
Paul H. Brookes Publishers
www.pbrookes.com/catalog/books/asq.htm
www.brookespublishing.com
1-800-638-3775

DIAGNOSTIC DEVELOPMENTAL ASSESSMENT TOOLS

The following tools generally require training for use:

Bayley Scales of Infant Development, second edition
Age 1 through 42 months
Psychological Assessment Resources, Inc. (PAR)
www.parinc.com
1-800-331-8378

Gesell Developmental Screening Inventory (Revised)
Birth through school age
Order from Lorraine Coulson
E-mail: lrcoulson@ualr.edu
1-501-565-7627

Home Observation for Measurement of the Environment (HOME) Scale
Betty Caldwell and Robert Bradley
www.ualr.edu/~crtldept/home4.htm
Order from Lorraine Coulson
E-mail: lrcoulson@ualr.edu
1-501-565-7627

RESOURCE BOX

Developmental Management of Infants—cont'd

Nursing Child Assessment Satellite Training (NCAST) Scales
Feeding and Teaching Scales (birth through 3 years)
Personal Environmental Assessments (manual only needed)
Sleep Activity Record (manual only needed)
www.ncast.org
1-206-543-8528

Neonatal Behavioral Assessment Scale
The Brazelton Institute
www.brazelton-institute.com/
1-617-355-4959
1-800-323-9540

PARENT AND PROVIDER EDUCATIONAL RESOURCES

Brazelton TB, Sparrow JD: *Touchpoints three to six: your child's emotional and behavioral development*, Cambridge, MA, 2001, Perseus Publishing Services.

Bright Futures
Project of National Center for Education in Maternal and Child Health
www.brightfutures.org
1-202-784-9770

Goldberg S: *Baby and toddler learning fun*, Cambridge, MA, 2001, Perseus Publishing Services.

Holland K: *Johnson's your baby from birth to 6 months*, New York, 2002, DK Publishing.

Mackonochie A: *Your baby's first year: month by month*, New York, 2001, Lorenz Books.

Masi W, Leiderman RC: *Gymboree baby play*, San Francisco, 2001, Creative Publishing International.

Reach Out and Read National Center
www.reachoutandread.org
1-617-629-8042

Satter E: *How to get your kid to eat...but not too much*, Palo Alto, CA, 1987, Bull Publishing Company.

Schmitt B: *Your child's health: the parent's guide to symptoms, emergencies, common illnesses, behavior, and school problems*, New York, 1991, Bantam Books.

Shelov S, Hannemann R: *Caring for your baby and young child: birth to age 5*, Elk Grove Village, IL, 1999, American Academy of Pediatrics.

Weissbluth M: *Healthy sleep habits, happy child*, New York, 1999, Fawcett Books, Ballantine Publishing Group.

Zero to Three
www.zerotothree.org
1-202-638-1144 (office)
1-800-899-4301 (ordering publications)

Some primary care practices have providers with the expertise to manage minor developmental problems, and in consultation with a specialist, may take an initial "wait-and-see" approach. An NP with expertise in developmental, sleep, feeding, or behavioral assessments and parenting issues can be a valuable resource, conducting ongoing assessments as the infant grows and helping parents implement interventions to foster healthy development. If the infant is referred, the NP works with parents to connect them to community resources and to advocate for necessary services, as well as continuing to provide the infant with primary care.

REFERENCES

Anders TF, Goodlin-Jones BL, Zelenko M: Infant regulation and sleep-wake state development, *Zero to Three* 19:5-8, 1998.

Barnard K: *Beginning rhythms: the emerging process of sleep wake behaviors and self regulation*, Seattle, 1999, NCAST, University of Washington.

Carey WB: Let's give temperament its due, *Contemp Pediatr* 15:91-113, 1998.

Diagnostic Classification Task Force: *Diagnostic classification 0-3: diagnostic classification of mental health and developmental disorders of infancy and early childhood*, Arlington, VA, 1995, Zero to Three/National Center for Clinical Infant Programs.

Dixon SD, Stein M, editors: *Encounters with children: pediatric behavior and development*, St Louis, 2000, Mosby.

Green M, Palfrey J, editors: *Bright Futures: guidelines for health supervision of infants, children, and adolescents*, ed 2, revised, Arlington, VA, 2002, National Center for Education in Maternal and Child Health.

Jellinek M, Patel BP, Froehle MC, editors: *Bright Futures in practice: mental health—volume I. Practice guide*, Arlington, VA, 2002a, National Center for Education in Maternal and Child Health.

Jellinek M, Patel BP, Froehle MC, editors: *Bright Futures in practice: mental health—volume II. Tool kit*, Arlington, VA, 2002b, National Center for Education in Maternal and Child Health.

Martin JA et al: Births: final data for 2001, *National Vital Statistics Reports*, 51, Dec 18, 2001. Available at *www.cdc.gov/nchs/default.htm* (accessed Jan 4, 2003).

Minino AM, Smith BL: Deaths: preliminary data for 2000, *National Vital Statistics Reports*, 49, Oct 9, 2001. Available at *www.cdc.gov/nchs/products/pubs/pubd/nvsr/49/49-13.htm* (accessed Jan 4, 2003).

Shonkoff JP, Phillips DA, editors: *Committee on Integrating the Science of Early Childhood Development, Board on Children, Youth, and Families: from neurons to neighborhoods: the science of early childhood development*, Washington, DC, 2000, National Academies Press.

Steward D, Steward M: The observation of Anglo-Mexican and Chinese-American mothers teaching their young sons, *Child Dev* 44:329-337, 1973.

7 Developmental Management of Toddlers and Preschoolers

Mary A. Murphy

Developmental changes in the second through fifth years of life are more subtle than those in the first year, yet they are highly significant. Children enter toddlerhood as babies, dependent on parents and caregivers for their very survival, and leave as accomplished children with elaborate and sophisticated skills. Ready to enter the social world of school and community, 5-year-olds have a sense of self that will shape the quality of their character as older children, adolescents, and adults. Children begin this process of change by refining abilities acquired in the first year, learning, for example, to walk smoothly with control and speed, to run and climb, and to combine words into phrases and sentences. They add to their repertoire of skills, growing stronger, bigger, and more socially, emotionally, and intellectually capable. This chapter reviews some of the many changes that occur for toddlers (usually defined as a child age 12 to 24 months) and preschoolers (a child age 2 to 5 years), as well as the nurse practitioner's (NP's) role when working with these children and their families.

DEVELOPMENT OF TODDLERS AND PRESCHOOLERS

Physical Development

Physical and physiologic changes in toddlers and preschoolers continue at a much slower pace than in the first year of life (see Table 12-8 for a review of yearly gains in weight, height, and head circumference). The average 2-year-old weighs 26 to 28 lb (12.5 to 13.5 kg), with boys being slightly heavier than girls, and is 34 to 35 inches (85 to 90 cm) tall. Head circumference in the average 2-year-old is 19 to 19.5 inches (48 to 50 cm). Most toddlers have no palpable fontanels by 12 months; for all children, the anterior fontanel should be completely closed by 18 to 19 months. During the fourth and fifth years, skeletal growth continues as additional ossification centers appear in the wrist and ankle and additional epiphyses develop in some of the long bones. For the 4- to 5-year-old, the legs grow faster than the head, trunk, or upper extremities. Changes related to body systems are highlighted in Table 7-1. More detailed discussion of development, issues, and disease processes in each of these systems can be found in Units 3 and 4 of this text.

Motor Skills Development

Motor skills development is divided into two components—gross and fine. Gross motor refers to the development and use of the large muscles. Fine motor includes hand and finger development and oral-motor development. See Table 6-1 for a review of gross and fine motor milestones by age.

In addition to the eight general developmental principles listed in Chapter 5, there are six principles specific to

TABLE 7-1 Physical Development of Toddlers and Preschool-Age Children

Body System	Developmental Changes
Dental	By 12 months, the child usually has six to eight primary teeth. By 2 years of age, the child has a complete set of 20 primary teeth. By 3 years of age, the second molars usually erupt. During the second year, calcification begins for the first and second permanent bicuspids and second molars. Most growth and calcification of the permanent teeth occurs within the gums; it is not visible.
Neurologic	Continued myelinization and cortical development occur; brain development is influenced by multiple factors (Shonkoff & Phillips, 2000). Brain growth, combined with musculoskeletal development, allows children to perform more complex physical tasks. Fine motor movements are more detailed and sustained: • 2-year-olds can easily manipulate fingers to stack two blocks. • 3-year-olds can create a tower of eight or more blocks. • 4-year-olds can easily build a 12-block step design. • 5-year-olds can grasp a pencil appropriately to copy simple geometric designs accurately and write their name in block letters. Gross motor skills are smoother and more coordinated. Sensory function is more mature. Visual acuity is 20/70 for 2-year-olds; 20/30 for 5- to 6-year-olds.
Cardiovascular	Little change occurs in the second and third year. By the fifth year the heart has quadrupled in size since birth. By age 5 years, the heart rate has decreased to 70 to 110 beats per minute. Normal sinus arrhythmia may continue, and innocent murmurs are common. The hematologic system should produce only adult hemoglobin. The hemoglobin level stabilizes at 12 to 15 g/dl.
Pulmonary	Abdominal respiratory movements continue until the end of the fifth or sixth year. Respiratory rate steadies and slows to about 30 breaths per minute.
Gastrointestinal	By 2 years of age, the salivary glands reach adult size. The stomach becomes more bowed and increases its capacity to about 500 ml. Many children still require a nutritious snack between meals, because of small stomach size. During the second year, the liver matures and becomes more efficient in vitamin storage, glycogenesis, amino acid changes, and ketone body formation. The lower edge of the liver may still be palpable. By 4 to 5 years of age, the gastrointestinal system is mature enough for the child to eat a full range of foods. Stools are more like those of adults.
Renal	Kidneys begin descending deeper into the pelvic area and grow in size. Ureters remain short and relatively straight. A 2-year-old may excrete as much as 500 to 600 ml of urine a day. A 4- to 5-year-old excretes between 600 and 750 ml daily.
Endocrine	Quiescent time for sexual growth, with few physical or hormonal changes. Growth hormone stimulates body growth.

fine motor development that relate to the toddler and preschool years (Dixon & Stein, 2000):

1. Primitive reflexes must disappear before voluntary behaviors appear (e.g., children do not walk until involuntary stepping disappears).
2. Development is proximal to distal (e.g., children reach before they grasp).
3. Development is ulnar to radial (e.g., children pick up objects with the little finger side of the hand before they use the thumb side of the hand).
4. The hand develops supination before pronation (e.g., children use the palm up to place objects in their mouth).
5. Grasp develops before release (e.g., a newborn reflexively grasps a rattle and a 12-month-old is able to grasp and voluntarily release the rattle).
6. Fine motor development in the hand moves from flexion to extension and involuntary to control. The pincer grasp appears before release movements. Use of the dominant hand may appear as early as 8 to 12 months but generally emerges between 2 and 4 years. The

4-year-old can thread small beads on a chain; grasp a pencil appropriately to copy some letters (v, h, t, o); draw a person with head and features, legs, trunk, and arms; use scissors to cut on a line; fasten buttons; and eat with a fork. By 5 years, these movements expand to copying a square and additional letters (x, l, a, c, u, y), writing some letters spontaneously, producing identifiable pictures, counting fingers on one hand, and using all eating utensils appropriately.

Gross motor development follows four general principles:

1. Skills are built on neuromotor tone (e.g., a 1-year-old with hypotonia has difficulty standing, stepping, and walking).
2. Reflexive behavior progesses to volitional behavior (e.g., children move from a stepping reflex to a controlled walk).
3. More efficient behavior is easier and requires less energy (e.g., it is easier to walk than to crawl).
4. Speed and accuracy increase with practice (e.g., a wide-based, awkward waddle develops into a narrow-based, smooth, controlled walk).

The following are gross motor behaviors that an average 5-year-old could demonstrate:

- Walk with control
- Step easily over a balance beam
- Climb—stairs with alternate feet both up and down to any height, up ladders
- Run—around corners, stop voluntarily, lightly on toes
- Ride a tricycle using the pedals to pedal
- Show more control in throwing, catching, bouncing, and kicking a ball
- Skip using alternate feet
- Easily walk a narrow line
- Move rhythmically to music

Communication and Language Development

Language uses symbols for thoughts; thus it emerges with Piaget's preoperational stage of development. Beginning around 2 years of age, toddlers use words to convey their thoughts and feelings. Once the process begins, it develops rapidly. Cognitive development is a basic requirement for language development because the child must decipher the rules of language independently, problem solve to understand the communication of others, and create symbols that can be understood by others and that reflect his or her ideas and emotions. The development of language requires mastery of the following:

- Oral-motor ability to articulate sounds
- Auditory perception to distinguish words and sentences
- Cognitive ability to understand syntax, semantics, and pragmatics
- Psychosocial-cultural environment to motivate the child to engage in language use

Language milestones are evident in two general categories—receptive and expressive language. These are presented for infants and children younger than 5 years of age in Table 6-2.

Articulation

Articulation skills are practiced daily, and by 24 months of age speech sounds are 25% intelligible to a stranger. The intelligibility rate jumps to about 66% between 24 and 36 months of age, with 90% intelligibility by age 3 years. By 4 years of age, speech should be completely intelligible with the exception of particularly difficult consonants; by 5 years the tongue-contact sounds of n, t, d, k, g, y, and ng are more intelligible. Some sounds, such as the zh sound, are not added until 6 to 8 years of age. Figure 7-1 identifies sounds articulated by children at specific ages.

During the second year, the child practices playful changes in pitch and loudness. Three- and 4-year-olds can

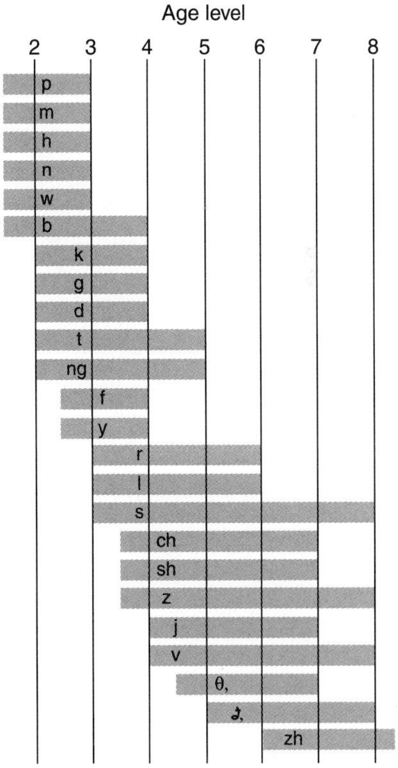

FIGURE 7-1 Norms for development of speech sounds. θ, *th* as in *thin*, ð, *th* as in *this*. (From Van Riper C, Erickson RL: *Speech correction: an introduction to speech pathology and audiology*, ed 9, Needham Heights, MA, 1996, Allyn & Bacon, p 98. © 1996 by Allyn & Bacon. Reprinted by permission.)

show normal hesitance in speech or stuttering. These dysfluencies should pass if ignored and are no longer expected in 5-year-olds.

Children usually progress through a regular sequence of mispronunciations as they learn new articulation skills. At first, they simply omit the new sound, and then they try to substitute a more familiar sound for the new one (e.g., the "w" for "r" substitution, as in "wabbit" for "rabbit"). Distortion is followed by "addition" as the child adds an extra sound (e.g., "gulad" for "glad"). Knowing each of these steps allows the examiner to reassure the parent that the child is developing normally or needs monitoring.

Lexicon

Lexicon refers to vocabulary. Size of vocabulary is influenced by many factors, including environment, stimulation, intelligence, bilingualism, culture, and personality. Children usually understand more words than they are able to express, and addition of words to their expressive vocabulary comes with continued practice. Girls usually say their first word between 8 and 11 months, boys about 14 months. Most 2-year-olds have more than 200 words in their vocabulary, and most 4- to 5-year-olds add approximately 50 words a month to their vocabulary. Five-year-olds should be able to define some words with other words (e.g., "cup" is "you drink with it," or "chair" is "to sit on").

Syntax

Syntax, or grammar, refers to the structure of words in sentences or phrases. The ability to construct sentences that convey meaning is a complex skill, proceeding through several stages in children: receptive, holophrastic, and telegraphic speech. Much of this skill is developed between 8 months and 3.5 years. By 8 months of age, children are developing receptive language; that is, they understand others who use a new word or structure before they are able to use it themselves. When asked "Where is the ball?" an 8-month-old searches for the ball. Between 12 and 18 months, children begin to use holophrases or single words to express whole ideas. The child says "milk" to mean the whole sentence, "Give me a glass of milk." A complex idea is expressed in one succinct word. Holophrastic sentences are denominative (labeling) or imperative (commanding).

Around 18 months of age, children begin using telegraphic speech, which is more complex and possesses two classes: pivot and open. The pivot class consists of a few frequently used words, and the open class contains newly learned words. Thus the child may use the pivot word "daddy" with open-class words for "daddy eat," "daddy all gone," or "daddy sleep." From this stage, which lasts 2 to 3 months, the child further subdivides the pivot class into articles, demonstrative pronouns, and a second pivot class. The second pivot class is subdivided into adjectives and possessives, and a third pivot class, and so on as the child developmentally progresses from simple to more complex language. Sentence structure also becomes more complex as children move from active sentences, to questions, to passive and negative construction, and then add plurals (3 years of age) and past tenses (4 years of age) to their grammar. Three- to four-word sentences should be evident by 3 years, and by 5 years of age, the child's syntax is close to adult style, including use of future tense and complete sentences of five to six words in length.

Semantics

Semantics, or the study of word meaning, is learned in stages from global to more specific. Words used in any language have both denotative (the specific, concrete referent of the word) and connotative (a broader range of feelings aroused by the word) meanings. Development of semantics is an ongoing process covering the years into young adulthood. Even though children may be quite adept at using words correctly, they may have only a vague, diffuse connotative understanding of these words.

Bilingualism

Parents may choose to raise their children bilingually or monolingually. Bilingualism may help preserve the family culture and heritage. Studies show that bilingual children have greater mental flexibility. They may also have enhanced employment and lifestyle opportunities. Maintaining bilingualism requires time and effort as the child learns to read and write and maintain fluency in both. For families anxious to integrate culturally in a society with a different language, emphasizing skill in the language of the new community may be viewed by the family as a first priority (Chiocca, 1998).

Simultaneous bilingualism occurs when children hear and learn two languages from infancy. These bilingual children should be equally competent in both languages by age 3 years. Sequential bilingualism occurs when the child, usually 3 years of age or older, learns one language and then is immersed in another. Children learning sequentially may have more apparent differences in their skills from language to language until they have developed proficiency in both.

Bilingual preschoolers experience no delays in development of their vocabulary and are proficient in sorting one language from the other, although they may "code switch" to the other language for clarity as they talk. They switch languages depending on whom they are speaking with and the circumstances. Some even translate for others, seeming to understand that not everyone speaks or understands both languages. Ultimately, whether a second or even third language is learned simultaneously or sequentially, most children have one dominant language.

Social and Emotional Development

Theories

Theories of child development described in Chapter 5 form the basis for social and emotional development of toddlers and preschoolers. Freud viewed toddlers as progressing through an anal stage in which they find pleasure in manipulation of the anal area. He argued that toddlers control their environment by manipulating control of bowels and bladder. According to Freud, the preschool years represent a tremendously active stage, with the child's development evolving around the Oedipus complex, with love for the parent of the opposite sex and fear of the parent of the same sex.

Erikson believed that toddlers develop a sense of autonomy and move away from total dependence into more interdependence. During this process, toddlers discover themselves and explore their own bodies and their expanding world. With their increased mobility, they move away from their parents for short periods of time and look at the world outside their beds, houses, and yards. According to Erikson, preschoolers begin to develop a sense of initiative, learning new skills and exploring the larger outside world.

Kohlberg investigated moral development of children and described 12- to 18-month-old children as "amoral," with an ability to follow commands only occasionally. He believed that 2-year-old children, in a preconventional stage, can follow commands more frequently. Preschool-age children are in a conventional stage of morality, able to follow commands consistently as they work to maintain approval of adults and to behave as "good" children are expected to do.

Temperament, another theoretic perspective important to child development, is discussed in Chapter 21. Resilience and vulnerability are two other characteristics under current discussion in the literature. *Resilience* (sometimes called *hardiness*) is a person's capacity to survive intact, both psychologically and physically, despite adversity. *Vulnerability*, in contrast, refers to a person's sensitivity and inclination to decompensate in the face of life stressors. These characteristics are also found in children and affect outcomes in life experiences as stressors come and go. Many children demonstrate remarkable resilience despite significant risks.

Psychosocial changes in toddlers and preschoolers are remarkable. Emotions and cognition are interconnected so that assessment of any one area of development is somewhat arbitrary. Toddlers no longer spend most of their time sleeping; rather they are up, running about, verbalizing, and demanding to join in family activities. These are years of intense learning about and managing feelings, such as love, happiness, anger, frustration, aggression, and jealousy. They learn the words that go with these feelings and, with guidance, the appropriate behaviors. A major developmental milestone for this age is the achievement of a sense of independence and autonomy.

Social Interaction

Learning how to interpret and manage feelings is a challenge for both toddlers and their parents, as illustrated in the birthday announcement from one set of parents: "Roses are red, violets are blue. Watch out world, Charlene is two!!!" Toddlers need a great deal of love, warmth, and comfort, primarily from their parents and caregivers. Toddlers learn to give love and find satisfaction in pleasing their parents. They learn to respond to kisses, hugs, and cuddles they have received by giving kisses, hugs, and cuddles in return. Toddlers who make these early attempts at giving love and are rejected or ignored soon stop trying and begin to find pleasure elsewhere. Toddlers with sensory issues learn to avoid some gestures unless they are in control and decide they can handle the pressures, tactile feelings, or sensory feelings (Kranowitz, 1998). Some toddlers find that thumb sucking, rhythmic body movements, and body manipulation are more pleasurable and reliable than person-to-person contacts. Maternal depression has a significantly negative effect on the development of normal infant engagement behaviors that can persist into the toddler and preschool years (Murray & Cooper, 1997). This can lead to serious social problems later. Even at this young age, problems of sibling jealousy and possessiveness emerge. These are based on the child's emerging sense of self-identity (Sturner & Howard, 1997b).

Preschoolers develop a broader understanding of the nature of social interactions. They discover that love is not all taking but comes with certain obligations and responsibilities. They develop ideas about giving and sharing. The 4- to 5-year-old moves away from the extremely self-centered attitude of earlier toddlerhood. Parents are viewed as the epitome of wisdom, power, integrity, and goodness. If early stages of the love relationship have not been satisfied, preschoolers can show more fears, inhibitions, explosive behavior, and demands for attention.

By preschool years children begin to show some interest in table manners, being polite, saying "Thank you" without a reminder, sharing, saying (and meaning) "I'm sorry," and taking turns. These social skills are learned daily interactions at home, school, and church, from parents, peers, relatives, and neighbors. Children learn to read social clues of others' behavior (e.g., the voice tone, slight facial expression, posture), and correct their own behavior. Some children, frequently boys, find these clues vague and difficult to learn, and parents can help by explaining and discussing them.

Dependence versus independence is an important struggle for toddlers and preschoolers, and the road from depending on a parent for everything to doing some things for oneself is rocky and uneven. Children at this age vacillate between being a big boy or big girl and mommy's baby. They take great pride in doing as many things as possible for themselves, yet they need to feel totally secure in their parents' care. Toddlers like to have a choice in matters and quickly learn the power of the word "no." They can become extremely negative, practicing the power of "no" every day for months. As toddlers practice making choices, they are clumsy, awkward, and frequently wrong. This can be very frustrating for them, and their outraged responses can be equally annoying for their parents. With time, they become more skilled, make better choices, have more successes, and feel more powerful. They no longer have to work so hard to show others their power, and the negative stage passes.

On some days toddlers cling to mother's skirt, not letting her out of sight; on other days the child can play for short periods in the next room, trotting back every so often to see, touch, and hear the mother and be reassured by her presence. Gradually the periods of separation lengthen and the child needs only to hear the mother's voice or to check occasionally for security. Separation anxiety is frequent during these years and can be traumatic for both parents and child. Preschool children are much less dependent on their parents and frequently can tolerate physical separation for several hours. Peer dependence begins to be important.

Preschool-age children respond more verbally than toddlers and are able to perform many more self-care tasks—feed themselves using appropriate utensils, blow their own noses, and go to the bathroom unassisted. Interactions become easier and more enjoyable as the child learns to verbally express needs and feelings.

The preschool years teach the child the social skills of living with others—how to express temperament, demonstrate behavioral control, manage stresses, seek supports, articulate feelings, and foster family relationships. Emotionally, preschool children continue to be self-centered but become more aware of the responsibilities of being part of the family and group; sharing; contributing; knowing right from wrong; beginning to control emotional states; delaying gratification; managing frustration, separations, fears, anxieties, and anger; and demonstrating patience. This is often a time when conflict and worries decrease and family life is relatively calm.

Sibling Interaction

Young children need to learn to share. This is most easily done when they live in a family with siblings. Opposite gender, temperament, insecure attachment, family discord, corporal punishment, and perceptions of unequal treatment affect interaction patterns between siblings. Many toddlers or preschoolers regress when a new baby arrives. On the other hand, older children can experience excitement, love, and enhanced self-esteem when the new baby arrives. Parents need to promptly limit any aggression expressed by the older child, provide love and attention, and talk about feelings. When older children fight, parents need to describe the situation and provide even-handed control. Blaming a child, except in clear-cut instance of misbehavior, is usually unproductive. Promoting support, loyalty, and friendship are important goals for sibling interactions (see Chapter 19).

Morality

Morality, or the ability to know right from wrong, is still based on external control during the toddler years, stemming from children's love of their parents and a desire to please them. Parent teaching generally focuses more on helping the child to make safe decisions than moral ones. Toddlers cannot be expected to make correct choices if left alone in potentially dangerous situations, because their internal sense of conscience is rudimentary and judgment is absent. Any room with electrical sockets, knobs for technical equipment, open windows, or hot food represents a risk. As toddlers gain language skills, they begin to echo the parent's firm "No," but they do not understand the full meaning of the term. By 24 months, many toddlers show beginning internalization by saying "No" to themselves and stopping the act; they may continue with the act as they talk to themselves, still saying "No."

For the 4- to 5- year-old, morality becomes more internally controlled. Instead of basing all decisions on the knowledge of the consequences of the act (e.g., "If I take a cookie, I will be sent to my room"), older children show an elementary understanding of what is right and wrong, fair or unfair. They begin to think ahead and are able to plan and control their urges, thus avoiding punishment. Four-year-olds can internalize some demands from their parents, and feelings of guilt can be elicited after some transgressions.

Peer Relationships

Toddlers may be fascinated by children of their own age, and can demonstrate curiosity by examining the other child closely, poking and probing; but they generally do not engage with their peers in an interactive way. Parallel play is the norm. Preschoolers learn to interact with peers as their social world grows. Play becomes more interactive, cooperative, and shared, with use of more symbolic language. Imaginary play leads to "let's pretend," role-playing, and creation of imaginary friends. Fantasy and make-believe are very important during these years. The play activities of children are culturally influenced. Farver and Shin (1997) videotaped the play of Korean American and Anglo American 4- and 5-year-old children, looking for frequency of pretend play, communicative strategies, and pretend play themes. Although there were no differences in the frequency of pretend play, the Korean American children included everyday activities and family role themes, whereas the Anglo American children enacted more environmental danger and fantasy themes. As they played together, the Anglo American children described their own actions, rejected their playmates' suggestions, and used directives. In contrast, the Korean American children described their partner's actions; used tag questions at the end of statements, such as "Right?" or "OK?"—semantic ties that expanded on the statements just made by the other child; articulated statements of agreement; and made polite requests.

Shared or cooperative play makes simple games of hide-and-seek and tag possible. Games with complicated rules can be frustrating to the preschooler, who prefers simple table games with the option of making up the rules as the game proceeds. Cheating in order to win is common, because the boundaries of acceptable play are not yet clear and the earliest stages of moral behavior are only beginning to emerge.

Body Image

Toddlers are often highly concerned about body image. They realize that they are separate persons and begin to take notice of their own bodies. They may become fascinated with the different parts of the body and how they work. Bodily injury becomes a concern, and cuts and bruises elicit much discussion. Toward the end of the second year, children may notice the inner feelings of their bodies (e.g., the urge and tension to move the bowels, the release and relaxation resulting from going to the bathroom, the discomfort of hunger, and the pleasure of eating). These are abstract feelings that toddlers cannot put into words, but can show with actions. Toddlers quickly learn the pleasure of control in these situations and show it when they say, "Yes, I will go to the bathroom," or "No, I won't!" Toddlers discover the delights of control over others and themselves. This increases their sense of power but can also lead to misunderstandings and hurt feelings if their parents do not read their moods properly.

During the preschool years, the sense of separateness increases and children are more aware that they are different from their surroundings, their families, and their friends. They begin to realize that other persons also have feelings, fears, and doubts. They reexamine themselves, and worries over a lost tooth or a skinned knee are common. Curiosity about their bodies and those of others generates a wealth of innocent questions that generally require a simple answer. They learn that genital manipulation brings pleasure, and masturbation peaks around 3 to 4 years of age.

Fears

As the 2- to 3-year-old's world expands and the ability to fantasize develops, fears can appear about things that might happen. "Magical thinking," characteristic of preschoolers, can accentuate these fears. Early fears include fear of separation, strangers, water, loud noises, crowds, the dark, and animals. Four- to 5-year-olds add wild animals, masks, and aggressive actions to the list. Adults should not dismiss the fears as trivial, but offer reassurance with words and their presence; this helps children work through the anxiety and tension they feel. Preschool children may still express fear of the dark or of harm to their bodies, but if the fears do not decrease with time, the child and family need referral for counseling. By 4 years of age, children can identify nightmares as "not real," although they may still be afraid. Fears may be expressed in a variety of ways: flight, requests for help, sudden shyness, irritability, hyperactivity, frustration, or aggressive actions (Dixon & Stein, 2000).

Cognitive Development

Cognitively, toddler thinking is highly concrete. According to Piaget (see Table 5-1), 1-year-olds are still in the sensorimotor stage, demonstrating many repetitive responses, showing increased ability to solve problems, and beginning trial-and-error experiments. They become more differentiated from the environment. They search for a hidden object where they last saw it, showing their increasingly thorough understanding of object permanence. From 18 to 24 months of age, children begin to use mental imagery and infer a cause when they can see only the effect.

By the end of the second year, children enter the preoperational stage with preconceptual and intuitive thinking.

Primitive conceptualization processes begin with the development of symbolic thinking. A block becomes a car; words become symbols for ideas. The 3-year-old continues to develop symbolic thinking, such as drawing and acting out elaborate play scenarios. However, children at this age generally are unable to take another's perspective and continue to view the world egocentrically from their own worldview. Attending to one characteristic at a time is another feature of preschool thinking. For example, the child will try to fit a jigsaw puzzle piece using either color or shape but not both. Parents have difficulty understanding the thoughts of preschool children. On the surface, preoperational thinking has many characteristics that resemble adult thinking, and parents are often deceived into believing that children are able to think as adults do. Preschool children, for example, are developing the use of language and the ability to symbolize concepts mentally. Some of their verbalizations appear quite precocious, as evidenced by the 3-year-old who stares out the window and then states, "Look, Mommy, the trees are saying yes and no!" In fact, preschool children continue to be concrete and egocentric in their thinking, and their logic is the source of many communication problems between parents and children. Table 7-2 identifies major characteristic of the thinking of preschool children and gives examples of each.

TABLE 7-2 ***Examples of Preschool Children's Thinking Using Piaget's Preoperational Stage***

Characteristic	Example
Egocentricism	"It's snowing, so I can go play in it."
Unable to abstract to see other's viewpoint	If John is holding a doll with its face toward Ann, Ann thinks John can also see the doll's face.
Mental symbolization of the environment	"The wind is crying." "The (flushing) toilet is an angry animal."
Incomplete understanding of sequence of time	Knows names of time components: today, tomorrow, yesterday, minutes, days, weeks, etc., but uses them inconsistently: "I'm not going to take a nap yesterday." Yesterday means any time before now; tomorrow means any time in the future. Historical events are conceptualized in terms of the present: "Mommy, do you know George Washington?"
Developing sense of space: from experiencing space as a part of their activity to moving through it to understanding space in terms of detail and direction	Frequently used words: in, on, up, down, at, under.
Evolving ability to categorize or order objects and phenomena	Early preschooler: no understanding of concept of class or groups; undisturbed to see new Santa Claus on every corner. Cluster phenomena: when asked to sort a series of blocks, the child may cluster a small, medium, and large block as a "baby," "mommy," and "daddy" block. By 4-5 yr, child is able to consistently use one or two categories to arrange objects in some order (color, number, form, or size).
Developing ability to establish causality (realism, animism, artificialism)	*Realism*: Child thinks self to be personally responsible for results; present in infancy. *Animism*: 2- to 3-year-olds think objects possess innate person-like qualities that cause results: "The chair made me fall down." *Artificialism*: 3- to 4-year-olds think things are caused by some controlling force that controls the world.
Transductive reasoning: from particular to particular	If the child does not like one particular vegetable, he or she will not like another particular fruit: "I can't eat my banana because my potatoes are burned."
Developing sense of conservation of quantity, weight, mass	Preschooler is usually unable to conceptualize that change in shape does not affect quantity, weight, or mass of an object. Generally, 50% of 5-year-olds have mastered conservation of quantity and 50% of 6-year-olds have mastered conservation of weight or mass.

Language development through the toddler and preschool years remains one of the most sensitive indicators of cognitive development, and assessment tools plot language ability as a way of measuring cognitive levels. Social development and adaptive or relationship skills are strongly affected by cognitive development and vice versa (Shonkoff & Phillips, 2000). Differentiation of the self from others, with increasing sensitivity not only to the rules and norms for social interaction but also to the perception of the perspectives and feelings of others, requires ever increasing cognitive capability. Finally, quality of play can be used as an indicator of cognitive development. Through play, children manipulate and learn to control their environment in safe yet stimulating ways.

ASSESSMENT OF TODDLERS AND PRESCHOOLERS

Developmental assessment is an essential part of each health maintenance visit and can include both screening and diagnostic testing. Its goal is to monitor the growth and development of the child and determine at an early stage if problems exist. The process begins by building rapport with the parents, encouraging them to share developmental concerns, and listening to their comments with care and attention. Data are collected through parent interview, use of screening or assessment tools, observation of the interactions between child and parents (this can often be more revealing than formal developmental testing), physical examination, and laboratory or other diagnostic measures. In contrast, diagnostic assessments are done when a more individualized approach is required to decide if a developmental problem exists and how to manage it.

Screening

The child's development and progress should be reviewed periodically by the NP in a variety of areas. General screening tools provide a quick, inexpensive method of identifying potential problems. They are generally viewed as appropriate for all children, although culture and experience can affect outcomes and must be taken into consideration. In each area of screening, NPs ask questions directly of the parent, make sure they have understood the parent, and follow up with more probing questions as appropriate to clarify any concerns. Table 7-3 lists a variety of developmental screening

TABLE 7-3 ***Screening Tools for Toddler and Preschoolers***

Screening Tool	Appropriate Age; Screening Time	Characteristics
ASQ: Ages and Stages Questionnaire: A Parent Completed Monitoring System	4-60 mo; 10-20 min	30 individual questions FM, GM, adaptive social/personal
BDI: Battelle Developmental Inventory Screening Test	0-8 yr; 10-15 min	96 standardized items, personal/social, adaptive, motor communication, cognitive
CDI: Child Development Inventories	15 mo-6 yr; 10-20 min	Questions: social, self-help, GM, FM, language, preacademic
DASE: Denver Articulation Screening Exam	2.5-7 yr; 5 min	30 repeated words
DENVER II: Denver Developmental Screening Test	Birth-6 yr; 20-30 min	Standardized items in FM, GM, language, social
ESI-R: The Early Screening Inventory—Revised	3-6 yr; 15-20 min	Parent interview
First STEP: Developmental Profile II	Birth-9.5 yr; 20-40 min	Parent interview Physical, self-help, communication, social academic
HSQ: Home Screening Questionnaire	0-3 and 3-6 yr; 15-20 min	Parent questionnaire, 80 questions on environment
PEDS: Parent's Evaluation of Developmental Status	Birth-8 yr; 2 min	Parent interview with open-ended questions
PDQ-II: The Prescreening Developmental Questionnaire	0-9 mo, 9-24 mo, 2-4 yr, 4-6 yr; 5-10 min	Parent questionnaire, FM, GM, social, language
TABS: Temperament and Atypical Behavior Scale	Birth-6 yr; 15-20 min	Parent interview, 55 questions on detached, hypersensitive/hyperactive, underreactive, dysregulated behaviors
SSP: Short Sensory Profile	Birth-adulthood; 15-20 min	Parental questions in seven areas: tactile sensitive, taste/smell sensitivity, movement, underresponsive, auditory filtering, low energy/weakness, visual/auditory

FM, Fine motor; *GM*, gross motor.

tools, and the Resource Box in Chapter 6 provides information on how to obtain these tools.

Physical Development

Toddlers and preschool children should be screened for certain physical parameters with every well-child check, including anthropomorphic measures and, after age 3, blood pressure. Vision; hearing; dentition; and tuberculosis, lead, and cholesterol screening are recommended at certain ages or for those children at risk (see Chapter 1 for American Academy of Pediatrics [AAP] recommendations for health supervision visits).

The following questions can be used to assess behavior related to physical development:

Question	Purpose/Outcomes/ Goals of Question
Ask how the child usually feels	Invites discussion of somatic issues and complaints
Ask if the child appears similar to other children of the same age	Assesses parent perceptions of physical development; developmental milestones
Ask about bodily functions	Provides parents with provider's framework for systematically assessing child; can be especially helpful for children with a chronic illness
Ask if any illness has interfered with daily activities	Assesses possible chronic medical problem and effects on development
Ask about daily habits: toilet training, sleeping, eating	Assesses parent understanding of readiness, child's cues, changing behaviors, and current status

Motor Skills Development

Toddlers and preschoolers continue to develop and refine their motor skills, driven by curiosity, desire for independence, and endless energy. Gross and fine motor skills are best assessed by standardized screening tests such as the Denver Developmental Screening Tool II.

Fine motor development is evaluated by assessing finger, hand, and oral movements; gross motor skills are evaluated by assessing the child's ability to crawl, sit, walk, run, hop, skip, and climb. The quality of the child's movements during these activities is important to note as well.

The following questions can be used to assess behavior related to motor skills development:

Question	Purpose/Outcomes/ Goals of Question
Ask how the child gets from place to place (e.g., walks, climbs, runs, rides tricycle)	Assesses gross motor skills
Ask how the child feeds self (e.g., cup, bottle, utensils)	Assesses fine motor skills
Ask about play activities	Assesses gross and fine motor skills

Communication and Language Development

Communication is a vital part of being a happy, functioning human being, and assessment of language is important during the early childhood. About 80% of the essential information about language comes from a careful history, only 15% from a physical examination, and the remaining 5% from diagnostic testing. Listening to children and talking with their parents is essential, but the NP should also remember that parents may not be fully sensitive to speech problems because they are accustomed to hearing the child's current speech.

Language screening is divided into expressive and receptive language skills (see Table 6-2). Because language and cognitive skills are intricately interwoven, most intelligence tests have language sections that can be useful in assessing the total child. Expressive language screening places emphasis on articulation and vocabulary. Receptive language looks at comprehension, repetition, and follow-up of language heard (e.g., child's ability to follow directions). Language skills can be screened using tools such as the Early Language Milestones (ELM) test or the Denver Articulation Screening Exam (DASE) (Table 7-4).

The following questions can be used to assess behavior related to communication and speech development:

Question	Purpose/Outcomes/ Goals of Question
Ask how the child communicates needs and desires	Assesses verbal and nonverbal communication strategies, vocabulary, and expressive language
Ask what the child understands	Evaluates cognitive level and receptive language
Ask how the child responds to simple commands; to two- or three-step commands	Evaluates receptive language; evaluates short-term memory, and auditory sequencing
Ask if child uses plurals, pronouns, phrases, and sentences	Indicates increased understanding of more complex structures

TABLE 7-4 Speech and Language Evaluation Tools

Evaluation Tool	Age Assessed and Test Characteristics	Source
Clinical Linguistic and Auditory Milestone test (CLAMS/CAT)	0-36 mo Interview and some observation (Capute et al, 1986) Tests language and problem-solving skills to help clearly identify between the two	Arnold J. Capute Assoc. Professor of Pediatrics Johns Hopkins University School of Medicine E-mail: capute@kennedykrieger.org
Denver Articulation Screening Examination (DASE)	3-6 yr Screens articulation only (not a complete assessment)	Denver Developmental Materials, Inc. 1-800-419-4729
Fluharty Preschool Speech and Language Screening Test	2-6 yr Direct testing Vocabulary, articulation, comprehension, repetition (expressive) (Fluharty, 1974) Riverside Publishing Co.	8420 Bryn Mawr Ave. Chicago, IL 60631 1-800-323-9540
Early Language Milestone Scale (ELM)	0-36 mo Tests visual and auditory receptive, auditory expressive History, testing, observation 3-5 min (Coplan et al, 1982)	Pro-Ed 8700 Shoal Creek Blvd. Austin, TX 78757-6897 1-800-897-3202 1-502-451-3246 *www.proedinc.com*
REEL—Receptive and Expressive Emergent Language	0-36 mo Interview or direct observation of expressive and receptive language	Riverside Publishing Co. 8420 Bryn Mawr Ave. Chicago, IL 60631 1-800-323-9540
Clinical Evaluation of Language Fundamentals—Preschool (CELF)	3-6 yr Assesses receptive and expressive language	The Psychological Corporation (Publisher) 1-800-211-8378 *www.depts.washington.edu/soccomm/tests/celf.html*
Clinical Evaluation of Language Fundamentals—School Age (CELF-3)	6-21 yr Assesses receptive and expressive language	The Psychological Corporation (Publisher) 1-800-211-8378 *www.depts.washington.edu/soccomm/tests/celf.html*
Goldman-Fristoe Test of Articulation	2-16 yr Assesses articulation skills	American Guidance Service Publishing 1-800-328-2560 *www.agsnet.com*
Peabody Picture Vocabulary Test	2.5-40 yr Screens for receptive vocabulary	American Guidance Service Publishing 1-800-328-2560 *www.agsnet.com*

Ask if child is intelligible to adults; to peers	Indicates increased articulation ability

Social and Emotional Development

Assessment of psychosocial and emotional development addresses children's roles in the family, success in making friends and working with peers, self-esteem, and feelings of contentment and security. As previously suggested, social development is related to cognitive development with capacities to "read" situations, interpret the roles and behaviors of others in relation to self, and develop self-control and self-monitoring skills.

The following questions can be used to assess behavior related to psychosocial and emotional development:

Question	Purpose/Outcomes/ Goals of Question
Ask the extent to which the child has developed independence in eating, dressing, and toileting	Assesses adaptive skills, comfort with own abilities
Ask how child acts within family, with other family members	Assesses child's development of roles with the family system; attachment should be evident

Ask how parent guides child's behavior without always saying "No"	Evaluates adaptability, creativity, repertoire of parent's skills in response to child's behaviors
Ask about responses to discipline and limit-setting	Assesses child's understanding of limits of appropriate behavior, social rules, and self-control
Ask about child's reaction to strangers and new vs. familiar situations	Evaluates child's ability to deal with increasingly complex social situations
Ask about tantrum behavior	Evaluates responses to stress, development of independence, and social control
Ask what child does for play	Indicates social and emotional well-being
Ask how child acts around peers	Considers social development with peers and development of appropriate play
Ask about friends' names and shared activities	Indicates child is developing social circle and increasing opportunities for practicing new social skills
Ask if the child seems to understand the feelings of others	Assesses empathy
Ask about child's fears and how parent manages them	Evaluates parents' responses to child's emotional stresses and understanding of child's view and feelings
Ask about imaginary friends and fantasy	Allows child to explore emotions and developing roles in a safe way

Cognitive Development

Cognitive development is primarily expressed through motor activities in children younger than 2 years of age (Piaget's sensorimotor stage). After age 2, the child begins to use symbol systems and language as thinking moves into the preconceptual stages. The following questions can be used to assess behavior related to cognitive development:

Questions Asked of 1- to 3-year-olds	Purpose/Outcomes/ Goals of Questions
Ask about typical day: with whom does child play, in what type of activities does child engage	Assesses complexity of manipulation of objects, parallel and cooperative play, role-playing
Ask name, age, gender	Three-year-olds should know beginning facts
Ask about ability to follow simple instructions	Assesses ability to retain and process instructions and respond to input
Ask about language development, both receptive and expressive	Assesses progress in decoding, encoding, and using a language system effectively
Ask about nature of interaction with family members, peers, and others	Indicates understanding of social systems and norms

Questions Asked of 4- to 5-year-olds	Purpose/Outcomes/ Goals of Questions
Ask general information questions (e.g., colors, numbering objects)	Assesses general fund of knowledge
Ask what makes the sun come up	Illustrates child's belief about causality
Ask about concepts of time	Assesses understanding of a relatively sophisticated concept
Ask about spontaneous play (e.g., with puppets or dolls), imaginative use of play materials (e.g., clay, crayons, other toys)	Assesses imagination and magical thinking
Ask child to draw a person	50% of 4-year-olds draw a three-part person; by 5 years of age, child can draw an eight-part person
Ask about involvement in preschool, how child behaves when there	Assesses language, social, and play development in relation to peers in a setting where expectations differ from those at home

Diagnostic Assessment

Once a child has been identified through screening to have a possible problem, more definitive diagnostic testing or referral to an appropriate specialist is necessary. Some diagnostic assessment tools commonly used in this age-group are listed in the Resource Boxes in Chapter 6.

ANTICIPATORY GUIDANCE FOR TODDLERS AND PRESCHOOLERS

Anticipatory guidance for toddlers and preschoolers is directed at helping parents and children transition from a highly dependent relationship to one in which the child has established a sense of autonomy with an evolving understanding of the self as a separate, creative, and powerful being. In addition, parents learn new skills of communicating and interacting with their children. The toddler and preschool years can be frustrating at times, but the ultimate outcome of good communication and relationships that support the potential of both child and parent is worth the effort. NPs can offer anticipatory guidance in all areas of growth.

Regulation and Sleep/Wake Patterns

- Discuss the need to assist toddlers and preschoolers to transition from one state to another. Use of a comfort object (e.g., teddy bear), as well as consistent schedules and rituals (e.g., bedtime) can help.
- Explain that children's ability to process information and control themselves at this age can be overwhelmed if they have too much stimulation.
- Explain that some children may have sensory integration problems that require even more modulation of their environment.
- Discuss how to help children identify and name their feelings. This ability will help them to more successfully organize and integrate the sensations they are experiencing and respond appropriately (Brazelton & Sparrow, 2001).
- Encourage parents to provide opportunities for children to have some control in daily activities (e.g., can select the story to be read at bedtime), while maintaining important rituals.
- Discuss sleep problems that may appear at this time, including sleep resistance, bruxism, nightmares, and somnabulism (see Chapter 16).
- Encourage parents to provide naps if necessary, but not to force them on children.

Strength and Motor Coordination

- Discuss the importance of play as a way for toddlers and preschoolers to practice their developing physical, social, and emotional skills.
- Encourage parents to provide their children with a variety of play activities that use both fine and gross motor skills, such as the following:
  - Take children to a park to run, throw balls, play on the swing set, and roll on the grass.
  - Provide children with pencils, crayons, paper, paints, utensils, blocks, and Legos.
- Explain how parents can incorporate practice of motor skills into daily routines (e.g., have child help pour the milk, hold the cup, or squeeze the toothpaste; encourage child to do own buttons, snaps, and zippers).
- Emphasize the need for constant adult supervision of children's activities.
- Discuss how parents can make the environment safer for their child: securing doors and windows; removing toxic substances and dangerous objects; providing toys that are developmentally appropriate and safely constructed.
- Reinforce teaching about car seat use and explain to parent need for larger car seats and booster seats.

Feeding and Self-Care

- Provide parents with information about healthy foods and nutritional needs of their child (see Chapter 12). Three meals and two nutritious snacks per day are encouraged, if possible.
- Discuss parents' responsibility to provide their children with healthy foods and to allow children to make choices among healthy food options. Young children may go on "food jags," refusing some foods or requesting the same food day after day. Parents need to make sure the food eaten is nutritious.
- Explain how changes in toddlers' eating habits are caused by developmental changes (e.g., child has a decrease in appetite, is easily distracted, demonstrates more curiosity about what is going on around him or her than in eating, is more interested in using gross motor skills than in sitting still).
- Explain nonnutritive value of food and eating (e.g., finger foods stimulate fine motor and cognitive development, as well as child's sense of control and independence; eating together as a family can strengthen relationships and develop social skills).
- Encourage self-feeding to help child gain new skills.
- Encourage parents to structure family meal times that are pleasant and interactive; this may mean offering the toddler foods that can be eaten in short periods of sitting. Avoid making meals a power struggle.
- Discuss weaning (if not already done by 12 months).
- Explain the importance of the child gaining mastery of self-care (e.g., toileting, bathing, dressing) and the valuable role the parent plays as teacher in the process. Assist parents to cope with the frustration or tensions generated by toddlers and preschoolers wanting to "do it myself!"

Communication and Language

Encourage parents to stimulate their child's language skills by doing the following:

- Reading to children daily, using short, simple stories or picture books (see information on Reach Out and Read [ROAR] program in Resource Box, Chapter 6)
- Modeling appropriate language
- Talking to their child, explaining in clear, simple language what is happening around the child; this helps increase vocabulary and the child's understanding of the world
- Listening with care and responding actively to the child's verbalizations
- Providing the child with opportunities to interact verbally with other children and adults
- Explaining to parents that children need constant reinforcement of their speech and language efforts, but that nonverbal language, especially touch, continues to be crucial
- Giving parents an opportunity to explain their expectations for their child; discouraging parental pressure on child to perform (e.g., use of flash cards, requirement that child articulate sounds correctly), but pointing out that daily activities provide a wealth of opportunities to practice language skills
- Reassuring parents that language errors of young children will usually disappear as the child grows, and that reading to, listening to, and talking interactively with the child are the best ways to learn
- Instructing parents that children learn receptive language first, then expressive; and that children may not fully understand the meaning, especially connotative meaning, of what they are hearing or saying (e.g., a 4-year-old may innocently use a swear word picked up at preschool); parents should explain clearly, simply, and unemotionally which words are appropriate and in which settings
- Having parents limit television viewing to 1 to 2 hours or less of appropriate programs per day

Social and Emotional Growth

The emotional development of toddlers is an area in which parents may need a great deal of anticipatory guidance and support. The balance between dependence and independence is constantly in flux for toddlers and their parents, and conflict can develop as a result of inconsistent and extreme behavior. "Behavior around others is comprised of the quality of relationships, social skills and emotional development, temperament, family discipline, biologically determined behavioral disposition, and contextual stresses and supports. Controlling emotional states, including delayed gratification, and tolerating frustration, separations, and fears without breaking down emotionally, are lifelong tasks that should be mastered during the toddler and preschool period" (Sturner & Howard, 1997b, p. 328). In helping families with this process, NPs should do the following:

- Reemphasize the role of parents in guiding their child's social and emotional growth. Parents must actively engage with their children, showing interest in their activities and giving them instruction on appropriate behavior (see Table 6-3).
- Encourage parents to give their children opportunities to expand social skills and form important attachments outside the immediate family by doing the following:
    - Providing toys that the child can use creatively
    - Allowing children to explore, guiding them to activities that are fun
    - Allowing child to make choices when possible; do not give child a "choice" when there really is none (e.g., "Do you want to go to bed?")
    - Discussing differences among people openly and positively
    - Helping child identify, name, and express feelings, both positive and negative
    - Teaching the child to manage anger and resolve conflicts without violence
    - Discussing television programs and movies to help children distinguish fantasy from reality
    - Taking children on trips to places of interest in the community
    - Arranging play times with other children; encouraging cooperative play (e.g., tag, hide-and-seek)
    - Reinforcing positive child behavior ("catching the child being good")
    - Making the limits of what is expected of the child clear and able to be achieved; try for consistency
- Discuss parenting and discipline (see Chapters 5 and 18).
- Clarify each parent's expectations of child's behavior.
- Discuss how parents plan to resolve differences in expectations.
- Differentiate discipline and teaching from punishment.
- Provide information to parents related to child development and what parents can expect their child to be able to do. Recommend parenting classes that provide information on developmental milestones, anticipated changes, and management strategies as children grow.
- Encourage parents to show affection in the family.

- Explain to parents that myths or fables can be important ways of teaching children abstract concepts such as love, sharing, and giving.
- Instruct parents on the need to provide a feeling of safety and security for children. Parents can do the following:
  - Support use of comfort or transitional objects to allay fears (e.g., blanket, toy)
  - Consider use of a night light
  - Provide reassurance if nightmares or fears occur; respond to child's fears
  - Explain about "good" and "bad" touches to private parts
  - Reinforce that the child can always come to parent for comfort

Cognitive and Environmental Stimulation

- Explain to parents that toddlers and preschoolers are concrete and preoperational in their thinking. As a result, parents need to be ready to explain things over and over patiently, without expecting the child to understand the adult's interpretation clearly. Also, children may use words to convey thoughts and feelings, but many responses are repetitive and trial-and-error problem solving is usually crude. They frequently attend to only one aspect of a problem, giving partial answers.
- Emphasize that parents should avoid putting their own meaning on the child's behavior or statements. For example, the child's statement, "What if you just bought a new house, and I was allergic to something in the house? I guess you'd have to get rid of me," should not be interpreted to mean the parents have somehow failed to show the child how much they love him or her. Rather, the child can be exploring the concepts of place, ownership, belonging, size, or importance. In the child's mind, a house is much bigger than he or she is and may be more important. An appropriate response from the parent might be, "No, we'd probably have to get a new house or take out whatever you are allergic to. Even if we just bought it, you are more important than any house, and we wouldn't want to lose you."
- Reassure parents that "Why?" will not always be the child's most frequent question. Toddlers and preschoolers are actively exploring meaning in their world, and have learned that asking "Why?" brings them more information—as well as attention. As parents answer them, children begin to show threads of symbolic and more abstract thought.

COMMON DEVELOPMENTAL ISSUES FOR TODDLERS AND PRESCHOOLERS

Temper Tantrums

Description

Temper tantrums are episodes in which the child is frustrated and angry and loses control of his or her feelings. The tantrum may be as mild as whining and pouting, or it may be a full-blown display of crying, yelling, flinging oneself on the floor, kicking, and screaming. About 5% of children hold their breath until they pass out (Sturner & Howard, 1997b).

Incidence and Etiology

Temper tantrums are common, with as many as 50% to 80% of children experiencing them; they usually peak at about 18 to 28 months. Tantrums stem from the child's striving for power and control and the sudden loss of both. There are so many activities that toddlers want and struggle to do, but are not developmentally ready to perform. Being tired or hungry exacerbates the frustration children can feel when their wishes are thwarted.

Management

Ultimately, children will learn how to regulate the self, to identify a feeling and manage the actions appropriately to that feeling, and will thus "outgrow" the temper tantrums of toddlers. Management, therefore, means helping children master self-regulation and learn that there are better ways to handle frustration; this is a process that requires parents to engage in many of the interactions discussed earlier in this chapter (see Anticipatory Guidance for Toddlers and Preschoolers). Management also requires that parents deal with the immediate event of the tantrum itself. Some parents are aghast that their child would show such a violent display of emotions; others can be frightened. Parents' responses usually depend on their comfort level. Some parents go to the child and hold, comfort, and distract him or her; some remove the child from the stimulation of the moment, putting him or her in "time out"; and some physically restrain the child in a "bear hug" until the crying and thrashing about behavior subsides. Generally, the most effective measures are thought to be the following:

- Ignore the child's behavior (give no physical or eye contact).
- Ensure that the child is safe and will not be injured.

Prevention

NPs can prepare parents for the possibility of temper tantrums by discussing them at the 12-month visit. They should describe the developmental stages the child will be progressing through (autonomy, independence, and preoperational thinking) and explain how those stages can contribute to high levels of frustration for the child. When parents understand the dynamics of tantrums, they can minimize the likelihood that they will occur. Parents can do this by not putting children in positions that they cannot easily handle, providing support for the child or redirecting the child early in the emotional cycle if frustration appears to be building, and making sure that external factors (e.g., hunger, sleepiness) are managed well. NPs should also give parents an opportunity to discuss how they would like to handle the tantrum should it come. Parents should be counseled to avoid hitting or spanking the child because it only teaches the child that hitting is permitted if you are an adult and when emotions are high, and the hitting can quickly escalate to abuse.

Child Care and Preschools

Many parents return to work during the first year of their child's life and must make arrangements for child care. In 1999 more than 64% of mothers with preschool-age children and 60% of mothers whose youngest child was under 2 years of age were working outside the home (House Ways and Means Committee, 2002). By 2001 approximately 56% of 3- to 5-year-olds participated in "center-based" early childhood care, such as Head Start, preschool, and nursery schools (Wirt & Livingston, 2002). Many other children are in day care settings. Table 19-9 outlines important criteria for parents to consider when making choices about day care placement.

Entering a setting outside the home that has a teacher, curriculum, and learning expectations can be a stressful experience. Suddenly parents find their child compared to 20 other children. A child with developmental delays (e.g., speech, motor, physical) may be singled out as different, not fitting in, or a behavior problem. Preschool and kindergarten was originally intended to help the child learn separation, sharing, listening, paying attention, and some simple social skills. But curriculum planning has changed over the years and kindergarten children are expected to show preacademic skills such as writing, counting, and letter and word recognition, as well as the preschool social skills of paying attention and sitting still.

School readiness criteria are outlined in Table 8-6. Parents can make more appropriate decisions about their child's ability to handle the demands of a structured preschool setting by considering school readiness factors, as well as the following points:

- Social skills (e.g., ability to separate from parent for several hours)
- Language skills, both expressive and receptive
- Physical size of the child
- Energy level of child (e.g., able to participate actively)
- Neurologic maturation required for fine and gross motor activities (e.g., writing, cutting, coloring, climbing, running, walking)
- Neurologic maturation of sensory and cognitive function (e.g., visuospatial perception, tactile maturation, auditory processing, attending skills, memory)

Toileting

Toileting skills and training are a major milestone for a child and the parents. It is a complex developmental skill that many children master effortlessly, but some children and families need guidance and support along the way (see Chapter 14).

Safety

As children grow and develop, their world expands and exposes them to ever increasing dangers. Safety should be a topic of every well-child visit and needs to be addressed from the developmental age of the child. Toddlers are not to be trusted, even for a moment, but it is easier to monitor their environment because it is generally restricted to the house, the yard, or the parent's side. For preschoolers the world is bigger and more dangerous and includes the house, the yard, the neighborhood, the preschool, and traveling (e.g., car, bike, scooters). See Chapter 11 for a discussion of causes and management of unintentional injuries.

RED FLAGS FOR TODDLERS AND PRESCHOOLERS

Although a wide range of normal development may be seen when assessing children, the NP needs to be alert to developmental red flags, signs of delayed or abnormal development. In addition to obvious abnormalities, minor problems that are left untreated can develop into major concerns; minor signs and symptoms that persist can indicate a more serious underlying problem; or a major problem can occur as a one-time event (e.g., child who sets a fire). Some children and families are at high risk and need careful monitoring and guidance to detect problems at an early stage or to prevent their occurrence (e.g., very early premature infants, families with history of violence, families with chronic medical or mental health problems, some single-parent families). The warning signs, or red flags, can be found in Table 7-5. Children who demonstrate these behaviors should be referred. Immediate referral is required for children who stop eating, demonstrate cruelty to animals or other people, are self-harmful, start fires, or talk of harming themselves, their peers, or others.

Physical Disorders

Physically, children should be monitored for missing or delayed milestones. Most growth or milestone charts give a range that is normal, and when the child falls outside that limit, there should be investigation, screening, and referral, if appropriate. When children are following a normal progression for weight and begin to level off or fall below that range, it should not be ignored. If a child begins to have symptoms—stops eating, complains of tiredness, is not as active as usual, or the parents state that the child has regressed—it is time to investigate.

Cognitive Disorders

Mental and cognitive delays are more difficult to recognize and categorize without the help of a screening tool or more in-depth assessment. These tools rank children on the basis of a standardized score or against standardized criteria (e.g., word definition). Children with scores below 85 on intelligence scales, for example, predictably have more difficulty in school. Significant discrepancies between test scores taken over time also suggest problems. The causes of delay must be carefully assessed as well, because some children may have a neurologic limitation, whereas others may be delayed as a result of material or environmental deprivation. Identifying the causes can help providers plan effective interventions.

Language Disorders

Description

Language delays or disorders are problems in learning the systems of communication and, when present, can affect other areas of development, especially social and emotional development. Children with language delays have delays in receptive and expressive language. They can start saying words late, talk very little as toddlers, and have prolonged stages of normal stuttering, distortion, and substitution.

Etiology

Language delays are caused by cognitive, familial, environmental, or cultural factors. Because language development is the best indicator of cognitive development, language delays can reflect serious issues needing developmental and educational intervention. Language delays or disorders may occur if the child does not hear, is not immersed in a language-rich environment, or has a psychologic disorder such as severe deprivation or autism. Speech disorders, in particular, are often associated with physical problems (e.g., cleft lip, cleft palate, cerebral palsy, hearing impairments), or they can be idiopathic.

Assessment

Language evaluation must involve assessment of the total child, including physical, cognitive, social, emotional, and perceptual characteristics. Both expressive and receptive language must be evaluated.

Findings Related to Expressive Skills

The inability to use the symbols of language may be characterized by the following:

- Improper use of words and their meanings
- Inappropriate grammatical patterns
- Improper use of speech sounds
- Speech disorders involve problems producing correct speech sounds and may be characterized by difficulty in the following:
  - Producing speech sounds (articulation)
  - Maintaining speech rhythm (fluent speech)
  - Controlling vocal production (voice)

Management

Management of children with language disorders requires a clear understanding of the nature of the problem and referral to a specialist (e.g., pediatric speech pathologist) to make that determination is often the first step. Deficits identified in Table 7-5 are cause for referral for additional testing. Other criteria that warrant referral include the following:

- There is excessive, indiscriminate, irrelevant verbalizing after age 18 months.
- The child is not talking by age 2 years.
- There is consistent and frequent omission of initial consonants, which are generally mastered by early in the second year; the child uses mostly vowel sounds after 1 year.
- Sentence structure is consistently faulty after age 5 years.
- There are many substitutions of easy sounds for difficult ones after age 5 years.
- Word endings are consistently dropped after age 5 years.
- There are unusual confusions, reversals, or telescoping in connected speech.
- There is a loss of previously acquired language skills.
- The child stops talking.
- The child reacts to his or her own speech with embarrassment or withdrawal.

TABLE 7-5 *Red Flags of Development: Toddlers and Preschoolers*

Age	Growth/Rhythmicity/ Sleep/Temperament	Psychosocial/ Emotional Skills	Cognitive and Visual Abilities	Language and Hearing	Fine Motor/Feeding/ Self-Care	Gross Motor/Strength/ Coordination
15 mo	No nighttime ritual Difficulty with transitions Parents express concern about temperament or control issues	Problems with attachment to caregiver	Lack of object permanence	Lack of consonant production Does not imitate words No gestures/pointing	No self-feeding	No attempts at walking
18 mo	Poor sleep schedule Problems with control/ behavior	Does not pull person to show something	Primary play: mouthing of toys No finger exploration of objects Lack of imitation	Unable to follow simple directions (e.g., "no," "jump")	Does not try to scribble spontaneously Unable to use spoon	Not yet walking or frequently falls when walking
24 mo (2 yr)	Less than 4 times birth weight or falling off growth curve Poor sleep schedule Awakens at night; unable to put self back to sleep	Absent symbolic play No evidence of parallel play Displays destructive behaviors Always clings to mother		Use of noncom-municative speech (echolalia, rote phrases) Unable to identify five pictures Unable to name body parts No jargon History of >10 episodes of otitis media	Unable to stack four to five blocks Still eating pureed foods Unable to imitate scribbles on paper Unable to dump pellet from bottle	Unable to walk downstairs holding a rail Persistent waddle walk Persistent toe-walking
30 mo	Resistance to regular bedtime Beginning behavior issues	Problems with biting, hitting playmates, parents	Does not try to get toy with stick	No two-word sentences Unable to name some body parts	Unable to feed self Unable to tower six blocks Unable to imitate circle shape Unable to imitate vertical stroke	Unable to jump in place Unable to kick ball on request
36 mo (3 yr)	Problems with toilet training Unable to calm self	Not able to dress self Does not understand taking turns		Unable to give full name Unable to match two colors Does not use plurals Does not know two to three prepositions Unable to tell a story Unclear consonants Unintelligible speech Unable to construct a sentence	Unable to build a tower of 10 blocks Holds crayon with fist Unable to draw circle	Unable to balance on one foot for 1 sec Toeing in causes tripping with running

48 mo (4 yr)	Lack of bedtime ritual Behavior concerns: withdrawn or acting out Stool holding Problems with toilet training	Unable to play games, follow rules Unable to follow limits/rules at home (e.g., put toys away) Cruelty to animals, friends Interest in fires, fire starting Persistent fears or severe shyness Inability to separate from mother	Unable to count three objects Unable to recall four numbers Unable to identify what to do in danger, fire, with a stranger Consistently poor judgment	Difficulty understanding language Problems understanding prepositions Limited vocabulary Unclear speech	Lack of self-care skills—dressing, feeding Unable to button clothes Unable to copy square	Unable to balance on one foot for 4 sec Unable to alternate steps when climbing stairs
60 mo (5 yr)	Continued sleep problems Concerns with night terrors Hair pulling—scalp or eyelashes	Difficulty making and keeping friends; no friends Difficulty understanding sharing, school rules, organization of daily activities Cruelty to animals, friends Interest in fires, fire starting Bullying or being bullied Prolonged fighting, hitting, hurting Withdrawal, sadness, extreme rituals	Unable to count to 10 Unable to identify colors Difficulty following three-step command	Speech pattern not 100% understandable Cannot identify a penny, nickel, or dime Abnormal rate or rhythm of speech	Unable to copy triangle Unable to draw a person with a body	Difficulty hopping, jumping

- The child's voice is monotone, extremely loud, largely inaudible, or of poor quality.
- Pitch is not appropriate to the child's age and gender.
- Hypernasality or lack of nasal resonance occurs.

SUMMARY

Child development has been compared to a rose stem: an elegant spiral with smooth parts and thorns, the positive with the negative, the stressful with the placid. By monitoring children over time, both parents and providers learn that children have ups and downs as they develop. The "terrible twos" are followed by the "terrific threes," the "fierce fours" by the "fantastic fives." Normal growth and development changes happen with the parent's presence and guidance. Deviations, delays, and voids need to be assessed, monitored, and managed to foster optimal growth and achieve the goal of a functional, happy, productive adult. Participating in the process of his or her child's growth can be one of a parent's treasures. Having the support of an NP can make it easier and smoother.

REFERENCES

Brazelton TB, Sparrow JD: *Touchpoints three to six, your child's emotional and behavioral development*, Cambridge, MA, 2001, Perseus Publishing.

Capute AJ et al: The Clinical Linguistic and Auditory Milestone Scale (CLAMS): identification of cognitive defects in motor-delayed children, *Am J Dis Child* 140:694-698, 1986.

Chiocca E: Language development in bilingual children, *Pediatr Nurs* 24:43-47, 1998.

Coplan J et al: Validation of an early language milestone scale in a high-risk population, *Pediatrics* 70: 677-683, 1982.

Dixon S, Stein M: *Encounters with children: pediatric behavior and development*, St Louis, 2000, Mosby.

Farver J, Shin Y: Social pretend play in Korean- and Anglo-American preschoolers, *Child Dev* 68:544-556, 1997.

Fluharty NB: The design and standardization of a speech and language screening test for use with preschool children, *J Speech Hear Disord* 39:75-88, 1974

House Ways and Means Committee: *Child care. Green book. Almanac of policy issues*, Washington, DC, 2002, US House of Representatives.

Kranowitz CS: *The out-of-sync child: recognizing and coping with sensory integration dysfunction*, New York, 1998, Peerigee.

Murray L, Cooper P: Postpartum depression and child development, *Psychol Med* 27:253-260, 1997.

Shonkoff JP, Phillips DA, editors: *From neurons to neighborhoods: the science of early childhood development*, Washington, DC, 2000, National Academy Press.

Sturner R, Howard B: Preschool development. I. Communicative and motor aspects, *Pediatr Rev* 18:291-301, 1997a.

Sturner R, Howard B: Preschool development. II. Psychosocial/behavioral development, *Pediatr Rev* 18:327-336, 1997b.

Wirt J, Livingston A: *The condition of education 2002 in brief*, NCES 2002-011, Washington, DC, 2002, US Department of Eduction, National Center for Eduction Statistics.

8

Developmental Management of School-Age Children

Barbara Jones Deloian,
Bonnie Gance-Cleveland

School-age children are busy, active, curious, and creative. With guidance and encouragement, they eagerly apply the skills they learned as toddlers and preschoolers as they move into more structured school, home school, or community settings. Their physical abilities advance and they may join organized sports activities, as well as engage in casual play with friends or siblings. Cognitively and emotionally, school-age children face daunting challenges. They must master the intellectual skills of reading, writing, mathematics, science, and other academic work. They are also expected to become skilled socially, separating from home and family, establishing friendships, negotiating with siblings and other family members, and working on developing a sound sense of who they are as unique members of the community.

School-age children pass through several phases on their way from preschool innocence to the complexity of adolescence. The school-age years can be divided into early childhood (5 to 7 years), middle childhood (8 to 10 years), and late childhood (11 to 12 years) (Dixon & Stein, 2000). Children in each of these phases demonstrate different developmental goals and achievements. Each school-age child is unique, and patterns of "normal" development have broad parameters. The goals of school-age children's development include laying the groundwork for achievement, creating a sense of self-worth, developing the ability to contribute to the group, and, ultimately, gaining satisfaction with life.

Nurse practitioners (NPs) must be familiar with theoretic models of psychosocial development in this age-group, as well as the physical parameters of growth. Parents often turn to their health care provider for understanding and guidance. Some authors have characterized the school-age period as one of quiescence, but a remarkable amount of growth takes place and the route is not always smooth. NPs can support children and their families to successfully achieve during these important years.

DEVELOPMENT OF SCHOOL-AGE CHILDREN

Physical Development

School-age children gain strength and coordination and become more physically capable, setting the stage for participation in sports, dance, gymnastics, and other activities. Social status among children is often based on physical competence; therefore the child's feelings about physical development can be as important as the physical growth itself.

The rate of growth of school-age children increases significantly from that of the toddler and preschooler and occurs in "spurts." The child can literally "grow out of his or her clothes" in a matter of weeks (see Table 12-8). The best way to evaluate an individual child's growth is to monitor his or her progress for height, weight, and body mass index (BMI) on a growth chart. Head circumference increases slowly. By middle childhood the brain is about 90% of its adult size. Full adult size is reached by about age 12 years. Myelination of the brain, which is responsible for information processing, is not complete until early adulthood. The cerebral cortex (responsible for intelligence) and the frontal lobe (responsible for problem solving and decision making) are the last to develop. The increasing maturation of the brain allows children to complete increasingly complex skills and have greater control over their bodies (Shonkoff & Phillips, 2000) (see Chapter 28). Organ development is complete. Usually school-age children have decreased fat; however, recent national data indicate that in 1999 and 2000, 15.3% of children 6 to 11 years old were overweight, and 11.1% of children between 6 and 18 years old were obese (Ogden et al, 2002; Wang, 2001). Most middle childhood children sleep about 12 hours per night (range 8 to 14 hours) without naps, particularly during the school year. Night terrors or sleepwalking may emerge (see Chapter 16).

A comprehensive discussion of the physical growth of school-age children can be found in general pediatric texts. The following section looks briefly at significant changes in body systems; discussion of the health issues and disease processes related to these systems can be found in Units 3 and 4 of this text.

Skin and Lymph

The lymphatic system is at its peak of development. Tonsils and adenoids are their largest at around 6 years of age and then later atrophy. Few skin changes are noted until children reach prepubescence, when the sebaceous glands become more active. Uncontrollable blushing caused by vasomotor instability may be a concern with the transition to early adolescence.

Head, Eyes, Ears, Nose, and Mouth

By early childhood the head becomes smaller in proportion to the rest of the body. Head trauma continues to be a significant risk, and helmets and choices in sporting activities should be discussed with parents (see Chapter 15 for guidance in choosing sports activities for different age-groups).

The sinus cavities are not fully developed and are highly sensitive to exposure to smoke, allergens, and infections. Frequent upper respiratory infections or sinus headaches can affect the overall well-being of the child and his or her ability to attend to the tasks of childhood.

During middle childhood, visual acuity changes from farsighted (hyperopic) to 20/20 or normal. The fovea of the retina is fully developed by 6 to 7 years of age; until this occurs, a child may need large-print books to see well at a close distance. Discriminating between letters such as d, b, p, and q is also much easier in larger letters. In middle childhood, a child is much more able to see individual objects in a complex background; this allows for an extended discriminatory attention span and less distractibility. Poor control of eye movements or vision may go undetected because the child does not recognize that there is a problem. Therefore vision screening is important at this age.

The eustachian tube grows longer, narrower, and more slanted during middle childhood. Some children develop hearing defects caused by chronic ear infections, and screening for hearing is critical during middle childhood. Hearing and language are closely correlated as children gain an ability to discriminate differences in sounds and voice pitch. They also duplicate phonetic sounds and understand the translation of these sounds. Learning a second language at this time is much easier than during adulthood, but not as easy as in the toddler and preschool years.

The first primary teeth are shed and the first permanent teeth erupt between 5 and 6 years of age, starting with the central incisors. After this, approximately four teeth per year are replaced, one set in the lower jaw and one set in the upper. Malocclusion can be noted in middle childhood when the upper and lower teeth do not meet properly horizontally or vertically. Significant problems may cause concerns with appearance, chewing, or speech. Crossbite may also be noted when lower teeth cross over the upper teeth when the mouth is closed. This necessitates early orthodontia before the bones of the maxilla are fused (see Chapter 34 for in-depth discussion).

Respiratory

Overall body growth and maturation provide the foundation for the increased efficiency and maturation of the respiratory system. The lungs gradually descend into the thoracic cavity, and alveolar development is complete at about 8 years of age. The tidal volume increases during middle childhood, allowing for an increase in physical activities. The increase in lung growth also results in more adultlike breath sounds with a rate of 18 to 30 breaths per minute.

Cardiovascular

By 5 years of age, the heart is four times larger than at birth, allowing for greater resilience and tolerance for activity. By 7 years of age, the left ventricle thickens and the overall muscle mass is two to three times greater than the right ventricle. Blood pressure increases to 90/60 to 108/60 mm Hg. Cardiac volume continues to increase, and although the heart rate varies with each child's age, gender, size, and activity level, it declines gradually to 60 to 100 beats per minute.

Gastrointestinal

The gastrointestinal system of the school-age child has matured but is susceptible to the interplay of both hereditary and environmental factors. Symptomatic complaints such as stomachaches, diarrhea, and constipation are common and require a sensitive evaluation of both physical and psychosocial factors. By middle childhood, the digestive system is of adult size and functioning. Drinking sufficient water and eating adequate amounts of fiber are important to prevent problems of constipation. Stools are usually passed once or twice a day and well formed.

Genitourinary

By 6 years of age, urinary elimination patterns are established for more than 90% of children. The bladder capacity expands and neurologic function matures, so most children stay dry during the day with only occasional enuresis. Continuing nocturnal enuresis should be thoroughly evaluated. Encopresis or enuresis can be problematic for some children (as many as 5% to 10% of children in middle childhood). By late childhood these issues should be resolving and if not, a thorough evaluation should be completed (see Chapter14).

Puberty usually begins during late childhood, between ages 10 and 12 years for girls and 11 and 14 years for boys, but can be normal for either sex at any time after age 8. Some children have no evidence of secondary sexual characteristics (e.g., axillary perspiration, breast budding) at all during late childhood, which can be within normal limits. Stronger personality traits (including aggression in boys), feelings, and moods may be noted as bodily changes begin to appear.

Musculoskeletal

Throughout childhood the skeletal system develops as the epiphyses of the bones grow, become thinner, and eventually disappear or "fuse." At this point, no further skeletal growth can occur. Bone age can be estimated by using x-rays to determine how many epiphyses are fused. During childhood, the spine becomes straighter, even though posture may be worse. Legs become straighter, often correcting knock-knee, toeing-in, or toeing-out deformities. The school-age child's bones are still immature, and fractures of the growth plate can easily occur. Facial bones are actively changing, particularly with growth of the nasal accessory sinuses.

Immune System

The immune system matures rapidly during middle childhood, though there is a high incidence of infections during the first years of school due to an increased number of exposures to sick children and poor hygiene. By late childhood the maturity of the immune system and the body's ability to localize infection has improved. Allergic conditions may become more common and severe.

Motor Skills Development

In middle childhood, gross motor skills continue to be refined, allowing children to run, jump, climb, hop, skip, tandem walk, alternate their foot patterns, and use an overhand motion. Activities that require balance and coordination such as riding a bicycle, swimming, and roller skating demonstrate children's expanding skills. In late childhood, gross motor skills become more controlled and purposeful. Skills are perfected with much practice. A sense of competition is high as children try to outlast or outperform one another.

Mastery of fine motor skills includes finer dexterity and better control of scissors and writing tools such as crayons and pencils. In early childhood, children become adept at dressing themselves, including being able to tie knots and manage buttons and zippers. Their drawings become more recognizable, showing details of eyes, ears, and other body parts. Self-care skills (e.g., combing hair, brushing teeth) are also improved. In late childhood, hand-eye coordination improves and the child is able to use each hand independently with speed and smoothness. During this time, skill in playing musical instruments emerges.

Communication and Language Development

The child's language patterns provide insight into the status of the neurologic system, as the maturing brain is capable of increasingly complex language skills. Both receptive and expressive language skills improve. Six-year-olds have a well-developed vocabulary and are able to retrieve words quickly. They have simple syntactic abilities and can follow simple directions. The language demands of school can be challenging for 6-year-olds. First, they may not be accustomed to attending to total auditory stimuli as in the classroom environment. Second, they are still mastering connotative and semantic skills such as understanding the concepts "before" and "after," relative clauses (e.g., "the cat was chased by the dog"), and the structures of sentences. These factors can make it difficult for them to follow complicated directions or cope with the increased demand to recall information within a specific time frame. Narrative skills can be poor and reading may be difficult. The expressive language of 6-year-olds should be fully intelligible. Stuttering has usually resolved by school age, but may be seen if young children are overly eager to express themselves. Stuttering should be ignored at this age.

Seven-year-olds' receptive language is strong; they generally have language decoding mastered and are working on encoding information. They can use previous knowledge, organize it, and verbally express or write it down.

They are able to solve word problems. Expressively, mastery of articulation may not be achieved until 7 or 8 years of age with the sounds of l and th.

Eight- to 9-year-olds have had significant syntactic growth and demonstrate better use of pronouns, allowing them to understand convoluted sentences. Comparatives are learned, and the child is able to distinguish qualities such as more/less, near/far, and heavy/light. By age 8 years, children can follow complex directions. They are beginning to tell jokes because they understand different meanings of words. In their expressive language, children have better narrative abilities and significantly improved storytelling and summarization skills needed for such activities as explaining a task to other children. Vocabulary grows, and there are gradual improvements in grammar (e.g., noted by the use of past and future tenses and plural forms of nouns, particularly irregular nouns and verbs).

At 10 years of age, children are able to discuss ideas and understand inflections and metaphors. Their ability to understand these ambiguities of sentence structure, word meaning, and language contributes to their increasing ability to enjoy jokes and riddles. Using concrete operational thinking, they can also analyze and interpret language and become more aware of the inconsistency in spoken languages. Children in late childhood understand that the literal meaning of words may not be the only meaning. By age 12 years, children should be able to answer questions involving sophisticated concepts. Expressively, their sentences should be grammatically correct and they have more detail in their verbal skills. The ability to express emotions also develops. Language has become a means of socializing, and fewer gestures are used. Language can become a game as children make up words and participate in story telling using proper sequence and pronouns.

Social and Emotional Development

Theories

Psychosocial theories of development illustrate many critical tasks for school-age children, who are in the process of learning to interact with and master their environment. The stages through which children progress as they become more socially and emotionally mature are sequential and have been built on since birth, with each being a prerequisite for the next (Table 8-1) (see Table 5-1 and discussion in Chapter 5 on theoretic models of development).

In Freud's theory, school-age children (6 to 11 years old) are in the latency period. In this stage, sexual urges are submerged and energy can be put into acquiring cultural skills and forming friendships.

Erikson posited that school-age children are in the stage of industry versus inferiority. He believed that children in this stage are internally motivated to compete, achieve, and obtain recognition. They are eager to learn but can feel inferior, develop a sense of failure, and lose interest in learning if their efforts to achieve are unsuccessful.

In Piaget's developmental theory, school-age children are in the concrete operations stage, capable of logical thought processes described in Box 8-1. Children's ability to mentally manipulate the world, relationships, and viewpoints of others is facilitated when they have the opportunity to physically manipulate concrete materials (e.g., using paints, paper, and glue; building things; making dams and forts of mud, snow, or rocks).

The information-processing model provides another useful conceptual framework for understanding cognitive development in school-age children. For effective cognitive work, young people must recognize salient cues in the environment, organize their thoughts, consider relationships with other information, use short- and long-term memory retrieval and storage skills, make decisions based on the analysis of information, take action, and use feedback to further their learning.

Kohlberg (1981) provided a theory of moral development based on the child's evolving ability to think and reason. Kohlberg's model is divided into three levels of conscience, each with two stages (see Table 5-1 and Table 8-1). He did not correlate these stages to children's ages, but most experts agree that Level I, the Preconventional Stage, occurs during early childhood (approximately 4 to 8 years of age). At this level, moral reasoning is determined by the consequences of behavior: to avoid punishment, receive rewards, or meet one's needs. There is some consideration of the feelings of others but only as it serves one's needs. At Level II, the Conventional Stage (ages 9 to 12 years), children act first to please others (Stage 3) and later to conform to authority (Stage 4). In late childhood, children begin to move into Level III, the Postconventional Stage.

Social Interaction

The earliest school-age milestone in the psychosocial area occurs when children learn to separate easily from family, allowing them to go to school. As they move into the community, they develop their own sense of self. This sense of self includes their role and feelings of belonging to a family. During the school-age years, children maintain their attachments with parents but also develop secondary attachments with other adults outside the home. Having good relationships with adults outside the home is especially important when the family is not wholly functional—not responsive and supportive—to the child (Schor, 1998).

TABLE 8-1 ***Developmental Characteristics of the School-Age Child***

Approximate Stages/Ages	Psychosexual Development	Social/Emotional Development	Cognitive and Problem-Solving Development	Moral Development
Early childhood (5-7 yr) (carried over from the toddler and preschool years to about 6 yr of age)	*Phallic Stage (Freud):* Attachment to the parent of the opposite sex. Usually sexual identity occurs at the end of this phase, and sexual urges are submerged.	*Initiative vs. Guilt (Erickson):* Moving into a larger social environment and thus are able to initiate activities on their own. Begin to learn to modulate their own behaviors through development of a consciousness as to what is appropriate for parents and society.	*Preoperational Period (Piaget)*: Representative language and early reasoning. Problem solving intuitive rather than logical. Thought process involves magical thinking, egocentrism, centration, syncretism, juxtaposition, animism, artificialism, participation, and irreversibility.	*Preconventional Stage (Kohlberg):* Stage 1: Reasoning based on rewards and punishment or the consequences of behavior. Stage 2: Begins to base behaviors on own needs and at times the needs of others. Reciprocity is concrete. Others' feelings are secondary.
Middle childhood (7-10 yr)	*Latency Stage (Freud):* The superego or conscious is internalized. Energy is put into acquiring cultural and social skills. Guidelines established by the family are followed.	*Industry vs. Inferiority (Erickson):* Begins to appreciate individual interests and skills and seeks to become a successful member of a group. Internal motivation to achieve, compete, and obtain recognition. If unsuccessful, learning motivation is lost.	*Early Concrete Operational (Piaget)*: Begins to use logic and become more objective using an external point of view. Thinking becomes dynamic, decentralized, using conservation, transitivity, seriation, classification, and reversibility. The ability to understand size, shape when the physical properties can be manipulated.	*Conventional Stage (Kohlberg):* Stage 3: Begins to act to please others. Stage 4: Begins to conform to rules.
Late childhood (10-12 yr) (carried into adolescence)	*The Genital Stage (Freud):* Reemergence of sexual impulses.	*Industry vs. Inferiority (Erickson):* Continuation of socialization with other children and groups. Development of hobbies and interests outside of school allows recognition of individual worth.	*Late Concrete Operational (Piaget)*: Able to conceptualize size, shape, quantity, space, and thus able to problem solve using abstract thought. Able to classify items into a hierarchical system. *Formal Operational (Piaget)*: Distinguished by the ability to use abstract thinking, complex reasoning, flexibility, and hypothesis formation. Become more aware of contractions, falsehoods, and shortcomings in previous beliefs. Become aware of how others think of them.	*Postconventional Stage (Kohlberg):* Stage 5: Begins to appreciate that their behaviors benefit society. Stage 6: Begins to form principles from conscience, even if they differ from what is generally acceptable in society. Look for rationale in rules. Respect for authority and maintaining social order.

BOX 8-1 *Piaget's Concrete Operational Stage: Characteristics of Thought Process*

Decentration—can focus on more than one aspect of a situation at a time (e.g., keeping track of both color and shape when working on a jigsaw puzzle)
Conservation—can understand that some aspects of things, such as weight, remain the same despite changes in appearance
Transitivity—can deduce new relationships from sets of earlier ones
Seriation—can sequence in order (e.g., ordering triangle shapes from smallest to largest)
Classification—can group objects on the basis of common features (e.g., separating out all the triangles from circles, squares, and stars)
Reversibility—can mentally reverse a process or action (e.g., ice can melt to water and then refreeze)

Peer Relationships. A major task of school-age children is to develop competence in social relationships. "Friendships promote resilience, enhance self-image, fill emotional needs, and help compensate for stresses in other areas of life" (Coleman & Lindsay, 1998, p. 111). Studies have shown that attraction to gang involvement may occur during late childhood for youth without a positive social support group (Taylor et al, 2002).

Relationship skills include initiating interactions, keeping them going, resolving conflicts, and terminating interactions positively. However, many other factors are necessary for children to be successful with their peers—understanding the meaning in social situations, being socially responsive, using the jargon of the group, making use of previous interactions to repeat successful behaviors, being appropriately assertive, and being empathetic (Coleman & Lindsay, 1998).

Social acceptance is especially important at this age. Friends are generally chosen because of shared skills, interests, personality, and loyalty. Children come to see themselves in the eyes of their friends. As early as age 7 years, some children are more concerned about a friend's opinion than about adults' opinions. They develop "best friends" and dress and talk like their peers. A special-friend phase should occur at around 10 years of age. This is an intense attachment to a same-sex child. With that friend, the child expands the self, learns altruism, shares feelings, and learns how others manage problems. Talking on the telephone and sleepovers become more common. These early friendships are the basis for later relationships. Family conflicts can arise when peer activities and expectations conflict with family rules and values.

Children's temperaments affect the way they interact with peers, teachers, family, and others in their environment. Emotional problems during these years often follow frustrations, losses, and situations in which the child's self-esteem is threatened or the child is faced with adversity.

Morality

Although there is variability in moral development, by age 7 years, most children can name a site for their conscience (heart or brain), and, consistent with concrete thinking, school-age children tend to be rather rigid in their views of right and wrong. They can understand the relationships between responsibility and privileges and realize that choices between right and wrong behaviors are within their control. Some children at this age act appropriately to get a direct reward, whereas others do their duty, viewing moral behavior as following the rules of higher authority (see Table 8-1).

The ability to reason through difficult situations with a variety of factors operating is heavily dependent on cognitive development, however, and school-age children do not have the cognitive maturity to cope with all situations. The school environment, where rules and values differ from those of the immediate family, must be confronted and negotiated daily. This presents a challenge to the child's concepts of right and wrong. Social pressures also may make it difficult to choose actions that the child believes are right. The pressures of gangs, drugs, and peers push many children to make decisions about their activities and behaviors before they are developmentally ready. Furthermore, the values of the family are challenged as the child learns that other families make decisions and have beliefs that are different from their own.

Body Image

School-age children can appear to be totally oblivious of their bodies (e.g., the 9-year-old who does not change his shirt for 3 days), perhaps because they are so busy with their daily lives. In fact, children at this age are extremely curious about changes happening to them as they grow, and they are sensitive to others around them. Highly literal in their thinking, they can be very frank with questions to people they trust (e.g., "Grandma, why are you growing a moustache?"). At the same time, they are learning the importance of social politeness—what is appropriate in certain situations and how to behave themselves—so they may be uncomfortable or shy about new or unusual situations. Modesty is characteristic of school-age children.

Sexual exploration, including masturbation, is common. Children in early childhood, 5 to 7 years of age, often play "doctor," and in middle childhood, children will compare their bodies with friends of the same sex.

Physical growth and neurologic maturation give children the ability to master many new skills in which they use their bodies. Young swimmers, runners, skateboard enthusiasts, and soccer players all emerge at this time. Their achievements—and failures—help them define who they are and are the basis for their evolving self-image. This is the age when children learn that they are "as clumsy as the day is long," or "a born horse-back rider," or "really smart but not very good at sports." The images they have about their bodies come from the experiences they have and from the feedback from family, peers, teachers, and others in the community. This feedback can help clarify their understandings and allow the child to gain in self-confidence and feelings of worth (see Chapter 18).

Coping Skills

As a part of the process of developing relationships with others, school-age children refine their ability to identify, label, and manage their feelings. However, their experiences are limited and their cognitive abilities still expanding; they continue to need help labeling complex emotions such as sadness, depression, worry, and envy. They also need help in consciously managing those and other feelings in acceptable ways.

An important coping skill learned by school-age children is impulse control. Without impulse control, random behavior occurs; on the other hand, overly controlled children appear hostile, uncreative, or both. By age 7 years, children should have developed sufficiently to function in a variety of settings (e.g., home, school, playground) with increasing competence.

School-age children face a variety of stressors in society today, including violence, early responsibilities, and lack of support in school. Violence is a constant problem for many, not only in neighborhoods where they live and play, but in the schools where they go to learn. Some children are given heavy responsibility at a young age: When parents work, many children must care for themselves after school. Latchkey children remain alone, housebound, and unsupervised, until adults return at the end of the day. Some also have responsibility for caring for younger siblings. Many schools lack resources to maintain small class sizes or offer special programs for children with learning difficulties. As a result, children are passed on from grade to grade without remediation of their fundamental learning problems, and with the stigma of failure.

Children with chronic illnesses or disabilities may have trouble adapting to their disorders during the school-age years and may need special help to foster independence and a sense of self-esteem (Vessey & Mebane, 2000). Latchkey children with chronic illnesses are especially vulnerable because they may need to make decisions about their health care without adult advice. For example, they may need to know whether they should have more medication or need to complete a treatment. Such children need to understand their illness, medications, where to go for emergency care, how to write down instructions or messages, and how to follow important rules (Vessey & Jackson, 2000). Children mature at different rates in their ability to manage their self-care throughout the school-age years. A child's capacity for self-care of chronic illnesses depends on the illness, its stability, and the child's age and cognitive skills.

Cognitive Development

In early childhood, children transition from a preoperational mode of thinking that uses intuitive problem solving to early concrete operational thinking. When they make this transition, children are more likely to be ready for school. Magical thinking and egocentric logic fade, and concepts of conservation, transformation, reversibility, decentration, seriation, and classification emerge. By middle childhood, children need to be able to understand relationships of mass and length and multiple variables relating to objects. School-age children should be able to classify or group materials in relation to other information they have. By late childhood, children should have well-developed concrete operational thinking. They should be able to focus on more than one aspect of a problem and use logical thinking.

These concrete operational abilities allow children to read, write, and communicate thoughts effectively. Learning about the world, its people, and the views and values of others becomes possible. With the ability to understand the viewpoints of others and the decline of egocentricity, logical thinking and new social skills appear. Empathy, or the ability to share and understand another's feelings, emerges, and with it, the capacity for making deep friendships.

School-age children should be developing a sense of personal competence as they experience success in school.

ASSESSMENT OF SCHOOL-AGE CHILDREN

Some authorities have questioned the value of screening tests and the physical examination because few physical problems are identified in school-age children (4%) and parents may experience some overconfidence when a child "passes" the physical examination (Hoekelman, 2001). The real value of preventive health visits may be in the monitoring, screening, and anticipatory guidance related to developmental, behavioral, and emotional issues. It is by reviewing the child's progress, offering suggestions, and validating parent's efforts that NPs can best assist families as they move through the school-age years. Table 8-2 summarizes some key points to discuss with children and their families.

Developmental surveillance (see Chapter 5) is an essential aspect of each contact with the school-age child because visits are less frequent during the school years. Most visits are for minor acute illnesses rather than health maintenance. Data must be collected on the child's physical, nutritional, neurodevelopmental, psychosocial, behavioral, and emotional status. As with all children, assessment of the family system is crucial; for the school-age child, it is particularly important to evaluate how well the family is nurturing the child while supporting the child's efforts to separate, become more independent, and create a unique self in the community.

The assessment process begins by building rapport with the parents and the child. Direct questions first to the child, encouraging him or her to share aspects of daily routines, family experiences, school activities, and sensitive developmental concerns. Parents can then be invited to expand on data collected, providing information not only about the child's abilities but also about interactions between child and parents.

Screening

Developmental screening tools and questionnaires may be useful in the NP's busy practice. These tools allow the child, parent, and teachers to provide specific information about a child's development, behaviors, and emotional status. They also document a baseline status, highlight potential need for referrals, and evaluate the effectiveness of intervention strategies. Differing parental, school, and child perceptions about specific issues may be noted. However, the information can provide the NP with insights into areas needing further investigation and those that may require counseling, therapy, or other intervention strategies. The Resource Box at the end of this chapter provides a list of different developmental and behavioral screening tools (also see Chapter 6 Resource Box; some tools used in infant years are appropriate for school-age children). Table 8-3 provides key indicators for developmental referrals.

In addition, the American Academy of Pediatrics (AAP) recommends six routine health visits for children during the school years at 5, 6, 8, 10, 11, and 12 years (AAP, 2000) (see Chapter 1, Figure 1-5 for specific recommendations).

Physical Development

A traditional history should be obtained and physical examination conducted and findings documented (Table 8-4). Growth measurements (weight, height, BMI) and blood pressure should be evaluated and compared with age-appropriate norms at each visit. Hearing and vision should be screened annually. Hemoglobin or hematocrit

TABLE 8-2 ***Topics for Preventive Health Visit***

5 to 7 Years	8 to 10 Years	11 to 12 Years
Adaptation to school	Progress at school	Progress in school
After-school activities	After-school activities	After-school activities
Development of peer relationships	Peer relationships—friendships, bullying, or victimization	Peer relationships
Family relationships	Family relationships	Family relationships
Activities that support positive self-esteem	Sexual education	Community safety; membership in gangs
Problem solving away from home, without parents immediately available	Community safety; joining gangs	Activities that support positive self-esteem
	Activities that support positive self-esteem	Problem solving away from home—avoiding drugs, alcohol, and smoking
	Problem solving away from home	Handling emotions—sadness, anger, worries
	Handling emotions—sadness, anger, worries	Completion of basic education in sexuality and reproductive health

TABLE 8-3 ***Developmental Red Flags: School-Age Child***

Age	Psychosocial/Emotional Skill	Cognitive and Visual Abilities	Language/Hearing	Fine Motor	Gross Motor
6 yr	Problems with peer relationships Latchkey: stays home alone Unable to state special quality about self Flat affect, depression, withdrawn Cruelty to animals, friends Interest in fires/firesetting	School problems with grades, behavior, interest in school Unable to sit still in class Unable to give age Watching television more than 2 hr per day Unable to name interests	Language partially unintelligible	Unable to copy "+" Picture of self includes less than 8 parts	Unable to catch a ball
8 yr	Lack of hobbies Lack of best friend Cruelty to animals, friends Interest in fires/firesetting Flat affect, depression, withdrawn	Unable to state days of the week Unable to add and subtract Unable to identify right and left	Unable to read simple phrases Unable to relate simple story	Unable to copy a diamond and square Unable to print name Unable to tie shoes Picture of self includes less than 12-16 parts	Unable to walk a straight line Poor coordination/endurance/strength
10 yr	Lack of team sports or extracurricular activities at school Lacks understanding of rules Poor peer influence, interest in gangs Cruelty to animals, friends Interest in fires/firesetting Flat affect, depression, withdrawn	Lack of operational thinking: cause and effect, relationships of whole and parts, nonegocentric thinking	Problems with reading and math	Difficulty holding pencil with penmanship/cursive writing	Problems throwing or catching
12 yr	Risk-taking behaviors: smoking, alcohol, sex Problems about sexuality Cruelty to animals, friends Interest in fires/firesetting Flat affect, depression, withdrawn	Difficulty with school work Lack of organizational skills for homework	Problems understanding/following through with verbal instructions Problems with reading comprehension	Problems getting written homework done because of difficulties holding pencil or doing paper-and-pencil tasks	Unable to list strengths and physical things he or she likes to do

TABLE 8-4 *Guidelines for the History and Physical Examination of the School-Age Child*

Assessment Area	Findings
Chief complaint	Common concern (e.g., school performance: inattention, fidgeting, difficulty completing tasks, stays on tasks forever, forgetful, angry, frustrated, poor academic performance, moody, irritable, talks excessively)
Subjective Data/History	
Birth history	Early development, including feeding, sleep/wake cycles, colicky or fussy baby, poor suck; Apgar scores; length of hospitalization; oxygen or phototherapy
Past medical history	Illnesses that may explain the child's problems (e.g., otitis media, chronic illness, vision problems, dental problems, food allergies, reflux, or undiagnosed pain); chronic conditions such as asthma, congenital cardiac conditions; hospitalizations or surgeries
Past development	Early developmental progress, especially in language and social skills (e.g., toilet training)
Interim history	Onset of problems; description of when it occurs; note child's use of alcohol, drugs, and cigarettes; systems review related to any chief complaint
Daily activities	Daily sleep/wake pattern, routines and schedule, amount of passive activities (TV) vs. active play and recreational activities; note family routines, family activities, family expectations of the child, and child's ability to complete chores or jobs around the house
Temperament/ personality	Identify difficulty with change and transitions, establishing routines, or finishing tasks; difficulty with mood, new situations, making or keeping friends
School history	School progress, subjects liked/disliked, peer relationships, match with teacher and school philosophy
Family history	Family and home routines and environment, family support systems, activities, involvement in social and school activities, parent's knowledge of child's friends and involvement with child's friends; family history of medical problems or congenital anomalies
Family review of systems	Family history of attention-deficit hyperactivity disorder, learning problems, mental retardation, autism, emotional or psychiatric problems, sleep problems, drug or alcohol abuse, diabetes, obesity, asthma, or allergies
Objective Data/Physical Examination	
Measurements/ vital signs	Child's growth percentiles, especially if below the 5th percentile; note head circumference for all children (even adolescents); note BMI and blood pressure and compare with norms for age of child; hematocrit
General	Child's overall appearance, cooperation, parent-child interaction, parent's responsiveness to the child, and the child's responsiveness to the parent
Skin and lymph	Rashes, lesions, edema, and shape of the nails, hemangiomas, hirsutism, fat tissue, and skin folds; note enlarged lymph nodes, or mottling of the skin
Head, eyes, ears, nose, mouth	*Head:* Unusual skull shape, hair swirls/unruly hair, and hairline; identify any problems with the temporomandibular joint
	Face: Flat midface, short mandible, asymmetric facial movements, and unusual facies
	Eyes: Eye position (hyperteliarism/hypoteliarism), asymmetries, small epicanthal folds or palpebral fissures; lid: ptosis; conjunctiva: clarity; pupils: PERRLA and cover test, especially for strabismus; EOM: visual fields, nystagmus; fundus: light reflex, vessels, disc, and macula
	Nose: Size, shape, bridge, and anteverted nostrils
	Mouth/lips/fulcrum/tongue: Thin upper lip, micrognathia/retrognathia, long philtrum, maxohypoplasia, or malocclusion; tongue: fasciculations, symmetry, suck, swallow, and strength
	Teeth: Enamel, shape, dentition, and signs of bruxism
	Palate: Pharynx, palate shape, size of tonsils, movement of uvula, gag reflex
	Neck: Asymmetric strength of movement, swallow, trachea, lymph; thyroid: position, asymmetry, movement
Chest	Shape, pectus excavatum, and short xiphoid
Breasts	Tanner stage; asymmetry or extra numerary nipples
Lungs	Inspiratory and expiratory wheezing or absence of breath sounds; peak flow if history of asthma
Cardiac	PMI, heart sounds, murmurs, and thrills; pulses: equality, symmetry, and strength

TABLE 8-4 Guidelines for the History and Physical Examination of the School-Age Child—cont'd

Assessment Area	Findings
Abdomen	Bowel sounds, abdominal shape and movements, umbilicus position, tenderness, masses, organ size, bladder distention or bowel distention
Musculoskeletal	Note size of muscles, symmetry, hypertonia or hypotonia, range of motion, posture, joints, dactyly *Back:* Evaluate spine for scoliosis, cysts, dimples, hair tufts, and CVA tenderness *Upper/lower extremities:* Evaluate active and passive strength (tone), symmetry, hyperextension of fingers and joints, and presence of tremors; movement: observe body while sitting, standing, running, walking, jumping, skipping, hopping, and kicking; note hip dysplasia, foot position, palmar creases, short fifth finger, incurved fifth finger, tapered phalanges, nail hypoplasia, flexion of elbow
Genitourinary/ gynecologic	Evaluate anatomy and Tanner stage *Male:* Note testes size, placement; note if circumcised or not; evaluate for hydrocele, hernia, or hypospadias *Female:* Note hypoplastic labia; evaluate for hernia

BMI, Body mass index; *PERRLA*, pupils equal, round, reactive to light and accommodation; *EOM*, extraocular movements; *PMI*, point of maximum intensity; *CVA*, costovertebral angle.

is done during early childhood (5 years) and again during late childhood and into adolescence (11 and 12 years). Immunization status is an important aspect of these preventive health visits. Tanner staging should be a part of the physical examination because school-age children can begin pubertal changes as early as 8 years of age and some endocrine problems may emerge in the school years. Also, evaluation for specific conditions listed in Box 8-2 can provide direction for the NP in the physical examination.

BOX 8-2 Physical Conditions to be Identified in the School-Age Child

- Cataracts
- Congenital heart disease
- Congenital hip dysplasia
- Cryptorchidism
- Genetic syndromes
- Glaucoma
- Lymphadenopathy
- Scoliosis
- Tumors (benign and malignant)

Motor Skills Development

Strength and coordination can be evaluated using a systematic musculoskeletal and neurologic examination as identified in Table 8-5. Concerns about balance, coordination, strength, and mobility should be followed up depending on attention, school performance, and overall developmental function. Problems in this area may account for school performance or learning problems.

Communication and Language Development

Assessment of communication and language development is ongoing during the health care visit as the NP talks directly with the child, probing for the child's level of understanding (e.g., can child follow directions? Does the child understand explanations given by the NP?); listening to the child's articulation, vocabulary, sentence structure, and grammar; and noting the child's ability to interact socially with the examiner, the parent, and others in the setting. The child can be asked to write something on a sheet of paper to screen writing skills. Assessment is also based on reports from the parent.

Social and Emotional Development

Assessment of social and emotional development includes examining children's roles in the family, success in making friends and working with peers, self-esteem, and

TABLE 8-5 Guidelines for Neurodevelopmental Assessment of the School-Age Child

Assessment Area	Findings
Overall impression	Behavior, attentional skills and distractibility, motor activity level, impulsivity, degree of cooperativeness, strategies for and persistence in task completion, problem solving, organizational skills, ability to follow directions and ask for assistance.
Cerebral	State control, attention, behavior, orientation, cooperation, participation, and separation from parents. Are judgment, orientation, memory (short- and long-term ability to remember eight familiar objects in "memory box"), affect, and calculation age appropriate or immature?
Cranial nerves	Note any asymmetries or oral-motor dyspraxia.
Cerebellar functioning	*Fine motor movements:* Evaluate for dysfunctions, including problems with balance, fine motor control (rapid alternating movements), and pincer or pencil grasp. *Coordination:* Evaluate coordination, including balance (Romberg, balance on one foot), tandem walk (heel-toe walk), duck walk, and coordination while throwing and catching a ball (use a small ball with older children).
Sensory functioning	Evaluate problems recognizing body parts or body position, sensitivity to touch, asymmetric or poor graphesthesia (letters/numbers) or stereognosis (objects).
Gross motor function	Evaluate overall gait, coordination for age while skipping, running, walking on balance beam. Appropriateness for age. Note posture, ability to sit in chair straight vs. leaning on desk. Ability to stand for periods of time without leaning on something.
Extraneous movement/ tremors	Evaluate for synkinesis (motor overflow), dyskinesis (incomplete or fragmented movements), mild dyspraxic movements, dysdiadochokinesia (inability to perform rapid movements), motor impersistence.
Auditory perceptual abilities	Evaluate discrimination, processing, integration, memory, and comprehension or auditory information. Evaluate ability to follow twofold and fivefold directions. Note directionality and consistent or inconsistent use of right or left eye, hand, foot. Note ability to remember series of spoken words and numbers forwards and backwards, and ability to understand/comprehend a written paragraph. Note expressive language ability (word retrieval, formulation, and articulation). Evaluate conversation spoken spontaneously through story or history. Evaluate ability to define words appropriate for age.
Visual perceptual abilities	Identify memory recall (short and long term), visual discrimination, visuospatial perception, visual memory for objects, visual discrimination of subtle differences in words (e.g., ten and tin), object assembly, and decoding.
Organization	Observe problem solving of math problems.
Visual motor integration and coordination	Note ability to copy a design (+, 0, square or triangle) and handwriting. Evaluate picture of a person drawn by the child for age appropriateness.
Learning style	Evaluate concrete/abstract thinking, sequential/stimulus processing, thought integration, perseveration, ritual/routine; control; adaptation to changes; modulation of behaviors; exaggeration (overdo/underdo) activities.

feelings of contentment and security. It is important to watch the interaction between parents and child during the examination. *Bright Futures: Guidelines for Health Supervision of Infants, Children, and Adolescents* (Green & Palfrey, 2002), *Bright Futures in Practice: Mental Health,* volume I, *Practice Guide* (Jellinek, Patel, & Froehle, 2002a), and *Bright Futures in Practice: Mental Health,* volume II, *Tool Kit* (Jellinek, Patel, & Froehle, 2002b) provide resources for screening in this area (also see Ecomap, Chapter 3).

Cognitive Development

Assessment of cognitive development is difficult in school-age children. Generally, standardized paper-and-pencil tests are more accurate than clinical judgments. Knowledge about the child's performance compared with that of peers in the classroom, the child's grades, and information from conferences with teachers provide some data. Often a psychologist is asked to test children cognitively if more definitive information is needed.

Diagnostic Assessment

If problems are suspected, additional testing can be performed (e.g., wrist radiographs can establish bone age; intelligence testing can establish cognitive abilities). Further endocrine, nutrition, genetic, or other assessments may be necessary if the child does not meet the norms for physical growth.

ANTICIPATORY GUIDANCE FOR SCHOOL-AGE CHILDREN

Anticipatory guidance should be an individualized discussion with parents that helps them understand, respond to, and guide their child's behavior and development. Some discussion points are identified in this section. The lists are not intended to be used exhaustively at visits but to illustrate how parents can apply developmental concepts in everyday living. If problems emerge from discussions in these areas, the NP is referred to the appropriate chapter for ideas for assessment and management (e.g., sleep problems are discussed in Chapter 16).

Parent Development

Parents, too, must change when their children enter school, and it is not always an easy transition. Some parents feel as if they have "lost" their child, watching him or her move from dependence on the family to participation in a new world of which the parent is not a part. Other parents look forward to the new opportunities facing the child and the family. For most, school entry is a mixed blessing.

Parents see their children confronted with a new social system that in many ways evaluates the work that the parents have done over the previous years: Are the children prepared for self-care throughout the day? Can they toilet; independently choose and eat a lunch; negotiate travel from home to school to classroom and home again; express needs to school personnel; participate appropriately in the classroom; make friends; and have enough self-control to resist peer pressures to act against family rules and expectations? If the child "fails" to meet the expectations of school entry, parents can feel guilty or responsible.

Parents are expected to support the school's standards, and research indicates that parents' educational expectations for their children help determine the child's school success (Ganzach, 2000). As school-age children move through the years from 6 to 12, parents must continue to extend freedoms along with adding new responsibilities. They need to provide opportunities that allow children to experience and master new challenges, as well as adjust family patterns of nutrition, sleep, activities, health maintenance, safety, and communication to fit with the child's needs and emerging skills. Parents must reinforce and support the positive self-esteem and self-image of these vulnerable young people. Spending time with their children in positive, reinforcing ways is essential.

Regulation and Sleep/Wake Patterns

Family routines provide a support to the daily life of the child and help the child self-regulate. If children have routines that they can rely on, they are more comfortable exploring in new areas and trying new skills. Family routines strengthen the relationship between parent and child, provide family stability and continuity, and serve as a buffer during times of change and transition (Kubicek, 2002). They may also serve as protection against risk factors such as divorce, alcoholism, substance abuse, or violence. Suggestions the NP can make to parents include the following:

- Encourage the family to establish and recognize traditions or family activities that are special (e.g., birthday celebrations, Sunday afternoon walks, videos and popcorn on Saturday night).
- Help parents explore ways to adapt the child's new schedule in an effort to maintain previous routines or readjust routines to meet the new schedule (e.g., if the child must meet a school bus at an early hour, making a school lunch the night before can become part of a new evening routine).

School-age children who do not receive adequate sleep often demonstrate irritability, fatigue, poor attention, and poor learning. Bedtime is still difficult and delay tactics are not uncommon. Parents can be encouraged to do the following:

- Continue a regular nighttime routine to transition from active daytime play to evening quiet play.
- Set a regular time for morning awakening, giving the child extra time to come fully awake without being rushed.
- Minimize stimulation (e.g., scary television programs) before bedtime.

Strength and Motor Coordination

Because of the maturity of the central nervous system and cognitive advances, most children are physically capable. Most enjoy playing hard so that they can develop physical skills, strength, and coordination. Parents can support this growth if they do the following:

- Encourage children's participation in daily exercise.
- Provide for activities that are fun, involve family or peers, and require cognitive or social skills, including rules, strategies, and skills.
- Include children's friends in family activities (e.g., hiking, skiing, swimming).
- Support children's interest in preferred physical activities that are healthful; personal achievement in an activity can be crucial to children's self-image.

- Encourage hobbies and activities that foster fitness and increased motor skills.
- Encourage activities that require training, commitment, and effort, especially for older children.
- Help children avoid the stress of overactivity.
- Limit activities that include TV, video games, or computer time.
- Let the children "own" the activity (e.g., Little League baseball games should be fun for the children, not a contest among parents over whose child is the best).
- Explore ways children with physical limitations can participate in preferred activities and with their peers.

Nutrition, Self-Care, and Safety

Nutrition

School-age children have good appetites. Diets can be deficient in iron or vitamin C, however, and high-fat snack foods can become a habit, with resulting obesity. Choosing nutritious foods while away from home and learning to eat new foods are areas for learning. Because food is not readily available all day at school, eating well at breakfast and dinner becomes especially important. High-calorie snacks and other high-calorie foods have contributed to obesity in school-age children, and monitoring and weight control programs are needed at earlier ages (see Chapter 12). Parents should be advised to do the following:

- Ensure that the child has three nutritious meals and two nutritious snacks daily.
- Know that food jags are common.
- Establish an eating routine, with at least one daily meal together as a family. Maintain family meals as much as possible to preserve family time and share interests and experiences from the day's activities.
- Monitor food choices and opportunities to determine best foods.
- Teach children to understand the importance of eating healthy foods.
- Encourage participation in meal planning, food shopping and selection, and preparation.
- Discuss making nutritious choices at fast food restaurants.

Self-Care

For school-age children, learning to take responsibility for their own health begins with simple goals and moves to more complex decision-making strategies. For example, children may begin by deciding to have a fruit or vegetable at each meal and then progress to helping plan some meals and participate in their preparation. Other areas in which children take increasing responsibility are dental health, hygiene and grooming, snacking, and exercise. Children at this age see health in positive terms and equate it with being able to participate in desired activities (Story, Holt, & Sofka, 2002). Parents can do the following things to assist the child's achievement in self-care:

- Explain the relationship between good health and self-care.
- Supervise personal hygiene such as brushing teeth, combing hair, and doing nail care; for older school children, supervision is minimal, with an occasional reminder.
- Set clear limits on expectations for cleanliness, healthy exercise, hours of sleep, and other health promotion behaviors.
- Recognize that children may be "noncompliant" as a means of exerting independence; a discussion about decision making and healthy choices may be needed to resolve the issue.
- Be flexible.
- Provide children with opportunities to experiment with appropriate healthy behaviors that allow them to develop self-expression (e.g., school-age children can enjoy new hair styles or having their hair dyed).
- Encourage shared decision making and self-care during illnesses and for chronic disease management.
- Give children an opportunity to ask questions about sexuality, drugs, alcohol, and tobacco; encourage discussion about these topics as a family; teach about puberty changes.
- Model healthy behaviors.

Safety

Unintentional injuries are common among school-age children. Often their growing bodies allow them to get themselves into situations that they cannot get out of without help. They need guidance and direction to be safe and make safe choices. Although parents do not provide the constant supervision they did for toddlers and preschoolers, it is important that they work with their school-age child to ensure safety. The NP can provide guidance to parents and encourage them to do the following:

- Help children learn "survival skills" (e.g., name, telephone number, address, use of 911, how to ask adults for help, what to do if lost).
- Require use of protective gear when riding bicycles, skateboards, or scooters.
- Wear seatbelts.
- Encourage use of sunscreen (sun protection factor 15 or higher) before going outside to play.
- Teach children to swim; supervise their activities near water.

- Educate children about hazards, both physical and social (e.g., pedestrian traffic on busy streets; facts about pregnancy, intercourse, and sexually transmitted diseases; what to do if they find a weapon).
- Get rid of firearms or ensure that they are unloaded and locked, with ammunition in a different location.
- Help children to think about safety aspects of activities; talk about safety.

Social and Emotional Growth

Finding support in his or her family system and peer group while establishing individuality and independence is the hallmark of successful social and emotional growth for the school-age child. Project Cornerstone, a program of the Search Institute, identifies building blocks, or assets, needed for children to grow up as healthy, caring, and responsible individuals (Search Institute, 2003). NPs can help foster that growth by encouraging parents to do the following:

- Enhance goal setting with charts, calendars, and tally sheets. Care should be taken not to reward children too much, because this can decrease motivation. Let children set goals while parents monitor activities and point out options.
- Appreciate the products of the child's work at home and at school; encourage successful activities.
- Play and work together as a family to teach children how to work together with their classmates and to function as a team; children should maintain their responsibilities to the family (e.g., jobs or chores around the house).
- Share family history and visits with relatives to help children be proud of their heritage.
- Help children feel that the home base is secure so that they are confident in moving to other domains.
- Make home rules and expectations clear, and use consistency in applying them.
- Discuss the reasons for family values and rules, and the differences that the child may face when away from home.
- Provide positive expressions of love, concern, and pride to promote a sense of belonging to the family.
- Provide opportunities for children to make and develop friendships with a variety of children, teaching them how to initiate, sustain, and terminate relationships with friends.
- Include the child's friends in some activities and outings.
- Provide social skills training and supervised social success experiences.
- Teach children how to read social cues.
- Help children learn to communicate well with other adults.
- Recognize that children may identify with a special person, such as a movie star or athlete.
- Provide fantasy play opportunities to allow children to deal safely with their emotions and concerns and to develop their creativity.
- Help children identify and appropriately express their emotions.
- Provide guidance for how to appropriately express feelings of aggression and emerging sexuality.
- Discuss sexual values.
- Support participation in activities that allow channeling feelings of aggressiveness plus giving a sense of group accomplishment.
- Recognize that parents are role models and that children internalize parental values as they begin to form a conscience.
- Model positive conflict resolution and good communication.
- Teach anger management and conflict resolution skills.
- Provide children with opportunities for appropriate behavior when values are challenged (e.g., "You can say, 'No, my Mom won't let me do that,' and then walk away").
- Teach respect for authority and rules away from home.
- Help children with decision making and accepting consequences of actions.
- Recognize that having a strong sense of self-esteem helps "inoculate" children against some of the negative peer pressures children may experience.
- Help children learn delayed gratification and increase their frustration tolerance. However, parents need to remain sympathetic.

Cognitive and Environmental Stimulation

The school is a major source of intellectual stimulation and an arena in which the child experiences cognitive growth. Expectations for performance increase over the school years with examinations, graded papers, and homework assignments. Reading becomes a tool to attain and master knowledge rather than being an end in itself. Thus poor readers begin to experience broader academic failure and can become increasingly frustrated. Unless these children are provided with social and remedial support, they may see school as an unpleasant burden, develop feelings of failure, and look for validation through nonacademic experiences. Social supports can help children cope with this stress, and interacting with healthy, interested, and caring adults is the strongest support children can have.

The family also provides the child with stimulation for cognitive growth, and parents can be counseled to do the following:

- Read to the child and have the child read to the parent.
- Stimulate thinking with the younger child about comparisons (e.g., changes in shape, volume, directions to and from school) to facilitate cognition at the concrete operations level.
- Discuss variables in objects or situations as experienced, seen on television, or read about to help move the child's thinking away from the earlier egocentric style.
- Provide opportunities to gain knowledge through books, outings, classes, and family discussions.
- Engage children in experiences with other languages, music, and cultural groups.
- Explore and explain the environment and community to the child to promote broader understanding of the world.
- Establish a regular homework time and place to help the child maximize time for cognitive practice.
- Establish an environment that encourages children to focus and complete tasks with limits clearly defined.
- Provide help early if children experience school problems to lessen secondary problems with emotions and conflict.
- Volunteer at the child's school or participate in school activities for parents.
- Recognize academic achievement because success motivates further work.
- Stay involved with school assignments and evaluate progress to support the child's work.
- Encourage problem-solving efforts.
- Provide more complex opportunities to plan and complete projects that use school skills, such as planning and cooking meals, planning family outings, and managing money and a budget.

COMMON DEVELOPMENTAL ISSUES FOR SCHOOL-AGE CHILDREN

First-Grade School Readiness

Description

School entrance is based on chronologic rather than developmental age. As a result, readiness problems occur for some children. School entry is stressful for all children, but immature children have increased stress because the expectations for performance are beyond their abilities and they have poorly developed coping resources. Children who lack necessary skills to meet school demands and expectations can be unsuccessful, and early school failure has significant negative consequences.

School participation requires skills to perform self-care, interact with a variety of new people, act with a sense of responsibility, and emotionally separate from the family and home base. Children need to meet school standards, which may be different from those at home. There is a social expectation to gain an awareness of "the group"—an ability to go along with the group while meeting some personal needs through the group's achievements.

Studies in the early 1990s indicated that teachers thought that 35% of children were not ready for school. Their concerns centered around deficiencies in language richness, emotional maturity, general knowledge, social confidence, moral awareness, and physical maturity (Boyer, 1993). Socially and economically disadvantaged children are at greatest risk (Byrd, 1998).

Clinical Findings

History

- *Child experiences:* Evaluate opportunities for participating in activities away from home, following directions, playing with other children, habits, and interest in school.
- *Parents and family:* Assess the parents' feelings about their child's entering school. Reluctance on their part may be communicated to their child, a message that does not facilitate the child's positive regard for this anticipated event. Ask about family activities, sibling school experiences, traumatic events, or separation on the part of the child or parents.
- *Home environment:* Inquire about daily routines, family activities together, parent- versus child-initiated activities for learning.
- *Developmental progress:* Ask about the child's developmental opportunities and skills in communicating needs, fine motor and gross motor activities, behaviors, fears, separation from parents, play with other children.

Physical Examination

The child should have a complete physical examination with special focus on the following:

- Neurologic development, including sensory, cognitive, and language
- Height, weight, BMI, blood pressure
- Dental health
- Immunization status

Diagnostic Tests

- Hearing
- Vision
- Urine
- Hematocrit

Other Testing or Evaluations

Developmental Evaluation. Normative skills are included in Table 8-6.

Ancillary Studies. Screening tests to evaluate school readiness have established norms and are generally reliable in predicting developmental outcomes (Table 8-7). They should be used to consider all areas of readiness and to provide an explanation of readiness for parents. Test results should be evaluated in conjunction with history, observation, family situation, and previous experiences.

Management

Preventive strategies for high-risk children begin before the school-age years and include enrollment in preschool, interactive reading with the child from an early age to promote language mastery, increased time for young children to play with peers and engage in creative play activities, and interaction with caring adults (Byrd, 1998).

TABLE 8-6 ***Basic First-Grade School Readiness Skills***

Language skills	Counts 10 or more objects Uses complete sentences of at least five words Uses future tense Gives first and last name Recognizes four colors Defines five to seven words Communicates needs Recalls parts of a story Follows three-part commands Understands number concepts
Personal and social skills	Separates easily from parent Dresses without supervision Plays interactively with other children Has toilet skills Follows instructions Feels support from other adults
Fine motor and adaptive skills	Copies geometric shapes (circle, square, triangle) Draws a person (six parts with distinct body) Prints some letters Classifies similar objects
Gross motor skills	Hops on one foot Catches bounced ball Walks backward heel/toe Balances on each foot 6 sec

Ensuring school readiness involves sharing data with school counselors and teachers, parents, and primary care providers, and offering anticipatory guidance in the following areas:

- Teach and encourage parents to assist their child with skills that will be needed for school (e.g., knowing colors and numbers, behavioral expectations).
- Encourage parents to visit the school, meet the teacher, and discuss their child's characteristics with the teacher.
- Instruct parents to rehearse school activities with their child before school begins (e.g., getting to school, finding class, eating meals, going to the bathroom, asking for help, getting home, and following the rules).
- Help parents deal with their own stress of separation. Review their expectations of the child and identify what will be new and different.
- Provide parents with available community and school resources they may need to access to meet the developmental needs of their child.
- Encourage children to start school with their age-appropriate group. Children who are not ready often need extra support at school, and they would benefit by spending another year at home.
- Be an advocate for parents and children with identified deficits to ensure that the school adequately assesses both strengths and weaknesses of children and develops a program of study that maximizes children's strengths.
- Counsel parents that deficits identified in a child's readiness may occur with the best of parenting.
- Develop a care plan with parents to address deficits in a comprehensive way while preserving the child's self-esteem.
- Monitor the child's progress through the year, advocating as necessary.

Learning Problems

Description

Learning problems can be a hidden handicap that appears during the school-age years. Ability to manage school learning expectations requires growth in four areas: basic processing of information, memorization, increased attention span and recall of important events, and beginning problem-solving skills.

Knowledge (the sum of what children know) rapidly expands as a result of schoolwork, experiences at home, and activities with friends. The organization of knowledge improves as school-age children grow older and integrate knowledge into existing concepts. Self-awareness, reflected by children's ability to predict performance, develops slowly and in areas in which children have the most knowledge (Table 8-8).

TABLE 8-7 ***Screening Tests to Evaluate School Readiness***

Denver Developmental Screening Test II	Denver Developmental Materials, Inc. PO Box 371075 Denver, CO 80237-5075 1-800-419-4729	Divided into four areas: Gross motor Language Fine motor Personal/social
VMI-4 (Beery, K. 1996)	Pro-Ed 8700 Shoal Creek Blvd. Austin, TX 78757-6897 1-800-897-3202 1-502-451-3246 Website: *www.proedinc.com*	Test of visual motor integration
Pediatric Examination of Educational Readiness (PEER) and Pediatric Examination of Educational Readiness at Middle Childhood (PEERAMID)	Educators Publishing Service, Inc. 31 Smith Place Cambridge, MA 02138-1007 1-617-547-6706 Fax: 1-617-547-0412 Website: *www.epsbooks.com*	Combined neurodevelopmental, behavioral, and health assessment

TABLE 8-8 ***Developmental Changes in Thinking Skills***

Component	Developmental Changes	Examples
Basic skills	Improvements in the speed and efficiency of memory, attention, language processing, motor implementation	Longer digit span Ability to work for longer stretches of time The use of adultlike logical principles The development of reading skills
Strategies	Use of active, complex strategies to improve basic skills	Greater spontaneous use of strategies Wider repertoire of strategies Greater likelihood of generalization to new areas
Knowledge	Expansion of what is known and greater organization of knowledge	Development of hobbies and special areas of interest More complex network of concepts
Metacognitive awareness	Development of explicit self-conscious knowledge about how to think	Ability to predict success or failure Ability to plan and to modify strategies

From Feldman H: Development of thinking skills in school-aged children, *Pediatr Ann* 18:358, 1989.

Although children with learning problems generally have difficulties with basic thinking skills, they may have specific problems in linguistic skills, attention, and organizational skills; higher cognitive functions, such as memory and sensory function; motor capacities; visuospatial analysis and neuromotor function; and social awareness and behavior (Tanner, 1995).

Clinical Findings

History. A complete, in-depth history is needed to examine underlying or related issues because learning difficulties are attributed to many different causes. The history will often provide the most information about how a child's learning is affecting aspects of the child's life. It should also identify areas of strength on which the child and family can build strategies for managing the learning difficulties, including the following:

- *Medical history:* prenatal history, neonatal history, recurrent or chronic medical conditions, allergies, medications, hospitalizations, syndromes; congenital, neurologic, metabolic, or endocrine conditions; current illnesses; vision and hearing problems

- *Developmental history:* achievement of developmental milestones, especially in language; experiences for achieving developmental skills at home or in preschool, daily routines and preferred play activities; temperament and behavioral concerns of the parents; ability of the child to handle transitions and change; child's initiation of activities versus parent-guided activities
- *Family medical history:* family history of difficulties in school or school dropout, learning difficulties, mental retardation, genetic disorders, and overall family members' functioning
- *Family social history:* family stressors, violence, utilization of community resources, problem-solving and decision-making skills, financial resources

Physical examination. A complete physical examination, with special attention to the neurodevelopmental assessment (see Table 8-5) should be performed.

Diagnostic Testing or Evaluations

- *School records:* Information needs to be obtained from the school system to evaluate the child's school performance and to review any educational testing that has been done. Testing must provide a picture of the child's strengths and weaknesses, revealing the cognitive styles that teachers and parents will be most successful in tapping. The Pediatric Examination of Educational Readiness at Middle Childhood (PEERAMID), a neurodevelopmental examination for 9- to 14-year-olds, may be administered (Levine et al, 1988).
- *Psychologic testing:* The school may or may not have the capacity for psychologic evaluations. Often parents must ask for this, and they may need to seek outside evaluations. Schools are required, under Public Law 94-142, to provide appropriate education to all children identified with developmental delays.
- *Cognitive testing:* The school's ability to provide cognitive and learning evaluations may be limited, requiring the parents to seek outside testing. An evaluation for a learning disorder is not complete without this information.
- *Developmental assessment:* A multidisciplinary developmental evaluation through a developmental program may be needed to provide the most appropriate plan of care for an individual child. Additional testing may be recommended such as genetics testing with chromosome studies, neurologic radiographs, and endocrine and metabolic testing.

Differential Diagnosis

The following diagnoses need to be considered in children with learning problems:

- Vision problems
- Hearing problems
- Mental retardation—genetic syndrome, neurologic insult, or malformation
- Cognitive developmental delay
- Speech or language delay
- Depression
- Neurologic problems
- Attention-deficit hyperactivity disorder (ADHD)
- Autism
- Toxin-related delay (e.g., lead, fetal alcohol syndrome)
- Medication-related delay (e.g., anticonvulsant, antihistamine)
- Substance abuse

Management

NPs can encourage parents to obtain an early diagnosis and identify and access appropriate school programs. Some children qualify for special educational support. Parents need to review educational plans, provide an environment rich with experiences for children, and set realistic goals. They also need to act as advocates for their children during every school year, because classrooms and teachers change. Parents should work to correct secondary problems such as poor self-esteem, hopelessness, or depression. Finally, parents need to be encouraged to avoid the use of the many unsubstantiated cures for learning disabilities. See Chapter 17 for further discussion of ADHD and other cognitive-perceptual problems.

School Refusal (Phobia)

Description

School refusal is a term that was introduced in the 1970s to describe the heterogeneity of its causes. The prevalence ranges from 0.4% to 18% of all school-age children. The disorder includes, but is not limited to, separation anxiety disorder, simple and social phobias, and depression. The criteria for a diagnosis include the following: (1) severe difficulty attending school or refusal to attend school; (2) severe emotional upset when attempting to go to school; (3) absence of significant antisocial disorders; and (4) staying at home with the parent's knowledge (Marino, 2001). Children may request to stay home from school with a variety of physical complaints, including stomachaches, headaches, dizziness, fatigue, or a combination of these. The symptoms gradually improve as the day progresses and often disappear on weekends. Unexcused school absences peak with the beginning of school attendance and again at 11 to 12 years of age.

Clinical Findings

History. Because child, parent, family, and school environmental factors may all play into the causes of school refusal, an in-depth history exploring these areas is needed. Specific areas include the following:

- Frequent somatic complaints or sleep difficulties
- Parents' ambivalent feelings about children's attendance at school, evidence of overindulgence or overprotection
- Difficult home situation; for example, children may try to stay at home, knowing that their mother drinks excessively when alone
- Recent or anticipated loss or separation
- School environment and evidence of bullying, violence, humiliation, lack of privacy, mismatch with teacher

Physical Examination. A complete physical examination and any indicated laboratory testing should be done to rule out specific indications of organic disease.

Diagnostic Testing and Evaluations. Laboratory testing that is symptom specific, noninvasive, and cost-effective to rule out organic disease is appropriate to assure child and parents that the problem is taken seriously. Both parent and child may then be more willing to accept the lack of organic disease and work toward addressing the underlying psychologic issues and cooperating in the development of a treatment plan.

- Depression and anxiety questionnaires (see Chapter 21)
- ADHD evaluation tools (see Chapter 17)

Differential Diagnosis (Marino, 2001)

- Somatic illness or overresponse to minor illness. Avoid overresponding with excessive diagnostic testing.
- Depression: isolation from peers, withdrawal from activities, sleep disturbances, erratic moods, poor self-esteem, and decreased activity level.
- ADHD and conduct disorder. The child who is unsuccessful in school, either academically or socially, may try to withdraw from the school environment.
- Anxiety disorder. This is the most common reason for school refusal, usually manifesting as an inability to cope with anxiety, especially anxiety stemming from separation.
- Sexual or physical abuse. Children who are being abused or who experience violence either at home or at school can feel intimidated to the point that they refuse to attend school.
- Chronic physical illness with poor adaptation.
- Learning disability with poor adaptation.
- Substance abuse.
- Pregnancy.
- Family dysfunction.
- Truancy.

Management

Intervention is generally successful when behavioral measures are combined with supportive counseling of parents. The physical complaints must be reasonably evaluated to rule out organic disease without excessive medical attention or diagnostic testing. Once the possibility of organic disease is set aside (or a plan is established to evaluate somatic problems), children must go to school. Generally, once they are at school, symptoms resolve.

- Support parents in getting children to school and insist on full attendance.
- Notify school personnel and encourage them to support and expect children's attendance and intervene to improve any situations related to children's anxiety.
- Assess home situation and identify issues that must be handled. Provide referrals as needed for family and parent problems for counseling, social service, or other resources.
- Referral for psychiatric care should be initiated immediately if no improvement occurs within 2 weeks (Van Buskirk, 1999).
- Criteria for mental health referral include the following (Munro, 2001):
    - Unresponsive to pediatric management
    - Out of school for 2 months
    - Onset in adolescents
    - Psychosis
    - Depression
    - Panic reactions
    - Parental inability to cooperate with plan

Recurrent Physical Symptoms

Description

Complaints of recurrent symptoms such as headaches, abdominal pain, and limb pain are frequent in school-age children. There is no good medical explanation for these symptoms, but the frequency of complaints in school-age children suggests a correlation with developmental factors. Children with recurrent symptoms often have parents with increased psychosocial problems and preoccupation with somatic complaints. Often, children receive a great deal of attention for these symptoms.

Clinical Findings

History

- Vague and intermittent complaints of abdominal pain, headaches, nausea, or malaise but absence of significant findings on physical examination

- Normal function between episodes
- No symptoms of vomiting, diarrhea, or constipation
- Family member with similar symptoms
- Stress in school or home environment (e.g., new social situation, school, teacher, examination, peer group conflict, moving, family illness or loss, parental or self-initiated pressure for achievement or perfection)

Physical Examination. No evidence of organic disease.

Differential Diagnosis

- Chronic, recurrent abdominal pain (see Chapter 33): consider irritable bowel syndrome, lactose intolerance, acid peptic disease, inflammatory bowel disease, sickle cell anemia, porphyria, hereditary angioedema, systemic lupus erythematosus, and dysmenorrhea in adolescent females (see Chapter 36)
- Neurologic conditions (see Chapter 28 for discussion of headaches)
- School refusal

Management

The following are keys to management of recurrent symptoms:

- Try not to "medicalize" the problem with a barrage of tests if the initial history and physical examination do not indicate systemic symptoms.
- Encourage the child to keep a food or pain diary.
- Reassure the child and expect normal participation in activities.
- Refer for mental health counseling if symptoms persist.
- Discuss coping strategies to deal with stressors.
- Discuss family strategies that are supportive but that do not reinforce the illness behavior.

RESOURCE BOX

Screening and Assessment Tools for the School-Age Child

Tools	Ages	Reference	Reporter	Item No.	Strengths	Weaknesses
Pediatric Symptoms Check List (PSC)	6-12 yr	Jellinek, Murphy, Robinson (1988); Jellinek, Murphy, Little (1999)	Parent report for ages 6-16. List of behaviors followed by never, sometimes, often.	35	Measures psychosocial dysfunction. Normative data, reliable, valid. Specificity of 68% and sensitivity of 95%.Used extensively in pediatric populations	Not for older adolescents. No depression-specific subscore, measures global dysfunction.
Child Behavior Check List (CBCL)		Jensen, Watanabe, Richters, et al (1996); Stancin, Palermo (1997)	Parent report for ages 4-18. Checklist.	138	Multidimensional. Widely accepted and used providing normative data for age and gender. Reliable and valid. Studied in many languages and countries. Often used to validate other screens.	Requires 20-25 min. Not easily scored. Computer scoring recommended. May not be feasible for mass screening. Subscales may have lower sensitivity than total scores.

Continued

RESOURCE BOX

Screening and Assessment Tools for the School-Age Child—cont'd

Tools	Ages	Reference	Reporter	Item No.	Strengths	Weaknesses
Child's Depression Inventory (CDI)	7-16 yr (used up to 18 yr)	Brooks, Kutcher (2001); Myers, Winters (2002)	Child selects one of three statements.	27	Well studied, reliable, and internally consistent.	CDI scores vary with age and sample, making cutoff scores difficult for mass screening. Some studies failed to distinguish between depressed and nondepressed children. Does not ask if suicide was attempted.
Child Depression Inventory—Parent (CDI-P)	6-16 yr	Wierzbicki (1987)	Parent selects one choice from three statements.	27	Ability to ask a second informant. Studied in a nonclinical population.	Noted to be an experimental screen in 1987. Validity of the CDI-P based on the validity of the instruments from which it was derived (CDI and BDI).
Psychosocial Screening (PSC—Youth)	9-14 yr	Gall, Pagano, Desmond, et al (2000)	Self-report. List of behaviors followed by never, sometimes, often.	35	Addresses psychosocial impairment. Used in nonclinical populations.	Fewer validation studies than the parent version.
Children's Depression Rating Scale (CDRS)—Revised	6-12 yr	Brooks, Kutcher (2001)	Interviewer based; 14 items for parents, 3 items based on child observation.	17	Reliable. Valid. Combines multiple informants. Interviewer does not need to be qualified clinician. All depressive symptoms.	Takes more than 30 min to complete. Recommended method is for trained interviewer to speak separately with parent, child, and another adult such as the teacher. Involves training.

RESOURCE BOX

Websites

American Academy of Pediatrics
www.aap.org

Bright Futures
www.brightfutures.com

Child Development Institute
1-714-998-8617
www.childdevelopmentinfo.com/

NAPNAP
www.napnap.org

National Academy for Child Development
www.nacd.org/resources

Search Institute
www.search-institute.org

REFERENCES

American Academy of Pediatrics, Committee on Practice and Ambulatory Medicine: Recommendations for preventive pediatric health care, *Pediatrics* 105:645, 2000.

Boyer E: Ready to learn: a mandate for the nation, *Young Children* 48:54-57, 1993.

Brooks SJ, Kutcher S: Diagnosis and measurement of adolescent depression: a review of the commonly utilized instruments, *J Child Adolesc Psychopharmacol* 11:341-376, 2001.

Byrd R: School readiness: more than a summer's work, *Contemp Pediatr* 15:39-53, 1998.

Coleman W, Lindsay R: Making friends: helping children develop interpersonal skills, *Contemp Pediatr* 15:111-129, 1998.

Dixon S, Stein M: *Encounters with children: pediatric behavior and development*, St Louis, 2000, Mosby.

Feldman H: Development of thinking skills in school-aged children, *Pediatr Ann* 18:358, 1989.

Gall G et al: Utility of psychosocial screening at a school-based health center, *J Sch Health* 70:292-298, 2000.

Ganzach Y: Parents' education, cognitive ability, educational expectations and educational attainment: interactive effects, *Br J Educ Psychol* 70(pt 3):419-441, 2000.

Green M, Palfrey JS: *Bright Futures: guidelines for health supervision of infants, children, and adolescents*, Arlington, VA, 2002, National Center for Education in Maternal and Child Health.

Hoekelman RA, editor: *Primary pediatric care*, ed 4, St Louis, 2001, Mosby.

Jellinek MS et al: Use of the Pediatric Symptom Checklist to screen for psychosocial problems in pediatric primary care, *Arch Pediatr Adolesc Med* 153:254-260, 1999.

Jellinek MS et al: Pediatric Symptom Checklist: screening school-age children for psychosocial dysfunction, *J Pediatr* 112:201-209, 1988.

Jellinek MS, Patel BP, Froehle MC, editors: *Bright Futures in practice: mental health*, vol I, *Practice guide*, Arlington, VA, 2002a, National Center for Education in Maternal and Child Health.

Jellinek MS, Patel BP, Froehle MC, editors: *Bright Futures in practice: mental health*, vol II, *Tool kit*, Arlington, VA, 2002b, National Center for Education in Maternal and Child Health.

Jensen PS et al: Scales, diagnoses, and child psychopathology: II. Comparing the CBCL and the DISC against external validators, *J Abnorm Child Psychol* 24:151-168, 1996.

Kohlberg L: *The philosophy of moral development*, San Francisco, 1981, Harper & Row.

Kubicek LF: Fresh perspectives on young children and family routines, *Zero to Three* 22:4-20, 2002.

Levine M et al: Neurodevelopmental readiness for adolescence: studies of an assessment instrument for 9- to 14-year-old children, *Dev Behavior Pediatr* 9:181-188, 1988.

Marino RV: School absenteeism and school refusal. In Hoekelman RA, editor: *Primary pediatric care*, St Louis, 2001, Mosby.

Munro R: Mental health: recovery is a state of mind, *Nurs Times* 97:12, 2001.

Myers K, Winters NC: Ten-year review of rating scales. II. Scales for internalizing disorders, *J Am Acad Child Adolesc Psychiatry* 41:634-659, 2002.

Ogden CL et al: Prevalence and trends in overweight among US children and adolescents, 1999–2000, *JAMA* 288:1772-1773, 2002.

Schor E: Guiding the family of the school-aged child, *Contemp Pediatr* 15:75-93, 1998.

Search Institute: Cornerstone Project. Available at *www.search-institute.org* (accessed Feb 23, 2003).

Shonkoff JP, Phillips DA, editors, Committee on Integrating the Science of Early Childhood Development, Board on Children, Youth, and Families: *From neurons to neighborhoods: the science of early childhood development*, Washington, DC, 2000, National Academies Press.

Stancin T, Palermo TM: A review of behavioral screening practices in pediatric settings: do they pass the test? *J Dev Behav Pediatr* 18:183-194, 1997.

Story M, Holt K, Sofka D, editors: *Bright Futures in practice: nutrition*, ed 2, Arlington, VA, 2002, National Center for Education in Maternal and Child Health.

Tanner J: Neurodevelopmental variation in school-aged children, *Compr Ther* 21:499-506, 1995.

Taylor CS et al: Individual and ecological assets and positive developmental trajectories among gang and community-based organization youth, *New Dir Youth Dev Fall* 95:57-72, 2002.

Van Buskirk D: School refusal. In Dershewitz R, editor: *Ambulatory pediatrics*, ed 2, Philadelphia, 1999, JB Lippincott.

Vessey JA, Jackson PA: School and the child with a chronic condition. In Jackson PA, Vessey JA, editors: *Primary care of the child with a chronic condition*, St Louis, 2000, Mosby.

Vessey JA, Mebane DJ: Chronic conditions and child development. In Jackson PA, Vessey JA, editors: *Primary care of the child with a chronic condition*, St Louis, 2000, Mosby.

Wang Y: Cross-national comparison of childhood obesity: the epidemic and the relationship between obesity and socioeconomic status, *Int J Epidemiol* 30:1136-1137, 2001.

Wierzbicki M: A parent form of the Children's Depression Inventory: reliability and validity in nonclinical populations, *J Clin Psychol* 43:390-397, 1987.

9 Developmental Management of Adolescents

Ardys M. Dunn, Judith W. Fisher

The changes a young person experiences during the transition from childhood to young adulthood are dramatic. The extent of physiologic growth and maturation rivals that occurring during infancy. Social and psychologic changes are also extreme, and these changes can create a tenuous sense of balance during this phase of development. The common question on the mind of most adolescents is, "Am I normal?" Anticipatory guidance and reassurance during well-child care are perhaps the most valuable services a health care provider can offer the adolescent. This chapter focuses on the normal physical and psychosocial growth and development of adolescents, and provides practitioners with a framework for structuring care of the adolescent client.

DEVELOPMENT OF ADOLESCENTS

Puberty is the term for the biologic process that ultimately leads to fertility. The hormonal regulatory systems in the hypothalamus, pituitary, gonads, and adrenal glands undergo major changes between the prepubertal and adult states. Accompanying these changes are rapid growth in height and weight, development of secondary sex characteristics, and onset of fertility (Fig. 9-1) (see Chapters 26 and 36). Limits of normal can be difficult to define and are best understood as approximations rather than precise parameters. However, even though the timing (tempo) of adolescent development is variable, the sequence of events is orderly (Fig. 9-2).

Adolescence refers to the psychosocial and emotional transition from childhood to adulthood. The physical changes of puberty are accompanied by significant cognitive and psychosocial development that affects how adolescents view themselves and how the world views adolescents. Successful development in adolescence culminates in achievement of goals that can provide the basis for a healthy and productive adult life (Table 9-1).

Physical Development

Tanner Stages

Pubertal growth and maturation can be divided into five stages ranging from prepubertal (sexual maturity rating [SMR] 1) to adult (SMR 5). These divisions are termed *Tanner stages* (Tanner, 1962) (Figs. 9-3 and 9-4). Pubertal changes occur on a continuum, with individual differences in timing or tempo.

Female Stages. Females enter puberty earlier than males do and thus lose a year or so of the slow, but steady, prepubertal growth that males experience. For girls, puberty usually progresses sequentially in the following pattern:

- Ovaries increase in size; no visible body changes occur.
- Breast budding (thelarche) occurs, on average, at 11 years of age, with 95% of normal girls having initial breast development between 9 and 13 years of age. Most girls (85%) experience the development of breast buds approximately 6 months before the appearance of pubic hair. However, some females have pubic hair before the development of breast buds. The timing of onset of breast development in females has no relationship to breast size at the completion of puberty.
- Rapid linear growth usually begins shortly after the onset of breast budding and reaches its peak about a year later. Most girls experience peak height velocity (PHV) at

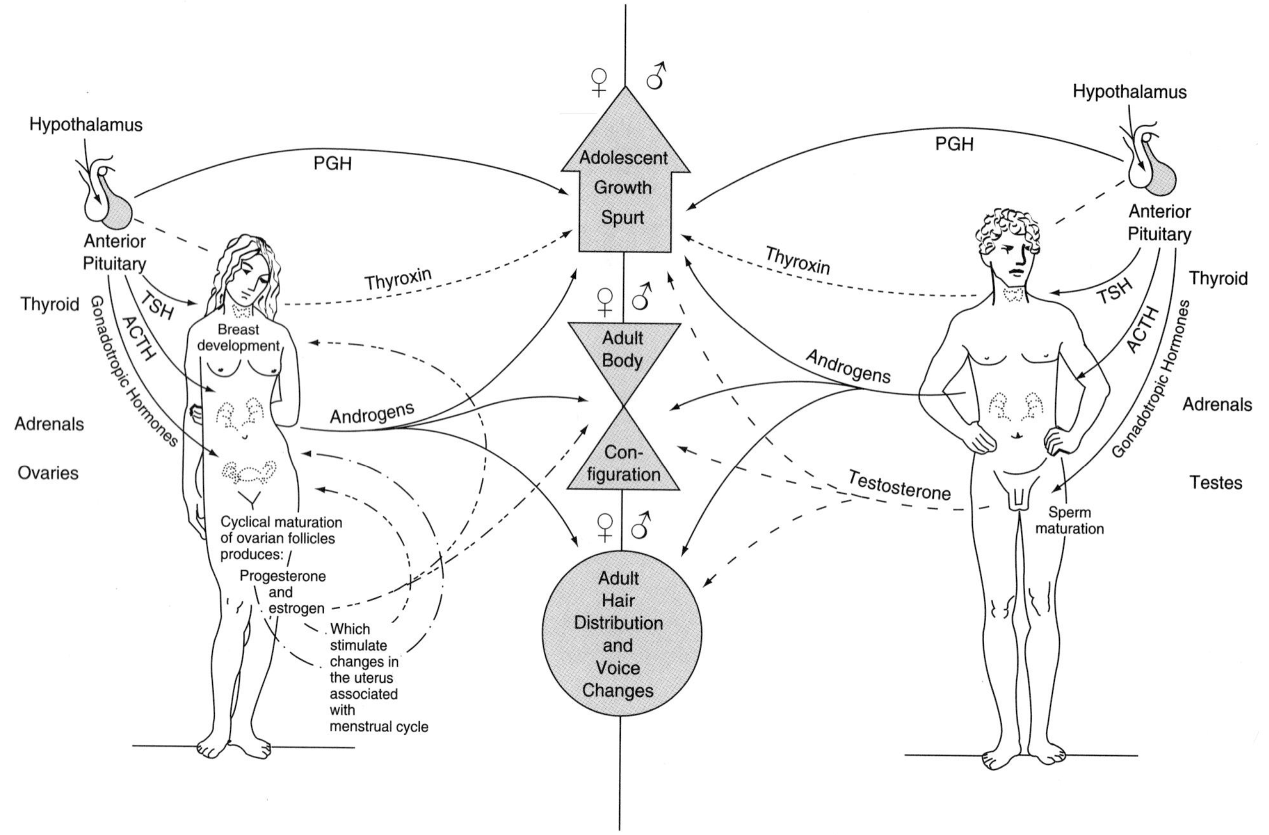

FIGURE 9-1 The endocrine system at puberty. *ACTH,* Adrenocorticotropic hormone; *PGH,* pituitary growth hormone; *TSH,* thyroid-stimulating hormone. (From Valadian I, Porter D: *Physical growth and development from conception to maturity,* Boston, 1977, Little, Brown.)

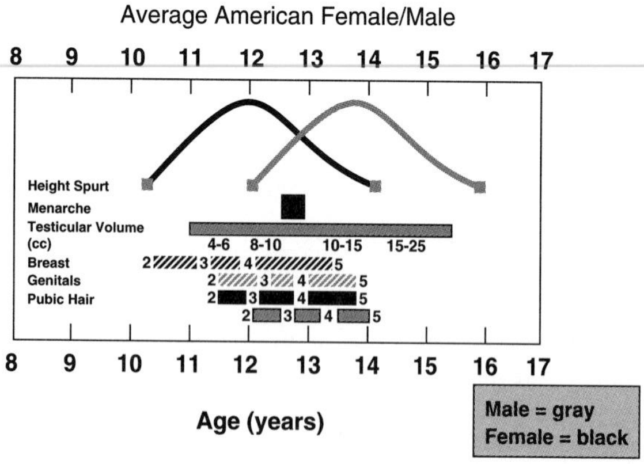

FIGURE 9-2 Sequence of pubertal events. Breast, genital, and pubic hair development indicate Tanner stages 2 to 5. (Adapted from Division of Adolescent Medicine, Children's Hospital Medical Center, Cincinnati, OH, 1995.)

about SMR 3, generally between ages 11 and 12, and PHV is completed by age 13. Early developers may experience a height spurt between ages 9 and 10, whereas late developers may not experience a height spurt until between the ages of 13 and 14. Final height is determined by the amount of bone growth at the epiphyses of the long bones. Growth stops when hormonal factors shut down the epiphyseal plates.

- Appearance of pubic hair (adrenarche or pubarche), which commences at about 11.5 years of age, is related to adrenal rather than gonadal development, not to thelarche; therefore it is less valid than other secondary sex characteristics in assessing sexual maturation.
- First menstrual period (menarche) occurs. The average age of menarche is 12.5 years, with more than 95% of girls experiencing menarche between 10.5 and 14.5 years of age. The mean age of menarche is highly dependent

TABLE 9-1 ***Adolescent Development and Related Anticipatory Guidance***

Area of Development	Anticipatory Guidance
Physical	
Experience growth from prepubescence to sexual maturity Reach adult parameters of height and physical growth by late adolescence Become comfortable with one's body	Teach child about body functions (e.g., menstruation, nocturnal emissions) of both sexes Provide prevention counseling regarding substance abuse, safety, and unintentional injuries (e.g., bicycle helmet use, seat belts, gun storage) Offer reassurance that physical findings are normal; explain what to expect; listen to adolescents' concerns; encourage sports participation and body fitness
Cognitive	
Move from concrete thinking to ability to reason abstractly Develop personal value system and moral integrity	Emphasize value of successful completion of school Engage adolescent in conversation, explain procedures, and answer questions Encourage discussion of what the adolescent feels is important and what the adolescent finds of value Help the adolescent develop skills in conflict resolution and avoidance Discuss respect for rights, needs, and opinions of others
Psychosocial	
Establish independence from parents Develop sense of self-identity Create new relationships with peers and other adults	Explain to parents an adolescent's need for privacy and that not joining in all family activities is not a sign of rejection Discuss the notion that increased independence also requires increased responsibility Encourage adolescents to take responsibility for their own health care Encourage adolescent to take on new challenges; discuss plans for the future (e.g., school, work, family) Discuss importance of activities with peers; identify healthy ways to be part of a group Encourage the adolescent to participate in community activities Provide information and opportunity to discuss questions regarding sexuality, how to differentiate between "love" and "infatuation," how to be sexually responsible, and how to protect against pregnancy and sexually transmitted diseases

on ethnic, socioeconomic, and nutritional factors. Menarche generally occurs 1.5 to 2.5 years after thelarche. An average of 17% of body fat is generally needed for menarche, and about 22% is needed to initiate and maintain regular ovulatory cycles. It may be 18 to 24 months after menarche before females establish regular ovulatory cycles. To some degree, menstrual cycles may be affected by the athletic activity of the female (Warren & Perlroth, 2001).

Changes in the body composition of females also occur during puberty, and adolescent girls will benefit from the nurse practitioner's (NP's) reassurance that these changes are normal. Girls often have asymmetric breasts and need assurance that breasts become more or less the same size within a few years after the onset of breast budding. The female body shape changes (to the glee or chagrin of teenagers) as girls progress through puberty; broadening of the shoulders, hips, and thighs becomes apparent. Girls experience a continuous increase in proportion of fat to total body mass during puberty. They enter puberty with approximately 80% lean body weight and 20% body fat. By the time puberty ends, lean body mass drops to about 75%. As mentioned, body fat is an important mediator for the onset of menstruation and regular ovulatory cycles.

Male Stages. Physical body changes of puberty generally occur sequentially in males as follows:

- Growth of the testes occurs approximately 6 months before the development of pubic hair in most males. If testicular enlargement does not precede other changes, the NP should consider whether the youngster is taking exogenous anabolic steroids. Once puberty begins, the left testis generally hangs lower than the right.
- Pubic hair development follows a pattern similar to that of girls (see Fig. 9-4).
- First release of spermatozoa (spermarche) generally occurs in midpuberty at a mean age of 13.5 to 14.5 years. However, it can occur at any stage of development from SMR 2 to 5.
- Elongation and widening of the penis usually begins in SMR 3 and continues through SMR 5 (see Fig. 9-4).

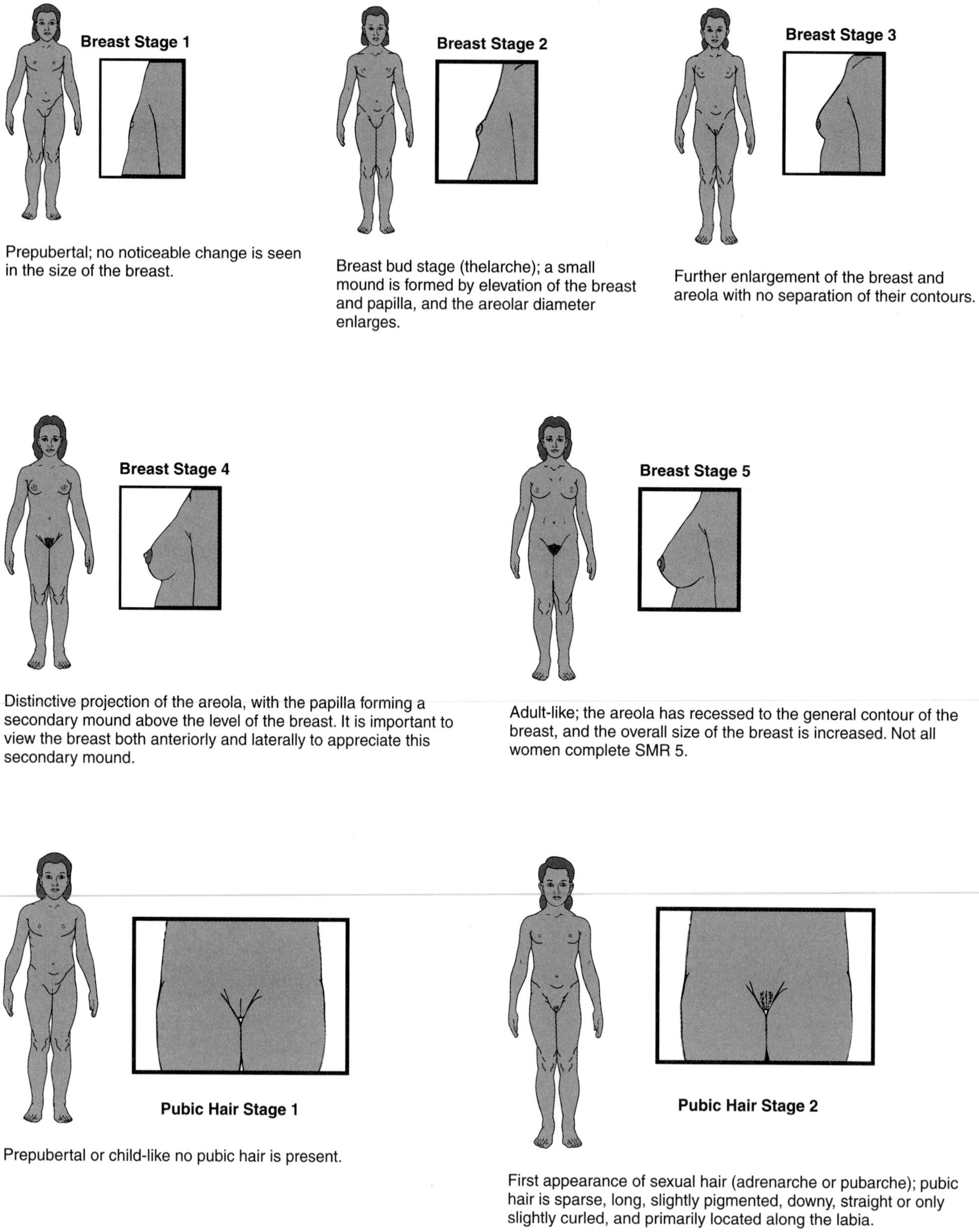

Breast Stage 1
Prepubertal; no noticeable change is seen in the size of the breast.
Breast Stage 2
Breast bud stage (thelarche); a small mound is formed by elevation of the breast and papilla, and the areolar diameter enlarges.
Breast Stage 3
Further enlargement of the breast and areola with no separation of their contours.
Breast Stage 4
Distinctive projection of the areola, with the papilla forming a secondary mound above the level of the breast. It is important to view the breast both anteriorly and laterally to appreciate this secondary mound.
Breast Stage 5
Adult-like; the areola has recessed to the general contour of the breast, and the overall size of the breast is increased. Not all women complete SMR 5.
Pubic Hair Stage 1
Prepubertal or child-like no pubic hair is present.
Pubic Hair Stage 2
First appearance of sexual hair (adrenarche or pubarche); pubic hair is sparse, long, slightly pigmented, downy, straight or only slightly curled, and primarily located along the labia.

FIGURE 9-3 Tanner stages: female. (Adapted from Division of Adolescent Medicine, Children's Hospital Medical Center, Cincinnati, OH, 1995.)

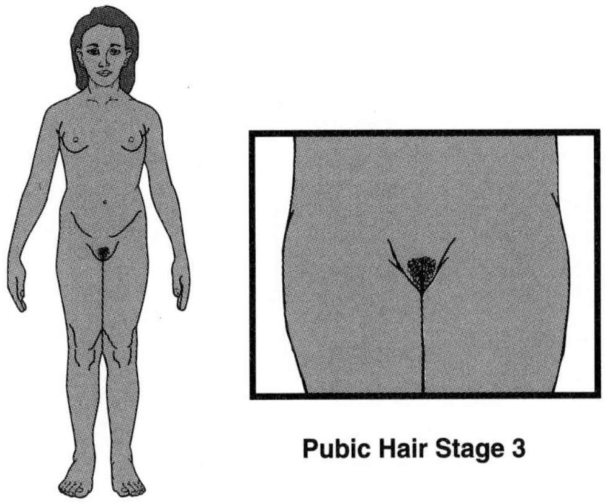

Pubic Hair Stage 3

Pubic hair is coarser, darker, and more curled; spreads over the middle of the pubic bone.

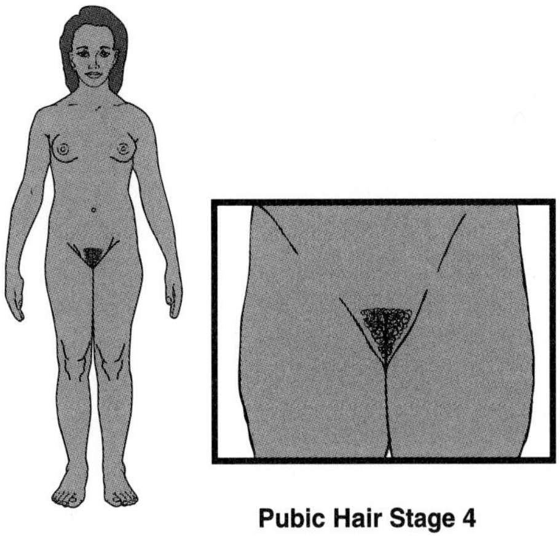

Pubic Hair Stage 4

Pubic hair is adult-like in appearance but not in distribution; does not extend onto the thighs.

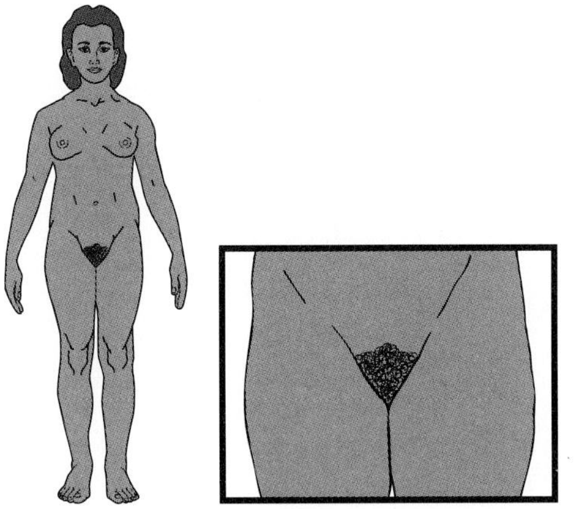

Pubic Hair Stage 5

Pubic hair is adult-like in appearance and extends onto the thighs; may extend in the midline in the shape of a broad-based triangle. Generally, females reach pubic hair stage 5 before reaching breast stage 5.

FIGURE 9-3 cont'd

- Rapid growth in height occurs. The PHV for males tends to occur late in middle puberty to early in late puberty. Boys generally lag about 2 years behind girls, but the height spurt can begin as early as 10.5 years or as late as 16 years. One fifth of normal adolescent males do not reach their PHV until SMR 5, and there is some evidence that late maturers may achieve greater PHV (Iuliano-Burns, Mirwald, & Bailey, 2001). Males can continue to grow, although minimally, well beyond their teenage years.
- Change in the male voice occurs; this coincides with the PHV.
- Development of axillary, facial, and body hair occurs. Axillary hair generally does not appear before SMR 4 pubic hair. Facial hair appears only after SMR 4 pubic hair and does so in an ordered sequence. It starts at the outer corners of the upper lip and moves inward, then appears on the upper parts of the cheeks and middle of the lower lip, and finally grows along the sides and lower border of the chin. The extent of body hair is determined to a large extent by genetic factors. Body hair develops gradually after facial hair. The hair changes should not, however, be used as a parameter for assessing pubertal maturation related to changes in the endocrine system.

As with girls, the body composition of adolescent boys changes, and the NP can be an invaluable source of information and reassurance. In contrast to females, males

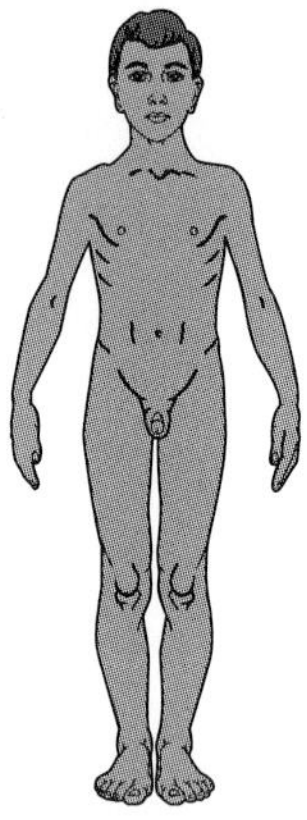
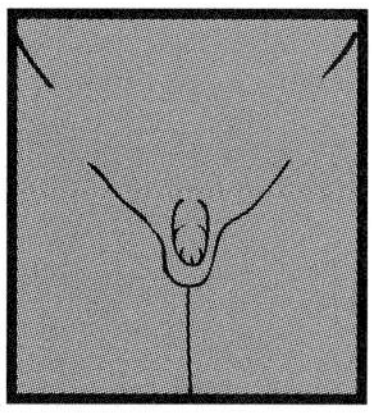

Pubic Hair Stage 1

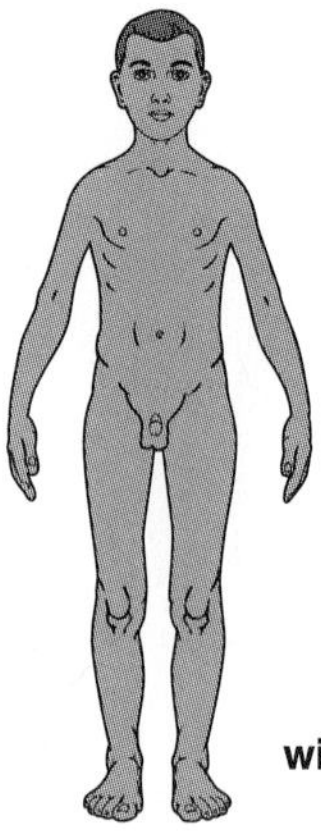
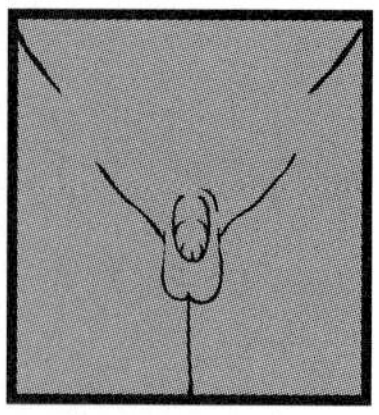

Pubic Hair Stage 1 with Early Testicular Maturation

Prepubertal; no pubic hair is present; penis, testes, and scrotum are child-like in size. The prepubertal testis is generally less than 4 ml in volume and less than 2.5 cm in greatest diameter.

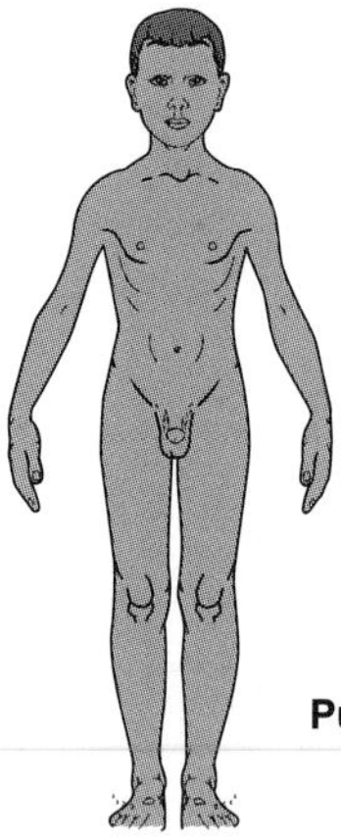
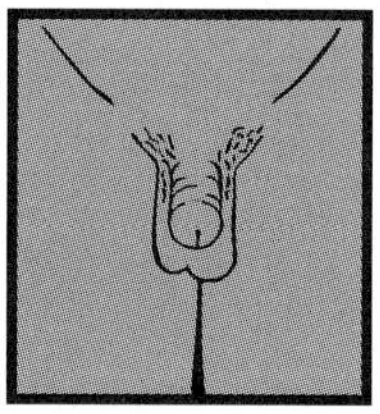

Pubic Hair Stage 2

First appearance of sexual hair (adrenarche or pubarche); sparse growth of fine, downy hair along the base of the penis. Enlargement of the scrotum and testes begins, but the penis usually does not enlarge. The scrotal skin reddens.

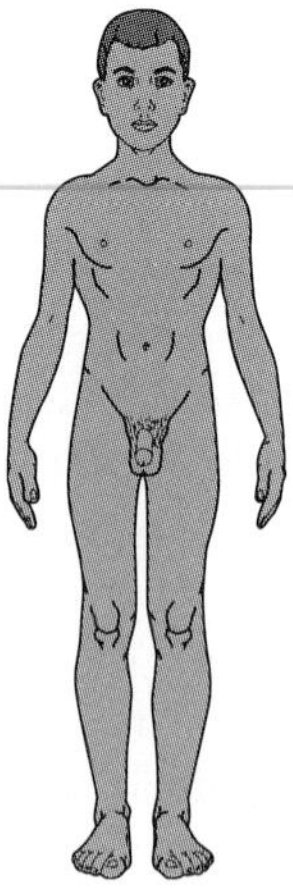
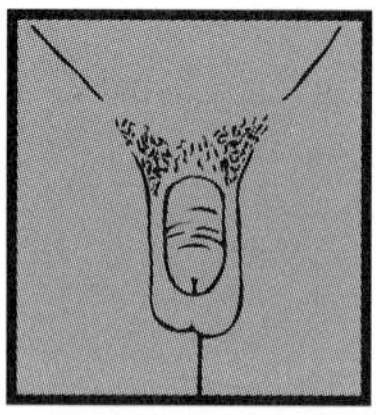

Pubic Hair Stage 3

Pubic hair is darker, coarser, and curlier and extends over the middle of the pubic bone. Further growth of the testes and scrotum occurs, with enlargement of the penis, mostly in length.

FIGURE 9-4 Tanner stages: male. (Adapted from Division of Adolescent Medicine, Children's Hospital Medical Center, Cincinnati, OH, 1995.)

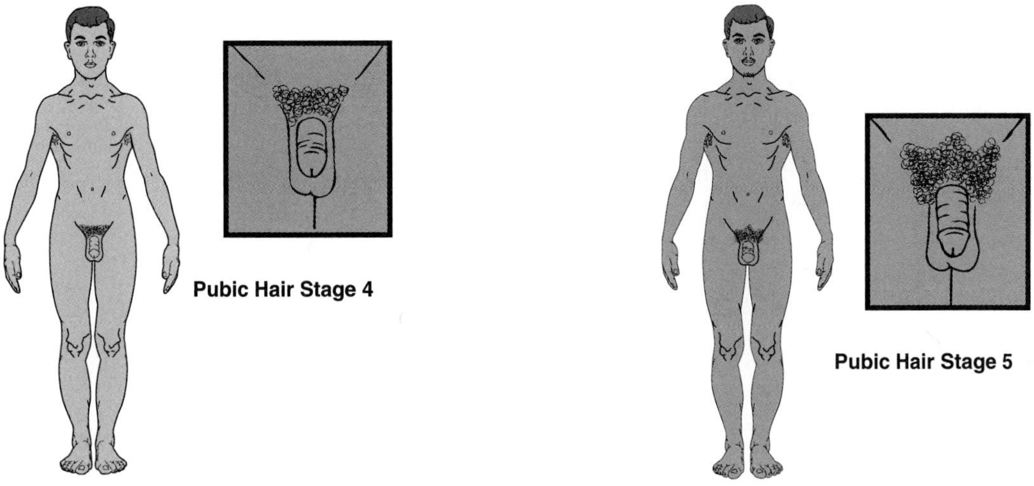

Pubic hair is adult-like in appearance and extends onto the thighs; may extend toward the umbilicus. Genitals are adult-like in size. Growth of the penis is generally complete before full development of the testes or pubic hair.

Pubic hair is adult-like in appearance but not in distribution; does not extend onto the thighs. Growth of the testes (10 to 15 ml) and scrotum continues. The penis increases in size, especially in width, because of growth of the corpora cavernosa in response to testosterone.

FIGURE 9-4 cont'd

generally experience progressive loss in the relative amount of body fat through puberty, along with an increase in muscle mass.

Some changes associated with puberty may be unwelcome. For males, approximately half the population experiences a transient enlargement of breast tissue called *gynecomastia.* Gynecomastia generally lasts 12 to 18 months and resolves completely in nearly all cases by late puberty. However, in a small percentage of males, some palpable breast tissue may persist. Acne starts in early puberty, and by midpuberty many males have moderate to severe acne, which becomes somewhat worse by the end of puberty. In cases of persistent gynecomastia or severe acne, the history should include questions to the patient regarding the use of alcohol, marijuana, and anabolic steroids, all of which can exacerbate these conditions.

Psychosocial, Emotional, and Cognitive Development

Principles of Adolescent Psychosocial, Emotional, and Cognitive Development

Although each child develops in a unique fashion, all adolescents have specific cognitive, emotional, and psychosocial developmental milestones to achieve as they transition from childhood to adulthood. These milestones include the following:

- Feeling a sense of belonging in a valued group
- Acquiring skills and mastering tasks that are important to the valued group
- Developing a sense of self-worth
- Developing at least one reliable relationship with another
- Demonstrating cognitive potential

The adolescent's ability to achieve these goals depends in part on brain functioning. Although full-sized, the adolescent brain continues to develop. In particular, the prefrontal cortex, which coordinates executive functions of abstract thinking, reasoning, judgment, self-discipline, ethical behavior, personality, and emotions, is experiencing rapid growth. As with the infant brain, a process of pruning and reinforcement occurs, based on the stimuli, activities, and experiences of the teenager. The brain is subject to chemical, hormonal, physical, and biologic changes.

The adolescent brain appears to be particularly vulnerable to schizophrenia and to addiction. Schizophrenia most often appears in the second decade of life, during late adolescence or early adulthood, and is characterized by disturbances in memory and concentration, a decreased sense of connectedness, and changes in emotional responses. The individual often experiences hallucinations or hears voices. Though its cause is unknown, schizophrenia may be due to previous brain damage, and there is some indication that the cortex of the brain is slightly thinner in individuals with this disease.

Drugs, including alcohol, have a significant negative impact on the adolescent brain, damaging the neural circuitry in the "reward" or motivation pathways, and shutting down the body's ability to respond to stimuli that normally generate feelings of pleasure. In essence, the drug becomes the only thing that leads to pleasurable feelings, and a craving for the drug is "etched" into the brain—the individual becomes addicted. Genetic structures of individuals vary, however, and not all brains respond to drugs in this way, but the adolescent brain, due to its rapid growth, is highly vulnerable.

A wide variety of normal behavior characterizes the process of psychosocial, emotional, and cognitive development. Three general principles may be used to understand the changes seen in adolescent development:

- Transition is continuous and generally smooth.
- Disruptive family conflict is not the norm.
- The quality of thinking changes from concrete to formal operational thinking.

Smooth Transition. The first principle of adolescent psychosocial development is that the transition from adolescence to adulthood is continuous and generally smooth. A commonly held myth is that adolescence is a period of "storm and stress." This view was originally described by G. Stanley Hall in 1904 (Hall, 1904). Although his argument was not based on research, his ideas continue to be popular and influential today. It is important to remember that this period of development is only one of many transitional phases in life and may not be a difficult period for many.

Family Relationships. The second principle of adolescent psychosocial development is that the biologic, cognitive, and emotional changes experienced by adolescents prompt a reworking of family relationships. Some degree of adolescent-parent conflict is to be expected because of this reworking of relationships, but disruptive family conflict is not the norm. Despite societal changes, mundane, everyday issues such as what clothes to wear, hairstyles, household chores, curfew, and friends continue to be the usual sources of parent-adolescent conflict. It may also help to remind parents that verbal debate, or "arguing," is a normal behavior of teens that reflects their use of more abstract thinking skills. It is a way of practicing abstract thinking and engaging parents. However, the parent should not become too deeply engaged because the adolescent rarely is, and the "arguments" tend to blow over fairly quickly (Box 9-1).

Families should not be experiencing one crisis after another. If family crises are the norm, one should be concerned. When true turmoil exists, it usually represents psychopathology and will not be simply "outgrown." Careful assessment and treatment are required. Behavior that results in negative consequences is cause for concern (e.g., red hair dye grows out, but being expelled from school has long-term consequences).

Cognitive Changes. The third principle of adolescent psychosocial development reflects change in cognitive abilities. Adolescents develop what is referred to as *formal operational thinking*, which is characterized by the use of propositional thinking and abstract reasoning. The principal difference between concrete and formal operational thinking is the ability to reason using verbal manipulation rather than in terms of concrete objects. In early adolescence, thinking tends to be very concrete. The classic example is an adolescent who when asked, "Are you sexually active?" responds, "No, I just lie there." Or when

BOX 9-1 *Tips for Parents: Adolescent Survival Guide*

1. Start with clear rules and expectations before children are teenagers. State expectations and future consequences before trouble has occurred (e.g., before the dance, not when the teen comes home late).
2. Be firm and follow through.
3. Try to be flexible and allow teenagers to negotiate. Discussing principles and negotiating solutions are valuable life skills for the future. Do not negotiate rules that are nonnegotiable.
4. Fighting and arguing are typical, often employed by teens as they practice their developing reasoning skills. Often, teens are engaged more recreationally than emotionally. Therefore when the patient is tired, disengage and walk away. Try not to take what they say personally.
5. Teenagers want parents to be involved, concerned, and asking questions. They just may not know it.
6. Know who their friends are and call those parents from time to time. Compare household rules if possible.
7. Be involved at their school if possible. Try to meet their teachers and stay in contact with them.
8. Continue to involve teenagers in family activities, even when they no longer want to. Bringing friends along will help.
9. Keep promises made to teens. This builds trust and respect and makes you a role model.

asked, "What brings you here to see me today?" answers, "The bus."

Younger children think in concrete fashion. Around age 14 and throughout adolescence, most teenagers acquire increasing sophistication in abstract thought. They learn to conceptualize about past and future events and to relate actions to consequences. During this process, adolescents begin to:

- Consider values. The ones they challenge most are those with which they are most familiar (e.g., in the past they always attended church on Sundays or always went to their grandmother's for Sunday dinner, but now they do not want to).
- Understand concepts of good and evil and understand human nature (e.g., not all authority figures are good people).
- Be aware of contradictions between what is said and what is done (e.g., parents may tell their children not to smoke or drink even though they do, or they may tell them to wear their seat belts although they do not).
- Understand the significance of the concept of time (past, present, future) and begin thinking about what they will be doing in the future (e.g., college, technical school, job, marriage, and family).

Although most teenagers become able to translate experiences into abstract ideas and think about the consequences of actions, approximately one third do not achieve more fully sophisticated thinking abilities even as adults. Environmental influences on the brain, both in adolescence (e.g., drug use or drinking by teenagers) and previously (e.g., prenatal alcohol exposure—even in children not diagnosed with fetal alcohol syndrome) affect the adolescent's thinking capacity (Mattson et al, 1999). Parents can help adolescents refine their critical thinking skills by arguing points of principle, but not taking emotional positions (Elkind, 1984).

Emotional Changes of Adolescence

Hormones present during puberty cause emotional as well as physical changes. As with physical growth and development, emotional changes appear differently in males than in females. Some males may experience an association between an increase in testosterone and sad and anxious affects, as well as acting out, aggressive behavior, and sexual activity.

Some emotional changes that occur in males are not directly associated with hormonal changes. Research has shown that boys with adultlike physiques are given more leadership roles, are more proficient in sports, are perceived as more attractive and smarter than their peers, and are more popular than others in their age-group. In general, they also demonstrate high self-esteem in early adolescence. Late-maturing boys who are short and childlike in appearance until 15 or older tend to show more personal and social maladjustment over the entire course of adolescence. They tend to be insecure, suggestible, and vulnerable to peer pressure. Members of this group may be seen as weak, immature, and often less competent than average. Males, as they progress through puberty, typically develop a more positive self-image and mood, whereas females may feel a diminished sense of attractiveness as their bodies mature. Boys tend to be more satisfied with their body image and often want to gain weight, whereas girls are more likely to express dissatisfaction with changes in their body and want to lose weight. This dissatisfaction with body image tends to develop earlier than adolescence (in one study of third graders, 17% of boys and 24% of girls had dieted or were dieting to lose weight [Robinson et al, 2001]), and efforts to change weight continue into the teen years (McCabe & Ricciardelli, 2001).

The emotional affect and behavior of pubescent females differ in other ways from those of boys. Early-maturing girls have more problems in adaptation than do girls who are late maturing (Ge, Conger, & Elder, 2001). Often, these early bloomers get "bumped up" to an older group of peers and become the objects of sexual attention from older males. The developing body of early-maturing females may not match their chronologic age or emotional maturity. For instance, a female fifth grader who is as tall as her teacher stands out from her peers. This difference can influence her behavior and place some females at risk for early sexual involvement, smoking, and drinking (Kaltiala-Heino et al, 2001; Lanza & Collins, 2002).

Egocentrism of Adolescents

Changes in the quality of adolescent thinking coupled with physical and emotional changes give rise to a form of egocentrism. This change may result in a rather self-centered, but not necessarily selfish, view of the world. Although there are recommendations that this prototype requires more research for validation (Vartanian, 2000), four major types of adolescent egocentrism that even adults exhibit at times are generally recognized (Elkind, 1984):

- *Imaginary audience:* Everyone is thinking about them.
- *Personal fable:* They are special.
- *Overthinking:* They make things more complicated than they are.
- *Apparent hypocrisy:* Rules apply differently to them than to others.

Imaginary Audience. Abstract thinking allows teenagers to wonder what others are thinking about. At the same time, adolescents are obsessed by the physical changes brought about by puberty. These changes and their new thinking abilities create the notion that everyone is thinking about the same thing that they are (i.e., them). Teenagers may believe that one can read minds and know what others are thinking. For example, a boy who goes to the drugstore to purchase a condom may feel that he is "on stage," the object of everyone's scrutiny. An adolescent wearing orthopedic braces may think that everyone is staring at him. A young girl who has a pimple on her nose may feel that it is the first thing others see when they look at her.

Personal Fable. The second type of egocentrism is the personal fable. If everyone is watching you and thinking about you (thanks to the imaginary audience), you must be someone special. The personal fable is the concept that the laws of nature do not apply to oneself and that one's thoughts and feelings are totally unique. Common examples include adolescents who believe that they will never grow old, cannot get pregnant (especially the first time), cannot get a sexually transmitted infection despite engaging in unprotected intercourse, or will not suffer long-term consequences from substance use. The personal fable has a positive aspect as well, in that it provides adolescents with a sense of importance, purpose, and hope.

Overthinking. Overthinking involves making things more complicated than they need to be. An example might be an adolescent who attributes complicated motives to simple oversights (e.g., an adolescent boy who thinks that his parents would not have divorced if only he had helped more with the chores around the house, or an adolescent girl who breaks up with her boyfriend because she assumes that he does not like her because he did not compliment her on her new red dress).

Apparent Hypocrisy. Apparent hypocrisy is the notion that rules apply differently to adolescents than they do to others. For example, an adolescent girl may believe that she should have free access to her parent's clothes and electronic equipment (such as the stereo or home computer), whereas her parents entering her room to borrow a tape constitutes an invasion of privacy.

DEVELOPMENTAL SCREENING AND ASSESSMENT

Approaches to Assessment of Adolescents

Throughout infancy and the preschool and school years, the focus of the health care visit is always clearly the parent or caregiver and the child as a unit. This dyad changes with adolescence. Teenagers must be evaluated independently of their parents, and discussions about developmental issues occur with the adolescents themselves. Nonetheless, parents remain concerned and should ideally be involved in their child's health care.

Effective interviews with adolescent clients are based on the use of good general interviewing techniques: demonstrating respect for the client; establishing parameters of what can be accomplished during the visit; using appropriate body language, active listening, and communication techniques; and working with the client to develop a realistic, individualized treatment plan. The message given by the NP is that the teenager and his or her concerns are important, that no judgments will be made, and that the NP and teenager are a team, working together to achieve the healthiest outcome possible.

Preserving confidentiality with the teenager while acknowledging the importance of parents to the child's development is essential. Adolescents should be reassured that the NP will not share information with the child's parent or caregiver (general confidentiality), unless the adolescent agrees. At the same time, NPs must inform the teenager that there are limits to confidentiality (limited confidentiality). As "mandatory reporters," NPs are required by law to report information that puts the child in danger (e.g., physical or sexual abuse; some states require reporting teen sexual activity, even if consensual, if an age difference of 3 or more years exists between the couple). NPs should also inform the adolescent that information that compromises the health of the child or others (e.g., threat of potential suicide, violence, evidence of an eating disorder) will be disclosed. If adolescents perceive that their provider will maintain confidentiality, they are more likely to disclose more sensitive, relevant information; and it has been found that when providers discuss the limits to their confidentiality, teens continue to disclose (Ford et al, 1997).

NPs may believe that involving parents or other significant adults in the adolescent's care is essential. However, that decision is not always the NP's to make alone; the adolescent must be actively included in decisions about sharing information with others. For many sensitive health issues, the NP will need to help the teenager understand and evaluate the risks and benefits of involving family members. NPs must also provide guidance and support on how to best inform the family, if that is the final choice. This approach can help protect a teen from the parent who may be abusive or unsafe. It also can reduce the problem of parents who are upset if they feel they are denied information about the child they love and for whom they feel responsible.

The American Medical Association (AMA) has developed a thorough interview format for teens in their published AMA Guidelines for Adolescent Preventive Services

(GAPS) program (Elster & Kuznets, 1994). The HEADSS technique can be used to assess risk behaviors of adolescents (see discussion later in this chapter).

For teenagers who are hesitant to discuss sensitive issues, a questionnaire or checklist may be an effective way to collect information (Wilf-Miron et al, 2000). Questionnaires used to identify adolescent strengths have also been created by the Search Institute and have been used by communities to enhance adolescent self-concept (see Chapter 18).

Physical Development

Adolescents should have height, weight, body mass index (BMI), and blood pressure measured at each health maintenance visit. Assessment of the growth trajectory with grids to identify growth norms is essential. Additionally, the Tanner stage should be recorded at each visit to evaluate progression of the pubertal changes initiated by the endocrine system. Testicular growth can be directly assessed by palpation of the testes in the scrotum and comparison of their size with a standardized orchiometer. Self-assessment is generally reliable, and adolescent males can be asked to evaluate their own level of development if provided with standards against which to compare themselves. Varicocele, or enlarged veins palpable in the scrotum, may develop at sexual maturity and are not cause for alarm unless a discrepancy in testicular size is noted on examination. Gynecomastia in boys should be noted. Scoliosis may develop rapidly at this age, and assessment should be done annually. The thyroid gland should be palpated because goiter may appear in this age-group. Additionally, the teen should be questioned about attitudes regarding physical growth and development. Dissatisfaction with body appearance might warrant further probing to elicit unhealthy behavior (e.g., bingeing and purging, steroid use).

Cognitive Development

Assessment should include questions about school attendance, school performance, and educational or career goals. Successful school performance can be an important predictor for adolescent well-being and healthy behaviors (Bryant et al, 2000). Children who are behind a grade have a 20% to 30% greater chance of dropping out of school. School failure could be viewed as "failure to thrive in adolescence" (Reiff, 1998). Chronic absenteeism, class skipping, and other types of school avoidance may indicate an underlying mental health problem and should be assessed in depth. Objective assessment of cognitive development, as with school-age children, requires formal psychologic testing, which is best done through schools.

Social and Emotional Development

Key areas to assess in relation to social and emotional development include adolescents' emerging independence from family, relationships with peers, and goals for the future (an area that older teenagers should address more specifically than younger adolescents).

Adolescents should be interviewed about school, family, and peer relationships; safety (e.g., use of seat belts); exposure to violence, abuse, or weapons in their home or community; mental health issues such as mood, depression, anger problems, or suicidal ideation; sexuality, sexual activity, and sexual orientation; and involvement in risk behavior such as tobacco, alcohol, and prescription or street drug use and eating disorders.

Parent Assessment

As at other developmental stages of childhood, parents are also changing in response to the adolescent's pressure on the family. Parents, too, need advice, support, and encouragement.

GAPS (Elster & Kuznets, 1994) also offers recommendations for health guidance for parents. The parent interview should occur on three occasions during adolescence: early, middle, and late. The interview should consist of parents' concerns about adolescents relating to

- Health problems
- Physical development
- Social and emotional development
- Parenting issues
- Changing family structures

If problems exist in the parent's view or a discrepancy and potential conflict emerge in the interviews, the NP should bring the teen and parent together to clarify the concern and offer counseling.

ANTICIPATORY GUIDANCE DURING ADOLESCENCE

One simple way to understand adolescence is to divide it into three psychosocial developmental phases: early, 11 to 14 years old or junior high school; middle, 15 to 17 years old or high school; and late, 18 to 21 years old or college, work, or vocational-technical school.

Each phase is characterized by certain behavior. Understanding such behavior can assist in identifying behavior of concern to the adolescent or family. Within each developmental phase, adolescents deal with issues of autonomy, body image, peer group involvement, and identity development.

Early Adolescence (11 to 14 Years)

Parameters of Normal Development

Early adolescence is the most difficult adjustment period for young people (Larson et al, 2002). Rapid changes are occurring simultaneously in all parts of the adolescent's life; cognitive skills may not be able to keep pace with physical changes; emotional reactions may overwhelm the child's ability to understand and cope. Early adolescents are often confused, even frightened, by the changes they are experiencing. They can be difficult people to be around, and the responses their behavior elicits from parents and other adults may be exactly the opposite of the support, caring, and understanding they desperately need.

Young adolescents begin to renegotiate relationships with parents and other significant adults and develop more intimate contacts with their peers. At the same time, lacking experience and social skills, they may not yet be a part of an adolescent subculture, and can be very lonely. At this stage teenagers can appear to be antiadult, preferring to spend more time with friends than with family, and suddenly finding their parents to be an embarrassment. This behavior is a normal and healthy step toward maturity and a first step toward independence. One way of demonstrating independence is to challenge parental authority. The adolescent may become more argumentative and disobedient, refuse to do chores, and want to renegotiate rules (e.g., curfews, allowance, household responsibilities).

Wide mood swings—from euphoria to sadness—can occur within a matter of minutes. Normative fluctuations of mood are linked to adolescent developmental processes and are characterized by their transient nature, commonly measured in hours or days. These emotional fluctuations can and should be distinguished from the unremitting, long-standing mood and behavior changes of serious depressive disorders.

During this period, adolescents become extremely conscious of their bodies as they adjust to the physical changes they are experiencing. They begin to spend more time in front of the mirror combing their hair, checking their skin, and putting on makeup. Clothes and appearance become more important for all teenagers in this group, including those with a developmental delay or chronic handicap.

The most important question for an early adolescent is, "Am I normal?" Health care providers for adolescents must never lose sight of this concern. Early adolescents often use their friends as the measure by which they determine standards of normal appearance. They become overly sensitive and critical of their own appearance, certain they are too tall, too short, too fat, too thin, too developed, or not developed enough. NPs should allay anxiety during an adolescent's examination by actively affirming normalcy.

As their thinking abilities develop, teenagers daydream frequently. Parents and teachers need to be reminded that daydreaming is cognitive work for adolescents and that they need time to participate in this activity. At the same time, adolescents should be given the opportunity to use their growing reasoning skills to actively solve problems, explore values, and examine principles on which they make decisions.

Early adolescents set idealistic goals that change frequently. One day they want to be an engineer and the next day a pilot or a parent who stays home to raise children. Typically, these adolescents experience a drop in academic performance in junior high school, which is related to motivation rather than ability. Much of adolescents' time is used in the development of new friendships as a greater number of opportunities become possible.

Adolescents have a desire for greater privacy. They often spend more time in their room alone listening to music or talking on the phone. They magnify their problems and believe that no one could possibly understand what they are feeling.

Early adolescents begin to develop their own value system. They may try value systems other than the one that they have learned from their family, often leaving family members befuddled or even threatened. However, once adolescence is complete, young adults often have a modified value system very similar to the one with which they grew up.

The onset of secondary sex characteristics increases anxieties about menstruation, wet dreams, masturbation, and size of the breasts or penis. This is an opportune time to dispel myths (e.g., masturbation causes blindness and acne) and to provide anticipatory guidance (e.g., a premenarchal girl often has vaginal leukorrhea, which is generally a clear, mucoid discharge). Same-sex friendships occur, usually with one best friend. These strong friendships may lead to fleeting same-sex experimentation and the further development of a sexual identity. Contact with the opposite sex is usually in groups (e.g., middle school dances with boys on one side of the gym and girls on the opposite side). The peer group serves the purpose of aiding continued identity development.

Sexual feelings emerge, and behavior includes masturbating, telling dirty jokes, making lewd remarks to others, demonstrating interest in watching explicit sexual scenes in the media, or looking at magazines of nude individuals.

The type of sexual experimentation may vary greatly, depending on the adolescent's subculture. For example, by this age some teenagers have already experienced sexual intercourse or pregnancy, whereas others have not even held hands.

Developmental Anticipatory Guidance

Anticipatory guidance should be an individualized discussion with teenagers that helps them understand, respond to, and take responsibility for their own behavior and development. Separate discussions need to be conducted with parents to help them understand and support their child's maturation and need for independence. In these discussions, the NP should clarify what values and expectations parents have for their child, and how the teenager perceives those expectations. Some discussion points are outlined here. These topics are not all-inclusive, nor are they intended to be covered exhaustively at each visit. They can be used by the NP to apply developmental concepts in everyday living. If problems emerge from discussions in these areas, the NP is referred to the appropriate chapter for ideas for assessment and management (e.g., sexuality issues are discussed in Chapter 20).

Physical and Sexual Development

- *Rapid physical growth:* Knowing what to expect and understanding the implications of growth (e.g., for injury) help adolescents become more comfortable with their bodies.
- *Physical activity:* Finding ways to enjoy lifelong physical activity (e.g., team, club, or individual sports) is an important part of adolescence.
- *Sexuality:* Discussion should include the following:
  - Menstruation and its management
  - Masturbation and nocturnal emissions
  - Pubertal development of the opposite sex
  - Anticipated sexual changes
  - Abstinence counseling
  - Protection against sexually transmitted diseases and pregnancy

Cognitive Development

- Discuss with the adolescent how meeting academic responsibilities is a priority activity that needs to be integrated with other activities.
- Discuss with the adolescent how changes in cognitive abilities may contribute to "overthinking" or a sense of confusion; encourage him or her to do "reality checks" with a trusted adult.

Social and Emotional Development

- *Family interaction:* Not joining the family for all activities should not be interpreted by parents as rejection of the family.
- *Feelings:* Learning to identify feelings is the first step in understanding that "feelings" influence body processes.
- *Peers:* Peer interaction is important for all teenagers.
- *Dating relationships*: Healthy relationships are based on mutual respect.
- *Diversity:* Maturation involves understanding and appreciating multicultural differences.
- *Independence and responsibility:* Developing increased independence and accepting responsibilities at home and school and in the community are essential to maturation.
- *Privacy:* Some privacy within the home should be expected.

Self-care

- *Accident prevention:* Correct and consistent use of helmets, seat belts, and proper sports equipment should be taught and encouraged.
- *Weapons:* Access to guns and other weapons should be restricted, with emphasis on safety and responsibility.
- *Abusive behavior:* Counseling should be provided on the following:
  - Avoiding gang involvement
  - Preventing the use of drugs, cigarettes, and alcohol
  - Stopping substance use for those who are using
  - Avoiding date rape or other abusive relationships

Middle Adolescence (15 to 17 Years)

Parameters of Normal Development

Parental conflict peaks as middle adolescents continue to argue and renegotiate issues such as curfew, allowance, going to parties or movies, and dating. Rules and expectations must be clear by this stage. Physical development is nearing completion. Middle adolescents have less concern about body changes but increased interest in making themselves more attractive. As body attractiveness increases in importance, teenagers spend more time with hairstyles, clothes, and, for some, dieting or activities to build muscle mass. Teenagers with apparent handicaps have no less concern about their body image and participate in the same activities to improve their appearance.

Middle adolescents defy the limits of their bodies, and many have periods of excessive physical activity followed by periods of lethargy. They cannot seem to find the energy to get out of bed on the weekends to help the family with chores, but if one of their friends asks them to wash cars to raise money for a local charity, they are out the door with lightning speed.

Middle adolescence is the essence of adolescence and its subculture. Picture in your mind's eye what typical adolescents look like and how they behave (e.g., jocks, nerds, skaters, druggies, Goths). What are they wearing? How do they act? What language are they using to communicate to adults and to one another? The picture that probably comes to mind is that of a middle adolescent. Middle adolescents stand out for their unique appearance. Peer group involvement is intense and includes the establishment of a dress code, communication style, and code of conduct. They tend to be more nonadult than antiadult, a characteristic of early adolescents. By this time, more than twice as much of adolescents' time is spent with peers as with adults. The need for peer contact is no less important for teenagers with developmental disabilities, chronic handicaps, or both. However, peer involvement may be more limited for this group for any number of reasons (e.g., ostracism by the peer group, parental overprotectiveness, lack of social skills).

Sexual drive emerges, and middle adolescents begin to explore their ability to attract a partner. Dating activity and sexual experimentation and intercourse are beginning at younger ages. Frequently, physical urges precede emotional maturity, and societal pressure to experiment with sex is great. Adolescents of today are much more sexually tolerant than their predecessors. They are more sexually active than their parents were at the same age, and may be more sexually active than adolescents of any earlier time, including their older siblings. Ambivalence about desire for pregnancy is not uncommon, especially among adolescents lacking clear future goals.

Intellectual ability and creativity increase in middle adolescents. Practicing these skills of reasoning, logic, and decision making strengthens the adolescent's ability to establish healthy patterns as an adult. They demonstrate increased concern with neighborhood issues and certain societal issues, such as war or peace and the environment.

Because of the developing egocentrism and the concept of personal fable, with feelings of omnipotence, invulnerability, and immortality, risk taking and behavioral experimentation intensify. This stage may include smoking, use of alcohol, sexual activity, or drinking and driving.

Developmental Anticipatory Guidance

Physical and Sexual Development

- *Physical growth:* Rapid growth and increasing skill allow adolescents to engage in a wider variety of activities.
  - Recommend fitness and sports activities; discuss the dangers of performance-enhancing drugs.
  - Recommend involvement in other activities (e.g., clubs, hobbies).
  - Discuss nutrition and the relationship between good nutrition and health and a positive body image.
- *Sexuality:* Provide discussion and counseling about the following:
  - Implications of sexual intercourse
  - Postponement of coitus or the choice of abstinence
  - Prevention of sexually transmitted diseases
  - Birth control, including emergency methods
  - Breast or testicular self-examination

Cognitive Development

- Discuss the importance of completing schooling and making plans for the future.
- Acknowledge and validate more abstract reasoning.

Social and Emotional Development

- *Family interactions:*
  - Families should set reasonable limits for adolescents' behavior.
  - Families need to show interest in teenagers' work, interests, and activities.
- *Peers:* Adolescents should establish relationships with peers based on mutual respect, not promiscuous behavior.
- *Independence and responsibility:* Discuss how the adolescent is:
  - Learning to constructively resolve conflicts and manage feelings of anger
  - Learning to identify symptoms of stress and use of stress-reducing techniques

Self-care

- *Accident prevention:* Encourage correct and consistent use of helmets, seat belts, and proper sports equipment.
- *Weapons:* Access to guns and other weapons should be restricted, with emphasis on safety and responsibility.
- *Abusive behavior:* Counseling should be provided on the following:
  - Avoiding gang involvement
  - Preventing the use of drugs, cigarettes, and alcohol
  - Stopping substance use for those who are using
  - Avoiding date rape and other abusive peer relationships

Late Adolescence (18 to 21 Years)

Parameters of Normal Development

Many late adolescents are preparing for high school graduation or entry to college. They are working, entering the military, marrying, or participating in a vocational or technical training program. These are all examples of normal behavioral autonomy. This period of late adolescence is a time when decisions are made about how to contribute to society as a responsible adult.

By now, adolescents usually relate to the family as adults. Relationships with parents and family are gradually renegotiated to a more adult-adult basis. The role of the parent during late adolescence should be one of support.

By the end of late adolescence, this status has optimally progressed to autonomy for adolescents in the context of continuing strong affectional ties to the family.

Late adolescents have attained an adult level of reasoning skills. They are generally capable of understanding the consequences of their actions and behavior and can make complex and sophisticated judgments about human relationships. They no longer base their judgments about people on overt behavior but have a good understanding of inner motivations, including multiple determinants of an action. Of course, this most mature level of cognition is not used by teenagers or adults all the time, and some never reach this level of cognitive maturity.

A substantial number of late adolescents have established their sexuality and entered into an intimate, committed partner relationship. Selection of a partner is based more on individual preferences and less on the peer group's values.

Much of the final shaping of identity centers on adolescents' perceptions of their future options as adults. Among contemporary late adolescents, roughly half attend college and the other half enter the adult world of work. In many significant ways, the years in college offer a "moratorium," a time to engage in further consolidation of identity. College life offers both maximal autonomy and a structured, supportive environment in which to complete developmental tasks in what could be considered a prolonged adolescence. Those adolescents who enter the workforce and leave home immediately out of high school have quite different tasks and experiences. Their identity may be consolidated earlier because they do not have the added time and supportive structures of the college experience to delay facing the issues of earning a living, forming a family, and accepting other adult responsibilities. For adolescents who are unsuccessful in the educational system or the workplace (underemployed or unemployed), identity may be established by joining peers in gangs or by becoming socially isolated, both of which have negative implications for achieving healthy adult roles.

Developmental Anticipatory Guidance

Physical and Sexual Development

- *Physical growth:* Exercise, nutrition, and rest are important to optimal physical growth; encourage adolescent to incorporate them into lifestyle.
- *Sexuality:* Discussion and counseling should be provided about the following:
  - Implications of sexual activity—sexual feelings for the same or opposite sex should be discussed with a trusted adult or health professional
  - Postponement of coitus or the choice of abstinence
  - Prevention of sexually transmitted diseases
  - Birth control, including emergency methods
  - Breast or testicular self-examination

Cognitive Development

- Discuss the importance of completing academic work.
- Validate choices made to achieve positive future goals and plan for the future—college, vocational training, military, and job or career.

Social and Emotional Development

- *Family interactions:*
  - Closer relationships with and an interest in the family should be reemerging.
  - Families need to be supportive of independence efforts.
- *Peers:*
  - Intimate relationships are established.
  - Respect for the rights, needs, and views of others is a measure of maturity.
- *Independence and responsibility:* Adolescents should be encouraged to do the following:
  - Take on new challenges that increase self-confidence.
  - Identify talents and interests to be pursued.
  - Continue to clarify values and beliefs. Ethical and behavioral role modeling behavior is valued.
  - Develop skills in conflict avoidance; resolution reflects cognitive growth and maturity.
  - Learn to manage stress.
  - Find a balance between job and school or vocational training.

Self-care

- *Accident prevention:* Encourage correct and consistent use of helmets, seat belts, and proper sports equipment.
- *Weapons:* Access to guns and other weapons should be restricted, with an emphasis on safety and responsibility.
- *Abusive behavior:* Counseling should be provided on:
  - Avoiding gang involvement
  - Preventing the use and selling of drugs, cigarettes, and alcohol
  - Stopping substance use for those who are using
  - Avoiding date rape and other abusive relationships
- *Health care:* Assist the adolescent to learn about health insurance, how to enter and use the health care system, and to take responsibility for self-care.

COMMON DEVELOPMENTAL ISSUES FOR ADOLESCENTS

Risk Behavior

Description

Risk behavior consists of actions that jeopardize adolescents' physical, psychologic, or emotional health. It is a paradox of adolescence that developmental tasks (i.e., gaining independence, developing one's own values, becoming comfortable with one's body, and establishing meaningful relationships) may be achieved (albeit in negative ways) through risk-taking behavior (Alsaker, 1996). Adolescents needing peer affiliation and striving for increased autonomy are likely to explore, experiment, and otherwise push the limits of their personal experience—often in ways that put them at risk for health-compromising outcomes. However, many adolescents engage in risk behaviors without apparent negative outcomes. Is an adolescent who is sexually active but uses condoms on a regular basis engaged in risk behavior? Is an adolescent who goes to a party on the weekend and has a beer or smokes marijuana at risk? On the other hand, some teenagers who seem at high risk do not engage in risk behavior. What factors keep them from doing so?

Etiology

Although it is normal for behavioral experimentation to occur during this time, adolescents vary tremendously in their ability to think abstractly about the consequences of risky behavior. Their thinking is often characterized by the notion that "it can't happen to me" (personal fable). Although adolescents have an increase in abstract cognitive skills, thinking related to emotionally charged topics (e.g., substance use, sex, school performance, peer pressure) is often less sophisticated. An adolescent who is drinking may be doing so in part to be accepted by friends or to feel a sense of independence and maturity. Because the behavior meets important developmental needs, it may be difficult for the adolescent to look at it objectively and relinquish it. In addition, the impact of alcohol on brain function further limits the adolescent's reasoning ability.

Environmental factors, both social and physical, can influence adolescents' decisions to take risks. Factors that contribute to the adolescent engaging in risk behaviors include, but are not limited to, the following:

- Poverty
- Poor academic performance or low intellectual function
- Impulsivity or attention-deficit hyperactivity disorder
- Role models for deviant behavior (e.g., parents who abuse drugs or engage in criminal behavior)
- Low self-esteem
- Sense of hopelessness or helplessness
- Child abuse or other types of early emotional trauma
- Depression or other mental-emotional disorders
- Illiteracy or lack of job skills

Protective Factors

Protective forces may help counter the effects of risk factors and help adolescents make healthier lifestyle choices. Parent monitoring and direction in the child's life has a particularly strong protective influence (DiClemente et al, 2001; Nelson, Patience, & MacDonald, 1999; Pettit et al, 2001), and community support of positive adolescent behavior appears to minimize risk taking (see Chapter 18). Examples of possible protective factors are:

- High self-esteem
- Sense of future
- Academic success
- Parental direction
- Involvement in the family
- An interested adult
- Community involvement

Adolescents with multiple risk factors and few protective factors are more likely to engage in risk behavior, with potential health- and life-threatening results. These adolescents need prompt attention and assessment to determine the likelihood of negative outcomes. Conversely, resilient adolescents who are doing well, despite multiple risk factors, should be acknowledged and applauded.

Assessment

All adolescents should be assessed for their level of risk-taking behavior. The provider's approach to a discussion of sensitive issues should include ensuring confidentiality, providing privacy, using constructive communication strategies, and establishing rapport.

The HEADSS technique for assessment is cited as a method of assessing risk behavior. Areas for assessment include home, education/employment, activities, drugs, sexuality, and suicide/depression (Ehrman & Matson, 1998). NPs should also be alert for red flags at each developmental stage because delays in development may contribute to negative behavior (Table 9-2).

Clinical Findings

The following are considered examples of risk behavior:

- Substance use or abuse
- Poor academic performance
- Unprotected sexual intercourse
- Drinking and driving
- Delinquency or involvement with gangs
- Violence-related behavior such as carrying weapons

The consequences of such behavior can be addiction, school failure, pregnancy and sexually transmitted diseases, accidents, convictions for driving under the influence, incarceration, or death. Engaging in chronic risk-taking behavior often arrests developmental progression toward adult emotional maturity.

TABLE 9-2 *Developmental Red Flags: Adolescent*

Age	Physical and Sexual Development	Psychosocial Development	Cognitive Development
Early adolescence (11-14 yr)	Difficulty reading close or distant Female kyphosis/scoliosis Less than Tanner stage 2 Female short stature or lack of height spurt Poor nutrition, poor oral health, caries, malocclusion Loss of appetite Chronic disease such as heart disease, diabetes, or a family member with a chronic or lifelong illness No physical activity; overweight Sleep disturbance Sexual experimentation	Social habits: Early experimentation with drugs or alcohol (including tobacco) Relationships: Permissive or authoritarian parental style No participation in home chores History of family violence School fights No close or "best" friend Friends or siblings in gangs Cruelty to animals Sexuality: Sexual orientation worries Mood: Pervasive sad mood, feelings of hopelessness, suicidal thoughts or gestures, history of previous suicide attempt Flattened affect without expressions of joy, sorrow, or excitement Excessive worrying or rumination Self-concept: Believes self to be "ugly" or "fat"; is dieting despite normal body size and shape Negative feelings of self-worth Does not fantasize or dream about adult career	Low IQ Behind in grade or failing classes Chronic absenteeism or class skipping Attention problems Lack of organizational skills for homework Disruptive behavior Unable to identify feelings Unable to control own behavior (e.g., anger, impulsivity)
Middle adolescence (15-17 yr)	Difficulty reading close or distant Male kyphosis/scoliosis Less than Tanner stage 4 Male short stature or lack of height spurt Male muscular growth without testicular maturation Male persistent gynecomastia and acne Female primary or secondary amenorrhea Poor nutrition, poor oral health, caries, malocclusion Loss of appetite Chronic disease such as heart disease, diabetes, or a family member with a chronic or lifelong illness No physical activity; overweight Sleep disturbance Unprotected sexual intercourse Multiple sexual partners	Social habits: Recurrent experimentation or frequent use of drugs or alcohol; blackouts Drinking and driving Relationships: Excessively oppositional, defiant of all authority Abusive dating relationships School fights No identified peer group Gang association or involvement Sexuality: Sexual orientation worries Mood: Pervasive sad mood, feelings of hopelessness, suicidal thoughts or gestures, history of previous suicide attempt Flattened affect without expressions of joy, sorrow, or excitement Excessive worrying or rumination Self-concept: Believes self to be "ugly" or "fat"; is dieting despite normal body size and shape	Low IQ Behind in grade or failing classes Chronic absenteeism or class skipping Attention problems Disruptive behavior Unable to differentiate emotional states from physical states Unable to control own behavior (e.g., anger, impulsivity) Poor judgment

Continued

TABLE 9-2 ***Developmental Red Flags: Adolescent—cont'd***

Age	Physical and Sexual Development	Psychosocial Development	Cognitive Development
		Negative feelings of self-worth No life goals Does not fantasize or dream about adult career	
Late adolescence (18-21 yr)	Difficulty reading close or distant Less than Tanner stage 4 or 5 Poor nutrition, poor oral health, caries, malocclusion Loss of appetite Chronic disease such as heart disease, diabetes, or a family member with a chronic or lifelong illness No physical activity; overweight Sleep disturbance Unprotected sexual intercourse Multiple sexual partners	Social habits: Substance abuse Drinking and driving Relationships: Lacks intimate relationships Abusive dating relationships Unable to separate from peer groups Unable to separate from parents Gang association or involvement Unable to keep a job Sexuality: Sexual orientation worries Mood: Pervasive sad mood, feelings of hopelessness, suicidal thoughts or gestures, history of previous suicide attempt Flattened affect without expressions of joy, sorrow, or excitement Excessive worrying or rumination Self-concept: Believes self to be "ugly" or "fat"; is dieting despite normal body size and shape Negative feelings of self-worth	Low IQ Behind in grade or failing classes Dropout Attention problems Disruptive behavior Persistent egocentrism Unable to control own behavior (e.g., anger, impulsivity) Unable to reason or plan based on future/abstract concepts Poor judgment Chronic health care seeking for psychosomatic complaints

Management

Interventions should be considered when the adolescent's behavior threatens the accomplishment of developmental tasks or the adolescent's health, safety, and well-being. Generally, when adolescents' behavior supports the achievement of developmental tasks, such behavior should be encouraged. Adolescents who pierce their noses, shave half their heads, and spend evenings with friends, for example, may be irritating to parents, but their behavior can help them establish their autonomy, identity, and ability to relate to others. On the other hand, such behavior may be an indicator of more serious problems. Tattoos and body piercings, especially among younger adolescents, have been shown to have a strong correlation with high-risk behaviors (Carroll et al, 2002). It is important to understand the meaning of the behavior for the adolescent. Teenagers are more likely to engage in risk behaviors if they are neglected, feel hopeless or powerless, and lack self-esteem.

The approach used when providing care to teenagers differs from that used with younger children. Earlier, parents were central to the success of interventions. Although parents are still critical to successful intervention, the NP must recognize that the teenager makes the decisions, and the NP may need to mediate between the two at times. The NP's role is to provide the adolescent with information and guidance to make the best decisions possible.

Generally, high-risk teenagers require numerous services. NPs need to know their state laws regarding adolescent health issues, how to access community resources, and how to use other professionals collaboratively. The following list identifies basic services that at-risk teenagers may need:

- Food resources for teenage parents and their offspring
- Temporary shelters for teenagers
- Counseling and mental health services for teenagers and their families

RESOURCE BOX

Adolescents

Adolescent Health Transition Project
Resource for adolescents with special health care needs, chronic illnesses, physical or developmental disabilities
http://depts.washington.edu/healthtr/
1-206-685-1358

Alliance of Professional Tattooists, Inc. (APT)
Organization for education of health professionals and the public
www.safe-tattoos.com

American Academy of Family Physicians
www.aafp.org/
1-800-274-2237

American Academy of Pediatrics
www.aap.org/
1-847-434-4000

Centers for Disease Control and Prevention (CDC)
www.cdc.gov/health/adolescent.htm

Kids Counsel: Center for Children's Advocacy
Legal resources, information, and advocacy for children and adolescents
www.kidscounsel.org/kidscounsel/
1-860-570-5327

Search Institute
www.search-institute.org

Society for Adolescent Medicine
www.adolescenthealth.org/
1-816-224-8010

BOOKS FOR PARENTS

Greydanus DE, editor: *Caring for your adolescent: ages 12-21*, Elk Grove Village, IL, 1991, AAP.

Ingersoll BD, Goldstein S: *Lonely, sad and angry: a parent's guide to depression in children and adolescents*, Plantation, FL, 2001, Specialty Press.

Lopez RI: *The teen health book: a parent's guide to adolescent health and well-being*, New York, 2002, WW Norton.

Slap GS, Jablow MM: *Teenage health care: the first comprehensive family guide for the preteen to young adult years*, New York, 1994, Pocket Books.

- Foster care services for teenage parents and their offspring
- Local medical and social work services
- Local juvenile justice system and protective services
- Drug rehabilitation programs for teenagers
- Alternative school and vocational education programs
- Sports, fitness, and community activities for teenagers
- Support programs for teenagers, such as Big Brothers or Big Sisters

Advocating for children and adolescents at risk; involving their families, communities, and schools; and helping young persons identify an individual who cares for them and trusts them are important actions an NP can take.

SUMMARY

As adolescents struggle with issues of autonomy, body image, peer relationships, and, ultimately, identity, parents and health care providers must be aware of and sensitive to the phase of development and the range of normal behavior. Both risk and protective factors must be assessed accurately. Intervention requires weighing the balance of risk versus protective factors, the actual behavior, and the potential threat to health and well-being. At-risk situations cannot always be avoided; therefore adolescents and their families need anticipatory guidance and strategies for managing risk. The desired outcome is for the teen to emerge into adulthood with a healthy mind, body, and identity.

REFERENCES

Alsaker FD: Annotation: the impact of puberty, *J Child Psychol Psychiatry* 37:249-258, 1996.

Bryant AL et al: Understanding the links among school misbehavior, academic achievement, and cigarette use: a national panel study of adolescents, *Prev Sci* 1:71-87, 2000.

Carroll ST et al: Tattoos and body piercings as indicators of adolescent risk-taking behaviors, *Pediatrics* 109:1021-1027, 2002.

DiClemente RJ et al: Parental monitoring: association with adolescents' risk behaviors, *Pediatrics* 107:1363-1368, 2001.

Ehrman WG, Matson SC: Approach to assessing adolescents on serious or sensitive issues, *Pediatr Clin North Am* 45:189-204, 1998.

Elkind D: *All grown up and no place to go: teenagers in crisis*, Reading, MA, 1984, Addison-Wesley.

Elster A, Kuznets N: *AMA guidelines for adolescent preventive services (GAPS)*, Baltimore, 1994, Williams & Wilkins.

Ford CA et al: Influence of physician confidentiality assurances on adolescents' willingness to disclose information and seek future health care: a randomized controlled trial, *JAMA* 278:1029-1034, 1997.

Ge X, Conger RD, Elder GH: Pubertal transition, stressful life events, and the emergence of gender differences in adolescent depressive symptoms, *Dev Psychol* 37:404-417, 2001.

Hall G: *Adolescence: its psychology and its relations to physiology, anthropology, sociology, sex, crime, religion and education*, Englewood Cliffs, NJ, 1904, Prentice-Hall.

Iuliano-Burns S, Mirwald RL, Bailey DA: Timing and magnitude of peak height velocity and peak tissue velocities for early, average, and late maturing boys and girls, *Am J Human Biol* 13:1-8, 2001.

Kaltiala-Heino R et al: Early puberty and early sexual activity are associated with bulimic-type eating pathology in middle adolescence, *J Adolesc Health* 28:346-352, 2001.

Lanza ST, Collins LM: Pubertal timing and the onset of substance use in females during early adolescence, *Prev Sci* 3:69-82, 2002.

Larson RW et al: Continuity, stability, and change in daily emotional experience across adolescence, *Child Dev* 73:1151-1165, 2002.

Mattson SN et al: Executive functioning in children with heavy prenatal alcohol exposure, *Alcohol Clin Exp Res* 23:1808-1815, 1999.

McCabe MP, Ricciardelli LA: Parent, peer, and media influences on body image and strategies to both increase and decrease body size among adolescent boys and girls, *Adolescence* 36:225-240, 2001.

Nelson BV, Patience TH, MacDonald DC: Adolescent risk behavior and the influence of parents and education, *J Am Board Fam Pract* 12:436-443, 1999.

Pettit GS et al: Antecedents and behavior-problem outcomes of parental monitoring and psychological control in early adolescence, *Child Dev* 72:583-598, 2001.

Reiff MI: Adolescent school failure: failure to thrive in adolescence, *Pediatr Rev* 19:199-207, 1998.

Robinson TN et al: Overweight concerns and body dissatisfaction among third-grade children: the impacts of ethnicity and socioeconomic status, *J Pediatrics* 138:158-160, 2001.

Tanner J: *Growth at adolescence*, Oxford, 1962, Blackwell.

Valadian I, Porter D: *Physical growth and development from conception to maturity*, Boston, 1977, Little, Brown.

Vartanian LR: Revisiting the imaginary audience and personal fable constructs of adolescent egocentrism: a conceptual review, *Adolescence* 35:639-661, 2000.

Warren MP, Perlroth NE: The effects of intense exercise on the female reproductive system, *J Endocrinol* 170:3-11, 2001.

Wilf-Miron R et al: Using a Health Concerns Checklist as a bridge from reason for encounter to diagnosis of girls attending an adolescent health service, *Pediatrics* 106:1065-1069, 2000.

UNIT 3

Approaches to Health Management in Pediatric Primary Care

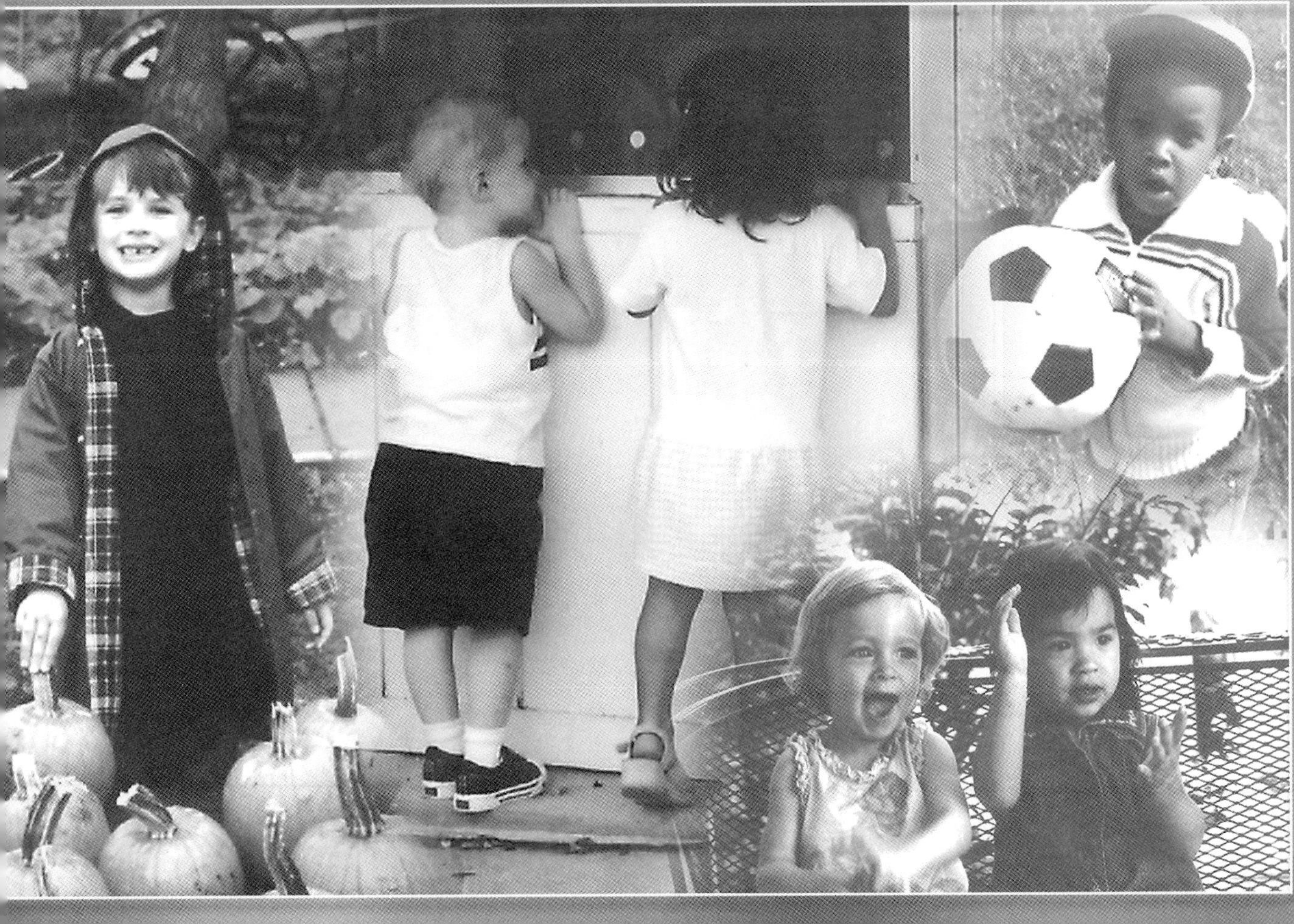

10 Introduction to Health Promotion

Catherine E. Burns

Health care is considered by many to be a birthright, and health is highly valued by all cultures in the world. Although valued, health is often compromised by behaviors of daily living. Lifestyle choices are the major causes of morbidity and mortality in infants, children, and adolescents in the United States. Thus the majority of life-threatening and debilitating conditions of children are preventable. The goals of *Healthy People 2010*, the health promotion and disease prevention objectives for 2010 (U.S. Department of Health and Human Services, 2000) focus on essential lifestyle and behavioral factors related to health. If these goals are to be met, proactive, comprehensive health promotion and disease prevention strategies directed at individuals, families, and communities are absolutely essential.

The nurse practitioner (NP) is in an excellent position to influence the health care outcomes of the nation through work in the health promotion arena. Teaching and modeling healthy behaviors help children learn to promote their own health, and, because many health problems of children are carried into adulthood, working with children has long-term health effects on the whole population. The broad perspective used by NPs serves as a framework to encompass all the factors that have an impact on health. The use of functional health patterns, a construct unique to nursing, focuses one's practice directly on lifestyle and health behaviors. Consistent and vigorous attention to issues of nutrition, activity, coping and stress tolerance, accident prevention, and other factors of lifestyle has as much or more impact on achievement of national goals as time spent managing minor illnesses that occur in daily practice.

To provide maximal support for achievement of the nation's health goals, however, a much broader array of professionals and citizens must be involved. Nurses, teachers, health educators, city planners, legislators, the industrial community, volunteers, and others from all levels of society need to guide development of an infrastructure that supports health care for all. Although this section of the book focuses on management of individual children within families, a broader perspective on community intervention and support for health also needs to be maintained. When opportunities to work with communities on their primary health care issues arise, the NP is strongly encouraged to become involved.

This chapter introduces the functional health patterns unit of the book. In this chapter, models that predict health behavior, factors that influence health promotion behaviors, functional health patterns used to describe the lifestyle domains that health promotion strategies must address, and specific management strategies for use with children and families are presented and discussed. Subsequent chapters in this unit examine each functional health pattern and its relationship to health.

MODELS TO PREDICT HEALTH BEHAVIOR

Four models are often used to predict health behaviors: the health belief model, the self-efficacy model, the health promotion model (Pender, 1996), and the transtheoretic (stages of change) model of behavior change (Prochaska, 1995; Prochaska, Diclemente, & Norcross, 1992; Prochaska et al, 1994; Sarkin et al, 2001). These models address issues of motivation, the first step toward action. They provide guidance for assessment of the motivation of the client, as well as cues to plan efforts that will encourage the client to take positive action.

Health Belief Model

This model explains behavior that seeks to prevent disease better than behavior that attempts to promote health. According to this model, people engage in preventive behaviors if they have a reason or motive to do so and if they hold certain beliefs. They must meet the following criteria:

- Feel vulnerable or susceptible to the disease or health problem
- Believe that the disease will have negative consequences for them if they get it
- Be convinced that taking some action will reduce the risk
- Accept that the benefits of action outweigh the costs

The health belief model can be illustrated by assessing the motivation for toothbrushing behavior: the client must believe that caries are possible; that tooth loss, pain, or disfigurement would be unfortunate consequences of caries; that brushing teeth can prevent caries; and that the benefits of brushing outweigh the inconvenience, time, and costs of maintaining a supply of toothbrushes and toothpaste over time. This is a simple example. Getting a teenager to change the cholesterol content in his or her diet after considering the consequences of heart disease in later life is not so easy.

Self-Efficacy Model

Bandura's (1977) concept of self-efficacy augments the health belief model. Self-efficacy is the belief that the self is capable of acting effectively. "Expectations of personal efficacy determine whether coping behavior will be initiated, how much effort will be expended, and how long it will be sustained in the face of obstacles and aversive experiences." Bandura thought that two kinds of expectations were important. First, one estimates one's capacity to do what is required—expectation that the behaviors used can achieve the goal. This expectation is based on performance accomplishments in the past, vicarious modeling experiences (watching the consequences of someone else's efforts), and verbal persuasion (someone saying, "You can do it"), with emotional arousal providing additional energy for action. Second, the outcome expectations (i.e., estimations that particular behaviors will lead to intended outcomes) need to be considered. In other words, the person needs to believe that if he or she performs as well as expected, the outcome will be influenced favorably, being contingent on the actions taken rather than being independent of them.

Health Promotion Model

Pender (1996) developed a much more comprehensive model with a focus on health promotion rather than on disease prevention. The model consists of two main domains—cognitive-perceptual factors and modifying factors—that explain participation in health promotion behaviors (Fig. 10-1). The cognitive-perceptual factors include all the concepts in the health belief and self-efficacy models, locus of control notions, and individuals' definitions of health and their own health status estimates. Modifying factors in the model include demographic, biologic, behavioral, and situational factors, as well as interpersonal influences. Together, the two groups of factors are important in helping a person decide whether to engage in health promotion behaviors. This model has been developed by a nurse and used most often by nurses.

Transtheoretic Model

The transtheoretic model is the newest of the four models. It incorporates elements from health belief and self-efficacy theories to develop a model that can be used to describe the stages of change that individuals go through as they initiate behaviors that promote health. The model describes 5 stages of change, 10 processes that facilitate movement from one stage to another, and 4 patterns that individuals use to progress through the various stages (Fig. 10-2) (Prochaska et al, 1992).

Stages of Change

The stages are precontemplation, contemplation, preparation, action, and maintenance. Shifts in attitudes and behaviors occur at each stage. The time required in each stage depends on the individual and the task to be attempted.

Precontemplation. At this stage, the individual does not acknowledge that a serious problem exists, although a wish to change may be expressed. Resistance to change is the hallmark of this stage, and the reasons not to change are most clear to the individual.

Contemplation. Awareness of the problem exists, and the individual struggles with the costs and energy required for change. Many individuals remain stuck in this phase.

Preparation. Planning begins in this stage. Small behavior changes may occur in preparation for commitment to the actual plan.

Action. Behaviors to eliminate the problem occur in this stage. These may include initiating new behaviors, accessing resources, modifying the environment, and mitigating barriers.

Maintenance. Plans occur here to prevent relapse, consolidate gains, and establish new behaviors as long-term changes. Maintenance occurs after at least 6 months in the action stage.

Patterns of Change

Most people are not able to proceed through all five stages in a linear way. Rather, there are relapses back to the precontemplation stage. Environmental barriers, external

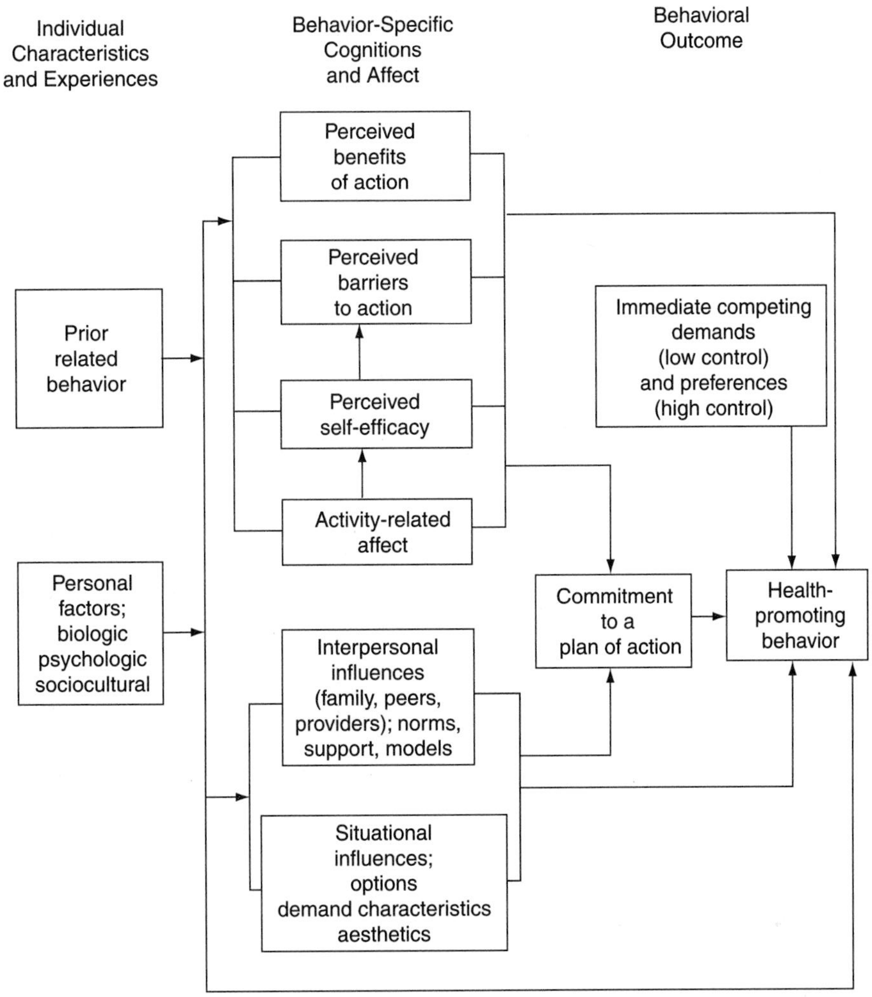

FIGURE 10-1 Health promotion model. (From Pender N: *Health promotion in nursing practice*, ed 3, Norwalk, CT, 1996, Appleton & Lange.)

pressures to change beyond the individual's own desires, or problems with maintenance of steps not mastered at earlier stages can contribute to relapses. *Recycling* is defined as regression to the contemplation or preparation stages. The person spirals through small increments of change, recycling and moving forward again. Success with the change is increased with effort, action, and mastery of the tasks of each stage.

Many dieting, smoking cessation, and drug rehabilitation programs fail to sustain changes because assessment of readiness and readiness training to assist individuals to move through stages successively is not included in the initial plans. Drug and alcohol programs are frequently imposed externally on individuals (e.g., court-ordered drug treatment). As soon as the pressure is relieved from the source, the individual relapses because changes are not internally driven.

Decisional Balance

Another component of the model is the cognitive exercise of weighing the pros and cons of change. In the precontemplative stage, the cons of no change must predominate over the pros of change (i.e., "If I don't change, I'll get cancer). To sustain behavior in the action stage and move to the maintenance stage, the pros of change must outweigh the cons of returning to old ways (i.e., "No smoking is cheaper than when I smoked"). Because most people at risk for health problems are in a precontemplative stage, programs need to be designed to move them to the contemplative stage. Also, programs designed to maintain changes made are important.

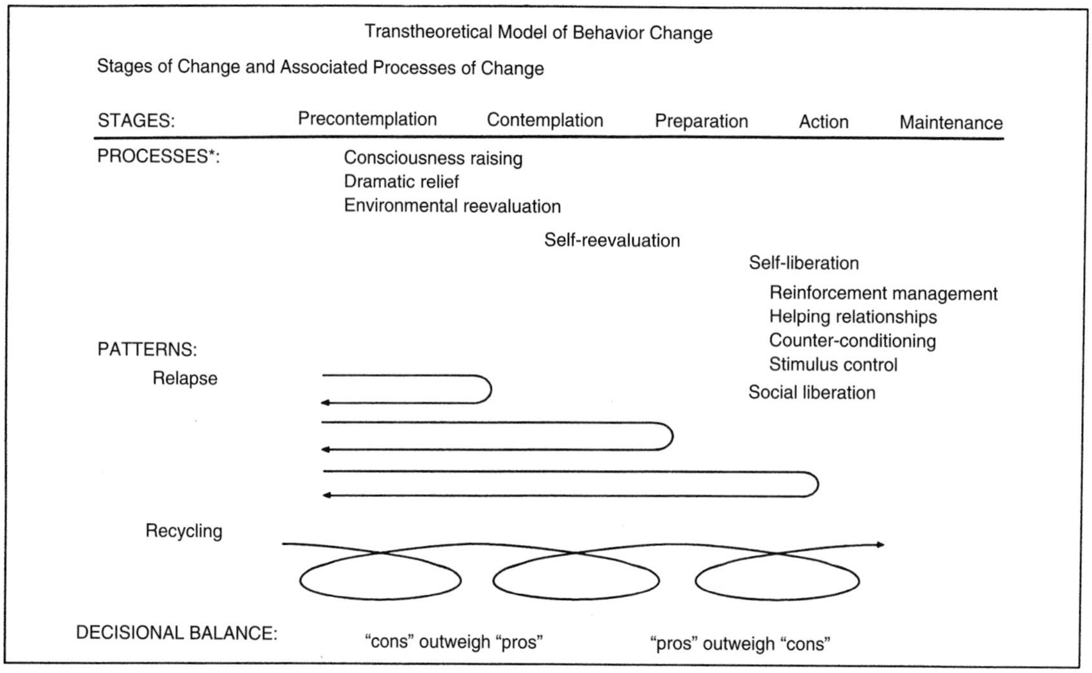

Explanations of Processes of Change	Associated Interventions
Consciousness raising: gathering information about self and problem†	Observation of others, confrontations Classes, bibliotherapy, interpretations
Dramatic relief: feeling and expressing feelings related to problem	Role play, psychodrama, grief work
Environmental reevaluation: assessing one's behavior on environment	Documentary information, empathy, training
Self-reevaluation: exploring one's feelings about self and the problem	Value clarification, imagery Corrective emotional experience
Self-liberation: choosing to act, changing belief in ability to change‡	Decision-making training Making resolutions, commitment-enhancing techniques
Social liberation: increasing alternatives and support for health behaviors	Empowerment and advocacy activities, policy interventions
Reinforcement management: establishing a reward system	Overt and covert reinforcement, contingency contracts
Helping relationships: trusting and sharing problem with a caring person*	Therapeutic alliance, buddy system, self-help/support groups
Counter-conditioning: substituting alternatives for problem behavior	Relaxation, desensitization, assertive skills, self-affirmations
Stimulus control: avoiding triggers of problem behavior	Restructuring environment, avoidance techniques, cue identification

*Most frequently used. Used more frequently for psychologically distressing problems.
†Second most frequently used.
‡Third most frequently used. Used more frequently for weight control.

Adapted from Prochaska, DiClemente, and Norcross,1992.

FIGURE 10-2 Transtheoretic (stages of change) model. (Adapted from Prochaska J, Diclemente C, Norcross J: In search of how people change: applications to addictive behaviors, *Am Psychol* 47:1102-1114, 1992.)

Integration of the Models

Elder and colleagues (1999) suggest that primary care providers can readily integrate the main themes of these various theoretic models in planning management for health behavior change with patients. The various models all include the following themes that a person must have to be successful:

- Have a strong positive intention or predisposition to perform the behavior
- Face a minimum of information-processing physical, logistical, and social- environmental barriers to performing the behavior
- Perceive herself or himself as having the requisite skills
- Believe that material, social, or other reinforcement will follow the behavior
- Believe that there is a normative pressure to perform and none sanctioning the behavior
- Believe that the behavior is consistent with the person's self-image
- Have a positive affect regarding the behavior
- Encounter cues or enablers to engage in the behavior at the appropriate time and place

What is less well known is how these various factors develop in children and how and at what ages they will influence health-related behaviors. These same factors can also be used with parents of children, who are responsible for many of the health behaviors of their children, and also with the health care providers, who may or may not feel that they have the requisite teaching and knowledge skills to influence their clients' health-related behaviors such as smoking or lack of physical activity.

INFLUENCES ON CHILDREN'S HEALTH PROMOTION BEHAVIORS

Children's health promotion behaviors are influenced by their own understanding of health and illness, the views and behaviors of their family, and community variables. The latter include direct effects of standards and practices in child care, school, and other community settings, as well as indirect effects, such as cultural and community values related to health.

Children's Concepts of Health and Illness

Children's concepts of health and illness must be considered within a developmental framework. Cognitive development is often used as a framework to analyze children's understandings of health and illness. Expectancy theory (from Bandura's work)—children's perceived vulnerability to health problems and the relationship of health problems to health behaviors—is also useful. Many studies offer evidence of children's views, but the knowledge base is relatively weak, with more research needed in the area. NPs need to understand the health beliefs of their young patients, as well as their goals, hopes, priorities, health interests and concerns, perceptions about seriousness of problems, feelings of vulnerability to health problems, and perceptions of benefits and barriers to taking action.

One model for understanding children's cognitive processing of health information, used more in the 1970s and 1980s, is Piaget's theory of cognitive development (see Chapter 5). Following this framework, preschoolers are in Piaget's preoperational stage of cognitive development. They have an egocentric view of health. Children at 3 to 5 years of age are just learning about the differences between being sick versus being well for themselves and their family members. They have little understanding of their internal bodies. Their lack of understanding of time and transformations means that the process of healing, for example, is not clearly understood.

School-age children are in the concrete operations cognitive development stage. They can list specific acts and rules used to maintain health and generally need overt signs of illness or health to recognize the health status of a person.

Adolescents, who are in the formal operations stage, are able to understand the difficulties of defining health (e.g., a person who looks well but has a cancerous tumor inside versus a person whose mobility is limited but is actually healthy). Teenagers understand the difference between the sick role and actual pathology, are sensitive to feeling states, and differentiate mental health from physical health. Nevertheless, the provider should not consider adolescents ready for explanations at an adult level because they vary in their utilization of formal operations thinking with age and issue.

Yoos (1994) offered an alternative view in which she argues that children's understanding may be better enhanced by use of a novice-expert model. Accordingly, with more experience and knowledge, children can incorporate more elaborate concepts into an understanding of how the body works, contagion, differences between physical and mental well-being, and the like. Similarly, adults may be cognitively sophisticated but demonstrate very elementary understanding of specific conditions based on lack of experience and knowledge rather than inability to process information. NPs should provide information based on the child's current base of knowledge and experience. If NPs assume, on the basis of a child's age, that he or she has a certain level of knowledge, experience, or cognitive abilities, they may fail to provide the most useful information to the child.

A significant health factor for adolescents is their risk-taking behavior. Questions the NP must consider when caring for teenagers include the following: What is the adolescent's perception of risk? When do teenagers identify behaviors as risky but choose to engage in them anyway for the perceived social value?

Other Determinants of Health Behavior of Children

A variety of studies have considered the determinants of health behavior of school-age children and adolescents, not just their cognitive understanding of health or illness.

Family Involvement with Health of Children

The family is the basic unit of health care management. The family influences lifestyles and the health status of its members. The NP needs to understand family dynamics, especially the influence of the mother; decision-making patterns; and parenting styles, including autonomy and rewards for children and reasoning used to teach children. The psychologic characteristics of the family, belief that members can make a difference, and the role of the family as a natural support system are all important in planning effective health promotion strategies. Knowledge of the family's composition, health, lifestyles, nutrition, economic resources, and recent changes is helpful. Exercise, diet, hygiene, and rest patterns are family routines affecting the health of individual members.

A variety of studies provide some information about the health promotion practices of families for their children. Chapter 11 identifies factors that facilitate families' choosing health promotion behaviors.

Peers

In a review article, LaGreca, Bearman, & Moore (2002) identify a variety of studies that support the proposition that peers offer support, influence adherence to treatment regimens, and affect both health promotion and health risk behaviors. For example, in adolescents with diabetes, friends provide more support for certain aspects of treatment such as exercise and emotions. On the negative side, peer smoking is the best predictor of adolescent smoking.

Community Involvement with Health of Children

The community influences health promotion behaviors of families with children. The community provides options for health care, an economic base for family survival and prosperity, social norms, and regulation of the environment and behaviors of citizens. The community also provides many direct services, including schools, day care centers, social services, community organizations, and health care centers, that support or impede family efforts to maintain the health of the members (Earls & Carlson, 2001).

Use of community resources benefits families positively if recommendations for access and utilization are appropriate and timely. As discussed in Chapter 11, appropriate use of community resources is an expected behavior in the maintenance and management of functional health patterns. Use of community standards and health values can effectively influence behaviors of individual families. According to Rogers' (1983) diffusion theory, innovators are the first to adopt new ideas in a community. They are followed by early adopters, then the early majority, the late majority, and finally late adopters. When between 10% and 25% of the population adopt an idea, it diffuses through the rest of the population. Thus, for example, when the use of bicycle helmets reaches a critical mass of 10% to 25%, use should become common enough so that the remaining families are persuaded to buy helmets and expect their children to use them.

In summary, many factors influence the health behaviors of children and their families. NPs helping families change lifestyle and behaviors to promote health need broad understandings of the health perspectives of their clients, as well as an awareness of age, sex, education, and peer and community influences.

FUNCTIONAL HEALTH PATTERNS—THE BEHAVIORS OF HEALTH

The functional health patterns that Gordon (1987) has used to describe the domain of nursing practice serve as the framework for the chapters in this unit. The patterns describe the health-related behaviors in which people engage. These functional health patterns are universal, applying to all humans regardless of age, sex, culture, health status, or other factors. All people need to eat, sleep, and eliminate, for example. Each pattern is described as follows:

Health perception–health management pattern: Describes client's perceptions of personal health and health care behaviors, prevention, and compliance with prescriptions for management of health and illness problems.

Nutrition-metabolic pattern: Describes patterns of food and fluid intake. Includes choice of foods and food supplements, eating habits, and schedules.

Elimination pattern: Describes patterns of bowel and bladder excretion. Includes schedule and habit patterns and use of laxatives or other methods to facilitate excretory functions.

Activity-exercise pattern: Describes patterns of activity and exercise, including type of activity, schedule of participation, vigor, effect on leisure, physical state, and meaning of activity to the client.

Sleep-rest pattern: Describes patterns of sleep and rest, including schedule, habits, aids to sleep, and perceived feelings of renewal, fatigue, or exhaustion.

Cognitive-perceptual pattern: Describes sensory-perceptual and cognitive patterns, including adaptations to hearing, vision, or other perceptual losses; includes the process of finding meaning from environmental stimuli and the effectiveness of efforts to compensate for deficits. Pain perception is a component.

Self-perception–self-concept pattern: Describes patterns of perception and valuing of the self, as well as evaluation of strengths and weaknesses and sense of self-worth.

Role-relationships pattern: Describes pattern of roles and responsibilities of the client and patterns of relationships with family and others.

Sexuality-reproductive pattern: Describes patterns of satisfaction or dissatisfaction with sexuality and sexual relationships. Involves perception and development of sexual identity, as well as reproductive expectations, behaviors, and outcomes.

Coping–stress tolerance pattern: Describes patterns of coping with the range of stresses experienced. Includes strategies used, effectiveness, support systems, and perceived ability to control and manage difficult situations.

Values-beliefs pattern: Describes patterns of values and beliefs that influence daily living activities, guide decision making, and provide meaning to life. Involves religious and spiritual activities, as well as personal values and beliefs.

Screening and Assessment of Functional Health Pattern Disorders

The same diagnostic reasoning methods are used by the NP to manage both health and illness issues. One must look at risk factors, comorbidities, etiology, differential diagnosis, and options for management that are acceptable to the client.

Screening for the presence of lifestyle and health behavior problems is a first step for NPs. In pediatric practice, the majority of screening is done in the clinical interview. Questions are asked about sleep, nutrition, elimination, play, discipline, utilization of primary care services, and others. Questionnaires can be used to ask about diet, smoking, exercise, use of seat belts, and feelings of satisfaction with self and health status. The clinical interview is more than taking a history of medical problems. It involves learning about concerns and worries, as well as goals, lifestyle, family life, and cultural background. It produces information to put the child and family into a context necessary to plan for care. For instance, if a family has little money, decisions about care need to factor in the inability to pay for services, medications, or equipment.

If information generated by the clinical interview is appropriate, given the child's age and other factors, no further probing of the area is done. On the other hand, if an answer to a screening question is atypical, the NP begins the assessment mode to identify the nature, severity, duration, and effects of the problem to plan appropriate interventions. For example, if a mother notes that she has not been very happy lately, the Beck Depression Scale might be administered to assess whether she is depressed or not. Assessment might involve use of daily diaries of food intake, activity, or sleep/wake patterns. Screening methods are used for all children of a given age in the practice, whereas assessment is individualized and should yield information about the extent of the problem and comorbidities for a given client. The goal of assessment is development of a plan of care to manage the problem effectively and efficiently.

Health supervision using a clinical preventive services model involves regular visits timed to offer periodic screening opportunities. The visits need to be scheduled infrequently enough to be economical but frequently enough to identify changes in the patterns of growth and development or early physiologic, psychologic, or social problems that might be detrimental to the child's health. Health supervision includes the clinical interview, developmental and educational surveillance, observation of parent-child interaction, physical examination, and screening procedures such as measuring height, weight, head circumference, body mass index (BMI), vision, hearing, blood pressure, and hemoglobin or hematocrit. The purpose of the health supervision visit is to assess strengths and weaknesses in health. The content of health supervision visits throughout infancy, childhood, and adolescence is addressed in Chapters 2 and 11. The details of screening, assessment, and management of functional health problems identified are found in the remaining chapters of this unit.

Nursing Diagnoses—A Way to Label Functional Health Pattern Problems

Nursing diagnoses developed by the North American Nursing Diagnosis Association (NANDA) provide a way to label, describe, and categorize the problems that NPs manage in the nursing part of their role. One advantage to the use of nursing diagnoses lies in systematically identifying the health problems that NPs manage with labels that allow data retrieval for evaluation of practice outcomes and research purposes. Unfortunately, nursing diagnoses are generally not reimbursed. However, using the labels in charting ensures that the range of services that NPs provide is explicit. Without labeling the problems of sleep, nutrition, coping, and so forth, no one knows what the NP does while in the room with the patient and family aside from managing medical problems. The services provided become invisible, and the perception is left that NPs are slower in managing diseases than other primary care providers are. To be valued, the NP's total work must be recognized. The use of nursing diagnosis labels can make the work in the health promotion domain of functional health patterns more visible.

Nevertheless, nursing diagnoses are not used systematically by all NPs. The first problem is that some NANDA diagnoses are not stated specifically enough for clinical application, although they identify an area of patient difficulty. For example, "sleep pattern disturbance" does not tell the NP whether the issue involves getting to sleep, staying asleep, or waking early. Each problem would be managed differently. Second, many senior NPs (those who are more likely to teach students) were educated as NPs before the development of nursing diagnoses. Thus students might not see role models using the system. Third, nursing diagnoses are not reimbursed, although some ICD-9-CM (International Classification of Diseases, 9th revision, clinical modificaiton) diagnoses (see inside back cover) can be substituted. Fourth, there is a misconception on the part of some NPs that they should use nursing labels for medical diagnoses. NPs should use medical diagnoses for the pathophysiologic problems and nursing diagnoses for the problems of lifestyle and health behaviors not covered by medical diagnosis labels. The use of both sets of labels makes the scope of practice of the NP explicit. Therefore, for example, "impetigo" is best for describing the skin infection but "alteration in parenting" alerts other professionals to look at parenting behaviors.

In the functional health patterns chapters (Chapters 11 to 22), nursing diagnoses that might be appropriate to label problems in a particular pattern are identified for those who wish to use them. However, the content of each chapter is organized conceptually around the nature of the pattern and not the nursing diagnosis framework.

MANAGEMENT STRATEGIES FOR HEALTH PROMOTION

This section discusses some management strategies for promoting health and working with functional health pattern problems. To provide excellent health promotion care, the NP must

- Give consistent, credible health messages
- Merit trust and confidence
- Understand clinical preventive service recommendations and provide preventive services consistent with those recommendations
- Have working relationships with other health care providers, social services, and educational professionals in the community
- Ensure that the clinic setting creates an environment consistent with good health and is developmentally appropriate
- Use motivational, patient education, and behavioral strategies effectively

In the Nursing Interventions Classification (NIC), McCloskey and Bulechek (2000) classify nursing interventions into six domains: (1) physiologic: basic; (2) physiologic: complex; (3) behavioral; (4) safety; (5) family; and (6) health system (Box 10-1). For the problems of functional health patterns and health maintenance and promotion, interventions in domains 1, 3, 4, 5, and 6 are most appropriate. The interventions of domain 2 (physiologic: complex) are most appropriate for the disease/pathophysiologic problems NPs manage. This text does not formally use the NIC. However, it is a useful tool when developing management strategies relevant to specific problems. For example, the interventions most specifically designed to result in behavioral changes desired for health promotion and disease prevention include those in NIC domain 3 (behavior therapy, cognitive therapy, communication enhancement, coping assistance, patient education, and psychologic comfort).

Patient Education

Patient education is the most commonly used strategy for guiding patients to increase health promotion behaviors and manage lifestyle problems. Primary health education involves instructing clients about ways to avoid contracting preventable diseases, ways to change lifestyle to reduce risks, and methods to maintain a healthy environment. Secondary health education teaches people to recognize early illness and prevent disease progression, whereas tertiary health education relates to instruction of patients about their specific illnesses, treatments, and available health services and resources (Watts & Breindel, 1981).

Friere (1973) adds a sociopolitical dimension to learning that community health nurses find helpful. According to his model, education should be self-generated rather than simply receptive, with empowerment and liberation identified as outcomes for individuals who engage in the educational process. Education occurs after the student and the teacher first come to a common understanding

BOX 10-1 ***Nursing Interventions Classification: Domains and Classes of Interventions***

1. *Physiologic, basic:* Care that supports physical functioning
   A. Activity and exercise management
   B. Elimination management
   C. Immobility management
   D. Nutrition support
   E. Physical comfort promotion
   F. Self-care facilitation
2. *Physiologic, complex:* Care that supports homeostatic regulation
   A. Electrolyte and acid-base management
   B. Drug management
   C. Neurologic management
   D. Perioperative care
   E. Respiratory management
   F. Skin/wound management
   G. Thermoregulation
   H. Tissue perfusion management
3. *Behavioral:* Care that supports psychologic functioning and facilitates lifestyle changes
   A. Behavior therapy
   B. Cognitive therapy
   C. Communication enhancement
   D. Coping assistance
   E. Patient education
   F. Psychologic comfort promotion
4. *Safety:* Care that supports protection against harm
   A. Crisis management
   B. Risk management
5. *Family:* Care that supports the family unit
   A. Childbearing care
   B. Child-rearing care
   C. Life span care
6. *Health system:* Care that supports effective use of the health care delivery system
   A. Health system mediation
   B. Health system management
   C. Information management
7. *Community:* Care that supports the health of the community
   A. Community health promotion
   B. Community risk management

From McCloskey JC, Bulechek GM, editors: *Nursing interventions classification (NIC)*, ed 3, St Louis, 2000, Mosby.

about the relationship between individual health problems and the social context of those problems. Part of the education focuses on addressing the social issues, such as barriers to care, that affect the management of the specific problem at hand.

Patient Education Process

Patient education is the method used to provide patients and families with the knowledge they need to make decisions related to their health and to carry out self-care activities that will positively affect their health or allow them to manage their diseases.

The core methodology for patient education for individuals and groups is reviewed here and summarized in Box 10-2.

1. *Set the climate for learning.* Patients, families, or groups need to be in an environment that is comfortable, free of distractions, and provides cues that learning activities

BOX 10-2 *The Patient Education Process*

1. Set the climate for learning—make introductions, provide comfortable environment.
2. Establish a structure of mutual planning—identify learner and nurse practitioner goals.
3. Assess the learner's style of learning, level of knowledge and competency, readiness, physical and developmental capabilities, attitudes, and feelings.
4. Plan—provide knowledge, role modeling, practice, discussion. Various aids facilitate teaching—books, pamphlets, diagrams, videos, and models. The plan is formulated with objectives specifying the behaviors that the learner should exhibit to demonstrate learning.
5. Manage the learning intervention—use methods and resources for instruction with the patient or family (or both) to implement the plan.
6. Evaluate the outcomes—judge achievement of objectives and then reformulate the plan to move the learner to the next level.

will occur. Introductions and a mutually agreed-on time limit are helpful. For example, mothers who are worried about being home when the school bus drops off their children attend poorly to teaching, no matter how skilled the NP is.

2. *Establish a structure of mutual planning.* Identify learner and NP goals. If learning is to be successful, the client must recognize a need for new knowledge. It becomes the NP's responsibility to identify the client (child, parent, class) need. Getting the client to express questions is the most direct way to identify client needs. The NP can also ask about the client's health goals. Sometimes it is necessary to provide information alerting clients to potential or emerging problems if lifestyle or behavior changes do not occur. In other words, the client does not always come to the NP with preestablished goals or needs; however, the client must agree with the NP that change is necessary in order for the mutual planning requirement of patient teaching to be met.
3. *Assess the learner.* Assessment includes readiness, attitudes and feelings, style of learning, level of knowledge and competency, and physical and developmental capabilities. Use of one of the health belief models identified earlier can provide the necessary information about the readiness and attitudes and feelings factors. Questions in the following areas may be useful:

   Readiness
   - Does the client ask questions?
   - Does the client have multiple stresses in his or her life that would inhibit concentration on learning?
   - Is the client coping with survival issues, such as chronic poverty, unemployment, or rehabilitation from substance abuse, that inhibit learning?
   - When is the best time to meet with the client, given other daily expectations?

   Attitudes and Feelings
   - Have there been past attempts at learning with successful outcomes?
   - Does the client have a sense of control over his or her future, as demonstrated by an ability to set and achieve goals, a positive feeling about life, and an ability to care for himself or herself adequately?
   - Does the client have worries, depression, or a life situation that would decrease learning?
   - Does the client feel vulnerable?
   - Does the client feel that actions could make a difference?
   - Does the client feel that the benefits of taking action outweigh perceived costs?
   - Does the client feel capable of taking the necessary actions?

   Style of Learning
   - What are the preferred modalities of learning for the client? (e.g., "Do you learn best by reading or listening?" "Does watching a videotape help you learn?")
   - What does the client already know about the subject?
   - Judging from the developmental level of the client, how concrete or abstract can the teaching be?
4. *Plan.* The plan is formulated using objectives that specify the behaviors that will demonstrate learning. Objectives need to be realistic, achievable, and relevant to the goals of the client. Both short-term and long-term objectives are written if the goals are not achieved in one teaching session. The use of both types of objectives helps the client and NP set priorities and stage education in achievable steps. Generally in routine pediatric visits, objectives are verbally stated, not written, but both client and NP should agree on what is to be achieved. Various aids facilitate learning—books, pamphlets, diagrams, videos, and models. Modalities for learning that are most appropriate for the client should be used. Methods for

teaching include formal classes, role playing, demonstration and return demonstration, lecture and discussion, reading, viewing videos, or other activities. The plan should facilitate clear presentation of material to the client, provide for frequent reinforcement and feedback, and include some kind of active involvement of the client. Passive listening does not ensure learning.

5. *Manage the learning intervention.* During implementation of the teaching plan, the process is carefully orchestrated to actively engage the client in successful learning. Progress is constantly evaluated, new information added, success reinforced, the pace of feedback assessed, the pace adjusted, and outcomes and achievement of objectives evaluated.
6. *Evaluate the outcomes.* Judge achievement of objectives and then reformulate the plan to move the client to the next level. Learning is evaluated using a variety of methods, such as asking questions that require use of new knowledge to answer, watching for new behaviors, and looking for feelings of achievement and expressions of new understanding.

Patient Education with Children and Adolescents

Teaching children includes all the aforementioned steps, as well as careful assessment of the child's developmental level, because the concepts the child can learn vary with cognitive abilities. Children's attention spans are often short; therefore information needs to be presented in smaller bites, with frequent reinforcement and opportunities for doing rather than just listening. Reading skills may not be developed, so verbal and demonstration strategies are more effective for younger children. Terminology might need to be adjusted to use simpler words and concepts. Verbal and nonverbal reinforcement and feedback need to be appropriate for the child. The use of star charts is a good way to reinforce behaviors visually and concretely. Such strategies are consistent with school-age children in Piaget's concrete operations cognitive stage.

For adolescents, assessment of developmental level is also important. The young adolescent (13 to 14 years of age) understands and engages in learning differently from the 18-year-old. Motivators for teenagers do not include knowledge of long-term effects. The use of several modalities, such as discussions with peers, reading, reviewing, and viewing audiovisual media, is helpful. Advice needs to be practical. Teenagers do best when they are viewed as decision makers who need information to make good choices. Identification of strengths and weaknesses is always important. The use of peer groups can be extremely effective.

There are many good examples of health education for youth and adolescents that have been successful. For example, the Pathways program is an obesity prevention program for American Indian schoolchildren that uses social learning theory and a variety of individual, behavioral, and environmental factors (Davis et al, 1999). Hulton (2001) has used the stages of change model of Prochaska to help adolescents with sexual abstinence behaviors. Harrell and colleagues (1996) have studied a school-based intervention to reduce cardiovascular disease risk factors among elementary-level schoolchildren (the Cardiovascular Health in Children [CHIC I] study). Goldberg and colleagues (2000) have studied a multipronged intervention to help prevent anabolic steroid use among adolescents while also promoting health behaviors among the participants. This group also used social learning theory principles.

Patient Education with Parents

When working with parents, the provider must keep in mind that parents are experts for their child and home environment, whereas the health care provider has more knowledge about children as an aggregate. Thus collaboration between parents and providers produces the best outcomes for the child at hand. Adult education has some unique aspects. First, adults usually want knowledge to help them make decisions for change, not just to gain knowledge per se. Furthermore, they usually have expectations or goals and ideas about activities that will help them. Finally, adults may have to unlearn previous knowledge that is outdated or irrelevant to the situation at hand.

Roberts (1981) developed a model of levels of parent education that is useful to NPs (Table 10-1). The model

TABLE 10-1 Levels of Parent Education

Parent Need Level	Nursing Intervention
I. No obvious needs	"Prospective mode"—providing anticipatory guidance
II. Parents uneasy or engaging in some child care practices that may cause difficulties in the future	"Resource mode"—responding to specific issues of parenting
III. Parents have obvious needs, because children display difficulties	"Collaborative mode"—taking more direct actions to support family
IV. Parents' resources inadequate to meet the needs of their children	"Protective mode"—protecting the children and sometimes the parents

Adapted from Roberts E: A model for parent education, *Image Journal of Nursing Scholarship* 13:89, 1981.

identifies four levels of parental needs with related levels of responses by nurses. When parents have no obvious needs (level I), they may gain from anticipatory guidance. The nurse's role is one of providing prospective advice and information for future use. When parents feel uneasy about some aspect of child rearing (level II), the nurse begins to serve as a resource to help with the specific issue. At level III, problems overtly affect children in particular areas. The nurse, at this point, moves into a collaborative mode, taking more direct action to support the family rather than merely offering advice for the parents to use. For example, the nurse might begin to make telephone calls to arrange consultation appointments for the family or arrange transportation as needed. Finally, at level IV, the parents' resources are inadequate to meet the child's needs, so the nurse moves into a protective mode on behalf of the child.

Parent teaching is most effective at levels I and II. At level III, the parent generally needs more than teaching. At level IV, the activities of the nurse are designed to support the child first.

Anticipatory Guidance

Anticipatory guidance is a particular form of patient teaching. It is used when the NP wants to be sure that the patient and family have information for decision making about issues predicted to arise at some time in the future, usually between the current and the next scheduled visit. With the rapid growth and developmental changes occurring in childhood, anticipatory guidance is essential if competent child-rearing practices are to be maintained and developed. Skilled anticipatory guidance involves a process outlined in Box 10-3. The process involves a finely tuned cooperative discussion with the client about issues of client concern. It is not a rote recitation of information automatically provided at a specified visit. Skilled anticipatory guidance is individualized teaching, with outcomes mutually agreed on by provider and client. Part of the skill of the NP relates to making issues of anticipated change in the child relevant to the parent so that those issues can become topics for guidance.

BOX 10-3 *Anticipatory Guidance Steps*

1. Scan. Discover the problem
2. Formulate. Explore the issue, specify, and name it.
3. Appraise. Patient decides whether the issue is worth working on—readiness and willingness.
4. Negotiate. Develop willingness on part of both parties.
5. Plan. Divide labor, plan action, and follow up.
6. Implement.
   Orient—develop or change feelings about the issue.
   Guide—identify actions to occur.
   Develop decision-making rules and problem-solving strategies.
   Practice.
7. Evaluate.

Providing Data

Often, providing data about a child's status to the parents or adolescent is a powerful yet easy patient education intervention. The height and weight grid and developmental screening or laboratory test scores with interpretation are often significant motivators or reinforcers for the work that parents have been doing. The key is interpretation of information so that the parents know how their child compares with the appropriate norms. Data provided should include both normal outcomes and areas of concern.

Role Modeling

Social learning theory suggests that modeling is an effective way for people to learn. Modeling appropriate parenting techniques can be most effective, especially when the parent then rehearses the desired behaviors with positive reinforcement. McCloskey and Bulechek (2000) classify interventions in this area as behavior therapy. The NP must be careful to create a situation in which parents are left feeling competent—that they are doing a fine job rather than that someone else could do it better. Parents need to feel new confidence as a result of working with the NP and trying out new behaviors. Parenting classes and support groups often provide more time for role modeling and practice of new behaviors than can occur during a primary care visit. Several visits are often needed to help parents learn new responses to children's behavior. Part of the developmental process requires that parents make decisions about when to use new responses they are learning.

Contracting

Establishing a contract with a client or family is an effective intervention that is interactive and collaborative in style. It requires shared responsibility and control on the part of patient and provider. Contracting can involve either contingencies (rewards) for completion of the client's actions to meet the contract or noncontingencies with the implied reward of better health consequences for progress made. It is important to make the contract with all the parties involved.

The contracting process involves three major phases. Phase one includes mutual identification of needs and problems and mutual agreement on goals, resources, and a plan of action. In phase two, the provider and client divide up the labor and responsibilities, establish a time frame, and then implement the plan. Mutual evaluation and renegotiation occur along the way. In phase three, the contract is terminated. A key factor is to keep the goals achievable.

Bibliotherapy

Promoting use of reading materials can be an excellent intervention in primary care. Books or pamphlets provide information that is well organized and presented in a manner that facilitates its retention. Furthermore, written materials allow patients or families to pace their learning at their own rate, and they serve as a familiar source of reference when needs arise at unexpected times. Redman (1993) refers to printed teaching material as a "frozen language that is selective in its description of reality (which is both a strength and a weakness). It encourages limited feedback but is constantly available." The good reader uses reading materials efficiently, scanning for important words, stopping to summarize the material learned, and using illustrations to enhance the meanings derived from the text. On the other hand, the unskilled reader either spends an inordinate amount of time trying to master the material at hand or sets aside the task, usually without letting the NP know of the difficulties encountered. Thus the reading levels of the client and the materials must be considered.

Reading also provides vicarious role models for both children and parents, acts as a support by acknowledging the feelings and problems encountered by others with similar problems, and expands perspectives on various health-related issues. Stories can help children, especially adolescents, explore new ideas, clarify their own feelings and perceptions, and serve as an impetus for change.

Health System Interventions

McCloskey and Bulechek (2000) identify another domain of nursing interventions that address health system utilization problems. Families with children have many complex needs, which are often met by different organizations such as governmental agencies; health care resources, including clinics, screening programs, health promotion programs, and hospitals; and volunteer programs.

Referrals should be considered whenever there is need for expertise, a more accessible resource, more time for intervention than is available in the current setting, or special types of intervention such as a support group, class, or practice opportunities. Managed care settings, in some cases, seem to discourage use of referrals. However, solving problems efficiently and effectively, even if that means using another resource, is generally a cost-effective intervention.

Identifying and using various community resources requires knowledge and skills that some families do not have. Locating services and helping families learn to use them might be necessary. Transportation, financial resources, the process for entering the system, and the services that can be anticipated are all factors to be discussed with families.

SUMMARY

Health promotion management is as important to the health of children as is illness management. The process of diagnosis and treatment is the same for both domains of NP practice. Interventions for both health promotion and disease management include preventive and therapeutic strategies, with patient education essential to ambulatory management. The clients include children and their parents, as well as other family members or foster parents. For adolescents, the client increasingly becomes the adolescent as the independent decision maker.

Because children change so rapidly, their functional health patterns are stable for only short periods of time. The patterns need continual reassessment in light of developmental progress. Parents also need continuing information and new skills such as teaching behaviors to manage their children's evolving health care needs adequately. In addition, a multitude of factors such as family practices and attitudes, peer influences, and community effects influence the health behaviors of children. Thus, in many ways, health promotion care for children is more difficult than is management of their physical status. Developing skill as a manager of health promotion for clients is no easy task, but it is worth the effort. It is in the area of functional health pattern management that the unique contributions of NPs to the health care of their clients are confirmed.

REFERENCES

Bandura A: Self-efficacy: toward a unifying theory of behavioral change, *Psychol Rev* 84:191-215, 1977.

Davis S et al: Pathways: a culturally appropriate obesity-prevention program for American Indian schoolchildren, *Am J Clin Nutr* 69:796s-802s, 1999.

Earls F, Carlson M: The social ecology of child health and well-being, *Annu Rev* 22:143-166, 2001.

Elder J et al: Theories and intervention approaches to health-behavior change in primary care, *Am J Prev Med* 17:275-284, 1999.
Friere P: *Education for critical consciousness*, New York, 1973, Seabury Press.
Goldberg L et al: The adolescents training and learning to avoid steroids program: preventing drug use and promoting health behaviors, *Arch Pediatr Adolesc Med* 154:332-338, 2000.
Gordon M: *Nursing diagnosis: process and application*, New York, 1987, McGraw-Hill.
Harrell J et al: Effects of a school-based intervention to reduce cardiovascular disease risk factors in elementary-school children: the Cardiovascular Health in Children (CHIC) study, *J Pediatr* 128:797-805, 1996.
Hulton L: The application of the transtheoretical model of change to adolescent sexual decision-making, *Issues Compr Pediatr Nurs* 24:95-115, 2001.
LaGreca A, Bearman K, Moore H: Peer relations of youth with pediatric conditions and health risks: promoting social support and healthy lifestyles, *J Dev Behav Pediatr* 23:271-280, 2002.
McCloskey J, Bulechek G, editors: *Nursing interventions classification*, ed 3, St Louis, 2000, Mosby.
Pender N: *Health promotion in nursing practice*, ed 3, Norwalk, CT, 1996, Appleton & Lange.
Prochaska J: Disease management needs new paradigms, *J Gen Intern Med* 10:472-473, 1995.
Prochaska J, DiClemente C, Norcross J: In search of how people change: applications to addictive behaviors, *Am Psychol* 47:1102-1114, 1992.
Prochaska J et al: Stages of change and decisional balance for 12 problem behaviors, *Health Psychol* 13:39-46, 1994.
Redman B: *Patient education*, ed 7, St Louis, 1993, Mosby.
Richardson S: Child health promotion practices of parents, *J Pediatr Health Care* 2:73-78, 1988.
Roberts F: A model for parent education, *Image* 13:86-89, 1981.
Rogers EM: *Diffusion of innovations*, New York, 1983, Free Press.
Sarkin J et al: Applying the transtheoretical model to regular moderate exercise in an overweight population: validation of a Stages of Change Measure, *Prev Med* 33:462-469, 2001.
US Department of Health and Human Services: *Healthy people 2010: understanding and improving health*, ed 2, Washington, DC, 2000, US Government Printing Office.
Watts A, Breindel C: Health education: structural vs. behavioral perspectives, *Health Political Educ* 2:47-57, 1981.
Yoos L: Children's illness concepts: old and new paradigms, *Pediatr Nurs* 20:134-140, 1994.

11

Health Perception and Health Management Pattern

Ardys M. Dunn

OVERVIEW

Children's health depends on a multitude of factors, including appropriate nutrition, stimulation, exercise, rest, and emotional and social nurturance. In addition to healthy lifestyle behaviors, prevention and management of illness and injury is essential to children's growth and development. This chapter discusses ways in which nurse practitioners (NPs) can work with parents, children, and families to ensure that decisions made and actions taken regarding health management are best suited to growing children's needs. The chapter explores factors that influence the health behavior of children and their families and summarizes the health maintenance needs of infants, toddlers, preschoolers, school-age children, and adolescents.

Definition of Health Perception and Health Management Pattern

The health perception and health management functional health pattern provides a framework for assessing children's health status and the behaviors that contribute to health. Questions relevant to health perception and management include the following: How is health perceived? What characteristics of children contribute to their health status (e.g., is there an underlying chronic illness or genetic disorder)? What decisions have families made and what actions have been taken to bring children to their current level of health? What resources to support good health are available to families? How can providers intervene to support healthy behaviors or to help change those that are unhealthy?

Significance for Nurse Practitioner Practice

Effective health management requires a commitment to good health, prevention of illness and injury, knowledge of ways to achieve optimum health, and access to and use of necessary health care resources. This functional health pattern is most concerned with the primary level of prevention—that is, actions taken to promote health or protect against specific factors that threaten health, or both.

Use of this functional health pattern gives NPs a better understanding of why certain decisions about health care are made. For example, in some communities, fewer than 50% of children younger than 2 years of age are fully immunized. Parents do not bring their children for regular well-child examinations or for scheduled immunizations. These behaviors could be attributed to many factors, such as the parents' belief that immunizations are unnecessary or even dangerous, or to a lack of knowledge about community health resources that provide immunizations. Transportation, child care problems, and lack of financial resources can contribute to a parent's failure to bring children for regular well-child visits. By assessing factors that influence the decisions families make, the NP can intervene more effectively so that parents and children will actively engage in positive health management.

Standards of Practice

Bright Futures: Guidelines for Health Supervision of Infants, Children, and Adolescents (Maternal and Child Health Bureau, 2002) provides a comprehensive framework of preventive care standards for NPs, including the following:

- Preventive services visits, including health history and complete physical examination for
  - Infants at 2, 4, 6, and 9 months
  - Toddlers at 1 year, 15 and 18 months, and 2, 3, and 4 years
  - Young children at 5, 6, 8, and 10 years
  - Older children and adolescents, annually between 11 and 21 years
- Immunizations based on Advisory Committee on Immunization Practices (ACIP) and American Academy of Pediatrics (AAP) *Red Book* (2000) guidelines
- Screening, risk assessment, appropriate referral for formal assessment, and timely intervention for problems related to
  - Hearing, vision, iron-deficiency anemia, lead, hyperlipidemia, hypertension, dentition, sexual maturity rating, and sexually transmitted diseases (STDs).

The Bright Futures project has extensive materials for pediatric primary care providers that focus on primary care, nutrition, oral health, physical activity, and mental health (see Resource Box for contact information).

Guidelines for Adolescent Preventive Services (GAPS) recommendations (American Medical Association, 1997) for the care of adolescents related to this functional health pattern include the following:

- Recommendations for delivery of health services:
  - Annual age and developmentally appropriate preventive services visits for children ages 11 to 21 years, sensitive to individual and sociocultural differences; three complete physical examinations
  - Established office policies regarding confidential care of adolescents, including how parents will be involved, clearly communicated to adolescent and parent
- Recommendations for health guidance:
  - Provide health guidance to parents or other adult caregivers at least once during early adolescence, once during middle adolescence, and, preferably, once during late adolescence, with a goal of promoting parents' understanding of physical growth, as well as psychosocial and psychosexual development; parents' active involvement in health care decisions; reduction of injuries
  - Annual guidance regarding dietary habits, healthy diets, and safe weight management; the benefits and encouragement of physical activity; responsible sexual behaviors; and avoidance of tobacco, alcohol, and other abusable substances, as well as anabolic steroids
- Recommendations for screening:
  - Annual screening for hypertension, risk for hyperlipidemia and adult coronary heart disease, eating disorders and obesity, tobacco use, alcohol and substance use, and use of over-the-counter or prescription drugs, including anabolic steroids, for nonmedical purposes
  - Annual interviews discussing involvement in sexual behaviors; screen sexually active adolescents for STDs; offer confidential human immunodeficiency virus (HIV) screening to adolescents at risk for HIV infection, and screen sexually active female adolescents or those older than 18 for cervical cancer (Papanicolaou [Pap] test)
  - Annual interviews about behaviors or emotions indicating severe depression or risk of suicide; history of emotional, physical, and sexual abuse; and learning or school problems
  - Annual tuberculin skin test if the adolescent is at risk for tuberculosis
- Recommendations for immunizations:
  - Prophylactic immunizations according to ACIP guidelines

The AAP Committee on Practice and Ambulatory Medicine (2001b) and the U.S. Preventive Services Task Force (2002) have each developed recommendations and periodic schedules of preventive services for children (see Fig. 1-5 for a listing of recommended services).

NORMAL PATTERNS OF HEALTH PERCEPTION AND HEALTH MANAGEMENT

Health perceptions are the ways in which a person thinks about and defines health-related experiences. Health management involves the actions taken to deal with these experiences. It is based on health perceptions and reflects the judgments of individuals and families, the ways they solve problems, and the decisions or choices they make. Positive health management assumes that wise decisions are made. It also assumes that resources are available for families to implement these decisions. This section discusses normal patterns of behavior.

Components of Health Perception

By exploring a family's health perceptions, the NP can begin to see reasons behind the decisions made by a particular family. Components of health perception include how individuals perceive and feel about their general state of health, past, present, and future; and the belief that there is a relationship between health status and health practices. Elements of health perception are also discussed under Models to Predict Health Behavior in Chapter 10.

Perception of Health

How parents, caregivers, and children themselves perceive and feel about children's health status is shaped by several interrelated variables, including

- Perception of one's susceptibility to the condition
- Severity of the condition
- Extent to which the condition has an impact on one's ability to function
- Knowledge about the condition
- Knowledge about how children's developmental stages affect their response to illness
- Developmental stage of the child
- Cultural or social cues about the condition

Health perceptions are reflected in health behaviors (Table 11-1).

Belief That Health Practices Affect Health Status

The degree to which parents and children believe that they can influence their health status varies. In general, individuals and families with an internal locus of control believe that their behavior affects their health status. They are motivated to take action, seek information, and set goals, believing that such behaviors will make a difference in the outcome. Even when confronted with the stress and uncertainty of illness, they are active problem solvers, engaged in the process of decision making. Families with an internal locus of control often are able to more effectively cope with their child's illness (Dunn et al, 2001; Engstrom, 1999). In contrast, many individuals and families with an external locus of control tend to believe that factors outside their control determine illness outcomes. These families are passive and dependent, lack motivation to engage in self-care, or fail to follow through with recommended treatments. Rather than actively seeking to change the condition, they let things happen to them.

A variety of factors appear to affect the extent of belief in one's ability to control health outcomes (Steptoe & Wardle, 2001). Age and sex are two factors noted in children, with older children and girls having a more internal locus of control. Additionally, families who are usually self-directed can experience excessive stress related to their child's illness or other life circumstances and may temporarily feel inadequate to cope.

Components of Health Management

Health management is a process of seeking to maintain and promote health. It includes making decisions, taking action, and using resources within a particular environment.

TABLE 11-1 ***Relationship between Health Perception and Health Behaviors***

Variable Affecting Health Perception	Related Health Behaviors
Perception of susceptibility	Increased sense of susceptibility contributes to taking precautions (e.g., immunizations) and seeking early treatment.
Severity of condition	Severity of condition usually, but not always, results in health-seeking behaviors; if signs and symptoms are subtle or appear minor, care may be delayed. Minor conditions with alarming signs (e.g., urticaria) may be responded to aggressively.
Impact on ability to function	Decreased function motivates health-seeking behaviors (e.g., child with minor illness may not be brought for care unless the condition disrupts sleep or eating patterns).
Knowledge about condition	Increased understanding of condition usually increases family's ability to manage, either by seeking appropriate health care or providing self-care. Increased education has not always contributed to health promotion activities.
Knowledge regarding child development	Knowledge of child development gives parents ability to anticipate behavior and recognize variations of normal. Parents who lack knowledge of child development may interpret normal behavior as problematic, or may not perceive atypical behavior as a problem.
Developmental stage of child	Children's conceptualization and response to illness vary by developmental stage (see Chapter 10).
Cultural or social cues	Cultural beliefs shape health perceptions (see Chapter 4). Messages or cues may be mixed (e.g., children are encouraged not to smoke, yet movie stars are increasingly shown lighting up cigarettes) and can lead to positive and negative health behaviors.

Decision Making

When confronted with health issues, families are expected to take some action. The actions taken, however, do not always make sense to providers. For example, some parents choose to use harsh forms of discipline to manage their children's behavior, or they elect not to bring their children for regular well-child visits despite the need for immunizations or care of a chronic illness. The decisions behind these actions are a result of an active process tying together the subjective content of health perceptions with the objective reality of health behavior. Although the ways in which people make decisions vary greatly, forms of decisions may fall into categories in which the following occur:

- The decision maker examines and reexamines all options and selects one but may alter the choice if new information or variables arise.
- The person making the decision looks at options but is comfortable making a quick decision without excessive reflection.
- The person making the decision is overly concerned, shifts back and forth from one option to another, and never focuses on one as viable.
- The person elects not to make a decision, procrastinating or avoiding the situation entirely.

A family's decision making is influenced by many factors, including the following:

- Social support structures
- Perception of health status
- Emotional competence of family members, which may be situational (e.g., the family is confronted with a condition that severely disrupts their emotional or psychologic health, such as severe, unexpected trauma to a child)
- Past experience
- Education and knowledge level
- Cognitive abilities of family members
- Values and cultural perspectives
- Economic conditions
- Environment
- Information and advice from the health care provider

The decisions that a family makes lead directly to the health practices and behaviors in which they engage.

Health Behaviors

Several behaviors are expected by health care providers of families within this functional health pattern:

- Establishing an ongoing relationship with a primary health care provider
- Using health and community resources to promote health
- Demonstrating lifestyles that promote health and prevent illness and injury

Establishing a Primary Caregiver Relationship. It is expected that the family will establish an ongoing relationship with a primary health care provider, ensuring that the child receives regular physical and developmental evaluations; health maintenance care, such as immunizations; early intervention for minor acute health problems; and information and guidance related to growth and development issues of the child and the family. Having a regular provider also offers the family a stable contact and access to health care resources in case the child requires hospitalization, surgery, or long-term care.

Using Health and Community Resources to Promote Health. A second behavior expected of a positive health management pattern is that families use health care services in the most effective and efficient manner possible. This includes identifying and accessing appropriate social, community, family, and health-related resources, as well as interacting appropriately with providers during the health visit. Many community resources are available to families; for example, school nurses or school-based clinics provide case management or primary care in the school setting. The NP can inform parents about these resources, explain their purpose, and encourage parents to communicate with school personnel about children's health needs. School-based health services are especially important for children with chronic illnesses.

Social supports offer a buffer against the stress of daily living, allowing the individual and family to respond more positively to both usual and unexpected events. Families isolated from a social network find it much more difficult to structure health maintenance into their lives or to cope with a child's illness. Connection to a network of community resources (e.g., schools, day care, recreational facilities) also provides structure to support families in daily living activities.

The way parents use health care services may be based on their past experiences. Past experience reinforces beliefs about what causes illness, what is the most appropriate treatment, and how effectively parents can care for their children. For example, if parents of an ill child have once managed a fever successfully, they are more likely to feel confident coping with a fever in the child's current condition. If they believe that their child remains free of illness as a result of their care, they are more likely to continue health promotion activities. In contrast, if the child is healthy or ill, despite what the parents do, they can be more inclined to depend on the practitioner for advice or care or to not seek care at all.

Families need both economic and experiential resources for optimal health management. The cost of health care services or deficits in health care insurance coverage are barriers to access, contributing to delay or neglect in seeking essential treatment. There must also be a sufficient number of providers and health care services in the community. For many children, economic barriers prevent access to health care, but for others, adequate resources are simply not available.

Demonstrating Healthy Lifestyles. Healthy families are expected to demonstrate lifestyles that enhance health and prevent illness and injury. Health, disease, illness, and injury are the results of multiple physical, psychologic, and environmental factors, some of which are beyond the control of individuals and families. In many cases, however, health status is influenced by the lifestyle choices that are made. There are specific categories of behavior in which change has an impact on health status (Box 11-1). In addition, individuals can take actions that significantly change their external environment, thus influencing forces that affect their health and the health of family members.

Environment

Environmental conditions relate to health management on two levels: first, the nature of the environment affects health status (see Chapter 42); and, second, as noted earlier, resources to support health may or may not be present in the physical environment. Environmental factors such as urban crowding, air and noise pollution, streets with heavy traffic, inadequate housing, poor nutrition, lack of appropriate stimulation (e.g., no playgrounds or recreational facilities), violence, and physical and emotional stress are experienced by many children. In addition, families with limited economic resources have limited access to health care services, and frequent moves prevent families from establishing ongoing connections with a health care provider.

BOX 11-1 ***Lifestyle Choices that Affect Health Status***

- Nutrition
- Smoking
- Alcohol use
- Drug use
- Exercise
- Motor vehicle use
- Sexual behavior
- Social/interactional patterns (family and community relations)
- Coping and stress management skills

Rural environments often lack health-related resources, with few providers, clinics, or hospital services easily available. Children living in rural settings are also at high risk of injury because of exposure to animals, farm machinery, pesticides, herbicides, unsafe transportation, and other physical hazards (AAP Committee on Injury and Poison Prevention and Committee on Community Health Services, 2001; Gerberich et al, 2001).

Children with Special Needs

Health management of children with special needs is challenging. Children with chronic illness receive expert illness care from a number of specialists, but their primary care needs are often neglected. Primary care NPs can serve to coordinate health maintenance care with ongoing specialty illness management. Communication and collaboration with the child's specialty physician are essential, as is clear communication with the parents about the role of each provider in the child's care.

NPs also need to adapt normal intervention techniques when providing primary care to children with chronic illness. The regular immunization schedule may need to be adjusted, for example, or special techniques for obtaining height and weight or vital signs might be necessary. Parents and children should be assisted to develop ways to meet daily living needs consonant with the child's abilities. Children with physical handicaps, for example, require special intervention to meet activity and exercise needs for growth and development.

ASSESSMENT OF HEALTH PERCEPTION AND HEALTH MANAGEMENT PATTERN

Assessment of this functional health pattern focuses on health perception, health management, and decision making.

History

Components of Health Perception

Perception of Health. Health perception is assessed by examining the family's health belief structure and knowledge levels. During the initial intake history, the focus is on the family's general perception of health. At subsequent visits, questions look at the particular condition (e.g., "Tell me what this illness means to you"). General assessment questions include the following:

- How would you describe your child's health right now?
- Compared with other children, how healthy would you say your child is?
- What does it mean for you to say that your child is "healthy"?

- How do you describe good health in your family?
- Do you have any questions or concerns about your child's health, growth, or development?
- How important is it to you to have a regular health care provider?
- What makes you decide to call your health care provider or take your child in for an examination (e.g., as a way to stay well, for a serious problem such as a high fever, an accident, or a problem you've never seen before or one that won't go away)?
- What do you know about this current condition?
- Has your child had a problem like this before?
- How do you expect your child to respond when sick? To this particular sickness?
- What things can you do to help your child cope with being sick?

Belief That Health Practices Affect Health Status. General intake questions can give the NP important information about whether the family and child believe that their health practices affect outcomes. These include the following:

- Has your child ever had this type of problem before?
- What have you done for it in the past?
- What do you do or have you done that you believe makes a difference in how your child responds to illness?
- What kind of personality would you say your child has? How would you describe your child's temperament?
- When confronted with sudden changes in plans or a disruption of normal routine, feelings often change. What kinds of feelings do you have when this happens? How do you deal with those feelings?
- Describe the feelings you have when your child gets ill. How do you deal with those feelings?
- How do you think those feelings affect the way you handle your child's health and illness?

Locus of control can also be assessed using classic rating scales such as Rotter's (1966) internal-external scale, the health locus of control scale (Wallston et al, 1976), the perceived health competence scale (Smith, Wallston, & Smith, 1995), or the multidimensional health locus of control scale (Wallston, Wallston, & DeVellis, 1978). Measures of the effect of locus of control on a particular health condition, such as weight and injury treatment, have been explored (Halloran et al, 1999; Holt, Clark, & Kreuter, 2001).

Components of Health Management

Decision Making. Assessment of the family's decision making examines how active the family is in making decisions about child's health care, the process used, and the factors that influence those decisions. Questions in this area include the following:

- What do you do when your child has health problems?
- Who makes decisions about health care in your family?
- How do you make those decisions? Do you talk things over? Do you get advice from others?
- Why do you think that you make decisions in that way?
- What are the most important things that you consider when making a decision about health care for your child?
- What is most difficult for you when you have to make decisions related to your child's health?

Health Behaviors and Use of Resources. The following questions refer to actions taken and resources used to promote health and healing:

- Do you have a regular health care provider for your child?
- What health care resources are available to you? Is there a primary care provider you can get to conveniently? Clinics? Pharmacies?
- When was the last time your child visited a regular health care provider or dentist?
- What makes it hard for you to follow the advice of your health care provider?
- What immunizations has your child received?
- What have you done to protect your child from injuries? What are your patterns of seat belt use?
- Does your child have any special health problems? How do you manage them?
- There has been much focus on healthy lifestyles lately, such as eating right and exercising. What does your family do regularly to stay healthy?
- Does anyone in your family (adolescents, you yourself) smoke, drink, or use drugs? How often? What kind? Are there other things that your family does that you think are bad for your children's health?
- How does your family fit into your neighborhood? Do you feel like part of the community? Do you have relatives or neighbors on whom you can call if you need help or advice?
- Who cares for your child when you are not at home and the child is not in school?
- How are you managing household, work, school, and other child care responsibilities during this illness? What is most difficult for you?
- Having sick children can create a financial strain on families. Is this a problem for your family? What is the most difficult part?
- How comfortable do you feel managing this illness? Have you had experience in the past that helps you manage?

Environment. Environmental conditions are difficult to assess during a clinic visit, even if the parent is open, cooperative, and willing to share information. If there is a question about the health of the child because of possible environmental problems, it may be appropriate to arrange for a community health nurse to visit the family at home to gain a thorough understanding of the family environment.

Questions that can be asked in the clinic include the following:

- Do you use booster seats, seat belts, or child restraints when riding in a car?
- Where does your child play? Do you believe it is safe? Why?
- Is your home childproof? If you have firearms, are they unloaded and locked? Are pools fenced and gated?
- How do you heat or cool your home? Is it comfortable?
- Is there any danger of falls? Does your child get enough to eat? Is he or she dressed warmly for cold weather? Do you have a working smoke alarm?
- What would you do if your child had a health emergency? Do you have a car, or is there a friend, family member, or neighbor close by who could help you?
- What other conditions in your child's environment do you think could be a health risk?

Children with Special Needs. Assessment of the health perception and management pattern for children with special needs encompasses all the categories just discussed, as well as questions such as the following:

- What does it mean for you to say that your child is "healthy"?
- How did you feel when your child's problem was diagnosed? What did you do? What coping strategies do you currently use as you care for your child?
- How has managing a chronic illness changed your family functioning? How does your family function?
- Who is providing specialty care to your child? Do you believe this is adequate? What other special needs do you believe your child has that require care?
- How comfortable are you in providing home care? What would you need to be more comfortable?
- How are your child's regular health needs met—that is, those not directly related to the chronic illness, such as immunizations?
- What resources do you know about that can help you understand and manage your child's illness?
- What special physical arrangements have you made to accommodate your child's illness? At home? In the car? At school or day care?

MANAGEMENT STRATEGIES FOR POSITIVE HEALTH PERCEPTION AND HEALTH MANAGEMENT

Parents and NPs work together to manage children's health. Each has a responsibility to ensure that children are receiving the best possible care. This section discusses areas of intervention relevant to health perception and health management.

Providing Health Maintenance for Children by Developmental Age

Health supervision visits for children are more than simple physical checkups. Visits with the NP also allow assessment of home, family, and social life, teaching about growth and development, and problem solving related to issues that affect children's health status. The visits can be used to enhance children's sense of independence and positive self-concept and to encourage children to make healthy lifestyle decisions. As children mature, they should be actively involved in the visit, with the NP asking them questions directly and providing appropriate feedback to their responses. In addition to screening interventions recommended by the AAP Committee on Practice and Ambulatory Medicine (2001) (see Fig. 1-5), the health supervision visit examines the child's daily living and functional health patterns as identified in Table 11-2.

Facilitating Communication between Families and Nurse Practitioners

Effective communication between families and NPs requires sensitivity and skill. Families must be given the message that their values and beliefs are important, that NPs recognize they are making their best effort to do the right thing, and that those efforts are to be applauded. If families are listened to, they are more likely to participate in health care decision making and be more invested in the process and outcome. Communication is facilitated by two strategies in particular, one focused on content and the other on process. These strategies relate to health promotion as well as illness management.

First, NPs, parents, and children must develop a mutual understanding of the perspectives that each brings to the encounter (Kleinman, Eisenberg, & Good, 1978). To do this, family members must be encouraged to explain their understanding of the child's illness, as well as their expectations for its outcome and the role each player has in working toward that outcome. NPs must explain their perspective, usually biomedical, focusing on similar areas of concern: cause, symptoms, pathophysiology, nature and course of the illness, and treatment. Kleinman, Eisenberg, & Good (1978) outlined a set of questions to elicit information about a family's health beliefs. These questions can be adapted and used with parents when asking about their child's illness (see Table 4-3). With this information in hand, NPs, parents, and children can compare similarities and differences between their perspectives and create a mutually agreed-on plan of care.

TABLE 11-2 ***Health Supervision Visits: Daily Living and Functional Health Patterns***

	Infant	Toddler	Preschool Child	School-Age Child	Adolescent
Parent-child interaction	• Degree of mutual and reciprocal response between infant and parents • Emotional status of parents • Appropriateness of parental response to infant's cues	• Parental confidence in role • Emotional status of parents • Appropriateness of parental response to toddler's cues • Degree of affection demonstrated between toddler and parents • Parental encouragement of independence, yet active involvement with child	• Consistency in parents' behavior • Emotional status of parents • Appropriateness of parental response to child's cues • Degree to which parents provide affection, praise, and emotional support and encourage child to express feelings • Parental encouragement of independence, yet active engagement with child	• Clear, consistent, but flexible expectations expressed by parents • Appropriate limits set by parents • Degree to which parents provide attention, affection, praise, approval, and emotional support and encourage child to express feelings • Degree to which parents support independence, yet participate with child in activities • Degree to which child demonstrates self-confidence, industriousness, cooperation, and consideration	• Parental confidence and pleasure in role • Open communication with mutual respect for privacy • Parental encouragement of independence and activities with peers • Reasonable and consistent limits • Active parental interest in adolescent's activities, friends, school performance • Parental pride and pleasure in adolescent's achievements
Developmental assessment to determine extent to which child has achieved milestones and received emotional nurturing	• See Chapters 6 and 18	• See Chapters 7 and 18	• See Chapters 7 and 18; look for child who is friendly, secure, cooperative, proud, and happy • Conduct speech evaluation	• See Chapters 8 and 18 • Conduct speech evaluation	• See Chapters 9 and 18
Nutrition/metabolic	• Choice of feeding, breastfeeding versus bottle feeding (see Chapter 13) • When to introduce solids; management of feeding problems or special nutritional needs (see Chapter 12) • Fluoride beginning at 6 mo as indicated according to fluoride level in water source	• Management of self-feeding, feeding problems, or special nutritional needs (see Chapter 12) • Pattern of dentition, need for good oral hygiene (see Chapter 34) • Fluoride as indicated • Skin care: apply sun screen whenever child is exposed to sun	• Need for well-balanced diet • Parents' responsibility to provide nutritious foods, pleasant atmosphere for meals, and healthy role models for child; child's responsibility to select appropriate foods from those provided (see Chapter 12) • Pattern of dentition, need for dental assessment (see Chapter 34)	• Healthy food selections with child making more independent choices (see Chapter 12) • Daily dental hygiene (see Chapter 34) • Fluoride as indicated • Skin care: apply sun screen whenever child is exposed to sun	• Nutritional needs, dietary patterns with adolescent making choices (see Chapter 12) • Body image and self-perception as they relate to eating habits • Good oral hygiene, regular dental care (see Chapter 34), orthodontia

	• Skin care: apply sun screen whenever child is exposed to sun		• Fluoride as indicated • Skin care: apply sun screen whenever child is exposed to sun		• Fluoride until age 16, as indicated • Skin care: apply sun screen whenever child is exposed to sun • Acne management as appropriate
Sleep and rest: sleep needs, patterns, and changes as child grows (see Chapter 16)	• Importance of bedtime ritual, infant cues for sleep and wake states • Position infant on back for sleep	• Importance of bedtime ritual	• Typical night fears, night terrors	• Sleepwalking and night terrors	• Sleep needs during rapid growth of adolescence
Activity and exercise (see Chapter 15): injury prevention (see Tables 11-4 through 11-7)	• Physical developmental needs and skills of infant	• Set limits and provide safe environment for expression of physical needs and developing skills	• Set limits and provide safe environment for expression of physical needs and skills • Active, pretend and fantasy play; discourage passive activities such as watching television • Child's tendency to become overtired, often needing parent's help to calm down	• Encourage regular physical activity • Bicycle, skateboard, pedestrian, swimming safety • Balance of nutrition with exercise to achieve appropriate weight gain • Scoliosis in child age 10-12 years	• Regular physical activity, participation in fitness and organized sports activities • Scoliosis evaluation • Sports fitness and safety
Elimination (see Chapter 14)	• Diapering, infant patterns of stooling and urination	• Toilet training	• Management of occasional "accidents" in toilet-trained child • Good hygiene, handwashing	• Good hygiene, handwashing • Explain relationship between nutrition, exercise, and elimination	• Good hygiene, handwashing • Explain relationship between nutrition, exercise, and elimination
Sexuality (see Chapter 20)	• Infant's sense of physical comfort and pleasure related to stimulation of genitalia • Parents to express their perceptions of sexuality in infant and child • Testes and inguinal canal for abnormalities	• Toddler's sense of physical comfort and pleasure related to genital stimulation, masturbation • Parents to express their perceptions of sexuality; ways parents communicate with toddler about sexuality	• Child's natural curiosity related to sexuality • Parents to answer questions at age-appropriate level • Concept of "good" and "bad" touch; private body parts	• Children's natural curiosity and exploration related to sexuality • Parents to answer questions at age-appropriate level, set appropriate limits for sexual activity in child • Sexual maturation (SM) stage (Tanner)	• Developing sense of sexual identity, masturbation, degree of intimacy with others • Sexual responsibility to self and others, how to say "no" and how to deal with potential sexual abuse or "date rape" • Prevention of sexually transmitted diseases and pregnancy; birth control options • Sexual maturation stages, gynecomastia in boy

Continued

TABLE 11-2 *Health Supervision Visits: Daily Living and Functional Health Patterns—cont'd*

	Infant	Toddler	Preschool Child	School-Age Child	Adolescent
					• Pelvic examination in sexually active girl, girl with menstrual problems, or those with history of mother taking diethylstilbestrol (DES) • Breast and testicular self-examination • Folic acid 400 μg/day for girl
Role relationships (see Chapters 3 and 19)	• Infant's interaction with siblings and other family members; impact child has on family system, place of child in family	• Discipline strategies • Interaction of toddler with siblings, other family members; impact child has on family system, place of child in family • Day care needs and plans	• Discipline strategies • Interaction of child with siblings, other family members; impact child has on family system, place of child in family • Day care needs and plans • School readiness for older preschool-age child	• Increasing child's participation in family activities, taking more responsibility for tasks in household • Nature of child's interaction in school and with peer group • Parents encourage and participate in hobbies, reading, other activities with child and peer group	• Increasing independence in adolescents; responsibilities at home, school, or workplace • Need to keep communication open among adolescent, peers, and parents
Self-concept/ self-perception (see Chapter 18)	• Infant's developing an awareness of self as separate from parents and others	• Importance of giving child positive feedback on achievements • Parents to relate to child in warm, loving manner; avoid harsh words, punitive and inconsistent parental behavior	• Parents to give children choices, allowing children to express selves and participate in family tasks • Children's sense of absolutes at this age; discourage teasing and threats • Parents to participate in child's activities (e.g., school field trips)	• Parents to give child attention and positive reinforcement of choices, allowing child to express self and expecting participation in family tasks	• Opportunities to discuss changes in self and to openly ask questions about development • Parents to give adolescent positive attention, reinforcement for healthy choices and appropriate activities, allowing adolescent privacy, and expecting reasonable participation in family activities

Coping and stress tolerance; for all ages, examine the following: • Family support network • Knowledge of community resources • Knowledge of child development • Level of parenting skills	• Parents' health habits (e.g., smoking, exercise, diet) may affect child	• Discipline styles and options • Parent to guide and instruct child's positive social behavior (e.g., sharing, not hitting or biting)	• Discipline styles and options; need to set limits • Parents to help child name and identify feelings and ways the child can manage feelings	• Discipline styles and options; need to set limits • Parents to praise child's efforts at self-control, management of feelings • Depression assessment	• Discipline styles and options • Parents to provide appropriate limits while fostering independence • Adolescent's emotional states related to rapid growth and changes of puberty • Depression assessment
Values and beliefs	• Parents' expectations of self and child as family grows	• Parents to identify their value and belief framework; how they demonstrate their beliefs to their child	• Parents to provide opportunities for child to express ideas, feelings, and emotions • Child included in family spiritual activities	• Parents to provide opportunity for child to explore understanding of emotions, values, and beliefs in more formal settings (e.g., religious institutions, spiritual activities)	• Adolescent, as part of normal process of developing self-identity, may appear to reject family values • Encourage adolescent to discuss values and beliefs

A second strategy that strengthens communication and contributes to families having a greater sense of control in the situation relates to the process of the client-provider interaction. Marshall (1988) asserted that, in order to arrive at the appropriate interpretation of what the clinical situation means, clients and providers must engage in a process of interpretation at the conversational level. This "conversational cooperation" is enhanced when family members and the NP do the following:

- Use cooperative turn-taking in the conversation.
- Use similar patterns of conversation, such as open-ended questions or narrative discussion; communication is at risk, for example, if parents are using a narrative form of discussion and the NP is using close-ended questions.
- Listen for the images clients use in speech patterns and try to respond in kind. Parents may use visual, auditory, or kinesthetic imagery when they talk, and may better understand providers who respond with similar imagery. For example, the parent may state, "I don't see any change . . ."; the provider responds, "You're looking for . . . ". Or the parent states, "I want to do something . . . ," and the provider answers, "You'd like to take some action . . ." (Howard, 1998).
- Confirm assumptions.
- Develop a clear understanding of differences in perspectives or meaning of the illness.
- Remain open to alternative explanations and solutions, not limited to following an isolated path of clinical reasoning.
- Explain or provide the context of pronouns used; for example, if NPs say, "I'll check on that for you," they should be sure the parent understands what "that" means.

Helping Families Develop Sound Decision-Making Skills

The health decisions people make may not necessarily be shaped by the health education they receive. Nevertheless, health education is viewed as an essential component of intervention. The manner in which information is given, however, may be as important as the information itself. NPs who work with parents to establish effective communication, to generate mutual understanding of problems, and to listen actively to feelings, perceptions, fears, and anxieties are more likely to be heard by parents when they offer information or suggestions for care. Developing this level of rapport is important, because it is the information that NPs provide that allows parents to identify, evaluate, select, and implement options for care. NPs also serve an essential role in structuring the forum for parents to discuss feelings, clarify points of confusion, and receive validation for their choices in this decision-making process. The process of making health care decisions includes the following steps:

- Identify the problem being confronted. Review the facts and feelings one has about the problem.
- Generate alternative solutions to the problem.
- Evaluate the alternatives. Which are feasible? Which are cost effective? What are the consequences of each? Which best fits the family's belief system?
- Select a solution.
- Develop and implement a plan of action based on that solution.
- Review the outcomes of the decision and the action taken.

For this process to function well, families must be able, or be assisted, to communicate effectively, understand abstract concepts, and mobilize resources. Children should be encouraged to participate in the process consistent with their developmental abilities. Adolescents, especially, are at a stage at which they can make many decisions independently of their parents. NPs serve a vital role in helping families and children develop sound decision-making skills.

Helping Families Gain Access to Health Care Resources

Access to health care resources is influenced by a number of factors. Strategies to increase parents' ability to access resources occur on two levels: (1) giving parents the information to more easily and appropriately gain access and (2) removing barriers to access.

Giving Parents Information to Gain Access

Teaching Telephone Triage. The nature of the telephone interaction between parent and NP can be a critical factor in accurately interpreting a child's condition, deciding on appropriate measures of care, and establishing confidence and trust. See Chapter 23 for a discussion of how pediatric care providers can work with parents to use the telephone in the management of illnesses.

Identifying Resources. NPs serve as advocates by helping families locate local, regional, or national health care resources to meet their health needs. It is important that NPs develop and maintain a resource list relevant to their practice. Using a resource list facilitates making referrals and recommendations to parents; it gives the clear message that the family is not alone with their concern, that help is available, and that the NP is a knowledgeable ally in the family's effort to maintain good health.

Assisting in Contact of Support Networks. As an advocate, NPs make every effort to encourage independent action and decision making by families, but if the family's coping abilities are compromised, it is not enough simply to give the name of a resource or contact to the family. In these situations, NPs may need to contact the resource themselves or assist the family to make the contact. For some families in crisis, it is appropriate to refer them to a community or mental health nurse for assistance in establishing and maintaining contact with a supportive network.

Removing Barriers to Access

Among the primary barriers to health care access are cost, geography, and lack of essential infrastructure services such as transportation and child care. NPs are aware of the relationship between the high cost of care and the failure of children to receive regular well-child care. Lack of primary care resources in rural and isolated areas also prevents families from obtaining regular care. Without adequate transportation or child care services, the cost of seeking well-child care, or even treatment of minor acute problems that worsen without medical intervention, often outweighs the benefits perceived by the family.

NPs can work with parents and social workers to identify resources in the community that help overcome some of these barriers. For example, transportation may be available through some managed care plans or local volunteer organizations (e.g., churches), or a relative may have time to care for other children while the parent takes one child to the clinic. For other barriers, however, the solution lies in making changes in the way health care services are organized and financed. This task goes far beyond the primary care setting, but it is nonetheless the responsibility of NPs to be aware of and to participate in the process of restructuring and reorganizing the health care system within their community.

ALTERED PATTERNS OF HEALTH PERCEPTION AND HEALTH MANAGEMENT

Ineffective Use of Health Care System

Description

Ineffective use of the health care system includes seeking care primarily when children are ill or when there is an external mandate (e.g., when immunizations are required to attend school), using emergency departments for routine care needs, using outpatient services for emergency care, not establishing an ongoing relationship with a primary care provider, underutilizing health care resources, or failing to comply or follow up with prescribed regimens. A key element of noncompliance is that the child or caregivers actively choose not to adhere to health recommendations despite knowledge of the benefits and risks.

Etiology

Ineffective use of the health care system can have many causes. Among these are long-standing patterns of misuse, knowledge deficit about how to gain access to and use the system, and knowledge deficit about health and illness, such as the seriousness of illness in children. Access to care can be limited by social, physical, or economic barriers. Health care in the United States is largely connected to employment, and the unemployed or those with low incomes may not be able to afford insurance. In addition, some employees receive no health insurance coverage benefits or, for others, insurance coverage is inadequate. The Medicaid program reimburses providers for primary health care services for families whose income is low enough to qualify for welfare, but reimbursement is often less than the cost of the services provided; as a result, some providers refuse care to Medicaid clients.

Cultural perceptions of care and the perception that health care providers do not understand or value the family or their cultural beliefs can discourage use of health care services. Values, beliefs, and perceptions of risk and benefits contribute to the choices made. For example, a client may refuse chemotherapy for leukemia, believing that there is greater risk associated with the treatment than with the disease itself. Finally, a lack of health care resources can contribute to incomplete care. Rural and poor urban communities often lack health facilities or the facilities there are understaffed, leaving residents with inadequate care.

Clinical Findings

The following are found with ineffective use of the health care system:

- No regular provider for child
- History of lack of continuity or fragmented care
- Use of emergency department for nonemergent conditions
- Lack of follow-up care for child seen in emergency department
- Failure to adhere to prescribed medical treatment or standards for well-child health supervision after having adequate information for decision making
- Child at risk for delayed or ineffective treatment or both
- Poor health status of children as a result of untreated illness or other health problem
- Underimmunization
- Parents' dissatisfaction with health care providers

Differential Diagnosis

- Dysfunctional family systems related to cognitive, emotional, or psychologic variables

Management

Interventions vary depending on the reasons families ineffectively use the system.

Lack of an Identified Primary Care Provider

- Assist the family to establish a permanent relationship with a provider.
- Encourage and reinforce positive, ongoing communication with the primary care provider.
- As a primary care provider, the NP should establish a positive, accepting environment of trust and mutual respect, encouraging the family and child to take an active role in health care.
- Assist the child and family to develop an understanding of the importance of regular care.

Barriers to Health Care Services

- Inform families of health care resources available in the community.
- Teach the family how to access and use health care services most effectively.
- Assist families to identify strengths and resources within their social and family network.
- Refer to social services or other resources to deal with financial concerns.
- Work with community, local, state, and federal leaders to change the way health care services are organized and financed.

Knowledge Deficit about Children

- Assess knowledge level of families related to development and health care needs of children.
- Educate parents about normal growth and development of children.
- Provide anticipatory guidance about variations of normal.

Knowledge Deficit Related to Illness

- Explain what can be expected during minor illnesses or with conditions that change the child's health status. For example, what signs and symptoms might be seen with an ear infection or following routine immunizations? What physiologic changes can be expected in the child with an acute asthma attack? What factors might precipitate an asthma attack? Discuss what the caregiver can do to manage the condition in the home. For example, what can the parent do to control a fever if one should occur? How can the family manage the child's environment to minimize the possibility of an asthma attack?
- Strengthen the family's ability to make appropriate decisions regarding care of ill children in the home. Support active participation in decision making and provide information needed to care for children in the home.
- Establish a plan with the family about when and who to call for help. Although minor conditions can often be managed and more serious conditions prevented by actions taken in the home, many problems require professional intervention or advice. Families should be encouraged to initiate contact with the NP when they have questions and doubts about their child's condition. Parents should be given clear instructions on when to use the telephone, when to bring the child back to the office, or when to use the emergency department (see Tables 23-4 and 23-5).

Noncompliance with Health Requirements

- Develop a partnership with the family around health care decision making.
- Ensure that clients are active participants, invested in the decisions made.
- Assist the family to identify the bases of their decision making.
- Identify differences between families' and NPs' approaches to health care.
- Clearly state when and why the NP disagrees with the client's decisions. In some cases, clients and NPs can "agree to disagree" on one issue, finding others on which they can work together. In other cases, NPs can feel so strongly about an issue that they need to refer clients to another provider or intervene as an advocate for the child.
- Provide positive reinforcement for healthy decisions.

Risk-Taking Behaviors

Description

Risk-taking behaviors include activities that threaten the health and well-being of the child or adolescent. Although these include behaviors such as substance abuse, unprotected sexual activity, abuse, and violence, this section focuses on smoking in adolescents. Smoking appears within a cluster of risk-taking behaviors, and adolescent smokers are more likely than their nonsmoking peers to use marijuana and hard drugs, sell drugs, have multiple drug problems, drop out of school, and experience early pregnancy and parenthood. These adolescents are also at higher risk for low academic achievement and behavioral problems at school, stealing and other delinquent behaviors, and use of predatory and relational violence (Ellickson, Tucker, & Klein, 2001).

Etiology and Incidence

During the 1990s, cigarette smoking among non-Hispanic black, non-Hispanic white, and Hispanic high school students increased significantly in three assessed areas:

"lifetime smoking (defined as having ever smoked cigarettes, even one or two puffs), current smoking (defined as smoking on >1 of the 30 days preceding the survey), and current frequent smoking (defined as smoking on >20 of the 30 days preceding the survey)." From 1997 to 2001, however, there was a significant decline in smoking among high school students. Approximately 28.5% of high school students were smokers in 2001 (down from 36.4% in 1997), and 13.8% were frequent smokers in 2001 (down from 16.7% in 1997) (Centers for Disease Control and Prevention [CDC], 2002). These data do not include teenagers who were not attending high school between 1997 and 2001, an estimated 5% of the adolescent population (CDC, 2002). Smoking is more common among older, Caucasian teens, and it is positively related to tobacco industry advertising (Federal Trade Commission, 2001), portrayal of smoking in films (Sargent et al, 2001), and parent smoking (Fleming et al, 2002). A study of younger children indicates that smoking is related to access in the home and whether a sibling or close peer smokes (Johnson et al, 2002).

Clinical Findings

In the clinical setting, adolescents' smoking patterns are best assessed through direct questioning. At every visit, children should be asked whether they or their friends smoke or use other forms of tobacco. Biochemical tests to measure tobacco by-products (e.g., carbon monoxide in serum or expired alveolar air; urine cotinine, a primary metabolite of nicotine; and thiocyanate, a detoxification product of hydrogen cyanide in tobacco smoke) are used primarily in the research setting and are not appropriate as a diagnostic tool in primary care.

Increased incidence of respiratory disease in children, including asthma, is a clinical finding in smokers or in families in which parents smoke (see Chapter 42).

Management

Management of adolescent tobacco use takes place on two levels: (1) primary, with a goal of preventing the child from starting to use, and (2) secondary, with a goal of cessation (Table 11-3). Many adolescents experiment with tobacco use but stop after a short period before becoming addicted to nicotine. Nicotine addiction appears to occur over about a 2-year period (Elster & Kuznets, 1994), giving providers an opportunity to intervene early for more effective cessation.

Prevention may be facilitated by increasing costs of tobacco products, implementing school-based programs (VanDyke & Riesenberg, 2002), using population-focused antismoking campaigns (Farrelly et al, 2002), and supporting positive parenting styles (O'Byrne et al, 2002).

Many children are exposed to nicotine in utero or to secondhand smoke of parents or other caregivers. This not only puts them at risk for health and learning problems (Higgins, 2002), but children who live in a family with smokers are more likely to become smokers themselves. Therefore, although pediatric NPs are not the parents' primary caregivers, they can encourage parents to make the decision to stop smoking, support efforts to decrease

TABLE 11-3 ***Primary and Secondary Prevention/Tobacco Use Cessation Strategies for Adolescents***

Primary Prevention	Secondary Prevention
Provide multimedia, multisite health information, not limited to schools	Ask at every visit whether adolescent or friends use tobacco
Emphasize skills to avoid peer pressure	Inform adolescent of health risks of tobacco use and process by which one becomes addicted to nicotine; emphasize that it is easier to stop early
Focus on adolescents' developmental need to belong to a social group	Develop mutual understanding of problem
	Determine realistic stop-use date
	Help adolescent identify barriers to stopping and ways to overcome those barriers
	Provide information about self-help and support groups; encourage adolescent to try to stop smoking with a friend
	Provide nicotine patches protocol if adolescent feels this will help
	Schedule follow-up visits to monitor progress; reinforce positive efforts
	Assess parents' tobacco use patterns; provide information and support to stop use

smoking behaviors, and refer the parents for smoking cessation that involves the following:

- Asking about smoking at every medical visit
- Advising all smokers to stop
- Assisting patients with stop-smoking contracts and self-help and motivating materials
- Setting a quit-smoking date and prescribing nicotine gum
- Arranging follow-up visits to reinforce the intervention (Elster & Kuznets, 1994)

In addition, medical practices could implement population-based interventions to help their clients stop tobacco use. These include tracking and monitoring smokers, providing insurance coverage for tobacco-cessation services, educating employees not to use tobacco, and lobbying for public antismoking campaigns and increased taxes on tobacco products.

Unintentional Injuries

Description

Unintentional injuries are traumatic events that are unanticipated and accidentally caused (see Chapter 40 for a more complete discussion of injuries in children).

Etiology and Incidence

Unintentional injury in children results from many factors, including the presence of hazards in the environment, unsafe or risky behaviors, and inadequate adult supervision. Injuries are one of the most serious health problems faced by the pediatric population, and morbidity secondary to injury is significantly more common than mortality. The nature and severity of childhood injuries vary by age, gender, race, and socioeconomic status (Behrman, Kliegman, & Jenson, 2004). After 1 year of age, motor vehicle trauma is the major cause of pediatric mortality in the United States. Mortality and morbidity related to falls, poisoning, drownings, near-drownings, fires and burns, and trauma secondary to weapons are significant in children. Male children are more likely to experience injury than female children. Native American children have the highest rate of injuries, followed in order by black, Hispanic, white, and Asian children. Children from lower socioeconomic groups experience more injuries than those from higher income groups. Injury rates are also high for many sports (see Chapter 15).

Clinical Findings

Clinical presentation of injuries varies, depending on the nature and extent of the trauma experienced. A thorough history of the child with an injury is essential, and the following information should be gathered to construct a clinical picture:

- Description of environment in which injury took place
- Condition of child before injury
- Actions of child and others immediately before injury
- Mechanism of injury
- Extent of supervision by adults
- First aid management at scene of injury

Differential Diagnosis

The differential diagnoses for unintentional injuries include the following:

- Child abuse and neglect
- Suicide attempt
- Disease condition that makes the child more susceptible to injuries (e.g., osteogenesis imperfecta or hemophilia)

Management

Prevention is the key treatment. A discussion of safety issues needs to be incorporated into the NP's anticipatory guidance at every well-child and adolescent visit, clarifying how the potential for injury, as well as the type of injury, varies by the child's age and developmental level. Effective management of unintentional injuries requires that parents understand how, at each age, developmental characteristics influence children's behavior and put them at risk for injury. Once aware of how children may be at risk, parents can more clearly see how they can intervene to prevent an injury from occurring. Tables 11-4 through 11-7 outline major injuries, developmental characteristics of children, the risks for injury these present, and strategies for intervention that parents can use to decrease the potential for injury (National Center for Injury Prevention and Control, 2002a).

Efforts to prevent injury include the following:

- Restructure the environment to make it safer.
  - Place devices in the environment (e.g., automobile restraint systems, fenced swimming pools [Box 11-2 on p. 207]) to protect children.
  - Remove hazards from the environment (e.g., child-proof the home).
  - Adjust environmental conditions (e.g., lower the water heater temperature).
- Mandate and enforce behavior or use of devices that protect the child (e.g., bicycle helmets, seat belts).
- Implement school policies and procedures to ensure that playground equipment and activities are well maintained and suited for children's developmental abilities.
- Teach children age-appropriate safe behavior to decrease risks of motor vehicle accidents, burns, drowning, poisoning, weapons, and falls.

TABLE 11-4 *Primary Injury Prevention Related to Developmental Characteristics of Infants*

Unintentional injuries account for 67% of all external causes of infant mortality and are the seventh-leading cause of infant death in the United States; 59.7% of all injury-related deaths in infants are caused by asphyxiation, 18.4% are caused by motor vehicle trauma, and 8.5% are caused by drowning (National Center for Injury Prevention and Control, 2002a).

Age and Developmental Characteristics	Potential Injuries	Strategies for Prevention
Birth to 6 mo		
Poor head control at younger ages	Injury to neck	Handle child with care when picking up or moving Support neck of young infant Supervise other children when they are playing with infant Never jiggle or shake infant
Reflex behavior; especially strong suck reflex in early months Skin thin and sensitive	Aspiration of foreign objects Suffocation Friction burns Burns	Keep occlusive materials, especially plastic, out of child's bed Check toys, mobiles for sharp, detachable parts, strings, or cords Handle child with care when picking up or moving Do not hold infant in lap when drinking hot beverage or smoking Set water heater thermostat below 120° F
	Sunburn	Use cover-up (e.g., hat) whenever child is exposed to sun; avoid exposure
Poor body temperature control	Hypothermia Hyperthermia	Dress infant appropriately Never leave child alone in car
Rolls, turns, and scoots	Falls	Do not leave infant alone on bed, changing table, or other area from which infant may fall Use playpen as safe area
	May slide between mattress and crib slats	Make sure mattress fits tightly against bed railings; railings are no more than $2\frac{3}{8}$ inches apart
	Slips in bath	Place washcloth under infant in bath; stay with infant during bathing
	Motor vehicle trauma Burns	Correctly use approved child safety restraint units in cars Install smoke detectors in home and check batteries routinely
Age 6 to 12 mo		
Grasps and mouths objects	Aspiration of foreign objects Suffocation	Keep small, sharp objects off floor and play area, out of reach Check toys for detachable parts Keep balloons, plastic wrappers, and plastic bags out of reach
	Poisoning	Use childproof caps on medications Keep medications out of reach in locked cabinet Keep household, garden, and car products out of reach Supervise children's activity Keep poison control numbers near telephone and alert older siblings and babysitters about them
Sits, rolls, scoots, crawls, may stand while holding support, cruises, may walk	Falls	Do not use walkers Supervise children's activities Survey home for all accident hazards, sharp objects, table edges, stairs, loose rugs; remove those possible, provide protection of infant for others; use gates
	Drowning	Keep pool or water ponds behind closed and locked gates Never leave children alone in bath Use playpen as a safe area
Pulls and reaches	May pull objects down onto self	Remove tablecloths, dangling cords, appliances that may be in infant's reach
	Burns	Do not drink hot beverages or smoke when holding infant

Continued

TABLE 11-4 *Primary Injury Prevention Related to Developmental Characteristics of Infants—cont'd*

Age and Developmental Characteristics	Potential Injuries	Strategies for Prevention
Developing fine pincer grasp	Electrocution	Insert plastic plugs in electrical outlets
	Swallowing, aspiration, or insertion of foreign body in body orifices	Keep small objects out of reach
	Motor vehicle trauma	Correctly use approved child safety restraint units in cars
	Fire	Install smoke detectors in home and check batteries routinely Install carbon monoxide detectors in home

TABLE 11-5 *Primary Injury Prevention Related to Developmental Characteristics of Toddlers and Preschoolers*

Injuries cause more death and disability than all contagious diseases combined; 36.7% of all deaths in children age 1 to 4 years are injury related; 30.8% of all injury-related deaths are due to motor vehicle trauma, and 27% of injury-related deaths are caused by drowning (National Center for Injury Prevention and Control, 2002a).

Developmenatal Characteristics	Potential Injuries	Strategies for Prevention
Increased fine motor skills: • Can open doors, gates, drawers, bottles, boxes • Increased curiosity	Poisoning	Use childproof caps on medications; keep medicines locked in cabinet out of reach Keep household, garden, and car products locked or out of reach Place Mr. YUK stickers on toxic materials Have telephone number of poison control center readily available
Increased gross motor skills and control: • Able to walk, run, climb, throw objects, ride tricycle • Engages in more active play outdoors, with peers	Falls	Confine play to fenced area Supervise play, especially in areas where climbing occurs Use gates or screens to block off stair; lock windows and doors
	Sunburn	Use sunscreen whenever children are exposed to sun
	Motor vehicle trauma	Use approved child safety restraints Provide tricycle/bicycle helmet Teach children sidewalk, street, and highway safety Never let children cross street alone or play unsupervised on sidewalks near streets
	Contusions and bites	Supervise interactive play of children Teach children how to share, control temper; use adult interaction or distraction to stop harmful behavior or tantrum trauma
Increased curiosity; reaches, stretches, and pulls	Burns, scalding	Turn handles of cooking utensils away from outer edge of stove Use caution in kitchen with children about Adjust hot water thermostat to 120° F Keep matches out of reach

TABLE 11-5 ***Primary Injury Prevention Related to Developmental Characteristics of Toddlers and Preschoolers—cont'd***

Developmenatal Characteristics	Potential Injuries	Strategies for Prevention
Increased curiosity, desire to explore Easily distracted, lacks judgment, unaware of danger of heights, water, fire, toxic materials, electricity, weapons, animals, or strangers	Drowning Other injuries	Fence swimming pools Supervise use of swimming and wading pools Never leave children unattended in a car or alone at home Do not allow children to play near running machinery, mowers, cars, or tools Provide plastic covers for electrical outlets; teach children safety with electrical appliances and cords Do not allow children to use pointed objects in play Do not allow children to run or walk with sticks, lollipops, or other such objects Remove weapons from the house, or keep in locked cabinet, with guns unloaded; store ammunition in separate, locked area Teach children to avoid strange animals, especially ones that are eating
	Abuse	Teach stranger safety
Easily distracted, not always attentive	Choking, aspiration	Do not give foods that can be easily aspirated, such as nuts, gum, popcorn, hotdogs, grapes Supervise mealtimes and snacks

TABLE 11-6 ***Primary Injury Prevention Related to Developmental Characteristics of School-Age Children***

Motor vehicle and pedestrian accidents, burns, drowning, and choking are the most common fatal injuries (National Center for Injury Prevention and Control, 2002a); 42.5% of all deaths in children age 5 to 9 years are injury related; 38.2% of all deaths in children age 10 to 14 years are injury related.

Developmental Characteristics	Potential Injuries	Strategies for Prevention
Motor skills improve; becomes more physically agile and coordinated	Motor vehicle trauma as passenger, pedestrian, or cyclist	Use approved safety restraints in car Provide bicycle helmet and insist on its use Teach importance of seat belt and helmet use Teach bicycle safety Do not allow children to ride tricycles or bicycles with training wheels in the street Prohibit use of all-terrain vehicles Teach pedestrian safety
Is adventurous and more independent, looks for new challenges; may accept dares	Falls	Use knee pads, elbow pads, wrist support, and helmets when skateboarding
	Drowning	Teach to swim; teach rules of water safety: swim in a supervised area with a buddy, check depth before diving, use life preservers in boats
Engages in sports and strenuous exercise Enjoys physical activity Works hard to improve skills Can strain self with excessive activity	Sprains and strains, fractures, and other bodily injuries	Encourage child to be active and stay conditioned; if engaged in organized sports, provide supervised strength training Ensure use of properly fitted equipment for each sport and safe playing area

Continued

TABLE 11-6 ***Primary Injury Prevention Related to Developmental Characteristics of School-Age Children—cont'd***

Developmental Characteristics	Potential Injuries	Strategies for Prevention
Engages in group activities, subject to peer approval Is curious and exploring Easily distracted by environment Accepts explanations and is responsive to reasoning	Burns	Teach children dangers of flammable and toxic materials; how to handle them safely Supervise use of matches Develop a family plan for fires
	Poisoning Choking	Keep hazardous materials out of reach, in locked location; supervise their use Teach first aid, what to do in case of burns, choking, or poisoning Keep poison control center telephone number readily available
	Sunburn	Use sunscreen whenever children will be exposed to sun
	Abuse	Teach child to memorize telephone number and address, use of 911 Warn child never to go with or accept things from strangers

TABLE 11-7 ***Primary Injury Prevention Related to Developmental Characteristics of Adolescents***

In 2000, 5251 adolescents age 15 to 19 died as a result of motor vehicle trauma in the United States, nearly 78% of all unintentional injury deaths among teenagers; 1 in 50 teens is hospitalized for motor vehicle injury every year; sports injuries are the most common nonfatal injury (Hambidge et al, 2002; MacDorman et al, 2002; National Center for Injury Prevention and Control, 2002a).

Developmental Characteristics	Potential Injuries	Strategies for Prevention
Able to legally drive motor vehicles	Motor vehicle trauma as passenger, pedestrian, or cyclist	Use approved safety restraints Take driver's education classes Use bicycle helmet Encourage to learn how to maintain bicycle Teach proper use of all-terrain vehicles Reinforce pedestrian safety Emphasize danger of driving, drinking, and drug use; support peer group efforts to control inappropriate behavior
Increased physical strength and ability	Falls	Use knee pads, elbow pads, wrist support, and helmet when skateboarding Use helmet when cycling
Perception of invulnerability; may take risks	Drowning	Teach to swim Reinforce rules of water safety: swim in a supervised area with a buddy, check depth before diving, use life preservers in boats and when water skiing
More participation in structured sports activities	Sprains, strains, fractures, and other bodily injuries	Encourage adolescent to stay active and conditioned, engage in supervised strength training
Use of complex equipment, tools, weapons	Burns Bodily injury Choking	Teach first aid and cardiopulmonary resuscitation: what to do in the event of injuries, burns, choking, or poisonings Teach gun safety; ask if families of child's friends have weapons in their homes

TABLE 11-7 *Primary Injury Prevention Related to Developmental Characteristics of Adolescents—cont'd*

Developmental Characteristics	Potential Injuries	Strategies for Prevention
Strong peer influence	Poisoning (drug and alcohol abuse)	Teach dangers of drug and alcohol use
Need for independence and peer approval Able to problem solve, reason, and think abstractly		Provide an opportunity to discuss values, perceptions, fears, and needs related to high-risk behaviors; discuss how adolescent deals with anger and violence, as well as how to prevent trauma related to violence; encourage healthy options

BOX 11-2 *Pool Safety Recommendations*

Use four-sided fencing that children cannot climb over. Fences should have gates that close and latch automatically around all pools.
Have *constant* adult supervision while children are playing in water (i.e., no distractions for adult—talking on telephone, mowing lawn, reading, etc.).
Never drink alcohol or allow teenagers to use alcohol while swimming or supervising children.
Do not run, push, shove, or play around pools.
Do not eat or chew gum while in a swimming pool.
Learn to swim. Children age 4 and over should be enrolled in swim classes if available.
Learn cardiopulmonary resuscitation (CPR).
Do not use air-filled swimming aids (e.g., "water wings") in place of life preservers.
Check water depth before entering the pool. American Red Cross recommends 9 feet depth for diving or jumping.
Post CPR instructions and 911 number in the pool area.
Keep lifesaving equipment (e.g., pole, life preserver, rope) in a visible, safe, easily reached spot in the pool area.

From Carl R, Leo H, Cox E: Recreational water safety in Wisconsin, *Wis Med J* 100:43-46, 2001; National Center for Injury Prevention and Control: *Drowning prevention*, Atlanta, 2002b, Centers for Disease Control and Prevention. Available at *www.cdc.gov.ncipc/factsheets/drown.htm* (accessed Dec 5, 2002).

- Advocate for school curricula that teach safety at every grade level.
- Provide health education regarding safety and protection, including first aid and safety and cardiopulmonary resuscitation techniques for both children and adults.
- Teach importance of adult supervision of children's activities.
- Encourage and instruct about proper training for sports in children and adolescents.
- Provide parents with poison control center telephone numbers.

Management of Motor Vehicle Trauma

Motor vehicle trauma continues to be the leading cause of death among children in the United States, with significant mortality and morbidity rates in all age-groups. In 2001, 2197 children 0 to 14 years of age died in motor vehicle crashes, and approximately 267,000 were injured. Alcohol was a contributing factor in 23% of pediatric motor vehicle fatalities. Fifty percent of children killed were passengers in a car of a drinking driver; 104 children were passengers in a car hit by a drinking driver; and 81 children were pedestrians or cyclists hit by an alcohol-impaired driver (National Center for Statistics and Analysis, 2002).

When correctly used, child restraint systems (CRSs) can prevent fatalities from motor vehicle trauma and can reduce the number and severity of injuries to children (National Highway Traffic Safety Administration [NHTSA], 2000; Sweitzer et al, 2002). Nonetheless, many children ride unrestrained or incorrectly restrained. In states with primary seat belt enforcement laws (i.e., drivers can be stopped and cited by law enforcement for failure to wear a seat belt) versus those with secondary enforcement laws (i.e., drivers can be cited if they are stopped for another traffic violation and are not wearing a seat belt), seat belt usage is significantly higher (Davis et al, 2002; Phelan et al, 2002). Understanding how important seat belts are to health also increases usage among college students (Steptoe et al, 2002).

In addition to not using restraints, a number of common errors have been found in the way CRSs are used (Box 11-3). As many as 85% of children have been found to have their restraint improperly positioned or adjusted (Taft, Mikalide, & Taft, 1999). Providers should assess the parents' use of CRSs and correct errors. This may mean accompanying parents to the parking lot to observe how children are placed in the restraint. Use of CRSs should be reviewed at each well-child visit, and children should be involved in the discussion from a very early age. Both parents and children should receive positive reinforcement for proper use of CRSs. Current information from the National Highway Traffic Safety Administration on which restraint system is appropriate for the size, age, and condition of the child should be shared with parents (see Resource Box).

Airbags were developed to prevent serious injury in the event of a motor vehicle accident. Designed to protect a 165-pound, 5-foot, 9-inch-tall man who is not wearing a seatbelt in a 30 mph frontal crash, airbags have caused fatalities in infants and children (Sato, Ohshima, & Kondo, 2002) and can be equally hazardous for small adults. Based on the nature of these fatalities, children younger than 12 years of age should not ride in the front passenger seat if an airbag can be deployed. The optimal position for children is in the center back seat, with infants weighing less than 20 pounds placed in a rear-facing child seat (Table 11-8).

Pedestrian injuries or injuries involving bicycles, skateboards, and automobiles are common in children (Injuries and deaths among children, 2002). The NP should ask children about their pedestrian safety habits during the well-child visit, and educational efforts to instruct children on pedestrian safety and age-appropriate safe use of cycles or boards should be supported. In addition, children of all ages need adult supervision related to motor vehicles. Adult supervision is especially important for younger children who are unaware of the dangers, and the NP should discuss this issue with parents at each well-child visit.

Adolescents, especially new drivers, are often involved in motor vehicle accidents because of their inexperience, immature judgment, or a tendency to take risks. Legislation has been passed in some states, Victoria, Australia, some Canadian provinces, and New Zealand to restrict adolescent driving. "Graduated licensing" legislation requires teenagers to complete driver education classes, restricts their driving to certain times of day, or prevents them from driving with other teenagers in the car. As adolescents gain experience and age, restrictions on driving decline. Successful implementation of the law depends on parents acting as advocates for safety and supporting their adolescents' compliance with the regulations. NPs also can reinforce the message to teenagers that driving is a privilege that requires skill and maturity.

BOX 11-3 *Common Errors in the Use of Child Restraint Systems*

- Seat belt is not tight enough.
- Rear-facing seat is not positioned at a 45-degree angle.
- Harness straps are not snug (infant may be wrapped in a "cocoon" of blankets).
- Harness straps in infant, rear-facing seat are not at or below shoulders of infant.
- Harness straps in child, forward-facing seat are not at or above shoulders of child.
- Retainer clip in child, forward-facing seat is not at armpit level.
- Seat belt is not in locked mode.
- Infant less than 1 year old is placed in forward-facing position.

Management of Firearms Safety

Injuries among children related to firearms have decreased significantly in the recent past, especially among older children (MacDorman et al, 2002). In 2000, 1549 children ages 15 to 19 years in the United States died due to an assault with a gun (a 9.3% decrease from 1999); 897 committed suicide using a firearm (an 8.2% decrease from 1999); and accidental gun fatalities ranged from 0.4% among 1- to 4-year-olds to 1.2% among 10- to 14-year-olds (a 33.3% decrease from 1999) of all unintentional injury deaths. Nonetheless, gun-related injuries still represent a serious health problem and have been identified as a public health issue requiring community-based solutions (Zakocs, Earp, & Runyan, 2001). NPs should work with families and community agencies to decrease gun-related injuries by doing the following:

- Including questions about children's access to guns in primary care assessment data
- Educating parents and children about gun safety
- Supporting parents' efforts to reduce children's exposure to guns (e.g., encouraging parents to ask other parents if they have guns in their households, and not allowing their children to play in unsafe households)
- Advocating at the community level for responsible sale, storage, and use of guns
- Advocating to reduce violence in media

TABLE 11-8 *Vehicle Child Restraint Systems: Recommendations for Use*

Age of Child	Weight of Child	Type of Restraint	Seat Position
Birth-1 yr	Up to at least 20-22 lb	Infant only or rear-facing convertible Harness straps at or below shoulder level	Rear-facing seat only In rear seat
Over 1 yr (toddler)	Over 20 lb; up to 40 lb	Convertible/forward-facing seat Harness straps at or above shoulder level	Forward-facing seat In rear seat
Ages 4-8	Over 40 lb; height less than 4 ft 9 in	Belt positioning booster seat	Forward-facing seat In rear seat
Older children	Height greater than 4 ft 9 in	Belt positioning without booster seat	Forward-facing seat In rear seat until age 12
Children with Special Needs			
Very small infants	Less than 5-7 lb	Infant only; maximum distance from crotch strap to back of seat is 5.5 in; height of harness straps should be less than 10 in If too small for infant seat, use side-lying car bed with restraints	Rear-facing seat or side-lying car bed In rear seat
Children with physical disabilities	Birth to adolescent (systems available for children up to 130 lb)	SpelCast (Snug Seat) is designed for children in spica cast; Snug Seat Car Bed (Snug Seat) for infants up to 21 lb who cannot ride seated semi-upright; a number of systems are designed for older, heavier children (National Highway Traffic Safety Administration, Resource Box)	

NURSING DIAGNOSES RELATED TO HEALTH PERCEPTION AND HEALTH MANAGEMENT: *Functional Health Pattern*

Diagnoses relate to concepts of therapeutic regimen management, health-seeking behaviors, health maintenance, and home maintenance:

- Decisional conflict
- Deficient knowledge (specify)
- Effective therapeutic regimen management
- Ineffective therapeutic regimen management
  - Ineffective family therapeutic regimen management
  - Ineffective community therapeutic regimen management
- Ineffective health maintenance
- Ineffective home maintenance management
- Health-seeking behaviors (specify area of concern)
- Impaired adjustment
- Noncompliance
- Risk for injury
- Self-care deficits—bathing, dressing/grooming, feeding, toileting

From North American Nursing Diagnosis Association: *NANDA nursing diagnoses: definitions and classification 2001-2002*, Philadelphia, 2001, The Association.

RESOURCE BOX

Health Perception and Management

HEALTH PERCEPTION AND HEALTH MANAGEMENT

Bright Futures
1-202-784-9556
www.brightfutures.org
Materials for health professionals on healthy child assessment and health promotion

Health Perception and Management in Nursing Care to Children
www.accd.edu/sac/nursing/r2201/plinks1.html
Links to several parent-child focused resources

Kids Health (Nemours Foundation)
http://kidshealth.org
Patient and parent educational information

GENERAL SAFETY RESOURCES

National SAFE KIDS Campaign
1-202-662-0600
www.safekids.org

Children's Safety Network (funded by U.S. Maternal and Child Health Bureau)
1-888-434-4624
www.childrenssafetynetwork.org

Consumer Products Safety Commission
1-800-638-2772
www.info@cpsc.gov

National Program for Playground Safety (funded by CDC)
1-800-554-7529
www.uni.edu/playground

WATER SAFETY

American Red Cross
www.redcross.org/services/hss/tips/healthtips/safetywater.html

United States Lifesaving Association (USLA)
www.usla.org

FIREARMS

Handgun Control and Center to Prevent Handgun Violence
www.handguncontrol.org
www.cphv.org
Two groups lobbying and educating to establish gun regulations

Join Together Online
www.jointogether.org
Educational materials, funding advice

Violence Policy Center
www.vpc.org
Legislation and litigation activities

American Academy of Pediatrics: Firearm Injury Prevention Training Project
www.aap.org/advocacy/firearms.htm

Common Sense about Kids and Guns
www.kidsandguns.org

RESOURCES FOR PATIENTS

Craig-Shashko AL, Katcher ML: Firearm injury prevention: Internet resources for the health care provider, *Wis Med J* 100:26-31, 2001.

Annotated bibliography that lists a variety of public health and advocacy websites related to firearm injury prevention

MOTOR VEHICLE SAFETY

National Highway and Transportation Safety Administration
www.nhtsa.dot.gov/people/injury/childps
Statistics on injuries; guidelines for use of restraint systems: Proper Child Safety Seat Use Chart

CHILD RESTRAINT SYSTEMS

Snug Seat
www.snugseat.com
Side-facing car bed for infants who cannot sit upright; restraint for child in spica cast, both rear and forward facing; car seats for larger children with special needs

Car seats for larger children with special needs
www.adaptivemall.com
Produced by Columbia, Sammons Preston, and Snug Seat

REFERENCES

American Academy of Pediatrics: *Red book*, ed 25, Elk Grove Village, IL, 2000, American Academy of Pediatrics.

American Academy of Pediatrics Committee on Injury and Poison Prevention and Committee on Community Health Services: Prevention of agricultural injuries among children and adolescents, *Pediatrics* 108:1016-1019, 2001.

American Academy of Pediatrics Committee on Practice and Ambulatory Medicine: Recommendations for preventive pediatric health care, *Pediatrics* 105:645, 2001.

American Medical Association: *Guidelines for adolescent preventive services (GAPS): recommendations monograph*, Chicago, 1997, American Medical Association.

Behrman RE, Kliegman RM, Jenson HB, editors: *Nelson textbook of pediatrics*, ed 17, Philadelphia, 2004, WB Saunders.

Carl R, Leo H, Cox E: Recreational water safety in Wisconsin, *Wis Med J* 100:43-46, 2001.

Centers for Disease Control and Prevention, Office on Smoking and Health and Division of Adolescent and School Health, National Center for Chronic Disease Prevention and Health Promotion: Trends in cigarette smoking among high school students—United States, 1991-2001, *MMWR* 51:409-412, 2002.

Davis JW et al: Motor vehicle restraints: primary versus secondary enforcement and ethnicity, *J Trauma* 52:225-228, 2002.

Dunn ME et al: Moderators of stress in parents of children with autism, *Community Ment Health J* 37:39-52, 2001.

Ellickson PL, Tucker JS, Klein DJ: High-risk behaviors associated with early smoking: results from a 5-year follow-up, *J Adolesc Health* 28:465-473, 2001.

Elster A, Kuznets N: *AMA guidelines for adolescent preventive services (GAPS)*, Baltimore, 1994, Williams & Wilkins.

Engstrom I: Inflammatory bowel disease in children and adolescents: mental health and family functioning, *J Pediatr Gastroenterol Nutr* 28:S28-S33, 1999.

Farrelly MC et al: Getting to the truth: evaluating national tobacco countermarketing campaigns, *Am J Public Health* 92:901-907, 2002.

Federal Trade Commission: *Cigarette report for 1999*, Washington, DC, 2001, Federal Trade Commission.

Fleming CB et al: Family processes for children in early elementary school as predictors of smoking initiation, *J Adolesc Health* 30:184-189, 2002.

Gerberich SG et al: Injuries among children and youth in farm households: Regional Rural Injury Study—I, *Inj Prev* 7:117-122, 2001.

Halloran EC et al: The relationship between aggression in children and locus of control beliefs, *J Genet Psychol* 160:5-21, 1999.

Hambidge SJ et al: Epidemiology of pediatric injury-related primary care office visits in the United States, *Pediatrics* 109:559-565, 2002.

Higgins S: Smoking in pregnancy, *Curr Opin Obstet Gynecol* 14:145-151, 2002.

Holt CL, Clark EM, Kreuter MW: Weight locus of control and weight-related attitudes and behaviors in an overweight population, *Addict Behav* 26:329-340, 2001.

Howard BJ: Working with difficult families. Paper presented at the 1998 Pediatric Update, Portland, OR, Nov 1998.

Injuries and deaths among children left unattended in or around motor vehicles—United States, July 2000-June 2001, *MMWR* 51:570-572, 2002.

Johnson CC et al: Fifth through eighth grade longitudinal predictors of tobacco use among a racially diverse cohort: CATCH, *J Sch Health* 72:58-64, 2002.

Kleinman A, Eisenberg L, Good B: Culture, illness and care: clinical lessons from anthropologic and cross-cultural research, *Ann Intern Med* 88:251-258, 1978.

MacDorman MF et al: Annual summary of vital statistics—2001, *Pediatrics* 110:1037-1052, 2002.

Marshall RS: Interpretation in doctor-patient interviews: a sociolinguistic analysis, *Culture Med Psychiatry* 12:201-218, 1988.

Maternal and Child Health Bureau, Health Resources and Services Administration: *Bright Futures: guidelines for health supervision of infants, children, and adolescents*, ed 2, revised, Arlington, VA, 2002, National Center for Education in Maternal and Child Health.

National Center for Injury Prevention and Control: *Ten leading causes of death, United States 2000, all races, both sexes*, Atlanta, 2002a, Centers for Disease Control and Prevention. Available at *http://webapp.cdc.gov/cgi-bin/broker.exe* (accessed Dec 8, 2002).

National Center for Injury Prevention and Control: *Drowning prevention*, Atlanta, 2002b, Centers for Disease Control and Prevention. Available at *www.cdc.gov.ncipc/factsheets/drown.htm* (accessed Dec 5, 2002).

National Center for Statistics and Analysis: Traffic safety facts 2001—children, 2002. Available at *www.nhtsa.dot.gov* (accessed Nov 27, 2002).

National Highway Traffic Safety Administration: *Traffic safety facts 2000: occupant protection*, Washington, DC, 2000, National Highway Traffic Safety Administration.

North American Nursing Diagnosis Association: NANDA nursing diagnoses: definitions and classification 2001-2002, Philadelphia, 2001, North American Nursing Diagnosis Association.

O'Byrne KK, Haddock CK, Poston WS: Parenting style and adolescent smoking, *J Adolesc Health* 30:418-425, 2002.

Phelan KJ et al: Pediatric motor vehicle related injuries in the Navajo Nation: the impact of the 1988 child occupant restraint laws, *Inj Prev* 8:216-220, 2002.

Rotter JB: Generalized expectancies for internal versus external control of reinforcement, *Psychol Monogr* 80:1-25, 1966.

Sargent JD et al: Effect of seeing tobacco use in films on trying smoking among adolescents: cross sectional study, *BMJ* 323:1-6, 2001.

Sato Y, Ohshima T, Kondo T: Air bag injuries—a literature review in consideration of demands in forensic autopsies, *Forensic Sci Int* 128:162-167, 2002.

Smith MS, Wallston KA, Smith CA: The development and validation of the perceived health competence scale, *Health Educ Res* 10:51-64, 1995.

Steptoe A, Wardle J: Locus of control and health behaviour revisited: a multivariate analysis of young adults from 18 countries, *Br J Psychol* 92 (pt 4):659-672, 2001.

Steptoe A et al: Seatbelt use, attitudes, and changes in legislation: an international study, *Am J Prev Med* 23:254-259, 2002.

Sweitzer RE et al: Children in motor vehicle collisions: analysis of injury by restraint use and seat location, *J Forensic Sci* 47:1049-1054, 2002.

Taft CH, Mikalide AD, Taft AR: *Child passengers at risk in America: a national study of car seat misuse*, Washington, DC, 1999, National SAFE KIDS Campaign.

US Preventive Services Task Force: *Guide to clinical preventive services*, ed 2, ed 3, McClean, VA, 2002, International Medical Publishing.

VanDyke EM, Riesenberg LA: Effectiveness of a school-based intervention at changing preadolescents' tobacco use and attitudes, *J Sch Health* 72:221-225, 2002.

Wallston BS et al: Development and validation of the health locus of control (HLC) scale, *J Consult Clin Psych* 44:580-585, 1976.

Wallston KA, Wallston BS, DeVellis R: Development of multidimensional health locus of control (MHLC) scales, *Health Education Monogr* 6:160-170, 1978.

Zakocs RC, Earp JA, Runyan CW: State gun control advocacy tactics and resources, *Am J Prev Med* 20:251-257, 2001.

12 Nutrition

Ardys M. Dunn

OVERVIEW

Definition of Nutrition Pattern

Nutrition is a complex science that includes the study of how food, nutrients, and other substances found in foods interact with the body to foster growth and health or contribute to disease. Nutrition examines the processes by which organisms ingest, digest, absorb, transport, utilize, and excrete food substances. In addition, knowledge of nutrition requires an understanding of social, economic, cultural, and psychologic implications of food and eating. Adequate nutrition is essential for normal growth and development of children and plays a critical role in maintenance and restoration of good health. Nutrition affects children's ability to interact with their environment. The effect of nourishment on children's behavior can be immediate and dramatic, as with the hungry, irritable infant who eagerly nurses and falls asleep; or nutrition can have long-range implications, as in the relationship between childhood cholesterol levels and adult coronary heart disease.

Significance for Nurse Practitioner Practice

The primary roles of the nurse practitioner (NP) in relation to nutrition are to assess accurately the nutritional status of children, to determine parents' and children's knowledge related to nutrition, to identify ways in which food is managed and used, and to ensure that children are adequately nourished. The NP's interventions, aimed at helping children and families meet nutritional requirements and preventing problems related to poor nutrition, are based on certain assumptions, including the following:

- Children's nutritional needs vary as they grow.
- Children's nutritional needs are influenced by their state of health.
- A wide range of food choices and feeding behaviors are used to meet nutritional needs.
- Recommended dietary allowances are guidelines only.
- Parents and other caregivers are responsible for providing food choices that are nutritionally adequate and for establishing healthy eating patterns; to do so, they must be well informed.
- The NP is a source of information regarding nutrition, feeding patterns, and health.
- The NP works with a network of specialists (e.g., registered dietitians) to manage children's nutrition.

Standards for Preventive Care

A number of recommendations have been developed related to nutrition. *Bright Futures in Practice: Nutrition* (Story, Holt, & Sofka, 2002) provides an overview of nutritional guidelines, discussion of issues and concerns related to pediatric nutrition, and tools for providers to assess and manage nutrition in children. The U.S. Preventive Services Task Force (1996) recommends that practitioners counsel parents about the nutritional requirements of infancy and childhood, and the American Medical Association notes that "all adolescents should receive health guidance annually about dietary habits, including the benefits of a healthy diet and ways to achieve a healthy diet and safe weight management" (Elster & Kuznets, 1994). Nutrition recommendations for children emphasize that

- Breast milk is the best food for infants
- Children's diets should include a wide variety of foods
- Iron-rich foods are essential, especially for infants and adolescents
- Fat intake, particularly saturated fats and cholesterol, should be limited
- Calories and carbohydrates should be appropriate to metabolic needs
- Sugar intake should be limited
- Extra calcium, iron, and folic acid are important nutrients in adolescent girls' diets
- Children's diets should include adequate fiber and sodium

NORMAL PATTERNS OF NUTRITION

General Considerations

Energy

Energy intake, measured in kilocalories, should meet the basic needs of body metabolism, growth, and activity. Resting energy expenditure (REE), a concept used interchangeably with basal metabolic rate (BMR), is the largest source of energy consumption in the body. Growth, a second source of energy consumption, is greatest in infancy and again during adolescence. Finally, activity, exercise, and other metabolic demands increase the level of calories needed to maintain good health. The body meets these energy demands, or estimated energy requirements (EER), by using stored energy sources or by consuming necessary nutrients and calories. EER for healthy children can vary significantly by age (Table 12-1).

Macronutrients (protein, carbohydrates, and fats) and alcohol provide the calories necessary to meet the body's energy needs. There is wide latitude on how much of each macronutrient is necessary for optimal nutrition; the body will utilize whichever is present for its energy needs. Of critical importance is whether basic energy needs are met and whether other essential nutrients (e.g., vitamins, minerals), as well as calories, are consumed. Table 12-2 presents recommended macronutrient intake based on age for children who are of average height, weight, and physical activity level. Macronutrient intake is expressed in recommended grams per day and in the form of "acceptable macronutrient distribution range" (AMDR). AMDR is the percent of the total daily energy intake recommended for that macronutrient and is considered to be a range that provides adequate overall nutrition while minimizing risks for chronic disease associated with an excess or deficit of the macronutrient (Food and Nutrition Board, Institute of Medicine, 2002).

Energy needs are influenced by a number of variables. Illness can affect metabolism and increase the body's need for energy. The growth demands of infancy and puberty and

TABLE 12-1 ***Daily Estimated Energy Requirements (EER) of Infants, Children, and Adolescents: Calculations (EER = Total Energy Expenditure [TEE] + Energy Deposition)***

Age	Formula
0-3 mo	EER = (89 × weight of infant [kg] − 100) + 175 (kcal for energy deposition)
4-6 mo	EER = (89 × weight of infant [kg] − 100) + 56 (kcal for energy deposition)
7-12 mo	EER = (89 × weight of infant [kg] − 100) + 22 (kcal for energy deposition)
13-35 mo	EER = (89 × weight of child [kg] − 100) + 20 (kcal for energy deposition)
Boys 3-8 yr	EER = 88.5 − (61.9 × age [yr]) + (PA × [26.7 × weight (kg) + 903 × height (m)]) + 20 (kcal for energy deposition)
Girls 3-8 yr	EER = 135.3 − (30.8 × age [yr]) + (PA × [10.0 × weight (kg) + 934 × height (m)]) + 20 (kcal for energy deposition)
Boys 9-18 yr	EER = 88.5 − (61.9 × age [yr]) + (PA × [26.7 × weight (kg) + 903 × height (m)]) + 25 (kcal for energy deposition)
Girls 9-18 yr	EER = 135.3 − (30.8 × age [yr]) + (PA × [10.0 × weight (kg) + 934 × height (m)]) + 25 (kcal for energy deposition)

Physical activity coefficient (PA) varies by gender, age, and body weight as follows:

Physical Activity Level Category (see below)	Physical Activity Coefficient Boys, 3-19 yr	Physical Activity Coefficient Girls, 3-19 yr
Sedentary	1.0	1.0
Low active	1.13	1.16
Active	1.26	1.31
Very active	1.42	1.56

Physical Activity Level (PAL) Category	Walking Equivalence (mi/day* at 2-4 mph) for *Heavy weight (120 kg)*	*Middle weight (70 kg)*	*Light weight (44 kg)*
Sedentary	None	None	None
Low active	1.5	2.2	2.9
Active	3.0-5.3	4.4-7.3	5.8-9.9
Very active	7.5-17.0	10.3-23.0	14.0-31.0

*The low, middle, and high mi/day values apply for relatively heavy-weight (120 kg), mid-weight (70 kg), and light-weight (44 kg) individuals, respectively.

TABLE 12-2 ***Recommended Daily Allowance or Adequate Intake* of Nutrient by Age, for Children of Average Height, Weight, and Physical Activity Level***

	Age								
Nutrient	**0-6 mo**	**7-12 mo**	**1-3 yr**	**4-8 yr**	**Boys 9-13 yr**	**Boys 14-18 yr**	**Girls 9-13 yr**	**Girls 14-18 yr**	**Pregnant <18 yr**
Protein, g	9.1*	13.5	13	19	34	52	34	46	71
Protein (AMDR)	ND	ND	5-20	10-30	10-30	10-30	10-30	10-30	10-35
Carbohydrates, g	60*	95*	130	130	130	130	130	130	175
Carbohydrates (AMDR)	ND	ND	45-65	45-65	45-65	45-65	45-65	45-65	45-65
Fats, total, g	31*	30*	—	—	—	—	—	—	—
Fats, polyunsaturated fatty acids (linoleic acid), g	4.4*	4.6*	7*	10*	12*	16*	10*	11*	13*
Fats, total (AMDR)			30-40	25-35	25-35	25-35	25-35	25-35	20-35
Vitamin A (RAE) μg	400*	500*	300	400	600	900	600	700	750
Thiamin (B_1), mg	0.2*	0.3*	0.5	0.6	0.9	1.2	0.9	1.0	1.4
Riboflavin (B_2), mg	0.3*	0.4*	0.5	0.6	0.9	1.3	0.9	1.0	1.4
Niacin (NE), mg	2*	4*	6	8	12	16	12	14	18
Pyridoxine (B_6), mg	0.1*	0.3*	0.5	0.6	1.0	1.3	1.0	1.2	1.9
Folate, μg	65*	80*	150	200	300	400	300	400	600
Vitamin B_{12}, μg	0.4*	0.5*	0.9	1.2	1.8	2.4	1.8	2.4	2.6
Vitamin C, mg	40*	50*	15	25	45	75	45	65	80
Vitamin D, μg	5*	5*	5*	5*	5*	5*	5*	5*	5*
Vitamin E, mg	4*	5*	6	7	11	15	11	15	15
Vitamin K, μg	2.0*	2.5*	30*	55*	60*	75*	60*	75*	75*
Calcium, mg	210*	270*	500*	800*	1300*	1300*	1300*	1300*	1300*
Fluoride, mg†	0.01*	0.5*	0.7*	1*	2*	3*	2*	3*	3*
Iron, mg	0.27*	11	7	10	8	11	8	15	27
Zinc, mg	2*	3	3	5	8	11	8	9	12

Adapted from Food and Nutrition Board, Institute of Medicine: *Dietary reference intakes for energy, carbohydrates, fiber, fat, fatty acids, cholesterol, protein, and amino acids (macronutrients),* Washington, DC, 2002, Institute of Medicine.
*Adequate intake.
†Fluoride supplement is not necessary if the water supply contains ≥0.6 parts per million fluoridation.
AMDR, Acceptable macronutrient distribution range; ND, not deteminable; *RAE,* retinol activity equivalents. To calculate RAE from RE (retinol equivalent) of provitamin A carotenoids in foods, divide the RE by 2. For preformed vitamin A in foods or supplements or for provitamin A carotenoids in supplements, 1 RE = 1 RAE.

variations in activity levels require higher caloric intake. Energy needs vary from one individual to another; an athletic adolescent girl, for example, needs more calories than a teenage boy who has a sedentary lifestyle. Healthy individuals maintain a balance between the body's energy demands and caloric intake. Currently, many children have limited physical activity and are at risk for excess weight gain. These children should be encouraged to engage in regular physical exercise to balance energy use and caloric intake.

Water and Electrolytes

Water. Water is the primary component of body tissue, and maintaining fluid balance is essential to good health. Because of the wide variation of healthful intake and output, there is no specific recommended daily requirement for water (Manz, Wentz, & Sichert-Hellert, 2002). Infants present special concerns. Factors such as their large skin surface per unit of body weight, the immaturity of their renal system to process solutes, their high daily water turnover (up to 15% of body weight), and their inability to express thirst make them uniquely susceptible to rapid variations in water balance.

Water loss is influenced also by illness, activity level, altitude, and temperature and dryness of ambient air. If a child is vomiting and has diarrhea, water loss can be significant, leading to dehydration and other complications.

A child who exercises strenuously, especially in a warm, dry environment, requires additional water intake. When more than 10% of body weight is lost without replacement, dehydration can become life threatening.

Sodium. Sodium functions primarily to regulate extracellular fluid volume. It also regulates osmolarity, acid-base balance, and the membrane potential of cells and is involved in the cell membrane transport pump, exchanging with potassium in intracellular fluid. Sodium loss occurs with vomiting, diarrhea, and perspiration.

Sodium requirements vary with the rate of extracellular fluid expansion, which is most rapid in infants and very young children. With the older child, it is not necessary to add sodium to the diet, even for children who exercise and perspire heavily. In fact, the typical North American diet far exceeds minimum requirements for sodium intake, with most sodium coming from salt added during processing and manufacturing of foods.

Potassium. Potassium serves to maintain intracellular homeostasis and contributes to muscle contractility and transmission of nerve impulses. Severe potassium deficit (hypokalemia) can lead to cardiac arrhythmias and death. Excessive potassium (hyperkalemia) can cause cardiac arrest. The urinary and gastrointestinal systems function to regulate potassium levels, and extreme imbalances are almost always due to disease processes or medication rather than to dietary factors. Potassium requirements are related to increases in lean body mass and are proportionally higher during the rapid growth of infancy and adolescence than during middle childhood. Fruits, vegetables, and fresh meat have high potassium content.

Chloride. Chloride functions in conjunction with sodium to maintain fluid and electrolyte balance. Loss of chloride occurs through the same routes as sodium loss: vomiting, diarrhea, and perspiration. The major source of chloride is salt (NaCl or KCl) added to foods during processing. There is no recommended daily allowance for chloride, but adequate amounts are ingested with a normal diet.

Protein

Protein is a fundamental component of all body cells. Dietary protein is broken down into amino acids, which are necessary for the synthesis of body cell protein and nitrogen-containing compounds and are required in some enzyme and hormone activity, cell transport, and tissue growth and development. Nine amino acids, called "indispensable" or essential amino acids, are not synthesized by the body and must be provided for in the diet. The body requires sufficient caloric intake to use dietary protein for protein synthesis. Depending on their age, children should receive approximately 5% to 30% of daily calories from proteins (see Table 12-2).

Protein and amino acid deficiencies rarely appear alone but follow other dietary deficits. Extreme stress and disease processes can deplete nitrogen, contributing to tissue wasting and creating an increased demand for protein. Growth needs of the premature infant require higher levels of protein intake than those of infants born at term. The demand for protein is not generally increased with normal activity except as needed to build additional muscle tissue during body conditioning or during some illnesses.

Carbohydrates

Carbohydrates are the body's major dietary source of energy. It is recommended that more than half (45% to 65%) of children's body energy requirements be supplied by carbohydrates (Food and Nutrition Board, Institute of Medicine, 2002). In addition to providing energy, adequate carbohydrate intake is essential to facilitate protein synthesis. Carbohydrates are either simple sugars (the monosaccharides and disaccharides of sucrose, fructose, and lactose found in fruits, vegetables, milk, and prepared sweets) or complex carbohydrates (starches found in cereal grains, potatoes, legumes, and other vegetables). Most dietary carbohydrates should be in the complex form. If dietary carbohydrates are extremely limited or absent (e.g., with a ketogenic diet used to manage intractable seizures of epilepsy; see Chapter 28), the body lipolyzes stored triglycerides, oxidizes fatty acids, and breaks down dietary and tissue protein. This process contributes to accumulation of ketone bodies.

Fats

Lipids, fats, and fatty acids are used by the body to provide energy, to facilitate absorption of the fat-soluble vitamins (A, D, E, and K), and to maintain integrity of cell membranes and myelin. Essential fatty acids, all of which are found in most vegetable oils, are not produced by the body and must be included in the diet.

Major pediatric organizations recommend that there be no restrictions on fat intake for children less than 2 years of age; that children over 2 years of age gradually adopt a diet of 30% (maximum) and 20% (minimum) of total calories from fats, with less than 10% of total calories in the form of saturated fat; and that daily diets have no more than 300 mg of cholesterol (American Academy of Pediatrics Committee on Nutrition, 1998; Joint Working Group of the Canadian Paediatric Society [CPS] and Health Canada, 2001). The Food and Nutrition Board of the Institute of Medicine (IOM) recommends that children 3 and under receive 30% to 40% of total calories from fats; children over 3 should have a diet in which 25% to 35% of total calories come from fats. Saturated fats, trans-fatty acids, and cholesterol in the diet are unnecessary and their intake should be minimized, with zero intake of trans-fatty acids (Food and Nutrition Board, IOM, 2002). Children should be encouraged to eat a variety of foods, including many complex carbohydrates, and to engage in vigorous physical activity.

In some cases, excessively restricted fat and caloric intakes have contributed to loss of essential nutrients and resulted in growth failure (Lifshitz & Tarim, 1996). However, low-fat diets for children (20% to 28% of energy from fat), when properly supervised to ensure that there is an adequate intake of nonfat nutrients, can contribute to healthful growth (Clauss & Kwiterovich, 2002; Rask-Nissila et al, 2002).

It appears that a moderate approach to fat restriction and an emphasis on avoiding trans-fatty acids and saturated fats while including unsaturated fats, especially omega-3 fatty acids, in the diet is in order. Lower-fat diets (approximately 28% fat as a source of energy) in children age 8 to 10 years (Van Horn et al, 2003) and in children between 7 and 36 months who also had high vitamin and nutrient intake (Niinikoski et al, 1997) have been shown to reduce cholesterol levels safely without affecting normal growth and development. The NP should strive for balance when counseling parents about fat in their children's diets. A diet with about 30% of calories from fat easily provides for energy and growth needs; below 20% total fat, the child can be at nutritional risk.

Vitamins

A number of fat-soluble and water-soluble vitamins are essential for good health. Table 12-2 lists recommendations for daily vitamin intake. Table 12-3 identifies specific metabolic functions, dietary sources, and signs of deficiency or excessive intake of these vitamins.

Fat-Soluble Vitamins. Several characteristics of the fat-soluble vitamins (A, D, E, and K) have implications for dietary assessment and management:

- They can be stored for long periods of time in body tissues. As a result, temporary dietary deficiencies may not affect the body's growth and development. If stores are depleted and nutritional intake is inadequate, signs of vitamin deficiency appear. If intake is excessive, as can occur with supplementation, toxic effects can appear.
- They are absorbed in the intestines along with fats and lipids in foods. Low-fat diets, as well as increased intestinal motility or malabsorption syndromes, may put individuals at risk for vitamin deficiency.
- They are fairly stable when heated, as in cooking. Food preparation does not destroy fat-soluble vitamins as readily as water-soluble vitamins.
- They require bile for absorption. Conditions that compromise the hepatobiliary system put the individual at risk for decreased vitamin absorption.
- They do not contain nitrogen and do not act as coenzymes in cellular metabolism of nutrients.

Water-Soluble Vitamins. Unlike fat-soluble vitamins, water-soluble vitamins (C and B complexes) are stored in very small amounts in the body. If water-soluble vitamin intake is above that needed by the body, absorption (primarily in the jejunum) decreases and excess vitamins are excreted. As a result, daily intake of water-soluble vitamins is necessary and there is little risk of toxicity from large doses. The B vitamins also contain nitrogen and serve as essential coenzymes in the body's metabolism of nutrients.

Minerals and Elements

Major minerals are defined as those present in the body in amounts greater than 5 g. Calcium, magnesium, and phosphorus are considered major minerals. Dietary reference intakes (DRI) have been set for boron, calcium, chromium, copper, fluoride, iodine, iron, magnesium, manganese, molybdenum, nickel, phosphorus, selenium, silicon, vanadium, and zinc (Food and Nutrition Board, IOM, 2002). Table 12-2 identifies recommended allowances for calcium, fluoride, iron, and zinc.

Peak bone density is directly related to calcium intake during the years of bone mineralization. Most mineralization takes place by the time an individual is 20 years old, but recent research indicates that calcification can continue for several years. To ensure maximum peak bone density, dietary calcium needs remain high until about 25 years of age. Breastfed infants or those who are fed an approved infant formula receive sufficient calcium and should not be given a supplement.

Minerals and essential trace elements, their functions, dietary sources, and signs of deficiency or excess are presented in Table 12-4. Foods rich in iron are listed in Table 12-5.

Use of Vitamin and Mineral Supplements

National surveys reveal that many U.S. children have suboptimal nutrient intakes. A national sample of more than 3000 children, ages 2 to 19 years, concluded that less than 1% meet all of the national standards for recommended dietary intake. Sixteen percent met none of the recommendations (Munoz et al, 1997). School-age children, especially girls, are at high risk for vitamin and mineral deficits (Suitor & Gleason, 2002).

Recommended daily requirements for most foods should be evaluated over a 3-day period (i.e., children do not need to eat a recommended dietary allowance [RDA] for all foods

Text continued on p. 222

TABLE 12-3 *Vitamins: Function, Dietary Sources, Interactions, Deficiency, and Excess*

Vitamin	Function	Dietary Sources	Interactions Affecting Absorption or Utilization	Signs of Deficit	Signs of Excess
Fat-Soluble Vitamins					
Vitamin A	Vision, cellular differentiation and growth, reproductive and immune system function	Liver, fish liver oils, fortified milk, eggs, carrots, dark-green leafy vegetables	Absorption and utilization are facilitated by dietary fat, protein, and vitamin E Absorption of vitamin A is hindered by lack of protein, iron, or zinc	Anorexia, dry skin, keratinization of epithelial cells of respiratory tract, night blindness, corneal lesions, increased susceptibility to infections	Headache, vomiting, double vision, hair loss, dry mucous membrane, peeling skin, liver damage Toxic at 10 times the RDA No toxicity with excessive intake of carotenoids (e.g., carrots)
Vitamin D	Bone growth and development; regulates intestinal absorption of calcium and phosphorus	Sunlight, artificial ultraviolet light, fortified food products, especially milk	Utilization compromised in patients with renal failure Increased exposure to sunlight increases intake Darker skin and aging skin inhibit synthesis	Inadequate bone mineralization, rickets or skeletal malformations, delayed dentition	Anorexia, nausea, vomiting, diarrhea, weakness, hypercalcemia, hypercalciuria, calcium deposits in soft tissue, permanent renal or cardiovascular damage
Vitamin E	Antioxidant, traps free radicals, prevents oxidation of polyunsaturated fats	Vegetable oils, margarine, nuts, wheat germ, green leafy vegetables	Low serum levels have been associated with prematurity and congenital defects of the hepatobiliary system (e.g., cystic fibrosis, biliary atresia)	Macrocytic anemia and dermatitis in infants; neurologic defects in severe malabsorption	Unknown, if any
Vitamin K	Forms proteins that regulate blood clotting	Green leafy vegetables, milk, dairy products, liver	Inhibited by long-term antibiotic use, hyperalimentation, chronic biliary obstruction, or lipid malabsorption syndromes	Defective coagulation of blood, hemorrhages, liver injury	Vitamin K–responsive hemorrhagic condition, especially if patient is being treated with anticoagulants
Water-Soluble Vitamins					
Vitamin C	Essential for collagen formation and function; promotes growth and tissue repair; enhances iron absorption; improves wound healing	Vegetables and fruits, especially citrus fruits, broccoli, collard greens, spinach, tomatoes, potatoes, strawberries, peppers	Vitamin C is easily lost in food storage and preparation owing to exposure to heat, oxygen, and water Exposure to cigarette smoke increases vitamin C requirement	Scurvy, cracked lips, bleeding gums, slow wound healing, easy bruising	Unknown; excessive vitamin is excreted in urine

Thiamine (vitamin B_1)	Necessary for carbohydrate metabolism; promotes normal appetite and digestion	Whole grains, brewer's yeast, legumes, seeds and nuts, organ meats, lean cuts of pork	Availability inhibited by presence of thiaminase (found in raw fish); alcohol contributes to thiamine deficiency	Beriberi: muscle weakness, ataxia, confusion, anorexia, tachycardia, heart failure in infants	None by oral intake; excess excreted in urine
Riboflavin (vitamin B_2)	Necessary for oxidation-reduction reactions, essential for function of vitamin B_6 and niacin; helps maintain integrity of skin, tongue, and lips	Dairy products, meat, poultry, fish; enriched or fortified grains, cereals, and breads; green vegetables such as broccoli, spinach, asparagus, turnip greens	Positive nitrogen balance contributes to function of riboflavin	Oral-buccal cavity lesions, generalized seborrheic dermatitis, scrotal and vulval skin changes, normocytic anemia, dimness of vision	None known
Niacin	Essential for energy metabolism, glycolysis, fatty acids; maintains nervous system, integrity of skin, mouth, tongue	Meats, fortified grains, legumes Milk, eggs, and meats contain tryptophan	Requires riboflavin for absorption and utilization Grains treated with lime have more biologically available niacin Dietary tryptophan converts to niacin	Pellagra: dermatitis, diarrhea, inflammation of mucous membranes, indigestion	No known toxicity with dietary doses; heat rush flushing with excessive doses
Vitamin B_6 (pyridoxine)	Essential for metabolism of amino acids, lipids, nucleic acids, and glycogen	Chicken, fish, kidney, liver, pork, red meat, eggs, unrefined rice, soybeans, oats, whole wheat, peanuts, walnuts	Riboflavin enhances function Increased protein intake increases requirements for vitamin B_6 Processing of foods destroys vitamin B_6	Seen in combination with other B-complex vitamin deficiencies; dermatitis, anemia, convulsions, neurologic symptoms, and abdominal distress in infants	Ataxia, sensory neuropathy when taken in gram quantities for months or years
Folate (folacin)	Essential for amino acid metabolism and nucleic acid synthesis; red blood cell formation	Liver, yeast, dark-green leafy vegetables, legumes, fruits, oranges, brewer's yeast, milk	Only about 25% of folate in foods is directly bioavailable for absorption in intestine; more efficiently absorbed if serum levels are low Boiling milk destroys about 50% of folate present	Poor growth, megaloblastic anemia in severe cases; macrocytic anemia, glossitis, gastrointestinal disturbances; increased risk of neural tube defects in infants of folate-deficient mothers	None known in dietary doses; excessive folic acid supplementation may inhibit uptake of phenytoin and contribute to seizures in epileptic cases controlled by phenytoin
Vitamin B_{12}	Essential for metabolism, adequate red blood cell formation	Animal products: meat, eggs, and milk; shellfish	Absorbed in ileum; intrinsic factor mediated In strict vegetarians, the vitamin excreted in the bile is reabsorbed	Megaloblastic anemia, neurologic symptoms, sore tongue, weakness	None known

RDA, Recommended dietary allowance.

TABLE 12-4 ***Minerals and Trace Elements: Function, Dietary Sources, Interactions, Deficiency, and Excess***

	Function	Dietary Sources	Interactions Affecting Absorption or Utilization	Signs of Deficit	Signs of Excess*
Minerals					
Calcium	Development of bone tissue; vital role in nerve conduction, membrane permeability, blood clotting, and muscle contraction	Milk and milk products, green leafy vegetables, broccoli, kale, and collards, soft bones of fish, foods processed or fortified with calcium	Absorption enhanced in the presence of vitamin D, adequate protein intake, during periods of rapid growth, and if dietary intake of calcium is low	Decreased bone strength, increased risk for fractures	Constipation, increased risk for urinary stone formation; risk for decreased renal function
Phosphorus	Essential for bone integrity and general metabolism; provides essential energy during the metabolic process	Almost all foods, especially meat, poultry, fish, milk, cereal grains; food additives in processed foods	Aluminum hydroxide in antacids prevents absorption	Bone loss, weakness, malaise, anorexia, and pain	None known
Magnesium	Activates enzymes, facilitates cell metabolism, maintains electrical potential of cell membranes, enhances transmission of nerve impulses, assists to maintain adequate serum levels of calcium and potassium	Nuts, legumes, whole (unmilled) grains, green vegetables; bananas provide some magnesium	High-fiber diet may reduce absorption slightly	Nausea, muscle weakness, irritability	None in healthy individual; with impaired renal function, excess may contribute to nausea, vomiting, hypotension, bradycardia, central nervous system depression
Iron	Formation of the heme molecule; used in oxygen transport	Meat, eggs, vegetables, cereals, foods fortified with iron additives; Table 12-5 identifies a number of iron-rich foods	Absorption is enhanced if iron stores or daily intakes are low; presence of ascorbic acid increases absorption Heme iron in meats is more bioavailable than non–heme iron from grains, fruits, and vegetables Absorption inhibited if the iron-rich food is ingested with milk or caffeine or in presence of phytic acid, oxalic acid, and tannic acid	Anemia Children are particularly susceptible to iron deficiency during periods of rapid growth combined with low dietary iron intake: from about 6 mo to 4 yr of age and during early adolescence; adolescent girls are at risk owing to menstruation	Iron poisoning, can be fatal; for a 2-year-old, a fatal dose is approximately 3 g; for adolescents and adults, 200-250 mg/kg may be fatal
Zinc	Cellular metabolism, growth, and repair	Meats, animal products, seafood (especially oysters), eggs	Absorption may be decreased if taken with high-fiber diet	Anorexia, growth retardation, skin changes, immunologic abnormalities	Gastrointestinal disturbances, vomiting, acute toxicity, impaired immune response

Iodine	Production of thyroid hormones	Water, seafood, airborne water from ocean mist, iodized salt, food processing related to milk and bread	None known	Thyroid dysfunction ranging from simple goiter to cretinism and mental retardation	Thyrotoxicosis; goiter, rare and not seen in children with intake up to 1 mg/day; toxic levels not known
Trace Elements					
Selenium	Unknown	Seafood and organ meats; may be in grains grown in soil containing selenium	Intake linked to vitamin E intake; if vitamin E is adequate, selenium is likely to be also; may need to supplement in lactating women Total parenteral nutrition (TPN) feedings contribute to deficiency	May be related to muscle weakness and pain, cardiomyopathy (Keshan's disease) in young children	Nausea, abdominal pain, diarrhea, fatigue, nail and hair changes or loss; toxic levels not known
Copper	Normal growth	Organ meats, seafood, nuts, seeds; infants store copper in liver during gestation	TPN feedings contribute to deficiency; high vitamin C, molybdenum, or zinc intake may reduce retention or bioavailability	Bone loss, anemia, neutropenia, growth impairment	Liver disease, gastrointestinal symptoms, diarrhea, vomiting
Manganese	Unknown, may be related to reproductive health, normal growth	Whole grains and cereals	Increased absorption during third trimester of pregnancy	Unknown, may be related to growth retardation	Unknown, may be related to learning disabilities, anemia
Fluoride	Prevents dental caries, enhances bone health	Fluoridated water, tea, meat and bones of marine fish, potatoes, wheat germ	Processing foods in fluoridated water or cooking with Teflon increases content; cooking foods in aluminum reduces fluoride	Dental caries, may be related to poor bone health	Mottling of teeth, kidney disease, bone disease, may affect muscle and nerve function
Chromium	Assists in glucose metabolism	Brewer's yeast, calves' liver, American cheese, wheat germ	TPN feedings can contribute to deficiency	May be related to impairment of glucose tolerance	Unknown, requires further study
Molybdenum	Enzyme function	Milk, beans, breads, cereals	TPN feedings can contribute to deficiency	Unknown	Related to loss of copper, may lead to goutlike symptoms

*Nearly all trace minerals are toxic in large quantities, because many are metals.

TABLE 12-5 ***Iron-Rich Foods***

Food	High Levels (>5 mg/serving)	Moderate Levels (2-4 mg/serving)	Low Levels (<2 mg/serving)
Breads, grains, cereals, seeds*	Almonds (1 cup, whole, oil roasted) Cashews (1 cup, dry roasted) Pumpkin seed kernels (1/4 cup, roasted) Fortified cereals Mixed nuts (1 cup, dry roasted with peanuts) Brown glutinous rice (1 cup, cooked) Sunflower seeds (1 cup, dry roasted) Watermelon kernels (1 cup, dried) Wheat germ (1 cup, toasted)	Bagel (1, egg or plain) Bread, Indian fry (1 piece) Breadstick (10, plain, without salt) Filberts (1 cup, dried) Gingerbread (1 piece) Muffin (1 wheat) Peanuts (1 cup, dried) White rice (1 cup, enriched, regular, cooked) Waffles (2 each) Walnuts (1 cup, dried)	Biscuits (1 each) Bread (1 slice, whole wheat) Egg noodles (1 cup, cooked) English muffin (1 each) Pancakes (1 each) Peanut butter (2 tbsp) Oatmeal (1 cup, cooked)
Fruits*	Apricot (1 cup, dried halves)	Avocado (1 whole) Currants (1 cup, dried Zante) Fig (10 each, dried) Pear (10 each, dried halves) Prune juice (1 cup) Raisins (1/2 cup)	Apple (1 medium, unpeeled) Apple juice (1 cup) Banana (1 medium) Dried mixed fruit (2 oz) Orange (1 medium) Orange juice (1 cup)
Vegetables*	Kidney beans (1 cup, cooked, fresh) Lentils (1 cup, cooked) Soybeans (1 cup, cooked) White beans (1 cup, cooked) Spinach (1 cup, cooked) Tofu (1/2 cup)	Black beans (1 cup, cooked) Garbanzo beans (1 cup, cooked) Refried beans (1 cup, canned) Beet greens (1 cup, cooked) Potatoes (1 medium, with skin, baked) Peas (1 cup, fresh, cooked) Snow peas with pods (1 cup, raw or cooked) Molasses (2 tbsp, blackstrap) Spinach (1 cup, frozen, cooked)	Kidney beans (1 cup, canned) Green beans (1 cup, raw or cooked) Broccoli (1 cup) Carrots (1 cup) Corn (1/2 cup) Lettuce (1 cup) Potato (1/2 cup, baked, with skin) Spinach (1 cup, raw) Sweet potatoes (1 cup, fresh, boiled, mashed) Tomatoes (1 cup fresh) Tomato juice (1 cup, canned) Turnip greens (1 cup, cooked)
Meats, poultry, fish, other protein sources†	Clams (3.5 oz, 5 each, or 1 cup) = 22 mg Fe Oysters (3.5 oz) Beef heart meat (3.5 oz, cooked) Beef liver (3.5 oz, simmered) Veal liver (3 oz, simmered) Chicken liver (3.5 oz, cooked) Turkey liver (3.5 oz, cooked)	Ground beef (3 oz, cooked lean) Catfish (1 piece, floured, fried) Tuna (1 cup, canned, water packed) Lamb (3.5 oz, cooked)	Roast beef (3 oz, lean) Chicken (1 cup, dark or light meat) Egg (1, whole) Halibut (1 piece, baked or broiled) Ham (1 cup, roasted) Bacon (3 pieces, cooked) Pork (3 oz, lean shoulder roast)

Adapted from Hands ES: *Food finder: food sources of vitamins and minerals*, ed 3, Salem, OR, 1995, ESHA Research; Hands ES: *Nutrients in food*, Philadelphia, 2000, Lippincott Williams & Wilkins.
Fe, Iron.
*Iron in plant foods is better absorbed when eaten with vitamin C or meat products.
†Iron in meat, poultry, and fish is more bioavailable than iron in other food sources.

every day to be healthy). Vitamin and mineral supplements are not necessary for children who consume a varied, healthy diet, and caution should be used to prevent oversupplementation, especially since safe upper limits have not been identified for some elements (Food and Nutrition Board, IOM, 2002). Children at risk for nutritional deficit, however, may benefit by supplementation with multivitamins. Risk factors for vitamin and mineral deficiency may include economically deprived families, neglect or abuse, anorexia, poor and capricious appetites, fad diets, dietary restrictions to manage obesity, pregnancy, and vegetarian diets. Preterm or low-birth-weight babies and children with chronic illness also may need supplementation.

Age-Specific Considerations

Newborns and Infants

Energy. Rapid growth in infancy requires high caloric intake. Table 12-1 can be used to calculate the energy needs of infants to meet demands of metabolism and growth. Breast milk or infant formulas meet all energy needs for infants until age 4 to 6 months.

Fat. For proper myelinization to occur, infants must have adequate fat intake. Children younger than age 2 years can require more than 30% dietary fat for neural development. The lipid content of breast milk and formulas meets infants' dietary requirements. During the second year of life, cow's milk can be included in children's diets. Because the majority of fat in the diet is derived from milk and milk products, skim milk is not recommended for infants. The American Academy of Pediatrics recommends whole milk for children between 12 and 24 months of age, although 2% milk, as part of a varied diet, can contribute to adequate fat intake and has no negative affect on growth or body composition (Wosje, Specker, & Giddens, 2002).

Vitamins. Vitamin and mineral supplements, except iron, are usually not necessary for healthy term infants who are breastfed or formula fed and who receive mixed feedings of cereal, fruits, vegetables, and proteins after 4 to 6 months of age. Breastfed infants and infants who receive a formula not fortified with vitamin D (which is rare), need supplementation. Infants also should have an adequate source of vitamin C, especially after 4 to 6 months of age. A multivitamin supplement is recommended for infants at nutritional risk as a result of lifestyle, economic status, or recurrent illness.

Iron. Iron deficiency is the leading cause of anemia in children, and iron supplementation is appropriate in some cases. Term infants who are breastfed usually have adequate iron supplies until 4 to 6 months of age. Premature or low-birth-weight infants, infants who are exclusively breastfed beyond 4 to 6 months of age, and infants who are fed cow's milk before age 12 months are at high risk for iron deficiency anemia. Iron-fortified cereals and iron-fortified formulas are excellent sources of dietary iron supplements for infants 6 to 12 months of age. Earlier supplementation may be necessary for breastfed premature infants.

Fluoride. The most recent guidelines from the American Dental Association recommend beginning fluoride treatment at 6 months of age (American Dental Association, 2002). See Chapter 34 for recommended fluoride dosages.

Infant Formulas. Breast milk is the ideal food for newborns and infants and should be encouraged whenever possible. Most iron-fortified infant formulas provide adequate nutrition and, for some families, may be an appropriate alternative. Box 12-1 outlines the nutritional content of various commercial formulas and breast milk.

Occasionally, infants demonstrate intolerance to formula, showing irritability, weight loss or slow gain, emesis, diarrhea, constipation, other gastrointestinal problems, or atopic dermatitis. The NP must work closely with parents to identify a formula tolerated by the infant, being careful to allow sufficient time for the baby to respond to a new formula as it is introduced. This can be a time- and energy-consuming process in which parents need support, reassurance, and encouragement. Referral to a registered dietitian can be helpful. See the discussion on food intolerances (Altered Patterns of Nutrition) later in this chapter for management of the lactose- or protein-intolerant infant.

Introduction of Solids. A number of variables converge at about 6 months of age that make this an appropriate time to introduce solids into infants' diets:

- Infants' sucking patterns have changed sufficiently to allow mastery of chewing and swallowing.
- Infants can sit with some support, and they are able to purposefully move their heads.
- Infants are able to grasp, pick up, and bring objects to their mouths.
- Iron stores present at birth are being depleted.
- Growth demands require nutrients other than those provided in milk alone.
- Developmental needs (cognitive, sensory, and motor) are stimulated by new foods, textures, smells, and tastes, as well as use of utensils.

The specific foods that parents provide for their children vary by cultural and family customs, and there are no set recommendations as to a sequence by which to introduce solids. Commercial baby foods provide adequate nutrition, but labels should be examined to determine their content, especially looking at calories, fats, additives, salt, and sugar. Home-prepared foods, such as mashed bananas, applesauce, pureed squash, cooked peas, and blenderized meats, can provide adequate nutrition if the diet is well balanced. Box 12-2 lists some principles to keep in mind when beginning solids. The period in which solid foods are first offered can be a creative, frustrating, learning-filled time for both children and caregivers, and NPs can offer suggestions and guidance to make feeding a positive

BOX 12-1 *Categories of Infant Formulas Available**

- Premature formulas (hospital and transitional)
  - Higher caloric content more nutrient dense than regular cow's milk–based formulas
  - Protein source: human milk, nonfat cow's milk, whey
- Cow's milk–based formulas
  - Standard formula for healthy term infants
- Nutrient-dense cow's milk–based formulas
  - Similar to premature formula, but with less phosphorus and calcium; some preparations have up to 27 kcal/oz (vs. 20 kcal/oz in regular formula and 24 kcal/oz in premature formula)
- Hypoallergenic formulas
  - Partially hydrolyzed whey-based formulas
  - Soy-based formulas (protein source: soy protein isolate with L-methionine)
  - Casein hydrolysate formulas
  - Amino acid–based formulas
- Formulas with long-chain polyunsaturated fatty acids
  - More closely approximates human milk with content of docosahexaenoic acid (DHA, an omega-3 fatty acid) and arachidonic acid (ARA, an omega-6 fatty acid)
  - Benefit of enhanced visual and mental development not confirmed by research (Fewtrell et al, 2002)
- Formulas for feeding beyond 4-6 months of age, supplemented with solids
- Nutrient-dense formulas for older child
  - Caloric content up to 30 kcal/oz; other nutrients increased over regular infant formula
- Specialized formulas
  - Higher caloric content (24-30 kcal/oz); nutrient dense; free amino acid and peptide-based formulas
- Protein supplements
- Nitrogen-free calorie supplements
- Oral electrolyte solutions

*For names of formulas and detailed description of formula content, see Hattner J, Kerner J: *Approximate composition of pediatric formulas*, Stanford, CA, 1997, Stanford University Medical Center/Lucile Packard Children's Hospital, Department of Nutrition and Food Services.

BOX 12-2 *Principles for the Introduction of Solids into the Infant's Diet*

Introduce one food at a time, waiting 3 to 5 days before offering another in order to assess for adverse reaction.
Offer rice cereal, the least allergenic of cereal grains, as the first food.
Introduce fruits, vegetables, and other cereals in any sequence desired.
Feed only iron-fortified cereals.
Avoid allergenic foods (e.g., wheat, nuts [especially peanuts], shellfish, egg whites, citrus) before 12 months of age.
Prepare food appropriate to child's developmental abilities (e.g., strained, mashed, or finger foods).
Use commercially prepared or home-prepared foods.
Provide a variety of foods.
Help child develop healthy patterns of eating:
  Be alert and responsive to child's cues when eating.
  Use a spoon to feed solids.
  Offer about 1 tbsp per year of age as a serving for infants; for older children, about one fourth to one half an adult serving.
  Never force a child to eat.
  Include the child in family meal times.

experience. Lessons learned here can influence eating habits for a lifetime.

Toddlers and Preschoolers

Energy and Protein. The growth rate of toddlers and preschoolers is slower than that of infants, resulting in decreased energy needs per unit of body weight. But because of increased size and activity, these children require an increased number of total calories. Addition of muscle mass also demands a continued high protein intake.

Establishing Eating Habits in Early Childhood. Good nutrition for children is not simply a matter of meeting dietary requirements. When providing nutritional counseling, NPs must also consider the eating habits of children and families. The toddler and preschool years are critical to establishing lifelong patterns of eating, and many eating problems, including obesity, are, in part, due to poor eating habits learned in early childhood.

Children learn how and what to eat by observing adults around them and by responding to what adults provide for them to eat. Learning eating habits can be a positive growth experience for both children and parents. Among other things, children learn about textures, smells, and colors, as well as taste. They learn physical skills of fine motor control, cognitive skills of relationships between action and consequence (the dog will eat whatever is dropped on the floor), and interactional skills of social exchange among family members.

Use of Vitamin and Mineral Supplements. Evaluate a child's intake over the course of a week. If children persist with extremely limited food choices or picky eating behavior, they might benefit from a children's multivitamin plus mineral supplement.

School-Age Children

Energy and Protein. Energy and protein needs of school-age children vary greatly, depending on body size, growth patterns, and activity and exercise levels. Protein needs increase in older children as they acquire more muscle mass. Boys older than 10 years need between 2500 and 3000 calories a day, whereas girls require about 2200 calories daily (see Table 12-1).

Eating Habits. Food likes and dislikes carry over from the preschool years. There is great variation in appetite and intake as a result of uneven growth and activity levels. School-age children have a tendency to skip meals and are more likely to snack as they become engrossed in activities. This tendency is exacerbated in families with hectic schedules, unstructured mealtimes, and reliance on fast foods. Parents can identify healthful "fast" foods (e.g., homemade burritos, stir-fry chicken, peanut butter sandwiches, string cheese and a bagel on the way to soccer practice) that fit a busy school-age child's schedule.

School-age children are particularly at risk for excessive weight gain if caloric intake exceeds energy needs, and problems with obesity begin at this age (see discussion of obesity later in this chapter).

Use of Vitamin and Mineral Supplements. Poor eating habits place school-age children at risk for deficiencies in iron, thiamine, vitamin A, and calcium. Teaching children about specific nutrient sources and encouraging healthy eating habits can prevent many problems, and supplementation with a daily multivitamin is usually not necessary.

Adolescents

Energy and Protein. The growth rate of adolescents is remarkable (Table 12-6), and the description by some parents that their children never seem to stop eating is apt. High levels of energy are needed to support adolescents' rapid growth, and if children participate in sports or other exercise programs, additional caloric intake can be needed. Adequate protein intake is essential to produce muscle mass. The average intake of protein in the U.S. diet is significantly above the RDA, so additional supplementation is usually not necessary.

Eating Habits. Eating habits of adolescents are influenced by their increasing independence and social activity, perceptions of body image, and physical growth patterns. Adolescents often have erratic eating patterns, skip meals, eat high-fat, high-calorie, low-nutrient snack foods, and consume calories late in the day.

Use of Vitamin and Mineral Supplements. Thiamine, riboflavin, niacin, folate, iron, zinc, and calcium needs increase during adolescence (see Table 12-2). Most adolescents who eat a well-balanced diet need no supplements, but their irregular eating habits put them at risk for deficits.

Pregnancy in Adolescence. Pregnancy presents an added complication to the normal adolescent nutrient intake. Nutrition needs are high for the pregnant teenager, particularly if she is younger than 15 years old, in the midst of her pubertal growth spurt. During this period, teenagers' bodies are still growing and compete with their fetuses for nutrients. Infants born to teenage mothers are at higher risk for prematurity, low birth weight, chronic illness, disabilities, and death. Proper nutrition and early prenatal care can increase the chance of a successful pregnancy.

The nutrition needs of pregnant teenagers are the highest at a time when it is most difficult to meet them. Irregular eating patterns typical of adolescents contribute to poor nutritional status. Calcium; iron; zinc; vitamins A, D, and B_6; riboflavin; folic acid; and total calories—all of which are

TABLE 12-6 ***Average Weight, Height, and Head Circumference Gains in Infancy through Adolescence***

Age	Weight	Height	Head Circumference	Comments
Infant (mo)	Average weekly gain:	Average monthly gain:	Average monthly gain:	
0-3	210 g (8 oz)	3.5 cm	2.0 cm	Regain or exceed birth weight by 2 wk
3-6	140 g (5 oz)	2.0 cm	1.0 cm	Birth weight doubles by 4-6 mo
6-12	85-105 g (3-4 oz)	1.2-1.5 cm	0.5 cm	
Toddler	Average yearly gain:	Average yearly gain:	Average yearly gain:	
1-3 yr	2-3 kg (4.4-6.6 lb)	12 cm	3.0 cm	Height at 2 yr approximately half of adult height
Preschool-age child				
3-6 yr	2 kg (4.5 lb)	3-7 cm	1.0 cm	
School-age child				
6-12 yr	3-3.5 kg (7 lb)	6 cm	2-3 cm during entire period	Growth is discontinuous, in spurts lasting about 8 wk, occurring 3-6 times a year
Preadolescent/ adolescent	Average total gain:	Average yearly gain:		Weight gain follows linear growth, with several months delay; adolescents first grow taller, then fill out
Girl, 10-14 yr	17.7 kg (39 lb)	6-8.3 cm		95% linear growth achieved by onset of menarche
Boy, 12-16 yr	22.2 kg (50 lb)	6-9.5 cm		95% linear growth achieved by 15 yr

Adapted from Behrman RE, Kliegman RM, Jenson HB, editors: Nelson textbook of pediatrics, ed 17, Philadelphia, 2002, WB Saunders.

essential to fetal growth—are often found to be inadequate in the diets of female adolescents (Lytle et al, 2002).

When managing the pregnant teenager, the NP should carefully assess dietary intake and counsel the adolescent to eat a varied and healthful diet. A prenatal multivitamin and mineral supplement, including iron and folic acid, is advised, and calcium supplements can be indicated. The pregnant teenager should strive for a total of 1300 to 1500 mg of calcium through diet and supplements each day. Daily folic acid intake of 0.4 mg is recommended for all adolescent girls, increased to 0.6 mg during pregnancy (Food and Nutrition Board, IOM, 2002).

Weight gain in pregnant teens should be carefully monitored. Healthy teens should gain the amount they would normally gain in 9 months if they were not pregnant plus the upper limit of normal pregnancy weight gain. This amounts to about 35 to 48 lb total weight gain. Adolescents who begin pregnancy when overweight should gain less (Gorrie, McKinney, & Murray, 1998). For those adolescents who meet income guidelines (185% of poverty level), the federal supplemental food program for women, infants, and children (WIC) is a valuable resource. In addition to providing nutritious foods, the program offers nutrition education and counseling.

ASSESSMENT OF NUTRITIONAL STATUS

The goals of nutritional status assessment are to determine dietary adequacy and to identify deviation from normal growth and development. Data collected include a history of food and fluid intake, physical findings, and laboratory and diagnostic indicators.

History

Questions to elicit a history of nutritional status can be grouped into several categories:

- Food and fluid intake:
  - Nutritional status of mother during pregnancy.
  - Type of feeding method used during infancy. If not breastfed, formula name and preparation. Any problems? When weaned? When solids started? Any allergies or intolerances noted?
  - Current nutritional intake of child (if child is still an infant, ask more specifically about frequency and amounts of feedings in 24-hour period).
  - Type of foods and fluids.
  - Amounts eaten (may use 24-hour recall, 3-day diet history, or length of time child is at breast).

   - Additional intake (e.g., vitamin, fluoride, or iron supplements).
- Eating patterns:
   - Frequency of eating (nursings, meals, snacks).
   - Feeding patterns or behaviors for both child and family.
   - Bottle feeding: Is bottle propped? Does child take bottle to bed at night or at naptime? Who feeds child?
   - Breastfeeding: On demand or scheduled? How flexible is mother to demands of infant? Is mother working? Is breast milk frozen and fed by someone other than mother?
   - Describe mealtimes: Does family sit down together? Are meals prepared at home? Does child eat at school? How often are "fast foods" eaten? What amount of time is spent eating? How long does it take to feed child?
   - Does family eat out frequently?
- Reactions to and attitudes about foods:
   - Any reaction to particular foods (e.g., vomiting, diarrhea, rash).
   - Food preferences or dislikes.
   - Cultural factors: What beliefs or attitudes does family have about how and what child should eat or how family should eat?
   - What is child's attitude about foods and eating?
   - Feeding abilities of child. For example, does child choke, gag, vomit, or refuse certain foods, perhaps due to texture or smell?
- Management of foods in the family:
   - Who plans, purchases, and prepares food and meals for family?
   - Economic and environmental factors that influence how food is managed. For example, are finances adequate to supply nutritious foods? Is there a refrigerator? Does family have a car to carry larger amounts of food from store? Is there a full-service grocery store in the neighborhood? What is the socioeconomic status of family? Is food shopping budgeted? Are food stamps or other supplemental programs used?
- Health status affected by nutrition:
   - Special considerations for children or family related to food. For example, does child have a chronic illness that requires a special diet? Are any medications being taken?
   - Elimination patterns.
   - Dental status and care of teeth.
   - Patterns of wound healing, infections, colds, and mild illnesses.
   - Any change in hair, nails, skin, or mucous membranes?
   - Tolerance for hot or cold weather?
   - Growth, activity, and exercise pattern. For example, has child been growing as parent expects? Has there been a history of unusual weight gain or loss? Does child have energy to play?
   - Family history: hypertension, diabetes, hyperlipidemia, obesity, heart disease, allergies, eating disorders.

Physical Examination

The physical examination should include the following:
- Body temperature
- Height, weight, and head circumference measurements (see growth charts, Appendix B; also see Table 12-6 for average weight and height gains expected during childhood); arm circumference and triceps and subscapular skinfold caliper measurements for children at risk for obesity or malnutrition
- Body mass index (BMI) (see growth charts, Appendix B)
- Skin condition (clear, smooth, firm, with good turgor)
- Muscle tone, posture, skeletal development (body erect, tone good)
- Hair (smooth, full, shiny; no dryness, broken ends, bare patches, or discoloration)
- Mucous membranes, eyes (moist, shiny, no dark circles, conjunctiva pink)
- Teeth (eruption appropriate to age, gums healthy, no bleeding)
- Neck (thyroid, parotid glands of normal size)
- Abdomen (flat, soft)
- Cardiovascular (no murmur; normal heart size; skin warm, pink, less than 3-second capillary refill; peripheral pulses equal, strong)
- Neurologic/behavior (alert, active, reflexes present, no complaints of headache, neuritis)

Laboratory and Diagnostic Tests

Laboratory and diagnostic tests are performed as indicated:
- Hemoglobin or hematocrit
- Iron/ferritin levels (see Chapter 27)
- Serum levels for various elements: albumin, nitrogen balance, minerals
- Bone radiographs for suspected iodine, vitamins C and D, or copper deficiency, or to compare bone age with height age (age at which 50% of children reach the patient's height)

MANAGEMENT STRATEGIES FOR OPTIMAL NUTRITION

NPs can work to ensure that dietary intake adequately supports optimal growth and development through nutritional education, counseling, and anticipatory guidance. Information and guidance are provided regarding children's nutritional requirements, eating behaviors, and strategies and foods used to provide adequate nutrition.

Children's Nutritional Requirements

Parents are not always aware of the nutritional needs of their children. NPs should explain the nutritional requirements of children and offer anticipatory guidance about how physical growth and development create demands for specific nutrients. Information about which foods are good sources of these nutrients can also be given. The relationship between disease and inadequate dietary intake should be discussed.

The Food Guide Pyramid

The Food Guide Pyramid is a useful tool for educating families and children of all ages about a healthful diet. The Food Guide Pyramid illustrates the proportions of a healthy diet and emphasizes a foundation of grains, fruits, and vegetables. The Oregon Dairy Council has adapted the Food Guide Pyramid to identify foods that are nutrient dense, as well as serving sizes. Called "Pyramid Plus," this adaptation is presented in Fig. 12-1. Additional Food Guide Pyramids have been created that may be used by various ethnic groups and those who eat a vegetarian diet (Fig. 12-2).

MILK & MILK PRODUCTS	MEAT & MEAT ALTERNATIVES	VEGETABLES	FRUITS	BREADS & CEREALS
Supplies: **Calcium,** riboflavin, protein	Supplies: **Iron, protein,** niacin, thiamine, zinc, B_{12}	Supplies: **Folic acid, vitamins A and C,** fiber	Supplies: **Folic acid, vitamins A and C,** fiber	Supplies: **Fiber, complex carbohydrate,** thiamine, iron, niacin
Amount recommended: 2–3 servings each day	Amount recommended: 2–3 servings each day	Amount recommended: 3–5 servings each day	Amount recommended: 2–4 servings each day	Amount recommended: 6–11 servings each day
★★★★	★★★★	★★★★	★★★★	★★★★
nonfat plain yogurt, nonfat milk, nonfat cream cheese, 1% milk, buttermilk, low-fat cheese, 2% milk	fish, shellfish, poultry (light meat, skinless), turkey, ham, beef (round and sirloin, well trimmed), pork (tenderloin, well trimmed), veal (leg and shoulder, well trimmed), lentils	red and green bell peppers, bok choy, spinach, leaf lettuce, broccoli, carrots, cauliflower	papaya, strawberries, kiwi, orange, grapefruit, orange juice, cantaloupe, mandarin oranges, mango	barley, bulgur, bran or whole grain cereals, popcorn (air-popped or lite microwave), whole grain breads, oatmeal, whole grain pasta, corn or whole wheat tortilla
★★★	★★★	★★★	★★★	★★★
part-skim ricotta cheese, whole milk, regular-fat cheese, low-fat chocolate milk, low-fat fruit yogurt, nonfat frozen yogurt	beef (rib, chuck, flank, and ground), ham (lean), tofu, veal and lamb (leg and loin), poultry (dark meat with skin), pork (loin and rib), Canadian bacon, poultry sausage, dried beans and peas, eggs	cabbage, chard, asparagus, kale, vegetable juice, brussels sprouts, iceberg lettuce, sweet potato, tomato, snow peas, zucchini, okra, winter squash, green beans	honeydew, raspberries, apricots, rhubarb, pineapple, watermelon, pineapple juice, blueberries	brown rice, bran muffin, whole grain crackers, soft pretzel or breadstick, English muffin, enriched pasta, popcorn (oil-popped)
★★	★★	★★	★★	★★
pudding, custard, low-fat frozen yogurt, ice milk	hot dogs, pork sausage, chicken nuggets, fish sticks, nuts and seeds	beets, cucumber, celery, jicama, artichoke, peas, mushrooms	peach, banana, plum, cherries, frozen fruit juice bar, canned fruit	flour tortilla, bagel, enriched breads, enriched rice, pancakes, waffles, graham crackers, saltines, sweetened cereal, dry pretzels or breadsticks
★	★	★	★	★
milkshake, cottage cheese, ice cream, nonfat sour cream	peanut butter, bologna	eggplant, corn, avocado, potato	pear, apple, dried fruit, grapes, raisins	cornbread, fruit or nut bread, biscuit, stuffing, croissant

FIGURE 12-1 Pyramid Plus. Based on the U.S. Department of Agriculture Food Guide Pyramid, Pyramid Plus emphasizes foods from five major food groups. Each food group is important for the nutrients it provides, and no one food group is more important than another. For a healthy diet, you need foods from each group in the amounts recommended. The "Plus" in Pyramid Plus is nutrient density, a guide to the nutrient value of individual foods. Within each group, foods are listed according to the amount of key nutrients per calorie each provides. Key nutrients are listed in **bold** type. Four-star foods have the most nutrition per calorie. Generally, four-star foods are also lowest in fat. One-star foods should not be viewed as bad foods—they are merely less nutrient dense. The most effective way to reduce fat, sugar, and calories without compromising nutrition is to cut back on sometimes foods, those foods that provide little or no nutrition. Young adults (11 to 24 years of age) and pregnant and breastfeeding women need four servings of milk and milk products each day. (Adapted from Nutrition Education Services/Oregon Dairy Council, 1994.)

Sometimes Foods: Alcoholic beverages, bacon, bouillon, butter, cakes, candy, coffee, cookies, condiments, snack crackers, cream, regular-fat cream cheese, doughnuts, french fries, fruit-flavored drinks, gelatin dessert, gravy, honey, jam, jelly, margarine, mayonnaise, nondairy creamer, olives, onion rings, pickles, pies, potato chips, salad dressings, sauces, seasonings, sherbet, soft drinks, sour cream, sugar, tea, tortilla chips, vegetable oils

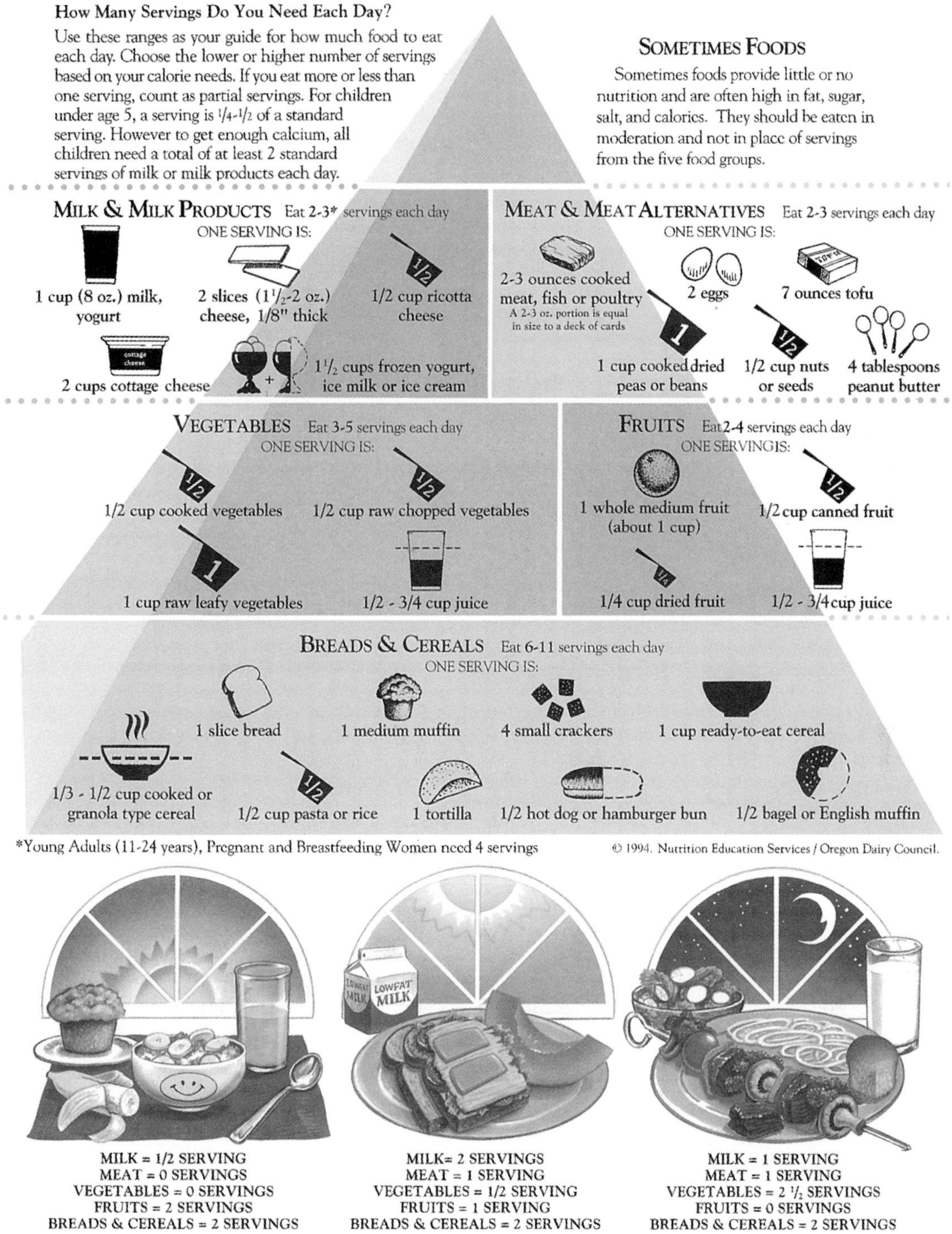
How Many Servings Do You Need Each Day?
Use these ranges as your guide for how much food to eat each day. Choose the lower or higher number of servings based on your calorie needs. If you eat more or less than one serving, count as partial servings. For children under age 5, a serving is 1/4-1/2 of a standard serving. However to get enough calcium, all children need a total of at least 2 standard servings of milk or milk products each day.
SOMETIMES FOODS
Sometimes foods provide little or no nutrition and are often high in fat, sugar, salt, and calories. They should be eaten in moderation and not in place of servings from the five food groups.
MILK & MILK PRODUCTS Eat 2-3* servings each day
ONE SERVING IS:
1 cup (8 oz.) milk, yogurt
2 slices (1 1/2-2 oz.) cheese, 1/8" thick
1/2 cup ricotta cheese
2 cups cottage cheese
1 1/2 cups frozen yogurt, ice milk or ice cream
MEAT & MEAT ALTERNATIVES Eat 2-3 servings each day
ONE SERVING IS:
2-3 ounces cooked meat, fish or poultry
A 2-3 oz. portion is equal in size to a deck of cards
2 eggs
7 ounces tofu
1 cup cooked dried peas or beans
1/2 cup nuts or seeds
4 tablespoons peanut butter
VEGETABLES Eat 3-5 servings each day
ONE SERVING IS:
1/2 cup cooked vegetables
1/2 cup raw chopped vegetables
1 cup raw leafy vegetables
1/2 - 3/4 cup juice
FRUITS Eat 2-4 servings each day
ONE SERVING IS:
1 whole medium fruit (about 1 cup)
1/2 cup canned fruit
1/4 cup dried fruit
1/2 - 3/4 cup juice
BREADS & CEREALS Eat 6-11 servings each day
ONE SERVING IS:
1 slice bread
1 medium muffin
4 small crackers
1 cup ready-to-eat cereal
1/3 - 1/2 cup cooked or granola type cereal
1/2 cup pasta or rice
1 tortilla
1/2 hot dog or hamburger bun
1/2 bagel or English muffin
*Young Adults (11-24 years), Pregnant and Breastfeeding Women need 4 servings
© 1994. Nutrition Education Services / Oregon Dairy Council.
LOWFAT MILK
MILK = 1/2 SERVING
MEAT = 0 SERVINGS
VEGETABLES = 0 SERVINGS
FRUITS = 2 SERVINGS
BREADS & CEREALS = 2 SERVINGS
MILK= 2 SERVINGS
MEAT = 1 SERVING
VEGETABLES = 1/2 SERVING
FRUITS = 1 SERVING
BREADS & CEREALS = 2 SERVINGS
MILK = 1 SERVING
MEAT = 1 SERVING
VEGETABLES = 2 1/2 SERVINGS
FRUITS = 0 SERVINGS
BREADS & CEREALS = 2 SERVINGS

FIGURE 12-1 cont'd

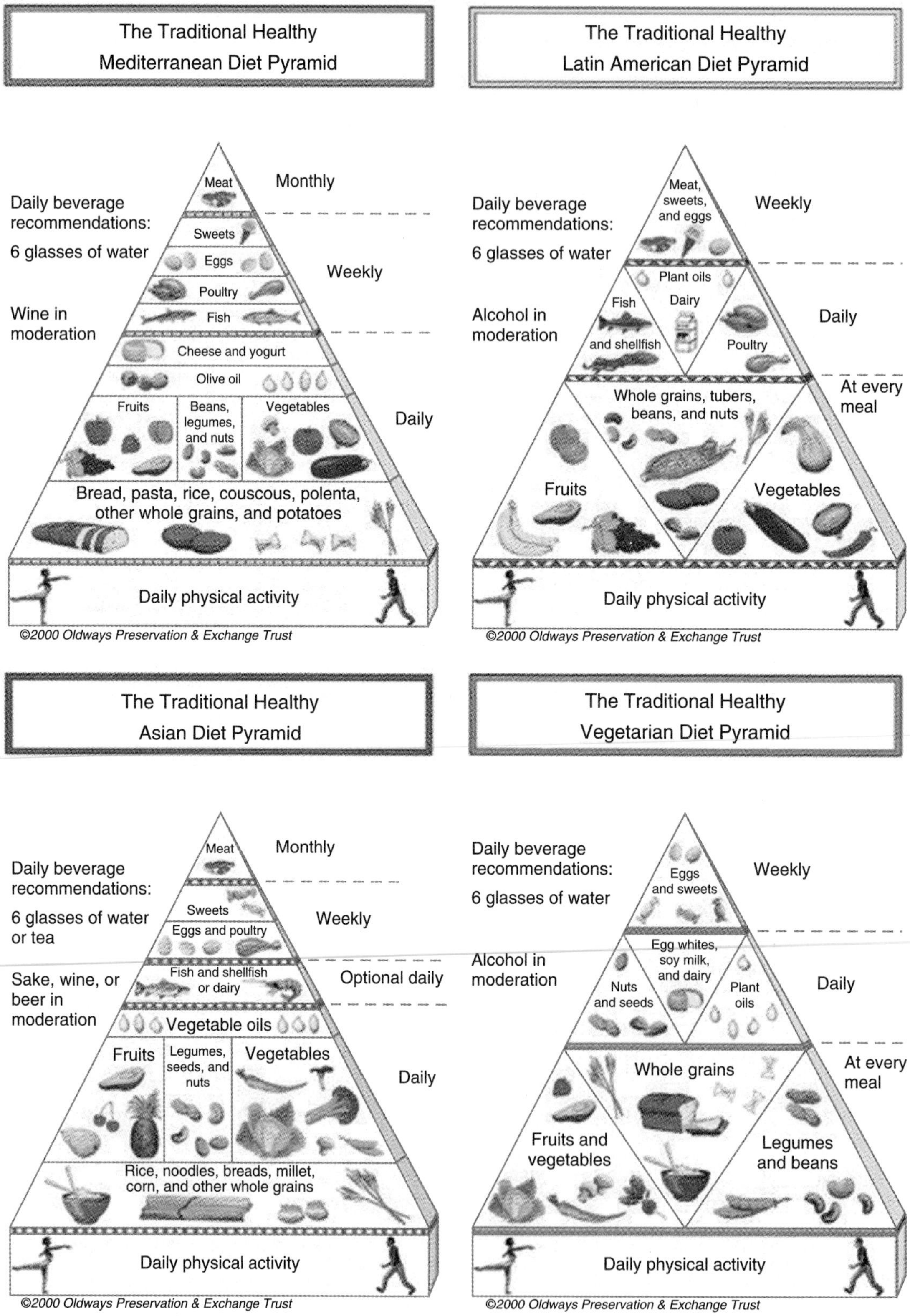

FIGURE 12-2 Four traditional healthy Food Guide Pyramids. (Copyright 2000, Oldways Preservation and Exchange Trust, www.oldwayspt.org.)

The first level of the pyramid consists of grains, which are rich in B vitamins, minerals, fiber, and complex carbohydrates and provide vital fuel for the body. Bread, cereal, rice, and pasta serve as energy staples of a low-fat, nutrient-dense diet. In general, the more active the child, the more carbohydrate is needed in the diet to fuel muscle work.

The second level of the Food Guide Pyramid features the fruit and vegetable groups. The groups are separated because of the different nutrients each provides. Most vegetables are virtually fat free and are rich in fiber, vitamins A and C, folic acid, iron, and magnesium. A minimum of three servings is recommended each day. Fruits and fruit juices provide important amounts of vitamin A, vitamin C, fiber, and potassium. A minimum of two servings daily is recommended, with emphasis placed on fiber-rich fresh fruit.

Protein and dairy foods remain important sources of essential nutrients, and two to three servings, the equivalent of 5 to 7 ounces of cooked lean meat, poultry, or fish per day, are recommended. Although rich in B vitamins, iron, zinc, and protein, some meats in this group contribute high levels of fat and cholesterol to the diet. Moderation is the key to making wise choices from this group, and smaller amounts of protein contribute to better health.

As with meats, some dairy products contribute significant fat, saturated fat, and cholesterol to the diet. However, there is a wide array of low-fat and nonfat dairy products available. Nonfat or 1% milk, nonfat yogurt, low-fat cheeses, and reduced-fat ice milk and frozen yogurt all offer the nutritional benefits of milk with less fat. The dairy group is a notable source of calcium, riboflavin, and protein. Three daily servings of dairy products are recommended for children.

The tip of the Food Guide Pyramid, which comes with the caution "use sparingly," includes foods typically labeled "junk foods" with "empty calories," such as soda, candy, cookies, butter, margarine, jam, and jelly. These foods provide taste and calories but little in the way of nutrition. Just as the tip of the Food Guide Pyramid is a small piece, these "tip" foods should be a small piece of the diet. But overly restricting these foods, especially in children, can contribute to unhealthy attitudes and eventual eating disorders. Moderate intake of sweets and fats can help meet the caloric and taste requirements of active youngsters.

Serving sizes change as children grow. A general principle to keep in mind is to serve 1 tablespoon of food per year of age. Thus, for children younger than 5 years of age, one serving is about one fourth to one third of an adult serving. Children's appetites vary, however, and parents should be alert to cues that the child wants more or less of any particular food.

Eating Behaviors

As noted, basic eating patterns are established in the toddler and preschool years; these patterns tend to continue through the child's life. Children learn eating behaviors by observation and instruction, and parents are the primary teachers in this process. Often that teaching is done without conscious reflection or planning on the part of parents. Studies indicate that children tend to eat what their parents do, and that parents who exert overt pressure on their children to eat less fat or more fruits and vegetables—without changing their own habits—actually contribute to poor eating patterns (Fisher et al, 2002; Lee & Birch, 2002).

In the process of developing the child's eating habits, adults have the responsibility to provide a variety of healthy, nutrient-rich foods in an environment that makes eating pleasant and comfortable. Children have the responsibility to decide the amount and kinds of food (from those the parent has provided) to be eaten.

An example of parents not meeting their responsibility to their children occurs when they provide foods with "empty" calories rather than those containing essential nutrients. Parents may rationalize by stating, "That's all my child will eat, and I know she needs the energy," or "But he cries and carries on if I don't give it to him." If children learn early that healthy, nutrient-filled foods are readily available, and that mom and dad enjoy them, they will enjoy them as well. If "empty calorie" foods are occasionally available, but are not the foundation of the child's diet, children learn to make better choices about how to fit these foods into a healthful diet. The NP can have parents do a "pantry evaluation" to see what types of snack foods are available for their children. If "empty calorie" foods are not available, children will not eat them.

Parents may also try to decide what and how much their child should eat (e.g., making a child sit at the table to finish his vegetables). Appetite fluctuations and preferences are typical of children, and parents should be aware that children may appear to eat less than the parent thinks is sufficient or too much of one particular food to the neglect of others. If parents punish a child for not eating or force a child to eat, they have taken away the child's responsibility to choose. In response, the child may develop an aversion to certain foods, overeat, or act out in other ways. Mealtimes can become contests of will between parents and children, creating feelings and patterns of interacting that extend far beyond the dinner table. Parents need to find out what healthy foods their children enjoy (it is perfectly alright to eat only carrots and broccoli!) and make those available. If provided a nutritious variety of foods they like, children tend to select those necessary for their healthy growth, in terms of both amount of calories and other nutrients.

NPs can help parents make the process more positive by having them examine their own values and patterns related to eating, identify and reinforce those they would like to foster in their children, and eliminate those they see as negative. The NP can inform parents about age differences and offer suggestions for effectively managing the eating experience. Parents should be encouraged to provide the following:

- Positive examples of healthy intake; parents are the child's role model
- An adequate supply of a wide variety of age-appropriate, nutritious foods
- Limits, but not prohibitions, on consumption of non-nutritious sugars and "tip" foods
- Food prepared in a form that stimulates children's appetites
- Regular, structured mealtimes; this may only be one meal a day
- A pleasant, relaxed environment for mealtimes
- Clear, developmentally appropriate expectations for children's behavior at mealtimes
- Developmentally appropriate access to and instruction in the use of utensils
- Appropriate supervision during mealtimes
- Healthy, age-appropriate snacks
- Developmentally appropriate opportunities to participate in preparing and serving meals
- Adequate exercise, sleep, and rest to stimulate appetites

The introduction of new foods can create tension between parents and children, with children refusing to try or rejecting new tastes or textures. Parents should be informed that this is a normal reaction for many children. Strategies that can be used to increase the chances of children accepting a new food include the following:

- Offer the food when children are hungry
- Allow children to taste a little of the food rather than eating a full portion
- Expose children to the food by preparing and serving the food without expecting them to eat it
- Provide an example of parents eating and enjoying the food
- Prepare the food the way children prefer: few spices, lukewarm, recognizable
- Associate food with pleasant experiences
- Never force food on children

Physical Activity

Physical activity is integrally related to healthy nutrition. Increased activity creates a demand for more calories and nutrients; more sedentary behavior means the body needs fewer calories. The epidemic of obesity among children in the United States (see discussion later in this chapter) is a result, in large part, of children's low physical activity level. Figure 12-3 presents an integration of the Food Guide Pyramid with a Physical Activity Pyramid and can be used by NPs to proactively counsel children about the importance of being active (Reinhardt & Brevard, 2002).

Vegetarian Diets

An increasing number of individuals are adopting a meat-free lifestyle. Vegetarian diets are nearly as varied as the children who eat them and may be initiated based on religious, ecologic, or health beliefs; economic necessity; or other reasons. A recent study of over 3000 Midwestern children found that adolescents, especially adolescent boys, who were on a vegetarian diet were at risk for eating disorders (Perry et al, 2001).

Description

Individuals who are vegetarians fall into one of the following categories:

- Vegans, or strict vegetarians, eat only foods of plant origin, including fruits, vegetables, grains, nuts, seeds, and legumes (e.g., beans, peas, lentils, tofu, and peanuts).
- Lacto-vegetarians include milk and dairy products in their diet, as well as all plant-based foods.
- Lacto-ovo-vegetarians consume eggs, dairy products, and all plant-based foods in their diet.
- "Sometimes" vegetarians have a diet that consists predominantly of plant-based foods, but they occasionally eat fish, chicken, or some seafoods.

For children who are lacto- or lacto-ovo-vegetarians, or who from time to time eat nonred meat, it is not difficult to achieve adequate amounts of protein, vitamins, and minerals needed for proper growth and development. The diet of these children is often closer to the model of the Food Guide Pyramid and is more likely to meet the *Healthy People 2010* goals than that of their red meat–eating peers (Perry et al, 2002). If they continue to follow a plant-based diet into adulthood, vegetarian children can expect to have a lower incidence of obesity, high blood pressure, heart disease, and perhaps cancer.

On the other hand, the child who eats a strict vegan diet faces greater difficulty meeting protein and nutrient needs. A high incidence of vitamin B_{12} deficiency and suboptimal zinc status has been noted in these children, and they may be at risk for developmental retardation. If girls who are vegetarian become pregnant, the fetus is also at risk for vitamin B_{12} deficiency, with potentially permanent neurologic damage.

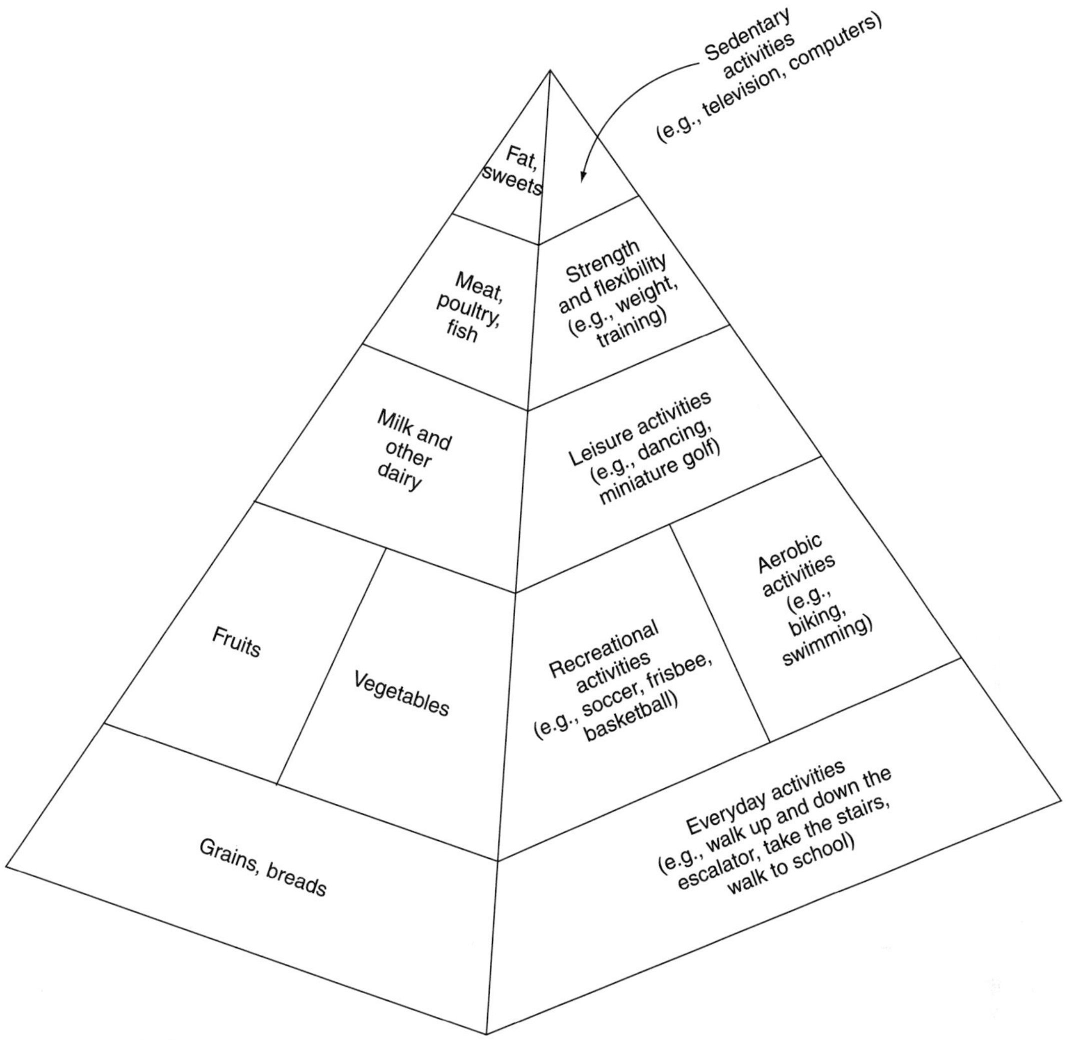

FIGURE 12-3 Physical Activity Pyramid. (Data from Reinhardt WC, Brevard PB: Integrating the Food Guide Pyramid and Physical Activity Pyramid for positive dietary and physical activity behaviors in adolescents, *J Am Diet Assoc* 102:596-599, 2002.)

Management

Careful diet planning is needed for children who are vegetarian in order to achieve optimal growth and development (Messina & Mangels, 2001; Sabaté, 2001). Plant sources of protein are considered "incomplete" because they lack the full array of amino acids needed to synthesize new tissue. To ensure adequate intake of essential amino acids, these children need to consume plant-based proteins that "complement" each other and that together provide a complete protein. The daily diet needs to include these complementary proteins, but not necessarily in the same meal. Examples of foods that provide complete proteins include combinations of legumes and grains, nuts, or seeds (e.g., peanut butter/wheat bread, beans/rice, lentils/rice, lentils/sunflower seeds, peas/rye or wheat, or tofu/almonds).

Vitamin B_{12}, in the form of a supplement or in a fortified food (such as fortified soy milk or nutritional yeast), is required for the child who is a vegan, because bioavailable vitamin B_{12} is present only in animal-based foods. Use of algae as a source of vitamin B_{12} may be counterproductive, because vitamin B_{12} from algae does not appear to be bioavailable and may, in excess, actually block vitamin B_{12} metabolism (Dagnelie, 1997). The child who eats a strict vegan diet can also require supplemental riboflavin, zinc, iron, calcium, and vitamin D (Table 12-7).

TABLE 12-7 Vitamins and Minerals at Risk for Deficit in Strict Vegetarian (Vegan) Diets

Vitamin and Minerals at Risk for Deficit	Usual Sources	Alternative Sources in Vegan Diet
Vitamin D	Animal products: egg yolk, butter, liver, salmon, sardines, tuna; sunlight	Fortified cereals, milk, or margarine; sunlight (20-30 min/day, 2-3 times per wk)
Vitamin B_{12}	Animal products only: meat, fish, eggs, dairy products	Fortified soy milk, fortified soy-based meat substitutes, nutritional yeast, fortified cereals, vitamin supplements
Riboflavin	Milk and meat are best sources; also in eggs, dried yeast, grains, dark-green leafy vegetables, avocado, broccoli	Brewer's yeast, wheat germ, beans, almonds, soybeans, tofu, dark-green leafy vegetables, avocado, broccoli, orange juice
Calcium	Milk is best source; also in some fruits, nuts, dark-green leafy vegetables	Fortified soy milk, dried fruits, almonds, sunflower seeds, filberts, whole sesame seeds, green leafy vegetables (avoid spinach, swiss chard, beet greens, whose oxalic acid hinders calcium absorption)
Iron	Iron in meat sources is more bioavailable than iron in plants; lentils, beans (cooked black, soy, garbanzo, lima) are good sources	All legumes, almonds, pecans, dates, prunes, raisins, fortified cereals, white or brown rice; absorption is enhanced by ascorbic acid–rich foods
Zinc	Meats, animal products, seafood (especially oysters), eggs; found in whole grains, brown rice, nuts, spinach; however, best plant sources also contain phytic acid, which inhibits zinc absorption	Whole grains, brown rice, almonds, wheat germ, tofu, pecans, spinach

Because plant-based diets tend to be high in fiber and low in calories, the child may fill up before consuming sufficient calories and nutrients. Children eating a vegetarian diet are advised to eat frequent meals and snacks, concentrating on nutrient-dense foods to achieve adequate energy and nutrient intake.

Nutrition assessment of the child with a vegetarian diet should include regular growth measurements, diet recall and analysis, and laboratory assessment of vitamin B_{12}, zinc, and iron status.

It is important that the NP offer advice and counseling within the context of the child's and family's belief system. But in extreme cases, such as a highly restrictive macrobiotic diet resulting in growth failure or if the child is using vegetarianism as a form of eating disorder, intervention on behalf of the child is necessary, with referral to appropriate health professionals and agencies.

ALTERED PATTERNS OF NUTRITION

Overview

An estimated 10% to 20% of the general pediatric population is affected by chronic illness and handicapping conditions that affect nutritional status (American Dietetic Association, 1995). Special health care needs affecting these children include chronic disorders, chronic illnesses, developmental disabilities, developmental special needs, and handicapping conditions.

Chronic conditions requiring specialized nutrition care are increasing, largely because of expanded screening programs, increased survival rates in children with certain chronic disorders, and improved prognosis for the very small (less than 1500 g), underdeveloped neonate. Increased rates of pediatric human immunodeficiency virus (HIV) infection and prenatal exposure to drugs and alcohol also have enlarged the population of children with special health care needs.

Nutrition and feeding problems are concerns for all children with special needs or disabilities. As many as 80% of children with developmental delay have feeding problems (Manikam & Perman, 2000). Nutrients often found to be inadequate in children with developmental disorders include iron; calcium; niacin; folic acid; vitamins A, C, and D; calories; and fluid.

The nutrition management of children with special health care needs requires input from a multidisciplinary team and is best managed by providing interventions directed at a specifically diagnosed feeding problem.

Physical, occupational, and speech therapists, particularly speech pathologists, can assess head and trunk control, positioning, body mechanics, and oral-motor skills as they relate to feeding. Depending on the child's symptoms and diagnosis, gastroenterologists, allergists, endocrinologists, and other specialists may need to participate in the child's care; surgical as well as medical intervention may be necessary (Manikam & Perman, 2000; Schwarz et al, 2001). For children who are socially or economically deprived, or both, social workers and psychologists are central to appropriate assessment, counseling, and referral to outside services and agencies. The family should be included as an integral component of the team.

In addition to coordinating the medical management of children with special health care needs, the NP must be prepared to carefully assess the nutritional status of this population. Children who meet the criteria outlined in Box 12-3 should be referred to a registered dietitian for comprehensive nutrition assessment and treatment.

Disorders Requiring Increased Caloric Intake

Description

A common nutrition problem in children with special health care needs is inadequate weight gain and delayed growth. Inadequate caloric intake should be suspected in any child with a weight-to-age ratio below the 10th percentile on standardized growth charts. For children who are genetically small or have a disabling condition that limits growth, a weight-to-length ratio or weight-to-height ratio below the 10th percentile indicates suboptimal nutrition.

Incidence and Etiology

The actual incidence of children requiring an increased caloric intake is not known, but it occurs commonly. An estimated 15% to 25% of children seen for developmental disabilities are underweight or growth retarded, or both (Ekvall, 1993).

Caloric needs of children are influenced by multiple factors, and a number of conditions put children at risk for insufficient caloric intake, including the following:

- Conditions in which activity level is increased, either by purposeful or by involuntary muscle work, such as athetoid cerebral palsy, attention-deficit hyperactivity disorder, or chronic lung conditions
- A hypermetabolic state, sometimes complicated by secondary malabsorption, which may be present in the child who has acquired immunodeficiency syndrome (AIDS), cancer, or frequent infections or who has recently had surgery
- Psychosocial factors such as inadequate resources, poor feeding relationship with caregiver, and improper dilution of formula, which can lead to delayed growth and require increased calories for the child's catch-up growth
- Oral-motor impairment or chronic conditions, such as congenital heart disease, which can contribute to fatigue and poor feeding
- Low-birth-weight or premature infants
- Medical treatment (e.g., a child receiving corticosteroid treatment for Crohn's disease)
- Conditions in which malabsorption occurs (e.g., cystic fibrosis)

BOX 12-3 ***Suggested Criteria for Nutrition Referral***

- Markedly overweight or underweight (height or length for weight below the 5th or above the 95th percentile)
- Mechanical feeding difficulties or neuromotor dysfunction
- Feeding skills below those anticipated for developmental level or mental age
- Unusual food habits (e.g., pica or food faddism)
- Inadequate or imbalanced dietary intake, according to dietary history or 24-hour recall
- Nutrition treatment central to medical management (e.g., inborn errors of metabolism, diabetes, malabsorption syndromes, allergy)
- Overt physical signs of nutritional deficiency (e.g., extremely underweight, anemia)
- Emotional disturbances and associated feeding and nutrition problems (e.g., anorexia nervosa, autism)
- At high risk for compromised nutritional status (e.g., takes stimulant or anticonvulsive drugs, family below poverty level, inadequate housing, pregnant adolescent)

Adapted from Ekvall SW, Ekvall VK, Frazier T: Dealing with nutrition problems of children with developmental disorders, *Topics Clin Nutr* 8(4):51-57, 1993.

Clinical Assessment and Findings

History. A thorough history should be taken, assessing for the following:

- Type and amount of foods and liquids consumed (e.g., nutrient content and consistency)
- Amount of food that falls from utensils, cups, or bottles during feeding and is not ingested
- Physical effort and time required for meal
- Any impaired oral functions (e.g., tongue thrust, drooling, difficulty chewing, choking, or aspiration)
- Position of child during feeding
- Family's pattern of feeding child (e.g., time, place, utensils used)
- Child's apparent food likes and dislikes

Physical Examination. Anthropometric measures are reliable indicators of a child's growth and development, especially if accurately measured and compared over time. Appendix B provides standard growth and BMI charts, as well as growth charts for premature infants. These charts can be used to determine whether the child is following a consistent growth curve. Growth charts specific to children with Down syndrome, myelomeningocele, Prader-Willi syndrome, sickle cell anemia, and Turner syndrome have also been developed (see Resource Box). Anthropometric measures taken at each visit can include the following:

- Height
- Weight
- Weight-to-height ratio
- Basal metabolic index
- Head circumference
- Arm circumference
- Skinfold measurements

A feeding evaluation can be included in the physical examination, particularly for the child with oral-motor or behavioral problems associated with eating. Such an evaluation is usually conducted by a multidisciplinary team of primary health care provider, physician specialist such as a gastroenterologist, dietitian, speech pathologist, and physical or occupational therapist (or both). In this type of assessment, parents or caregivers are asked to replicate the home experience, using the same types of foods, utensils, and positioning. If possible, the parents should videotape the child eating at home, and providers should review the video with them. By observing the interaction between the child and the caregiver during feeding, the health care team can more accurately assess feeding success and problems, as well as emotional or psychologic issues related to feeding.

Laboratory Studies. Laboratory studies are done as indicated:

- Hematocrit or hemoglobin
- Serum ferritin and transferrin levels
- Metabolic screening (chemistry screen)

Initial basic workup for failure to thrive (FTT) includes the following:

- Complete blood count (CBC) with reticulocytes
- Thyroid studies
- Chemistry screen
- Urinalysis, with culture and sensitivity
- Stool for ova and parasites
- Stool culture for enteric pathogens (e.g., *E. coli*)
- Bone age

Clinical Findings. When a child is malnourished, regardless of etiology, the nutritional insult follows a predictable course. In the early stages, the child maintains or begins losing weight. If poor intake continues, the child's linear growth slows or ceases. Finally, head circumference, indicating compromised brain development, levels off.

Other signs of inadequate nutrition include the following:

- Anemia
- Pallor
- Fatigue
- Vulnerability to infections
- Delayed healing
- Behavior problems
- Inactivity
- Irritability
- Poor academic performance, poor vocabulary
- Perceptual difficulties

Management

The management of the child with delayed growth or poor weight gain varies with the underlying cause of the problem and can require the intervention of specialists. Although the NP can coordinate the plan of care, a team approach to management is optimal.

A child with an increased activity level, a metabolic condition that increases energy requirements, or a condition that decreases the body's ability to absorb nutrients needs to receive caloric- and nutrient-dense meals and snacks at 2- to 4-hour intervals.

A child with a chronic disease that decreases the appetite (e.g., AIDS, cancer) needs creative approaches that consider food preferences, optimal times of day for snacks and meals, and family dynamics that encourage eating.

A child with a condition that affects oral-motor control will need special equipment, specific feeding techniques, proper positioning, and use of foods and liquids with appropriate consistency to improve oral intake.

A child who is not receiving enough food because of neglect, inadequate financial resources, or other psychosocial factors requires referral to appropriate health care professionals and social services. The community health nurse can be an invaluable resource for these children.

Although feeding by the oral route is preferable from a developmental perspective, tube feedings may be indicated. Frequently, a medical crisis precipitates the use of supplemental tube feedings.

Premature or low-birth-weight infants (particularly those with a poor suck) frequently require supplemental feedings. Breastfeeding is both possible and desirable for these infants, and ensuring that they receive higher-fat hindmilk is important; pumping may be necessary (see Chapter 13). Human milk fortifiers or premature formulas that increase the caloric density from 20 kcal/oz to 24 kcal/oz are often fed to premature neonates. Regular infant formulas can be mixed to increase the kcal/oz ratio from 20 kcal/oz to 24 kcal/oz or 27 kcal/oz, and nutrient-dense formulas for older infants and children are available (see Box 12-1). Care must be taken that infants do not receive too much protein in concentrated infant formulas, because the breakdown and excretion of excess protein by the kidneys may place an excessive demand on the renal system.

Practical suggestions for increasing calories, protein, and nutrients needed for weight gain and growth are outlined in Box 12-4. A "complete" multivitamin and mineral supplement is also recommended, because it contains the entire spectrum of these nutrients and can usually be chewed or crushed and mixed into soft foods.

Increasing intake of calories, protein, and nutrients to age-specific norms is not sufficient for children who are underweight or growth retarded. Catch-up growth requires an excess of calories and protein until growth is normalized. A method for calculating calories and protein required for catch-up growth is presented in Box 12-5. Calculations for catch-up growth in children with chronic diseases that contribute to poor weight gain (e.g., cystic fibrosis) can be found in more detailed nutrition texts.

Additionally, some chronic conditions require more complex treatment. Early treatment with growth hormone may be helpful for some children (Simon et al, 2002).

Frequent monitoring of the child with inadequate caloric intake is necessary. Infants should be weighed at least weekly and length and head circumference measured once a month. Children older than 2 years of age should be measured for height and weight at least once a month.

BOX 12-4 *Suggestions for Increasing Energy Intake*

- Use readily available, economical foods that are familiar to the child.
- Fortify milk by adding 1 cup of nonfat dry milk powder to 1 qt of whole milk. Drink or use to prepare cooked cereals, creamed soups, pancakes, pudding, milkshakes (do *not* use with children younger than 2 years of age).
- Add additional margarine or cheese to potatoes, vegetables, casseroles, rice, pasta, cooked cereals, etc.
- Encourage high-calorie snacks such as fruit juice, dried fruits, nuts, bananas, cheese cubes, pudding or custard, cereal with whole milk, fruit yogurt (alone or as a dip for fruit), cheese or peanut butter on crackers, olives, sliced or mashed avocado (as a dip for vegetables or crackers).
- Add instant breakfast mixes to whole milk.
- Use commercially prepared formula with high caloric content.
- Use commercial liquid supplements such as Pediasure or Pediasure with fiber (Ross Laboratories) for children with lactose intolerance.
- Establish regular times for meals and snacks, 2 to 4 hours apart. Do not allow the child to nibble continually on small amounts of food.
- Keep mealtimes relaxed and pleasant. Avoid scolding, nagging, or force feeding.
- Allow the infant or child to provide cues regarding hunger and satiety.

Complications

The child with inadequate caloric intake often displays a multitude of other nutrient deficiencies. A direct connection has been established between inadequate nutrition and mental and physical abilities. In the child with a chronic medical condition, compromised nutrition contributes to frequent illness, medical complications, and impaired development.

The etiology of growth retardation is multifactorial, including genetic disorders, in utero insults (e.g., maternal infection, fetal alcohol syndrome), neurologic impairments, metabolic disorders, and environmental deprivation. In many of these physiologic disorders, restoring nutritional status does not ultimately resolve growth deficits. In the case of environmental deprivation, the success of catch-up growth depends on the timing, length, and severity of the nutritional insult.

BOX 12-5 *Estimating Catch-up Growth Requirements**

$$\text{Catch-up growth requirement (kcal/kg/day)} = \frac{\text{Calories required for weight age (kcal/kg/day)} \times \text{Ideal weight for age (kg)}}{\text{Actual weight (kg)}}$$

1. Plot the child's height and weight on the CDC growth charts.
2. Determine at what age the present weight would be at the 50th percentile (weight age).
3. Determine recommended calories for weight age (see Table 12-1).
4. Determine the ideal weight (50th percentile) for the child's present age.
5. Multiply the value obtained in step 3 by the value obtained in step 4.
6. Divide the value obtained in step 5 by actual weight.

Estimated protein requirements during catch-up growth can be calculated similarly (see Table 12-2):

$$\text{Protein requirement (g)} = \frac{\text{Protein required for weight age (g)} \times \text{Ideal weight for age (kg)}}{\text{Actual weight (kg)}}$$

Adapted from Rathbun JM, Peterson KE: Nutrition in failure to thrive. In Grand RJ, Sutphen JL, Dietz WH, editors: *Pediatric nutrition*, Boston, 1987, Butterworth.

*Guidelines are used to estimate catch-up growth requirements. Precise individual needs vary and are mediated by medical status and diagnosis.

CDC, Centers for Disease Control and Prevention.

Complications of treatment must also be considered for children with caloric deficits. The NP must be alert to negative effects of a sudden change to a high-calorie, high-protein diet. As discussed previously, a dramatic increase in protein can increase renal solute load to the point where a child is at risk for dehydration. The child on a high-protein diet should be counseled to drink adequate fluids. Diarrhea can result from an abrupt increase in carbohydrates owing to their high osmolality. Gradually changing the child's diet can decrease these negative effects.

Disorders Requiring Decreased Caloric Intake

Description

Health conditions that contribute to decreased metabolic activity in children require changes in nutritional intake. If children's caloric intake exceeds their metabolic needs, excessive weight gain, even obesity, can occur, placing the child at risk for additional health problems. The assessment and management of obesity is discussed later in this chapter as an eating disorder. This section looks specifically at medical conditions that contribute to excessive weight gain.

Incidence and Etiology

Any disorder or disability that reduces energy output places the child at risk for obesity. Obesity is common, for example, in children with Prader-Willi syndrome, myelomeningocele, or Down syndrome.

The child with Prader-Willi syndrome is hypotonic and may demonstrate dysphagia and failure to thrive as an infant. By 3 to 4 years of age, the child becomes hyperphagic, lacking the internal regulation responsible for satiety. In addition to abnormally high food intake, children with Prader-Willi syndrome are short in stature.

Obesity occurs in 50% of children with spina bifida. Energy expenditure in nonambulatory children with myelodysplasia is estimated at only 25% to 50% of that of children who are walking (Ekvall, 1993).

Most children with Down syndrome have short stature, and before age 3 years, children with Down syndrome may have a low weight-to-height ratio. The Down syndrome growth chart should be used to evaluate height and weight. As a result of a lower resting metabolic rate or hypothyroidism, the child with Down syndrome requires fewer calories than children without the syndrome, and obesity is common, but not inevitable. Healthy eating and exercise habits begun in early childhood can help prevent obesity.

Clinical Assessment and Findings

History. The history should assess for the following:

- Level of physical activity in which child engages (see Table 12-1)
- Diet recall (3 day)
- Mealtime patterns
- Concerns and attitudes of parents and child regarding weight gain
- Previous interventions or attempts to control weight

Physical Examination. Key components of the physical examination include the following:

- Weight-to-height or weight-to-length ratio
- Triceps skinfold measurement
- Midarm circumference
- Body frame type
- Muscle mass
- BMI

Laboratory Studies. Laboratory studies include those for thyroxine and circulating thyroid-stimulating hormone to rule out hypothyroidism. Because of sequelae associated with obesity, children should be monitored at least annually for the following:

- Hypertension
- Blood sugar
- Complete lipid profile
- Liver function

Clinical Findings. The following clinical findings indicate level of obesity:

- Weight-to-height ratio greater than 75% on growth chart may indicate mild obesity.
- Weight-to-height ratio greater than 95% on growth chart may indicate significant obesity.
- Triceps skinfold measurement greater than 85% of norm is a diagnostic criterion for obesity in children.
- BMI in 85th percentile may indicate obesity.

A child's growth pattern is evaluated over time. A child who is consistently in the 85% weight-to-height ratio may be genetically programmed to be big, whereas a child who suddenly zooms from the 60% to the 90% weight-to-height ratio can be developing a weight problem.

Management

Children with medical conditions that decrease caloric need often require special management. The goal of nutrition management is to ensure that the child receives adequate nutrients without excessive caloric intake.

Because of the reduced energy expenditure of children with impaired mobility, Prader-Willi syndrome, spina bifida, Down syndrome, or other such disorders, caloric intake needs to be restricted. A referral to a registered dietitian is recommended to establish an appropriate caloric level and eating plan individualized to each child's growth needs.

A complete multivitamin with mineral supplement is recommended, because a restrictive diet can result in nutrient deficiencies.

Whenever possible, children with a disorder that is associated with decreased caloric need should be encouraged to increase their energy expenditure through physical activity. The goal is to both increase calories used and increase the child's level of fitness. A team approach, involving a physical or recreational therapist, or both, is advised when developing exercise strategies for these children.

In some cases, access to food needs to be rigidly enforced (e.g., in children with brain dysfunction affecting hypothalamic control or Prader-Willi syndrome). The family, school, and other care environments need to provide limited access to food, which may include locks on refrigerators, cupboards, and garbage cans.

Frequent monitoring is necessary in order to assess compliance and devise alternate strategies as indicated; weekly weight and monthly height measurements are recommended.

Support for families and children is essential. Despite the best efforts, many children gain excess weight. The NP needs to model and encourage a positive, accepting attitude toward the child, independent of weight gain or loss.

Disorders Requiring Restricted or Supplemental Diets

Description

The body's ability to absorb and metabolize nutrients is compromised when hormone, enzyme, or cofactor activity necessary for metabolism is either excessive or deficient or when physiologic conditions limit absorption of nutrients. Under these conditions, nutritional intake must be adjusted to maximize the body's ability to use foods. Diet restrictions or supplemental nutrients, or both, can be essential for optimal growth and development.

Table 12-8 lists several metabolic conditions seen in the primary care setting that affect children's nutritional status. A number of defects of absorption or transport affect nutritional status in children; most are rare, but the NP may be part of the team managing the care of a child with inflammatory bowel disease (Crohn's disease or ulcerative colitis), short bowel syndrome, or celiac disease.

Incidence and Etiology

Most metabolic disorders are rare, although type 1 diabetes mellitus affects about 1.9 in 1000 school-age children, and cystic fibrosis is seen in 1 in 3500 white infants. An estimated 1 in 70 individuals in the United States is a carrier of phenylketonuria (PKU); only about 1 in 10,000 persons has this autosomal recessive disease.

The etiology of metabolic disorders can differ from one individual to another. Some disorders are considered to be inborn errors of metabolism (e.g., PKU). Genetic conditions other than inborn errors of metabolism, autoimmune diseases, surgical intervention, drugs and medications,

TABLE 12-8 Metabolic Conditions Affecting Nutrition in Children

Excessive Hormone/Enzyme Production	Deficient Hormone/Enzyme Production
Pancreas	
Reactive hypoglycemia	Diabetes mellitus
Organic or fasting hypoglycemia	Cystic fibrosis
Thyroid	
Hyperthyroidism	Hypothyroidism
Graves' disease	
Parathyroid	
Hyperparathyroidism	Hypoparathyroidism
Adrenal Cortex	
Cushing syndrome	Addison's disease
Corticosteroid therapy	
Inborn Errors of Metabolism	
	Phenylketonuria (deficiency of phenylalanine hydroxylase)
	Maple syrup urine disease
	Tyrosinemia
	Galactosemia

tumors, and infectious disease also contribute to metabolic dysfunction and problems of absorption or transport. For some individuals, a genetic predisposition to the disorder can be triggered by environmental factors, and the disorder appears later in life.

Clinical Assessment and Findings

Clinical findings related to specific disorders are discussed in Unit IV. If nutrition is inadequate in children with these chronic conditions, clinical signs and symptoms worsen, pathophysiologic processes of the disorder accelerate, and growth is attenuated.

Management

Disorders of absorption and metabolism are usually managed with specialized diagnostic tests and treatments and require the efforts of a coordinated health care team. Although not a cure for disease, nutrition is an essential component of treatment plans and can make a critical difference in the child's outcome. The goals of nutritional intervention include the following:

- Provide adequate nutrients for normal growth and development
- Maintain optimal level of health
- Prevent or delay development of complications associated with disease progression (e.g., diarrhea, fistulas)
- Prevent or delay need for more aggressive intervention (e.g., surgical bowel resection)

Nutritional intervention in chronic disorders can be extremely complex. Referral to a registered dietitian is necessary, and the NP should consult frequently with the dietitian when providing primary care to the child.

In some conditions, dietary restrictions are lifelong requirements; success of dietary intervention depends on the child's and family's willingness to adhere to the plan of care. Cooperation is enhanced if the child and family are actively included in decision making and if meal plans are developed that minimize disruption to the family's lifestyle while maximizing flexibility and normalcy for the child. Families and children must be given ample opportunity to express their concerns and frustrations regarding the child's condition. The NP's support, empathy, and encouragement can be vital elements in determining how well a family copes with the child's chronic condition.

Certain principles of nutrition related to disorders of absorption and metabolism guide the dietitian, NP, and family as they create diet plans. Boxes 12-6 through 12-9 outline these principles for several specific conditions.

Complications

See Unit IV for complications of specific disorders. Additionally, pregnant women with phenylalanine levels greater than 10 mg/dl are at great risk of injuring their fetus. When phenylalanine levels exceed 20 mg/dl, 90% of infants will have intrauterine growth retardation, microcephaly, and mental retardation. Approximately 1 in 30,000 women in the general population has a phenylalanine level high enough to damage her fetus or contribute to a spontaneous abortion, but not necessarily high enough to hurt her. All pregnant women should be questioned about a history of PKU or special diets during childhood, and maternal PKU should be considered in any woman who has delivered a microcephalic offspring or experienced spontaneous abortion.

Disorders Requiring Physical Alterations in Diet Management

Description

Physical conditions such as cleft lip or palate, esophageal atresia, cerebral palsy, gastroesophageal reflux, and pyloric stenosis can create difficulty sucking, chewing, swallowing, or retaining food and liquids in the gastrointestinal tract.

BOX 12-6 *Principles for Dietary Management of Diabetes Mellitus*

- Individualize diet. There are many types of meal planning systems for diabetics; identify one that works best for child and family.
- Space food intake to account for type of insulin used.
- Structure diet to include foods that everyone else eats; do not be overrestrictive; use insulin coverage to allow child to eat as typical a diet as possible.
- Vary specific nutrient intakes depending on child's age, size, and activity level.

General guidelines for nutrients include the following:

Energy

- Intake is essentially same as for child without diabetes; energy demands vary with growth spurts, exercise.
- Maintain plasma glucose as near normal physiologic range as possible.

Carbohydrates

- Obtain 55% to 60% of total calories from carbohydrates. Complex carbohydrates are recommended; limit simple sugars; small amounts can be acceptable as part of a mixed meal.
- Emphasize consistent intake of carbohydrates from day to day.
- Include 25 to 40 g per 1000 kcal/day of fiber; increase fiber as complex carbohydrates are increased.
- Increase carbohydrates 10 to 30 g/hr (depending on level of exertion) for intensive exercise; best effect if intake is several hours preceding exercise.

Protein

- Same as for child without diabetes.

Fat

- Same as for child without diabetes.

Vitamins and Minerals

- Same as for child without diabetes; if diabetes is poorly controlled, supplements are recommended.

Sweeteners

- Noncaloric sweeteners such as aspartame and saccharine are acceptable but not encouraged; no long-term adverse effects of artificial sweeteners have been noted.
- Caloric sweeteners such as fructose, sucrose, glucose, sorbitol, and mannitol can be used (with caution) as a substitute for carbohydrate calories.
- Excess sorbitol intake can contribute to diarrhea.

Incidence and Etiology

Most of these conditions are congenital in nature, and a combination of environmental, hereditary, and behavioral factors appears to influence their development. Stenoses, atresias, or fistulas can also be secondary to environmental trauma such as a chemical burn. Incidence varies by condition, with approximately 1 in 750 white children born with cleft lip and 1 in 2500 with cleft palate in the United States each year. Boys are more likely to have a cleft lip with or without a cleft palate, and Asian children are most likely and black children least likely to have clefts (Behrman, Kliegman, & Jenson, 2004). Pyloric stenosis, occurring in about 3 in 1000 births, is four times more common in boys, especially first-born; it is more frequent in children with Down syndrome and white children of Northern European heritage. It is rare in Asian children. Esophageal atresia occurs in 1 in about 4000 live births. In more than 90% of cases, it is accompanied by a tracheoesophageal fistula (Behrman, Kliegman, & Jenson, 2004).

Gastroesophageal reflux (GER) is common in normal individuals following a meal and can be exacerbated by increased intraabdominal pressure (as with crying, coughing, defecation, or external pressure from movement or position). GER in infants can occur during, immediately after, or several hours after a feeding. Children with insufficient lower esophageal sphincter tone are especially susceptible to GER.

BOX 12-7 *Principles for Dietary Management of Cystic Fibrosis*

- Nutrients needed (high protein, high fat, high energy) may cause physical distress; work with family to help them understand the balance between comfort and adequate nutrition sought.
- Small, frequent meals, eaten slowly, are better tolerated.
- Consume nutrient-dense foods; avoid "empty calories."
- Increase fluid intake to prevent dehydration and help liquefy secretions.
- Assess intake on a 3- to 5-day diet record rather than daily.

General guidelines for nutrients include the following:

Energy

- Energy needs are increased as a result of malabsorption of nutrients, extra effort needed for respirations and frequent pulmonary infections.
- Vary caloric intake for each child, depending on condition, activity, and growth.

Carbohydrates

- Obtain 40% to 50% of total calories from carbohydrates. Simple sugars may be better tolerated than complex carbohydrates.
- Include extra fiber; increase fiber as complex carbohydrates are increased.

Protein

- Higher need than for children without cystic fibrosis; 15% to 20% of caloric intake should be in proteins.
- Breastfed children may need supplements (e.g., casein hydrolysates).

Fat

- Increase to level of tolerance, as much as 40% to 50% of total caloric intake.
- Use medium-chain triglyceride oils to enhance absorption and decrease steatorrhea.
- Use corn or soy oil and include absorbable linoleic acid in diet to ensure essential fatty acid intake.

Vitamins and Minerals

- Daily multivitamin supplement and water-soluble preparation of vitamins A, D, and E are advised; 50 to 100 μg/day of vitamin K is recommended.
- Daily calcium supplements are necessary.
- Normal diet is usually adequate to replace sodium lost through excessive sweat; can use salt tablets (intake is more easily monitored than adding salt to diet) if exercise or fever leads to profuse sweating.

Supplements

- Pancreatic enzymes are indicated.
- Other supplements include casein hydrolysates and powdered or liquid nutrient-dense preparations.

Reflux becomes symptomatic early in life, peaks at about 4 months of age, and spontaneously resolves for most children by 12 to 24 months of age (Behrman, Kliegman, & Jenson, 2004).

Children with cerebral palsy or other neurodevelopmental problems can have difficulty chewing or maintaining coordinated suck-swallow skills. GER is also a common problem in children with cerebral palsy, and if the etiology for food refusal cannot be determined, GER may be a likely explanation.

Clinical Assessment and Findings

History. A thorough history of the infant's feeding patterns, incidence of gagging or vomiting, timing of emesis in relation to feeding, character and quantity of emesis, and associated symptoms is essential. Parents also should be asked about treatments they have tried and whether they have been successful.

Physical Examination. Clinical signs can be present at birth, and a diagnosis of the underlying condition, such as cleft lip or palate, can be made in the delivery room.

BOX 12-8 *Principles for Dietary Management of Phenylketonuria*

- Intervene promptly. Infants who begin treatment before 3 weeks of age do not suffer mental retardation secondary to phenylketonuria (PKU).
- All children require phenylalanine in their diet.
- Recommended daily intake of phenylalanine decreases with age. Dietary restrictions continue for life.
- Most foods contain phenylalanine (approximately 5% of all protein is phenylalanine).
- The goal of PKU dietary therapy is to prevent excess phenylalanine accumulation in the body.
- Involve older children in preparation of nutritional supplements.
- Supplements may be more palatable if served as frozen drinks or flavored with juices or fruits.

General guidelines for nutrients include the following:

Energy, Carbohydrate, Fat, Vitamin, and Mineral

- Requirements are same as for child without PKU. Restrictions on high-phenylalanine carbohydrates.
- Daily multivitamin is recommended.
- Nutrient requirements not met by commercial formulas must be supplemented by a phenylalanine-deficient food.

Protein

- Same protein requirements as for child without PKU.
- Phenylalanine intake is restricted. Dietary intake to maintain serum phenylalanine levels between 2 and 10 mg/dl in children. Plasma phenylalanine levels greater than 6 mg/dl should be controlled with dietary therapy.
- Low/minimal phenylalanine-deficient medical foods are necessary to meet protein requirements.

BOX 12-9 *Principles for Dietary Management of Inflammatory Bowel Disease*

- Restrict irritating and poorly absorbed foods (e.g., carbonated beverages, fried foods).
- Decrease intake of foods that stimulate peristalsis (e.g., high-fiber foods) during inflammatory periods. High-fiber foods, especially those that retain water, can be introduced as clinical signs and symptoms decrease.
- Small, frequent meals are better tolerated.
- Vary specific nutrient intakes depending on child's age, size, activity level, and severity of disease. Mild disease can still require supplemental formulas; severe disease can require enteral elemental nutrition via tube feeding, or total parenteral nutrition.
- Condition can be complicated by lactose or gluten intolerance.

General guidelines for nutrients include the following:

Energy

- Teens need 40 to 50 kcal/kg of ideal body weight per day; younger children need up to 120 kcal/kg of ideal body weight per day.

Protein

- Greater than 1.5 g/kg of ideal body weight per day.

Fat

- Low fat (40 g/day) intake is necessary.
- Emulsified fats or medium-chain triglycerides (commercial preparation) are better tolerated.

Vitamins and Minerals

- Take a 100% to 150% daily multivitamin with minerals supplement.
- May need additional vitamin and mineral supplements (e.g., water-soluble vitamins, vitamin B_{12} intramuscularly), folic acid, iron, zinc, copper, calcium, potassium, and magnesium.

Roentgenography and endoscopy are diagnostic techniques used to confirm atresias or fistulas. Some conditions, such as pyloric stenosis, occur later in the neonatal period.

Management. The treatment goals related to conditions that require biomechanical or physical intervention include the following:

- Provide adequate nutrients for normal growth and development
- Provide increased calories to add more weight if needed before surgical procedures
- Strengthen infant's resistance to infection
- Prepare infant to tolerate stress of surgical procedures
- Facilitate healing processes postoperatively
- Ensure correct development and use of oral-facial and oropharyngeal muscles and structures
- Minimize disruption of family processes
- Prevent development of feeding problems

Some conditions require surgical correction of the underlying condition. In many cases (e.g., a simple cleft lip), initial surgical intervention is sufficient and the child progresses normally. In others, especially for the child with serious or multiple anomalies, long-term treatment is required. However, the treatment itself can lead to problems that require further management. For example, correction of esophageal atresia, tracheoesophageal fistulas, or presence of a tracheostomy can result in scarring and strictures, which, in turn, put the child at risk for impaired swallowing, choking, and aspiration. See Table 12-9 for strategies related to feeding in children with cleft lip or palate.

GER usually can be managed in the outpatient setting. Most babies "spit up," especially when burped or placed in certain positions directly after a feeding. A small regurgitation of undigested formula or breast milk is usually not of concern, but GER puts the infant at risk for esophagitis, pulmonary infection, and failure to thrive. See Table 12-10 for specific suggestions related to managing GER.

The NP must also support parents emotionally and psychologically as they care for their children. Parents of a child with birth anomalies can suffer shock, loss, or disappointment and may find it difficult to accept their child; they can experience a wide range of feelings, including guilt, rejection, or anger. Difficult feeding or uncertainty about the child's long-term prognosis adds additional pressure to parents who are already facing an extremely

TABLE 12-9 ***Strategies for Feeding in Children with Cleft Lip or Palate***

Age	Problem Presented	Management Strategy
Infants	Poor suction when nursing Nasal regurgitation	Individualize position used to feed infant; semiupright (60-90 degrees) position is often most effective. Breastfeed if possible; experiment with nipple position: position nipple toward side of mouth, do not put nipple into cleft. Use of longer, soft, or cross-cut nipples and squeezable bottles assists in infants with weak suck. Use of prosthetic device may be helpful. Wean child by 12 mo of age. Tube or gavage feedings may be necessary in severe cleft.
	Swallows air Fatigue	Burp frequently. Allow sufficient time for feeding; work toward providing adequate nutrients in 30 min.
Toddlers	Risk of aspiration Nasal regurgitation	Encourage use of cup, spoon, finger foods as developmentally appropriate. Avoid small, hard, sticky foods that can lodge in palate opening; supervise feeding.
School-age children and adolescents	Malocclusion Difficulty coordinating chewing, swallowing, and breathing Aspiration	Dental referral and treatment are essential. Teach child how to chew, swallow, and breathe, not to talk and chew at the same time. Cut food into small pieces; child can take sips of water while eating. Inform parents that child will chew with mouth open.
	Anorexia secondary to decreased sense of taste/smell	Plan diets that stimulate appetite; provide child's favorite foods.

TABLE 12-10 *Strategies for Feeding in Children with Gastroesophageal Reflux*

Condition	Management Strategies
Mild	Keep child in slightly upright position (10-15 degrees) after feeding; do not elevate head too much because it will cause scrunched over or slouched position that puts pressure on abdomen. Burp frequently during feeding. Thicken formula with rice cereal if bottle feeding to decrease episodes of vomiting.
Moderate to severe	Position infant on left side or supine after feeding; use folded and rolled blankets to keep child in position. Prone position should be used only if complications of gastroesophageal reflux outweigh risk of sudden infant death syndrome (SIDS) (Rudolph et al, 2001). Consult with pediatric gastroenterologist. Medication may be indicated (see Chapter 33). Surgical referral may be necessary in cases that do not respond to medical management.

stressful situation. Creating a positive feeding experience can facilitate a healthy parent-infant bond. The NP can intervene in the following ways:

- Encourage parents to express their feelings
- Listen without judging, acknowledging those feelings
- Demonstrate techniques that increase feeding success
- Explain the child's condition, treatments, and prognoses, both short and long term
- Emphasize how the parent can be involved in the child's progress
- Encourage parents to make decisions related to their child's care; provide suggestions and guidance as the child grows, as treatment is carried out, and as needs change

Complications. Aspiration, failure to thrive, poor parent-child bond, esophagitis, and esophageal strictures are complications of difficulty in feeding.

Eating Disorders

An eating disorder is defined as "a situation where the time spent eating (or not eating) in response to an external stimulus is greater than the time spent eating in response to internal hunger cues" (Hahn, 1998). Anorexia nervosa and bulimia are two eating disorders seen in the pediatric population. Obesity can also be considered an eating disorder since many people who are obese focus on food and its external cues rather than their body's messages about hunger and satiety.

Anorexia Nervosa and Bulimia

Description. Individuals with anorexia nervosa claim to feel fat even when underweight or emaciated, have an intense fear of becoming obese (the fear does not decrease as weight loss progresses), and actively seek to reduce their weight further. Anorexia nervosa is also characterized by weight loss to a body weight that is 15% less than ideal body weight for age with no known physical illness that would account for such loss and, in girls, absence of at least three consecutive menstrual cycles when they are expected to occur (Behrman, Kliegman, & Jenson, 2004).

Bulimia is defined as a pattern of binge eating, followed by attempts to lose weight through self-induced vomiting, severely restricted diets, fasting, and use of laxatives or diuretics. Bulimia may be present in children of normal weight as well as in children who are overweight.

Incidence and Etiology. Anorexia nervosa occurs most often in adolescent girls (about 1 in 100), although approximately 10% of anorexics are males; a bimodal distribution of the condition is present, with peaks at 14.5 and 18 years. Initially found only in middle- and upper-class girls in the United States, anorexia has been diagnosed in all social classes and in some other countries (Behrman, Kliegman, & Jenson, 2004). Bulimia peaks in later adolescence, at about age 18 to 19 years, with binge eating occurring approximately 2 years before purging begins (Stice et al, 1998).

A specific cause for these eating disorders is unknown, though a number of etiologic theories are suggested, including psychodynamic, biologic, behavioral, sociocultural, and family systems theories. A relationship between eating disorders and child sexual abuse is evident, but further research on the specifics of that relationship is necessary (Smolak & Murnen, 2002). Poor attachment, insecurity, and fear of abandonment have been identified as factors contributing to eating disorders in some young women (Ramacciotti et al, 2001). Bulimia appears to have a significant element of learned behavior, acquired through modeling among peers (Stice et al, 1998), and negative affect may lead to purging (Tyrka et al, 2002).

Clinical Assessment and Findings. Diagnosing anorexia or bulimia can be difficult. Some clinical findings characteristic of these eating disorders are also seen in the healthy adolescent. For example, it is not uncommon for a 14-year-old girl who is neither anorexic nor bulimic to express concern about her body appearance, stating that she is too fat or ugly. Additionally, adolescents with anorexia or bulimia, and their families, can work hard to hide their condition, denying problems or presenting a mature, self-sufficient, and successful facade. Early in the disease process, the family system may appear to be coherent, making it difficult to collect accurate data about family relations and behavior patterns that contribute to eating disorders.

Assessment using the Eating disorder Screen for Primary care (ESP) or the SCOFF questionnaire has been found to be highly reliable in the primary care clinical setting (Box 12-10).

Clinical Assessment and Findings—Anorexia Nervosa

History. The history should assess for the following:

- FTT as a child
- Amenorrhea
- Dizziness, syncope
- Expresses pleasure with weight loss
- Denies hunger
- States, "I feel fat," even though not overweight
- Preoccupied with food; often fixes elaborate meals but does not eat; has rituals associated with food
- Attempts to lose weight through diets, exercise, or self-induced vomiting
- Hides eating habits, lies about intake
- Displays social isolation and mood changes: irritable, sullen, hostile, introverted, unhappy, intolerant of others, can have suicidal ideation
- Has fixed, highly structured schedule, inflexible to change

Physical Examination. The physical examination may reveal the following:

- Growth parameters: decreased height-to-weight ratio; weight 25% below ideal for age and height
- Abdomen: pain and distention, decreased bowel sounds
- Skin: dry, rough, cracked, yellowish or grayish color; mucous membranes dry, dull; edema
- Hair: thin, brittle, dull, can have alopecia, bristle hairs on scalp, lanugo on body
- Muscles: weak, decreased definition and mass
- Sensory: lack of concentration, drowsy, confused, irritable, apathetic
- Vital signs: decreased temperature, pulse, respirations, blood pressure for age and weight

BOX 12-10 *Screening Questions for Eating Disorders*

SCOFF Questions*

†Do you make yourself **Sick** because you feel uncomfortably full?
†Do you worry you have lost **Control** over how much you eat?
Have you recently lost more than **One** stone (14 lb or 7.7 kg) in a 3-month period?
Do you believe yourself to be **Fat** when others say you are too thin?
Would you say that **Food** dominates your life?

Eating Disorder Screen for Primary Care (ESP) Questions

‡Are you satisfied with your eating patterns? (No = abnormal answer)
†Do you ever eat in secret? (Yes = abnormal answer)
‡Does your weight affect the way you feel about yourself?
§Have any members of your family suffered with an eating disorder?
†Do you currently suffer with or have you ever suffered in the past with an eating disorder?

SCOFF questions from Luck AJ et al: The SCOFF questionnaire and clinical interview for eating disorders in general practice: comparative study, *BMJ* 325:755-756, 2002. ESP questions from Cotton MA, Ball C, Robinson P: Four simple questions can help screen for eating disorders, *J Gen Intern Med* 18:53-56, 2003.
*One point for every "yes"; a score of 2 indicates a likely case of anorexia nervosa or bulimia.
†Best questions for ruling in an eating disorder. Cotton and colleagues (2003) recommend using these four questions as basic screening tool; needs to be tested further on large-scale population for validation.
‡Best questions for ruling out an eating disorder.
§Question was not helpful in distinguishing eating disorders; recommend deleting from screening tool.

Laboratory. Laboratory studies are done as indicated:
- Hematocrit, hemoglobin, transferrin (decreased amounts)
- Serum glucose, albumin, electrolytes (decreased); may have hypernatremia
- Liver enzymes (elevated liver function)
- Thyroid function (low thyroxine)
- Creatine phosphokinase (elevated)
- Electrocardiogram (ECG) (abnormalities)

Clinical Assessment and Findings—Bulimia

History. The history may include
- Excessive concern about weight
- Weight fluctuation
- Pattern of strict dieting followed by eating binges
- Plans for binge eating
- Frequent overeating, often used as a coping mechanism to manage stress
- Guilt expressed about eating
- Self-induced vomiting after bingeing; hematemesis
- Pattern of hiding information about bingeing and purging
- Complaints of frequent diarrhea or constipation
- Gregarious behavior but evidence of mood swings, especially depression
- Other destructive behaviors: shoplifting, substance abuse
- Family history of chaos, abuse, sexual abuse

Physical Examination. The physical examination may indicate
- Usually normal weight, can range from obese to severely underweight
- Tooth decay, lost enamel
- Enlarged parotid glands
- Skin: dry, rough, cracked, sores on mucous membranes of mouth and around fingernails, broken blood vessels in face; edema
- Weakness, fatigue
- Cardiac arrythmias
- Decreased blood pressure for age or weight

Laboratory. Laboratory studies are done as for anorexia nervosa.

Differential Diagnosis (Anorexia and Bulimia). The differential diagnoses for anorexia and bulimia include
- Diabetes
- Hyperthyroidism
- Inflammatory bowel disease
- Malignancy/central nervous system neoplasm
- AIDS
- Pregnancy
- Systemic lupus erythematosus
- Depression
- Substance abuse

Management. Management of children and adolescents with anorexia nervosa or bulimia is difficult, in part because the child, family, and even the health care provider often deny the significance of the problem. Diagnosis can be delayed and treatment inadequate. Because the issue is not food but, rather, sociopsychologic dynamics of control in the child's life, effective treatment is complex and long term (American Dietetic Association, 2001). Treatment must include both psychologic and physiologic interventions, and referral to psychiatric therapists and medical specialists can be essential. The multidisciplinary team dealing with a child with an eating disorder can experience high levels of stress and uncertainty (Garcia de Amusquibar, 2000). Specific treatment modalities vary, depending on the age of the child (Robb, 2001), the severity of the condition, and causal factors, and can include the following:
- Hospitalization to stabilize fluids, electrolytes, and nutrient intake
- Medications and supplementation
- Antidepressants (e.g., fluoxetine)
- Estrogen
- Progesterone
- Minerals (potassium, calcium, phosphate, zinc, magnesium, iron)
- Folate
- Individual psychotherapy
- Group psychotherapy
- Family therapy
- Nutritional counseling
- Assertiveness training
- Body work: relaxation, biofeedback, movement therapy

Complications. The complications of anorexia nervosa or bulimia include
- Death, usually secondary to cardiac arrhythmia, hypokalemia, congestive heart failure, or suicide
- Alcohol and drug addictions
- Osteoporosis
- Gastrointestinal disturbance: ulcers, motility disorders
- Fertility problems
- Gynecologic problems related to prolonged amenorrhea
- Growth retardation
- Dehydration

Obesity

Description. Excessive adipose tissue is the hallmark of obesity. A gain in adipose tissue can be related to an increase either in the size of fat cells (hypertrophy) or in the number of fat cells (hyperplasia). Childhood-onset obesity that is hyperplastic in nature is especially difficult to control, because fat cells can be reduced in size but not in number. Ideal body weight–to–height ratio and BMI are used to define parameters of obesity. Ideal body weight is calculated based on the Centers for Disease Control and Prevention (CDC) growth charts (Table 12-11).

TABLE 12-11 ***Calculation of Ideal Body Weight from Centers for Disease Control and Prevention Growth Charts****

% Ideal Body Weight for Healthy Children	Interpretation
>120%	Overweight
90%-110%	Normal
80%-90%	Mildly underweight
70%-79%	Moderately underweight
<70%	Severely underweight

*% Ideal body weight = Current weight divided by weight at 50th percentile for current stature multiplied by 100.

In adults, normal BMI ranges from 18.5 to 24.9, and an individual is defined as obese if BMI is 30 or greater. For children older than 2 years of age, use of BMI for groups may be appropriate, but it must be used cautiously to assess individual children (see Appendix B). Some children are genetically large boned and have a body weight or BMI in excess of the norm for their age, gender, and height without having excess fat; athletic adolescents may have a higher BMI as a result of heavier muscle mass with little body fat.

Incidence and Etiology. Although studies indicate a decline in dietary fat intake since 1990, rates of childhood obesity have increased dramatically. The National Heart, Lung, and Blood Institute found that the percent of overweight girls in California, Ohio, and Washington, D.C., populations nearly doubled in the 10 years of the Institute's Growth Study. Black girls were more likely to be overweight and obese than whites, with 30.6% versus 22.4% overweight at age 9 and 56.9% versus 41.3% overweight at age 19. Nearly 18% of black girls and 7.7% of white girls were obese at age 9, and one third of black girls and almost 20% of white girls were obese at age 19 (Kimm et al, 2002). Older children who are obese and obese children who have an obese parent are more likely to be obese as adults (Whitaker, 2002).

Obesity results from a complex relationship between genetics, environment (e.g., exercise, caloric intake), and the body's response to environmental factors (e.g., neurohormonal regulation of the body's set point). Biologic factors (e.g., the hormone leptin as a regulator of body weight or satiety) and genetics may affect one's susceptibility to obesity. The contribution that genetics versus environment makes in the obese child is not entirely clear, because, just as parents pass on genetic traits, they also influence lifestyle habits and set patterns associated with eating and activity. A young child whose mother has a BMI of 27 or more is at risk for obesity (Bergmann et al, 2003). Some of that risk may lie with genetic factors, but the dietary and exercise habits in which parents engage and model for their children also contribute to obesity. Other risk factors or predictors of obesity include maternal smoking during pregnancy, bottle feeding, low socioeconomic status, binge eating in response to overvaluation of body image, social stresses to be thin, depression, and low self-esteem (Bergmann et al, 2003; Stice, Presnell, & Spangler, 2002).

Sedentary activity contributes to obesity, and American children are participating less in physical activity and more in sedentary behavior. A National Institute of Child Health and Human Development study found that one group of third-grade children participated in less than 25 minutes per week of moderate physical activity during physical education classes (Nader, 2003). The Youth Risk Behavior Surveillance for the United States in 1999 indicated that about two thirds of all students, and just over half of girls (less than half of black girls), reported that they had participated in vigorous physical activity for at least 20 minutes on more than 3 of the previous 7 days. Only about one quarter of students participated in moderate physical activity (more than 30 minutes on more than 5 of the last 7 days) (CDC, 2000). Children with chronic conditions that limit physical activity are especially susceptible to excessive weight gain.

Watching television, playing computer games, and talking on the telephone are all examples of sedentary behaviors in which children engage. Nationally, children ages 2 through 18 spend an average of over 4 hours a day watching videos or television, playing video games, or using the computer. One third of these children watch television for more than 3 hours a day, and 17% watch television for more than 5 hours a day (Kaiser Family Foundation, 1999). Older children, blacks, and boys tend to watch more television (CDC, 2000).

A positive relationship has been noted between the time spent watching television and levels of body weight and fat for some children (Lowry et al, 2002). Besides replacing active play, the exposure to television advertising increases the likelihood that children will snack on low-nutrient-dense foods.

Psychosocial factors also contribute to the increased incidence of obesity, particularly in regard to family dysfunction. Children who suffer neglect or abuse or have an overcontrolling parent may turn to food for comfort and solace.

Clinical Assessment and Findings

History. Overweight children may actually eat less than their normal-weight counterparts, but they tend to have lower energy output (Rocandio, Ansotegui, & Arroyo, 2001). Therefore the history must look at patterns of eating and exercise for both the child and the family system, including the following:

- Dietary intake
- Total caloric intake
- Fat intake as percentage of total calories
- Carbohydrate intake as percentage of total calories
- Nutrient adequacy of diet
- Exercise pattern
- Parental obesity
- Time of onset of obesity
- Family history of diabetes
- Episodes of sleep apnea
- Social adjustment, peer group, friends
- Family readiness to participate in a weight management treatment program

Physical Examination. A complete physical examination is necessary to determine the child's level of fitness, looking especially at the following:

- Blood pressure
- Vital signs
- Height and weight
- Ideal body weight (see Table 12-11)
- BMI
- Tricep skinfold
- Midarm circumference
- Skin (for acanthosis nigricans)

Laboratory

- Fasting lipid screen
- Fasting glucose tolerance test may be indicated in children with a family history of diabetes
- Thyroid screen, thyroid-stimulating hormone, T4

Differential Diagnosis. The differential diagnosis includes medical conditions such as hypothyroidism, Down syndrome, and Prader-Willi syndrome that contribute to obesity in children.

Management. The primary goal of weight management in children is to normalize weight, not reduce weight. Because most children are in a rapid growth and development phase, recommendations for treating obesity center on slowing the rate of weight gain, thereby allowing children to grow into their weight. Restricting fat and calories in infants is not recommended because of the rapid neurologic development occurring at this age.

Treatment goals include supporting the child and family as they change lifestyle patterns that lead to excessive weight gain. Even though children must be monitored for height and weight on a regular basis, progress should be measured by other parameters as well. Improved dietary habits, increased physical activity, and enhanced self-esteem are significant endpoints that should be acknowledged and praised by the family and health care team alike.

The American Dietetic Association (1999) recommends that children should develop healthful eating patterns, including adequate fiber, no excessive fat intake, and the nutrients recommended for their age. Children should also increase their level of activity.

A Maternal and Child Health Bureau committee of pediatric obesity experts (Barlow & Dietz, 1998) recommends the following:

- Use of either weight loss or weight maintenance strategies, depending on child's age, baseline BMI percentile, and presence of medical complications
- Early treatment (in infancy if child is obese)
- Family-centered treatment, with emphasis on parenting skills
- Increased activity
- Decreased high-fat and high-calorie foods
- Stepwise interventions with a goal of long-term change
- Ongoing support for families

When counseling obese children and their parents, the NP is advised to emphasize a family-centered approach. When the entire family changes to a more healthful diet and engages in regular physical activity, the obese child has a much greater chance at weight normalization. This approach also tends to be positive rather than punitive and thereby helps raise the child's self-esteem. Parents who overly restrict their children's intake, or who demand that children eat even when not hungry, actually contribute to the problem of overeating and obesity (Fisher & Birch, 2002). Box 12-11 provides useful approaches and suggestions to use when counseling obese children and their families.

BOX 12-11 *Guidelines for Managing Childhood Obesity*

- Do not put child on a diet. Instead, gradually modify the entire family's eating habits. For example, serve fruit as a substitute for dessert, switch to nonfat or 1% milk, experiment with low-fat recipes and methods of food preparation, and use reduced-fat margarine, salad dressings, and other low-fat condiments. Serve nutritionally dense foods that reflect the Food Guide Pyramid, including whole grains, fruits, vegetables, lean protein foods, and low-fat dairy products.
- Do not force children to clean their plates. They should eat only until they are full.
- Schedule and enforce regular times for meals and snacks. Do not skip meals. Do not allow childen to nibble throughout the day.
- Have low-calorie, nutritious snacks readily available, such as air-popped popcorn, pretzels, low-fat yogurt, frozen fruit juice bars, skim milk, low-sugar cereals, fresh fruit, and raw vegetables.
- Do not have high-calorie snacks readily available (e.g., potato chips, cookies, cakes, pies, ice cream, candy, soda pop, and doughnuts).
- Promote physical activity. Make daily exercise a priority. Encourage family participation, individual exercise, and team sports and structured activities with peers.
- Limit television viewing. Children who watch 4 or more hours of television per day are twice as likely as other children to become obese. Children are more sedentary when they watch television, and frequent food advertising has been linked to increased snacking.
- Scale back television watching slowly, replacing time with activities, hobbies, or chores.
- Praise and reward children for the progress they make in reaching nutrition, activity, self-esteem, or weight goals.
- Emphasize the uniqueness of each child, pointing out special talents, abilities, and positive qualities.

Complications. Children who are obese are at much higher risk for related conditions, including hypertension, impaired glucose tolerance, sleep apnea, orthopedic problems (e.g., slipped capital epiphysis), social rejection, and lowered self-esteem. In the child with a physical disability, obesity can further impair mobility and reduce energy expenditure.

Adverse Food Reactions

Description

A distinction is made between *food allergy*, a hypersensitivity to a food or food additive with either an immediate or a delayed immune system response (e.g., anaphylactic reaction to ingestion of nuts), and *food intolerance*, a nonimmunologic inability to process or tolerate the food product (e.g., PKU secondary to the body's inability to metabolize phenylalanine) (Fig. 12-4). Both are considered adverse reactions to food.

Incidence and Etiology

Many individuals believe they have a food allergy or intolerance. This perception, however, may not be accurate. Only about 1% to 2% of individuals meet the criteria of having "either a positive double-blind, placebo-controlled food challenge or an unequivocal report of a reaction with the typical features of an immunoglobulin E (IgE)–mediated severe allergic or anaphylactic reaction" (Hourihane, 1998). Eight foods—cow's milk, hen's eggs, peanuts, soya, wheat, fish, crustacea, and tree nuts (including almonds and cashews)—account for nearly 90% of actual IgE-mediated allergic reactions (Burks, James, & Hiegel, 1998). Any food, however, can cause reactions in a specific individual, and food is the most common cause of anaphylaxis in children (Clark & Ewan, 2003). Factors contributing to adverse food reactions include the following:

- *Heredity.* A child with one parent with a food allergy has a 30% to 35% chance of developing the condition; if both parents have food allergies, the child's chances increase to 65%. Children born with a metabolic disorder (e.g., deficient lactase enzyme) can have adverse reactions to specific foods.
- *Immature gastrointestinal tract.* Before 7 months of age, the infant gastrointestinal tract is more permeable to large molecules, including most food proteins.
- *Compromised gastrointestinal tract.* As a result of injury or illness, the gastrointestinal system can be more permeable to allergens such as large proteins.
- *Type of food.* Some foods are more allergenic than others, and some individuals have greater sensitivity to certain foods.
- *Allergic load or tolerance level.* Conditions such as illness, stress, surgery, or trauma can place excessive metabolic demands on the body. An individual who is susceptible

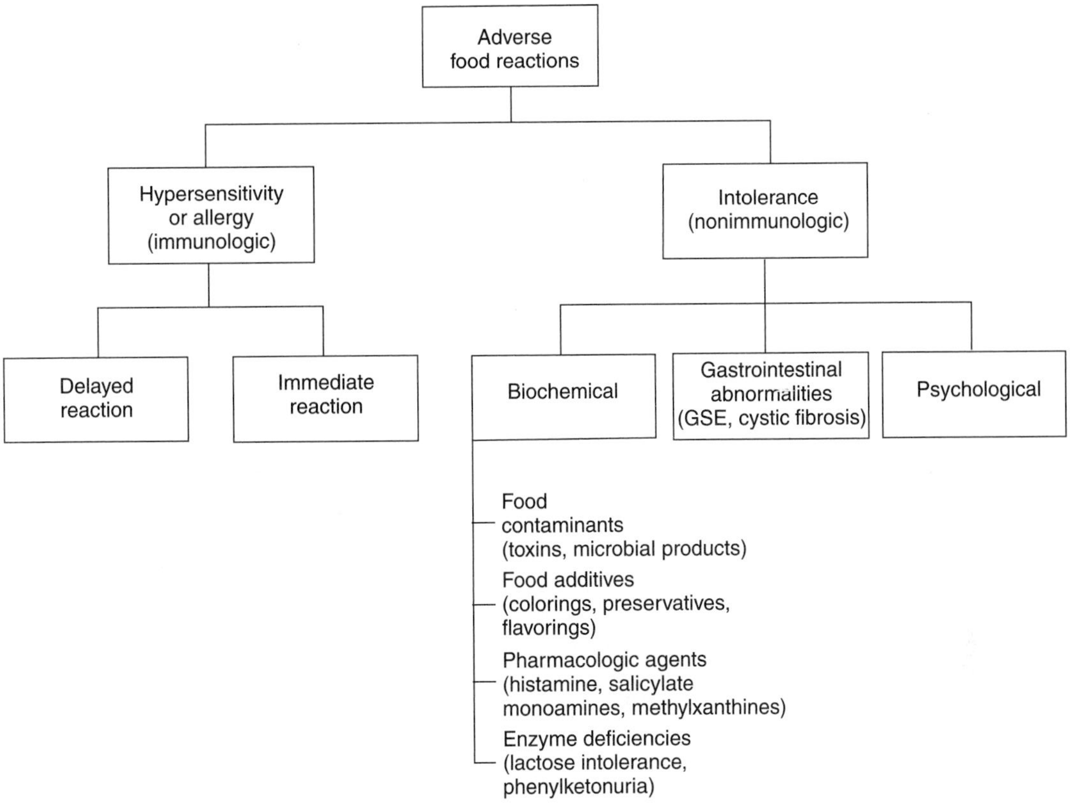

FIGURE 12-4 Adverse food reactions. (From Davis J, Sherer K: *Applied nutrition and diet therapy for nurses*, Philadelphia, 1994, WB Saunders.)

to food intolerance or allergy can have a reaction when these conditions are present. Additionally, frequent exposure or exposure to large quantities of the allergen can lead to a reaction.

Clinical Assessment and Findings

The goals of clinical assessment are to determine whether an adverse food reaction is present, distinguish between an allergy and a food intolerance, determine the degree of severity of the problem, and identify the source or sources of the problem. This process is extremely challenging and can require referral to a registered dietitian or use of a team approach with NP, dietitian, and allergist for a more in-depth diagnostic workup. The basic examination includes the history, physical examination, laboratory studies, and food elimination and challenge.

History. The history should assess the following:

- Is there a family history of allergies, especially a history of reaction to certain foods?
- Does the child have a history of symptoms frequently seen in food allergies (e.g., respiratory distress, eczema, urticaria, rashes, colic, vomiting, diarrhea), unaccompanied by other signs of illness or history of exposure to infectious agents?
- Does the child have a history of symptoms following ingestion of food?
- Description of symptoms
- Time of onset of symptoms related to food intake
- Type and quantity of food ingested
- Description of other factors that are present and may contribute to or aggravate an allergic response (e.g., stress, environment, exercise)
- What is the child's diet history? When and what types of foods were introduced into the diet?

Describe the child's usual intake. A food diary is an excellent mechanism for obtaining these data and includes the following:

- All foods and fluids ingested for at least 3 days
- How food is prepared (e.g., commercially, at home, fried, baked)
- How food is stored and fed to the child
- All medications

Physical Examination. Signs and symptoms of adverse food reactions vary by type and severity, from a mild local reaction to life-threatening anaphylaxis, making it difficult to diagnose the condition definitively. Table 12-12 lists possible clinical manifestations of food allergies or intolerances by body system, and Table 12-13 relates clinical features of a reaction to the level of severity of the child's condition. The most critical problem in food allergies is respiratory compromise, which may mimic asthma (Clark & Ewan, 2003).

Laboratory Studies. Laboratory studies assist in distinguishing between food allergies and intolerances. Tests include

- Serum IgE and eosinophil count (elevated serum IgE and eosinophilia greater than 400/mm^3 are related to allergies)
- Skin tests
- Radioallergosorbent tests
- Metabolic screening tests (e.g., PKU)

Food Elimination and Challenge. When a food has been identified as a potential source of the problem, the process of elimination and challenge is used to confirm the diagnosis. Referral to an allergist or immunologist for such a challenge is necessary. The suspected foods are completely eliminated from the child's diet for at least 2 weeks and reintroduced one at a time. An allergy or intolerance is confirmed if symptoms cease when the food is eliminated

TABLE 12-12 ***Possible Clinical Manifestations of Food Allergies or Intolerances by Body System***

System	Symptoms
Respiratory system	Chronic rhinitis Asthma Croup Cough Serous otitis media Bronchitis
Gastrointestinal system	Swelling of lips, mouth, throat Nausea, vomiting Diarrhea Colic Protein-losing enteropathy Bloating, flatulence Constipation Gastrointestinal blood loss Malabsorption
Integumentary system	Eczema Pruritus Atopic dermatitis Rashes Urticaria
Central nervous system	Headaches (sinus, migraine) Fatigue Drowsiness, listlessness Irritability Depression Excessive sweating
Circulatory system	Hypotension Cardiac arrhythmias Anaphylaxis Pallor

From Davis J, Sherer K: *Applied nutrition and diet therapy for nurses*, Philadelphia, 1994, WB Saunders.

TABLE 12-13 Severity of Allergic Reactions to Foods

Severity	Clinical Manifestations
1. Mild	Localized cutaneous erythema/urticaria/angioedema/oral pruritis
2. Mild	Generalized erythema/urticaria/angioedema
3. Mild	At least 1 or 2 (above) plus gastrointestinal symptoms/rhinoconjunctivitis
4. Moderate	Mild laryngeal edema/mild asthma
5. Severe	Marked dypsnea; hypotension

Adapted from Clark AT, Ewan PW: Food allergy in childhood, *Arch Dis Child* 88:79-81, 2003.
/, and/or.

and then reappear as it is reintroduced. If multiple foods are suspected or if the potential reaction to a food is severe, the process of elimination and challenge in the outpatient setting may not be feasible, and the child may need to be hospitalized for diagnostic evaluation.

Differential Diagnosis

The differential diagnoses for food allergy and food intolerance include

- Reactions related to other environmental allergens
- Asthma due to other causes
- Psychologic reactions to feeding
- Malabsorption syndromes
- Chronic diarrhea

Management

Care of children with adverse food reactions aims to maintain nutrition levels adequate for normal growth and development, prevent nutrient deficits, avoid exposure to offending food or foods, and respond appropriately to episodes of exposure. Achieving these goals requires the coordinated efforts of pediatric allergists, dietitians, the primary care provider, and teachers or child care providers, as well as children and their families.

Once a child has been assessed as to the severity of the condition (see Table 12-13), a treatment plan can be made. Epinephrine is prescribed for children with moderate or severe allergies. Children, their parents, and other caregivers should be educated on intramuscular injection using pre-prepared Epipens. Antihistamines are prescribed for children with mild allergies, unless there is a history of a reaction to trace amounts of the allergen or the child has asthma from another cause. In these cases, epinephrine is appropriate (Clark & Ewan, 2003). Children with food allergies should wear a medical-alert (Medic Alert) bracelet or necklace.

Education of families, children, and adults who are responsible for the child's well-being is critical; the NP can do outreach to teachers, schools, and day care centers with information about how to understand and safely manage the child's condition, as well as be an ongoing source of suggestions, support, and advocacy for parents.

Balancing nutrient requirements with the need to restrict certain foods can be challenging. Not only must the restricted food be replaced with one of equivalent nutrient value, the physical signs of allergies (e.g., diarrhea, vomiting, eczema) can create a need for extra nutrients to maintain health and foster growth. The NP, family, and child should work with a dietitian to structure dietary care.

Once the offending food has been identified, elimination or rotation diets can be planned. Elimination diets seek to remove the food completely. Elimination of the food is required for highly allergenic foods. This can be difficult, especially when purchasing processed or prepared foods or eating in restaurants. Table 12-14 lists foods that are likely to contain more common allergens. With a rotation diet, items in "food families" are rotated every 4 to 5 days, reducing the potential food allergy load and allowing the child to tolerate a more diverse diet. Strict rotation diets appear to be most effective when the child has multiple, mild food allergies.

Because food allergies and intolerances, especially to foods such as milk and eggs, are often outgrown, it may be appropriate to carefully challenge the child with most offending foods every year or two. There is some research to indicate that children may not outgrow their allergy, but its immediate effect is masked as the child grows. Obvious and immediate problems are gone, but long-term problems may occur (Hodson, 1992). Many fatalities related to food allergies occur among older children, teenagers, and young adults. Some foods appear to remain allergenic for longer periods (e.g., seafood). If the child's reaction has been serious or even life threatening, the parents may decide to continue to avoid the food. Children with allergies to nuts should never be challenged.

Management of food intolerances secondary to metabolic disorders is discussed earlier in this chapter (see Disorders Requiring Restricted or Supplemental Diets).

Complications

Complications of adverse food reactions include the following:

- Anaphylaxis
- Convulsive coughing and sneezing, leading to aspiration or choking

TABLE 12-14 *Common Foods Containing Allergens*

Foods Likely to Contain	May Be Listed on Label As	Substitutes
Milk		
Milk	Milk	Soy milks
Buttermilk	Milk solids	Nut milks
Hot chocolate	Buttermilk solids	Milk-free shakes
Many nondairy products	Curds	Some nondairy creamers
Many baked goods	Whey solids	Baked goods without milk
Many baking mixes	Whey	Most French breads
Granola	Casein	Bagels, saltines
Cheese	Lactalbumin	Soy cheese
Prepared meats (hot dogs, luncheon meats)	Caseinate	Kosher-prepared meats
Macaroni and cheese	Cream	Products labeled parve or pareve
Canned spaghetti	Sodium caseinate	Foods prepared without milk or butter (e.g., potatoes, scrambled egg casseroles)
Potatoes mashed with milk or butter		
Vegetables in cream, cheese, or butter sauces		Milk-free margarines, salad dressings, sauces, and gravies
Many margarines		Milk-free sherbets, ices, and sorbets
Many salad dressings		Frozen tofu desserts
Imitation sour cream		Cornstarch puddings with fruit juice
Some gravies		Jello
Ice cream		
Some sherbets		
Yogurt		
Puddings		
Egg		
Eggnog	Albumin	Egg-free baked goods and specialty items
Root beers	Egg white	Pasta, rice, potatoes, egg-free substitutes
Many baked goods	Egg white solids	Prepared meats and imitation seafood without egg products
Pancakes, waffles, French toast	Egg yolk	
Egg noodles	Yolks	Soups without egg products
Eggs		Imitation mayonnaise, sauces, and salad dressings prepared without egg products
Most egg substitutes		
Many prepared meats (hot dogs, luncheon meats, imitation seafood)		Cornstarch, tapioca puddings prepared without eggs
		Baked goods prepared without eggs
Many batter-dipped foods		
Noodle soups		
Mayonnaise		
Hollandaise sauce		
Many salad dressings		
Tartar sauce		
Custards		
Puddings		
Boiled frostings		
Meringues		
Macaroons		
Marshmallow products		
Fondants and other candies		
Wheat		
Instant breakfast	Wheat	Breads and other wheat-free baked goods
Postum	Flour	Wheat-free cereals, Rice Chex, Cream of Rice
Many baked goods	Wheat bran	Rice cakes and crackers
Most baking mixes	Wheat germ	Rye crackers
Pancakes, waffles	Wheat starch	Cornmeal coating
Many cereals	Gluten	Corn tortillas

TABLE 12-14 *Common Foods Containing Allergens—cont'd*

Foods Likely to Contain	May Be Listed on Label As	Substitutes
Many crackers	Graham flour	Rice, corn pasta
Breaded foods	Enriched flour	Meat products without wheat added
Wheat tortillas	Durum flour	Gravies and sauces thickened with cornstarch, potato starch
Pasta, noodles	Vegetable gums	Homemade baked goods made without wheat
Prepared meat products, hot dogs, luncheon meats	Modified food starch	Worcestershire sauce
Gravies and sauces thickened with flour	Vegetable starches	Salt
Cakes, cookies, pies	Malted cereal syrup	Popcorn, corn chips
Soy sauce	Hydrolyzed vegetable protein	
Pretzels	Semolina	
Beer, including nonalcoholic beer		
Soy		
Soy formula	Soy	Casein hydrolysate formula
Soy milks	Soy flour	Milk or nut milks
Nondairy creamers	Soy protein	Homemade breakfast shake
Instant breakfast	Soy protein isolate	Breads, cereals, and crackers made without soy
Many baked goods	Hydrolyzed vegetable protein	
Many baking mixes		
Corn		
Carbonated beverages	Corn	Flavored seltzer
Many sweetened fruit drinks	Cornstarch	Fruit juice
Instant breakfast	Corn syrup	Homemade breakfast shake
Many bread products	Corn oil†	Breads, crackers, and cereals made without corn products
Many cereals	Corn sweeteners	Wheat tortillas
Many crackers	Corn syrup solids	Processed meats made without corn products
Some baking and pancake mixes	High-fructose corn syrup	Peanut butter without added sweeteners
Corn tortillas	Maltodextrin	Foods without corn sweeteners or other corn products added
Some processed meats	Vegetable oil†	Other oils
Imitation seafood		Soy-free margarines or butter
Imitation cheese		Homemade dressings made without corn oil
Peanut butter with corn syrup added		Fresh fruit or packed in own juice
Canned spaghetti and sauces		Sugar, pure maple syrup, or honey
Canned baked beans		Pure fruit spreads
Canned soups		Frozen desserts without added corn sweeteners
Au gratin potato mixes		Featherweight baking powder
Vegetable starch		Flour or potato starch
Vegetable gums		
Soybean oil*		
Vegetable shortening*		
Hydrogenated oils*		
Corn oil†		
Corn oil margarine†		
Salad dressing†		
Pancake syrup		
Jellies and jams		
Popsicles and ice cream		
Most baking powders		
Catsup and barbecue sauce		

Adapted from Mahan LK, Escott-Stump S: *Krause's food nutrition and diet therapy*, ed 10, Philadelphia, 2000, WB Saunders.
*Tolerated by most people with soy allergy. Caution is advised for those with a history of anaphylaxis.
†Tolerated by most people with corn allergy. Caution is advised for those with a history of anaphylaxis.

- Malnutrition
- Gastrointestinal dysfunction
- Secondary skin infections
- Disruption of family processes

Prevention

The best treatment for food allergies and intolerances is prevention. Ideally, all infants should be breastfed for a minimum of 4 to 6 months and for 12 months if possible; infants who have been identified as being at high risk for adverse reactions, especially allergies, should be exclusively breastfed until 6 months of age (Chandra, 1997). If formula is used, avoid soy-based or cow's milk–based formula for high-risk infants. Specially prepared formulas such as Nutramigen, Pregestimil, or Alimentum can be appropriate substitutes. The first foods introduced should be hypoallergenic (e.g., rice cereal, squash, bananas). At least 3 to 5 days are allowed between each new food introduced so that any adverse reaction has time to occur. Cow's milk, wheat, corn, and citrus fruits should be avoided completely before 12 months of age.

Breastfeeding mothers of infants at high risk for allergies should avoid allergenic foods as well (e.g., cow's milk, nuts, fish), because the proteins from these foods may be passed to the infant via breast milk. Garlic, onions, cabbage, and broccoli also have been noted to cause gastrointestinal reactions in infants.

Effect of Medications on Nutritional Status

Description

Medications are designed to alter the body's biochemistry in an effort to produce a healing effect. Biochemical processes inherent in drug therapy have implications for the individual's nutritional status. Some medications deplete essential nutrients from the body; others interfere with the body's ability to metabolize nutrients; still others have an adverse affect on the appetite or cause nausea. Although a medication can have an immediate effect on an individual, adverse changes in nutritional status are most often seen after prolonged therapy.

Incidence and Etiology

Drug-induced malnutrition results from drug-related alterations in the body's ability to absorb, distribute, metabolize, utilize, or excrete nutrients and their metabolites (Wynne, Woo, & Millard, 2002). Absorption is affected by characteristics of the molecule being absorbed (size, ionization, lipid solubility), gut motility (too rapid as with diarrhea or too slow as with Hirschsprung's disease), and environment of the gastrointestinal tract (e.g., gastric pH, lack of intrinsic factor). As medications change gastrointestinal motility or environment, they influence the absorption of nutrients.

Distribution of nutrients is affected by plasma protein-binding capabilities, total body water content, and relative fat content in the body. For example, if a drug that binds highly with plasma protein is taken for long periods of time, or if a child has low serum albumin, nutrients have to compete for protein-binding sites.

Metabolism occurs primarily in the liver, and drugs can either inhibit or stimulate hepatic enzyme activity, thus influencing the body's ability to metabolize nutrients for use at the cellular level.

The relationship of medications and nutrients in terms of excretion is less marked than with absorption, distribution, and metabolism, but drugs can have an effect on renal function, especially tubular reabsorption, which has an impact on nutritional status.

Clinical Assessment

Nutritional assessment of children on medication includes the general parameters discussed earlier, such as anthropometric measures, physical examination, and diet history. Specific attention should be paid to those nutrients for which drug therapy places the child at risk of deficiency.

Management

Management involves ongoing assessment and anticipatory intervention to prevent nutritional problems for children on drug therapy. Referral to a dietitian can be helpful. General interventions include the following:

- Alter dietary intake to include more foods containing nutrients affected.
- Supplement diet with required vitamins or minerals, or both.
- Administer medications in a manner that minimizes their impact on nutrition.
- Consider alternative medications and treatment modalities.

See Table 12-15 for dietary suggestions related to specific classes of medication. This list is limited, and a comprehensive pharmacology reference should be consulted for specific drugs.

Complications

Malnutrition, slowed growth, delayed healing, and drug toxicity are complications of the effects of medication on nutritional status.

TABLE 12-15 *Nutritional Risk of Selected Drugs*

Drug Category or Name	Nutritional Risk	Nutritional Intervention
Antibiotic (e.g., chloramphenicol)	Inhibits vitamin K–producing intestinal microflora Increases excretion of riboflavin Nausea, vomiting, diarrhea Decreases absorption of calcium, fat, and protein Decreases lactase activity Suppresses bone marrow (chloramphenicol) May cause aplastic anemia	Use acidophilus tablets, acidophilus milk, or yogurt to replace gastrointestinal organisms Supplement with vitamin C, B-complex vitamins, vitamin B_{12}, biotin, vitamin K, or well-balanced vitamin and mineral supplement Use lactose-reduced milk
Barbiturate (e.g., phenobarbital)	Breaks down vitamin D May cause calcium deficiency, rickets, or osteomalacia May decrease serum folate, vitamin B_{12}, pyridoxine, magnesium May cause nausea, vomiting, constipation	May need vitamin D and calcium supplements Give drug with meals Give high-fiber and high-fluid diet If folic acid supplementation is indicated, administer cautiously
Antihistamine (e.g., cimetidine, diphenhydramine)	Decreases gastric acid secretion, increases pH Decreases absorption of iron, folate, vitamin B_{12} May lead to hyperglycemia May disrupt vitamin D metabolism	
Corticosteroid	Increases protein catabolism and gluconeogenesis; decreases protein synthesis, contributing to nitrogen wasting Stimulates appetite May cause hypokalemia, hyperglycemia, hypernatremia, hypocalcemia associated with osteoporosis May elevate serum lipids	If edema occurs, restrict sodium intake High doses require calcium and vitamin D supplements Supplement with vitamin B_6, vitamin C, and folic acid Increase dietary protein Monitor weight and restrict calories if there is excessive weight gain
Digoxin	May cause anorexia and nausea, weight loss May cause hypokalemia May increase urinary excretion of magnesium and calcium	Increase dietary potassium Evaluate need to increase dietary magnesium and calcium
Isoniazid	Interferes with enzyme pathway for creation of niacin Increases excretion of vitamin B_6 and folic acid May cause nausea and vomiting Decreases absorption of vitamin E Increases absorption of iron May cause hyperglycemia	Give pyridoxine supplement Increase foods high in folate, niacin, vitamin B_6, and magnesium Avoid foods with histamine and tyramine, such as tuna, mackerel, sardines, dry sausages and meats, imitation and hard cheeses, meat and protein extracts, and excessive amounts of caffeine (Davis & Sherer, 1994)
Methotrexate	Folate antagonist, contributes to folate deficiency May cause stomatitis, anorexia, diarrhea Decreases absorption of vitamins A, D, E, and K, β-carotene	Give mineral oil Supplement with multivitamin given midway between times mineral oil is administered Give folate
Oral contraceptive	Increases vitamin A and calcium absorption Causes low serum vitamin C; possibly contributes to low levels of vitamins B_1, B_{12}, B_6, B_2, folate, magnesium, zinc	Increase intake of vitamins C, B_1, B_{12}, B_6, B_2, folate, magnesium, zinc

Continued

TABLE 12-15 *Nutritional Risk of Selected Drugs—cont'd*

Drug Category or Name	Nutritional Risk	Nutritional Intervention
Phenothiazide	Increases excretion of riboflavin	
Hydantoin, phenytoin	May cause nausea, vomiting, constipation May cause hyperglycemia Impairs metabolism and absorption of folate; may lead to megaloblastic anemia Inactivates vitamin D; can lead to osteomalacia Decreases serum vitamin K	Supplement with vitamin D, vitamin K, folate, but excessive folate levels can decrease action of anticonvulsants Administer drug with, or immediately after, a meal
Supplements		
• Calcium	If taken with iron supplement, only calcium carbonate does not affect iron absorption; if taken with fluoride, absorption of both is decreased	
• Zinc	Greater than 1500 mg/day: decreases copper absorption, possibly leading to anemia-related fatigue	
• Iron	Causes nausea, possibly anorexia	
• Theophylline	May cause vitamin B_6 deficiency	Give pyridoxine supplements

Controversies in Pediatric Nutrition

Cow's Milk in Children's Diets

During the first year of life, the use of unmodified cow's milk is contraindicated because of its high protein content, its inappropriate nutrient composition, and the risk of gastrointestinal bleeding and allergic reactions. Instead, infants should receive breast milk or an approved iron-fortified infant formula that closely matches the composition of breast milk. Although most pediatric providers agree on this recommendation, there is some debate about the use of cow's milk in the toddler's diet.

In most cases, children older than 1 year of age can safely drink cow's milk, and it can be recommended as a rich source of protein, calcium, riboflavin, and vitamin D. The calcium and vitamin D are present in highly absorbable forms, and the protein is highly bioavailable. Cow's milk is an easy and sure way for children to receive these essential nutrients. For some children, cow's milk has a detrimental effect; parents may wonder whether the nutrition benefits of cow's milk are worth possible health risks; if the protein and nutrients found in milk are included in the child's diet with other foods, milk may not be necessary.

A small number of children, estimated at less than 5%, have a true milk allergy, evidenced by skin rashes, digestive disturbances, or respiratory symptoms and confirmed by allergy testing. Most of these children eventually outgrow their milk allergy as they mature.

Another condition that can limit dairy product intake by children is lactose intolerance, a condition caused by a lack of the enzyme lactase, normally present in the small intestine. Lactose intolerance is rare in infants but common in older children and adults from Asian, Native American, black, and Hispanic ethnic groups, and an acquired lactose intolerance may follow an episode of viral gastroenteritis in children. The condition causes symptoms of bloating, flatulence, abdominal cramps, and diarrhea between 15 minutes and 2 hours after the consumption of foods containing lactose. Children with low lactase levels may be able to digest small amounts of milk and other dairy products. Yogurt, aged cheese, and fermented dairy products, which are much lower in lactose than milk, are usually better tolerated. Commercial preparations are also available (e.g., Lactaid) that break down the lactose in milk.

Effects of Sugar

Widely perceived as causing hyperactive behavior among children, controlled scientific studies have failed to demonstrate a link between sugar and behavior or cognitive performance (Krummel, Seligson, & Guthrie, 1996; Wolraich, Wilson, & White, 1996). Anecdotal reports from parents

RESOURCE BOX

Nutrition Issues

ALLERGIES

Allergy Information and Referral Hotline
1-800-822-2762

Asthma and Allergy Foundation of America
1-800-727-8462
www.aafa.org

Food Allergy Center
Program of Alpha Nutrition
1-800-937-7354
www.nutramed.com/allergy/foodallergy.htm

The Food Allergy Network
1-800-929-4040
www.foodallergy.org

EATING DISORDERS

American Anorexia Bulimia Association, Inc.
212-575-6200

Anorexia Nervosa and Related Eating Disorders (ANRED)
Affiliated with National Eating Disorders Association (NEDA)
1-800-931-2237 (NEDA)
www.anred.com

National Association of Anorexia Nervosa and Associated Disorders
Hotline: 1-847-831-3438

Shapedown
Child and adolescent obesity weight control program
1-415-453-8886
www.shapedown.com

National Eating Disorders Centre (Canada)
1-866-633-4220
www.nedic.ca

DIABETES

American Diabetes Association
1-800-342-2383
www.diabetes.org
English and Spanish-speaking assistance

Juvenile Diabetes Research Foundation International
www.jdrf.org

GASTROINTESTINAL DISEASES

Celiac Sprue Association/United States of America, Inc.
1-402-558-0600
www.csaceliacs.org

Celiac Disease Foundation
1-818-990-2354
www.celiac.org

Canadian Celiac Association
1-800-363-7296
www.celiac.ca

Crohn's and Colitis Foundation of America
www.ccfa.org

Gluten Intolerance Group
1-206-246-6652
www.gluten.net

PULMONARY DISEASES

Cystic Fibrosis Foundation
1-800-344-4823
www.cff.org

GROWTH CHARTS FOR CHILDREN WITH SPECIAL CONDITIONS

In Hall J, Frostr-Iskenius UG, Allanson JE: *The handbook of normal physical measurements*, Oxford, 1989, Oxford University Press.

- Achondroplasia height and head circumference, male and female
- Marfan syndrome height
- Noonan syndrome height
- Prader-Willi height
- Williams syndrome height
- Arthrogryposis-amyoplasia, height and distal heights, male and female
- Multiple ptergium height, male and female
- Diastrophic dysplasia height
- Pseudoachondroplasia height
- Spondyloepiphyseal dysplasia congenita height
- Turner syndrome

From Child Development and Rehabilitation Center, Genetics Clinic, 1-503-494-8307:

- Myelomeningocele height and weight, male and female, ages 2-18 years
- Asian children, height and weight, male and female, ages 0-6 years (also see www.fcc.org)

From Cystic Fibrosis Foundation, 1-800-FIGHT-CF:

- Cystic fibrosis growth chart

From Platt OS: Sickle cell anemia, *N Engl J Med* 311:7, 1984:

- Sickle cell anemia growth chart

Continued

RESOURCE BOX

Nutrition Issues—cont'd

OTHER

About Face USA
Craniofacial conditions
1-800-665-3223
www.aboutfaceusa.org

American Cleft Palate Association
1-800-242-5338
www.cleftline.org

Human Nutrition Information Service/USDA
Public Affairs Staff
1-301-504-5719
www.nal.usda.gov/fnic/

National Center for Nutrition and Dietetics (NCND)
The American Dietetic Association
1-312-899-0040 (Chicago)
1-202-775-8277 (Washington, DC)
Consumer Nutrition Hotline: 1-800-366-1655
www.eatright.org

American School Food Service Association
1-703-739-3900
www.asfsa.org

National Association of School Nurses, Inc.
1-866-627-6767 (Western office)
1-877-627-6476 (Eastern office)
www.nasn.org

NURSING DIAGNOSES RELATED TO NUTRITION: *Functional Health Pattern*

Diagnoses are related to the following concepts: infant feeding pattern, swallowing, nutrition, fluid volume.

- Anorexia (not a NANDA diagnosis)
- Bulimia (DSM-IV diagnosis)
- Ineffective infant feeding pattern
- Impaired swallowing
- Imbalanced nutrition: less than body requirements
- Imbalanced nutrition: more than body requirements
- Readiness for enhanced nutrition
- Deficient fluid volume
- Risk for deficient fluid volume
- Excess fluid volume
- Risk for fluid volume imbalance
- Readiness for enhanced fluid balance
- Nausea

Source: North American Nursing Diagnosis Association: *NANDA nursing diagnoses: definitions and classification 2003-2004*, Philadelphia, 2003, North American Nursing Diagnosis Association.

and teachers reinforce the misconception that sugar adversely affects behavior in children. This misconception may stem from the association between sugar consumption and activities (e.g., birthday parties, Halloween) that often result in excitable behavior among children.

The role of the NP is to educate and reassure parents that moderate sugar consumption rarely results in adverse behavior. High-sugar diets are to be avoided, however, because these foods tend to replace more nutrient-dense foods and contribute to dental caries if eaten frequently throughout the day. Current dietary recommendations are that 10% or less of calories should come from sugar. For the average child who consumes 2000 calories daily, this would amount to 50 g or about 10 teaspoons each day.

Chocolate and Acne

Chocolate is often thought to initiate or worsen acne. Again, no controlled scientific studies have ever established a link between intake of chocolate and the incidence or severity of acne.

REFERENCES

American Academy of Pediatrics Committee on Nutrition: Cholesterol in children, *Pediatrics* 101:141-147, 1998.

American Dental Association: *Fluoridation facts*, Chicago, 2002, American Dental Association.

American Dietetic Association: Position of the American Dietetic Association: dietary guidance for healthy children aged 2 to 11 years, *J Am Diet Assoc* 99:93-101, 1999.

American Dietetic Association: Position of the American Dietetic Association: nutrition intervention in the treatment of anorexia nervosa, bulimia nervosa, and eating disorders not otherwise specified (EDNOS), *J Am Diet Assoc* 101:810-819, 2001.

American Dietetic Association: Position of the American Dietetic Association: nutrition services for children with special health needs, *J Am Diet Assoc* 95:809-812, 1995.

Barlow SE, Dietz WH: Obesity evaluation and treatment: Expert Committee recommendations. The Maternal and Child Health Bureau, Health Resources and Services Administration and the Department of Health and Human Services, *Pediatrics* 102:E29, 1998.

Behrman RE, Kliegman RM, Jenson HB, editors: *Nelson textbook of pediatrics*, ed 17, Philadelphia, 2004, WB Saunders.

Bergmann KE et al: Early determinants of childhood overweight and adiposity in a birth cohort study: role of breast-feeding, *Int J Obes Relat Metab Disord* 27:162-172, 2003.

Burks AW, James JM, Hiegel A: Atopic dermatitis and food hypersensitivity reactions, *J Pediatr* 132:132-136, 1998.

Centers for Disease Control and Prevention: Youth Risk Behavior Surveillance—United States, 1999, *MMWR* 49(SS05):1-96, 2000.

Chandra RK: Five-year follow-up of high-risk infants with family history of allergy who were exclusively breast-fed or fed partial whey hydrosylate, soy, and conventional cow's milk formulas, *J Pediatr Gastroenterol Nutr* 24:380-388, 1997.

Clark AT, Ewan PW: Food allergy in childhood, *Arch Dis Child* 88:79-81, 2003.

Clauss SB, Kwiterovich PO: Long-term safety and efficacy of low fat diets in children and adolescents, *Minerva Pediatr* 54:305-313, 2002.

Cotton MA, Ball C, Robinson P: Four simple questions can help screen for eating disorders, *J Gen Intern Med* 18:53-56, 2003.

Dagnelie PC: Some algae are potentially adequate sources of vitamin B-12 for vegans, *J Nutr* 127:379, 1997.

Davis J, Sherer K: *Applied nutrition and diet therapy for nurses*, ed 2, Philadelphia, 1994, WB Saunders.

Ekvall SW, editor: *Pediatric nutrition in chronic diseases and developmental disorders: prevention, assessment, and treatment*, New York, 1993, Oxford University Press.

Elster AB, Kuznets NJ: *AMA guidelines for adolescent preventive services (GAPS): recommendations and rationale*, Baltimore, 1994, Williams & Wilkins.

Fisher JO, Birch LL: Eating in the absence of hunger and overweight in girls from 5 to 7 y of age, *Am J Clin Nutr* 76:226-231, 2002.

Fisher JO et al: Parental influences on young girls' fruit and vegetable, micronutrient, and fat intakes, *J Am Diet Assoc* 102:58-64, 2002.

Food and Nutrition Board, Institute of Medicine: *Dietary reference intakes for energy, carbohydrates, fiber, fat, fatty acids, cholesterol, protein, and amino acids (macronutrients)*, Washington, DC, 2002, Institute of Medicine.

Garcia de Amusquibar AM: Interdisciplinary team for the treatment of eating disorders, *Eat Weight Disord* 5:223-227, 2000.

Gorrie T, McKinney E, Murray S: *Foundations of maternal-newborn nursing*, Philadelphia, 1998, WB Saunders.

Hahn NI: When food becomes a cry for help: how dietitians can combat childhood eating disorders. Interview with Monika M. Woolsey, *J Am Diet Assoc* 98:395-398, 1998.

Hands ES: *Food finder: food sources of vitamins and minerals*, ed 3, Salem, OR, 1995, ESHA Research.

Hands ES: *Nutrients in foods*, Philadelphia, 2000, Lippincott Williams & Wilkins.

Hattner J, Kerner J: *Approximate composition of pediatric formulas*, Stanford, CA, 1997, Stanford University Medical Center/Lucile Packard Children's Hospital.

Hodson AH: Empirical use of exclusion diets in chronic disorders: discussion paper, *J R Soc Med* 85:556-559, 1992.

Hourihane JO'B: Prevalence and severity of food allergy—need for control, *Allergy* 53(suppl):84-88, 1998.

Joint Working Group of the Canadian Paediatric Society (CPS) and Health Canada: *Nutrition recommendations update: dietary fat and children*, Ottawa, reaffirmed Feb 2001.

Kaiser Family Foundation: *Kids and media at the new millenium (monograph)*, Menlo Park, CA, 1999, Kaiser Family Foundation.

Kimm SY et al: Obesity development during adolescence in a biracial cohort: the NHLBI Growth and Health Study, *Pediatrics* 110:c54, 2002.

Krummel DA, Seligson FH, Guthrie HA: Hyperactivity: is candy causal? *Crit Rev Food Sci Nutr* 36:31-47, 1996.

Lee Y, Birch LL: Diet quality, nutrient intake, weight status, and feeding environments of girls meeting or exceeding the American Academy of Pediatrics recommendations for total dietary fat, *Minerva Pediatr* 54:179-186, 2002.

Lifshitz F, Tarim O: Considerations about dietary fat restrictions for children, *J Nutr* 126(suppl):1031s-1041s, 1996.

Lowry R et al: Television viewing and its associations with overweight, sedentary lifestyle, and insufficient consumption of fruits and vegetables among US high school students: differences by race, ethnicity, and gender, *J Sch Health* 72:413-421, 2002.

Luck AJ et al: The SCOFF questionnaire and clinical interview for eating disorders in general practice: comparative study, *BMJ* 325:755-756, 2002.

Lytle LA et al: Nutrient intake over time in a multi-ethnic sample of youth, *Public Health Nutr* 5:319-328, 2002.

Mahan LK, Escott-Stump S: *Krause's food, nutrition, and diet therapy*, ed 10, Philadelphia, 2000, WB Saunders.

Manikam R, Perman JA: Pediatric feeding disorders, *J Clin Gastroenterol* 30:34-46, 2000.

Manz F, Wentz A, Sichert-Hellert W: The most essential nutrient: defining the adequate intake of water, *J Pediatr* 141:587-592, 2002.

Messina V, Mangels AR: Considerations in planning vegan diets: children, *J Am Diet Assoc* 101:661-669, 2001.

Mitchell MK: *Nutrition across the lifespan*, ed 2, Philadelphia, 2003, WB Saunders.

Munoz KA et al: Food intakes of US children and adolescents compared with recommendations, *Pediatrics* 100:323-329, 1997.

Nader PR: Frequency and intensity of activity of third-grade children in physical education, *Arch Pediatr Adolesc Med* 157:185-190, 2003.

Niinikoski H et al: Growth until 3 years of age in a prospective, randomized trial of a diet with reduced saturated fat and cholesterol, *Pediatrics* 99:687-694, 1997.

North American Nursing Diagnosis Association: *NANDA nursing diagnosis: definitions and classification 2003-2004*, Philadelphia, 2003, North American Nursing Diagnosis Association.

Nutrition Education Services/Oregon Dairy Council: *Pyramid Plus: a star-studded guide to food choices for better health*, Portland, OR, 1994, Nutrition Education Services/Oregon Dairy Council.

Perry CL et al: Adolescent vegetarians: how well do their dietary patterns meet the *Healthy People 2010* objectives? *Arch Pediatr Adolesc* 156:431-437, 2002.

Perry CL et al: Characteristics of vegetarian adolescents in a multiethnic urban population, *J Adolesc Health* 29:406-416, 2001.

Ramacciotti A et al: Attachment processes in eating disorders, *Eat Weight Disord* 6:166-170, 2001.

Rask-Nissila L et al: Effects of diet on the neurologic development of children at 5 years of age: the STRIP project, *J Pediatr* 140:328-333, 2002.

Rathbun JM, Peterson KE: Nutrition in failure to thrive. In Grand RJ, Sutphen JL, Dietz WH, editors: *Pediatric nutrition*, Boston, 1987, Butterworth.

Reinhardt WC, Brevard PB: Integrating the Food Guide Pyramid and Physical Activity Pyramid for positive dietary and physical activity behaviors in adolescents, *J Am Diet Assoc* 102:596-599, 2002.

Robb AS: Eating disorders in children. Diagnosis and age-specific treatment, *Psychiatr Clin North Am* 24:259-270, 2001.

Rocandio AM, Ansotegui L, Arroyo M: Comparison of dietary intake among overweight and non-overweight schoolchildren, *Int J Obes Relat Metab Disord* 25:1651-1655, 2001.

Rudolph CD et al: Pediatric GE reflux clinical practice guidelines, *J Pediatr Gastroenterol Nutr* 32(suppl 2):S1-S31, 2001.

Sabaté J: *Vegetarian nutrition*, Boca Raton, FL, 2001, CRC Press.

Schwarz SM et al: Diagnosis and treatment of feeding disorders in children with developmental disabilities, *Pediatrics* 108:671-676, 2001.

Simon D et al: Treatment of growth failure in juvenile chronic arthritis, *Horm Res* 58(suppl 1):28-32, 2002.

Smolak L, Murnen SK: A meta-analytic examination of the relationship between child sexual abuse and eating disorders, *Int J Eat Disord* 31:136-150, 2002.

Stice E et al: Age of onset for binge eating and purging during late adolescence: a 4-year survival analysis, *J Abnorm Psych* 107:671-675, 1998.

Stice E, Presnell K, Spangler D: Risk factors for binge eating onset in adolescent girls: a 2-year prospective investigation, *Health Psychol* 21:131-138, 2002.

Story M, Holt K, Sofka D, editors: *Bright Futures in practice: nutrition*, ed 2, Arlington, VA, 2002, National Center for Education in Maternal and Child Health.

Suitor CW, Gleason PM: Using dietary reference intake–based methods to estimate the prevalence of inadequate nutrient intake among school-aged children, *J Am Diet Assoc* 102: 530-536, 2002.

Tyrka AR et al: Prospective predictors of the onset of anorexic and bulimic syndromes, *Int J Eat Disord* 32:282-290, 2002.

US Preventive Services Task Force: *Guide to clinical preventive services*, ed 2, Baltimore, 1996, Williams & Wilkins.

Van Horn L et al: A summary of results of the Dietary Intervention Study in Children (DISC): lessons learned, *Prog Cardiovasc Nurs* 18:28-41, 2003.

Whitaker RC: Understanding the complex journey to obesity in early adulthood, *Ann Intern Med* 136:923-925, 2002.

Wolraich ML, Wilson DB, White JW: The effect of sugar on behavior or cognition in children. A meta-analysis, *JAMA* 274:756-757, 1996.

Wosje KS, Specker BL, Giddens J: No differences in growth or body composition from age 12 to 24 months between toddlers consuming 2% milk and toddlers consuming whole milk, *J Am Diet Assoc* 102:53-56, 2002.

Wynne AL, Woo TM, Millard M: *Pharmacotherapeutics for nurse practitioner prescribers*, Philadelphia, 2002, FA Davis.

13 Breastfeeding

Pamela J. Hellings

OVERVIEW

Breast milk provides the ideal food for newborns and infants and supports infant nutrition essential for optimal growth and development. In addition, the parents and the infant receive psychologic, physical, and emotional benefits that last a lifetime. A high priority should be placed on promoting and supporting breastfeeding whenever possible.

Breastfeeding is a learned skill for both the mother and the infant. Nurse practitioners (NPs) have an important role in assessing the mother's knowledge level and in providing information and support to increase the skills of the mother-infant dyad during the transition to a successful breastfeeding experience. More generally, NPs play an important part in the promotion, education, outreach, support, and management of breastfeeding. NPs can teach about the benefits of breast milk so that families can make educated choices about infant feeding. They can provide classes to increase knowledge in order to avoid common problems or assist in the decision to seek consultation for problems. Additionally, the NP's willingness to take the time required to determine the cause of a breastfeeding problem, to develop a plan to address the problem, and to support the family through difficulties may make the difference in continuation of breastfeeding. Among health care professionals, the NP can play a major role by contributing to hospital, clinic, and community committees, advisory boards, and task forces that develop policies to promote and support breastfeeding; advising and educating colleagues on breastfeeding issues; teaching breastfeeding content to students in the health professions; and serving as an expert contact for the media on issues related to breastfeeding. In all these activities, the NP serves an important leadership function in promoting and supporting breastfeeding.

Breastfeeding Recommendations

Major health professional organizations, including the National Association of Pediatric Nurse Practitioners (2001) and the American Academy of Pediatrics (1997), recommend breastfeeding for the first year of life. Despite these strong recommendations, much work remains to be done to meet this goal, and NPs can make a major contribution to the success of breastfeeding efforts.

The Baby-Friendly Hospital Initiative

In 1991 a worldwide effort to recognize hospitals that provide optimal lactation support was developed by the World Health Organization (WHO) and the United Nations International Children's Emergency Fund (UNICEF) (UNICEF, 1992). This effort, known as the Baby-Friendly Hospital Initiative, bases assessment of the quality of a lactation program on 10 steps for successful breastfeeding, delineated in a joint WHO/UNICEF statement (WHO/UNICEF, 1989). Every facility that provides maternity services and care for newborn infants should

- Have a written breastfeeding policy that is routinely communicated to all health care staff
- Train all health care staff in skills necessary to implement this policy
- Inform all pregnant women about the benefits and management of breastfeeding
- Help mothers initiate breastfeeding within a half hour of birth
- Show mothers how to breastfeed and how to maintain lactation even if they are separated from their infants
- Give newborn infants no food or drink other than breast milk, unless medically indicated
- Practice rooming-in (i.e., allow mothers and infants to remain together) 24 hours a day
- Encourage breastfeeding on demand
- Give no artificial teats or pacifiers (also called dummies or soothers) to breastfeeding infants
- Foster the establishment of breastfeeding support groups and refer mothers to them on discharge from the hospital or clinic

Benefits of Breastfeeding

With rare exception, breast milk is the ideal food for the human infant. Each mammalian species provides milk uniquely suited to its offspring, and milk from the human breast is no exception. It is a living fluid rich in vitamins, minerals, fat, proteins (including immunoglobulins and antibodies), carbohydrates (especially lactose), enzymes, and cellular components, including macrophages and lymphocytes, as well as many other constituents that offer ideal support for growth and maturation of the human infant. Even as complementary foods are added after 5 to 6 months, breast milk continues to make an important nutritional contribution. Amazingly, as the infant grows and develops, the properties of the breast milk change. The sequence of colostrum, transitional milk, and mature milk meets the changing nutritional needs of the newborn and infant. In addition, some of the constituent properties in the milk are different from one time of the day to another and change with the passage of time over the months of the infant breastfeeding experience. Thus the milk of a mother of a 9-month-old has different concentrations of fat, protein, and carbohydrate, as well as different physical properties such as pH, when compared with the milk of the mother of a 1-month-old.

Breastfed babies have additional protection against bacterial, viral, and protozoan illnesses. Despite some methodologic difficulties, various studies have documented decreases in the incidence and severity of allergies and gastrointestinal and respiratory diseases, including ear infections, diarrhea, and pneumonia (Blaymore Bier et al, 2002; Oddy, 2001). Breast milk supports the growth of *Lactobacillus bifidus* in the intestine of the breastfed infant and creates an environment that discourages the growth of pathogens such as *Salmonella* and *Shigella*. Lactoferrin, an iron-binding protein, inhibits the growth of certain iron-dependent bacteria in the gastrointestinal tract.

There are also benefits for the mother that include more rapid return to nonpregnant state, establishment of the strong bond associated with successful nursing, and decreased risk for premenopausal ovarian cancer and breast cancer (Collaborative Group on Hormonal Factors in Breast Cancer, 2002; Siskind et al, 1997).

Breastfeeding also provides an economic incentive as a free and plentiful source of excellent infant nutrition. The cost of formula and other necessary supplies can exceed $1000 each year.

Contraindications to Breastfeeding

In addition to all the beneficial nutrients that are provided to the infant during breastfeeding, certain infections and many drugs or medications can also be passed to the infant via breast milk. Although rare, contraindications to breastfeeding occur in some of these situations. In addition, a small number of infant conditions also preclude breastfeeding. Contraindications to breastfeeding include the following:

- A human immunodeficiency virus (HIV)–positive mother (living in a developed nation)
- Maternal abuse of cocaine and intravenous drugs
- Maternal exposure to radioactive compounds
- Regular maternal use of drugs such as lithium, anticancer drugs, thiouracil, iodides or bromides, and ergot compounds
- Herpetic lesions on the mother's nipples, areolas, or breast
- Maternal diagnosis and treatment of cancer
- Infant with galactosemia

Special Situations

Additional circumstances require special consideration regarding the advisability or management of breastfeeding. These circumstances include the following:

- Significant maternal or infant illness affecting the ability to feed
- Maternal illness such as tuberculosis, chickenpox, or hepatitis B
- Invasive breast surgery, in particular breast reduction in which the areola was removed and reattached
- Documented history of milk supply problems

CHARACTERISTICS OF HUMAN MILK

Components of Human Milk

The uniqueness of human milk to support the growth and development of the human infant cannot be overestimated. Scientists continue to find new components and to clarify the purposes of known components. Over 200 constituents of milk have been identified (Lawrence & Lawrence, 1999).

Colostrum

Colostrum production begins at about 20 weeks of gestation. The pregnant woman may notice a small amount of yellow discharge on her nipple or clothing. After delivery of the baby, production of colostrum increases to 2 to 20 dl per feeding. This thick, rich, yellowish fluid has fewer calories than mature milk does (67 versus 75 kcal/100 ml) and is lower in fat (2% versus 3.8%). It is rich in immunoglobulins, especially IgA, and other antibodies. In addition, it is higher in sodium, chloride, protein, fat-soluble vitamins, and cholesterol than mature milk and facilitates the passage of meconium. Because of the outstanding contribution to the infant's immunologic status, colostrum is often referred to as the infant's "first immunization." Colostrum provides everything that a normal term newborn needs for the first few days of life, and no routine supplementation is needed.

Transitional Milk

Transitional milk appears several days after delivery. Significant variability is seen in the constituent properties of transitional milk between mothers and within samples from the same mother. However, as a general rule, transitional milk has more lactose, calories, and fat and less total protein than colostrum does.

Mature Milk

Mature milk gradually replaces transitional milk by about the second week after delivery and provides, on average, 20 kcal/oz.

Water. Approximately 90% of human milk is water. Breast milk can meet the fluid needs of the infant without any supplementation, even in tropical and desert climates.

Fat/Lipid Content. Various fats/lipids make up the second greatest percentage of constituents of human milk. They are also the most variable component, with differences noted within a feeding, between feedings, in feedings over time, and between different mothers. On average, the fat content is approximately 3.8% and contributes 30% to 55% of the kilocalories in human milk. During feeding, the fluid content of the mammary gland becomes mixed with droplets of fat in increasing concentration. Thus the fat content is higher at the end of the feeding (hindmilk) than it is at the beginning (foremilk). The type and amount of fat in the maternal diet are thought to affect the type of lipid but not the total amount of fat found in the mother's breast milk.

The cholesterol content varies little in human milk and is approximately 240 mg/100 g of fat. Changes in the maternal diet do not produce changes in these cholesterol values. Breastfed infants have higher plasma cholesterol levels than do formula-fed infants. Recent research suggests, however, that breastfeeding may have a protective effect against cardiovascular disease, because adults tend to have lower cholesterol levels if they were breastfed (Owen et al, 2002).

Currently, research is being conducted on how fatty acids such as docosohexaenoic acid (DHA) and other long-chain polyunsaturated acids (e.g., LC-PUFA) are regulated during breastfeeding and the role they play in brain and retinal growth (Heird, 2001).

Protein. Approximately 0.9% of the contents of human milk is protein. When milk is heated or exposed to enzymes as in digestion, a clot, or casein, is formed. The clear portion that remains is known as whey. In human milk, 60% to 70% of the protein is whey, which primarily consists of β-lactalbumin and lactoferrin, and 30% to 40% is casein. In contrast, cow's milk is 20% β-lactalbumin and 80% casein, with distinct chemical differences between the casein found in cow's milk and that found in human milk. The curds of human milk are more easily digested by the infant. Other proteins include immunoglobulins, nonimmunoglobulins, and lysozyme—a nonspecific antibacterial factor.

Carbohydrates. The primary carbohydrate of human milk is lactose, which is synthesized by the mammary gland from glucose. Lactose is highly concentrated in human milk (6.8 versus 4.9 g/100 ml in cow's milk) and appears to be essential for growth of the human infant. In addition, lactose enhances the absorption of calcium, a potentially important role because of the relatively low level of calcium in human milk.

Vitamins and Minerals. Human milk has more than adequate amounts of vitamins A, E, K, C, B_1, B_2, and B_6. However, the level of vitamin D intake may not be adequate in breastfed infants who lack exposure to sunlight because of weather, living conditions, or being swaddled with the head covered. Thirty minutes per week of exposure to the sun while dressed in a diaper only or 2 hours per week clothed (as long as the head is not covered) provides adequate vitamin D for a breastfed infant (Specker et al, 1985). Sunscreen blocks Vitamin D absorption. The American Academy of Pediatrics (AAP) recommends a supplement of 200 IU per day for all breastfed infants unless they are weaned to at least 500 ml per day of vitamin D–fortified formula or milk (Gartner, Greer, & the Section on Breastfeeding and Committee on Nutrition, 2003).

Iron is found in low levels in human milk. However, iron absorption from human milk is highly efficient, with 49% of the available iron absorbed in contrast to 4% from formula. A full-term infant who is exclusively breastfed for 4 to 6 months is not at risk for iron deficiency anemia.

Zinc, another mineral identified as important to the human infant, is readily available in human milk and has an absorption rate of 41% versus 31% from cow's milk protein formulas and 14% from soy formulas.

ANATOMY AND PHYSIOLOGY

Pregnancy brings about the final stage of mammogenesis—growth and differentiation of the mammary gland and development of the structures to support breast milk production. Estrogen, progesterone, placental lactogen, and prolactin all play a role in mammogenesis. By approximately 20 weeks, the breast is capable of milk production. The actual production of breast milk is triggered by the fall in progesterone concentration after birth of the baby. Placental retention inhibits milk production because of the influence of progesterone and other hormones.

Suckling by the infant plays an important role in the establishment and maintenance of lactation. The amount of milk produced is dependent on stimulation of the breast, removal of milk from the breast, and release of hormones. The concept of "supply and demand" is an important one for NPs and parents to understand. Suckling stimulates the hypothalamus to decrease prolactin-inhibiting factor, thus permitting release of prolactin by the anterior pituitary, leading to a rise in the level of prolactin. The hypothalamus also stimulates the synthesis and release of oxytocin by the posterior pituitary (Fig. 13-1).

Prolactin levels are directly proportional to the level of suckling by the infant. In addition, baseline levels vary greatly from one woman to another. Prolactin is more important to the initiation than to the maintenance of lactation.

Oxytocin reacts with receptors in the myoepithelial cells of the milk ducts to initiate a contracting action that results in forcing milk down the ducts. This action leads to an increase in milk pressure called the *letdown reflex* or *milk ejection reflex*. Oxytocin also aids in maternal uterine involution.

Under the influence of the hormones mentioned previously, the mammary gland undergoes a dramatic change with an increase in size and rapid growth of the lobuloalveolar tissue. The alveoli are the site of milk production and combine in numbers of 10 to 100 to form lobuli. Twenty to 40 lobuli combine into lobes, and 15 to 25 lobes empty into a lactiferous duct. The ducts transport the milk to the nipple (Fig. 13-2).

The nipple and surrounding areola serve as a visual and tactile target to assist with latch-on. The size and shape of the woman's breast and areola vary greatly. Fortunately, the size of the breast is not a predictor of breast milk volume. Even women with very small breasts can successfully breastfeed. The NP should be alert, however, for the occasional presence of insufficient glandular tissue, which is characterized by the absence of breast changes associated with pregnancy, a unilaterally underdeveloped breast, or conical-shaped breasts (Neifert, Seacat, & Jobe, 1985).

The size, shape, and position of the nipple also vary among women. The nipple may be everted (protuberant from the breast), flat, or inverted. It is not always possible to detect an inverted nipple by observation only. The "pinch test" may be needed to identify nipples that invert with tactile stimulation to the areola. To accomplish the

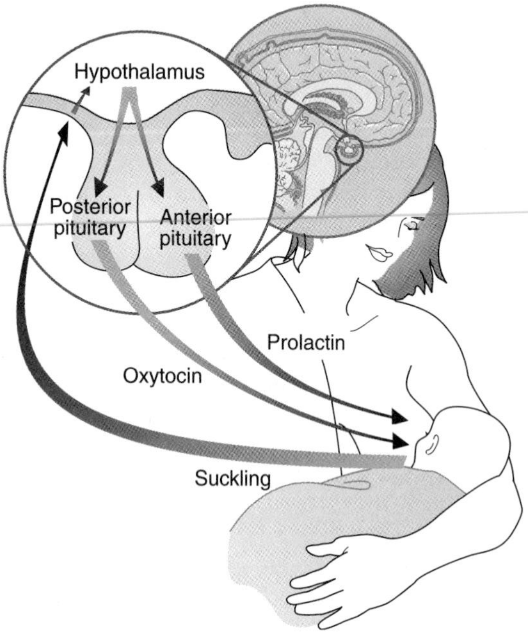

FIGURE 13-1 Neuroendocrine loop.

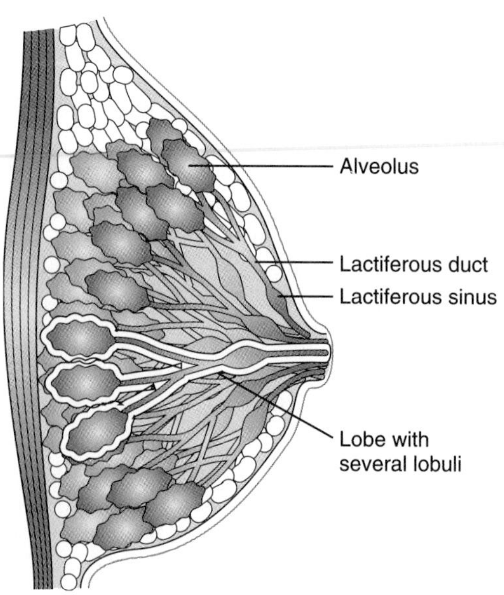

FIGURE 13-2 Anatomy of the breast.

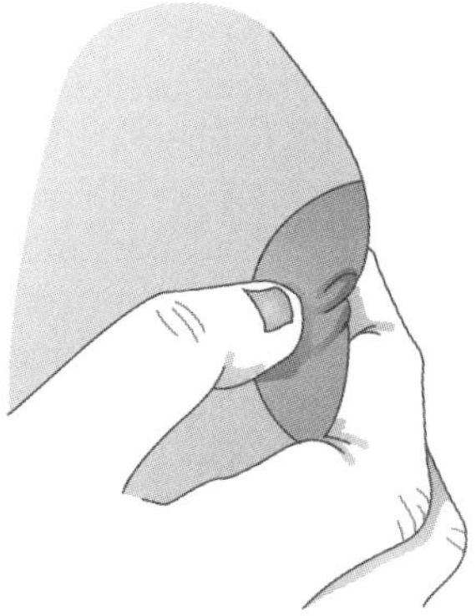

FIGURE 13-3 Pinch test.

pinch test, the NP places the thumb and forefinger on opposite sides of the areola about 1 to 1.5 inches back from the nipple-areolar junction. Gentle compression as though bringing the two fingers together will result in the nipple becoming more everted or inverted. This assessment should be conducted prenatally on every patient (Fig. 13-3). Management of inverted nipples is discussed later in this chapter.

Despite the complexity of the anatomic and physiologic processes, the great news is that breastfeeding can proceed for the mother and the baby with little or no awareness on their part of these considerations!

ASSESSMENT OF THE BREASTFEEDING DYAD

Prenatal assessment focuses on maternal expectations for breastfeeding; knowledge about breastfeeding, especially techniques for getting off to a good start; and identification of any contraindications to breastfeeding. A nipple evaluation should be completed. All pregnant women should be assessed, not just primiparas. In the early postpartum period, assessment focuses on the transition to breastfeeding and should include observation of a feeding. In addition, signs of progress for successful breastfeeding should be reviewed, and the names and phone numbers of contact persons should be given to mothers for follow-up or questions.

Maternal History

In general, subjective data should be collected about the following areas:

- Overall health, including documentation of any chronic illnesses or allergies
- Previous breastfeeding experience
- Routine use of over-the-counter, prescribed, or recreational/street drugs, including tobacco
- Surgical interventions, especially to the breast or thoracic region
- Nutritional status
- Family and community support for breastfeeding
- Pregnancy history, especially any complications or need for medications
- Labor and delivery history, including medications, procedures, or complications

Infant History

Subjective data are gathered on the infant in the following areas:

- Overall health status
- Congenital conditions such as cardiac, respiratory, or orofacial conditions
- Trauma or complications during delivery
- Medications received during labor and delivery or in the early postpartum period
- Activities including circumcision, use of bilirubin lights, or use of bottle/cup/tube feeding
- Gestational age
- Early responses to feeding attempts

Maternal Examination

Examination of the mother should focus on an evaluation of the breast in the following areas:

- Type of nipples—everted, flat, or inverted
- Presence of surgical scars on the breast or thoracic area
- Any nipple bruising or bleeding

Infant Examination

Evaluation of the infant's oral-motor skills and structures serves as the basis for the examination. The infant should be able to suck smoothly and evenly as a finger is inserted into the infant's mouth. The examiner's finger should be inserted beyond the gum line nearly to the soft palate to assess the wavelike motion of the tongue as the infant draws the finger in for suckling. The hard and soft palate should be intact, without palpable clefts or submucosal clefts. The infant should be able to extend the tongue over the lower gum with no evidence of a tight frenulum. In the process of the examination, the infant's state of alertness and readiness for feeding are also observed.

POSITIONS FOR BREASTFEEDING

Getting off to a good start begins with positioning the baby at the breast in a way that is comfortable for both the mother and baby and that allows for good latch-on. The three most common positions are the cradle, side-lying, and football hold positions.

Principles of Correct Positioning

Several principles are common to all of the various positions for breastfeeding. These principles include the following:

- Both the mother and the baby should be comfortable.
- The infant should be positioned "face-on" at nipple height so that no head turning or tilting is required. The nipple should be directed toward the center of the infant's mouth.
- The infant should be lying on the side, not the back.
- The infant's body should be in good alignment, with a straight line from the ear to the shoulder to the hips.
- The infant's top and bottom lips should be flanged out (Fig. 13-4).
- The infant's tongue should extend forward over the lower gum line and cup around the nipple and areola.
- Good latch-on results in quiet feedings. No "clicking" or "popping" sounds should be heard from the infant. After mother's milk is in, audible swallowing, like a "glug" or air blowing out the baby's nose, should be heard.

Cradle Position

The cradle position (also called the Madonna or cuddle position) and its variation known as the cross-cradle position begin with the mother sitting upright or leaning slightly forward with her feet on the floor or stool or her legs crossed in front of her. The infant is held with the mouth at nipple height, and the mother and infant are in a tummy-to-tummy arrangement. The mother uses her free hand to support the breast, if needed, while keeping her fingers well back from the areola so that she does not interfere with latch-on. The "cigarette hold" or pinching of the breast tissue should not be used. In the regular cradle position, the baby's head is supported in the crook of the elbow on the same side as the breast being suckled (Fig. 13-5). In the cross-cradle position, the baby's head and shoulders are supported by the opposite hand. This position often works well for a premature infant because it provides extra support to the head and shoulders.

After positioning the baby, the mother should touch the baby's lower lip with her nipple to stimulate mouth opening. As the mouth opens, the mother should bring the baby close so that the lips come up and over the nipple and back onto the areolar tissue and the nipple rests on top of the baby's tongue. Once the baby appears latched on, the mother can check the lips for a flanged, open placement. At this point the baby is very close to the breast, with the tip of the infant's nose touching it. Mothers often need to be shown that the baby is able to breathe without a need to press down on the breast tissue. If the baby appears to be pushed into the breast, the infant's buttocks should be brought closer into the tummy-to-tummy position. As the mother looks down at her baby, she should see a straight line from the baby's ear, to the shoulders, to the hips. Once

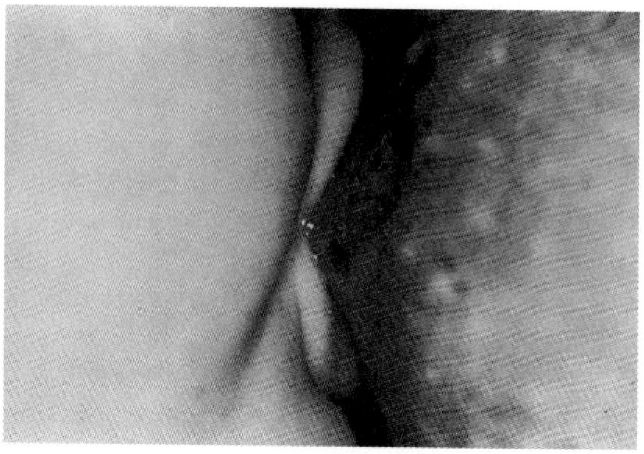

FIGURE 13-4 Lip position. (Courtesy of UNICEF.)

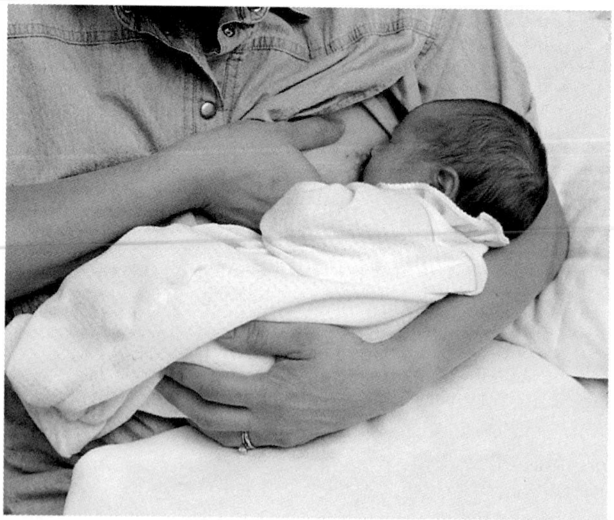

FIGURE 13-5 Cradle hold. The mother positions the infant's head at or near the antecubital space and level with her nipple with her arm supporting the infant's body. Her other hand is free to hold the breast. Once the infant is positioned, pillows or blankets can be used to support the mother's arm, which may tire from holding the baby. (From McKinney ES et al: *Maternal-child nursing,* Philadelphia, 2002, WB Saunders.)

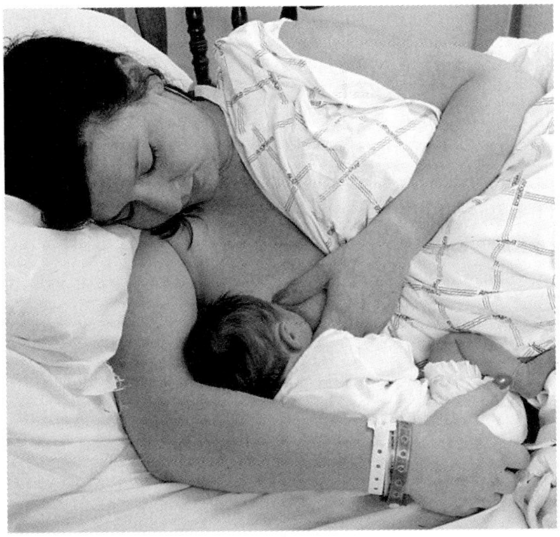

FIGURE 13-6 The side-lying position avoids pressure on episiotomy or abdominal incisions and allows the mother to rest while feeding. She lies on her side, with her lower arm supporting her head or placed around the infant. A pillow behind her back and between her legs provides comfort. Her upper hand and arm are used to position the infant on the side at nipple level and hold the breast. When the infant's mouth opens to nurse, the mother leans slightly forward or draws the infant to her to insert the nipple into the mouth. (From McKinney ES et al: *Maternal-child nursing,* Philadelphia, 2002, WB Saunders.)

the baby is suckling well, the mother can usually remove the hand that was supporting her breast and use it to cradle the baby in her arms. She can also relax back from the forward-leaning position that she used at the beginning.

Side-Lying Position

The side-lying or other lying-down variations are often helpful when the mother is uncomfortable sitting up or wishes to nap or sleep with her baby. In the early days of learning to achieve latch-on, the side-lying position is not easy to use because the mother cannot see her breast and nipple quite as well. In the hospital, a nurse should be available to help the mother and infant. At home and with practice, the mother and infant can achieve latch-on without assistance.

In the side-lying position, the mother lies on her side, cradles her infant in her elbow, and supports the infant's back and neck. The mother or the nurse should arrange one to two pillows under the mother's head and shoulders and a rolled towel or blanket along the infant's back to keep the infant in a side-lying position. As in the cradle position, the mother may support her breast with her upper hand (Fig.13-6).

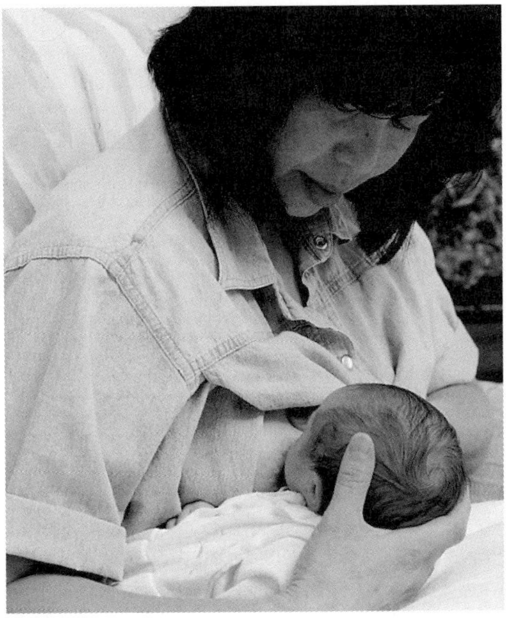

FIGURE 13-7 Football hold. The mother supports the infant's head in her hand, with the infant's body resting on pillows alongside her hip. This method allows the mother to see the position of the infant's mouth on the breast, helps her control the infant's head, and is especially helpful for mothers with heavy breasts. This hold also avoids pressure against an abdominal incision. (From McKinney ES et al: *Maternal-child nursing,* Philadelphia, 2002, WB Saunders.)

Football Hold

In the football hold, the infant is supported off to the side of the mother. This position is often used by a mother who has had a cesarean delivery because it does not require that the infant be positioned along her abdomen. In addition, this position can be used by a mother of multiples when she would like to feed two babies at once. Finally, mothers with flat or inverted nipples are often able to achieve latch-on more easily with this position.

One or two firm pillows should be placed at the mother's side to help support the infant. The baby is in a side-lying position and flexed at the hips, with the buttocks back against the chair or couch. As in other positions, the mother may support her breast to assist with latch-on and remove her hand once the baby is suckling well (Fig. 13-7).

DYNAMICS OF BREASTFEEDING

Early Feedings

The first breastfeeding should take place as soon after birth as possible. Full-term neonates often have an alert period for 30 to 60 minutes after delivery that is ideal for the first feeding practice. This first feeding can take place in the delivery area, if necessary, and should be encouraged by all in attendance. This early feeding will not delay, to any significant extent, any procedures required such as weighing and measuring the infant, instilling ointment or drops in the infant's eyes, and giving vitamin K injections. These procedures can be done one at a time in the delivery room or at the bedside after return to the room. The mother and infant should remain together as much as possible, with rooming-in preferable. The family needs to be encouraged and supported in making their wishes known to the staff about their desire to promote close contact and initiate breastfeeding. In addition, the NP should advocate changes in institutional policy to support the needs of breastfeeding families.

The infant usually goes into a deep sleep after the initial alertness and is difficult to wake for feeding practice. Parents should be instructed to watch for any awakening behavior such as opening eyes or movement in the bed. Many newborns will not cry at this point, so parents need to be alert for these signs of feeding readiness. Full-term infants are born with stores of fluid and energy to carry them through this time of infrequent feeding and low volume of colostrum. During this period the infant is making the transition to the nonuterine environment. The stomach, liver, and kidneys are gearing up for the larger volumes of higher-fat food that will come in a few days. It is not necessary to provide water, dextrose in water, or formula calories to a healthy, full-term neonate. In addition, the use of a rubber or silicone nipple that does not work like the breast in delivering milk may lead to nipple confusion.

During this transition time, assistance and support from an individual knowledgeable in breastfeeding can be helpful to the mother and infant as they practice latch-on and suckling. The infant should be encouraged to go to each breast for at least 10 to 15 minutes of active suckling, although some infants may spend even longer. The infant's behavior is much more important during this time than the clock. However, an infant who falls asleep in 5 minutes should be stimulated to continue active suckling. Attention to proper positioning and technique becomes important as the frequency and duration of the suckling behavior increase. A mother is unlikely to get sore or cracked nipples when her infant is latched on correctly. These early feedings are excellent "practice" sessions both for the mother, who gains confidence in her breastfeeding ability, and for the infant, who gets first colostrum and then milk for the efforts at suckling.

The goal of discharge planning is to maintain successful breastfeeding and includes the following:

- Review proper positioning.
- Review signs of good latch-on.
- Review signs of infant progress indicating adequate nutrition (Table 13-1).
- Arrange daily follow-up for 2 to 3 days after discharge.
- Provide a phone contact for questions and concerns.
- Encourage the mother to contact breastfeeding resources whenever she has questions.

These early efforts to provide contact and support during the transition to home can make all the difference in maintaining breastfeeding. Problems encountered during engorgement, sleep deprivation, and times of uncertainty or lack of confidence can be addressed quickly and directly rather than after a bottle has been introduced or the mother's nipples are cracked and bleeding.

Frequency and Duration of Feedings

After the first 24 hours, the infant should be going to the breast 8 to 12 times (or every 2 to 3 hours) in 24 hours for approximately 20 to 45 minutes at each feeding. Frequent suckling stimulates milk production and establishes a regular routine early on. Exclusive breastfeeding for the first month should be encouraged to ensure the establishment of an adequate milk supply and avoid any nipple confusion. Parents need to be alert for an infant who sleeps for 4 to 5 hours at a time or who goes to sleep at the breast in 5 minutes. These infants must be actively wakened and stimulated for feeding.

If the mother and infant must be separated for one or more feedings or supplements are medically necessary, they may be given with a dropper, a cup, or a 5-French feeding tube placed at the breast. Proper instructions, close supervision, and follow-up are needed for each of these methods, and they should not be used routinely.

Urine and Stool Output Guidelines

Urine

In the first 2 days of life as the volume of breast milk is increasing, the infant may urinate only one to three times in 24 hours. By day 3 the infant should have four or more wet diapers in 24 hours and then four to six wet diapers per 24 hours by day 4. Over time, the infant should have a minimum of six to eight wet diapers in a 24-hour period. The urine should be light yellow with no strong odor. If the parents are anxious or if they have a question about breastfeeding progress, a diary of wet diapers can be kept to aid in the accurate assessment of progress. Parents need to be alerted, however, to the difficulty of doing accurate diaper counts with disposable diapers and may elect to insert a tissue liner into the diaper or to use cloth diapers for the first few weeks. Ultra-absorbent diapers should be avoided when close monitoring of output is necessary.

TABLE 13-1 *Signs of Infant Progress: A Handout for Parents*

	First 8 hr	8-24 hr	Day 2	Day 3	Day 4	Day 5	Day 6 On
Milk supply	You may be able to express a few drops of milk.		Milk should come in between the second and fourth day.			Milk should be in. Breasts may be firm or leak milk.	Breasts should feel softer after nursing.
Baby's activity	Baby is usually wide awake in first hr of life. Put to breast within ½ hour of birth.	Wake your baby. Babies may not awaken on their own to feed.	Baby should be more cooperative and less sleepy.	Look for early feeding cues: rooting, lip smacking, hands to face. Note that baby swallows regularly while nursing.			Baby should appear satisfied after feeding.
Feeding routine	Baby may go into a deep sleep 2-4 hr after birth.	Feed your baby every 1½ -3 hr or as often as wanted.	Feedings should be at least 8-10 times each day.			May go up to 5 hr between feedings (once in a 24-hr period).	
Breastfeeding	Baby will wake up and be alert and responsive for several more hours after the initial deep sleep.	Nurse at both breasts as long as baby is actively suckling and mother is comfortable.	Try to nurse on both sides at each feeding, aiming for 10-15 min each side. Expect some nipple tenderness.	Consider hand-expressing or pumping a few drops of milk to soften the nipple if the breast is too firm for the baby to latch on.	Nurse at least 10-15 min each side every 2-3 hr for the first few months of life.		Mother's nipple tenderness is decreased or gone.
Baby's urine output		Baby must have at least one wet diaper in first 24 hr.	Baby should have at least one wet diaper every 8 hr.	Wet diapers should increase to four to six in 24 hr.	Baby's urine should be light yellow.	Baby should have six to eight wet diapers per day of colorless or light yellow urine.	
Baby's stools		Baby should have a black-green stool (meconium stool).	Baby may have a second very dark (meconium) stool.	Baby's stools should be changing from black-green to yellow.		Baby should have three to four yellow, seedy stools per day.	The number of stools may slowly decrease after 4-6 wk.

From Thilo EH, Townsend SF: Early newborn discharge: have we gone too far? *Contemp Pediatr* 13:29-46, 1996.

Stool

In the first 24 hours after delivery, the baby should have at least one meconium stool followed by another on day 2. By day 3, stools are beginning to make the transition to the characteristic loose, yellow, seedy stools of breastfeeding, and the infant should begin having two to three stools in 24 hours. That number may continue to increase in the first few weeks of life. Some infants stool with every feeding. After the first month, the pattern may change again as some infants begin to stool less frequently and may go several days between stools. As long as the infant is healthy and gaining weight, there is no problem. However, infrequent stooling, especially in the first month, should stimulate a feeding history and possibly a weight check to make sure that the infant is getting enough breast milk.

Pumping

Routine pumping is unnecessary for breastfed infants whose mothers are available for a feeding every 2 to 4 hours. However, if the mother and infant must be separated for more than one or two feedings, pumping should be part of the plan to assist with milk production. If the mother and infant are separated right after birth, pumping should begin as soon as possible, within the first 24 hours. The mother should pump six to eight times in 24 hours for 15 minutes if she is using a double-pump setup or 10 minutes per breast if she is using a single-pump setup. She should be encouraged to save even the smallest amounts of colostrum to be given to her infant.

Hand expression and manual pumps work well for infrequent or short-duration pumping. However, a hospital-grade, piston-style pump that permits pumping both breasts at the same time is ideal for a mother who will have to pump for several weeks or months. No pump works as well as an infant in stimulating production, but frequent pumping goes a long way toward establishing a milk supply and provides the mother a concrete, healthful contribution to her sick or preterm infant. As the volume of milk goes up over the first few days, the mother can see the success of her efforts. She should be counseled about the increase in production in contrast to the small volume of colostrum produced in the first few days.

Collection and Storage of Breast Milk

A mother who is pumping should be reminded to wash her hands well before she begins pumping and to use clean containers for collection and storage. In addition, the pump parts should be thoroughly cleaned after each use. Many of the pump parts can go through a dishwasher, but the directions that come with the pump should be consulted for specific instructions on cleaning.

Milk collected from pumping should be stored in clean plastic bottles or disposable milk bags. It is preferable to store breast milk in small amounts so that only the amount that is needed is defrosted and used. Milk that has been defrosted and not used within 24 hours should be discarded. Pumped breast milk should be refrigerated as soon after pumping as possible and can be stored there for 24 to 48 hours. If it is not going to be used in that time, it should be immediately frozen. In a refrigerator freezer that maintains a steady temperature, breast milk can be stored for up to 3 months. Breast milk can be stored for more than 6 months in a freezer where 0° F is routinely maintained. The bottles or bags should be labeled with the date of collection so that the oldest milk can be used first. If the milk must be transported to the hospital or day care facility, it should be placed in ice or on a blue ice unit to minimize the amount of warming or thawing.

Infant Weight Gain

Normal newborn infants lose 5% to 10% of their birth weight in the first few days of life. It is helpful for parents to be aware of both the birth and discharge weights. Once the maternal milk volume increases, the infant begins to gain weight in the range of 0.5 to 1 oz per day or 4 to 7 oz per week. Most breastfed infants have regained their birth weight by 2 weeks. One criterion for failure to thrive is lack of return to birth weight by 3 weeks. Breastfed infants usually double their birth weight by 5 to 6 months of age and triple it by 1 year.

An early study of the growth patterns and nutrient intake of a cohort of breastfed and formula-fed infants has presented evidence that breastfed babies gain at a slower rate after the first 3 months (Dewey et al, 1992). More recent research indicates that breastfed infants may grow more rapidly initially, then slow their weight-for-age gain between 3 and 12 months. In this study, length-for-age gains fell below the reference by 6 months, but caught up by 12 months, and head circumference showed no significant difference at any age (Kramer et al, 2002).

An infant who has followed the growth grid curves until 3 or 4 months and then falls slightly may be growing at a normal rate for a breastfed infant. In the absence of growth grids specifically designed for breastfed infants, an important consideration in assessing an apparently slowly gaining infant is developmental progress and other measures of growth. Characteristics of a healthy, but slowly growing, breastfed infant include the following:

- Active and alert state
- Developmentally appropriate progress
- Age-appropriate height and head circumference
- Good skin turgor and color
- Sufficient output of at least six wet diapers and several stools per day
- Contented and satisfied behavior after feeding

Growth Spurts

Just when the parents begin to think that breastfeeding is going well, the first growth spurt occurs and can once again arouse their concern. The term *growth spurt* is often used to describe those recurring times during breastfeeding when the baby's growth exceeds the breast milk supply at that moment. For 2 to 4 days the infant feeds more frequently to increase milk production. However, an inexperienced parent may interpret this behavior as a sign of inadequate milk production and begin supplementation. This practice leads to inadequate breast milk volume, whereas allowing and even encouraging frequent breastfeeding results in an appropriate increase in milk production. Once the level of milk production has risen, the infant returns to the normal feeding pattern. Growth spurts tend to occur every 3 to 4 weeks, but parents seem to notice them less as time goes on. The behavior becomes an expected part of the breastfeeding experience.

Weaning

The decision about the time for weaning is an individual one. Breastfeeding should be encouraged for at least 1 year, but individual circumstances may dictate a different choice for a family. Sometimes weaning is led by the mother and other times by the infant. Typically, a natural weaning process occurs as other foods become a part of the infant's diet and the infant begins to participate in self-feeding. When a family inquires about the ideal time to begin weaning, the NP can counsel them to consider factors such as the following:

- Beliefs and desires of individual family members
- Developmental readiness of the infant
- Nutritional replacements for breast milk
- Social and environmental issues affecting the decision

Whether weaning occurs as a planned or unplanned activity, it is best to implement it gradually. If necessary, the mother can use a breast pump to gradually decrease milk production and avoid breast engorgement, blocked ducts, and discomfort. A good approach is to pump when uncomfortable and pump only to comfort, not to empty. In situations where weaning was not an anticipated or planned event, the NP may help the mother deal not only with the act of weaning but also with her feelings about it. Some mothers grieve the early loss of the breastfeeding experience.

In an effort to avoid premature weaning, the NP should maintain close communication with families, especially those who are more likely to wean early. Early identification and support of these families may assist them to continue breastfeeding for a longer period. Factors associated with early weaning include the following:

- Younger, poorer mothers
- Lower maternal education
- Early return of the mother to work outside the home
- Lack of support from family or health professionals
- Previous breastfeeding failure

Maternal Nutritional Needs during Breastfeeding

Maternal nutritional needs increase during lactation. Characteristics of a good diet include the following:

- A minimum of 1800 calories
- An additional 500 calories over the nonpregnant diet
- Generous intake of fruits and vegetables, whole grain breads and cereals, calcium-rich dairy products, and protein-rich meats, fish, and legumes
- Rich sources of calcium, zinc, folate, magnesium, and vitamin B_6
- Culturally appropriate foods
- Supplementation with calcium or prenatal vitamins or both only if the diet is poor (Institute of Medicine, 1991)

The mother should be encouraged to eat well for her own sake to keep herself healthy and to meet the energy demands of nursing. In addition, an adequate intake of fluid is necessary, but excessive use of fluids does not increase breast milk production. A good guideline for adequate fluid intake is maternal urine that is light yellow and has no strong odor. Eligible mothers and infants should be referred to the Women's, Infant's, and Children's (WIC) Special Supplemental Food Program for nutritional counseling, as well as for food supplements. Most WIC programs offer food supplements for the breastfeeding mother's diet because she does not need formula for the infant. Even with a diet that is adequate in nutrients and calories, a gradual maternal weight loss of 1 to 2 lb per month usually occurs. In fact, breastfeeding is the ideal way for a mother to return to her prepregnancy weight.

No foods need to be routinely excluded from the maternal diet unless there is evidence that a particular food bothers the infant or the infant appears to be allergic to it. Sometimes the food does not need to be eliminated but merely decreased. Maternal intake of cow's milk products has been associated with colic, and some highly allergic babies are sensitive to their mother's intake of saturated fats (Hoppu, Kalliomaki, & Isolauri, 2000). When a mother has markedly decreased or eliminated cow's milk from her diet, another source of calcium must be identified. Certain foods such as onions and garlic may change the flavor and odor of the milk but do not negatively affect its quality. The nutrient characteristics of breast milk are fairly stable. One positive way to look at the variety of foods in the diets of mothers from all over the world is to acknowledge that infants are getting early exposure to the foods of their culture.

Increased alcohol intake does not improve lactational performance, and in fact, intake of an amount over 0.5 g/kg of maternal body weight (two cans of beer, 8 oz of wine, or 2 to 2.5 oz of liquor) can impair the milk ejection reflex (Institute of Medicine, 1991). The occasional use of small amounts of alcohol need not be avoided, but regular use should be discouraged.

Large amounts of caffeine from coffee, sodas, or chocolate should be discouraged because caffeine is associated with jitteriness in the infant and may have a negative effect on the iron content of the breast milk. However, the equivalent of one to two cups of coffee per day should pose no problem (Institute of Medicine, 1991).

Returning to Work

Women who return to work outside the home after initiating breastfeeding should be encouraged to continue breastfeeding and be supported in their decision with accurate information about how to manage both work and breastfeeding. The mother can be assisted to investigate her work environment by use of tools such as a breastfeeding assessment worksheet that reviews type of work performed and where, space for pumping and storing, and individuals and policies that support her intention (Bar-Yam, 1998). The ideal work environment provides the following:

- Breaks or lunch time (or both) in which the mother can pump or go to the infant
- A private, convenient location for pumping with access to a sink for washing up and a refrigerator for storage
- Supportive colleagues and supervisors

In addition to providing information regarding pumping, storing, and transporting breast milk; introducing the bottle; and handling the challenges of multiple demands (Box 13-1), NPs can support community initiatives that promote these conditions in employment settings. Women are more likely to continue breastfeeding if they have workplace support (Wyatt, 2002).

Employers also benefit from breastfeeding mothers. In one study (Cohen, Mrtek, & Mrtek, 1995), a comparison of infant illnesses that resulted in 1 day of maternal absence from work demonstrated that 75% occurred in formula-fed babies. In addition, in the 28% of infants who experienced no illnesses, 86% were breastfed.

BOX 13-1 *Advice for Mothers on Returning to Work*

Before Delivery

Communicate plans to employer
Discuss options with other employees who have continued to breastfeed after returning to work
Investigate pumps, including rental or purchase
Read about working and breastfeeding

During Maternity Leave

Practice method of expression will be using at work
Begin freezing milk
Introduce bottle after breastfeeding well established (usually around 3 to 4 weeks)
Offer bottle one or two times a week

After Return to Work

Try to relax and avoid stress
Have a picture of your baby at the pump
Pump two to three times per day
Plan on 15 to 30 minutes to complete pumping
Wear clothes for easy access to breasts and to hide leaks

Feeding Breast Milk

Warm or thaw milk in warm water
Do not use microwave because milk heats unevenly and presents a risk for burns
Refrigerate thawed milk for no more than 24 hours
Do not add milk to a bottle that has already been used

Important Reminders

Wash hands before and after pumping
Wash pump parts with dish detergent and rinse well after each use

From Meek JY: Breastfeeding in the workplace, *Pediatr Clin North Am* 48:461-474, 2001.

Findings such as these may increase the likelihood that an employer will establish programs to support breastfeeding employees.

MEDICATIONS FOR BREASTFEEDING MOTHERS

Frequently, women question whether they can take certain medications while they are breastfeeding. Concerns relate primarily to two areas—the effect of the drug on maternal milk supply and the effect of the drug on the infant. General guidelines for maternal drug recommendations include the following:

- Give drugs that are normally safe for infants or have been tested in infants.
- Avoid long-acting forms of a drug.
- Schedule feeding at times when the drug level is lowest. Often, breastfeeding immediately after taking the drug is the safest time.
- Observe the infant for changes in feeding pattern, fussiness, vomiting/diarrhea, or rash.
- Consider all appropriate options and select the drug with the lowest level in breast milk.
- Avoid drugs that inhibit prolactin release such as estrogen, antihistamines, and ergot compounds.
- Be cautious about herbal preparations.

The American Academy of Pediatrics Committee on Drugs (2001) has developed eight categories of drugs grouped by their risk factors for breastfeeding. Four of these groups are summarized in Table 13-2, including drugs that

- Are contraindicated
- Require temporary cessation of breastfeeding
- Have an unknown effect on nursing but may be of concern
- Have been associated with significant effects on some infants and should be used with caution

A good drug reference should be available to the NP. Four excellent resources are shown in Box 13-2. Decisions about drug selection are difficult, especially when contraindicated drugs are being considered, but the consequences of weaning and loss of breast milk for the infant must be included in the deliberations.

TABLE 13-2 ***Medications Affecting Breastfeeding***

Contraindicated Drugs	Drugs Requiring Temporary Cessation of Breastfeeding	Drugs Whose Effect Is Unknown	Drugs Associated with Significant Effects: Give with Caution
Amphetamine Cocaine Cyclophosphamide Cyclosporine Doxorubicin Heroin Marijuana Methotrexate Phencyclidine (PCP)	Radioactive compounds such as • ^{64}Cu • ^{67}Ga • ^{111}In, ^{123}I, ^{125}I, ^{131}I • Radioactive sodium • ^{99m}Tc, $^{99m}TcO4$ Need to stop breastfeeding for a minimum of 5 half-lives of the durg Milk samples can be screened by radiology departments for radioactivity before resuming breastfeeding	Antidepressants • Amitriptyline • Amoxapine • Bupropion • Clomipramine • Desipramine • Dothiepin • Doxepin • Fluoxetine • Fluvoxamine • Imipramine • Nortriptyline • Paroxetine • Sertraline • Trazodone Antianxieties • Alprazolam • Diazepam • Lorazepam • Midazolam • Perphenazine • Prazepam • Quazepam • Temazepam	Acebutolol 5-aminosalicylic acid Aspirin Atenolol Bromocriptine Clemastine Ergotamine Lithium Phenindione Phenobarbital Primidone Sulfasalazine

Continued

TABLE 13-2 Medications Affecting Breastfeeding—cont'd

Contraindicated Drugs	Drugs Requiring Temporary Cessation of Breastfeeding	Drugs Whose Effect Is Unknown	Drugs Associated with Significant Effects: Give with Caution
		Antipsychotics • Chlorpromazine • Chlorprothixene • Clozapine • Haloperidol • Mesoridazine • Trifluoperazine Others • Amiodarone • Chloramphenicol • Clofazimine • Lamotrigine • Metoclopramide • Metronidazole • Tinidazole	

From American Academy of Pediatrics Committee on Drugs: The transfer of drugs and other chemicals into human milk, *Pediatrics* 108:776-789, 2001.

BOX 13-2 Drug References

American Academy of Pediatrics Committee on Drugs: The transfer of drugs and other chemicals into human milk, *Pediatrics* 108:776-789, 2001.

Hale TW: *Medications and mothers' milk*, Amarillo, TX, 2002, Pharmasoft Medical Publishing. Updated and reprinted every other year. Order from 800-378-1317 or *www.ibreastfeeding.com*. Excellent, inexpensive reference.

Lawrence RA, Lawrence RM: *Breastfeeding: a guide for the medical profession*, ed 5, St Louis, 1999, Mosby.

Wynne AL, Woo T, Millard M: *Pharmacotherapeutics for nurse practitioner prescribers*, Philadelphia, 2002, FA Davis.

COMMON BREASTFEEDING PROBLEMS

Flat or Inverted Nipples

Description

A nipple can look as though it is inverted, but a "pinch test" is necessary to determine what happens to the nipple during breastfeeding (see the previous description and Fig. 13-3 for the technique). If the nipple pulls in, it is considered to be inverted. If the nipple does not pull in or everts with compression, it is considered to be flat. In most cases the nipple everts when compressed.

Inverted nipples can make it more difficult for the infant to latch on in the early days because it is harder to pull the nipple into the mouth for suckling. As the baby continues to breastfeed, the nipple tissue elongates, and with time, the problem usually becomes less severe and successful breastfeeding is possible.

Flat nipples do not generally change over time, but the infant develops a style to more easily latch on successfully.

Etiology

Adhesions cause retraction or inversion of the nipples. Flat nipples are often found in women with larger breasts.

Differential Diagnosis

The differential diagnosis for flat or inverted nipples is dimpled, fissured, or unusually shaped nipples.

Management

Prenatal. If the patient is not at risk for preterm labor, breast shells can be used during the third trimester for inverted nipples. The obstetrician or nurse midwife should be notified before their use. Shells are plastic, dome-shaped devices with small holes for ventilation. An opening in the portion that lies against the skin fits over the nipple,

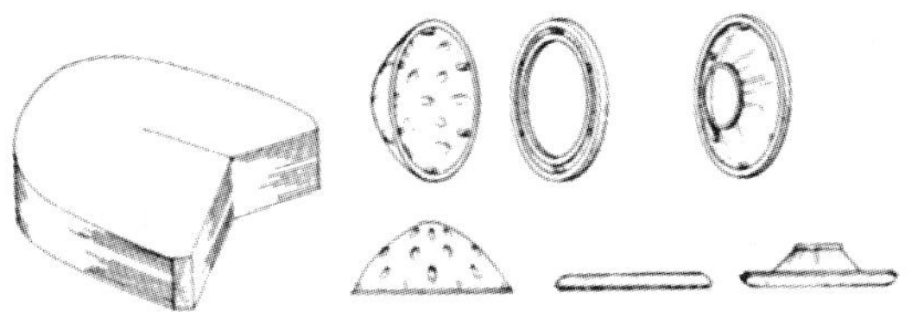

FIGURE 13-8 Breast shells. (Courtesy of Medela, Inc.)

and gentle suction during use helps stretch the nipple tissue (Fig. 13-8). The bra cup holds the shell comfortably in place, and the use of shells during the last trimester generally helps stretch out adhesions in preparation for breastfeeding.

Postpartum. The NP should stay with the mother during early feeding attempts; give extra praise, reassurance, and support; and emphasize the need for extra patience and persistence. Encourage use of the football hold position during feedings, and have the mother lean slightly forward as she latches the baby on.

The mother should do the following:

- Wear breast shells between feedings.
- Manually pull or roll the nipple immediately before latch-on.
- Use a breast pump for 1 or 2 minutes before latch-on.
- Put a cold cloth or ice on the nipple for a few seconds.
- Avoid pacifiers and bottle nipples until the infant is 4 to 6 weeks of age.
- If supplementation is medically indicated, use a syringe, dropper, feeding tube, or supplemental nutrition system (Fig. 13-9).

Although there are strong arguments against the use of nipple shields, in some cases mothers have used nipple shields successfully (Brigham, 1996), and their use has been shown to increase milk intake by preterm infants (Meier et al, 2000). Every mother-infant dyad should be uniquely assessed and managed, and for some infants, use of a thin, silicone nipple shield may be preferable to no breastfeeding at all. Monitoring of infant weight is essential to ensure adequate weight gain. Cleansing and drying both the shields and breast after feeding is important to prevent skin breakdown and infection.

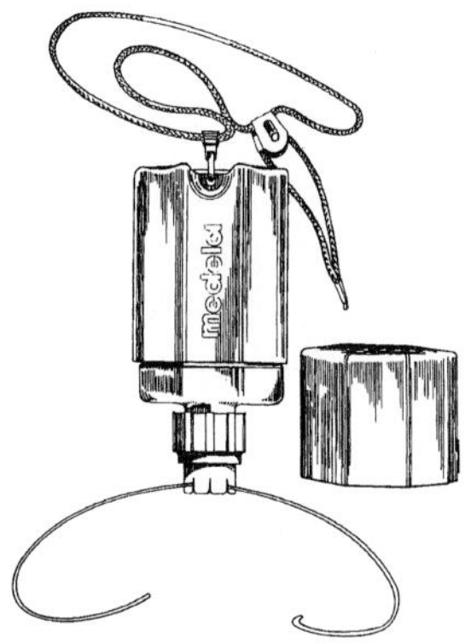

FIGURE 13-9 Supplemental nursing system. (Courtesy of Medela, Inc.)

Complications

Complications of flat or inverted nipples include the following:

- Frustration
- Loss of self-confidence
- Inadequate infant nutrition and its sequelae
- Severe maternal engorgement, plugged ducts, or mastitis

Sore Nipples

Description

Soreness of the nipples is pain caused by irritation or trauma to the nipples and areola, often accompanied by a breakdown in skin integrity.

Etiology

Sore nipples have many causes, including the following:

- Improper latch-on and positioning at the breast
- Prolonged negative pressure
- Inappropriate suction release from the breast
- Use of or sensitivity to nipple creams and oils
- Incorrect use of breastfeeding supplies (e.g., pumps, shells, shields)
- Thrush (candidiasis)
- Leaking nipples that are not properly air-dried

Clinical Findings

The nipples, areolae, and breasts are tender, bruised, raw, cracked, bleeding, blistered, discolored, swollen, or traumatized.

Differential Diagnosis

The differential diagnoses for sore nipples include the following:

- Mild tenderness, which is sometimes described by new mothers as they are getting used to the infant's suckling
- Breast or nipple trauma from another cause
- Thrush (candidiasis)
- Mastitis
- Abscess
- Milk plugs at the nipple pores

Management

The following measures can be taken to manage sore nipples:

- Assess breastfeeding at an early feeding. Prevent the problem by demonstrating and reinforcing the proper latch-on technique and positioning of the infant.
- Counsel mothers to seek help early for more than mild tenderness. Nipples can be damaged by constant high negative pressure and do not "toughen up" as breastfeeding progresses. Cracking and bleeding are not normal.
- Rub a few drops of colostrum or hindmilk onto the nipple and areola after every feeding and let it air-dry.
- Expose the nipples to air for short periods several times a day.
- Use breast shells to prevent the bra or clothing from rubbing against the nipple.
- Nurse from the least sore side first.
- Use short, frequent feedings.
- Pump the affected breast if pain is too severe to allow nursing.
- Use mild analgesics as necessary.
- Refer to a lactation specialist as appropriate.

Severe Engorgement

Description

Severe engorgement is characterized by extremely full, sore, swollen breasts beyond the normal fullness experienced as the milk comes in.

Etiology

Engorgement is caused by milk stasis in the breast from inadequate emptying.

Clinical Findings

The following are seen in severe engorgement:

- Painful, hard, lumpy, swollen breasts
- Breasts usually warm to the touch
- Nipples flattened by the swelling
- Bruising or trauma to the nipples and areolae

Differential Diagnosis

The differential diagnosis for severe engorgement is bilateral mastitis.

Management

The following measures can be taken to manage engorgement:

- Take a hot shower or wrap the breasts with warm, wet compresses for 5 to 10 minutes before nursing. Disposable diapers can be wet with hot water and then wrapped around each breast and "tabbed" to hold them in place. The plastic liner holds the heat in longer than an ordinary washcloth or towel does.
- Gently massage the entire breast or use an electric pump with intermittent suction on the minimal setting for several minutes after using wet heat.
- Manually express milk before feeding to soften the areola and make it easier for the infant to latch on properly.
- Nurse frequently and make certain that latch-on and position are correct and audible swallowing is heard.
- Avoid long stretches between feedings in the early weeks as the milk supply is being established. Pump the breasts if a feeding will be missed.

Mastitis

Description

Although rarely seen in the postpartum hospital setting, mastitis is an infection of the breast that can occur at any time during lactation. Occasionally, it has been identified during the third trimester of pregnancy.

Etiology

Staphylococcus aureus is most commonly associated with mastitis, but *Escherichia coli* and, more rarely, various streptococci are also found (Foxman et al, 2002). Predisposing factors include the following:

- Stress, fatigue
- Cracked nipples, plugged ducts
- Constricting, improperly fitting bra
- Inadequate emptying of the breast
- Sudden weaning or a significant decrease in the number of feedings
- Using a manual pump

Clinical Findings

The following are seen in mastitis:

- Malaise
- Breast tenderness or pain
- A reddened, warm lump in any quadrant, sometimes associated with red streaking
- Flulike symptoms, including fever, chills, and body aches

An old adage is that the "flu" in a breastfeeding woman is mastitis until proved otherwise.

Management

Recommendations for treatment of mastitis include the following:

- Penicillinase-resistant penicillin or a cephalosporin that covers *S. aureus*. Currently, dicloxacillin is most commonly

recommended to treat mastitis. Treatment should be maintained for 10 to 14 days.
- Fluconazole has been used for candidia-caused mastitis (Chetwynd et al, 2002).
- Rest (extremely important).
- Nurse frequently, or if pain is severe, pump milk carefully from the affected breast. Breast milk is not infected and is fine for the infant.
- Do not wean abruptly because of the possibility of mastitis progressing into an abscess.
- Take warm showers or use warm wet compresses.
- Increase fluids.
- Use analgesics as necessary (Foxman et al, 2002; Lawrence & Lawrence, 1999).

Complications

Abscess and septicemia are complications of mastitis.

Nipple Confusion

Description

Nipple confusion is not commonly discussed in research literature but has been seen anecdotally by experienced clinicians. If babies accustomed to bottle feeding are offered the breast, they use the same sucking pattern as with a bottle: They thrust their tongues up against their mother's nipple, which makes it difficult to obtain adequate nourishment and may contribute to maternal sore nipples. They may cry, fuss, or push away with their arms during attempts to nurse.

Etiology

Different oral-motor skills are used in breastfeeding and bottle feeding, and infants who have been given a bottle or pacifier sometimes attempt to breastfeed as though they were bottle feeding. Nipple confusion cannot be predicted and may occur in some infants after a single bottle feeding (Newman, 1990). Thus, unless absolutely necessary, early bottle feeding should be avoided in the breastfeeding infant.

Clinical Findings

The following are seen in nipple confusion:
- Ineffective suckling at the breast
- Breast refusal
- Sore, red, or bruised maternal nipples

Differential Diagnosis

The differential diagnoses for nipple confusion are other causes of fussiness and refusal to feed.

Management

The following are recommended to manage nipple confusion:
- Avoid all rubber bottle nipples and pacifiers for the first 4 to 6 weeks.
- Retrain the infant to suck correctly at the breast by correct positioning at the breast, proper latch-on technique, suck training to repattern tongue movements, and supplementation via alternative methods if required.
- Avoid nipple shields.
- Consult with a lactation specialist as indicated.
- If supplements are medically indicated, give with an eyedropper, spoon, syringe, or cup or through a 5-French feeding tube (attached to a 20- or 30-ml syringe) taped to the areola or breast. The end of the tubing protrudes slightly past the end of the nipple so that the tube, nipple, and areola are in the infant's mouth.

As with management of inverted nipples, some infants who experience nipple confusion may continue to refuse the breast despite the best efforts of mothers and lactation specialists. When confronted with a decision of whether to continue to attempt to offer the breast (and maintaining a conflictive and frustrating interaction between the mother and baby), discontinue breastfeeding altogether, or use a thin, silicone nipple shield and encourage the infant to suckle at the breast, mothers may decide to try the nipple shield. In some cases, they are successful at getting latch-on and suckling until the breastfeeding difficulties can be resolved (Brigham, 1996). However, infant weight gain must be monitored to ensure continued growth.

Complications

The following are complications of nipple confusion:
- Failure to thrive
- Hyperbilirubinemia
- Colic and crying
- Prolonged feedings
- Sore and cracked nipples
- Plugged ducts
- Mastitis
- Frustration

Breast Milk Jaundice

Description

Breast milk (late onset) jaundice is an elevated serum indirect bilirubin concentration with the peak level occurring on or after the seventh to tenth day of life in an infant drinking an adequate amount of breast milk with no other signs of liver pathology.

Etiology and Incidence

The exact cause of breast milk jaundice is unknown; however, an enzyme may be present in some mothers' milk that inhibits the action of glucuronyl transferase and increases intestinal absorption of bilirubin. Breast milk jaundice is more common in Asian and North American Indian infants. Siblings with the same mother are often affected. True breast milk jaundice is uncommon and estimated to occur in less than 1 in 200 births (Lawrence & Lawrence, 1999).

Clinical Findings

Physical Examination. The following are seen with breast milk jaundice:
- Healthy and thriving infant
- Adequate stooling and voiding
- Appropriate weight gain
- Appearance of elevated bilirubin levels between the seventh and tenth day of life
- Bilirubin peaks around day 10 to 15
- Persistence into the third month of life

Diagnostic Tests. The following tests are usually indicated:
- Serum bilirubin
- Urine and other cultures, which are sometimes necessary to rule out infection

Differential Diagnosis

The differential diagnosis for breast milk jaundice is pathologic jaundice.

Management

In breast milk jaundice, breastfeeding should be continued unless clinical signs of pathologic jaundice are observed. See Chapter 39 for a discussion of pathologic jaundice. The family should be reassured that breast milk jaundice is not harmful.

Thrush

When oral candidiasis is diagnosed in the infant or found on the nipple/areolar areas of the nursing mother, both members of the dyad should be treated. See Chapter 34 for a discussion of thrush.

Poor Weight Gain

Description

Problems associated with poor weight gain occur at two different times and represent different challenges for management. During the newborn period, initiation of breastfeeding may not proceed normally and the infant may actually continue to lose weight or, at best, gain very slowly. After the newborn period, infants may gain weight more slowly than expected given normal parameters for their age.

Etiology

Poor weight gain has a number of contributing factors, including the following:
- Infrequent or inadequate feeding because of poorly managed breastfeeding or environmental or social circumstances in the family system
- Inadequate milk production
- Genetic predisposition
- Infection
- Organic disease
- Physical anomaly that prevents good suckling or swallowing

Clinical Findings

The following may be seen in poor weight gain:

Infant Factors
- Continued weight loss after 5 to 7 days of age
- Failure to regain birth weight by 2 to 3 weeks of age
- Failure to maintain an ongoing weight gain of 0.5 to 1 oz/day
- Weight below the third percentile for age (this finding can be a pattern over time or a sudden change)
- Lethargic, sleepy, inactive, unresponsive infant
- Newborn or young infant sleeping longer than 4 hours between feedings
- Dry mucous membranes
- Poor skin turgor

Technique Factors
- Ineffective latch-on or sucking
- Short time at the breast (the infant is removed before nursing is finished, thus reducing access to hindmilk and total consumption)
- Infant kept on a preset schedule despite cues for more feeding
- Infant given water between feedings to "get through" to the next feeding
- Infant encouraged or allowed to sleep through the night before 8 to 12 weeks of age
- Fewer than eight feedings in 24 hours
- Infant fed in a distracting environment
- In older infants, breastfeeding offered after solids are given
- Infant in a day care setting that does not facilitate breastfeeding

Maternal Factors

- Does not initially respond to infant's cues for feeding or does not recognize that waking is needed to establish feeding
- Uses nipple shields
- Hectic schedule with limited time for breastfeeding
- Recent illness or significant weight loss
- Uses oral contraceptives or other hormones

Differential Diagnosis

The differential diagnoses for poor weight gain are a pattern of slower but normal weight gain in healthy breastfed infants and failure to thrive.

Management

The following measures should be taken to manage poor weight gain:

- Complete a thorough history to elicit information regarding infant and maternal factors.
- Conduct a thorough assessment of breastfeeding techniques to accurately determine the extent to which mismanagement is a cause.
- Provide instruction, encouragement, and reinforcement for correct breastfeeding techniques.
- Refer for treatment of physical or organic causes.
- Be alert for any infant who has lost too much weight and is unable to feed with vigor at the breast; such infants require an immediate infusion of calories for energy.
- Use a supplemental system at the breast if supplementation is required (see Fig. 13-9).
- Encourage and reassure the parents.

Complications

Complications of poor weight gain include developmental delay, poor bonding, and severe dehydration. In situations of early failure to establish breastfeeding, some infants may appear to be in a septic state and require hospitalization for rehydration and further evaluation.

NURSING DIAGNOSES RELATED TO BREASTFEEDING

- Effective breastfeeding
- Interrupted breastfeeding
- Ineffective breastfeeding

Source: North American Nursing Diagnosis Association: *NANDA nursing diagnoses: definitions and classification 2003-2004*, Philadelphia, 2003, North American Nursing Diagnosis Association.

RESOURCE BOX

Breastfeeding

Ameda-Egnell
1-800-323-8750
www.ameda.com
Breast pumps and breastfeeding products

Human Milk Banking Association of North America
www.cdc.gov/breastfeeding/compend-milkbanks.htm
Guidelines and information on human milk banking; as a clearinghouse for member milk banks; currently lists five regionally located human milk banks in United States; one in Mexico; one in Canada

International Board of Lactation Consultant Examiners (IBLCE)
1-703-560-7330
www.iblce.org
International board certification program for lactation consultants

International Lactation Consultant Association (ILCA)
1-919-861-5577
www.ilca.org
Annual conference with continuing education programs and peer-reviewed professional journal, *Journal of Human Lactation*

Lactation Education Resources
1-703-691-2069
www.leron-line.com
Education materials and training course

Lactation Institute (with Pacific Oaks College)
1-818-995-1913
www.lactationinstitute.org
Degree programs for lactation consultant preparation, educational materials for families and health care providers, lactation educator program, specialized treatment center

Continued

RESOURCE BOX

Breastfeeding—cont'd

Lactation Study Center
Department of Pediatrics
University of Rochester Medical Center
1-585-275-0088
www.cdc.gov/breastfeeding/compend-bhlsc.htm
Poison center and information on medications and breastfeeding

La Leche League International
1-800-525-3243 (LA-LECHE)
www.lalecheleague.org
Educational materials for breastfeeding families, annual workshops for lactation consultants and primary care providers

Medela, Inc.
1-800-435-8316
www.medela.com
Breast pumps and breastfeeding products, referral hotline for consumers, corporate lactation program

National Alliance for Breastfeeding Advocacy
1-410-995-3726
www.naba-breastfeeding.org
Continuing education programs, educational materials for families and health care providers; links to other breastfeeding resources and advocate groups

Nursing Mothers Counsel
www.nursingmothers.org
Support group for mothers

Rocky Mountain Drug Consultation Center
1-800-332-3073
www.rmpdc.org
Pharmaceutical and over-the-counter medication and drug information and consultation services for health care providers; information on poisoning

Wellstart
1-619-295-5192
www.wellstart.org
International educational programs, curricula, materials, speakers, conferences

WHO Global Data Bank on Breastfeeding
www.who.int/nut/db_bfd.htm
International information and links on infant, child, and maternal nutrition; links to WHO-UNICEF Baby-Friendly Hospital Initiative

REFERENCES

American Academy of Pediatrics: Breastfeeding and the use of human milk, *Pediatrics* 100:1035-1039, 1997.

American Academy of Pediatrics Committee on Drugs: The transfer of drugs and other chemicals into human milk, *Pediatrics* 108:776-789, 2001.

Bar-Yam N: Workplace lactation support, part I: a return-to-work breastfeeding assessment tool, *J Hum Lact* 14: 249-254, 1998.

Blaymore Bier JA et al: Human milk reduces outpatient upper respiratory symptoms in premature infants during their first year of life, *J Perinatol* 22:354-359, 2002.

Brigham M: Mothers' reports of the outcome of nipple shield use, *J Hum Lact* 12:291-297, 1996.

Chetwynd EM et al: Flucanozole for postpartum candidal mastitis and infant thrush, *J Hum Lact* 18:168-171, 2002.

Cohen R, Mrtek M, Mrtek R: Comparison of maternal absenteeism and infant illness rates among breastfeeding and formula feeding women in two corporations, *Am J Health Promot* 10:148-153, 1995.

Collaborative Group on Hormonal Factors in Breast Cancer: Breast cancer and breastfeeding: collaborative reanalysis of individual data from 47 epidemiological studies in 30 countries, *Lancet* 360:187-195, 2002.

Dewey KG et al: Growth of breast-fed and formula-fed infants from 0 to 18 months: the DARLING study, *Pediatrics* 89: 1035-1041, 1992.

Foxman B et al: Lactation mastitis: occurrence and medical management among 946 breastfeeding women in the United States, *Am J Epidemiol* 155:103-114, 2002.

Gartner LM, Greer FR, the Section on Breastfeeding and Committee on Nutrition: Prevention of rickets and vitamin D deficiency: new guidelines for vitamin D intake, *Pediatrics* 111:908-910, 2003.

Heird W: The role of polyunsaturated fatty acids in term and preterm infants and breastfeeding mothers, *Pediatr Clin North Am* 48:1731-1788, 2001.

Hoppu U, Kalliomaki M, Isolauri E: Maternal diet rich in saturated fat during breastfeeding is associated with atopic sensitization of the infant, *Eur J Clin Nutr* 54:702-705, 2000.

Institute of Medicine Subcommittee on Lactation: *Nutrition during lactation*, Washington, DC, 1991, National Academy Press.

Kramer MS et al: Breastfeeding and infant growth: biology or bias? PROBIT Study Group, *Pediatrics* 110:343-347, 2002.

Lawrence RA, Lawrence RM: *Breastfeeding: a guide for the medical profession*, ed 5, St Louis, 1999, Mosby.

Meier PP et al: Nipple shields for preterm infants: effect on milk transfer and duration of breastfeeding, *J Hum Lact* 16: 106-114, 2000.

National Association of Pediatric Nurse Associates and Practitioners: NAPNAP position statement: breast-feeding, *J Pediatr Health Care* 15:22A, 2001.

Neifert M, Seacat J, Jobe W: Lactation failure due to insufficient glandular development of the breast, *Pediatrics* 76:823-828, 1985.

Newman J: Breastfeeding problems associated with the early introduction of bottles and pacifiers, *J Hum Lact* 6:59-63, 1990.

Oddy WH: Breastfeeding protects against illness and infection in infants and children: a review of the evidence, *Breastfeed Rev* 9:11-18, 2001.

Owen CG et al: Infant feeding and blood cholesterol: a study in adolescents and a systematic review, *Pediatrics* 110:597-608, 2002.

Siskind V et al: Breastfeeding, menopause, and epithelial ovarian cancer, *Epidemiol* 8:188, 1997.

Specker B et al: Sunshine exposure and serum 25-hydroxyvitamin D concentrations in exclusively breast-fed infants, *J Pediatr* 107:372-376, 1985.

UNICEF: Baby-Friendly Hospital Initiative, Part II. Hospital level implementation. In *UNICEF guidelines*, Geneva, 1992, UNICEF.

WHO/UNICEF: *Protecting, promoting and supporting breastfeeding: the special role of maternity services: a joint WHO/UNICEF statement*, Geneva, 1989, World Health Organization.

Wyatt SN: Challenges of the working breastfeeding mother: workplace solutions, *AAOHN J* 50:61-66, 2002.

14 Elimination Patterns

Ardys M. Dunn

Patterns of elimination include skin, bowel and bladder habits, and excretory function. These serve as indicators of how well the gastrointestinal (GI), renal, urinary, and integumentary systems are functioning. This chapter discusses normal bowel and bladder function, normal developmental activities such as toilet training, and behaviors that are often self-limited in young children, but that can require intervention (e.g., encopresis and enuresis). Problems related more directly to GI and renal pathophysiology are presented in Chapters 33 and 35. Dermatologic conditions are discussed in Chapter 37.

Healthy children demonstrate an extremely wide range of "normal" elimination behavior, and nurse practitioners (NPs) have a responsibility to help parents understand the parameters of those norms. This can be a challenge because cultural and social expectations about elimination vary greatly, causing some parents to believe that their child has a problem when none exists. Also, developmental processes such as toilet training can lead to problems if not appropriately managed. NPs must conduct thorough and accurate assessments, provide anticipatory guidance for parents about what to expect as their child develops, help parents facilitate healthy bowel and bladder function, and refer for more complicated conditions.

STANDARDS

The American Academy of Pediatrics (AAP) recommends routine urinalysis at 5 years of age and a dipstick test for leukocytes at least once in adolescence or annually for all sexually active male and female adolescents (AAP, 2000). The U.S. Preventive Services Task Force (1996) does not recommend "routine screening for asymptomatic bacteriuria in...persons (other than pregnant women)." The guidelines for adolescent preventive services (GAPS), from the American Medical Association (AMA), recommend screening for urine leukocyte esterase in adolescent males as one way to assess for sexually transmitted diseases (AMA, 1997). The AAP recommends that toilet training begin at about 2 years of age (Shelov & Hannemann, 1999).

NORMAL PATTERNS OF ELIMINATION: BOWEL AND URINARY

Infants

Bowel Patterns

Bowel patterns of infants are related to the frequency and amount of feeding and differ between bottle-fed and breastfed babies. Breastfed infants commonly have many small stools per day in the first weeks of life. As children grow, fewer stools are typical, with some older breastfed infants having a stool once a day or as infrequently as once every 10 to 14 days. The stools are usually soft, sticky or watery, and light yellow, and have a "sour" but not unpleasant odor and a curdlike texture. Iron supplements can darken the stool and make it firmer.

Bottle-fed babies have two to four stools each day in the first month. As patterns become established, the number of stools decreases and older bottle-fed infants may have one to three stools each day. Stools of bottle-fed infants are firmer, darker, and smellier than those of breastfed infants. They may be brown, greenish, or dark yellow, depending on the type of formula and whether iron supplements are given. They are soft and semiformed. The stools of both breastfed and bottle-fed babies become firmer and darker as solid foods are introduced.

Urinary Patterns

Urination is associated with fluid intake and increases as infants take more fluids. Healthy, well-hydrated infants, whether breastfed or bottle-fed, should urinate a minimum of 6 times a day but can void, in small amounts, 15 to 20 times a day. Fever in infants can quickly lead to dehydration, with less frequent urination.

Infants are not capable of voluntary bowel and bladder control because these functions are dependent on myelination of the pyramidal tracts in the spinal cord, a process probably completed between 12 and 18 months of age. Infants 9 to 12 months old generally have regular patterns; they may have a bowel movement early in the morning or after feeding, or stay dry for several hours and urinate immediately after waking from a nap.

Toddlers and Preschoolers

Bowel Patterns

Toddlers and preschoolers usually have a regular pattern of elimination. Although they typically have one to three stools a day, it is not unusual for children in this age-group to defecate every other day or every third or fourth day. It is a myth that healthy children must have a bowel movement every day. Constipation is defined as a hard stool, passed with difficulty, infrequently—every third day (Behrman, Kliegman, & Jenson, 2004). Normal stools have an unpleasant odor and are soft, formed, and various shades of brown, depending on the child's diet.

Urinary Patterns

By the time children are 2 years of age, renal function is fully developed. Fluid intake, environmental conditions, perspiration, fever, and diarrhea with significant fluid loss influence the urinary pattern of toddlers and preschoolers. They typically urinate 8 to 14 times a day. Cold weather, excitement, and stress lead to increased frequency. Children generally do not void during sleep after 18 months (Jansson et al, 2000).

School-Age Children

Bowel Patterns

Elimination patterns in school-age children approximate those of adults. Depending on a child's intake, bowel movements occur from one to three times a day to once every 2 to 3 days. Stool is soft, formed, and brown and has an odor. School-age children should be completely toilet trained, although occasional soiling of underwear occurs as a result of poor hygiene or because children do not respond quickly to cues to defecate. It is important to remember children's increasing needs for independence and privacy during the school-age years and incorporate consideration of those needs into management of toileting.

Urinary Patterns

School-age children have essentially the same capacity as adults to produce urine—between 650 and 1500 ml in a 24-hour period—but the kidneys are still small and accommodate a smaller urine volume at any one time than those of adults. Children normally void five to six times a day. Girls appear to have slightly larger bladder capacity than boys. Dysfunctional voiding (too little = 1 to 3 times a day; too much = 8 to 12 times a day), daytime incontinence, or nocturnal enuresis warrants further evaluation, especially because these conditions can be associated with infection, dehydration, or sexual abuse.

Adolescents

Bowel and Bladder Patterns

Gastrointestinal and renal function is at adult levels in adolescents, and patterns of elimination are similar to those of adults. Abnormal variation can occur in teenagers who have eating disorders. Adolescents are also susceptible to the demands of schedules, stress, and irregular eating patterns. The need for privacy and personal space might inhibit normal elimination in public places such as school or dormitory restrooms. Sexual activity can contribute to changes in bowel or bladder function, including infections or constipation.

ASSESSMENT OF PATTERNS

Assessment of elimination patterns begins with a thorough health history, with questions being asked of the parent or the child, depending on the child's age and ability. As variations of normal behavior become evident, relevant follow-up questions should be asked to clarify and complete the patient's health picture.

Health History

Description of Current Status

The patient's current elimination status can be assessed with the following questions:

- How often does your child urinate? How many wet diapers does your baby have in a 24-hour period?
- How often does your child have a bowel movement? Describe what the stools look and smell like. How does your child act when having a bowel movement?
- Describe anything unusual about your child's elimination habits. Does your child resist going to the bathroom?
- Describe your child's toileting habits. For example, at what time of day does your child have a bowel movement?
- Do you use any medications, including over-the-counter preparations or home remedies, to help your child with bowel movements?

- How do you think the process of toilet training will happen? (Ask parents of a 9- to 12-month-old child.)
- Is your child toilet trained? When did training begin? Describe the process. How often do "accidents" happen? How do you (parent) feel toilet training is progressing?
- What names do you use in your family for stool and urine, for body parts, and for the process of using the toilet?

Birth History

Determine whether any problems with the child's urine or stool were present at birth. For example, did the baby pass a meconium stool within 48 hours after birth? How soon after birth did the baby urinate?

Review of Systems

The review of systems should include the following questions:

- Has your child ever been constipated or had diarrhea? Was that condition related to anything in particular (e.g., a particular illness, a certain food, or change in diet)? Is it chronic or only occasional? If chronic, did it start after a particular incident (e.g., illness, during toilet training)? How does the parent define constipation and diarrhea?
- Has your child ever had a urinary tract infection? Describe. Any workup (e.g., ultrasonography, urethrogram)?
- Has your child had any illness, injury, or operation related to the bowel or bladder? Describe.
- Does your child have a physical condition or chronic illness that affects voiding or bowel movements?
- What medications, including over-the-counter preparations, does your child take?

Family History

Determine whether any family members, including parents, have had problems with urination or bowel movements and obtain a description of those problems (e.g., chronic constipation or diarrhea, bedwetting). Has there been any travel or residence outside the United States?

Environmental and Psychosocial

Environmental and psychosocial issues should be assessed:

- How do you, as a parent, feel about the issue of toileting?
- How do you interact with your child around toileting issues?
- How do you deal with toileting "accidents"?
- What plans do you have for managing toilet training?
- Describe your child's typical diet.
- Tell me about the toileting facilities at your child's house/day care/school. How do you think they affect your child's toileting habits?

Physical Examination

The physical examination includes external examination of the perineum, anus, and urinary meatus and auscultation and palpation of the abdomen for bowel sounds, softness, masses, peristalsis, and tenderness.

Laboratory and Diagnostic Tests

A urinalysis is done as indicated, including once as a screening during the preschool years, at about age 5 years, and again during adolescence. Annual urinalysis for leukocytes is recommended for sexually active adolescents (AAP, 2000).

MANAGEMENT STRATEGIES FOR NORMAL PATTERNS

Toilet Training

Toilet training occurs in the toddler and preschool years and is usually complete by age 4. Successful toilet training requires sensitivity, understanding of development, good communication, hope, humor, and patience. In addition to becoming self-sufficient in their toileting, children should also learn that elimination is a natural and necessary process. As self-toileting is mastered, both parents and children should experience pride and satisfaction in having worked together to accomplish an important developmental task.

The NP plays an important role in providing anticipatory guidance to parents (Kinservik & Friedhoff, 2000). NPs should introduce the topic of toilet training at the 9-month visit and again at 12, 15, and 18 months; assess for parents' expectations and plans; and provide ample opportunity for discussion of realistic toileting outcomes. Because true voluntary sphincter control is a function of psychologic and social, as well as physiologic, development, children are not usually ready for toilet training until 18 to 24 months of age or even older (Schum et al, 2002). Although every child is unique, and readiness cues should ultimately be used to decide when to begin training, parents should be discouraged from attempting to toilet train their children before 24 months. If begun too early, the process can be very stressful, and at least one study has shown that children with primary encopresis had more difficult and disruptive toilet-training experiences than those without (Fishman et al, 2002). In contrast, a study by Bakker and associates (2002) found that children with bedwetting problems tended to be trained later than those without problems; this study suggests, however, that a structured yet flexible approach to training that is

TABLE 14-1	*Guidelines for Assessing Readiness to Toilet Train*
Child's physical skills	Has voluntary sphincter control
	Stays dry for 2 hr, may wake from naps still dry
	Is able to sit, walk, and squat
	Assists in dressing self
Child's cognitive skills	Recognizes urge to urinate or defecate
	Understands meaning of words used by family in toileting
	Understands what the toilet is for
	Understands connection between dry pants and toilet
	Is able to follow directions
	Is able to communicate needs
Child's interpersonal skills	Demonstrates desire to please parent
	Expresses curiosity about use of toilet
	Expresses desire to be dry and clean
Parental skills	Expresses desire to assist child with training
	Recognizes child's cues of readiness
	Has no compelling factor that will interfere with training (e.g., new job, move, family loss)

BOX 14-1 *Management of Toilet Training*

- Keep child as clean and dry as possible:
 - Change diapers frequently.
 - Use training pants when child stays dry for several hours during the day; use diaper at night.
- Talk to child about toilet training:
 - Praise child for asking you to have diaper changed.
 - Explain connection between being clean and dry and using toilet.
 - Encourage child to use toilet, especially before going out to play, going on a trip, before naps, and at bedtime.
- Teach child how to use toilet:
 - Allow child to observe while parents or older siblings use toilet.
 - Demonstrate how to sit on toilet, use toilet paper, flush, and wash one's hands.
- Provide practice time for child:
 - Provide a potty chair or portable toilet seat.
 - Allow child to sit on potty chair with clothes or diaper on.
 - Encourage child to use potty chair while parent uses regular toilet.
 - Have child sit on potty chair without diapers for 5 to 10 minutes at a time.
 - Practice at times a child usually urinates or defecates.
- Provide a comfortable, safe-feeling environment:
 - Seat child facing backward on a regular toilet or provide a footstool to rest the feet on.
 - Never flush the toilet when child is sitting on it.
 - Stay with child for safety reasons.
- Give consistent, positive feedback:
 - Praise child for trying, as well as for success.
 - Be understanding of child's refusal to use toilet.
 - Never demand performance.
 - Never make child sit on toilet if child resists.
 - Ignore or minimize undesired behavior.
 - Never scold or punish if a child wets or soils.

responsive to the child's cues is likely to be most successful. Guidelines for assessing toilet-training readiness include physical, cognitive, interpersonal or psychologic, and parental skills (Table 14-1).

Typically, children are trained first for nocturnal bowel control, then daytime bowel control, daytime bladder control, and finally nocturnal bladder control. Girls tend to be trained earlier than boys; average times for completing training are around 3 to 4 years of age, with a range of up to a year for individual children as normal. Average ages for girls and boys to accomplish other tasks of toilet training are as follows (Schum et al, 2002):

- Showing an interest in using the toilet: girls, 24 months; boys, 26 months
- Telling parents of their need to use the toilet: girls, 26 months; boys, 29 months
- Staying dry for at least 2 hours: girls, 26 months; boys, 29 months
- Staying dry during the day: girls, 32.5 months; boys, 35.0 months

When children and parents are ready to begin toilet training, several management techniques are helpful (Box 14-1). If children resist training, the project should be put on hold for a few weeks before trying again. If toddlers seem to be toilet trained for a brief period and suddenly regress to wetting and soiling consistently, they should be placed back in diapers and the process begun again within a few weeks.

Toilet training is one of the tasks toddlers master on their way to independence, and NPs should work with parents to ensure that the process does not become one of a power struggle for control (Kinservik & Friedhoff, 2000). Parents can become extremely frustrated if their expectations do not match the abilities and performance of their children, and the incidence of child abuse related to toilet training is high. Berkowitz (2000) notes that issues around toileting are the second most prevalent factor precipitating fatal child abuse. The NP can play a crucial role in making the experience a positive one and preventing abuse by giving parents information about child development, techniques for managing the process, and support and encouragement for their efforts.

ALTERED PATTERNS OF ELIMINATION

The following discussion focuses on four relatively common conditions of childhood related to elimination: stool toileting refusal, encopresis, enuresis, and dysfunctional voiding. These conditions are considered here as developmental problems of normal urinary and bowel habits. If assessment reveals indication of pathology, further investigation and different management, including referral, are necessary.

Stool Toileting Refusal

Description

Stool toileting refusal is present when a child demonstrates a pattern of successfully using the toilet to urinate but refusing to use the toilet for bowel movements. These children will usually defecate in a diaper, training pants, or "pull-ups." In some cases, children will retain stool, or defecate outside the toilet. Encopresis without constipation also fits this description: The child defecates outside the toilet when beyond the age of expected training.

Incidence and Etiology

The incidence of stool toileting refusal has not been recently documented. Taubman (1997) found that 22% of healthy children between 18 and 30 months of age experienced at least 1 month of stool toileting refusal. The presence of younger siblings in the household and the parents' inability to set limits for the child appear to be related to refusal. Although children who displayed stool toileting refusal tended to have "a more difficult temperament" than did children who were toilet trained (Blum, Taubman, & Osborne, 1997), they did not have any more behavior problems. Constipation and painful bowel movements, a possible result of stool toileting refusal, may also be a cause of the problem.

Clinical Findings

History. Parents or caregivers report that the child demonstrates the following:

- Bladder control but refusal to defecate on the toilet
- A regular pattern of bowel movements
- Signs that a bowel movement is imminent

Physical Examination. The physical examination will be unremarkable if the child has a pattern of regular bowel movements.

- Examine the anus for fissures or irritation that may cause a child to refuse to defecate.
- Check for signs of stool retention:
  - Abdominal distention
  - Abdominal tenderness on palpation
- Palpation of a mass in the sigmoid colon or at the midline in the suprapubic area (impaction).

Differential Diagnosis

The differential diagnosis includes stool withholding, constipation, and encopresis.

Management

Behavioral management is appropriate for younger children. Return them to diapers and reintroduce toilet training in about a month or when the child indicates interest. Some children prefer not to wear diapers all the time, but will ask to have one put on when they feel the urge to defecate. After having a bowel movement, they ask to be changed and return to wearing training pants. This pattern may continue for several weeks or months. For older children, schedule daily times for the child to sit on the toilet for 5 to 10 minutes; have these times be positive, never punitive or forced. Never flush the toilet while the child is sitting on it. Provide incentives and give positive feedback when the child successfully uses the toilet for bowel movements (Kuhn, Marcus, & Pitner, 1999). If the child has constipation, fecal impaction, or both, initial bowel cleanout is necessary, in conjunction with increased fiber and fluid in the diet. Mineral oil, suppositories or medication may be useful (see Table 14-2 for management of a child with encopresis with constipation).

Complications

Refusal to use the toilet for bowel movements may lead to stool withholding, constipation, and impaction, conditions that result in primary encopresis. Psychologic complications include embarrassment, shame, conflict, and stress between children and parents, especially as the child becomes older. Child abuse can be a significant complication (Berkowitz, 2000).

Patient Education and Prevention

Prevention through appropriate toilet training is key (see Box 14-1). If a child refuses to defecate on the toilet, use of punishment or force can complicate the problem. Parents should be alert for signs of constipation (hard stools, fewer than three bowel movements per week) and should

TABLE 14-2 ***Management of Children with Encopresis with Constipation***

Treatment Phase	Treatment Program	Comments
Catharsis	In the home: four 3-day cycles (12 days total): • Day 1: Fleet enema (adult size) • Day 2: Bisacodyl suppository • Day 3: Bisacodyl tablet (children >3 yr old) • Day 13: Bisacodyl tablet Return to clinic Follow-up addominal radiograph to confirm catharsis	Goal of catharsis is to empty the bowel; there are no absolute best ways to achieve this. Catharsis may need to occur in the hospital if • Retention is severe. • Home compliance is poor. • Parents prefer admission. • Parents should not administer enemas for psychologic reasons. Enema should be fully expelled to prevent hypertonic dehydration The child may have watery or soft stools for several days after catharsis; parents and patient should be informed that ongoing maintenance is essential for the bowel to return to fully normal functioning (see Fig. 14-1). Initial improvement can be falsely reassuring and may contribute to poor compliance with maintenance regimen.
Maintenance	**Medications** Stool softener: Mineral oil, starting at 2 tbs bid; titrate dose to facilitate soft stools without mineral oil leakage Daily multivitamin to counteract possible decreased absorption of fat-soluble vitamins Oral laxatives: Polyethylene glycol 3350 (PEG), 0.8 g/kg titrated up or down to maintain soft stools Milk of magnesia, 6-12 yr: 15-30 ml/day **Behavioral changes** Toilet sitting 3-4 times a day for 10 min; at least twice a day for 10 min each time Increased physical activity **Dietary changes** Increased fluids (other than milk), increased fiber in diet, consider limiting constipating foods Document every bowel movement: time, quality, amount, location Regular visits to provider at 2 wk, 1 mo, 3 mo, 6 mo	Goals of maintenance: • No soiling; prevent reimpaction • Regular, soft bowel movements (at least every other day; >3/wk) • Increased ability to sense the urge to defecate Laxatives may be substituted for or used alternately with stool softeners. PEG has been shown to be effective in treatment of constipation when used alone (Pashankar & Bishop, 2001) and more effective than lactulose (Gremse, Hixon, & Crutchfield, 2002). Use of senna is not recommended. Toilet sitting should be scheduled at times the child is most likely to have a bowel movement (e.g., on wakening, after meals). Plan on 6 months of treatment before bowel regains full function
Follow-up	Regular visits (about every 4-10 wk) depending on severity and need of family Telephone availability to discuss progress and adjust doses Counseling or referral as appropriate for psychosocial and developmental issues Continued education of normal bowel function (see Fig. 14-1)	Goals of follow-up visits: • Monitor compliance. • Provide encouragement and support. • Detect and treat relapse early if it occurs.

Data from Levine MD, Carey WB, Crocker AC: *Developmental-behavioral pediatrics,* ed 3, Philadelphia, 1999, WB Saunders; Felt B et al: Guideline for the management of pediatric idiopathic constipation and soiling, *Arch Pediatr Adolesc Med* 153:380-385, 1999.

encourage fluids, fiber, and exercise to facilitate bowel movements and prevent encopresis.

Encopresis and Constipation

Description

Encopresis is defined as stool incontinence after an age when children should be able to control bowel movements, usually 4 years of age. Primary, or continuous, encopresis is present in children who have never been toilet trained. Secondary, or discontinuous, encopresis is seen in those who were previously trained but who begin to soil. There are two subtypes of encopresis: encopresis with constipation, associated with stool retention, constipation, and incontinence overflow; and encopresis without constipation. In encopresis with constipation, stool retention over time leads to distention of the colon and stretching of the rectum, ineffective peristalsis, decreased sensory threshold in the rectum, and weakened rectal and sphincter muscles. Stool becomes dry, hard, and difficult to evacuate (can be impacted), and bowel movements can be painful. Soft, semiformed or liquid stool from higher in the colon can leak around retained stool and pass through the rectum, causing soiling. Encopresis with constipation is involuntary, and the child is often unaware of the actual incontinence. Children with encopresis with constipation may either refuse or be willing to use the toilet.

Those few children with encopresis without constipation have voluntary bowel movements, but in their clothing or other inappropriate places.

Incidence and Etiology

Encopresis may be more common than believed because many families hesitate to inform their health care provider about it. In the school-age child, it is more common among boys than girls (Behrman, Kliegman, & Jenson, 2004). The etiology of encopresis is unclear and appears to differ among children. Both physiologic and psychosocial factors are involved. Often there is a history of an acute stool problem (e.g., child had an illness that caused dehydration and constipation) that was not adequately managed, leading to a cycle of constipation—painful defecation—stool retention—more severe constipation—more painful defecation—more stool retention and so on.

Physiologic. Physiologic factors related to constipation and encopresis include the following:

- Inadequate fluid intake
- Dehydration caused by illness and fever or during active play in hot weather
- A change in diet such as the introduction of solids or increased carbohydrates and decreased fiber
- Inappropriate use of laxatives, suppositories, or enemas by parents who do not understand normal bowel patterns in children and infants
- Stool retention and constipation secondary to the following:
  - Painful bowel movements
  - Anal fissures
  - Paradoxic constriction of the external anal sphincter muscle during attempted defecation
  - Neurogenic conditions (e.g., aganglionic colon [Hirschsprung's disease], cerebral palsy, myelomeningocele)
  - Endocrine and metabolic conditions (e.g., hypothyroidism)
  - Medications (e.g., codeine, iron supplements)

Psychosocial. Psychosocial factors related to constipation and encopresis include the following:

- Major family or life adjustments such as loss of a parent, sibling, or other significant person
- Inappropriate toilet-training techniques; children who are pushed might rebel in the only way they can, by refusing to cooperate
- Irregular toileting patterns, often caused by travel, unfamiliar bathrooms, lack of regular routine
- Physical abuse and sexual abuse

Clinical Findings

History. The history can include the following:

- Stained underwear
- Report of fewer than three bowel movements per week
- Difficult or painful defecation
- Large-caliber or hard stool
- Child suddenly becoming still during play, attempting to hide when urge to defecate is felt
- Child attempting to retain stool (e.g., crossing legs, grimacing, or shifting from one foot to another)
- Reports of a bloated sensation, abdominal pain, or both
- Odor of stool from leakage into underwear
- Streaks of bright blood on toilet paper or underwear
- Enuresis
- Urinary tract infections
- Anorexia

Physical Examination. The physical examination should assess for the following:

- Overflow soiling
- Abdominal distention
- Abdominal tenderness on palpation
- Impactions felt on digital rectal examination (rectal examination may be deferred if the history and other

signs allow for a clear diagnosis, because it can be traumatic for the child)
- Mass felt at the midline in the suprapubic area
- Anal fissures
- Neurologic signs: abdominal, cremasteric, anal wink reflexes, deep tendon refexes (DTRs) in lower extremities

Laboratory and Diagnostic Tests. X-rays and laboratory tests to identify structural or organic causes of constipation are not routinely necessary (Loening-Baucke, 2002), but can be appropriate if clinical suspicion is high or primary treatment for encopresis is unsuccessful. Results of an abdominal radiograph can indicate accumulation of stool in the sigmoid colon (see Chapter 33).

Differential Diagnosis

The differential diagnoses for encopresis with constipation are as follows:
- Anorectal stenosis
- Spina bifida occulta
- Hirschsprung's disease
- Mental retardation
- Hypothyroidism
- Hypercalcemia
- Cerebral palsy
- Other organic causes of constipation
- Normal red-faced grunting and straining of infants on defecation

Management

Treatment of children with encopresis differs depending on whether they have impactions, are constipated, or have normal bowel movements but defecate in places other than the toilet. In all cases, the goals of treatment are to establish a regular bowel routine, "demystify" the problem, alleviate blame, and gain cooperation for treatment plans (Felt et al, 1999; Levine, Carey, & Crocker, 1999).

Box 14-2 outlines approaches to treating a child with encopresis without constipation (also see management of stool toileting refusal earlier in this chapter).

Children who have encopresis with constipation present a greater challenge. A clear message to children and parents should be that the dynamics of encopresis (retention, stretching, decreased peristalsis, impaction, leaking) are not voluntary—no one is to blame; they can be reversed through bowel rehabilitation; correcting them will take hard work, cooperation, and time; and the NP will work with the family to ensure success.

Table 14-2 provides guidelines to treating a child with encopresis with constipation, including appropriate medications. Figure 14-1 can be used to educate parents and children about the bowel rehabilitation process involved in the treatment plan.

Management of encopresis is often multidisciplinary, combining medical and psychologic interventions (Borowitz et al, 2002; Loening-Baucke, 2002). Psychologic counseling of both the child and family may be necessary. In some cases, referral to a psychologist or behavioral pediatrician is appropriate. Because this problem often occurs in school-age children, the NP may need to consult with the school nurse to ensure that the child receives appropriate medications, hygiene management, and essential psychologic and emotional support.

If primary treatment is unsuccessful, review compliance. If compliance is good, consider other diagnoses; referral for evaluation of alternative diagnoses or to a gastroenterology subspecialist for more focused management may be appropriate.

BOX 14-2 Management of Children with Mild Encopresis without Constipation

- Monitor diet:
  - Ensure adequate fiber and water intake.
  - Decrease milk to 16 oz/day; limit cheese, rice, applesauce, bananas.
  - Provide 2-4 oz prune juice daily.
- Avoid use of stool softeners or laxatives.
- Encourage child to take responsibility for own toilet habits.
- Use incentives or rewards to reinforce positive behavior.
- Establish a regular toileting routine.

Complications

Persistent encopresis is an unpleasant condition, and children with encopresis often experience ridicule and shame. Age-group peers frequently treat children with scorn, hostility, and rejection. Teachers and other adults might be disgusted by children with encopresis, and parents, dealing with anger, guilt, embarrassment, and helplessness, find their children and the condition extremely difficult to manage. Social, interpersonal, and family relations are at grave risk.

Patient Education and Prevention

The best treatment of encopresis is prevention. If constipation or encopresis is caused by an underlying anatomic or organic cause (e.g., Hirschsprung's disease, occult spina

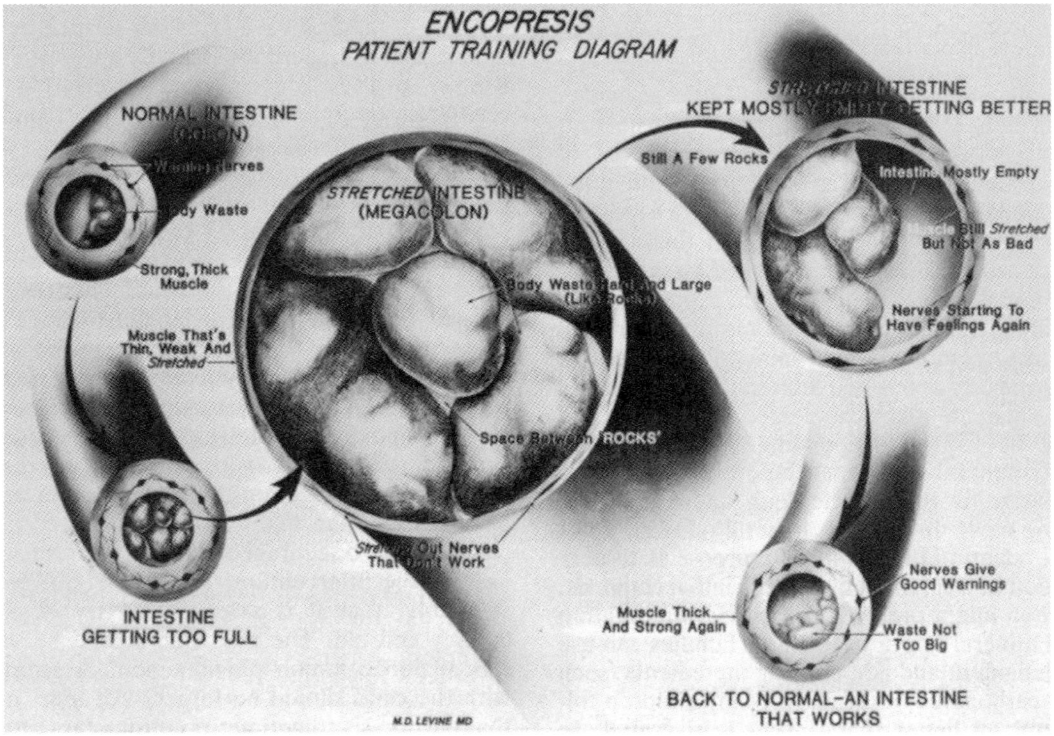

FIGURE 14-1 Encopresis: patient training diagram. (From Levine MD, Carey WB, Crocker AC: *Developmental-behavioral patterns*, ed 3, Philadelphia, 1999, WB Saunders.)

bifida, hypothyroidism), early diagnosis and referral is essential. It is important for the pediatric provider to understand the relationship between constipation and encopresis, recognize conditions that may contribute to each, and provide parents with anticipatory guidance related to dietary and toileting management of their children to prevent their occurrence. It is equally important to provide support during treatment. Although parents should be informed that treatment may be required for months or years, NPs should emphasize that by following a clear, consistent, aggressive treatment protocol, the condition can be managed. Finally, the NP, parents, and child must work together to prevent recurrence of symptoms after successful treatment.

Enuresis

Description

Enuresis is defined as involuntary or unintentional urination at an age when voluntary control should be present. Children who have never established control have primary enuresis. Secondary enuresis is present when children have been dry for more than 6 to 12 months and begin wetting. Nocturnal enuresis, also called monosymptomatic nocturnal enuresis (MNE), is incontinence during sleep. Diurnal enuresis occurs during waking hours. There is no consensus on what frequency of wetting justifies a diagnosis of enuresis. The DSM-IV specifies 2 wet nights per week and the International Classification of Diseases (ICD) specifies 1 night per month as the threshold for enuresis. Parents may ask for help if their child has as few as 1 to 3 wet nights per month, a number that some use as a standard for "cure or full response to therapy" (van Gool, 2002).

Some children who have MNE without an organic cause (i.e., anatomic defects, infections) appear to have problems being roused from sleep when they need to void (Brunell et al, 2001). The need to void can be due to either normal urine volume with a small bladder capacity, or normal bladder capacity with a large urine volume. In either case, the bladder signals the need to void, the child is difficult to rouse, and wetting occurs. Wetting appears to occur most frequently in the first two thirds of the night (Wolfish, 2001).

Incidence and Etiology

The age at which urinary continence is normally achieved varies greatly. As a result, the prevalence of enuresis is difficult to assess. Boys are more likely to have nocturnal enuresis than girls, and black children have a greater incidence of enuresis than white children. Generally, enuresis is not considered to be outside the range of normal limits before 5 to 6 years of age. Approximately 7% of 5-year-old boys and 3% of 5-year-old girls have enuresis; 3% of 10-year-old boys and 2% of 10-year-old girls. At age 18, it is 1% for boys but very rare in girls (Behrman, Kliegman, & Jenson, 2004).

Approximately 95% of voiding problems are functional, whereas the remainder may represent an organic condition. Primary nocturnal enuresis has an organic etiology in only about 1% of cases (Behrman & Kliegman, 2002). The actual cause of enuresis is difficult to determine, and it differs among children. A number of factors have been found to be associated with enuresis, including the following:

- Familial disposition. Chromosomal linkages have been found for enuresis (Loeys et al, 2002; von Gontard et al, 2001). It is estimated that 77% of children with enuresis have two parents with a history of enuresis; 50% of children have one parent with a history of enuresis; and for 15% of children with enuresis, neither parent has a history of enuresis.
- Inappropriate toilet training, especially when parents are overly demanding or punitive of the child.
- Stress and family disruptions such as a divorce, move, or a new member.
- Neurologic developmental delay in which the child is unable to inhibit bladder contraction.
- Small bladder capacity. A bladder capacity of 300 to 350 ml is necessary for a child to sleep through the night without incontinence. In some children, bladder capacity appears normal during the day but is reduced at night (Yeung et al, 2002).
- Sleep arousal patterns. Although studies show little overall difference in the sleep of children with and without enuresis (Bader et al, 2002), children who "sleep deeply" appear more prone to nocturnal bedwetting (Wolfish, 2001).
- Detrusor instability, in which the child has learned to inhibit sphincter relaxation and prevent complete emptying of the bladder, combined with delayed arousal from sleep and polyuria can be a factor in nocturnal enuresis.
- Hormonal regulation. Some children with enuresis may have lower levels of antidiuretic hormone (ADH), contributing to nocturnal polyuria (Pomeranz et al, 2000; Tomasi et al, 2001).
- Chronic constipation.
- Stress incontinence.

Clinical Findings

History. With daytime enuresis, parents often report that the child

- Demonstrates an immediate urgency to void
- Becomes restless or jiggly, crosses the legs, or holds the penis or pubic area
- May smell of urine

Nocturnal enuresis is characterized by the following:

- Spot urination (the child wakes after beginning to urinate and is able to stop the stream)
- Bedwetting

Parents should be asked about the following:

- History of enuresis, treatment, and age of resolution for other family members, including parents
- Frequency of wetting
- Time of wetting (daytime or nighttime)
- Volume of urine voided
- Type of urinary stream
- Any urgency, dysuria, polyuria, or dribbling
- History of toilet training; age began, how handled (was child ever dry? For how long?)
- Presence of other behavior problems
- Changes in the home, family, or school environment
- Affect on child and parents
- Manner in which family deals with the enuresis (e.g., is child punished?)

Physical Examination. The physical examination includes the following:

- Assess the external genitalia for signs of irritation, infection, labial fusion, meatal stenosis.
- Assess for bladder capacity; can have parents collect and measure urine over 3 days.
- Observe the size and velocity of the urine stream.
- Check for fecal impaction.
- Examine the abdomen for masses, especially at the suprapubic midline and in the left lower quadrant.
- Examine the lower back for dimples, hair tufts.
- Assess for neurologic function, DTR.

Laboratory and Diagnostic Tests. A urinalysis, with culture, is recommended in all children with enuresis. More sophisticated testing is usually not necessary (Cayan et al, 2001; van Gool, 2002).

Differential Diagnosis

The differential diagnosis includes daytime or extraordinary urinary frequency syndrome, a benign condition of excessive (more than 8 to 12 per day, often as frequent as every 15 to 30 minutes) urination seen in previously toilet-trained children. Daytime urinary frequency syndrome has no known cause but may be associated with viral cystitis or urethritis, stress, and hypercalciuria. Though considered self-limited because it does not typically respond to medication, daytime frequency syndrome can persist for months or even years. Treatment with pelvic floor exercise (Kegel) and biofeedback has shown promise (in one study more than 85% of children improved), but further research is indicated (Glazier et al, 2001).

Organic causes of enuresis must be identified; the most common is urinary tract infection, which occurs in 1% to 2% of cases. Urinary tract infections may be related to encopresis, and a child with enuresis should be examined for fecal impaction and a history of soiling. Wetting can also be due to a primary detrusor instability. Other organic causes to consider include the following:

- Diabetes mellitus
- Diabetes insipidus
- Sickle cell disease, in which treatment by means of forced fluids may lead to increased urine output
- Chronic renal failure, in which the kidneys are unable to concentrate urine
- Structural anomalies such as vesicoureteral reflux, ectopic ureter (constant leakage is noted)
- Neurologic abnormalities, including neurogenic bladder
- Hypercalciuria
- Obstructive uropathy
- Vaginitis
- Sleep apnea

Management

Although most children maintain urinary continence after toilet training is established, wetting is a common phenomenon, and parents should be reassured that it rarely indicates disease. A thorough physical examination to distinguish between organic and nonorganic causes is the first step in treatment. Organic conditions are treated as appropriate; referral may be necessary.

Treatment of functional enuresis (i.e., from nonorganic causes) takes several forms because the condition is heterogeneous. A combined approach using alarms, behavioral and motivational therapy, and medication is often indicated, and such a "full-spectrum" treatment plan has been shown to be highly effective (Van Kampen et al, 2002). Successful treatment has been correlated to family functioning and requires active involvement of both parents and children. Families should be active in deciding what treatment is most appropriate and when it should be implemented.

Outcomes of treatment are categorized as full response (greater than 90% reduction in wet nights), partial response (50% to 90% reduction in wet nights), or no response (less than 50% reduction in wet nights). A cure is a full response that continues 6 months or longer after treatment has ended (van Gool, 2002).

Because functional enuresis is largely self-limited, there is consensus to delay aggressive treatment until the child is 6 to 8 years of age. Strategies for use with a 6-year-old or older child include the following:

- *Bladder control training (urotherapy).* Because many children with enuresis have low functional bladder capacities, the goal of urotherapy is to increase children's awareness of the need to urinate and to give them more control of the urination process. Urotherapy involves increasing daytime urination by encouraging children to urinate frequently, *not* holding urine until the micturation urge is felt. Urotherapy trains children through visualization exercises to imagine what it feels like to have the urge to urinate and encourages them to practice urinating. Proper posture (sitting upright, feet on floor; standing erect) while urinating is important in order to be more sensitive to cues of a full bladder and to control urination. This approach is used effectively for children with hyperactive bladders, may make medication unnecessary for many children, and warrants further clinical research (Kruse, Hellstrom, Hjalmas, 1999; Robson & Leung, 2002).
- *Enuresis alarm.* Behavioral modification involves the introduction of a stimulus that leads to a desired response from the subject. An electric alarm with a bell or buzzer is triggered as the child begins to wet and reflexively, urination stops. The child must then use the toilet. Initially, children may not rouse and parents must take them to the toilet, even though the child may not be fully awake. Wet bed linens and pajamas are then changed and the alarm is reset. Subsequently, as the alarm is triggered and the child is roused, the child learns to associate a full bladder and the beginning of urination with waking and toileting. Low functional bladder capacity and difficulty arousing the child are factors that limit the success of alarms (Butler & Robinson, 2002). Although this method has a significantly higher success rate than other methods (Mellon & McGrath, 2000), some children, especially older children, may object to continued use, others may relapse without the external stimulus, and parents must be committed to getting up with the child for up to 3 months of treatment.
- *Motivational therapy.* This strategy assumes that children will take responsibility for the problem and for learning how to resolve it. The family is expected to provide supportive reinforcement for positive behavior, such as use of a "star chart," rewards, and praise. Children are taught to be increasingly sensitive to their body's cues to

urinate, encouraged to void in the toilet, and reinforced, either emotionally, materially, or both, for success. This therapy is emotionally time consuming and requires a high level of healthy communication between parents and children. Provider support of both parents and children is essential. Children should be seen by the provider every 2 weeks; 70% to 90% show improvement. Hypnosis, self-hypnosis, and acupuncture also may have promise, but require more clinical research (Mellon & McGrath, 2000; Serel et al, 2001).

- *Drug therapy.* Drug therapy is often used in conjunction with other strategies and usually has high initial success rates. Unfortunately, it is expensive and extremely high relapse rates can occur when the drug is discontinued. However, it can be extremely useful for overnight stays (e.g., camp), when staying dry is very important to the child. Medications used for MNE include desmopressin, imipramine, and oxybutynin (Table 14-3 and Appendix A).

Desmopressin, available in tablet and nasal spray forms, has an antidiuretic effect and appears to be effective in children with large nocturnal urine production and normal nocturnal bladder capacity. Some researchers suggest that desmopressin, combined with use of an enuresis alarm, could lead to nearly 100% correction of nocturnal enuresis (Mellon & McGrath, 2000). There is a high relapse rate associated with short-term therapy, but long-term therapy has been found to be very safe (Tullus et al, 1999).

Imipramine is a tricyclic antidepressant whose action related to enuresis is not entirely clear. It may change sleep patterns, have an anticholinergic effect on the bladder, or have an antidiuretic effect (Tomasi et al, 2001). Because of serious side effects, most significantly cardiac death, and a low long-term response rate, imipramine is not considered a first-line medication and is not used by some providers (Mikkelsen, 2001). The panel of the First International Consultation on Incontinence, sponsored by the World Health Organization (WHO) and the International Union Against Cancer (UICC), does not recommend use of imipramine in the treatment of enuresis (Abrams, Khoury, & Wein, 1998). If all other treatments are ineffective, or if the child is diagnosed with hyperactivity disorders, imipramine can be used (Hjalmas, 1999).

TABLE 14-3 ***Drug Therapy for Children with Monosymptomatic Nocturnal Enuresis***

Medication	Dosing	Comments
Desmopressin acetate (DDAVP)	Oral: 0.2 mg tablets once daily at bedtime; can be adjusted up to maximum of 0.6 mg/day Nasal spray: 20 μg (2 sprays) intranasally at bedtime; can be adjusted up to 40 μg/day or down to 10 μg/day	Not recommended in children younger than 6 yr When switching from nasal spray to tablets, give first oral dose 24 hr after last intranasal dose When using nasal spray, administer one-half dose per nostril Changes in nasal mucosa (e.g., with upper respiratory infection) may compromise absorption; in these cases, administer an antihistamine or decongestant 30-60 min before using or consider oral form Caution must be used with patients who are hypertensive or have a potential for fluid-electrolyte imbalance (e.g., children with cystic fibrosis susceptible to hyponatremia) Use least amount effective Take on empty stomach; avoid caffeine, chocolate, Nutrasweet, and carbonated beverages Children must be wakened to urinate within 10 hr of taking the medication
Imipramine hydrochloride	Dosing: 0.9-1.5 mg/kg/day (Zaontz & Welch, 2002) Initially, 25 mg daily 1 hr before bedtime. After 1 wk can increase to 50 mg for children 6-12 yr, 75 mg for children older than 12 yr	Not recommended in children younger than 6 yr Administer with great care Use least amount effective Has serious side effects and a high level of toxicity; has been fatal to patient or siblings in some cases Requires electrocardiogram before and after treatment has started to rule out cardiac conduction disorder
Oxybutynin chloride	5 mg bid, maximum of 5 mg tid	Not recommended in children younger than 5 yr Effective in children with daytime enuresis

Oxybutynin chloride is an anticholinergic drug that relaxes the smooth muscle of the bladder, allows increased urine retention, and reduces frequency. It is sometimes used in conjunction with desmopressin, and it appears to be most effective as a treatment for MNE if the child also has daytime incontinence (Neveus, 2001).

Children taking medications on a regular basis should have a drug "holiday" every 3 to 6 months to assess the need for continued pharmacotherapy. If wetting recurs, medication can be continued at the effective dosage for another 3 to 6 months. After 1 month without wetting, medications can be tapered over a 2- to 4-week period, decreasing the dose (e.g., from 0.6 to 0.4 mg/day of desmopressin), decreasing dosing by 1 day a week, then to every other day. Some providers discontinue medication abruptly (Brunell et al, 2001).

Complications

Enuresis contributes to poor self-esteem and disrupted family interactions and threatens the child's ability to establish strong peer relationships. Children with nocturnal enuresis tend to demonstrate externalizing behaviors such as aggression and acting out (Kodman-Jones, Hawkins, & Schulman, 2001). Self-concept is lower in girls than boys and in older children, and more treatment failures are related to lower self-concept (Theunis et al, 2002; Wolanczyk et al, 2002).

Patient Education and Prevention

Supportive education of parents, positive reinforcement of children's efforts, and use of the toilet-training techniques described earlier can help prevent enuresis. For 3- to 5-year-old children, a nonjudgmental attitude of "benign neglect" in the face of accidents is the best approach.

Dysfunctional Voiding

Description

Dysfunctional voiding, or pediatric unstable bladder, is characterized by poor initiation of micturition, poor inhibition of voiding, or incomplete emptying of the bladder.

Incidence and Etiology

The cause of dysfunctional voiding is unknown, but it is believed to be primarily related to voiding immaturity. Detrusor instability or hyperactivity may be a factor. Constipation, urinary tract infection, and structural abnormalities must be considered. It is more common in girls and is usually seen in children 4 to 8 years of age.

Clinical Findings

History. Because of the various problems characteristic of dysfunctional voiding, children have a history of differing symptoms, including the following:

- Infrequent voiding
- Sudden daytime incontinence after having been dry
- Urgency
- Frequency
- Inability to stop the voiding stream
- Occasional nocturnal enuresis, but usually daytime wetting
- Constipation or enuresis
- Urinary tract infection

Physical Examination. A complete physical examination should be done.

Laboratory and Diagnostic Tests. Invasive diagnostic procedures are not routinely necessary (Schewe, Brands, & Pannek, 2002). The following tests are indicated:

- Urinalysis
- Urine culture and sensitivity
- Renal and bladder ultrasound if structural abnormalities are suspected; an abnormal ultrasound can show a normal upper renal system and a thick-walled bladder

Differential Diagnosis

The differential diagnoses for dysfunctional voiding are as follows:

- Urinary tract infection
- Structural abnormality, such as abnormal sphincters, ectopic ureter, duplicated urethra, or urethral valves
- Neurogenic bladder
- Vesicoureteral reflux
- Trauma or abuse
- Urethritis (may be caused by chemicals in soaps, bubble baths)

Management

The goal of management is to prevent or break the cycle of urinary dysfunction, infection, and/or irritable bladder. Intervention includes the following:

- Treat any urinary tract infection if present (see Chapter 35 for a discussion of infections).
- Retrain the bladder. This process works well with 6- to 8-year-olds and requires a motivated child (see Box 14-3 for suggestions on bladder retraining).
- Treat pelvic floor dysfunction, if appropriate (e.g., Kegel exercises with biofeedback) (Herndon, Decambre, & McKenna, 2001).
- Treat constipation if present.

BOX 14-3 *Bladder Retraining for Dysfunctional Voiding*

Establish a schedule for voiding. Have child go to the bathroom every 2-4 hr, whether urgency is felt or not.

Void with relaxation. Have child take a deep breath and relax sphincter when exhaling; use a straw to breathe through. Have child try grasping fingers together and pulling them apart.

Void to completion. Teach child to use Credé maneuver or manual pressure over suprapubic area to complete voiding.

Double void. After voiding completely, have child wait on toilet 2-3 min and attempt to void again.

NURSING DIAGNOSES RELATED TO ELIMINATION: *Functional Health Pattern*

- Bowel incontinence
- Constipation
  - Risk for constipation
  - Perceived constipation
- Encopresis (not a NANDA diagnosis)
- Enuresis (not a NANDA diagnosis)
- Urinary incontinence
- Readiness for enhanced urinary elimination

Source: North American Nursing Diagnosis Association: *NANDA nursing diagnoses: definitions and classification 2003-2004*, Philadelphia, 2003, North American Nursing Diagnosis Association.

RESOURCE BOX

Resources for Enuresis and Encopresis

National Enuresis Society/National Kidney Foundation
1-800-WAKE DRY
www.kidney.org/patients/bedwet.cfm
www.peds.umn.edu/Centers/NES/

National Kidney and Urologic Diseases Information Clearinghouse
Urinary Incontinence
www.niddk.nih.gov/health/urolog/pubs/uichild/uichild.htm

ENURESIS ALARMS

www.wetbuster.com/alarms.htm
List of alarm options, with prices listed, available from a variety of corporations in countries around the world, including the following:

Nite train'r Alarm
Koregon Enterprises
1-800-544-4240
www.nitetrain-r.com

Nytone
Nytone Medical Products
1-801-973-4090
www.nytone.com

Palco Wet-Stop Alarm
Palco Laboratories
1-800-346-4488
www.wetstop.com

Potty Pager
Ideas for Living, Inc.
1-800-497-6573
www.pottypager.com

Sleep Dry
StarChild/Labs
1-800-346-7283
www.sleepdryalarm.com

ENCOPRESIS

http://hsc.virginia.edu/cmc/tutorials/constipation/encopre.htm
Clinical information for providers and parents regarding constipation and encopresis

www.keepkidshealthy.com
General information for parents about pediatric conditions, including encopresis and enuresis.

- Treat symptoms with anticholinergics such as oxybutynin chloride. Oxybutynin chloride is not recommended for use in children younger than 5 years; the dose in children older than 5 years is 2.5 to 5 mg every day or twice a day. Recently, tolterodine has been used in children with fewer side effects than oxybutynin, though it is not as effective as time-release oxybutynin (Reinberg et al, 2003). Tolterodine dosage in children 5 to 10 years of age is 1 mg twice a day; in older children, up to 4 mg twice a day (Hjalmas et al, 2001; Munding et al, 2001).

- Teach parents or child to perform intermittent catheterization if appropriate. Self-catheterization has been effective in decreasing dysfunctional voiding and promoting continence (Pohl et al, 2002).

Patient Education and Prevention

Effective toilet training can prevent urinary retention, especially if children learn to be sensitive and responsive to cues to urinate. Parents should be instructed to be alert to signs of dysuria. If urination is painful, children often struggle to retain urine or void incompletely. Early treatment for urinary tract infections is essential to prevent renal dysfunction.

REFERENCES

Abrams P, Khoury S, Wein A, editors: Conservative management in children. *Proceedings from the First International Consultation on Incontinence, June 28–July 1, 1998*, St. Helier, Jersey, United Kingdom, 1998, Health Publication, Ltd.

American Academy of Pediatrics Committee on Practice and Ambulatory Medicine: Recommendations for preventive pediatric health care, *Pediatrics* 105:149-150, 2000.

American Medical Association: *Guidelines for adolescent preventive services (GAPS): recommendations monograph*, Chicago, 1997, American Medical Association.

Bader G et al: Sleep of primary enuretic children and controls, *Sleep* 25:579-583, 2002.

Bakker E et al: Results of a questionnaire evaluating the effects of different methods of toilet training on achieving bladder control, *BJU Int* 90:456-461, 2002.

Behrman RE, Kliegman RM, editors: *Nelson essentials of pediatrics*, ed 4, Philadelphia, 2002, WB Saunders.

Behrman RE, Kliegman RM, Jenson HB, editors: *Nelson textbook of pediatrics*, ed 17, Philadelphia, 2004, WB Saunders.

Berkowitz CD: *Pediatrics: a primary care approach*, ed 2, Philadelphia, 2000, WB Saunders.

Blum NJ, Taubman B, Osborne ML: Behavioral characteristics of children with stool toileting refusal, *Pediatrics* 99:50-53, 1997.

Borowitz SM et al: Treatment of childhood encopresis: a randomized trial comparing three treatment protocols, *J Pediatr Gastroenterol Nutr* 34:378-384, 2002.

Brunell PA et al: *Taking a closer look at primary nocturnal enuresis. Monograph: infectious diseases in children*, sponsored by Aventis Pasteur, 2001.

Butler RJ, Robinson JC: Alarm treatment for childhood nocturnal enuresis: an investigation of within-treatment variables, *Scand J Urol Nephrol* 36:268-272, 2002.

Cayan S et al: Is routine urinary tract investigation necessary for children with monosymptomatic primary nocturnal enuresis? *Urology* 58:598-602, 2001.

Felt B et al: Guideline for the management of pediatric idiopathic constipation and soiling, *Arch Pediatr Adolesc Med* 153:380-385, 1999.

Fishman L et al: Early constipation and toilet training in children with encopresis, *J Pediatr Gastroenterol Nutr* 34:385-388, 2002.

Glazier DB et al: Utility of biofeedback for the daytime syndrome of urinary frequency and urgency of childhood, *Urology* 57:791-793, 2001.

Gremse D, Hixon J, Crutchfield A: Comparison of polyethylene glycol 3350 and lactulose for treatment of chronic constipation in children, *Clin Pediatr* 41:225-229, 2002.

Herndon CD, Decambre M, McKenna PH: Interactive computer games for treatment of pelvic floor dysfunction, *J Urol* 166:1893-1898, 2001.

Hjalmas K: Desmopressin treatment: current status, *Scand J Urol Nephrol Suppl* 202:70-72, 1999.

Hjalmas K et al: The overactive bladder in children: a potential future indication for tolterodine, *BJU Int* 87:569-574, 2001.

Jansson UB et al: Voiding pattern in healthy children 0 to 3 years old: a longitudinal study, *J Urol* 164:2052-2054, 2000.

Kinservik MA, Friedhoff MM: Control issues in toilet training, *Pediatr Nurs* 26:267-272, 2000.

Kodman-Jones C, Hawkins L, Schulman SL: Behavioral characteristics of children with daytime wetting, *J Urol* 166:2392-2395, 2001.

Kruse S, Hellstrom AL, Hjalmas K: Daytime bladder dysfunction in therapy-resistant nocturnal enuresis. A pilot study in urotherapy, *Scand J Urol Nephrol* 33:49-52, 1999.

Kuhn BR, Marcus BA, Pitner SL: Treatment guidelines for primary nonretentive encopresis and stool toileting refusal, *Am Fam Physician* 59:2171-2178, 2184-2186, 1999.

Levine MD, Carey WB, Crocker AC: *Developmental-behavioral pediatrics*, ed 3, Philadelphia, 1999, WB Saunders.

Loening-Baucke V: Encopresis, *Curr Opin Pediatr* 14:570-575, 2002.

Loeys B et al: Does monosymptomatic enuresis exist? A molecular genetic exploration of 32 families with enuresis/incontinence, *BJU Int* 90:76-83, 2002.

Mellon MW, McGrath ML: Empirically supported treatments in pediatric psychology: nocturnal enuresis, *J Pediatr Psychol* 25:193-214, 2000.

Mikkelsen EJ: Enuresis and encopresis: ten years of progress, *J Am Acad Child Adolesc Psychiatry* 40:1146-1158, 2001.

Munding M et al: Use of tolterodine in children with dysfunctional voiding: an initial report, *J Urol* 165:926-928, 2001.

Neveus T: Oxybutynin, desmopressin and enuresis, *J Urol* 166:2459-2462, 2001.

Pashankar DS, Bishop WP: Efficacy and optimal dose of daily polyethylene glycol 3350 for treatment of constipation and encopresis in children, *J Pediatr* 139:428-432, 2001.

Pohl HG et al: The outcome of voiding dysfunction managed with clean intermittent catheterization in neurologically and anatomically normal children, *BJU Int* 89:923-927, 2002.

Pomeranz A et al: Night-time polyuria and urine hypo-osmolality in enuretics identified by nocturnal sequential urine sampling—do they represent a subset of relative ADH-deficient subjects? *Scand J Urol Nephrol* 34:199-202, 2000.

Reinberg Y et al: Therapeutic efficacy of extended release oxybutynin chloride, and immediate release and long acting tolterodine tartrate in children with diurnal urinary incontinence, *J Urol* 169:317-319, 2003.

Robson WL, Leung AK: Urotherapy recommendations for bedwetting, *J Natl Med Assoc* 94:577-580, 2002.

Schewe J, Brands FH, Pannek J: Voiding dysfunction in children: role of urodynamic studies, *Urol Int* 69:297-301, 2002.

Schum TR et al: Sequential acquisition of toilet-training skills: a descriptive study of gender and age differences in normal children, *Pediatrics* 109:E48, 2002.

Serel TA et al: Acupuncture therapy in the management of persistent primary nocturnal enuresis—preliminary results, *Scand J Urol Nephrol* 35:40-43, 2001.

Shelov SP, Hannemann RE: *Caring for your baby and young child*, Elk Grove Village, IL, 1999, American Academy of Pediatrics.

Taubman B: Toilet training and toileting refusal for stool only: a prospective study, *Pediatrics* 99:54-58, 1997.

Theunis M et al: Self-image and performance in children with nocturnal enuresis, *Eur Urol* 41:660-667, 2002.

Tomasi PA et al: Decreased nocturnal urinary antidiuretic hormone excretion in enuresis is increased by imipramine, *BJU Int* 88:932-937, 2001.

Tullus K et al: Efficacy and safety during long-term treatment of primary monosymptomatic noctural enuresis with desmopressin. Swedish Enuresis Trial Group, *Acta Paediatr* 88:1274-1278, 1999.

US Preventive Services Task Force: *Guide to clinical preventive services*, ed 2, Baltimore, 1996, Williams & Wilkins.

van Gool JD: Enuresis and incontinence in children, *Seminars in Pediatric Surgery* 11:100-107, 2002.

Van Kampen M et al: High initial efficacy of full-spectrum therapy for nocturnal enuresis in children and adolescents, *BJU Int* 90:84-87, 2002.

von Gontard A et al: The genetics of enuresis: a review, *J Urol* 166:2438-2443, 2001.

Wolanczyk T et al: Attitudes of enuretic children towards their illness, *Acta Paediatr* 91:844-848, 2002.

Wolfish NM: Sleep/arousal and enuresis subtypes, *J Urol* 166:2444-2447, 2001.

Yeung CK et al: Reduction in nocturnal functional bladder capacity is a common factor in the pathogenesis of refractory nocturnal enuresis, *BJU Int* 90:302-307, 2002.

Zaontz M, Welch V: Enuresis: state of the art. Presentation at National Association of Pediatric Nurse Practitioners Annual Educational Conference, March 16, 2002.

15 Activities and Sports for Children and Adolescents

Catherine E. Burns, Catherine G. Blosser

Maintenance of activity is a basic health need of all people, including infants, children, and adolescents. Activity promotes motor and cognitive development, psychologic well-being, and physical health. Activity also promotes psychologic development through promotion of self-esteem as the child masters new skills and learns to interact with others in mutual activities. Activity is essential for optimal functioning of the body; body systems are influenced by the metabolic, physical, and neurologic responses needed to execute and maintain a healthy level of activity. Further, activity patterns become long-term lifestyle habits that either promote or compromise health of the individual in the future.

The trend toward obesity in youth is one staggering consequence of inactivity. Cardiovascular heart disease, depression, and diabetes are imminent long-term consequences of inactivity and obesity (Janz, Dawson, & Mahoney, 2002; Metzl, 2002). The increase in chronic disease rates caused by hypernutrition and inactivity has also caught the attention of the World Health Organization (WHO). A report by WHO member states in 2002 requested collaboration "with WHO in developing a global strategy on diet, physical activity and health for the prevention and control of non-communicable diseases" (WHO, 2002).

Results of health-related surveys illustrate the magnitude of the problem in the United States. The number of students in grades 9 through 12 enrolled in daily school physical education in 2000 decreased from prior years and moved away from the *Healthy People 2000* target of 50%. According to the WHO Health Behavior in School-aged Children Study, children in the United States, when compared with children of similar ages in 27 other countries, (1) were less likely to report regular exercise; (2) reported more males than females exercising; (3) were less likely to eat fruits and vegetables and more likely to eat potato chips, French fries, chocolate, soda pop, and sweets; and (4) had the highest rate of dieting behavior, with one half of 11-year-olds and two thirds of 15-year-olds reporting that they "should" diet or "were dieting" (WHO, 2000). Activity declines significantly between ages 10 and 16 years, especially in girls (Strauss et al, 2001). In another study of preadolescents' physical activity, Trost and colleagues (1999) found that physical activity self-efficacy, agreement with social norms related to physical activity, and involvement with community physical activity organizations were important predictors of boys' physical activity. Only physical activity self-efficacy was a predictor of girls' physical activity.

Healthy People 2000 outcome data also showed that the greatest increase in prevalence of overweight was in the 12- to 19-year-old age-group (National Center for Health Statistics, 2001). Yet, in 1995, only 30% of nurse practitioners (NPs) asked about exercise and only 14% discussed an exercise plan with patients. Nevertheless, those percentages were the highest among all providers surveyed (Clark & Ferguson, 2000). Galuska and colleagues (1999) surveyed pediatricians about a variety of preventive health topics. In their study, 41% to 59% reported always discussing physical activity with children from 2 to 18 years of age. These numbers could be improved further. The NP can play an integral role in assessing and promoting activities for health at all ages. The outcomes influence the health of children and their families in many ways.

CLINICAL PREVENTIVE SERVICES GUIDELINES AND STANDARDS FOR PHYSICAL ACTIVITY AND FITNESS IN CHILDREN

Healthy People 2010 Guidelines for Physical Activity and Fitness

Healthy People 2010 includes objectives for physical activity and fitness in children (USDHHS, 2000). These include the following:

1. Increase the proportion of adolescents who have engaged in moderate physical activity for at least 30 minutes on 5 or more of the previous 7 days.
2. Increase the proportion of adolescents who engage in vigorous physical activity that promotes cardiorespiratory fitness 3 or more days per week for 20 or more minutes per occasion.
3. Increase the proportion of the nation's public and private schools that require daily physical education for all students.
4. Increase the proportion of adolescents who participate in daily school physical education.
5. Increase the proportion of adolescents who spend at least 50% of school physical education class time being physically active.
6. Increase the proportion of adolescents who view television 2 or fewer hours on a school day.

American Medical Association Guidelines for Adolescent Preventive Services

The American Medical Association's (AMA's) Guidelines for Adolescent Preventive Services (GAPS) addresses the issue of physical activity for young people, including the following (AMA, 1997):

1. All adolescents should receive health guidance annually about the benefits of exercise and should be encouraged to engage in safe exercise on a regular basis.
2. All adolescents should receive health guidance annually to promote the reduction of injuries. This should include "counseling to promote appropriate physical conditioning before exercise."

Sports Injuries

Thirty million children participate in organized sports, and many others participate in a recreational sport (e.g., bicycling, skateboarding). Although activity is encouraged for good health, athletic participation is also a risk factor for serious injury in youth. A Centers for Disease Control and Prevention estimate is that more than 775,000 children under 15 years of age visit emergency departments yearly for sports-related injuries. Another estimate is that 3 million youth are seen in hospital emergency departments annually for sports-related injuries and another 5 million are seen annually by physicians and sports-related clinics (Micheli, Glassman, & Klein, 2000). Though these injuries are rarely fatal, approximately 25% are regarded as serious. In the District of Columbia, 17% of sports injuries occur in six sports—baseball/softball, basketball, biking, football, skating, and soccer (Cheng et al, 2000). Traditionally, football, gymnastics, and wrestling have involved the most injuries. Since the increase in popularity of pole-vaulting and cheerleading (especially for females), these sports have eclipsed football for producing the most catastrophic injuries (Hergenroeder, 2002).

One of the goals of this chapter is to provide information to help young people engage in healthy sports and activities while minimizing the risks of injury. The preparticipation physical examination plays an important role in identifying those at most risk for injury. Preparticipation examinations are not required for many recreational activities of children and adolescents. The NP also needs to evaluate the risks for youngsters participating in nonorganized recreational activities such as in-line skating, skateboarding, cycling, swimming, and skiing and recommend age-appropriate fitness activities for all children.

Choosing Age-Appropriate Fitness Activities

Although the focus of this chapter is on sports for older children and adolescents, it is recognized that younger children also need daily activity and play to promote their growth and development. Table 15-1 provides the NP with information to counsel parents on age-appropriate physical activities by age-groups. All children, regardless of disability or chronic health conditions, benefit from fitness activities.

For school-age youth and adolescents with health problems wanting to participate in organized sports, the process for decision making about the appropriateness of various sports is more complex. First the young person's health is assessed. The provider then reviews the recommendations for participation in various sports for given health conditions. Finally, a decision is made about the client's participation (Fig. 15-1). The NP may wish to consult with the appropriate specialist working with the patient's particular health condition before recommending any specific modification or adaptation to a fitness regimen.

TABLE 15-1 ***Appropriate Fitness Activities by Age-Group***

Age-Group	Strengths/Development Factors	Fitness Activities	Family Fitness Fun
Infant-toddler	Enjoys playing with family and others Enjoys moving Enjoys playing with objects Is curious and explores environment Moves in new ways when challenged with interesting activities Mastering basic motor milestones		
2-3 yr	Participates in and enjoys many physical activities Enjoys playing with family and others	Unstructured play: running, swinging, climbing, playing in sandbox, supervised water play. Most children are not ready for organized or competitive sports.	Walking, playing, and running in the backyard
4-5 yr	Mastering more complex motor activities—running, jumping, skipping, throwing, climbing, kicking, balancing	Roll large balls, play catch, ride bike with training wheels away from traffic, swimming, dancing, skiing, skating. Judgment, safety awareness, and coordination skills are limited. Enroll in swimming lessons.	Walking, playing, running, tennis, skiing, dancing, ice-skating, hiking
6-12 yr	Participates in and enjoys many physical activities Develops a positive attitude toward physical activity Wants to improve motor skills Is developing a sense of responsibility for own health Has positive role models for physical activity Has opportunities for participation in physical activities 5-6 yr: mastering fundamentals of skilled movements 7-9 yr: refining skills such as distance throwing and accuracy 10-11 yr: beginning complex skills (e.g., basketball); integrating cognitive skills with motor skills for sports (e.g., rules, strategy, team roles)	Abilities developed sufficiently for participation in organized sports, but muscles and tendons are short, tight, and easily injured due to growth. Noncompetitive sports include swimming, ice-skating, gymnastics, dance, and martial arts. Avoid sports specialization until >10 yr. Weight lifting at age 11 (with supervision) helps build muscles to minimize later injury. Monitor for eating disorders for those in gymnastics, wrestling, or dance. Number of pitches should be limited (<75 per game) among 9- to 12-year-olds to prevent shoulder or elbow injury (Lyman, 2001).	Walking, bike riding, camping, hiking, tennis, skiing, dancing, ice-skating, swimming Do not use trampolines
13-18 yr	Participates in physical activities Enjoys physical activities Wants to improve skills but feels competent Takes responsibility for own health Has positive role models for physical activity Mastering complex skills for some sports or recreational activities	Any activity, including competitive sports, skateboarding, in-line skating, rock climbing, snowboarding, weight training (with supervision); exercise at least 30 min, three times a week.	Walking, cycling, camping, hiking, tennis, skiing, dancing, ice-skating, swimming

Data from American Medical Association: Fitness, 1999. Available at *www.medem.com/MedLB*; Faigenbaum A, Micheli L: Preseason conditioning for the preadolescent athlete, *Pediatr Ann* 29(3):156-161, 2000; Patrick K et al: *Bright Futures in practice: physical activity*, Arlington, VA, 2001, National Center for Education in Maternal and Child Health.

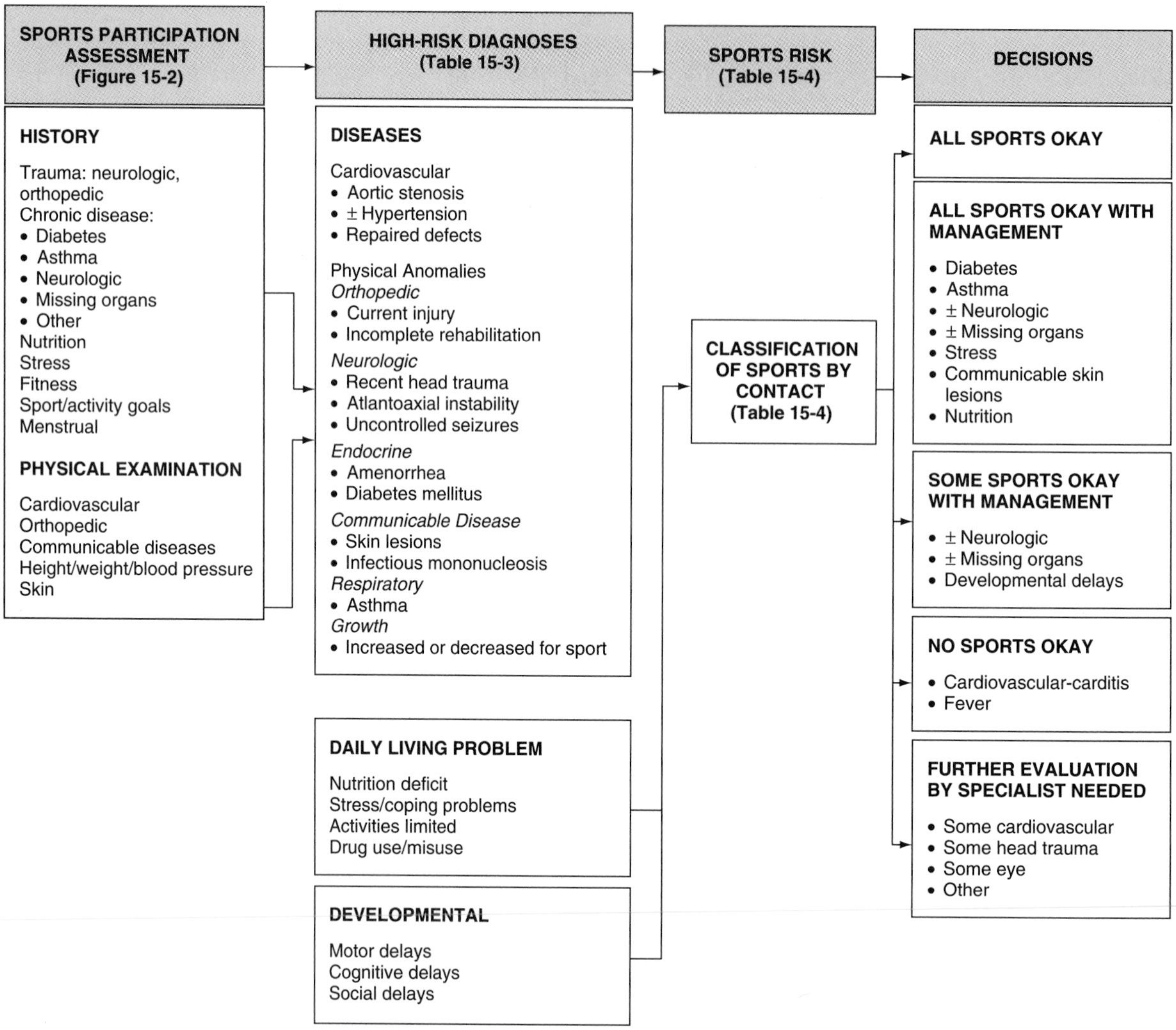

FIGURE 15-1 Decision making for sports participation.

ASSESSMENT

The Preparticipation Sports Examination

The preparticipation sports examination (PPE) is one of the most common reasons for youths and adolescents to seek primary health care. Approximately 10% of patients will have findings that need further evaluation or referral before participation, and 2.6% will have significant enough findings (neurologic, musculoskeletal, or vascular) to warrant exclusion from sports participation (Feinstein, 2002). For the majority of youth, this examination is their only health assessment for the year (Glover, Maron, & Matheson, 1999). The American Heart Association recommends sports examinations every 2 years through high school, once on entering college, and, thereafter, yearly blood pressure and interim history (Sudden Death Committee, 1998). The examinations should be done at least 6 weeks before the season begins to allow time for follow-up of problems before engagement (Feinstein, 2002). For the NP to avoid any malpractice liability, it is important that the PPE be done according to customary and standard practices for this type of examination; all history and physical findings must be fully documented in case of sudden death occurrences (Greene, 2000).

The PPE historically served as a vehicle to provide liability protection, satisfy insurance regulations, and detect cardiovascular risks for sudden death. Over the years, other objectives have been identified that include the following (Glover, Maron, & Matheson, 1999):

- Detection of injuries and illnesses that might lead to the recognition of the need for further evaluation and treatment
- Opportunity to recommend alternative sports activities, as appropriate, or to exclude the person from certain sports
- Identification of lifestyle risk factors and promotion of healthy choices
- Documentation of athletes' age and grade-level eligibility
- Collection of medical data for emergencies
- Opportunity to recommend ways to improve athletic performance
- Interaction with youth for a variety of health-related issues

Ideally, the sports physical examination should be an individually scheduled appointment with the child's primary care provider. However, mass screenings are common in many school districts as an efficiency measure or because some youth may not be able to afford the examination or may have difficulty getting to such appointments. The mass screenings can be designed with stations for each part of the examination or organized with one-station visits for each child. However, there is a loss of continuity from history to physical examination and minimal opportunity to use the visit for health-promotion purposes. Altemeier and Robinson (2000) have questioned the quality of such assembly-line screenings. For NPs working in school-based clinics, the sports physical can provide an opportunity to begin to introduce clinic services to the students and to encourage them to return for other health-related services. Communication with parents, coaches, and trainers is essential, whatever process for conducting the examinations is selected.

The psychosocial implications of sports participation need to be clearly identified both for practitioners and for the children and families with whom they work (Table 15-2).

TABLE 15-2 *Psychosocial Implications of Sports Activities*

Positives	Negatives
Fitness	Stress
Social skills	Meeting adult goals
Family activity and involvement	Potential for injuries
Self-esteem	Child may be made to feel inadequate; negative attributes may be emphasized
Confidence	
Coordination and physical skills	
Fun and recreation	

Risk Factors

When assessing the young person for participation in sports, any history or physical findings in the following areas should be of special concern:

- Previous trauma, especially musculoskeletal or central nervous system injuries
- Cardiovascular disease, hypertension (greater than 99th percentile), or exertional syncope
- Asthma or other allergic reactions
- Seizure disorder
- Infectious mononucleosis
- Skin infection
- Anatomic abnormalities or Down syndrome
- Obesity

Recommendations for sports participation, if any of these conditions exist, are discussed later in this chapter. Specific conditions are listed in Table 15-3. Table 15-4 classifies various sports by risk.

TABLE 15-3 *Medical Conditions and Sports Participation***

Condition	May Participate?
Atlantoaxial instability (instability of the joint between cervical vertebrae 1 and 2) *Explanation:* Athlete needs evaluation to assess risk of spinal cord injury during sports participation.	Qualified yes
Bleeding disorder *Explanation:* Athlete needs evaluation.	Qualified yes
Cardiovascular diseases: Carditis (inflammation of the heart) *Explanation:* Carditis may result in sudden death with exertion.	No

Continued

TABLE 15-3 ***Medical Conditions and Sports Participation—cont'd***

Condition	May Participate?
Hypertension (high blood pressure) *Explanation:* Those with significant essential (unexplained) hypertension should avoid weight lifting and power lifting, bodybuilding, and strength training. Those with secondary hypertension (hypertension caused by a previously identified disease) or severe essential hypertension need evaluation.	Qualified yes
Congenital heart disease (structural heart defects present at birth) *Explanation:* Those with mild forms may participate fully; those with moderate or severe forms, or those who have undergone surgery, need evaluation.	Qualified yes
Dysrhythmia (irregular heart rhythm) *Explanation:* Athlete needs evaluation because some types of dysrhythmia require therapy or make certain sports dangerous, or both.	Qualified yes
Mitral valve prolapse (abnormal heart valve) *Explanation:* Those with symptoms (chest pain, symptoms of possible dysrhythmia) or evidence of mitral regurgitation (leaking) on physical examination need evaluation. All others may participate fully.	Qualified yes
Heart murmur *Explanation:* If the murmur is innocent (does not indicate heart disease), full participation is permitted. Otherwise, the athlete needs evaluation (see "congenital heart disease" and "mitral valve prolapse" above).	Qualified yes
Cerebral palsy *Explanation:* Athlete needs evaluation.	Qualified yes
Diabetes mellitus *Explanation:* All sports can be played with proper attention to diet, hydration, and insulin therapy. Particular attention is needed for activities that last 30 min or more.	Yes
Diarrhea *Explanation:* Unless disease is mild, no participation is permitted, because diarrhea may increase the risk of dehydration and heat illness (see "fever" below).	Qualified no
Eating disorders: anorexia nervosa, bulimia nervosa *Explanation:* These patients need both medical and psychiatric assessment before participation may be allowed.	Qualified yes
Eyes: functionally one-eyed athlete, loss of an eye, detached retina, previous eye surgery, or serious eye injury *Explanation:* A functionally one-eyed athlete has a best corrected visual acuity of <20/40 in the worse eye. These athletes would suffer significant disability if the better eye was seriously injured, as would those with loss of an eye. Some athletes who have previously undergone eye surgery or had a serious eye injury may have an increased risk of injury because of weakened eye tissue. Availability of eye guards approved by the American Society for Testing Materials (ASTM) and other protective equipment may allow participation in most sports, but this must be judged on an individual basis.	Qualified yes
Fever *Explanation:* Fever can increase cardiopulmonary effort, reduce maximum exercise capacity, make heat illness more likely, and increase orthostatic hypotension during exercise. Fever may rarely accompany myocarditis or other infections that may make exercise dangerous.	No
Heat illness: history of *Explanation:* Because of the increased likelihood of recurrence, the athlete needs individual assessment to determine the presence of predisposing conditions and to arrange a prevention strategy.	Qualified yes
Human immunodeficiency virus (HIV) infection *Explanation:* Because of the apparent minimal risk to others, all sports may be played that the state of health allows. In all athletes, skin lesions should be properly covered, and athletic personnel should use universal precautions when handling blood or body fluids with visible blood.	Yes
Kidney: absence of one *Explanation:* Athlete needs individual assessment for contact, collision, and limited-contact sports.	Qualified yes
Liver: enlarged *Explanation:* If the liver is acutely enlarged, participation should be avoided because of risk of rupture. If the liver is chronically enlarged, individual assessment is needed before collision, contact, or limited-contact sports are played.	Qualified yes
Malignancy *Explanation:* Athlete needs individual assessment	Qualified yes

TABLE 15-3 *Medical Conditions and Sports Participation*—cont'd*

Condition	May Participate?
Musculoskeletal disorders *Explanation:* Athlete needs individual assessment.	Qualified yes
Neurologic disorders: history of serious head or spine trauma, severe or repeated concussions, or craniotomy *Explanation:* Athlete needs individual assessment for collision, contact, or limited-contact sports, and also for noncontact sports if there are deficits in judgment or cognition. Research supports a conservative approach to management of concussion.	Qualified yes
Convulsive disorder: well controlled *Explanation:* Risk of convulsion during participation is minimal.	Yes
Convulsive disorder: poorly controlled *Explanation:* Athlete needs individual assessment for collision, contact, or limited-contact sports. Avoid the following noncontact sports: archery, riflery, swimming, weight lifting, power lifting, strength training, or sports involving heights. In these sports, occurrence of a convulsion may be a risk to self or others.	Qualified yes
Obesity *Explanation:* Because of the risk of heat illness, obese persons need careful acclimatization and hydration.	Qualified yes
Organ transplant recipient *Explanation:* Athlete needs individual assessment.	Qualified yes
Ovary: absence of one *Explanation:* Risk of severe injury to the remaining ovary is minimal.	Yes
Respiratory: pulmonary compromise, including cystic fibrosis *Explanation:* Athlete needs individual assessment, but generally all sports may be played if oxygenation remains satisfactory during a graded exercise test. Patients with cystic fibrosis need acclimatization and good hydration to reduce the risk of heat illness.	Qualified yes
Asthma *Explanation:* With proper medication and education, only athletes with the most severe asthma have to modify their participation.	Yes
Acute upper respiratory infection *Explanation:* Upper respiratory obstruction may affect pulmonary function. Athlete needs individual assessment for all but mild disease (see "fever" above).	Qualified yes
Sickle cell disease *Explanation:* Athlete needs individual assessment. In general, if status of the illness permits, all but high-exertion, collision, or contact sports may be played. Overheating, dehyration, and chilling must be avoided.	Qualified yes
Sickle cell trait *Explanation:* It is unlikely that individuals with sickle cell trait (AS) have an increased risk of sudden death or other medical problems during athletic participation except under the most extreme conditions of heat, humidity, and, possibly, increased altitude. These individuals, like all athletes, should be carefully conditioned, acclimatized, and hydrated to reduce any possible risk.	Yes
Skin: boils, herpes simplex, impetigo, scabies, *molluscum contagiosum* *Explanation:* While the patient is contagious, participation in gymnastics with mats, martial arts, wrestling, or other collision, contact, or limited-contact sports is not allowed. Herpes simplex virus probably is not transmitted via mats.	Qualified yes
Spleen: enlarged *Explanation:* Patients with acutely enlarged spleens should avoid all sports because of risk of rupture. Those with chronically enlarged spleens need individual assessment before playing collision, contact, or limited-contact sports.	Qualified yes
Testicle: absent or undescended *Explanation:* Certain sports may require a protective cup.	Yes

Used with permission of the American Academy of Pediatrics. From American Academy of Pediatrics Committee on Sports Medicine: Medical conditions affecting sports participation, *Pediatrics* 107(5):1205-1209, 2001. Copyright 2001 by the American Academy of Pediatrics.

*This table is designed to be understood by medical and nonmedical personnel. In the "Explanation" section, "needs evaluation" means that a physician with appropriate knowledge and experience should assess the safety of a given sport for an athlete with the listed medical condition. Unless otherwise noted, this is because of the variability of the severity of the disease or of the risk of injury among the specific sports listed in Table 15-4.

TABLE 15-4 Classification of Sports by Contact

Contact/Collision	Limited Contact	Noncontact
Basketball	Baseball	Archery
Boxing*	Bicycling	Badminton
Diving	Cheerleading	Bodybuilding
Field hockey	Canoeing/kayaking (white water)	Canoeing/kayaking (flat water)
Football	Fencing	Crew/rowing
• Flag	Field	Curling
• Tackle	• High jump	Dancing
Ice hockey	• Pole vault	Field
Lacrosse	Floor hockey	• Discus
Martial arts	Gymnastics	• Javelin
Rodeo	Handball	• Shot put
Rugby	Horseback riding	Golf
Ski jumping	Racquetball	Orienteering
Soccer	Skating	Power lifting
Team handball	• Ice	Race walking
Water polo	• In-line	Riflery
Wrestling	• Roller	Rope jumping
	Skiing	Running
	• Cross-country	Sailing
	• Downhill	Scuba diving
	• Water	Strength training
	Softball	Swimming
	Squash	Table tennis
	Ultimate frisbee	Tennis
	Volleyball	Track
	Windsurfing/surfing	Weight lifting

Used with permission of the American Academy of Pediatrics. From American Academy of Pediatrics Committee on Sports Medicine: Medical conditions affecting sports participation, *Pediatrics* 94:757-760, 1994. Copyright 1994 by the American Academy of Pediatrics.
*Participation not recommended.

History

Coaches and others need to be aware of the athlete's health status in case problems arise during participation. Many medical history forms are available that are used to identify children with health conditions that might be adversely influenced by participation in a sport. A newer health history and physical examination form (Fig. 15-2) used by the Ohio High School Athletic Association (2002) expands on a prior form offered by the American Academy of Family Physicians in 1997. Many of the questions on the form relate to the risk factors listed earlier.

For a more holistic view, the NP should also ask questions about the following:

- The particular sports activity planned
- Extent of participation
- Level of competition
- Training schedule
- Coaching and supervision
- Hazardous playing and field conditions
- Plans for the activity in the future
- Health promotion and preventive strategies planned
- Planned nutrition
- Preparticipation conditioning
- Risk behaviors such as increased alcohol consumption, driving while intoxicated, lack of seat-belt use, lack of helmet use, lack of contraception use, use of drugs or performance-enhancing substances (including steroids, creatine, gamma-hydroxybutyrate [GHB], gamma-hydroxybutyrolactone [GBL], 1,4-butanediol [BL], and dehydroepiandrosterone [DHEA]), smoking, unprotected sexual activity, and numbers of sexual partners
- Family involvement and support
- Psychologic issues
  - Stress management during the competitive season
  - Measures for success
  - Recent life changes
  - Strategies to maintain schoolwork

Physical Examination

The physical examination should consist of two parts, the musculoskeletal examination and the general physical examination. The 2-minute orthopedic screening examination, which includes 12 simple steps, is recommended (Fig. 15-3). The examination focuses on musculoskeletal alignment, flexibility, and proprioception, which are effective measures of abnormalities and injury sequelae. The additional musculoskeletal examination is done in conjunction with the regular physical examination (see Fig. 15-2). Table 15-5 describes the components that should be included for different organ systems.

Laboratory Examination

Urinalysis and hematocrit or hemoglobin are not recommended as part of the sports preparticipation examination. Although these can be useful for evaluation of a specific disease, there is no true indication from a health screening perspective. For adolescent girls, iron deficiency anemia is common enough that it may be appropriate to screen for the condition. Urine drug screening and human immunodeficiency virus (HIV) testing may be required by certain elite amateur or professional organizations. Voluntary testing should be encouraged if the athlete has any risk factors.

Ohio High School Athletic Association
Preparticipation Physical Examination Form

(Please type or print)

Student's Name ______________________________ **Birth Date** ________ **Sex** ______ **Grade** ______

Last First Middle

City ________________ **School** ________________ **Place of Birth** ________

Student's Address ______________________________

Street City Zip Telephone

Parent(s) or Guardian(s) Name ______________________________

Address (if different than student) ______________________________

Street City Zip Telephone

Family Physician's Name, Address, Telephone ______________________________

History

This section is to be carefully completed by the student and his/her parent(s) or legal guardian(s) before participation in interscholastic athletics in order to help detect possible risks.

Explain "YES" answers below. Circle questions you don't know the answer to.

	Yes	No
1. Have you had a medical illness or injury since your last checkup or sports physical?	☐	☐
Do you have an ongoing or chronic illness?	☐	☐
2. Have you ever been hospitalized overnight?	☐	☐
Have you ever had surgery?	☐	☐
3. Are you currently taking any prescription or nonprescription (over-the-counter) medications or pills or using an inhaler?	☐	☐
Have you ever taken any supplements or vitamins to help you gain or lose weight or improve your performance?	☐	☐
4. Do you think you are in good health?	☐	☐
5. Do you have any allergies (for example, to pollen, medicine, food, or stinging insect)?	☐	☐
6. Have you ever had a rash or hives develop during or after exercise?	☐	☐
Have you ever passed out during or after exercise?	☐	☐
Have you ever been dizzy during or after exercise?	☐	☐
Have you ever had chest pain during or after exercise?	☐	☐
Do you get tired more quickly than your friends do during exercise?	☐	☐
Have you ever had racing of your heart or skipped heartbeats?	☐	☐
Have you had high blood pressure or high cholesterol?	☐	☐
Have you ever been told you have a heart murmur?	☐	☐
Has any family member or relative died of heart problems or of sudden death before age 50?	☐	☐
Is there a family history of heart problems in a close relative younger than age 50 (examples are enlarged heart, cardiomyopathy, long QT interval, abnormal EKG, abnormal heart rhythm)?	☐	☐
Have you had a severe heart infection (for example, myocarditis or pericarditis)?	☐	☐
Is there a family history of Marfan's Syndrome?	☐	☐
Has a physician ever denied or restricted your participation in sports for any heart problem?	☐	☐
7. Have you ever had a severe viral infection within the last month (for example, mononucleosis)?	☐	☐
8. Do you have any current skin problems (for example, itching, rashes, acne, warts, fungus or blisters)?	☐	☐
9. Have you ever had a head injury or concussion?	☐	☐
Have you ever been knocked out, become unconscious or lost your memory?	☐	☐
Have you ever had a seizure?	☐	☐
Do you have frequent or severe headaches?	☐	☐
Have you ever had numbness or tingling in your arms, hands, legs or feet?	☐	☐
Have you ever had a stinger, burner or pinched nerve?	☐	☐
10. Have you ever become ill from exercising in the heat?	☐	☐
11. Do you cough, wheeze or have trouble breathing during or after activity?	☐	☐
Do you have asthma?	☐	☐
Do you have seasonal allergies that require medical treatment?	☐	☐
12. Do you use any special protective or corrective equipment or devices that aren't usually used for your sport or position (for example, knee brace, special neck roll, foot orthotics, retainer on your teeth, hearing aid)?	☐	☐
13. Have you had any problems with your eyes or vision?	☐	☐
Do you wear glasses, contacts or protective eyewear?	☐	☐
14. Have you ever had a sprain, strain or swelling after injury?	☐	☐
Have you broken or fractured any bones or dislocated any joints?	☐	☐
Have you had any other problems with pain or swelling in muscles, tendons, bones or joints?	☐	☐

If yes, check the appropriate box and explain below.

☐Head	☐Upper Arm	☐Hand	☐Knee
☐Neck	☐Elbow	☐Finger	☐Shin/calf
☐Back	☐Forearm	☐Hip	☐Ankle
☐Chest	☐Wrist	☐Thigh	☐Foot
☐Shoulder			

	Yes	No
15. Do you want to weigh more or less than you do now?	☐	☐
Do you lose weight regularly to meet weight requirements for your sport?	☐	☐
16. Do you feel stressed out?	☐	☐

17. Record the dates of your most recent immunizations (shots) for:

Tetanus ____________ Measles ____________

Hepatitis B ____________ Chickenpox ____________

18. FEMALES ONLY

When was your first menstrual period? ____________

When was your most recent menstrual period? ____________

How much time do you usually have from the start of one period to the start of another? ____________

How many periods have you had in the last year? ____________

What was the longest time between periods in the last year? ____________

19. ALL PARTICIPANTS

Explain "Yes" answers here: ______________________________

We consent to the participation of the above-named student in the interscholastic program of his/her school including practice sessions and travel to and from athletic contests. We also agree to emergency medical treatment as deemed necessary by the physician(s) designated by school authorities. **We have read and understand the OHSAA Athletic Eligibility Information Bulletin.**

______________________ ______________________ ____________

Student Signature Parent or Guardian Signature Date

The student has family insurance ___ Yes ___ No; If yes, family insurance co. name, policy #: ______________________

NOTE: History and Consent Must be Completed Prior to Physical Examination

Modified from the form approved by the American Academy of Family Physicians, the American Academy of Pediatrics, the American Medical Society for Sports Medicine, the American Orthopaedic Society for Sports Medicine and the American Osteopathic Academy of Sports Medicine.

FIGURE 15-2 Preparticipation physical examination form. (Modifed from the form approved by the American Academy of Family Physicians, the American Adademy of Pediatrics, the American Medical Society for Sports Medicine, and the American Osteopathic Academy of Sports Medicine.)

Physical Examination

(Please type or print)

Student's Name ______________________________ **Birth Date** ____________
Last First Middle

Height ________ **Weight** ________ **% Body Fat (optional)** ________ **Pulse** ________ **BP** _____/_____

Vision R 20/ ________ **L 20/** ________ **Corrected: Y N** **Pupils: Equal** _____ **Unequal** _____

	Normal	Abnormal Findings	Initials*
MEDICAL			
Eyes/Ears/Nose/Throat			
Lymph Nodes			
Heart			
Pulses			
Lungs			
Abdomen			
Genitalia (males only)			
Skin			
MUSCULOSKELETAL			
Neck			
Back			
Shoulder/Arm			
Elbow/Forearm			
Wrist/Hand			
Hip/Thigh			
Knee			
Leg/Ankle			
Foot			

*Station-based examination only

Clearance

☐ **Cleared**

☐ **Cleared after completing evaluation/rehabilitation for:** ______________________________

☐ **Not cleared for:** ______________________ **Reason:** ______________________

Recommendations: ______________________________

I certify that I have on this date examined this student and that, on the basis of the examination requested by the school authorities and the student's medical history as furnished to me, I have found no reason which would make it medically inadvisable for this student to compete in supervised athletic activities **(Note exceptions above).**

____
Physician's Name and Address (stamp or print)
If the Physician's Assistant (P.A.) or Advanced Nurse Practitioner (A.N.P.) performed the exam, name and address of collaborating physician or physician group:
____

____
Examiner's Signature **Date**

____
Examiner's Telephone Number

NOTE: History and Consent Must be Completed Prior to Physical Examination

FIGURE 15-2 cont'd

EXAMINATION PARAMETERS

- Appropriate for interscholastic, intramural, and extramural sports activities.
- A screening evaluation created to direct attention to problems but *not* evaluate the problems.
- Identifies the following conditions that might be adversely affected by athletic participation:
  a. Congenital problems
  b. Acquired problems

HISTORY Questions such as the following are to be answered by the athlete and signed by BOTH the athlete and parent:

- Have you ever had an illness, condition, or injury that required you to go to the hospital, either as a patient overnight or in the emergency room or for x-rays; required an operation; caused you to see a doctor; caused you to miss a game or practice?
- Are you now or have you been under the care of a physician for any reason?
- Do you currently have any medical problems or injuries?
- Have you ever had a broken bone, joint sprain or ligament tear, muscle pull, head injury, neck injury or nerve pinch, dislocated joint, back trouble or problems?

ACTIVITY 1

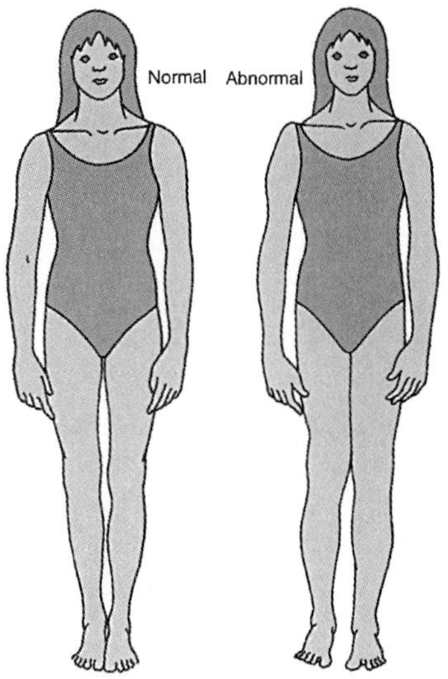

INSTRUCTIONS Stand straight with arms at sides.

OBSERVATIONS Symmetry of upper and lower extremities and trunk.
Common abnormalities:
1. Enlarged acromioclavicular joint
2. Enlarged sternoclavicular joint
3. Asymmetrical waist (leg length difference or scoliosis)
4. Swollen knee
5. Swollen ankle

ACTIVITY 2

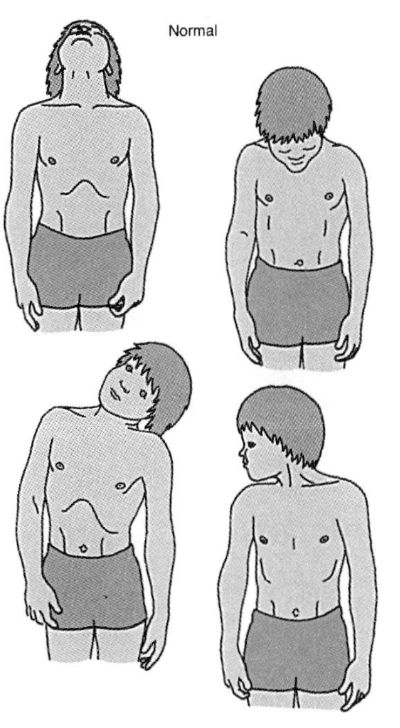

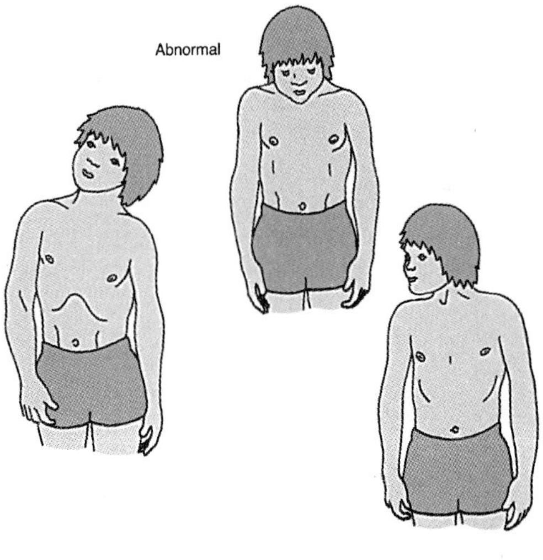

INSTRUCTIONS Look at ceiling; look at floor; touch right (left) ear to shoulder; look over right (left) shoulder.

OBSERVATIONS Should be able to touch chin to chest, ears to shoulders and look equally over shoulders.
Common abnormalities (may indicate previous neck injury):
1. Loss of flexion
2. Loss of lateral bending
3. Loss of rotation

FIGURE 15-3 The orthopedic physical examination for sports participation. (Used with permission of Ross Products Division, Abbott Laboratories, Columbus, OH 43216. From *For the Practitioner: Orthopaedic Screening Examination for Participation in Sports.* © 1981 Ross Products Division, Abbott Laboratories.)

ACTIVITY 3

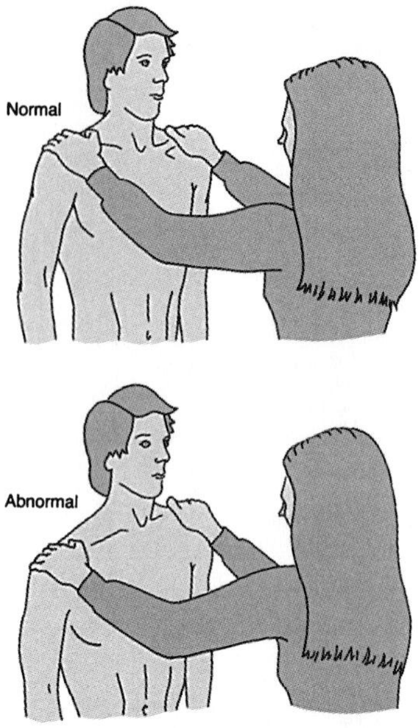

INSTRUCTIONS Shrug shoulders while examiner holds them down.

OBSERVATIONS Trapezius muscles appear equal; left and right sides equal strength.
Common abnormalities (may indicate neck or shoulder problem):
1. Loss of strength
2. Loss of muscle bulk

ACTIVITY 4

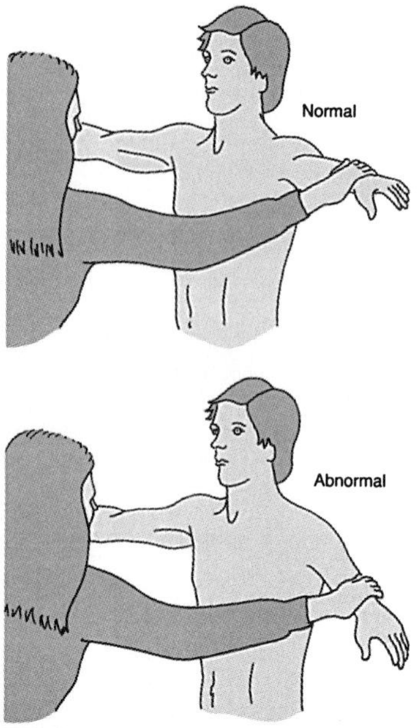

INSTRUCTIONS Hold arms out from sides horizontally and lift while examiner holds them down.

OBSERVATIONS Strength should be equal and deltoid muscles should be equal in size.
Common abnormalities:
1. Loss of strength
2. Wasting of deltoid muscle

ACTIVITY 5

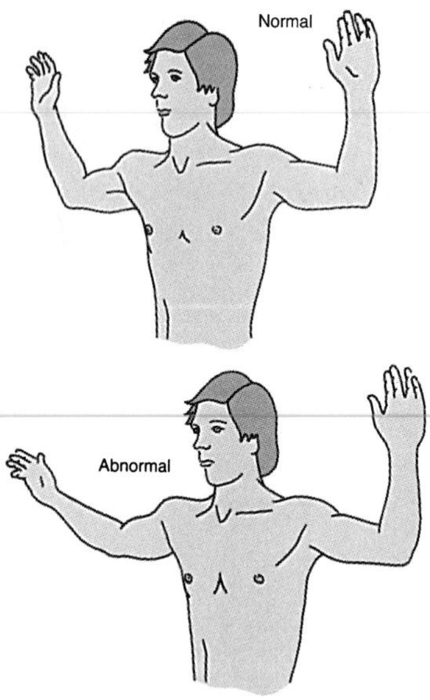

INSTRUCTIONS Hold arms out from sides with elbows bent (90°); raise hands back vertically as far as they will go.

OBSERVATIONS Hands go back equally and at least to upright vertical position.
Common abnormalities (may indicate shoulder problem or old dislocation):
1. Loss of external rotation

ACTIVITY 6

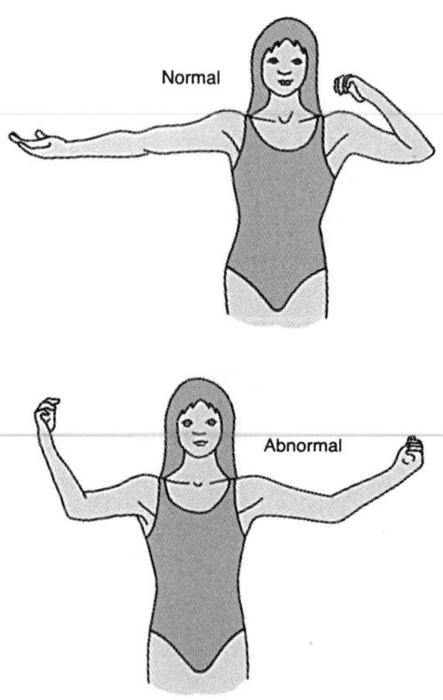

INSTRUCTIONS Hold arms out from sides, palms up; straighten elbows completely; bend completely.

OBSERVATIONS Motion equal left and right.
Common abnormalities (may indicate old elbow injury, old dislocation, fracture, etc.):
1. Loss of extension
2. Loss of flexion

FIGURE 15-3 cont'd

ACTIVITY 7

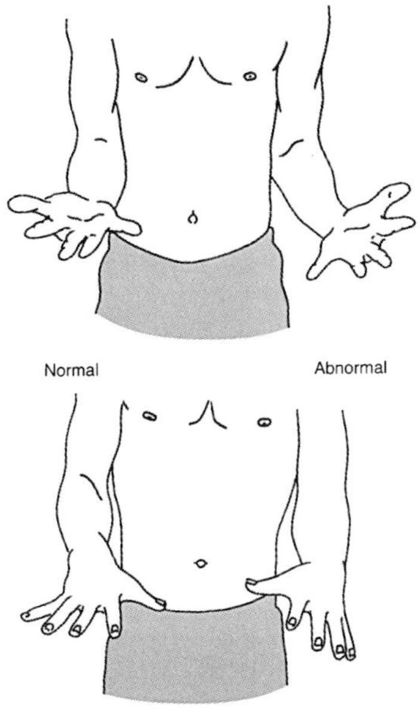

INSTRUCTIONS Hold arms down at sides with elbows bent (90°); supinate palms; pronate palms.

OBSERVATIONS Palms should go from facing ceiling to facing floor. Common abnormalities (may indicate old forearm, wrist, or elbow injury):
1. Lack of full supination
2. Lack of full pronation

ACTIVITY 8

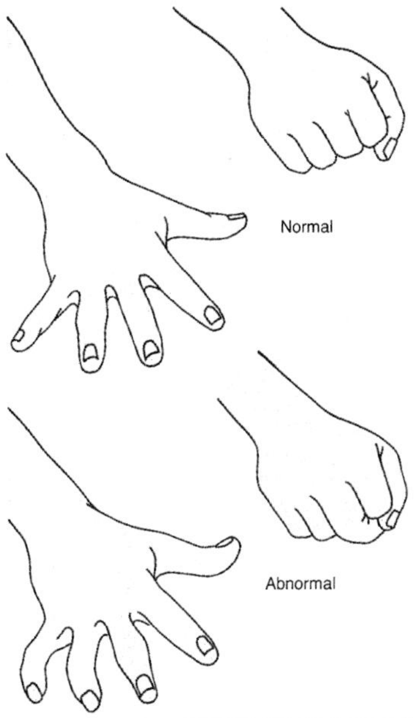

INSTRUCTIONS Make a fist; open hand and spread fingers.

OBSERVATIONS Fist should be tight and fingers straight when spread. Common abnormalities (may indicate old finger fractures or sprains):
1. Protruding knuckle from fist
2. Swollen and/or crooked finger

ACTIVITY 9

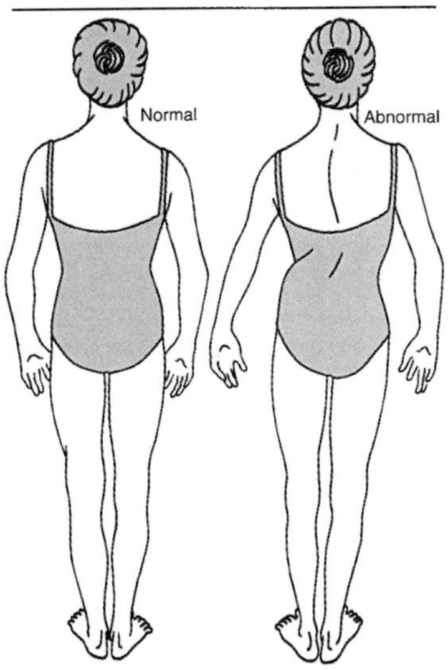

INSTRUCTIONS With back to examiner stand up straight.

OBSERVATIONS Symmetry of shoulders, waist, thighs, and calves. Common abnormalities:
1. High shoulder (scoliosis) or low shoulder (muscle loss)
2. Prominent rib cage (scoliosis)
3. High hip or asymmetrical waist (leg length difference or scoliosis)
4. Small calf or thigh (weakness from old injury)

ACTIVITY 10

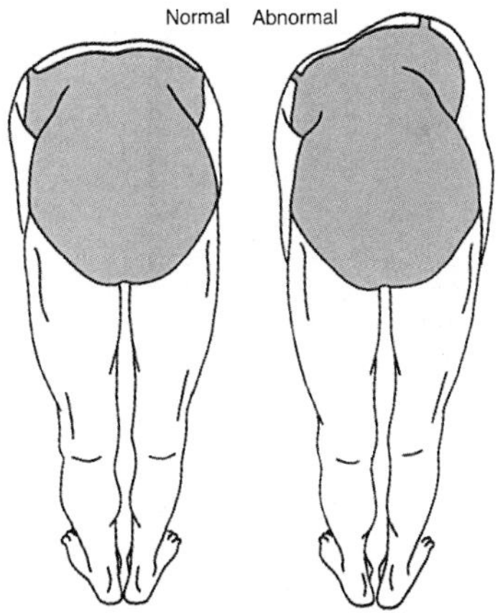

INSTRUCTIONS Bend forward slowly as to touch toes.

OBSERVATIONS Bends forward straightly and smoothly. Common abnormalities:
1. Twists to side (low back pain)
2. Back asymmetrical (scoliosis)

FIGURE 15-3 cont'd

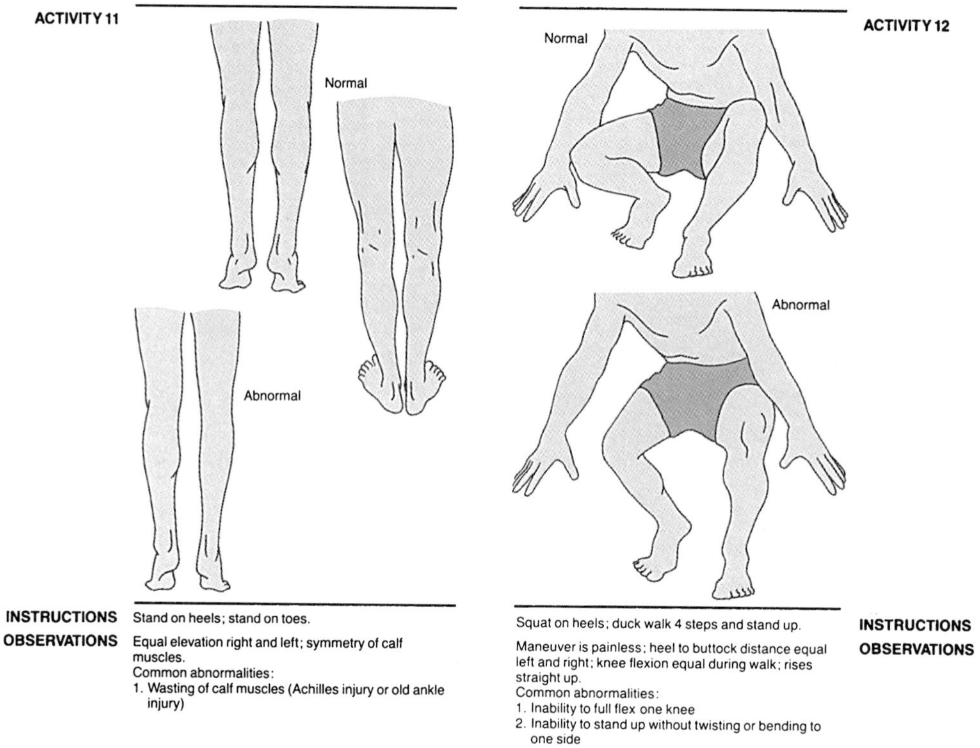

ACTIVITY 11
Normal
Abnormal
INSTRUCTIONS Stand on heels; stand on toes.
OBSERVATIONS Equal elevation right and left; symmetry of calf muscles.
Common abnormalities:
1. Wasting of calf muscles (Achilles injury or old ankle injury)
ACTIVITY 12
Normal
Abnormal
INSTRUCTIONS Squat on heels; duck walk 4 steps and stand up.
OBSERVATIONS Maneuver is painless; heel to buttock distance equal left and right; knee flexion equal during walk; rises straight up.
Common abnormalities:
1. Inability to full flex one knee
2. Inability to stand up without twisting or bending to one side

FIGURE 15-3 cont'd

TABLE 15-5 *Example of an Appropriate Preparticipation Physical Examination*

Examination Feature	Comments
Blood pressure	Must be assessed in the context of participant's age, height, and sex.
General appearance	Measure for excessive height and observe for evidence of excessive long-bone growth (arachnodactyly, arm span > height, pectus excavatum) because these suggest Marfan syndrome.
Eyes	Important to detect vision defects that leave one of the eyes with >20/40 corrected vision. Lens subluxations, severe myopia, retinal detachments, and strabismus are associated with Marfan syndrome.
Cardiovascular	Palpate the point of maximal impulse for increased intensity and displacement, which suggest hypertrophy and failure, respectively.
	Perform auscultation with the patient supine and again with the patient standing or straining during Valsalva maneuver.
	Femoral pulse diminishment suggests aortic coarctation.
Respiratory	Observe for accessory muscle use or prolonged expiration, and auscultate for wheezing. Exercise-induced asthma will not produce manifestations on a resting examination and requires exercise testing for diagnosis.
Abdominal	Assess for hepatic or splenic enlargement.
Genitourinary	Hernias and varicoceles do not usually preclude sports participation, but the sports examination can also serve as an appropriate time to screen for testicular masses if the athlete is not receiving regular general examinations.
Musculoskeletal	The two-minute orthopedic examination (see Fig. 15-3) is a commonly used systematic screen. Consider supplemental shoulder, knee, and ankle examinations.
Skin	Evidence of *molluscum contagiosum*, herpes simplex infection, impetigo, tinea corporis, or scabies would temporarily prohibit participation in sports where direct skin-to-skin competitor contact occurs (e.g., wrestling, martial arts).

From Kurowski K, Chandran S: The preparticipation athletic evaluation, *Am Fam Physician* 61:2683-2690, 2696-2698, 2000.

Classification of Sports for Risk

The American Academy of Pediatrics (AAP) has classified the most common sports activities into three types: contact/collision, limited contact, and noncontact (see Table 15-4). When used with Table 15-3, the clinician can make specific recommendations as to which sports are appropriate for young people with identified health problems.

Recommendations for Participation in Sports for Children with High-Risk Conditions

Table 15-3 summarizes the AAP's recommendations for sports for youth with specific health conditions. Tables 15-3 and 15-4 should be available in the clinic setting. They lend credibility to sports participation recommendations and should serve as guidelines for recommendations the NP makes to students and their families. Although families and schools will make their own choices, the recommendations should be recorded in both the student's permanent record and the form returned to the school or sports facility. The goal is to find safe, healthful activities for all children, not to restrict their activities unnecessarily. Several high-risk conditions are discussed in the following section.

HIGH-RISK CONDITIONS FOR SPORTS PARTICIPATION

Previous Trauma

Musculoskeletal

All musculoskeletal injuries require individual assessment and decision making. Sprains, subluxations, dislocations, muscle contusions, and overuse injuries can result in pain and changes to joints, ligament stability, range of motion, strength, and endurance. Referral to an orthopedist may be required. Before returning to sports participation, the athlete must be able to demonstrate the following (Kurowski & Chandran, 2000):

- Absence of joint effusion
- Full range of motion
- At least 80% to 90% of normal strength
- Ligament stability
- Endurance and motor skills without pain

If these conditions are not met, repeated injury can be anticipated from residual musculoskeletal deficiencies (Hergenroeder, 2002). Successfully returning to sport participation does not solely depend on the absence of pain; correct rehabilitation is a more important factor (Metzl, 2002).

Neurologic

An estimated 300,000 sports- or recreation-related traumatic brain injuries occur annually in the United States (Brain Injury Association, 2002; Wilson, Carlin, & Tyburski, 2002). Head and neck injuries cause 70% of sports-related traumatic deaths and 20% of permanent disabilities (Proctor & Cantu, 2000). Central nervous system trauma is important to assess, because repeated concussions are often progressively more serious. Various neurologic assessment and concussion management protocols have evolved (American Academy of Neurology Quality Standards Subcommittee, 1997) (Tables 15-6 and 15-7).

TABLE 15-6 *Recognizing a Concussion in Athletes*

Symptoms	Signs Frequently Observed (Note Early vs. Late)
Early (minutes to hours)	Vacant stare (befuddled facial expression)
Headache	Delayed verbal and motor responses (slower to answer questions or follow instructions)
Dizziness or vertigo	Confusion/distractibility (easily distracted and unable to follow through with normal activities)
Unawareness of surroundings	Disorientation related to time, place, date (walking in wrong direction; unaware of time, date, place)
Nausea or vomiting	Slurred, incoherent speech (making disjointed or incomprehensible statements)
Late (days to weeks)	Gross incoordination (stumbling, unable to walk tandem/straight line)
Light-headedness	Emotions out of proportion to situation (appearing distraught, crying for no apparent reason)
Persistent mild headache	Memory deficits (asking same question repeatedly; cannot remember words, numbers for 5 min)
Poor attention/concentration	Any period of loss of consciousness (paralytic coma, unresponsive to stimuli)
Memory dysfunction	
Fatigue	
Irritability/low frustration tolerance	
Sleep disturbance	

From American Academy of Neurology Quality Standards Subcommittee: Practice parameter: the management of concussion in sports (summary statement), *Neurology* 48:581-585, 1997.

TABLE 15-7 ***Sideline Evaluation for Assessment of Head and Neck Trauma***

Mental Status Testing	
Orientation	Time, place, person, activity, situation before and after the trauma
Concentration	Digits said backward: 3–1–7, 4–6–8–2, 5–3–0–7–4
	Months of year said backward
Memory	Names of teams in prior contest
	Details of contest, such as plays or strategies used
	Recall of three words and three objects at 0 and 5 min
	Recent newsworthy events
Exertional Provocative Tests	
Exercises*	40-yard sprint
	5 push-ups, 5 sit-ups, 5 knee bends
Neurologic Tests	
Pupils	Symmetry and reaction
Coordination	Finger-nose-finger
	Tandem walk
Sensation	Finger-nose with eyes closed
	Romberg test

From American Academy of Neurology Quality Standards Subcommittee: Practice parameter: the management of concussion in sports (summary statement), *Neurology* 48:583, 1997.

*Any associated symptoms are abnormal, including headache, dizziness, nausea, unsteadiness, photophobia, blurred or double vision, emotional lability, or mental status changes.

For the young person with a history of any serious head injury or intracranial surgery, consultation with a neurosurgeon should occur before participation.

Athletes may suffer from *second-impact syndrome*, which can arise when a second brain injury occurs before symptoms of a prior head injury have resolved (generally within 72 hours to 1 week). Massive brain swelling with significant risk of mortality can result (Luckstead & Patel, 2002). Because of this possibility, properly identifying the concussion (see Table 15-6) and accurately excluding the athlete from competition based on set criteria (Box 15-1), as well as preventing early reinjury, are of utmost importance. Generally, athletes with a history of concussion who have been asymptomatic (no headache, dizziness, or sensory or mental changes) and who have no neurologic symptoms are allowed to participate in sports (Kurowski & Chandran, 2000).

After neck injuries, the athlete should be free of neck and arm pain, have a full range of neck motion, and have full neck strength. Neck radiographs and magnetic resonance imaging (MRI), if done, should not reveal abnormal position, disk disease, or spinal stenosis (Proctor & Cantu, 2000).

Burners, stingers, and transient quadriplegia must be asymptomatic before clearance for sports participation. Burners and stingers are nerve root or brachial plexus compression or traction injuries and generally cause unilateral symptoms. They may require cervical spine evaluation if recurrent or persistent. Transient quadriplegia is a much more significant problem and generally appears with bilateral symptoms. It is a contraindication for contact/collision sports until fully evaluated or if any objective structural problems are found. Youths with mild to moderate burners, stingers, or transient quadriplegia symptoms need careful evaluation and must be free of symptoms before sports clearance (Kurowski & Chandran, 2000).

Chronic Medical Conditions

Cardiac Disease

Most grade I–II/VI systolic murmurs without significant cardiovascular history do not need further evaluation. However, louder or diastolic murmurs, unusual loudness, or wide splitting of S2, and increased loudness with Valsalva maneuver or standing, require further evaluation. A history of syncope with exertion, palpitations, exertional chest pain or discomfort, or exertional shortness of breath, or a family history of Marfan syndrome, atherosclerosis (especially

BOX 15-1 *Recommendations for Management of Concussion* in Sports*

Grade 1 Concussion

Definition: Transient confusion, no loss of consciousness, and a duration of mental status abnormalities of <15 min.

Management: The athlete should be removed from sports activity, examined immediately and at 5 min intervals, and allowed to return that day to the sports activity only if postconcussive symptoms resolve within 15 min. Any athlete who incurs a second grade 1 concussion on the same day should be removed from sports activity until asymptomatic for 1 wk.

Grade 2 Concussion

Definition: Transient confusion, no loss of consciousness, and a duration of mental status abnormalities of ≥15 min.

Management: The athlete should be removed from sports activity and examined frequently to assess the evolution of symptoms, with more extensive diagnostic evaluation if the symptoms worsen or persist for >1 wk. The athlete should return to sports activity only after asymptomatic for 1 full wk. Any athlete who incurs a grade 2 concussion subsequent to a grade 1 concussion on the same day should be removed from sports activity until asymptomatic for 2 wk.

Grade 3 Concussion

Definition: Loss of consciousness, either brief (seconds) or prolonged (minutes or longer).

Management: The athlete should be removed from sports activity for 1 full wk without symptoms if the loss of consciousness is brief or 2 full wk without symptoms if the loss of consciousness is prolonged. If still unconscious or if abnormal neurologic signs are present at the time of initial evaluation, the athlete should be transported by ambulance to the nearest hospital emergency department. An athlete who suffers a second grade 3 concussion should be removed from sports activity until asymptomatic for 1 mo. Any athlete with an abnormality on computed tomography or magnetic resonance imaging brain scan consistent with brain swelling, contusion, or other intracranial pathology should be removed from sports activities for the season and discouraged from future return to participation in contact sports.

Data from Centers for Disease Control and Prevention: Sports-related recurrent brain injuries—United States, *JAMA* 277:1190-1191, 1997; American Academy of Neurology Quality Standards Subcommittee: Practice parameter: the management of concussion in sports (summary statement), *Neurology* 48:581-585, 1997; Kelly J: Reply from the authors: management of concussion in sports, *Neurology* 53(9):829, 1999.

*A *concussion* is defined as head-trauma–induced alteration in mental status that may or may not involve loss of consciousness. Concussions are graded in three categories. Definitions and treatment recommendations for each category are presented. Mental status abnormalities include impairment in orientation, immediate memory, concentration, or delayed recall.

premature), or sudden unexpected death in the young or middle-aged, should be evaluated for problems such as hypertrophic cardiomyopathy (formerly called idiopathic hypertrophic subaortic stenosis) regardless of physical examination findings (Kurowski & Chandran, 2000). See Box 15-2 for "red flags" that may predispose a sudden death occurrence. Hypertrophic cardiomyopathy is the primary cause of sudden death; the incidence is rare at 1:100,000 to 1:300,000 participants (Verst, 2000). Other cardiovascular causes of sudden death among teenagers engaged in athletic events include left and right heart valvular obstructive lesions, Marfan syndrome, ventricular tachycardia, coronary arterial abnormalities, congestive heart failure, large shunt lesions, and pulmonary hypertension. Individuals with myocarditis, pericarditis, fibrillation, long QT-interval syndrome, hypertrophic cardiomyopathy, severe aortic stenosis, or anomalous coronary artery disease should have activities restricted (Berul, 2000). Asking about use of anabolic steroids and cocaine is important, because both have cardiotoxic effects (Kurowski & Chandran, 2000). The *26th Bethesda Conference: Recommendations for Determining Eligibility for Competition in Athletes with Cardiovascular Abnormalities* (Mitchell, Haskell, & Raven, 1994) may serve as a useful reference for the NP. Specific exercise prescriptions can be developed under a cardiologist's direction for children with known cardiac disease.

Hypertension

Hypertension should be diagnosed only after elevated blood pressures have been demonstrated on three separate occasions with use of proper technique. Children with mild hypertension (95th to 99th percentiles for normal blood pressure ranges for age) should not be restricted from any sports. Those with severe hypertension (greater than 99th

BOX 15-2 *Sudden Death from Pulmonary Congestion: Warning Signs*

- Exertional dyspnea
- Fatigue
- Orthopnea
- Paroxysmal nocturnal apnea
- Chest pain
- Excessive, unexplained shortness of breath
- Long QT wave
- Syncope
- Near-syncope
- Light-headedness
- Palpitations
- Increase in systolic blood pressure
- History of death in family member or significant heart disease under age 50 yr

Adapted from Greene P: Pearls for practice: recognizing young people at risk for sudden cardiac death in preparticipation sports physicals, *J Am Acad Nurse Pract* 12(1):11-14, 2000.

percentile for age) should not be cleared for participation until the condition is evaluated and treated (Kurowski & Chandran, 2000). The AAP Committee on Sports Medicine and Fitness (1997) recommendations are similar but also recommend counseling of hypertensive youth to adopt healthful lifestyle behaviors, including avoidance of anabolic steroids, growth hormone, alcohol, tobacco, and high sodium intake. For some athletic governing bodies, use of diuretics and β-blockers is prohibited.

Asthma

Children with asthma should be encouraged, not discouraged, from participation in sports. It has been suggested that a free-run challenge test be part of the PPE to identify at-risk youth. The running test was found to be more predictive than peak expiratory flow rates in detecting such risk (Hammerman et al, 2002). Poorly controlled asthma will cause the following symptoms: persistent coughing, recurrent respiratory complaints or symptoms after participating in physical activity, and reluctance to participate or a low stamina level (Patrick et al, 2001).

Properly managed asthma should not cause such problems with exertion as were common in the past. The great majority of patients with asthma can engage in sports, even though most may experience exercise-induced asthma (EIA). Exercise-induced bronchospasm is found in up to 50% of children with asthma and in 11% of children with no previous asthma but with a history of allergies or a family history of asthma (Spooner, Saunders, & Rowe, 2002). Progressive airway obstruction generally occurs after physical activity ceases, with peak airway resistance occurring 5 to 10 minutes after activity stops and resolving within 30 to 60 minutes. There is a refractory period for 50% of people that lasts up to 2 hours after an EIA episode. This period either allows the person to exercise without recurrence or to experience a lessened EIA event. Doing warm-up drills before vigorous exercise can help athletes use this refractory period to their benefit. Breathing cold, dry air is more irritating than warm, humid air. Thus swimmers are known to experience less EIA, whereas hockey players and figure skaters have high incidences of the condition. EIA is generally not life threatening.

Recommended management includes using both pharmacologic and nonpharmacologic regimens. The use of a short-acting β_2-agonist bronchodilator (inhaled albuterol, pirbuterol, or terbutaline taken 15 minutes before exercise) or an antiinflammatory (e.g., cromolyn sodium or nedocromil sodium) is needed by most (Mayers & Rundell, 2000). The inhaled β_2-agonists are effective in 80% to 95% of users for up to 4 hours; long-acting bronchodilators (salmeterol) can act for up to 9 to 12 hours. Cromolyn and other mast cell release inhibitors are effective in 70% to 87% of users (Stricker, 2000).

Warm-up drills for 10 to 60 minutes before the sports event can prevent or lessen EIA episodes by maintaining airway warmth and moisture. Covering the mouth and nose with a scarf or mask when exercising in cold air achieves the same purpose. Athletic conditioning also helps improve muscle and exercise efficiency. Warming down, or gradually decreasing exercise at the end of a session, also seems to help decrease the magnitude of the attack. Teachers and coaches should be aware of exercise-induced asthma. Many children with well-controlled asthma experience some airway obstruction after exercise (American Academy of Allergy, Asthma and Immunology, 2002).

Seizures

Children and adolescents with seizure disorders can participate in most sports. They should be excluded from certain sports only if having a seizure would put them or others at significant risk (e.g., high diving, rock climbing, gymnastics). If the seizures are poorly controlled, they should be excluded from contact or collision activities or hazardous sports (e.g., archery, riflery, swimming, weight lifting). Decisions about participation in specific sports should be made with information about the severity, frequency, etiology, and degree of control of the seizures and may need to include an evaluation by a neurologist (Kurowski & Chandran, 2000). Benefits of participation include some evidence of a reduction in number of seizures, improved ambulation or other motor function, and enhanced self-esteem (Patrick et al, 2001).

Diabetes Mellitus

Children with diabetes, whether insulin dependent or not, should be the least restricted of all those with chronic diseases. Exercise is an essential component of their management. The child should be well controlled before entering a sports program and should have immediate access to a home blood glucose monitoring system. Assistance from a diabetic educator or the physician who plans the child's insulin therapy, nutrition, and exercise regimen is important. It is important to know that exercise can delay the hypoglycemic response from insulin.

Children with diabetes should not participate in physical activity if they have retinal hemorrhages present, they are ill or have an infection, or their blood glucose is less than 100 mg/dl or greater than 250 mg/dl with urine ketones present, or greater than 300 mg/dl without urine ketones (Patrick et al, 2001). Medical identification, proper nutrition, injection of insulin into body parts that are less active, consideration of timing of insulin, and adjustment of the dosage will help avoid diabetic problems. Keep high-carbohydrate foods available for the athlete to avoid hypoglycemia. Provision of fluids for adequate hydration is also advised.

Acute Infections

Infectious Mononucleosis

The risk of splenic rupture with mononucleosis needs to be considered. Ultrasonography may reveal splenomegaly that is not clinically palpable. Splenic rupture has not been reported longer than 4 weeks after resolution of clinical symptoms, so this can be a good guideline to follow for deciding when the young person can return to contact sports, assuming that splenomegaly is not present on examination.

Skin Infections

Skin infections are a special consideration for wrestlers. The incidence of contracting *herpes gladiatorum* from exposure to a person with a herpes simplex infection ranges from 20% to 50%. Lesions should be healed before wrestling is resumed. For other sports, bandaging may be sufficient to prevent transmission. Athletes with impetigo or other streptococcal or staphylococcal infections should be on antibiotics for at least 48 hours or until significant improvement is seen before participating in contact or collision sports. Scabies, lice, and *molluscum contagiosum* preclude participation in contact or collision sports, especially in sports in which mats are used and in sports such as baseball, in which equipment is shared. Tinea infections can also be passed from athlete to athlete.

Human Immunodeficiency Virus and Other Blood-Borne Viral Pathogens

The risks of infection via skin or mucous membrane exposure to blood or other infectious body fluids is extremely low (AAP Committee on Sports Medicine and Fitness, 1999). Thus infected athletes should be allowed to participate in all sports. Their health status is to be treated with confidentiality, and universal precautions should be practiced in all sports. Hepatitis B virus (HBV) immunizations should be encouraged. The AAP 1999 policy provides additional measures for the protection of all.

Physical Anomalies

Hernia

Hernias should be repaired. However, the teen with a hernia need not be restricted from sports participation but should be aware of the symptoms of incarceration.

Absence of Paired Organs

Sports that involve objects, sticks, or racquets, or aggressive play, such as football or basketball, have greater risks for eye injuries. Baseball is the most dangerous eye sport. Face shields are now required for hockey, and the incidence of serious injuries in this sport has dramatically decreased. Eyewear is available for all sports except those such as boxing and full-contact martial arts.

The child with one eye or best-corrected vision in one eye worse than 20/40 should be required to wear molded polycarbonate sport frames with 3 mm–thick polycarbonate lenses for all sports involving rapidly moving objects, bats, or racquets. For collision sports involving headgear, such as football, hockey, or lacrosse, the same frames and lenses should be worn under the cage shield or mask. These children should not participate in sports in which the use of eye protection is not possible. A history of detached retina is significant, and participation should be limited to nonstrenuous sports until consultation with an ophthalmologist is complete.

Those with a single polycystic or abnormally located kidney should be excluded from contact or collision sports (Kurowski & Chandran, 2000).

Young men with a single testicle can be adequately protected with the use of a hard-cup athletic supporter for contact and collision sports, as well as those in which objects are projected at high speed. Although somewhat uncomfortable to wear, most affected men comply if the risks of sterility are explained (Kurowski & Chandran, 2000). Girls with one ovary are not restricted because of the protected location of the organ.

Atlantoaxial Instability

Children with Down syndrome can have a bony anomaly and ligament laxity that causes instability where the skull and the first two cervical vertebrae articulate. The incidence of this atlantoaxial instability is between 10% and 30%. Routine radiographic screening has traditionally been recommended for these children; those with atlantoaxial separation greater than 4.5 mm or a neural canal width less than 14 mm were excluded from certain sports. Removal of this recommendation, by the American Academy of Pediatrics Committee on Sports Medicine and Fitness in 1995, has been challenged by other physicians in the Down syndrome field (Brockmeyer, 1999; Cohen, 1998; Pueschel, 1998). Clearance for Special Olympics still requires radiographic screening. Any other youths with known problems in this area should not engage in contact or collision sports or limited-contact or impact sports (see Table 15-4) or in such sports as diving. They may, however, engage in most of the noncontact sports listed in Table 15-4. An MRI is done if instability is detected by radiograph. Surgical fusion may be indicated. The risk of spinal cord injury cannot be minimized.

Risks for the Female Athlete

Females are less likely to suffer sudden death that males. However, there are some issues specific to females that the NP needs to be aware of. Such awareness affords the opportunity to provide vital preventive health care. Referred to as the *female athlete triad* (anorexia, amenorrhea, and osteoporosis), this progressive array of symptoms is becoming a common finding as more females participate in sports. Stress fractures are 12 times more likely to occur in female runners than in male runners. Amenorrheic female athletes can suffer from osteoporosis (Kurowski & Chandran, 2000). The symptoms occur along a continuum rather than in unison; therefore the identification of the early existence of an eating disorder or weight loss from a PPE history or examination should alert the NP to take a more thorough history and initiate early treatment (Metzl, 2002). Females participating in running and aesthetic sports such as gymnastics, cheerleading, dance or ballet, and figure skating seem more prone to eating disorders. Primary or secondary amenorrhea or stress fractures are also good clues to the possible existence of the triad.

A recent report by Maffulli and Baxter-Jones (2002) disproved the notion that intensive sport training delays the growth and sexual maturation of young female athletes. This concern has been repeatedly raised at every World Olympics in regard to female gymnasts. However, the aforementioned report credits the differences in growth and maturation more to the genetic makeup of the individual rather than to extended, intensive training.

MANAGEMENT STRATEGIES TO SUPPORT ACTIVITY PATTERNS FOR CHILDREN AND ADOLESCENTS

NPs can address a variety of health-oriented issues to support children and adolescents participating in physical activities. Injury management should not be the goal! These are summarized in Box 15-3 and discussed in greater depth in this section. Injury management is addressed in Chapter 40.

BOX 15-3 *Primary Care Sports Participation Management*

Diseases

- Control symptoms of specific diseases or conditions
- Rehabilitate injuries
- Prevent injuries, heat illnesses
  - Hydration
  - Protective equipment
  - Correct footwear
  - Proper training
  - Safe environment
  - Educated coaching

Daily Living

- Nutrition
  - Balanced diet
  - Adequate calories
  - Hydration
- Stress management
  - Realistic expectations
  - Stress reduction for performance
  - Supportive coaching
  - Supportive parenting
- Balanced home, school, recreation goals and outcomes
- Drug-free performance

Development

- Sports and activities are selected for success within capacity
- Supportive training/coaching

Counseling Families about Sports for Their Children

Physical activity needs to be encouraged from infancy. Playing outside and engaging in family physical activities serve important developmental needs. When children enter school, sports opportunities become organized, so children and their families need to make specific decisions and choices about the sports in which they want to participate. At this time, it is important to identify the parent who has sports goals for the child that may be meeting the parent's needs more than the child's. For the prepubertal child entering sports, the goals should be healthful activity, learning basic skills, and mastering the rules of the game. All children do not mature at the same rate. The skills of several children of the same age can be widely discrepant, and the performance of a 16- or 17-year-old is very different from that of the same child at age 12.

The following are some basic concepts to keep in mind for counseling:

- Noncontact team sports participation can begin at about age 6 years but should be guided by the child's development and individual interest. Contact sports such as basketball, soccer, and wrestling can be added at age 8 years. Collision sports such as tackle football and ice hockey should be delayed until 10 years (Preventing sports injuries in kids, 1998).
- The child who is an exceptional athlete may still have maturation difficulties in social and psychologic areas. Finding a balance in supporting the development of an athletically gifted child can be difficult given the stress this child may face in the competitive arena.
- Children with handicaps can participate in sports. They should make the choice of which sport with advice about the health effects that can result, as well as the conditioning that may be necessary.
- Children with academic problems should not be denied participation in sports. Sports can be the best arena for boosting self-esteem for the child who does not experience success in the classroom. Helping the child find a balance between academic work and sports participation is essential.
- Boys and girls can play together, especially in the prepubertal years. Differences in height and weight can make it unsafe for smaller girls to compete in contact sports with boys after puberty.
- Injuries occur in some sports more often than in others. Football, hockey, gymnastics, and wrestling are especially high-risk activities. Good supervision and appropriate equipment can help minimize some of the risks.
- Families need to support physical activity for children, provide opportunities for children to engage in a variety of activities, role model healthy physical activity, and supervise to ensure safety and a positive experience for each child.

Injury Prevention

A variety of strategies can be used to reduce the incidence and severity of injuries. Safety rules for games are designed to reduce injuries, especially for contact sports; protective equipment such as head and mouth protection makes a significant difference; maintenance of playing fields, floors, and equipment is important; coaches need to teach good techniques and guide athletes through adequate warm-up and stretching exercises before and after the game; and support personnel need to be qualified to manage acute trauma and cardiopulmonary resuscitation. Design changes may prevent equipment-related injuries (Cheng et al, 2000). Heat related illnesses and dehydration can be avoided. Many injury prevention interventions are best considered in terms of the specific sport or recreational activity at hand.

Avoiding Injury: The Readiness Factor

Readiness can be addressed from two perspectives, developmental readiness and preseason conditioning readiness. Of course, physical and cognitive development for play begins in infancy and should continue throughout the life span. Patel, Pratt, and Greydanus (2002) discuss developmental readiness for organized sports participation, an issue for many children and their parents. They note that children are not able to compare their abilities to those of others until age 6, do not understand the competitive nature of sports until age 9, and do not understand the complex nature of tasks involved in a given sport until age 12 years. Sports participation involves not only physical but also cognitive and social readiness.

Preseason conditioning, or preparatory muscle conditioning, for children is receiving more notice as a method for decreasing overall injuries and the severity of injuries; lessening overuse injuries (stress fractures, bursitis, tendonitis) and the amount of time needed for rehabilitation; and improving performance (Faigenbaum & Micheli, 2000). Such conditioning is not sport specific but entails activities geared toward improving strength, flexibility, and endurance; it is not intended to be confused with weight lifting or bodybuilding. It should begin at least 8 weeks before sports participation with no more than a 10% increase each week in training time, amount of distance covered, or number or repetitions performed. An estimated

50% of overuse injuries could be prevented with such supervised youth strength training programs.

Coaches and fitness instructors should be certified and be knowledgeable about age-specific training techniques and safety; adult training techniques should never be applied to children.

Traumatic Injury Prevention

Strains and Sprains. These injuries are most related to basketball injuries (Taylor & Attia, 2000).

- Do preseason stretching
- Tape site of previous injury
- Warm up body temperature before stretching
- Maintain playing surfaces
- Use proper footwear
- Limit practice time

Knee braces do not have sufficient scientific evidence to recommend them for pediatric athletes. However, their use seems to provide subjective relief and thus they are prescribed clinically. They should not replace rehabilitation and surgery, if required (AAP, Martin, Committee on Sports Medicine and Fitness, 2001).

Fractures. These injuries are most related to rollerblading and in-line skating (Taylor & Attia, 2000).

- Do strength-conditioning exercises
- Use proper techniques
- Take safety precautions
- Use protective gear that fits well, such as wrist guards

Laceration/Contusions/Abrasions. These injuries are most related to baseball (contusion/abrasion) and ice hockey (lacerations) (Taylor & Attia, 2000).

- Protective equipment is essential.

Head and Neck. Greatest risks for injury are from cycling, diving, equestrian sports, football, gymnastics, ice hockey, wrestling, and cheerleading. Risks increase with age (Luckstead & Patel, 2002; Proctor & Cantu, 2000).

- Have appropriate supervision
- Adhere to safety rules of the game
- Strengthen neck muscles
- Use appropriate equipment—helmets, face and mouth gear
- Follow management of concussion guidelines for return to sport after injury

Eye. Eye injuries are most commonly related to baseball and ice hockey.

- Use headgear and protective glasses

Overuse Injury Prevention

Stress Fractures

- Use soft running and playing surfaces
- Use proper footgear
- Do strengthening exercises
- Stop activity when pain occurs

Anterior Leg Pain Syndrome (Shin Splints)

- Stretch before and after activity
- Pronate and supinate feet while standing
- Use soft playing surface
- Use proper footwear—proper fit, impact-absorbing sole, support for hindfoot
- Avoid sudden increase in activity
- Limit forceful, extensive use of foot flexors

Plantar Fasciitis

- Use proper footwear (cushioned with fitted heel counters or lifts)
- Stretch calf and Achilles tendon
- Do ice massage after event
- Correct biomechanical errors
- Limit hills and speed work; increase soft-surface running

Blisters

- Wear socks
- Wear properly fitted shoes
- Use powder, petroleum jelly, or a product such as Second Skin on reddened or at-risk areas

Heat and Humidity

Heat is acquired both endogenously and exogenously when environmental temperature exceeds body temperature. Heat is dissipated through evaporation, conduction, convection, and radiation; heat is dissipated only through evaporation when environmental temperature exceeds body temperature, and this, only when humidity is 75% or less. There is no evaporation at 90% to 95% humidity. Because children have a higher metabolic rate at a given submaximal walking or running speed, they produce more heat. This higher metabolic load, in addition to several other pediatric physiologic factors, including poor sweating capacity, larger surface-to-mass ratio, and an immature cardiovascular system, results in a shorter tolerance for exercising in hot climates and greater susceptibility to heat stress for children.

Hard exercise increases metabolic rate 8 to 10 times, with increases of core body temperature of 1° to 1.5° C in 20 minutes. Heavy uniforms or sweat suits reduce evaporation further. Younger children dehydrate sooner and have higher core temperatures than adults do under the same conditions. Therefore they are at greater risk for heat illness, heat exhaustion, and heat stroke. The AAP Committee on Sports Medicine and Fitness (2000a) recommends that activities lasting 30 minutes or more be reduced whenever the humidity or the temperature is high.

Acclimatization requires gradual heat stress over a period of at least 2 weeks. Acclimatization allows the individual to dissipate more heat through evaporation with decreased sodium concentration in sweat and thus exercise longer and harder in heat without loss of excessive electrolytes. Children require more time to acclimatize and may need 8 to 10 exposures of 30 to 45 minutes each to make the adjustment. The AAP Committee on Sports Medicine and Fitness (2000a) recommends one exposure per day.

Very young children with a higher surface-to-mass ratio, those with fever, and those who are dehydrated are at greater risk for heat illnesses. Children with a variety of chronic illnesses are also at risk. Fever, vomiting, diarrhea, diabetes insipidus, and diabetes mellitus may increase risk through fluid losses. Decreased sweat production may occur with spina bifida, quadriplegia, scleroderma, severe eczema, and sunburn, among other conditions. Excessive sweating as with cystic fibrosis and some cardiac conditions can increase fluid losses. Diminished thirst sensation increases the likelihood of dehydration, and obesity, especially related to lack of conditioning, predisposes to heat illness. Certain drugs can also increase heat production or decrease sweating. Of course, environmental factors such as high temperature, high humidity, and excessive clothing will also increase the risk of heat illnesses (Hoffman, 2001).

Heat Illnesses (Hyperthermia)

Heat Cramps. Prickly heat, heat edema of hands and feet, and heat syncope are early indicators of the body's responses to excessive heat. Heat cramps is one of the mildest form of heat illness. Symptoms include painful muscle spasms of extremities and abdomen during or after strenuous exercise with profuse sweating. The cramps are brief (less than 1 minute), intermittent, and painful contractions, especially of the lower extremities, abdomen, and shoulders. They may occur after intense exercise and are thought to be related to electrolyte depletion. The subject is thirsty but well oriented and alert. Salted liquid (a sports drink or 0.5 to 1 teaspoon of salt in 1 quart of water) taken by mouth over 1 to 2 hours or normal saline given intravenously, rest in a cool area, and several days of avoidance of the activity causing the cramps is the treatment (Hoffman, 2001). Heat cramps occur most commonly when athletes are not adequately conditioned for participation at high temperature or humidity, or both.

Heat Exhaustion. Heat exhaustion is the most common heat illness of athletes. It occurs with excess sweating in a hot, humid environment. It is a reversible condition, whereas heat stroke causes irreversible damage to tissues. Symptoms include cramps, as well as headache; fatigue; weakness; dizziness; and possibly nausea, anorexia, or diarrhea. The core temperature may rise above 38° C but is usually less than 40° C. Mentation is generally normal; dry tongue and mouth, as well as weight loss, may occur. Cardiovascular symptoms may result from volume loss and include tachypnea and orthostatic hypotension. Malaise, myalgias, vertigo, chills, visual disturbances, and cutaneous flushing may also occur. The skin is ashen, cold, and clammy because of sodium depletion, or hot and dry from water depletion. Mild shock may be present, but there are no major central nervous system dysfunctions. Management includes rest in a cooler environment; cooling measures, such as removing clothing and fanning to enhance evaporation and spraying or sponging the skin with water; and oral or intravenous fluids. The child should be allowed unrestricted access to salty foods. Emergency department monitoring is preferred. If the athlete is confused or refuses to drink, intravenous fluids are needed. A patient with the latter symptoms may need hospitalization (Hoffman, 2001).

Heat Stroke. Heat stroke is a medical emergency with morbidity rates from 17% to 70%. It can occur over several days as with a heat wave or rapidly with exertion. In either case, rapid cooling is essential because the high body temperature damages tissues and alters heart, lung, brain, kidney, and other organ system functions. The classic triad of symptoms is hyperpyrexia, severe central nervous system disturbance (coma), and anhidrosis. Rectal temperature over 40° C, headache, chills, nausea, vomiting, muscle cramps, ataxia, and incoherent speech occur. Sweating may or may not be present, depending on the degree of depletion of fluids that has occurred. Tachycardia and hypotension can occur. Loss of consciousness, circulatory failure, coagulopathy, and renal and hepatic failure occur as body systems decompensate. Rapid transport to an emergency department is essential for administration of intravenous fluids; rapid cooling with ice water immersion or lavages; and support of respiratory, cardiovascular, and renal functions. While waiting for transport, the patient should be placed in a cool environment, clothing should be removed, and water should be applied to the body with fanning to increase evaporation. Ice packs are to be avoided because melting ice dissipates less heat than evaporation does. Fluids should be given orally if the athlete is alert. Antipyretics will not be useful (Hoffman, 2001).

Preventive Measures. Preventive measures for heat illnesses are listed in Box 15-4. They include efforts to decrease metabolic effort, increase evaporation, and increase hydration. Children are also at risk in hot water such as saunas. Acclimatization is helpful for young athletes.

Nutrition

Adolescents are growing at a rate second only to that of infants. Thus the nutritional intake of adolescent athletes must meet both growth and activity needs. The AAP

BOX 15-4 *Strategies to Prevent Heat Illnesses*

Athletes should wear lightweight, dry, permeable clothing.
Athletes should be fully hydrated before activity begins.
Athletes should drink cool water at a rate of 100-150 ml every 15 min for activities lasting more than 30 min.
Athletes should have scheduled rest periods in the shade.
Athletes should be gradually acclimatized to heat over 7-10 days, if possible.
Athletes at greater risk should be observed carefully. Risk factors include cystic fibrosis; hyperthyroidism; obesity; previous heat stroke; general health problems; poor conditioning; diabetes; kidney disorders; and medications such as diuretics, antihistamines, antidepressants, and others.
Activities should be scheduled in early morning or evening to avoid direct sunlight and hottest time of day.
Activity should cease if any signs and symptoms of heat illness develop.

Committee on Sports Medicine and Fitness (2000b) recommends the following:

- Calories to support energy requirements for the sport, as well as normal growth
- A balanced diet using the Food Guide Pyramid (no particular dietary constituents should be emphasized)
- Adequate iron to provide adequate stores for growth, as well as oxygen transport during activity
- Calcium following recommendations for all youth—1200 to 1500 mg/day

Depending on the sport, calorie requirements for activity exceed baseline needs by 1500 to 3000 calories. The recommended diet for the athlete is the same as for all people—high in carbohydrates (50% to 60% of calories), 25% to 30% of calories from fats, and 15% to 20% of calories from protein. Normal growth of children requires an intake of 60 kcal/kg of ideal body weight per day. Vitamins and minerals do not need to be supplemented except in women who have a diet low in both calcium and iron.

Short-term, high-intensity activities, such as high jumping or diving, involve use of anaerobic fuel sources, whereas longer-term activities, such as running or cross-country skiing, involve use of aerobic sources. Carbohydrates are used in both anaerobic and aerobic metabolic states, but fats and proteins are used only aerobically. Most of the carbohydrate intake should come from nutritional foods such as fruits and vegetables, grains, and milk sugars rather than refined sugars. Nutrition recommendations are summarized in Table 15-8.

In general, ingesting carbohydrate before activities has no effect on performance, and carbohydrate loading has not been studied in children. Carbohydrate intake during physical activity lasting more than 1 hour improves performance. After competition, carbohydrate intake is again

TABLE 15-8 *Nutrition Recommendations for Athletes*

Nutrient	Recommendations
Calories from carbohydrates/fat/protein	Maintain same as for all people: 50%-55% carbohydrate, 30% fat, 15%-20% protein Do not decrease caloric intake during sports season May need added 500 to 3000 calories to meet activity requirements
Vitamins and minerals	Same as for all people Adolescent girls may need to bring calcium and iron intake up to recommended range Do not take salt tablets; they can increase dehydration
Carbohydrates	5-10 g/kg body weight is recommended intake Use nutritious foods such as fruits, vegetables, grains, and milk sugars Carbohydrate intake during prolonged activity may increase performance Carbohydrate intake of 100 g in first 30 min after performance is recommended to promote muscle glycogen resynthesis and rapid reloading
Protein supplements	None needed; hypercalciuria with calcium loss and dehydration can occur if protein intake is too high
Fluids	Plain water before, during, and after activity Athletic drinks containing electrolytes may be helpful for endurance athletes and those who sweat heavily (not preadolescents) 8 oz fluid every 15-20 min for events lasting more than 30 min Replace water loss after activity at 2 cups per pound of weight lost Avoid caffeine drinks because they can increase diuresis

important to improve muscle glycogen resynthesis, which is most rapid in the first few hours after exercise. Consuming 100 g of carbohydrate in the first 30 minutes after performance is recommended. This can be in the form of snacks or liquids (Patrick et al, 2001). Weight gain of mostly muscle mass occurs primarily through eating extra carbohydrate calories and exercising. Carbohydrate intake must meet basic needs plus replacement for exercise energy expenditure to ensure normal growth.

Protein requirements are easily met with normal diets of 1 g/kg of body weight. No protein supplements are needed. In fact, hypercalciuria with calcium loss and dehydration can occur if protein intake is too high because the excess nitrogen, and hence water, is excreted. Intense endurance sports and strength training probably requires an additional 0.5 to 1 g/kg per day. Youths who eat too much protein may not consume adequate carbohydrates and fats.

Weight loss by adolescent athletes can be a dangerous practice. Wrestlers may try to make weight, runners sometimes vomit to run lighter, and female gymnasts may practice significant nutritional control to maintain size. Dancers, divers, figure skaters, and cheerleaders also control weight for appearance advantages. Bodybuilders, rowers, distance runners, and swimmers also often try to control their weight. Starvation can lead to suppressed growth hormones, can interfere with pubertal gonadal hormone changes, and may result in eating disorders. Nutritional counseling is essential, with a reminder that muscle weighs more than fat and that weight gain during adolescence with growth is normal.

Weight loss by energy restriction (reduced calories) significantly reduces anaerobic performance by wrestlers. Further, wrestlers on high-carbohydrate refeeding diets tend to recover their performance, whereas those on moderate-carbohydrate diets do not (Rankin, Ocel, & Craft, 1996). Wrestlers, coaches, and parents may sign a contract requiring that the child eat three meals a day, that fluid be available at all times, and that no artificial means be employed to remove fluids from the body (e.g., sauna or sweat suit, laxatives, diuretics, diet pills, licit or illicit drugs, nicotine, prolonged fasting, overexercising, or vomiting) (AAP Committee on Sports Medicine and Fitness, 1996).

The young person can avoid dehydration by drinking cool, flavored water before, during, and after the activity. Athletic drinks containing electrolytes can help replace losses for endurance athletes performing under extreme conditions or for those who sweat profusely, but they are generally unnecessary. In fact, the principal effect of added sodium may be to make the athlete more thirsty so that he or she drinks more (Ryan-Krause, 1998). For the preadolescent who does not sweat well, use of electrolyte solutions is definitely not warranted. Exercise in the mature adolescent can cause fluid losses of more than 1 L per hour. The athlete should drink 16 oz of water 2 hours before the activity. For events lasting more than 30 minutes, 8 ounces of water must be consumed every 15 or 20 minutes. Because the first sensations of thirst occur only after dehydration has already begun, drinking needs to begin before the need is felt. Furthermore, performance is reduced by the amount of dehydration present; by the time the athlete feels thirsty, he or she already is at less than peak performance. A weight loss of more than 4% of body weight puts the athlete at risk for heat cramps, heat illness, heat stroke, and even death. After competition, rehydration is important. Generally, drinking 2 cups of water for each pound of weight lost is adequate. Small amounts of sodium such as are found in sports drinks enhance rehydration, but additional sodium supplements are not recommended. Drinking fluids with caffeine should be avoided, because these beverages increase urine output, causing further dehydration. Use of separate fluid containers for each child participating may help monitor the intake of each while decreasing the risk of disease spread. (See Table 15-8 for nutrition recommendations for athletes.) Scheduling fluid breaks and rotating players more frequently may also help avoid dehydration.

Stress and Sports: Keeping Activities Fun

Children and adolescents need to enjoy sports and to find that they reduce rather than induce stress if they are going to include vigorous physical activity in their lifestyles. The athletic environment should foster psychologic as well as physical well-being. It is part of the NP's role to assess the psychologic dimensions of sports participation and intervene when problems appear. Most children will benefit from participation in a variety of sports and recreational activities, both in terms of reducing repetitive movements that can increase overuse injury risks and to avoid premature commitment to a sport for excellence. Children should experience happiness and success from their sports participation (Metzl, 2002).

Athletic stress arises as a result of the interactions between situational factors, personality factors, and motivational factors. Situationally, athletes need to have sufficient developmental and psychologic resources to meet the demands of the event. Cognitively, athletes make an appraisal of the situation. They assess the demands and their resources, the consequences of success or failure, and their personal interpretation of the consequences. A person with low self-confidence might assess a particular event as more stressful than would a person with high self-confidence even if both have equal skills. Stress occurs when the assessment yields perceived negative outcomes. There is also a physiologic component to stress. When the athlete becomes overexcited, performance decreases. Finally, stress is related to the coping and behavioral responses the athlete uses. In part, these will be related to his or her developmental level.

The consequences of excessive athletic stress can be withdrawal from sports, decreased enjoyment, decreased performance, and negative physical effects, including interference with eating and sleeping or possible increase in injuries.

Management of Athletic Stress

First, cognitive interventions can be taken to manage athletic stress. The following are key points that may be helpful to youngsters and their families:

- Winning is not everything or the only thing.
- Failure is not the same thing as losing.
- Success is not winning but rather striving for victory (the effort).
- Preferred goals include the following:
  - Regular physical activity to promote health
  - Participation in organized sports to acquire basic motor skills, learn social skills for teamwork, learn sportsmanship, and have fun (AAP Committee on Sports Medicine and Fitness, 2001).

Second, the organization and administration of sports programs can make a difference in the pleasure experienced by young athletes. Some positive strategies include the following:

- Establishing different skill and competition levels
- Organizing homogeneous groups by age and size
- Not scoring games, keeping season records, or calculating individual statistics
- Directly altering games to increase opportunities for success, such as playing T-ball instead of pitched softball, lowering the basket, decreasing the length of games, using a smaller playing field, and changing some rules, such as no press defense in basketball or no stealing in baseball

Third, coaching roles and relationships can be modified. Coach-effectiveness training has been shown to positively influence athletes' feelings of self-esteem, player attitudes, appreciation of the coach, and relationships among the players. Coaches should use positive control techniques, reframe winning into success for effort, and work on team cohesion and development of positive desire. Coaches may also need to support the injured athlete's need for reduced training and rehabilitation. Coaches should not overtrain athletes because this results in fatigue and a sense of being "stale." Again, reduced training may be needed (AAP Committee on Sports Medicine and Fitness, 2000b; Hergenroeder, 1998).

Fourth, parents need to focus on supporting their children rather than identifying with them. Parental success and feelings of self-worth should not derive from having a child who wins at sports. Neither should the family build its identity around the young athlete to the extent that poor performance becomes a family catastrophe (Hergenroeder, 1998).

Finally, stress management training can be recommended for the child who anticipates giving a significant amount of energy and commitment to a sport over several years.

Drugs and Supplements

Anabolic-Androgenic Steroids

Endogenous anabolic-androgenic steroids (AASs) start adolescent development in the prepubertal male. Exogenous anabolic-androgenic drugs used by teenage athletes are derivatives of testosterone. The term *androgenic* refers to the effects on the male reproductive tract and the development of secondary male sexual characteristics. Anabolic effects are changes that occur in nonreproductive tissues, such as closure of bony epiphyses, changes in the larynx, and increases in muscle bulk and strength. Aggressive male behavior is also thought to be related to androgenic effects.

Reports of anabolic steroid use by adolescents have been seen in the literature since the 1980s. Current prevalence rates range from 4% to 12% for boys and up to 2.5% for girls (Congeni & Miller, 2002). Risk factors identified include the following:

- Male
- Using illegal drugs
- Participating in school sports, especially strength-dependent ones

Other reported risk factors include higher socioeconomic status, poor body image, self-reported violence and aggression, and a family history of drug abuse (Congeni & Miller, 2002).

Teenagers may use oral or injected forms of testosterone, alkylated testosterones (oral), and other agents, such as testosterone esters (injected) and derivatives. Generally, these drugs are taken in cycles of use lasting 4 to 12 weeks each. Sometimes adolescents use more than one type at a time ("stacking") or alternate use to prevent developing tolerance. They increase the dose incrementally and then taper the dose at the end of a cycle ("pyramiding").

Clinical effects include acne, seborrhea, weight gain, deepening voice, and gynecomastia. With higher doses, some of the more serious side effects include priapism (sustained penile erection), edema, testicular atrophy, and liver dysfunction. Premature epiphyseal closure can leave the teenager shorter than expected. Hepatotoxicity is most related to the 17-alkylated derivatives. In adolescent females, AASs cause menstrual irregularities and breast atrophy, clitorimegaly, hirsutism, male pattern baldness, amenorrhea (may be partially reversible after termination of use), and deepening of the voice with larynx changes. Some of these changes in both males and females are irreversible. Behavioral changes are not clearly documented in the literature, but some investigators report psychologic dependence on the drugs—that is, preoccupation with drug use, inability to stop despite psychologic effects, drug craving, mood swings with attempts to stop, violent behavior, heightened aggression, and mood swings with depression possibly severe enough to be linked with suicide. Depression as a withdrawal symptom has been well described (Congeni & Miller, 2002).

Anticipatory guidance and education are essential in this area. Education needs to include both benefits and risks, and the educator needs to be well informed to be credible. Educational programs that offer alternatives to taking anabolic steroids can be helpful. Nutrition and strength-training techniques are important aspects of these programs (Congeni & Miller, 2002).

Androstenedione and Dehydroepiandrosterone

Androstenedione ("andro") and dehydroepiandrosterone (DHEA) are precursors to endogenous testosterone production—sometimes called prohormones. DHEA is converted to androstenedione and then to testosterone. Of themselves, they have few anabolic-androgenic steroid effects; they are intended to trigger those effects by the user's body. They are available over the counter; their use, however, has not been well studied. Baseball star Mark McGwire used andro at the time he broke a home run record, but generally studies do not demonstrate enhanced performance outcomes.

The research is, as yet, incomplete, without documentation of effects at different dosages. Early studies show only significant increases in estrogen but not testosterone levels. Adverse effects are not well known (Congeni & Miller, 2002; Johnson, 2001).

Creatine and Other Supplements

Synthetic creatine is an over-the-counter supplement used to enhance performance. In two studies, only 5.6% to 8.2% of high school athletes reported its use (Metzl et al, 2001; Smith & Dahm, 2000). Another study reports high school use at 16% (Ray et al, 2001).

Creatine is an amino acid stored in muscle as phosphocreatine. During intense exercise, it is broken down to release initial energy for muscle contraction. The normal daily requirement is about 2 g for a 70 kg person. Some comes from animal protein and some is synthesized by the body. Supplementation increases muscle stores and results indirectly in greater muscle mass and weight gain. Athletes generally take 20 to 25 g per day for 4 to 6 days and then a maintenance dose of 2 to 5 g per day. It has been shown in studies to increase performance for high-intensity strength work and repeated sprints, as in football. The exercise must be maximal and anaerobic and last long enough to deplete the stores nonusers would have. If the duration of the activity is too long, however, other sources of energy supplant the creatine effects. Athletes for some other sports report poorer performance, perhaps because of excess weight gain. Weight gain is the only proven side effect (Schnirring, 1998). Unanswered questions in pediatrics include the following (Congeni & Miller, 2002; Johnson, 2001):

- Minimal dose for beneficial effect
- Effects and benefits in children
- Effects on endogenous synthesis
- Long-term health effects—especially on the renal system
- Ethics of societal rewards for performance enhanced by an exogenous substance

Recreational Activity Safety

Swimming

All children should learn to swim. This is essential to their safety near water environments. Swimming is an excellent sports activity that can be engaged in throughout life.

Bicycling

Bike riding can be an excellent aerobic activity. However, children need to wear helmets, learn to handle their bicycles with skill, and know the rules of the road for bicyclists. Wearing a helmet decreases the severity of injury (Laroque et al, 1999)

In-line Skating

In-line skating is a fun activity that can be risky if children do not wear helmets, knee pads, wrist guards, gloves, and elbow pads. In one study, 49% of in-line skating injuries were fractures and 86% of the fractures were to the wrist (Hassan & Dorani, 1999). Children need to learn to skate only in safe environments and to watch for traffic, irregular pavements, and other hazards. Because 37% of all in-line skating injuries involve the wrist and 67% of these are fractures, wrist guards are essential (AAP Committee on Injury and Poison Prevention and Committee on Sports Medicine and Fitness, 1998).

Skiing and Snowboarding

There are approximately 600,000 skiing injuries per year, with beginners three to five times more likely to be hurt than advanced skiers. Much of the decrease in injury rates over the past 20 years has been the result of improvements in equipment. Children should have formal training, as well as well-fitting boots and poles with bindings appropriately adjusted.

Snowboarding results in fewer knee injuries than found in skiing, whereas ankle injuries are more frequent because soft-shell boots protect the ankle less well than ski boots do. Snowboarders have twice as many upper limb injuries than skiers. Fitness training can reduce fatigue injuries. Lessons can help both skiers and snowboarders learn proper techniques and principles of slope safety.

Skateboarding and Scooters

The ankle, wrist, and face are the most common areas injured, accounting for 38% of skateboard injuries. Irregularity of the riding surface is often the etiologic factor for the accident. Younger children are at greater risk, as are males. Scooter injuries often occur on the street or sidewalk, from collision with motor vehicles, and are related to poor braking and mechanical problems (Markovsky et al, 2002). As with in-line skating, recommended equipment includes helmet, knee and elbow pads, and wrist guards. The AAP recommends education to learn the activity properly. Learning in a supervised environment with a smooth surface and no traffic can be helpful. The AAP Committee on Injury and Poison Prevention (2002) recommends that children be 10 years of age or older to ride skateboards without supervision.

Trampolines

Although the AAP recommended that trampolines be banned from schools and competitive sports in 1977, trampolines are still popular for home recreational use by children. Injury rates increased 98% from 1990 to 1995, with an estimated 249,400 trampoline accidents treated in emergency departments during that period (Smith, 1998).

RESOURCE BOX

Activities and Sports Resources for Professionals and Parents

American Academy of Pediatrics
www.aap.org
Pediatric health care focus with a committee on sports medicine that sets standards for children and sports

American College of Sports Medicine
www.acsm.org
Diagnosis, treatment, and prevention of sports-related injuries and advancement of research related to exercise

American College of Sports Dentistry
Dental Arts Building
Nine Linden St.
Worcester, MA 01609
Organization dedicated to the prevention of sports-related injuries to the head, face, mouth, and related oral structures

American Orthopaedic Society for Sports Medicine
1-847-292-4900
Fax: 1-847-292-4905
Provides a variety of pamphlets on nutrition for sports, heat and athletic performance, flexibility, designing weight programs, and preparticipation physical examination; provides a resource directory for disabled athletes from their Committee on Athletes with Disability

American Sport Education Program
1-800-747-5698
Provides information on sports and youth

International Center for Sports Nutrition
502 S. 44th St., Suite 3012
Omaha, NE 68105
Association to stimulate research related to nutrition and human performance

National SAFE KIDS Campaign
1-202-662-0600
www.safekids.org

National Youth Sports Foundation, Inc. (NYSSF)
1-617-277-1171
www.nyssf.org
An educational and research organization dedicated to promoting safety and well-being for children participating in sports; fact sheets and bibliographies available

Sports, Cardiovascular and Wellness Nutritionists
1-303-799-1950
Nutrition professionals with expertise in sports nutrition, health promotion, and fitness; associated with the American Dietetic Association

NURSING DIAGNOSES RELATED TO ACTIVITY AND EXERCISE: *Functional Pattern*

- Activity intolerance
- Deficient diversional activity
- Impaired physical mobility

From North American Nursing Diagnosis Association: *NANDA nursing diagnoses: definitions and classification 2003-2004*, Philadelphia, 2003, North American Nursing Diagnosis Association.

The median age for injury was 10 years. Ninety-three percent of these accidents occurred at home. Injuries from trampoline use can be grouped as follows: injuries to extremities (70%), face injuries (11%), head and neck trauma (10%). Annually, about 1400 children require hospitalization for their injuries. Quadriplegia and death have been well described. The number of injuries seen in emergency departments doubled between 1990 and 1995. Trampolines cannot be recommended for home use because there is no protective equipment that is helpful, and spotters cannot help when children collide or bounce out of reach (Smith, 1998).

REFERENCES

Altemeier W, Robinson D: Preparticipation screening by assembly line, *Pediatr Ann* 29(3):139-140, 2000.

American Academy of Allergy, Asthma and Immunology (AAAAI): Tips to remember: exercise-induced asthma. Available at *www.aaaai.org* (accessed June 5, 2002).

American Academy of Family Physicians et al: Preparticipation physical evaluation. In American Academy of Family Physicians, American Academy of Pediatrics, American Medical Society for Sports Medicine, et al: *The physician and sportsmedicine*, ed 2, Minneapolis, 1997, McGraw-Hill.

American Academy of Neurology Quality Standards Subcommittee: Practice parameter: the management of concussion in sports (summary statement), *Neurology* 48:581-585, 1997.

American Academy of Pediatrics Committee on Injury and Poison Prevention: Skateboard and scooter injuries, *Pediatrics* 109:542-543, 2002.

American Academy of Pediatrics Committee on Injury and Poison Prevention and Committee on Sports Medicine and Fitness: In-line skating injuries in children and adolescents, *Pediatrics* 101:720-721, 1998.

American Academy of Pediatrics Committee on Sports Medicine and Fitness: Atlantoaxial instability in Down syndrome: subject review, *Pediatrics* 96:151-154, 1995.

American Academy of Pediatrics Committee on Sports Medicine and Fitness: Promotion of healthy weight control practices in young athletes, *Pediatrics* 97:752-753, 1996.

American Academy of Pediatrics Committee on Sports Medicine and Fitness: Athletic participation by children and adolescents who have systemic hypertension, *Pediatrics* 99:637-638, 1997.

American Academy of Pediatrics Committee on Sports Medicine and Fitness: Human immunodeficiency virus and other blood-borne viral pathogens in the athletic setting (RE98221), *Pediatrics* 104:1400-1403, 1999.

American Academy of Pediatrics Committee on Sports Medicine and Fitness: Climatic heat stress and the exercising child and adolescent, *Pediatrics* 106:158-159, July 2000a.

American Academy of Pediatrics Committee on Sports Medicine and Fitness: Intensive training and sports specialization in young athletes, *Pediatrics* 106:154-157, July 2000b.

American Academy of Pediatrics Committee on Sports Medicine and Fitness: Organized sports for children and preadolescents (RE0052), *Pediatrics* 107:1459-1462, 2001.

American Academy of Pediatrics, Martin T, Committee on Sports Medicine and Fitness: Technical report: knee brace use in the young athlete, *Pediatrics* 108(2):503-507, 2001.

American Medical Association, Department of Adolescent Health: GAPS recommendation monograph, 1997.

American Medical Association: Fitness, 1999. Available at *www.medem.com/MedLB* (accessed June 11, 2002).

Berul C: Cardiac evaluation of the young athlete, *Pediatr Ann* 29(3):162-165, 2000.

Brain Injury Association: Sports and recreation. Available at *www.biausa.org* (accessed June 12, 2002).

Brockmeyer D: Down syndrome and craniovertebral instability: topic review and treatment recommendations, *Pediatr Neurosurg* 31(2):71-77, 1999.

Cheng T et al: Sports injuries: an important cause of morbidity in urban youth, *Pediatrics* 105(3):E32, 2000.

Clark M, Ferguson S. The physical activity and fitness of our nation's children, *J Pediatr Nurs* 15(4):250-252, 2000.

Cohen B: Atlantoaxial instability: what's next? *Arch Pediatr Adolesc Med* 152(2):199-222, 1998.

Congeni J, Miller S: Supplements and drugs used to enhance athletic performance, *Pediatr Clin North Am* 49:435-461, 2002.

Faigenbaum A, Micheli L: Preseason conditioning for the preadolescent athlete, *Pediatr Ann* 29(3):156-161, 2000.

Feinstein R: Preparticipation physical examinations. In Burg F et al, editors: *Gellis and Kaan's current pediatric therapy*, ed 17, Philadelphia, 2002, WB Saunders.

Galuska DA et al: Are health care professionals advising obese patients to lose weight? *JAMA* 282(16):1581-1582, 1999.

Glover D, Maron B, Matheson G: The preparticipation physical examination: steps toward consensus and uniformity, *Physician Sportsmed* 27(8), 1999. Available at *www.physsportsmed.com* (accessed Oct 19, 2003).

Greene P: Pearls for practice: recognizing young people at risk for sudden cardiac death in preparticipation sports physicals, *J Am Acad Nurse Pract* 12(1):11-14, 2000.

Hammerman S et al: Asthma screening of high school athletes: identifying the undiagnosed and poorly controlled, *Ann Allergy Asthma Immunol* 88(4):380-384, 2002.

Hassan I, Dorani B: Rollerblading and skateboarding injuries in children in northeast England, *J Accident Emergency Med* 16:348-350, 1999.

Hergenroeder A: Prevention of sports injuries, *Pediatrics* 101:1057-1063, 1998.

Hergenroeder A: Sports medicine. In Finberg L, Kleinman R, editors: *Saunders manual of pediatric practice*, ed 2, Philadelphia, 2002, WB Saunders.

Hoffman J: Environmental emergencies: heat-related illness in children, *Clin Pediatr Emergency Med* 2:203-210, 2001.

Janz K, Dawson J, Mahoney L: Increases in physical fitness during childhood improve cardiovascular health during adolescence: the Muscative study, *Int J Sports Med* 23 (suppl 1):S15-S21, 2002.

Johnson W: Nutritional supplements and the young athlete: what you need to know, *Contemp Pediatr* 18: 63-74, 2001.

Kurowski K, Chandran S: The preparticipation athletic evaluation, *Am Fam Physician* 61:2683-2690, 2696-2698, 2000.

Laroque D, Barlow B, Durkin M: Prevention of youth injuries, *J Natl Med Assoc* 91(10):557-571, 1999.

Luckstead E, Patel D: Catastrophic pediatric sports injuries, *Pediatr Clin North Am* 49(3):581-591, 2002.

Lyman S et al: Longitudinal study of elbow and shoulder pain in youth baseball pitchers, *Med Sci Sports Exerc* 33(11): 1803-1810, 2001.

Maffulli N, Baxter-Jones A: Intensive training in elite young female athletes: effects of intensive training on growth and maturation are not established, *Br J Sports Med* 36(1):13-15, 2002.

Mankovsky A et al: Evaluation of scooter-related injuries in children, *J Pediatr Surg* 37: 755-759, 2002.

Mayers L, Rundell K: *Current comment: exercised-induced asthma*, written for American College of Sports Medicine, Jan 2000. Available at *www.acsm.org* (accessed Oct 19, 2003).

Metzl J: Expectations of pediatric sports participation among pediatricians, patients, and parents, *Pediatr Clin North Am* 49(3):497-504, 2002.

Metzl J et al: Creatine use among young athletes, *Pediatrics* 108(2):421-425, Aug 2001.

Micheli L, Glassman R, Klein M: The prevention of sports injuries in children, *Clin Sports Med* 19(4):156-161, June 2000.

Mitchell J, Haskell W, Raven P: Classification of sports. 26th Bethesda Conference: recommendations for determining eligibility for competition in athletes with cardiovascular abnormalities, *Med Sci Sports Exerc* 26(suppl):S242-S245, 1994.

National Center for Health Statistics: *Healthy people 2000 final review*, Hyattsville, MD, 2001, Public Health Service.

Ohio High School Athletic Association (OHSAA): Preparticipation physical examination form. Available at *www.ohsaa.org* (accessed Aug 8, 2002).

Patel D, Pratt H, Greydanus D: Pediatric neurodevelopment and sports participation. When are children ready to play sports? *Pediatr Clin North Am* 49:505-531, 2002.

Patrick K et al: *Bright Futures in practice: physical activity*, Arlington, VA, 2001, National Center for Education in Maternal and Child Health.

Preventing sports injuries in kids, *Patient Care Nurs Pract*, pp 24-36, June 1998.

Proctor M, Cantu R: Head and neck injuries in young athletes, *Clin Sports Med* 19(4):693-715, Oct 2000.

Pueschel S: Should children with Down syndrome be screened for atlantoaxial instability? *Arch Pediatr Adolesc Med* 152(2):123-125, 1998.

Rankin J, Ocel J, Craft L: Effect of weight loss and refeeding diet composition on anaerobic performance in wrestlers, *Med Sci Sports Exerc* 28:1292-1299, 1996.

Ray T et al: Use of oral creatine as an ergogenic aid for increased sports performance: perceptions of adolescent athletes, *South Med Assoc J* 94:608-612, 2001.

Ryan-Krause P: The score on high-tech sports nutrition for adolescents, *J Pediatr Health Care* 12:164-166, 1998.

Schnirring L: Creatine supplements face scrutiny, *Phys Sports Med* 26:15-23, 1998.

Smith G: Injuries to children in the United States related to trampolines, 1990–1995: a national epidemic, *Pediatrics* 101:406-412, 1998.

Smith J, Dahm D: Creatine use among a select population of high school athletes, *Mayo Clin Proc* 75:1257-1263, 2000.

Spooner C, Saunders L, Rowe F: Nedocromil sodium for preventing exercise-induced bronchoconstriction, *Cochrane Database Syst Rev* 2:CD001183, 2002.

Strauss R et al: Psychological correlates of physical activity in healthy children, *Arch Pediatr Adolesc Med* 155:897-902, 2001.

Stricker P: Swimming: a case-based approach to exercise-induced asthma and rotator cuff tendonitis, *Pediatr Ann* 29(3):166-170, 2000.

Sudden Death Committee: Cardiovascular preparticipation screening of competitive athletes: addendum, *Am Heart Assoc* 97:2294, 1998.

Taylor B, Attia M: Sports-related injuries in children. Comment, *Acad Emerg Med* 7:1424-1427, 2000.

Trost SG et al: Correlates of objectively measured physical activity in preadolescent youth, *Am J Prev Med* 17:120-126, 1999.

US Department of Health and Human Services: *Healthy people 2010: understanding and improving health*, ed 2, Washington, DC, 2000, US Government Printing Office.

Verst A: Get in the game: principles of the preparticipation physical, *Adv Nurse Pract* 8(8):66-68, 2000.

Wilson R, Carlin A, Tyburski J: Sports concussion: implications of the exam after head injury, *Consultation in Primary Care* 42(2):230-234, 2002.

World Health Organization: Cross-national study on health behavior in school-aged children from 28 countries: findings from the United States, *J Sch Health* 70(6):227-228, 2000.

World Health Organization: *Diet, nutrition and the prevention of chronic diseases: report of a Joint WHO/FAO expert consultation*, WHO Technical Report Series 916. Geneva, Switzerland, 2002.

16 Sleep and Rest

Catherine E. Burns

Many of the common pediatric sleep disorders are related to sleep development issues. In their review of sleep studies, Howard and Wong (2001) note that 20% to 30% of children experience sleep problems. The highest incidence of disorders may occur in children 1 to 2 years of age (Zuckerman, Stevenson, & Bailey, 1987). They also found that 18% of 3-year-olds had trouble getting to sleep, whereas 22% had trouble with night waking. Perhaps of more importance, they found that 41% of children with sleep problems at 8 months of age still had problems at 3 years of age. Other studies show that 20% to 30% of children have problems with sleep, and these represent one of the most common concerns of parents (Dahl, 1998).

A number of psychologic and physiologic factors are related to sleep problems in infants and children. It is important to recognize that sleep problems of infants and children are interrelated with family problems, such as those stemming from maternal depression, social stresses, or problems such as child abuse, or a combination of these. Pediatric sleep problems may produce sleep deprivation in the caregiver. They may also result in behavioral problems or significant physiologic problems, including cardiovascular disruptions. Sleep problems may result from a variety of other problems, including the following:

- Physical factors
  - Ear infections
  - Neurologic disorders
  - Hypothyroidism
  - Obesity
  - Tonsillar and adenoid hypertrophy
  - Pain
  - Blindness
  - Orofacial anomalies
  - Asthma
- Psychologic factors
  - Developmental stage
  - Separation anxiety (Blum & Carey, 1996)
  - Depression, anxiety, or other mental health problems (Anders & Eiben, 1997; Lavigne et al, 1999)
  - Stress
  - Substance abuse
- Family factors
  - Parental mismanagement of sleep routines
  - Maternal depression
- Environmental and temperamental factors
  - Temperament characteristics, including low sensory threshold, negative mood, and decreased adaptability
  - Environmental factors, including sleeping arrangements, altered daily routines, and feeding practices
  - Toxins or substance abuse

As with all other primary care problems in pediatrics, the provider must be vigilant for a myriad of potential etiologies and recognize that the family disruption caused by a rebellious or noisy nonsleeper in a household may be significant. Attention to cultural definitions of normal sleep habits also is essential.

Nurse practitioners (NPs) should be concerned with sleep in children because this will be an extremely frequent topic for discussion with parents. Second, insufficient sleep affects many areas of child well-being, including both physical and mental health issues. Science has yet to determine the reason that humans need to sleep. "There are numerous links between sleep and the regulation of attention, arousal, affect, and social behavior, and insufficient sleep has a strong impact across these domains" (Dahl, 1998).

NORMAL SLEEP STAGES AND CYCLES

Normal sleep can be divided into two distinct phases: rapid eye movement (REM) sleep and non–rapid eye movement (non-REM) sleep. Non-REM sleep can be further divided into four distinct stages based on changes in electroencephalographic (EEG) patterns.

Rapid Eye Movement Sleep

REM sleep is considered to be the dreaming phase. Although nerve impulses to the spinal cord and muscles are blocked, leaving the body paralyzed except for minor twitching, the respiratory, eye, and middle ear muscles remain active. The child may smile in a transitory way or make short utterances. Breathing and heart rates become irregular and relatively rapid. Reflexes, kidney function, hormonal secretions, and auditory sensitivity are all altered. The rapid eye movements of this phase are of particular interest. People awakened during REM sleep may report dreams at the time. Children as young as 2 years of age have reported dreams during REM sleep. The function of REM sleep is unclear. Newborns enter the sleep cycle with REM sleep (sometimes called "active sleep" in neonates), but after a few months non-REM sleep occurs first. Because REM sleep is associated with arousals and because REM sleep predominates in the first year of life, infants are likely to have problems with maintenance of sleep. Some mothers are concerned about their infants' restless sleep when, indeed, it is only REM sleep that they are observing.

REM sleep occurs in approximately 90-minute cycles with the longest REM episode occurring just after the body temperature reaches its lowest point during the night, around 5 AM. Thus, in older children and adults, most REM sleep occurs later in the night.

Non–Rapid Eye Movement Sleep

The four phases of non-REM sleep become distinguishable within 6 months of birth. After 3 months of age, non-REM sleep is the first type of sleep entered by the infant from the awake phase and soon dominates the total sleep distribution. In the preschool and school-age years, non-REM stages III and IV predominate. These stages end with a REM phase. The parasomnias, including nightmares and sleepwalking, which are related to this transition from non-REM to arousal or REM phases, occur most commonly in children in these developmental stages.

Stage I

Stage I sleep is a state of drowsiness. There may be eye-rolling movements, decreased body movements, and perhaps opening and closing of the eyelids. Individuals may believe that they are awake, but they cannot report accurately events that occurred during this time. In mature individuals, stage I accounts for about 5% of sleep.

Stage II

Stage II sleep is somewhat deeper than that of stage I, although the person can still be easily aroused. Eye movements slow, as do breathing and heart rate. Muscles weaken. If aroused, the person may report thinking about things and may report dreams. Mature sleepers spend about 50% of their sleep in this stage, generally in the last half of the night.

Stage III

Stage III sleep is still deeper than that of stage II. The body is deeply relaxed, breathing is shallow, and heart rate is slow. Growth hormone appears to be secreted in larger amounts during stages III and IV of sleep (Behrman, Kliegman, & Jensen, 2004). About 15% to 20% of sleep takes place in stages III and IV, occurring earlier in the night. Stages III and IV sleep seem to develop at about 3 to 4 months of age; by 4 months quiet sleep makes up more of the total sleep than active sleep.

Stage IV

Stage IV is defined by the EEG pattern it produces. When the delta waves occupy 50% of the EEG pattern, stage IV sleep has begun. During both stage III and stage IV, the sleeper is hard to arouse. If awakened, the individual feels confused and disoriented. The transition from stage IV to waking is related to the etiology of several common pediatric sleep disorders, such as night terrors and sleepwalking (Dahl, 1998).

Sleep Cycles

Sleep onset is the time when the person enters stage I non-REM sleep. The sleep period begins with sleep onset and continues until full arousal occurs. The sleep cycle includes the repeated episodes of non-REM and REM sleep of the sleep period. Waking involves full alert and recall after the sleep period. Semiwakefulness or alerting to the immediate environment occurs easily in REM sleep or stages I or II in non-REM sleep. The child cycles between REM and non-REM phases throughout the night (Fig. 16-1). Both total amount of sleep and proportion of REM sleep decrease with age (Table 16-1).

REM sleep usually precedes a brief period of semiwakefulness, after which the individual descends again through the non-REM stages to REM, followed by another brief awakening. Later in the evening, the REM phase becomes more pronounced. In older children and adults, the periods of semiwakefulness may last for a few seconds to a few minutes. It may be the time when one turns over, looks at the clock, or adjusts the covers. The infant sometimes has difficulty returning to the next sleep cycle from this normal waking episode. Young infants have more sleep cycles per night than older individuals do, and each cycle has a brief waking that precedes the next sleep period. Therefore more opportunities for

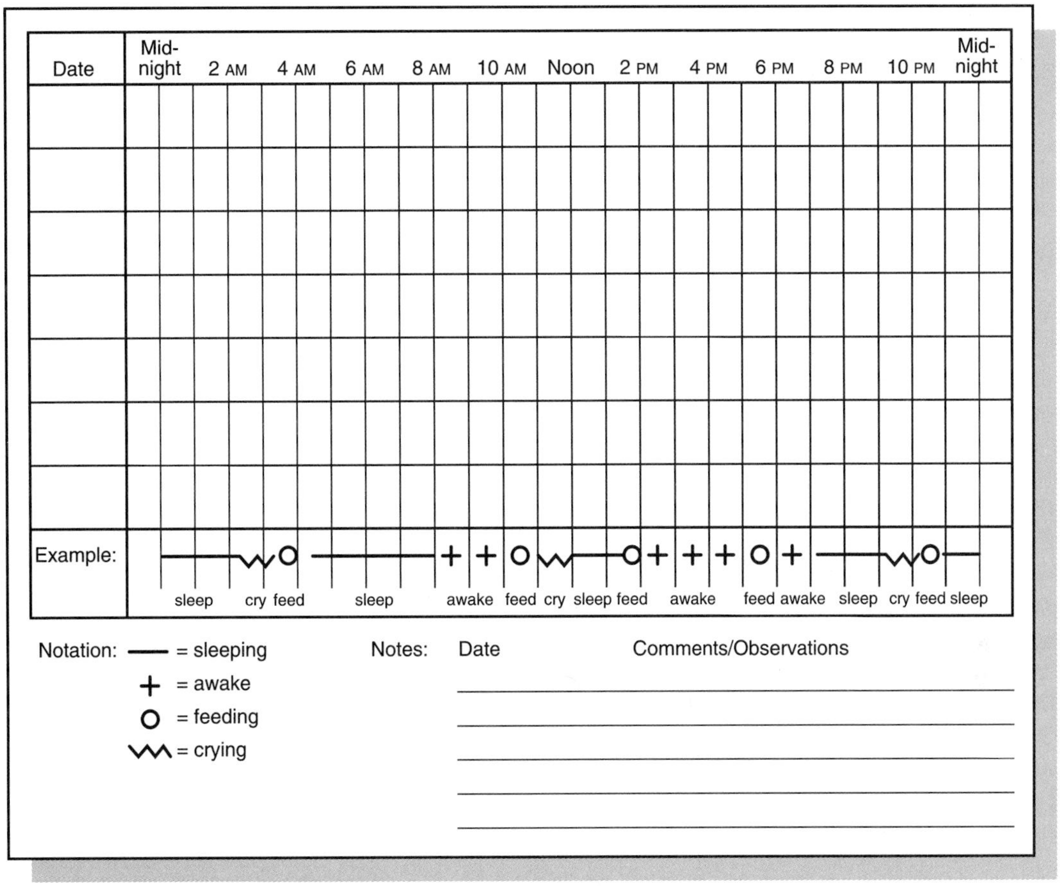

FIGURE 16-1 Example of sleep-activity-feeding record.

sleep disturbance can arise with infants. Children generally achieve adult sleep patterns by 3 years, and each cycle will last from 70 to 100 minutes (Howard & Wong, 2001).

Adolescents also experience sleep problems; the most common is difficulty falling asleep. Middle adolescents (14- to 16-year-olds) seem to have more sleep disturbances than younger or older teenagers. Chronic sleep deprivation is a common reason for sleepiness in adolescents (Dahl, 1998).

Knowledge of the sleep cycle pattern is helpful for the clinician. Most of the non-REM deep sleep occurs in the early night, so associated problems such as night terrors and sleepwalking occur then. Most REM sleep occurs in the second half of the night, so problems associated with REM sleep such as nightmares occur more in this phase. The short periods of wakefulness throughout the night are times when sleep-onset problems occur (Dahl, 1998).

Duration of Sleep

The typical neonate sleeps 16.5 hours each day. Half of this is daytime sleep. The longest neonate sleep period is 2.5 to 4 hours and can occur at any time during the 24-hour day. The neonate has only one or two sleep cycles during a sleep period, each lasting 50 to 60 minutes. By 3 months of age, the baby sleeps almost 15 hours, but the sleep times are more clearly organized into daytime wakefulness and nighttime sleep. Most 6-month-old infants sleep through the night and have morning and afternoon naps. At 1 year of age, most children sleep about 13.5 hours. The morning nap is generally given up between 12 and 24 months, but the afternoon nap may persist to age 4 or 5 years. By age 2 years, the child is probably sleeping 11 to 12 hours at night with a 1- to 2-hour nap after lunch. Six-year-olds sleep 10.75 hours per night on average. The average sleep requirement for adolescents is believed to be about 8 to 9 hours per night (see Table 16-1).

Circadian Rhythms and Establishment of Normal Sleep Patterns

Many biologic activities are set on a 24-hour cycle. These include sleep and wakefulness; body temperature regulation; hormonal activity; and respiratory, cardiac, renal, and

TABLE 16-1 ***Average Sleep by Age***

Age	Nighttime Sleep (hr)	Daytime Sleep (hr)
1 wk	8.25	8.25
1 mo	8.5	7.0
3 mo	9.5	5.5
6 mo	10.5	3.75
9 mo	11.0	3.0
12 mo	11.25	2.5
18 mo	11.5	2.0
2 yr	11.5	1.5
3 yr	11.0	1.0
4 yr	11.5	
6 yr	10.75	
9 yr	10.0	
12 yr	9.25	
15 yr	8.75	
18 yr	8.25	

Adapted from Howard B, Wong J: Sleep disorders, *Pediatr Rev* 22:327-341, 2001, p 335.

intestinal functions. People use a variety of cues to set the cycle, including daylight, darkness, meals, and activities. Parents need to make these cues clear to infants and children to help them establish healthful bedtime and sleep patterns. *Sleep hygiene* is a term used to define healthful sleep behaviors.

Melatonin secreted by the hypothalamus is responsible for the timing of physiologic processes, including the sleep/wake cycle. It is a product of tryptophan metabolism and is secreted into the general circulation by the pineal gland, an organ related to the visual system. Light suppresses melatonin production, and darkness is associated with the highest melatonin levels. In normal humans, melatonin begins to rise when the sun sets, is at highest levels at 2 AM, and falls to almost undetectable levels in the daytime. The day-night melatonin cycle is established between 4 and 6 months of age. Levels peak at 1 to 3 years of age and then decline with age. Maternal melatonin crosses the placental barrier and is secreted in breast milk. Exposure to bright light of even 1 minute at night will suppress melatonin for at least 40 minutes. Use of aspirin, ibuprofen, and other nonsteroidal antiinflammatory drugs during the night also suppresses melatonin synthesis. These drugs inhibit the lowering of body temperature during the night, another factor in melatonin production. Thus the cues of darkness and cool temperature should enhance sleep (DiLeo, Reiter, & Taliaferro, 2002).

Recio and colleagues (1997) suggest that if mothers are giving pumped milk to infants trying to establish a sleep/wake cycle, it is better to give night-pumped milk to the infant at night. An additional suggestion is to not turn on the lights brightly at night (for both mother and infant sleep support) but have the child nap in a lighter room during the day (DiLeo, Reiter, & Taliaferro, 2002).

Feeding Effects on Sleep

Breastfed infants need to eat more frequently than babies fed cow's milk. Probably this is due to the shorter emptying time for breast milk (Blum & Carey, 1996). Because of this, breastfed babies probably wake more frequently in the night. Bedsharing by mother and infant increases both the length and frequency of breastfeeding episodes in 3- to 4-month-old infants (McKenna, Mosko, & Richard, 1997). By 6 months of age, most babies can go for a 6- to 12-hour period without being fed. This extended period coincides with the longest sleep period. Thus, after 6 months of age, feeding in the night can be considered a learned behavior. Starting solids early to increase length of nighttime sleeping is a myth. Several studies have shown that solids do not help the baby sleep for longer periods.

Co-Sleeping

Sleep habits are strongly influenced by culture. Co-sleeping is common in many cultures and has been the human norm for many thousands of years. Co-sleeping by family members is probably more common worldwide than is separate sleeping as advocated in the United States. Warmth, protection, and a sense of well-being are undoubtedly facilitated by having babies sleep with their mothers or siblings. It is most common in black and Hispanic families. Co-sleeping is also common with father absence. One study found that infants between 11 and 15 weeks of age had more arousals from both stages I to II and III to IV when sharing the bed with their mothers than when sleeping alone; researchers interpreted this as perhaps a protection against sudden infant death syndrome (SIDS) (Mosko, Richard, & McKenna, 1997). Co-sleeping is not, in itself, a reason for sleep problems. However, some families allow the child to sleep with the adults because of problems with enforcing bedtimes, anxiety about leaving the child alone, problems with the quality of daytime interactions, or a desire to avoid the spouse. Sexual misuse of the child also needs to be considered. In these cases, intervention may be helpful to the family (Howard & Wong, 2001).

The American Academy of Pediatrics (AAP) Task Force on Infant Position and Sudden Infant Death Syndrome, in a 2000 statement, states that bedsharing should not be considered as a strategy to reduce SIDS risk. If a mother chooses to sleep with her infant, care should be taken to avoid using soft sleep surfaces—quilts, blankets, pillows, comforters, or other similar materials should not be placed under the infant. The bedsharer should not smoke or use substances that impair arousal. Finally, parents should understand that safety standards are in place for the design of infant cribs, but there are no standards for adult beds, so entrapment might be possible (AAP Task Force on Infant Position and Sudden Infant Death Syndrome, 2000). Parents who plan to co-sleep should have an "exit plan" such as ending the practice at 6 months, before the child will protest excessively (Howard & Wong, 2001).

School-age children who want to co-sleep may have significant emotional problems such as separation anxiety, which may require counseling.

Bedtime Routines

Good sleep hygiene requires an environment that is dark, quiet, and slightly cool; a regular schedule for waking, nap lengths, and bedtime; sleep-conducive activities in the child's life that include non–fear-inducing stories, videos, or television; quiet activities before bedtime; and consistent parenting methods that are quieting before bedtime (Howard & Wong, 2001). Many authors believe that children from earliest infancy should be put into bed awake so that they learn to put themselves to sleep with self-soothing behaviors such as thumb sucking (Adair & Bauchner, 1993; Blum & Carey, 1996; Ferber, 1996; Howard & Wong, 2001). Bringing an inanimate transitional object to bed is a sleep aid for many children, from 3 months on. The transitional object may change from time to time, at least among infants (Burnham et al, 2002). Other sleep hygiene principles include avoiding hunger and excessive fluids at bedtime or during the night, and avoiding stimulating drugs and foods such as caffeine, coffee, and chocolate in the evening.

Some sleep problems, such as trained night feeding and trained night crying, are learned. Sleep-onset problems can also be learned (Blum & Carey, 1996; Ferber, 1996). For instance, the child who is always rocked to sleep in mother's arms and then moved to the crib when asleep learns that the place to go to sleep is in mother's arms. During arousals in the night, the child then looks for those arms and not the sides of the crib to move into the next sleep cycle.

Sleep Positioning

Studies have provided strong evidence that positioning young infants on their backs significantly decreases the incidence of SIDS. The current recommendation of the AAP is to have all infants sleep in a side-lying or supine position at naps and at bedtime during the first 6 months of life unless there is some specific medical contraindication to that position. The AAP also recommends use of a crib, avoidance of soft materials in the sleep environment, avoidance of bedsharing, and avoidance of overheating the infant (AAP Task Force on Infant Position and Sudden Infant Death Syndrome, 2000). A 1997 study in Washington, D.C., found that almost half of licensed day care centers had caregivers who were unaware of the relationship between sleep position and SIDS (Gershon & Moon, 1997). Further education needs to be directed to this group to decrease this risk factor for young infants. Current risk factors for SIDS in the United States include very low birth weight infants, infants of smoking mothers, unmarried mothers, African American infants, and infants in large families who received limited prenatal care (Paris, Remler, & Daling, 2001; Pollack & Frohna, 2002).

A 1997 study of 343 infants found that infants sleeping on their sides or supine were significantly less likely to be rolling over at their 4-month checkup visits (Jantz & Blosser, 1997). Whether this is a result of reluctance of parents to put their infants on their stomachs during the day or whether it stems from other developmental effects of back sleeping is unclear. The AAP recommends that parents place the baby on its stomach sometimes while awake to encourage upper body motor development and to avoid positional plagiocephaly (AAP Task Force on Infant Position and Sudden Infant Death Syndrome, 2000).

ASSESSMENT

Assessment of sleep patterns requires an understanding of the developmental progression of sleep patterns, a comprehensive history, and a physical examination. Assessment of sleep patterns should be included in all well-child visits. Before a decision is made that a sleep problem exists, the provider must be sure to determine whether the child's sleep pattern is problematic for the caregiver. Late bedtimes, early rising, night waking, co-sleeping, and so on may be upsetting to some parents but not to others. Only sleep problems identified by the parent should be addressed, or cases in which there is evidence that the child's sleep patterns are disruptive to his or her health and well-being. Of course, preventive counseling is always in order. The nurse practitioner must be careful not to impose his or her ideas of the best night's sleep habits onto the family.

History

The practitioner asks the parents, "Are you satisfied with your child's current sleep behaviors?" The normal sleep pattern, the general health history, the parents and family, and the sleep environment are assessed for factors that may affect sleep and rest.

Normal Sleep Pattern

1. Nighttime and daytime sleep hygiene patterns include the following:
   - Quality and quantity of sleep
   - Sleep hours, including naps
   - Awake time when parents are also awake
   - Longest night sleep interval
   - Number and frequency of feedings (for infants less than 3 months old), day and night
   - Description of the state changes of the child, moving from wakefulness to sleep and then to waking again
   - Cues given by the infant or child to indicate need for sleep or rest
   - Daytime sleepiness
   - The routines used for getting the child to sleep and the child's behavior at these times
2. Sleep problem history includes the following:
   - Nighttime waking and the routine for managing these episodes
   - Nightmares and night terrors
   - Walking, talking, head banging, rocking
   - Snoring and breathing cessation during sleep
   - Jerks and twitches during sleep
   - Daytime sleepiness
   - Inappropriate sleep and awake times
   - Enuresis
   - Age when problem began and circumstances
   - Aggravating and relieving factors
   - Effects on daily living for child and family
   - Caffeine intake (child or breastfeeding mother)
3. The environment is assessed for sleeping, noise, light, temperature, safety, and co-sleeping pattern.
4. Parental work patterns that affect sleep are assessed (shift work and night child care).

General Health History

1. Indicators of the health and well-being of the child: Energy and alertness for daily activities need evaluation. The child with chronic inadequate sleep may appear to the parents to be functioning well. However, with more sleep, the parents will notice a decrease in irritability and better performance in many arenas.
2. Past medical history and review of systems: Medical problems of the child are often associated with sleep difficulties. Ear infections, medications such as bronchodilators, some neurologic problems, respiratory conditions, or anything that causes pain can affect sleep.
3. Developmental problems can affect the child's ability to learn appropriate sleep behaviors.
4. Depression or other psychiatric problems may be significant in older children with sleep problems.
5. Substance/medication/tobacco use, including caffeine drinks and alcohol, can affect sleep.

Parental and Family Assessment

1. Indicators of the health and well-being and rest of the caregiver; maternal depression has been clearly associated with children's sleep disruptions.
2. Parental knowledge and beliefs about infant and child sleeping patterns. Parental understanding of the relationships between illness, temperament, and sleep should be explored (Blum & Carey, 1996; Jimmerson, 1991).
3. Parental ability to modulate the child's sleep and rest state.
4. Family sleep routines and expectations.
5. Recent changes in family living arrangements.
6. Divorce, separation, or other family stresses.
7. Extent of disparity of problem with family's cultural expectations (Anders & Eiben, 1997).
8. Family history of sleep disorders (Howard & Wong, 2001).

Box 16-1 provides questions to include in a sleep assessment (Howard & Wong, 2001).

Physical Examination

It is important that a general physical examination be performed to detect signs of illness or pain. Signs of fatigue, irritability, or inattention may be associated with lack of adequate rest. Other clinical findings associated with sleep problems include upper respiratory infection, gastroenteritis, teething, pinworms, and injuries. Gastroesophageal reflux may affect sleep (Blum & Carey, 1996). Children with seizure disorders or other neurologic problems may have sleep-related problems. The degree of nighttime difficulty with airway resistance and obstruction cannot be accurately evaluated by assessing the size of tonsils and adenoids (Dahl, 1998).

Diagnostic Studies

A 24-hour, 7-day chart for the parents to record the child's sleep patterns may be useful for assessing the problem and establishing a baseline from which to evaluate improvement over time (Fig. 16-2). Sleep EEG studies are occasionally warranted. Nocturnal polysomnography may be needed to diagnose obstructive sleep apnea and other conditions.

STRATEGIES FOR PREVENTION AND MANAGEMENT OF SLEEP PROBLEMS

Usual management strategies include counseling parents, modifying diet, ignoring nocturnal crying, and scheduling awakenings. Sedation is sometimes helpful as a temporary measure. A study from New Zealand demonstrated that written instructions for parents about management of sleep problems were highly effective (Seymore et al, 1989). Deeper fears, depression, or family stresses may require counseling.

Parenting tips for managing the infant's state changes are helpful, and successful parenting strategies should be supported. A variety of parental behaviors help prevent sleep problems in children (Table 16-2).

Parent education about the development of normal sleep patterns in children and "sleep hygiene" patterns they need to teach their children are helpful (Mindell, 1999). For most infants and children, establishing a bedtime routine is probably the most important thing that parents can do. The routine should begin at a regular time with quieter activities and then sleep-routine activities. Often this routine includes a bath; changing into pajamas; brushing teeth; and sharing a story, song, or prayer. Lights should be turned out, although a hall light or nightlight may be reassuring to the child. Infants and preschoolers often need to take a "transition object," such as a toy or blanket, to bed with them. Establishing consistent wake-up and naptime routines and schedules are also useful strategies.

BOX 16-1 *Sleep Assessment*

Does your child have trouble falling asleep?
How old was he or she when this problem started?
What is the bedtime routine and how does the child respond?

- Bedtime regularity and time
- Where does child sleep?
- Length of time between last feeding and bedtime
- Length of time between going to bed and sleep onset
- Needs for body contact, bottle or pacifier, television or radio noise, or other stimuli to induce sleep

What is the nap(s) routine?

- Need for other stimuli to induce sleep
- Waking before or after 4 PM at last nap

Total sleep time per 24 hours?

If Night Waking

Age of onset?
Regular or intermittent problem?
When is first waking (<30 min, 60-90 min, >3 hr)?
Caregiver response to waking?

- Feed child
- Body contact with caregiver

Child's emotion on waking?
Daytime sleepiness greater than expected?
Other behavioral or emotional problems?
Health or developmental problems?
Medicines, caffeine drink intake, street drug use, smokes?

Adapted from Howard B, Wong J: Sleep disorders, *Pediatr Rev* 22:327-341, 2001.

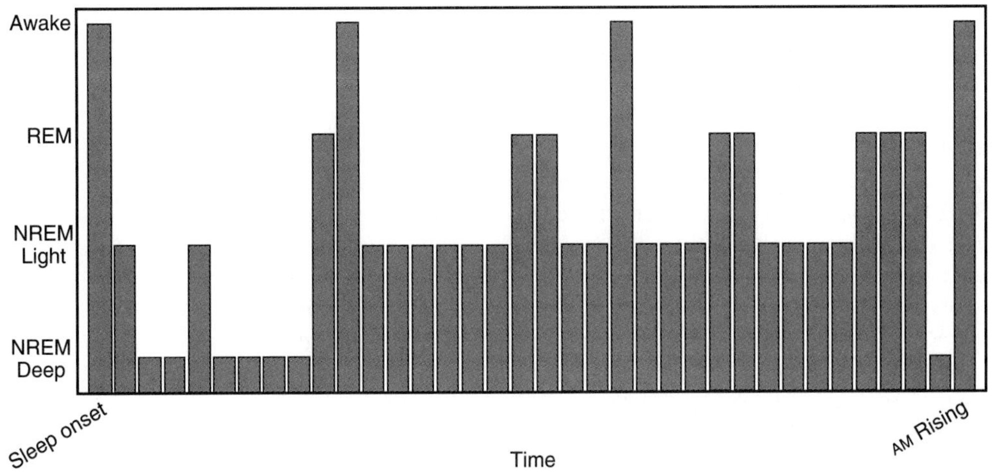

FIGURE 16-2 Schema of typical night sleep pattern of sleep states and stages. *REM*, rapid eye movement; *NREM*, non–rapid eye movement. (From Adair R, Bauchner H: Sleep problems in childhood, *Curr Probl Pediatr* 23[4]1:150, 1993.)

TABLE 16-2 ***Prevention of Sleep Problems***

Newborn	
During the day	Respond to crying; hold the baby when fussy Hold the baby frequently to avoid fussy episodes Schedule feedings at least 2 hours apart
During the night	Put the baby to bed while drowsy but still awake Feed the baby at the parents' bedtime and then let the baby awaken for feedings and feed with little stimulation, dim lights, no play Avoid bringing the baby into the parents' bed unless co-sleeping is the family norm
Age 2-4 Months	
During the night	Move the baby to a separate bedroom unless this is not the cultural norm for the family Try to delay and then discontinue middle-of-the-night feedings No bottles in the crib Continue to keep middle-of-the-night feedings (if they are still occurring) as nonstimulating occasions
Age 6-12 Months	
During the night	Keep soft toy animal, doll, or blanket in the crib for snuggling Leave the bedroom door open and respond to any fears quickly and with reassurance
Age 1 Year and Older	
During the night	Keep bedtimes friendly and predictable occasions Always respond to nighttime fears with reassurance and comfort Allow the child to take increasing responsibility for self-management of body functions, including sleep Expect the child to remain in bed during the night

Helping parents to understand their child's temperament can be a useful intervention. For example, for the child who is less adaptable or who has tendencies to withdraw from new situations, changing the sleep routine in any way may be particularly difficult. For children who are "difficult" (irregular, intense, with frequent negative moods), parents should be informed that sleep schedules and needs will be unpredictable, and reactions to parental interventions may be intensely resistant. Strategies parents have used with success in the past should be identified and similar parenting activities adapted for managing sleep difficulties. Children with low sensory thresholds also have more problems with night waking because they are more sensitive to light, sound, temperature, and tactile stimulation (Carey, 1974). All these stimuli must be considered by parents who are trying to promote sleep onset and maintenance behaviors in their children.

Family stressors need to be recognized and dealt with. Posttraumatic stress disorder, abuse, domestic violence issues, or other psychologic problems in children may also be factors requiring family and individual counseling.

Medication is not generally recommended for childhood sleep problems. Hypnotic drugs such as benzodiazepines are discouraged because of the problems with dependence. They are sometimes used for arousal disorders, but effectiveness is variable. Antihistamines have not been studied for effectiveness when used for long periods. Tricyclic drugs are sometimes used, especially for arousal disorders where other treatments are inadequate. Medication may be helpful when the sleep problem is the result of underlying physical or psychiatric disorders (Stores, 1996).

COMMON SLEEP PROBLEMS

The line between normal and problematic sleep may be somewhat fuzzy. The NP needs to identify that the child's sleep patterns are problematic for the caregivers and family or are resulting in problems for the child's health and well-being. The International Classification of Sleep Disorders (American Sleep Disorders Association, 1990) is more complex than the system used in this chapter and refers to both adult and child sleep problems. It classifies sleep problems as *dyssomnias*, or problems of insufficient, excessive, or inefficient sleep; *parasomnias*, or problems that intrude on the sleep state; and medical/psychiatric sleep disorders. This section identifies problems as found in Table 16-3.

TABLE 16-3 ***Summary of Common Pediatric Sleep Problems and Interventions***

Sleep Problem	Clinical Findings	Differential	Intervention
Dyssomnias			
Night waking	Needs help during the night to enter the next sleep cycle	Medical problem, pain, hunger, trained night feeder Depression	Always put the child to bed while still awake; keep day and nighttime cues very clear; do not reinforce calling out/crying behavior; try scheduled wakening technique
Sleep refusals	Toddler/preschooler refuses to settle down when put to bed	Fears, separation anxiety, sleep needs less than parents' expectations Temperament irregular or low sensory threshold Emotional stress	Maintain consistent sleep routine and expectations; use transitional objects
Trained night feeder	Infant awakens predictably to be fed after age 4 mo	Night wakening, pain or medical problem, feeding needs	Move the child onto a 3-4 hr feeding schedule in the day; at first feed the infant only once after the parents' bedtime; then, either eliminate the feeding or progressively decrease the volume of that feeding
Delayed sleep phase	Child goes to bed late and awakens late	Sleep refusal Depression	Have the child awaken progressively 15 min earlier until appropriate bedtimes and waking times result
Advanced sleep phase	Child goes to bed early and awakens early		Progressively have the child stay up later; awakening will occur later
Unpredictable schedule	Child goes to bed and awakens at random times	Family on erratic schedule; inconsistent parent expectations; excessive naps	Keep predictable eating, activity, and sleeping schedules for the family; maintain consistent expectation for bedtime and awakening but allow child to stay awake in bed if not disruptive to others
Parasomnias			
Nightmares	Child awakens in fear/crying, has memory of event; is interactive while upset; occurs in latter half of the night; slow return to sleep	Night terrors; seizures; stress if nightmares occur frequently	Soothe and reassure the child; a nightlight or flashlight that the child can use may help if afraid of the dark
Night terrors and sleepwalking (variant)	Child awakens screaming/crying but is not interactive with the parent at the time; has no memory of the event; occurs in the first third of night; rapid return to sleep; sleepwalking is variant	Nightmares; seizures; physical exhaustion	Protect the child from injury if he or she is thrashing about or walking; help the child to lie down to return to sleep; protect child from stairways and other unsafe places sleepwalker might go
Medical/Psychiatric Problems			
Depression	Insomnia or hypersomnia with other symptoms of depression	Other psychiatric disorder; dyssomnia or parasomnia disorder	Manage the psychiatric condition first
Obstructive sleep apnea	Snoring with apneic periods against increased respiratory efforts, restless sleep, daytime sleepiness/fatigue	Central apnea, benign snoring, seizure disorder	Refer to sleep studies and possible adenotonsillectomy

Dyssomnias

Dyssomnias are disorders of sleep related to the process of going to sleep, putting oneself back to sleep from an arousal, and sleeping on a regular basis at a reasonable time.

Sleep-Onset Association Problems (Night Waking)

Description. The child is unable to enter the sleep cycle easily unless a particular routine is carried out. For the infant, the problem results in frequent night waking and crying, most often between midnight and 5 AM.

Etiology. This is learned behavior, often seen in infants who fall asleep while being rocked and who are then put in their beds (Dahl, 1998).

Incidence. Sleep-onset association problems are common. Studies identify incidence patterns ranging from 10% of 8-month-olds, to 44% of 6- to 12-month-olds, to 20% of 9-month-olds, to 20% to 40% of 12- to 24-month-olds (Adair & Bauchner, 1993). Mindell (1999) notes the frequency of night waking in a variety of studies to be 20% to 25% of children ages 1 to 5 years.

Clinical Findings. The history reveals a baby or child who has frequent night awakenings. When the parent goes to the child and repeats a particular intervention, the child falls asleep promptly.

Differential Diagnoses. The differential diagnoses for sleep-onset association problems are pain or a medical condition affecting sleep, fear in an older child, and inappropriate expectations related to the amount of sleep the child needs. Too early bedtime, day-night reversal, trained night feeding, trained night waking, and gastrointestinal reflux are other possible causes to be addressed. Obstructive sleep apnea, nightmares, and mood disorders can also cause night waking (Howard & Wong, 2001).

Management. The infant or child must learn to go from the arousal phase into the next sleep cycle independently in the night. The parent must learn to change the responses given during the night. Two strategies have been recommended in the literature:

1. Put the child down to sleep at night while he or she is awake. When the child awakens and cries in the night, the parent should go to him or her briefly to give comfort and reassurance but not to hold, rock, or feed. The parent's response must be supportive and comforting but should not reinforce a return to old patterns of infant behavior or parental response. This technique is termed *extinction.* Going "cold turkey" (not going to the child at all from the very beginning) is difficult for parents to do, although children learn to return to sleep alone within a few nights, crying for shorter periods each time. Waiting for progressively longer intervals before going to the child over several nights may work if the parents can maintain compliance (graduated extinction) (Blum & Carey, 1996; Mindell, 1999).
2. Alternatively, use a planned or scheduled awakening approach. The first night, the parent should go to the child 30 minutes before night awakening is expected. The child is awakened, rocked for a few minutes, and then left again. When spontaneous awakenings stop, scheduled awakenings are gradually delayed 30 minutes more each night. If the child then awakens spontaneously, he or she learns to wait for the parents to come, knowing it will happen, and gradually learns to return to sleep. This pattern seems to be less stressful for parents and is as effective in teaching independent sleep onset within 6 weeks as is delayed comforting (Blum & Carey, 1996; Mindell, 1999).

It may be easier to work on development of self-sleep during naps first, and then transfer this behavior to nighttime. Most infants use sleep aids such as a blanket or stuffed animal to assist with self-soothing (Burnham et al, 2002).

Ineffective management strategies include use of diphenhydramine medication, which will provide moderate improvement, but the sleep problems can be expected to return when medication is stopped (Mindell, 1999).

Sleep Refusal

Description. In toddlers and preschoolers, the problem is one of difficulty with bedtime settling. "Sleeping alone through the night without parental intervention is a learned process" (Dahl, 1998, p. 80).

Incidence. A variety of studies report that approximately 20% of children between 15 and 48 months of age engage in bedtime resistance. Bedtime resistance was identified in 25% of patients age 2 to 13 years, with 29% of preschoolers experiencing the problem (Hedger-Archbold et al, 2002).

Etiology. The child may experience an inability to make the transition from daytime activities to nighttime sleeping. Separation anxiety is a problem for some, as are nighttime fears.

Clinical Findings. The child makes repeated attempts to obtain parental attention (e.g., demanding snacks, asking for a drink, requesting another story, leaving bed to return to family activities, watching activities from afar).

Differential Diagnosis

Infant: Sleep association problem, hunger, circadian rhythm disorder

Preschooler: Sleep association problem, circadian rhythm disorder, limit setting, bedtime fears

School age and adolescent: Sleep association problem (TV or radio on); circadian rhythm disorder; anxiety at bedtime related to daytime stresses, exposure to violence, chaotic household, family stresses, sexual/physical abuse (Howard & Wong, 2001)

Management. For the toddler or preschooler who exhibits sleep refusal try the following regimen:

1. Use a sleep log to chart the child's pattern initially. It can then be used to mark progress toward the goal.
2. Maintain the bedtime routine and use transitional objects and a quiet environment for sleep.
3. Set limits on the child's demands for attention. The parent should leave the room at the end of the bedtime routine, expecting good behavior. If the child arises, return the child to bed, saying, "It is time for bed," each time the child gets up (Blum & Carey, 1996).
4. Be sure that the child is not being expected to sleep earlier or for longer periods than expected for his or her age.
5. For children older than 3 years of age, positive rewards, such as sticker charts, may help (Ferber, 1996). Stresses and fears must be addressed.
6. If the child has bedtime fears, leaving may increase the problem. In these cases, the parent may sit quietly in the room until the child falls asleep. When the child can fall asleep easily this way, the parent should move to the bedroom door and eventually out of sight. The child needs to understand that the parent will only remain in the room if there are no tantrums and the child stays in bed (Blum & Carey, 1996).

Trained Night Feeder

Description. The child learns to nurse or feed at night with regularity. Ferber (1996) sees this as a problem of (1) feeding, which generates excessive fluid and increases wet diapers and associated discomfort, and (2) a disruption of circadian rhythms as a result of nutrient input into intestinal and hormonal systems, which are in a resting physiologic state.

Etiology. Night feeding in volume, frequent daytime feedings (grazing), feeding until asleep, and leaving a bottle in the bed are all causes of this sleep disturbance.

Incidence. Trained night feeding is a common problem.

Clinical Findings. With this disturbance, middle-of-the-night feedings occur in a child older than 4 months of age.

Differential Diagnosis. The differential diagnosis is night waking not related to feeding.

Management. Three strategies are recommended:

1. Lengthen the time between daytime feedings.
2. Feed the child only once after the feeding given at the parent's bedtime.
3. Discontinue bottles in bed either cold turkey or, less stressfully, by gradually decreasing the volume of each feeding after the infant is on a 3-hour feeding schedule in the daytime.

The problem should resolve in 1 to 2 weeks (Ferber, 1996).

Complications. Night feedings should not be withheld from children who are not thriving for other reasons and who need the nutrition of another nighttime feeding.

Sleep-Cycle Problems (Circadian Rhythm Disorders)

Delayed Sleep Phase

Description. The sleep cycle begins at a late hour and is followed by a late awakening. This is commonly an adolescent problem.

Etiology. The child's internal clock for sleep and rest is not consistent with appropriate hours for sleep. Excessive naps or late morning waking may be related factors, especially for school-age children and adolescents.

Differential Diagnosis. The diagnoses are prolonged bedtime routine and oppositional disorder, which both involve active resistance to going to bed rather than inability to fall asleep.

Management. Three approaches are suggested:

1. Keep the nighttime routine in place but awaken the child earlier each morning in 15-minute increments.
2. For the adolescent or older child who is off schedule by many hours (e.g., at the end of summer, when beginning the school year will require getting up earlier), it could take weeks to back up the cycle appropriately using 15-minute increments. In this case, it is better to go forward in time. In other words, have the child remain awake until the next evening and then go to bed at the desired hour, beginning the desired routine from that point.
3. Have the child or family keep a sleep log to document gradual change (Howard & Wong, 2001).

Advanced Sleep Phase

Description. The sleep cycle begins too early with correlated early rising.

Management. Meals, naps, and bedtime should be delayed until the desired times. The early waking resolves itself.

Inappropriate or Unpredictable Schedules

Description. Some people have a poorly organized sleep/wake cycle. This is described by some as a temperament problem of rhythmicity.

Management. The routines of eating, activities, and sleeping should be kept as regular as possible. The older child may need to learn to play quietly in bed until others awaken or until a clock radio goes off. At night, the child may need to learn to read or listen to music in bed when bedtime comes.

Parasomnias: Night Terrors, Sleepwalking, and Nightmares

In parasomnias, behaviors intrude on ongoing sleep rather than representing disruptions of the sleep process such as going to sleep, waking in the night, or sleeping on an inappropriate schedule. In general they are more common in males, and children with one type of parasomnia are more likely to exhibit symptoms of another at some point.

Positive family histories are common. Parasomnias are divided into arousal disorders, sleep/wake transition disorders, REM parasomnias, and miscellaneous (Anders & Eiben, 1997). The arousal disorders include sleep terrors and sleepwalking and are discussed next. Both occur 1 to 3 hours after sleep onset when the child transitions from non-REM stage IV to REM sleep. Both occur sporadically, may be triggered by excessive fatigue or unusual stress, and can be considered as problems that the child will outgrow rather than needing a specific intervention. Nightmares are a REM parasomnia, and bruxism is a miscellaneous parasomnia (Anders & Eiben, 1997). Laberge and colleagues (2000) report high anxiety scores among 11- to 13-year-olds with various parasomnia disorders.

Night Terrors or Sleep Terrors

Description. Night terrors are defined as a partial awakening from non-REM sleep stage III or IV in which the child is not fully conscious and aware of surroundings. Episodes occur 60 to 90 minutes after onset of sleep and may last from less than a minute to 5 minutes or more.

Etiology. These are related to the transition from the stage IV non-REM sleep to the REM sleep cycle and are not psychologic or developmental problems. Excessive fatigue or unusual daytime stresses may precipitate attacks in some children, but they are not considered mental health problems. A full bladder is also considered a trigger factor.

Incidence. Night terrors are most common in 3- to 6-year-olds, although they occur in children from 18 months to adolescence. Incidence has been reported at 3% of children, mostly from 18 months to 6 years.

Clinical Findings. The child usually sits up screaming but cannot be reasoned with or consoled. Indeed, the child does not even seem to hear the caregiver. The child can have pallor, pupil dilation, piloerection, tachycardia, and sweating, all symptoms of an autonomic discharge (Anders & Eiben, 1997; Howard & Wong, 2001). The child may speak incoherently and may thrash about. The child is not awake or aware of the surroundings and does not remember the episode in the morning. It is the caregiver who is disturbed, not the child. Episodes may occur in bouts of up to 20 per night for a few weeks and then disappear, with possible later recurrences.

Differential Diagnosis. The differential diagnosis is nightmares or seizures with stiffening, jerking, or drooling.

Management. The child should be helped to lie down again and should be soothed back to sleep. Emptying the bladder at bedtime should be routine. Waking the child 30 minutes before the expected episode each night for about a week may interrupt the pattern. The child should be protected from injury, and baby-sitters should be prepared for these episodes. An afternoon nap may change the sleep stages at night (Anders & Eiben, 1997; Howard & Wong, 2001).

Sleepwalking (Somnambulism)

Description. Sleepwalking is a variation of night terrors in which the manifestation is walking rather than sitting up and screaming. It occurs with arousal from stage IV sleep, usually 1 to 2 hours into sleep.

Etiology. The cause is the same as that for night terrors; it is an arousal disorder in stage IV. It can be triggered by excessive fatigue, changes in routines, or daily stress.

Incidence. Sleepwalking is more common in boys and tends to be outgrown. It occurs in 15% of children at one time or another.

Clinical Findings. The child arises and walks about without being fully alert and responsive. The child may fall or bump into things, wander in illogical places, or urinate outside the toilet.

Differential Diagnosis. The diagnosis is dissociative state or seizure.

Management. The child needs to be led back quietly to bed. A gate may need to be placed across the bedroom door if the sleepwalking becomes frequent. Doors may need to be secured to ensure that the child does not wander into unsafe areas. Stairways are particularly dangerous to the sleepwalking child (Howard & Wong, 2001). An afternoon nap may also be helpful in altering the stage IV pattern (Anders & Eiben, 1997).

Nightmares, Monsters, and Other Nighttime Fears

Description. Nightmares are classified as a REM parasomnia disorder. Nightmares occur as the child awakens from REM sleep, remembering dreams that are disturbing. Occasional nightmares are normal and benign. The child is awake, frightened, and able to describe the fears.

Differential Diagnosis. The differential diagnosis for nightmares is night terrors, in which the child is not fully conscious. The significance and severity of other nighttime fears need to be assessed. Separation anxiety in toddlers, domestic violence, or a scary event may make nighttime frightening.

Management. Parents should give comfort, reassurance, and a sense of security and not dismiss the fear as imaginary. The child may need to have the parent lie down with him or her for a period of time, or the child may even get into bed with the parent. However, this should not become habitual.

Monsters may be kept away by keeping on a nightlight, by using a flashlight to "sweep them away," or by keeping the bedroom door open.

Behavioral strategies or counseling may be required if nighttime fears are frequent or the degree of fear is exceptionally severe.

Head Banging and Bruxism

Sleep/wake transition disorders include sleep talking, nocturnal leg cramps, and rhythmic movement disorders such as head banging and body rocking, which usually occur with sleep onset. One study reported that at 9 months of age, 58% of infants exhibited at least one of several repetitive behaviors that included head turning, head banging, or rocking (Klackenberg, 1982). Generally the incidence reduces to about 22% at 2 years. Most disappear by age 5 years. No interventions are considered necessary aside from ensuring the child's safety (Anders & Eiben, 1997).

Sleep bruxism is stereotypic grinding or clenching of the teeth during sleep. There may be some relationship to stress. It frequently appears between ages 10 and 20 years, although there is a short-lived infant version. Seizure disorder would be a differential diagnosis. Dental referral may be useful (Anders & Eiben, 1997).

OBSTRUCTIVE SLEEP APNEA

Description

Obstructive sleep apnea syndrome is a serious problem for some infants and children because it is an indicator of severe airway obstruction. It is "a disorder of breathing during sleep characterized by prolonged partial upper airway obstruction and/or intermittent complete obstruction (obstructive apnea) that disrupts normal ventilation during sleep and normal sleep patterns" (American Thoracic Society, 1996). It should be distinguished from primary snoring, which is snoring without obstructive apnea, frequent arousals from sleep, or gas exchange abnormalities.

Etiology

Collapse of the pharyngeal airway with increased airway resistance above the collapsing segment causes sleep apnea. The child makes repeated vigorous attempts to breathe. Snoring is associated with these efforts but will not be heard if obstruction is complete. Arousal may occur, and with it, upper airway muscle tone improves. The cycle may repeat many times during the night. The condition may also be partial, called *obstructive hypoventilation.* Other factors may include the following (Marcus, 1998; Rosen, 1999):

- Large adenoids or tonsils or both
- Nasal deformities
- Abnormally small oropharyngeal structures as in Pierre Robin syndrome
- Craniofacial structural problems such as midface hypoplasia
- Factors affecting neural control such as generalized hypotonia, central nervous system injury, and brain stem dysfunction, which includes cerebral palsy and muscular dystrophy (these conditions relate to incoordination of upper airway muscles)
- Idiopathic or genetic cause—Prader-Willi syndrome, sickle cell disease, mucopolysaccharidosis
- Obesity

Incidence

Sleep apnea may occur in approximately 2% of 4- to 5-year-olds (AAP Section on Pediatric Pulmonology, Subcommittee on Obstructive Sleep Apnea Syndrome, 2002; Anders & Eiben, 1997). Snoring occurs in 3% to 12% of preschool-age children (AAP Section on Pediatric Pulmonology, Subcommittee on Obstructive Sleep Apnea Syndrome, 2002). Corbo and colleagues (2001) report a prevalence of 5.6% in school-age and adolescent children, with obese boys 15 years and older having higher rates.

Clinical Findings

History

Sleep screening should be a part of all routine health care visits (AAP Section on Pediatric Pulmonology, Subcommittee on Obstructive Sleep Apnea Syndrome, 2002). The following should be assessed:

- Disrupted sleep patterns (timing, restlessness, positions, diaphoresis, behavior while asleep)*
- Snoring (pitch, periods of silence, intensity, onset, frequency, duration)*

*These findings are associated with obstructive sleep apnea in AAP Section on Pediatric Pulmonology, Subcommittee on Obstructive Sleep Apnea Syndrome (2002).

- Observed increased breathing effort (rib cage retraction, paradoxic chest wall movement) or apnea*
- Alertness and functioning when awake*
- Associated conditions (e.g., craniofacial syndromes, tonsillar hypertrophy)*
- Growth and development*
- Factors indicating high-risk patient: infant, patient with craniofacial disorder, Down syndrome, cerebral palsy, neuromuscular disorder, chronic lung disease, sickle cell disease, central hypoventilation syndromes, or genetic/metabolic/storage disease*

Physical Examination

The physical examination should include the following:

- Vital signs, including blood pressure*
- Height and weight for failure to thrive or obesity*
- Complete ear, nose, and throat examination, including tonsils and adenoids, midfacial hypoplasia, retrognathia or micrognathia, patency of nasal passages, tongue size, signs of cleft palate*
- Cardiac functioning for evidence of cor pulmonale, to include increased pulmonic component of the second heart sound indicating pulmonary hypertension*
- Observation for digital clubbing, pectus excavatum
- Muscle tone

Laboratory Evaluation

Tape recording the apneic episodes may be helpful in assessing the problem. The child needs to be referred for a variety of sleep studies, as well as electrocardiogram and echocardiogram if the problem is severe. Radiographs of the head and neck are usually not helpful. Nocturnal polysomnography is the "gold standard" diagnostic technique. Nocturnal pulse oximetry, videotaping, and daytime nap polysomnography are useful if the results are positive but do not rule out obstructive sleep apnea syndrome if negative (AAP Section on Pediatric Pulmonology, Subcommittee on Obstructive Sleep Apnea Syndrome, 2002).

Differential Diagnosis

The differential diagnoses are seizure disorder and central apnea, which are characterized by no airflow and no respiratory effort. Central apnea is a brainstem problem that is more commonly seen in premature or newborn infants (Anders & Eiben, 1997). Primary snoring also needs to be considered.

*These findings are associated with obstructive sleep apnea in AAP Section on Pediatric Pulmonology, Subcommittee on Obstructive Sleep Apnea Syndrome (2002).

NURSING DIAGNOSES RELATED TO SLEEP AND REST: *Functional Health Pattern*

- Disturbed sleep pattern
- Sleep deprivation
- Fatigue
- Readiness for enhanced sleep
- Risk for sudden infant death syndrome

From North American Nursing Diagnosis Association: *NANDA nursing diagnoses: definitions and classification, 2003-2004*, Philadelphia, 2003, North American Nursing Diagnosis Association.

Management

The child should be referred for sleep studies and possible adenotonsillectomy (the first-line treatment) or other surgical strategies. Nasal continuous positive airway pressure (CPAP) has also been used. Drugs are ineffective. Avoidance of indoor pollutants may be helpful. Weight loss may help if the child is obese. Oxygen therapy does not prevent the problems of the condition and may worsen hypoventilation. Patients undergoing surgical intervention should be reevaluated. High-risk children need to be referred to a pediatric specialist because they are at increased surgical risk and require more complex management (AAP Section on Pediatric Pulmonology, Subcommittee on Obstructive Sleep Apnea Syndrome, 2002).

Complications

Cardiac problems, including cor pulmonale resulting from hypoxic episodes, right ventricular hypertrophy, pulmonary hypertension, heart failure, systemic hypertension, and polycythemia can occur (AAP Section on Pediatric Pulmonology, Subcommittee on Obstructive Sleep Apnea Syndrome, 2002; Marcus, 1998). Neurologic problems, including failure to thrive, developmental delay, learning problems, hyperactivity, excessive daytime sleepiness, and morning headache, have been reported; however, some studies have not been well controlled, including snoring children without objective evaluation, control groups, or sleep studies to distinguish those with apnea from those without sleep-disordered breathing (AAP Section on Pediatric Pulmonology, Subcommittee on Obstructive Sleep Apnea Syndrome, 2002; Chervin et al, 2002).

REFERENCES

Adair R, Bauchner H: Sleep problems in childhood, *Curr Probl Pediatr* 23:147-170, 1993.

American Academy of Pediatrics Section on Pediatric Pulmonology, Subcommittee on Obstructive Sleep Apnea Syndrome: Clinical practice guideline: diagnosis and management of childhood obstructive sleep apnea, *Pediatrics* 109:704-712, 2002.

American Academy of Pediatrics Task Force on Infant Position and Sudden Infant Death Syndrome: Changing concepts of sudden infant death syndrome: implications for infant sleeping environment and sleep position (RE9946), *Pediatrics* 105:650-656, 2000.

American Sleep Disorders Association: *International classification of sleep disorders: diagnostic and coding manual*, Lawrence, KS, 1990, Allen Press.

American Thoracic Society: Standards and indications for cardiopulmonary sleep studies in children, *Am J Respir Crit Care Med* 153:866-878, 1996.

Anders T, Eiben L: Pediatric sleep disorders: a review of the past 10 years, *J Acad Child Adolesc Psychiatr* 36:9-20, 1997.

Behrman R, Kliegman R, Jenson H, editors: *Nelson textbook of pediatrics*, ed 17, Philadelphia, 2004, WB Saunders.

Blum N, Carey W: Sleep problems among infants and young children, *Pediatr Rev* 17:87-93, 1996.

Burnham M et al: Use of sleep aids during the first year of life, *Pediatrics* 109:594-601, 2002.

Carey W: Nightwaking and temperament in infancy, *J Pediatr* 84:756-758, 1974.

Chervin R et al: Inattention, hyperactivity, and symptoms of sleep-disordered breathing, *Pediatrics* 109:449-456, 2002.

Corbo G et al: Snoring in 9- to 15-year-old children: risk factors and clinical relevance, *Pediatrics* 108:1149-1154, 2001.

Dahl R: The development and disorders of sleep, *Adv Pediatr* 45:73-90, 1998.

DiLeo H, Reiter R, Taliaferro D: Chronobiology, melatonin, and sleep in infants and children, *Pediatr Nurs* 28:35-39, 2002.

Ferber R: Childhood sleep disorders, *Neurol Clin* 14:493-511, 1996.

Gershon N, Moon R: Infant sleep position in licensed child care centers, *Pediatrics* 100:75-78, 1997.

Hedger-Archbold K et al: Symptoms of sleep disturbances among children at two general pediatric clinics, *J Pediatr* 140:97-102, 2002.

Howard B, Wong J: Sleep disorders, *Pediatr Rev* 22:327-341, 2001.

Jantz J, Blosser C: A motor milestone change noted with a change in sleep position, *Arch Pediatr Adolesc Med* 151:565-568, 1997.

Jimmerson K: Maternal, environmental, and temperamental characteristics of toddlers with and toddlers without sleep problems, *J Pediatr Health Care* 5:71-77, 1991.

Klackenberg G: Sleep behavior studied longitudinally: data from 4-16 years in duration, night awakening and bedtime, *Acta Paediatr Scand* 71:501-506, 1982.

Laberge L et al: Development of parasomnias from childhood to early adolescence, *Pediatrics* 106:67-74, 2000.

Lavigne J et al: Sleep and behavior problems among preschoolers, *J Dev Behav Pediatr* 20:164-169, 1999.

Marcus C: Does your child snore? *Contemp Pediatr* 15:101-115, 1998.

McKenna J, Mosko S, Richard C: Bedsharing promotes breastfeeding, *Pediatrics* 100:214-219, 1997.

Mindell J: Empirically supported treatments in pediatric psychology: bedtime refusal and night wakings in young children, *J Pediatr Psychol* 24:465-481, 1999.

Mosko S, Richard C, McKenna J: Infant arousals during mother-infant bedsharing: implications for infant sleep and sudden infant death syndrome research, *Pediatrics* 100:841-849, 1997.

Paris C, Remler R, Daling J: Risk factors for sudden infant death syndrome: changes associated with sleep position recommendations, *J Pediatr* 139:771-779, 2001.

Pollack H, Frohna J: Infant sleep placement after the back to sleep campaign, *Pediatrics* 109: 608-614, 2002.

Recio J et al: Synchronizing circadian rhythms in early infancy, *Med Hypotheses* 49:229-234, 1997.

Rosen C: Clinical features of obstructive sleep apnea hypoventilation syndrome in otherwise healthy children, *Pediatr Pulmonol* 27:403-409, 1999.

Seymore F et al: Reducing sleep disruptions in young children: evaluation of therapist-guided and written information approaches: a brief report, *J Child Psychol Psychiatry* 30:913-918, 1989.

Stores G: Practitioner review: assessment and treatment of sleep disorders in children and adolescents, *J Child Psychol Psychiatry* 37:907-925, 1996.

Zuckerman B, Stevenson J, Bailey V: Sleep problems in early childhood: continuities, predictive factors, and behavioral correlates, *Pediatrics* 80:664-667, 1987.

17 Cognitive-Perceptual Patterns

Kathleen Shelton, Catherine E. Burns

Cognition and perception are interrelated activities engaged in by all humans. Gordon (1987) describes the cognitive-perceptual functional health pattern to include "the adequacy of sensory modes, such as vision, hearing, taste, touch, or smell, and the compensation or prostheses utilized for disturbances. Also included are the cognitive functional abilities, such as language, memory, and decision-making." Gordon notes that "to hear, see, smell, taste, and touch are human functions taken for granted until deficits arise." Little has been written about children in terms of the cognitive-perceptual pattern per se. However, attention-deficit hyperactivity disorder (ADHD), deafness, blindness, and autism are all pediatric problems that involve use of sensory modes and are related to cognition, language, and the functional abilities of day-to-day life; that is, they represent problems within the cognitive-perceptual pattern.

Facilitating the developmental progress of children should be an overriding concern for families and health care providers. Cognition is an essential component of development. Assisting children and families to minimize the effects of perceptual problems on cognition, and thus development as a whole, is an important role of the nurse practitioner (NP). In this chapter, selected cognitive-perceptual problems of children are addressed as they relate to functioning in daily life.

STANDARDS FOR CARE

Healthy People 2010: Health Promotion and Disease Prevention Objectives for the Year 2010 (U.S. Department of Health and Human Services, 2001) supports the need for primary care for children with cognitive and perceptual problems. *Healthy People 2010* includes the following objectives:

1. Reduce blindness and visual impairment in children and adolescents age 17 years and under (28-4).
2. Increase the proportion of newborns who are screened for hearing loss by age 1 month, have audiologic evaluation by 3 months, and are enrolled in appropriate intervention services by 6 months (28-11).

The American Medical Association's (AMA's) guidelines for adolescent preventive services (GAPS) (Elster & Kuznets, 1994) recommend that "all adolescents should be asked annually about learning or school problems." Learning disability, ADHD, medical problems, and other factors are identified as areas for further assessment if the young person is not successful in school.

CONCEPTUAL BACKGROUND

Normal Cognitive-Perceptual Patterns

Cognition and general knowledge represent the accumulation and reorganization of experiences that result from participating in a rich learning setting with skilled and appropriate adult interventions. From these experiences, children construct knowledge of patterns and relations, cause and effect, and methods of solving problems of everyday life.

For children to develop, they must perceive and process information from varied stimuli. External stimuli include visual, auditory, proprioceptive, tactile, and other modalities, whereas internal stimuli include emotions, associations, fantasies, visceral-autonomic sources, and memory sources (Levine, Carey, & Crocker, 1999). When children experience problems perceiving their environment, both animate and inanimate, development is at risk. For example, the deaf child who fails to hear sounds or learn a communication system early in life can develop faulty language and experience decreased knowledge acquisition and storage skills, reading difficulties, and social difficulties.

Learning requires feedback related to behaviors exhibited. Feedback provides information to the child, positive reinforcement for correct responses to stimuli, and negative reinforcement for behaviors that are not appropriate. Parents, peers, and others provide important feedback to the child. For the child with perceptual problems, not only is the initial cue missed but also the feedback cues, which the child needs in order to know whether his or her response was appropriate. This feedback is an essential component of the learning process.

Information-Processing Theories

Information processing is thinking or problem solving. The collection of information-processing theories can serve as a useful framework for understanding learning from the perspective of cognitive and perceptual processes. The theories collectively focus on information presented, processes used to transform information, and memory limits that constrain the amount of information that can be represented and processed. Unlike Piaget's learning model, information-processing theories try to develop a complete theory of cognition, are relatively specific, and are testable. Information-processing theorists sometimes use computer models to develop and test their ideas.

Atkinson and Shiffrin (1968) have provided a broad theory of information processing. They proposed a system with structural and process components. Structural features include a sensory store with both visual and auditory registers, a short-term store, and a long-term store. There are also several processes or actions essential to the system. Rehearsal activity is used to keep information in the short-term store—the working memory. Automatic processing activities transform information outside the direct control of the individual to retain information not consciously remembered. One can see immediately that blind or deaf children will have difficulty with the two registers, visual and auditory, with deficits in one and the necessity for greater skill in the other. Children with ADHD or autism can have serviceable visual and auditory registers but have difficulty screening input from the registers appropriately or have problems using the processes of rehearsal and automatic processing effectively and efficiently, or both.

The task environment or the context in which the child acts is also important. For example, a particular solution to a problem may create moral conflicts and thus alter the child's options. Encoding is also important. It involves identification of critical information in a situation and use of it to create internal representations (Levine, 2000). If children fail to identify or comprehend critical elements or do not know how to encode them efficiently, they do not learn from potentially useful experiences. A key role of parents and teachers is to help children learn to identify critical cues and encode and process the information so that it becomes useful knowledge.

Levine, Carey, & Crocker (1999) and Levine (2000) applied information-processing concepts to the clinical understanding and management of pediatric learning disorders. Their information-processing model (Fig. 17-1) asserted that selective attention is a gateway between the availability and perception of stimuli and the representational and storage processes the child mobilizes to use the information. A great deal of information in the form of various stimuli may be available to the child. Selective attention begins the processes of information management—taking in, manipulating, storing, and responding.

Perception and attention are closely related phenomena. Perception is awareness of stimuli, whereas attention serves as a filtering process to focus on the most important perceptions at the moment. The primary care provider needs to assess both perceptual and selective attention skills of cognition.

Cognitive-Perceptual Developmental Patterns

Infants

The infant uses perceptions in a highly literal way to develop cognition as explained by Piaget's sensorimotor stage. The infant watches, listens, tastes, smells, and manipulates objects in the environment in order to learn. Eye-hand coordination is important; achieving object permanence as a concept is essential.

Toddlers and Preschoolers

Toddlers continue to develop cognitively in the sensorimotor stage, whereas preschoolers, sometime after age 2 years, move into the preoperational stage. In this egocentric phase, they continue mentally to construct models that explain how the world works. However, they are unable to do several critical operations, including the following: considering several variables at once; recognizing that others have different perceptions; classifying proficiently; and understanding that some objects are inanimate, without intention and ability to act. Visual and auditory perceptions and selective attention are key factors in toddler learning. Language development assists them to encode and store information for retrieval and use.

School-Age Children

School-age children have increased perceptual skills. They have mastered the concept that others may have a different perception of the world from theirs, an especially important step that helps them understand the world from psychosocial perspectives. Piaget described their thought processes as concrete operations. In other words, they

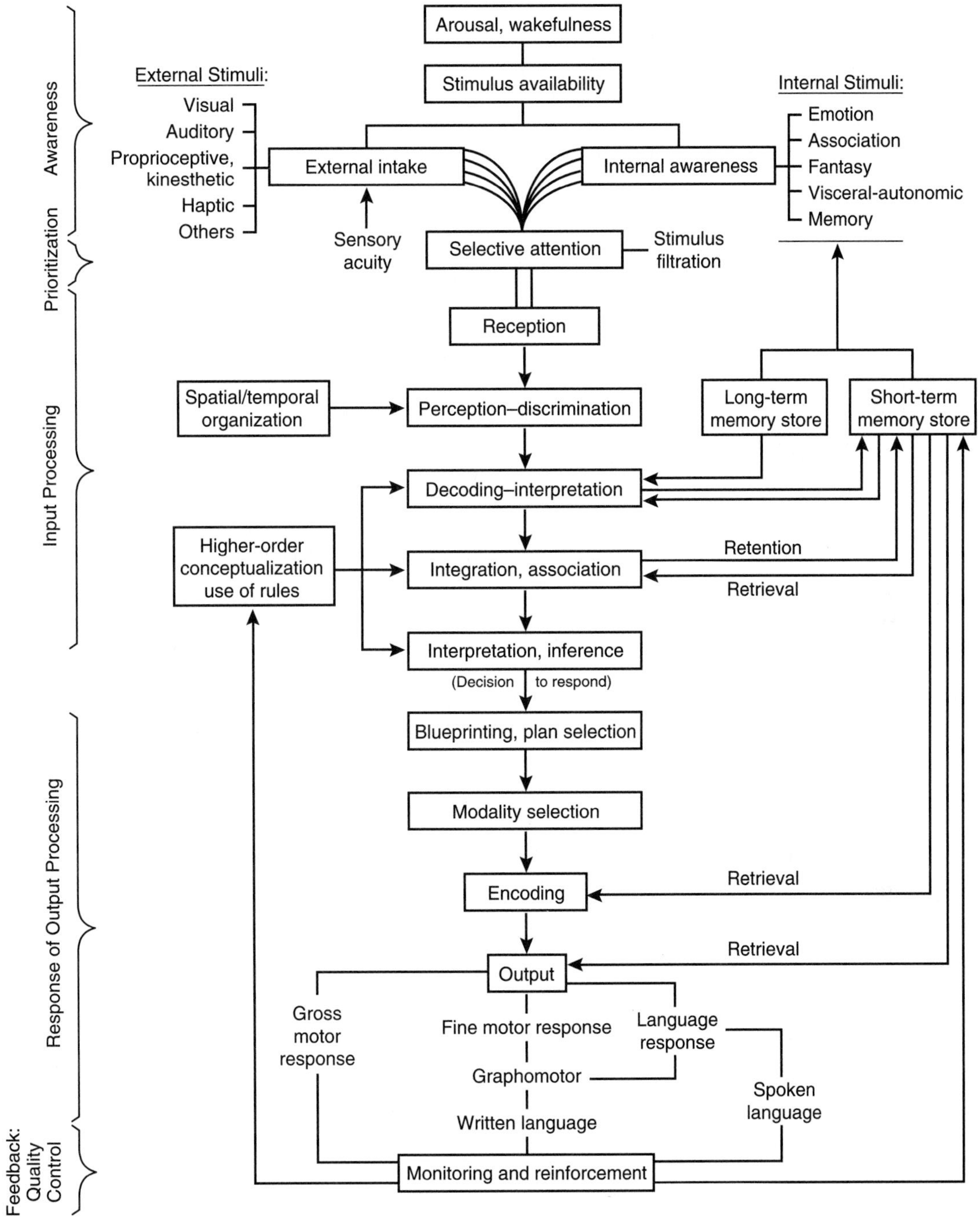

FIGURE 17-1 Information-processing model. (From Levine M, Brooks R, Shonkoff J: *A pediatric approach to learning disorders*, New York, 1980, Wiley, p 480.)

reason best when physically manipulating variables so that the senses are directly stimulated rather than manipulating variables abstractly as they reason out problems. Reading becomes another type of coded language that allows further broadening of experience beyond that which is directly observable.

Adolescents

Most adolescents can use formal operational thinking, including the capacity to reason from hypotheses and to identify various possible outcomes. Cognitive and perceptual skills are considered mature. (Of course, both adolescents and adults do not always use formal operational reasoning.)

The developmental milestones for children with cognitive-perceptual problems are altered from these normal patterns. A summary of some of the differences in blind and deaf children is found in Table 17-1. Children with ADHD often achieve motor milestones on time but may experience delays in speech, social, and emotional areas of development.

Delays or Alterations in Cognitive-Perceptual Developmental Patterns

Although most children develop according to normal patterns, developmental delays, specific deficits, and alterations in cognitive-perceptual patterns sometimes occur. Developmental delays from environmental deprivation or neglect are frequently reversible once identified. Other forms of developmental delays may result from prenatal or perinatal events, genetic dispositions, environmental toxins, trauma, or other insults to normal developmental patterns. Mental retardation results in mild, moderate, or severe cognitive deficits. The spectrum of learning disabilities may mimic alterations in cognitive-perceptual development; however, learning disabilities do not necessarily indicate lower intelligence. Instead, the challenge is to identify how the child can learn and to provide adequate experiences. It is not within the scope of this text to address the many disabling conditions involving cognitive-perceptual patterns; however, the NP can play an active role on an interdisciplinary team for diagnosis and management of developmental delays by providing care coordination, health maintenance monitoring, and family education and support (Gedaly-Duff, Stoeger, & Shelton, 2000).

Effects of Cognitive-Perceptual Pattern Problems on the Family

Family caregiving of children with impairments of all types is a related area that the NP must understand. Families adapt to achieve caregiving demands while trying to maintain family integrity. This adaptation is sometimes stressful. Because children with chronic conditions are rarely institutionalized, society relies on families to provide complex and time-consuming care.

How families cope with chronic disabling conditions and developmental delays is of interest to nursing researchers. Knafl and colleagues (1996, 2001) identified the following family management styles when a child had a chronic or disabling condition: thriving, accommodating, enduring,

TABLE 17-1 ***Developmental Milestones of Blind and Deaf Infants and Children***

	Blind	Deaf
Infants (0-1 yr)	Tend to lie quietly in crib. Attachment problems possible due to decreased social cues and visual following. Decreased use of hands and bringing hands to midline, decreased prone position, decreased facial expressions. Head control normal but delayed pull to sit; creep, stand, and walk delayed about 4 mo. Creeping delayed until reaching on sound cue is achieved. Increased separation anxiety may begin by 6 mo. Increased echolalia (Ryan, 1988). Sensorimotor delays common. Delayed object permanence.	Sensorimotor stage normal. Language development: deaf children exposed early to sign language develop language similarly to hearing children exposed to spoken language (Meadow-Orlans, 1990). Deaf children exposed to both spoken and sign language learn both and progress as hearing children (Meadow, 1980). Deaf children exposed only to spoken language have language delays (Gregory & Mogford, 1981). Language output decreased around 6-9 mo.
Toddlers (12 mo-2 yr)	Decreased aggression but increased tantrums and motor behavior when frustrated. Continued delayed object permanence. Walks at 17 mo on average. "Blindisms" appear—rocking, swaying, head turning (Phillips & Hartley, 1988).	Sensorimotor stage normal.
Preschoolers (3-5 yr)	Decreased social skills, decreased self-help skills. "I" sense of self delayed to 4 yr (Phillips & Hartley, 1988).	May have preoperational delays (Quigley & Kretschmer, 1982). Symbolic play may be delayed if language skills are decreased.
School-age children (6-12 yr)	Reading and mobility delays. Conservation delayed to 9 years (Tobin, 1972).	May have concrete operations delays (Quigley & Kretschmer, 1982). Decreased self-concept.
Adolescents (13-19 yr)	Delays may continue or adolescent may finally achieve developmental level with achievement in academic and social maturity areas.	Increased adjustment problems and decreased social maturity (Meadow, 1980), decreased self-concept. May have formal operations delays.

struggling, and floundering. Each management style described how parents perceived the child (normal, problematic, tragic), the parenting philosophy and view of illness, and their perception and approach to managing the illness. For example, parents who embraced a thriving family management style viewed the illness from a "life goes on" perspective and normalized the child's illness as best they could. They had a parenting philosophy that was able to accommodate the illness into parenting activities and a confident mindset, and they were proactive in their management approach.

Other typologies have been described for families with children with other cognitive-perceptual problems. Kendall (1998) described four types of families of children with ADHD along a trajectory: the chaotic family, the ADHD-controlled family, the surviving family, and the reinvested family. Other studies of families living with ADHD indicate considerable disruption to family routines and an inability to achieve some sense of "normalcy"; some families describe family life as a "nightmare," despite outward indicators (intact marriage, stable residence, adequate income, resources to manage the ADHD, etc.) that the family is doing well (Shelton, 2001). Families of learning-disabled children have been described as healthy, split, chaotic, and blaming (Ziegler & Holden, 1988).

One role of NPs with families with a child with a chronic condition is to help them understand the behaviors that are developmentally appropriate and not disease/treatment related (Deatrick, Knafl, & Murphy-Moore, 1999). Another mechanism for helping family members to understand a child's deficits in cognitive-perceptual patterns is to read age-appropriate books together. Local children's librarians can provide reading lists of books about children with many kinds of health problems. The Resource Box at the end of the chapter provides information about other national resources.

ASSESSMENT OF COGNITIVE-PERCEPTUAL PATTERNS

Normal Patterns

Assessment of normal cognitive-perceptual patterns is discussed earlier in this chapter and elsewhere in this book. Developmental assessments appropriate to the age of the child and hearing and vision screening are the usual modes of assessment.

Assessment of Children with Cognitive-Perceptual Problems

No matter what the particular type of problem, an assessment should include three aspects:

1. Diagnosis or monitoring, or both, of the child's health from a primary care perspective
2. Evaluation of parent and family responses to the problem
3. Evaluation of the child's development

The details of these assessments vary with the condition. A variety of special assessment tools are available and are generally administered by experts. Some assessment tools for children with ADHD are listed in Table 17-2. Mislabeling of

TABLE 17-2 ***Checklists Specific to Attention-Deficit Hyperactivity Disorder***

The following scales have been recommended by the American Academy of Pediatrics Committee on Quality Improvement and Subcommittee on Attention Deficit Hyperactivity Disorder (2000) as clinical options for evaluating children with attention-deficit hyperactivity disorder (ADHD). Use of broadband scales is not recommended in the diagnosis of children with ADHD, although they may be useful for other purposes.

Study	Scale	Age
Connors (1997)	Connors Parent Rating Scale—1997 Revised Version: Long Form, ADHD Index Scale	6-17 yr
Connors (1997)	Connors Teacher Rating Scale—1997 Revised Version: Long Form, ADHD Index Scale	6-17 yr
Connors (1997)	Connors Parent Rating Scale—1997 Revised Version: Long Form, DSM-IV Symptoms Scale	6-17 yr
Connors (1997)	Connors Teacher Rating Scale—1997 Revised Version: Long Form, DSM-IV Symptoms Scale	6-17 yr
Breen & Altpeter (1991)	Barkley's School Situations Questionnaire—Original Version, Number of Problem Settings Scale	6-11 yr
Breen & Altpeter (1991)	Barkley's School Situations Questionnaire—Original Version, Mean Severity Scale	6-11 yr

All scales cited in Green M et al: *Diagnosis of attention deficit hyperactivity disorder: technical review 3*, AHCPR pub 99-0050, Rockville, MD, 1999, US Department of Health and Human Services, Agency for Health Care Policy and Research.

children can occur when tools for sighted or hearing children, for instance, are adapted intuitively for children with visual or auditory disabilities.

MANAGEMENT STRATEGIES

Children and families with problems in this domain generally need support in four areas: social and adaptive skills, education, social support, and multidisciplinary health care team consultations.

Social and Adaptive Strategies

Social and adaptive care relates to helping children achieve maximal independence in living and learning to get along with family and others in a variety of social environments. The family delivers most of this care, but some parents need help with knowing what social and adaptive developmental steps children should master at various ages. Sorting out what "normal" children do at given ages versus what the handicapped child is doing requires thoughtful analysis. Particular strategies to help the impaired child learn new skills are often learned by trial and error or can be gleaned from parents of children with similar handicaps. Physical therapists, occupational therapists, and teachers with special education to help children with cognitive perceptual impairments can be important resources. The NP can serve as case manager, help parents explore other ideas, or act as a conduit to help parents find others who have solved similar problems.

Educational Strategies

Children with ADHD, deafness, blindness, and other problems are entitled to special education opportunities to maximize their learning potential. Two federal laws, the Americans with Disabilities Act (ADA), passed in 1990, and the Individuals with Disabilities Education Act (IDEA), reauthorized in 1997, provide mandates for services for children with cognitive-perceptual problems. These laws provide mechanisms for parents and teachers to use to facilitate optimal learning opportunities for students with cognitive-perceptual difficulties.

- The Individualized Educational Plan (IEP) is designed for children who demonstrate a gap between learning potential and actual academic performance. The IEP is mandated for children with medical conditions that interfere with academic success and arises from the IDEA.
- The "Section 504 Plan" provided within the Americans with Disabilities Act is a civil rights protection to facilitate academic success in students whose disability might otherwise make them ineligible for a public education. Many children with ADHD and learning disabilities who do not have cognitive deficits but do have significant behavioral or emotional problems that interfere with learning are eligible for the Section 504 Plan.

School programs need to be individualized. When children reach school age, decisions are made collaboratively between parents and school personnel about the best placement of the child, whether in a mainstream classroom, in a special classroom, or in a combination of settings. Blind and deaf children sometimes attend special schools designed to meet their needs in either residential or day programs. Children with ADHD or learning problems are usually managed in regular schools. Annual planning of the educational program is often a frustrating experience for parents because school resources and teacher experience vary from year to year.

In addition to school-based programs, infant stimulation opportunities are extremely important for blind and deaf children, and early-intervention preschool programs are essential.

Information for parents about these legal rights and provisions can be found on websites about ADHD and learning disabilities and governmental websites at the Centers for Disease Control and Prevention (CDC), National Institutes of Health (NIH), and National Institutes of Mental Health (NIMH) (also see Resource Box).

Social Support Strategies

Living with a child with a cognitive-perceptual problem, whether the problem is blindness, deafness, hyperactivity, learning difficulties, or other, generally requires that the family develop a structure and organization to support the child without becoming overprotective or intrusive, and an environment that offers consistency for the child. For many families, maintenance of family organization and consistency is difficult.

Social support has been shown to provide significant benefits to families with children with health problems of all sorts. National organizations provide information and expert advice, and local groups can facilitate direct help. Connecting families to others with similar experiences is helpful. Further, the extended family, especially grandparents, can provide significant tangible support to families working to cope with the stresses (financial, temporal, energy, and emotional) of caring for a child with special needs. Siblings may also need support. NPs can be helpful in organizing, supporting, and providing referrals to community support groups. Often national support groups provide expertise to communities that wish to establish a local chapter.

Multidisciplinary Team Strategies

The use of a variety of specialists can provide the best resources for children with special needs. Generally, these include medical specialists, physical and occupational therapists, social workers, and specially educated teachers. The NP helps families identify appropriate teams, serves as a case manager among the parties, and ensures that primary health care needs are integrated with the special services provided (Levine, 2000).

COGNITIVE-PERCEPTUAL PROBLEMS OF CHILDREN

Attention-Deficit Hyperactivity Disorder

Description

ADHD is the most commonly diagnosed behavioral problem in childhood. The cardinal features of this disorder are inattention, distractibility, impulsivity, and overactivity (American Psychiatric Association [APA], 1994). These primary behaviors and their secondary manifestations have an impact on every aspect of life for affected children. The intensity and effect of ADHD behaviors vary widely among children. Behaviors can also change over time in response to normal maturational influences. ADHD is now regarded as a chronic condition that continues into adulthood. ADHD in adolescence requires particular attention because of the increased demands on students at school and the decreasing abilities of adolescents with ADHD to succeed in school without interventions (Evans, Raggi, & Paolitto, 2002; Robin, 2002).

In an attempt to unify the understanding about ADHD, Barkley (1997) outlined a theoretical model of ADHD. The essential impairment is a deficit in behavioral inhibition, disrupting the developmental process of learning to self-regulate behaviors. Instead, external behaviors of inattention, distractibility, impulsivity, and hyperactivity, which may be age appropriate in young children, persist into school age and adolescence and result in the inability to regulate behavior internally as the child matures.

Attention. Attention includes the ability to maintain concentration for an appropriate period of time and to resist attending to competing stimuli. Without these abilities, children and adolescents appear distracted at times when they are expected to concentrate on something else. Attention also implies skill at picking out salient versus trivial information and choosing effective problem-solving strategies. Lacking this component of attention leads to missing the point in academic and social situations and doing things the hard way without careful thought about how to plan and solve a problem.

Distractibility. Distractibility is a by-product of inattention that results when one pays attention to multiple stimuli at one time or in rapid succession. Difficulty maintaining enough mental effort to complete a task is related to distractibility. These characteristics lead to inconsistent performance in school and lost interest in activities and social plans.

Impulsivity. Impulsivity, acting before thinking, is described in the *Diagnostic and Statistical Manual of Mental Disorders*, fourth edition (DSM-IV) (APA, 1994), in part by the behaviors manifested: impatience; difficulty delaying responses, such as blurting out answers in class or interrupting conversations; and blundering without following directions.

Hyperactivity. Hyperactivity describes the cluster of behaviors of overactivity, including fidgeting, an inability to remain seated when expected, and moving "as though driven." These behaviors interfere with attention. They are also regarded as disruptive to group activities and create negative social consequences for the child with ADHD.

Longitudinal studies on ADHD, research using the newest imaging technology, and new conceptualizations about the nature of ADHD suggest that common ADHD behaviors occur when executive functions in the cortex of the brain fail to inhibit impulsive and hyperactive behaviors (Flick, 2002). This research also indicates that those with inattention without impulsivity and hyperactivity may have a disorder distinct from what is now called ADHD. There is no biologic marker for ADHD.

Etiology

ADHD has multiple etiologies, and many are controversial (Barkley, 1998). Most findings are correlational rather than causal. A variety of antecedent factors seem to cause a disturbance in a final common pathway in the nervous system. Neurologic and physiologic factors associated with ADHD include perinatal hypoxic and anoxic insults, other injuries at birth, delayed brain maturation, imbalances in neurotransmitter functions, and differences in cerebral blood flow patterns. Elevated lead levels, cigarette smoking, and ingestion of alcohol or drug use during pregnancy are three environmental factors implicated with ADHD (Mick et al, 2002). A frequently found positive family history of ADHD implies a familial, if not genetic, predisposition (Hechtman, 1996). Extensive studies have failed to find connections between food additives or refined sugar and ADHD (Milich, Wolraich, & Lindgren, 1986).

Incidence

Psychiatric studies give the incidence of ADHD as 3% to 5% (Goldman et al, 1998). In a 2002 study (Rowland et al, 2002), the incidence was much higher—5% for girls and 15% for boys. ADHD is more commonly diagnosed in boys than girls, with a ratio of 3:1 found in several studies. Confusion around diagnostic criteria and the unique manifestation of symptoms in each child contributes to wide discrepancies in reported incidence.

Attention-Deficit Hyperactivity Disorder and Family Functioning

The effects of ADHD often produce stress in families, day care, and school environments. At home, family functioning and activities of daily living are most disrupted. Parents are often frustrated and exhausted. Frequently, there is increased physical fighting between the child with ADHD and his or her siblings or parents. Tolerance for this aggressive behavior results in the absence of successful family interventions. A cycle develops whereby families minimize the degree of aggression and violence as a coping strategy. Correlational studies indicate that increasing age and severity of ADHD symptoms are associated with more negative effects on family functioning (Robin, 2002). Of course, some families cope better than others.

A family study has identified developmental trajectories for the child with ADHD, the parents, and other family members (Kendall, 1998) and indicates that early interventions are necessary to prevent the escalation of family violence, the deterioration of family functioning, and negative effects on all family members. Even when families appear to be "doing well," parents still report that family life with an ADHD child is frequently a "nightmare" (Shelton, 2001).

Children with Attention-Deficit Hyperactivity Disorder at School

Children with ADHD may be unsuccessful in developing meaningful relationships with peers and other adults. Social interactions at school may involve aggressive behaviors, leading to exclusion from group activities or isolation and withdrawal on the part of the child with ADHD. Developmental tasks of adolescence frequently are negatively affected by ADHD.

The school experience comprises both educational and social aspects. Inattention, distractibility, and hyperactivity can interfere with learning directly by disrupting the child's ability to concentrate and complete work. Indirectly, the social consequences of the disruption produced by ADHD symptoms may alienate and frustrate the child, the teacher, and classmates, which reinforces the cycle of difficulty with learning, low self-esteem, and lack of satisfying friendships.

Assessment

DSM-IV criteria must be met and differential diagnoses ruled out to confirm the diagnosis and to plan treatment for this highly individualized problem. If problems have been identified by different observers and noted since early childhood, ADHD is more likely to be diagnosed. Children who display impulsive and hyperactive behaviors are more likely to be evaluated at a younger age than children who display inattentive and distractible behaviors. The American Academy of Pediatrics (AAP) has published practice guidelines for the diagnosis and treatment of ADHD (AAP Committee on Quality Improvement and Subcommittee on Attention Deficit Hyperactivity Disorder, 2000, 2001).

Proper diagnosis of ADHD is labor intensive and cannot be done adequately in a short office visit. Frequently, during the office visit parents express concerns about ADHD characteristics. Information must then be gathered from other settings, such as school or other structured activities, and a detailed medical, social, and family history is taken from the parents at a follow-up visit. After this information is gathered, the child should be examined, and in some cases referred for further testing by a psychologist, an occupational therapist, or a learning specialist, before a final diagnosis is made. Structured interviews may be helpful in discriminating ADHD from other comorbid conditions.

History. Questioning in a direct and nonjudgmental way often invites children and parents to share sensitive information. DSM-IV criteria for ADHD signs and symptoms are found in Table 17-3. Suggestions for a complete history of the child who may have ADHD are found in Table 17-4. A developmental and functional health pattern is assessed, and a family/social/environmental history is taken.

The history must include assessment of the following:

- Family history: ADHD, neurologic problems, learning difficulties, or psychologic problems
- Birth history: prenatal history, maternal health; use of medications, recreational drugs, alcohol, and tobacco during pregnancy; birth anoxia, difficult delivery, postpartum complications, and postnatal history
- General health history: consider especially neurologic status, vision, hearing, and chronic diseases
- Developmental history: milestones achieved
- Behavioral history: child behavior, parenting methods
- Social/environmental history: stress and family coping

TABLE 17-3 *DSM-IV Criteria for Attention-Deficit Hyperactivity Disorder*

Domain	Criteria
Essential features	Symptoms occur in two or more settings (home, work, school, in public) *and* there is clear evidence of significant impairment in social, school, or work settings Symptoms have persisted for more than 6 mo Symptoms have been present before age 7 yr
Inattention traits	At least *six* of the following symptoms of inattention are present: • Fails to tend to details, makes careless mistakes routinely in work and schoolwork • Has difficulty sustaining attention on a task at work or at play • Does not seem to listen when spoken to • Fails to follow instructions or fails to complete tasks (not due to oppositional behavior or failure to understand instruction) • Has difficulty organizing tasks and activities • Often avoids or puts off tasks requiring sustained mental effort • Often loses things necessary for performing tasks • Is easily distracted by extraneous stimuli • Is often forgetful in daily activities
Hyperactivity/impulsivity traits	At least *six* of the following symptoms of hyperactivity/impulsivity are present: • Often squirms in seat or fidgets with hands or feet • Often leaves seat when remaining in seat is expected • Often runs, climbs, or moves restlessly in situations when it is inappropriate • Often has difficulty playing or enjoying quiet leisure activities • Is often described as "on the go" or "driven" • Often talks excessively • Often answers before question is completed or blurts out answer • Has difficulty taking turns • Often interrupts or intrudes in others' activities

TABLE 17-4 *Attention-Deficit Hyperactivity Disorder History*

Assessment Area	Suggested Topics to Explore
Chief complaint/history of present problem	Major areas of concern First awareness of problem Beliefs about causation of problem Previous evaluations and results Medication history for behavioral, emotional, or learning problems
Birth history*	Prenatal history, maternal health; use of medications, recreational drugs, alcohol, and tobacco during pregnancy Birth anoxia, difficult delivery Postpartum complications, birth defects Neonatal behavior: feeding, sleep, temperament problems
General health*	Neurologic status, vision, hearing, chronic diseases Hospitalizations, prolonged illness Frequent injuries Poisoning or lead or environmental exposures Outbursts of uncontrollable sounds/words

Continued

TABLE 17-4 *Attention-Deficit Hyperactivity Disorder History—cont'd*

Assessment Area	Suggested Topics to Explore
	Tics, habit spasms, uncontrollable twitches Ongoing medications
Attention/hyperactivity symptoms history	Attention: paying attention, sustaining attention, listening, following through, organization, reluctant to engage in activities that need sustained attention, loses things, distracted, forgetful Activity: fidgets, leaves seat, runs/climbs when inappropriate, has difficulty with quiet games, talks excessively, has problems waiting turn, interrupts, "on the go"
Developmental history*	Milestones: motor, personal-social, language, cognitive Strengths (e.g., personality, activities, friendliness) Weaknesses
Behavioral history*	Frequency with which child complies when told to do something Methods used at home to improve behavior and effectiveness Parenting skills training Parental agreement about child management Counseling history for child or family (or both)
Academic history	Child's progress at each grade level Adjustment problems at school Difficulties with specific skills: reading, writing, spelling, math, concepts Performance problems—attention, grades, participation, excessive talking, disturbing others, fighting, abusive language, not completing work School assistance: tutoring, counseling, special help
Functional Health Patterns	
Feeding	Not able to sit through a complete meal Messy and clumsy with utensils, dishes, and glasses Inadequate caloric intake can be result of symptoms and further exacerbated by medications used to treat ADHD Gastric distress may be a side effect of stimulant medication
Sleeping	Difficulty falling asleep, night waking, needs less sleep than other family members Complains about fatigue interfering with completion of tasks
Activity	Difficulty maintaining routines for activities of daily living
Cognitive	Level of performance is below potential for achievement Tends to miss the point of conversations and activities Often does things the hard way in absence of established routines
Self-concept	Struggles with low self-esteem, moodiness
Role relationships	Inadequate social and relational skills Lies, steals, plays with fire, hurts animals, is aggressive with other children, talks back to adults
Coping/stress tolerance	Low tolerance for frustration Outbursts of temper Moody, worried, sad, quiet, destructive, fearful/fearless, self-deprecating Somatic complaints
Social/environmental history*	Family stress and coping patterns Home, day care, and school environments Family social risk factors: recent moves, financial stress, parental job losses, births, deaths, divorces, remarriages, alcohol and drug use, involvement with law enforcement, weapons in the home
Family history*	ADHD, neurologic problems, learning difficulties Mental health history of close family members, health or behavior problems in other family members
Teacher history	Obtain information from school about child's problems, strengths, weaknesses, academic management of issues

*These must be included in the assessment.

Physical Examination. The physical examination should include the following:

- Complete health history and physical examination
- Neurologic examination
- Minor congenital anomalies (e.g., fetal alcohol syndrome features)
- Auditory screening
- Visual screening
- Growth parameters
- Signs of anemia, chronic illness, or allergy

Other Studies. Additional studies may be needed, including the following:

- Neurodevelopmental examination with fine and gross motor skills test
- Brief mental status examination and screening for learning disabilities
- Laboratory work, including tests for anemia and lead, as well as a thyroid screen and levels of anticonvulsants if indicated by history and physical examination
- Behavior checklists completed by parents and teachers (see Table 17-2)
- Psychoeducational tests to identify children with cognitive, language, or visual-spatial-motor problems

It is difficult to diagnose children with ADHD who are younger than 4 years of age when the characteristic features of ADHD may still be age appropriate. Often, the diagnosis is made in young children only when behaviors are extreme.

Differential Diagnosis

Other diagnoses to consider include normal variation; giftedness; language disorder; mental retardation; migraines; lead poisoning; hearing loss; thyroid dysfunction; visual disturbance; genetic disorders such as fragile-X syndrome; seizure disorder; Tourette's syndrome; psychologic disorders such as anxiety, bipolar disorder, oppositional defiant disorder, conduct disorder, posttraumatic stress disorder, or depression; substance abuse; pervasive developmental disorder; environmental disorders (e.g., child abuse, family stress, domestic violence, parenting disruptions, parental psychopathology, inappropriate educational setting); and learning disabilities. Careful differentiation is needed to identify proper pharmacologic and psychotherapeutic interventions (Jensen et al, 2001).

Primary ADHD can exist simultaneously with family situations that predispose children to exhibit behaviors similar to those seen in children with ADHD. With increased evidence that domestic violence, family dysfunction, and child abuse can mimic ADHD, it is important to do an in-depth family assessment to ensure accuracy of the diagnosis and to intervene when domestic violence and child abuse are occurring. Primary ADHD is the only form that is properly treated with medication; therefore it is important to make an accurate diagnosis of ADHD to develop an appropriate management plan.

Primary Attentional or Behavioral Problems. These children have attentional problems that are chronic, permeate most areas of the child's life, and meet the DSM-IV diagnostic criteria (see Table 17-3). ADHD characteristics represent maladaptation and are often not consistent with age-specific developmental expectations. This type of inattention is also associated with concurrent difficulties with planning, self-monitoring, and completing tasks. Medication used to treat ADHD is targeted to this category of attentional problems and works well in about 70% to 80% of children in this group (Greenhill et al, 2001).

Situational Attentional or Behavioral Problems. These problems develop in specific situations and often reflect inappropriate environmental expectations. They do not permeate all settings. Problems with boredom, distractibility, and hyperactivity can be traced or related to family social problems; difficult temperament leading to a poor fit between child, parent, and school; parent-child relational problems; environmental overstimulation; and inappropriate reward systems. These children are still able to accomplish age-specific developmental tasks despite inattention and hyperactivity and do not meet the criteria for an ADHD diagnosis. Stimulant medication is not recommended when attentional or behavioral problems are situational.

Secondary Attentional or Behavioral Problems. These problems result from underlying deficits in cognitive abilities; specific learning disabilities; undetected vision and hearing problems; medical problems such as mild cerebral palsy, seizure disorders, allergies, and asthma; and side effects to medications used for such conditions. The gifted child who is bored may also fit some of the behavioral patterns listed here but should be quickly identified as not having ADHD. Other significant and perhaps undiagnosed emotional problems, including unresolved anger, depression, anxiety, oppositional defiant disorder, conduct disorder, autism, and abuse, may exist. These children do not meet the DSM-IV criteria for ADHD and should be diagnosed according to their other diagnostic features.

Comorbidity

A number of children with ADHD also have a concurrent diagnosis for learning disabilities (35%) or a psychiatric disorder such as anxiety (25%), depression (25%), oppositional defiant disorder, or conduct disorder (50%). A mental health specialist should evaluate children for comorbid conditions. The management of ADHD needs to include strategies for prioritizing needs and interventions in concert with these other conditions. If more than one health care provider is involved because of comorbid conditions, the NP may serve as case manager to keep family members and other health care professionals informed and to coordinate treatment plans and services.

Management

The clinical practice guideline (AAP Committee on Quality Improvement and Subcommittee on Attention Deficit Hyperactivity Disorder, 2001) provides the rationale and strategies for careful management of children with ADHD. It acknowledges the lack of in-depth education on ADHD that primary care providers may have and stresses the importance of continuing education in this area. A toolkit was developed and is available from AAP to assist primary care providers in the diagnosis and management of ADHD in an office practice. The AAP guideline stresses the importance of regular monitoring, and it suggests that monitoring should be focused on specific outcomes and that information regarding these outcomes be regularly obtained from parents, the child, and teachers (Stein, 2002). See Fig. 17-2 for the AAP algorithm.

Medication. Stimulant medication is often the most effective intervention. Medications should be used in conjunction with behavioral, family, cognitive-behavioral, and other interventions (Table 17-5). The landmark MTA Cooperative Group study (1999) has supported the use of medications and behavioral therapy.

Methylphenidate and amphetamines are the most commonly used drugs for treating children with ADHD (Kratochvil, 2003; Wender, 2001). In response to the AAP clinical practice guideline (AAP Committee on Quality Improvement and Subcommittee on Attention Deficit Hyperactivity Disorder, 2001), journals are providing excellent continuing education about medication management (Adesman, 2002; Wender, 2001, 2002). New formulations of these two basic classes of medications are now available and provide more flexibility and individual tailoring of medications for children and adolescents. Stimulants have been shown to increase attention span, gross and fine motor coordination, and compliance while decreasing impulsiveness, hyperactivity, and aggression.

Both short- and long-acting medications are available. The short-acting forms provide greater flexibility to maximize positive behaviors at important times of the day. Usually, they are given at breakfast and again at lunch. The long-acting forms last 6 to 8 hours, getting a child through the school day. The potencies may differ between the two forms. Some families mix the forms, giving, for instance, the long-acting form for the day and then a short-acting dose to last until bedtime (Adesman, 2002; Wender, 2001, 2002).

Careful monitoring of children on medications for ADHD is necessary to minimize side effects. Antidepressants, stimulants, and allergy and asthma medications (especially over-the-counter preparations) should not be taken simultaneously without proper education; moreover, physicians should prescribe each medication with awareness of the other drugs the patient is taking. All medications for acute illnesses should be prescribed only with full knowledge of potential interactions with medications for ADHD and concurrent problems.

It is common for medication regimens to need periodic adjustment or complete change as the child grows. Increase in body weight or other medical conditions requiring medication may indicate the need to reassess the medication plan for ADHD. Social and emotional maturation may decrease or eliminate the need for medication in late childhood and adolescence. Changes in family or school schedules may necessitate a long-acting preparation or an adjustment in the timing of doses. For example, once a medication regimen has been established in early elementary grades, the plan may be successful for several years. As the child approaches middle school, the symptoms of greatest concern to the school and family may have changed or the child may decide he or she no longer wants to take medication.

- Ask the parents and the child at regular intervals about how the medication is working and if they perceive a need to make adjustments.
- Assess the need to adjust medication at the beginning of each school year and at times when major changes are occurring in the family that affect the family system (e.g., births, deaths, divorces, remarriages, residential moves, death of pets, significant illness or injury).

The new drug atomoxetine (Strattera) is a nonstimulant drug that may be used as a first-line medication. Other nonstimulant medications may help children who respond poorly to an adequate trial of stimulants. This may be due to their comorbid conditions. These medications are used cautiously because some are not yet approved by the Food and Drug Administration (FDA) for these uses, but controlled studies and clinical data support their trial. Tricyclic antidepressants, including imipramine, desipramine, and nortriptyline, are used. Bupropion is an antidepressant that has been used. Antihypertensives, such as clonidine and guanfacine, have also been used (Adesman, 2002).

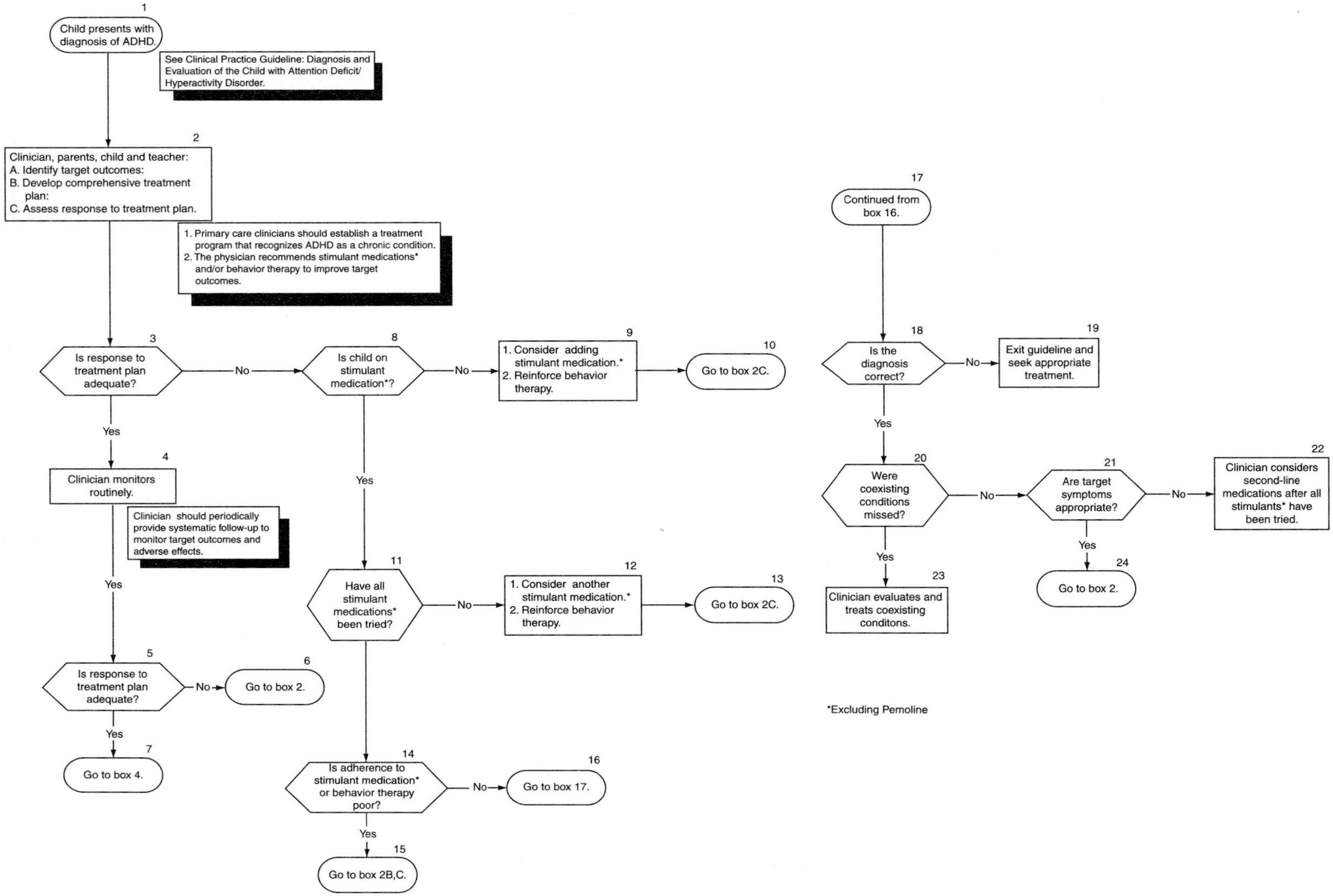

FIGURE 17-2 Algorithm for the treatment of the school-age child with attention-deficit hyperactivity disorder. (From American Academy of Pediatrics: Clinical practice guideline: treatment of the school-aged child with attention-deficit/hyperactivity disorder, *Pediatrics* 108:1035, 2001.)

TABLE 17-5 *Medications Used to Manage ADHD Symptoms*

Medication	Side Effects	Monitor	Comments
Stimulants			
Methylphenidate (Ritalin, Metadate CD Concerta, Ritalin LA)	Anorexia, insomnia, stomachache, headache, irritability, "rebound," flattened affect, social withdrawal, crying, tics, weight loss, reduced growth rate	Height, weight, blood pressure, pulse	Do not chew or cut sustained-release tablets in half Avoid decongestants
Dextroamphetamine (Dexedrine, Dextrostat)	Anorexia, insomnia, stomachache, headache, irritability, "rebound," tics, stereopathy, weight loss, reduced growth rate	Height, weight, blood pressure, pulse	Avoid decongestants Risk of abuse
Four mixed amphetamine salts (Adderall, Adderall XR)	Same as dextroamphetamine		8-10 hr effect Tablet can be split Potential for abuse
Nonstimulants (Not Approved by FDA for ADHD Use)			
Imipramine (Tofranil)	Constipation, fatigue, stomach upset, dry mouth, blurry vision, dizziness, tachycardia	Baseline ECG ECG and blood level with dose change Blood pressure, pulse	May affect cardiac conduction rate Increased levels with methylphenidate Use with ADHD-related tics, enuresis, anxiety
Desipramine (Norpramin)	Tachycardia, dizziness, fatigue, stomach upset, dry mouth, blurry vision, constipation	Baseline ECG ECG and blood level with dose change Blood pressure, pulse	May affect cardiac conduction rate Increased levels with methylphenidate Use with ADHD-related tics, enuresis, anxiety
Nortriptyline (Pamelor)	Dry mouth, constipation, weight gain	Baseline ECG ECG and blood level at steady state Blood pressure, pulse	Use with ADHD-related tics, enuresis, anxiety
Bupropion (Wellbutrin)	Agitation, dry mouth, insomnia, headache, nausea, constipation, tremor		Lowers seizure threshold Contraindicated in patients with eating disorders or tics
Clonidine (Catapres)	Sedation, dizziness, nausea, orthostatic hypotension, clinical major depression, nightmares	Blood pressure at baseline, after dose adjustment and follow-up	Sedation decreases over time Rebound hypertension if stopped abruptly Not first-line agent
Guanfacine (Tenex)	Sedation, dizziness, nausea, orthostatic hypotension, insomnia, agitation, headache, stomachache	Blood pressure at baseline, after dose adjustment and follow-up	Not first-line agent
Atomoxetine (Strattera)	Slight diastolic blood pressure and heart rate increase	Weight decreases significantly in first 9-12 wk, then expect catch-up and parallel growth curve	Nonstimulant, nonadrenergic mechanism Twice-daily dosing Superior to placebo at 1.2 to 1.8 mg/day Once-daily dosing may be effective

ADHD, Attention-deficit hyperactivity disorder; *ECG*, electrocardiogram; *FDA*, Food and Drug Administration.

Family Education about Diagnosis. Families need to be well educated about the disorder because a large part of the treatment for ADHD involves parent-management techniques. The chronic nature of ADHD has a tremendous impact on family functioning. Conversely, family factors play a part in the outcomes for children with ADHD. Parents often have to educate others about the special needs of their child. Because children with ADHD manifest a great variety of behaviors, parents become the experts who ultimately manage the problems and affect the outcome for their child.

Family education must be ongoing and reflect the developmental maturation of the child and unique expression of ADHD within each child and family. When the diagnosis is shared with parents, it is best to arrange for adequate time to educate families about ADHD, parenting strategies, community resources, and medication management. Parents are better able to pay attention to this information when the child is not present in the room; it is helpful if parents arrange a separate appointment for this discussion or bring a family helper to stay with the child in the waiting area. Educational needs at the time of diagnosis usually emphasize the broad scope of ADHD and address the parents' most pressing concerns. As parents and children adjust to the progression of this condition, their needs for education become more individualized to reflect the particular needs of the family. In addition, features of ADHD appear differently in early and middle childhood and adolescence. Parents and the children themselves need periodic assessment to ascertain which developmental tasks are being met and how education and support to accomplish those tasks should be focused.

Another perplexing but predictable situation arises when behavioral modifications that have worked for a period of time seem to become ineffective. Education about how normal growth and development interacts with the symptoms of ADHD should be updated as children move through developmental stages.

- Designate at least one visit (or more) per year to assess developmental milestones, acknowledge gains in skills and abilities, and plan strategies with the family to address any developmental lags.
- Routinely ask how the child's behavior is affecting the family. Plan with the family how to address the needs of the child with ADHD without eclipsing the needs of other family members.
- Routinely ask about significant changes within the family that may affect general family functioning. Individualize behavioral modifications for all family members to facilitate adjustment to changes within the family.

Family Support. Support is necessary initially to help parents understand the complexity of the diagnosis, to deal with feelings of shock or confusion, and to cope with guilt. The diagnosis of a child is often the first clue to the eventual diagnosis of an older sibling or a parent who is experiencing similar difficulties. National support groups with local affiliates can offer understanding and specific expertise in managing daily problems that come from living with the diagnosis (see Resource Box). Support groups are often helpful around the time of the initial diagnosis. Many families use support services initially and then discontinue attending. Families need to know that they may return to such groups during times of increased stress as children move through developmental stages or other family stressors appear. Family therapy is sometimes useful and is frequently used for short terms with goals specific to the family's current situation.

- Periodically assess the need for family support.
- Ask families if there is aggressive behavior toward family members.
- Encourage family members to offer support to other families experiencing ADHD.
- Make referrals to professionals who are experienced with clients who have ADHD and their families.

Nutrition. Monthly height, weight, body mass index, and blood pressure checks may be needed to monitor growth and potential weight loss as side effects of stimulant medications. When possible, give the morning dose before breakfast. Saltines offered with the morning dose of stimulant medication can decrease complaints of stomachaches. Providing instant breakfast drinks to supplement calories when the child has low calorie intake because of difficulty sitting through meals may be helpful.

Ask the child about his or her favorite foods and level of appetite. Diet therapy has not proven to be effective, and ADHD children should not be put on special diets. Efforts to control the child's diet can put strains on the family. Guilt can result when inevitable indiscretions occur. If the whole family goes on the diet, some members may become resentful of the affected child. Further, once the child enters school, it is very difficult for the family to fully control the child's diet.

Sleep. Many children and adults with ADHD do not require as much sleep as other people. Sleep problems should be addressed in a comprehensive assessment and a parent training program. Ritualized bedtime routines are important to ADHD families; detailed instruction in massage, deep breathing, and relaxation techniques is sometimes helpful. It is necessary to ascertain the safety of children with ADHD who remain awake after other family members go to bed. Sleepwalking and night prowling sometimes cause safety concerns and should be addressed.

- Periodically ask if the child is sleeping well and staying in bed the entire night. Determine whether a safety plan is needed for night prowling.

Individual Educational Plan. When ADHD affects a student's academic performance, schools have a role in the management of ADHD (Hannah, 2002). Individual educational plans (IEPs) are usually necessary for ADHD children. Special accommodations at school are provided by the reauthorization of the Individuals with Disabilities Education Act (IDEA). These plans should always include academic learning objectives, as well as behavior modification objectives. NPs who are familiar with state and federal laws and local educational resources can guide parents as they work with the school to develop the child's plan.

Frustration is common in ADHD students, their families, and school personnel. Inform parents that special assessments and evaluations can take 6 to 8 months of a school year, and children may be without special services during this entire time. IEP objectives are written in educational terms and may need to be restated in behavioral terms that children, parents, and classroom teachers can readily understand and implement. A helpful suggestion for parents is to ask that they be given a list of who is responsible for each aspect of the IEP. This spells out what is expected of the parents and individual teachers over the course of the year. Midterm or midyear monitoring of the IEP objectives is advised. A case manager may be helpful for children and adolescents who are not succeeding in school by the first grading period of each school year. School nurses and NPs in clinical settings often are well positioned to coordinate the medical, behavioral, and educational needs of children with ADHD.

- Ask parents what the IEP objectives are for the current school year and if they understand and support them. Help them identify whom to contact for clarification.
- Make sure that medication slips required by schools are completed and available at the time prescriptions are renewed. This simple office routine can provide significant help to parents and schools. Keep in mind that learning and language problems can coexist with ADHD. Therefore psychoeducational testing is essential to develop an appropriate educational plan. (Box 17-1 provides suggestions for classroom adaptations.)
- Routinely ask if there are any problems when a child must take medication at school.

Psychologic Interventions. The MTA Cooperative Group study (1999) supports behavioral therapy along with medications. Social skills training and cognitive-behavioral training are helpful when social skills deficits exist. However, recent reconceptualizations of ADHD suggest that this disorder is not caused by lack of knowing what behavior is appropriate, but by lack of ability to act on what is known. In addition, counseling may help with problems related to anxiety, self-esteem, and depression.

Children with ADHD may be overwhelmed by the number of adults involved with managing their symptoms. When this situation occurs, professionals should prioritize treatment recommendations in the following ways:

- Ask parents whether there is confusion or conflict about the management strategies of the professionals involved with their child to determine the best way to address these problems.
- Ask about daily and weekly schedules to determine whether the child has plenty of time for normal activities of childhood, including time to do nothing and daydream.
- Periodically assess the child and adolescent for anxiety or depression. Ask if other family members are in need of psychologic assessment or support.

Advocacy. Families often need assistance in accessing educational services. Primary care providers are often in a position to exercise some influence in the local schools when services are not forthcoming. Some NPs specialize in the care and support of ADHD children and families. Those who monitor medications and provide family support should undertake these tasks only with adequate knowledge and experience and the availability of consultation with ADHD experts.

Case Management Issues. NPs may be in a unique position to offer case management services to ADHD families. Coordination of medical supervision, school programs, and family therapy or parent training programs is necessary for families to manage ADHD successfully.

- Ask whether the family thinks that the efforts to manage their child's ADHD are coordinated.

Complications

Children with ADHD can develop depression, problems with self-esteem, and failure to meet school educational expectations secondary to their attention and hyperactivity problems. Medication interactions and side effects are also potential complications for children with ADHD. Children with concurrent diagnoses of emotional disorders and chronic illness are at greatest risk for complications involving medication interactions. Often, different physicians prescribe medications; side effects can be missed because they mimic symptoms already present in a confusing and complicated disorder.

BOX 17-1 *Suggestions for Classroom Adaptations for Children with Attention-Deficit Hyperactivity Disorder*

Memory and Attention

- Seat the child close to the teacher
- Keep oral instructions brief with repetitions
- Provide written directions
- "Walk" the child through assignments to be sure they are understood
- Break tasks and homework into small tasks
- Use visual aids
- Teach active reading with underlining and active listening with note taking
- Provide remedial help in small sessions
- Teach subvocalization to aid memorizing

Impulse Control

- Remind the child to slow down
- Teach the child to monitor quality of work before turning it in

Classroom Atmosphere

- Provide a structured classroom with clear expectations
- Use moderate, consistent discipline
- Rely on positive reinforcement for good behavior

Organizational Skills

- Establish a daily checklist of tasks
- List homework assignments in a special notebook with the due date and needed resources
- Follow up on homework not turned in

Productivity Problems

- Divide work sheets into sections
- Reduce the amount of homework and written classwork
- Cut down on the number of math problems to be completed

Written Expression

- Give extra time to complete written tests and assignments
- Provide help with handwriting
- Allow child to dictate reports and take tests orally
- Reduce the quantity of written work required
- Do not reduce grades for untidy work, spelling errors, poor handwriting

Self-Esteem

- Reward progress
- Encourage performance in areas of child's strength
- Avoid humiliation
- Give hand signals only the child can see as private reminders of appropriate behavior

Social Relationships

- Provide feedback about behavior involving other children
- Make sure other children do not feel that the child with ADHD is doing less or allowed unacceptable behavior; change the rules for all children, if necessary

Adapted from Baren M: Managing ADHD, *Contemp Pediatr* 11:33, 1994.

A cumulative effect can be seen when relationships at home, school, and in the community deteriorate, putting the child or adolescent with ADHD at risk for engaging in delinquent or socially unacceptable behaviors. High school dropout rates for adolescents with ADHD are significantly higher than those in the general population, as are rates for juvenile offenses, underemployment, and imprisonment in adulthood (Goldstein, 1997; Rasmussen, Almvik, & Levander, 2001).

Learning Disorders

Description

Learning disorders, or learning disabilities as psychologists prefer, are diagnosed when an individual's achievements on individually administered standardized tests in reading, writing, or mathematics are below the expected performance based on age, education, and intelligence level (Gottesman & Kelly, 2000).

A group of disorders characterized as learning disorders share the following factors:

- The disorders are manifested by significant difficulties in acquiring and using listening, speaking, reading, writing, reasoning, and mathematic skills.
- The problems are always present in the individual and are assumed to be caused by central nervous system dysfunction.
- The disorders may occur with other handicapping conditions such as sensory impairment, mental retardation, or emotional disturbance; cultural differences; or educational deficits, but not resulting from those conditions or influences.

Etiology and Incidence

Learning disorders may result from a variety of genetic, constitutional, or neurodevelopmental factors. Any factor that disrupts central nervous system function may result in a learning disorder. The incidence is thought be 10% to 15% of the population.

Clinical Findings

Language processing, visual and auditory processing, memory, motor coordination, and spatial and temporal orientation difficulties are hallmarks of the condition, although a given child will probably not have difficulties in all areas.

- Reading: difficulty decoding unfamiliar words, poor comprehension and retention, slow reading rate
- Mathematics: difficulty remembering number facts, solving practical problems
- Writing: poor and labored handwriting, faulty spelling, grammar and syntax errors

Assessment

The assessment is much as for children with ADHD. It will include identification of risk factors, observation for characteristics of learning disorders, and consideration of other causes for the learning problems.

History

- Parent interview:
  - Functioning at home versus school
  - Coping with school
  - Birth and past medical history for risk factors
  - Developmental history
  - Family history of learning problems and level of academic achievement
  - Ability to attend to and complete tasks
  - Strengths and weaknesses of the child
  - Psychologic/behavioral/stress responses to the problems
- School review:
  - Teacher's report of academic performance, behavioral information
  - Any academic test results
- Patient assessment:
  - Child's description of the problems
  - Child's perception of the cause of the problems
  - Child's experiences at school with teachers, peers, homework

Physical Examination

- Behavioral observations
- Hearing and vision evaluation
- Physical examination, especially for neurologic problems

Differential Diagnosis

Visual or hearing problem, school absence, environmental deprivation in preschool, ADHD, mental retardation, and emotional disturbance are included in the differential diagnosis.

Management

- *Educational:* In 1997 the IDEA mandated that all public schools assess and educate children with learning disabilities. The school should have a multidisciplinary team available to evaluate the child's needs and develop an IEP. The team should include a school psychologist, an educator, a special educator, a social worker, and a language specialist.
- *Parent support:* Community agencies and national organizations can provide assistance and support (see Resource Box). Parents may also need advocacy help and sometimes legal help.
- *Assistive technologies:* Read-aloud devices from text and computer programs to help remediate deficiencies may

be helpful. Calculators and word processors may help circumvent handwriting problems.

Deafness

Description

Deafness as a cognitive-perceptual problem is discussed here. Other information related to hearing screening and ear problems is found in Chapter 30. Deafness is classified as conductive or sensorineural. Conductive deafness is caused by a mechanical interruption of the sound waves from the external ear to the inner ear. It can sometimes be corrected through medical or surgical management. Hearing aids can be useful in assisting transmission of sound waves. Sensorineural deafness indicates inability of the inner ear or nerve to respond to sound waves. Sensorineural deafness can involve some frequencies more than others, resulting in a distortion of sound that is not helped by amplification. Central deafness is the least common hearing condition seen in children and is a problem between the brainstem and cortex in which sounds are heard but not understood. Mixed types also occur.

Etiology and Incidence

Deafness is categorized as profound, severe, or less than severe. Profound deafness is deafness in which only sounds higher than 90 dB are perceived (41% of deaf children). Severe deafness is deafness to sounds 71 to 90 dB (19% of deaf children). Less than severe deafness is deafness to sounds less than 71 dB (33% of deaf children). The prevalence rate of newborns and infants with profound hearing loss is estimated to range between 1 and 3 per 1000 live births (AAP, 1999; Van Naarden, Decouflé, & Caldwell, 1999).

Conductive deafness results from damage, inflammation, obstruction, or malformation of the outer or middle ear, or a combination of these. Sensorineural hearing loss is caused by damage or malformation of the inner ear or auditory nerve and accounts for 90% of all cases of serious and profound hearing loss in children (Van Naarden, Decouflé, & Caldwell, 1999). Heredity, encephalitis, intrauterine infections, exposure to loud noise, ototoxic drugs, and premature birth with anoxia, severe jaundice, or intraventricular hemorrhage are also causes of both conductive and sensorineural hearing loss. Syndromes involving renal, cardiac, musculoskeletal, dermatologic, neurologic, and ophthalmologic systems can include deafness. Approximately 30% of prelingual deafness is related to a genetic syndrome (Jeng & Robin, 2002).

Assessment

The AAP (1999) recommends universal hearing screening of all neonates. Methods may include evoked otoacoustic emissions (EOAE) and auditory brainstem response (ABR), either alone or in combination (Thompson et al, 2001). Because infants and toddlers are treated by health care professionals on multiple occasions, there are many opportunities for screening and paying close attention to parental concerns about their child's hearing. Early identification and intervention in children with hearing impairments significantly affects the child's development, language acquisition, and academic achievement.

- For children with possible deafness, the NP should do a thorough assessment as described in Chapter 30 for hearing loss.
- A variety of hearing tests are described in Chapter 30.
- Vision screening should be done because deaf persons need good sight. Also, Usher syndrome, which includes deafness and later retinitis pigmentosa, may need to be identified.
- Development needs to be monitored regularly, especially in linguistic and cognitive areas.

Differential Diagnosis

Cerumen impaction, otitis media with effusion, and chronic suppurative otitis media with perforation of tympanic membrane are differential diagnoses. Consider tumor with sensorineural loss. For the child with significant hearing loss, comorbidities may exist, including developmental and communication problems, family disruptions, depression, genetic disorders, and others.

Management

Multidisciplinary Team. The use of a multidisciplinary team working with the family provides the best support for the child with a hearing impairment. The team should include a primary care provider, a physician, an audiologist, a speech and language pathologist, a sign language specialist, a teacher of the deaf, and others as needed. From an information-processing perspective, much of the management of the deaf child is directed at providing stimuli that the infant and child can use to understand and interact with the environment. Visual stimuli are used as the primary substitute for auditory deficits. Language serves not only as a communication device but also as a system for storing and using information.

Amplification Devices and Their Care. Identification and amplification before 6 months makes a significant improvement in speech and language abilities of hearing-impaired children (Behrman, Kliegman, & Jenson, 2004). Different types of hearing aids have different purposes. The body box is used for children younger than 3 years of age and for those in need of more powerful or durable amplification. Postauricular devices are used for older children. Ear molds need a good fit (sometimes revised every 3 to 6 months with growth) and careful cleaning to avoid clogging. By ages 4 to 6 years, ear molds are changed yearly. Batteries last only about 100 to 150 hours and are toxic if ingested.

External otitis media can be avoided with use of petroleum jelly to decrease friction and adjustment of molds to reduce irritation. Ear molds should be washed with soap and water each night. If an infection occurs, it can usually be managed by using an antibiotic ointment and leaving the molds out for 1 to 2 days. For fungal infections, antifungal drops should be used and molds left out for 3 to 5 days.

Cochlear implants are used with some children who will not benefit from traditional hearing aids. They help children access some sounds in the environment, but positive outcomes involve multidisciplinary teams of specialists (Arts, Garber, & Zwolan, 2002).

Communication Needs. Communication needs can be supported by the use of text telephone devices, smoke alarms and doorbells with lights instead of alarms, a hearing ear dog, and other communication systems in the child's environment.

Family Support. Often there is stress for the family when the diagnosis is made. Siblings may need support as they cope in a family with a child identified as having a disabling condition (Bat-Chava & Martin, 2002). Parents often need counseling, support, and information related to their acceptance and parenting of the identified child. Grandparents and extended family can also need information and support.

Children with hearing impairments are at higher risk than the general population for child maltreatment and neglect (Sullivan & Knutson, 1998). The most prevalent form of maltreatment among deaf children is child neglect (Sullivan, Brookhouser, & Scanlan, 2000). Children with hearing impairments often demonstrate more behavior problems than their peers and need mental health services with professionals experienced in treating children with disabilities. Periodic screening for family stress and child maltreatment is an important part of well-child care.

Education. Children identified with hearing loss by 6 months of age who received early intervention services had better language development than children identified later (Yoshinaga-Itano et al, 1998). Deaf children need opportunities to learn by using their strongest modalities. Language and communication needs are paramount. There are several schools of thought related to education of the deaf. Oralists focus on amplification, speech reading, and speech training. They do not support exposure to sign language. Those who believe in the total communication approach counter that the use of sign language links the deaf to the deaf community and increases their acquisition of language and functioning in adulthood. Total communication methods include amplification, sign language, finger spelling, speech reading, and speech training. Parents are sometimes pressured by professionals or other deaf people to accept one approach over the other.

Parents also need education to communicate with their child effectively. One study indicates that two thirds of children learn sign language, but only one half of parents learn the same language. Lederberg and Everhart (1998) found that mothers of deaf 2-year-olds primarily communicated with their children by speech, even though the children did not visually attend. Thus, in some families, parents and children cannot fully communicate with one another. Early education for deaf children should begin in infancy. Educational services need to be family centered and culturally sensitive. American Sign Language (ASL) is the language the deaf use with one another, and it provides the strongest link with the deaf community for the child.

Interpreter Services. If children sign, they should be provided with an interpreter during health care visits. Deaf children may have inadequate health care information and knowledge because of poor communication between provider and child.

Genetic Counseling. Refer families for genetic counseling if the problem is inheritable.

Blindness

Description

Blindness varies from inability to distinguish light from darkness to *partial vision*, defined as visual acuity between 20/70 and 20/200 best corrected. *Legal blindness* is defined as distant visual acuity of 20/200 in the better eye or a visual field that includes an angle not greater than 20 degrees.

Children with visual impairments experience developmental delays. Table 17-1 shows a summary of milestones to be expected.

Etiology and Incidence

Blindness is caused by a variety of pathologic conditions, including congenital cataracts, congenital glaucoma, high refractive errors, retinopathy of prematurity (ROP), detached retina, neurologic conditions involving cranial nerve II, cortical blindness, and optic atrophy. ROP is the most common cause of severe visual impairment. Retinoblastoma, trauma, infection, hydrocephaly, and genetic conditions are also etiologic factors.

About 1 in 500 children in the United States has partial vision, whereas about 35,000 children are legally blind (Behrman, Kliegman, & Jenson, 2004). Up to 30% to 70% of visually handicapped children have additional handicaps, including mental retardation, deafness, seizures, and cerebral palsy (Mervis, Yeargin-Allsopp, & Winter, 2000).

Assessment

Primary care providers need to remember that the blind child needs special cues to understand the environment. Talk softly to the infant or child before touching and look for a variety of body cues rather than visual or facial signals. Be gentle in touching because the child has no warning that contact is coming. For older children, address the child by name, describe what you plan to do and how, warn the child of contacts or discomforts anticipated, and let the child touch or examine instruments when possible.

Signs and Symptoms of Blindness. Characteristics to assess include the following:

- History of failure of the infant to follow a moving object, or wandering eyes
- Poking the eyes or waving the hands in front of the face
- Nystagmus
- Failure to blink at a camera flash in front of the face
- Failure to fix and follow by 6 weeks
- Photophobia or chronic tearing
- History of prematurity with diagnosis of ROP
- Fixed strabismus or intermittent strabismus persisting longer than 6 months
- Lack of smiling in response to visual stimuli

The following should also be assessed:

- Family history of genetic visual impairments
- Family issues and environment
- General medical history
- Developmental history (attachment, midline play, reaching, gross motor skills, language skills)

Physical Examination. The physical examination should include a search for the following:

- Enlarged or cloudy cornea
- Abnormal or absent red reflex
- Lack of pupillary reflex
- Nystagmus
- Neurologic disorder

Other Tests. An ophthalmologic examination and developmental testing are also done.

Differential Diagnosis

See the etiologic factors discussed earlier.

Management

Multidisciplinary Team. The primary care provider, ophthalmologist, special certification teacher, and orientation and mobility specialist are among the important team members for visually impaired children and their families. Genetics counselors, social workers, and other specialists can also be useful.

Family Support. As noted, families with blind children adapt in a variety of ways. Because visual cues are so important in language and social interactions, the family of the blind child may experience difficulties with attachment resulting from failure of eye contact and facial expressiveness. For instance, smiling is not recognized or imitated by the blind infant. Families of children with visual impairment may benefit from specialized anticipatory guidance designed to facilitate development throughout childhood.

Parent support groups are valuable, and national organizations provide reading materials that are very helpful (see Resource Box). Sometimes families benefit from counseling.

Education. Public school educational programs for the visually impaired child include several distinct models. Infant early education and developmental preschool programs are essential. When children are ready to enter elementary school, full-time classes for blind children are sometimes available. These are taught by teachers with special certification to work with the blind. Some schools have resource-room programs where the child spends part of the day with a specially trained teacher, and the remainder of the day in a regular classroom. Some school districts provide itinerant programs in which a specially trained teacher works with several teachers in regular classrooms, consulting with them about the learning needs of the visually handicapped children involved. Schools for the blind are generally reserved for children with multiple handicaps.

IEPs need to be developed annually, with input from both parents and school officials. When the child enters school, psychologic assessments need to be done using tests designed for blind children to ensure correct educational placement and appropriate educational support systems.

Educational programs for visually handicapped children need to include some extra components. Blind children begin learning Braille when sighted children learn to read. They learn to write Braille in the early elementary grades by using a special typewriter. By fourth grade, blind children should also learn to use a regular typewriter. Developing additional listening skills and gaining proficiency in the use of computers with aids are also essential skills. The Optacon is a handheld device that translates printed text into tactile displays. Children are ready to use this device at about 10 years of age. The ViewScan can be used by partially sighted individuals to enlarge type size for reading text on a screen.

Daily living skills include dressing, eating, hygiene, use of the telephone, and handling money. An orientation and mobility specialist teaches the visually handicapped child to travel with a sighted guide, use a cane, and use public transportation.

Physical education and fitness are as important to visually impaired children as to other children. Generally, individual sports, such as gymnastics and swimming, are more successful endeavors for a blind child than team sports, even if the child is partially sighted.

Developmental Interventions. Some strategies that parents can use to promote development in their visually impaired infant or child are found in Table 17-6.

Autism, Autistic Spectrum Disorder, Asperger Syndrome, Pervasive Developmental Disorders

Description

Autism is a lifelong disability that usually becomes apparent in the first 3 years of life. Communication and social interactions are impaired. Development is uneven, with occasional talent in a limited area such as music or mathematics coupled with severe deficits in other areas. Many autistic children have other impairments, such as mental retardation (70%) or seizures. The disorder varies considerably in severity (Tanguay, 2000).

Most children with autism have the following characteristics:

- Disturbances in development of physical, social, and language skills
- Abnormal responses to sensory stimuli, usually sound; abnormal sensory responses to pain, heat, and cold; tendency to taste and smell objects
- Restricted and repetitive patterns of behavior
- Speech, language, and nonverbal communication disturbances (the child may talk but have difficulty communicating; e.g., speech may be echolalic)
- Abnormal ways of relating to people, objects, and events
- Sleep disturbances (common among children with autism)

Milder forms of autistic spectrum disorder (ASD) are Asperger syndrome and pervasive developmental disorder—not otherwise specified (pdd-nos). Asperger syndrome consists of qualitative impairments in development of social interactions. Language is not as severely impaired as it is with autism. Clinical findings include repetitive movements and restricted obsessional interests. The person with Asperger syndrome may appear "eccentric" to others. Whether this condition is a distinct diagnosis or a milder form of autism with higher functioning has not been determined (Behrman, Kliegman, & Jenson, 2004). See Box 17-2 for "red flags" for autism screening.

Incidence and Etiology

The incidence rate for autism is about 1:1000 children (AAP Committee on Children with Disabilities, 2001). It is four times more likely to occur in male children. There is good evidence of a genetic link for some types of autism (10%). Other causes include prenatal infections, such as congenital rubella or cytomegalovirus, as well as neonatal infections. The etiology is unknown for most cases. A hypothesized relationship with measles-mumps-rubella (MMR) vaccine has not been supported (AAP Committee on Children with Disabilities, 2001).

Assessment

Fewer than 10% of children are diagnosed when behavior difficulties are first addressed by health care professionals and most families report little help after multiple visits (Report of the Quality Standards Subcommittee, 2000).

Infants. An autistic infant may be a passive, nonengaging, quiet, floppy infant or a difficult, colicky, stiff baby with poor eye contact. Attachment problems appear. There is failure to respond to name or gestures. Usually, autism is not identified in infancy.

Toddlers. During the toddler stage, parents are convinced that something is wrong with their child. Language delays, lack of social relatedness, and severe behavior problems are common. Expressive language is delayed. Socially, the child exhibits detachment, decreased eye contact, a lack of fear, and poor creative play skills. Tantrums that persist; repetitive movements; a preference to line, stack, or spin toys; and insistence on routines are commonly observed behaviors. Use of echolalia is persistent.

Preschoolers. Language delays include lack of meaningful speech, decreased gestures, and gaze disturbances. Social interaction disturbances, such as lack of fear of strangers, invasion of the territory of others, preference to be alone, and lack of social awareness, are often seen. Persistent and insistent behaviors are common. Symbolic play is limited. The child may have precocious or average development of rote memory skills but often without comprehension of concepts.

School-Age Children. School-age children with autism often lack reciprocal friendships and continue with language, social, and behavioral problems. Transitions from place to place and activity to activity are difficult. Behaviors are ritualistic.

Adolescents. Adolescents usually continue with similar behaviors. Rote learning is possible, but comprehension lags. It should be noted, however, that some high-functioning autistic children are mainstreamed and do very well in

TABLE 17-6 ***Developmental Interventions for Visually Impaired Infants and Children***

Age	Psychosocial	Cognitive	Motor
Birth-4 mo	Hold and talk to the infant to promote recognition through tactile and auditory modalities.	Stimulate the hands and mouth. Provide a cradle gym so that reaching and touching give feedback. Provide toys with feedback such as sound, interesting textures, or tastes.	Encourage the prone position at times while awake, a position that blind children do not generally like, because they have no reinforcement visually for lifting the head. Also encourage head turning. Bring the hands into midline. Exercise the legs and massage during baths and diaper changes. Put bells on booties.
5-8 mo	Stranger anxiety occurs early. Parents need to be available. Provide predictable routines.	Provide finger foods. Provide new temperatures, textures, toys with various sounds and sensations. Talk to the child. Call attention to music and other sounds in the environment.	Encourage play out of doors and on the floor. Dance and move the child actively.
9-12 mo	Provide routines that are predictable. Touch and voice are all-important. Cuddle.	Encourage reaching to find a sound source. Provide toys that respond to the actions of the child to develop cause-and-effect concepts. Name and describe the activities and items in the environment.	Encourage creeping about, which will occur after the child can reach for a sound. Help to stand and cruise. Touch and name body parts.
13-24 mo	Stranger anxiety continues. Reassure toddler of return. Regression and tantrums are frustration responses. Guide behavior into more appropriate responses. Reduce frustrations when possible.	Continue to work on object permanence concept, which is delayed. Noncontingent sounds such as television or radio are not helpful.	Walking should begin. Crab walking is a common problem that needs to be eliminated. Walking with the child's feet on the adult's can help develop the reciprocal pattern. "Blindisms" may appear and can be altered with teaching. Walk together both indoors and outdoors.
2-5 yr	Interactions with peers and sighted children. Establish behavioral limits as with sighted children. Teach self-help skills—hygiene, feeding, dressing.	Teach games with directional concepts. Provide experiences in a variety of settings—park, grocery, etc.	Develop motor skills—walking, climbing, swimming.
6-10 yr	Continue to develop social skills and develop self-esteem through opportunities to be successful in activities. Provide opportunities to be with other children. Continue to develop self-help skills.	School with additional supports for the visually impaired. Braille and computer education.	Specific mobility training.

Data from Lewis V: *Development and disability*, Philadelphia, 2003, Blackwell; Teplin S: Visual handicaps. In Green M, Haggerty R, editors: *Ambulatory pediatrics*, Philadelphia, 1999, WB Saunders.

BOX 17-2 *Red Flags for Autism Screening*

- Failure to meet childhood developmental milestones
- Sibling with autism
- Problems with eye contact
- Child does not respond to his or her name
- Not babbling or gesturing by 12 months
- No single words by 16 months
- No two-word (not echolalic) phrases by 24 months
- Loss of any language or social abilities at any age

Data from Report of the Quality Standards Subcommittee of the American Academy of Neurology and the Child Neurology Society: Practice parameter: screening and diagnosis of autism, *Neurology* 55:468-479, 2000.

regular classrooms. Mildly affected persons may have social relationship problems.

History. Developmental history is essential. A family history may reveal other members with pervasive developmental disorder, autism, speech delay or language deficits, mood disorders, or mental retardation. The review of systems should investigate seizures, hearing loss, head injury, and meningitis.

Physical Examination. The child should be checked for general appearance of genetic syndromes and neurologic findings of focal abnormalities.

Other Tests. Evaluation of the child for autism is best done at a specialty center. It is a diagnosis by exclusion. A developmental test, a behavioral assessment, an electroencephalogram (EEG) if needed for seizures, DNA testing for fragile-X syndrome or other syndromes, lead screening especially if pica is present, and a hearing test may be conducted if the case indicates a possible link. Several screening tests for autism are undergoing refinement. Computed tomography scans and magnetic resonance imaging are not routinely indicated (AAP Committee on Children with Disabilities, 2001).

Differential Diagnosis

Two levels of diagnosis are required: the first in primary care for screening and early identification; the second, by specialists, to investigate identified children and differentiate autism from other developmental disorders (Report of the Quality Standards Subcommittee, 2000).

Gifted child, elective mutism, obsessive-compulsive disorder, Tourette's syndrome, schizophrenia of childhood, conduct disorder, mental retardation, Rett syndrome, hearing impairment, lead poisoning, phenylketonuria, tuberous sclerosis, and fragile-X syndrome are all differential diagnoses for autism. Asperger syndrome includes characteristics of mild autism but without language or developmental delays. Children with ADHD may appear rigid, whereas children with autism may seem poorly focused.

Management

Management of children with ASD is complex and will require a multidisciplinary approach. A focus on interactive patterns is the mainstay of management of autism. Children need social skills training, early and intense developmental work, and assistance with learning. Early intervention programs offer diverse approaches for autistic children; it is important to match the aim of interventions to the individual needs of each child for optimal outcomes (Erba, 2000).

Behavior. The most important aspect of management is behavioral training. The target behaviors vary according to age, developmental level, and disruptiveness of behaviors. Reasonable goals need to be set (AAP Committee on Children with Disabilities, 2001).

Education. Extensive assessment and early, intense intervention are necessary to maximize educational abilities and enhance learning for children with autism. Planning for care requires cognitive testing to identify the child's strengths and weaknesses, in addition to social, behavioral, and language assessment. Early intervention programs for preschoolers, school-based special education, and information and assistance for school personnel are essential.

When special abilities are discovered in children with autism, attempts should be made to encourage opportunities for success in these areas. Although these children may not be successful in many educational activities, this should not preclude their participation in areas where they have talents or excel. A child with musical or mathematic gifts may not be able to complete other grade-level work or tolerate the social demands required to demonstrate his or her special abilities. Accommodations to advance children in the areas of their unique abilities are necessary, and parents and school personnel will need to become skilled advocates for the child. Protection from unrealistic expectations of social competence is often necessary to help the child with autism to succeed. "The long-term goal should be to permit the child to function as effectively and comfortably as possible in the least restrictive environment" (Bauer, 1995, p. 32).

Medications. None work well. Haloperidol is sometimes used, but it can have serious side effects, including dyskinesias. Usually, autistic children do not benefit from stimulant medications. Fluoxetine (Prozac) may be helpful for some if they are also depressed. Because 25% of autistic children also have seizures, they may be given anticonvulsants.

Diet. No significant effects result from special diets.

Family Counseling and Support. Families need a great deal of support and training to manage children with autism. They may benefit from assistance from members of the Autism Society of America (see Resource Box).

Because many unproved treatment programs are touted for children with autistic behavior, parents need to be given information about programs that have proved useful and those that have not. Consideration of possible harm to child or family, scientific validation, individual assessment, and integration as a holistic part of the child's total program are factors for parents to consider before adopting a new treatment approach.

- The family and siblings may need supportive counseling and referral because of the considerable stress found in families with children with autism.
- Long-term care needs to be addressed because few autistic children become fully independent employed adults,

RESOURCE BOX

Resources for Cognitive-Perceptual Problems of Children

ATTENTION-DEFICIT HYPERACTIVITY DISORDER (ADHD)

Children and Adults with Attention Deficit Disorders (CHADD)
www.chadd.org
600 local chapters, educational literature, newsletter available with membership

ADD Warehouse Catalog
www.addwarehouse.com
Distributors for all ADHD literature published for children, parents, professionals, and educators

National Attention Deficit Disorder Association
www.add.org

DEAFNESS

Alexander Graham Bell Association for the Deaf (AGBAD)
1-202-337-5220/5221 (voice/TTY)
www.agbell.org

American Society for Deaf Children
1-800-942-2732 (hotline)
www.deafchildren.org

Cochlear Implant Club International
1-202-895-2781 (voice/TTY)

Imagery Language and Visual Communication
www.handspeak.com

National Association of the Deaf (NAD) and American Association of the Deaf-Blind
1-301-587-1788
www.nad.org
www.aadb.org

National Information Center on Deafness, Gallaudet University
www.gallaudet.edu/~nicd/

SEE (Signing Exact English) Center for Advancement of Deaf Children
1-562-430-1467 (voice/TDD)
www.seecenter.org

Telecommunications for the Deaf
1-301-589-3786 (voice)
1-301-589-3006 (TTY)
www.tdi-online.org

BLINDNESS

American Council of the Blind (ACB)
www.acb.org

American Foundation for the Blind
www.afb.org

Blind Children's Fund (BCF)
www.blindchildrensfund.org

National Association for Parents of Children with Visual Impairments (NAPVI)
PO Box 317
Watertown, MA 02471
1-800-562-6265
1-617-972-7441
Fax: 1-617-972-7444
www.spedex.com/napvi/
A national organization that enables parents to find information and resources for their children who are blind or visually impaired, including those with additional disabilities

National Federation of the Blind
Division for Parents of Blind Children
1800 Johnson St.
Baltimore, MD 21230
www.nfb.org

AUTISM

Autism Research Institute
www.autism.com/ari

Autism Society of America
www.autism-society.org

Continued

RESOURCE BOX

Resources for Cognitive-Perceptual Problems of Children—cont'd

ALL CHILDREN WITH DISABILITIES

National Information Center for Children and Youth with Disabilities
www.nichcy.org
Source for age-appropriate books

National Family Association of the Deaf-Blind
1-800-255-0411
www.nfadb.org

National Institute on Deafness and Other Communication Disorders
1-301-496-7243 or 1-800-241-1044 (voice)
1-301-402-0252 or 1-800-241-1055 (TTY)
www.nidcd.nih.gov

NURSING DIAGNOSES RELATED TO COGNITIVE-PERCEPTUAL: *Functional Health Pattern*

Diagnoses are related to the following concepts: environmental interpretation, sensory perception, and cognition—knowledge, memory, and thought processes.

- Confusion (acute or chronic)
- Deficient knowledge (specify)
- Disorganized infant behavior
  - Risk for disorganized infant behavior
  - Readiness for enhanced infant behavior
- Disturbed sensory perception (specify sense)
- Disturbed thought processes
- Impaired environmental interpretation syndrome
- Impaired memory

From North American Nursing Diagnosis Association: *NANDA nursing diagnoses: definitions and classification 2003-2004*, Philadelphia, 2003, North American Nursing Diagnosis Association.

although the prognosis for children with autism is highly variable and very difficult to predict. Those who are highly functioning as children will do best as adults.

Alternative Therapies. Autism is a chronic disorder. To date, there is no cure. Neither is there scientific evidence that supports alternative interventions (AAP Committee on Children with Disabilities, 2001).

Sensory Integration. Children who have been diagnosed with autistic disorder often demonstrate sensory processing impairments manifested in their daily activities. Deficits in sensory processing or sensory integration are often seen in the child's difficulty modulating his or her responses to movement, touch, or auditory stimuli. Clinicians frequently combine play and developmentally based interventions with the sensory integrative approach. Sensory integration involves the organization of sensation for use and is a complex set of processes in the central nervous system that include modulation, perceptual, and praxic functions. Although efficacy studies of sensory integration are mixed, a sensory integrative approach used within a comprehensive occupational therapy program may, with continued research, provide an important feature of service for the child with autistic disorder (Ayres, 1972; Mailloux, 2001).

REFERENCES

Adesman AR: New medications for treatment of children with attention deficit hyperactivity disorder: review and commentary, *Pediatr Ann* 31:514-521, 2002.

American Academy of Pediatrics: Newborn and infant hearing loss: detection and intervention, *Pediatrics* 103:527-530, 1999.

American Academy of Pediatrics Committee on Children with Disabilities: The pediatrician's role in the diagnosis and management of autistic spectrum disorder in children, *Pediatrics* 107:1221-1226, 2001.

American Academy of Pediatrics Committee on Quality Improvement and Subcommittee on Attention Deficit Hyperactivity Disorder: Clinical practice guideline: treatment of the school age child with attention deficit hyperactivity disorder, *Pediatrics* 108:1033-1044, 2001.

American Academy of Pediatrics Committee on Quality Improvement and Subcommittee on Attention Deficit Hyperactivity Disorder: Diagnosis and evaluation of the child with attention deficit hyperactivity disorder, *Pediatrics* 105:1158-1170, 2000.

American Psychiatric Association: *Diagnostic and statistical manual of mental disorders*, ed 4, Washington, DC, 1994, American Psychiatric Association.

Arts HA, Garber A, Zwolan TA: Cochlear implants in young children, *Otolaryngol Clin North Am* 35:925-943, 2002.

Atkinson R, Shiffrin R: Human memory: a proposed system and its control processes. In Spence K, Spence J, editors: *Advances in the psychology of learning and motivation research and theory*, vol 2, New York, 1968, Academic Press.

Ayres A: *Sensory integration and learning disorders*, Los Angeles, 1972, Western Psychological Services.

Barkley R: *ADHD and the nature of self control*, New York, 1997, Guilford Press.

Barkley RA: *Attention-deficit hyperactivity disorder: a handbook for diagnosis and treatment*, New York, 1998, Guilford Press.

Bat-Chava Y, Martin D: Sibling relationships of deaf children: the impact of child and family characteristics, *Rehabilitation Psychology* 47:73-91, 2002.

Bauer S: Autism and the pervasive developmental disorders: part 2, *Pediatr Rev* 16:168-176, 1995.

Behrman R, Kliegman R, Jenson H: *Nelson's textbook of pediatrics*, ed 17, Philadelphia, 2004, WB Saunders.

Breen MJ, Altpeter TS: Factor structures of the Home Situations Questionnaire and the School Situations Questionnaire, *J Ped Psych* 16:59-67, 1991.

Deatrick J, Knafl K, Murphy-Moore C: Clarifying the concept of normalization, *J Nurs Sch* 31:209-214, 1999.

Elster A, Kuznets N: *AMA guidelines for adolescent preventive services (GAPS)*, Baltimore, 1994, Williams & Wilkins.

Erba HW: Early intervention programs for children with autism: conceptual frameworks for implementation, *Am J Orthopsychiatry* 70:82-94, 2000.

Evans S, Raggi V, Paolitto A: School based treatment of adolescents with ADHD, *ADHD Report* 10:10-16, 2002.

Flick G: Controversies in ADHD, *Adv Nurse Pract*, Feb 2002, pp 34-43.

Gedaly-Duff V, Stoeger S, Shelton K: Working with families. In Nickel RE, Desch LW, editors: *The physician's guide to caring for children with disabilities and chronic conditions*, Baltimore, 2000, Brookes.

Goldman L et al: Diagnosis and treatment of attention-deficit/hyperactivity disorder in children and adolescents, *JAMA* 279: 1100-1107, 1998.

Goldstein S: Attention deficit/hyperactivity disorder: implications for the criminal justice system. *Law Enforcement Bull* 6, 1997. Available at *www.fbi.gov/library/leb/1997/june973.htm* (accessed).

Gordon M: *Nursing diagnosis: process and application*, New York, 1987, McGraw-Hill.

Gottesman R, Kelly M: Helping children with learning disabilities toward a brighter adulthood, *Contemp Pediatr* 17:42-61, 2000.

Greenhill L et al: Impairment and deportment responses to different methylphenidate doses in children with ADHD: the MTA titration trial, *J Am Acad Child Adolesc Psychiatry* 40:180-187, 2001.

Gregory S, Mogford K: Early language development in deaf children. In Kyle WJ, Deucher M, editors: *Perspectives on British sign language and deafness*, London, 1981, Croon Helm.

Hannah JN: The role of schools in attention deficit hyperactivity disorder, *Pediatr Ann* 31:507-513, 2002.

Hechtman L: Families of children with attention deficit hyperactivity disorder: a review, *Can J Psychiatry* 41:350-360, 1996.

Jeng L, Robin N: Progress in understanding the genetics of impaired hearing, *Contemp Pediatr* 19:79-96, 2002.

Jensen P et al: ADHD comorbidity findings from the MTA study: comparing comorbid subgroups, *J Am Acad Child Adolesc Psychiatry* 40:147-158, 2001.

Kendall J: Outlasting disruption: process of reinvesting in families with ADHD children, *Qual Health Res* 8:839-857, 1998.

Knafl K et al: Family response to childhood chronic illness: description of management styles, *J Pediatr Nurs* 11:315-326, 1996.

Knafl K, Dietrick J, Kirby A: Normalization promotion. In Craft-Rosenberg M, Denehy J, editors: *Nursing interventions for infants, children, and families*, Thousand Oaks, CA, 2001, Sage.

Kratochvil C: Improving ADHD outcomes: the role of newer agents, *Contemp Pediatr* (suppl), Jan 2003.

Lederberg A, Everhart V: Communication between deaf children and their hearing mothers: the role of language, gesture, and vocalizations, *J Speech Lang Hear Res* 41:887-899, 1998.

Levine M: Neurodevelopmental dysfunction in the school-aged child. In Behrman R, Kliegman R, Jenson H, editors: *Nelson textbook of pediatrics*, ed 16, Philadelphia, 2000, WB Saunders.

Levine M, Carey W, Crocker A: *Developmental-behavioral pediatrics*, ed 3, Philadelphia, 1999, WB Saunders.

Mailloux Z: Sensory integrative principles in intervention with children with autistic disorder. In Roley S, Blanche E, Schaaff R, editors: *Understanding the nature of sensory integration in diverse populations*, Philadelphia, 2001, Harcourt.

Meadow K: *Deafness and child development*, Berkeley, 1980, University of California Press.

Meadow-Orlans KP: Research on developmental aspects of deafness. In Moores DE, Meadow-Orlans KP, editors: *Educational and developmental aspect of deafness*, Washington, DC, 1990, Gallaudet University Press.

Mervis C, Yeargin-Allsopp M, Winter S: Aetiology of childhood visual impairment, metropolitan Atlanta, 1991–93, *Paediatric Perinatal Epidemiol* 14:70, 2000.

Mick E et al: Case-control study of attention-deficit hyperactivity disorder and maternal smoking, alcohol use, and drug use during pregnancy, *J Am Acad Child Adolesc Psychiatry* 4:378-385, 2002.

Milich R, Wolraich M, Lindgren S: Sugar and hyperactivity: a critical review of empirical findings, *Clinical Psychology Review* 6:493-513, 1986.

MTA Cooperative Group: A 14-month randomized clinical trial of treatment strategies for attention-deficit hyperactivity disorder. The MTA Cooperative Group. Multimodal treatment study of children with ADHD, *Arch Gen Psychiatry* 56:1073-1086, 1999.

Phillips S, Hartley JT: Developmental differences and interventions for blind children, *Pediatr Nurs* 14(3):201-204, 1988.

Quigley S, Kretschmer R: *The educational of deaf children: issues, theory, and practice,* Baltimore, 1982, University Park Press.

Rassmussen K, Almvik R, Levander S: Attention deficit hyperactivity disorder, reading disability, and personality disorders in a prison population, *J Am Acad Psychiatry Law* 29:186-193, 2001.

Report of the Quality Standards Subcommittee of the American Academy of Neurology and the Child Neurology Society: Practice parameter: screening and diagnosis of autism, *Neurology* 55:468-479, 2000.

Robin AL: Attention deficit hyperactivity disorder in adolescents, *Pediatr Ann* 31:485-491, 2002.

Rowland A et al: Prevalence of medication treatment for ADHD among elementary school children in Johnson County, NC, *Am J Public Health* 92:231-234, 2002.

Ryan: Hearing and speech assessment. In Ballard R, editor: *Pediatric care of the ICN graduate,* Philadelphia, 1988, WB Saunders.

Shelton K: The family experience with school when an adolescent has ADHD. Unpublished doctoral dissertation. Oregon Health and Science University, 2001.

Stein MT: The role of attention deficit hyperactivity disorder diagnostic and treatment guidelines in changing physician practices, *Pediatr Ann* 31:496-504, 2002.

Sullivan P, Brookhouser P, Scanlan J: Maltreatment of deaf and hard of hearing children. In Hindley P, Kitson N, editors: *Mental health and deafness,* London, 2000, Whurr.

Sullivan PM, Knutson JF: Maltreatment and behavioral characteristics of youth who are deaf and hard of hearing, *Sexuality and Disability* 16:295-319, 1998.

Tanguay PE: Pervasive developmental disorders: a 10-year review, *J Am Acad Child Adolesc Psychiatry* 39(9):1079-1095, 2000.

Thompson DC et al: Universal newborn hearing screening: summary of evidence, *JAMA* 286:2000-2010, 2001.

Tobin: Conversation of substance in the blind and partially blind, *Br J Edu Psychol* 142:192-197, 1972.

US Department of Health and Human Services: *Healthy people 2010: health promotion and disease prevention objectives for the year 2010,* Washington, DC, 2001, US Government Printing Office.

Van Naarden K, Decouflé P, Caldwell K: Prevalence and characteristics of children with serious hearing impairment in metropolitan Atlanta, 1991-1993, *Pediatrics* 103:570-575, 1999.

Wender EH: Managing stimulant medication for attention deficit hyperactivity disorder, *Pediatr Rev* 22:183-189, 2001.

Wender EH: Managing stimulant medication for attention deficit hyperactivity disorder: an update, *Pediatr Rev* 23(7):234-236, 2002.

Yoshinaga-Itano C et al: Language of early- and later-identified children with hearing loss, *Pediatrics* 102:1161-1171, 1998.

Ziegler R, Holden L: Family therapy for learning disabled and attention deficit disordered children, *Am J Orthopsychiatry* 58:196-210, 1988.

18 Self-Perception

Nancy Barber Starr

All people—children and adults—have mental pictures of themselves that steer the course of their lives. This mental picture, or self-perception, begins to develop at birth, emerges in childhood, and is refined and crystallized in adolescence, but it continues to evolve throughout life. Significant relationships, temperament, heredity, and experiences in life all influence self-perception. Self-perception has to do with how individuals act, think, and feel about themselves, their abilities, and their bodies. It is also influenced by the response of others to them. This perception, in turn, influences the attitudes each person takes and the choices each person makes throughout life. A positive self-perception is a precious gift that provides the confidence and energy to take on the world, to withstand crises, and to focus outside one's self. It enhances the building of relationships and giving to others. People with a negative self-perception are handicapped, focused on their own needs, trying to get and prove their self-worth. A negative self-perception drains energy, interferes with building relationships, and often leaves the person feeling like a victim.

Over the last several decades much research has focused on low self-esteem and its potential effect on "a host of social ills, from poor academic performance and marital discord to violent crime and drug abuse" (Goode, 2002). Recent research, however, debunks the idea that a positive self-esteem prevents many of these behaviors, and cites other psychologic factors, such as narcissism or self-absorption, and the use of external measures (e.g., academic performance or appearance) as much more important in determining or predicting negative behaviors or outcomes (Goode, 2002).

Assessing self-perception is not a straightforward task but is interwoven with other data that the nurse practitioner (NP) collects. It may be helpful to think of self-esteem as including cognitive, affective, and behavioral aspects (Reasoner, 2002). The cognitive element emerges as an individual thinks about the discrepancy between the ideal self and the perceived self. The affective component refers to the feelings that emerge when considering that discrepancy. The behavioral aspect is seen in traits such as assertiveness, resilience, and being decisive and respectful of others. Routine anticipatory guidance, education, and counseling, individualized to the child and family, give the NP the opportunity to facilitate the development of positive self-perception and to assist in avoiding potential problems. Self-perception problems are often hidden within somatic complaints and require an awareness and sensitivity to the child or adolescent in order to identify and deal with them. If done successfully, the child's life can be significantly affected.

STANDARDS OF CARE

Bright Futures in Practice: Mental Health (Jellinek, Patel, & Froehle, 2002) focuses on preventive and early recognition of psychosocial problems and mental disorders. The comprehensive practice guide and toolkit have a section in each developmental chapter that focuses on the sphere of self functioning and its appropriate assessment and management. Goals in *Healthy People 2010* (U.S. Department of Health and Human Services, 1999), the *Guide to Clinical Preventive Services* (U.S. Preventive Services Task Force, 1996), the *AMA Guidelines for Adolescent Preventive Services (GAPS)* (Elster & Kuznets, 1994), and the *Put Prevention into Practice (PPIP): Clinician's Handbook of Preventive Services* (U.S. Public Health Service, 1998) all address screening for depression and potential suicide. These are potential complications of a negative self-esteem and should be considered by the NP working with children and adolescents (see Chapter 21 for an in-depth discussion of these topics).

NORMAL PATTERNS OF SELF-PERCEPTION

Components of Self-Perception

The term *self-perception* may be used interchangeably with terms such as *self-concept, self-esteem*, and *self-image*. The term *body image* refers to one's picture of and feelings regarding the body.

Self-perception, being personal and subjective, includes both a description of the self and an evaluation of that description. The description a person draws and the evaluation a person makes come from thoughts and feelings, beliefs and convictions, observations, understanding, insight, and awareness received both from the self and from others. The three key components of self-perception are significance, worthiness, and competence (Box 18-1).

Significance refers to having a sense of belonging; feeling loved and lovable; feeling secure, cared for, and supported; and being accepted and understood unconditionally for who one is, not what one does. This is the most important component in developing and maintaining a healthy self-esteem.

Worthiness refers to being whole on the inside, feeling valuable and acceptable, meeting personal moral standards, and respecting and feeling good about oneself.

Competence refers to feeling capable, confident, adequate, in control, and able to approach new tasks and to deal with life optimistically, hopefully, and with courage. Competence is one part of resilience—the inner strength to cope with any challenge one faces in life (Brooks, 2002). Competence is measured in terms of cognitive, physical, or social skills.

Children who feel significant, worthy, and competent confidently initiate activities, explore the environment, take risks, and rebound from disappointments. Appreciating themselves, they are able to reach out to and interact with others, accepting and offering love, respect, and encouragement. Perry (2001) describes an active learning process beginning with a child's natural curiosity that leads to mastery and accomplishment, thereby growing a child's self-esteem and resilience (Box 18-2).

Children who do not feel significant, worthy, and competent look increasingly to external measures such as those listed in Box 18-3 to try to create a positive self-perception. Physical attractiveness and intelligence are two measures frequently used in society to evaluate people. Financial status, state of physical health, temperament, coping style, and an overly protective environment are other factors that affect self-perception. However, undue or excessive emphasis on external measures causes children to compare themselves with others, adopting the description and evaluation others make of them. "Most of us are what we think others think we are" (Dobson, 1999), or, "Self-attitudes develop in response to how children think others see them" (Hunsberger, 1994, p. 520). Children whose self-perception is based on a comparison of themselves with others feel and describe themselves as insecure, inferior, and inadequate. Attempting to prove themselves, they often become both bossy and aggressive, or people pleasers and approval seekers.

BOX 18-1 *Key Components of Self-Perception*

Significance: I am loved!
Worthiness: I am OK! I like and respect myself!
Competence: I can do it!

BOX 18-2 *Enhancing Self-Perception: The Cycle of Learning*

- Curiosity results in exploration.
- Exploration results in discovery.
- Discovery results in pleasure.
- Pleasure leads to repetition.
- Repetition results in mastery.
- Mastery results in new skills.
- New skills lead to confidence.
- Confidence contributes to self-esteem.
- Self-esteem increases sense of security.
- Security results in more exploration.

From Perry BD: Creating novelty, *Scholastic Parent and Child* 9:67-68, 2001.

Developmental Stages

The development of children's self-perception is closely tied to normal growth and development. Each stage of growth and development provides opportunities for learning about the self and interacting with and observing others and the environment. Transient periods of low self-esteem as a child masters new skills or sets new goals are a normal part of development. Self-perception can change as a result of relationships or experiences or can be maintained in spite of contrary evidence (e.g., the adolescent cheerleader who is loved and is successful in school

BOX 18-3 *External Measures Used to Build Self-Perception*

Physical appearance or attractiveness: How do I look?
Intelligence: What do I know?
Performance: How do I do?
Importance: Who do I know?
Financial status: What and how much do I have?
Control: What and whom do I control?

and relationships, yet is anorexic and feels she is never "good enough").

One theoretic perspective that can be useful clinically is to view the development of self-perception as occurring in two stages (Box 18-4). The first stage, emergence of the self, occurs in infants, toddlers, and preschool-age children. Parents and caretakers play a key role during this stage. Infants are learning that they are separate individuals who affect others by their behavior. This is best accomplished in a supportive environment where the infants come to view the world (their parents and caretakers) as responsive to their needs, both physical and emotional. Toddlers, with their new motor, cognitive, and language skills, learn to explore their capabilities and limits and make others aware of their needs, desires, and concerns. They thrive with positive acceptance, praise, and guidelines that set limits while allowing them to make choices. Preschoolers begin to use "I" to describe their own activities. They become aware of discrepancies in abilities and discover their whole body, including the differences in sexes. The early feelings of competence begin to emerge, and preschoolers can be coached through early problem solving. Preschoolers internalize parents' demands and move away from seeing the self as the center of the world. Siblings and peers play an increasingly important role in the preschooler's life.

The second stage of self-development, refining the self, occurs in school-age children and adolescents. Friendships and peers, and the time spent in various activities, play an increasing larger role in shaping the child's character and personality, and thus self-perception. Cultural stereotypes such as those found in magazines, television, billboards, and the Internet all influence the child's perception of society's "ideal" self. School-age children are preoccupied with evaluating themselves on the basis of external evidence: cognitive and physical skills, achievements, physical appearance, social abilities and acceptance, and a sense of control. They are particularly prone to comparing themselves to others, making them more vulnerable to social pressure. Any deviation from normal is subject to criticism and ridicule.

Self-perception continues to be refined during early adolescence, solidifying in later adolescence. Early adolescents are still highly dependent on cultural stereotypes and peer acceptance, with physical and emotional changes being the main focus of self-evaluation. Body image formation, a crucial element in shaping identity, is finalized at this stage. Any defect, disability, or discrepancy between what is seen and what is visualized as ideal is magnified and significant in the adolescent's eyes. By late adolescence, a more established view of the self should be in place, with acceptance of that identity—physical, social, and spiritual. Teenagers with positive self-perception have values, goals, and competencies that guide them into adulthood. Areas to be evaluated in the adolescent include academic/scholastic achievements, physical/athletic achievements, peer/social acceptance, physical attributes, interpersonal acceptance (close friendships, romantic appeal), moral behaviors as compared with internal standards, sense of control over personal accomplishments, relationships, and participation in activities.

BOX 18-4 *Developmental Stages of Self-Perception*

Emergence of Self (First Stage)

- Infants—learn that they are separate individuals who affect others by their behavior, view the world as responsive or unresponsive to their needs.
- Toddlers—explore their capabilities and limits, and make others aware of their needs, desires, and concerns.
- Preschoolers—begin to use "I," become aware of discrepancies in abilities, discover their bodies, begin to do simple problem solving, move from seeing themselves as the center of the world.

Refining the Self (Second Stage)

- School-age children—evaluate self on the basis of external evidence, compare themselves with others, criticize and ridicule deviations from normal.
- Early adolescents—finalize body image, focus on physical and emotional changes with peer acceptance determining self-evaluation.
- Late adolescents—refine and crystallize self-perception (physical, social, spiritual) with values, goals, and competencies guiding their future in place.

Data from Kump T: Self-esteem: why little kids need BIG egos, *Healthy Kids*, Oct/Nov 1998, pp. 53-58; Hunsberger M: Fostering self-esteem. In Betz CL, Hunsberger M, Wright S, editors: *Family centered nursing care of children*, ed 2, Philadelphia, 1994, WB Saunders; Sieving RE, Zirbel-Donisch ST: Development and enhancement of self-esteem in children, *J Pediatr Health Care* 4:290-296, 1990.

Boys consistently score higher than girls on measures of self-esteem during adolescence. One study of adolescent self-esteem examined eight domains identified across a number of instruments: personal security, home/parents, peer popularity, academic competence, attractiveness, personal mastery, psychologic permeability, and athletic competence (Quatman & Watson, 2001). Of the eight domains, only peer popularity and academic competence showed no significant difference between genders, though boys still exceeded girls in all eight. Parent and home life, personal security, academic competence, and personal mastery were the four domains that strongly influenced global self-esteem. Low priority was assigned to athleticism. The authors concluded that boys seem to have an "at-homeness" in the world, both in the home and outside, where they feel confident and masterful, not undone by adversity. In contrast, girls felt significantly less confident and masterful, more psychologically vulnerable.

Developmental Assets

Developmental assets are basic life skills and attributes that are critical building blocks to help a child or adolescent grow into a caring, competent, contributing, and responsible adult. Developmental assets assist a young person to make wise decisions; they increase in value over time, provide a sense of security, and are resources to draw on over and over; and they are cumulative. The more assets a young person has, the more likely he or she is to make wise decisions and choose positive lifestyles while avoiding risky behaviors or dangerous activities. Developmental assets have been identified and revised by the Search Institute based on nationwide surveys of more than 100,000 young people in 200 communities (Benson, Galbraith, & Espeland, 1998a). There are two categories of assets: (1) external assets, things in the environment (home, school, community) that support, nurture and empower, set boundaries and expectations, and make constructive use of time; and (2) internal assets, attitudes (commitment to learning and a positive identity), positive values, and social competencies that belong in the head and heart of every child (Benson, Galbraith, & Espeland, 1998a). Forty developmental assets have been described (Table 18-1). Most children and adolescents have only 18. Girls tend to have more assets than boys do in a ratio of 19.5 to 16.5, and younger children have more assets than older ones do (Benson, Galbraith, & Espeland, 1998a). The Search Institute believes that young people should have at least 31 assets.

Ten developmental deficits, or roadblocks to building assets, have also been identified by the Search Institute (Benson, Galbraith, & Espeland, 1998a). The more deficits a child has, the more likely he or she is to make negative choices and decisions. The deficits are as follows:

1. Spending 2 hours or more a day alone at home without an adult
2. Putting a lot of emphasis on selfish values
3. Watching more than 2 hours of television a day
4. Going to parties where friends drink alcohol
5. Feeling stress or pressure most or all of the time
6. Being physically abused
7. Being sexually abused
8. Having a parent with an alcohol or drug problem
9. Feeling socially isolated from people who provide care, support, and understanding
10. Having numerous close friends who often get into trouble

Environmental Influences

Significant relationships in a child's life, temperament, traits endowed by heredity, and experiences in everyday life are all environmental factors that influence the development of self-perception.

Significant relationships include parents or parent figures, siblings and other family members, and ongoing caretakers. As children get older, peers and authority figures also have an influence. Constant unconditional acceptance and love, empathy, and an attitude of understanding, coupled with appropriate limits and boundaries, are the most important interactions these significant others offer. Time spent with and encouragement given to the child, both in being together and in doing things, as well as in sharing life's happenings (listening, talking, and problem solving), are also essential ingredients (see the Parenting Pyramid discussed in Chapter 5). The sturdy base built by positive relationships is a key component in the child's developing positive self-esteem. By feeling, seeing, and hearing these continual reinforcements, children internalize or know that they are significant, worthy, and competent. In contrast, a study of French-Canadian children who experienced verbal aggression (rejection, demeaning, terrorizing, criticizing, or insulting) showed significantly lower self-esteem. These children perceived themselves as less competent, less comfortable, and less worthy. They were also more prone to depression (Solomon & Serres, 1999). Peers and authority figures serve to confirm or deny what is taught at home.

Temperament may also play a role in the child's development of self-perception. This is particularly the case when there is a mismatch of temperaments, especially between parent and child, or when a child has traits that are labeled difficult or challenging. If these traits are understood and managed correctly, the child's self-esteem can be positively affected. (See Kurcinka [1998] for an in-depth

TABLE 18-1 *40 Developmental Assets*

Category	Asset Name and Definition
External Assets	
Support	*Family support*—Family life provides high levels of love and support.
	Positive family communication—Young person and her or his parent(s) communicate positively, and young person is willing to seek advice and counsel from parent(s).
	Other adult relationships—Young person receives support from three or more nonparent adults.
	Caring neighborhood—Young person experiences caring neighbors.
	Caring school climate—School provides a caring, encouraging environment.
	Parent involvement in schooling—Parent(s) are actively involved in helping young person succeed in school.
Empowerment	*Community values youth*—Young person perceives that adults in the community value youth.
	Youth as resources—Young people are given useful roles in the community.
	Service to others—Young person serves in the community 1 hr or more per week.
	Safety—Young person feels safe at home, at school, and in the neighborhood.
Boundaries and expectations	*Family boundaries*—Family has clear rules and consequences and monitors the young person's whereabouts.
	School boundaries—School provides clear rules and consequences.
	Neighborhood boundaries—Neighbors take responsibility for monitoring young people's behavior.
	Adult role models—Parent(s) and other adults model positive, responsible behavior.
	Positive peer influence—Young person's best friends model responsible behavior.
	High expectations—Both parent(s) and teachers encourage the young person to do well.
Constructive use of time	*Creative activities*—Young person spends 3 hr or more per week in lessons or practice in music, theater, or other arts.
	Youth programs—Young person spends 3 hr or more per week in sports, clubs, or organizations at school or in the community.
	Religious community—Young person spends 1 hr or more per week in activities in a religious institution.
	Time at home—Young person is out with friends "with nothing special to do" two or fewer nights per week.
Internal Assets	
Commitment to learning	*Achievement motivation*—Young person is motivated to do well in school.
	School engagement—Young person is actively engaged in learning.
	Homework—Young person reports doing at least 1 hr of homework every school day.
	Bonding to school—Young person cares about her or his school.
	Reading for pleasure—Young person reads for pleasure 3 hr or more per week.
Positive values	*Caring*—Young person places high value on helping other people.
	Equality and social justice—Young person places high value on promoting equality and reducing hunger and poverty.
	Integrity—Young person acts on convictions and stands up for her or his beliefs.
	Honesty—Young person tells the truth even when it is not easy.
	Responsibility—Young person accepts and takes personal responsibility.
	Restraint—Young person believes it is important not to be sexually active or to use alcohol or other drugs.
Social competencies	*Planning and decision making*—Young person knows how to plan ahead and make choices.
	Interpersonal competence—Young person has empathy, sensitivity, and friendship skills.
	Cultural competence—Young person has knowledge of and comfort with people of different cultural/racial/ethnic backgrounds.
	Resistance skills—Young person can resist negative peer pressure and dangerous situations.
	Peaceful conflict resolution—Young person seeks to resolve conflict nonviolently.
Positive identity	*Personal power*—Young person feels that he or she has control over "things that happen to me."
	Self-esteem—Young person reports having a high self-esteem.
	Sense of purpose —Young person reports that "my life has a purpose."
	Positive view of personal future—Young person is optimistic about her or his personal future.

discussion.) However, if temperament is not understood, the child may carry negative perceptions and labels that adversely affect his or her self-perception (see Chapter 21 for a discussion of temperament).

The role of heredity in the development of self-perception is due to family traits over which the child has no control. Aspects such as appearance, intelligence, and family characteristics, including alcoholism, mental illness, and disfiguring disease, are to be considered. Conditions in which the child exists, such as poverty and homelessness, also are important (Costello et al, 2003). Family traits and attributes either contribute to a positive self-perception or may become barriers to be overcome.

The effect of race on self-esteem has been much studied over the last 50 years, with initial studies seeming to demonstrate that blacks had lower self-esteem. In 2000, Chapman & Mullis studying racial differences in adolescent coping and self-esteem found no difference between the self-esteem of white and black adolescents. Additionally, Gray-Little and Hafdahl (2000) performed a meta-analytic synthesis of 261 studies on self-esteem. Comparisons based on more than one-half million respondents showed that black children, adolescents, and young adults had higher self-esteem scores than their comparable Caucasian counterparts. The authors, however, caution against using race as an independent variable in assessing self-esteem.

Children's social experiences provide an opportunity to observe the world, test skills and abilities, interact with others, and try various roles. Positive experiences such as success in solving problems, working out difficulties, and learning to carry on after setbacks contribute to significance, worth, and competence, encouraging further exploration and risk taking. Negative experiences cause children to retreat or attempt to compensate through other means.

ASSESSMENT OF SELF-PERCEPTION

The goal of assessing self-perception is to know how children describe and evaluate themselves and to identify the sources that provide the input they use to develop their self-concept. These assessments then lay the groundwork for planning interventions for the child and family. Corresponding assessment of the parents' and caretaker's self-perception is important. Assessment of self-perception is not a simple task. It cannot be observed directly or obtained from questioning alone, but must be inferred from observed behavior, self-statements or self-ratings, and other relevant information. Self-rating, observational scales, draw-a-person tests, and puppet interview are possible means of assessment. The puppet interview is an indirect interview with a large hand puppet for 5- to 7-year-olds (Verschueren, Buyck, & Marcoen, 2001). The draw-a-person test, used with younger children, asks the child to draw a picture of himself or herself, and also a picture of another child. A comparison of the two drawings often gives an idea of the child's self-perception. Somewhere between fourth and sixth grades, self-esteem inventories can be considered. Davis-Kean and Sandler's (2001) comprehensive meta-analysis of measures of self-esteem for young children offers helpful information if the reader is interested in measures for young children. A variety of measures are available for adolescents (see Schott & Bellin, 2001, for one example).

History

General Questions

Ask the following questions (Spratt, 2002):

- What does your child think she or he does well?
- How does your child respond to failure?
- Does your child have close friends?
- How does your child respond to new challenges?
- How does your own style (e.g., personality, patience, energy level, talents) compare with your child's?
- Are you setting reasonable or attainable expectations for your child?

Components of Self-Perception

Significance

- Does the child feel loved, lovable, cared for, secure, supported, accepted, understood?
- Is this conditional or unconditional? Is this based on who the child is or what the child does?

Worthiness

- Does the child feel valuable, acceptable?
- Are self-respect and self-liking evident?
- What beliefs or convictions does the child have? Do they match the child's lifestyle?

Competence

- Does the child feel capable, adequate, optimistic overall?
- Does the child approach new tasks with confidence?
- What are the child's cognitive, physical, and social strengths?

Developmental Stage

Infant

- Does the infant recognize self as separate from others?
- Does the infant realize his or her effect on others?

Toddler

- Does the toddler explore capabilities and limits?
- Does the toddler make others aware of needs, desires, and concerns?

Preschooler

- Does the child use "I"? Describe activities? Discover his or her body?

- Does the child internalize parental demands? Move away from self as center of world?
- Are siblings and peers increasingly important? How does the child think, feel, and act about self?

School-Age Child

- How does the child describe and evaluate self, including body image? Is the evaluation in comparison to peers?
- How does this view compare with the child's perceptions of peers' evaluation?
- What cognitive and physical skills and achievements are described?
- What friends, social abilities, and activities are described?
- Is there a sense of control over life? Confidence in self?

Early Adolescent

- How does the adolescent describe and evaluate himself or herself? What role do peers play?
- How are physical attributes described (body image)?
- What are academic, physical, and social activities and achievements?
- How do moral behaviors compare with internal standards?
- Is there a sense of control over personal activities, accomplishments, and relationships?

Late Adolescent

- How does the adolescent describe and evaluate self?
- What choices are being made? What values, goals, and plans are expressed? Is there a sense of optimism about that direction?

Developmental Assets

To determine how many and what assets a child has, two checklists (Boxes 18-5 and 18-6), one for children and adolescents and another for parents, have been developed (Benson, Galbraith, & Espeland, 1998a). It is suggested that

BOX 18-5 *Developmental Assets: A Checklist for Kids and Teens*

Check each statement that is true for you.

1. I feel loved and supported in my family.
2. I can go to my parents or guardians for advice and support. I have frequent in-depth conversations with them.
3. I know three or more other adults (besides my parents or guardians) whom I can go to for advice and support.
4. My neighbors encourage and support me.
5. My school provides a caring, encouraging environment.
6. My parents or guardians help me succeed in school.
7. I feel valued by adults in my community.
8. I am given useful roles in my community.
9. I serve in my community 1 hour or more each week.
10. I feel safe at home, at school, and in my neighborhood.
11. My family has clear rules and consequences for my behavior, and they monitor my whereabouts.
12. My school has clear rules and consequences for behavior.
13. Neighbors take responsibility for monitoring my behavior.
14. My parents or guardians and other adults in my life model positive, responsible behavior.
15. My best friends model responsible behavior.
16. Both my parents or guardians and my teachers encourage me to do well.
17. I spend 3 hours or more each week in lessons or practice in music, theater, or other arts.
18. I spend 3 hours or more each week in school or community sports, clubs, or organizations.
19. I spend 1 hour or more each week in religious services or participating in spiritual activities.
20. I go out with friends with nothing special to do two or fewer nights each week.
21. I want to do well in school.
22. I like to learn new things.
23. I do 1 hour or more of homework each school day.
24. I care about my school.
25. I read for pleasure 3 hours or more each week.
26. I believe that it's really important to help other people.
27. I want to help promote equality and reduce world poverty and hunger.

Continued

BOX 18-5 ***Developmental Assets: A Checklist for Kids and Teens—cont'd***

28. I act on my convictions. I stand up for my beliefs.
29. I tell the truth—even when it's not easy.
30. I accept and take personal responsibility for my actions and decisions.
31. I believe that it's important not to be sexually active or to use alcohol or other drugs.
32. I'm good at planning ahead and making decisions.
33. I'm good at making and keeping friends.
34. I know and am comfortable with people of different cultural, racial, and ethnic backgrounds.
35. I resist negative peer pressure and avoid dangerous situations.
36. I try to resolve conflicts nonviolently.
37. I believe that I have control over many things that happen to me.
38. I feel good about myself.
39. I believe that my life has a purpose.
40. I'm optimistic about my future.

From Benson PL, Galbraith J, Espeland P: *What kids need to succeed*, Minneapolis, MN, 1998, Free Spirit Publisher.

BOX 18-6 ***Developmental Assets: A Checklist for Parents***

Check each statement that is true for you or your child.

1. I give my child a lot of love and support.
2. My child can come to me for advice and support. We have frequent in-depth conversations.
3. My child knows three or more other adults whom he or she can go to for advice and support.
4. Our neighbors encourage and support my child.
5. My child's school provides a caring, encouraging environment.
6. I'm actively involved in helping my child succeed in school.
7. My child feels valued by adults in our community.
8. My child is given useful roles in our community.
9. My child serves in our community 1 hour or more each week.
10. My child feels safe at home, at school, and in our neighborhood.
11. Our family has clear rules and consequences for behavior. We monitor each other's whereabouts.
12. My child's school has clear rules and consequences for behavior.
13. Our neighbors take responsibility for monitoring my child's behavior.
14. I model positive, responsible behavior, and so do other adults that my child knows.
15. My child's best friends model responsible behavior.
16. I encourage my child to do well, and so do my child's teachers.
17. My child spends 3 hours or more each week in lessons or practice in music, theater, or other arts.
18. My child spends 3 hours or more each week in school or community sports, clubs, or organizations.
19. My child spends 1 hour or more each week in religious services or participating in spiritual activities.
20. My child spends two or fewer nights each week out with friends "with nothing special to do."
21. My child wants to do well in school.
22. My child likes to learn new things.
23. My child does 1 hour or more of homework each school day.
24. My child cares about her or his school.
25. My child reads for pleasure 3 hours or more each week.
26. My child believes that it's really important to help other people.
27. My child wants to help promote equality and reduce world poverty and hunger.
28. My child acts on his or her convictions. My child stands up for his or her beliefs.
29. My child tells the truth—even when it's not easy.

BOX 18-6 *Developmental Assets: A Checklist for Parents—cont'd*

30. My child accepts and takes personal responsibility for her or his actions and decisions.
31. My child believes that it's important not to be sexually active or to use alcohol or other drugs.
32. My child is good at planning ahead and making decisions.
33. My child is good at making and keeping friends.
34. My child knows and is comfortable with people of different cultural, racial, and ethnic backgrounds.
35. My child resists negative peer pressure and avoids dangerous situations.
36. My child tries to resolve conflicts nonviolently.
37. My child believes that he or she has control over many things that happen to him or her.
38. My child feels good about herself or himself.
39. My child believes that his or her life has a purpose.
40. My child is optimistic about her or his future.

From Benson PL, Galbraith J, Espeland P: *What kids need to succeed*, Minneapolis, MN, 1998, Free Spirit Publisher.

parents and children complete the lists separately, then sit down and share each other's responses. These checklists become helpful tools for parents and children to compare their perceptions, identify strong and weak areas, and plan for areas of growth.

Environmental Influences

Family Structure

- Who makes up the family? Significant others? Caretakers? What is the family like?
- What is the family's social and financial status?
- What is the physical living situation?
- Does anyone in the family have any physical disease? Any mental or social disease (e.g., mental illness or retardation, alcoholism)?

Parental Influences

- Who plays the parental role? How do parents describe themselves? Perceive their role?
- How does the parent describe the child? How valued is the child? How is that shown?
- What are parental expectations for the child? Is the child given age-appropriate guidance, responsibilities, freedoms?

Significant Others Outside Family

- Who are they? Peers? Teachers? Neighbors? Authority figures? Social supports? Networks? Mentors?
- What are the relationships like?

Temperament Issues

- What temperament traits does the child have?
- How does the parent describe the child? React to the child? Interact with the child?

Environment

- What is the child's environment like? What experiences or opportunities are there? Within the family? In the neighborhood? More formally (e.g., play groups, extracurricular activities)?
- What opportunities are there to test skills and abilities? Interact with others? Try new roles? Is this encouraged?
- How protected is the child?

Discipline

- How is the child disciplined? What methods are used? Is guidance given?
- Are limits and consequences clear?
- Is the child allowed to try and not be rescued?

Communication

- What messages is the child receiving (e.g., "you are a helper," or "you are a bad boy")?
- Is he or she listened to? Are feelings acknowledged?
- What does the child say about himself or herself (e.g., describes self as "good" or "bad," "smart" or "dumb")?

Observations during the History and Examination

Direct questioning about all the areas previously listed gives the NP information about the child. However, equally important is observation of the child and interactions between the child and the accompanying person throughout the office visit.

- What is the relationship between the two?
- What actual words are said? With what tone of voice?
- What kind of nonverbal interaction occurs? What kind of physical interaction?
- Is the child encouraged to answer questions and perform tasks? Is rescuing occurring? Is guidance given?
- What expectations are voiced?
- How is discipline conducted within the examination setting? What limits are set?

Box 18-7 lists risk factors for low self-perception.

BOX 18-7 *Risk Factors for Low Self-Perception*

1. *Physical alterations, including body image.* Chronic illness (visible or not), disfiguring disabilities, sensory disabilities, obesity, anorexia
2. *Mental/emotional alterations.* School problems such as slow learner, semi-illiterate, underachiever, culturally deprived, late bloomer, difficult temperament, emotional or mental illness or abuse
3. *Environmental/relational alterations.* Disrupted families and family relationships or inability to meet basic needs, unrealistic expectations or faulty thinking, temperament or personality misfits, social disorders, stress, past experiences of failure, rejection, criticism

MANAGEMENT STRATEGIES FOR DEVELOPING POSITIVE SELF-PERCEPTION

Anticipatory guidance, education, and counseling are strategies the NP uses to guide and direct the family, child, and adolescent in developing healthy self-perception. If problems are significant, referral for more in-depth counseling is necessary.

While working with the child and family, specific strategies to improve self-perception are chosen, keeping in mind that familial, generational, ethnic, and cultural practices influence the choice and use of strategies. A multitude of books on developing children's self-esteem are available, a few of which are listed in the references (Benson, Galbraith, & Espeland, 1998a, 1998b; Day & Day-Ferraz, 1997; Dobson, 1999; Hart, 1990; Jones & Jones, 1998; Kump, 1998; Kurcinka, 1998; Kvols, 1997; Rosemond, 2001).

Facilitate Good Parenting

- Parental self-perception, either positive or negative, has a significant effect on the child's self-perception. Parents should be encouraged to understand and accept themselves, acknowledge their strengths and accept their uniqueness, take care of themselves, treat themselves with respect, and be aware of their own feelings.
- Parental roles include being available to the child both physically and emotionally, teaching the child, modeling behavior, and helping the child learn to relate to others. This is done by meeting basic needs (e.g., feeding, getting up at night, bathing), as well as spending time together, enjoying the child, having fun, touching, talking, and watching.
- Value children. Appreciate and praise who they are rather than what they do. Show belief in their ability to learn, improve, and grow. Look in their eyes when you talk to them. Recognize their unique means of self-expression. Delight in their discoveries. Contribute to their collections. Identify their strengths, focus on their efforts, structure situations for success, and offer thanks for what they do. Avoid shame, criticism, and humiliation.
- "Know your children" (Dobson, 1999). See what they see, feel what they feel, hope what they hope. This provides needed empathy. Children have their own personality, temperament, dreams, and opinions and need to be known, loved, accepted, and respected for who they are.
- Be there. Presence endorses the child's involvement and reinforces the importance of their efforts. Do things with them, not just for them. Show up at their concerts, games, and events. Visit their schools.
- Take time; avoid being hurried, especially during times of transition. Preschedule times just to be together. Play with your children and let them set the pace (Webster-Stratton, 1997). Spend at least 20 minutes each day giving them undivided attention. Consider whether dawdling, acting out, or feeling bad may be related to being hurried and lack of emotional support (Jellinek, Patel, & Froehle, 2002).
- Know their friends. Encourage positive involvement with friends and activities. Help find the right niche (e.g., length of time, type of activity) that fits the child. Show an interest in friends (e.g., host a sleepover, take a group to the zoo). Steer them away from less constructive friends and activities.
- Avoid comparing children. Children are individuals who grow and develop in their own way and at their own rate. Celebrate their accomplishments. Tell them how terrific they are. Their individuality needs to be respected, and comparisons to siblings or peers should be avoided.
- Let go. Develop a gradual, planned granting of freedom and responsibility, beginning in infancy and ending in late adolescence. Letting go involves offering trust, providing opportunities, giving choices, instilling confidence, and refraining from rushing to aid a struggling child. As part of this process, each year the child should make more decisions and assume more routine responsibilities than during the prior 12 months (Dobson, 1999).

Refer to Chapter 5 (section on parent development and parent-child interaction) and Table 21-3 for further information and strategies.

Maintain Appropriate Expectations of the Child

- Attempt to keep expectations involving tasks, toys, and roles appropriate to the child's age. Expectations that are too high lead to pressure on children and a constant feeling of failure even when children are doing their best. Expectations that are too low diminish children's value and make them feel as if the parent has no faith in them. Expecting their best can even be overly demanding because no one can consistently "do their best" all the time (Spratt, 2002).
- Set expectations that are appropriate to the child's unique qualities. Each child's individual personality, temperament, strengths, and weaknesses must be considered. Parent-driven versus child-driven expectations need to be identified. Although this is a sensitive issue, knowing where expectations begin (with parent or child) and how they fit the child and family is important. Recognize differences between parent's style and abilities and child's.
- Clearly state expectations so that both the child and parent alike can avoid frustration, distrust, and further problems.
- Develop resilience in children by learning to view failure or mistakes as chances to learn. Mistakes are accepted and expected. Realistically assessing performance, emphasizing strengths, and discussing strategies that could lead to success prepare children to approach future obstacles and disappointments (Spratt, 2002).

Use Discipline Techniques That Enhance Self-Esteem

- The goal of discipline is to teach children, not punish them. The manner and intent of providing discipline are as important as the techniques used.
- Identify limits and consequences clearly and follow through. Knowing clearly what is expected provides security for the child. Encourage flexible limit setting (e.g., "You have to wear a coat, but you can choose the blue or red one") (Jellinek, Patel, & Froehle, 2002).
- Help the child learn to choose acceptable behaviors and learn self-control. Establish house rules. Catch the child being good and offer praise. Be sincere.
- Foster problem solving to build confidence. This begins by providing opportunities to make choices and decisions. The steps to problem solving (stating the problem, expressing needs, considering alternatives, agreeing on a solution, and implementing and following through with the agreed-on solution) need to be used and taught. Part of the process means taking time and waiting to let the child work through the process.
- Avoid rescuing children. Allowing them to persevere, learn, and work through frustration empowers them for further success. Rescuing (providing unrequested assistance too soon) must be differentiated from guiding, encouraging, and being an ally to the child. Respect the child's choices.
- Provide guidance to understand the self and the surrounding world, to develop a conscience, and to steer clear of potential problems. This helps the child learn independence.

Communicate Positively

- Listen to children. Good listening means taking them seriously, being interested, and letting them finish what they are saying. Show love by giving hugs and back rubs, by stroking hair, or by giving positive facial expressions. Say "I love you" often and in a variety of ways. Refer to Table 21-3 for further strategies.
- Be aware of the words used, as well as the tone of voice, the intent of the words, and body language. Avoid negative messages that are sent in comparisons, put-downs ("You are such a baby"), humiliation ("You can't do anything right"), labeling ("You're such a slob"), and fault finding.
- Praise and encourage children often, especially as they undertake new challenges or roles. Say "thanks" for their cooperation. Catch them doing well (e.g., "I like the way you..."). Acknowledge their help (e.g., "I appreciate..."). Love their person (e.g., "I love being with you...") (Hall, 1998).
- Help children identify, handle, and express their feelings by accepting and acknowledging those feelings. Avoid trying to change them or stop them by denial or reassurance. Listen. Parents should share their own feelings and failures. Intervention may take place at the thought and behavior level after feelings are brought forward.
- React with "I" statements, not "you" judgments, to separate performance from worth and validate children's behavior while still allowing behavior to be modified.
- Be aware of children's "self-talk." What children say to themselves not only reflects what they believe but also gives further definition to who they are. Positive

statements enhance self-perception and minimize stress children feel. "Stinkin' thinking" (Hart, 1990) or negative statements reflect low self-perception and require intervention.
- Nurture curiosity and exploration to encourage mastery of new skills and help children reach their potential (Perry, 2001).

Provide Helpful Strategies for the Child and Adolescent

- Support early and ongoing self-assertions as means of children expressing themselves (Kump, 1998). For example, allow your preschooler to wear the outlandish outfit chosen unless it is totally inappropriate (a bathing suit in November), or your school-age child to create the menu one night a week.
- Find and build on the "island of competence" (Brooks, 1995; Kump, 1998). Every child has an interest, ability, or skill that can be developed and displayed to provide the child with a sense of success and a defense from failure. Identify what the child is interested in and good at, and encourage and praise those skills, talents, efforts, and achievements. Seven kinds of intelligence have been identified: linguistic, mathematic, spatial, musical, bodily, interpersonal, and intrapersonal (Dobson, 1999), and any or all can be used to build and affirm the child's island of competence.
- Help your child compete (Dobson, 1999). A child needs encouragement to develop skills, opportunities to use the skills, and second chances when failure occurs. A child is empowered by having an ally in these endeavors.
- Help your child develop a sense that he or she can affect the outcome of events in life. Children feel more effective if they feel they are contributing. Provide opportunities to make choices, solve problems, and develop responsibilities (Spratt, 2002).
- Encourage a healthy connectedness. Children need to belong to and feel that they are a part of their family, as well as groups outside their family through social activities and links within their community, ethnic group, or geographic area.
- Promote a sense of ownership. Children who are given responsibility for themselves and their actions are also given a sense of control over their life.
- Keep a close eye on the classroom (Dobson, 1999). Problems in the classroom are often symptoms of other problems in a child's life. Temporary rough spots are normal and must be distinguished from more pervasive problems that require intervention.
- Offer genuine encounter moments (GEMs) (Hall, 1998). This refers to a mutually agreed on time that is set apart for 100% attention and love, focused attention, or direct involvement. The child takes the lead in how the time is spent.
- Defuse feelings of inferiority (Dobson, 1999). Throughout the school years and adolescence, comparisons are the norm, and feelings of inferiority often result. Children aware of this fact who have learned to compete and compensate are more likely to believe in themselves despite feelings of inferiority.
- Prepare for adolescence (Dobson, 1999). A special time set aside to talk with preadolescents about the coming physical, social, and hormonal changes helps prepare them to handle the transitions with greater ease.

Encourage Asset Building

Fostering developmental assets can positively change a young person's life. Because all young people need assets, and building assets is an ongoing process, everyone (the child, parents, teachers, health care providers, and community members) can be involved in developing assets in the young people around them. Relationships are critical to building assets. Consistent messages about what is important in life and what is expected from the young person are essential. Intentional redundancy, hearing the same positive messages over and over again from many different people, is also important. One way for anyone to start developing assets in a young person is to use checklists (see Boxes 18-5 and 18-6) to help identify an area in which to begin to build one or more assets. The Search Institute has many resources and programs to assist individuals and communities to build assets in young people. For information on how to contact the Search Institute, see the Resource Box. Two particularly helpful books, *What Kids Need to Succeed* and *What Teens Need to Succeed* (Benson, Galbraith, & Espeland, 1998a, also available in Spanish), define each asset and give ideas for building that asset in the home, school, community, and congregational setting.

It is possible to overcome the deficits in a young person's life. Five areas identified by the Search Institute (Benson, Galbraith, & Espeland, 1998a) that are helpful in overcoming deficits are

1. Getting involved in structured, adult-led activities
2. Setting boundaries and limits
3. Nurturing a strong commitment to education
4. Providing support and care in all areas of life, not just the family
5. Cultivating positive values and concern for others

SPECIFIC SELF-PERCEPTION PROBLEMS IN CHILDREN

Self-Esteem Problems

Description

When a child's sense of significance is disturbed, self-esteem problems arise. The child has a loss of confidence, and feelings of insecurity are evidenced. Counterproductive coping strategies may be used (Table 18-2). Disruptive behavior, social withdrawal, poor academic achievement, and delinquency are associated with poor self-esteem (Jellinek, Patel, & Froehle, 2002). This may, over time, emerge as aggressive behavior that eventually leads to violence.

Etiology

Self-esteem problems arise when children are unsure of belonging and of being loved, cared for, and accepted. Love is often conditional, with acceptance coming for what they do rather than who they are. Emotional maltreatment (abuse or deprivation) is an extreme example of this (see Chapter 19). Self-esteem problems may be situational or transient, or they may be chronic. Girls with low self-esteem are three times more likely to initiate sexual intercourse than girls with high self-esteem (Spencer et al, 2002). Interestingly, neither children with idiopathic short stature (Theunissen et al, 2002) nor adolescents who were extremely low birth weight (less than 1000 g) (Saigal et al, 2002) showed significant difference in self-esteem from controls.

Assessment

The child with self-esteem problems seeks attention, importance, and security. Because of the desire for acceptance and love, these children are often people pleasers. Position and status are attempts to prove importance. Attention seeking may be extreme, causing aggression and leading to behavior problems. There may be a history of rejection or a dysfunctional family. Parental insensivity, fatigue and time pressure, guilt, and rivals (e.g., siblings) may all contribute. Self-destructive behaviors (e.g., suicide, eating disorders, teen pregnancy) may be present (Goode, 2002). Self-absorption or obsession with external markers of self-worth may be evident (see Table 18-2).

Differential Diagnosis

Differential diagnoses include personal identity problems, role performance problems, and body image problems.

Management

Unconditional love, acceptance, belonging, and security are needs that are not being met. Refer to the management strategies discussed previously for specific strategies to achieve these, especially "parental roles," "know your children," and "limits and consequences."

Complications

Anxiety, behavior problems, depression, suicide, eating disorders, teen pregnancy, and violence are complications of self-esteem problems.

Personal Identity Problems

Description

When children are uncertain of their worth, personal identity is shaky and feelings of inferiority are manifested. Children may feel confusion about who they are.

TABLE 18-2 *Counterproductive Coping Strategies: Signs of Low Self-Esteem*

Behavior	Example
Quitting	Ending a game before it is over to avoid losing
Avoiding	Not even trying something for fear of failure
Cheating	Copying answers from someone else on a test
Clowning around	Acting silly to minimize feeling like a failure
Controlling	Telling others what to do
Bullying	Putting others down to hide feelings of inadequacy
Denying	Minimizing the importance of a task
Rationalizing or making excuses	Blaming the teacher for failing a test

From Brooks R: Self-esteem. In Parke S, Zuckerman B, editors: *Behavioral and developmental pediatrics*, Boston, 1995, Little, Brown.

Etiology

Personal identity problems arise when children do not receive respect as individuals and are not valued for who they are. This results in their questioning their worth and makes them wonder if they truly are OK. The child relies on others to define self, never knowing for sure who he or she is. This leads to internalizing others' negative perceptions. Potential parental factors that contribute to these feelings of inferiority include insensitivity to the child in words or attitude, fatigue and time pressure, guilt, and rivals for love.

Assessment

Children with personal identity problems do not feel good about themselves and often lack evidence of self-respect and self-liking, feeling as if they have not lived up to adult expectations. They may talk about themselves in degrading terms. There is a struggle to prove "I am OK." Coping may take the form of withdrawal, fighting, clowning, denying there is a problem, or striving for conformity (Dobson, 1999). There may be a history of the child being criticized, embarrassed, shamed, or humiliated, or a history of familial mental illness or abuse.

Differential Diagnosis

Self-esteem problems, role performance problems, and body image problems are differential diagnoses for personal identity problems.

Management

Self-respect, self-value, and feeling good about oneself are needs that are not being met. See the earlier discussion of management strategies for specific strategies to achieve these, especially "value children," "maintain appropriate expectations of the child," and "defuse feelings of inferiority." Helping the child learn to compensate can conquer low self-esteem (see section on finding the "island of competence"). Nondirective or experiential play therapy may be useful to help the child discover self and experience growth (Galligan, 2000). Time must be made to spend with the child in one-on-one interaction.

Complications

Depression, guilt, anger, and hostility are complications of personal identity problems.

Role Performance Problems

Description

When children are unable to perform expected activities or behaviors because of physical, mental, or cognitive disability, or they feel incompetent, role performance problems emerge and feelings of inadequacy often result. A typical scenario involves a child with school problems.

Etiology

Role performance problems arise when children do not feel adequate, confident, and in control and can occur in cognitive, social, and physical areas.

Assessment

Children with role performance problems may retreat and be hesitant to approach new opportunities and experiences. They may be perfectionists, always striving to prove competence: "I can do it." A history of "failure," or being a slow learner, semiliterate, an underachiever, a late bloomer, or culturally deprived, may be found

Differential Diagnosis

Self-esteem problems, personal identity problems, body image problems, and actual physical, mental, learning, or cognitive problems are differential diagnoses for role performance problems.

Management

Competence, confidence, adequacy, and being in control are needs that are not being met. See the previous discussion of management strategies for specific strategies to achieve these, especially "letting go," finding the "island of competence" (a key), and "help your child compete." Working with the school to achieve these goals is helpful.

Complications

Complications of role performance problems include depression, withdrawal, and somatic complaints.

Body Image Problems

Description

Discrepancy between how children's bodies are and how they want them to be results in body image problems. The discrepancy may be temporary or permanent, seen or unseen, occurring in terms of size, function, appearance, or potential. Attitudes, feelings, and fantasies all play a role in body image. Eating disorders are one example of a body image problem.

Etiology

Disturbance in body image arises from sources as varied as physical illness or disability, chronic illness, emotional disturbances, abuse, or attitudes conveyed by others. Body image problems are most common in adolescence, when teenagers are most concerned about physical appearance in comparison to that of their peers, but they also occur in younger children. An example of a younger child's body image disturbance can be seen when a child is unable to cope with the inability to master his or her environment because of a fracture and the subsequent immobilization.

Assessment

Children with disturbed body image may have concerns related to body size, function, appearance, or potential. These may be noted by questioning or techniques such as puppet interview or draw-a-person. A body esteem questionnaire for adolescents is available (Mendelson, Mendelson, & White, 2001).

Possible behaviors include the following:

- Lack of maternal identification (aspiring to be like one's mother); maternal identification positively correlates with self-esteem and negatively correlates with eating problems and body dissatisfaction (Hahn-Smith & Smith, 2001)
- Refusing to look at or touch the altered or missing part
- Preoccupation with the loss or change
- Feeling of shame and embarrassment
- Distorted perception of a normal body
- Fear of rejection or unwanted attention from others
- Overexposure or hiding of body part
- Actual or perceived change in structure and function of body or body part

Differential Diagnosis

Self-esteem, personal identity, or role performance problems are differential diagnoses for body image problems.

Management

The discrepancy between the real and the desired body, as well as the cause of the discrepancy, must be identified. Severity and cause of the discrepancy guide the intervention. If the discrepancy is developmental and not severe, education and counseling should help. If the problem is significant, referral for psychiatric care is often necessary.

Practices to develop appropriate ideas about appearance and value include the following (Hostetler, 2001):

- Explore parental feelings about appearance. Look for ways to broadcast healthy attitudes.
- Prompt children to determine where attitudes originate. Appreciate concern about physical appearance, but discuss extremes. Favorite television shows or movies are good starting points.
- Teach that happiness and beauty do not go hand in hand. Discuss feeling beautiful (outward changes) and being beautiful (inward growth).
- Celebrate each family member's uniqueness. Focus on personality traits and attitudes about life, school, and people, not on externals.

Other interventions that are helpful include the following:

- Encourage regular physical activity. One study (Ransdell et al, 2001) showed improved physical self-perception in adolescent girls and their mothers when they participated in a physical activity intervention together.
- Point out ways the child/adolescent is on target developmentally, and identify what can be expected over the next year. Emphasize the fact that there is a high degree of variability in development.
- Identify areas where assistance is needed.
- Refer to counselors, dietary therapy, occupational therapy, or physical therapy as appropriate.
- Visit school or social arenas before a child with health problems returns to that setting to educate and prepare the setting for the child.
- Involve the child in a peer group with similar problems.
- Provide ongoing support and encouragement from primary care provider with focus on positive aspects of body and functioning.
- Verbalize acceptance.
- Use play therapy to encourage verbalization.
- Teach new ways of handling situations to accommodate for loss or change.
- Discuss ways to camouflage (e.g., wig or scarf for hair loss).
- Compliment behaviors that indicate acceptance.

NURSING DIAGNOSES RELATED TO SELF-PERCEPTION: *Functional Health Pattern*

Diagnoses are related to the following concepts: identity, loneliness, self-esteem, and body image.

- Disturbed personal identity
- Powerlessness
  - Risk for powerlessness
- Hopelessness
- Risk for loneliness
- Chronic low self-esteem
  - Situational low self-esteem
  - Risk for situational low self-esteem
- Disturbed body image
- Readiness for enhanced self-concept

From North American Nursing Diagnosis Association: *NANDA nursing diagnoses: definitions and classification 2003-2004*, Philadelphia, 2003, North American Nursing Diagnosis Association.

RESOURCE BOX

Resources for Building Self-Perception

Bright Futures
www.brightfutures.org
A national initiative to promote and improve the health and well-being of infants, children, and adolescents; volume 1: *Mental Health Series*; volume 2: *Tool Kit*

Verb
www.verbparents.com (also: www.verbnow.com for tweens [9- to 13-year-olds])
From the U.S. Department of Health and Human Services, Centers for Disease Control and Prevention; geared toward keeping 9- to 13-year-olds active and increasing their self-esteem

Redleaf Press
www.redleafpress.org
Books, videos, and resources for early childhood that are developmentally and culturally appropriate and free of stereotypes

Ms. Foundation for Women
www.ms.foundation.org
From the creators and sponsors of Take Our Daughters to Work, an "empowering" GirlWorld site with information on organizations, publications, and websites for girls and their parents

National Association for Self-Esteem (NASE)
www.self-esteem-nase.org
Includes a book list, links to other sites, and lots of information on self-esteem

Free Spirit Publishing, Inc.
1-612-338-2068
1-800-735-7323
www.freespirit.com
Publishes books and other learning materials for children and teens, parents, educators, counselors, and everyone else who cares about kids

Search Institute
1-877-240-7251
www.search-institute.org
E-mail: si@search-institute.org
These researchers of developmental assets have multiple resources for individuals, schools, communities, and congregations; includes books, handouts, newsletter, and programs

Raising Resilient Children Foundation
www.raisingresilientkids.com
Disseminates information that assists adults to raise, support, and develop stress-hardy children; books, videos, articles, and a resiliency quiz

Winners on Wheels
www.wowusa.com
Provides an innovative learning environment to promote academic, social, and emotional development for children in wheelchairs

Resilience, Self-Esteem, Motivation, and Family Relationships
www.drrobertbrooks.com
Monthly newsletter, books, and on-line articles

Arthur M. Blank Family Foundation
www.blankfoundation.org
Supports programs and organizations that create and enhance self-esteem and increase awareness about cultural and community issues among young people

Marsh Media
www.marshmedia.com
Books and videos to help kids grow up safe, healthy, and with a sense of self-worth

Soy Unica! Soy Latina!
www.soyunica.org
Bilingual initiative for Hispanic girls ages 9 to 14 (and their mothers/other caregivers) by the Substance Abuse and Mental Health Services Administration (SAMHSA) designed to help build and enhance self-esteem, mental health, and decision-making and assertiveness skills, and to prevent the harmful consequences of alcohol, tobacco, and illicit drugs

BOOKS THAT TEACH SELF-ESTEEM

Brave New Girls by Jeanette Gadeberg (Fairview Press, 1997) for ages 9 years and older
Corduroy by Don Freeman (Viking, 1968) for ages 3 to 8 years
I Like Being Me: Feeling Special, Appreciating Others and Getting Along by Judy Lalli (Free Spirit, 1997) for ages 4 to 8
Leo the Late Bloomer by Robert Kraus (Harper Collins, 1971) for ages 4 to 8 years
On the Day You Were Born by Debra Frasier (Harcourt Brace, 1991) for ages 2 years and older
Those Can-Do Pigs by David McPhail (Dutton, 1996) for ages 5 to 9 years

REFERENCES

Benson PL, Galbraith J, Espeland P: *What kids need to succeed,* Minneapolis, MN, 1998a, Free Spirit Publisher.

Benson PL, Galbraith J, Espeland P: *What teens need to succeed,* Minneapolis, MN, 1998b, Free Spirit Publisher.

Brooks R: Self-esteem. In Parke S, Zuckerman B, editors: *Behavioral and developmental pediatrics,* Boston, 1995, Little, Brown.

Brooks R: *What is resilience?* Available at *www.raisingresilientkids.com* (accessed Oct 30, 2002).

Chapman PL, Mullis RL: Racial differences in adolescent coping and self-esteem, *J Genet Psychol* 161(2):152-160, 2000.

Costello EJ et al: Relationships between poverty and psychopathology, *JAMA* 290(15):2023-2029, 2003.

Davis-Kean PE, Sandler HM: A meta-analysis of measures on self-esteem for young children: a framework for future measures, *Child Dev* 72(3):887-906, 2001.

Day J, Day-Ferraz T: *Children believe everything you say: creating self-esteem with children,* United Kingdom, 1997, Harper Collins.

Dobson J: *The new hide or seek: building self-esteem in your child,* Grand Rapids, MI, 1999, FH Revell.

Elster AB, Kuznets NJ: *AMA guidelines for adolescent preventive services (GAPS),* Baltimore, 1994, Williams & Wilkins.

Galligan AC: That place where we live: the discovery of self through creative play experience, *J Child Adolesc Psychiatr Nurs* 13(4):169-176, 2000.

Goode E: Deflating self-esteem's role in society's ills. Available at *www.nytimes.com/2002/10/01/health/psychology/0125TE.html?ei = 1&en = d2809ed774* (accessed Oct 2, 2002).

Gray-Little B, Hafdahl AR: Factors influencing racial comparisons of self-esteem: a quantitative review, *Psychol Bull* 126(1):26-54, 2000.

Hahn-Smith AM, Smith JE: The positive influence of maternal identification on body image, eating attitudes, and self-esteem of Hispanic and Anglo girls, *Int J Eat Disord* 29(4):429-440, 2001.

Hall H: Ways to enhance your child's self-esteem. Presentation at the NAPNAP National Conference, Chicago, 1998.

Hart L: *The winning family: increasing self-esteem in your children and yourself,* Oakland, CA, 1990, LifeSkills Press.

Hostetler B: Looking beyond looks: helping your child look beyond their physical appearance, *Focus on the Family,* July 2001, pp 20-21.

Hunsberger M: Fostering self-esteem. In Betz CL, Hunsberger M, Wright S, editors: *Family-centered nursing care of children,* ed 2, Philadelphia, 1994, WB Saunders.

Jellinek M, Patel BP, Froehle MC, editors: *Bright futures in practice: mental health,* vol 1, *Practice guide,* vol 2, *Toolkit,* Arlington, VA, 2002, National Center for Education in Maternal and Child Health.

Jones A, Jones AE: *104 activities that build: self-esteem, teamwork, communication, anger management, self-discovery, and coping skills,* Richland,WA, 1998, Rec Room Publishing.

Kump T: Self-esteem: why little kids need BIG egos, *Healthy Kids,* Oct/Nov 1998, pp 53-58.

Kurcinka MS: *Raising your spirited child,* New York, 1998, Harper-Perennial.

Kvols KJ: *Redirecting children's behavior,* ed 3, Seattle, 1997, Parenting Press.

Mendelson BK, Mendelson MJ, White DR: Body esteem scale for adolescents and adults, *J Pers Assess* 76(1):90-106, 2001.

Perry PD: Creating novelty, *Scholastic Parent and Child* 9:67-68, 2001.

Quatman T, Watson CM: Gender differences in adolescent self-esteem: an exploration of domains, *J Genet Psychol* 162(1): 92-117, 2001.

Ransdell LB et al: Daughters and mothers exercising together (DAMET): a 12-week pilot project designed to improve physical self-perception and increase recreational physical activity, *Women Health* 33(3/4):101-116, 2001.

Reasoner R: *The true meaning of self-esteem,* 2002. Available at *www.self-esteem-nase.org/whatisself-esteem.shtml* (accessed Sept 19, 2002).

Rosemond J: *Parent power and the six point plan for raising happy healthy children,* Kansas City, MO, 2001, Andrews McMeel Publishers.

Saigal S et al: Self-esteem of adolescents who were born prematurely, *Pediatrics* 109(3):429-433, 2002.

Schott ER, Bellin W: The relational self-concept scale: a contest specific self-report measure for adolescents, *Adolescence* 36(141):85-103, 2001.

Sieving RE, Zirbel-Donisch ST: Self-esteem in children, *J Pediatr Health Care* 4:290-296, 1990.

Solomon CR, Serres F: Effects of parental verbal aggression on children's self-esteem and school marks, *Child Abuse Negl* 23(4):339-351, 1999.

Spencer JM et al: Self-esteem as a predictor of initiation of coitus in early adolescents, *Pediatrics* 109(4):581-584, 2002.

Spratt E: Assessing and reinforcing your child's self-esteem. In Jellinek M, Patel BP, Froehler MC, editors: *Bright futures in practice: mental health,* vol 2, *Tool kit,* Arlington, VA, 2002, National Center for Education in Maternal and Child Health.

Theunissen NCM et al: Quality of life and self-esteem in children treated for idiopathic short stature, *J Pediatr* 140(5):507-515, 2002.

US Department of Health and Human Services: *Healthy people 2010,* 1999. Available at *http://web.health.gov/healthypeople* (accessed Sept 15, 2002).

US Preventive Services Task Force: *Guide to clinical preventive services,* ed 2, Baltimore, 1996, Williams & Wilkins.

US Public Health Service: *Put prevention into practice (PIPP): clinician's handbook of preventive services,* ed 2, McLean, VA, 1998, International Medical Publishers.

Verschueren K, Buyck P, Marcoen A: Self-representations and socioemotional competence in young children: a 3-year longitudinal study, *Dev Psychol* 37(1):126-134, 2001.

Webster-Stratton C: *The incredible years: a trouble-shooting guide for parents of children aged 3-8,* Toronto, 1997, Umbrella Press.

19 Role Relationships

Ardys M. Dunn, Margaret A. Brady

OVERVIEW

Understanding family dynamics and role relationships is essential in the delivery of primary care to children and adolescents. The nurse practitioner (NP) must be sensitive to the roles that parents or caregivers, siblings, extended family members, and peers have in shaping the developing child. Likewise, the community is an extension of the family and serves as a major component in the widening circle of influence that affects children's and adolescents' lives. Chapter 3 outlines important considerations and appropriate tools to be used when assessing family systems. This chapter discusses the family life cycle and family variations, as well as the assessment and management of situations or events that the NP is likely to encounter in a primary care setting related to violence, family relationship problems, child maltreatment or neglect, and sibling rivalry. Preventive interventions for role relationship problems that are directed at the population as a whole (universal interventions) and specific individuals or groups at risk (selective interventions) are identified. Advice about securing nurturing, safe, and developmentally appropriate child care is discussed.

Family Life Dynamics

Healthy families are cohesive and adaptable, with positive communication patterns (Friedman, Bowden, & Jones, 2003). Family cohesion is an indication of the emotional bonding between family members and can range from the extremes of very low (disengaged) to very high (enmeshed) bonding, with moderate to high (connected) bonding representing the middle ground. Family adaptability is the ability of a family system to change its power structure, role relationships, and relationship rules in response to situational and developmental stress. The range of adaptability varies from very rigid (very low) to chaotic (very high), with a middle ground between structured and flexible. A key element in adaptability is the ability to change when appropriate. Communication patterns range from positive communication skills that convey messages such as empathy, reflective listening, and supportive comments to negative communication skills that reflect double messages, double binds, or criticism and that minimize opportunities to share feelings. Communication is one of the most crucial elements within any interpersonal relationship. Family cohesion and adaptability are threatened and thwarted with negative communication patterns.

Each family has its own unique pattern of growth and development, and family systems evolve and change, demonstrating different dynamics depending on the stage of the family's life cycle. Just as a child goes through stages of development, so do family units. Family life with young infants and preschool children is vastly different from family life with school-age children, with early versus late adolescents, or with young adults. Also, different types of family units—nuclear, single-parent, divorced, or blended—will express different styles or patterns of family life.

Dimensions of Family Functioning

Regardless of how a family is classified or typed, common themes exist within all families, and five key dimensions have a significant impact on family functioning, contributing to cohesiveness, adaptability, and positive communication. To assist parents and children across the family life cycle and during times of stress, the NP must carefully assess these elements, which include family

- Resources
- Stresses
- Values
- Structures
- Coping styles

Family resources include a social support network of extended family members, friends, and community; as well as financial and other material assets. Families with limited resources or social support networks are more vulnerable to stressful life events than are families with resources and support systems in place.

Potential family stresses and changes are numerous and include financial strains, illness, marital strain, family transitions, losses, and lack of effective coping strategies. Life brings transitions that necessitate change. Many transitions are normal, some are anticipated, and others are unexpected; all can have a significant impact.

Values shared by family members provide a framework to guide, explain, and understand events being experienced, and within which to find comfort, joy, and solace. Spiritual beliefs are one example of values that can support a family in its everyday life and in times of challenge.

Family roles and structures vary greatly, from one family to another, within an individual family, and as family members grow and develop. Role responsibilities and structures often change in response to external demands experienced by the family.

The way in which demands are met, transitions handled, and concerns resolved depends on the family's ability to cope. Positive or effective coping is characterized as a creative response to a change or stressor that results in a new behavior or attitude. Coping styles reflect habitual patterns of action. In contrast, coping efforts refer to specific actions taken as a direct result of a specific situation.

The Interactive Family Life Cycle

The family life cycle is interactive, both within the family and between the family and its community. Within the family, each member influences all others in the family and is likewise affected by them. Maladaptive patterns of interaction among family members can place a child and family at risk for negative outcomes. For example, if the family unit does not provide a protective, supportive, and loving environment to nurture the child or fails in its responsibility to help the child learn self-discipline and the ability to socialize with others, the child often develops maladaptive behaviors.

In addition, children are at risk for developing mental health problems as a result of environmental factors such as living in poverty, living in a community with a high crime rate, living in a home marked by marital conflict or domestic violence, living in a home in which they or their siblings are the victims of child maltreatment or neglect, or having a parent who abuses alcohol or other substances or has mental illness.

In contrast to at-risk factors, there are factors that are protective and foster child resiliency. Certain temperaments, a caring relationship, and effective parenting can counter the negative effects of adverse risk factors and contribute to a child's positive mental health. The degree of satisfaction as a married couple and as parents is an important outcome measure of how well the family is functioning as a family unit. Single-parent households may face many challenges that can have a negative impact on the family unit, but are enhanced by developing nurturing relationships in both the parent's and the child's life.

ASSESSMENT OF FAMILY RELATIONSHIPS AND DYNAMICS

In addition to issues that may arise with "typical" family relationships, NPs are likely to encounter parent- or child-initiated concerns, situations, and events related to relationship problems, child maltreatment or neglect, and violence. Families and children who are either experiencing or who are at risk for these stressful situations must be identified. Also, family strengths and attributes that sustain and help families effectively deal with stress are important factors to evaluate in the assessment process. In an assessment of family dynamics, the health care provider must investigate the relationships among child, parent or caretaker, and social and environmental factors. Each factor must be analyzed separately, with its various component parts identified. The interactive effect of these factors must then be explored. The goal of assessment is to determine factors that have a negative impact on the child's ability to achieve his or her optimum level of physical, social, cognitive, or emotional growth and development, as well as factors that support healthy growth.

The following list of significant child, parent or caregiver, and social and environmental factors is not exclusive, but can be used to alert the NP to areas that need further investigation.

Significant points to identify as part of the child factor are the following:
- Chronologic age and developmental level
- Present or past history of physical, emotional, or cognitive problems
- Personality traits and characteristics, as well as temperament
- Prior maltreatment or significant negative life events
- Special care needs
- School performance

Significant points to identify as part of the parent or caregiver factor are these:
- Physical, intellectual, or emotional abilities, illnesses, or limitations
- Level of involvement in child care and life events of child
- Awareness of, responsiveness to, and availability to the child

- Level of parenting skills and pattern of communication
- Structure of family—two-parent family, single-parent household, or other patterns
- History of maltreatment as a child
- A victim or perpetrator of domestic violence
- Previous parental history of child neglect or maltreatment
- Current drug use in the home or previous history of substance abuse (drugs or alcohol, or both)
- Financial resources
- Child-rearing practices experienced as a child
- Beliefs about discipline and corporal punishment

Significant points to identify as part of social and environmental factors are the following:

- Type and strength of family social support network or social isolation of a family
- Peer group relationships
- Sibling assessment
- Cultural belief system
- Environmental condition of home
- Community characteristics—both needs and assets
- Availability and accessibility of community support systems and partnerships
- Stresses, crises, or conflicts in the home environment
- Stresses in neighborhood environment

MANAGEMENT FOR HEALTH PROMOTION AND DISEASE PREVENTION

Primary care providers are often approached by parents with concerns about developmental or role relationship issues that can be managed with healthy parenting and good communication (see Chapters 5 through 9 and Chapter 18). The NP, as a supportive health care professional, is in a strategic position to prevent problems and empower parents and children by providing anticipatory guidance, education, resources, and opportunities for counseling. NPs must always remember to emphasize the need for preventive services for children and their parents and families.

The NP is typically involved in universal preventive interventions and, depending on background and education, can be involved in selective and indicated preventive interventions. Universal preventive interventions are directed at enhancing the parent-child relationship and are an essential part of routine pediatric health care supervision. Universal interventions address the population as a whole and stress wellness promotion, improving communication, and strengthening relationships. Selective preventions are directed at individuals or groups at risk for the development of mental health or relationship problems, or both. Indicated preventions are for high-risk individuals who are experiencing symptoms or who have biologic markers for mental illness. Selective and indicated preventions often employ a multidisciplinary approach, with community resources and other professionals from various social fields joining together. The NP must develop a plan of action with goals and outcome measures and specific criteria that indicate when there is need for referral to a mental health or other professional.

Healthy People 2010: Understanding and Improving Health addresses issues of violence and abusive behavior and their negative effect on children, families, and society (U.S. Department of Health and Human Services [USDHHS], 2000). Child maltreatment is recognized as a significant public health problem, and data indicate that the vast majority of child abuse (84%) is perpetrated by parents (Children's Bureau, 2002). The target goal of *Healthy People 2010* for maltreatment of children is 10.3 per 1000 children under age 18 years, and for child maltreatment fatalities, 1.4 per 100,000 children under age 18 years (USDHHS, 2000). National, state, and local efforts must be dedicated to reducing preventable death and disability and to enhancing the quality of life for all children. Health professionals in their individual practice settings and as a collective group must commit time and talents to improving the quality of life by incorporating health promotion and disease prevention as integral components of health care for children and their families.

CHALLENGES TO FAMILY RELATIONSHIPS

Separation and Divorce

Description

Divorce or the separation of parents has a profound effect on family life and can lead to major disruption and disequilibrium in the lives of children. Custodial and visitation arrangements for children are variable. Joint custody is an option that allows both parents the opportunity to participate in mutual decision making about their child's life and welfare. Various living arrangements and visitation rights are possible with joint custody. There are instances in which single custody is in the best interest of the child, however, and the noncustodial parent may have sporadic contact with the child and limited involvement in the child's life.

Research studies investigating the psychologic consequences of divorce on children have reported varying data on its negative effect. In one study, divorce was not specifically related to psychopathology in children (McMahon et al, 2003). A 10-year review of the literature indicates that, although children from divorced families have more adjustment problems than children whose parents do not

BOX 19-1 *Child-Related Assessment Factors in Divorce*

Developmental Stage of Children

- Age and developmental stage of children greatly affect their response to separation and divorce of parents.
- Common reactions of children to divorce by age-group:
  - 2-5 yr: Regression, irritability, sleep disturbances, aggression
  - 6-8 yr: Open grieving and feelings of rejection or being replaced; whiny, immature behavior, sadness, fearfulness
  - 9-12 yr: Fear and intense anger at one or both parents
  - ≥13 yr: Worried about own future, depressed, or acting-out behaviors (e.g., truancy, sexual activity, alcohol or drug use, suicide attempts)

Common Issues for Children of Divorcing Parents

- Continued tension, conflict, and fighting between parents
- Litigation disputes over custody and visitation arrangements
- Abandonment by one parent or sporadic visitation (decreased availability) vs. denial of visitation
- Diminished parenting resulting from such factors as availability issues or emotional inaccessibility, distress, or instability
- Limited social support system outside nuclear family
- Feelings of loneliness or emotional abandonment, or both

BOX 19-2 *Parental and Family Unit Assessment Factors in Divorce*

Impact of Divorce on Parent

Psychologic functioning of parent and availability to child are often negatively affected.

Feelings of bitterness and acrimony toward divorcing spouse are common.

Feelings of helplessness and depression can overwhelm parent, who may no longer be able to maintain household standards or standards of behavior for child.

Economic Consequence of Divorce

Often devastating economic hardships and decline in living standard are problems that families (especially women) face as a result of divorce.

Nonpayment or delinquency in payment of child support is a widespread problem.

divorce, those problems may arise from the conflictive relationships existing before the divorce, rather than the divorce per se (Kelly, 2000). Children's fear of abandonment may be a critical factor in their degree of successful adaptation to divorce (Wolchik et al, 2002b). There also are data to support that children can adapt to and successfully cope with marital separation and divorce with no long-term negative effect, especially if family conflict is minimized or they have significant nurturing support, such as with a grandparent (Cohen, 2002; Lussier et al, 2002; Wolchik et al, 2002a).

Incidence

In recent years the rate of divorce has decreased slightly in the United States. The Centers for Disease Control and Prevention (CDC) reported a divorce rate of 4.0 per 1000 marriages in 2001, down slightly from 4.2 per 1000 in 2000, but significantly higher than the 3.5 per 1000 in 1970 (Bramlett & Mosher, 2002). Parents who marry at younger ages are more likely to experience divorce. Approximately one of three first marriages will end in divorce within 10 years, and one of five first marriages will end in divorce within 5 years (Bramlett & Mosher, 2002). Thus, though divorce occurs in marriages with children of all age-groups, the children in divorcing families tend to be younger.

Assessment

The goal of assessment of the family experiencing separation or divorce is to determine the needs and strengths of the family, and use that information to assist them to healthy coping. Areas to investigate include the following:

- Developmental stage of the children
- Common psychosocial reactions to divorce likely at that stage
- The psychosocial impact of the divorce on the parents
- The economic consequences of divorce on the family unit
- Family assets and resources, both internal and external to the family unit (Boxes 19-1 and 19-2)

Management

Anticipatory guidance given to parents who are in the process of separating and divorcing should cover four main topics:

- The need to prepare the child for the impending separation, if possible
- The need to give ongoing explanations about the divorce and custody issues, plus assurances that the child will be taken care of and is loved

- Suggestions about self-help measures
- Indications when referral for mental health counseling is needed (Table 19-1)

Patient Education and Prevention

The goal of health education for children and parents experiencing divorce is to help restore a sense of wholeness and integrity in children's lives. NPs must stress those factors that have been shown to significantly affect whether the child will experience a healthful adjustment to the divorce (Box 19-3). Successful efforts implemented during initial periods of disequilibrium and reorganization will strengthen normal development and prevent future psychologic trauma. In an early research study, Wallerstein (1983) identified six psychologic tasks that children of divorce must master beginning from the time of parental separation and culminating in young adulthood. These tasks continue to be relevant for children whose parents are divorced. If these psychologic tasks are not achieved, the child's mastery of normal developmental tasks associated with growing up is negatively affected. Long-range and preventive interventions need to focus on helping the child to achieve these tasks or goals:

- Acknowledge the reality of the marital breakup.
- Disengage from parental conflict and distress and resume customary pursuits.
- Resolve loss of familiar daily routine, traditions, and symbols, and the physical presence of two parents.
- Resolve anger and self-blame.
- Accept the permanence of the divorce.
- Achieve realistic hope regarding relationships—the capacity to love and be loved.

The NP should offer support and may schedule additional visits or telephone contacts with the family to monitor their adjustment. Be careful not to use terminology that is offensive such as "broken home," "intact family," and "child

TABLE 19-1 ***Key Anticipatory Guidance Issues for Families Experiencing Divorce or Separation***

Anticipatory Guidance Issue	Discussion Points with Parents
Advise parents to prepare the child for the impending breakup.	If possible, tell the child in advance of the breakup. Children who are told before the separation occurs handle the situation more calmly than those who are given no preparation and wake up to find the parent gone.
	Discussions should focus on supporting the child's needs for reassurance and stability, not on blame, recriminations, or the parent's needs.
Explain to parents the need to discuss the following key issues with their children:	Assure children they will continue to see the departing parent if this is true.
	Explain what divorce means in language appropriate to the child's cognitive and developmental level; offer an explanation of reasons for the divorce in the same terms.
	Reassure children that they did not cause the divorce, that they cannot correct their parents' unhappiness in the marriage, and that the divorce is the parents' decision.
	Explain what the family structure will look like afterward, and what imminent changes will be necessary in the way the family functions.
	Explain the visitation arrangements as soon as they are established.
	Reassure children that they will be cared for, and they are not being abandoned by either parent, unless a parent has disappeared or refuses involvement.
	Tell children that feelings of sadness, anger, and disappointment are normal; that they should not "take sides" but love both parents.
Suggest self-help measures:	Children and parents may benefit from attending divorce recovery workshops, classes about families in transition, or peer support groups.
	School counselors, religious groups, or community and social service agencies may be resources for children and parents.
Discuss when referral for mental health counseling might be indicated.	Children often demonstrate internalized or externalized psychosocial problems (e.g., sadness, depression, acting-out behaviors, drug use, promiscuous sexual behavior, anger, violence) in response to divorce. Professional counseling can be an essential part of the recovery process, depending on the nature of symptoms, their severity, and how long they continue without improvement.
	Referral to individual or family counseling with mental health providers may be appropriate.

BOX 19-3 *Factors Affecting a Child's Ability to Achieve Healthy Adjustment to Divorce in His or Her Family*

The opportunity for continued participation of the noncustodial or visiting parent in the child's life on a regular basis
The ability of the custodial parent to handle and successfully parent the child
The ability of parents to separate their own feelings of anger and conflict and resolve their own hostility toward the other parent so that the child's need for a relationship with both parents is met
The child does not become involved in parental conflict and does not feel rejected
The availability of a social support network
The ability of parents to meet the child's developmental needs and to help the child master the developmental tasks before him or her
The child's overall personality and personal assets, as well as deficits

of divorce." In addition, look at each family as a unique situation and avoid negative stereotyping (e.g., "deadbeat dad" or "angry mom"). In addition, help the family cope by focusing on their positive strengths and ability to be resilient.

Single-Parent Families

Description

A *single-parent family* is defined as a household in which there is one parent only (no spouse) and one or more children under age 18 years. In some cases, other people related by birth (e.g., a brother or sister), marriage (e.g., a sister-in-law), or adoption may live in the household; unrelated (e.g., a friend) adults or children may also live with the family. Single-parent families are distinguished from *multigenerational families*, which are defined as families with a single parent or a married couple living with their children, their parents, their in-laws, or their grandchildren. Being a single parent is often a difficult, challenging role. Children living in single-parent households generally experience significantly lower standards of living and family income than children in two-parent households.

Incidence

The traditional two-parent family has gradually declined over the past few decades, although it is still the norm for families with children. According to the 2000 census, 51% of all U.S. households are headed by a married couple, and 23.5% consist of a married couple with children under age 18. Just over 7% of all households (7.2%) have a female head-of-household (no spouse present) with children under age 18, and 2.1% are single-parent families with a male head-of-household (Simmons & O'Neill, 2001). These data represent an increase from 1990, when 6.6% of households with children were headed by single mothers. The incidence of single-parent families varies by geographic, racial, and ethnic demographics. The south-central United States and large urban areas have more single-parent families; the midwestern United States has fewer single-parent families. Approximately 10% of children living in Mississippi or Washington, D.C., live in single-parent families; the rate in North Dakota and Iowa is nearly half that, 1 in 19 children (Simmons & O'Neill, 2001). Black and Hispanic children are more likely than white children to be members of single-parent households.

Numerous circumstances lead to single-parent households, including unemployment, divorce, births to unmarried mothers, abandonment of the family by a parent, incarceration of a parent, or death of a parent.

Assessment

Several key areas are important to assess when working with single parents and their children. They can be divided into parent- and child-related factors. Parent-related factors include the following:

- Availability of emotional support from a social network such as extended family members, friends, or church and community groups
- Presence of financial difficulties and economic hardships, which are often major concerns
- Living situation and insurance coverage
- Availability and quality of child care for parents who must work
- Opportunities for the single parent to have a social life and relationships or personal time

- Emotional and physical well-being of the parent; the capacity to parent when exhausted or overwhelmed
- Ability of the parent to maintain consistency in discipline, as well as a positive outlook and commitment to parenting (e.g., does the parent have the energy and temperament to parent in a consistent fashion?)
- Availability of financial and emotional support from a noncustodial parent

Child-related factors to assess include the following:

- Availability of emotional support from a social network such as extended family members and friends
- Role of the child in the family; responsibilities to care for siblings and opportunities to participate in activities outside of home
- Relationships with custodial parent (e.g., is the child the single parent's primary source of emotional support or contact?)
- Location of and relationship with the noncustodial parent (e.g., is it supportive or conflictive?)
- Availability of opportunities to accomplish age-appropriate developmental tasks (e.g., is child doing well in school? Does he or she have friends? Is child participating in sports or club activities?)
- Signs of problem behavior at school, at home, or with social activities, or the presence of children in the home with special needs (e.g., developmental disability, cognitive delay, or chronic illness)

Management

Many single families cope well with the demands they face, benefiting from advice, anticipatory guidance, encouragement, and support of the NP. On an individual level, several critical factors promote successful child rearing in single-parent homes. They involve the availability of a social support network and positive communication patterns (Box 19-4). Social organizations such as Big Brothers and Big Sisters offer a supportive role model for children in single-parent families. Parents Without Partners is a national organization that offers social activities and support for single parents (see Resource Box).

If parents request specific help or demonstrate signs of being exhausted, depressed, overwhelmed, burdened, or socially isolated, a referral to more specialized services such as counseling may be appropriate. Similar signs in children plus deviant behaviors, emotional adjustment problems, or school disciplinary, academic, or behavioral problems can be indicators for mental health referral. The type of referral depends on the nature of the problem, the severity of symptoms, and the continuance of symptoms or problems without signs of improvement. Referrals can include individual or family counseling with mental health practitioners (see Management section under Separation and Divorce).

BOX 19-4 *Significant Determinants for Successful Child Rearing in a Single-Parent Home*

- Support persons in the child's life who
  - Collaborate with the single parent
  - Develop quality relationships with the child
  - Are available for the child
- Adults in child's community who provide support, including
  - Teachers
  - School officials
  - Health care providers
  - Support person(s) for the parent
- Capacity of parent to communicate with child in open, direct, and understanding manner
- Ability of parent to recognize child's need for and to provide opportunities for enjoyment and accomplishment outside the home
- Economic stability and well-being that is adequate to meet family's needs

Patient Education and Prevention

Although individual families may be helped to gain better coping skills, significant positive change in the quality of life of single-parent families depends on restructuring and increasing economic, educational, and family support resources in the community. NPs should become informed of the impact that social service legislation has on the families they serve, and provide information to policy makers to help them make more appropriate decisions. One example is the 1996 Personal Responsibility and Work Opportunity Reconciliation Act (PRWORA), which required single parents on welfare to enter the workforce. In concert with the Temporary Assistance to Needy Families (TANF) legislation, the PRWORA was intended to assist parents to find employment and improve their income and the lives of their children. Unfortunately, the legislation has led to an increase in the number of children in poverty, Hispanic welfare recipients, urban poor, and black nonwelfare families who are low income. It has also led to a decrease in the number of low-income single parents acquiring some college education and a decrease in number of low-income families with health insurance (Peterson, Song, & Jones-DeWeever, 2002).

Remarriage: The Blended Family

Description

The *blended family* is a term used to describe family reorganization or reconstitution associated with remarriage. Often children from two families are involved in becoming one "blended" household. Because of past negative connotations of the term *stepfamily*, the currently preferred term is *blended family*.

Incidence

The majority of women and men who divorce or are widowed remarry. Children whose parents are divorced spend an average of 5 years in single-parent households. With remarriage, children become members of blended families. Blended families can present unique parenting challenges in family adaptation, cohesiveness, coping, and role relationships.

Assessment

The introduction of a stepparent and possibly stepsiblings can be beneficial for a child or can be a time of difficult adjustment. The majority of children within blended families gradually adjust well to their new family situations. However, role relationship problems do arise related to the special needs of reconstituted families. The NP must remember several important points when assisting blended families during times of transition or problems. They include the developmental stage of the children, the common psychosocial issues that these children experience, and characteristics of problem behaviors in blended families (Box 19-5).

Management

The goal of primary care interventions is to foster positive parenting behaviors, protect the development of the stepchild, and enhance family functioning. A careful assessment of any behavioral concern should be done. Whether the family is given guidance and followed closely by the primary care provider or given a referral to mental health services depends on the presence of significant behavioral problems or pathology. NPs should investigate community services that assist blended families, such as a self-help group for stepparents or a parenting group. Written information about and telephone numbers of community resources should be maintained in a handbook or resource guide kept in the practice setting.

BOX 19-5 *Assessment of Children in Blended Families*

Developmental Stage of Child

Age and developmental stage of child greatly affect child's response to the remarriage and ability of child to cope with change and new family relationships.
Early adolescence is often a time of greatest difficulty in adjustment to remarriage.
A mother's subsequent pregnancy is often a time of increased frequency and intensity of problems with young children.

Common Issues for Children in Blended Families

Complex relationship with new family members
Altered relationships with own family members and possible feelings of betraying other biologic parent or being torn between parents
Possible relocation and separation from family members and friends
Continued or new tensions between parents and tensions between stepparents; rivalries between parents and stepparents
Jealousy among stepsiblings
Establishing new family traditions and values
Continuing to respect earlier family history, traditions, and loyalties that may be in conflict with new family ties
Unrealistic expectations by child of stepparent
Unrealistic expectations by stepparent from child for instant love, respect, and obedience
Tensions within blended family household, creating anxiety and fear of another family breakup

Characteristics of Problem Behaviors in Blended Families

Problems can occur both at home and at school.
Children in divorced and blended families experience more behavioral, social, emotional, and educational problems than do children from nondivorced families.
Parental conflict more than family structure is the critical factor that influences both marital and family adjustment.

Patient Education and Prevention

Counseling and guidance before remarriage that looks at coping with transition in a blended family should be explored with parents. Relationships develop and are created over time. Many children go on to develop strong and meaningful attachments to their stepparents if the relationship is cultivated over time with careful sensitivity to the needs of the child.

Adoption

Description

Adoption is the legal process that gives children permanent family membership other than that of their birth parents. Birth parents terminate their rights, and the adoptive parents are awarded legal custody. The adoption process has changed greatly in the past two decades from that of the traditionally married couple adopting a newborn. Single-parent adoption; subsidized adoption of children with special needs; independent, identified, and international adoptions; surrogacy arrangements; and open adoptions are examples of the changing pattern of adoption. Public and private agencies, independent adoption through attorneys, and foreign adoption services are potential avenues to assist in the placement of children.

Incidence

Since 1975, with the dissolution of the National Center for Social Statistics, there have been no federal agencies or nonprofit organizations that collect data on the annual number of total adoptions in the United States. Statistics are kept on the adoption of foster children. It is known that adoption rates have declined markedly over the past 20 years as more unwed women elect to keep their babies and not place them for adoption. Adoption of children from minority backgrounds continues to be a problem because of the limited availability of adoptive parents of the same race or ethnic group.

Assessment

Important information that the NP should attempt to ascertain when assisting adoptive families includes the following:

- Legal arrangements and circumstances surrounding adoption process
  - What, if any, contact will the birth parent or parents have with the child?
  - When will the adoption be finalized? How long is the waiting period?
  - Are there support services available for the adoptive family if an agency is arranging the adoption?
- Knowledge of medical and psychosocial history of birth parents and child
  - Was the presence of any inherited diseases or mental illnesses reported about the birth parents? Does the child have any known or suspected medical problems?
  - Is information about the pregnancy, delivery, and neonatal period or subsequent medical problems available?
  - Children adopted from foreign countries can be at risk for medical problems. Routine recommended screening tests are outlined in Box 19-6.
- Availability of social supports for adoptive parents and older child
  - The presence of a social support network is important. Adoptive parents face the same parenting challenges as biologic parents do when their child passes through the various developmental stages of childhood. In addition, adoption is a special circumstance and can present special challenges to parents.

Management

Often parents will request a preadoption consultation. This is an ideal time to review many of the identified issues. Other families may be in a foster care situation, considering adoption. Support through this process, before adoption is finalized, is crucial because there may be many ups and downs to contend with. Once adoption is finalized, close monitoring and support by the NP during the initial adoption period are important. Scheduling of additional or more frequent health supervision visits is appropriate even when all appears well, but especially if high-risk situations or conditions are identified. If problems arise, prompt referral to mental health or social service agencies is imperative. Children with known special needs who are adopted are often eligible for federal and state financial support and services. Excellent books about adoption for adults and children are available in local bookstores. The NP should select and recommend those books that best fit the needs of the parents and children in the practice.

Patient Education and Prevention

In considering adoption, the parent or parents often benefit from a preadoption visit to the health care provider who will take care of their child. Parents often have many questions to ask about the initial adoption period and the establishment of a family relationship. Adoption is a lifetime commitment. Issues that the NP should address with parents include the following:

- There should be a gradual disclosure of the adoption to the child.

BOX 19-6 *Recommended Screening Tests for Children Adopted from Foreign Countries*

- Newborn metabolic screening panel (all infants)
- Complete blood count with differential, platelet count, and indices
- Thyroid function tests (if not done as part of newborn screen)
- Urinalysis
- Lead level
- PPD, despite any previous BCG vaccination; if positive obtain chest x-ray
- Stool for ova and parasites and *Giardia* antigen
- Hepatitis B panel, including surface antibody and antigen and core antibody
- Hepatitis C antibody
- Syphilis serology
- HIV-1, HIV-2 enzyme-linked immunosorbent assay (ELISA), with confirmatory Western blot; if positive for children under 18 months, further evaluation is necessary
- Developmental, dental, hearing, and vision screening
- Hemoglobin electrophoresis (Asian, Latin American, and African children)
- G-6-phosphate dehydrogenase assay (Asian, Mediterranean, and African children)
- Malaria (peripheral blood smear) (children from tropical or subtropical regions and those with fever of unknown origin)
- Polycythemia, familial or congenital (central European and Russian children)
- Rickets (radiograph) (Chinese children)
- Lactose intolerance (black, Latino, American Indian, and Asian children)

BCG, Bacille Calmette-Guérin; *HIV*, human immunodeficiency virus; *PPD*, purified protein derivative.

- Discussions of the adoption should be open, keeping in mind the child's developmental stage, cognitive abilities, and emotional needs.
- Discussions with the parents should address any myths, concerns, or fears that the parents might have about adoption and their adopted child.
- Parents need to understand that their child's wish to know about or seek out the biologic parents is not a rejection of them.
- Adolescence can be difficult for adoptive children as they seek their own identity and deal with the fact that they are adopted. If teenagers wish to seek out their biologic parents, they should be encouraged to wait until they are older.

Teenage Parents

Description

Teens who become pregnant and give birth face the challenge of raising an infant at a period in their lives when they are seeking to learn who they are and what they are about. The phrase often used to describe teen mothers is "children having children." Adolescent pregnancy is linked with poor educational and vocational outcomes for the mother, which, in turn, is associated with socioeconomic disadvantage. Some teens can successfully parent their infant if given support. Maternal age is an important predictor of successful parenting; however, preexisting family and individual factors that lead a teenager to become a mother before completing the educational and developmental tasks necessary for adult life are more relevant predictors of successful parenting.

Incidence

In 2001 the birth rate for teenagers was 45.3 live births per 1000 women ages 15 to 19 years. In the past decade, the teen birth rate declined 24% (Ventura, Hamilton, & Sutton, 2003).

Assessment

Key issues to address in assessment of at-risk status vary depending on the stage of the teen. Assessment issues related to each of these stages are separately addressed.

Before-Pregnancy Issues. Adolescent sexuality is an issue that should be discussed as a routine part of every health care encounter (see Chapter 20). Early identification and targeting of at-risk teens (both female and male) for intervention is an important role of the NP. Predictors of teen motherhood include the following:

- Sexual molestation as a child
- Abuse or neglect in childhood
- Being a child of an addicted parent or family history of mental illness

- Lack of family involvement; an intolerable home situation
- Poor academic achievement or school dropout
- Loss of a parent by death, separation, divorce, or foster placement
- Living in an impoverished social environment where adolescent pregnancy is commonplace and accepted

Addressing issues that arise during pregnancy, at birth, and postpartum can contribute to a more successful pregnancy outcome and prevent problems from appearing later in the child or teen parent's life.

Pregnancy

- Disclosure of pregnancy to family, the baby's father, peers, or other significant people. Who has the teen told about the pregnancy? Are they supportive? Many teens and their families are in turmoil during the pregnancy.
- Access to prenatal care and compliance with pregnancy health supervision. Does the teen need to access federal- and state-sponsored programs for medical financial coverage and general assistance?
- Adjustment to the emotional and physical changes of pregnancy.
- Preparation and plans for the delivery and after the baby is born: current living arrangements; plans for future living and child care arrangements, returning to school or work, and financial support.

Birth and Postpartum

- Preparation for childbirth and postpartum care.
- Identification of who is available to give emotional support and physical help at this critical time.
- Infancy.
- Adolescent mother-infant attachment. Is there evidence of healthy attachment, or emotional or physical neglect?
- Confidence of teen mother to care for her infant.
- Conflicts between the teen's needs and those of her infant. Is the mother more interested in reestablishing her adolescent lifestyle, or caring for her infant?
- Living arrangements. With whom and where are the teen mother and baby living?
- Plans for birth control.
- Degree of involvement of the social support network in the mother's and infant's life. Is the baby's father invested in the child? Is the teen mother's or father's family supportive, overprotective, or not involved?
- Return to school or the workforce. What are the child care arrangements? How has this affected the teen mother and baby?

Later Years. Toddler years are challenging, particularly for teens who themselves are survivors of abuse or neglectful parenting. Typically, the teen mother and young child, if living with family, move out on their own or with the mother's partner. The NP needs to assess the following:

- Mother's ability to cope with the normal inquisitive and provocative behaviors of her toddler
- How well the family unit is functioning
- Progress made by the mother toward reaching her life goals

As the child gets older, the teen mother is thought of as a young mother. Children of these mothers, especially those who are poor and living in urban settings, are more likely than their peers to have behavioral problems. When their own children are adolescents, they find this a difficult period, and often they become young grandmothers as the teen pregnancy circle is perpetuated.

Management

Key points in management include the following:

- Maintain regular and frequent contact with the teen mother during her pregnancy and during the child's infancy and early childhood.
- Refer to a community health nurse for home visits early in pregnancy and postpartum. This intervention has proven most successful in delaying subsequent pregnancy and improving healthy parenting and family life (Olds, 2002).
- Provide referrals for resources and community agencies that can assist teen mothers (e.g., parenting classes or literature; support groups; special clinic programs that see both infants and teen mothers; Women, Infants, and Children [WIC] program).
- Remember that both the teen mother and the infant or child have their own separate needs for health supervision and guidance.
- Provide a supportive environment for the teen mother. Have a plan for follow-up so that teen mothers do not get lost in the system.
- Involve other family members (e.g., grandparents, the father) in discussions about child-rearing issues depending on the teen's wishes.
- Emphasize the strengths of the teen mother and praise her positive efforts.
- Intervene early when warning signs of potential neglect or abuse are evident.

Other Variations in the Family Unit

There are a number of variations in the family unit that reflect changes in American family life and the diversity of parental experiences. Each of these situations is unique and requires a thorough assessment. Key issues to consider when working with these families follow.

Children Living with Grandparents or Extended Family Members

In 2001, approximately 5.5 million children lived with their grandparents, some in multigenerational households that included their parents as well. Approximately 2.4 million grandparents were responsible for their own grandchildren under age 18 years; nearly half a million of these grandparents lived below the poverty level, and many others were at or just above the poverty level (U.S. Census Bureau, 2001). NPs should be alert to the following factors as they work with grandparents who are primary caregivers:

- Often, children have lived with one or two biologic parents before either voluntary or court-ordered placement with the grandparent. Such children frequently bring with them a history of significant stress, hardship, and emotional turmoil.
- Children can be involved in continuing conflict with their biologic parent or parents and may experience emotional reaction to separation from or abandonment by the parent or parents.
- Children can experience the loss of friends, schoolmates, and familiar surroundings.
- Caring for children can be an overwhelming responsibility, especially for older relatives or grandparents; the parenting experience can be physically, emotionally, and financially draining on relatives.
- Children need a supportive environment and consistency in discipline.
- Such families need significant support from social service agencies, the educational system, and health care providers.

Children Living in Foster or Group Homes

The number of children in foster homes is increasing, and meeting their psychosocial needs is a growing problem in the United States. Census data report that more than 200,000 children were in foster care placement in March 2000 (U.S. Census Bureau, 2003), but this may be an underestimate, because foster care is a transient arrangement. The Administration for Children and Families (ACF) states that on September 30, 1999, there were 568,000 foster children in the United States (ACF, 2001). On any given day, well over 550,000 U.S. children are likely to be in foster care (Casey Family Programs, 2003).

- Children are generally placed in protective custody because of concerns of neglect, physical abuse, sexual abuse, or other forms of child maltreatment or because their parents are unable to care for them.
- Children frequently have a history of significant stress, hardship, and emotional turmoil in their family life.
- Children can experience multiple placements and separation from siblings.
- Foster children are often involved in family reunification programs and are placed back with their parents under the supervision of the child protective services, with home-based family preservation services available to monitor the situation, assist the parents, and safeguard the children.
- Foster children are placed under legal mandates in foster homes that mirror the children's ethnic, racial, and cultural identities as much as feasible.
- Foster children often receive erratic health care before and after their placement; a medical passport can be used as a means to keep track of medical problems, treatments, and special needs.
- Foster children have special needs, should be followed closely, and should receive preventive health services.
- Children are emancipated from the foster care system at age 18 years and need to be prepared for this major life change.

Children Living with Homosexual Parents

- Children living with homosexual parents may be the "biologic products" of former heterosexual relationships, or they may have been adopted, or they may have been conceived by artificial technology. Perrin (1998) reports that between 6 and 10 million children currently live with one parent who is lesbian or gay. These families reflect every ethnic, racial, and socioeconomic group in the United States.
- Children of homosexual parents show no significant differences in their emotional and social adaptation, self-esteem, gender identity, sexual behavior, or sexual orientation than their counterparts raised with heterosexual parents (Anderssen, Amlie, & Ytteroy, 2002; Golombok et al, 2003; Hunfeld et al, 2002).
- Children can experience problems because of teasing or social isolation and stigmatization by peers, secrecy of parents, or negative reaction of the noncustodial biologic parents.
- Children do well if parents are committed to their children, are sensitive to the children's needs, and are patient.
- Children do well if the homosexual stepparent is supportive of the other parent and the child or children. Some states allow adoption by the nonbiologic parent; this is called *co-parent adoption.*
- Children find it easier to deal with questions posed about their parents if they learn about their parents' sexual orientation during childhood rather than during adolescence.
- Children are not at risk to develop a homosexual identity based on their living situation.

Children Living with Two Parental Figures Who Are Unmarried

- Children can be the biologic children of two adults who decide not to marry but live together (cohabitation), the biologic children of one of the adults but not the other, or children who live with their guardian and the guardian's unmarried partner.
- In each of these family situations, the development of a high-quality parent-child relationship, consistency in discipline, and a continued commitment to the child are hallmarks of successful parenting and child rearing.
- Children face significant developmental risks if they sense a lack of permanence or certainty in their lives; if family life is characterized by conflict or poverty; or if there is inconsistency in who lives in the home, frequent breakups, new adult relationships, or frequent changes in living arrangements.
- Children can be torn emotionally if other significant adults in the children's lives (other biologic parents, grandparents, or other extended family members) express distress about the relationship between the unmarried adults.
- Many families who cohabit live in poverty, and the outcome for children may be no better or even worse than living in low-income single-parent families (Acs & Nelson, 2002).

Homeless Children and Their Families

The homeless family and homeless children are an increasing special-need population. Approximately 3.5 million Americans experience homelessness in any given year, and nearly 39% percent, or 1.35 million, are children (Urban Institute, 2000). Only about 35% of homeless children live in shelters, where they can be counted. Others (an estimated 34%) double up with friends or family or live in motels or other locations (23%); they may not be recognized as homeless and thus are denied access to educational services (National Coalition for the Homeless, 2002). Characteristics of these children include the following:

- Living in poverty because of low income and inadequate social support services (e.g., housing, job training, educational opportunities)
- Families with a history of substance abuse, domestic violence, mental illness, or unexpected family or economic crisis
- A significant minority representation, with the majority of these children being younger than 5 years of age
- A teen population composed of runaway and "throwaway" adolescents who are often victims of physical and sexual abuse and neglect, or teens alienated from their parents for multiple reasons
- Living in a variety of environments, such as a car, motel, makeshift shelters of cardboard or tents, or homeless shelters; often children and parents in families are separated
- Three times more likely to be placed in remedial classes in school and to become school dropouts (National Coalition for the Homeless, 2001)

Health care problems for which these children are at high risk include the following:

- Early initiation of and sustained substance abuse
- Diseases linked to poverty, including tuberculosis, multiple caries, impetigo
- Sexually transmitted diseases (STDs) for runaway teens who prostitute themselves
- Emotional health problems; social isolation
- Those who attend school may be ostracized by other children because of their unkempt appearance, poor hygiene, or substandard living conditions (National Coalition for the Homeless, 2001).

Children with Chronic Illnesses

Common chronic illnesses in children include allergies (e.g., asthma and eczema) and neurologic conditions (e.g., seizure disorders or cerebral palsy). Although the incidence of childhood diabetes is increasing, and celiac disease may be more common than once thought, pediatric chronic illnesses tend to cover a wide range of conditions and are relatively rare. Approximately 4% to 5% of children seen in health care facilities have a mild chronic condition, and another 4% to 5% have a moderate to severe chronic illness (Neff et al, 2002). Demands on families of children with chronic illnesses are constant and challenging. NPs can be a resource as families develop ways to maximize family function and enhance the growth of all family members. NPs can also assess family systems for the risk of stress and its consequences, such as maltreatment of the child. The Family Impact of Childhood Disability (FICD) scale has been found to predict future parenting stress of both mothers and fathers (Trute & Hiebert-Murphy, 2002). Chapter 23 provides a discussion of critical issues for NPs to consider when working with families of children with chronic disease.

OTHER CHALLENGES TO THE FAMILY UNIT

Sibling rivalry, multiple births, and death are challenges to the family unit that can cause a period of disequilibrium. Sibling rivalry is a familiar problem, with tales of sibling rivalry recorded in early historical writings. With advances in reproductive technology and the use of fertility drugs, multiple births of two or more infants are much more common, particularly to women over 30 years of age. Many families are faced with death of grandparents, parents, siblings, and others in the child's social network.

Sibling Rivalry

Birth or Adoption of a New Infant

The birth or adoption of a sibling is often an occasion marked by some degree of unrest and distress for an older sibling. Many parents dread the possibility of jealousy on the part of an older child, and frequently voice concern about transient behavioral regressions occurring after a new infant is brought home. The developmental stage of the older sibling at the time of the new sibling's arrival is an important consideration in helping parents prepare their older child for the new sibling and in dealing with rivalry behaviors afterward. For example, the 2-year-old who is working on developing autonomy often feels highly vulnerable with the appearance of a new sibling. However, many school-age children experience feelings of sibling rivalry, which may continue in varying degrees as the children grow and develop.

Anticipatory guidance about this common challenge is critical. The NP needs to prepare parents before the arrival of the new sibling for the possibility of sibling rivalry and guide them in managing this situation.

Assessment. The key issues to discuss with parents about sibling rivalry after the arrival of a new infant are whether the older child has

- Manifested regressive behaviors since the new sibling arrived (e.g., bed wetting, return to the bottle, temper tantrums) and, if so, what they are
- Made negative comments about the new sibling or become more demanding of the parents
- Voiced psychosomatic complaints

In addition, the NP should ask parents to describe how they have reacted to the older sibling's behaviors or verbal comments and if and how they have disciplined the child.

Management

Management strategies include the following:

- Before delivery or adoption:
  - Explain to parents that sibling rivalry is a common, probably universal response of older siblings at the time of the arrival of a younger sibling and continues throughout childhood.
- Encourage parents to do the following:
  - Tell child about pregnancy or adoption and new baby, using time frame and language appropriate to child's developmental stage.
  - Investigate possibility of sibling preparation classes for older siblings.
  - Be honest with older child (e.g., tell child that it will be a long time before the baby can play with him; that mom will be tired and busy).
  - Include older child in preparations for new baby and in excitement of the event (e.g., have child visit mother and baby in hospital if possible).
- After the infant or child comes home:
  - Help parents plan ways to spend special time with the older sibling, so that he or she feels appreciated and valued (e.g., plan to do simple activities around the house or amusing outdoor activities, such as going to the park).
  - Emphasize the need to see the individuality of each child and his or her uniqueness.
  - Explain the need for tolerance when a child younger than 4 years exhibits regressive behaviors such as toileting accidents; wanting the bottle or pacifier again; willful destruction of toys, books, or valuables; or temper tantrums.
  - Reassure the parents that regressive behavior associated with the arrival of a new sibling is not a reflection of poor parenting.
  - Educate parents about teaching children to distinguish between acceptable and unacceptable behaviors.

See Box 19-7 for additional suggestions for parents.

BOX 19-7 ***Clues for Parents for Coping with Rivalry between Siblings***

Do

Allow children to vent negative feelings
Encourage children to develop solutions
Anticipate problem situations
Foster individuality in each child
Spend time with children individually
Compliment children when they are playing together
Tell children about the conflict you had with your siblings when you were children
Define acceptable and unacceptable behaviors

Don't

Take sides
Serve as a referee
Foster rivalry by comparing siblings or their accomplishments
Use derogatory names
Permit physical or verbal abuse between siblings

From Berkowitz CD: Sibling rivalry. In Berkowitz CD, editor: *Pediatrics: a primary care approach*, Philadelphia, 1996, WB Saunders, p. 98.

Sibling Rivalry between Older Children

To assess sibling rivalry, ask parents to

- Describe sibling behaviors that concern them—fighting, verbal abuse, bickering
- Identify any precipitating events or situations that seem to elicit negative behaviors between the siblings
- Identify how rivalry behaviors between siblings was handled in the past

Multiple Births

There are several important points to cover in anticipatory guidance for parents who experience multiple births. Characteristically, these children

- Often develop a special sibling relationship marked by loyalty and cooperative play
- Have periods in which they get along well or quarrel with each other just as other siblings do
- Work out relationships among themselves and function more independently, needing less parental attention
- May develop their own language among themselves as young children
- Display sibling rivalry, especially if they are fraternal rather than identical twins

Advise parents who have multiple births to do the following:

- Breastfeed if possible. Twins can be breastfed at the same time or one right after the other. Develop a plan to rotate breastfeeding if the mother has more than two infants.
- Organize the home for daily activities and plan ahead to have sufficient supplies such as bottles, diapers, and car seats.
- Schedule daily activities to accomplish all that needs to be done—this is crucial.
- Take time out for themselves and as a couple.
- Keep a sense of humor.
- Promote individuality of each child (e.g., discipline and praise as individuals, build a one-to-one relationship with each child).
- Seek out support people to help (e.g., enlist the aid of extended family members) during early infancy when the tasks of physically caring for multiple infants can be overwhelming.
- Contact support groups such as the National Organization of Mothers of Twins Clubs, Inc. (see Resource Box).

If an older sibling or siblings are in the family, be cognizant of their needs and feelings during this time of major family transition. Suggestions for strategies to handle this are discussed in the section on arrival of a new sibling.

A Death in the Family

Death in families is traumatic and disruptive. If the death is natural and "expected" (e.g., an elderly, ill, or frail grandparent), families may be more prepared and able to cope more effectively. Nonetheless, loss of a loved one who has been special to the child, even if expected, can be devastating. If a parent or sibling dies, the remaining children and parent may be unable to cope well. Parents, however, need to incorporate caring for their children into their own grieving of a family loss. This responsibility can be overwhelming and requires sensitive and intensive support from health care professionals. The NP can help parents understand and respond to their children's needs, as well as support parents in their own grief. The NP can explain the following to parents:

- Children's perceptions of death vary by age and developmental stage.
- Children's response to a death depends on both their understanding of death and the cues they receive from adults and other children around them.
- Children must grieve their loss, and often are disruptive, "acting out" their anger, fear, and sense of loss or guilt.
- The grief process is a long-term one, with both parents and children needing to "reprocess" their feelings about the loss at subsequent stages of development (e.g., parents often will become saddened when they reflect that their child would "be starting first grade this fall . . .").

Parents should be encouraged to do the following:

- Give clear, honest, age-appropriate information to their children; correct misconceptions.
- Encourage children to express and share their feelings about the person who has died and about their response to the death (e.g., they may be angry or feel guilty). Drawing, painting, or making collages are all ways children can express their feelings of loss.
- Comfort their children and empathize with their feelings.
- Permit children to participate in rituals, funerals, memorials, or other ceremonies; prepare them for what they can expect.
- Keep as consistent a family routine as possible (e.g., school, meals, bedtimes).
- Take time for themselves.
- Seek out support and counseling as appropriate.

Although the NP can be an invaluable resource for support to the family, referral for grief counseling is often helpful; a mental health referral also may be appropriate; and many books are available to help children understand and cope with a family death.

CHILD CARE

Selecting a child care provider and a setting that offers safe, nurturing, and developmentally appropriate child care are challenges for many parents. The individual needs of the child together with parental needs for work coverage and flexibility must be matched with the philosophy and constraints of the child care setting. The NP is often called on to advise parents about how to select a suitable provider. The four-step approach developed by the Administration for Children and Families, U.S. Department of Health and Human Services, is recommended as a guideline for parents (Box 19-8; also see Resource Box).

BOX 19-8 *Guidelines for Selecting a Child Care Provider: A Four-Step Approach*

Step 1: Interview Potential Child Care Providers and Observe the Program or Setting

Ask questions about

1. Cost—cost calculation per hour, daily, weekly, monthly; any late fees; policy about fee structure and rules (e.g., if the child is absent)
2. Enrollment—number of children enrolled in the program, the maximum daily capacity of setting
3. Child factors—age of the children served in the setting/program
4. Daily activities or program plan—structured vs. unstructured activities
5. Accreditation and licensing regulations related to the provider or setting; review copy of any license or certificate
6. Caretaker issues—credentials and experience (e.g., academic degrees, course, cardiopulmonary resuscitation certification)
7. Policies—open visiting, illness in the child, emergency care, nutrition and feeding policies
8. Preventable illness prevention—immunization requirements for child and staff

Carefully observe the environment:

1. Look at provider-child interactions—check for evidence of nurturing, responsive, comforting interactions
2. Look at safety issues of the physical environment—the play areas, toileting and diaper changing areas, outdoor environment, napping and eating areas
3. Assess the quality of the learning materials and toys (from an educational and safety perspective)

Step 2: Check References

1. Talk to parents with children enrolled in the program or being cared for by the provider; ask about their experience relative to how the providers handled the care (discipline) and whether they were nurturing and responsive to parents as well as the child; ask about reliability and consistency of the providers
2. Talk to local child care resource and referral program or licensing office; Child Care Aware (1-800-424-2246) provides information about the nearest child care resource and referral programs

Step 3: Make a Decision Based on Specific Criteria

1. The child will be happy with this care provider and have a safe, nurturing, and developmentally appropriate environment.
2. If the child has special needs, these will be met.
3. The values of the provider and parents are compatible.
4. The child care is affordable.

Step 4: Be an Involved Parent

1. Regularly talk to the provider about how the child is doing.
2. Talk to the child daily about activities and experiences at the facility.
3. If possible, visit the setting unannounced and observe at various times of the day.
4. Communicate with other parents and become involved in child care events as much as possible.

From US Department of Health and Human Services, Administration for Children and Families: March 1999. Previously available at *www.acf.hhs.gov/programs/ccb/faq/4steps.htm* (website no longer accessible, 2003).

ROLE RELATIONSHIP PROBLEMS

Violence

Description

Violence is the outcome of aggressive behavior that becomes destructive and results in physical injury to people or damage to property. Violence has been acknowledged as a major social and public health problem, and it has become a way of life for many of today's youth, who are either perpetrators, victims, or witnesses of violent acts (see Chapter 21 for additional discussion).

Certain key features are characteristic of violence:

- *Continuity.* Once it is used as a coping mechanism, violence becomes a habit that is hard to break.
- *Reciprocity.* Violence generates violent behavior in others, increasing tension and eliciting negative responses.
- *Sameness.* One form of violence becomes as acceptable as another. As its use becomes more common, violence permeates all of one's life.
- *Addiction.* Violence gives a sense of power and control that, though temporary, is addictive.
- *Limitations of options or alternative actions.* Reasoning is difficult in violent situations, and problem-solving abilities are not used.
- *Escalation.* Violence begets more frequent and more intense violence, with potential for serious sequelae.

Five main categories of violence can have an impact on children and their families:

- Domestic violence, including child abuse, corporal punishment, sibling violence, and spousal abuse
- Predatory violence (e.g., a crime or assault)
- Peer violence, such as fighting and gang violence
- Sexual assault and rape
- Dating violence

NPs are likely to become involved with young people who are involved as witnesses, victims, or perpetrators of crime related to one or more of these five categories.

Etiology

There is no one cause of violent behavior. Violence has certain antecedents (e.g., a situational crisis); risk factors have been identified that increase the likelihood of violent behavior (e.g., abuse of alcohol); and there are developmental and environmental factors that contribute to violence (e.g., impulsivity in young children; poverty and limited resources). Not all individuals exposed to such factors resort to violence, however. Violence is in large part a learned behavior, and what children are taught, by example and instruction, will become part of their method of interacting as they grow.

Effective management of violence in families and communities depends on understanding major influences and key risk factors that contribute to or sustain violence. These include the following (Commission for the Prevention of Youth Violence, 2000):

- *Behavioral influences.* Children who demonstrate violent behavior are more likely to have a history of aggression, conduct disorder, and school problems (Borowsky, Ireland, & Resnick, 2002). They may be easily frustrated, have difficulty making transitions, and have no sense of a future or hope for a better life.
- *Biologic influences.* A review of the literature indicates that maternal nutrition, smoking during pregnancy, and neurologic immaturity, especially related to prefrontal brain development, may be important factors in aggressive behavior in children (Raine, 2002).
- *Economic influences.* Over 16% of American children live in poverty (defined in 2003 as an income of less than $17,603 for a family of four), and in Washington, D.C., the rate is nearly twice that (over 30%) (Children's Defense Fund, 2002). Factors associated with poverty (poor housing, malnutrition, transience, and lack of connectedness to schools and community) are also risk factors for aggressive behavior (Borum, 2000).
- *Societal, familial, and environmental influences.* Family violence, unstable home life, poor parenting, rejection by peers, exposure to violence in the media and at school, easy access to weapons, alcohol and other drugs, and lead poisoning are some of the social and environmental factors that contribute to aggressiveness and violence in children and youth.

Key risk factors associated with youth violence include the following:

- Alcohol and other drug use
- Child maltreatment
- Gang membership
- Access to guns
- Media violence
- Violence among peers and intimate family members

Boys are more likely to perpetrate violence and are more often victims of violence, except for sexual assault, though more girls are engaging in aggressive behaviors (Simmons, 2002). Aggressiveness, bullying, and violent behavior increases with age, peaking around 15 years of age.

Incidence

Homicide and injury to another are typically the end results of violence. Although murders of children have decreased significantly in the past few years (the good news), they continue to be the fourth leading cause of death for 1- to 4-year-olds, 5- to 9-year-olds, and 10- to 14-year-olds and the second leading cause of death among 15- to 19-year-olds. In 2000 firearm-related death rates, including homicides, suicides, and accidents for children ages 5 to 14 and 15 to 19 years old, were 4.9% and 18% of total deaths, respectively (MacDorman et al, 2002). From 1987 through 1994, there was a 155% increase in firearm homicides for youth ages 15 to 19 years (CDC, 1996). From 1999 to 2000, that rate declined by 9.3% (MacDorman et al, 2002). Although there are major differences in rates of violence-related injuries and death by ethnic groups, the majority of homicides involve people who know each other and are of the same race. The typical scenario is played out as follows: An argument occurs, alcohol or drugs have been consumed, a weapon is available, and a homicide is the end result.

Youth are often the innocent victims of a crime or assault and at the same time perpetrators of crime; most know the other person or persons involved. Young people are more likely than those over 24 years of age to be victims of assault, and there has been a steady decline in youth crime since a peak in 1993 (Snyder & Sickmund, 1999).

Assessment

The assessment of youths who are victims or perpetrators of violent crime should focus on certain key pieces of historical information and the presence of risk factors to help determine the potential for future violence. If possible, the youth and parent(s) should be interviewed separately.

- History of the episode
  - What seemed to cause the incident?
  - Did the child or family know who was involved, or was this a random event?
  - Were alcohol or drugs involved?
  - Did either the victim or the perpetrator have or threaten to use a weapon? If yes, what type of weapon?
- Past history
  - Have there been prior incidents of violence or assault?
  - What is the usual pattern of drug or alcohol use?
  - Does the child have a history of mental health problems, or was the youth a victim of child abuse?
  - Does the youth have a criminal or police history?
  - Is there gang involvement or membership, or do friends carry weapons?
  - Does the youth have access to or carry a weapon or weapons?
- Family and social history
  - How is the youth supervised by his or her parent(s)?
  - Is there a family history of child abuse, substance abuse, domestic violence, mental illness, or a criminal record?
  - Are there handguns or rifles in the home?
  - Is the youth attending school? If yes, have there been any academic or behavioral problems?
  - Does the youth have a job? How is free time spent? Are the youth's friends in gangs or in trouble with the law?
  - Are siblings involved in gangs? Do they have a criminal history? Have any family members ever been victims, witnesses, or perpetrators of crime?

Management

The NP is likely to become involved with (1) the health care management of minor trauma resulting from assault, (2) counseling after an incident of violence or threat of violence, and (3) the prevention of youth violence. In brief, the following are the key points in the management of minor assaults:

- Treatment of minor trauma or referral
- Alcohol and drug screening
- Reporting the incident to law enforcement
- Referral to social worker or mental health professional

Prevention of Youth Violence

Prevention of youth violence requires use of a public health model that addresses the complexity of causes and risk factors behind the problem. Some suggested approaches follow. NPs are able to address many of these issues as they give individual family and child care in the primary care setting. Others require more active involvement in the community as a child and family advocate.

Primary Prevention

- Strengthen families:
  - Provide parents with skills for effective parenting (see Chapters 5 through 9 and 18).
  - Support parents to be actively involved with their children, and to supervise youths and their activities.
  - Connect families to needed community service resources.
  - Educate parents about the impact of violence on their children; discuss ways to minimize exposure; teach about gun safety.
- Strengthen developmental competencies of youth:
  - Educate youths about violence at an early age.
  - Teach anger management and strategies for avoiding a fight (role playing).
  - Teach self-defense strategies such as teaching youths martial arts and the use of mace.
  - Discuss ways to manage a difficult or potentially violent situation (Boxes 19-9 and 19-10).
- Improve the environment:
  - Support diversity training and bullying prevention programs in public schools.
  - Support after-school programs for youth and work for community commitment to youth programs.
  - Make neighborhoods and schools safe places for youth.

BOX 19-9 ***Practical Hints for Talking with Teens about How to Keep Out of Trouble***

Do not carry a weapon; instead, "fight clean" (i.e., discuss the issue in conflict). Carrying weapons only makes one less safe; pulling out a weapon begins a cycle of retaliation.
Do not go into harm's way. Avoid being around fights because the cycle of escalation and retaliation often involves innocent people.
Avoid being caught alone; stay with friends.
Do not be provoked into fighting. Words are said and names are called, not because the names are true, but rather to provoke anger and a fight.
If one becomes involved in a fight, try to end the incident on equal ground; that way, anger is more likely to be diffused. The person who wins often takes on the aggressor role; the loser then becomes the scapegoat. Thus violence continues and becomes cyclic.
Suggest discussions with friends about ways to handle potential situations in which a gun or knife might be brandished.
Do not join gangs or associate with individuals who turn to violence as a way of settling differences.

BOX 19-10 ***Talking with Teens about Date or Gang Rape***

Both males and females can be victimized.
Alcohol intoxication or the use of drugs is a major factor in date rape. Prevention includes not placing oneself in harm's way by using such substances.
Manipulative verbal threats and physically trapping the victim are common tactics used by perpetrators.
Reluctance to report gang or date rape is common. However, keeping the rape a secret only leads to self-doubt and delays healing. The teen should report the rape immediately and seek professional counseling.

 - Involve the community in a commitment to preventing violence.
 - Address the issues of media violence and of condoning violence as a way of life.
 - Regulate alcohol sales and use.
 - Legislate control of handguns.
 - Limit access to and carrying of weapons.

Secondary Prevention

- Care for children exposed to or threatened by violence:
  - Treat any physical or emotional problems in the primary care setting. Early intervention can prevent more serious problems later; referral may be necessary.
  - Provide home visits for new babies, especially those in low-income and teen-mother families.
  - Create support groups for children who have suffered trauma or loss (e.g., school counseling for traumatic experiences).
  - Refer families to community support programs such as Big Brothers Big Sisters of America (see Resource Box).
- Screen for potential problems:
  - Assess for violence risk factors at all health supervision and illness visits.
  - Screen for alcohol abuse problems.
  - Ask about weapons in the home—their presence, use, storage, and access.

Tertiary Prevention. Treatment and rehabilitation programs for offenders, and treatment for victims and their families, can be difficult and costly and can yield mixed results. It is essential to prevent violence by strengthening families and communities so that violent behavior is no longer an acceptable option.

Child Maltreatment

Description

Child maltreatment or child abuse includes physical abuse, physical neglect, sexual abuse, mental injury or emotional maltreatment, and threat of harm. The acts of inflicting injury (commission) and allowing injury to occur (omission) are key determinants in defining abuse.

Incidence and Etiology

In 2000, child protective services agencies in the United States received approximately 3 million reports of child abuse and neglect concerning the welfare of about 5 million children. Two thirds of these reports were investigated, and one third of those investigated were substantiated, finding abuse or neglect (or both) present. A total of 879,000 children, or 12.2 per 1000 children, were found to be victims of maltreatment. This is a small increase over 1999, though numbers had been decreasing slightly each year since 1993, when 15.3 children per 1000 suffered abuse. Approximately 1200 children died of abuse in 2000; 44% of those were less than 1 year old, and 85% were less than 6 years old (U.S. Department of Health and Human Services, Administration on Children, Youth, and Families [USDHHS, ACYF], 2002).

As children become older, abuse decreases. In 2000 there were 15.7 cases of abuse per 1000 children age birth to 3 years and 5.7 cases per 1000 among 16- and 17-year-olds. Rates for overall abuse of boys and girls were similar: 11.2 and 12.8 per 1000 children, respectively. The majority of victims were white (51%); 25% were African American; 15% were Latino; 2% were Native American; and 1% were Asian or Pacific Islander (USDHHS, ACYF, 2002).

Abuse, as with violence, can be a multigenerational, learned means of coping or disciplining children. Situational stress, drug or alcohol use, poverty, and limited social supports can aggravate the problem. Family structure is a risk factor for abuse; young children who live in families with a parent and an unrelated adult male have been found to be eight times more likely to be killed than children who live in two-parent or single-parent homes (Stiffman et al, 2002).

Assessment

See Box 19-11 for behavioral signs that should be investigated in a child suspected of having been abused.

Management

All categories of child abuse endanger the child's physical or emotional health and development. Although the severity of injury is always an important consideration in treatment and disposition of the child, it does not determine, per se, whether intervention should occur. The burden to report minor injury or emotional maltreatment is just as great as the burden to report significant trauma resulting in grave bodily injury.

NPs delivering primary care to children are in a unique position to identify children who are maltreated and to institute strategies for primary prevention aimed at high-risk families. Each state has its own laws related to the various categories of child maltreatment. Nurses are mandated reporters in all states and must report known or suspected child abuse. Both civil and criminal immunity is ensured to mandated reporters who are acting within their professional role when making a required or authorized report. If the history or physical examination is suspicious for child abuse and the child is not in acute danger, the NP only need notify the child abuse registry. If the child requires protection and is in imminent danger, both the police and the child abuse registry must be called. Most states have a system of cross-reporting cases with their social service agency, usually referred to as child protective services, responsible for child abuse investigations and law enforcement. NPs should contact the department of social services or the office of the attorney general in their state for written guidelines about individual state reporting laws and procedural policies related to child abuse. The telephone number for reporting suspicion of child abuse should be readily available in each practice setting. In addition, consultation with experts in the field of child maltreatment is appropriate for those situations that are problematic or questionable for the NP.

It has been pointed out that the philosophy "I am not my brother's keeper" should never be applied to children. Children are a vulnerable, easily traumatized, powerless group, and it is the responsibility of all those who work with them to provide protection and care and to be "our children's keepers" (Johnson, 2002).

BOX 19-11 *Behavioral Signs Associated with Child Maltreatment*

- Overly compliant or exhibits exaggerated fearfulness
- Clingy and indiscriminate attachment
- Extremes in behavior (aggressive/passive)
- Apprehensive when other children cry
- Wary of physical contact with adults
- Frightened of parents or of going home, or both
- Exhibits drastic behavioral changes in and out of parental or caregiver presence
- Depressed, hypervigilant, withdrawn, apathetic, antisocial; exhibits destructive behavior
- Suicidal (suicide attempts or plans) or engages in self-mutilation
- Overprotective of parents or caregivers
- Displays sleep or eating disorders

Physical Abuse

Description

Any act that results in nonaccidental physical injury to a child is physical abuse. Physical abuse often occurs when the parent or caregiver is frustrated or angry. In these instances, the injury is frequently due to shaking, striking, or throwing the child and can involve unreasonably severe corporal punishment or unjustifiable punishment. Physical injury also can represent intentional, deliberate assault such as burning, biting, cutting, poking, twisting limbs, or torturing. Children who suffer physical abuse are younger, more likely to have a preexisting medical condition, and more severely injured than children who experience unintentional injuries (DiScala et al, 2000).

Incidence

Approximately 170,000 children, or 2.3 of every 1000 children, suffered physical abuse in 2000. This constitutes 19.3% of all abused children (USDHHS, ACYF, 2002).

Assessment

Determining the presence of physical abuse can be difficult. A child or parent may disclose a history of an inflicted injury, or there may be behavioral or physical findings. Behaviors are not definitive signs of physical abuse but are important areas to investigate for additional information. Specific physical findings are often the key to a diagnosis of nonaccidental injury resulting from physical abuse. The provider should have a high level of suspicion if there are discrepancies in the history of the injury, the child's age and developmental capabilities, and the type and severity of injury.

History. The history should assess for the following:

- Child states that injury was caused by abuse.
- Injury is unusual for a specific age-group.
- Injuries are unexplained or implausible (e.g., parent or caregiver cannot explain injury, is vague about how the injury occurred, gives discrepant accounts of what happened, or blames someone else); explanation does not match the type or mechanism of injury; or child is not developmentally capable of reported injurious behavior.
- Parent or caregiver delays seeking care for child or seeks inappropriate care.
- Child or parent or caregiver, or both, hides injury (e.g., child wears excessive layers of clothing), or child is kept out of school.
- There is presence of triggering behaviors such as inconsolable, colicky crying in an infant, toilet-training accidents, or sleeping or discipline problems that may have led to a violent response by a caregiver.
- There is a report of a crisis or stressful time for the family (e.g., financial difficulties) or domestic violence.
- There is a problem with substance abuse in the family.

Physical Findings. Key considerations of abuse that should guide the physical examination include the following:

- Location of the physical injury
- Type of injury (Tables 19-2 and 19-3)
- Presence of multiple injuries

Diagnostic Studies. These should include (1) blood coagulation studies (platelet count, bleeding time, prothrombin time, and partial thromboplastin time) on any child who is severely bruised or has a history of "easy bruising" and suspicious bruises (see Table 19-4 for general dating of contusion injuries) and (2) radiographic studies. A child with limited range of motion or bony tenderness on examination should have a local radiologic evaluation. A radiologic skeletal survey should be ordered for any child with soft tissue findings who is nonverbal or unable to give a clear history (usually younger than 4 to 5 years) or for infants suspected of failure to thrive (FTT). The minimum radiologic survey is a skull series, long bones, and ribs. Bone scan, computed tomography scan, and magnetic resonance imaging study should be ordered on the basis of physical findings or symptoms. Serum calcium, phosphorus, and alkaline phosphatase levels are useful measurements if bone disease is suspected. Ultrasonography is useful if visceral injury is suspected. Other studies are ordered depending on physical findings (Behrman & Kliegman, 2002).

TABLE 19-2 Common Sites of Injury in Physical Abuse of Children

Location of Injury*	Common Physical Finding
Head area	Eyes—bilateral black eyes
	Earlobe—pinch and pull marks
	Cheek—slap marks, squeeze marks
	Upper lip and frenulum—lacerations or bruises
	Scalp—bare and broken hair, bruises
Neck	Choke marks
Trunk	Chest—bite marks, fingertip encirclement marks
	Buttocks and lower back—paddling and strap marks
Genitals	Pinch marks, penile wrapping with constrictive materials
Extremities	Upper arms—grab marks
	Ankles or wrists—tethering, friction burn marks
	Feet—pin or razor tattoo marks

*The shins, elbows, and knees are the most typical sites of accidental, non–child abuse, injuries. Bruises, cuts, and abrasions are most commonly seen. The back surface of the body, from knees to neck, is the most common site of intentional, abusive injuries.

Differential Diagnosis

Differential diagnoses are identified by type of intentional physical injury:

- Soft tissue injuries:
  - Normal bruising from accidental injuries that typically involve the knees, anterior tibia, and forehead
  - Mongolian spots and allergic shiners

TABLE 19-3 Common Characteristics of Physical Abuse by Type of Injury

Type of Injury	Key Considerations
Bruises—surface and soft tissue	Pattern, shape, outline Location Number Stages of coloring
Burns—superficial or deep	Location: burns on palms, soles, flexor surface of thighs or perineum are pathognomonic for abuse Patterns, such as sharply demarcated or circumferential (e.g., sock, glove, zebra, branding, doughnut or cigarette shape)
Bites	Pattern such as doughnut or double-horseshoe shape; adult >3 cm between canine teeth; can be on any part of the body
Abrasions and lacerations	Location Number "C" or "U" shape typical of belt buckle mark
Central nervous system	Radiographic findings (e.g., subdural hematomas, subarachnoid hemorrhages, skull fractures, suture spread), retinal hemorrhages
Shaken infant syndrome	Retinal hemorrhage, subdural hematoma, posterior rib and metaphyseal fractures
Internal organs	Liver, bowel, spleen, pancreas, kidney damage consistent with blunt-force trauma May be no visible marks or bruises on abdomen May have symptoms of shock Internal injury is second leading cause of death in child abuse
Skeletal	Spiral fractures of long bones, avulsion of metaphyseal tips, multiple rib fractures in different stages of healing, subperiosteal proliferation reaction, unexplained fracture; fractures from birth injuries heal by 4 mo
Poisoning/ingestion of medication	Deliberate poisoning, or exposure to substance abuse via breast milk, passive inhalation of marijuana
Munchausen-by-proxy syndrome	Creates a fictitious illness or induces illness in child; signs and symptoms stop when perpetrator no longer has unsupervised contact with child

  - Bleeding disorders
  - Cultural practices such as "coining," sometimes practiced by Southeast Asian groups
- Burns: impetigo, bullous impetigo, or toxic epidermal necrolysis (scalded skin syndrome)
- Fractures: osteogenesis imperfecta and rare bone diseases such as scurvy, congenital syphilis, and neoplasms
- Head injuries: bruising from falls

TABLE 19-4 General Dating of Contusion Injury

Bruise Characteristic	Age of Bruise
Swollen, tender	0-2 days
Red/purple/blue	0-5 days
Green	5-7 days
Yellow	7-10 days
Brown	10-14 days
Clear	2-4 wk

Most infant falls do not result in head injury. Falls from beds or sofas do not cause skull fractures, and less than 1% of infants in a large study suffered concussion or skull fracture because of a fall (Warrington, Wright, & Team, 2001).

Management

Medical treatment of specific types of injuries is discussed in Unit 4 of this text under the appropriate illness-related heading. If physical abuse is suspected, certain general management strategies should be followed. The NP must

- Report suspicions of child maltreatment to child protective services or law enforcement agencies, or both.
- Carefully document findings and any statements made by parent or caregiver or child, or both.
- Secure photographic documentation of soft tissue injury or burn injury; this can be done by law enforcement personnel or health care providers, as appropriate.
- Refer for appropriate medical treatment of injuries depending on type and severity of injury.

- Refer for psychologic counseling; this is generally handled by child protective services. The need for long-term or intermittent therapy often depends on the individual child, the severity of the physical injury, and other life events.

Patient Education and Prevention

Prevention of physical abuse involves the following steps:

- Screen for parental history of abuse during childhood, history of domestic violence, and absence of a social support network in the family. Pursue positive screens.
- Identify at-risk families and children. At-risk families include those with any of the following characteristics:
  - Prior history of child maltreatment, drug abuse, violent behavior, or serious mental illness
  - Evidence that the mother is not showing attachment to her infant, makes negative remarks about the child, or lacks basic parenting knowledge, skill, and motivation
  - Evidence of spanking of young infants
  - Isolated parent who lacks social support network
  - History of infant or child death resulting from child maltreatment (categorized as extremely high risk)
- Make early referrals for supportive service, including social service referrals, parenting classes, self-help groups (e.g., Parents or Alcoholics Anonymous plus battered women's services), respite care, public health nurse visits, or a combination of these.
- Provide close primary care supervision and ill-child follow-up visits of at-risk families and children.
- Use a multidisciplinary team approach to manage at-risk or high-risk families. A team approach gives objectivity to a situation.
- Report immediately to child protective services if abuse is suspected.
- Gain the support of community child abuse prevention programs.

Neglect

Description

Physical neglect refers to the negligent treatment or maltreatment of a child that can harm or threaten harm to a child's health or welfare. Neglect by the parent or caregiver can be severe or more subtle in its effects. Severe neglect includes instances in which the parent or caregiver fails to protect the child from dangers such as severe malnutrition (may be seen clinically as medically diagnosed nonorganic FTT); willfully places the child in a situation in which the child's health is endangered (e.g., exploitation requiring a child to engage in criminal behavior); or intentionally fails to provide adequate clothing, shelter, education, or medical care. General neglect refers to failure to meet the child's basic needs such as adequate food, clothing, shelter, medical care, or supervision where no obvious physical injury to the child occurred as a result. A key factor in neglect is the extreme or persistent presence of these conditions in the child's home.

Incidence

In 2000, approximately 7.8 per 1000 children (62.8% of all abused children) suffered neglect (USDHHS, ACYF, 2002).

Assessment

Assessment should focus on the key issue of whether the child's safety and welfare are threatened. General indicators of neglect are divided into child, home, and supervision factors (Box 19-12). In the primary care setting, NPs can more accurately assess child factors (i.e., child's appearance and general status, as well as access to needed dental and health care) than home factors or the degree of adult supervision provided, though questions and discussion about the home situation can be included in the history.

BOX 19-12 *General Indicators of Neglect: Child, Home, Supervision Factors*

Child

Dirty, malnourished, poor hygiene, inadequately dressed for weather
Inadequate medical and dental care (has multiple caries)
Always sleepy (chronic fatigue) or hungry

Home

Fire hazards or other unsafe conditions
No heating or plumbing
Nutritional quality of the food inadequate
Meals not prepared; food spoiled in refrigerator or cupboards

Supervision

Child has history of repeated physical injuries or ingestion of harmful substances with evidence of poor supervision by adult caregiver
Child cared for by another child
Child left alone in the home, car, or anywhere without supervision (typically defined as a child younger than 12 years of age who is left unsupervised during the daytime, or child age 16 to 18 years left unsupervised by an adult at night)

Referral to a public health nurse for home assessment may be necessary, and a report of child neglect to child protective services may lead to investigation. Child protective workers look at home factors with a focus on a safe and sanitary environment. To determine degree of adult supervision, factors such as the child's age and level of functioning, the length of time the parent was away, where the parent went, whether the parent left a plan of supervision (e.g., relative or adult living next door or nearby who was readily available to the child), and how often the child has been left alone are investigated. Most child protective services hold parents to the standard of a "reasonable or prudent" parent, and economic factors are also considered when making judgments about parents' efforts to provide adequately for their children.

Differential Diagnosis

Differentiating willful neglect from neglect resulting from poverty, mental retardation, or mental illness is necessary. Educational neglect differs from truancy (i.e., child is sent to school but never arrives) in that the parent makes no provisions for the child to attend school.

Management

Referral to child protective services is needed in cases of neglect. NPs can also refer families to public health and social service agencies.

Emotional Maltreatment

Description

Emotional maltreatment or mental injury is harm to a child's ability to think, reason, or feel. Emotional maltreatment may take two forms: emotional abuse or emotional deprivation. Parents who subject children to cruel statements and acts, or who reject, terrorize, ridicule, isolate, and corrupt the child, are perpetrating emotional abuse. Torture, confinement, exposure to violence (witnessing domestic violence), and deprivation of food and water are extreme examples.

Failure to adequately nurture children with support and affection so that the child can develop a healthy personality is an example of emotional deprivation. Parents or caregivers who do not provide the normal experiences necessary for a child to feel loved, wanted, secure, or worthy are depriving their child of the emotional security that is critical for positive self-esteem.

Emotional maltreatment may contribute to psychologic FTT, speech or sleep disorders, or a wide range of behavioral and emotional problems in children (e.g., withdrawal, aggressiveness, neediness, conduct disorders). The issue of consistency or recurrence of negative parental behaviors, as well as willful cruelty or unjustifiable emotional punishment, is a key indicator of emotional maltreatment.

Etiology and Incidence

Parents or caregivers can ignore or reject their child for any number of reasons, including drug use, psychiatric disturbances, personal problems, or other preoccupying situations. Poor coping skills, high stress levels, a history of emotional maltreatment, and poor parenting can contribute to the parent's behavior. Children with chronic illness, or those who are "different" than their siblings, may become scapegoats in the family system.

Approximately 1 in 1000 children (7.7% of all abused children) suffer emotional maltreatment (USDHHS, ACYF, 2002).

Assessment

Behavioral indicators often lead to suspicions of emotional maltreatment but can also be due to other causes; therefore a careful history is important. Interviewing both parent or caregiver plus any child older than 3 years of age is essential. A range of behavioral indicators can be exhibited by children who are emotionally deprived or abused. Physical indicators of emotional maltreatment such as psychosocial FTT are assessed for degree of severity, as well as etiology. The assessment includes the history, physical examination, and diagnostic studies.

History. The history can include the following:

- Past history—might be suggestive of neglect (e.g., little or no health care supervision, immunizations not up to date, earlier removal of a sibling for neglect)
- Interview with mother—might reveal mother's negative feelings toward child, a state of feeling overwhelmed or depressed, plus feelings of being deprived or unloved; mother may be cognitively delayed
- Behavior problems with child in school, among peers (e.g., bullying, being picked on, withdrawal)
- Feeding and dietary history—can be helpful in distinguishing accidental feeding or formula-preparation error from neglect and organic or psychologic causes; dietary history should be obtained but might not be truthful
- Inquire about financial hardships related to inability to provide for basic needs, especially food

Physical Findings. Physical assessment of emotional maltreatment can be difficult. Assessment of psychosocial FTT is one means of assessing emotional maltreatment. *Psychosocial FTT* is defined as a condition in which children younger than age 5 years have growth persistently and significantly below the norms for their age and sex with no organic cause. Infancy is the major period of time when FTT due to nonorganic causes is diagnosed. Children older than 2 years of age can often get their own food. However, purposeful starvation in older children by their caregiver does happen. FTT can be related to both physical and psychosocial factors; and both should be considered, because they may be concurrent. The physical assessment in FTT includes the following (see Chapter 33):

- Weight-for-height ratio. Will be less than normal in FTT; short stature with a proportional weight can reflect chronic malnutrition or a genetic or endocrine-based problem.
- Growth trajectory. Child fails to maintain normal growth trajectory.
- Signs of general neglect: poor hygiene such as filthy fingernails, clothes, body, rampant diaper rash, or untreated impetigo. Child may have flattened occiput from lying in one position.
- Appetite. Child may be ravenous; NP should try to observe the caregiver feed the infant.
- Child's behavior. Child may avoid eye contact, resist being cuddled, or have an expressionless face.
- Mother-child interaction. Parent may indicate a lack of attachment or presence of anger or dislike of child; may belittle, tease, or verbally abuse child.
- Associated developmental delays resulting from little psychosocial stimulation.

Diagnostic Studies. Diagnostic evaluation by a mental health professional is needed to determine whether the behaviors or psychopathology, or both, in the child are due to parental emotional abuse or deprivation.

If the child has FTT, dietary management should be undertaken for 1 week to determine whether there is significant weight gain before laboratory studies are ordered to rule out organic causes of FTT (see Chapter 33).

Differential Diagnosis

Intentional mental injury should be distinguished from that caused by parental deficits such as cognitive, psychologic, and economic limitations. Psychopathology in the child resulting from other causes is also in the differential diagnosis.

The differential diagnoses for emotional maltreatment resulting in FTT include accidental feeding or formula errors and organic causes of FTT, such as endocrine, metabolic, gastrointestinal, cardiovascular, genetic, neurologic, infectious, and renal conditions.

Management

Because emotional maltreatment is generally difficult to prove, the NP must carefully document what was said in the interview or what behavioral indicators were found. Referral to a community health nurse for in-home assessment is appropriate if the NP has concerns. Referral to a mental health professional for evaluation should be considered. Reporting concerns to the appropriate child protective services agency is essential, as is close supervision of these families. Family therapy may be necessary, and parents can benefit from parenting support and education, as well as social service support to cope with demands on the family system (e.g., child care, nutritional education, access to economic resources). The child may need to be placed in foster care.

If a child has FTT, the condition must be treated clinically. Hospitalization may be required. Demonstration of adequate weight gain while out of the home (either in hospital or foster care) is diagnostic. Dietary management should include an appropriate diet for age that provides 120 kcal per 24 hours times median weight (in kilograms) for measured length. Most children younger than 6 months of age with caloric-deprivation FTT gain weight by 2 to 3 days; children 6 to 24 months gain weight by 2 to 17 days (Behrman & Kliegman, 2002). Close and long-term health care supervision and follow-up plus psychosocial intervention and local case management by child protective services are needed.

Patient Education and Prevention

Prevention of emotional maltreatment and psychosocial FTT generally involves the same prevention strategies as identified in the section on physical abuse and neglect. Early recognition and intervention are key to preventing subsequent mental health problems. The importance of frequent health visits to monitor height and weight for infants who are falling behind is essential to prevent significant growth and development problems.

Sexual Abuse

Description

Sexual abuse or *sexual maltreatment* is defined to include acts of sexual assault or sexual exploitation of minors, or both. These acts can occur over an extended period of time or involve a one-time incident; they may or may not involve force; they can involve threats of physical harm to a child or others in the family, or involve emotional entrapment of the child; and they can often involve a secret between the victim and the perpetrator. The perpetrator is usually known to the child and is often a "trusted" adult. A growing group of perpetrators are adolescents who commit sexually aggressive acts on young children.

Sexual assault of children includes a range of acts including rape, rape in concert, incest, sodomy, lewd or lascivious acts on a child younger than 14 years of age (e.g., fondling or touching of genital areas and breasts or inappropriate kissing), oral copulation, and penetration of genital or anal openings by a foreign object. Sexual exploitation includes activities such as pornography depicting minors and promoting prostitution by minors. Proving sexual abuse in young children is difficult.

Incidence

In 2000, 1.2 per 1000 children suffered sexual abuse, which represents 10.1% of the total number of child abuse and neglect cases. Reported abuse among girls is more prevalent than among boys—1.7 per 1000 girls in 2000, compared with 0.4 per 1000 boys (USDHHS, ACYF, 2002). Multigenerational abuse is common in cases of child sexual abuse.

Assessment

Chapter 36 discusses the examination of the genitalia in girls. The child or adolescent who has been sexually assaulted by a stranger usually discloses the abuse and comes in for an immediate evaluation. This type of assessment is straightforward and involves the usual taking of a history and performing the medical examination with collection of possible evidence. If the incident occurred within 72 hours, evidence (e.g., semen, nail scraping, and pubic hair) is collected, and testing for sexually transmitted diseases should be done. These children are often seen in the emergency department of a local hospital or at a special center that treats victims of child sexual abuse.

The NP in a primary care setting is likely to become involved in a child sexual abuse case in any of the following circumstances: there is a spontaneous disclosure by the child; a parent voices concerns about the possibility of abuse or reports a disclosure by the child; there are suspicious physical or historical findings, or both; or laboratory tests indicating STDs are positive. In many instances, sexual abuse occurs over several years before the child discloses.

If possible, the assessment of the child should be done by a health care provider who is an expert in the field of sexual abuse of children. The assessment of a child who has been molested in the past but whose molestation has only recently been disclosed, or who is suspected of being sexually abused, should focus on three areas: behavioral indicators, physical indicators, and the interview of the child.

Behavioral Indicators

- Loss of bowel and bladder control
- Regressive behaviors such as newly manifested clinging and irritability in young children, thumb sucking, renewed need for a security object
- Night terrors, inability to sleep alone, bed wetting after having been dry at night
- Overeating or lack of appetite; compulsive behaviors or unusual fears and phobias
- Change in school performance; loss of concentration or easy distractibility
- Sexualized behavior or play inappropriate for developmental level
- Depression or inactivity, poor peer relationships, poor self-esteem, acting out, excessive anger
- Runaway, suicide attempts, prostitution or promiscuity, substance abuse, teen pregnancy, psychosomatic gynecologic and gastrointestinal complaints

Behavioral indicators per se are not diagnostic of sexual molestation but indicate a need for a thorough investigation.

Physical Indicators—Nonspecific

- Pain on urination; vaginal or penile discharge; vaginal, rectal, or penile bleeding; enuresis and encopresis
- Urethral or lymph gland inflammation; genital or perianal rashes; labial adhesions
- Pain in anal, gastrointestinal, pelvic, and urinary areas
- Genital injuries or signs such as bruising, scratches, bites, grasp marks, swelling of the genitalia that are unexplained or inconsistent with history

Physical Indicators—Specific

- Blunt-force trauma (lacerations, bruising, abrasions, tears) to the genital or rectal areas, or both, that is inconsistent with the history, or these same findings with a history of sexual contact or penetration
- Commonly encountered STDs (by probability of sexual abuse in prepubertal infants and children from certain to uncertain):
  - Certain—gonorrhea (by culture) and syphilis if not perinatally acquired
  - Probable—chlamydia (culture is only reliable diagnostic method), condyloma acuminatum (if not perinatally acquired), *Trichomonas vaginalis*, herpes type 2
  - Possible—herpes type 1 (in the genital area)
  - Uncertain—bacterial vaginosis

Pregnancy and semen are certain indicators of sexual abuse in young children.

Lack of Significant Physical Findings

- Most child victims of sexual abuse do not have any significant physical findings.
- Lack of findings is often the result of delayed disclosure and the nature of the abuse.
- Most sexual abuse of young children does not involve penetrating trauma.

Interview of the Child. The purpose of the health provider interview with the child is to collect adequate information to decide whether to report the case. A social worker, psychologist, or law-enforcement person with experience in evaluating sexually abused children will conduct a detailed interview after the case is reported.

When talking with a child who is disclosing sexual abuse, or who you suspect was or is being sexually abused, be nonjudgmental, use language that the child understands, identify the words the child uses for the genital and rectal areas, have the child tell you what happened in his or her own words, and ask open-ended questions. Do not ask leading questions.

If the child gives a spontaneous or clear disclosure of sexual abuse during a primary care visit, report the case. Children rarely lie about such matters. Always think, "How would a child that age know about such sexual details?" Consider separate questioning of the child and parent or caregiver if the child is 4 years or older.

Recanting a disclosure of sexual abuse is not uncommon because of fear of what disclosure can bring to the family or child.

Diagnostic Studies. Any sexual abuse of children that involves oral, genital, rectal, or penile contact or penetration within the previous 72 hours requires that appropriate forensic specimens be collected. In addition, the rectal, throat, urethral, or endocervical areas should be cultured for *Neisseria gonorrhoeae* and *Chlamydia trachomatis.* Blood testing for syphilis should be obtained. In selected cases, additional diagnostic tests for human immunodeficiency virus (HIV), hepatitis B, herpes simplex, bacterial vaginosis, human papillomavirus, and *T. vaginalis* can be performed if indicated.

Testing for STDs in children who were molested in the past (more than 72 hours previously) is a judgment call. Recent exposure and the possibility of penile contact are key indicators for whether specimens need to be collected for possible STDs. Testing for *N. gonorrhoeae, C. trachomatis,* and syphilis should be considered in all children with a history of sexual abuse. A colposcopic examination of the genital and rectal areas by an expert in the field is often requested by law enforcement agencies to determine whether there is evidence of acute traumatic or past healed injury to the genital or rectal areas.

Differential Diagnosis

Differential diagnoses include straddle injury to the genitalia or rectal area, which produces labial ecchymosis, abrasions, or tears; penetrating vaginal trauma from accidental injury such as jumping from dresser onto bedpost (needs careful investigation); perinatally acquired STDs or STDs acquired through close contact but not sexual abuse; lichen sclerosus, poor hygiene, and pinworm infestation, resulting in vulvar skin irritation; and foreign body (frequently toilet paper) and other nonsexually transmitted bacteria causing vaginal discharge.

Management

An immediate forensic examination for a chain of evidence is required if the child gives a history that sexual abuse including ejaculation occurred within 72 hours. Specimen collection for semen, STDs, pregnancy, and other evidence is done according to the local law enforcement protocol for child or adolescent rape. If possible, the child should be referred to health providers who are skilled in performing this special examination on children and adolescents. An expert in the medical examination of children suspected of being sexually abused should evaluate the child if the incident or incidents occurred more than 72 hours before the disclosure. A psychosocial interview with an expert in the field of child sexual abuse is often part of the evaluation.

If the NP is the first health care provider to see the child, he or she is likely to become involved in the following management issues:

- Careful documentation of the history and physical examination findings for medical-legal purposes
- Reporting of the case to law enforcement and social service agencies as required by law
- Referral for medical and psychosocial evaluation by experts in the field of child sexual abuse
- Referrals for crisis counseling of the child and other family members as needed
- Prescribing medication for treatment of STDs; follow-up STD cultures or blood work as indicated
- Referrals for therapy, as well as support and encouragement, for the child and family

Patient Education and Prevention

Prevention of later psychologic problems related to child sexual abuse and revictimization are key issues. Prevention of sexual abuse involves the following steps:

- Instruct parents and caregivers about the need for early and consistent education of their children about good, bad, and questionable touching of private parts; how to say no or the use of self-defense techniques (e.g., yelling, kicking, or fighting back) if someone inappropriately touches them; to tell a responsible adult; and not to keep secrets. Parents should again bring up this subject as their child progresses through the various developmental stages. Young children who have been molested by a trusted adult often do not disclose for many years because they were threatened not to tell anyone or they interpreted the sexual activity (if it is not painful) as a sign of affection from the trusted adult and not as

RESOURCE BOX

Role Relationships

Administration on Developmental Disabilities
www.acf.hhs.gov/programs/add/
1-202-690-6590
Federal government site with links to information, advocacy, and policy related to children with special needs

American Professional Society on the Abuse of Children
www.apsac.org
1-312-554-0166
Professional education and resources

Big Brothers Big Sisters of America
www.bbbsa.org
Youth service organization whose website connects to state programs

Brave Kids
www.bravekids.org/
1-888-653-2393
Support for families with children with chronic illness; links to resources for health professionals on a wide range of chronic illnesses; material in Spanish

Center to Prevent Handgun Violence
www.handguncontrol.org
1-202-898-0792
National lobbying and activist group

Child Care Aware
www.childcareaware.org
1-800-424-2246
Information on child care resources

Community Directory of International Adoption Medical Clinics
www.comeunity.com/adoption/health/clinics.html
Resource list of clinics and doctors in the United States and Canada specializing in international adoption health

Dougy Center for Grieving Children
www.dougy.org
1-503-775-5683
National center for grieving children and families; counseling, therapy, informational resources

International Adoption Clinic
www.peds.umn.edu/iac/
1-612-624-1164
Clinic at the University of Minnesota; provides counseling and expert advice for parents and providers, as well as clinical screening for recently arrived children

Kempe Children's Center
www.kempecenter.com/
Resources for professionals and families working with child abuse

Kids Health
www.kidshealth.org
Support group, information for parents, kids, and adolescents

The Lesbian and Gay Parenting Handbook
A resource book for parents by April Martin; published by HarperPerennial, 1993

Medical Passports for Adopted Children
www.in.gov
The state of Indiana has legislation providing for medical passports for adopted children; search the state website for "medical passport"

Mothers of Supertwins (MOST)
www.mostonline.org
1-631-859-1110
Triplets and more

National Adoption Center
www.nationaladoptioncenter.org/
1-800-862-3678 (TO-ADOPT)

National Adoption Information Clearinghouse
U.S. Department of Health and Human Services
Administration for Children and Families
www.calib.com

National Center on Secondary Education and Transition
www.ncset.org
1-612-624-2097
Educational and occupational opportunities for youth with disabilities; links to other resources

National Child Care Information Center
www.nccic.org
1-800-616-2242
Project of Child Care Bureau, a national resource for information regarding child care delivery system; links to other resources

National Clearinghouse of Child Abuse and Neglect Information
Department of Health and Human Services (DHHS)
www.calib.com/nccanch
1-800-394-3366

RESOURCE BOX

Role Relationships—cont'd

National Coalition for the Homeless
www.nationalhomeless.org/
1-202-737-6444

National Committee for Prevention of Child Abuse
www.childabuse.org
1-312-663-3520

National Foster Care Coalition
www.nationalfostercare.org
1-202-467-4441
Coalition of groups to support foster care program; affiliated with Casey Family Programs

National Foster Parent Association, Inc.
www.nfpainc.org
1-800-557-5238
Support and advocacy group for foster parents and children

National Organization of Mothers of Twins Clubs, Inc.
www.nomotc.org
1-877-540-2200
Information, resources, and support for families with multiple births

National Organization of Single Mothers
www.singlemothers.org/

National Resource Center on Child Sexual Abuse
www.janela1.com/vh/docs/v0000388.htm
1-800-KIDS-007
Funded by DHHS; professional training and resources

National Resource Center for Health and Safety in Child Care
http:/ /nrc.uchsc.edu/
1-800-598-5437 (KIDS)
Funded by U.S. Maternal and Child Health Bureau; information for parents, providers, day care centers

North American Council on Adoptable Children
www.nacac.org
1-651-644-3036
Adoption information and resources for older and foster children

Parents Without Partners
www.parentswithoutpartners.org
1-561-391-8833
International nonprofit educational organization for single parents and their children

Rape Abuse and Incest National Network
www.rainn.org
National Sexual Assault Hotline:
1-800-656-4673 (HOPE)

Stepfamily Association of America, Inc.
www.saafamilies.org/
1-800-735-0329

Twins and Multiple Births Association
www.tamba.org.uk
United Kingdom organization with international links

Zero to Three
www.zerotothree.org
Information on child care options

molestation. Later, feelings of guilt, fear, and betrayal can emerge when children realize they were molested.

- Emphasize to parents that they must not place their child in high-risk situations (e.g., a parent who was abused by her father may have kept this a secret, blaming herself for what happened; she may erroneously believe that the perpetrator will not sexually abuse her child and leaves her daughter with him). Counsel that children are never safe around a pedophile.
- Provide families with information and educational reading materials about the topic of sexual abuse of children. Teaching should be tailored to the child's cognitive and learning abilities.
- Report promptly any suspicion of sexual abuse.
- Refer for individual and family counseling if sexual abuse is confirmed or suspected.
- Support efforts to target high-risk groups for intervention to avoid the continued spread of child abuse (e.g., adolescents who have exhibited sexual curiosity beyond the bounds of normal or have experimented with but not yet victimized younger children).
- Support public education efforts and community child sexual abuse prevention programs.
- Educate parents about the need to talk to their children about their daily activities, especially what their children did during the time they were not with the parents.

NURSING DIAGNOSES RELATED TO ROLE RELATIONSHIPS: *Functional Health Pattern*

Diagnoses are related to the following concepts: caregiving, parenting, family processes, role performance, and social interaction.

- Caregiver role strain
- Impaired parenting
  - Risk for impaired parenting
- Interrupted family processes
- Interrupted family processes: alcoholism
- Risk for impaired parent/infant/child attachment
- Ineffective role performance
- Parental role conflict
- Impaired social interaction
- Readiness for enhanced communication

From North American Nursing Diagnosis Association: *NANDA nursing diagnoses: definitions and classification 2003-2004*, Philadelphia, 2003, North American Nursing Diagnosis Association.

REFERENCES

Acs G, Nelson S: *The kids are alright? Children's well-being and the rise in cohabitation*, Washington, DC, 2002, The Urban Institute. Available at *www.urban.org/url.cfm?ID = 310544* (accessed Oct 20, 2003).

Administration for Children and Families, National Clearinghouse on Child Abuse and Neglect: *Foster care national statistics April 2001*, Washington, DC, 2001, Department of Health and Human Services.

Anderssen N, Amlie C, Ytteroy EA: Outcomes for children with lesbian or gay parents. A review of studies from 1978 to 2000, *Scand J Psychol* 43:335-351, 2002.

Behrman RE, Kliegman RM: *Nelson essentials of pediatrics*, ed 4, Philadelphia, 2002, WB Saunders.

Berkowitz CD: Sibling rivalry. In Berkowitz CD, editor: *Pediatrics: a primary care approach*, Philadelphia, 1996, WB Saunders.

Borowsky IW, Ireland M, Resnick MD: Violence risk and protective factors among youth held back in school, *Ambul Pediatr* 2:475-484, 2002.

Borum R: Assessing violence risk among youth, *J Clin Psychol* 56:1263-1288, 2000.

Bramlett MD, Mosher WD: Cohabitation, marriage, divorce, and remarriage in the United States, *Vital Health Stat* 23(22), 2002.

Casey Family Programs: Foster care info. Available at *www.casey.org/fostercareinfo/index.htm* (accessed 2003).

Centers for Disease Control and Prevention: *National summary of injury mortality data 1987-1994*, Atlanta, 1996, National Center for Injury Prevention and Control.

Children's Bureau, Administration on Children, Youth and Families: *National Child Abuse and Neglect Data System (NCANDS) summary of key findings from calendar year 2000*, Washington, DC, 2002, Department of Health and Human Services.

Children's Defense Fund: *The state of children in America's union: a 2002 action guide to Leave No Child Behind*, Washington, DC, 2002, Children's Defense Fund.

Cohen GJ, American Academy of Pediatrics Committee on Psychosocial Aspects of Child and Family Health: Helping children and families deal with divorce and separation, *Pediatrics* 110:1019-1023, 2002.

Commission for the Prevention of Youth Violence: *Youth and violence: medicine, nursing, and public health: connecting the dots to prevent violence*, Chicago, 2000, American Medical Association. Available at *www.ama-assn.org/ama/upload/mm/386/fullreport.pdf* (accessed Oct 20, 2003).

DiScala C et al: Child abuse and unintentional injuries: a 10-year retrospective, *Arch Pediatr Adolesc Med* 154:16-22, 2000.

Friedman MM, Bowden VR, Jones E: *Family nursing: research, theory and practice*, ed 5, Upper Saddle River, NJ, 2003, Prentice Hall.

Golombok S et al: Children with lesbian parents: a community study, *Dev Psychol* 39:20-33, 2003.

Hunfeld JA et al: Child development and quality of parenting in lesbian families: no psychosocial indications for a-priori withholding of infertility treatment. A systematic review, *Hum Reprod Update* 8:579-590, 2002.

Johnson CF: Child maltreatment 2002: recognition, reporting and risk, *Pediatr Int* 44:554-560, 2002.

Kelly JB: Children's adjustment in conflicted marriage and divorce: a decade review of research, *J Am Acad Child Adolesc Psychiatry* 39:963-973, 2000.

Lussier G et al: Support across two generations: children's closeness to grandparents following parental divorce and remarriage, *J Fam Psychol* 16:363-376, 2002.

MacDorman MF et al: Annual summary of vital statistics—2001, *Pediatrics* 110:1037-1052, 2002.

McMahon SD et al: Stress and psychopathology in children and adolescents: is there evidence of specificity? *J Child Psychol Psychiatry* 44:107-133, 2003.

National Coalition for the Homeless: Homeless families with children. NCH Fact Sheet no 7, June 2001. Available at *www.nationalhomeless.org/families.html* (accessed Oct 20, 2003).

National Coalition for the Homeless: How many people experience homelessness? NCH Fact Sheet no 2, Sept 2002. Available at *www.nationalhomeless.org/numbers.html* (accessed Oct 20, 2003).

Neff JM et al: Identifying and classifying children with chronic conditions using administrative data with the clinical risk group classification system, *Ambul Pediatr* 2:71-79, 2002.

North American Nursing Diagnosis Association: *NANDA nursing diagnoses: definitions and classification 2003-2004*, Philadelphia, 2003, North American Nursing Diagnosis Association.

Olds DL: Prenatal and infancy home visiting by nurses: from randomized trials to community replication, *Prev Sci* 3:153-172, 2002.

Perrin EC: Children whose parents are lesbian or gay, *Contemp Pediatr* 15(10):113-130, 1998.

Peterson J, Song X, Jones-DeWeever A: *Life after welfare reform: low-income single parent families, pre-and post-TANF*, Washington, DC, 2002, Institute for Womens Policy Research.

Raine A: Annotation: the role of prefrontal deficits, low autonomic arousal, and early health factors in the development of antisocial and aggressive behavior in children, *J Child Psychol Psychiatry* 43:417-434, 2002.

Simmons R: *Odd girl out: hidden culture of aggression in girls*, New York, 2002, Harvest Book Harcourt Brace.

Simmons T, O'Neill G: *Households and families: 2000 census*, Washington, DC, 2001, US Census Bureau, US Department of Commerce.

Snyder HN, Sickmund M: *Juvenile offenders and victims: 1999 national report*, Washington, DC, 1999, US Department of Justice, Bureau of Justice Statistics.

Stiffman MN et al: Household composition and risk of fatal child maltreatment, *Pediatrics* 109:615-621, 2002.

Trute B, Hiebert-Murphy D: Family adjustment to childhood developmental disability: a measure of parent appraisal of family impacts, *J Pediatr Psychol* 27:271-280, 2002.

Urban Institute, The: *A new look at homelessness in America*, Washington, DC, 2000, The Urban Institute.

US Census Bureau: Grandparents responsible for grandchildren <18 years of age. 2001 Supplementary Survey Summary Tables. Available at *www.census.gov*, 2001.

US Census Bureau: Table C2: household relationship and living arrangements of children under 18 years/1, by age, sex, race, Hispanic origin/2, and metropolitan residence: March 2000. Available at *www.census.gov/population/socdemo/hh-fam/p20-57/2000/tabc2.pdf* (accessed Oct 20, 2003).

US Department of Health and Human Services: *Healthy people 2010: understanding and improving health*, Washington, DC, 2000, US Government Printing Office.

US Department of Health and Human Services, Administration on Children, Youth, and Families: *Child maltreatment 2000*, Washington, DC, 2002, US Government Printing Office.

US Department of Health and Human Services, Administration for Children and Families: March 1999. Previously available at *www.acf.dhhs.gov/programs/ccb/faq/4steps.htm* (website no longer accessible, 2003).

Ventura SJ, Hamilton BE, Sutton PD: Revised birth and fertility rates for the United States, 2000 and 2001, *National Vital Statistics Report* 51:1-6, 2003.

Wallerstein JS: Children of divorce: the psychological tasks of the child, *Am J Orthopsychiatry* 53:230-243, 1983.

Warrington SA, Wright CM, Team AS: Accidents and resulting injuries in premobile infants: data from the ALSPAC study, *Arch Dis Child* 85:104-107, 2001.

Wolchik SA et al: Six-year follow-up of preventive interventions for children of divorce: a randomized controlled trial, *JAMA* 288:1874-1881, 2002a.

Wolchik SA et al: Fear of abandonment as a mediator of the relations between divorce stressors and mother-child relationship quality and children's adjustment problems, *J Abnorm Child Psychol* 30:401-418, 2002b.

20 Sexuality

Ardys M. Dunn, Jeanette M. Broering, Catherine G. Blosser

Sexuality is an integral part of the human experience for people of all ages and lifestyles. The sexual health of patients must therefore be a consideration for the primary care provider. To provide comprehensive primary health care, nurse practitioners (NPs) must understand how variations in health status relate to an individual's sexuality, assess an individual's sexual functioning and concerns as a part of health status, and make appropriate decisions for anticipatory guidance, intervention, or referral to resources. Much of the literature on sexuality deals with problems. This chapter focuses on health promotion, emphasizing that sexual development is a necessary and healthy part of human growth.

STANDARDS

The American Medical Association's *Guidelines for Adolescent Preventive Services (GAPS)* recommends a comprehensive primary and secondary prevention strategy for promoting healthy adolescent psychosexual development and preventing the negative consequences of sexual behaviors (American Medical Association, 1997). This strategy includes the following:

- Health guidance to promote a better understanding of psychosexual development
- Health guidance regarding responsible sexual behaviors, including abstinence
- Latex condoms to prevent sexually transmitted diseases (STDs), including infection with human immunodeficiency virus (HIV), and appropriate methods of birth control with instructions on how to use them effectively
- Annual interviews about involvement in sexual behaviors that may result in unintended pregnancy and STDs, including HIV infection
- Screening sexually active adolescents for STDs
- Confidential HIV screening of adolescents at risk for HIV infection
- Annual screening of sexually active females or females older than 18 years for cervical cancer by use of a Papanicolaou (Pap) test
- Annual interviews about a history of emotional, physical, and sexual abuse
- Universal vaccination of adolescents for hepatitis B
- Vaccinating all 11- to 12-year-olds for hepatitis B
- Vaccinating older, unimmunized adolescents with identified risk factors for hepatitis B infection
- Widespread use of hepatitis B vaccination because risk factors are not always easily identifiable among adolescents

NORMAL PATTERNS OF SEXUALITY

Definition of Sexuality, Sexual Health, and Sexual Identity

Parents, children, and adolescents have a right to information, education, and health care services that promote, maintain, and restore optimal sexual health. There is little consensus, however, regarding the scope of issues involved in the areas of sexuality and sexual learning. This lack of consensus is exacerbated by the lack of clarity in terminology. The definitions presented herein form the basis for the following discussion of sexuality in children.

Sexuality

The term *sexuality* is imprecise, referring variously to the process of development, a dimension of personality, and an expression of behavior (Roberts, 1980). *Sexuality* has been defined by the Sexuality Information and Education Council of the United States (SIECUS) as encompassing "the sexual knowledge, beliefs, attitudes, values, and behaviors of individuals. It deals with anatomy, physiology, and biochemistry of the sexual response system; with roles, identity, and personality; with individual thoughts, feelings, behaviors, and relationships. It addresses ethical, spiritual, and moral concerns, and group and cultural variations" (Haffner, 1990).

Sexual Health

Sexual health has been defined in a holistic perspective by the World Health Organization (1975) as the positive integration of somatic, emotional, intellectual, and social aspects of sexual being in ways that are positively enriching and that enhance personality, communication, and love. Sexual function, sexual self-concept, and sexual relationships are dimensions of sexual health.

Sexual function incorporates the biologic component of the human sexual response cycle and refers to the ability to give and receive sexual pleasure. Sexual self-concept is the psychologic component of sexuality, the image one has of oneself as a man or a woman, and the evaluation of one's adequacy in masculine and feminine roles. Sexual relationships refer to the social domain of sexuality and include the interpersonal relationships in which one's sexuality is shared with others.

Sexual Identity

Sexual identity as a component of sexuality evolves over the life span of an individual and encompasses four elements: biosexual identity, gender identity, sex role identity, and sexual orientation:

1. Biosexual identity ("What sex am I?") is determined from conception and is based on chromosomes. Morphologically, by 12 weeks of gestation, the anatomy of the fetus's gender can be observed. Gender assignment occurs during ultrasonography or at birth with the pronouncement of "It's a girl!" or "It's a boy!" From then, the process of gender role scripting begins.
2. Gender identity, or one's sexual self-concept, is the internal belief or sense of being male or female and is achieved in the toddler and preschool years.
3. Sex role identity ("How do I appear?") is characterized by the emergence of behaviors, attitudes, and feelings that are labeled as male, female, or neutral. This process begins at preschool age and continues into adulthood.
4. Sexual orientation ("Whom do I love?") refers to an individual's feelings of sexual attraction and erotic potential. Sexual orientation emerges over the life span, although it has been suggested that sexual attraction to one sex or the other is identified in late infancy and prepubertal childhood (Money, 1988).

Developmental Patterns of Sexuality

A full discussion of normal child development is found in Chapters 5 to 9. This section briefly emphasizes those components of development related to sexuality, especially those that are used in assessment of the child's health status (Table 20-1) (Smith, 1993).

Infant

Newborn infants are reflexive beings, responding to their physical environment without hesitation or cognition. Sexual reflexes are present prenatally and are easily stimulated in the infant. It is not uncommon to observe a penile or clitoral erection in the nursing child, for example, and infants clearly enjoy the sensual feelings of warm water or air on their naked bodies. As infants mature, self-stimulation is a natural part of exploring their environment and most frequently begins between 6 and 12 months of age. The sexual meaning attributed to such spontaneous or reflexive behavior is absent for the infant.

Healthy parent-infant bonding requires physical contact, as well as social interaction. Parents must hold, cuddle, stroke, talk to, look at, and respond to children if children are to develop a sense of trust, on which intimacy will be based in later years.

Toddler and Preschool Child

Toddlers are able to recognize and pronounce themselves as "I'm a girl" or "I'm a boy," but they can easily confuse gender in others and, sometimes, in themselves. Changing one's style of clothes, for example, can be perceived as a change in gender. Children cannot integrate gender identity into their self-concept until they understand that gender is a permanent condition, usually by age 3 or 4 years.

Children in this age-group are extremely curious about their environment (including their own and other people's bodies); they love to explore and experiment. They have a cognitive awareness of the pleasure self-stimulation gives them and frequently masturbate, but, as with infants, they attribute no erotic or sexual meaning to their actions. The combination of curiosity and lack of self-consciousness characteristic of toddlers can contribute to embarrassing social incidents for their parents. Sexual behavior among 3- to 6-year-olds has been found to be more open at home than in a more structured preschool setting (Larsson & Svedin, 2002).

The ways in which parents communicate about sexuality are important for the toddler and preschooler. Because children at this age interpret statements so literally and have "magical" thinking, their understandings of the physical self can be distorted and lengthy explanations about body functions can be misunderstood. Parents should give

TABLE 20-1 ***Sexual Function, Self-Concept, and Relationships during Childhood through Young Adulthood***

	Sexual Function	Sexual Self-Concept	Sexual Role/Relationship
Infancy	Orgasmic potential present Erectile function present	Gender identity reinforced	
Toddler	Genital pleasuring and exploration Sensual activity (e.g., hugging, stroking)	Association of sexuality and good/bad Distinction between self and others	Sex role differences learned Discrimination between male and female role models Sexual vocabulary learned
Preschool	Sex play—exploration of own body and those of playmates Self-pleasuring (masturbation)	Core gender identity solidified by age 3 years	Sex roles learned Parental attachment and identification
School age		Curiosity about sex Sexual fears and fantasies Interest in aspects of sexual development Self-awareness as sexual being	Same-sex friends Off-color humor related to sexuality
Adolescence, prepubertal	Menarche (female) Seminal emissions (male)	Concerns about body image	Same-sex friends Sexual experiences as part of friendship
Adolescence, early	Awkwardness in first sexual encounter Masturbation, petting May or may not be sexually active	Anxiety over inadequacy, lack of partner, virginity	Appropriate sex friendships Dating
Adolescence, late Young adult	May or may not be sexually active Experimentation with sexual positions, expressions Exploration of techniques	Responsibility for sexual activity Responsibility for sexual health (e.g., contraception, sexually transmitted disease prevention) Development of adult sexual value system, tolerance for others	Intimacy in relationships learned Giving and receiving pleasure learned Long-term commitment to relationship developed

children the message that they and their bodies—including its sexual parts—are valuable and important. Defining limits of appropriate and inappropriate behavior is also a parent's responsibility (e.g., it is not acceptable for a 3-year-old girl to discuss with a stranger on the bus the fact that she and her mother have "ginas" but her father and brother have penises). Clearly articulated limits help the child to better understand the social meanings given to sexuality.

School-Age Child

School-age children continue to have a high level of curiosity about sexuality, their bodies, and their environment and, aware of the pleasure stimulation gives, may actively seek sexual arousal. Masturbation and sex games are typical (e.g., playing "house" or "hospital"), and both homosexual and heterosexual encounters are commonly seen. Older school-age children are less sexual in their behavior than younger children (Friedrich et al, 1991). Younger school-age children tend to be modest about body exposure and may react negatively to nudity in the home; older children can demonstrate a certain "sexual prudery" that may, it is suggested, be a mechanism used to deal with negative messages received about sexuality (Money, 1988).

By the time children reach school age, or about 8 years of age, they begin to understand the significance of sexuality. They have often learned that "good" children do not demonstrate sexual behavior, that questions about sex are "dirty." In response, their sexual activity can become secretive or silly, and, unless parents actively communicate with their children, sexual lessons will be learned from peers, the media, jokes, and movies. Parents and teachers are in key positions to teach children that their sexual curiosity and feelings are normal and to help both boys and girls better understand how sexual development is an integral part of growing up.

Adolescent

Adolescence is a period of rapid physical, psychologic, and social change that presents a developmental challenge to both children and parents. In terms of sexuality, adolescents fit their sense of sexual being into their evolving self-image and personal identity; they learn about their bodies' (sometimes unexpected and embarrassing) sensual and sexual responses to stimulation, and they develop a sense of the moral significance of sexuality.

Privacy is essential for the adolescent to explore this emerging self, and activities such as group social functions, dating, participation in sports, and interactions at work and school provide opportunities to learn social and interpersonal skills of intimacy.

Learning how to communicate about sex, how to set limits, how to avoid misunderstandings, and how to say yes or no are important skills for adolescents. Equally important is the process of developing a set of sexual values. Whether the adolescent practices abstinence, has a double standard for men's and women's sexual behavior, or is exploitive or nurturing in close personal relationships is a reflection of the adolescent's sexual values.

ASSESSMENT OF NORMAL PATTERNS

Sexuality is an integral component of a child's development. Although for the majority of children the onset of the first sexual intercourse, or sexual debut, occurs in adolescence, sexual development, questions, and concerns are present throughout childhood.

Assessment of sexuality and sexual maturation should be integrated into the health history and physical examination at all health maintenance visits. Data suggest that adolescents are quite honest when responding to a self-report sexual questionnaire (Siegel, 1998).

History

Functions of the Sexual History

The sexual history is designed to achieve several purposes. First, it is used to collect information. Second, by including it within the health history, permission is given to the child, adolescent, or parent to ask questions and receive reliable information regarding issues of sexual concern. Third, it allows the NP to incorporate sexuality-specific education as a normal component of anticipatory guidance (Laube, 1982).

Types of Sexual Histories

The sexual history can be either comprehensive or problem oriented. The comprehensive sexual history is detailed, encompassing all aspects of sexual information about individuals, their family of origin, siblings, and peer relationships. It includes information about each phase of sexual development, body image, masturbation, learned attitudes, feelings about sexuality, sexual debut, sexual orientation, and a range of sexual behaviors. A comprehensive history is lengthy and may not be accomplished at the first visit or in a single interview, because it can be anxiety producing to have the client disclose such a level of detail during early visits, and clients can become fatigued by one lengthy interview.

In contrast, the problem-oriented sexual history usually focuses on the current complaint or assessment of specific behaviors such as the risk of exposure to pregnancy or the acquisition of STDs. Problem-oriented sexual histories are shorter, more direct, and specific to the issue at hand.

Approach to Taking a Sexual History

Taking a sexual history should be integrated as one part of the health history. In taking a sexual history, the interviewer should do the following:

- Convey an aura of comfort with the client and respond to the client without embarrassment.
- Give appropriate, factual information.
- Create a nonjudgmental environment.
- Use language that validates the client's understanding of terms and concepts. For example, when talking with adolescents, the question "Are you sexually active?" can denote a meaning of current activity on a planned and regular basis. The adolescent who has concrete cognitive abilities may respond negatively. However, the question "Have you ever had sex or are you currently having sex?" allows for a more inclusive description of sexual activity.
- Use open-ended questions. For example, use of phrases such as "explain how that happened," "what happened next," or "tell me about a typical date" elicit more complete information than do close-ended questions. Questions that contain "why" can require a level of analysis beyond the capabilities of children operating at a concrete level of cognition.
- In the questioning process, move from the least to most sensitive information.

Content of a Sexual History

The content of a comprehensive adolescent sexual and reproductive history is contained in Box 20-1. Box 20-2 lists questions for a problem-oriented sexual history. Questions for parents about their children follow. As the child grows, questions can be reworded and asked directly of the child or adolescent. Questions and the answers to them should be age appropriate (e.g., an 8- to 10-year-old should have some awareness of sexually transmitted disease, but a 4-year-old would not; it would not be necessary to ask the parent of a 2-year-old if the child has a healthy awareness of alternative sexual preferences).

- Does your child have meaningful interactions with men and women who have positive self-images?
- Do you have positive feelings about your child's gender?

BOX 20-1 *Comprehensive Adolescent Sexual and Reproductive History*

Background Data

Adolescent
- Age (birth date)
- Sex
- History of risky behaviors (e.g., drug history: onset, duration, and frequency of use of cigarettes, alcohol, other illicit drugs)

Parents
- Ages
- Religions
- Educational levels
- Occupations
- Marital status
- Affectional relationship (parent to parent)
- Child's feelings toward parent(s)

Childhood Sexuality

What were your parents' attitudes about sexuality when you were a child?
How did your parents handle nudity?
When do you first recall seeing a nude person of the same sex? Opposite sex?
Who taught you about sex, sex play, pregnancy, intercourse, masturbation, homosexuality, sexually transmitted disease, birth?
How often did you play doctor-nurse or other sex play with another child?
Tell me about any other sexual activity or experience that had a strong effect on you.

Adolescent Sexuality

Girls
- Onset of breast development?
- When did pubic hair appear?
- Onset of menstruation (age, regularity of periods; initially, now)?
- When was your last normal menstrual period (LNMP)?
- What hygienic methods are used (pads, tampons)?
- How were you prepared for menstruation? By whom?
- What were feelings about early periods? Later periods?
- Have you had unusual bleeding or pains?

Boys
- How were you prepared for adolescence? By whom?
- Age of first orgasm (ejaculation)?
- What were "wet dreams" like? How did they make you feel?
- When did pubic hair appear?

Body image
- How do you feel about your body?
- What about your breasts, genitals?
- How much time do you spend nude in front of a mirror?

Masturbation
- How old were you when you began?
- What are others' reactions to your masturbation?
- What methods do you use?
- What are your feelings about it?

Necking and petting
- How old were you when you began? How often?
- How many partners do you currently have?

Intercourse
- How often have you had intercourse?
- How many partners?
- How often do you initiate sex?
- How often do you currently have sex?
- How often have you had oral sex?
- Are your partners male, female, or both?
- Type of intercourse: penile-vaginal, orogenital, penile-anal, oral-anal

Contraceptive use
- What kinds of contraceptives have you used?
- What are you using now?
- Do you have any problems with contraceptives?
- Do you use condoms?
- How do you communicate about contraception with your partner?

Homosexuality
- What does it mean to be a lesbian, gay, or bisexual?
- Do you think you might be lesbian, gay, or bisexual?
- Do you think you need to have sex to find out? (Ryan & Futterman, 2000)
- Have you known any homosexual individuals?
- How often have you had homosexual feelings?
- How often have you been approached?
- How often have you had homosexual experiences? What kinds of experiences? What were the circumstances?

Seduction and rape
- When have you seduced someone sexually?
- When has someone seduced you?
- Have you been raped?
- Have you raped someone? How often have you forced someone to have sex?

Incest and abuse
- What kinds of touching did you receive in your home?
- From your mother? Father? Brother(s)? Sister(s)? Other relatives? Others?

Prostitution
- What feelings do you have about prostitution?
- Have you ever accepted money for sex?
- Have you ever had sex with a prostitute?

Sexually transmitted diseases (STDs)
- How old were you when you learned about STDs?
- Have you ever had an STD? Gonorrhea? Syphilis?

Continued

BOX 20-1 *Comprehensive Adolescent Sexual and Reproductive History—cont'd*

Adolescent sexuality—cont'd

Do you have any signs/symptoms now of STDs?

Pregnancy

- Have you ever been pregnant? At what age?
- How resolved—miscarriage, abortion, adoption, marriage, single parenthood?
- Do you think there is a chance you are pregnant now?
- Have you caused a pregnancy?

Abortion

- What are your feelings about abortion?
- Have you (or a partner) had an abortion? If yes, at what age? What were your feelings?
- What about your feelings now? What about your feelings immediately afterward? What about your feelings after 1 year?

Adapted from Laube HH: The use of a sexual history with adolescents. In Blum RW, editor: *Adolescent health care: clinical issues*, New York, 1982, Academic Press; Neinstein L, editor: *Adolescent health care: a practical guide*, Philadelphia, 2002, Lippincott Williams & Wilkins.

BOX 20-2 *Adolescent Sexual Problem History*

- Describe the sexual concern, problem, issue, or difficulty that you have.
- How do you feel about discussing this problem?
- How long have you had it? When did this problem begin?
- What do you think caused you to have this problem?
- What might be contributing to this problem?
- What kinds of things have you done to treat or solve this problem?
- What health professionals have you seen?
- What, if any, medication have you taken or are you taking?
- Have you talked to a friend or relative?
- Have you read any books to solve this problem? What books?

Adapted from Laube HH: The use of a sexual history with adolescents. In Blum RW, editor: *Adolescent health care: clinical issues*, New York, 1982, Academic Press.

- Is your child aware of physical sexual differences between men and women?
- What does your child know about his or her body parts? Does he or she know the correct terminology for body parts?
- What does your child know about sexuality? About gender differences?
- What does your child know about how babies are born and cared for (e.g., pregnancy, childbirth, breastfeeding)?
- What does your child know about STDs and acquired immunodeficiency syndrome (AIDS)?
- Does your child (older than 8 years of age) have a healthy awareness of alternative sexual preferences?
- How do members of your family demonstrate affection?
- Does your child seek and receive positive touching from others?
- Does your child experience a variety of sensory stimuli?
- Does your child have friends (same or opposite sex)? In what types of interactions do they engage? Is exploration (e.g., masturbation, playing "doctor") occurring? How is it handled?
- How does your child express sexuality? In play? By touching? Verbally?
- What sorts of questions does your child ask about sex?
- How do you respond to your child's sexual behavior and questions?
- What do you know about human sexuality? What are your feelings and attitudes about it?
- Does the child's school provide appropriate information about sexuality and reproduction?
- Is your child at risk for sexual abuse?

Physical Examination

The physical examination serves to identify normal (and variations of normal) sexual anatomy, stage of sexual development (Tanner stages), and pathology. The physical examination should include examination of the breasts, female genitalia and pelvis (in sexually active adolescents or when a pathology is suspected), male genitalia, and rectum, as indicated. Laboratory studies, including a Pap test, cultures or blood work for STDs, and genetic studies to determine gender, are performed as indicated. Analysis of smears and cultures in more than 10,000 patients between 10 and 19 years of age found an unusually high level of infectious processes, leading researchers to stress the importance of "early cervical Pap smear screening in the sexually active pediatric and adolescent population" (Mount & Papillo, 1999). NPs are frequently asked to determine whether a child has been sexually abused. Knowing variations of normal genital anatomy is important in making this assessment (see Reece, 1994, for specific variations; also see Chapter 19 for discussion of sexual abuse in children).

The physical examination should be performed with care and sensitivity to the child's or adolescent's feelings. A girl's first gynecologic examination can influence her attitude toward future gynecologic care, and subsequent examinations can reinforce positive or negative feelings toward her body. Very young children and toddlers make no distinction between examination of external genitalia and other body parts; young school-age children can be extremely modest, act embarrassed, and resist taking off their clothes for the examination. Older school-age children and adolescents can misinterpret the examination procedures and may feel violated or abused. By providing clear explanations of procedures, using straightforward techniques, and involving the child in the examination (e.g., asking if the child wishes to have the parent or another adult present), the NP can better achieve the fine balance necessary to perform a thorough, respectful examination (Kahn & Emans, 1999).

MANAGEMENT STRATEGIES OF NORMAL PATTERNS

The NP has two primary goals related to management of sexual development in children: to help children achieve healthy sexual identity and function and to provide support for parents to enable them to guide their children through the process of sexual development. By counseling parents about children's sexual development, both goals can be achieved. In particular, the NP must

- Assess the parent's level of understanding regarding normal physical and psychosocial sexual development in children
- Provide or clarify information as needed
- Provide strategies and support for teaching children about sexuality
- Assist the parent to connect to community-based resources

Setting the Stage

When working with children, the NP focuses on establishing and maintaining a positive relationship, based on mutual trust and respect, in which the child is validated and feels comfortable revealing concerns and asking questions. In addition to using a constructive approach to taking a sexual history, a positive relationship can be achieved by doing the following:

- Asking questions to give the message that the child is expected to be changing and is aware of and curious about those changes (e.g., "How are you feeling?" "How's your body?" "Do you notice that you're getting taller?")
- Asking questions to give the message that sexual changes are to be expected and are as normal as other body changes (e.g., "Have you noticed your breasts getting any bigger?" "Boys' penises begin to get longer and wider as they become teenagers. Have you noticed any changes in yours?")
- Asking questions to give the message that you care about the child's feelings (e.g., "How does that make you feel?" "Do you wonder sometimes about what's happening to your body?")
- Listening thoughtfully and carefully to the child's input
- Responding positively by answering the child's questions as fully as possible; being nonjudgmental, calm, friendly, and open; and having a sense of humor, yet taking the child seriously
- Using growth charts to give the message that this child is special (e.g., explain the child's personal development, discuss what the numbers of height and weight mean)
- Using appropriate teachable moments during the health visit (e.g., when examining a 3-year-old for inguinal hernia, the NP can discuss appropriate and inappropriate touching with the child and his or her parent)
- Providing accurate information and referral resources as appropriate
- Respecting the child's need for privacy (e.g., knocking before entering the examination room, providing appropriate gowns, examining the child semiclothed)
- Maintaining confidentiality as appropriate, especially with an adolescent; however, children of any age may give information that need not be shared with the parent

Sex Education

For the child, developing healthy sexuality means gaining knowledge about physical changes; shaping a positive gender identity; clarifying one's sexual identity as a boy or a girl; establishing close, intimate relationships with others; and demonstrating the ability to make healthy judgments about sexuality and sexual activity. It is the parents' responsibility to facilitate this learning. Human sexuality, however, is an emotionally charged issue for many parents, and they can find it difficult to be comfortable with their child's normal, innocent curiosity about sex, gender, and body parts and functions. The questions a child asks and the behaviors displayed can embarrass some parents, who may respond in a manner that frightens, shames, or confuses the child. Each parental response helps shape the child's perception of sexuality:

Although we may not like it, children are born as sexual beings, and parents, whether or not they are aware of it, are constantly providing lessons in sex education. The way parents respond to a child's innate sexuality and allow it to unfold is the core of a child's sex education. This response does more to mold that child's mature sexual behavior than all the information or misinformation parents may provide.

Parents should be encouraged to take advantage of teaching opportunities in normal childhood sexual play and to answer questions simply and directly, at the child's level of understanding (Box 20-3).

The content of sex education is controversial, but a comprehensive approach includes emphasis on human development, relationships, decision-making skills, sexual behavior, sexual health, and society and culture (SIECUS National Guidelines Task Force, 1996) (Table 20-2).

In most states, schools have a responsibility to provide sex education to children. Curricula that address the content outlined in Table 20-2 (e.g., "Reducing the Risk," a program intended to be incorporated into a family education offering) have been shown to have a positive impact on adolescent sexual behavior, contributing to a delay in initiating sexual intercourse, an increased use of protection against STDs and pregnancy by those who were sexually active, and an increase in parent-child communication on sexuality issues. The sex education curricula in most states, however, may not be as comprehensive as the SIECUS guidelines, and children may not be taught all they need to learn.

Contraception

Contraceptive Counseling

For NPs to provide reproductive health and contraceptive services to adolescents requires significant and specific knowledge. An in-depth discussion is beyond the scope of this text; however, several excellent management references are available (Carpenter & Rock, 2000; Hatcher et al, 1998; Neinstein, 2002). NPs who provide contraceptive counseling to adolescents should understand that the successful use of a contraceptive device requires a complex process of knowledge, decision-making skills, and public behaviors. To use contraceptives successfully, an individual must master the following:

- *Knowledge.* The person must acquire, process, and retain accurate information regarding the specific methods of birth control under consideration. For most adolescents, this means mastery of a barrier method such as condoms, spermicides, or diaphragm to prevent an STD, as well as a variety of hormonal methods for contraceptive purposes.
- *Ability to plan for the future.* Planning for the future requires self-admission that the adolescent will have sex in the future, as well as the ability to take the steps necessary to use a method consistently and correctly. Adolescents must be willing to use the chosen method of

BOX 20-3 ***Approaches to Teaching Your Child about Sex***

Discuss sex in a matter-of-fact way.
Avoid lecturing about sex. Keep the topic short and to the point, remembering the child's attention span.
Include values, emotions, feelings, and decision making in your discussion. Do not focus only on biologic facts.
Do not worry about telling children too much about sex. They tune out what they do not understand.
When your child uses "four-letter words," calmly explain what they mean and why it is not appropriate to use them. Do not laugh or joke about your child's four-letter words because this can serve as encouragement.
Use correct terminology when talking about body parts.
Discuss anticipated changes of puberty before they occur. Do not wait until your child is a teenager.
Discuss menstruation with boys as well as with girls.
Be direct in bringing up topics of sexually transmitted diseases, including acquired immunodeficiency syndrome (AIDS).
Encourage questions. Never embarrass children or tell them they are too young to understand or that they will learn that when they grow up.
If you do not know the answer to your child's question, say so, and then look it up. Ask your nurse practitioner or other pediatric primary care provider.
Check with your child to be sure your answer is understood. Make sure you answer the question that is asked, and give your child a chance to ask more questions.

Adapted from Masters WH, Johnson VE, Kolodny RC: *Human sexuality,* ed 5, New York, 1995, HarperCollins College Publishers.

TABLE 20-2 Comprehensive Sexuality Education

Content Area	Examples
Human development	Differences in anatomy between the sexes
	Puberty, menstruation
	Pregnancy and where babies come from
Relationships	Families
	Dating
	Respect for others and self
	Marriage and lifetime commitments
Personal skill	Communication
	How to say no
	How to be affectionate
	Importance of responsible behavior
	Judgment and decision making
	How to talk with parents about sexual questions
Sexual behavior	Appropriate limits on behavior
	Abstinence
	Masturbation
	Sexuality throughout life
Sexual health	Sexually transmitted diseases (STDs)
	Contraception
	Reproductive health
Society and culture	Gender roles
	Sexuality in the law and religion
	Sexual diversity
	Sexuality in the arts and media

From National Guidelines Task Force: *Guidelines for comprehensive sexuality education: kindergarten–12th grade.* Reprinted with the permission of the Sexuality Information and Education Council of the United States (SIECUS), 130 W. 42nd Street, Suite 350, New York, NY, 10036. Copyright 1991.

contraception consistently, not just when it is convenient to do so.

- *Willingness to acquire needed contraceptives publicly.* The adolescent must be willing and able to be public with requests for contraceptives; for example, to purchase condoms at a local pharmacy or to seek services at the local clinic, school-based health facility, or private practice.
- *Communication skills.* Adolescents must have the ability to communicate with another person such as their partner, health care provider, or salesperson about birth control needs. Communication also involves adolescents' willingness and ability to articulate how they feel about sexual activity, how it affects them, and the thinking behind their decision to be sexually active. Successful communication with partners appears to contribute to safer sex practices (Cobb, 1997).

Initial Screening to Assess for Appropriate Contraception

History. Examine developmental maturity and cognitive status, chronologic age, and the coexistence of other risk-taking behaviors. Obtain a thorough personal and family medical history with attention to absolute and relative contraindications for oral contraceptives; ask about first- or second-degree relatives with type 2 diabetes; ask about personal history of polycystic ovarian syndrome (PCOS).

Physical Examination

- Height and weight; body mass index (BMI)
- Blood pressure
- Thyroid examination
- Breast examination, including Tanner staging
- Auscultation of heart and lungs
- Abdominal examination
- Pelvic examination
- Skin examination for acanthosis nigricans

Laboratory Studies

- Pap smear
- Cultures for gonorrhea and chlamydia
- Potassium hydroxide (KOH) and saline preparation when indicated by presence of abnormal vaginal discharge
- Complete blood count or hemoglobin and hematocrit and rubella titer as indicated
- Venereal Disease Research Laboratories (VDRL) test or rapid plasma reagin (RPR) with known STD, particularly condylomas or genital ulcers
- Hyperlipidemia screen measuring serum cholesterol and triglycerides initially (fasting or nonfasting) and lipid profile if initial screen is elevated; screen if first-degree relative, especially a female relative, had a myocardial infarction before age 50 years or if client is a smoker or is hypertensive, with a history of first-degree relative with a myocardial infarction before age 65 years
- Fasting glucose if BMI greater than 85th percentile for age and sex, weight for height, or weight greater than 120% of ideal for height plus any two of following risk factors for type 2 diabetes:
    - Sign of insulin resistance of conditions associated with insulin resistance (acanthosis nigricans, hypertension, dyslipidemia, PCOS)
    - American Indian, African American, Latino, Asian/Pacific Islander
    - Family history of type 2 diabetes in first-or second-degree relative
    - HIV

Hormonal Methods of Contraception (Coitus-Independent Methods)

Protocol for Initial use of Oral Contraceptive Pills

The initial use of an oral contraceptive pill (OCP) requires special attention to dosing, preparation, timing, patient education, and follow-up.

Dosing. Initial dosing for an OCP should be at 30 to 35 μg estrogen, with low progestin potency per tablet. There are 20 μg combination OCPs available, should an ultra–low dose estrogen formulation be desired. The selection of an OCP can also be individualized based on menstrual characteristics or patient sensitivity. For example, a client with a history of cystic acne can be tried on an OCP where the progestins are desogestrel or norgestrel, or on Ortho Tri-Cyclen or Estrostep, the only oral contraceptives with Food and Drug Administration (FDA) approval for use in acne. For clients with hirsutism, a low androgenic potency pill is used. For clients who miss pills, using a monophasic pill provides more protection against escape ovulation than a triphasic pill (this client should also have a prescription for emergency contraception). Adolescents who demonstrate estrogen sensitivity can be tried on a more androgenic pill such as Lo/Ovral, Nordette, Triphasil, or Loestrin. For short-term therapeutic considerations, such as treatment of dysfunctional uterine bleeding, a 50 μg preparation with increased progestational activity (e.g., Ovral, Ortho-Novum 1/50, or Norinyl 1 + 50) is used. Otherwise, it is important to use the lowest possible dose of estrogen.

Preparation. Given the vast selection of products available to the NP, Hatcher and associates (1998) developed a flow chart to assist clinicians in choosing a combined oral contraceptive with low-dosage estrogen. The selection process contains four steps:

1. Does the adolescent have a contraindication to estrogen use?
2. If yes, consider the use of a progestin-only formulation.
3. If the client can use estrogen, the NP can select between numerous products, considering the following:
    - The number of micrograms of estrogen in the preparation
    - Availability of the pill
    - Ease of understanding the packaging of the pill
    - Price of the pill to the adolescent and possibly the clinic
    - Previous adverse event or experience the adolescent may have experienced in reaction to a specific preparation
4. Consider other clinical factors such as acne, nausea or vomiting, or both; spotting or breakthrough bleeding; and absence of withdrawal bleeding.

Timing. Ideally, oral contraceptives should not be started until the adolescent has had three to six regular periods after menarche, but sexually active or other high-risk teens can be put on OCPs even before menarche. Oral contraceptives can be started 3 to 4 weeks postpartum or after a first-trimester therapeutic abortion (Nelson & Neinstein, 2002a).

Patient Education. Emphasize correct and consistent use of the OCP. Remember that adolescents may not perceive the daily ingestion of an OCP as a medication.

Follow-up Management. Provide an emergency follow-up number, and instruct the client on indications for calling. Schedule a return appointment. The return visit gives the NP an opportunity to assess the physiologic effects of the OCP, as well as the adolescent's acceptance and use of this particular contraceptive method.

Adolescents tend to be acutely aware of and sensitive to body changes and processes. As a result, they may incorrectly interpret physical signs, exaggerate the effects of oral contraceptives on their bodies, and discontinue the OCP use without consulting their health care provider. At the follow-up visit, the NP should reemphasize the noncontraceptive benefits of the OCP, have the client discuss concerns about the OCPs, discuss the lower risks of OCPs compared with those of pregnancy, and review and reclarify directions and side effects.

The use of the acronym ACHES can help guide assessment questions but should be used carefully to help the teenager understand more clearly the advantages and risks of OCPs without unduly concerning her:

- **A**bdominal pain. Have you experienced abdominal pain (severe)?
- **C**hest pain. Have you noticed chest pain (severe), cough, or shortness of breath?
- **H**eadaches. Do you have headaches (severe), dizziness, weakness, or numbness?
- **E**ye problems. Have you had a change in vision (loss or blurring) or other eye problems or speech problems?
- **S**evere leg pain. Have you had any severe leg pain, especially in the calf or thigh?

Also, interview the client for STD exposure, drug compliance, satisfaction with medication, and perceived side effects. Physical examination parameters during the return visit include weight, blood pressure, and laboratory follow-up.

Estrogen/Progesterone Preparations of Oral Contraceptive Pills

Types of Preparations. Two basic preparations are available: a combination formulation that contains estrogen (less than 50 μg) and progestin in a low dose, and a progestin-only minipill. Most women in the United States use the combination formulation, either monophasic or triphasic. Progestin-only pills are prescribed for women for whom estrogens are contraindicated (e.g., lactating women or women over 40 years). They should not be prescribed in nonlactating adolescents because of higher rates of irregular bleeding and failure (Cullins & Huggins, 2000) (see Table 20-3 for summary of available formulations).

Mechanisms of Action

- Prevention of ovulation through hypothalamic and pituitary secretion secondary to estrogenic and progestational activity
- Alteration of cervical mucus, creating hostile environment for sperm
- Alteration of endometrial lining
- Alteration of tubal motility

TABLE 20-3 ***Oral Contraceptive Pills Available in the United States***

Group	Product Name (Manufacturer)	Type of Estrogen (μg/d)	Type of Progestin (mg/d)
Progestin only			
	Micronor (Ortho-McNeil)	NA	Norethindrone 0.35 mg
	Nor-QD (Watson—*generic*)	NA	Norethindrone 0.35 mg
	Ovrette (Wyeth-Ayerst)	NA	Norgestrel 0.075 mg
Monophasic			
20 μg estrogen	Alesse-21 (Wyeth)	EE, 20	Levonorgestrel, 0.1
	Alesse-28	EE, 20	Levonorgestrel, 0.1
	Loestrin 21 1/20 (Parke-Davis)	EE, 20	Levonorgestrel, 0.1
	Loestrin FE 1/20	EE, 20/75 mg ferrous fumarate (7 d)	Levonorgestrel, 0.1
	Microgestin FE 1/20 (Watson—*generic)*	EE, 20/75 mg ferrous fumarate (7 d)	Levonorgestrel, 0.1
	Mircette (Organon)	EE, 20	Levonorgestrel, 0.1
30 μg estrogen	Desogen (Organon)	EE, 30	Desogestrel, 0.15
	LevLen-21 (Berlex)	EE, 30	Levonorgestrel, 0.15
	Levlen-28	EE, 30	Levonorgestrel, 0.15
	Levora 0.15/30-21 (Watson—*generic*)	EE, 30	Levonorgestrel, 0.15
	Levora 0.15/30-28	EE, 30	Levonorgestrel, 0.15
	Loestrin 21 1.5/30 (Parke-Davis)	EE, 30	Norethindrone, 1.5
	Loestrin FE 1.5/30	EE, 30/75 mg ferrous fumarate (7 d)	Norethindrone, 1.5
	Lo/Ovral (Wyeth)	EE, 30	Norgestrel, 0.3
	Lo/Ovral-28	EE, 30	Norgestrel, 0.3
	Low-Ogestrel (Waston—*generic*)	EE, 30	Norgestrel, 0.3
	Nordette-28	EE, 30	Levonorgestrel, 0.15
	Ortho-Cept 28 (Ortho-McNeil)	EE, 30	Desogestrel, 0.15
	Yasmin 28 (Berlex)	EE, 30	Drospirenone, 3.0 (spirolactone progestin)
35 μg estrogen	Brevicon 28 (Watson)	EE, 35	Norethindrone, 0.5
	Demulen 1/35-21 (Pharmacia)	EE, 35	Ethynodiol, 1.0
	Demulen 1/35-28	EE, 35	Ethynodiol, 1.0
	Modicon 21 (Ortho-McNeil)	EE, 35	Norethindrone, 0.5
	Modicon 28	EE, 35	Norethindrone, 0.5
	Necon 0.5/35-21 (Watson—*generic*)	EE, 35	Norethindrone, 0.5
	Necon 0.5/35-28	EE, 35	Norethindrone, 0.5
	Necon 1/35 21 (Watson)	EE, 35	Norethindrone, 1.0
	Necon 1/35 28	EE, 35	Norethindrone, 1.0
	Nelova 0.5/35E 28 (Warner Chilcott—*generic*)	EE, 35	Norethindrone, 0.5
	Norinyl 1 + 35 28 (Watson)	EE, 35	Norethindrone, 1.0

Continued

TABLE 20-3 ***Oral Contraceptive Pills Available in the United States—cont'd***

Group	Product Name (Manufacturer)	Type of Estrogen (μg/d)	Type of Progestin (mg/d)
	Nortrel 0.5/35 21 (Barr)	EE, 35	Norethindrone, 0.5
	Nortrel 0.5/35 28	EE, 35	Norethindrone, 0.5
	Nortrel 1/35 21 (Watson)	EE, 35	Norethindrone, 1.0
	Nortrel 1/35 28	EE, 35	Norethindrone, 1.0
	Ortho-Cyclen 28 (Ortho-McNeil)	EE, 35	Norgestimate 0.25
	Ortho-Novum 1/35 21 (Ortho-McNeil)	EE, 35	Norethindrone, 1.0
	Ortho-Novum 1/35 28	EE, 35	Norethindrone, 1.0
	Ovcon /35 21 (Warner Chilcott)	EE, 35	Norethindrone, 0.4
	Ovcon /35 28	EE, 35	Norethindrone, 0.4
	Zovia 1/35E 21 (Watson)	EE, 35	Ethynodiol, 1.0
	Zovia 1/35E 28	EE, 35	Ethynodiol, 1.0
50 μg estrogen	Demulen 1/50-21 (Pharmacia)	EE, 50	Ethynodiol, 1.0
	Demulen 1/50-28	EE, 50	Ethynodiol, 1.0
	Necon 1/50 21 (Watson)	EE, 50	Norethindrone, 1.0
	Necon 1/50 28	EE, 50	Norethindrone, 1.0
	Norinyl 1+50 28 (Watson)	EE, 50	Norethindrone, 1.0
	Ogestrel 0.5/50-28 (Watson)	EE, 50	Norgestrel, 0.5
	Ortho-Novum 1/50 28 (Ortho-McNeil)	EE, 50	Norethindrone, 1.0
	Ovcon /50 (Warner Chilcott)	EE, 50	Norethindrone, 1.0
	Ovral-28 (Wyeth)	EE, 50	Norgestrel, 0.5
	Ovral (21)	EE, 50	Norgestrel, 0.5
	Zovia 1/50E-21 (Watson)	EE, 50	Ethynodiol, 1.0
	Zovia 1/50E-28	EE, 50	Ethynodiol, 1.0
Biphasic			
35 μg estrogen	Necon 10/11-21 (Watson—*generic*)	EE, 35	Norethindrone 0.5 mg (10 d); 1.0 mg (11 d)
	Necon 10/11-28	EE, 35	Norethindrone 0.5 mg (10 d); 1.0 mg (11 d)
	Ortho-Novum 10/11 21 (Ortho-McNeil)	EE, 35	Norethindrone 0.5 mg (10 d); 1.0 mg (11 d)
	Ortho-Novum 10/11 28	EE, 35	Norethindrone 0.5 mg (10 d); 1.0 mg (11 d)
Triphasic			
20 μg estrogen	Estrostep 21 (Parke-Davis)	EE, 20 (5 d), 30 (7 d), 35 (9 d)	Norethindrone, 1.0 mg
	Estrostep Fe	EE, 20 (5 d), 30 (7 d), 35 (9 d); 75 mg ferrous fumarate (7 d)	Norethindrone, 1.0 mg
	Tri-Levlen 21 (Berlex)	EE, 30 (6 d)	Levonorgestrel, 0.05 (6 d)
		EE, 40 (5 d)	Levonorgestrel, 0.075 (5 d)
		EE, 30 (10 d)	Levonorgestrel, 0.125 (10 d)
	Tri-Levlen 28	EE, 30 (6 d)	Levonorgestrel, 0.05 (6 d)
		EE, 40 (5 d)	Levonorgestrel, 0.075 (5 d)
		EE, 30 (10 d)	Levonorgestrel, 0.125 (10 d)
	Triphasil-21 (Wyeth)	EE, 30 (6 d)	Levonorgestrel, 0.05 (6 d)
		EE, 40 (5 d)	Levonorgestrel, 0.075 (5 d)
		EE, 30 (10 d)	Levonorgestrel, 0.125 (10 d)
	Triphasil-28	EE, 30 (6 d)	Levonorgestrel, 0.05 (6 d)
		EE, 40 (5 d)	Levonorgestrel, 0.075 (5 d)
		EE, 30 (10 d)	Levonorgestrel, 0.125 (10 d)
	Trivora-28 (Watson)	EE, 30 (6 d)	Levonorgestrel, 0.05 (6 d)

TABLE 20-3 *Oral Contraceptive Pills Available in the United States—cont'd*

Group	Product Name (Manufacturer)	Type of Estrogen (μg/d)	Type of Progestin (mg/d)
Progestin only			
		EE, 40 (5 d) EE, 30 (10 d)	Levonorgestrel, 0.075 (5 d) Levonorgestrel, 0.125 (10 d)
	Ortho-Novum 7/7/7 21 (Ortho-McNeil)	EE, 35 (21 d)	Norethindrone 0.5 (7 d) Norethindrone 0.75 (7 d) Norethindrone 1.0 (7 d)
	Ortho-Novum 7/7/7 28	EE, 35 (21 d)	Norethindrone 0.5 (7 d) Norethindrone 0.75 (7 d) Norethindrone 1.0 (7 d)
	Tri-Norinyl-28 (Watson)	EE, 35 (21 d)	Norethindrone 0.5 (7 d) Norethindrone 1.0 (9 d) Norethindrone 0.5 (5 d)
	Ortho Tri-Cyclen 28 (Ortho-McNeil)	EE, 35 (21 d)	Norgestimate 0.18 (7 d) Norgestimate 0.215 (7 d) Norgestimate 0.25 (7 d)

Adapted from American Hospital Formulary Service: *Drug information 2002*, Bethesda, MD, 2002, American Society of Health-System Pharmacists; Association of Reproductive Health Professionals (ARHP): Clinical proceedings August 2001. Understanding low-dose oral contraceptives. Available at *www.arhp.org* (accessed Mar 25, 2003).
EE, Ethinyl estradiol; d, days; μg, micrograms; *mg*, milligrams; *NA*, not applicable.

Theoretic and Use Effectiveness

- Lowest expected failure rate is 0.1%.
- Typical first-year failure rate in all women is 8% (Speroff & Darney, 2001).
- Unmarried, poor, minority women have failure rates of 10% to 20% (Speroff & Darney, 2001).

Benefits

- High rate of effectiveness
- Simple method to use
- Ease of discontinuing use
- Rapid reversal of effects after discontinuing medication
- Beneficial effects on the menstrual cycle

Medical Benefits. For women younger than age 20 years, the estimated death rate while on an OCP is 0.3 per 100,000 nonsmoking users (2.2 per 100,000 smoking users), as compared with that of childbirth, for which the estimated maternal death rate is 7 per 100,000 live births (Rosenfeld & Coupey, 2000).

- Reduction of premenstrual symptoms (e.g., dysmenorrhea)
- Reduction of anemia
- Decreased incidence of pelvic inflammatory disease (PID), which results in less morbidity in the areas of chronic pelvic pain, decreased incidence of ectopic pregnancies, and less infertility
- Probable protection against recurrent formation of ovarian cysts (Speroff & Darney, 2001)
- Reduction of endometriosis
- Reduction of ovarian and endometrial cancer
- Ortho Tri-Cyclen and Estrostep are approved by FDA for treatment of acne
- Decreased effect on high-density lipoproteins (with use of triphasics)
- Decreased effect on blood pressure (with use of triphasics)
- Decreased effect on carbohydrate metabolism (with use of triphasics)

Disadvantages of Triphasic OCP

- Confusion about color of package
- Increased incidence of breakthrough bleeding as compared with straight preparations
- No studies reliably document long-term effect on lipids
- Less flexibility of use by the prescribing person (e.g., difficult to use for periods greater than 21 days or for management of ovarian cysts, endometrial bleeding, or dysfunctional uterine bleeding)
- Some adolescents find the triphasic preparation confusing, especially if they forget to take a pill

Disadvantages of Progestin-Only OCP

- Irregular bleeding
- Effectiveness decreases dramatically if even one pill is missed; manufacturer recommends that progestin-only pills be taken at the same time every day and that a backup method of control be used if even one pill

is missed or taken more than 3 hours late (Andolsek, 2001)
- May increase acne

Failure/Lack of Efficacy. Reasons for failure of OCPs include the following:
- Method failure or method ineffectiveness
- Patient failure/user effectiveness—50% to 70% of women still use OCPs 1 year after initiation, with most discontinuing for nonmedical reasons
- Concurrent drug interaction such as with anticonvulsants, rifampin, or oral antifungals; antibiotics may predispose to escape ovulation (Speroff & Darney, 2001); with anticonvulsants, prescribe any OCP with at least 35 μg of estrogen or greater; with rifampin, use a backup method; otherwise, consider an alternative method to an OCP
- OCPs can increase the action of diazepam, Librium, tricylics, and theophylline

Evra Contraceptive Patch

The Evra patch is a 20 cm^2 transdermal adhesive patch comprised of progestin (17-deacetylnorgestimate) and ethinyl estradiol. It is placed on the trunk, buttock, or arm once a week for 3 weeks and removed for 1 week to allow for a withdrawal bleed. The advantage of the patch is that it does not require the user to remember a daily OCP. Disadvantages include the visibility of the patch, which precludes privacy of method, and the need to remember to replace the patch when indicated. It costs about the same (except for generic forms of OCPs) and has the same precautions and side effects as OCPs.

Nuva Ring

The Nuva Ring is a self-administered contraceptive, consisting of a soft, flexible, 2 inch transparent plastic ring with a hole in the middle. It is 0.125 inch thick and is impregnated with both estrogen and progestin. It is inserted vaginally once a month on or before the fifth day of menses, left in place for 3 weeks, removed for 1 week to allow for a withdrawal bleed, and then reinserted. Placement over the cervix is not necessary. As long as it is in contact with the vagina, it is working. If used as instructed, the failure rate is 1% to 2%. Advantages include it being coitus independent; it does not involve the use of messy creams or jells; and it is only dealt with once a month. It does not provide protection against STDs, there is some initial breakthrough bleeding, and the user must be comfortable inserting and removing the device and be able to adhere to the usage schedule.

Subdermal Implant Contraception

Implanon joins Norplant as an implanted form of progestin-only contraception. Implanon is a 3-year subdermal implant that has a newer form of progestin (etonogestrel). The advantage of an implant is that it provides long-acting contraception. Disadvantages include surgical insertion and removal procedures and side effects, such as irregular bleeding, weight gain, and acne. It is a more successful method for mature adolescents committed to long-term contraception.

Injectable Contraception

Medroxyprogesterone Acetate (Depo-Provera)

Protocol for Initial Use. Always evaluate for pregnancy before giving initial dose. A single 150 mg injection inhibits ovulation for 13 weeks. Dosage adjustment for body weight is not necessary. It is preferable to deliver the initial injection before day 5 of the menstrual cycle to minimize pregnancy potential. Injections are usually given at 12-week intervals. If more than 13 weeks have transpired between injections, evaluate for pregnancy before giving the injection.

Mechanism of Action
- Inhibits ovulation by inhibiting luteinizing hormone surge (normal ovulation occurs 6 months after the last injection; 25% will take up to 1 year to return to the normal menses pattern) (Speroff & Darney, 2001)
- Creates shallow, atrophic endometrium, unsuitable for implantation
- Increases thickening of cervical mucus, decreasing sperm penetration

Theoretic and Use Effectiveness

The lowest expected pregnancy rate is 0.3 per 100 women-years.

Benefits
- Typical failure rate: 3% (Speroff & Darney, 2001)
- One-time dosing every 3 months
- Good method for adolescents who want to keep their contraception private from family and friends
- Inhibits intravascular sickling; increases hemoglobin and red blood cell survival rate
- Beneficial effect on duration and quality of lactation in lactating females
- Gynecologic benefits (e.g., decreases in PID, ectopic pregnancy, and endometriosis)

Disadvantages
- Menstrual irregularities
- Amenorrhea or decreased menstrual flow
- Weight gain
- Headache
- Breast tenderness
- Acne
- Hirsutism
- Psychologic effects such as moodiness, depression, change in libido

- Increased risk for low birth weight in infants exposed in utero
- Evidence of bone density loss in adolescents; osteoporosis
- Intramuscular injection

Patients Appropriate for Depo-Provera. Depo-Provera is a contraceptive method of choice for patients with the following characteristics:

- Seeking a long-term, reversible, highly reliable, private method of contraception
- Those for whom use of estrogen is contraindicated (e.g., patients with a previous thromboembolic episode, lupus, sickle cell anemia)
- Those with seizures—improves control (Speroff & Darney, 2001)
- Those with poor compliance using other contraceptive methods
- Those with menstrual hygiene issues, such as individuals who are mentally retarded, because Depo-Provera often causes amenorrhea after two injections

Lunelle

Preparation. A combination estrogen-progesterone (5 mg estradial cypoinate and 25 mg of medroxyprogesterone [DMPA]) injectable preparation. The first injection is given within 5 days of menses and then every 28 days. The same selection process and follow-up management as OCPs are indicated.

Mechanisms of Action

- Same as for OCPs

Theoretic and Use Effectiveness

- 0.3% expected failure rate

Advantage

- Do not have to remember to take daily OCPs

Disadvantages

- Need to also use condoms to prevent STDs
- Need monthly injection; monthly office visit charges
- Side effects include weight gain, irregular bleeding, breast discomfort
- Issue same precautions as with OCPs regarding ACHES

Postcoital Hormonal Contraception or Emergency Contraception

Preparation. Emergency contraception (EC) is designed to be used after unprotected intercourse to prevent an unwanted pregnancy. Whichever EC regimen is used, it must be taken within 72 hours of intercourse. Preven and Plan B are FDA-approved emergency contraceptive "kits" marketed in the United States. Preven is a combination of estrogen and progestin; Plan B is a progestin-only method. Regular OCPs (combination) may also be used at recommended dosages; this regimen is referred to as the Yuzpe method. Progestin-only OCPs are another alternative (see Clinical Management).

Clinical Management. The client may have an advance prescription for self-administration that is available as needed. The prescription is intended for one-time-only prevention, such as after a sexual assault, when a condom breaks, or there has been a lapse in birth control method. EC is more effective when taken earlier after intercourse. Studies have shown that when readily available, the use of EC does not increase unprotected sex (Speroff & Darney, 2001). If a client has a need for EC within 72 hours after unprotected intercourse:

- Assess for pregnancy using rapid high-sensitivity urine pregnancy test. If last normal menstrual period has been within 1 month, a pregnancy test is not necessary.
- Have patient sign consent and follow-up agreement.
- If using the Yuzpe or Preven Kit method described below, administer antinausea medication one hour before the first dose of ECPs (recommended) or after the first dose of ECPs if nausea is severe or the patient vomits (e.g., 50 mg meclizine by mouth, which is available over the counter as Bonine and Dramamine 2)
- Use one of the following regimens, taken orally (Ott & Irwin, 2002; Speroff, 2003):
  - Yuzpe method (combination OCPs; dose is >100 μg ethinyl estradiol for two doses):
    1. Ovral or Ogestrel OCPs: two tablets within 72 hours, followed by two tablets 12 hours later
    2. Lo/Ovral, Nordette, Levlen, Low-Ogestrel, Levora, or yellow tablets of Triphasil, Trivora, or Tri-Levlen OCPs: four tablets, followed by four tablets 12 hours later
    3. Alesse or Levlite: five tablets, followed by five tablets 12 hours later
    4. Preven Kit (prepackaged combination estrogen/progestin): two tablets, followed by two tablets 12 hours later
  - Progestin-only methods:
    1. Plan B Kit (0.75 mg levonorgestrel): one tablet, followed by one tablet 12 hours later OR single dose of two tablets (1.5 mg levonorgestrel)
    2. Ovrette OCPs (0.075 mg norgestrel): 20 tablets, followed by 20 tablets 12 hours later
- Instruct patient to return for a pregnancy test if no menses occurs within 3 weeks.
- Instruct patient to abstain from intercourse until the start of her next cycle.
- Discuss a long-term birth control method; review current method and effectiveness for client.
- Schedule return visit in 3 to 4 weeks.

Mechanism of Action

- Delays ovulation

Side Effects. Side effects include nausea, vomiting, breast tenderness, headache, and dizziness.

Contraindications to Emergency Contraception

- Personal or family history of idiopathic thrombotic disease (Speroff & Darney, 2001)

Effectiveness. Preven has a 2% to 3% failure rate; Plan B has a 1% failure rate. The progestin-only methods have fewer side effects (Speroff & Darney, 2001).

Barrier Methods of Contraception (Coitus-Dependent Methods)

Condoms

Condoms are the most common barrier method of contraception. Used effectively, they can prevent pregnancy and STDs. Seventy-two percent of men and 68% of women ages 15 to 17 years old claim to use condoms (DuRant & Smith, 2002). Among all teens, the rate of condom use has increased 10% from 1988 rates (Nelson & Neinstein, 2002b).

More than 100 brands of condoms are available in an array of sizes (most are 170 by 50 mm), textures, lubricants, colors, and scents. Ninety-nine percent use latex condoms, and less than 1% use either natural skin or the newer polyurethane condoms. The polyurethane condoms are not subject to breakdown by petroleum-based lubricants, lack latex allergy precautions, and have an improved taste over latex. However, they are less elastic, which increases slippage and breakage. They should be reserved for those with latex allergies.

Protocol for Use

- Use every time!
- Apply correctly, allowing for 0.5-inch tip at end and removing any trapped air.
- Remove correctly after intercourse. Hold onto the condom while withdrawing the penis from the vagina to avoid the condom coming off in the vagina. Replace if used for oral or anal sex before intravaginal intercourse.
- Avoid use of petroleum-based lubricants, such as petroleum jelly, as well as shortening, and oil-based vaginal therapeutics such as Monistat or Femstat. Restrict the use of some of the sexual lubricants with latex or natural skin condoms, as well.
- Check expiration date on the package and make sure package is intact.
- Use only once and discard.
- Keep a prescription for EC handy.

Mechanism of Action

- Prevent sperm from entering vagina
- Spermicidal condoms inactivate motile sperm ejaculated into the condom; unknown whether a spermicidal condom is more effective in actual use than a nonspermicidal condom

Theoretic and Use Effectiveness

- First-year failure rate among typical users is 14% (Speroff & Darney, 2001).
- First-year failure rate among perfect users is 3%.
- Concomitant, perfect use of condoms with a spermicide has an estimated probability of contraceptive failure of 0.1%. This is equivalent to perfect-use failure rate with an OCP.

Benefits

- Encourages male participation
- Appeals to those who have episodic intercourse and for sexual debuts (Nelson & Neinstein, 2002b)
- Is inexpensive and accessible
- Use of lubricated condoms reduces mechanical friction and vaginal or penile irritation
- Decreases the risk of transmitting STDs
- Prevents development or enhances regression of cervical intraepithelial neoplasia
- Eliminates postcoital vaginal discharge
- Helps maintain erection for some men
- Has few contraindications

Disadvantages

- Condom breakage or slippage. Approximately 2% to 6% of condoms fail as a result of breakage or slippage.
- Natural-skin condoms are contraindicated if there is a risk of infection by sexually transmitted viruses (e.g., hepatitis B virus, human papillomavirus, herpes simplex virus, and HIV).
- Either partner may be allergic to latex.
- Male partner may fail to accept responsibility for use.
- Some men cannot maintain an erection when condom is used.

Other Barrier Methods

Diaphragm. Available for 100 years, there are currently four types of diaphragms in sizes from 50 to 105 mm, available by prescription only. For most adolescents, the 65 to 75 mm sizes are commonly prescribed. These are

- Flat spring (Ortho-White)
- Arching spring (Koroflex, Allflex, Ramses Bendex)
- Coil-spring rim (Koromex, Ortho, Ramses)
- Wide-seal rim (Milex)

The diaphragm can be placed in the vagina over the cervix up to 1 hour before intercourse and can be left in place for 24 hours, but it must be left a minimum of 6 to 8 hours. Reapplication of spermicide is required with subsequent intercourse.

Cervical Cap. The Prentif Cavity Rim Cervical Cap is the only type of cervical cap approved by the FDA for use in the United States. It comes in four sizes that properly fit 80% of women's cervices. The cap can be left in place for 48 hours, and subsequent intercourse within 6 hours or more requires additional intravaginal spermicide. Typical first-year failure rates are 18%. The cervical cap should probably be reserved for those adolescents who are older, more motivated to comply with contraception, and able to place and remove the device (Speroff & Darney, 2001). The association of abnormal Pap smear results with the use of the cervical cap is unresolved. FDA protocol recommends obtaining a Pap smear at the time of fitting, then 3 months after onset of use and annually thereafter.

Female Condom. The female condom is a device with an inner ring or dome that fits next to the cervix. An outer ring fits around the external opening to the vagina. The single-use condom acts as a barrier to prevent sperm from entering the vagina. Use is less than 1% in the United States (Rosenfeld & Coupey, 2000).

Protocols for Using Other Barrier Methods. These vary depending on the barrier method.

Theoretic and Use Effectiveness. Effectiveness of any of these methods is influenced by the patient's ability to use the method consistently and correctly, along with her own personal fertility characteristics. Patients who are younger than 30 years of age and have intercourse four or more times a week experience higher failure rates.

- Diaphragm failure rate is 16% to 18% in typical users (Rosenfeld & Coupey, 2000).
- Cervical cap failure rate averages 20% to 40% (Speroff & Darney, 2001).
- Female condom pregnancy rates are reported to be 18% to 25% (Rosenfeld & Coupey, 2000).

Benefits

- Diaphragms and female condoms help prevent transmission of STDs and decrease risk of PID, bacterial and viral infection, and cervical neoplasia.
- Female condoms are accessible over the counter.

Disadvantages

- Barrier methods are contraindicated if there is a history of toxic shock syndrome.
- Female condoms cost $3.00 versus $1.00 for male condoms and have a visible outer ring.
- Caps are contraindicated if there has been a full-term delivery within the last 6 weeks, if there has been a recent spontaneous or induced abortion, or if there is vaginal bleeding from any cause, including menstrual flow.
- Allergic reaction may occur in those sensitive to spermicide, rubber, latex, or polyurethane.
- Abnormalities in vaginal anatomy can interfere with satisfactory fit or placement of any of the devices.
- Diaphragm can cause recurrent urinary tract infections that do not resolve after diaphragm has been refitted.
- For diaphragms and caps, trained personnel may not be available to fit device or they may lack time to instruct patient adequately on use of method.
- Patient must be able to learn correct insertion and extraction techniques.
- Patient may not feel comfortable touching self, or may find procedure messy and unpleasant.

Spermicides

Protocol for Use

- Use every time!
- Keep adequate supply and store properly.
- Be alert to timing of product placement before intercourse. Place in vagina at appropriate time.
- Insert new application of product before every episode of repeated intercourse.

Mechanism of Action

Spermicides are a combination of an inert base or carrier (foam, cream, jelly, suppository, or tablet) with active spermicidal agent nonoxynol-9 or octoxynol, which kills sperm by permeating the cell membrane. Spermicides are marketed in various formats:

- Foams, creams, or jellies that can be used alone or in combination with a condom or diaphragm
- Spermicidal suppositories that are intended for use alone or with a condom; require a 10- to 15-minute wait before intercourse to allow the product to effervesce
- Vaginal contraceptive film that can be used alone or with a condom or diaphragm; film contains 72 mg of nonoxynol-9 in a thin sheet that is placed next to the cervix 5 minutes before intercourse

Theoretic and Use Effectiveness

- Estimate among perfect first-year users is 6% failure rate.
- Among typical users, failure is about 26% (Speroff & Darney, 2001).

Benefits

- Medically safe, with same efficacy as barrier methods or condoms
- Available over the counter without a prescription; no need to access medical system
- No need for partner involvement with decision making or implementation
- Used at midcycle to augment effectiveness of intrauterine device (IUD) or condom

- Used as backup option while waiting to start OCPs, for missed OCPs, or between relationships
- Emergency use when condom breaks (insert immediately)
- Effective against bacteria such as gonorrhea and chlamydia

Disadvantages

- Can cause allergic reaction in those sensitive to spermicidal agent or base
- Can be difficult for some people to learn correct insertion technique
- Abnormalities in vaginal anatomy can prevent correct placement or product retention (e.g., septum, prolapse, double cervix)

Contraceptive Methods Less Useful for Adolescents

The following methods are usually not recommended for use with sexually active adolescents because of higher failure rates, the need for more maturity, and proven and committed use of contraceptives:

- Periodic abstinence
- Fertility awareness or rhythm method, due to the more irregular cycles of adolescents
- Implanted contraception, due to intolerance of side effects and costs associated with early removal
- Progestin-only pills, unless indicated
- Intrauterine devices, due to increased risk of STDs and irregular bleeding

MANAGEMENT OF ALTERED PATTERNS

Sexual development is an integral part of children's whole development. Children's sense of self; personality; relationship to others and to the physical world; cognitive, emotional, and spiritual abilities; perceptions; and expressions are all influenced by and, in turn, influence their sexual development. If children experience problems with sexuality, all other aspects of development are affected. Issues of major concern include child sexual abuse (see Chapter 19) and adolescent pregnancy. Homosexuality, although an alternative rather than an altered pattern, is discussed later in this chapter, because the establishment of sexual orientation and intimacy often occurs during adolescence.

Adolescent Pregnancy

Description

Adolescent pregnancy occurs in girls or young women between ages 13 and 19 years, although pregnancy is possible for any girl who has begun ovulation. Pregnancy has been seen in girls before their first menstrual cycle and in those as young as 10 or 11 years of age.

Incidence and Etiology

See Chapter 1 for current statistics. The decrease in teen pregnancy is regarded as evidence of more effective contraceptive practices, delayed sexual debuts, and a decrease in sexual activity. Of teen pregnancies, approximately 56% end in live births, 14% in miscarriage, and 30% in therapeutic abortions (Neinstein & Farmer, 2002).

Research on adolescent pregnancy has established risk factors that may be helpful in identifying youth at risk for adolescent pregnancy. Periods of vulnerability to unwanted pregnancy in the sexual career of women have been described by using a developmental approach for known risk (Adler, 1984) (Table 20-4). A number of factors have been identified as predictors of failure or success with contraception. These include the following:

- Age. Adolescents 15 years of age and younger are at highest risk for pregnancy, because 46% report using no method of contraception at their first episode of intercourse. In comparison, only 17% of females age 19 years or older report using no method.
- Noncompliance with the first method chosen (previous method failure).
- Not acquiring a method of contraception at the first reproductive health visit.
- Frequency of family planning visits in the preceding 12 months. Increased compliance with clinic attendance appears to correlate with effective contraceptive use by client.
- Coital frequency. Adolescent females who have sexual intercourse more than six times per month are at greater risk of becoming pregnant.
- Length of time between first coitus and initiation of birth control use. The longer adolescents delay seeking services for contraception, the less likely they are to use a highly reliable method consistently and correctly.

Antecedent risk factors to unintentional pregnancy include the following:

- Early onset of sexual activity, especially before age 15 years
- Early onset of substance use, including cigarettes, alcohol, and illicit drugs
- Lesbian or bisexual; these females are as likely to have sex with males as heterosexuals, but their pregnancy rate is more than doubled (Meininger et al, 2002)
- Low educational expectation
- Low perception of life options
- Poor grades and academic achievement
- Behavior problems, including truancy and delinquency

TABLE 20-4 Developmental Risk Factors for Sexual Activity

Developmental Phase of Relationship	Associated Risk Factors
Early adolescence	No self-concept of being fertile (fecundity)
Initiation of a relationship	No self-concept of being fertile (fecundity)
	Feels conflict or guilt over planning to be sexually active
Developing relationship	Change from using coitus-dependent methods of contraception (condoms or spermicides), which have lower use effectiveness rates, to using coitus-independent (hormonal) methods, which have a reported higher use effectiveness rate; change involves learning new technique
	Change in relationship
	Shift in established communication skills from a known to an unknown partner
	Persons with immature interpersonal communication skills may be unprepared to negotiate the use of a contraceptive device with a new partner
Geographic mobility	Lack knowledge needed to access local systems of care that dispense contraceptive devices
Following each pregnancy	Lack understanding of reproductive physiology
	Unaware that ovulation may return within 2 wk after the termination of a pregnancy
	Perceive self to be at reduced risk of pregnancy

Adapted from Adler NE: Contraception and unwanted pregnancy, *Behav Med Update* 5:28-34, 1984.

- Negative peer influence
- Poor contraceptive compliance or failure with a contraceptive device
- Nonintact families (those without both biologic mother and father present)
- Depression
- Cultural values that favor adolescent pregnancy
- Prior history of sexual or physical abuse or violence at home (Neinstein & Farmer, 2002)

Assessment

History. The history should include the following:

- Menstrual history: last normal menstrual period, any oligomenorrhea or amenorrhea, hypomenorrhea or irregular period, intermenstrual spotting
- Sexual history (see Box 20-1)
- Associated symptoms: breast sensitivity, nipple tenderness (1 to 2 weeks after conception), fatigue, nausea, urinary frequency (2 weeks after conception)
- Patients often have vague unassociated complaints (e.g., headache, abdominal discomfort, dizziness)

Physical Examination. There are three classic signs of pregnancy, each of which can be observed during the pelvic examination:

- Hegar sign. Softening of the isthmus of the uterus (the area between the cervix and the uterine body). This may be observed before there is uterine enlargement.
- Chadwick sign. Dark-bluish or purplish discoloration of the vaginal and cervical epithelium, the result of increased blood supply to the pelvis. This is usually observed before uterine growth.
- Uterine enlargement. Occurs at 5 to 6 weeks and initially is due to changes in the uterine muscle rather than growing gestation. Uterine sizing is traditionally done by bimanual examination and recorded in weeks of estimated gestation.

Laboratory Studies. The following laboratory studies are done in cases of suspected pregnancy:

- Pregnancy testing. Quantitative serum human chorionic gonadotropin (HCG) is the most specific, accurate by 6 to 10 days after conception, and expensive. Quantitative serum HCG testing is indicated for serial measurements to evaluate ectopic pregnancy or molar pregnancy or to rule out gestational trophoblastic neoplasia (GTN). Urine testing is the chosen test for the ambulatory setting, because results can be obtained in 5 minutes and the test is highly accurate. Reliability allows for accurate results 6 to 8 days after ovulation or from 2 days after the last missed menstrual period.
- If pregnancy test is positive, laboratory diagnostics include the following:
  - Cervical cultures for *Neisseria gonorrhoeae* and *Chlamydia trachomatis*
  - Cervical cytology if indicated
  - Vaginal pH with saline and KOH wet mounts
- If the pregnancy is to be continued, additional serum testing, including syphilis serology, complete blood count, blood type and Rh status, rubella titer, screening

for hepatitis B serology, sickle cell in black females, Tay-Sachs in Mediterranean and Jewish females, and possibly for HIV infection.
- Urinalysis and urine culture.
- Possibly, pelvic ultrasonography to determine gestation accurately.

Differential Diagnosis

The differential diagnoses for pregnancy are as follows:
- Nonviable intrauterine pregnancy with partial spontaneous abortion
- Ectopic pregnancy
- Molar pregnancy to exclude GTN

Management

Prompt diagnosis assists with pregnancy planning, early onset of prenatal precautions (e.g., avoidance of medications, alcohol, and smoking), and medical care. Early care also allows women considering an abortion ample time for counseling, decision making, and obtaining an abortion in the first trimester, when the procedure is safest.

The NP should schedule a health visit to include pregnancy test, physical examination, and health counseling. If the pregnancy test is negative, counsel the adolescent regarding risk of potential pregnancy and reliable methods of contraception. If the pregnancy test is positive, schedule for a health visit to include the following:
- Pelvic examination to determine gestational age
- Counseling for pregnancy options, including continuing pregnancy and retaining custody of child, continuing pregnancy and placing child for adoption, or terminating pregnancy
- Assessment of need for involvement of social support system, including family, male partner, and any significant others; NP may need to serve as mediator for teenager in informing others
- Initiation of referrals as appropriate for the decision made:
  - If the choice is continuing pregnancy, refer to adolescent pregnancy program to initiate comprehensive medical, nutritional, psychosocial, and educational services
  - If adoption is the option of choice, refer to appropriate legal or social service agency, or both
  - If the choice is terminating pregnancy, refer to appropriate source for abortion
- Make additional referrals as indicated (e.g., Women, Infants, and Children [WIC] program or insurance coverage)

Public health–based research indicates that there is a significant positive effect on pregnancy, parenting, and child-rearing outcomes if home visits are made by public health nurses (Olds et al, 1997). Refer all pregnant teens to a public health nursing service (Koniak-Griffin et al, 2002).

Complications

Young age in a pregnant woman is an inherent risk factor, even with good prenatal care. Adverse outcomes are common in pregnant teenagers (DuPlessis, Bell, & Richards, 1997; Fraser, Brockert, & Ward, 1995) and include the following:
- Maternal
  - Anemia
  - Pregnancy-induced hypertension
  - Excessive weight gain
  - STDs
  - Cephalopelvic disproportion (CPD)
  - Puerperal complications
  - Potential social consequences (e.g., educational, economic, and occupational delay)
- Fetal/neonatal
  - Low birth weight
  - Intrauterine growth retardation
  - Prematurity
  - Sudden infant death syndrome (SIDS)
  - Minor acute infections
  - Perinatal death
  - Potential medical, social, behavioral, and educational sequelae

Prevention and Resources

Prevention goals include the following:
- Maintain sexual health
- Promote sexual responsibility
- Assist adolescents to make informed choices, recognizing educational, social, and economic impact of choices
- Delay onset of intercourse
- Provide contraceptive counseling and selection of a contraceptive device for any adolescent who has recently experienced a spontaneous abortion, as part of third-trimester health teaching before delivery, or at the time of an elective termination of pregnancy

These goals can be achieved by supporting a positive or protective environment, connecting the adolescent to an intervention program, and providing appropriate health care services. Common components of successful intervention programs have been described by Dryfoos (1990) as including the following:
- Intensive individualized attention
- Community-wide multiagency collaborative approaches
- Early identification of at-risk children
- Early intervention to prevent high-risk behavior
- Adequate staff training
- Social skills training for children
- Engagement of peers in interventions
- Parental involvement
- Link to the world of work

An environment that protects against pregnancy has been described (Fehring et al, 1998; Jaskiewicz & McAnarney, 1994) as

- Consistent and predictable
- Emphasizing educational achievement
- Having high parental education levels
- Having religious values

Appropriate health care services include the following:

- Confidential services with minimal or no financial barriers
- Easy availability (e.g., timed for easy access, on site at school, or easy transportation to site)
- Full range of contraceptive services for male and female adolescents (see section on contraception for specific methods)

Homosexuality

Description

Sexual orientation refers to a person's sexual responsiveness to partners of the same or opposite gender. The concept of sexual orientation includes at least three distinctive components: sexual imagery (fantasies or attraction), actual sexual behavior, and the person's self-identification as heterosexual, bisexual, or homosexual. Homosexuality is sexual orientation toward individuals of the same gender. It is not a mental disorder, nor is it a choice that individuals voluntarily make.

Incidence and Etiology

Sexual orientation received considerable attention after the release of data from the Kinsey studies of comprehensive sexual histories (Kinsey, Pomeroy, & Martin, 1949). Kinsey concluded that 4% of men in the cohort born between 1920 and 1930 were exclusively homosexual throughout their lives and 10% were more or less exclusively homosexual for at least 3 years. The estimates of the prevalence of homosexuality for American women were half those of corresponding male rates (Kinsey, Pomeroy, & Martin, 1953). Criticism has been raised as to whether Kinsey's data can be generalized, because the small convenience samples of students and tradesmen in the studies may have skewed findings. Adolescent-specific data on sexual orientation are sparse. Remafedi and associates (1992) surveyed a representative sample of 34,706 Minnesota junior and senior high school youths and reported that 10.7% were unsure of their sexual orientation, 88.2% described themselves as exclusively heterosexual, and 1.1% described themselves as bisexual or predominantly homosexual. Random-probability nationally based survey data on adolescent sexual orientation are absent.

The etiology of sexual orientation, either homosexual or heterosexual, is unknown. Sexual orientation appears to develop in phases, from the prenatal period through latency. Although the dynamics of its evolution are unknown, sexual orientation tends to be fixed by the end of the child's prepubertal years.

Because there is no scientific evidence to explain the development of sexual orientation, controversy continues as to "causes" of homosexuality. Some clinicians believe that it is a purely biologic phenomenon, largely determined in utero. The work of Bell, Weinberg, and Hammersmith (1981) served to rule out many psychosocial components when the researchers concluded that homosexuality does not result from a cold, distant father, poor peer relationships, sexual abuse, or sexual experimentation in childhood.

Assessment

Individuals with a homosexual orientation are diverse, and their behavior cannot be stereotyped. The daily lifestyles of those with a homosexual orientation and their ability to function in occupational, educational, and family structures are as varied as those of heterosexual individuals. The development of a homosexual orientation involves a process of acknowledging and integrating one's sexual identity.

A proposed model of homosexual identity formation includes sensitization, identity confusion, identity assumption, and commitment (Troiden, 1988).

- Sensitization occurs during childhood when individuals identify themselves as feeling different from others of the same gender. Girls describe themselves as "unfeminine," whereas boys often report feelings of disinterest in sports and a proclivity for artistic endeavors. Boys state that they are often called "sissies."
- Identity confusion usually occurs during adolescence when individuals begin to question whether they may be homosexual. On average, this occurs for males at age 17 years and for females at age 18 years. Feelings of inadequacy, insecurity, self-deprecation, poor self-esteem, and depression can result from unresolved identity confusion.
- Identity assumption is the stage at which the child assumes a homosexual identity that is shared with others. The age at which this occurs varies by gender, with males reporting an average age of 19 to 21 years and females 21 to 23 years. Exploration of the homosexual role can lead to multiple sexual experiences with accompanying risks of acquiring STDs, including HIV infection. In contrast, close, long-term relationships can develop. The late adolescent–young adult homosexual, sexually active male is at risk for having the same problems as his heterosexual counterpart.
- Commitment is an internalized pledge to live as a homosexual and enter into a same-sex relationship. This process can be referred to as "coming out." External disclosure to others who are not homosexual may vary, depending on what is perceived to be safe to the individual. A stigma management strategy of blending, or acting

in a "gender-appropriate" manner, may be adopted in an attempt to be safe in environments that are not tolerant or accepting of homosexuality.

Differential Diagnosis

The differential diagnoses for homosexuality are gender identity disorders and transvestism.

Management

A number of professional articles describe management issues for the primary care provider and characteristics of the primary care practice that youth who are homosexual prefer (Kreiss & Patterson, 1997; Meininger et al, 2002; Remafedi et al, 1992). It is important that the provider support and validate the adolescent throughout the process of developing his or her awareness of and commitment to a homosexual orientation. Specific interventions include the following:

- Providing a safe environment in which to access health care
- Providing appropriate counseling, nonjudgmental listening, assistance in problem solving, and communication between adolescent and others
- Educating about the high risk for STDs

Adolescents who are homosexual have indicated that there are qualities of the primary care provider that they find most helpful in supporting their health needs (Ginsburg et al, 2002). These include the following:

- Privacy
- Competence

RESOURCE BOX

Sexuality

American College of Obstetricians and Gynecologists
www.acog.org

Association of Reproductive Health Professionals
www.arhp.org
Interdisciplinary organization, research, and advocacy

Contraceptive Research and Development Program
www.conrad.org
General information on birth control methods, updates on research projects, and contraceptive technology workshops

Issues of Contraception Report
www.Contraceptiononline.org/contrareport/
To sign up for online mailings, contact
www.emron.com/TCR

JAMA Contraception Information Center
www.ama-assn.org/special/contra/contra.htm
Informational resource for health professionals

National Dissemination Center for Children with Disabilities
1-800-695-0285
www.nichcy.org

Reducing the Risk
1-800-321-4407
www.etr.org
Sex education program for high school students, available from ETR Associates

ReproLine
www.reproline.jhu.edu
Information and training for health professionals; maintained by JHPIEGO, an organization affiliated with Johns Hopkins University

Sexuality Information and Education Council of the United States (SIECUS)
1-212-819-9770 (New York)
1-202-265-2405 (Washington, D.C.)
www.siecus.org
Education and policy related to sexuality issues across the lifespan; English and Spanish

PREGNANCY

Planned Parenthood Federation of America
www.plannedparenthood.org
1-212-541-7800

HOMOSEXUALITY

Federation of Parents and Friends of Lesbians and Gays, Inc. (PFLAG)
www.pflag.org
1-202-467-8180
The national organization can provide referrals to local chapters

Family Pride Coalition
www.familypride.org
1-202-331-5015
Resources and links to legal and medical support

SEXUAL ASSESSMENT AND HISTORY TAKING

Davis CM et al: *Handbook of sexuality-related measures,* Thousand Oaks, CA, 1998, Sage Publications. Includes a wide range of standardized measurement tools and questionnaires with discussion of their use, reliability, and validity.

NURSING DIAGNOSES RELATED TO THE SEXUALITY: *Functional Health Pattern*

- Sexual dysfunction
- Ineffective sexuality patterns

From North American Nursing Diagnosis Association: *NANDA nursing diagnoses: definitions and classification 2003-2004*, Philadelphia, 2003, North American Nursing Diagnosis Association.

- Cleanliness
- Respect
- Honesty
- Nonjudgmental attitude

Counseling varies from one adolescent to another and can require referral to a psychologist. Several principles have been identified to guide counseling of homosexual adolescents (Schneider & Tremble, 1986):

- Homosexuality is not a barrier to developing and maturing into a happy, productive adult.
- Homosexual adolescents must not be allowed to use their sexual orientation as an excuse to ignore the responsibilities of growing up and maturing.
- Issues and concerns of homosexual youth are often the same as those of heterosexual youth.

Complications

A high incidence of mental health problems such as suicide ideation, suicide attempts, substance abuse, runaway behavior, school truancy, and other emotional trauma can occur among homosexual adolescents, especially if the normal process of developing one's homosexual identity has been conflictive and is not progressing toward resolution. The NP should assess for conflicts regarding sexual orientation as an etiologic factor if an adolescent has these clinical issues.

REFERENCES

Adler NE: Contraception and unwanted pregnancy, *Behav Med Update* 5:28-34, 1984.

American Medical Association: *Guidelines for adolescent preventive services (GAPS): recommendations monograph*, Chicago, 1997, American Medical Association.

Andolsek K: Contraception. In Rosenfeld J, editor: *Handbook of women's health: an evidence-based approach*, New York, 2001, Cambridge University Press.

Bell AP, Weinberg MS, Hammersmith SK: *Sexual preference*, Bloomington, IN, 1981, University Press.

Carpenter SE, Rock J, editors: *Pediatric and adolescent gynecology*, ed 2, Philadelphia, 2000, Lippincott Williams & Wilkins.

Cobb BK: Communication types and sexual protective practices of college women, *Public Health Nurs* 14:293-301, 1997.

Cullins V, Huggins G: Adolescent contraception and abortion. In Carpenter SE, Rock J, editors: *Pediatric and adolescent gynecology*, ed 2, Philadelphia, 2000, Lippincott Williams & Wilkins.

Dryfoos JG: *Adolescents at risk: prevalence and prevention*, New York, 1990, Oxford University Press.

DuPlessis HM, Bell R, Richards T: Adolescent pregnancy: understanding the impact of age and race on outcomes, *J Adolesc Health* 20:187-197, 1997.

DuRant R, Smith K: Vital statistics and injuries. In Neinstein L, editor: *Adolescent health care: a practical guide*, Philadelphia, 2002, Lippincott Williams & Wilkins.

Fehring RJ et al: Religiosity and sexual activity among older adolescents, *J Religion Health* 37:229-247, 1998.

Fraser AM, Brockert JE, Ward RH: Association of young maternal age with adverse reproductive outcomes, *N Engl J Med* 332:1113-1117, 1995.

Friedrich WN et al: Normative sexual behavior in children, *Pediatrics* 88:456-464, 1991.

Ginsburg KR et al: How to reach sexual minority youth in the health care setting: the teens offer guidance, *J Adolesc Health* 31:407-416, 2002.

Haffner DW: *Sex education 2000: a call to action*, New York, 1990, Sexuality Information and Education Council of the United States (SIECUS).

Hatcher RA et al: *Contraceptive technology*, ed 17, New York, 1998, Ardent Media.

Jaskiewicz JA, McAnarney ER: Pregnancy during adolescence, *Pediatr Rev* 15:32-38, 1994.

Kahn JA, Emans SJ: Gynecologic examination of the prepubertal girl, *Contemp Pediatr* 16:148-159, 1999.

Kinsey AC, Pomeroy WB, Martin CE: *Sexual behavior in the human male*, Philadelphia, 1949, WB Saunders.

Kinsey AC, Pomeroy WB, Martin CE: *Sexual behavior in the human female*, Philadelphia, 1953, WB Saunders.

Koniak-Griffin D et al: Public health nursing care for adolescent mothers: impact on infant health and selected maternal outcomes at 1 year postbirth, *J Adolesc Health* 30:44-54, 2002.

Kreiss JL, Patterson DL: Psychosocial issues in primary care of lesbian, gay, bisexual, and transgender youth, *J Pediatr Health Care* 11:266-274, 1997.

Larsson I, Svedin CG: Teacher's and parent's reports on 3- to 6-year-old children's sexual behavior—a comparison, *Child Abuse Negl* 26:243-245, 2002.

Laube HH: The use of a sexual history with adolescents. In Blum RW, editor: *Adolescent health care: clinical issues*, New York, 1982, Academic Press.

Masters WH, Johnson VE, Kolodny RC: *Human sexuality*, ed 5, New York, 1995, Harper Collins College Publishers.

Meininger E et al: Gay, lesbian, and bisexual adolescents. In Neinstein L, editor: *Adolescent health care: a practical guide*, Philadelphia, 2002, Lippincott Williams & Wilkins.

Money J: *Gay, straight, and in-between*, New York, 1988, Oxford University Press.

Mount SL, Papillo JL: A study of 10,296 pediatric and adolescent: Papanicolaou smear diagnoses in northern New England, *Pediatrics* 103:539-545, 1999.

Neinstein L, editor: *Adolescent health care: a practical guide*, Philadelphia, 2002, Lippincott Williams & Wilkins.

Neinstein L, Farmer M: Teenage pregnancy. In Neinstein L, editor: *Adolescent health care: a practical guide*, Philadelphia, 2002, Lippincott Williams & Wilkins.

Nelson A, Neinstein L: Combination hormonal contraceptives. In Neinstein L, editor: *Adolescent health care: a practical guide*, Philadelphia, 2002a, Lippincott Williams & Wilkins.

Nelson A, Neinstein L: Barrier contraceptives. In Neinstein L, editor: *Adolescent health care: a practical guide*, Philadelphia, 2002b, Lippincott Williams & Wilkins.

Olds D et al: Long-term effects of home visitation on maternal life course and child abuse and neglect, *JAMA* 278:637-643, 1997.

Ott M, Irwin C: Contraception. In Finberg L, Kleinman R: *Saunders manual of pediatric practice*, ed 2, Philadelphia, 2002, WB Saunders.

Reece RM: *Child abuse: medical diagnosis and management*, Philadelphia, 1994, Lea & Febiger.

Remafedi G et al: Demography of sexual orientation, *Pediatrics* 89:714-721, 1992.

Roberts EJ: *Childhood sexual learning: the unwritten curriculum*, Cambridge, 1980, Bollinger Publishing.

Rosenfeld W, Coupey S: Contraceptive counseling and prescription. In Coupey S, editor: *Primary care of adolescent girls*, Philadelphia, 2000, Hanley & Belfus, Inc.

Ryan C, Futterman D: Homosexuality. In Coupey S, editor: *Primary care of adolescent girls*, Philadelphia, 2000, Hanley & Belfus, Inc.

Schneider MS, Tremble B: Training service providers to work with gay or lesbian adolescents: a workshop, *J Counsel Dev* 65:98-99, 1986.

Sexuality Information and Education Council of the United States (SIECUS) National Guidelines Task Force: *Guidelines for comprehensive sexuality education: kindergarten–12th grade*, ed 2, New York, 1996, Sexuality Information and Education Council of the United States.

Siegel DM: Self-reported honesty among middle and high school students responding to a sexual behavior questionnaire, *J Adolesc Health* 23:2-28, 1998.

Smith M: Pediatric sexuality: promoting normal sexual development in children, *Nurse Pract* 18:37-44, 1993.

Speroff L, editor: Better methods for emergency contraception: abstract and commentary, *OB/GYN Clinical Alert,* 19(10):77, 2003.

Speroff L, Darney P: *A clinical guide for contraception*, ed 3, Philadelphia, 2001, Lippincott Williams & Wilkins.

Troiden RR: Homosexual identity development, *J Adolesc Health Care* 9:105-113, 1988.

World Health Organization: *Education and treatment in human sexuality: the training of health professionals*, Technical Report Series no 372, Geneva, 1975, World Health Organization.

21 Coping and Stress Tolerance: Mental Health Problems of Children and Adolescents

Gail M. Houck

Coping with a variety of challenges, potential threats, and adverse experiences is a central feature of human development. Influenced by temperamental and developmental differences, coping with stressful events and circumstances is crucial to children's immediate adjustment. The ways children cope can alter the course of their development and influence their responses to subsequent life events.

Most young children have experienced at least one major negative event by early adolescence. There are consistent relationships between stressful events and children's adjustment. Typically, higher levels of stress, whether caused by undesirable life events or daily circumstances, are associated with higher levels of behavioral symptoms. Problem behaviors, which are viewed as manifestations of children's responses to stress and as a reflection of their coping efforts, affect 10% to 30% of families with youngsters.

The nurse practitioner (NP) must assess children's adverse life experiences, as well as potential or actual behavioral problems that accompany them. Because preschool behavior problems tend to continue through the school-age years (Fagot & Leve, 1998; Mesman & Koot, 2000) and adolescent years (Tubman et al, 1993), and because they are linked to adult psychopathology, early identification and intervention in childhood behavior problems is crucial. Improvement in children with early behavior problems is related to reduction in occurrence of adverse life experiences or enhancement of children's environmental circumstances. If NPs take a proactive stance toward early intervention in children's stressful experiences and behavioral manifestations and toward the development of children's coping efforts, their subsequent development can be influenced in a positive direction.

DEVELOPMENTAL CONTEXT

To prevent mental health problems, the points during development when certain risk factors are most important must be identified. In fact, psychopathology can be considered a distortion in the normal developmental process when children lack integration of the cognitive, social, and emotional competencies crucial to adaptation at a given developmental period. Failure to achieve competencies at one developmental period makes adaptation more difficult at the subsequent period and affects adaptation throughout the life span. In short, early deviations or disturbances in functioning contribute to the emergence of later disturbed patterns.

Poor behavioral adaptation requires early intervention with a view toward prevention of later maladaptation. Two features of child development provide some optimism and direction for early intervention. First, children possess a self-righting and self-organizing tendency that encourages normal development in the face of pressure for deviation. A single instance of stress or a negative force at one traumatic point in time does not usually interfere with the child's development and adaptation. Rather, negative outcomes result from ongoing malfunction in the caregiving environment, such as poor parenting. Second, many factors—family changes, day care, foster care, reduced stress—mediate between early and later maladaptation to permit more positive outcomes. Changes in children's experiences allow the achievement of adaptive competencies and the successful negotiation of subsequent developmental tasks. Efforts that target children's coping problems and their behavioral manifestations by intervening with parenting and family environments at the earliest opportunity allow children to "self-right." The parent-child relationship and family functioning are critical to children's effective coping with inevitable stress.

TABLE 21-1 *Developmental Tasks and Issues by Age-group*

0 to 1 yr	Biologic regulation; formation of attachment
1 to 3 yr	Exploration of physical and social environment (with caregiver as secure base); development of self: separation, individuation, and autonomy; responding to external control of impulses
3 to 5 yr	Flexible self-regulation; self-reliance and initiative; gender concept; empathy; development of peer relationships
6 to 12 yr	Gender constancy; school adjustment; same-gender friendships; social understanding; sense of competence
13 yr and older	Perspective taking; loyal friendships; beginning heterosexual relationships; identity; emancipation

From Stroufe LA, Rutter M: The domain of developmental psychopathology, *Child Dev* 55:17-29, 1984.

STRESS DURING CHILDHOOD

The question of where stressors originate in relation to the child's and family's behavior is a crucial one from both theoretic and clinical perspectives. The origin of life events should be a concern of those who approach clinical work from a developmental perspective. There are four categories of life events that differ according to the independence of the event from the child's and family's behavior (Sandberg et al, 1998):

1. Rare events that represent chance or fate (floods, earthquakes, bombs)
2. Chronic adversities that tend to occur as part of societal structure or circumstances
3. Negative life events and chronic adversities that are family dependent or a function of parents' behavior
4. Events and stressors that stem from the person's (child's) own behavior

Of course, the child's perception of these events must be considered. Although change itself has been viewed as intrinsically stressful, more recent research shows that negative outcomes are largely confined to unpleasant or adverse experiences, especially those that continue over time (Sandberg et al, 1998).

Perceptions of events and reactions to them are filtered through children's developing cognitive, emotional, and social capacities. The relevance of life events and the child's vulnerability to their impact depend on the given developmental period. The salient tasks and issues that constitute each developmental period are listed in Table 21-1.

Developmental differences account, in part, for how some life events may be "nonshared" between siblings. An experience that is salient and perceived negatively by one child may be irrelevant to or perceived positively by another sibling. Experiences of short duration with immediate impact and no long-term consequences are relatively benign. In contrast, acute events with long-term impact or consequences carry psychosocial risk, and negative chronic experiences carry a long-term threat because they present ongoing or enduring factors that make the child vulnerable. On the whole, the most difficult life events are those that persistently alter personal relationships or foster negative self-evaluation, for example, divorce, family discord, and harsh or neglectful parenting styles.

CHILDHOOD COPING

Definition

Only in the last decade have perspectives on coping emerged that are more explicitly concerned with childhood and adolescence. *Coping* is defined as conscious volitional efforts to regulate emotion, thinking, behavior, physiologic reactions, and the environment in response to stressful events and adversity (Compas et al, 2001). These processes depend on the child's developmental level—biologic, cognitive, social, and emotional—which thereby contributes to both the resources available for coping and the limits on the types of available coping skills. According to this definition of coping, several distinctions must be made (Compas et al, 2001; Thomsen et al, 2002):

- Coping refers to responses to stress that involve volition and conscious effort and is distinguished from involuntary responses that are not under conscious control.
- Both voluntary and involuntary responses to stress can be further distinguished by a dimension of engagement (fight) and disengagement (flight).
- Voluntary engagement responses (coping) are distinguished by their goals, oriented toward achieving primary control (e.g., problem solving, emotional modulation) or secondary control (e.g., acceptance, distraction, positive thinking).
- Involuntary responses include physiologic reactivity and rumination.
- Coping mechanisms differ depending on resources, style, and situation. Resources are the personal and environmental characteristics that facilitate effective adaptation to stress. Personal characteristics that help shape children's coping responses include temperament and stress reactivity, as well as the developmental processes for self-regulation and coping. The nature of the social environment (e.g., a supportive network) also influences the development of coping strategies. Coping styles flow from personal and environmental resources and develop in response to particular types of stressful episodes.

Role of Temperament in Coping

Temperament serves as a foundation for coping. Temperament involves an individual's characteristic style of emotional and behavioral response across situations and has generally come to be accepted as inborn. Although biologic in origin, temperament characteristics evolve and develop over time and are influenced by and patterned in significant ways by the social environment. This view of temperament is clinically important because both short- and long-term psychosocial adjustments are shaped by the goodness of fit between the individual's temperament and the social environment. Goodness of fit refers to the congruence of a child's temperament with the expectations, demands, and opportunities of the social environment, including those of parents, family, and day care or school setting.

Infants' first coping efforts are determined by temperament and linked to reactivity and self-regulation. Physiologic reactivity includes individual differences in the threshold, dampening, and reactivation of autonomic arousal, and it varies across different emotions (Compas et al, 2001). Individual differences in temperament and reactivity affect the individual's initial automatic response to stress and thereby constrain or facilitate certain types of coping responses. Infants are also capable of regulating aspects of their autonomic arousal, behavior, and emotions, initially through involuntary, biologically based processes that are augmented by responses acquired through learning and experience in accordance with contextual cues. Coping continues to be influenced by the emergence of cognitive and behavioral capacities for regulation of the self in response to stress. Nonetheless, temperament is foundational and relatively stable from infancy through toddlerhood. Several dimensions of temperament have been proposed (Table 21-2). Overall, there appears to be consensus for three factors inherent in temperament: sociability (reactivity), activity, and emotionality (mood) (Jellinek, Patel, & Froehle, 2002).

TABLE 21-2 ***Temperament Dimensions***

Buss & Plomin (1984)	Thomas & Chess (1984)	Rothbart (1989)	Bates (1989)	Streleau (1983)
Activity	Activity level	Activity level	Attention regulation	Activity
Emotionality	Persistence	Attention span	Emotionality	Reactivity
Sociability	Rhythmicity (regulation)	Self-regulative functions	Adaptability	
	Mood (prevailing positive/negative)	Smiling and laughing	Reactivity	
	Intensity of response	Fear		
	Distractability or ease of soothing	Reaction to frustration		
	Approach vs. withdrawal to new stimuli	Soothability		
	Adaptability to new experiences	Reactivity		
	Threshold of responsiveness			

Data from Prior M: Childhood temperament, *J Child Psychol Psychiatry* 33:249-279, 1992.

Temperament Types

Three types of temperament have clinical utility and can be generalized cross-culturally: difficult, easy, and slow to warm up. Children with difficult temperaments tend to be characterized by an intense and negative mood, slow adaptability, withdrawal from new situations, and irregularity in biologic functions. Children with easy temperaments typically exhibit a prevailing positive mood, low intensity, ready adaptability, and regularity and predictability of biologic and behavioral patterns. In other words, these children are easygoing. Children with slow to warm up temperaments are characterized by initial quiet alertness and subdued emotionality. This reserve in the face of new situations and stimuli gives way to features of an easy or difficult temperament. There is no absolute standard for any of these classifications, and all features of temperament must be considered in the context of the parents' evaluations.

Temperament as a Risk Factor

Temperament predicts behavioral disturbance in preschool (Eisenberg et al, 2000; Mesman & Koot, 2002), elementary school (Mesman & Koot, 2002), and adolescence and young adulthood (Caspi et al, 1996). Difficult temperaments seem to be most consistently related to behavior disorders, although temperament alone is not a risk factor for maladjustment. Rather, temperament exerts an influence on children's psychosocial adjustment by way of its effect on caretaker-child interactions (Bates et al, 1998). Difficult temperamental features tend to engender parental criticism and irritability, as well as coercive interactions and restrictive parenting. Critical mediators of the role of temperament in the development of behavioral disorder include parental psychologic functioning, marital adjustment, child-rearing attitudes and practices, and social support factors. Although temperament is unrelated to intelligence quotient (IQ), it affects academic outcomes, and some children are clearly disadvantaged by their more difficult temperaments in the majority of school environments (Carey, 1998).

Temperament Management

The goal for the NP is to help parents achieve goodness of fit for their children. Specific strategies for intervening with temperament issues have been developed for parents. Strategies for helping parents respond effectively to their child's temperament at each developmental phase are outlined in *Bright Futures in Practice: Mental Health Practice Guide* (Jellinek, Patel, & Froehle, 2002), and can be readily integrated into well-child care. Those who care for children (e.g., parents, teachers, other caregivers) should be helped to

- Recognize the child's innate behavioral qualities as expressions of temperament. Perceptions about the child can be obtained through an interview about typical situations (e.g., changes in activities, new situations, changes in routines, new people) or by completing a standard temperament questionnaire.
- Understand how temperament is related to behavior and is not amenable to change. This means allowing parents, for example, to express their feelings about their child or their child's behavior, and assisting them to reframe their assessment more positively. Members of the extended family who often advise parents may need to be included to help alleviate feelings of failure.
- Develop temperament-based management strategies, especially ways to deal with the more challenging areas of temperament. Such strategies can be applied to new situations as the child develops and becomes more autonomous, including those that occur in toddlerhood and preschool, such as mealtime and bedtime or during school-related activities, such as doing homework.

Role of Development in Coping

Strategies that children use to cope vary according to their cognitive, motor, and affective capacities, social abilities, and feelings about themselves. Although little research has been conducted on the relationship between development and coping strategies, some general points can be made.

From birth to age 2 years, children are highly dependent on the primary caretaker, typically the mother, to cope effectively with the world. Dominant coping strategies include those behaviors and strategies that serve to meet the child's needs. The behaviors and strategies become more complex as autonomy and increasing sociability begin to emerge at about 1 year of age. Also at around 12 months of age, goal-directed behavior and a sense of causality reflect children's developing reasoning capacities. At about 15 to 18 months, capacities for fantasy and problem solving emerge, and language development facilitates shared communication.

From 2 to 6 years of age, several capacities emerge that help children learn about coping from parents: maintaining self-generated goals, modeling adult activities, naming and describing feelings, referring to the self as an objective entity, using language to share words and ideas, engaging socially with others, and reflecting on the self (self-awareness). Memory for events develops, with salient features retained and sometimes distorted. During this period, children can reason in familiar contexts about experiences but have difficulty reasoning with novel experiences. A search for causal explanations often results in magical thinking. Children's strategies for coping at this age include asserting themselves, engaging in limited problem solving, and using adults as resources for support and soothing. Symbolic play is a dominant medium for effective coping.

During middle childhood (6 to 12 years), more complex methods of emotion management and problem solving emerge (Compas et al, 2001). As cognitive and perspective-taking skills mature, school-age children can make logical inferences based on what is known. Dominant coping strategies include cognitive reframing, restructuring a problem situation, using self-talk to calm negative emotions, generating alternative solutions to solve problems, and taking overt and direct action to adapt to challenges (Compas et al, 2001). Children who are less adept at generating and using problem-focused coping strategies have more behavior problems. With increasing metacognitive skills, older school-age children and adolescents have a greater ability to match coping efforts to the expected characteristics of stress.

Stress and Ineffective Coping: General Behavior Problems

There are two broad categories of problem behaviors for preschool and school-age children: "internalizing" and "externalizing." Internalizing behavior is characterized by social withdrawal, depressive symptoms, sleep problems, and somatic problems. Internalizing disorders are conditions whose central feature is disordered mood or emotion. Externalizing behavior consists of aggressive and destructive behavior. Externalizing disorders are ones whose central feature is dysregulated behavior. Both behavior types demonstrate consistency from preschool through school age, with stability for the externalizing behavior most remarkable.

From 12% to 20% of young children are believed to exhibit behavior problems at some time during their early years in the home or school setting, or both. Transitory behavior symptoms might be argued as "normative," particularly in response to transient stresses, such as birth of a sibling, beginning school, or reaching developmental periods such as toddlerhood and adolescence. Whereas transitory behavior difficulties might not be cause for alarm, stable behavior problems in early childhood are good predictors for adverse long-term outcomes.

Behavior Problems as Risk Factors

Children with behavior problems in preschool do not simply outgrow their problems without intervention as many clinicians believe. The majority of preschoolers with behavior problems continue to have them in early grade school (Bates et al, 1998; Fagot & Leve, 1998; Mesman & Koot, 2000), especially those with externalizing behavior problems. These children are subsequently less competent and have greater pathology in adolescence and adulthood.

In an earlier epidemiologic study of the general population of children by Cohen and associates (1993), a 20% prevalence estimate for a psychiatric disorder rooted in behavioral problems was consistently identified with one third of 9- to 20-year-olds having received a diagnosis for at least a mild disorder. These estimates have held over the last decade, with at least 27% of children thought to have a mental health problem, 20% of children needing active mental health intervention, and 11% thought to have significant functional impairment (USDHHS, 2000). Pediatric behavior problems are common but usually remain undiagnosed or untreated; in fact, fewer than one in five children needing treatment are recognized (Cassidy & Jellinek, 1998).

Higher levels of stress, whether assessed in terms of negative life events or negative circumstances, predict higher levels of behavior problems, although these are certainly mediated or offset by children's voluntary engagement coping (Compas et al, 2001; Mesman & Koot, 2000). The level of family stress is related to the quality of the parenting (degree of nurturing and aversiveness) and the quality of the home environment, especially the degree of predictability and organization. When children with behavior problems improve (e.g., between preschool age and school age), a reduction in stressful life events and more optimal parenting and home environments have been found. These relationships between life events and psychosocial dysfunction do not appear to be influenced by gender or age (Fagot & Leve, 1998).

ASSESSMENT

Self-report, which is central to adult diagnosis, does not occur in children. The diagnosis of behavior problems usually depends on complaints by parents or teachers when the child's behavior is inconvenient, is embarrassing, or imposes on others. Assessment must therefore explore possible negative life events and circumstances, as well as behavioral symptoms, in the event that problems have yet to meet the nuisance criteria. The goal is not simply to relieve symptoms but to facilitate and strengthen long-term behavioral adaptation and progress in cognitive, social, and emotional development.

History

Recent Life Events

Assess recent events: "What important events or changes have occurred in your family in the past year?"

- Objectively defined events:
  - Moves
  - Changes in household composition (births, departures)
  - Separations from family
  - Illnesses and hospital contacts
  - Changes in parents' work
  - Changes in family relationships
  - Changes in school
  - Major traumatic incidents
  - Changes in routines
- Developmental context of events and whether most age mates would find the incident threatening or upsetting
- Contextual threat—short-term and long-term consequences:
  - Loss or risk of loss of attachment figure
  - Physical jeopardy
  - Witness to trauma
  - New role or responsibilities (psychologic challenge)
- Enduring change in life circumstances, for better or worse
- Consequent changes in the child's perception of self, family, or relationship security
- Extent to which events stem from the child's behavior (resulting in self-blame) or stem from the actions of other family members, especially parents (creating a sense of betrayal)

Chronic Experiences

Determine chronic events: "What sorts of difficulties in parenting or family life do you have on a daily basis?"

- Chronic conditions or circumstances:
  - Parental overprotection
  - Restrictive parenting
  - Control struggles
  - Ineffective conflict resolution
  - Lack of effective parental supervision
  - Parental failure to protect child in risky situations
  - Ineffective limit-setting strategies
  - Mental health problems of parents, especially maternal depression
  - Child's chronic illness or handicap
- Major life happenings with lasting influence:
  - Loss of parent by death or separation
  - Loss of sibling by death or separation
  - Chronic illness or handicap of any family member
  - Any hospitalization
  - Any separations (e.g., in home of relatives or foster care)
  - Victim of sexual or physical abuse
  - Witness of trauma
  - Major psychiatric illness in a parent
- Duration of experiences or circumstances

Behavioral Manifestations

Seek information about how the child's behavior problems manifest.

- Parental description of undesirable and desired behaviors
- Parental perceptions about the nature of the child's problems, including cause and severity as measured by frequency and duration
- Situational context that elicits or maintains problem behavior (setting, timing, who is present, triggers)
- Situational context in which the problem behavior does not occur
- Responses to and consequences of problem behavior

Parent and Family Assessment

The parent and family assessment includes the following:

- Parental knowledge and beliefs about child behavior problems
- As thorough a child and family history of behavior problems as is possible, especially given the role genetically driven biologic processes play in internalizing disorders (Kovaks & Devlin, 1998)
- Any indicators of parental psychopathology, particularly maternal depression (Sandberg et al, 1998)
- The parents' perception of the child, especially temperament
- The parents' knowledge and beliefs about harsh discipline or coercive parent-child interactions (Bates et al, 1998)
- The parents' knowledge and beliefs about the development of autonomy and self-esteem, especially in relation to parenting strategies (e.g., praise and affection) and conflict resolution
- Parental understanding of the relationship between life events and behavior
- Parental strategies to facilitate the child's coping, given developmental level and temperament

General Health History

The general health history should include the following:

- Prenatal history, including mother's use of substances
- Birth history, including complications or medical conditions
- Childhood illnesses
- Neurologic injuries or soft neurologic signs
- Developmental progress and achievement of milestones to reveal any existing vulnerability or risk status

Physical Examination

A complete physical examination and developmental screening should be included in the assessment. If warranted by suspicious or ambiguous findings, the child should be referred for a thorough developmental evaluation.

Diagnostic Studies

Laboratory

Pertinent laboratory tests (hemoglobin, blood lead level, urinalysis) rule out physical health problems with behavioral manifestations.

Structured Parental Reports

An assessment of temperament is useful for infants, toddlers, preschoolers, and school-age children (see the Resource Box for a list of assessment tools). A behavioral diary or log kept by parents, by the school-age child, and by the teacher informs the practitioner and family about the situational context for and severity of the behavior problem or problems. Often, this monitoring process itself serves as an effective intervention. Behavioral rating scales or checklists are valuable screening tools, especially because they usually have established reliability and validity and provide norms as a basis for comparison. The Child Behavior Checklist provides separate checklists for age-groups (2 to 3 years and 4 to 16 years), with norms provided by age and gender, and with separate report forms for parents and teachers. Other checklists with clinical utility include the Eyberg Child Behavior Inventory (ECBI) (Eyberg & Ross, 1978) for 2- to 16-year-olds and the Pediatric Symptom Checklist (PSCL) (Jellineck & Murphy, 1997) for 6- to 12-year-olds. Even if children's scores do not reach a clinical level by normative standards, attention must be paid to notably high scores, stable problem behavior, and attending circumstances.

Behavioral Observation

Behavioral observation of parent-child interactions and family dynamics can be made in the course of the assessment. Features to observe include the tone and quality of verbal communication, the emotional tone or warmth of the parent-child relationship, patterns of control and submissiveness, degree of involvement (e.g., enmeshed versus distant), acceptance and rejection, and affection. If necessary, children and their parents can be referred for further assessment, with concerns and observations documented.

STRATEGIES FOR MANAGEMENT

Pediatric primary care providers can manage selected coping and stress problems whereas others should be referred. Generally speaking, if the cause of the problem is a life event with acute, short-term consequences, such as the death of a pet or the loss of a friend, it is probably manageable in primary care settings. More enduring problems, such as loss of a parent, should be referred. The strategies that primary care providers can use effectively include primary, secondary, and tertiary prevention of behavior problems.

Primary Prevention

Primary prevention of behavior problems occurs through positive, nurturing parent-child relationships. It is crucial for children to experience a secure attachment relationship, with a sense of worth and lovableness, as a foundation for effective coping. Healthy parenting strategies are positive in tone and regard for the child, responsive to the child's autonomy and individuality, neutral in response to unwanted behavior, and attentive to the child's needs (Box 21-1). The development of self-regulation can be optimized by teaching-based

BOX 21-1 *Positive Parenting Strategies*

Attending to the Child Individually

Allow the child to make reasonable choices
Respond to child's bids for attention with eye contact, smiles, and physical contact
Comment on child's appropriate/desirable behavior frequently and positively throughout the day
Provide guaranteed special time daily: no interruptions, no directions, no interrogations
Avoid secondary gains for the child's minor transgressions by having no discussion, physical contact, perhaps even eye contact; be neutral and simply state the preferred behavior

Listen Actively

Paraphrase or describe what child is saying
Reflect the child's feelings
Share the child's affect by matching the child's body posture and tone of voice
Avoid giving commands, judging, or editorializing
Follow the child's lead in the interaction

Convey Positive Regard

Communicate positive feelings (e.g., love) directly
Give directions positively, firmly, specifically
Provide notice before requiring child to change activities
Label the behavior, not the child
Praise competency and compliance; say thank you
Apologize when appropriate
Avoid shaming or belittling the child
Strive for consistency

limit-setting strategies, with reasoning, explanations, and distractions, versus power-based strategies of behavior control (Houck & LeCuyer-Maus, 2001; Houck et al, 2002; Houck & LeCuyer-Maus, in press). A teaching-based style enhances the development of self-regulation without compromising the development of self-concept or social competence.

NPs can also assist parents to anticipate predictable life events that are likely to influence children, such as changes in day care or care providers, moves, or changes in schools. Children's developmental and temperamental needs must be assessed and strategies identified for facilitating the transition in a way that meets those needs. Parents can be educated to facilitate the uses of developmentally appropriate coping strategies available to children. Encouraging symbolic play or expression through developmentally appropriate media contributes to adaptive coping.

Secondary Prevention

Secondary prevention or early intervention is required for unanticipated life events. Such events occur, and behavior problems can emerge, even with positive parenting approaches. At the level of secondary prevention, appropriate parental management strategies must often be employed to deal effectively with the problem behavior (see Chapters 5 to 9 and Chapter 18). Harsh discipline or physical punishment is consistently linked to negative outcomes for children in terms of behavioral maladaptation, low self-esteem, and poor social competence. A variety of strategies, excluding coercive control efforts, must be explored, with emphasis placed on positive parenting strategies that are highly important in primary prevention.

Tertiary Prevention

Tertiary prevention and intervention are required for major losses and traumas, especially that of victimization through sexual or physical abuse, as well as marital problems, divorce, substance abuse, and parental psychopathology. Even in the absence of behavioral manifestations, a referral to a mental health specialist for further assessment and intervention is fruitful given the difficulties that can result and affect behavioral adaptation at a later point.

Referrals in these situations must be firmly presented with a direct appraisal of the circumstances that necessitate the referral. It is most helpful to frame the behavior problem as a "normal response to an unusual or stressful situation." The goal can be clarified as one that maximizes the child's development and growth. A release of information allows direct contact with the consultant to ensure follow-through. Ongoing follow-up is essential with children, families, and other professional providers. Table 21-3 presents information about common psychotropic medications that may be prescribed by mental health specialists for children and adolescents.

TABLE 21-3 *Understanding Common Pediatric Psychotropic Medications**

Prescribing Goals

- Lowest effective dose
- Minimal side effects: 1/2 daily dose the first wk; if no problems, advance to full dose
- Simple dosing regimens to facilitate child acceptance and minimize parent stressors
- Avoid need for ongoing laboratory and electrocardiographic (ECG) monitoring when possible

Drug	Pharmacology (Predominant Neurotransmitter Effects)	Indications	Concerns
Drugs for Depression			
Selective serotonin reuptake inhibitors (SSRIs) • Fluoxetine (Prozac) • Sertraline (Zoloft) • Paroxetine (Paxil) • Fluvoxamine (Luvox) • Citalopram (Celexa) • Escolalopram (Lexapro)	Complex series of changes in reuptake at multiple serotonin (5HT) receptors and autoreceptors may be responsible for the delay in therapeutic response Allow 4 wk to experience benefits before increasing dose Poor response to one SSRI does not indicate similar response to others Low toxicity	Depression Anxiety Obsessive-compulsive disorder (OCD) Panic disorder Social phobia	Low side effect profile, but may experience GI upset, headache with initial doses If increase in anxiety, diminish dose until benefits are experienced Infrequent—increased menstrual flow, dizziness with missed doses or discontinuation, paresthesias

TABLE 21-3 *Understanding Common Pediatric Psychotropic Medications—cont'd*

Drug	Pharmacology (Predominant Neurotransmitter Effects)	Indications	Concerns
	Once-daily dosing; starting and maintenance dose the same (escolalopram) "Cleanest" side effect profile of all SSRIs (escolalopram) Most rapid onset of benefit (escolalopram)		**Clinical Considerations of Side Effects**: Fluoxetine: generally activating; longest half-life advantage in poor or inconsistent compliance Paroxetine: generally deactivating; increased somnolence (23%); antianxiety effect (13%); weight gain common; withdrawal syndrome common Sertraline: generally "neutral" in activation/deactivation Citalopram: less activating with no active metabolites
Norepinephrine and dopamine reuptake blockers • Bupropion (Wellbutrin)	A unicyclic antidepressant whose action is primarily due to its active metabolite, hydroxybupropion which reaches higher concentrations in the brain Benefits seen within the first 2 wk; may be less likely to trigger mania ADHD application: Bupropion inhibits reuptake of norepinephrine and dopamine, whereas stimulants (methylphenidate, dexedrine, pemoline) cause release and inhibit reuptake of norepinephrine and dopamine Available in SR form: bid dosing for >200 mg, smoother response than the immediate-release form	Depression Anger ADHD when stimulants not appropriate	At daily doses of 450 mg or less of SR form, seizure incidence approximates that of other nontricyclic antidepressants; earlier guidelines for immediate-release form recommended doses of 5 mg/kg, Ensure that child can swallow SR tablets whole Generally well tolerated, initial transient effects May increase anxiety/arousal that (unlike SSRIs) does not diminish over time Dopamine reuptake inhibition increases activation More rapid onset of benefit than SSRI Once-a-day dosing often sufficient in SR form
Dual reuptake (serotonin-norepinephrine) inhibitors • Venlafaxine (Effexor)	Primarily inhibits reuptake of serotonin and norepinephrine; some dopamine reuptake inhibition at high doses Simulates beneficial actions of classic tricyclic antidepressants without the muscarinic/alpha-1 anticholinergic and antihistamine side effects Once-daily dosing of XR form Low toxicity	Depression, may be more effective in severe forms ADHD	Generally see benefits sooner than with SSRIs Generally well tolerated, possible initial transient GI side effects, headache Complaint of bad taste to immediate-release form not seen with XR form Norepinephrine reuptake generally at doses ≥150 mg/day "Withdrawal syndrome" common; discontinue slowly
Tricyclic antidepressants (TCAs) Tertiary amines • Imipramine (Tofranil) • Amitriptyline (Elavil)	Blocks serotonin and norepinephrine reuptake Muscarinic anticholinergic side effects include dry mouth, constipation, urinary retention, blurred vision	Depression Enuresis Insomnia ADHD	No longer first choice because available alternatives with fewer side effects and lower toxicity Require baseline and ongoing ECGs in children Lethal in overdose

Continued

TABLE 21-3 *Understanding Common Pediatric Psychotropic Medications—cont'd*

Drug	Pharmacology (Predominant Neurotransmitter Effects)	Indications	Concerns
• Clomipramine (Anafranil) Secondary amines • Desipramine (Norpramin) • Nortriptyline (Pamelor)	Alpha-1 anticholinergic side effects include orthostatic hypotension, dizziness Antihistamine side effects include sedation, weight gain		
Serotonin-2 antagonist/reuptake inhibitors • Trazodone (Desyrel)	Blocks serotonin-2 receptors and weakly inhibits serotonin reuptake Blocks alpha-1 adrenergic receptors (dizziness, orthostatic hypotension) Blocks histamine receptors (sedation, weight gain)	An antidepressant that is primarily used in children to improve sleep	Well tolerated at the low doses effective for insomnia Priapism is a rare side effect (1:15,000) Explain priapism to male clients/parents, requesting they notify prescriber if erectile changes occur
Drugs for Anxiety			
Serotonin-1A partial agonists • Buspirone (Buspar)	Acts directly to desensitize (downregulate) 5HT-1A receptors Delayed response, as with SSRIs	Anxiety	Alternative to benzodiazepines—nonsedating, no tolerance/withdrawal More effective when benzodiazepines have not been used previously May be used to augment SSRIs Not as effective as benzodiazepines for severe anxiety
Benzodiazepines • Clonazepam (Klonopin)	The benzodiazepine receptor is part of a complex of receptors modulating gamma aminobutyric acid's fast inhibitory effects on chloride ion channels in the brain There are multiple subtypes of benzodiazepine receptors, which accounts for the variety of benefits and side effects of benzodiazepines	Anxiety	Chronic administration results in dependence and withdrawal
Alpha-2 adrenergic agonists • Clonidine (Catapres) • Guanfacine (Tenex)	Acts like norepinephrine at alpha-2 receptors, reducing release of more norepinephrine	Anxiety Tourette's syndrome ADHD (Primary use is in adults for hypertension)	Reduces physiologic arousal (i.e., hypertension, tachycardia, dilated pupils), but not as effective at blocking emotional aspects of anxiety Useful in conjunction with Wellbutrin for ADHD impulsivity/hyperarousal Requires baseline cardiac evaluation, gradual taper up, and monitoring for blood pressure changes Inform client/parent of orthostatic hypotension symptoms and prevention (e.g., adequate fluids)—usually transient side effect Avoid sudden withdrawal of medication (rebound hypertension)

TABLE 21-3 ***Understanding Common Pediatric Psychotropic Medications—cont'd***

Drug	Pharmacology (Predominant Neurotransmitter Effects)	Indications	Concerns
			Clonidine: stronger effects on behavioral features of ADHD; risk of interdose rebound Guanfacine: longer acting; more receptor specific; less sedation with minimal changes to blood pressure or heart rate

Table contributed by Mary Beth Kaufman, MS, PMHNP, and Susan Hazel, MN, PMHNP. Data from Stahl S: *Essential psychopharmacology: neuroscientific basis and practical applications*, ed 2, Cambridge, 2000, Cambridge University Press; Maxmen JS, Ward NG: *Psychotropic drug fast facts*, ed 3, New York, 2002, WW Norton Co.

*This table is intended to provide clinical guidelines for understanding the uses and effects of commonly used medications for children and adolescents with mental health issues. Children who need these drugs should be under the care of a mental health specialist. For prescribing recommendations, refer to standard references.

ADHD, Attention-deficit hyperactivity disorder; *GI*, gastrointestinal; *SR*, sustained release; *XR*, extended release.

COMMON BEHAVIOR PROBLEMS

Fears, Phobias, and Anxieties

Fears and Phobias

Description. Fear is the occurrence of various avoidance responses to particular stimuli; it is a state of apprehension or response to a threatening situation. A phobia is a persistent, extreme, and irrational fear. The onset of fears occurs during the transition to toddlerhood.

Etiology and Incidence. Fears actually have a developmental function, and the nature of predominant fears varies with age. Childhood fears are a part of normal development. In a classic study by MacFarlane and colleagues (1954, as cited by Barrios & Hartmann, 1988), 90% of 2- to 14-year-olds were found to have at least one specific fear. A significant minority of children, however, have fears that interfere with their functioning. Specific phobias occur in about 5% of the population and in 15% of children referred for anxiety-related problems. Phobias are determined by multiple factors, with genetic influences, temperament, parental mental health problems, and individual conditioning histories converging in specific phobias (King & Ollendick, 1997).

Clinical Findings. Infants typically react defensively to loss of support, height, and unexpected stimuli. Toddlers experience separation anxiety and fear physical injury and strangers. Preschoolers fear imaginary creatures, animals, darkness, and being alone, and they also demonstrate some persistent separation anxiety. Fear of animals and darkness extends into school age, but safety, natural events, and school- and health-related fears dominate. In preadolescence and adolescence, fears of bodily injury, economic and political catastrophes, and social fears are central. Fear and phobic reactions typically involve symptoms of autonomic arousal. In phobias, the symptoms of autonomic arousal may evolve into panic attacks in addition to phobic avoidant reactions.

Differential Diagnosis. Distinction must be made between abnormal fears and normal developmental fears that encourage the acquisition of boundaries, caution, and safety. Clinical phobias are defined on the basis of persistence, magnitude, and maladaptiveness.

Management. Most fears are short lived, are not serious, and do not predict adult mental health problems. Parents absolutely must be cautioned against using fears as a form of behavioral control (e.g., threats of abandonment with toddlers) or as a strategy for discipline (e.g., leaving a preschooler alone in a dark room). The key to whether to refer for treatment is the impact of the fear on the child's functioning, developmental progress, learning experiences, and level of comfort. Various management strategies are available for treatment of phobias, including systematic desensitization, contingency management, cognitive-behavioral procedures, and family interventions (King & Ollendick, 1997).

Anxiety

Anxiety is distinguished from fear on the basis of its diffuse apprehension in response to less specific stimuli. It is a normal developmental response that is experienced by nearly every person at some point. Anxious responses include somatic symptoms mediated through the autonomic system, with physiologic changes such as increased heart rate and blood pressure, tremor, sweating, and enhanced vigilance and reactivity (Williams & Hodgman, 2001). Anxiety that persists at high levels and is reflected in maladaptive behavior warrants diagnosis and treatment. Children diagnosed with anxiety disorders tend to have multiple problems, are impaired in important areas of social functioning, and live with parents who experience symptoms of anxiety or mood disorders. Anxiety disorders typically appear earlier than behavior disorders, which, in turn, appear earlier than mood disorders (Kovacs & Devlin, 1998).

Risk factors include the following: (1) family history of anxiety, panic, social inhibition, or other disorders; (2) temperamental disposition for behavioral inhibition; and (3) social environment or life circumstances (e.g., parental distress/dysfunction or trauma), especially during vulnerable developmental periods (e.g., attachment or separation-individuation) (Williams & Hodgman, 2001). Youngsters with anxiety disorders are at high risk for subsequent anxiety disorders, for comorbid anxiety or mood disorders, and for adolescent substance use disorder. Anxiety disorders show distinct clustering in families (Kovacs & Devlin, 1998).

Separation Anxiety Disorder

Description. The essential feature of separation anxiety disorder is abnormal reactivity to real or imagined separation from major attachment figures, home, or familiar surroundings. Separation anxiety is a normal developmental phenomenon from about 7 months of age through the preschool years (Dashiff, 1995). Separation anxiety disorder, in which reactivity to separation interferes with daily activities and developmental tasks, manifests from 5 to 16 years of age; the mean age for clinical presentation is 9 years. Although the diagnosis has been reserved for children and not included in adult epidemiologic studies, there is growing evidence that adults with histories of school refusal exhibit a range of anxiety and depressive disorders, and that adult separation anxiety is associated with a history of childhood separation anxiety disorder (Silove, Manicavasagar, & Drobny, 2002). This diagnosis can be a precursor for agoraphobia or panic disorder in adolescence or adulthood (Masi, Mucci, & Millepiedi, 2001).

Etiology and Incidence. Separation anxiety is thought to evolve from a poor attachment relationship or the interaction among physiologic, cognitive, and overt behavioral factors in response to life events that threaten safety or primary relationships, or both. Separation anxiety is probably the most common anxiety disorder in school-age children and the most common reason for referral. Children are usually brought to the clinician when the disorder results in school refusal or somatic symptoms; about 80% of children with school refusal are thought to have separation anxiety disorder (Masi, Mucci, & Millepiedi, 2001). The rate decreases with age, being present in 13% of girls and 11% of boys at 10 to 13 years of age, 5% of girls and 1% of boys ages 14 to 16 years, and 2% of girls and 3% of boys ages 17 to 20 years (Cohen et al, 1993). Subsequent research with community and clinical samples has supported these observed differences in prevalence rates of childhood and adolescent separation anxiety (Compton, Nelson, & March, 2000).

Clinical Findings. The following are found in separation anxiety disorder:

- Developmentally inappropriate or excessive anxiety about separations (American Psychiatric Association [APA], 1994)
- Unrealistic worry about harm to self or attachment figures or about abandonment during periods of separation
- Reluctance to sleep alone or sleep away from home
- Persistent avoidance of being alone
- Nightmares about separation
- Physical complaints and signs of distress in anticipation of separation
- Social withdrawal during separations
- Environmental stress, parental dysfunction, and maternal depression are risk factors for separation anxiety disorder, especially with panic disorder or agoraphobia (Williams & Hodgman, 2001).

Differential Diagnosis. Anxiety can be a response to trauma or a manifestation of posttraumatic stress disorder. It is essential to attend to cues that a traumatic experience or situation (e.g., sexual or physical abuse) is the source of the symptoms of anxiety. Anxiety disorder not associated with separation is also a differential diagnosis. Common comorbidities with separation anxiety include social phobia and overanxious disorder, followed by major depression and behavior disorder (Compton, Nelson, & March, 2000; Kovacs & Devlin, 1998). In adolescence, comorbid substance use disorder increases in prevalence (Kovacs & Devlin, 1998).

Management. This is a family system or relationship-based problem that is preferably treated as such (Dashiff, 1995). The symptoms must be treated and then the sources of the problem pursued. The role of attachment figures must be noted. Refer the patient to a child therapist for early intervention. Psychoeducational, behavioral, and cognitive-behavioral approaches have been effective, with added benefits obtained from family intervention (Barrett, Dadds, & Rapee, 1996; Barrett et al, 2001; Mendlowitz et al, 1999; Williams & Hodgman, 2001). Pharmacotherapy should be used as an adjunct to nonpharmocologic intervention only if the child fails to respond to those treatments and considerable impairment in function is experienced. Selective serotonin reuptake inhibitors (SSRIs) are considered first-choice medications in separation anxiety disorder, in part because the adverse effects are limited (Masi, Mucci, & Millepiedi, 2001; see Williams & Hodgman, 2001, for review). Benzodiazepines are recommended only if a rapid reduction of symptoms is needed, until the SSRI becomes effective; this class of drug has an adverse effects profile and potential for abuse and dependence. Refer the patient to a child psychiatrist or mental health NP for a medication evaluation.

Generalized Anxiety Disorder

Description. Generalized anxiety disorder, or overanxious disorder, is cognitive and obsessive in nature. There are excessive anxiety, worry, and apprehensive expectations that are generalized about a number of events or activities. These anxieties are not focused on a specific object or situation, nor are they the result of a recent stressor. Children with generalized anxiety disorder are characterized as "worriers." The exact onset is not known, but older children and adolescents (9 to 18 years) tend to be represented (Coyle, 2001).

Etiology and Incidence. There is a familial association for anxiety that suggests a genetic vulnerability to anxiety as a consequence of social learning; twin studies suggest that shared environment is far less important than genetic factors (Kovacs & Devlin, 1998). Approximately 9% of all children have at least one anxiety disorder, and about one third of those with an anxiety disorder have more than one (Williams & Hodgman, 2001).

Clinical Findings. Major symptoms of generalized anxiety disorder are

- Worry about future events
- Preoccupation with past behavior
- Overconcern about competence
- Marked self-consciousness
- Somatic complaints without physical basis
- Need for reassurance

Additional symptoms include restlessness, fatigue, difficulty concentrating, irritability, tension, and disturbed sleep (APA, 1994). Comorbidity with other anxiety disorders or mood disorder is common (Kendall, Brady, & Verduin, 2001).

Differential Diagnosis. It is important to attend to cues that might point to traumatic experiences or conditions as the source of anxiety symptoms. Differential diagnoses are separation anxiety, adjustment disorder associated with a specific stressor, and attention-deficit disorder. The last does not involve worry about the future.

Management. Refer the patient to a child therapist for treatment of the manifest symptoms through relaxation techniques or cognitive-behavioral therapy (CBT). The source of anxiety must be pursued through individual or family counseling. Treatment outcomes are more positive when parents are involved in interventions that target familial contextual processes. If not addressed, family dysfunction and parental stress predict less favorable treatment outcomes for children (Crawford & Manassis, 2001). Younger children especially seem to benefit from a combination of cognitive-behavioral strategies and family intervention (Barrett, Dadds, & Rapee, 1996; Mendlowitz et al, 1999). Cognitive-behavioral therapy and CBT plus family management were found to be equally effective at long-term follow-up 6 years later (Barrett et al, 2001). Pharmacologic intervention may be warranted, especially if there is comorbid social phobia or separation anxiety disorder. Recent evidence points to the efficacy of the SSRIs, especially fluvoxamine (Coyle, 2001); it appears to be well tolerated and has short-term efficacy in pediatric patients (Cheer & Figgitt, 2002).

Obsessive-Compulsive Disorder

Description. Obsessions are recurrent thoughts, images, or impulses that are disturbing to the child and difficult to dislodge. They often involve a sense of risk or fear of harm to the child or family members; concerns for contamination are common. Compulsions are repetitive behaviors or mental acts that the child feels driven to perform to prevent harm or remove contaminants, such as washing (e.g., hands, objects, body), counting, or arranging objects. Recurrent worries, rituals, and superstitious games are common in children at various stages of development. These behaviors are attended by mild anxiety but do not cause distress. Abnormal compulsive behavior is distinguished by a sense of urgency or a profound discomfort until the ritual is completed. Children often deny the fear and lack recognition of the "senselessness" of the ritual and are thought to hide their illness (Rapoport et al, 2000). Obsessional thoughts are intrusive, recurrent, and disturbing and, unlike anxious worries, are generally unrelated to events or situations.

Etiology and Incidence. Obsessive-compulsive disorder (OCD) is more common than previously thought. Neurobiologic underpinnings include a role for serotonin and involve abnormalities in the basal ganglia and functionally related cortical structures. OCD appears to affect primarily preadolescents and adolescents, with boys more likely to have onset in preadolescence and girls more likely to have onset in puberty (Leonard et al, 2001). OCD is increasingly diagnosed in younger children, some as young as 2 years of age. The rate seems to be about 2.5% of the population (Valleni-Basile et al, 1994). Among adults with OCD, at least one third to one half had their illness as children or adolescents (Leonard et al, 2001). Familial transmission is evident (Kovacs & Devlin, 1998), although a poststreptococcal autoimmunity recently has been postulated as a potential cause of some childhood onsets (Leonard et al, 2001). Studies of OCD show that this condition is chronic, with high rates of comorbidity, typically with some other anxiety disorder, major depression, or substance use disorder (Kovacs & Devlin, 1998). Tic disorders, disruptive behavior disorders, and learning disorders are also common comorbid diagnoses (Leonard et al, 2001).

Clinical Findings. OCD is characterized by obsessions and compulsions, as previously defined. Children do not recognize that the obsessions or compulsions are excessive or unreasonable. No pleasure is derived from ritualistic activity. The obsessions and compulsions are time consuming and can significantly interfere with the child's or adolescent's normal routine, academic performance, and social functioning. Washing, checking, and ordering rituals are more common in children (APA, 1994).

Differential Diagnosis. If the obsessions or compulsions are a direct physiologic consequence of a specific medical condition, the diagnosis is anxiety disorder caused by a general medical condition. If a substance is etiologically related to the obsessions or compulsions, a substance-induced anxiety disorder is assigned. A diagnosis of OCD is warranted if the content of the obsessions and compulsions is unrelated to another disorder (e.g., social phobia, trichotillomania, body dysmorphic disorder). A major depressive episode is diagnosed if the obsessions are mood congruent (e.g., guilt), and generalized anxiety disorder is diagnosed if the obsessions are experienced as excessive worry about real-life circumstances (APA, 1994). In the case of acute onset or exacerbation of OCD, a thorough assessment of recent medical illnesses, including upper respiratory infections, is warranted (Leonard et al, 2001).

Management. Clinical and empirical evidence suggests that CBT, alone or in combination with pharmacotherapy using SSRIs, is effective treatment for OCD in children and adolescents (American Academy of Child and Adolescent Psychiatry [AACAP], 1998b). Anxiety management training and OCD-specific family interventions play an adjunctive role, especially in preventing the avoidant behavior that is a complication of OCD (Rapoport & Inoff-Germain, 1997). Recent findings support the efficacy of CBT with a structured family component. SSRIs are first-line pharmacologic agents, and refractory symptoms can be treated by augmentation with neuroleptics; clomipramine's usefulness is limited by side effects (Grados & Riddle, 2001).

Responses to Trauma: Posttraumatic Stress Disorder

Description

Childhood trauma is the result of one sudden traumatic event or exposure to repeated trauma over time, such as physical or sexual abuse. A single trauma is an unanticipated solitary event directed at the child or witnessed by the child, such as an act of violence that involves threat, injury, or death. It includes learning about unexpected or violent death, harm, or threat experienced by a family member or close friend (AACAP, 1998a). Repeated trauma or repeated exposure to a painful event, usually maltreatment (physical or sexual abuse, or both) or community violence is long standing. Ongoing maltreatment is typically accompanied by other family dysfunctions, including emotional abuse, neglect, and substance abuse. Exposure to trauma constitutes the first criterion for posttraumatic stress disorder (PTSD) (AACAP, 1998a).

PTSD describes a characteristic set of symptoms that develop following exposure to a severe stressor or trauma. A decade ago, Terr (1991) conceptualized stress responses according to whether the trauma was a single event ("one sudden blow" trauma) or variable, multiple, long-standing traumas such as ongoing maltreatment. Famularo and colleagues (Famularo et al, 1996) also described distinct symptoms between acute and chronic types of PTSD. According to the Diagnostic and Statistical Manual of Mental Disorders, 4th edition (DSM-IV), the duration of the symptoms distinguishes three subtypes:

- Acute PTSD—symptoms last less than 3 months
- Chronic PTSD—symptoms last greater than 3 months
- Acute stress disorder—symptoms appear within 1 month of exposure to extreme stressor; last less than 1 month

This latter distinction is probably most useful to the NP when referring a child or adolescent to mental health specialists for further assessment and treatment. According to the practice parameters for children and adolescents with PTSD (AACAP, 1998a), the child's response to trauma must include a specific number of symptoms from each of three broad categories for a diagnosis:

- Reexperiencing the trauma in some way (one symptom)
- Avoidance/numbing (three symptoms)
- Increased arousal (two symptoms)

Etiology and Incidence

As noted previously, there is a traumatic etiology for PTSD symptoms. Exposure to trauma is a key feature of the diagnosis. Unfortunately, there has been skepticism that children could suffer from PTSD. Parents and teachers frequently minimize traumatic impact, perhaps to relieve themselves of vicarious distress or to reassure themselves that children are not harmed, and others—including mental health professionals—have rationalized that children are too young to remember the trauma or too immature to be affected. However, the clinical descriptive and empirical literature has expanded, documenting PTSD symptoms and other psychologic difficulties experienced by children in various catastrophic situations and in situations of maltreatment (AACAP, 1998a). Substantial rates of PTSD have been documented for children in foster care who were sexually abused (64%) and who were physically abused (42%) (Dubner & Motta, 1999). As a result, the clinical manifestations of PTSD in children are better understood. Three factors have been found to consistently influence the severity of the response: severity of the trauma exposure, parental distress related to the trauma, and temporal proximity to the event (Foy et al, 1996).

Retrospective reports of adults with mental health problems indicate that stress disorder is more common than previously believed. Community-based studies revealed a lifetime prevalence rate of 1% to 14% (APA, 1994). However, more meaningful are prevalence rates among at-risk children, which range from 3% to 10%, and those for children exposed to community violence, which range from 24% to 35% (AACAP, 1998a). The rate of PTSD is high among those who have been physically and sexually abused, with estimates ranging from 25% to 75% of sexual abuse victims, depending on the perpetrator. The closer the perpetrator is in relation to the victim, the greater the trauma; for example, PTSD is more likely when the perpetrator is a member of the immediate family as opposed to an extended family member, family friend, or stranger.

The findings for gender differences in the development of PTSD symptoms following exposure to trauma have been inconsistent. The findings for age differences have also been inconsistent, with some researchers suggesting that there may be developmental differences in the clinical manifestation of symptoms rather than age-mediated differences in the prevalence rates. PTSD has been documented across cultural and ethnic groups, with cultural factors affecting how the symptoms are manifested.

Clinical Findings

The child's response to trauma must include a set of symptoms from each of three categories to warrant a diagnosis of PTSD (APA, 1994). Reexperiencing of symptoms (symptom required for diagnosis) include the following:

- Recurrent and intrusive memories of the trauma
- Nightmares without recognizable content or distressing dreams about the event
- Distress at exposure to cues that symbolize or resemble an aspect of the trauma, including physiologic reactivity

The trauma can be persistently reexperienced through repetitive play with themes of the trauma, frightening dreams, behavioral reenactment, or a combination of these. Sexualized (i.e., seductive) behavior is a hallmark sign of sexual abuse. Preschoolers display behavioral or physical symptoms that prompt the caregiver's or other adults' suspicions of sexual abuse.

Three of the following symptoms reflecting avoidance of stimuli associated with the traumatic event(s) and numbing of general responsiveness must not have been present before the trauma:

- Avoidance of reminders of the trauma
- Efforts to avoid thoughts, feelings, or conversations linked to the trauma
- Amnesia for an important aspect of the trauma
- Detachment or estrangement from others
- Emotional constriction (restricted range of affect)
- Diminished interest in or participation in usual activities
- A sense of a foreshortened future

Two persistent symptoms of increased arousal must be new to the child, present for at least 1 month, and cause clinically important distress or negatively affect functioning. These symptoms include the following:

- Sleep disturbances
- Hypervigilance
- Difficulty concentrating
- Exaggerated startle response
- Agitated or disorganized behavior
- Irritability or anger outbursts

As children mature, they are more likely to exhibit adultlike PTSD symptoms, especially adolescents. Those adolescents with chronic PTSD who have experienced prolonged or repeated traumatic stressors (i.e., maltreatment) may experience depersonalization and dissociative episodes, sadness and thoughts that life is too hard, rage directed against self or others, and internalizing or externalizing behavior problems. PTSD symptoms are related to adolescent suicidal ideation and behavior, and are not explained by depression or gender (Mazza, 2000).

Toddlers and preschoolers (18 to 28 months of age) retain fragments of memories to the extent that they have the verbal capacity to articulate them. Infants, toddlers, and preschoolers tend to have generalized anxiety symptoms: separation fears, stranger anxiety, fears of monsters or animals; sleep disturbance; preoccupation with certain words or symbols that may or may not have an obvious connection to the event; and avoidance of situations that may or may not have an apparent link to the trauma. Other symptoms to consider include play reenactment that is not especially repetitive, constriction of play, social withdrawal, or loss of acquired developmental competencies (Scheering et al, 1995).

School-age children may not become amnesic for the event or certain aspects of it; they may retain full, detailed memories. They may not have avoidant or numbing symptoms or visual flashbacks. Responses to exposure to a single traumatic event tend to be characterized by anxiety, with sleep disturbances. Reenactment of the trauma through play, drawings, or verbalizations is typical for this developmental stage (AACAP, 1998a). Disclosures by school-age children tend to be purposeful and unrelated to a precipitating event. However, repression and dissociation often preclude disclosure until adulthood.

Differential Diagnosis

The stressor must be of an extreme nature to warrant a diagnosis of PTSD, whereas the stressor can be of any severity in an adjustment disorder (e.g., moving, starting a new school, birth of a sibling, divorce); the clinician has some latitude in this determination (AACAP, 1998a). Acute stress disorder is distinguished by the symptom pattern occurring and resolving within a 4-week period after the traumatic event. Recurrent intrusive thoughts occur in OCD but are experienced as inappropriate and are not related to an experienced trauma as they are in PTSD. Flashbacks are also connected to the event and involve a feeling of reliving the event in PTSD, whereas hallucinations and other perceptual disturbances are unrelated to exposure to trauma. With depression or externalizing disorders, such as conduct disorder unrelated to trauma, memory is intact and psychic numbing and dissociation are not present. The most typical differential diagnosis is an anxiety disorder, which is distinguished by not being precipitated by a traumatic event.

Management

Assessment of PTSD in children requires careful and direct clinical interviews with the child and parents. If the identified traumatic event involves a parent as the perpetrator of child maltreatment or domestic violence, the nonoffending parent or other caretaker should be interviewed. During assessment, do not use prompting or leading questions. Instead, ask questions about whether someone has invaded the child's privacy, how it may have happened, and how the injuries came to be. Specific guidelines for such an interview can be found in AACAP (1998a). Enough of an assessment should be conducted to ascertain that a trauma has occurred, the nature of the trauma, and the consequent symptom pattern. A report to social service agencies is essential for children younger than 18 years of age. Referral to a child mental health specialist is crucial, even in the absence of a disclosure. Most child psychiatrists use medications to treat PTSD, preferring SSRIs and alpha-adrenergic agonists (Cohen, Mannarino, & Rogal, 2001). Crisis intervention is often necessary for child and parents. The NP should educate parents about trauma and PTSD. Child psychiatrists tend to additionally prefer psychodynamic or cognitive-behavioral approaches, and nonmedical therapists tend to prefer the modalities of cognitive-behavioral, family, and nondirective play therapy (Cohen, Mannarino, & Rogal, 2001). Symptom patterns persist, so consistent follow-up assessment is important.

Mood Disorders

Depression

Description. There are three categories of depression that may be assigned regardless of age: major depressive disorder, dysthymic disorder, and adjustment disorder with depressed mood (APA, 1994). A *major depressive disorder* is defined as a depressed or irritable mood or a markedly diminished interest and pleasure in almost all of the usual activities for a period of at least 2 weeks, or both. A *dysthymic disorder* is characterized by a depressed or irritable mood for the majority of days in the past year, as well as other symptoms, but not to the extent of a major depressive episode. *Adjustment disorder with depressed mood* typically occurs within 3 months after a major life stressor, involves less severe symptoms, and is relatively mild and brief.

Etiology and Incidence. Like that of other disorders, the rate of depression increases with age (Kovacs & Devlin, 1998; Pullen, Modrcin-McCarthy, & Graf, 2000). Depression is estimated to affect between 2% and 9% of school-age children; the rate increases to between 4% and 8% of adolescents (AACAP, 1998b; Shoaf, Emslie, & Mayes, 2001). This rate increase for adolescents is thought to be linked to biology (e.g., sexual maturation), social environment (e.g., greater social and academic expectations, greater exposure to negative events), and developmental factors (e.g., increased autonomy and abstract thinking) (AACAP, 1998b). Kovacs and Devlin (1998) concluded from their review of the empirical literature that gender differences in rates of depressive disorders are neither compelling nor consistent among children or young adolescents, whereas others found depression to be two times higher among adolescent girls (Birmaher et al, 1996; Obeidallah, McHale, & Silbereisen, 1996).

Vulnerability to depression involves an interplay of genetic, biologic/biochemical, and psychosocial forces (Jellinek & Syder, 1998). Genetic factors underlie the risk for major depression, especially for childhood onset. The offspring of depressed parents are three times as likely to be diagnosed with depression, with a peak incidence at 15 to 20 years of age (Weissman et al, 1997). Each successive generation is at greater risk for developing mood disorders, and they are manifesting at younger ages, especially mild to moderate depression (AACAP, 1998b). Three biologic theories of depression are used to understand the psychopharmacology of depression: impaired neurotransmission, endocrine dysfunction, and biologic rhythm dysfunction. Given this biologic predisposition, certain life events may trigger the onset of depression. These include loss of a parent or significant other, losses that attend a disability or injury, family dysfunction, and physical or sexual abuse. There is a high risk of recurrent depression in diagnosed children and adolescents that appears to persist into young adulthood. Major depression in childhood places children at risk for personality disorders as they transition to adulthood (Kasen et al, 2001).

An important feature of early-onset depressive illness is a switch from unipolar depression to bipolar depression. Psychiatric comorbidity with depression is to be expected (Rohde et al, 2001). The most common comorbidity with depression is an anxiety disorder (up to 70%), which co-occurs two to three times more often than conduct disorder (Shoaf, Emslie, & Mayes, 2001). Other disorders most frequently found with major depression include dysthymia, disruptive behavior disorders, and substance abuse/dependence. Comorbidity may also occur with a variety of medical conditions, especially those with a neurologic component, such as brain injury, learning disorder, migraine headaches, and epilepsy (Shoaf, Emslie, & Mayes, 2001).

Clinical Findings. Children and young adolescents with depression typically have difficulty in identifying or describing their emotional or mood states and are more likely to be irritable or act out behaviorally (National Institute of Mental Health [NIMH], 2000). Talking directly with the child or adolescent is essential because it is thought that half of depression cases are missed when parents alone are interviewed. The following depressive symptoms may exist:

- Depressed mood: sad, "blue," down, angry, bored
- Loss of interest and pleasure in usual activities
- Change in appetite/weight (loss or increase)
- Insomnia or hypersomnia
- Low energy and fatigue
- Difficulty concentrating; indecision
- Feelings of worthlessness or inappropriate or excessive guilt
- Recurrent thoughts of death or suicidal ideation

Tearfulness and depressed affect, observable psychomotor agitation or retardation, and somatic complaints are common. A diagnosis of major depressive disorder is made if there have been at least 2 weeks of depressed mood or loss of interest and at least four additional symptoms of depression. The symptoms cause considerable distress and impairment in social and academic functioning. Therefore it is important to assess the following:

- Recent life events and losses
- Family history of depression or other psychiatric disorders
- Family dysfunction
- Changes in school performance
- Risk-taking behavior, including sexual activity and substance use
- Deteriorating relationships with family
- Changes in peer relations, especially social withdrawal

Possible warning signs for suicide are listed in Table 21-4.

In infants, depressive symptoms may include anorexia with lack of expected weight gain, weight loss, or failure to thrive; sleep problems; apathy and social withdrawal; and developmental delays. Infants may not respond to extra efforts to sooth or engage them. Toddlers may lack energy, be too eager to please others, be excessively or unusually clingy or whiney, and have problems with separation, with a persistence and intensity atypical for toddlerhood. School-age children may manifest irritability, anger, or hostility, as well as externalizing behavior, such as hyperactivity, difficulty handling aggression, or reckless behavior. Frequent absences from school, perhaps because of school phobia, or poor performance and other school problems are common. On the other hand, school-age children may have internalizing symptoms such as boredom, lack of interest in playing with friends, social withdrawal, somatic complaints (stomachaches, headaches, muscle aches, or tiredness), eating or sleeping disturbances, and enuresis or encopresis. Some children who are depressed describe themselves in negative terms, whereas others, in an effort to compensate for feelings of poor self-worth, become preoccupied with attempting to please others. Depressive symptoms in adolescents additionally include impulsivity, fatigue, and hopelessness. Social withdrawal, with the appearance of shyness, boredom, or a lack of motivation, is common (Jellinek & Snyder, 1998). Substance abuse is a problem for about 20%.

Depression Scales. Both patient self-report and clinician-completed rating scales are available. The following are used in pediatrics:

- Child Behavior Checklist (CBCL; 4 to 18 years)
- Children's Depression Rating Scale—Revised (CDRS-R; 6 to 12 years)

TABLE 21-4 *Warning Signs for Suicide*

Area of Functioning	Signs*
Changes in behavior	Accident prone Drug and alcohol abuse Physical violence toward self, others, or animals Loss of appetite Sudden alienation from family, friends, co-workers Worsening performance at work/school Putting personal affairs in order Loss of interest in personal appearance Disposal of possessions Writing letters, notes, or poems with suicidal content Taking unnecessary risks Buying a gun
Changes in mood	Expressions of hopelessness or impending doom Explosive rage Dramatic swings in affect Crying spells Sleep disorders Talk about suicide
Changes in thinking	Preoccupation with death Difficulty concentrating Irrational speech Hearing voices, seeing visions Sudden interest (or loss of interest) in religion
Major life changes	Death of a family member or friend (especially by suicide) Separation or divorce Public humiliation or failure Serious illness or trauma Loss of financial security

From Oregon Health Division: Suicidal thoughts, suicidal deaths, *CD Summary* 46:24, 1997.
*These signs must be interpreted in context. Many of them are common outside the realm of presuicidal behavior.

- Reynolds Child Depression Scale (RCDS; 6 to 12 years)
- Children's Depression Inventory (CDI; 6 years to adolescent)
- Beck Depression Inventory (BDI; adolescents)
- Reynolds Adolescent Depression Scale (RADS; adolescents)
- Center for Epidemiologic Studies—Depression Scale (CES-D; adolescents)
- Depression Self-Rating Scale (adolescents)

From a recent review of depression rating scales for children and adolescents, the RCDS and the RADS were recommended for screening purposes (Myers & Winters, 2002). For clinical assessment, a combination of the clinician-administered CDRS-R along with the self-report CDI was recommended as the optimal approach (Myers & Winters, 2002). Although the CDRS-R was originally developed for children, it has been used widely with adolescents. The BDI and the CES-D are both good screening tools for adolescents.

Differential Diagnosis. Some medications (steroids, phenobarbital, antihypertensives) and certain chronic illnesses (hypothyroidism, multiple sclerosis, inflammatory bowel disease, and type 1 diabetes) predispose for mood disorder. If a substance (e.g., medication, toxin, or drug of abuse) is related to the mood disturbance, a substance-induced mood disorder is diagnosed. Infections and neurologic disorders can also mimic depression in children and adolescents. In general, a physical examination and screening laboratory tests are necessary to rule out potential organic etiologies.

Depressive symptoms in response to a psychosocial stressor are diagnosed as adjustment disorder, which has a good short-term prognosis and does not predict later dysfunction. With separation anxiety disorder, depressive symptoms usually arise only in the context of separation and resolve quickly with reunion; however, concomitant depressive disorder is not uncommon. A depressive episode with irritable mood can be difficult to distinguish from a manic episode with irritable mood; careful evaluation of the presence of manic symptoms (e.g., excessive activity, inflated self-esteem, little need for sleep, talkativeness) is required. Many adolescents and adults who develop mania had predominantly depressive symptoms in childhood. Family history of bipolarity is an important risk factor. Mood disturbance that reflects irritability rather than sadness or loss of interest must be differentiated; mood disorder can be overdiagnosed in youths with attention-deficit hyperactivity disorder (ADHD) (APA, 1994). Children with mood disorder do not usually manifest impulsivity. In addition, they typically have a normal attention span before the onset of symptoms.

Management. The first goal of management is determination of suicidal risk. In a follow-up study, approximately 37% of those with childhood-onset depression reported suicide attempts in the 12 years after they were diagnosed (Wolk & Weissman, 1996). Adolescent suicide represents 12% of total mortality rate for this age-group (AACAP, 1998b). Acute suicidal intent, which includes a plan, requires immediate psychiatric evaluation. Cumulative suicidal risks—prior suicidal behavior or attempts, depression, and alcohol or drug use—require psychiatric intervention as well, and immediate referral must be made. Attention must also be paid to the establishment of a safe environment (removal of firearms and lethal medications). Families of depressed adolescents may frequently be noncompliant with recommendations to remove guns from the home in spite of compliance with other aspects of treatment (Brent et al, 2000); vigilant follow-up in this regard is crucial. Other management strategies by the NP include provision of community resources, such as hotlines, and commitment to a no-suicide agreement by which the adolescent agrees to refrain from harming himself or herself and promises to notify the caretaker or care provider if suicidal ideation returns.

A major depressive episode requires intervention by a mental health specialist (NP or psychiatrist). Therapies typically include cognitive-behavioral strategies in a group or individual psychotherapy format (NIMH, 2000). There is a growing body of evidence for the effectiveness of CBT in groups for adolescence (Clarke et al, 1999). Often, family therapy or psychoeducation is indicated. A study of the long-term differential effects of cognitive behavioral therapy, systematic behavioral family therapy, and nondirective supportive therapy found all of these approaches to be effective with adolescents, with most (80%) recovering after a median time of 8 months (Birmaher et al, 2000). However, systematic behavioral family therapy has been found to have a greater impact on family conflict and parent-child relationship problems, whereas nondirective supportive therapy and CBT tend to improve anxiety symptoms more effectively (Kolko et al, 2000). Connectedness to school and family is considered a protective factor for emotional distress, violence, and suicide attempts among teens with learning disabilities (Svetaz, Ireland, & Blum, 2000).

A central issue in psychopharmacologic approaches is that children and adolescents are not usually included in clinical drug trial research; safety and efficacy data from the literature about adults are often extrapolated. In general, the use of tricyclic antidepressants (imipramine is approved for children age 12 years and older) is declining as the newer agents prove safer and more tolerable (AACAP, 1998b). In fact, available studies do not support the efficacy of tricyclic antidepressants for depression in young children (NIMH, 2000). The use of SSRIs in clinical practice is increasing, but there is limited research evidence documenting their safety and efficacy in depressed children and adolescents (AACAP, 1998b; Keller et al, 2001; NIMH, 2000). There is no compelling evidence for using monoamine oxidase inhibitors (MAOIs) in children. (See Table 21-4.)

Prognosis. More than 90% of depressed children and adolescents recover in 1 to 2 years. However, recurrences are common, from 40% to 70% (Shoaf, Emslie, & Mayes, 2001).

Bipolar Disorder

Description. Bipolar disorder is determined from a clinical course characterized by unusual shifts in mood, energy, and functioning and may begin with manic, depressive, or a mixed set of manic and depressive symptoms (NIMH, 2000). There is evidence that depression precedes mania early in the course of bipolar disorder in children and adolescents (Bowden & Rhodes, 1996), with bipolar disorder developing in 20% to 40% of depressed children and adolescents (AACAP, 1998b). It is a recurrent disorder in which nearly all of those (90%) who have a single manic episode will have future episodes. A characteristic pattern usually evolves for a particular person, with manic episodes preceding or following major depressive episodes. Most individuals with bipolar disorder return to a full level of functioning between episodes; 20% to 30% experience persistent mood lability and interpersonal difficulties (APA, 1994). Sometimes psychotic symptoms develop after several days or weeks of manic symptoms. Such features tend to predict that the individual with subsequent manic episodes will again experience psychotic symptoms.

Etiology and Incidence. There is evidence of a genetic influence for bipolar disorder from twin studies and adoption studies; bipolar disorder tends to cluster in families. Parents who are bipolar are at greater risk for having bipolar children. Although the lifetime prevalence of bipolar disorder varies from 0.4% to 1.6% (APA, 1994), there is concern that the prevalence of childhood onset (prepubertal) may be increasing (Geller, 1997). Nearly one third of bipolar adults identify significant psychiatric symptoms before age 14, most notably depression (Chang, Steiner, & Ketter, 2000). There is no differential incidence based on race, ethnicity, or gender. Children with ADHD seem to be vulnerable to bipolar illness (Lombardo, 1997) or it may be that attention-deficit disorder or ADHD is a misdiagnosed early sign of the mania to come (Akin, 2001). If children are also bipolar, treatment of ADHD with psychostimulants or antidepressants may precipitate a manic episode. Antidepressants in depressed children (6 to 12 years of age) may also precipitate mania and the onset of bipolar illness (Lombardo, 1997).

Clinical Findings. Bipolar disorder in childhood or early adolescence appears to be a different, more severe form of the illness than occurs with late adolescent or adult onset. The early-onset form is typically characterized by irritability and continuous, rapid-cycling, and mixed-symptom state that may also co-occur with disruptive behavior disorders (e.g., ADHD or conduct disorder); features of ADHD or behavior disorder are often early symptoms (NIMH, 2000). This prepubertal and early adolescent bipolar disorder is a fairly homogeneous phenotype, with no differences according to gender, puberty, or comorbid ADHD (Geller et al, 2000). In the later-onset form, the hallmark features are a classic manic episode, a more episodic pattern of mania and depression, and more stability between episodes. Symptoms include the following:

- Severe mood changes—extreme irritability or overly elated and silly
- Inflated self-esteem or grandiosity
- Increased energy
- Decreased need for sleep (sleeps few hours or no sleep for days without tiring)
- Talkativeness or compulsion to talk; frequent topic changes or cannot be interrupted
- Distractibility, with attention moving constantly from one thing to another
- Increase in goal-directed activity (socially or at school)
- Physical agitation
- Risk-taking behaviors or activities; taking "more dares"
- Hypersexuality in talk, thoughts, feelings, or behaviors (for those who have reached puberty)

In the context of a family history of bipolar disorder, these symptoms should definitely raise concerns for bipolar disorder in the child. The child or adolescent who has depression but also manifests symptoms of ADHD that seem severe (e.g., extreme temper outbursts and mood changes) should be evaluated by a child psychiatrist with experience in bipolar disorder (NIMH, 2000). Symptoms are manifested in relatively age-specific ways (Geller & Luby, 1997). With mania, children appear to the happiest of people and, as with adults, the happiness and laughter must be examined in the context of their history (usually negative). Grandiosity may manifest in efforts to correct teachers or critique their efforts, seeing themselves as above rules and laws, or devoting time to an activity for which they have no talent. Children's sleep difficulties are reflected in high activity levels before bed (e.g., rearranging the furniture) whereas adolescents need little sleep at all. Risk-taking behavior ranges from children climbing excessively high trees or hopping between rooftops to adolescents driving recklessly and speeding. In adolescents, manic episodes are more likely to include psychotic features and may be associated with school truancy, school failure, substance use, or antisocial behavior. No laboratory findings diagnostic of a manic episode have been identified, so a careful history and a thorough assessment are crucial.

Differential Diagnosis. A manic episode must be distinguished from a mood disorder caused by a medical condition (e.g., brain tumor) and a substance-induced mood disorder (e.g., laughing fits with marijuana, amphetamine highs followed by withdrawal "crashes," perceptual distortions/hallucinations of hallucinogens) (Geller & Luby, 1997). ADHD is also characterized by excessive activity, poor impulse control and judgment, and denial of problems that are found with a manic episode. ADHD is distinguished from a manic episode by its lack of clear onsets or episodes, absence of mood disturbances, and lack of psychotic features. However, recent evidence that children with ADHD are vulnerable to bipolar disorder and that pharmacologic treatments may precipitate manic episodes points to the need for very careful evaluation and referral to the provider who is treating the ADHD or, preferably, to a child psychiatrist or psychiatric–mental health NP who has experience working with bipolar disorder in youth.

Management. Referral to a child psychiatrist or child mental health NP is critical. The few researched options in the pharmacologic treatment of mania include lithium, valproate, carbamazepine, and low-dose chlorpromazine (Geller & Luby, 1997; NIMH, 2000). The use of lithium must be carefully monitored, especially given data that strongly support long-term maintenance on lithium to prevent relapse of bipolar symptoms (Geller & Luby, 1997). Psychoeducation and family counseling for the family are recommended to facilitate the understanding and management of this episodic disorder. This is especially important in light of recent research findings that living with an intact family improves the recovery rate for children and adolescents with bipolar disorder (Geller et al, 2001).

The Aggressive Child

Social Aggression

Description. Social aggression is a pattern of social behavior based primarily on aversive control of situations and others. Onset occurs in toddlerhood.

Etiology and Incidence. Acute, stressful life events or transitions can precipitate a brief period of social aggression. A range of antecedents have been found, including a history of maltreatment; inconsistent or harsh discipline, or both; lack of maternal responsiveness; separations from parents, shifts in parent figures, or parental rejection; and other enduring circumstances. Social aggression can be a precursor to conduct disorder or oppositional disorder. The incidence rate is thought to be higher than that for clinical diagnoses because most cases are untreated.

Clinical Findings. During preschool, social aggression manifests as oppositional or defiant behavior and is considered clinically significant if it interferes with normal developmental functioning. The pervasiveness, intensity, and persistence distinguish losing one's temper as an expression of developmentally appropriate self-assertions and frustration from being irritable, argumentative, defiant, and easily annoyed as precursors to oppositional defiant disorder (Keenan & Wakschlag, 2002). In the preschool period, children have a beginning understanding of the impact of their behavior on others and can control their behavior on the basis of internalized norms and developing self-regulation (Keenan & Wakschlag, 2002). When social aggression becomes a pattern, peer rejection is common. Aggressive behavior involves the following:

- Destruction of property
- Name calling
- Physical pestering
- Hitting, biting, kicking
- Frequent conflict with peers
- Temper tantrums
- Carrying expectations of others' hostility
- Misinterpreting social cues and responding aggressively
- Lack of problem solving in social situations

Differential Diagnosis. Oppositional disorder is directed primarily toward parents and teachers and is more defiant than aggressive in nature. Conduct disorder is a clear pattern of behavior established over a 6-month period, typically diagnosed at school age. However, there is growing evidence that preschool children manifest clinically significant disruptive behavior problems and that valid diagnoses of oppositional defiant and conduct disorder can be made. Typical and atypical problems can be differentiated, and, with a developmentally based DSM framework, children with these problems can be identified (Keenan & Wakschlag, 2002).

Management. It is important to ascertain whether a difficult temperament underlies the behavioral difficulty, especially in conjunction with a lack of fit with parental temperament. A difficult temperament may account for a child's being harder to discipline, having social behavior problems in school (e.g., poor fit with the teacher), or having poor academic achievement. In these situations, the use of positive parenting strategies does not have to change, but supportive counseling for the parents should be provided regarding temperament, its manifestations, and strategies for managing transitions and other difficult times or behaviors. A conference with the teacher may be valuable to provide similar information and to explore strategies to facilitate the child's learning and positive behavior (Carey, 1998).

When social aggression is a response to acute stress, the problem usually resolves if parents employ positive parenting strategies and facilitate developmentally appropriate coping efforts. If peer relationship development is hampered, close monitoring of and intervention with peer interactions by day care or preschool personnel, especially with the parents present for observations, enhance appropriate social behavior and competence. Changing schools in an effort to ameliorate problems is not advised, because children have been found to carry their social difficulties with them and assume the same roles in new groups. Teachers need to be supportive and facilitative.

When social aggression becomes a pattern of social behavior, referral for intervention is critical. Negative behavior in preschool playgroups is predictive of externalizing behavior problems in the classroom when children are in kindergarten (Fagot & Leve, 1998). Substantial research literature supports the stability and persistence of disruptive behavior and aggression from toddlerhood to school age (Keenan & Wakschlag, 2002). Early intervention is a must.

Conduct Disorder

Description. Conduct disorder (CD) is a repetitive and persistent pattern of behavior in which either the basic rights of others or major age-appropriate societal norms and rules are violated (APA, 1994). The onset of aggressive behavior is observed in toddlerhood. Early-onset conduct problems are diagnosed from 4 to 6 years of age; a formal diagnosis is typically made when the child is about 7 years of age or older.

Etiology and Incidence. The etiology of the disorder rests in chronic negative circumstances, as described for social aggression. Most common referrals for clinical treatment are for aggressive behavior patterns. Prevalence rates vary according to the age-groups and assessments used for classification. The rates range from 9.3% to 15.8% of boys from 10 to 18 years of age, and from 3.8% to 9.2% of girls in that age range; several studies have found odds of CD that were three to four times higher for boys than girls (Loeber et al, 2000). However, it is thought that the prevalence data do not accurately reflect the occurrence of conduct disorder for females because the diagnostic criteria emphasize physical aggression. The expression of behavioral disregulation tends to become notable during the transition from early to middle childhood and is mediated by changes in the structure and demands of the social environment—peers and school settings (Kovacs & Devlin, 1998). There is a high rate of comorbidity with major depression, and the joint presence of CD and depression increases the risk for substance abuse and suicide. ADHD is found to influence the development, course, and severity of CD; those with CD and comorbid ADHD have an earlier onset of disruptive behavior (Loeber et al, 2000).

Clinical Findings. In assessment, several factors are relevant to practitioners for their prognostic importance: how atypical the behaviors are for age or gender, how overt versus covert the behaviors are, the nature of any aggression, and the presence of early antisocial or psychopathy-related symptoms (Loeber et al, 2000). Physical aggression toward others is common, including the following:

- Hitting, kicking, fighting
- Physical cruelty to animals or people
- Physical destruction (including fire setting)
- Frequent temper tantrums
- A high rate of annoying behavior, such as yelling, whining, or threatening
- Disobedience to adult authorities
- Lying, cheating
- Covert stealing
- Truancy
- Running away from home

There is growing evidence that preadolescent and adolescent girls manifest CD more indirectly, using verbal and relational aggression, including alienation, ostracism, and character defamation directed at the relational bonds between friends (Loeber et al, 2000). With conduct disorder, social role functioning tends to be impaired, with poor academic performance, poor family and peer relationships, and poor self-management (Riley et al, 1998). For adolescent girls, CD is predictive of medical problems and substance abuse in early adulthood (Bardone et al, 1998).

Differential Diagnosis. Oppositional disorder is characterized by more disobedience than aggressiveness and is evidenced in preschool or early school age. Attention-deficit disorder, with which there is considerable overlap, is characterized by inattention, impulsiveness, and hyperactivity. Conduct disorder is distinguished from isolated acts of aggressive behavior by the repetitive and persistent pattern over at least 6 months (APA, 1994).

Management. If aggressive behavior is identified before a conduct disorder develops, prevention can be implemented. Successful programs typically address multiple risk domains, including a parent-directed component (parent education and support for positive parenting strategies and healthy, consistent approaches to discipline), social-cognitive skills training, proactive classroom management and teacher training, and group therapy (Burke, Loeber, & Birmaher, 2002). Once a conduct disorder is evident, referral for child and family intervention is crucial.

Among the most effective treatments are parent management training (Burke, Loeber, & Birmaher, 2002). Videotaped parent training programs, such as those developed by Webster-Stratton in the Parenting Clinic at the University of Washington School of Nursing, have been found to be effective in the treatment of conduct disorder. In a comparison of interventions, a combination of child training groups and parent training was found to produce the most significant improvements in child behavior 1 year later (Webster-Stratton & Hammond, 1997). For adolescents, the results are generally supportive of family therapy for conduct disorder, although there were some negative findings (Chamberlain & Rosicky, 1995). Collaboration between the family and the school is of critical importance, and the NP can assist with strategies in this regard. Isolated individual treatment has not been found to be superior to parent intervention programs, and, in fact, the results are thought to be rather modest (Burke, Loeber, & Birmaher, 2002). In conjunction with parenting interventions, problem-solving skills training as a way of building prosocial behavior has been found to be effective (Kazdin, 1997; Webster-Stratton & Hammond, 1997). Psychopharmacologic intervention tends to be reserved for explosive aggression and includes mood stabilizers, typical and atypical antipsychotics, clonidine, and stimulants; however, few randomized controlled trials have been performed (Burke, Loeber, & Birmaher, 2002). Effectiveness is not well established, and, given the high risk for substance abuse in those with CD, caution should be exercised in prescribing medications.

Oppositional Defiant Disorder

Description. Oppositional defiant disorder (ODD) is a pattern of negative, hostile, and defiant behavior that is excessive compared with other children of the same age. Precursors appear in early childhood, from 3 to 7 years of age. The disorder typically begins by 8 years of age.

Etiology and Incidence. Etiologic factors include many of the parenting and family dysfunctions identified for social aggression. Precursors to the disorder are common in early childhood, especially defiance and negativism. More common in boys before puberty, the gender distribution is approximately equal thereafter. Estimates for 10- to 13-year-olds include 10% of girls and 14% of boys, 15% of all 14- to 16-year-olds, and 12% of 17- to 20-year-olds. Data on gender differences in ODD during middle childhood and adolescence are inconsistent across studies, with most suggesting either slightly higher rates in boys or no gender differences (Loeber et al, 2000).

Clinical Findings. The essential feature of ODD is a recurrent pattern of behavior that is negativistic, defiant, disobedient, and hostile toward authority figures. Behavior is typically directed at family members, teachers, or peers whom the child knows well. The child manifests the following behaviors to an extent that leads to impairment:

- Actively defies or refuses adult requests or rules
- Is argumentative, angry, resentful, touchy, or easily annoyed

- Easily loses temper
- Blames others for own mistakes or difficulties
- Deliberately does things to annoy others

Children often see their own behavior as justifiable, not oppositional or defiant (APA, 1994).

Differential Diagnosis. Conduct disorder involves more serious violations of the rights of others.

Management. Attend to the early signs of defiant and oppositional behavior or aggression, or both, by educating parents about positive parenting strategies and by exercising consistent, healthy discipline, as with the management of conduct disorders. Because these children typically do not perceive themselves as having a problem and the etiology rests with the family system, referral for intervention is indicated. As described for conduct disorder, parent training programs are more successful, especially if multiple risk domains are targeted for intervention (Burke, Loeber, & Birmaher, 2002). Child training groups provide added benefit if combined with parent training groups. Again, collaboration with the school is important. These multiple approaches, conducted simultaneously, are most effective.

THE SHY CHILD

Shyness

Description

Shyness is a pattern of social inhibition with unfamiliar people, with novel objects, or in unfamiliar situations. Inhibition is evident in infancy as an inborn bias to respond to unfamiliar events with anxiety, distress, or disorganization. Shyness appears as a social behavior pattern in toddlerhood, with stability by early school age. Although most shy children do not develop later internalizing disorders, extremely shy toddlers may be at risk for becoming socially withdrawn in later childhood (Rubin et al, 1997) and for developing an anxiety disorder in adolescence (Prior et al, 2000).

Etiology and Incidence

Shyness is caused by a rather stable temperamental disposition toward withdrawal that is linked to family factors. Shyness is common. Behavioral inhibition in social situations may be adaptive if handled effectively by the parent and can be indicative of optimal self-regulation and development of conscience.

Clinical Findings

Retreat and withdrawal from social stimulation are noted in infancy. In toddlerhood, general inhibition persists, evidenced by irritability, withdrawal, and clinging to the mother in new situations. Shy children are slower to approach peers or initiate play with an unfamiliar child and often spend more time observing the situation and other children in play before engaging. School-age shy children continue to make fewer social approaches. They usually "warm up slowly" or may engage in solitary but appropriate play. Viewed by their peers as likable but shy, these children may be neglected by their peers. One or both parents usually identify themselves as shy.

Differential Diagnosis

Children with social withdrawal rather than shyness have a lower rate of social interaction overall and do not warm up to social situations.

Management

Parenting strategies that provide warmth, sensitivity, and responsiveness to the child's inhibition and shyness foster security in attachment relationships and facilitate social competence. In preschool and school-age children, insensitivity and a lack of responsiveness foster a sense of insecurity and predict social withdrawal, with associated internalizing disorders, including depression and adolescent anxiety (Prior et al, 2000). It is helpful to have parents prepare shy children for new situations by visiting the new settings, identifying a sensitive adult to whom they may turn with requests or concerns, and negotiating for them to be allowed to watch and observe before engaging in play or other activities.

Social Withdrawal

Description

Social withdrawal is a pattern of social behavior characterized by a low rate of social interaction with peers. Onset occurs in school-age children. Some withdrawn children avoid peers because of their own fearfulness, some simply prefer to play alone, and some are socially unskilled and are rejected by their peers (not allowed to play).

Etiology and Incidence

A rather stable inhibited temperament is usually antecedent and linked to a lack of family sensitivity and warmth, with consequent insecurity, or to a highly stressful experience or an exacerbation of stressful life events (Rubin et al, 1997). Social withdrawal is less common than shyness.

Clinical Findings

Socially withdrawn children have low interaction with peers; they make few social approaches and demonstrate limited or compliant (or both) responses to initiations by peers. These children tend to engage more often in solitary play. In group play, they are less communicative, deferential, submissive, and immature. Initially, socially withdrawn children may appear shy, but, unlike shy children, they do not warm up to social situations. Preschoolers are described as anxious and fearful. In early school age, similar patterns persist with poor social functioning. By middle childhood, social anxiety and low self-esteem are more prominent, and, by late childhood, depressive symptoms become evident (Kovacs & Devlin, 1998). Peer rejection is concomitant, and social problem-solving skills are poorly developed.

Differential Diagnosis

A differential diagnosis is depression, which is usually not diagnosed until the child is 10 years of age. Anxiety is another differential diagnosis and has been found in children as young as 6 years in relation to poor social functioning. The severity of symptoms may warrant a diagnosis of social phobia.

Management

The key is to intervene as early as possible to prevent negative consequences of poor social development. Addressing any acute or chronic life events alleviates the source of the problem. In addition, parent education and positive parenting strategies support efforts to restore social behavior. Confidence-boosting social experiences can be developed, such as opportunities to interact with or help younger playmates. Such situations provide opportunities for self-assertion and successful play. Similarly, assigning responsibilities in the social setting can serve to enhance the withdrawn child's social behavior (e.g., introducing and orienting a new child). Finally, structured intervention, such as assertiveness training and social skills training, might be necessary. Friendships have been found to mediate social withdrawal, especially in late childhood (10 years and older) (Fordham & Stevenson-Hinde, 1999). Small group interventions with socially withdrawn girls have been effective for developing social skills and friendships (Houck & Stember, 2002).

BEREAVEMENT

Description

Bereavement is the sad or lonely state resulting from loss or death. Grief is the effect of bereavement and typically involves distress, sorrow, and painful regret. Mourning is the psychologic process set in motion by loss of a loved one. The death of someone important to a child is considered one of the most stressful events to be experienced (American Academy of Pediatrics [AAP], 2000). For children and adolescents, death of a parent or sibling is the most profoundly disturbing.

Etiology and Incidence

The clinical picture of bereavement and grief depends, to some extent, on the concept of death. In toddlerhood, death is perceived as separation or abandonment, with no real cognitive understanding of death; the central issues are the sense of loss or abandonment resulting from disruption in caretaking or an attachment relationship. Preschoolers, up to 6 years of age, tend to perceive death as a continuation of life under different circumstances. Death is personified and perceived as a punishment (AAP, 2000). From 6 to 11 years of age, children grasp the irreversibility and finality of death, akin to the adult concept, although they struggle with understanding the specific loss of the loved one. Preadolescents and adolescents are able to be more abstract and philosophic about death. At any given developmental stage, a child can resolve the impact of the death only at that developmental level. Thus bereavement resurfaces and the significance of the loss needs to be reworked at each subsequent developmental stage. It is expected that most children and adolescents experience at least one significant loss before they reach adulthood. It is estimated that 5% of children lose one or both parents to death before age 15 years.

Clinical Findings

For a child, grief is a process that unfolds over time. Initially, children may seem emotionally unmoved, but the initial shock and denial will give way to depressive symptoms that can last for weeks or months (AAP, 2000). A normal reaction to loss, depressive symptoms include sadness, feeling depressed, poor appetite, weight loss, insomnia, crying, anxiety, guilt, and idealization of the person who died. Rage is a common reaction to the death of a parent, typically directed at the surviving parent and others in the immediate family. Angry behavior may be directed at peers as well, compounding a sense of inferiority and alienation. Fears of dying, disease, and growing old are often stimulated. Identification with the deceased is common and needs to be assessed to determine whether this furthers or inhibits development. Similarly, a fantasy connection to a dead parent can develop and may be helpful. Guilt and responsibility are typical issues for children but are less problematic for adolescents. Adolescents often manifest a sudden "maturity" along with numbness, regrets, disorganization, and despair before closure and reorganization are achieved. It is not unusual for adolescents to develop stronger ties with friends and to distance from family while grieving (AAP, 2000).

Differential Diagnosis

Children at high risk for pathologic bereavement or depression generally have a previous history of individual and family problems. Symptoms of bereavement that should concern the NP include the following:

- Long-term denial and avoidance of feelings
- Preoccupation with worthlessness
- Persistent anger
- Decline in school performance
- Social withdrawal
- Persistent sleep problems
- Hallucinations beyond transitory experience of hearing the voice of, or seeing the image of, the deceased

Management

Parent education can facilitate effective management of bereavement in children and adolescents. A first question is typically whether children and adolescents should attend the funeral or memorial service. Children need to be allowed to participate in the rituals around death as much as they choose (AAP, 2000). Such services and rituals provide even young children with an important way to grieve, especially if such involvement is supportive, appropriately explained, and congruent with the family's values. Children need parental help to understand the facts of death and to correct misunderstandings as they develop; children cannot understand, however, beyond their cognitive level. Parents often need to be reassured that their showing of feelings (disbelief, guilt, sadness, anger) is normal and helpful to children; sharing feelings about and memories of the family member who died is helpful as well (AAP, 2000). Sensitivity to the child's reactions of grief and restlessness is important, as is support for the child's assimilation and mastery of the loss and emotional experience. Children need to express and work through feelings and fantasies related to the loss; open communication is a must. There are many books about death, loss, and grieving available for children and adolescents that are geared to the various developmental levels. It is critical for children to have an attachment to an adult who can be an effective source of support and involvement, as well as a focus for reactions to loss (AAP, 2000). The child must be sensitively prepared for any changes occurring at the same time as the death, with the family advised to minimize these as much as possible. Any parental loss before age 5 years probably warrants treatment. Because bereavement resurfaces at subsequent developmental phases, early parental loss should be determined and current symptoms assessed as a possible manifestation of recurring bereavement issues. DeMaso, Meyer, and Beasley (1997) developed an excellent source for guidelines to assist parents with helping their children in response to a sibling's death.

SUBSTANCE ABUSE

Description

Substance use is a precursor to abuse or dependence, and regular use clearly increases the risk for developing a substance use disorder (SUD). However, the AACAP (1997) clarified in its practice parameters that the use of substances per se is not sufficient for a diagnosis of SUD. Substance abuse is a maladaptive pattern of the use of alcohol or drugs manifested in significant impairment or distress. The criteria for substance dependence in adults include tolerance, withdrawal, and compulsive drug use. For children and adolescents, tolerance and loss of control are not good indicators for a diagnosis. Instead, alcohol-related blackouts, craving, and impulsive sexual or risk-taking behavior tend to be more important criteria (AACAP, 1997). Onset is often in early adolescence, about 12 years of age. However, nearly half of problem drinkers are thought to have tried alcohol by age 10 and two thirds by age 13 (Finke & Bowman, 1997; Heyman & Adger, 1997).

Etiology and Incidence

The etiology of SUD is multifaceted (AACAP, 1997; Tweed, 1998; Weinberg et al, 1998). Many contributing factors exist, including the following:

- Genetic vulnerability (family history)
- Parental substance use
- Dysfunctional family relationships, such as rigidity, distant relationships, neglect or lack of supervision, history of abuse
- Negative life events
- Psychiatric conditions (e.g., conduct disorder, ADHD, depression)
- Ineffective coping (poor emotional regulation, poor problem-solving skills)

Precipitating life events tend to center around loss of relationships (e.g., parental separation, divorce, or death; death of a close friend) and chronic negative circumstances (e.g., parental substance abuse, maltreatment)

By the end of high school, 90% of students have tried alcohol and more than 40% have tried an illicit substance (AACAP, 1997; Tweed, 1998). The majority of adolescents who use drugs do not progress to abuse or dependence, and peer influence seems to be less significant to the etiology than previously thought (Weinberg et al, 1997). Boys tend to be more involved in both alcohol and drugs of all kinds than girls are at the same age (Finke & Bowman, 1997; Tweed, 1998). Generally, estimates reveal that, for both boys and girls, abuse of alcohol and other drugs is negligible from 10 to 13 years but doubles between midadolescence (12 to 16 years) and late adolescence (17 to 20 years), peaks between ages 18 and 25 years, and declines thereafter (Chassin, Pitts, & Prost, 2002).

Clinical Findings

Identifying an adolescent's problem with substance abuse requires a careful assessment, conducted with an accepting, nonjudgmental, nonthreatening, matter-of-fact attitude. The covert nature of substance abuse and the dynamic of denial make it crucial to avoid a critical tone. Also see Chapter 9 for discussion of how to assess and manage adolescent risk behavior.

History

Meeting with the adolescent and parents is helpful to explore changes they have observed. Interviewing the adolescent with the parents is a key strategy for obtaining information about etiologic factors and behavioral, cognitive, emotional, and physical changes in the adolescent. However, it is essential that the adolescent be interviewed alone at every visit (Heyman & Adger, 1997) to assess mental health and family issues.

When talking about substance use with an adolescent, it is important to begin with general questions that are not overly personal (Tweed, 1998). Begin by asking the adolescent about acquaintances who smoke, drink, or use drugs; whether anyone in the family has had problems with these; whether friends smoke, or use alcohol or drugs; and what the adolescent does with friends when they get together. It is helpful to ask about experimentation, under what circumstances it occurred, and the adolescent's feelings about it. To obtain a chronologic history of tobacco, alcohol, or drug use, it may be helpful to approach the subject by inquiring about prescription drugs and moving to illicit substances. The key is to remain nonjudgmental in order to elicit information that will indicate whether the adolescent is experimenting, a regular user, or dependent on substances. A helpful question asks about the adolescent's source of drugs or alcohol; the adolescent who uses substances provided by a friend or acquaintance is less advanced than one who purchases them directly.

A two-item conjoint screening test (TICS) for alcohol and other drug problems has been developed for adults, including 18- to 20-year-olds (Brown et al, 1997). The TICS asks "In the last year, have you ever drunk or used drugs more than you meant to?" and "Have you felt you wanted or needed to cut down on your drinking or drug use in the last year?" In a primary care setting, respondents who replied to both items with "no" had a 7.4% chance of having a current SUD, those with one positive response had a 45.5% chance of having a current SUD, and those with positive responses to both items had a 75% chance of having a current SUD. This may also be helpful for screening adolescents, because such assessments typically do not account for developmental differences in substance use patterns. Significant behavioral changes that may reflect drug use include the following:

- Lethargy, hyperactivity or agitation, hypervigilance
- Disinhibition; deviant or risk-taking behavior
- Repeated absences from school; suspensions from school
- Decline in academic performance
- Loss of interest in previously enjoyed activities
- Withdrawal from family and usual friends
- Change in friends to those involved in drugs and alcohol
- Angry or violent outbursts
- Early sexual activity

Parents may also be able to report on changes in personal habits, such as the following:

- Altered sleep pattern (lack of or excessive sleep)
- Loss of appetite
- Less attention to hygiene
- Use of eyedrops

Cognitive changes may include the following:

- Impaired concentration
- Changes in attention span
- Perceptual and overt changes in thinking (e.g., paranoia, delusions)

Mood changes include swings from depression to euphoria, nervousness, unreasonable anger, and frequent expressions of hopelessness or failure. Low self-esteem typically characterizes those who abuse substances.

Physical Examination

Physical signs that indicate a substance use problem include the following:

- Weight loss
- Red eyes, nasal irritation, hoarseness, chronic cough, wheezing
- Frequent "colds" or "allergies"
- Accidents, trauma, injuries
- Intoxication

Laboratory Studies

Urine toxicology can be helpful to verify adolescent truthfulness, although a positive drug screen does not indicate substance abuse or dependence but only indicates substance use. A negative drug screen does not rule out a substance use disorder. The approximate duration that drugs can be detected in the urine is as follows (AACAP, 1997):

- Stimulants—1 to 2 days
- Cocaine and its major metabolite—1 to 3 days
- Sedative-hypnotics—1 day to 1 week
- Barbiturates—2 to 4 weeks
- Quaaludes—2 to 3 weeks
- Opiates—1 to 2 days
- Marijuana—up to 30 days

Duration of detection from last substance use varies according to the laboratory and type of test used. The AACAP recommends that, to obtain a valid result, a positive result on immunoassay should be followed by confirmation with a more sensitive method, such as gas chromatography or mass spectrometry.

Differential Diagnosis

Substance abuse is distinguished from social drinking or nonpathologic substance use by the presence of compulsive use, craving, or substance-related problems (AACAP, 1997). Substance use disorders are comorbid most often with conduct disorder, depression, and anxiety (Weinberg et al, 1998).

Management

Exposure to tobacco and alcohol, as well as illicit substances, begins in early childhood. Heyman and Adger (1997) recommend that the pediatric primary care provider discuss parental modeling for the use of alcohol, tobacco products, and other substances in early childhood during routine well-child visits. Parents should be advised not to involve their child in their own substance use. Something as seemingly innocuous as "getting Dad a beer from the refrigerator" give the child practice in alcohol use. It becomes more important to provide education to school-age children and their parents about substance use and its consequences. For adolescents, a direct assessment and an interview about substance use are essential.

Substance abuse must be treated, and referral to a substance abuse program is crucial. However, the initial goal may be best defined as helping adolescents take positive steps toward changing their substance use and abuse behaviors (Tweed, 1998). If the adolescent denies any problem, efforts can be directed to helping the adolescent acknowledge problems. Clarifying reported negative consequences, creating doubts about substance use, and raising awareness of the risks related to current use are strategies that may be helpful. It is important to remain empathic and yet leave responsibility with the adolescent. If the adolescent has not reached a level of chronic use, harm reduction is the thrust of the intervention. Guide the adolescent to examine his or her substance use or abuse responsibly and identify ways to avoid harmful consequences.

If the adolescent has progressed to chronic substance use, a number of options exist. Outpatient or day treatment programs are effective for those who can live and be managed at home. For adolescents with serious addiction, comorbid psychiatric conditions, or suicidal ideation, residential treatment or hospitalization may be necessary. Given the prominence of family dysfunction and family life events in the etiology of the problem, family-based treatment

RESOURCE BOX

Resources for Assessment

TEMPERAMENT

Revised Infant Temperament Questionnaire
Carey WB, McDevitt SC: Revision of the infant temperament questionnaire, *Pediatrics* 61:735-739, 1978.

Toddler Temperament Questionnaire
McDevitt SC, Carey WB: The measurement of temperament in 3-7 year old children, *J Child Psychol Psychiatry* 19:245-253, 1978.

Middle Childhood Temperament Questionnaire
Hegrik RI, McDevitt SC, Carey WB: The Middle Childhood Temperament Questionnaire, *J Dev Behav Pediatr* 3:197-200, 1982.

Emotionality, Activity, Social Ability (EAS) Scale
Buss AH, Plomin R: The EAS approach to temperament. In Plomin R, Dunn J, editors: *The study of temperament: changes, continuities, and challenges*, Hillsdale, NJ, 1986, Erlbaum.

Continued

RESOURCE BOX

Resources for Assessment—cont'd

Dimensions of Temperament Survey
Lerner R et al: Assessing the dimensions of temperamental individuality across the life span: the Dimensions of Temperament Survey (DOTS), *Child Dev* 53:149-159, 1982.

Infant Characteristics Questionnaire
Bates J, Freeland C, Lounsbury M: Measurement of infant difficultness, *Child Dev* 50:794-803, 1979.

Temperament Inventory
Strelau J: *Temperament, personality, activity*, New York, 1983, Academic Press.

BEHAVIOR PROBLEMS

National Institute of Mental Health (NIMH) Anxiety Disorders website:
www.nimh.nih.gov/anxiety
1-88-88-ANXIETY
Child Behavior Checklist for ages 2 to 3 years
Child Behavior Checklist for ages 4 to 18 years
Youth Self-Report for ages 11 to 18 years
Teacher's Report Form for ages 5 to 18 years
Ordering information:
Child Behavior Checklist
1-802-656-8313

Behavior Screening Questionnaire
Richman N, Graham PJ: A behavioral screening questionnaire for use with three-year-old children: Preliminary findings, *J Child Psychol Psychiatry* 12:5-33, 1971.

Preschool Behavior Questionnaire
Behar L, Stringfield SA: Behavior rating scale for the preschool child, *Dev Psychol* 10:601-610, 1974.

Conners Parent Rating Scale
Sattler JM: *Assessment of children*, San Diego, 1986, Jerome M Sattler.

Eyberg Child Behavior Inventory
Eyberg SM, Ross AW: Assessment of child behavior problems: the validation of a new inventory, *J Clin Child Psychol* 7:113-116, 1978.

Pediatric Symptom Checklist
Jellineck MS, Murphy JM: The recognition of psychosocial disorders in pediatric practice: the current status of the Pediatric Symptom Checklist, *J Dev Behav Pediatr* 11:273-278, 1990.

Children's Depression Inventory
Kovacs M: *Children's Depression Inventory manual*, North Tonawanda, NY, 1992, Multi-Health Systems. Multi-Health Systems, 908 Niagra Falls Blvd., North Tonawanda, NY 14120-2060. Available at www.mhs.com.

Children's Depression Rating Scale—Revised
Poznanski EO, Mokros HB: *Children's Depression Rating Scale—Revised (CDRS-R)*, Los Angeles, 1999, Western Psychological Services.

Beck Depression Inventory
Beck A, Steer RA: *Beck Depression Inventory (BDI) manual*, ed 2, San Antonio, TX, 1993, Pscyhological Corporation. Pscyhological Corporation, 555 Academic Court, San Antonio, TX 78204-2498. Available at www.psychcorp.com.

Reynolds Child Depression Scale
Reynolds WM: *Reynolds Child Depression Scale (RCDS)*, Odessa, FL, 1989, Psychological Assessment Resources.

Reynolds Adolescent Depression Scale
Reynolds WM: *Reynolds Adolescent Depression Scale (RADS)*, Odessa, FL, 1987, Psychological Assessment Resources.

Center for Epidemiologic Studies—Depression Scale
Weissman MM, Orvaschel H, Padian N: Children's symptom and social functioning self-report scales: comparison of mothers' and children's reports, *J Nerv Ment Dis* 168:736-740, 1980.

Depression Self-Rating Scale
Birleson P: *Depression Self-Rating Scale (DS-RS)*, Royal Children's Hospital, Fleminton Road, Parkville, Victoria 3052, Australia.

programs are essential. Family-oriented therapies have been the most clinically researched, with family treatment, not family psychoeducation or family support groups, revealed as superior to other modalities (Weinberg et al, 1998). Follow-up assessments should include substance use issues, as well as other predictors of use: stress or negative life events, depression or negative affect regulation, and the presence of positive support within or outside of the family. Self-help or 12-step groups are thought to be an essential element in the recovery process.

NURSING DIAGNOSES RELATED TO THE COPING/STRESS TOLERANCE: *Functional Health Pattern*

Diagnoses are related to the following concepts: posttrauma responses, rape-trauma, fear, anxiety, sorrow, denial, adjustment, coping, self-mutilation, violence.

- Anticipatory grieving
- Anxiety
- Chronic sorrow
- Compromised family coping
  - Disabled family coping
  - Readiness for enhanced family coping
- Defensive coping
- Depressive episode (DSM-IV diagnosis)
- Dysfunctional grieving
- Fear
- Impaired adjustment
- Ineffective coping
  - Readiness for enhanced coping
- Ineffective community coping
- Readiness for enhanced community coping
- Ineffective denial
- Rape-trauma syndrome
- Relocation stress syndrome
- Risk for suicide
- Risk for violence (other-directed or self-directed)
- Self-mutilation
  - Risk for self-mutilation
- Substance misuse/abuse (not a NANDA diagnosis)

From North American Nursing Diagnosis Association: *NANDA nursing diagnoses: definitions and classification 2003-2004*, Philadelphia. 2003, North American Nursing Diagnosis Association.

REFERENCES

Akin LK: Pediatric and adolescent bipolar disorder: medical resources, *Medical Reference Services Quarterly* 20:31-44, 2001.

American Academy of Child and Adolescent Psychiatry: Practice parameters for the assessment and treatment of children and adolescents with substance use disorders, *J Am Acad Child Adolesc Psychiatry* 36(suppl):140S-156S, 1997.

American Academy of Child and Adolescent Psychiatry: Practice parameters for the assessment and treatment of children and adolescents with PTSD, *J Am Acad Child Adolesc Psychiatry* 37(10S):4S-26S, 1998a.

American Academy of Child and Adolescent Psychiatry: Summary of the practice parameters for the assessment and treatment of children and adolescents with depressive disorders, 1998b. Available at *www.aacap.org* (accessed Nov 7, 2003).

American Academy of Pediatrics, Committee on Psychosocial Aspects of Child and Family Health: The pediatrician and childhood bereavement, *Pediatrics* 105:445-447, 2000.

American Psychiatric Association: *Diagnostic and statistical manual of mental disorders*, ed 4, Washington, DC, 1994, American Psychiatric Association.

Bardone AM et al: Adult physical health outcomes of adolescent girls with conduct disorder, depression, and anxiety, *J Am Acad Child Adolesc Psychiatry* 37:594-601, 1998.

Barrett PM, Dadds MR, Rapee RM: Family treatment of childhood anxiety: a controlled trial, *J Consult Clin Psychol* 64:333-342, 1996.

Barrett PM et al: Cognitive-behavioral treatment of anxiety disorders in children: long-term (6-year) follow-up, *J Consult Clin Psychol* 69:135-141, 2001.

Barrios B, Hartmann C : Fears and anxieties. In Mash E, Terdal L, editors: *Behavioral assessment of childhood disorders*, ed 2, New York, 1988, Guilford Press.

Bates JE: Concepts and measures of temperament. In Kohnstamm GA, Bates JE, Rothbart MK, editors: *Temperament in childhood*, Chichester, England, 1989, Wiley.

Bates JE et al: Interaction of temperamental resistance to control and restrictive parenting in the development of externalizing behavior, *Dev Psychol* 34:982-995,1998.

Birmaher B et al: Childhood and adolescent depression: a review of the past 10 years, part I, *J Am Acad Child Adolesc Psychiatry* 35:1427-1439, 1996.

Birmaher B et al: Clinical outcome after short-term psychotherapy for adolescents with major depressive disorder, *Arch Gen Psychiatry* 57:29-36, 2000.

Bowden CL, Rhodes LJ: Mania in children and adolescents: recognition and treatment, *Psychiatric Ann* 26 (suppl): 430-434, 1996.

Brent DA et al: Compliance with recommendations to remove firearms in families participating in a clinical trial for adolescent depression, *J Am Acad Child Adolesc Psychiatry* 39:1220-1226, 2000.

Brown RL et al: A two-item screening test for alcohol and other drug problems, *J Fam Pract* 44:151-160, 1997.

Burke JD, Loeber R, Birmaher B: Oppositional defiant disorder and conduct disorder: a review of the past 10 years, part II, *J Am Acad Child Adolesc Psychiatry* 41:1275-1293, 2002.

Buss A, Plomin R: *Temperament: early developing personality traits*, Hillside, NJ, 1984, Erlbaum.

Carey WB: Let's give temperament its due, *Contemp Pediatr* 15:91-113, 1998.

Caspi A et al: Behavioral observations at age 3 years predict adult psychiatric disorders: longitudinal evidence from a birth cohort, *Arch Gen Psychiatry* 53:1033-1039, 1996.

Cassidy LJ, Jellinek MS: Approaches to recognition and management of childhood psychiatric disorders in pediatric primary care, *Pediatr Clin North Am* 45:1037-1052, 1998.

Chamberlain P, Rosicky JG: The effectiveness of family therapy in the treatment of adolescents with conduct disorders and delinquency, *J Marital Fam Ther* 21:441-459, 1995.

Chang KD, Steiner H, Ketter TA: Psychiatric phenomenology of child and adolescent bipolar offspring, *J Am Acad Child Adolesc Psychiatry* 39:453-460, 2000.

Chassin L, Pitts SC, Prost J: Binge drinking trajectories from adolescence to emerging adulthood in a high-risk sample: predictors and substance abuse outcomes, *J Consult Clin Psychol* 70:67-78, 2002.

Cheer SM, Figgitt DP: Spotlight on fluvoxamine in anxiety disorders in children and adolescents, *CNS Drugs* 16:139-144, 2002.

Chess S, Thomas A: *Origins and evolutions of behavior disorders*, New York, 1984, Guilford Press.

Clarke GN et al: Cognitive-behavioral treatment of adolescent depression: efficacy of acute group treatment and booster sessions, *J Am Acad Child Adolesc Psychiatry* 38:272-279, 1999.

Cohen JA, Mannarino AP, Rogal S: Treatment practices for childhood posttraumatic disorder, *Child Abuse Negl* 25:123-135, 2001.

Cohen P et al: An epidemiological study of disorders in late childhood and adolescence—I. Age- and gender-specific prevalence, *J Child Psychol Psychiatry* 34:851-867, 1993.

Compas BE et al: Coping with stress during childhood and adolescence: problems, progress, and potential in theory and research, *Psychol Bull* 127:87-127, 2001.

Compton SN, Nelson AH, March JS: Social phobia and separation anxiety symptoms in community and clinical samples of children and adolescents, *J Am Acad Child Adolesc Psychiatry* 39:1040-1046, 2000.

Coyle JT: Drug treatment of anxiety disorders in children, *N Engl J Med* 344:1326-1327, 2001.

Crawford AM, Manassis K: Familial predictors of treatment outcome in childhood anxiety disorders, *J Am Acad Child Adolesc Psychiatry* 40:1182-1189, 2001.

Dashiff CJ: Understanding separation anxiety disorder, *J Child Adolesc Psychiatr Nurs* 8:27-38, 1995.

DeMaso DR, Meyer EC, Beasley PJ: What do I say to my surviving children: emotional and behavioral adjustment following the death of a young family member, *J Am Acad Child Adolesc Psychiatry* 36:1299-1302, 1997.

Dubner AE, Motta RW: Sexually and physically abused foster care children and posttraumatic stress disorder, *J Consult Clin Psychol* 67:367-373, 1999.

Eisenberg N et al: Dispositional emotionality and regulation: their role in predicting quality of social functioning, *J Person Soc Psychol* 78:136-157, 2000.

Eyberg SM, Ross AW: Assessment of child behavior problems: the validation of a new inventory, *J Clin Child Psychol* 7:113-116, 1978.

Fagot B, Leve LD: Teacher ratings of externalizing behavior at school entry for boys and girls: similar early predictors and different correlates, *J Child Psychol Psychiatry* 39:555-566, 1998.

Famularo R et al: Persistence of pediatric posttraumatic stress after two years, *Child Abuse Negl* 20:1245-1248, 1996.

Finke LM, Bowman CA: Factors in childhood drug and alcohol use: a review of the literature, *J Child Adolesc Psychiatr Nurs* 10:29-34, 1997.

Fordham K, Stevenson-Hinde J: Shyness, friendship quality, and adjustment during middle childhood, *J Child Psychol Psychiatry* 40:757-758, 1999.

Foy DW et al: Etiologic factors in the development of posttraumatic stress disorders in children and adolescents, *J Sch Psychol* 34:133-145, 1996.

Geller B: "BPD and ADHD": commentary, *J Am Acad Child Adolesc Psychiatry* 36:720, 1997.

Geller B, Luby J: Child and adolescent bipolar disorder: a review of the past 10 years, *J Am Acad Child Adolesc Psychiatry* 36:1168-1176, 1997.

Geller B et al: Adult psychosocial outcome of prepubertal major depressive disorder, *J Am Acad Child Adolesc Psychiatry* 40:673-677, 2001.

Geller B et al: Diagnostic characteristics of 93 prepubertal and early adolescent bipolar disorder phenotype by gender, puberty and comorbid attention deficit hyperactivity disorder, *J Child Adolesc Psychopharm* 10:157-164, 2000.

Grados MA, Riddle MA: Pharmacological treatment of chilhood obsessive-compulsive disorder: from theory to practice, *J Clin Child Psychol* 30:67-79, 2001.

Heyman RB, Adger H: Office approach to drug abuse prevention, *Pediatr Clin North Am* 44:1447-1455, 1997.

Houck GM, LeCuyer-Maus EA: Maternal limit-setting patterns and toddler development of self-concept and social competence, *Issues Compr Pediatr Nurs* 25:21-41, 2001.

Houck GM, LeCuyer-Maus EA: Maternal limit-setting during toddlerhood, and delay of gratification and behavior problems at age five, *Inf Ment Health J*, 2003 (in press).

Houck GM, Stember L: Small group experience for socially withdrawn girls, *J Sch Nurs* 18:206-211, 2002.

Jellinek M, Patel BP, Froehle MC, editors: *Bright Futures in practice: mental health*, vol 1, *Practice guide*, Arlington, VA, 2002, National Center for Education in Maternal and Child Health.

Jellineck MS, Murphy JM: Screening for psychosocial disorders in pediatric practice, *Am J Dis Child* 142:1153-1157, 1997.

Jellinek MS, Snyder JB: Depression and suicide in children and adolescents, *Pediatr Rev* 19:255-264, 1998.

Kasen S et al: Childhood depression and adult personality disorder: alternative pathways of continuity, *Arch Gen Psychiatry* 58:231-236, 2001.

Kazdin AE: Practitioner review: psychosocial treatments for conduct disorder in children, *J Child Psychol Psychiatry* 38:161-178, 1997.

Keenan K, Wakschlag L: Can a valid diagnosis of disruptive behavior disorder be made in preschool children? *Am J Psychiatry* 159:351-358, 2002.

Keller MB et al: Efficacy of paroxetine in the treatment of adolescent major depression: a randomized, controlled trial, *J Am Acad Child Adolesc Psychiatry* 40:762-772, 2001.

Kendall PC, Brady EU, Verduin TL: Comorbidity in childhood anxiety disorders and treatment outcome, *J Am Acad Child Adolesc Psychiatry* 40:787-794, 2001.

King NJ, Ollendick TH: Treatment of childhood phobias, *J Child Psychol Psychiatry Allied Disciplines* 38:389-400, 1997.

Kolko DJ et al: Cognitive and family therapies for adolescent depression: treatment specificity, mediation, and moderation, *J Consult Clin Psychol* 68:603-614, 2000.

Kovacs M, Devlin B: Internalizing disorders in childhood, *J Child Psychol Psychiatry Allied Disciplines* 39:47-63, 1998.

LeCuyer-Maus EA, Houck GM: Mother-toddler interaction and the development of self-regulation in a limit-setting context, *J Pediatr Nurs* 17:184-200, 2002.

Leonard HL et al: Obsessive-compulsive disorders and related conditions, *Pediatr Ann* 30:154-160, 2001.

Loeber R et al: Oppositional defiant and conduct disorder: a review of the past 10 years, part I, *J Am Acad Child Adolesc Psychiatry* 39:1468-1484, 2000.

Lombardo GT: BPD and ADHD, *J Am Acad Child Adolesc Psychiatry* 36:719-720, 1997.

Masi G, Mucci N, Millepiedi S: Separation anxiety disorder in children and adolescents: epidemiology, diagnosis and management, *CNS Drugs* 15:93-104, 2001.

Mazza JJ: The relationship between posttraumatic stress symptomatology and suicidal behavior in school-based adolescents, *Suicide Life Threat Behav* 30:91-103, 2000.

Mendlowitz SL et al: Cognitive-behavioral group treatments in childhood anxiety disorders: the role of parental involvement, *J Am Acad Child Adolesc Psychiatry* 38:1223-1229, 1999.

Mesman J, Koot HM: Child-reported depression and anxiety in preadolescence: II. Preschool predictors, *J Am Acad Child Adolesc Psychiatry* 39(11):1379-1786, 2000.

Mesman J, Koot HM: Common and specific correlates of preadolescent internalizing and externalizing psychopathology, *J Abnorm Psychol* 109:428-437, 2002.

Myers K, Winters NC: Ten-year review of rating scales. II. Scales for internalizing disorders, *J Am Acad Child Adolesc Psychiatry* 41:634-659, 2002.

National Institute of Mental Health: Depression in children and adolescents: a fact sheet for physicians (NIH pub no 00-4744), 2000. Available at *www.nimh.nih.gov/publicat/depchildresfact.cfm* (accessed July 10, 2001).

Obeidallah DA, McHale SM, Silbereisen RK: Gender role socialization and adolescents' reports of depression: why some girls and not others? *J Youth Adolesc* 25:775-785, 1996.

Prior M et al: Does shy-inhibited temperament in childhood lead to anxiety problems in adolescence? *J Am Acad Child Adolesc Psychiatry* 39:461-468, 2000.

Pullen LM, Modrcin-McCarthy MA, Graf EV: Adolescent depression: important facts that matter, *J Child Adolesc Psychiatr Nurs* 13:69-75, 2000.

Rapoport JL et al: Childhood obsessive-compulsive disorder in the NIMH MECA study: parent versus child identification of cases, *J Anxiety Disord* 14(6):535-548, 2000.

Rapoport JL, Inoff-Germain G: Tourette syndrome. Medical and surgical treatment of obsessive-compulsive disorder, *Neurol Clin* 15:421-428, 1997.

Riley AW et al: Social role functioning by adolescents with psychiatric disorders, *J Am Acad Child Adolesc Psychiatry* 37:620-628, 1998.

Rohde P et al: Impact of comorbidity on a cognitive-behavioral group treatment for adolescent depression, *J Am Acad Child Adolesc Psychiatry* 40:795-802, 2001.

Rothbart MK: Temperament and development. In Kohnstamm GA, Bates JE, Rothbart MK, editors: *Temperament in childhood,* Chichester, England, 1989, Wiley.

Rubin KH et al: The consistency and concomitants of inhibition: some of the children, all of the time, *Child Dev* 68:467-483, 1997.

Sandberg S et al: Independence of childhood life events and chronic adversities: a comparison of two patient groups and controls, *J Am Acad Child Adolesc Psychiatry* 37:728-735, 1998.

Scheering MS et al: Two approaches to diagnosing posttraumatic stress disorder in infancy and early childhood, *J Am Acad Child Adolesc Psychiatry* 34:191-200, 1995.

Shoaf T, Emslie G, Mayes T: Childhood depression: diagnosis and treatment strategies in general pediatrics, *Pediatr Ann* 30:130-136, 2001.

Silove D, Manicavasagar V, Drobny J: Associations between juvenile and adult forms of separation anxiety disorder: a study of adult volunteers with histories of school refusal, *J Nerv Ment Dis* 190:413-415, 2002.

Streleau J: *Temperament, personality, activity,* New York, 1983, Academic press.

Svetaz M, Ireland M, Blum R: Adolescents with learning disabilities: risk and longitudinal study of adolescent health, *J Adolesc Health* 27:340-348, 2000.

Terr LC: Children traumatized in small groups. In Eth S, Pynoos RS, editors: *Posttraumatic stress disorder in children,* Washington, DC, 1991, American Psychiatric Press.

Thomas A, Chess S: *Temperament and development,* New York, 1977, Brunner-Mazel.

Thomsen AH et al: Parent reports of coping and stress responses in children with recurrent abdominal pain, *J Pediatr Psychol* 27:215-226, 2002.

Tubman JG et al: Temperament and adjustment in young adulthood: a 15-year longitudinal analysis, *Am J Orthopsychiatry* 62:564-574, 1993.

Tweed SH: Intervening in adolescent substance abuse, *Nurs Clin North Am* 33:29-45, 1998.

US Department of Health and Human Services: *Healthy people 2010,* 2000. Available at *www.health.gov/healthy people/* (accessed June 2000).

Valleni-Basile LA et al: Frequency of obsessive-compulsive disorder in a community sample of young adolescents, *J Am Acad Child Adolesc Psychiatry* 33:782-791, 1994.

Webster-Stratton C, Hammond M: Treating children with early-onset conduct problems: a comparison of child and parent training interventions, *J Consult Clin Psychol* 64:93-109, 1997.

Weinberg NZ et al: Adolescent substance abuse: a review of the past 10 years, *J Am Acad Child Adolesc Psychiatry* 37:252-26, 1998.

Weissman MM et al: Offspring of depressed parents, *Arch Gen Psychiatry* 54:932-940, 1997.

Williams T, Hodgman C: Medication for the management of anxiety disorders in children and adolescents, *Pediatr Ann* 30:146-153, 2001.

Wolk SI, Weissman MM: Suicidal behavior in depressed children grown up: preliminary results of a longitudinal study, *Psychiatr Ann* 26:331-335, 1996.

22 Values and Beliefs

Ardys M. Dunn

This functional health pattern examines values and beliefs and their impact on health. Increasingly, health care providers are aware of and actively investigating the ways in which beliefs, especially related to religion and spirituality, affect the health of individuals (Barnes et al, 2000; Boudreaux, O'Hea, & Chasuk, 2002; McEvoy, 2000; O'Hara, 2002). The nurse practitioner's (NP's) role is to assess social, cultural, and spiritual dimensions of the values and beliefs of children and their families; determine the impact of values and beliefs on health care decisions; and identify means to support those values, beliefs, and actions that promote health.

STANDARDS OF PRACTICE

Primary care providers are expected to give comprehensive care, which includes examining and treating all aspects of the individual—physical, emotional, psychosocial, and spiritual. Health care in the United States, however, has tended to focus on physical health and illness rather than integrate mental and emotional health. There are few guidelines for incorporating spiritual issues into care; this is especially true in the care of children.

The American Medical Association's (AMA's) *Guidelines for Adolescent Preventive Services (GAPS)* (Elster & Kuznets, 1994) includes the following points related to values and beliefs:

1. Preventive services should be appropriate for age and development and sensitive to individual and sociocultural differences.
2. All adolescents should receive health guidance annually to promote a better understanding of their physical growth, their psychosocial and psychosexual development, and the importance of being actively involved in decisions regarding their health care.
3. All adolescents should be asked annually about behaviors or emotions that indicate recurrent or severe depression or risk of suicide.

The U.S. Preventive Services Task Force (1996) does not set specific standards for values and beliefs. However, the Task Force does place emphasis on the importance of being alert to behavioral disorders, parent and family dysfunction, signs of child abuse or neglect, abnormal bereavement, and, among adolescents, depressive symptoms and suicide risk factors. Problems in these areas may reflect dysfunction or inappropriate development of values and beliefs.

The Spiritual and Child Health Initiative developed by the Department of Pediatrics, Boston Medical Center and Medical Anthropology (Barnes et al, 2000), has articulated guidelines for practice, suggesting that providers

- Anticipate patients will have spiritual or religious concerns
- Develop a self-awareness of their own spiritual and religious history and perspective
- Become broadly familiar with the religious worldview of the patient groups for whom they care
- Work with individual families and children to learn their specific values and beliefs
- Develop strategic interviewing skills
- Develop a resource list and network of local consultants
- Refer patients to appropriate spiritual care providers

These guidelines emphasize the importance of including discussions of spiritual and religious concerns in the provider-patient interaction, primarily in an effort to reach understanding, not necessarily agreement. Assessment of the patient and family should include this dimension because, based on the ethical principle of beneficence, providers have "a responsibility to be aware of and supportive of beliefs that are important to a patient in coping with his or her illness" (Boudreaux, O'Hea, & Chasuk, 2002). Issues of spiritual beliefs may be particularly important for families facing illnesses that seem unfair or that have no reasonable explanation.

NORMAL PATTERNS OF BEHAVIOR

Values and Beliefs: Definitions and Relationship to Behavior

Values have been defined as perceptions held about the worth or importance of a certain thing, person, or idea. Beliefs are attitudes representing whether one holds something to be true. Values and beliefs influence actions, both consciously and unconsciously. They are guides that individuals use as they make decisions. Values and beliefs are learned phenomena, and recognition and acceptance of shared values and beliefs are fundamental to the integrity of the individual, the family, and the social group (see Chapter 4). Although perceptions, attitudes, values, and beliefs are transmitted from one generation to another, they remain open to change and are responsive to social contexts and situations. Values clarification is the process by which one examines behavior in light of values and changing circumstances and asks why a certain action is taken or whether that action is consistent with the values one claims to have. Change in values, beliefs, and behavior can result from the process of values clarification.

Expected Patterns of Behavior Related to Values and Beliefs

The values and beliefs that children have are related to their developmental stage and are reflected in different behaviors at different ages. In general, healthy behaviors are expressions of positive values. In particular, the development of moral integrity, or conscience and spirituality, or faith, is expected of the healthy child.

As they develop moral and spiritual values, healthy children achieve a positive sense of self, internalize the cultural values and beliefs related to their social group, learn to value themselves and their contribution to the family and larger social system, and feel a sense of understanding and belonging to their community. Chapter 18 discusses stages and factors influencing the development of healthy self-perception in children. See Chapter 4 for a discussion of the cultural dynamics that occur as children grow within the context of family, cultural group, and society. This chapter examines the definition, assessment, and management of moral and spiritual development.

Children's responses to illness are also related to their values and beliefs. Research on adults indicates that there is a direct, though not necessarily causal, relationship between religiosity and health (Boudreaux, O'Hea, & Chasuk, 2002; Levin, 1994). A recent study of children with cystic fibrosis revealed that children, too, use a number of religious/spiritual strategies to cope with their illness (Pendleton et al, 2002). Having a spiritual foundation appears to strengthen a child's coping abilities.

Development of Moral Integrity or Conscience

Moral integrity involves demonstrating an understanding of right and wrong; engaging in reflection on ethical issues of justice and fairness; and expressing a sense of responsibility to oneself, others, and the environment. The development of moral integrity is enhanced if children believe that they and their contributions to the family and community are valued; if they are rewarded emotionally, psychologically, and intellectually for their participation in the community; and if their peer groups support positive behavior. Simply stated, children must believe that they make a difference and have a future.

Moral judgment is also dependent on the developmental stage of children. Developmental theorists have presented several perspectives on moral development in children:

- Freud asserted that children develop a conscience through identification with a significant caregiver and the processes of guilt and shame.
- Piaget claimed that children's moral development parallels their intellectual development and ability to reason.
- Kohlberg theorized that moral development proceeds sequentially through phases related to intellectual development and social interactions.
- Social learning theory states that positive role modeling teaches moral behavior.
- Developmental theories suggest that younger children have little sense of right and wrong and are often concrete in their thinking, whereas older children and adolescents are more likely to be reflective as they examine moral dilemmas, and they are able to articulate and understand motivation or conditions that influence behavior.

The variability of moral reasoning, based on cognition and developmental stages, is evident in the complex stage model or Defining Issues Test (DIT) developed at the University of Minnesota (Thoma, 2002). Other theorists have suggested that gender plays a significant role in the way children interpret situations and make choices based on moral judgment (Gilligan, 1990), and that even very young children demonstrate a moral awareness, though it is primarily experiential rather than reflective (Johansson, 2001).

Development of Spirituality

Spirituality has been defined as a unifying force that gives meaning to life, or "the feelings, thoughts, experiences, and behaviors that arise from a search for the sacred" (Larson,

TABLE 22-1 *Characteristics of Spirituality*

Inner Resources and Identity	Those who possess inner resources have a sense of wholeness, competence, and direction. They are capable of responding to crises or turmoil and draw on inner strengths to maintain a sense of stability and control.
Interconnectedness	Interconnectedness is the sense of being an integral part of the world, attached to others, to one's environment, and to a universal or supreme being.
Purpose or Meaning of Life	A sense of direction and meaning and a reason for existence are developed in the relationships individuals have with others and their world.
Transcendence	The ability to go beyond, or transcend, the experiences of daily life is evident in the expression of hope, meaning, and direction when an individual is faced with fear, inability to effect change, uncertainty, and ambiguity.

From Howden J: Development and psychometric characteristics of the Spirituality Assessment Scale, *Dissertation Abstracts International* 54, 1993, p 166.

Swyers, & McCullough, 1997). It is the acceptance of a nonmaterial higher power that encompasses all of life's affairs and is mediated through the individual's relationships to others, to the community, and to the environment. Although integral to religion, spirituality should not be confused with religious activities, rituals, and behaviors. Characteristics of spirituality are listed in Table 22-1 (Howden, 1993).

The development of spirituality in children has been conceived as paralleling cognitive and moral development. Table 22-2 presents that relationship and outlines age-specific interventions to enhance healthy growth (Stilwell et al, 1998; Walker, Hennig, & Krettenauer, 2000; Wolf, 2000). Infants and toddlers are engaged in the process of establishing autonomy or separateness of self from the parent, and becoming a part of a bigger culture (i.e., the family). Preschool and early school-age children gain an understanding of the meaning of life through fantasy play, active engagement with their environment, strong attachments to their parents, and growing relationships with their peers. Although they have achieved the task of defining themselves as separate individuals, their thinking and behavior in relation to faith issues is still an expression of the family's faith and practice. School-age children and adolescents define life's meaning within the context of their "self-sufficiency, competence, and role differentiation," and in their relationship to both peers and adults. Children at this age need to explore their understanding of the ultimate questions in life (Pasupathi, Staudinger, & Baltes, 2001). They are interested in issues such as life, death, war, evil, good, and creation, and develop wisdom as they discuss and think about these important matters.

ASSESSMENT

The goals of assessing values and beliefs include the following:

- Determine the nature of the child's and family's belief system.
- Identify ways that the family interacts to support these beliefs.
- Clarify how beliefs affect decisions and behaviors related to health care.

Because children are in the process of developing values and beliefs and because much of their development depends on their interaction with the parent or caregiver, assessment questions are often directed to or focused on the parent or caregiver.

Measures of spirituality are necessarily subjective, and spirituality is often included in the psychosocial assessment. Although as yet not validated by research, several models have been proposed for the assessment of spirituality. One model uses the mnemonic HOPE to focus clinical questions on the client's sources of **H**ope, peace, and comfort; participation in **O**rganized religion; **P**ersonal spiritual practices; and the **E**ffect these behaviors have on the client's medical care or end-of-life decisions (Anandarajah & Hight, 2001). Another model of collecting a spiritual history uses the mnemonic BELIEF: **B**elief system; **E**thics or values; **L**ifestyle behaviors (e.g., diet, rituals); **I**nvolvement in a spiritual community; religious **E**ducation; and **F**uture events, especially decisions about health that will be affected by religious beliefs (McEvoy, 2000). The Complementary Medicine Research Institute (2002) has developed the Spirituality Assessment Scale,

TABLE 22-2 *Developmental Outcomes and Appropriate Interventions Related to Values and Beliefs*

Area of Development	Infant (0-12 mo)	Toddler and Preschooler (1-5 yr)	School-Age Child (6-12 yr)	Adolescent
Moral integrity and conscience (right and wrong; sense of responsibility to oneself, others, and the environment)	Develops sense of trust in caregivers (Erikson, 1963); learns to adjust to family routine (e.g., sleeping, eating)	Believes rules are absolute; behaves well for fear of punishment or to receive rewards (Kohlberg, 1969); develops sense of autonomy, initiative, and purpose; differentiates self from others (Erikson, 1963)	Believes rules exist to keep order and protect people and that everyone benefits from them; behaves well to please others, to avoid guilt, and to maintain status of "good" child (Kohlberg, 1969); develops sense of industry, faith in self-competence; explores, creates, collects; understands cause and effect (Erikson, 1963)	Rules are based on ethical judgment; believes individual answers to personal conscience, has moral obligation to a social contract; behaves to maintain respect of self, peers, and larger community (Kohlberg, 1969); integrates personality and develops sense of identity, loyalty to group and significant others (Erikson, 1963)
Faith development	Primal or undifferentiated faith (Fowler, 1980); faith is trust (Aden, 1976); primary caregivers represent superordinate beings; infant develops object permanence, sense of trust, attachment, and sense of being nurtured	Intuitive-projective faith based on images, feelings, and symbols (Fowler, 1980); faith as courage and obedience: younger child learns to let go and take hold in order to affirm self, and older child develops more realistic perspective of self in relation to others, learns to balance self desires with demands of others; egocentric thinking may contribute to misconceptions; child begins to participate in family's religious practices and rituals	Mythic-literal faith, with concrete beliefs, rigid system of order and activities (Fowler, 1980); faith as assent, as child learns to master environment and become competent (Aden, 1976); child begins to explore ultimate issues, develop understanding of the meaning of life, develop and express moral decision making	Synthetic convention stage—ideas about spirituality are synthesized from peers, parents, and other significant adults, and life experiences (Fowler, 1980); faith as identity (Aden, 1976) as child seeks identity, understanding of self in the world; child demonstrates self-reflection, insight, sense of inner spiritual process and presence in the world, and continues to more fully develop understanding of ultimate questions, life's meaning
Experienced faith (infancy through early adolescence)	Children experience faith through relationships with others and others' faith traditions			

Affiliative faith (late adolescence)				Adolescent actively participates in a faith community, feels a sense of belonging, awe, and wonder; acknowledges authority of faith community
Parental Interventions to Foster Healthy Development				
	Respond to infant's physiologic and emotional needs promptly and adequately; demonstrate loving, gentle approach in communication and interaction	Treat child with respect and acceptance; set realistic limits on behavior; remove temptation from environment; provide positive role model; provide guided opportunities to interact with adults and other children as well as active play alone; be patient; involve child in family religious practices; begin to establish regular tasks for child in family activities	Treat child with respect and acceptance; set realistic limits on behavior; provide opportunities for active play alone and with other children; encourage group activity; allow children to make decisions as appropriate, helping them to explore meanings of feelings, events, and interactions; choose stories related to children's experience of moral dilemmas to explore right and wrong; regular tasks for child as member of family are established	Treat adolescent with respect and acceptance; set realistic limits on behavior; enforce family's moral standards; encourage involvement in family activities; allow children to make more of own choices regarding values and beliefs; allow experimentation in dress, hair, makeup as child develops sense of self; do not overreact to adolescent "crises," provide opportunities to discuss values, ethics, and moral behavior; provide support and encouragement for successes and failures in school, social, athletic, and work activities

primarily focused at adults, but which could be helpful for parents to complete. As the relationship between spirituality and health is investigated further, more valid and reliable measures are likely to be developed. The following discussion provides guidelines incorporating elements from these models for assessment in the primary care setting; questions should elicit information about the individual's subjective perceptions, as well as objective religious practices.

History

Moral Integrity or Conscience

The following points can guide the assessment:

- How does the child define right and wrong? How does the child's behavior reflect his or her moral understanding?
- What are family attitudes about right and wrong?
- How are parents teaching the child about right and wrong?
- What other influences affect the child's concept of right and wrong (e.g., day care, teachers and counselors, peer group)?
- How do parents set limits on the child's behavior?
- How does the child respond to discipline and limits?
- What messages do parents give about the value and importance of the child's contribution to the family and the community?
- What opportunities do parents give the child to make independent, age-appropriate decisions?
- What traditions and activities does the family have? How is the child included in these activities?

Spirituality

The following information should be identified in relation to spirituality:

General

- Tell me about your religious beliefs related to the following issues:
  - Family relations, gender roles, and children's and parents' responsibilities
  - Sexuality issues (e.g., homosexuality, premarital sex)
  - Dietary restrictions
  - Rituals (e.g., at mealtime or bedtime)
  - Use of drugs, alcohol, or tobacco
  - Medical treatment

Inner Resources and Identity

- What are your child's goals in life? Your family's goals?
- What are your child's strong points? Your family's strong points?
- What do you like about yourself? Your child? Your family?
- How important is faith in your child's life? In your life?
- What brings you, your child, and your family joy and peace? Where do you find hope and comfort?

Interconnectedness

- How do you feel about your child? About yourself? About your family?
- What do you do as a family to show love for each other?
- Who are significant people in your child's and your family's life?
- Whom do you ask for support when your family needs help?
- How do members of your family share feelings with others?
- Do you feel that you and your family are part of a community? Of a larger world or universe?
- Does the family belong to a religious or spiritual group?

Purpose or Meaning of Life

- What are your family's religious and cultural beliefs? What ethics or values are important in your family's life?
- What gives life meaning? What is the most important thing in life?
- How does your family express religious and cultural beliefs? How is your child involved?
- What religious rituals or practices contribute to a sense of spiritual fulfillment or peace?
- How do you teach your child about values and beliefs? How else does your child learn about values and beliefs?
- Are you comfortable talking about your beliefs with your child?

Transcendence

- How do members of your family deal with spiritual distress during a crisis?

Physical Examination

Observe the child's behavior, especially noting interaction with parents, other adults, and peers. The child exhibits the following behavior:

- Appears at ease, although behavior may vary (e.g., shy, quiet, active, talkative, engaging) depending on developmental level and temperament
- Responds to parent or caregiver cues; follows directions and conforms to limits set without demonstrating guilt or fear of punishment
- Shares toys
- Respects people and property
- Is not physically aggressive
- Is able to articulate moral reasoning (older child)
- Is able to articulate a faith statement, depending on spiritual, religious, and cultural background (older child)

MANAGEMENT OF NORMAL PATTERNS

Parents should function in the following ways:

- Be a loving, responsive, and accepting presence in their children's lives.
- Set realistic standards or limits for right and wrong behavior.
- State what is acceptable and what is unacceptable behavior.
- Provide a rationale for limits set; the explanation varies depending on the cognitive and developmental level of the child.
- Articulate personal values, beliefs, and faith statements for the child. Give clear, age-appropriate explanations of God and spiritual lessons.
- Be a role model for constructive and positive behavior.
- Give reinforcements for positive behavior and for attempts at positive behavior.
- Hold children accountable for negative behavior.
- Teach children strategies to avoid misbehavior; teach constructive coping skills.
- Use creative parenting strategies (e.g., distraction, diversional activities) to help children avoid misbehavior.
- Provide a developmentally appropriate environment to minimize children's misbehavior. It is usually easier to remove a breakable object from a table than to keep saying no or to discipline a child for breaking it.
- Provide opportunities for children to make age-appropriate decisions independently.
- Praise children in front of others.
- Do not give false praise.
- Articulate and reinforce messages that children belong and are valued for themselves, not just for their behaviors.
- Establish family traditions and projects that actively involve children (e.g., family outings, family value sessions, during which family members share a meal with directed conversation). Do not expect perfection.
- Involve children in the family's religious and cultural practices.
- Provide opportunities for the child to explore moral and ethical dilemmas and to develop possible solutions.
- Discuss moral and spiritual implications of events in the child's life (e.g., death of a grandparent, birth of a sibling, sharing, stealing, violence portrayed in media)

Nurse practitioners should do the following:

- Be aware of their own values and beliefs.
- Distinguish between moral and medical advice. Be willing to offer both, while recognizing that personal proselytizing is inappropriate in the provider-patient relationship.
- Recognize and appreciate differences between own and client's values.
- Provide an opportunity for parents to express values and beliefs and to discuss their child's moral and spiritual development.
- Provide information about parenting strategies, discipline, and effective communication between child and parents.
- Assist parents and child in values clarification as appropriate.
- Provide a role model of positive behavior.
- Offer an understanding, compassionate, and accepting presence.
- Modify the treatment plan as appropriate to meet spiritual needs.
- Refer the family for religious or spiritual counseling as indicated or requested.

ALTERED PATTERNS

Lack of Moral Integrity

Description

Although lack of moral integrity is not a clinically defined condition, some children demonstrate a lack of an age-appropriate capacity to respect others or the environment, to judge behavior as right or wrong, and to express empathy or remorse.

Etiology

The complexity of moral judgment makes it likely that a multitude of factors contribute to poor moral reasoning and antisocial behaviors. Research indicates that moral reasoning is related to children's interaction with parents and peers (Walker, Hennig, & Krettenauer, 2000). Moral development, based on a protective spirituality, is enhanced when children have positive adult-child interactions, characterized by respect, acceptance, value, and active participation of the children (Haight, 1998; Sutherland et al, 1997). Failure to treat children in this manner may contribute to lack of moral reasoning. Research also indicates that children whose mothers used power-assertive discipline (e.g., critical comments and physical coercion) tend to show less guilt when confronted with a hypothetical moral dilemma (Kochanska et al, 2002) and have more child conduct problems (Webster-Stratton, Reid, & Hammond, 2001).

Clinical Findings

Many behaviors seen are typical of normal children, depending on developmental and cognitive levels (e.g., lying, hitting, refusing to share), but the child expresses little or no remorse for negative behavior and demonstrates no internalization of a sense of justice, fairness, or right and wrong.

Differential Diagnosis

Attention-deficit hyperactivity disorder, conduct disorder, oppositional defiant disorder, and depression are differential diagnoses.

Management

In addition to strategies listed here, see the earlier discussion of management strategies for normal moral development. In extreme cases, referral for psychiatric management may be necessary.

- Tell stories to younger children.
- Use storytelling to explore moral and ethical issues (Binnendyk & Schonert-Reichl, 2002).
- Encourage interaction with older children who demonstrate higher levels of moral reasoning (Leman, 2002).
- Watch films and discuss books with adolescents.
- Assist child in values clarification process.

Complications

Antisocial behavior and delinquency are behavioral disorders in which lack of moral integrity is a key component.

Spiritual Distress

Description

Spiritual distress is "a disruption in the life principle that pervades a person's entire being and that integrates and transcends one's biological and psychosocial nature" (North American Nursing Diagnosis Association [NANDA], 2003). For children, issues of death and dying and serious illness are major reasons for seeking spiritual counsel. They are fearful and threatened, and often ask "why?" Comprehensive care involves support of a child's—and the family's—spirituality in order to prevent spiritual distress (Pfund, 2000).

Etiology

Because of the complex nature of spirituality, spiritual distress can result from a number of factors. These factors challenge the child's or family's belief system or contribute to separation from spiritual ties and can include the following:

- Trauma or violence
- Loss of significant other, especially parent or sibling
- Debilitating disease
- Chronic disease
- Separation of child from his or her family
- Recommended medical therapies in conflict with child's or family's religious or spiritual beliefs (e.g., Christian Science)
- Barriers in health care setting to practicing spiritual rituals
- Beliefs of health care providers, family members, or peers that conflict with those of child or parent

Clinical Findings

The following may be seen in spiritual distress:

- Depressive behavior (may be suicidal)
- Withdrawal
- No participation in usual religious practices
- Disparaging family's spiritual beliefs and values
- Questioning one's own value, meaning, and purpose of life
- Expressions of anger, resentment, fear of God, suffering, death
- Expressions of inner conflict and doubts about beliefs
- Expressions of sense of spiritual emptiness
- Sleep disturbance
- Behavior changes with mood swings
- Request for spiritual assistance

Differential Diagnosis

Depression, poor coping mechanisms, conduct disorders, and antisocial behavior are differential diagnoses for spiritual distress.

Management

The NP should take the following management steps:

- Identify situational factors that contribute to distress.
- Consult with parents as appropriate to identify family values and belief system.
- Assist parents to help their child process experiences contributing to distress. Referral may be necessary in cases in which child is experiencing significant psychologic trauma. An integrated team composed of psychologist, clergy, and parish nurse can be appropriate.
- Encourage child to participate in spiritual practices as desired.
- Encourage child to express feelings about spiritual distress.
- Encourage child to talk about beliefs and understandings of stressors such as death and illness.
- Answer questions honestly, according to the child's age and developmental level.
- Advocate for the child and parent when they express beliefs in conflict with those of other health care providers or other family members.

If parents refuse treatment for their child:

- Consider use of alternative methods of care.
- Provide opportunity for parents to discuss implications of decision and possible court order for temporary guardian who will give consent to treat the child.
- Provide opportunity for parents to express negative feelings.

NURSING DIAGNOSES RELATED TO VALUES AND BELIEFS: *Functional Health Pattern*

- Spiritual distress
- Readiness for enhanced spiritual well-being

From North American Nursing Diagnosis Association: *NANDA nursing diagnoses: definitions and classification 2003-2004*, Philadelphia, 2003, North American Nursing Diagnosis Association.

Complications

Depression, suicide, and conduct disorders are complications of spiritual distress.

REFERENCES

Aden L: Faith and the developmental cycle, *Pastoral Psychology* 24:215-230, 1976.

Anandarajah G, Hight E: Spirituality and medical practice: using the HOPE questions as a practical tool for spiritual assessment, *Am Fam Physician* 63:81-88, 2001.

Barnes LL et al: Spirituality, religion, and pediatrics: intersecting worlds of healing, *Pediatrics* 106:899-908, 2000.

Binnendyk L, Schonert-Reichl KA: Harry Potter and moral development in pre-adolescent children, *Journal of Moral Education* 31:195-201, 2002.

Boudreaux ED, O'Hea E, Chasuk R: Spiritual role in healing. An alternative way of thinking, *Prim Care* 29:439-454, 2002.

Complementary Medicine Research Institute: Spirituality Assessment Scale. Download available at *www.gbmhealing.org/downloads/spirituality assessment.pdf* (accessed 2002).

Elster AB, Kuznets NJ: *AMA guidelines for adolescent preventive services (GAPS): recommendations and rationale*, Baltimore, 1994, Williams & Wilkins.

Erikson EH: *Childhood and society*, ed 2, New York, 1963, Norton.

Fowler J: Moral stages and the development of faith. In Munsey B, editor: *Moral development, moral education, and Kohlberg*, Birmingham, AL, 1980, Religious Education Press.

Gilligan C: *Mapping the moral domain*, Cambridge, MA, 1990, Harvard University Press.

Haight WL: "Gathering the spirit" at First Baptist Church: spirituality as a protective factor in the lives of African American children, *Soc Work J Natl Assoc Soc Workers* 43:213-221, 1998.

Howden J: Development and psychometric characteristics of the Spirituality Assessment Scale, *Dissertation Abstracts International* 54, 1993, p 166.

Johansson E: Morality in children's worlds—rationality of thought or values emanating from relations? *Studies in Philosophy and Education* 20:345-358, 2001.

Kochanska G et al: Guilt in young children: development, determinants, and relations with a broader system of standards, *Child Dev* 73:461-482, 2002.

Kohlberg L: Stage and sequence: the cognitive-development approach to socialization. In Gastin D, editor: *Handbook of socialization: theory and research*, New York, 1969, Rand McNally.

Larson DB, Swyers JP, McCullough ME: *Scientific research on spirituality and health: a consensus report*, Rockville, MD, 1997, National Institute of Healthcare Research.

Leman PJ: Argument structure, argument content, and cognitive change in children's peer interaction, *J Genet Psychol* 163:40-58, 2002.

Levin JS: Religion and health: is there an association, is it valid, and is it causal? *Soc Sci Med* 38:1475-1482, 1994.

McEvoy M: An added dimension to the pediatric health maintenance visit: the spiritual history, *J Pediatr Health Care* 14:216-220, 2000.

North American Nursing Diagnosis Association: *NANDA nursing diagnoses: definitions and classification 2003-2004*, Philadelphia, 2003, North American Nursing Diagnosis Association.

O'Hara DP: Is there a role for prayer and spirituality in health care? *Med Clin North Am* 86:33-46, 2002.

Pasupathi M, Staudinger UM, Baltes PB: Seeds of wisdom: adolescents' knowledge and judgment about difficult life problems, *Dev Psychol* 37:351-361, 2001.

Pendleton SM et al: Religious/spiritual coping in childhood cystic fibrosis: a qualitative study, *Pediatrics* 109:E8, 2002.

Pfund R: Nurturing a child's spirituality, *J Child Health Care* 4:143-148, 2000.

Stilwell BM et al: Moral volition: the fifth and final domain leading to an integrated theory of conscience understanding, *J Am Acad Child Adolesc Psychiatry* 37:202-210, 1998.

Sutherland MS et al: Strengthening rural youth resiliency through the church, *J Health Educ* 28:205-218, 1997.

Thoma SJ: An overview of the Minnesota approach to research in moral development, *Journal of Moral Education* 31:225-236, 2002.

US Preventive Services Task Force: *Guide to clinical preventive services*, ed 2, Baltimore, 1996, Williams & Wilkins.

Walker LJ, Hennig KH, Krettenauer T: Parent and peer contexts for children's moral reasoning development, *Child Dev* 71:1033-1048, 2000.

Webster-Stratton C, Reid J, Hammond M: Social skills and problem-solving training for children with early-onset conduct problems: who benefits? *J Child Psychol Psychiatry* 42:943-952, 2001.

Wolf AD: How to nurture the spirit in nonsectarian environments, *Young Children* 55:34-36, 2000.

UNIT 4

Approaches to Disease Management

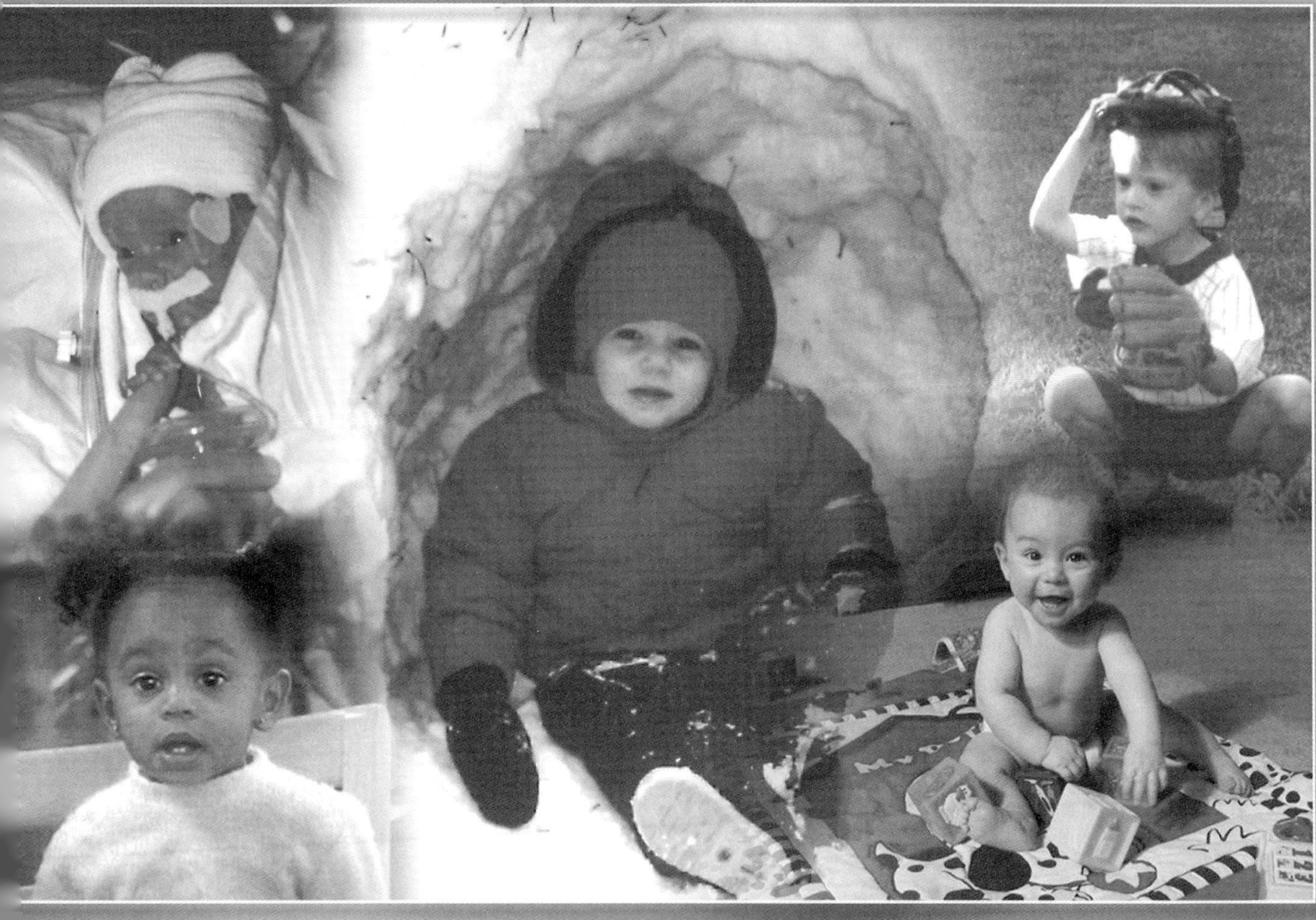

23 Introduction to Disease and Pain Management

Margaret A. Brady

APPROACHES TO ACUTE DISEASE IN CHILDREN

A major role of a primary care provider in pediatrics is to arrive at a diagnosis and to treat common illnesses of childhood with a management plan that is consistent with the community standard of practice. This process begins with a thorough assessment of the child and the presenting complaint. In caring for children with acute illnesses, the nurse practitioner (NP) must always remember that an accurate assessment of the ill child is contingent on the following five points:

1. Careful observation of the child
2. Attention to pertinent positive and negative historical and physical findings
3. Knowledge of physiologic functions and developmental considerations that vary by age
4. Consideration of the trajectory of the problem over time
5. Inclusion of the parents or caretakers and, if appropriate, the child as participants in the evaluation process

When satisfied that these five parameters have been given adequate attention, the NP forms an action or management plan that can include ordering basic laboratory and imaging studies and other special testing, if needed, to arrive at a final diagnosis. Extensive laboratory and other diagnostic tests are often not in the best interest of children, especially for those who would be best served by being referred to a pediatrician or pediatric specialist for diagnosis or treatment of their disease.

NPs are responsible for the assessment and management of children with common pediatric illnesses or conditions. The effectiveness of NPs in primary care is due in large part to their ability to educate patients and their families about the prevention of disease and the management of common illnesses. The patient-parent educational component of the management plan must be individualized but should always include the following essential points:

- Information about the length of time it can take before the child improves and symptoms wane; description of what the course of the disease or illness is likely to be
- Identification of specific signs and symptoms that indicate the need for immediate medical attention or for a return visit sooner than planned (examples for parents include a sick newborn, severe lethargy, tender abdomen, labored breathing, stiff or injured neck, bluish lips, purples "dots" on the skin, severe pain, child who cannot walk, or fever over 105° F [40.6° C])
- Instructions about when to return for a follow-up visit or telephone conference if needed
- Written instructions about any special treatment or therapy that is required
- Careful instructions about medication, both prescription and over-the-counter (OTC) drugs (see Use of Medication, later in this chapter)
- Specific information about any dietary needs or changes, special hydration needs such as electrolyte solutions or increase in fluid intake, plus any changes in eating patterns that can be expected
- Information about the etiology, transmission, and communicability of an infectious disease
- Information about the etiology and recurrence risks of noninfectious illnesses or medical condition
- Information about prevention and recurrence

- Determination of impediments that prevent the parent or the child from complying with the management plan (e.g., limited financial resources, inability to read, dysfunctional family, transportation problems) and discussion about steps to correct these difficulties
- Recognition and discussion of cultural practices and beliefs about illnesses, including the potential benefit or harm from specific folk medicine or complementary practices if used either alone or concurrently with prescribed or OTC medications
- Information for the working parent about resources for sick care in the community, if available in the area and affordable for the parent

In many situations, giving written information to parents about what signs and symptoms to expect with an illness or what warrants further evaluation and a return visit is essential. The NP should always assess the parents' or caregivers' understanding of instructions by asking them to repeat what they have been told. By doing this, any misunderstandings can be addressed. Be sure to have the family's current or contact telephone number in case a telephone contact needs to be made regarding the results of diagnostic tests that come back or to follow up on the child's condition.

It is important to allow time for the natural defense system of the body to fight disease. Premature and excessive pharmacologic therapy can result in needless iatrogenic disease and often serves to confuse the clinical picture. The drug of first choice—the one that is least harmful—should be given time to work. Prematurely changing to a new drug, adding additional drugs, and using more toxic drugs are dangerous practices.

For the most part, parents are alert to subtle changes in their children, so the NP should listen attentively when parents voice concerns about their children. Any sick child who is at high risk because of physical or social problems merits closer observation and follow-up than does the average thriving child who becomes ill. Finally, if the child returns and is not significantly improved or is more symptomatic, the NP should reassess the situation by carefully analyzing the symptoms, investigating problems related to compliance issues, and repeating the physical examination. The NP should rethink the original diagnosis and review likely differential diagnoses before deciding on another management plan.

Management of an ill child also can include a short stay in an outpatient clinic or private office for intravenous hydration, pulmonary therapy, medication, and close observation to determine whether the child's condition stabilizes. Hospitalization might not be needed if the child's condition stabilizes, the parent is reliable, the child can be monitored closely at home, the home has a telephone, and the parent has transportation available to return for follow-up or an emergency visit. However, before discharging an ill infant or child to home rather than admitting the child to the hospital, the NP must carefully assess the parent's ability to cope with a significantly ill child and to identify signs or symptoms of increasing illness.

The number of infants and young children in group day care is expanding as the number of women in the workforce increases. The disease pattern in this cohort of children is often related to group exposure to illnesses. The issue of multiple caregivers can complicate history taking. In these situations, obtaining accurate information about the manifestation or pattern of an illness can be difficult. Often, parents express feelings of guilt about being a poor parent because their child has been exposed at day care and they must work. Addressing these issues during the health encounter is often helpful for parents.

With the diversity of dialects spoken in the United States, language issues can be barriers to providing optimal health care. If a practice setting does not have access to an interpreter or native speaker, interpreter services can sometimes be obtained from local telephone services as a last resort. It is important that both the NP and the parent or caretaker can communicate with and understand each other.

APPROACHES TO CHRONIC DISEASE IN CHILDREN

It is estimated that between 5% and 15% of children experience a prolonged period of illness or disability, the severity of which varies, as does its interference with the child's usual daily activities (Liptak, 2001). Some chronic conditions are not permanent, serious, or obvious, whereas other conditions are nonreversible, serious, and readily apparent. There also can be great variability in both the presentation and the course of illness among children. Children with chronic medical or psychiatric conditions have special health needs. They and their families often face a range of problems that are as diverse as the conditions that cause these difficulties. A variety of genetic, congenital, and acquired conditions can lead to permanent or persistent problems that have a significant impact on the child's lifestyle and family functioning. Caring for children with chronic conditions also entails caring for their families (Hudson-Barr & Lambert, 2002). The NP must be cognizant of several key points when working with these children and their families:

- Prevention of special health problems is a primary goal of care and includes the following:
  - Early prenatal care for all pregnant women
  - Genetic counseling as indicated
  - Elimination of environmental triggers or toxins

- Early identification of the condition or disease is of paramount importance.
- Amelioration of any functional problem that is treatable is as essential as prevention of secondary complications.
- Early intervention whenever possible to prevent secondary psychosocial difficulties is crucial; the developmental aspects of long-term illness must be addressed.
- Counseling may be needed for the child and family to handle psychosocial and behavioral problems or to discuss their emotions and feelings.
- The child, the family, and school personnel must be consulted to ensure that the child is able to attain realistic developmental milestones.
- Appropriate educational support in school is a right.
  - Public law 94-142, the Education for All Handicapped Children Act of 1975, mandates an appropriate education for all school-age children with developmental disabilities in the least restrictive environment.
  - Public law 99-457 (1986) provides states with the opportunity to extend benefits of public law 94-142 to children from birth to 2 years of age.
- Early intervention from birth is optimal and encouraged.
- NPs should be prepared to participate in the child's individual education plan, if warranted, to ensure that school officials understand the often complex health care needs of the child.
- Each state has programs (Title V) to assist children with special health needs with medical care and linkage to social services, as well as state vocational rehabilitation programs and state school-to-work projects.
- Prevention of discrimination is a right and is mandated under legislation related to individuals with disabilities. The Americans with Disabilities Act (1990) is a law that provides federal protection in the areas of employment, transportation, public accommodations, and communication for individuals with disabilities. The scope of protection covers both private and public sectors. The Individuals with Disabilities Educational Act (IDEA) Amendments were signed into effect in 1997 to bridge the gap between what children with disabilities learn and what is required in regular curriculum (IDEA—public law 105-17).
- IDEA Section 504 of the Rehabilitation Act for students with disabilities in regular education/inclusive settings provides safeguards and support for reasonable accommodations in the school settings such as altered test schedules and settings, therapies, and support for medical issues.
- Advocacy for children with chronic conditions and their families includes assisting them to secure coordinated and comprehensive health care and community-based services as needed.
- Provision of primary care services—regular health maintenance supervision and anticipatory guidance—must not be overlooked.
- Social service support is essential to assist parents who need special services for their child and to help determine financial eligibility for Supplemental Security Income (SSI) or state program benefits for individuals with handicaps or specific chronic diseases.
- Recognizing that parents commonly seek cures by using alternative treatments or medications, some of which can potentially cause harm or have no proven effectiveness, is important.
- The time of diagnosis and periods of exacerbations of illness are viewed as times of crisis and added stress.
- Chronic sorrow is a phenomenon that involves feelings of sadness, anger, guilt, or failure that parents may experience at various times during their child's life. It is not pathologic and does not occur uniformly within families (Shepard & Mahon, 2002).
- The NP needs to develop a trusting relationship with these children and their families that is respectful and accepting of their varied emotional needs.

Medically fragile and technology-dependent children are living longer than in the past and are reaching adulthood mainly as a result of improved technology and major advances in medical and surgical care. These children require a multidisciplinary team approach to their care.

Although chronic illnesses are diverse in their severity and effect on the child, certain issues are often common concerns for children with chronic conditions and their families. They include the following:

- The high cost of treatment—the potential need for financial assistance
- Lack of, or difficulties and barriers in, acquiring health care insurance coverage
- Family lifestyle alterations that may be required of parents or siblings, or both, in caring for the child
- The need to overcome system barriers that families may face navigating through the maze of agency paperwork
- The need for supervised care by multiple health care providers and the frequent lack of coordination of services in providing continuity of care
- Unpredictability of the condition and the potential for complications, frequent medical visits, hospitalizations, and death
- The desire to be kept informed of their child's condition and progress
- Often daily treatments or procedures are required that may be embarrassing, painful, or time consuming

- The developmental impact that chronic disease can have on a child, especially during adolescence and early adulthood (periods of increased vulnerability)
- Longevity concerns—ability to live and function independently as an adult, including the need for career and vocational counseling
- The level of knowledge parents need about the pharmacologic management of pain and the disease process or other therapeutic treatments, including nutritional support for the at-home care of the child
- The impact of stress on emotional and psychologic well-being of the child and family members—parents or caregivers, siblings, and possibly the extended family support network
- Acceptance by peers
- Parental striving to successfully normalize their child's life—by acknowledging the child's condition and its impact on family lifestyle while actively engaging in accommodations in order to focus on the child and not the condition
- Dealing with feelings (e.g., anger, sorrow) while attempting to cope with chronic illness
- Developing advocacy skills for these children to access services through schools, state and community agencies, or special federally sponsored programs
- Securing special illness-related equipment (e.g., movement and mobility aids such as walkers, wheelchairs, or braces) or acquiring communication aids such as hearing aids or special computers with voices
- Finding respite care
- Legal conservatory issues and the concern about who will care for the child as an adult when parents are no longer capable of providing physical care or are deceased

A multidisciplinary team approach is best for children with complex chronic diseases. These teams offer the expertise of many individuals in a united approach. Involvement of a clinical social worker, a community health nurse, or a nurse case manager is important to secure essential community resources for child and family. The family should be part of the team and not viewed as only the recipient of interventions. All team members must remember to respect the knowledge that parents or caregivers have about their child, their child's condition, and how the child is likely to respond both physically and emotionally to new therapeutic interventions or treatments, situational changes, or exacerbations of illnesses (Shepard & Mahon, 2002). Empowerment of the child and family is a key concept that should be emphasized. Communications with parents should be open and honest. Parents should be treated with respect and dignity and allowed to vent their emotions and to use coping mechanisms that work for them.

Family support groups are often beneficial; they offer a chance to interact with others who have experienced many of the same challenges, difficulties, sorrows, and triumphs. Sibling issues and feelings such as anger, embarrassment, a sense of being overwhelmed with added responsibilities, or believing they need to be the protector for their brother or sister also must be addressed.

The NP must strive to help children with special health needs and their families achieve maximum functioning. The critical issue in health promotion and disease management for children with special health needs is to ensure an organized and coordinated approach to provide appropriate treatment for the child's specific chronic disease or condition and to ensure that the child's primary health care needs are met. Case management for children with special health needs is a system of care that includes (1) assessing needs, (2) planning comprehensive health care to provide for both physical and psychosocial needs, (3) facilitating and coordinating services, (4) following up and monitoring services given and the child's progress, and (5) empowering the child and family through education, counseling, and support (Liptak, 2001).

The NP's level or type of involvement in the treatment and management of a child with a specific chronic disease may vary depending on the unique situation of the child and family and the NP's subspecialty training and education. NPs can be involved in a variety of case management activities for these children in their practice setting. Strategies related to fostering the child's psychosocial development should be addressed at each health care encounter. Similarly, NPs should be alert to situations that may require their advocacy when children with special needs and their families are in a vulnerable position. Children with chronic conditions do well when family functioning is high and there is positive family adaptation.

ASSESSMENT

History and Physical Examination

Chapter 2 discusses the complete history and physical examination of children from infancy through adolescence. In addition, each of the pediatric disease management chapters in this unit focuses on key questions to ask in history taking and highlights significant findings to be alert to if found on physical examination. Careful attention must be given when analyzing the signs and symptoms of the illness, including the presentation of clinical findings, the course of the disease process, and its associated manifestations. The NP should listen to what parents say about their child. The physical examination is often a challenge when a young child is ill and uncooperative.

Patience is important when examining children who are sick. The sick child should be carefully assessed so that significant physical findings are not missed during a hurried or cursory examination.

Chapter 24 discusses an overall assessment and management plan for sick, febrile children. It also identifies specific infectious diseases and assessment criteria for illnesses or problems commonly seen in childhood. In general, with infectious diseases, the NP must remember that the age of a child is a significant factor to consider in any management plan. The immune response in infants ages 0 to 90 days is particularly poor because of their immature immune system. Infants and young children are at increased risk for overwhelming bacteremia with any infection. Similarly, in other noninfectious diseases and conditions, age often continues to remain a key factor in the assessment of the child. To assess the severity of illness in infants and young children, careful attention must be given to the following four key indicators during both the history and the physical examination:

1. Level of consciousness
2. Hydration
3. Respiratory status
4. Activity level (eating, sleeping, and changes in behaviors or activities)

Diagnostic Studies

When deciding whether to order diagnostic tests, the NP should keep the following goals in mind. Order only those tests that give the most information for the least money, and order a test only if it is a crucial factor in the establishment of a concrete diagnosis or if it is a critical element in the treatment plan. If radiographic or imaging tests are necessary, order the test that is the least invasive. There are several useful points to remember about common imaging tests:

- Conventional radiographs are
  - Useful diagnostic tools
  - The least expensive of the imaging tests
  - Readily available
- Computed tomography (CT) imaging
  - Provides excellent bone and soft tissue detail
  - Can be used with contrast material for special evaluations
  - Shows relationships well; images can be presented in the frontal, transverse, or sagittal planes or obtained in three-dimensional imaging
  - Requires sedation of infants and young children
  - Has greater radiation exposure
  - Is costly
- Magnetic resonance imaging (MRI)
  - Provides excellent images of soft tissue without exposure to ionizing radiation; bone imaging is poor
  - Is expensive
  - Often requires sedation or anesthesia in infants and young children, because immobilization is necessary
- Ultrasonography
  - Gives two-dimensional images and measurements of internal organ systems; however, air-filled lungs and gas-filled bowel loops are impenetrable to ultrasound
  - In the form of Doppler ultrasound, blood flow direction and velocity can be measured; a still picture of the image can be recorded as a permanent record, or sonography can be viewed as the image is being projected on a video screen
  - Is highly dependent on operator skill and experience
  - Does not require sedation
  - Involves no radiation exposure

Chapter 27 contains a detailed discussion of the complete blood count (CBC) and provides insight as to the information that can be gained from a CBC, as well as indications for ordering this basic laboratory study. Chapter 27 also discusses frequently ordered coagulation studies. Chapter 24 discusses the laboratory workup for young children with a fever of undetermined origin. All disease entities or conditions addressed in this text include information about diagnostic studies and laboratory tests. Diagnostic studies and tests are valuable but are only one part of the entire database. Tests should be ordered only when the results are necessary to guide clinical decision making.

USE OF MEDICATION

Pediatric patients are at increased risk for adverse drug reactions for numerous reasons such as the need for individualized doses based on patient's age, weight, and clinical condition and changing pharmacokinetic parameters at various ages and stages of maturational development. Selecting the appropriate pharmacologic agent to adequately treat an illness/condition and minimizing the risk of medication errors are important factors to consider. List current medications and dosages that the patient is taking, both prescription and OTC drugs, in a standard place in the patient's chart. Allergies to medications, with the identified adverse response, should be highlighted in a place that is easily visible.

Several key principles should guide the NP in the use of prescription drugs and OTC medications.

Safe Prescription-Writing Practices

Prescriptions should be written in a manner that conveys accurate information to the pharmacist and the patient or parent. The following suggestions are made to ensure safe prescription writing for children (Levine et al, 2001):

- Never place a decimal and a trailing 0 (zero) after a whole number, because the decimal point might not be read correctly (e.g., 3.0 ml can be mistaken for 30 ml).
- Place a leading 0 (zero) before fractions less than 1 (one). For example, write 0.3 ml rather than .3 ml, which can be confused with 3 ml if the decimal point is inadvertently missed.
- Never use dangerous abbreviations such as q.d. or qd (every day) or U or u (unit), which may be misinterpreted for q.i.d. or qid (four times daily) or 0 (zero), respectively. Write out in full the words "every day" or "unit." The abbreviation O.D. means right eye; never use O.D. as an abbreviation for once daily.
- Use the metric system only.
- Write legibly.
- Issue a complete prescription that contains all of the following:
  - Patient's full name, age (date of birth), and weight (for infants and young children)
  - Name of the drug, dosage, and strength
  - Instructions if a brand name drug is to be used rather than the generic drug option
  - Total amount or quantity to be dispensed
  - Route of administration (e.g., take by mouth, instill in both ears, insert in rectum, instill in right eye)
  - General instructions to the patient or parent about indications for or the purpose of taking the medication, how frequently, and for how long (e.g., take three times a day until completed, take every 4-6 hours as needed for pain for 3 days)
  - Special instructions to the patient or parent about the drug (e.g., give with food, do not give with dairy products) or other instructions (e.g., translate to the primary language of the parent if English is not spoken or read)
  - Number of refills
  - Instructions to fill with a measuring device or other essential delivery devices (e.g., spacer or aerochamber for an aerosolized medication)

In addition, some prescription plans or health care settings may require that a diagnosis and allergies to medication be listed on the prescription form. Do a SCRIPT analysis after you have written for any medication to review the pharmacologic management plan. SCRIPT is a useful acronym to remember and stands for the following:

- Side effects
- Contraindications
- Right medication, dosage, frequency, route, and duration
- Pediatric considerations
- Transmittal of all necessary information on the prescription

Prescribing Pharmacologic Agents

When prescribing pharmacologic agents or recommending OTC drugs, the NP must be knowledgeable of the pharmacokinetics of the drug, the usual dosage, its side effects, and the indications and contraindications for its use in children. The NP must have a clear purpose in mind for using a particular drug and should not prescribe or recommend agents because of pressure from a parent or any other individual. Keep the following points in mind when prescribing drugs or OTC medications:

- Lack of compliance in taking medications can be a major problem. Factors that affect compliance include the following:
  - The more often a drug must be given per day the greater the chance that a dose or doses will be missed.
  - Drugs that have a bitter or repulsive taste are difficult and sometimes impossible to get a child to take. For an extra cost, some pharmacies will sell flavoring products that increase palatability (e.g., FLAVORx).
  - The greater the number of drugs that a child is given, the greater the potential for a drug dose to be missed or the wrong drug taken.
  - Waking a child to take a medication is difficult for parents; prescribe round-the-clock dosing only when it is essential to maintain tight therapeutic drug levels.
- Poorly given or inadequate instructions increase the risk that the prescribed agent will be misused.
- Children with renal or hepatic dysfunction require dosing adjustments.

Educating Parents and Children about Pharmacologic Agents

The success of any pediatric health care encounter depends on the ability of the health provider to educate parents or children, or both. The NP is in a unique position to educate parents and children about preventive care and common childhood illnesses. Before patients and their parents or caregivers leave the health care setting, they should have a basic understanding about the pharmacologic effect of any medication or OTC drug that is prescribed or recommended. Points of information that the NP should emphasize include the following (Levine et al, 2001):

- The purpose of the drug, how much should be given, and the frequency of administration
- Instructions about the indications for using a drug that is given on an "as necessary" basis or under specific circumstances (e.g., a rescue plan for the child with asthma whose symptoms are worsening)

- Signs or symptoms that indicate that a drug is either effective or not producing the desired effect or effects
- Possible drug-drug or drug-nutrient interactions, precautions, or adverse reactions that can occur
- If applicable, any monitoring parameters that are required for safe administration of the drug or to maintain effective therapeutic blood levels (e.g., blood levels)
- Pregnancy risk factor of a drug and the need to screen for pregnancy when giving specific drugs to female teenagers
- For children who take multiple medications, the importance of always carrying with them an up-to-date list of medications (prescription, over the counter, herbal products, vitamins, and minerals), their strengths, and dosages, as well as a list of medications the child cannot take in case of an emergency or if the child is seen by another health care provider
- Tips to help parents administer medications that may be difficult to get the child to take (e.g., how to hold an infant or small child when administering a medication)

Some medications can be safely mixed to mask the flavor of unpleasant medications. However, be sure to counsel about any medication that may have untoward interactions with foods or should be administered on an empty stomach. The following is a listing of liquids or solid foods that may be suggested: chocolate syrup, ice cream, applesauce, frozen juice concentrates (orange, grape, lemonade), chocolate or strawberry syrup, chocolate pudding, regular or frozen yogurt, and jelly. Other suggestions are to have the child eat peanut butter crackers before taking a medicine, eat part of a flavored ice pop before and after taking medications, or chew on ice chips before or after the dose. Be sure to tell parents that they need to check with their NP to determine whether the medication can be taken with a food.

Return demonstration can be a useful adjunct to evaluate the ability of the parent or child to administer a drug or drugs in the desired fashion. Return demonstration is a desired teaching tool in many situations. Examples of such circumstances include the following:

- Administering oral suspensions to infants and young children
- Measuring small or exact dosages (e.g., when a syringe is needed to measure amounts)
- Giving injectable, intravenous, gastrostomy, or nasogastric tube medications
- Instilling ophthalmic drops or ointments or nasal sprays or drops
- Using a metered dose inhaler (MDI), spacers, or inhalation equipment
- Ensuring that parents with limited cognitive abilities can safely administer medication to their children
- Administering multiple medications to ensure that the correct dose of the correct medication is given (e.g., 3 ml of amoxicillin suspension and 1 ml of metoclopramide syrup and not the reverse)

Prescriptive Authority for Nurse Practitioners

NPs must be knowledgeable about the individual state regulations that govern their prescription-writing privileges. Some states do not use the term *prescribe* to identify what NPs do when writing medication prescriptions for patients. For example, in California, the term *furnish* is used to describe this activity. The individual state board of registered nursing identifies the terminology to be used for this activity and regulates (either as a single state regulatory entity or jointly with medicine or pharmacology state boards) the activities and procedures related to this particular function. Regulations about prescriptive activity vary from state to state. NPs are governed by individual state guidelines and are legally obliged to follow all state regulations and mandates related to any prescriptive authority granted to them.

EDUCATIONAL STRATEGIES

When educating parents and children about a particular illness or disease entity, the NP must use terms easily understood by the parent and child. The health professional must include information as appropriate to the individual situation about the following topics:

- Etiology of the disease if known, the epidemiology and communicability issues, and prevention guidelines if applicable
- The management strategy, including use of pharmacologic agents, nutritional counseling, and the need for special treatments
- How to use adaptive devices and how to perform in-home monitoring tests
- Need for laboratory, radiographic, or imaging tests and the meaning of results
- Specific information on the signs and symptoms that indicate either a worsening or an improvement in the child's condition or illness
- Issues related to administration of medications at school—appropriate forms completed and school personnel instructed on key issues related to pharmacologic therapy
- Specific directions about when to schedule follow-up appointments and the availability of the NP for telephone follow-up contact

The severity of the illness or disease and the child's age, maturity, and cognitive level are key factors that determine the child's degree of involvement in self-care activities related to acute illness and chronic disease management. Children should be taught basic health promotion and disease prevention behaviors from early childhood. Likewise, they should be involved in the management of their illness to the fullest extent possible considering their developmental capabilities. Health professionals frequently ignore or forget to include the school-age child or adolescent as a partner in the management plan. Children should be consulted regarding their responsibilities for self-care. The NP also might be called on to be a liaison with school personnel to optimize the child's educational and social experience at school.

Written instructions and easy-to-read handouts are useful for parents, caregivers, and children, whether the instructions deal with common illness management, complex treatment needs, or information about developmental milestones and anticipatory guidance issues. *Instructions for Pediatric Patients* (Schmitt, 1999) and *Health Care Advice: Patient Education for Children, Teens and Parents* (American Academy of Pediatrics, 2002) contain useful guidelines for parents or caretakers and are available in both English and Spanish versions. Whether a practice setting develops its own instruction sheets or uses information sheets from other resource texts, important issues are that the instructions should be written in the family's native language and at a reading level appropriate for the individual family.

There are a number of textbooks written for the lay public that are excellent resources to suggest to parents. The NP should develop a list of appropriate textbooks to give to parents based on the parent's literacy level and unique characteristics. Two informative texts that could be included on a recommended reading list are *Guide to Your Child's Symptoms* (Schiff & Shelov, 1997) and *What to Do When Your Child Gets Sick* (Mayer & Kuklierus, 1999), a basic reading level paperback book in both English and Spanish versions. These texts offer guidance about common infections of childhood, preventive pediatrics, common behavioral problems, and other frequently encountered pediatric concerns. Each practice setting should have its own list of books and supply of handouts, brochures, pamphlets, and other printed resources to share with families in their practice. All written materials either recommended or given to families should be congruent with the reading level of the family and their primary spoken language.

PREVENTION OF ILLNESS

Prevention of illness and communicable diseases is a significant responsibility for NPs providing primary health care services for children or managing the care of children with chronic diseases or conditions. Education of children and their parents or caretakers is a key component of all prevention programs or activities. NPs must be vigilant in their practice settings to prevent or reduce the possibility of exposure to communicable diseases and to control the spread of infectious diseases that are a threat to infants, children, and youth. Therefore NPs must strive to ensure the following:

- All children are appropriately immunized against vaccine-preventable diseases according to the recommendations of the Advisory Committee on Immunization Practices (ACIP), the American Academy of Pediatrics (AAP), and the American Academy of Family Physicians (AAFP).
- Communicable diseases are identified and treated appropriately and are reported in a timely fashion to public health departments as required by law.
- Health practices to prevent or control the spread of infectious disease are carried out in home care programs, out-of-home child care programs, schools and health care settings, and hospitals. Key practices include the following:
  - Use effective personal hygiene—handwashing to prevent fecal-oral and person-to-person skin contact spread of disease. Teach children the importance of washing their hands, especially after toileting and blowing their nose, and before eating.
  - Ensure appropriate environmental sanitation—disposing of waste (e.g., blood, urine, feces, vomit, saliva) together with proper cleaning and disinfection of equipment, toys, toilets, eating areas, and diaper-changing surfaces. There should be a regular schedule of cleaning, as well as cleaning when contaminated.
  - Reduce respiratory spread of disease—cover mouth when sneezing or coughing and dispose of tissue after wiping nose; discourage habits of touching the mouth, nose, and eyes; eliminate passive smoke and provide adequate ventilation.
  - Do not eat raw or undercooked eggs or meats.
  - Handle and prepare food using appropriate sanitation and storage.
  - Reduce exposure to communicable disease by separating sick children from well children.
- Educate youth about the prevention of sexually transmitted diseases.
- Educate young children and teenagers to not share food, liquids, personal hygiene products, cosmetics, hair coverings, grooming products, or towels with others.
- Discourage children from kissing pets.
- Provide preventive health guidance about avoiding secondhand smoke, especially in cars and other confined areas.

Out-of-home day care is a risk factor for the spread of infectious diseases. Day care in a small day care home is associated with less spread of infectious disease than is day care provided in a larger day care center. The American Public Health Association and the AAP, as part of a collaborative project, published *Caring for Our Children. National Health and Safety Standards: Guidelines for Out-of-Home Child Care Programs* (2002). This book outlines preventive health practices that promote a safe environment for infants and children and addresses the issues of disease prevention and management in family/group day care homes and child care centers. Preventing and controlling the spread of illness in these group settings are important issues in maintaining health.

PAIN IN CHILDREN

NPs must be familiar with the assessment and effective management of pain in the pediatric and adolescent population. Unrelieved pain has both negative physiologic and negative psychologic consequences. Pain can result from injury or disease process, or as a side effect of procedures or surgery. Early pain stimuli and experiences can produce long-term consequences for the child. Likewise, inadequate pain relief during initial procedures can decrease the effect of adequate analgesia during subsequent procedures. Therefore the current thinking is that pain management should be part of the treatment plan for even minor painful procedures, as well as when it is associated with more serious illness or injury (Zempsky & Schechter, 2000). The importance of effective pain management in children cannot be overemphasized. To this end, a joint statement was issued by the AAP and the American Pain Society (2001) reinforcing the need for health care providers to treat pain and suffering in all infants, children, and adolescents.

Assessment and management of minor pain in the primary care setting is the focus of this section. The NP should seek other references for the treatment of chronic pain in pediatric patients.

Key factors that can influence effective pain management in children include the following:

- Established pain is difficult to control; therefore prevention of pain is an important goal of pain management.
- Pediatric and adolescent patients and their families should be involved in pain assessment and management as much as possible.
- Culture and family learning patterns must be considered (e.g., beliefs about pain, folk remedies, how pain is expressed verbally, and language barriers).
- Genetic stressors may be responsible for differing levels of neurotransmitters or responses to medication.
- Physiologic and psychologic differences between individuals, memories, and possible prenatal and perinatal stressors can influence a child's perception of pain.
- Children with chronic pain may have a lower pain threshold than their healthy counterparts (Hudson-Barr & Lambert, 2002).
- Developmental issues (e.g., cognitive, emotional, and physical), age, and temperament significantly affect how pain is interpreted, expressed, and controlled.
- Cognitive issues that influence pain perception include the child's memory and level of understanding, ability to control what will happen, attachment of a meaning to the situation with regard to pain, and expectations of the intensity of the pain.
- Emotional issues that affect a child's pain perception include anxiety, fear, frustration, anger, and depression.
- Social issues, such as how others react (their behaviors) to the child in pain, can influence the treatment plan. Likewise, family harmony or conflict can influence a child's pain.
- Pain perception involves complex neural interactions that send out impulses or noxious stimuli generated by tissue damage. The physiologic process associated with pain is termed *nociception* and includes the following (Golianu et al, 2000):
  - Transduction—painful stimuli are translated into electrical signals at sensory nerve endings and forwarded to the spinal cord.
  - Transmission—the electrical impulses are forwarded through the sensory nervous system.
  - Modulation—alteration of information by endogenous mechanisms results in lessening or amplification of the initial signal.
  - Perception—the emotional and physical experience of pain.
- Pediatric or adolescent patients and their parents must be educated about the assessment and management of pain.
- For a variety of reasons (e.g., fear of getting a shot), some children do not report pain to health care providers.

The goal of acute pain management in pediatrics is to effectively control pain with minimum therapy side effects. Positive outcomes of good pain control are increased satisfaction for the child and parents, as well as facilitating the recovery process.

Pain Assessment

A systematic assessment of pain in children and adolescents begins by obtaining a pain history from the child or the parent. When talking with younger children, ask the parent what words the child uses for pain (e.g., "owie," "boo-boo," "ouchie," "hurting," "uncomfortable," "warm," or "stinging") and use these words with the child. Behavioral observations and physiologic findings provide additional information to complete a comprehensive pain assessment. The evaluation of pain in children needs to be multidimensional. The NP must collect data about what children say about their pain, assess for physiologic and emotional manifestations of pain, and investigate other pertinent factors that can contribute to the child's pain as listed earlier.

Clinical Findings

History

In assessing pain, the following information should be obtained:

- Pain history (symptom analysis):
  - Intensity (mild, moderate, severe, overwhelming)
  - Location (areas with pain and without pain)
  - Quality—how pain is described by child or parent (e.g., stinging, burning, "big ouchie") and any pain behaviors noted
  - Duration (how long has the pain been present)
  - Temporal features or chronology (when and how did the pain start, precipitating factors, any variations in intensity and quality)
  - Previous treatments or procedures
  - What makes the pain worse or better
  - Other associated symptoms, such as anxiety
- Past experience with pain, including child's memory of the painful experience and how the pain was treated.
- Cultural beliefs about pain and its treatment.
- Self-reports of pain in the verbal child (if possible, obtain pain history as noted). If needed, identify a tool that is reliable, valid, sensitive, and simple for the child to understand, and use the tool consistently. The use of self-report tools and other objective pain measures helps to objectively quantify pain before treatment and serves to evaluate the outcome of treatment. (See Table 23-1 for information about child pain scales and tools and Table 23-2 for a listing of interview tools and pediatric pain questionnaires.)

Behavioral Indicators

Behavioral observations include vocalizations (e.g., crying, whimpering, whining); social withdrawal; changes in sleep patterns (more or less); verbalizations; facial expressions of guarding, grimacing, vigilance, or anger; motor responses; body posture; and activity such as rubbing or touching the painful site, avoiding the painful site, or guarding the affected area (e.g., not letting anyone touch the abdomen). These may be the only cues of pain in preverbal or nonverbal children. Infants in pain sleep less, are irritable and agitated, do not feed as well or refuse to feed, and have increased muscle tone (Zempsky & Schechter, 2000).

Physiologic Indicators

Physiologic parameters (e.g., heart rate and blood pressure) are neither sensitive nor specific indicators of pain, particularly in children who experience chronic pain. Other physical indicators include such findings as diaphoresis and pallor. Pulse-oximetry readings may be decreased because of increased oxygen consumption. Other physiologic responses to pain can include changes in metabolic functioning (e.g., hypermetabolism, hyperglycemia, or lipolysis), decreased gut motility, sodium and water retention, and cytokine production (Golianu et al, 2000).

Management

If there is a known etiology or underlying disease causing the pain, treat its causes. Other measures also may be needed to control for pain symptoms. Principles of effective office-based pain management include the use of a combination of pharmacologic and nonpharmacologic measures.

Common nonpharmacologic measures include the following:

- Sensorimotor techniques for infants such as pacifiers, swaddling, holding, and rocking
- Cognitive/behavioral strategies such as relaxation procedures, music and play therapy, and preparatory information before painful procedures
- Physical strategies such as application of heat (if muscle spasm) or cold (if swelling, bleeding, or pain), massage, acupuncture, exercise, rest, or immobilization
- Distraction techniques such as having the child watch a video, practice imagery, perform self-hypnosis, look out the window, or play with a toy; praising the child; giving the child a party blower and asking the child to blow the pain away; providing stickers or stamps; gently stroking the child; or giving multiple injections (e.g., immunizations) at the same time

Pharmacologic measures used in primary care settings for acute pain include the following:

- Analgesic for mild to moderate pain: acetaminophen—10 to 15 mg/kg every 4 hours. Use of an antiinflammatory agent is more effective if inflammation is a key factor causing pain because acetaminophen has limited peripheral antiinflammatory action.
- Oral nonsteroidal antiinflammatory drugs (NSAIDs): The usual pediatric dosage for children weighing less than 50 kg is listed (Schechter, 2002; Taketomo, Hodding, & Kraus, 2002). See Appendix A for additional information about drugs, such as their availability in liquid, tablet, or gel form and the corresponding concentration (milligrams per dose) of the various preparations:
  - Aspirin—10 to 15 mg/kg every 4 hours up to a maximum of 90 mg/kg/day for children or 4 g/day for adults. However, because its use is contraindicated in most children due to its association with Reye's

TABLE 23-1 Common Pain Rating Scales Used to Measure Pain in Pediatric and Adolescent Patients

Pain Scale/Description	Instructions	Recommended Age/Comments
FACES Pain Rating Scale* (Wong, 1996; Wong & Baker, 1988): Consists of six cartoon faces ranging from smiling face for "no pain" to tearful face for "worst pain."	*Original instructions*: Explain to the child that each face is for a person who feels happy because he has no pain (hurt) or sad because he has some or a lot of pain. Face 0 is very happy because he does not hurt at all. Face 1 hurts just a little bit. Face 2 hurts a little more. Face 3 hurts even more. Face 4 hurts a whole lot. Face 5 hurts as much as you can imagine, although you do not have to be crying to feel this bad. Ask the child to choose the face that best describes how he or she is feeling. Record the number under the chosen face on the pain assessment record. *Brief word instructions*: Point to each face using the words to describe the pain intensity. Ask the child to choose the face that best describes his or her own pain and record the appropriate number.	Children as young as 3 years Using original instructions without affect words, such as *happy* or *sad*, or brief words resulted in same pain rating, probably reflecting child's rating of pain intensity. For coding purposes, numbers 0, 2, 4, 6, 8, 10 can be substituted for 0-5 system to accommodate 0-10 system. The FACES Pain Rating Scale provides three scales in one: facial expressions, numbers, and words.

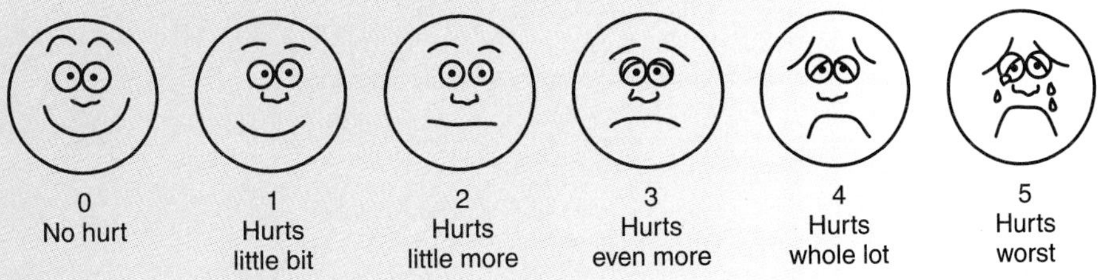
0
No hurt
1
Hurts
little bit
2
Hurts
little more
3
Hurts
even more
4
Hurts
whole lot
5
Hurts
worst

Pain Scale/Description	Instructions	Recommended Age/Comments
Oucher (Beyer et al, 1989): Consists of six photographs of child's face representing "no hurt" to "biggest hurt you could ever have"; also includes a vertical scale with numbers from 1-100; scales for African American and Hispanic children have been developed (Villarruel and Denyes, 1991).	*Numeric scale*: Point to each section of scale to explain variations in pain intensity: • "Zero means no hurt." • "This means little hurts" (pointing to lower part of scale, 1 to 29). • "This means middle hurts" (pointing to middle part of scale, 30 to 69). • "This means big hurts" (pointing to upper part of scale, 70 to 99). • "100 means the biggest hurt you could ever have." Score is actual number stated by child. *Photographic scale*: Point to each photograph on Oucher and explain variations in pain intensity using the following language: first picture from the bottom is "no hurt," second is "little hurt," third is "a little more hurt," fourth is "even more hurt than that," fifth is "pretty much or a lot of hurt," and the sixth is the "biggest hurt you could ever have." Score pictures from 0 to 5, with the bottom picture scored as 0. *General*: Practice using Oucher by recalling and rating previous pain experiences (e.g., falling off a bike). Child points to number or photograph that describes	Children 3 to 13 years. Use numeric scale if child can count to 100 by ones and identify larger of any two numbers, or by tens (Jordan-Marsh et al, 1994). Determine whether child has cognitive ability to use photographic scale; child should be able to seriate six geometric shapes from largest to smallest. Determine which ethnic version of Oucher to use. Allow the child to select a version of Oucher, or use the version that most closely matches the physical characteristics of the child.

Continued

TABLE 23-1 *Common Pain Rating Scales Used to Measure Pain in Pediatric and Adolescent Patients—cont'd*

Pain Scale/Description	Instructions	Recommended Age/Comments
	pain intensity associated with the experience. Obtain current pain score from the child by asking, "How much hurt do you have right now?"	
Poker Chip Tool[†] (Hester et al, 1998): Uses four red poker chips placed horizontally in front of the child.	Say to the child: "I want to talk with you about the hurt you may be having right now." Align the chips horizontally in front of the child on the bedside table, a clipboard, or other firm surface. Tell the child, "These are pieces of hurt." Beginning at the chip nearest the child's left side and ending at the one nearest the right side, point to the chips and say, "This (first chip) is a little bit of hurt and this (fourth chip) is the most hurt you could ever have." For a young child or for any child who may not fully comprehend the instructions, clarify by saying, "That means this one (first chip) is just a little hurt, this (second chip) is a little more hurt, this (third chip) is more yet, and this one (fourth chip) is the most hurt you could ever have." Do not give children an option for zero hurt. Research with the Poker Chip Tool has verified that children without pain will so indicate by responses such as "I don't have any." Ask the child, "How many pieces of hurt do you have right now?" After initial use of the Poker Chip Tool, some children internalize the concept of "pieces of hurt." If a child gives a response such as "I have one right now," *before* you ask or before you lay out the chips, record the number of chips on the pain flow sheet. Clarify the child's answer by words such as, "Oh, you have a little hurt? Tell me about the hurt."	Children as young as 4 years.
Word-Graphic Rating Scale[‡] (Tesler et al, 1991): Uses descriptive words (may vary in other scales) to denote varying intensities of pain.	Explain to the child, "This is a line with words to describe how much pain you may have. This side of the line means no pain and over here the line means the worst possible pain." (Point with your finger where "no pain" is, and run your finger along the line to "worst possible pain," as you say it.) "If you have no pain, you would mark like this." (Show example.) "If you have some pain, you would mark somewhere along the line, depending on how much pain you have." (Show example.) "The more pain you have, the closer to worst pain you would mark. The worst pain possible is marked like this." (Show example.) "Show me how much pain you have right now by marking with a straight, up-and-down line anywhere along the line to show how much pain you have right now." With a millimeter rule, measure from the "no pain" end to the mark and record this measurement as the pain score.	Children 4 to 17 years.

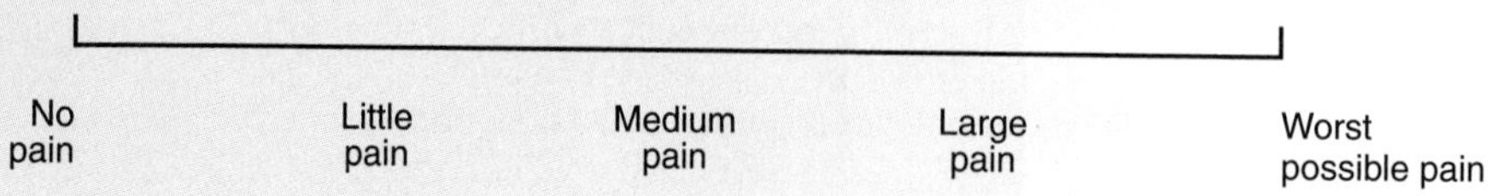

TABLE 23-1 *Common Pain Rating Scales Used to Measure Pain in Pediatric and Adolescent Patients—cont'd*

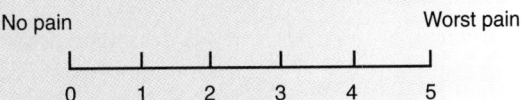

Pain Scale/Description	Instructions	Recommended Age/Comments
Numeric Scale: Uses straight line with end points identified as "no pain" and "worst pain" and sometimes "medium pain" in the middle; divisions along line are marked in units from 0 to 10 (high number may vary).	Explain to the child that at one end of the line is a 0, which means that a person feels no pain (hurt). At the other end is usually a 5 or 10, which means the person feels the worst pain imaginable. The numbers from 1 to 5 or 10 are for a very little pain to a whole lot of pain. Ask the child to choose a number that best describes his or her own pain. No pain — Worst pain 0 1 2 3 4 5	Children as young as 5 years, as long as they can count and have some concept of numbers and their values in relation to other numbers. Scale may be used horizontally or vertically. Number coding should be same as other scales used in a facility.
Visual Analogue Scale (Cline et al, 1992): Defined as a vertical or horizontal line that is drawn to a certain length, such as 10 cm, and anchored by items that represent the extremes of the subjective phenomenon, such as pain, that is measured.	Ask the child to place a mark on a line that best describes the amount of his or her own pain. With a centimeter ruler, measure from "no pain" end to the mark, and record this measurement as the pain score.	Children as young as 4.5 years, preferably 7 years. Vertical or horizontal scale may be used.
Color Tool (Eland, 1993): Uses markers for child to construct own scale that is used with body outline.	Present eight markers to the child in random order. Ask the child, "of these colors, which color is like . . .?" (the event identified by the child as having hurt the most). Place the marker (represents severe pain) away from the other markers. Ask the child, "Which color is like a hurt, but not quite as much as . . .?" (the event identified by the child as having hurt the most). Place the marker next to the marker chosen to represent severe pain. Ask the child, "Which color is like something that hurts just a little?" Place marker with the others. Ask the child, "Which color is like no hurt at all?" Show the four marker color choices to the child in order from worst to the no-hurt color. Ask the child to show on the body outlines where he or she hurts, using the markers. After the child has colored in the hurts, ask if they are current hurts or hurts from the past. Ask if the child knows why the area hurts if it is not clear to you why it does.	Children as young as 4 years, provided they know their colors, are not color blind, and are able to construct the scale if in pain.

From Hockenberry-Eaton M, et al: *Wong's nursing care of infants and children*, ed 7, St Louis, 2001, Mosby, pp 1052-1053.

* *Wong-Baker FACES Pain Rating Scale Reference Manual*, describing development and research of the scale, is available from the Mayday Pain Resource Center, City of Hope National Medical Center, 1500 East Duarte Road, Duarte, CA 91010; phone: 626-301-8941. Available at *www.elsevier.com/WOW.*

†Developed in 1975 by N. O. Hester, University of Colorado Health Sciences Center, School of Nursing, Denver, CO 80262. Also available in Spanish and French.

‡Instructions for Word-Graphic Rating Scale from Acute Pain Management Guideline Panel: *Acute pain management in infants, children, and adolescents: operative and medical procedures; quick reference guide for clinicians*, AHCPR pub no 92-0020, Rockville, MD, 1992, Agency for Health Care Policy and Research (now the Agency for Healthcare Research and Quality [AHRQ]), Public Health Service, US Department of Health and Human Services. Word-Graphic Rating Scale is part of the Adolescent Pediatric Pain Tool and is available from Pediatric Pain Study, University of California, School of Nursing, Department of Family Health Care Nursing, San Francisico, CA 94143-0606; phone: 415-476-4040.

TABLE 23-2 Structured Interviews, Pain Questionnaires, and Other Tools for Assessing Pain in Pediatric Patients: Used with Children Experiencing Long-Term, More Complex, or Intense Pain

Tool	Author
Adolescent Pediatric Pain Tool (APPT)	Savedra et al, 1989
Patient pain diary or journal	
Varni/Thompson Pediatric Pain Questionnaire	Varni, Thompson, & Hanson, 1987

syndrome, use only in the management of selected pediatric conditions (e.g., juvenile rheumatoid arthritis and Kawasaki disease).
  - Ibuprofen—4 to 10 mg/kg every 6 to 8 hours for infants and children; adolescent and adult, 200 to 400 mg/dose 3 to 4 times/day with 3.2 g/day maximum.
  - Naproxen (Naprosyn)—older than 2 years, 5 to 7 mg/kg every 8 to 12 hours; adolescents and adults for mild to moderate pain or dysmenorrhea; initial 500 mg dose and then 250 mg every 6 to 8 hours, maximum 1250 mg/day.
- Opioid agonists for moderate or severe pain:
  - Codeine—oral, 0.5 to 1 mg/kg every 3 to 4 hours. For younger patients, it is typically given as an acetaminophen and codeine elixir.
  - Hydromorphone (Dilaudid)—oral, young children 0.03 to 0.08 mg/kg/dose every 4 to 6 hours, maximum 5 mg/dose; older children and adults, 1 to 4 mg/dose every 4 to 6 hours with the usual adult dosage of 2 mg/dose.
  - Hydrocodone (in Lorcet, Lortab, Vicodin)—child dose not established; adolescent, 1 to 2 tablets or capsules every 4 to 6 hours. Is available in fixed combinations with acetaminophen.
  - Oxycodone (in Percocet, Percodan, Tylox)—oral, 0.05 to 0.15 mg/kg every 4 to 6 hours up to 5 mg/dose. Available in fixed combinations with acetaminophen. Adult dose is 1 or 2 tablets every 4 to 6 hours (4 g/day maximum).
  - Morphine—oral, 0.3 mg/kg every 3 to 4 hours; intravenous (IV) bolus, 0.05 to 0.1 mg/kg every 2 to 4 hours. This drug is not used commonly in primary care settings for the management of acute pain. IV necessitates close monitoring of vital signs and pulse oximetry.
- Topical analgesic creams such as eutectic mixture of local anesthetics (EMLA®) and iontophoresis delivery of drugs—used with procedures involving skin punctures.

An essential consideration in giving analgesics is whether there is a need to maintain certain serum concentration levels. In situations that require a steady-state serum concentration for pain relief (e.g., following same-day surgery, fractures), around-the-clock dosing of pain medications for 48 to 72 hours is preferable to "as needed" or prn dosing. "As needed" dosing is associated with drops in serum concentration levels. When the child is then given a prn dose of medication, a significant period of time may elapse before adequate analgesic effect occurs.

Pharmacologic measures used in primary care settings for chronic pain management include the following:

- NSAIDs, acetaminophen, and tricyclic antidepressants (TCAs) are the primary treatments used to treat chronic pain unrelated to disease or trauma. Assess for the efficacy of the pharmacologic therapy as follows:
  - Have the child or parent use a pain intensity rating scale and keep a diary of the child's activities and pain.
  - On follow-up visits, question whether symptoms have improved.
- Selective serotonin reuptake inhibitors, opioids, certain anticonvulsants, and other selected medications may be needed. The pain dosage for tricyclic antidepressants is lower than the dosage prescribed in the treatment of depression. Gabapentin is the anticonvulsant most frequently used to treat neuropathic pain. Children requiring these agents for the management of their chronic pain are best handled by referral.
- Nonpharmacologic techniques are frequently used as adjuvants to pharmacologic therapy. They include physical therapy, relaxation, massage, guided imagery, biofeedback, heat and cold, distraction, transcutaneous electric nerve stimulation (TENS), music therapy, acupuncture, and psychologic therapy. Invasive techniques such as neuroablative procedures and spinal cord stimulation are occasionally used as a last resort (DiMaggio, 2002).

Table 23-3 identifies common oral pain medications used in pediatrics and their doses to use as a quick guide. Table 23-4 outlines specific pain problems commonly seen in pediatrics, as well as their pain relief strategies.

TABLE 23-3 *Common Oral Pain Medications Used with Children and Their Doses*

Pain Medication	Dose (mg/kg)	Frequency
Acetaminophen	10-15	Q4-6hr (the safe maximum dose is 90 mg/kg/24 hr)
Ibuprofen	10	Q6hr
Codeine	0.5-1	Q4hr, maximum dose for children 60 mg/dose
Acetaminophen with codeine	0.5-1 (by codeine) and a safe dose of acetaminophen	Q4-6hr
Acetaminophen with hydrocodone	Dose is limited by appropriate dose of acetaminophen and hydrocodone (0.2 mg/kg)	Q4hr
Oxycodone	0.05-0.15	Q4-6hr
Acetaminophen with oxycodone	10-15 (by acetaminophen) OR 0.05-0.15 (by oxycodone)	Q4-6hr

Data from DiMaggio TJ: Pediatric pain management. In St Marie B, editor: *Core curriculum for pain management nursing*, St Louis, MO, 2002, WB Saunders.

TABLE 23-4 *Common Pediatric Pain Problems and Pain Relief Strategies*

Pediatric Pain Problems	Pain Relief Strategies
Otalgia	Acetaminophen or ibuprofen Auralgan otic gtts Warm oil in the ear Warmed compresses pressed against the ear
Pharyngitis	Acetaminophen or ibuprofen Antibiotics if GABHS Saltwater gargles Anesthetic lozenges for older child
Stomatitis	Ibuprofen Bland diet Saline mouth rinses for older children Benadryl/Maalox (in a 1:1 preparation) to coat the mucous membranes Viscous lidocaine (remember the potential for aspiration and toxicity) Sucralfate
Musculoskeletal injury	RICE—rest, ice, compression, and elevation Immobilization of affected area Cold for the initial 48-72 hr Nonsteroidal antiinflammatory drugs (NSAIDs)
Fractures and sprains	NSAIDs Narcotic analgesics if severe fracture or sprain Topical ibuprofen, ketoprofen, and felbimac have been shown to give relief in situations of soft tissue trauma, strains, and sprains; however, studies have involved only adults
Injection pain	Distraction and relaxation techniques Eutectic mixture of local anesthetics (EMLA) cream Ice Spot pressure (press down into muscle where shot is to be given)
Neonate and infant procedural pain	Sucrose orally Sucrose pacifier Acetaminophen

Data from Zempsky WT, Schechter NL: Office-based pain management, *Pediatr Clin North Am* 47:601-615, 2000.
GABHS, Group A β-hemolytic streptococci.

FEVER IN CHILDREN

Fever is a common phenomenon seen in children and involves neurologic, endocrine, and metabolic functions. It is a complex systematic inflammatory response. Cytokines are a critical factor in the fever and the inflammatory response. Viral infections are responsible for most fevers in children. Bacterial infection, malignancy, reaction to immunizations, and connective tissue disease are other known etiologic factors. Most pediatric sources define *fever* as a rectal temperature higher than 100.4° F (38° C) or an oral temperature higher than 100.0° F (37.8° C). In infants and young children, unless contraindicated for a medical reason, a rectal temperature should be obtained when critical clinical decisions must be made, because it more closely resembles body core temperature readings than do axillary, oral, or otic measurements. Because environmental conditions (e.g., swaddling an infant) may produce transient elevated temperatures, it may be necessary to take several readings to verify whether an elevated temperature is due to an environmental or a pathologic cause.

Those parents who have "fever phobia" need reassurance because they believe that temperatures greater than 104.0° to 104.2° F (40° to 40.1° C) cause brain damage or, if not treated, will go higher. Cellular damage does not occur until temperatures reach above 105.8° to 107.6° F (41° to 42° C). Fevers below 105.8° F (41° C), per se, are not associated with brain damage. Parents need to know that, except for temperatures over 104.0° F (40° C), fevers are a body defense mechanism. Fevers are thought to impart a beneficial effect by enhancing immunologic responses, such as increasing phagocytosis and leukocyte migration, and interfering with viral replication and virulence of some microbes. However, there are potential adverse effects from fevers, including increased metabolic rate with associated fluid loss, oxygen consumption, and increased caloric needs. High temperature can precipitate seizures in susceptible infants and young children. Associated symptoms of headache, malaise, anorexia, and irritability are uncomfortable for the child and always worrisome to parents (Koch, 2002).

Health care providers generally treat fevers depending on the severity of the fever or to provide comfort to the child. Parental concern can be a factor in a decision to use an antipyretic. Likewise, suppressing a fever in a young child who is ill can also assist in clinical decision making if the irritability, tachypnea, and tachycardia associated with a fever resolve after administration of an antipyretic. However, a febrile child's response to antipyretics should not be the sole criterion used to decide whether a pediatric patient is bacteremic or not (Koch, 2002).

Many health care providers treat fevers to provide comfort to a child and use pharmacologic agents when a temperature exceeds 102° F (38.9° C) and the child is uncomfortable or if the child has a persistent temperature above 101° F (38.3° C). Some clinicians use temperatures greater than 101.5° F (38.7° C) as their guide to treatment.

Management strategies for fever control include the following:

- Nonpharmacologic measures:
  - Provide adequate hydration.
  - Provide reassurance to parents and advice that not all fevers need to be treated.
  - Provide appropriate clothing—not bundled in additional clothing or coverings.
  - Provide ambient environment temperatures of around 72° F (22° C).
  - Sponge with tepid water for temperatures above 104° F (40° C). Sponging should be stopped if the child starts to shiver. Ice water baths and alcohol sponging should not be done.
- Pharmacologic measures—antipyretic agents (Koch, 2002; Taketomo, Hodding, & Kraus, 2002):
  - Acetaminophen, 10 to 15 mg/kg/dose every 4 to 6 hours, not to exceed five doses in 24 hours; temperature generally is reduced by 1° to 2° C within 2 hours. At a dose of 15 mg/kg/dose, it is as effective as ibuprofen at 10 mg/kg/dose. This is the drug of first choice.
  - Ibuprofen in children 6 months to 12 years: for temperature less than 102.5° F (39° C), 5 mg/kg/dose; for temperature greater than or equal to 102.5° F (39° C), 10 mg/kg/dose every 6 to 8 hours with a maximum daily dose of 40 mg/kg/day. The duration of fever response with ibuprofen may be longer than with acetaminophen. Thus the temperature remains lower for a longer period of time with ibuprofen.
  - Naproxen sodium is marketed as a "fever reducer." However, it has not been well studied as an antipyretic in children and should not be used for this purpose.
  - Alternating acetaminophen and ibuprofen has not proven beneficial in the management of fevers (Koch, 2002; Mayoral et al, 2000). The best approach is to use acetaminophen and switch to ibuprofen if the child fails to respond.

TELEPHONE MANAGEMENT OF ILLNESSES

Several excellent resources address telephone management of illnesses in children (Poole, 2002; Schmitt, 1998a, 1998b, 1998c). Many daytime telephone calls represent routine questions about common pediatric problems and can be effectively managed by office nurses with special training. NPs, with their specialty education and background in primary care, are frequently called on to give advice to parents over the telephone or are assigned to take telephone calls either during the daytime or after regular office hours. All NPs should ensure that their practice settings have developed a safe system for managing ill-child calls and follow-up calls on patients seen by the NP or physician.

Nonemergency calls to a practice about a sick child during the day are usually routed through a telephone receptionist, who can make an appointment, if appropriate, or transfer the call to a triage nurse or NP, who can determine the urgency of the need to see the child, give home care advice, or refer to the NP or physician for care. If home care advice is given, the triage person should use standards of care or telephone advice protocols addressing a particular set of symptoms, complaints, or a diagnosis that is agreed on for use in that particular setting.

Triage Categories

Schmitt's (1998b, 1998c) triage categories for sick calls are as follows:

- Life-threatening situation—call 911.
- Emergent—see patient immediately.
- Urgent—see patient within 4 hours.
- Urgent or uncomfortable patient—see the patient that day.
- Nonurgent—see the patient that day or the next day.
- Recurrent or persistent—see the patient within 2 weeks.
- Mildly ill—give home care advice.

The development of telephone protocols is a key factor to ensure an effective telephone management system for a busy practice setting. Schmitt (1998c) developed a quick reference for pediatric telephone protocols that can be reviewed for ideas about how protocols can be developed. Whatever protocols are used or developed in an individual practice setting, any management-by-telephone protocol should accomplish the following objectives:

- Allow the telephone triage person to manage ill-child calls safely.
- Provide a standard of care.
- Prevent omissions resulting from forgetfulness or fatigue.
- Prevent harmful triage or recommendations.
- Improve quality of care.

The NP who is doing telephone triage must be a perceptive, conscientious, and calm individual who carefully listens to the caller, asks selected questions, processes the information, determines the correct management protocol to use for a particular situation, gives the necessary instructions to parents, and writes notes in a log book. In addition, all these activities must be performed in a relatively short period of time. The sequence of steps that one must go through in using telephone protocols includes the ability to do all of the following:

- Collect data about the symptoms through open-ended and direct questioning.
- Identify the problem or main symptom.
- Determine a diagnosis or working assessment.
- Decide on a triage category for the patient.
- Select the correct protocol.
- Educate the parent about the plan of care.

Documentation

Documentation of the telephone call and disposition is an important element in a successful system for managing telephone calls for sick children. A documentation system, whether it consists of a log sheet or note pad, should be simple and brief. Written documentation serves several purposes, including the following:

- A medicolegal defense
- A method to review charts for quality improvement and assurance purposes
- An avenue to assist in complaint resolution if parents are upset about the advice given to them
- A tool to use when making follow-up calls to the family Important items to include in any telephone log include
- Date and time
- Patient data—name, age, sex, telephone number—and history of chronic disease or condition
- The chief complaint and a brief list of symptoms and signs, including their duration and frequency
- Diagnosis or working assessment
- Triage category
- Instructions given about follow-up
- List of medications and their dosage if prescribed by the NP
- An "other" section for any additional comments that are deemed important information

When using telephone protocols in a practice setting, training of all individuals who are doing telephone triage is essential and is the best method to ensure consistency in the use of the system. Staff sessions, designed to review the written documentation, are also useful teaching tools and should be encouraged. Perhaps the most important point to emphasize in training and about the use of any telephone management system is the need to assess the comfort of the parent with the advice given. Parents should be asked at the end of the telephone contact whether they are comfortable with the advice and plan. If the parent is not satisfied or is uneasy about the plan, physician or NP consultation should be an option. Finally, parents should be told to call back if their child's condition worsens or the problem persists too long.

Relating to Parents via the Telephone

There are several critical points about telephone management of common pediatric illnesses, conditions, or concerns. These include method of interaction, screening questions to ask, and points at which intervention is necessary. The individual should be receptive to the parent's call, using language and taking the necessary time to give the message that the call is as important to the provider as it is to the parent. Parents can be anxious and find it difficult to calmly state the problem. The individual also must be calm, direct, and comforting in order to help parents manage their child's illness.

Screening questions that should be asked of parents include the following:

- *Duration*: How long has the problem been present?
- *Description*: Tell me about the problem. What signs and symptoms are present?
- *Clinical changes*: How has the child's behavior or activity level changed (e.g., eating, sleeping, playing, interaction with peers and family members)?
- *Environmental problems*: Has there been any recent exposure, change, or stress in the child's environment?
- *Cause*: What does the parent believe is contributing to or causing this condition?
- *Management*: What has the parent done for the condition, and with what effect?
- *Feelings*: Does the parent feel anxious about how the child is behaving?

Questions should be asked in an effort to narrow the problem clinically and to assist the parent to be clear and focused. Questions should be clustered by area of concern, should move from most to least serious, and should follow a logical sequence based on initial data obtained.

After-hours or call centers are another avenue that pediatric practices use for handling sick calls after office hours. These centers employ nurses and NPs who use telephone protocols to guide parents in the management of their child's illness until their regular health provider is available. These call centers alleviate the burden of night call and are set up to use telephone protocols and a software program for documentation. It is incumbent on the pediatric health care providers within their practice setting to evaluate whether such a center would effectively meet their standards of care for after-hours management of children.

Educating Parents about Telephone Management of Illness

Practice settings should have a telephone call policy about sick calls and should acquaint parents with this policy. The policy should cover basic information about the office protocol for handling calls about sick children during office hours, well-child questions, prescription refills, nighttime (after-hours) calls, and weekend and holiday calls. Who screens calls, when calls are returned (e.g., during the noon hour or from 4 to 5 PM), and after-hours coverage are points to cover in the policy.

Parents should be encouraged to handle minor illnesses at home without unnecessary calling in for advice. Home instruction sheets for managing fevers (including dosage charts) and common childhood illnesses or books on common pediatric illnesses designed for parents are excellent resources to provide to parents (Schmitt, 1999). Pamphlets can be given to parents at anticipatory guidance visits. During illness visits, parents should be told what to expect when their child is ill, preparing them for the increasing temperature, vomiting, or diarrhea, as well as what to do if they occur.

Parents need to know what type of situations require a call for emergency medical services or the poison control center. If sick care is necessary after scheduled office hours, parents will need to give the following information about their child:

- The main symptoms
- Any chronic disease or health problem
- Temperature (and route it was taken)
- Approximate weight
- Names and dosages of current medications
- Type of insurance coverage

In addition, the parent should have the name and telephone number of the pharmacy available to give the provider (Schmitt, 1998c). Box 23-1 provides general rules for parents when calling a health care provider. Box 23-2 gives parental guidelines for deciding when to call.

BOX 23-1 *General Rules When Calling the Nurse Practitioner or Physician: Guidelines for Parents*

When calling for **nonurgent** matters, such as well-baby advice, prescription refills, or appointments, call during office hours whenever possible.

When calling for an **emergency**, tell the receptionist or answering service that your call is an emergency call.

Give the following **information on every call**: your child's name, age, sex, major problem, and telephone number where you can be reached.

Be ready to give **information related to your child's problem** as briefly and clearly as possible:

- What are signs and symptoms?
- How long has the problem existed?
- What have you done for the problem?
- How did your child respond to what was done?
- How do you feel about your child's condition? What is your intuition? Is your child getting better, or worse?

Be ready to give information about your **child's general health**:

Does your child have any chronic illnesses that need to be considered?
Is your child receiving medications for this problem or another problem? Has your child recently received immunizations?
Does your child have any allergies?

If you do not talk to your provider directly, **before hanging up**, ask when your call will most likely be returned.

If you do not receive a return call within a reasonable amount of time, **call back** to make sure your message was taken correctly.

If your provider decides not to examine your child, **before hanging up**, make sure you determine the following:

The most likely cause of your child's condition.
Which medicines or treatments should be given.
What signs or symptoms to watch for.
When you should call back for more advice or to report changes in your child's condition.

If you do not **understand the instructions** given, ask to have them repeated or call back for clarification.

If you are instructed to come to the office or go to an emergency department, make sure you have **clear directions** on how to get there. If you are too anxious to drive, ask a friend or neighbor to drive or call a taxi. If an ambulance is necessary, the provider may be able to call it for you.

Adapted from Brown JL: *Pediatric telephone medicine: principles, triage, and advice*, ed 2, Philadelphia, 1994, JB Lippincott.

BOX 23-2 *Deciding When to Call the Nurse Practitioner or Physician: Guidelines for Parents*

When to Call Immediately for an Infant Younger Than 3 Mo

Baby has the following symptoms:

Is lethargic (very sleepy or difficult to arouse), has poor color, or appears limp and unresponsive
Has a rectal temperature of 100.4° F (38° C) or higher
Refuses to eat three or four times in a row
Has repeated bouts of diarrhea or vomiting
Has a labored, wheezing, or grunting breathing pattern that lasts longer than 1/2 hr
Has an illness associated with a rash that looks like bleeding under the skin

Baby's eyes, hands, or feet have a yellow, jaundiced color or if the baby develops pumpkin-colored skin

You feel very nervous about your baby's illness or general condition

When to Call Immediately for an Older Child

Child has the following symptoms:

Seems unresponsive, does not make eye contact with you, or has cold and clammy skin that is not associated with vomiting
Looks much sicker than usual with a routine illness

Continued

BOX 23-2 *Deciding When to Call the Nurse Practitioner or Physician: Guidelines for Parents—cont'd*

Has an illness associated with a rash that looks like bleeding under the skin
Has any symptom that you believe to be unusual or frightening; this includes labored breathing, severe headache, or very high fever

When to Call Immediately after Trauma or Injury

Child has struck his or her head and has lost consciousness, has nausea or vomiting, or complains of severe headache; also call if there is mental confusion, unbalanced walking, poor coordination, loss of memory, or a discharge coming from one or both ears
There is a persistent swelling, tenderness, or deformity of the injured part
Child refuses to use an injured extremity for more than 1/2 hr
There is a deep puncture wound, a cut longer than 1/2 inch, or your child has not received a tetanus shot within the past 5-10 yr
There is injury to an eye that causes redness, pain, or tearing for more than 15 min
Child has been bitten by an animal and the bite has gone through the skin
You need first aid instructions for uncontrolled bleeding or other problems
You believe that your child may have swallowed a toxic or poisonous substance

When to Call about Symptoms

You are concerned about your child's general appearance
Symptoms seem to be getting progressively worse or last longer than expected
Fever of more than 101° F has persisted for longer than 24 hr
Cough, cold, sore throat, or runny nose has lasted longer than 48 hr
Vomiting has lasted longer than 8 hr or diarrhea longer than 24 hr, or when there is blood in the stool or vomit
Child has severe stomach pains lasting longer than 4 hr
Symptom seems more severe than it has in the past
Child has a rash or other problem and you are not sure what is causing it
You are not certain whether the child needs to be seen by the health care provider

Adapted from Brown JL: *Pediatric telephone medicine: principles, triage, and advice*, ed 2, Philadelphia, 1994, JB Lippincott.

REFERRALS AND CONSULTATIVE SERVICES

On many occasions, NPs identify clinical or behavioral problems that they are uncomfortable managing for any number of reasons, such as being out of the scope of their practice parameters or a problem that requires the expertise of a provider in a subspecialty practice. In these instances, patients should be referred to other providers for management of that problem. In other situations, the NP may wish to continue to manage the patient's care but seek consultation with other experts in the field. The NP uses this individual as a case consultant. Whether the NP refers the patient and family out to or consults with another health care expert, certain information must be shared with the referral or consultant provider in an organized, logical fashion. Guidelines for presenting this information are as follows:

- Give the patient's name, age, and actual or tentative diagnosis or chief clinical findings.
- Briefly discuss, in a sentence or two, why the patient or family is being referred to another provider or the reason that a consultation is being requested.
- Give a synopsis of the patient's history, clinical findings, prior management plan, and outcome of treatment if applicable.
- Identify any pertinent past medical history such as chronic illnesses or conditions.
- Provide pertinent family, educational, or social information, including insurance coverage if this is problematic.

If the NP is referring the patient out for problem-focused care, this should be made clear to the referral provider. In addition, guidelines should be established for when the patient should be seen again by the NP for primary care supervision and how information about the child's progress will be shared with the NP. If the child is to be seen by the NP for primary care services and at the same time by the referral provider for specialty care, coordination of responsibilities between the two providers relative to the need for follow-up testing, monitoring, treatments, or therapy should be identified.

The NP should maintain a listing of specialty providers in the local area who take referrals from the NP's work setting. The child's insurance coverage is often a major factor in referral and often prior authorization from an insurance carrier is needed for a referral. If the NP is employed in a large health maintenance organization, the NP should maintain a list of pediatric specialty providers in the organization. Important information to gather about these individuals includes their specialty or subspecialty practice area, evaluation of their effectiveness (can be an informal notation such as "great resource person"), and, if applicable, their fees for service (e.g., full fee or sliding scale) or which insurance plans will reimburse for their services.

Whether consulting formally or informally with another provider about the care of a particular patient, the NP should present information about the patient, as listed previously, and discuss potential management options. At the end of the consultation, the NP should summarize the key areas that were discussed and the recommendations that were agreed on. A notation about the consultation, the main discussion points, and the recommendations should be made in the patient's chart.

Often overlooked sources of free consultation are state and local public health departments or agencies and health-related professional organizations, as well as some major medical centers that provide telephone consultation about patients for providers in their service area. Again, a notation should be placed in the child's file if the case is discussed with a consultant in such an agency. Connecting with colleagues on the Internet is another option. Real-time chat sessions and E-mail exchanges are possible sources of consultation; however, information secured from unknown sources or not documented or referenced should be verified for accuracy.

When a patient is referred to another provider, the NP must explain the reason for the referral to the child and parent, how the transfer of care will be managed, and when the patient is to return to see the NP. The information should be presented in such a manner as to dispel fears of abandonment or giving up. The bond between the child, the parent, and the primary care provider is a strong relationship that individuals rely on. If the NP plans to seek a consultation, the child and parent should be informed by explaining the need for a second opinion or the desire to collaborate with others to ensure that nothing has been missed. After the consultation, parents should be informed about what was decided. Finally, the parent may seek consultation with another health care provider. If so, treat this as the parent's need to collaborate in the child's care and listen to the recommendation by this consultant. Be sure that the consultant's reports are filed in the child's chart.

TIPS REGARDING DOCUMENTATION: PATIENT VISIT AND FOLLOW-UP

There are several important rules for the NP to remember regarding documentation when charting. They include

- Being alert to a complaint or combination of complaints that are red flags for more serious illness (e.g., abdominal or chest pains, headache, syncope). Be sure to note pertinent positive and negative history and physical findings relative to these complaints when charting.
- Identifying differential diagnoses and ruling out the worst possible illness first. Be sure to gather enough data to either rule in or out the diagnosis based on history, physical findings, or diagnostic studies.
- Conveying the seriousness of the issue to the family or caretaker if there is the probability of a serious illness and the patient needs to return for additional visits or have diagnostic studies done. Be sure to document that conversation.
- Knowing patient or family risk factors and screening for them through diagnostic tests or history.
- Ensuring that there is a system in place in the practice setting to follow up and secure the results of diagnostic tests that were ordered. There should be a mechanism to ensure that the test or procedure was done and that the NP was given the results and documented reviewing them.
- Following up all abnormal test results. There should be a note placed in the patient's chart that the abnormal results were discussed (and with whom) and what the plan of action would be.
- Following up on referrals to other health care professionals or agencies and documenting the recommendations or treatments implemented from these referral sources.
- Revisiting an unresolved problem until it is resolved. This can be accomplished by
  - Rescheduling a follow-up examination.
  - Telephone contact with the family to determine if the complaint or illness has been resolved.

Chart audits should be a part of practice quality improvement. Look for such things as omissions of information, whether problems identified in earlier visits were addressed at subsequent visits until resolved, and compliance with routine health maintenance screenings.

RESOURCE BOX

National Organization for Rare Disorders (NORD)
55 Kenosia Avenue
PO Box 1968
Danbury, CT 06813-1968

1-203-744-0100
Toll free: 1-800-999-6673 (voicemail only)
TDD: 1-203-797-9590
Fax: 1-203-798-2291

NATIONAL AND LOCAL ORGANIZATIONS AND RESOURCES

Parents and their children with specific disease entities or health conditions can benefit from the educational materials, resources, and support that national health organizations provide. Learning to live with a chronic disease or handicapping condition presents a special challenge to families. Most national organizations provide written materials that parents and children can easily understand about the etiology, management, and treatment of the particular disease in question. These materials also help parents explain their child's condition to teachers and others. Many of these national organizations can guide parents and children to support groups with other families and children who are similarly challenged and to health professionals and other related groups who specialize in the treatment of a particular disease entity. Likewise, these organizations can assist parents in accessing unique services to benefit their children; for example, enrolling in special camps and sports activities, learning about the various legal rights of children with disabilities or handicapping conditions, and acquiring special adaptive equipment.

Many national and local health organizations and foundations provide educational materials and valuable information designed for health professionals about a variety of subjects related to their target population of children. For children with rare disorders, the National Organization for Rare Disorders (NORD) may be able to assist parents and offer information about the child's condition or disease. Often these national organizations can provide up-to-date information about new treatment modalities or management strategies. NPs should take advantage of the services that national health organizations and local chapters offer and inform parents about national organizations and local chapters that can assist them in meeting their child's special needs. In addition, every clinical or practice setting should have a listing of local community resources. One can make up a personal local resource guide and keep this information along with a listing of national organizations. Many such resources are listed at the end of each chapter in this textbook.

REFERENCES

American Academy of Pediatrics: *Health care advice: patient education for children, teens and parents*, Elk Grove Village, IL, 2002, American Academy of Pediatrics.

American Academy of Pediatrics and American Pain Society: Policy statement: the assessment and management of acute pain in infants, children, and adolescents (0793), *Pediatrics* 108:793-797, 2001.

American Public Health Association and the American Academy of Pediatrics: *Caring for our children. National health and safety standards: guidelines for out-of-home child care programs*, ed 2, Elk Grove Village, IL, 2002, American Academy of Pediatrics.

Beyer JE: *The Oucher: a user's manual and technical report*, Denver, CO, 1989, University of Colorado.

Brown JL: *Pediatric telephone medicine: principles, triage, and advice*, ed 2, Philadelphia, 1994, JB Lippincott.

Cline ME et al: Standardization of the visual analogue scale, *Nurs Res* 41:378-380, 1992

DiMaggio TJ: Pediatric pain management. In St Marie B, editor: *Core curriculum for pain management nursing*, St Louis, 2002, WB Saunders.

Eland J: Children with pain. In Jackson OB, Saunders RB, editors: *Child health nursing*, Philadelphia, 1993, JB Lippincott.

Golianu B et al: Pediatric acute pain management, *Pediatr Clin North Am* 47:559-587, 2000.

Hester NO et al: Putting pain measurement into clinical practice. In Finley GA, McGrath PJ, editors: *Measurement of pain in infants and children*, vol 10, Seattle, 1998, International Association for the Study of Pain Press.

Hudson-Barr DC, Lambert SA: Juvenile idiopathic arthritis. In Hayman LL, Mahon MM, Turner JR, editors: *Chronic illness in children*, New York, 2002, Springer.

Jordan-Marsh M et al: Alternate Oucher form testing gender, ethnicity, and age variations, *Res Nurs Health* 17:111-118, 1994

Koch WC: Fever. In Burg FD et al, editors: *Gellis and Kagan's current pediatric therapy*, ed 17, Philadelphia, 2002, WB Saunders.

Levine SR et al: Guidelines for preventing medication errors in pediatrics, *J Pediatr Pharmacol Therapeutics* 6:426-442, 2001.

Liptak GS: Physical disability and chronic illness. In Hoekelman RA, Adam HM, Nelson NM, et al, editors: *Primary pediatric care*, ed 4, St Louis, 2001, Mosby.

Mayer G, Kuklierus A: *What to do when your child gets sick*, Whittier, CA, 1999, Institute of Healthcare Advancement.

Mayoral CE et al: Alternating antipyretics: is this an alternative? *Pediatrics* 105(5):1009-1012, 2000.

Poole SR: *Developing a telephone triage and advice system for a pediatric office practice*, Elk Grove Village, IL, 2002, American Academy of Pediatrics.

Savedra MC et al: *Adolescent Pediatric Pain Tool (APPT) preliminary user's manual*, San Francisco, 1989, University of California.

Schechter WS: Pediatric pain management. In Burg FD, Ingelfinger JR, Polin RA, Gershon AA, editors: *Gellis and Kagan's current pediatric therapy*, ed 17, Philadelphia, 2002, WB Saunders.

Schiff D, Shelov S: *Guide to your child's symptoms*, Elk Grove, IL, 1997, American Academy of Pediatrics.

Schmitt BD: Calls about sick children: a triage system for the office, *Contemp Pediatr* 15(7):138-152, 1998a.

Schmitt BD: Calls about sick children: launching your own triage system, *Contemp Pediatr* 15(8):49-71, 1998b.

Schmitt BD: *Pediatric telephone protocols: the quick reference*, ed 2, Littleton, CO, 1998c, Decision Press.

Schmitt BD: *Instructions for pediatric patients*, ed 2, Philadelphia, 1999, WB Saunders.

Shepard MP, Mahon MM: Family considerations. In Hayman LL, Mahon MM, Turner JR, editors: *Chronic illness in children*, New York, 2002, Springer.

Taketomo CK, Hodding JH, Kraus DM: *Pediatric dosage handbook*, ed 9, Hudson, OH, 2002, Lexi-Comp, Inc.

Tesler MD et al: The word-graphic rating scale as a measure of children's and adolescent's pain intensity, *Res Nurs Health* 14:361-371, 1991.

Varni JW, Thompson KL, Hanson V: The Varni-Thompson pediatric pain questionnaire. I. Chronic musculoskeletal pain in juvenile rheumatoid arthritis, *Pain* 28:27-38, 1987.

Villarruel AM, Denyes MJ: Pain assessment in children: theoretical and empirical validity, *ANS Adv Nurs Sci* 14:32-41, 1991.

Wong: DL: The Wong-Baker FACES pain rating scale, *Home Health Focus* 2(8):62, 1996.

Wong D, Baker C: Pain in children: comparison of assessment scales, *Pediatr Nurs* 14:9-14, 1988.

Zempsky WT, Schechter NL: Office-based pain management, *Pediatr Clin North Am* 47:601-615, 2000.

24 Infectious Diseases

Catherine G. Blosser, Mark H. Goodman, Margaret A. Brady

Infections are a way of life for all children at one time or another. Viruses are the leading cause of most pediatric infections. Bacterial infections, particularly of the respiratory and gastrointestinal tracts, whether primary or secondary to viral illnesses, are also common problems. Most childhood illnesses resolve completely. The skilled nurse practitioner (NP) quickly needs to differentiate the insignificant illness from the more serious condition. In addition, parental anxiety and frustration in dealing with a sick child require the NP to communicate with, educate, and support the family during those trying times.

PATHOGENESIS OF INFECTIOUS DISEASES

Humans are host to a variety of microbes, most of which are harmless and, in fact, beneficial to the host. Microbial colonization occurs soon after birth. Normal host flora are protective in that they limit colonization of pathogenic organisms (Table 24-1).

An infectious process starts when a microorganism attaches to and invades host cells. For example, viruses attach and bind to the host cell surface structures by glycoproteins that are recognized by cell surface structures. Many microbes express factors that allow them to invade cells. In addition, there are other microbe–host cell interactions that permit colonization.

Illnesses occurring after colonization of viruses and bacteria result not only from cell lysis but also from cellular dysfunction or tissue destruction. For example, infection can cause an inflammatory response that is meant to defend the host against invasion by microbes but also results in destruction of both infected and adjacent tissue. This inflammatory response can occur at the local site of infection or can lead to systemic effects. With tissue infection, polymorphonuclear neutrophils (PMNs) and macrophages migrate to the site as part of the host immune response. Certain infections also have been associated with malignant changes. Chronic hepatitis B infection and Epstein-Barr viral infections are associated with hepatocellular carcinoma and Burkitt's lymphoma, respectively.

CLINICAL FINDINGS

The diagnosis of a common infectious disease in pediatric patients often is based solely on clinical findings. The history and physical examination constitute the cornerstones. The history must be comprehensive.

History

Important historical items for the NP to investigate include the following:

- Evolution of the symptoms—the order and timing of their presentation
- Epidemiology—looking for family, day care, school, or neighborhood contacts
- History of all recent and previous travel, and activities done while away
- Recent medical intervention or instrumentation—dental, gastrointestinal, genitourinary, vaccinations, transfusions
- Unusual occurrences, including loss of consciousness or trauma
- Possible drug use
- Contact with animals or animal by-products such as hides, waste, or blood
- Unusual dietary practices—ingestion of raw milk or meat
- Preexisting illness that may compromise the child
- Congenital anomalies that increase the likelihood of illness
- History of pica
- Medication history—previous and current medications used, including over-the-counter medications, herbal and folk remedies, and prescription medications
- Genetic background of family

TABLE 24-1 *Common Distribution Sites of Normal Microflora* Found in Humans*

Bacterium	Very Commonly or Commonly Found in These Locations	Notes
AEROBIC BACTERIA		
Gram Positive		
Staphylococcus		
S. aureus	Skin, hair, nasooropharynx, colon, cerumen	Rarely found in the vagina and conjunctiva; trachea, bronchi, lungs, and sinuses are normally sterile
S. epidermidis	Skin, hair, nasooropharynx, adult vagina, urethra, conjunctiva, ear (including cerumen)	Occasionally found in the vagina of prepubertal females; found in low numbers in "normal" urine, probably as result of contamination from urethra and skin areas
S. saprophyticus	Skin, hair, nasooropharynx, colon, cerumen	Occasionally found in urethra and conjunctiva
Streptococci	Mouth, nasal passages, nasopharynx	Group B uncommonly found in oropharynx and postpubertal vagina
S. faecalis (Streptococcus Group D, *Enterococcus faecalis)*	Colon, postpubertal vagina; occasionally found in mouth, urethra	
S. mitis	Skin, conjunctiva, nasooropharynx; less commonly in adult vagina and urethra	Uncommon in GI tract
S. mutans	Mouth; less common in pharynx	Has the potential of being a pathogen
S. pneumoniae (Pneumococcus, Diplococcus)	Conjunctiva, ear, mouth; rarely found in conjunctiva, ear; 20%-40% of population also have in nasopharynx	Has the potential of being a pathogen
S. pyogenes (Group A)	Skin, conjunctiva, ear, adult vagina	<10% also have in oropharynx as normal flora
S. viridans	Nasopharynx, mouth, skin	
Bifidobacterium bifidum	Colon	
Propionibacterium acnes	Skin	
Gram Negative		
Acinetobacter johnsonii	Skin, urethra, adult vagina	
Corynebacteria	Skin, cerumen, nasooropharynx, mouth, colon, urethra, adult vagina	
Citrobacter diversus	Colon	
Enterobacter	Colon, prepubertal vagina, mouth, axillary area	Has the potential of being a pathogen
Escherichia coli	Colon, vagina, mouth, urethra	Has the potential of being a pathogen
Haemophilus influenzae	Conjunctiva, ear, nasopharynx, but not commonly	Has the potential of being a pathogen
Klebsiella pneumoniae	Nose, colon, axillary area	
Lactobacillus spp.	Skin, ear, mouth, colon, adult vagina	
Moraxella catarrhalis	Nasopharynx	
Morganella morganii	Colon	
Mycobacterium spp.	Conjunctiva, ear, genital and axillary areas	
Mycoplasma	Nasooropharynx, colon, vagina	
Neisseria spp. (e.g., *N. mucosa*)	Nasopharynx (90%-100% of population)	*N. meningitidis* occurs in 5%-20% of the population as normal flora in anterior nares area
Proteus spp.	Colon, vagina, skin	
Pseudomonas aeruginosa	Nasopharynx and colon, but not common	Has the potential of being a pathogen
ANAEROBIC BACTERIA		
Bacteroides spp.	Skin, nasooropharynx, colon, adult vagina	Has the potential of being a pathogen
Clostridium spp.	Colon	Less commonly found in adult vagina, skin; can be found in small numbers in urine, but is probably a contaminant
Streptococci	Mouth, colon, adult vagina	
FUNGI		
Actinomyces spp.	Mouth, colon, skin	
Candida albicans	Skin, conjunctiva, mouth, colon, adult vagina	Can be found in voided urine but is a contaminant
Cryptococcus spp.	Skin	

TABLE 24-1 *Common Distribution Sites of Normal Microflora* Found in Humans—cont'd*

Bacterium	Very Commonly or Commonly Found in These Locations	Notes
PROTOZOA	Mouth, colon, adult vagina	
VIRUSES		500 species have been identified; the role of viruses as normal flora is undetermined

Data from Burton GR, Engelkirk PG: *Microbiology for the health sciences,* ed 5, Philadelphia, 1996, Lippincott Williams and Wilkins, p 177; Mikat DM, Mikat KW: *A clinician's dictionary guide to bacteria and fungi,* ed 4 (revised), 1983, distributed by Eli Lilly and Company, p 60-64; Tannock GW, editor: *Medical importance of the normal microflora,* Boston, 1999, Kluwer Academic Publishers, p 3-5; University of Wisconsin-Madison Department of Bacteriology: Bacteria 303—the bacterial flora of humans, 2002. (Available at *www.bact.wisc.edu/Bact303*; accessed December 2002).

*Normal microflora in humans are comprised of environmental organisms that colonize human body tissues. An individual's microflora depends upon genetics, age, sex, stress, nutrition, and diet. More than 200 species of bacteria are known to comprise the normal microflora. Skin microflora can also include yeast (*Malassezia furfur*), molds (*Trichophyton mentagrophytes* var. *interdigitale*, and mites (*Demodex folliculorum*). The spinal fluid, blood, and tissues are normally sterile; the cervix is normally sterile but can demonstrate flora similar to those in the upper area of the vagina. Antibiotics can have a minor to a major impact on the microflora (e.g., ampicillin has a major effect; erythromycin a moderate effect; and sulfonamides and penicillins minor effects).

- Hereditary diseases
- Cultural practices of family or community

Physical Examination

A complete physical examination must be undertaken. The specific examination procedures mentioned in other chapters concerning the various organ systems should be employed. Special attention should be given to the skin and mucous membranes for exanthemas and enanthemas.

Nonspecific signs of infection can include the following:

- Fever (temperature instability with severe infections in young children)
- Respiratory distress
- Vomiting or diarrhea (or both)
- Skin rashes, including petechiae
- Tachycardia, new-onset murmur
- Apnea and bradycardia (in infants)
- Irritability, high-pitched cry, bulging fontanel, convulsions
- Lethargy
- Weak suck or poor appetite
- Sweating
- Failure to thrive

DIAGNOSTIC AIDS

Laboratory Studies

The laboratory is only an adjunct to help confirm clinical suspicions. One can easily succumb to the lure of the laboratory and order all the tests necessary to rule out every illness in the differential diagnosis. This practice is ineffective and costly, and it can create confusion. Selective use of laboratory studies will help identify pathogens, predict results of treatment, and alert or track possible epidemics. If the NP has decided to do laboratory testing, the following guidelines will help ensure optimal results (Mitchell, 2002):

- Collect specimen directly from the site of active infection and sample several times (sputum sampling in children is rarely reliable).
- Take samples early in the infection.
- Sample before antibiotic treatment is initiated.
- Avoid contamination by preparing site and specimen well.
- Collect an adequate amount of the specimen.
- Transport promptly; know special handling requirements that are required or if refrigeration is needed. Contact the laboratory if in doubt about what type of collection system is indicated and how to handle the specimen once it is collected.

Common tests used to diagnose infectious diseases include the following.

Complete Blood Count

Bacterial and viral infections cause changes to the white blood cell count. Generally, bacterial infections cause leukocytosis with a differential left shift (e.g., increased polymorphonuclear leukocytes [polys] and bands). Viral infections usually cause leukopenia. There are some specific exceptions to this rule (e.g., pertussis causes an elevated white blood cell count with lymphocytosis). The clinical state of the patient is important in interpreting the complete blood count (CBC). Overwhelming sepsis, immunosuppressive drugs, and corticosteroids can alter the CBC and confuse the clinical picture.

Erythrocyte Sedimentation Rate

An elevated erythrocyte sedimentation rate (ESR), either zeta or Westergren method, suggests inflammation. Although not specific for infectious disease, it may suggest the need for further workup. It also is useful to evaluate treatment and resolution of many types of infections, such as osteomyelitis.

Cultures

Depending on the clinical presentation, one can obtain specimens for culture from all natural body orifices and, if necessary, create some additional ones (e.g., blood, cerebrospinal fluid [CSF], pleura, joints, and abscesses). Different types of bacteria, viruses, fungi, and parasites require different media. This can result in handling problems. One should notify the laboratory of clinical suspicions to ensure proper handling. Gram stains also can be performed on all body fluids and can help in the choice of proper antibiotics before the culture and sensitivity tests are available.

Skin Tests

Skin tests include the purified protein derivative (PPD) and Schick tests.

Serodiagnostic Tests

Staining Techniques. Specific antisera are combined with fluorescein dye. If a sensitive organism is present, antibodies congregate around it, and the resultant mixture illuminates. Gram stain remains a useful rapid test.

Serologic Tests. Specific antisera can cause an agglutination reaction. The tests are measured by dilutional factors. A fourfold rise is considered positive and suggests the diagnosis. There are false-positive and false-negative reactions owing to cross-reactivity of antisera.

Antibody Detection Techniques. Besides fluorescent staining techniques and serologic tests, other techniques of antibody detection include complement fixation, hemagglutination inhibition, and enzyme-linked immunosorbent assay (ELISA) testing.

Antimicrobial Sensitivity Testing. Standard zone diameters indicate sensitivity to or resistance of a microbe to a specific antibiotic.

Other Laboratory Tests

- Deoxyribonucleic acid (DNA) probes are DNA-segment specific, radioactively labeled reagents used to identify various bacteria.
- Enzyme immunoassay (EIA) tests are useful in helping to make a quick diagnosis (e.g., rotavirus and respiratory syncytial virus).
- Polymerase chain reaction (PCR) is a process that increases the amount of DNA sequences to be analyzed by multiplying copies of the original DNA segment.

Imaging Techniques

Radiographs can be useful in the diagnosis of infections. Chest radiographs, sinus series, and mastoid studies assist the NP in the evaluation of children with unusual or minimal findings. Radioactive scans are advantageous in the detection of osteomyelitis or abscesses. Computed tomography (CT) scans and magnetic resonance imaging (MRI) can detect abscesses or other purulent material collections.

GENERAL MANAGEMENT STRATEGIES

Principles for Preventing the Spread of Infections

Education of parents and children in the prevention of the spread of infectious diseases should be routinely done. Potential areas to cover include the following:

- The spread of respiratory disease may be decreased by handwashing, covering one's mouth when coughing, properly disposing of saliva-infected tissues, not sharing foods or liquids that someone else has eaten, and limiting exposure to ill contacts.
- Skin infections can be reduced by careful handwashing and limiting contact with fluid from skin lesions (e.g., covering lesions, if appropriate; use of separate towels for personal hygiene; keeping nails trimmed).
- Enteric infections are transmitted by the fecal-oral route; meticulous handwashing after toileting or changing diapers is critical. Attention to proper food handling and preparation to prevent growth of, or contamination with, bacteria, viruses, fungi, and parasites also is an area to discuss. Proper disposal of pet waste and washing of hands after contact with pets should be stressed.
- Parents of infants and young children in day care should be familiar with the day care setting's policies related to cleaning of toys and sleep equipment, toileting practices, diaper-changing procedures, routine handwashing procedures for both staff and children, ill-child procedures, and environmental sanitation procedures.

Principles Guiding the Judicious Use of Antimicrobial Agents

The increasing emergence of bacterial strains that are resistant to antimicrobial agents is worrisome. Between 1980 and 1992 there was a 48% increase in the number of antibiotics prescribed for children (Dowell et al, 1998).

Vancomycin-resistant enterococci, multidrug-resistant tuberculosis, and antimicrobial-resistant respiratory pathogens are now major threats to children who become infected with these organisms. Scientific data have shown that the key factor responsible for the emergence and spread of resistant organisms is the widespread use of antimicrobials, whether inappropriately or appropriately prescribed. A study by the Centers for Disease Control and Prevention's (CDC's) National Campaign for Appropriate Antibiotic Use reports that 40% of prescriptions for antibiotics are given for viral infections diagnosed in outpatient clinics (Besser, 2002). Parental pressure to prescribe unnecessary antimicrobials for the common cold, bronchitis, and viral pharyngitis is not an acceptable reason to prescribe an antibiotic. Parental education about the course and treatment of viral illnesses and the link of antimicrobial resistance to the overuse of antibiotics is a key point that NPs must address with parents. In addition, when antimicrobials are prescribed, completion of the prescribed course of therapy should be stressed. The use of antibiotics for prophylaxis is also being questioned, and caution is advised (Dowell et al, 1998).

PREVENTION OF INFECTION THROUGH THE USE OF VACCINES

Prevention is always better than treatment. Vaccination is the single best technique for the prevention of communicable infectious disease. Vaccines now exist to combat many childhood diseases (e.g., *Haemophilus influenzae* type b, *Streptococcus pneumoniae*, meningococcus, diphtheria, pertussis, tetanus, polio, measles, mumps, rubella, hepatitis A and B, influenza, varicella, and pneumococcus), but NPs still see some of these illnesses. Practitioners must continue to educate patients about the need to keep current with necessary immunizations. Failure to do so may result in avoidable epidemics.

Informed consent is critical when discussing the benefits and risks of vaccination. The National Childhood Vaccine Injury Act of 1986 (Public Law 99-660, amended by Public Law 101-239) became effective in 1988. This act has provisions that call for standardized consent forms. All practitioners are required to use these forms to fulfill their duty to warn the public. The act also requires that the vaccine lot number, site of inoculation, name of the person administering the vaccine, and parental signature are included in the medical record.

The National Childhood Vaccine Injury Act also requires health care providers to report selected adverse events that occur after immunization. These are discussed in detail later. The events are to be reported to the Vaccine Adverse Event Reporting System (VAERS), established by the U.S. Department of Health and Human Services. A standard confidential form for reporting suspected vaccine-related problems has been in existence since 1990. A VAERS staff member contacts the provider at 60 days and 1 year after the report to follow up on the patient's condition. The VAERS telephone number is 800-822-7967. Report forms are also available from the Food and Drug Administration (FDA) website (see Resources Box).

Vaccine Controversies

The Institute of Medicine's (IOM's) Immunization Safety Review Committee reported finding no general connection or insufficient causal evidence between the following: thimerosal and autism; attention-deficit hyperactivity disorder and speech/language delays; measles, mumps, rubella and autism; other neurologic events and bowel disease; and hepatitis B and demyelinating diseases of the central nervous system (CNS) and peripheral nervous system (multiple sclerosis, acute disseminated encephalomyelitis, optic neuritis, transverse myelitis, Guillain-Barré syndrome, and brachial neuritis [IOM, 2001a, 2001b, 2002b]). The IOM also looked at the role that multiple vaccines might play in causing type 1 diabetes or serious infections. After a review of dozens of scientific research studies, a causal relationship was dismissed. However, there was some mixed evidence between studies regarding a possible connection between asthma and diphtheria-tetanus-pertussis (DTP) vaccine (IOM, 2002a). The Immunization Safety Review Committee concluded that further research in all these areas was warranted given the public concern with vaccine safety, the threat of increased populations going unvaccinated because of these fears, and the resulting resurgence of preventable diseases.

Some vaccines had thimerosal, a preservative containing ethyl mercury, added to reduce bacterial growth. The elimination of thimerosal from all vaccines used in infants, children, and pregnant women has been recommended. Vaccines produced since July 2000 that are on the CDC's recommended list for childhood immunizations are regarded as being thimerosal free. There are a few that still contain trace amounts of thimerosal from the manufacturing process. Influenza vaccine is one that may still contain this preservative, but its use is recommended because the benefit is believed to outweigh any risk (IOM, 2001b; Stephenson, 2002).

Active Immunity

Inoculating a child with modified parts of a microorganism evokes an immune response. Whole organisms (live, attenuated, or killed), modified proteins, and sugars are used to prepare certain vaccines. The response to vaccination is often as protective as the natural infection. Antiinvasive, antitoxin, or neutralizing antibodies can be found soon after the vaccination is given. Some types of vaccines give lifelong immunity. Others require periodic boosters. The active and inert vaccine ingredients differ among manufacturers. One must be aware of these components because of a patient's possible hypersensitivity to the ingredients used. Live or attenuated vaccines usually confer broader and longer lived immunity than killed types. Killed and inactivated vaccines can provide systemic protection (immunoglobulin G [IgG] antibodies) but may fail to provide local mucosal antibody (IgA). Thus, although protected from systemic illness, a recipient of a killed vaccine can have local colonization or infection that can be a problem during an epidemic.

The American Academy of Pediatrics (AAP), the American Academy of Family Physicians (AAFP), and the Advisory Committee on Immunization Practices (ACIP) of the CDC annually approve a new unified recommended childhood immunization schedule (Table 24-2).

Maternal antibodies neutralize vaccines; therefore infants vaccinated in the first year of life require more inoculations than older children. Children who are not immunized in the first year of life should be vaccinated according to the schedule listed in Table 24-3. Missed vaccinations should be given when possible. One does not need to repeat the entire series again; just continue normally from that point. Vaccines given outside of the United States are acceptable as long as there is strict and reliable evidence of written proof (dates of administration, number of doses) and the age and spacing are the same as CDC recommendations. If in doubt, antibody titers can be checked. Generally, most vaccines used worldwide have been produced with adequate quality control and are reliable, but the handling can be suspect (AAP, 2003). If in doubt, immunize (children being adopted from overseas generally need all immunizations repeated). Proper storage of vaccines and correct immunization technique are critical for optimum results. The manufacturer's package inserts provide this information.

The ACIP has issued revisions to some of its prior recommendations (American Journal for NPS, 2002). These included the following:

- Vaccine doses may be given up to 4 days before prior minimum intervals or ages, to provide some schedule flexibility.
- If two live virus parenteral vaccines are given less than 28 days apart, the vaccine given second should be disregarded; repeat this second vaccine at least 4 weeks later.
- Administering rabies or hepatitis B vaccine in an incorrect site (e.g., gluteus) or via an inappropriate route (e.g., hepatitis B vaccine not given intramuscularly) decreases immunogenicity; the vaccine(s) would need repeating in such instances.
- Do not aspirate the syringe before injection (unproven necessity).
- Preterm infants whose mothers are hepatitis B surface antigen (HBsAg) positive, or whose status is unknown, should receive both hepatitis B vaccine and hepatitis B immune globulin (HBIG) within 12 hours of birth and three additional doses of hepatitis B vaccine at 1, 2, and 6 months.

Reportable vaccine-associated events related to all recommended childhood vaccines are identified in Table 24-4.

Diphtheria and Tetanus Toxoids with Pertussis Vaccine

Diphtheria and tetanus toxoids with acellular pertussis vaccine (DTaP) is now principally used in the United States rather than the whole-cell product, diphtheria and tetanus toxoids with pertussis vaccine (DTP). Whole-cell vaccines are still used in other parts of the world. DTP is a trivalent vaccine and is composed of the diphtheria and tetanus toxoids and killed whole-cell pertussis vaccine. DTaP is also composed of diphtheria and tetanus toxoids but has an acellular pertussis vaccine that lowers the side effects found with whole-cell vaccine. DTP is an acceptable alternative to DTaP. Scheduling for these vaccines is given in Tables 24-2 and 24-3. Universal immunization with DTaP (or DTP) is the only effective control measure for these illnesses. Diphtheria and tetanus toxoids are highly effective vaccines as proven by the rarity of these diseases in the United States. The usual dosage is 0.5 ml intramuscularly (IM). There are currently three licensed DTaP vaccines available in the United States: Tripedia, TriHIBit (a combination vaccine used as a fourth dose), and Infanrix. Previously licensed and available vaccines, Acel-Imune and Certiva, have been discontinued for sale in the United States by the manufacturer. All of these vaccines are equally effective but differ slightly in their ingredients.

Interchangeability of these vaccines has not been studied. When possible, one should continue the same vaccine for the first three primary doses. Any licensed product is acceptable for the fourth and fifth doses regardless of the product(s) used previously. If previously vaccinated using the whole-cell vaccine, future vaccines should be DTaP. Children younger than 7 years of age must be vaccinated with DT if there are contraindications to giving the pertussis vaccine. Td vaccine contains a smaller amount of diphtheria toxoid and is given to patients older than 7 years of age. Older children and adults require less stimulation for antibody production. If tetanus toxoid is required for contaminated wound management, consider using either DTaP, DT, or Td, as indicated, to provide adequate diphtheria immunity (Table 24-5).

There are a few relative contraindications to vaccinating a child with DTaP. The first is an immediate anaphylactic reaction and the second is encephalopathy within 7 days of receiving DPTaP or DTP. If DTaP or DTP was given and

TABLE 24-2 *Recommended Childhood and Adolescent Immunization[1] — United States, 2003*

Range of recommended ages | Catch-up vaccination | Preadolescent assessment

Vaccine	Birth	1 mo	2 mos	4 mos	6 mos	12 mos	15 mos	18 mos	24 mos	4–6 yrs	11–12 yrs	13–18 yrs
Hepatitis B[2]	HepB #1	only if mother HBsAg (-)										
		HepB #2			HepB #3				HepB series			
Diphtheria, Tetanus, Pertussis[3]			DTaP	DTaP	DTaP		DTaP			DTaP	Td	
Haemophilus influenzae Type b[4]			Hib	Hib	Hib	Hib						
Inactivated Polio			IPV	IPV	IPV					IPV		
Measles, Mumps, Rubella[5]						MMR #1				MMR #2	MMR #2	
Varicella[6]						Varicella			Varicella			
Pneumococcal[7]			PCV	PCV	PCV	PCV			PCV			
									PPV			
Vaccines below this line are for selected populations												
Hepatitis A[8]									HepA series			
Influenza[9]					Influenza (yearly)							

1. Indicates the recommended ages for routine administration of currently licensed childhood vaccines, as of December 1, 2002, for children through age 18 years. Any dose not given at the recommended age should be given at any subsequent visit when indicated and feasible. ▨ Indicates age groups that warrant special effort to administer those vaccines not given previously. Additional vaccines may be licensed and recommended during the year. Licensed combination vaccines may be used whenever any components of the combination are indicated and the vaccine's other components are not contraindicated. Providers should consult the manufacturers' package inserts for detailed recommendations.

2. **Hepatitis B vaccine (HepB).** All infants should receive the first dose of HepB vaccine soon after birth and before hospital discharge; the first dose also may be given by age 2 months if the infant's mother is HBsAg-negative. Only monovalent HepB vaccine can be used for the birth dose. Monovalent or combination vaccine containing HepB may be used to complete the series; 4 doses of vaccine may be administered when a birth dose is given. The second dose should be given at least 4 weeks after the first dose except for combination vaccines, which cannot be administered before age 6 weeks. The third dose should be given at least 16 weeks after the first dose and at least 8 weeks after the second dose. The last dose in the vaccination series (third or fourth dose) should not be administered before age 6 months. Infants born to HBsAg-positive mothers should receive HepB vaccine and 0.5 mL hepatitis B immune globulin (HBIG) within 12 hours of birth at separate sites. The second dose is recommended at age 1–2 months. The last dose in the vaccination series should not be administered before age 6 months. These infants should be tested for HBsAg and anti-HBs at 9–15 months of age. Infants born to mothers whose HBsAg status is unknown should receive the first dose of the HepB vaccine series within 12 hours of birth. Maternal blood should be drawn as soon as possible to determine the mother's HBsAg status; if the HBsAg test is positive, the infant should receive HBIG as soon as possible (no later than age 1 week). The second dose is recommended at age 1–2 months. The last dose in the vaccination series should not be administered before age 6 months.

3. **Diphtheria and tetanus toxoids and acellular pertussis vaccine (DTaP).** The fourth dose of DTaP may be administered at age 12 months provided that 6 months have elapsed since the third dose and the child is unlikely to return at age 15–18 months. **Tetanus and diphtheria toxoids (Td)** is recommended at age 11–12 years if at least 5 years have elapsed since the last dose of Td-containing vaccine. Subsequent routine Td boosters are recommended every 10 years.

4. ***Haemophilus influenzae* type b (Hib) conjugate vaccine.** Three Hib conjugate vaccines are licensed for infant use. If PRP-OMP (PedvaxHIB® or ComVax® [Merck]) is administered at age 2 and 4 months, a dose at age 6 months is not required. DTaP/Hib combination products should not be used for primary vaccination in infants at age 2, 4, or 6 months but can be used as boosters following any Hib vaccine.

5. **Measles, mumps, and rubella vaccine (MMR).** The second dose of MMR is recommended routinely at age 4–6 years but may be administered during any visit provided that at least 4 weeks have elapsed since the first dose and that both doses are administered beginning at or after age 12 months. Those who have not received the second dose previously should complete the schedule by the visit at age 11–12 years.

6. **Varicella vaccine.** Varicella vaccine is recommended at any visit at or after age 12 months for susceptible children (i.e., those who lack a reliable history of chickenpox). Susceptible persons aged ≥13 years should receive 2 doses given at least 4 weeks apart.

7. **Pneumococcal vaccine.** The heptavalent **pneumococcal conjugate vaccine (PCV)** is recommended for all children aged 2–23 months and for certain children aged 24–59 months. **Pneumococcal polysaccharide vaccine (PPV)** is recommended in addition to PCV for certain high-risk groups. See *MMWR* 2000;49(No. RR-9):1–37.

8. **Hepatitis A vaccine.** Hepatitis A vaccine is recommended for children and adolescents in selected states and regions, and for certain high-risk groups. Consult local public health authority and *MMWR* 1999;48(No. RR-12):1–37. Children and adolescents in these states, regions, and high-risk groups who have not been immunized against hepatitis A can begin the hepatitis A vaccination series during any visit. The two doses in the series should be administered at least 6 months apart.

9. **Influenza vaccine.** Influenza vaccine is recommended annually for children aged ≥6 months with certain risk factors (including but not limited to asthma, cardiac disease, sickle cell disease, HIV, and diabetes, and household members of persons in groups at high risk (see *MMWR* 2002;51[No. RR-3]:1–31), and can be administered to all others wishing to obtain immunity. In addition, healthy children age 6–23 months are encouraged to receive influenza vaccine if feasible because children in this age group are at substantially increased risk for influenza-related hospitalizations. Children aged ≤12 years should receive vaccine in a dosage appropriate for their age (0.25 mL if 6–35 months or 0.5 mL if ≥3 years). Children aged ≤8 years who are receiving influenza vaccine for the first time should receive 2 doses separated by at least 4 weeks.

Additional information about vaccines, including precautions and contraindications for vaccination and vaccine shortages, is available at http://www.cdc.gov/nip or at the National Immunization information hotline, telephone 800-232-2522 (English) or 800-232-0233 (Spanish). Copies of the schedule can be obtained at http://www.cdc.gov/nip/recs/child-schedule.htm. Approved by the **Advisory Committee on Immunization Practices** (http://www.cdc.gov/nip/acip), the **American Academy of Pediatrics** (http://www.aap.org), and the **American Academy of Family Physicians** (http://www.aafp.org).

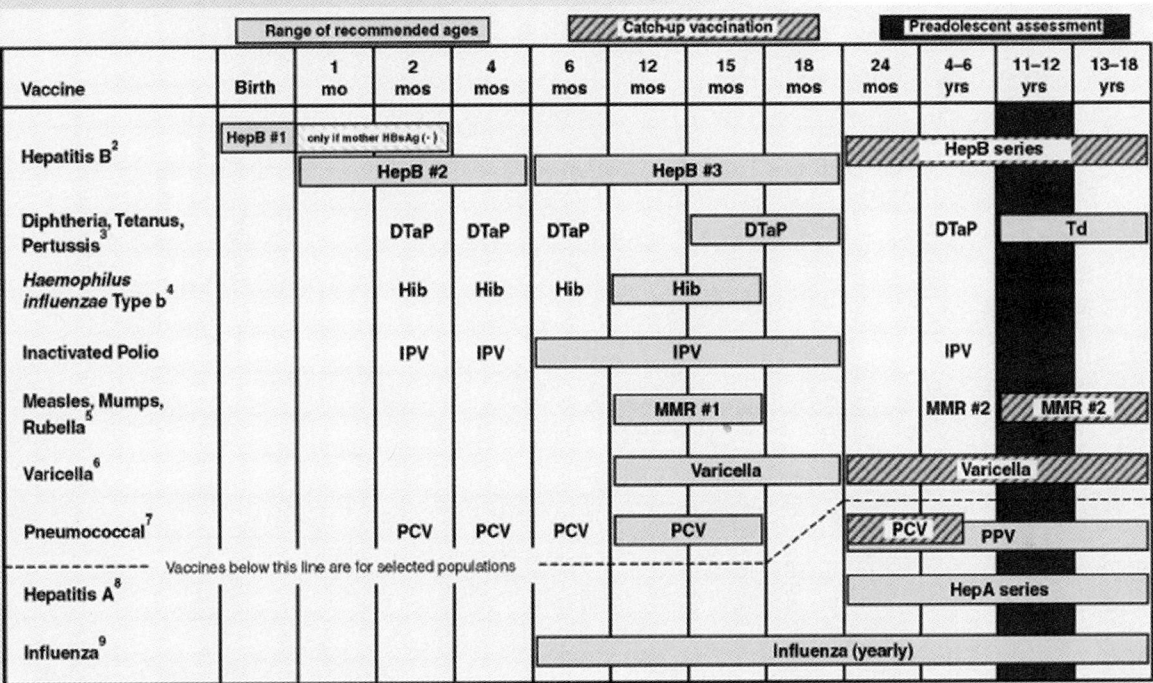

TABLE 24-3 *Catch-up Schedule for Children 4 Months to 18 Years of Age*

Dose One (Minimum Age)	Minimum Interval Between Doses				
	Dose One to Dose Two	**Dose Two to Dose Three**	**Dose Three to Dose Four**	**Dose Three to Booster Dose**	**Dose Four to Dose Five**
4 Months to 6 Years of Age					
DtaP (6 wk)	**4 wk**	**4 wk**	**6 mo**		**6 mo**[1]
IPV (6 wk)	**4 wk**	**4 wk**	**4 wk**[2]		
HepB[3] (birth)	**4 wk**	**3 wk** (and 16 weeks after first dose)			
MMR (12 mo)	**4 wk**[4]				
Varicella (12 mo)					
Hib[5] (6 wk)	**4 wk:** if first dose given at age <12 mo **8 wk (as final dose)**: if first dose given at age 12-24 mo **No further doses needed**: if first dose given at age ≥15 mo	**4 wk**[6]: if current age <12 mo **8 wk (as final dose)**: if current age ≥12 mo and second dose given at age <15 mo **No further doses needed**: if previous dose given at age ≥15 mo	**8 wk (as final dose)**: this dose only necessary for children age 12 mo to 5 yr who received three doses before age 12 mo		
PCV[7] (6 wk) or **PCV7**	**4 wk**: if first dose given at age <12 mo and current age <24 mo **8 wk (as final dose)**: if first dose given at age ≥12 mo or current age 24-59 mo **No further doses needed**: for healthy children if first dose given at age ≥24 mo	**4 wk**: if current age <12 mo **8 wk (as final dose)**: if current age ≥12 mo **No further doses needed**: for healthy children if previous dose given at age ≥24 mo	**8 wk (as final dose)**: this dose only necessary for children age 12 mo to 5 yr who received three doses before age 12 mo		
7 to 18 Years of Age					
	Td: 4 wk	**Td: 6 mo**		**Td**[8]: **6 mo**: if first dose given at age <12 mo and current age <11 yr **5 yr:** if first dose given at age ≥12 mo and third dose given at age <7 yr and current age ≥11 yr **10 yr**: if third dose given at age ≥7 yr	

IPV[9]: **4 wk** **HepB: 4 wk**	**IPV**[9]: **4 wk** **HepB: 8 wk** (and 16 wk after first dose)	**IPV**[2, 9]
MMR: 4 wk **Varicella**[10]: **4 wk**		

Adapted from CDC website: *www.cdc-gov/nip/recs/child-catchup* (accessed Nov 8, 2003).

[1]**Diphtheria and tetanus toxoids and acellular pertussis vaccine (DtaP)**: The fifth dose is not necessary if the fourth dose was given after the fourth birthday.

[2]**Inactivated polio (IPV)**: For children who received an all-IPV or all-OPV series, a fourth dose is not necessary if the third dose was given at age 4 years. If both IPV and OPV were given as part of a series, a total of four doses should be given, regardless of the child's current age.

[3]**Hepatitis B vaccine (HepB)**: All children and adolescents who have not been vaccinated against hepatitis B should begin the hepatitis B vaccination series during any visit. Providers should make special efforts to immunize children who were born in, or whose parents were born in, areas of the world where hepatitis B virus infection is moderately or highly endemic.

[4]**Measles, mumps, and rubella vaccine (MMR)**: The second dose of MMR is recommended routinely at age 4-6 years but may be given earlier if desired.

[5]***Haemophilus influenzae* type b (Hib)**: Vaccine is not recommended generally for children age ≥5 years.

[6]**Hib**: If current age is <12 mo and the first two doses were PRP-OMP (PedvaxHIB® or Comvax [Merck]®), the third (and final) dose should be given at age 12-15 months and at least 8 weeks after the second dose.

[7]**Pneumococcal conjugate vaccine (PCV)**: Vaccine is not recommended generally for children age ≥5 years.

[8]**Tetanus and diphtheria (Td) toxoids vaccine**: For children age 7-10 years, the interval between the third and booster doses is determined by the age when the first dose was given. For adolescents age 11-18 years, the interval between is determined by the age when the third dose was given.

[9]**IPV**: Vaccine is not recommended generally for persons age ≥18 years.

[10]**Varicella**: Give two-dose series to all susceptible adolescents age ≥13 years.

any of the following events occurred, they are listed as precautions to further administration of DTaP:

- Convulsion, with or without fever, within 3 days of immunization
- Persistent inconsolable screaming (longer than 3 hours) within 48 hours
- Collapse or shocklike state within 48 hours (referred to as hypotonic-hyporesponsive episodes)
- Unexplained temperature higher than 104.8° F (40.5° C) within 48 hours

DTaP, as previously noted, has a significantly lower probability of vaccine-associated reactions, such as moderate or high fever and local reactions. Most reactions to DTaP occur with the fourth or fifth dose. Reactions include swelling, erythema, and pain at the injection site, as well as fever. Reactions occur with mild intensity in 1% to 3% of recipients, usually within the first 48 hours, and resolve within days.

Children who have progressive developmental delay or a changing neurologic picture should be assessed on an individual basis. Those with stable encephalopathy (e.g., cerebral palsy or cognitive developmental delays) or controlled seizures can be immunized with pertussis. There are no studies that either conclusively prove or disprove a connection that specifically links DTaP (DTP) as a cause of brain damage. However, there can be confusion regarding the cause of some neurologic disorders. Infants and children who have or are suspected to have neurologic disorders or progressive degenerative diseases should have the pertussis vaccine

TABLE 24-4 ***Vaccine Adverse Event Report System (VAERS): Reportable Events following Vaccination****

Vaccine/Toxoid	Event	Onset Interval
Tetanus in any combination: DTaP, DTP, DTP-HIB, DT, Td, or TT	A. Anaphylaxis or anaphylactic shock	7 days
	B. Brachial neuritis	28 days
	C. Any sequelae (including death) of above events	No limit
	D. Events described in manufacturer's package insert as contraindications to additional doses of vaccine	See package insert
Pertussis in any combination: DTaP, DTP, DTP-HIB, P	A. Anaphylaxis or anaphylactic shock	7 days
	B. Encephalopathy (or encephalitis)	7 days
	C. Any sequelae (including death) of above events	Not applicable
	D. Events described in manufacturer's package insert as contraindications to additional doses of vaccine	See package insert
Measles, mumps, and rubella in any combination: MMR, MR, M, or R	A. Anaphylaxis or anaphylactic shock	7 days
	B. Encephalopathy (or encephalitis)	15 days
	C. Any sequelae (including death) of above events	Not applicable
	D. Events described in manufacturer's package insert as contraindications to additional doses of vaccine	See package insert
Rubella in any combination: MMR, MR, R	A. Chronic arthritis	42 days
	B. Any sequelae (including death) of above event	Not applicable
	C. Events described in manufacturer's package insert as contraindications to additional doses of vaccine	See package insert
Measles in any combination: MMR, MR, M	A. Thrombocytopenic purpura	7-30 days
	B. Vaccine-strain measles viral infection in an immunodeficient recipient	6 mo
	C. Any sequelae (including death) of above event	Not applicable
	D. Events described in manufacturer's package insert as contraindications to additional doses of vaccine	See package insert
Oral polio vaccine (OPV)	A. Paralytic polio (nonimmunodeficient/immunodeficient)	30 days/6 mo
	B. Vaccine-strain polio viral infection (same as above)	30 days/6 mo
	C. Any sequelae (including death) of above events	Not applicable
	D. Events described in manufacturer's package insert as contraindications to additional doses of vaccine	See package insert
Inactivated polio vaccine (IPV)	A. Anaphylaxis or anaphylactic shock	7 days
	B. Any sequelae (including death) of the above event	Not applicable
	C. Events described in manufacturer's package insert as contraindications to additional doses of vaccine	See package insert

TABLE 24-4 ***Vaccine Adverse Event Report System (VAERS): Reportable Events following Vaccination*—cont'd***

Vaccine/Toxoid	Event	Onset Interval
Hepatitis B	A. Anaphylaxis or anaphylactic shock	7 days
	B. Any sequelae (including death) of the above event	Not applicable
	C. Events described in manufacturer's package insert as contraindications to additional doses of vaccine	See package insert
Haemophilus influenzae, type b (conjugate)	A. Events described in manufacturer's package insert as contraindications to additional doses of vaccine	See package insert
Varicella	A. Events described in manufacturer's package insert as contraindications to additional doses of vaccine	See package insert
Rotavirus	A. Intussusception	30 days
	B. Any sequela (including death) of the above event	Not applicable
	C. Events described in manufacturer's package insert as contraindications to additional doses of vaccine	See package insert
Pneumococcal conjugate	A. Events described in manufacturer's package insert as contraindications to additional doses of vaccine	See package insert

Available from VAERS website: *http://vaers.org* (accessed Nov 6, 2003).
The Reportable Events Table (RET) reflects what is reportable by law (42 USC 300aa-25) to the Vaccine Adverse Event Reporting System (VAERS) including conditions found in the manufacturer's package insert. In addition, individuals are encouraged to report any clinically significant or unexpected events (even if you are not certain the vaccine caused the event) for any vaccine, whether or not it is listed on the RET. Manufacturers are also required by regulation (21CFR 600.80) to report to the VAERS program all adverse events made known to them for any vaccine.
*Effective date: Aug 26, 2002.
See text for definitions of abbreviations.

deferred until further assessment is complete. The decision to vaccinate should be based on the risk-benefit ratio. A family history of adverse immunization reactions should not preclude the use of DTaP in other family members. Children with a personal history of seizures are at greater risk for vaccine-related seizures, but this is not a contraindication. If the neurologic condition is stabilized, controlled, or resolved and pertussis vaccination is contraindicated, DT vaccination can be given. Children who are seropositive for pertussis do not need to receive further pertussis vaccinations.

DTaP and *H. influenzae* type b (HIB) vaccine have been combined in the vaccine TriHIBit. This vaccine is approved only for the fourth dose after a regimen of three doses of any other DTaP, whole-cell DTP, and primary HIB vaccine series has been given. Other conjugated HIB vaccines cannot be mixed with other DTaP products.

TABLE 24-5 ***Tetanus Prophylaxis in Wound Management***

Previous Tetanus Immunization	Clean Minor Wound	Dirty Wound
Uncertain or fewer than three doses	Td only*	Td* and TIG within 3 days
Three doses	Td (fourth dose)*	Td (fourth dose)*
More than three doses	Td* if last dose >10 yr ago	Td* if last dose >5 yr ago

*In children older than 7 years, use Td for vaccination. In children younger than 7 years of age, use DTaP (or DTP) or DT if pertussis is contraindicated.
See text for definitions of abbreviations.

Evidence from research studies suggests that controlling pertussis in young infants may depend on older children and adults receiving boosters with acellular pertussis vaccine (Steele, 2001a). Currently, the CDC has made no official recommendation.

Bacille Calmette-Guérin Vaccine

Bacille Calmette-Guérin (BCG) vaccine was developed in the early part of the twentieth century to prevent the spread of tuberculosis (TB). Studies of vaccine efficacy demonstrate inconsistent findings, but the vaccine is still recommended as a public health measure in developing countries with a high prevalence of TB. Two strains are currently licensed in the United States. Two meta-analyses of clinical and case-controlled studies proved the protective efficacy of BCG vaccine in children (greater than 80% protective), but the studies did not prove the efficacy in adolescents and adults.

In the United States, BCG is indicated only for infants and children with negative tuberculin skin testing and who (1) live with persons with infectious pulmonary TB who are untreated or ineffectually treated, cannot be removed from those persons, and are without a source of long-term primary treatment; or (2) live with persons who have drug-resistant forms of TB (to isoniazid and rifampin) and cannot be separated from those persons.

Health care workers in high-risk settings also may be candidates for BCG (CDC, 2000a).

BCG is given to infants from birth until 2 months of age without prior tuberculin testing as long as the child is not further exposed to tuberculosis. Older children must have a negative tuberculin test before the vaccine is given. The vaccine is given intradermally; the usual dose is 0.05 ml for a neonate and 0.1 ml for an older child. If given properly, a small papule forms at the site of injection. The papule enlarges, crusts, and lasts approximately 2 to 3 months. PPD testing should be repeated 2 months later. If the second PPD is not reactive, repeat the vaccination.

One percent to 10% of those vaccinated with BCG experience side effects. These include localized ulceration, axillary lymphadenopathy, or cervical lymphadenopathy. Osteomyelitis, meningitis, and death are rare reactions (World Health Organization [WHO], 2000). BCG is contraindicated in patients with immunologic disorders. Children who are receiving corticosteroids or other immunosuppressive agents should not be vaccinated. Although no fetal problems have been reported, pregnant women should not be inoculated with BCG. Approximately 100 million newborns are vaccinated each year with minimal side effects (WHO, 2000). A guideline for the use of BCG is available from the WHO.

Children with symptomatic human immunodeficiency virus (HIV) infection should not receive BCG. Asymptomatic HIV-infected children living in areas where the incidence of TB is low (e.g., the United States) should not be vaccinated. However, asymptomatic or suspected HIV-infected children living in areas where the incidence of TB is high should receive BCG as close to birth as possible. BCG vaccine can produce a mild to severe hypersensitivity reaction to tuberculin. It also can cause a false-positive reaction in children who receive tuberculin skin testing. Children with prior BCG vaccination should receive tuberculin skin testing. If the resultant induration is larger than 10 mm, treatment with isoniazid should be considered for those individuals who are foreign born, have lived in countries with high TB rates, had contact with persons with infectious TB, or have an occupation that requires close contact with susceptible individuals. If they are HIV positive and previously vaccinated with BCG, they are considered for treatment if the tuberculin skin testing is larger than 5 mm or they have had exposure to someone with infectious pulmonary TB (CDC, 2000a).

Polio Vaccine

Before January 2000, two forms of polio vaccine were licensed in the United States: live oral trivalent polio vaccine (OPV) and inactivated trivalent polio vaccine (IPV). The difference between the two vaccines is that IPV does not protect against intestinal infection with wild virus as does OPV.

Cases of vaccine-associated paralytic polio (VAPP) associated with the oral vaccine have occurred in vaccinees and close contacts. In immunologically normal or compromised children, the risk is 1 in 1.2 million after the first doses of vaccine. In both recipients and contacts, the risk is 1 in 2.4 million doses. The risk of paralysis is higher with administration of the first dose of vaccine and when immunocompromised persons are exposed to live polio vaccine (AAP, 2000). When polio was epidemic, these vaccine-induced cases were acceptable. The original IPV was less potent than the vaccine currently in use. The current strain of IPV is stronger (IPV-e, injectable poliovirus vaccine of enhanced potency).

The ACIP, AAP, and AAFP currently recommend an all-IPV schedule for routine childhood polio immunization. All children should receive four doses of IPV at 2 months, 4 months, 6 to 18 months, and 4 to 6 years (see Table 24-2). The dose of IPV is 0.5 ml IM. The need for booster dosages of enhanced IPV has not been determined. The contraindication to IPV is an anaphylactic reaction to either neomycin, polymyxin B, or streptomycin; it should be used in caution in pregnant women (AAP, 2003).

OPV is no longer distributed in the United States. However, if mass vaccination is needed to control outbreaks of paralytic polio, OPV would be considered a public health measure (AAP, 2003).

Haemophilus influenzae *Type B Vaccine*

Of the six serotypes of *H. influenzae*, type B (HIB) is the most virulent and is spread primarily through respiratory droplets. Until the advent of the first HIB polysaccharide vaccine in 1987, it was the cause of 95% of all *H. influenzae* invasive diseases. Type b disease was the most common etiology of bacterial meningitis in children under 5 years of age (mostly before 24 months of age). Mortality rate was 3% to 5%; neurologic sequelae rate was 15% to 30%. The issuance of this vaccine has resulted in a phenomenal 99% decrease in the incidence of HIB meningitis. Most new cases are in infants younger than 6 months of age; there have been no reported deaths (Kronemyer, 2002a).

The HIB vaccines consist of purified bacterial protein joined to a polysaccharide or oligosaccharide that is linked to a protein to enhance immunogenicity. PRP-D (ProHIBiT), HbOC (HibTITER), PRP-T (ActHIB or OmniHIB), PRP-OMP (PedvaxHIB), and combination HIB/hepatitis B (Comvax) are currently licensed HIB vaccines. HbOC, PRP-T, and PRP-OMP are given to infants beginning at 2 months of age. The vaccines are interchangeable for all doses (including booster), except that PRP-OMP requires only two doses in the primary series.

Most HIB vaccine failures have been seen in infants who received the two- to three-dose primary series too young (Kronemyer, 2002a). Therefore Comvax vaccine cannot be used at birth. PRP-D is licensed only for booster doses in children older than 12 months of age or for primary administration that starts at 15 months of age. Any child younger than 2 years of age who had invasive *H. influenzae* disease should be vaccinated with any of the conjugated HIB vaccines according to the schedule recommended for the child's age. This is because of the decreased natural immunity in this age-group. Unlike DTaP (or DTP) or polio vaccine, the number of doses of HIB vaccine changes depending on when the initial immunization is begun. The older the child is, the fewer doses the child receives. For all vaccines the dosage is 0.5 ml IM. Table 24-6 lists the HIB immunization schedule. CDC recommends that the same vaccine should be used for the primary series, but studies have not demonstrated a decline in antibody production if regimens involving different vaccine products are used. Any licensed single HIB vaccine may be used for the booster when the child is 12 to 15 months old. HIB vaccine is not given to children over 5 years of age given the rarity of *H. influenzae* infection after this age.

The HIB vaccines are safe. PRP-T (ActHIB, OmniHIB), and HbOC (HibTITER) use carrier proteins related to those components in the DTP vaccines. These formulations should not be used in children with suspected DTP reactions. PRP-OMP (PedvaxHIB) is the recommended vaccine. No severe side effects have been reported, but low-grade fever and local pain have been observed. There are no major contraindications to giving the vaccine. Follow manufacturer package inserts regarding the schedule for vaccinating children who are receiving chemotherapy or immunosuppressive agents. The caveat concerning use of vaccine during a febrile illness should be observed.

TABLE 24-6 Haemophilus influenzae *Type B Dosing Schedule*

Vaccine	Age (Mo) First Dose Given	Number of Doses	Schedule
HbOC/PRP-T	2-6	Four	Three at 2 mo intervals Fourth at 12-15 mo
	7-11	Three	Two at 2 mo intervals Third at 12-18 mo, given at least 2 mo after dose two
	12-14	Two	Two at 2 mo intervals
	15-59	One	One dose only
PRP-OMP	2	Three	If given at 2 and 4 mo, booster at 12-15 mo Otherwise, two at 2 mo intervals Third at 12-15 mo
	7-11	Three	Two at 2 mo intervals Third at 12-18 mo, given at least 2 mo after dose two
	12-14	Two	Two at 2 mo intervals
	15-59	One	None
Comvax (PRD-OMP/Hep B)	2-6	Three	Two at 2 mo intervals Third at 12-15 mo
HbOC-DTP	2-6	Four	

See text for definitions of abbreviations.

Children with immunologic disorders or certain chronic illnesses are at increased risk for invasive HIB. They also may have decreased ability to make HIB antibodies. Children with HIV infection, sickle cell disease, or functional or anatomic asplenia, or those who are receiving chemotherapy or immunosuppressive therapy, may require additional doses of HIB vaccine:

- Asplenia: If the child has received a complete primary series and booster, no additional vaccinations are needed. A child undergoing elective splenectomy for a medical condition may benefit from an additional dose of vaccine 7 to 10 days before the procedure.
- HIV infection, chemotherapy, immunosuppressive therapy, or IgG2 deficiency: There is not enough information at this time to determine whether additional doses of vaccine will be helpful. If these children have an incomplete course, they should be vaccinated to finish the series. Unvaccinated children older than 59 months of age should receive two doses of vaccine at least 1 to 2 months apart.

Measles-Mumps-Rubella Vaccine

Measles-mumps-rubella (MMR) is a trivalent vaccine. It is still possible, but often difficult, to obtain each component individually. The dosage is 0.5 ml subcutaneously (SC) for either MMR or its singular components. Since the monovalent and combined MMR vaccines have been available, the incidence of these diseases (including congenital rubella syndrome) has decreased more than 99% (CDC, 1998).

Measles. The Enders' live, attenuated Edmonston strain is the only licensed measles vaccine available in the United States. It is a chick embryo–prepared virus. Ninety-five percent of vaccinees develop antibodies to measles after the first dose (99% after two doses). The immunity is life long in most persons, but a second dose at entry to kindergarten or age 4 years is recommended. Children who do not receive the second dose at kindergarten should be revaccinated at the earliest possible time. Persons vaccinated with killed vaccine or live vaccine/IgG and those vaccinated before 12 months of age should be revaccinated.

The measles component is responsible for almost all the adverse reactions to the MMR vaccine. A fever of 103° F beginning approximately 1 week to 12 days after vaccination occurs in up to 15% of vaccine recipients. Those with fever usually have no other symptoms. Transient rashes occur about 5% of the time between 5 and 12 days after vaccination. Encephalopathy and encephalitis are rare complications of the vaccine (less than 1 per 1 million). They occur at a much lower rate than they do after the natural disease. Febrile convulsion is an infrequent occurrence in children after they receive the vaccine. In children with a history of seizure disorders, vaccinations are still recommended. The benefits outweigh the risks. Subacute sclerosing panencephalitis, once a consequence of wild-type measles infection, has declined with measles vaccination and is not caused by measles vaccination (Woods & Abramson, 2002). Allergic reactions to one of the components (e.g., neomycin, gelatin) and thrombocytopenia (seen 2 to 3 weeks after immunization) have been reported, but they are very rare occurrences.

Contraindications to measles vaccine include the following:

- Pregnancy: Women vaccinated with measles vaccine should not become pregnant for 3 months after MMR vaccination. If measles monovalent vaccine is given, the woman has to wait only 30 days before conceiving.
- Immunodeficiency or therapeutic immunosuppression: Patients with compromised immune systems should not receive any live vaccine. These include children receiving cancer therapy and children with other immunosuppressive disorders. The vaccine can be given to medically suppressed children at least 3 months after the therapy is stopped. Measles vaccine as part of MMR is recommended for both symptomatic and asymptomatic HIV-infected children who are not severely immunocompromised. Symptomatic HIV-infected children should be given IgG at the time of exposure to measles (unless they have received immune globulin intravenous [IGIV] within 3 weeks) because they may not be able to manufacture antibodies.
- TB: Measles vaccine can cause anergy to tuberculin skin tests. Skin testing can be done on the day of measles vaccination or postponed for 4 to 6 weeks.
- Allergy: Persons with anaphylactic reaction to either egg or neomycin or prior MMR vaccine should not be vaccinated without consulting with an allergist. If vaccination is warranted, it should be done with extreme caution. Persons with egg protein allergies or contact dermatitis from neomycin without anaphylaxis may be immunized (Woods & Abramson, 2002).
- Febrile illness: This is a relative contraindication. If fever suggests a serious illness, the child should not be vaccinated.
- Corticosteroids: Immunocompetent children on high-dose, long-term steroid therapy (longer than 14 days) should wait at least 1 month after discontinuing steroids before being vaccinated.

Immune globulin (IG) and blood products affect the body's ability to react to measles vaccine. Children who receive IG must be vaccinated according to the following schedule:

- Children who receive a relatively low dose of IG for tetanus or hepatitis (A or B) prophylaxis may be vaccinated with MMR 3 months after receiving IG.

- Children who receive rabies IG should wait 4 months before receiving MMR vaccination.
- Children (especially those who are immunocompromised) who receive large doses of IG in the range of 0.25 to 0.5 ml/kg for the prophylaxis of either varicella or measles should wait 5 to 6 months before being vaccinated with MMR.
- Children who are receiving replacement therapy or therapeutic IG in doses of 300 to 400 mg/kg per month should wait for approximately 8 months after the last dose of IG before receiving MMR vaccine.
- Children who receive adenine-saline red blood cells (RBCs), unwashed packed RBCs, whole blood cell transfusions, plasma, or platelets must wait 3, 5, 6, and 7 months, respectively, before being vaccinated with MMR.
- Children who are being treated for immune thrombocytopenic purpura or other disorders with a single dose of IG of 400 to 1000 mg/kg should be deferred from MMR vaccination for 8 to 10 months. With doses of IG of 1000 to 2000 mg/kg, MMR should be withheld for 10 to 11 months.
- Children who are to receive IG or blood products should receive any scheduled MMR vaccine 2 weeks before these products.

If exposure to measles is imminent, vaccination may be given after a shorter interval and a second dose of the vaccine given after the recommended time period.

Mumps. Live mumps virus vaccine is effective, with a 95% seroconversion rate. Immunity is usually life long. Reactions to mumps vaccine are rare. Febrile seizures, rash, pruritus, nerve deafness, encephalitis, purpura, and orchitis have been reported. Encephalopathy and encephalitis are rare complications of the vaccine. They occur at a much lower rate than they do after the natural disease. Contraindications are the same as for measles.

Rubella. RA 27/3 is the current vaccine licensed in the United States and is used principally to prevent congenital rubella. Seroconversion rate is 98%. Mild reactions to the vaccine include fever, lymphadenopathy, rash, arthritis and arthralgia (usually seen more in unvaccinated adolescent females with onset 7 to 21 days after vaccine), small peripheral joint pain, and paresthesia. Contraindications are the same as for the measles vaccine. Rubella vaccine can be given postpartum with RhoGAM. The vaccine should not be given to pregnant women. The fetus is at maximum theoretic risk of 1.4% to develop congenital rubella.

Hepatitis A Vaccine

Children serve as one of the largest vectors for hepatitis A (HA) disease. They are generally asymptomatic of the infection, and the illness can go unrecognized. One study showed that 20% to 40% of adults who became infected with HA disease had contact with an asymptomatically infected child under 6 years of age (CDC, 1999a). Therefore the primary focus of HA vaccine initiatives has been in children under 6 years of age. Another focus is in localities that have at least a twofold increase in HA infection over the national average, primarily in the western United States. These include Arizona, Alaska, Oregon, New Mexico, Utah, Washington, Oklahoma, South Dakota, Idaho, Nevada, and California. Children living in Missouri, Texas, Colorado, Arkansas, Montana, and Wyoming should also be considered for routine immunization given those states' higher than average HA incidence (AAP, 2003).

Havrix and Vaqta are the two inactivated HA vaccines licensed by the FDA for use in persons 2 years of age or older who are at risk for contracting HA disease. These vaccines have seroconversion rates of 100% and provide long-lasting immunity. HA vaccine can be administered simultaneously with other childhood vaccines but should be given at a separate injection site (intramuscular injection in the deltoid). The dosage is 0.5 ml for those 2 to 18 years of age; 1.0 ml if older than 19 years. The vaccine is contraindicated in those with an anaphylactic reaction to alum or 2-phenoxyethanol (Havrix only).

Current recommendations also target the following groups of individuals:

- Children 2 years of age or older who live in communities with high case rates—Native Alaskans, Native Americans, Hispanics, and those in contact with people from endemic countries (Mexico, Central America)—and children in day care centers with high rates of HA virus
- Homosexual and bisexual men
- Severe illness (e.g., chronic liver disease)
- Illicit drug users (using injectable or noninjectable drugs)
- Those with blood clotting disorders (e.g., hemophiliacs)
- Healthy persons who are older than 2 years of age at the health care provider's discretion
- Child care staff and attendees
- Custodial care workers
- Hospital care workers
- Food handlers

Table 24-7 lists the recommended HA vaccination schedule.

A new combined hepatitis A and B vaccine (Twinrix) was approved for use in 2001 for those older than 18 years of age. Three doses are needed. It is recommended for those with similar risk factors as listed previously. New studies have investigated the use of HA vaccine as a prophylaxis for preventing infection after exposure (Sagliocca et al, 1999). Though the vaccine has not been approved for this use,

TABLE 24-7 Recommended Doses and Schedules for Hepatitis A Vaccination

Vaccinee's Age (Years)	Vaccine	Dose	Volume per Dose (ml)	Number of Doses	Schedule
2-18	Havrix	720 ELU	0.5	2	Initial, 6-12 mo
≥19	Havrix	1440 ELU	1.0	2	Initial, 6-12 mo
2-18	Vaqta	25 U2	0.5	2	Initial, 6-18 mo
≥19	Vaqta	50 U2	1.0	2	Initial, 6-12 mo

Adapted from Centers for Disease Control and Prevention, National Immunization Program: Dosages and schedules for hepatitis A vaccines. Available at *www.cdc.gov.nip* (accessed Feb 16, 2003).
ELU, Enzyme-linked immunoassay units; *Havrix*, hepatitis A vaccine, inactivated, GlaxoSmithKline; *Vaqta*, hepatitis A vaccine, inactivated, Merck & Co., Inc.

some researchers view the Twinrix as potentially an effective way to prevent both diseases. The use of postexposure IG and HA vaccine given concurrently at different sites is acceptable (Woods & Abramson, 2002).

Hepatitis B Vaccine

Two recombinant hepatitis B (HB) vaccines are currently licensed in the United States: Engerix-B and Recombivax HB surface antigens. They are produced from common baker's yeast and differ in antigen concentration. They are equally immunogenic when used as directed according to manufacturer's guidelines. Seroconversion rate is 95%. Side effects are rare, but pain and soreness at the immunization site are common complaints; it should not be given to individuals who have had an anaphylactic reaction to baker's yeast. Pain at the injection site (3% to 29%) and low-grade fever (1% to 6%) are the most common reactions (Woods & Abramson, 2002). Table 24-8 lists recommended dosage and scheduling.

Although current recommendations call for universal immunization of all infants with HB vaccine and immunization for young children and adolescents not previously vaccinated, there are specific individuals who should also receive HB immunization (Woods & Abramson, 2002):

- Hemophiliac patients and other recipients of certain blood products
- Intravenous drug users
- Heterosexual persons with a history of multiple sex partners in the previous 6 months or with recent sexually transmitted diseases
- Sexually active homosexual or bisexual males
- Household and sexual contacts who are chronic carriers of hepatitis B virus (HBV) or who are hepatitis B surface antigen (HBsAG) positive
- Household members of adoptees from HBV-endemic, high-risk countries or children born to first-generation immigrants from such endemic areas

TABLE 24-8 Recommended Doses and Schedule for Hepatitis B Vaccination

	Vaccine Dose		
Vaccinee	Recombivax HB	Engerix-B	Schedule
Infants of HBsAg-negative mothers	5 μg (0.5 ml)	10 μg (0.5 ml)	0-2 mo, 1-4 mo, and 6-18 mo
Children 0-19 yr (not vaccinated)	5 μg (0.5 ml)	10 μg (0.5 ml)	1-2 mo, 4 mo, and 6-18 mo
Infants of HBsAg-positive mothers*	5 μg (0.5 ml)	10 μg (0.5 ml)	Day 0, 1-2 mo, and 6 mo
Infants of HBsAG status unknown mothers†	5 μg (0.5 ml)	10 μg (0.5 ml)	Day 0, 1-2 mo, and 6 mo
Patients ≥20 yr	10 μg (1 ml)	20 μg (1 ml)	Day 0, 4-6 mo (Recombivax HB only) Day 0, 1-2 mo, and 6 mo (Engerix-B)

*Give HBIG and HepB vaccine within 12 hours of birth; 0.5 ml HBIG should also be given at birth.
†Give HepB vaccine within 12 hours of birth, and give HBIG within first 7 days of life if mother found to be HBsAG positive.
See text for definitions of abbreviations.

- Alaskan Native and Asian/Pacific Islander children
- Specific infants, children, and other household contacts in populations of high HBV endemicity
- Staff and residents of institutions for the developmentally disabled
- Staff of nonresidential day care and school programs for the developmentally delayed if attended by a known HBV carrier; other attendants in certain circumstances
- Hemodialysis patients
- Health care workers and others with occupational risk
- International travelers who live for more than 6 months in areas of high HBV endemicity and who otherwise may be at risk
- Inmates of long-term correctional facilities

Engerix-B and Recombivax HB are not interchangeable vaccines, but either can be given with IG to ensure even better protection rates in postexposure vaccination.

Influenza Vaccine

Illness from the influenza virus causes approximately 20,000 deaths per year in the United States. Children serve as a major vector because of their own high rates of contractility; they shed virus at higher rates and for longer periods of time than adults (Woods & Abramson, 2002). After even one influenza illness, people remain susceptible to other influenza strains; severe epidemics have occurred historically.

There are now two routes of administration for influenza immunization. The recently approved live intranasally administered vaccine (HuMist, MedImmune, Wyeth) is anticipated to be more widely received, especially by children.

The inactivated influenza virus vaccine is a multivalent embryonic egg vaccine. Two types of trivalent influenza vaccines (TIVs) are made: whole and split cell. Only the split cell can be given to children younger than 13 years old. Two preparations are available: Fluzone (whole or split) and Fluvirin (purified surface antigen; used only in children older than 4 years of age). The vaccine is formulated yearly based on epidemiologic forecasts. Major changes in viral antigens occur at 10-year intervals. This process is called *antigenic shift*. Minor variations that occur are called *antigenic drift*. These changes within the virus can prevent the body's immune system from recognizing the altered strain and mounting an immunologic response. Because other common childhood viral agents can lead to diseases that look like influenza, the impact of the vaccine is less likely to be evident in children. The efficacy rate is 70% to 90% in children. The vaccine should be given at the beginning of October through mid-November (it can be started in September if vaccine is available), before the onset of the yearly influenza season that peaks between December and March. It can be given at the same time as any other routine immunization but in a different site and with a different syringe.

The ACIP has recommended that healthy children between 6 and 23 months of age and people in households with infants less than 6 months of age be vaccinated for the annual flu season (CDC, 2002b). However, the ACIP has not issued a stronger "universal recommendation" for this pediatric age-group because of the need for further data collection (Bechtel, 2002e). The recommendation for vaccination has largely been in response to the high hospitalization rates for influenza illness found in young children.

Two doses of inactivated vaccine, given 1 month apart, are required for children younger than 9 years of age who are first-time vaccine recipients. Only one dose is needed in subsequent years and for children age 9 years or older. Children 6 to 35 months of age receive 0.25 ml IM. Children older than 3 years require 0.5 ml IM.

Specific individuals who should also receive influenza vaccination include the following:

- High-risk children: children with chronic pulmonary disease (mild to severe asthma, bronchopulmonary dysplasia, cystic fibrosis) or hemodynamically significant heart disease, immunosuppressed children (should be off chemotherapy 3 to 4 weeks if possible), children with hemoglobinopathies such as sickle cell anemia
- Children with conditions such as diabetes mellitus, chronic renal disease, severe metabolic illness, symptomatic HIV, rheumatoid arthritis, and Kawasaki syndrome
- Children who are household contacts of high-risk patients
- Pregnant women at greater than 14 weeks of gestation; women in the early postpartum period during flu season
- Children who are on long-term aspirin therapy and who are at risk for developing Reye syndrome
- Residents of nursing homes and those in other chronic care facilities housing patients of any age with chronic medical conditions
- Persons 65 years of age or older
- Health care workers or others attending or living with high-risk persons

Young children, 6 to 24 months old, occasionally have fever in the first 6 to 24 hours after vaccination (10% to 35% incidence). Localized skin reactions are more common in adolescents and adults and occur in 10% of recipients. Asthmatic children have not demonstrated any increase in airway reactivity after the TIV. Data demonstrate a small increase in the risk of Guillain-Barré syndrome in adults (approximately 1 to 2 per 1 million recipients) (Woods & Abramson, 2002). Other side effects include tenderness, redness, and pain at the site of injection. Fever, malaise, myalgia, headache, and other flulike symptoms are also reported after immunization.

There are a few contraindications to the influenza vaccine. Children with severe anaphylactic reaction to egg rarely experience a similar type of reaction to TIV. If there is concern about this, an immediate-reacting IgE skin test using a dilution of influenza vaccine can be used to judge the potential risk of vaccination. If the skin test confirms hypersensitivity, the vaccine should not be given, unless the person has been desensitized. Children with a neurologic disorder characterized by progressive developmental delay or a changing neurologic picture should not receive influenza vaccine until the neurologic problem is stabilized. The occurrence of any neurologic symptom or sign after administration of influenza vaccine is a contraindication to further use.

The vaccine should not be given to a patient with a febrile illness. The use of influenza vaccine in pregnant women (greater than 14 weeks of gestation) is considered safe. Children who receive prolonged high-dose corticosteroid therapy (more than 2 mg/kg per dose or 20 mg of prednisone per day) may have impaired antibody response to the vaccine. Immunization should be deferred until the steroid dose is lowered. However, if it is not possible to lower the steroid dose before the influenza season starts, the influenza vaccine should be administered and no longer deferred.

FluMist, the intranasal trivalent cold-adapted influenza A and B strain vaccine, received FDA approval in June 2003. Clinical trials showed an efficacy of 87% against all culture-confirmed influenza cases (Bechtel, 2003). It is approved for use in healthy patients between 5 and 49 years of age. The vaccine comes in a 0.5 ml prefilled nasal sprayer. The dosages are as follows:

- Children 5-8 yr: two doses via intranasal spray, approximately 60 days apart, for the first flu season. This also applies to those who previously received the inactivated vaccine.
- Children 9-49 yr: one dose (0.25 ml into each nares)

The following are contraindications to FluMist:

- Do not give with other vaccines.
- Do not give live vaccines within 1 month.
- Do not give if patient has history of hypersensitivity to chicken eggs.
- Do not give to patients receiving aspirin or salicylates or those who are immunocompromised.

Clinical trials in children revealed an increased rate of asthma. For this reason, FDA approval was not granted for children less than 5 years of age. Because of the newness of this vaccine, health care providers are encouraged to report any suspected adverse reactions through VAERS (Pharmacology Consult Staff, 2003).

Varicella Vaccine

Varivax, a live, attenuated vaccine from the Oka strain of varicella virus, was licensed for use in the United States in 1995. The vaccine is reported to be well tolerated and immunogenic, and it is 85% effective in preventing varicella infection (CDC, 2002c). One study measured the impact of varicella vaccine in three states and demonstrated a decreased incidence of infection of 78% (Seward et al, 2002).

A small percentage of vaccinees (20% of children; 25% to 35% of adolescents and adults) develop localized pain, erythema, and tenderness. Others (6% to 10%) may develop a mild, generalized maculopapular rash or varicelliform eruption (with few lesions that are generally nonvesicular) after vaccination. The lesions are frequently around the site of injection; vaccine virus has been isolated from these lesions. On rare occasions (3 in 20 million doses), secondary transmission of virus to susceptible individuals can occur by recipients who developed such a rash following vaccination. However, these cases have resulted in minimal sequelae (CDC, 2002c). Given the low risk of secondary transmission, immunocompromised household contacts do not need to be isolated from recently vaccinated individuals (Woods & Abramson, 2002). Those that contract varicella infection after being immunized usually have minimal fever and fewer than 50 lesions, and recovery is more rapid than had they not been vaccinated.

Recommendations for vaccinating with varicella include the following:

- A one-time dose of vaccine for healthy children 12 to 18 months old who have not had chickenpox, given at the same time as MMR
- A one-time dose of vaccine for children 18 months to 13 years old who have not had chickenpox or been previously immunized
- Two doses of vaccine for children older than age 13 years who have never been immunized and who have no known history of chickenpox; give two doses 4 to 8 weeks apart

The vaccine is not recommended for the following individuals:

- Children with allergies to neomycin and gelatin.
- Children with cellular immunodeficiencies. It is approved for use in those with humoral immunodeficiencies, including leukemia and lymphoma, and other malignancies compromising bone marrow or lymphatics and congenital T-cell abnormalities. There is a research protocol for using the vaccine in children with acute lymphoblastic leukemia.
- Pregnant women; those contemplating a pregnancy should wait 1 month after receiving the vaccine before conceiving.
- Children receiving immunosuppression until free of such agents for 3 months and then only after consultation with subspecialists.
- Children with a first-degree relative with congenital hereditary immunodeficiency unless known to be immunocompetent.

- Children who have received blood products (including IG) within the last 5 months.

Unvaccinated children who are HIV infected should be considered for vaccination but only after consultation with subspecialists. If an immunocompromised child has been exposed to wild-varicella disease, the CDC recommends administering varicella vaccine within 3 to 5 days after exposure to prevent or minimize subsequent disease (CDC, 2002c). The vaccine is used in a similar manner to prevent known outbreaks and to modify the severity of disease.

Postexposure varicella-zoster immune globulin (VZIG) should be given to those for whom exposure poses significant risk. See the following section on passive immunity for further discussion.

A recent study by researchers from the Kaiser Permanente Vaccine Study Group found that MMR and varicella vaccine given concomitantly were as safe and effective as when given separately and avoided a potential to miss giving one of these vaccines (*Infect Dis Children* Editorial Staff, 2002). The AAP and ACIP are now advising clinicians to give these vaccines at the same time. A booster dose is not currently recommended, but further study may demonstrate its efficacy (AAP, 2003).

Heptovalent Pneumococcal Vaccine

There are 45 known serotypes of pneumococcus. *Streptococcus pneumoniae* is attributed to be the cause of most bacteremia or sepsis (85%), pneumonia (67%), sinusitis, meningitis (50%), and acute otitis media (up to 55%) in children. A vaccine, manufactured with the seven serotypes of pneumococcus most likely to cause 80% to 90% of such invasive diseases in children, was introduced in February 2000. It is a heptovalent pneumococcal conjugate vaccine (PCV7; Prevnar). A polysaccharide and an oligosaccharide serotype are conjugated with a modified diphtheria toxin. It is designed to cross-protect against some of the other serotypes and serogroups of pneumococcus.

In prelicensure trials, the vaccine proved to have a 94% efficacy against invasive bacteremia. Postlicensure results of the effectiveness of the vaccine have shown that on an average, a child fully immunized would make one third fewer visits to medical facilities for otitis media (8% decrease) (Black, 2002). Cases of pneumonia decreased 6% to 17% (Bechtel, 2002a). Another study found that the need for tympanostomy tubes was reduced by one fourth (Black, 2002). Similar success was seen with vaccine-type pneumococcus carried in the nasopharyngeal passage.

The vaccine is given at 2, 4, 6, and 12 to 15 months, IM at a different site from other vaccines given concurrently. There is some serotype priming after two doses, more complete priming after the third dose, but significant response after the booster (fourth) dose. Most reactions have been limited to local reactions (5% to 6%) and fever (up to 13%, and depends on concurrent vaccines given). The reactions lessen on the fourth dose. The first dose cannot be given before 6 weeks of age; low-birth-weight infants (less than 1500 g) should receive the initial dose when they are 6 to 8 weeks of chronologic age. Children younger than 23 months who did not receive PCV7 before 6 months should be caught up per the schedule enclosed in the vaccine package insert (Table 24-9). It is also recommended for children between 24 and 59 months who are at greater risk for contracting invasive pneumococcal infection (Box 24-1). Children with moderate risk should be evaluated on an individual basis. In making the judgment to vaccinate, the NP may consider such factors as social/economic disadvantage, crowded/substandard housing conditions or homelessness, excessive tobacco exposure, recurrent otitis media infections, prior tympanostomy tubes, or vaccine shortages necessitating prioritization (Woods & Abramson, 2002). PCV7 has received limited study for use in children at risk of invasive pneumococcal disease, and a single dose is not contraindicated (AAP, 2003).

Polysaccharide Pneumococcal

Before 2000, two pneumococcal vaccines were available to prevent invasive pneumococcal infection in children 2 years of age and older and adults (Pnu-Imune 23 and Pneumovax 23). These 23-valent pneumococcal vaccines (PPV23) are composed of purified, capsular polysaccharide antigens. The vaccination is given SC or IM once, dosing with 0.5 ml. Children younger than 2 years have shown poor immunogenicity with these vaccines. There is poor reduction of nasopharyngeal carriage; the vaccine has an efficacy rate of 63% in children 2 to 5 years old. The ACIP guideline for administering PPV23 is listed in the footnotes to Box 24-1.

Meningococcal Vaccine

Most outbreaks of meningococcal meningitis in the United States are caused by serogroup C (some outbreaks have been caused by serogroups B and Y). There is no vaccine for serogroup B. The meningococcal vaccine is a quadrivalent vaccine composed of serogroups A, C, Y, and W-135 *Neisseria meningitidis* (Menomune). It contains bacterial capsular polysaccharides of the respective groups and is not routinely given to children unless there is an epidemic or exposure. This vaccine is administered SC at a dose of 0.5 ml, is generally given as a single dose, and is for those 2 years of age and older. Children who should routinely receive meningococcal vaccine include those with functional or anatomic asplenia and terminal complement component or properdin deficiencies. It may be used as an adjunct to chemoprophylaxis. Children who are first

TABLE 24-9 ***Recommended Schedule for Use of Seven-Valent Pneumococcal Conjugate Vaccination***

Age at First Dose (mo)	Primary Series	Additional Dose
2-6	Three doses, 2 mo apart[a]	One dose at 12-15 mo[b]
7-11	Two doses, 2 mo apart*	One dose at 12-15 mo
12-23	Two doses, 2 mo apart[c]	—
24-59		
Healthy children	One dose	—
Children with sickle cell disease, asplenia, human immunodeficiency virus infection, chronic illness, or immunocompromising condition[d]	Two doses, 2 mo apart	—
Catch-up Schedule		
Age at Examination (mo)	**Previous PCV7 Vaccination History**	**Recommended Regimen**
7-11	One dose	One dose of PCV7 at 7-11 mo, with a second dose ≥2 mo later, at 12-15 mo
	Two doses	Same regimen
12-23	One dose before age 12 mo	Two doses of PCV7 ≥2 mo apart
	Two doses before age 12 mo	One dose of PCV7 ≥2 mo after the most recent dose
24-59	Any incomplete schedule	One dose of PCV7[e]

Modified from Centers for Disease Control and Prevention: Preventing pneumococcal disease among infants and young children, *MMWR Morb Mortal Wkly Rep* 49(RR09):1-38, 2000b.
[a]For children vaccinated at age <1 yr, minimum interval between doses is 4 wk.
[b]The additional dose should be administered ≥8 wk after the primary series has been completed.
[c]Minimum interval between doses is 8 wk.
[d]Recommendations do not include children who have undergone bone marrow transplantation.
[e]Children with certain chronic diseases or immunosuppressing conditions should receive two doses ≥2 mo apart.

immunized when they are younger than 4 years of age may be revaccinated after 2 to 3 years. The vaccine can be used for general vaccination during an epidemic.

The American College Health Association recommends that college students (freshmen living in dormitories are at higher risk) consider meningococcal vaccine to reduce their risk of this disease. Serotypes C and Y account for approximately two thirds of these college-age meningococcal infections. It also is given routinely to all military recruits in the United States. Travelers to areas where the disease is either epidemic or hyperendemic may benefit from vaccination if the outbreak is of a vaccine-preventable serogroup. The most common adverse reaction is localized erythema lasting 1 to 2 days (Woods & Abramson, 2002).

Lyme Disease Vaccine

Two vaccines (LYMErix and OspA) were previously produced for prevention of Lyme disease caused by the spirochete *Borrelia burgdorferi*. Both have been withdrawn by the manufacturers because of low demand (AAP, 2003). ImuLyme is currently awaiting FDA final approval. Vaccination dosing is started before the start of Lyme disease season, which is generally in April. Adverse reactions have included soreness (24%), redness and swelling at the injection site (2%), and myalgias/fever/chills within 48 hours of vaccination (3%), that lasted about 3 days. These symptoms were not severe. Vaccination has typically been for those between 15 and 70 years of age who resided, worked, or recreated in geographic areas of high to moderate risk of exposure to vector (AAP, 2000). The FDA has been considering lowering the age to children 5 years of age and older.

Anthrax Vaccine

The CDC obtained permission from the FDA to offer two regimens should anthrax become a threat. Either choice is believed to be efficacious and involves using the anthrax vaccine (three doses over 4-week period) plus antibiotics (for 40 days) or only taking antibiotics for 100 total days as

BOX 24-1 *Recommendation for Use of Seven-Valent Pneumococcal Conjugate Vaccine in Infants and Children (PCV7)*

Children Who Should Receive the Seven-Valent Pneumococcal Conjugate Vaccine

All children younger than 23 months old
Children 24 to 59 months old with the following:
- Sickle cell disease, other sickle cell hemoglobinopathies, congenital or acquired asplenia, splenic dysfunction*
- HIV*
- Immunocompromised or receiving immunosuppressive therapy or radiation therapy*
- Renal failure, nephrotic syndrome†
- Chronic illness: cardiac, pulmonary (excluding asthma unless on high-dose corticosteroid therapy), cerebrospinal fluid leaks, diabetes mellitus, cochlear implants†

Children Who Should Be Considered for the Seven-Valent Pneumococcal Conjugate Vaccine

All children 24 to 59 months old, with priority given to the following:
- Children of Native Alaskan, Native American descent‡
- Children of African American descent
- Children who attend group day care centers more than 4 hours per week

Adapted from Centers for Disease Control and Prevention: Preventing pneumococcal disease among infants and young children, *MMWR Morb Mortal Wkly Rep* 49(RR-09):1-38, 2000b; Centers for Disease Control and Prevention: Prevention of pneumococcal disease: recommendations of the Advisory Committee on Immunization Practices, *MMWR Morb Mortal Wkly Rep* 46(RR-8):1-24, 1997.
*These children should also receive one dose of the 23-valent polysaccharide vaccine (PPV23) at age greater than 2 years, and more than 2 months after the last dose of PCV7. They should be revaccinated with PPV23 after the initial PPV23 vaccine (if greater than 10 years, revaccinate in 5 years; if less than 10 years, revaccinate in 3 to 5 years).
†These children do not need to be revaccinated with PPV23.
‡These children may be considered for revaccination; refer to CDC guidelines.
See text for definitions of abbreviations.

postexposure prophylaxis. It is currently recommended for 18- to 65-year-olds in certain military positions and for laboratory workers working with *Bacillus anthracis.* Studies are ongoing regarding side effects of the vaccine (including birth defects), how many doses are needed, how protective the vaccine is, and how long the protection lasts (*Infect Dis Children* Editorial Staff, 2002). See further discussion under Infectious Agents Used in Bioterrorism later in this chapter.

Smallpox Vaccine

There are two brands of smallpox vaccine. Both contain freeze-dried, live vaccinia virus to protect against variola major and variola minor (Dryvax and another as yet unnamed one by Aventis). They were made 30 to 50 years ago and stockpiled. These vaccines are administered by pricking the skin 15 times with a small two-pronged needle. A telltale blister and subsequent scar at the injection site indicate a "take," or conferred immunity. Adverse effects include lymphadenopathy, fever, headache, arthralgias, inadvertent self-inoculation of other body sites, eczema vaccinatum (fatalities have been reported in individuals with a history of eczema), site necrosis, chills, and satellite lesions near the injection area. In some cases, acute illness can occur, such as postvaccinial encephalitis (seen mostly in children younger than 1 year and older adults not previously immunized). Given within 4 to 5 days after exposure, the vaccine can prevent death. If given within 72 hours after exposure, it will prevent or lessen symptoms of the disease (Unger, 2002).

Drug companies are applying new technologies to the development of a new generation of smallpox vaccine that would be safer and more effective (Bechtel, 2002c). In the event of a smallpox outbreak, current public health wisdom is against a mass, herd vaccination program. Containment will probably rely more on proven methods that entail the rapid identification and vaccination of cases, contacts, and contacts of contacts during incubation. This approach to controlling a wider outbreak is referred to as "search and containment" or "ring" vaccination. Quarantine is not efficient. Vaccination of clinicians will probably be needed in order to care for the sick and exposed. Other public health measures will focus on eliminating large gatherings of people (including closing public transportation), disseminating public health information, and the voluntary isolation of family cohorts (Oregon State Health Division, 2002).

Vaccines on the Horizon

Studies and research are underway regarding a plethora of new vaccines. One of these is a new, safe rotavirus vaccine that will contribute toward controlling the most common cause of diarrheal mortality in the world. The first rotavirus vaccine, RotaShield, was withdrawn from the market in late summer 1999 after a significant number of cases of intussusception were reported. Since then, further research has questioned the conclusion that the attenuated virus in the vaccine was the definitive cause (Bechtel, 2002b). Other vaccines under investigation include a shigella conjugate vaccine for children (currently undergoing clinical trials); vaccines for malaria, dengue fever, Hantavirus, HIV, West Nile virus, and Lassa fever; and improved polysaccharide-protein conjugate vaccines against meningococci and pneumococci. Other studies are ongoing to develop a conjugate group B streptococcus vaccine for pregnant women to provide passive immunity to their fetuses, a vaccine to cover more serotypes of *H. influenzae*, and live and subunit parainfluenza type 3 vaccines.

New vaccine delivery systems are being researched that include edible vaccines and needle-free injections. DNA technology is also being explored for use in encoding host immunogenic antigens (Woods & Abramson, 2002).

Passive Immunity: The Immunoglobulins

Passive immunization entails immunizing an individual with a solution of preexisting antibodies to prevent or amend an infectious disease. These antibodies are derived from sera from pooled human immune globulin (IG), illness-specific human IG, or IG formulated from animals. Passive immunization is reserved for patients who suffer from immunodeficiencies in whom a live or attenuated vaccine could be dangerous, or who have a problem making antibodies. IG is also indicated for nonimmunized or underimmunized patients who have been exposed to an infectious disease and whose incubation period is not long enough to allow complete active immunization. Patients at high risk for developing severe complications from an infectious disease should receive passive immunization when exposed. Some patients who suffer from disease-produced toxins benefit from antitoxin passive immunization. A poisonous snakebite, tetanus, diphtheria, and botulism are examples of this. Immune globulin manufactured in the United States is screened for HIV-1 and HIV-2, syphilis, human T-cell leukemia viruses (HTLV-1, HTLV-2, HTLV-III, lymphadenopathy-associated virus), and hepatitis B and C. Most adverse reactions from IG involve localized pain at the injection site but can also include flushing, headache, chills, sweating, and shock. It should not be given to people who have had prior adverse reactions to IG. The NP should be prepared for allergic reactions if IG is administered.

There are also some hyperimmune globulin preparations from human donors that provide "superimmunity" because of their high antibody levels to certain infectious diseases. Such products include those for hepatitis B (HBIG), rabies (RIG), tetanus (TIG), varicella-zoster (VZIG), botulinum antitoxin (BIG), and respiratory syncytial virus (RSV). Equine-derived antisera are available for botulism, tetanus, diphtheria, and rabies. These have more severe adverse reactions (including fatal anaphylaxis) associated with them. They should be used with caution and only after hypersensitivity testing to animal sera is completed by a specialist (Palmer & Feldman, 2002). Some of the more routine passive immunizations given to pediatric patients will be discussed.

Hepatitis A Immune Globulin

Hepatitis A prophylaxis is recommended for the following individuals:

- Household contacts and sexual partners of known cases
- Persons accidentally inoculated with a contaminated needle
- Newborn infants of infected, jaundiced mothers
- Persons with open lesions directly exposed to body secretions of known cases
- Children in schools where more than one case is reported
- All children and employees of day care centers where a case is reported
- Custodial care residents and staff in close contact with an active case
- Persons traveling to developing countries for less than 3 months

The dose of IG is 0.02 ml/kg IM preexposure or postexposure. It should be given within 2 weeks of exposure. It can be used in children younger than 2 years; products with thimerosal should be avoided for use in children and pregnant women. It is greater than 85% effective in preventing infection if given at the appropriate time. The dosage for those with continuous exposure to hepatitis A virus is 0.06 ml/kg every 5 months. Hepatitis A vaccine can be given concurrently with the IG, if warranted (Palmer & Feldman, 2002).

Hepatitis B Immune Globulin

Hepatitis B immune globulin (HBIG) prophylaxis is recommended for the following unvaccinated people:

- Newborns whose mothers are hepatitis B surface antigen (HBsAG) positive
- Household contacts younger than 12 months of age and all contacts if index case becomes a carrier

- Sexual partners of known cases
- Persons accidentally inoculated with a contaminated needle
- Individuals with percutaneous or permucosal exposure to body secretions of known cases

Newborns exposed to hepatitis B virus should receive 0.5 ml HBIG and hepatitis B (HepB) vaccine within 12 hours after birth, in different injection sites. Infants born to mothers not tested during their pregnancy should also receive HepB vaccine, and HBIG must be given within 7 days after birth if the mother tests positive for HBsAG. Sexual partners of known cases should receive 0.06 ml/kg HBIG (maximum dose, 5 ml) along with HepB vaccine up to 14 days after the last exposure. Repeat the vaccine at 1 and 6 months. Household contacts younger than 12 months should receive HBIG and three doses of vaccine. For children older than 12 months of age and other household contacts, follow the index case's antibody profile. If carrier status is determined, vaccinate all household members. For patients with percutaneous or permucosal exposure, give 0.06 ml/kg HBIG within 24 hours if possible. Follow up with HB vaccine within 7 days. Revaccinate at 1 and 6 months.

Measles Immune Globulin

Unvaccinated children, pregnant women, and the immunocompromised exposed to measles can be immunized with live attenuated vaccine if given within 6 days after exposure. The vaccine provides protection in most cases. The universal dosage of IG is 0.25 ml/kg (15 ml maximum dose). In immunocompromised individuals 0.5 ml/kg (15 ml maximum dose) is recommended. For patients who receive immune globulin intravenous (IGIV), use the same dosage as for IG given IM. Children with symptomatic HIV infection should receive 0.05 ml/kg IG regardless of vaccination status unless they were given IGIV within the previous 3 weeks. Asymptomatic children with HIV infection should be dosed at 0.25 ml/kg (15 ml maximum dose) when exposed to wild measles. Measles vaccine should not be given for 5 months to those who received the 0.25 ml/kg dose and for 6 months to those who received the 0.5 ml/kg dose.

Mumps Immune Globulin

Mumps vaccine is not effective in preventing infection after exposure. Mumps IG is also ineffective and is no longer manufactured.

Polio

Pooled human globulin may be considered for use in sudden virulent nursery outbreaks and in the immunocompromised or those with severe debilitating illnesses.

Respiratory Syncytial Virus Prophylaxis

Two products are on the market for use in infants at high risk for adverse outcomes after respiratory syncytial virus (RSV) infection: palivizumab (Synagis) and RSV-IGIV (Respigam). Palivizumab has the benefit of being administered IM rather than IV. It is given in monthly IM injections during RSV season (usually November through March or April) in dosages of 15 mg/kg, and is generally well tolerated. Palivizumab has been shown to be safe and effective in reducing RSV hospitalizations in high-risk infants. It does not interfere with routine immunizations, unlike RSV-IGIV, which requires revaccination with MMR and varicella (some suggest an additional dose of DTaP as well) 9 months after the last IGIV dose (Nelson, 2002). Both have a high cost-to-benefit ratio. Consider RSV prophylaxis for the following children (AAP, 2003):

- Infants born at less than 28 weeks of gestation, until they are 12 months of age
- Premature infants (less than 32 weeks of gestation)
- Children younger than 2 years of age with chronic lung disease (CLD) who required treatment for their CLD within 6 months of the onset of RSV season (including oxygen therapy)
- Infants born at 29 to 32 weeks of gestation if RSV season occurs before they are 6 months of age

Consider using RSV-IVIG in immunocompromised patients instead of palivizumab.

In clinical trials, there were no statistically significant differences in adverse side effects in infants treated with palivizumab versus placebo. IGIV has demonstrated more side effects. Both may be considered for use in children with immunodeficiencies.

Rubella Immune Globulin

In exposed persons (nonpregnant adult women, adult men, adolescents, and children), rubella is considered a benign disease. The routine use of IG after exposure in early pregnancy is not advised. The available evidence suggests that the use of IG modifies or suppresses the clinical manifestations of the disease without preventing the viremic stage. Live RA 27/3 vaccine given after exposure does not prevent illness. If a pregnant woman is exposed to rubella, either wild or as a result of being accidentally vaccinated within 3 months of conception, a blood specimen should be obtained as soon as possible. The presence of serum antibodies suggests that the fetus is not at risk (1.4% to 2% theoretic risk factor). If no antibody is detected, a second sample should be obtained 2 weeks later. A positive test indicates infection. A negative test calls for a third sample 2 weeks later. A positive test again indicates maternal infection. A negative test at 6 weeks after exposure indicates that maternal rubella infection has not occurred. IG is recommended only if termination of the pregnancy is not an option. IG may prevent or modify rubella infection; the dose is 0.55 ml/kg. The administration of IG and the absence of clinical manifestation of rubella infection in the mother do not guarantee that the child will be born without congenital rubella syndrome.

Tetanus Immune Globulin

Tetanus immune globulin (TIG) is recommended for individuals with tetanus-prone wounds who are undervaccinated (fewer than three tetanus toxoid vaccine doses) or whose vaccination status is unknown. The dose is 250 U given IM plus tetanus toxoid vaccine. For those with tetanus, TIG is recommended at 3000 to 6000 U given IM plus antibiotics (metronidazole or penicillin G). Immunodeficient patients, including HIV-infected patients, should be considered undervaccinated regardless of actual status. If TIG is not available, equine tetanus antitoxin (TAT) is used. TAT should not be used without hypersensitivity testing before the first dose. In cases of tetanus neonatorum, a smaller dose of 500 U is administered. Tetanus-prone wounds include those contaminated with dirt (especially if around horses), feces, or saliva; puncture wounds; avulsions; and wounds acquired as a consequence of missiles, burns, crushing, or frostbite. Minor, clean wounds are not included for consideration of TIG; if the patient is undervaccinated, a tetanus toxoid vaccine should be given.

Varicella-Zoster Immune Globulin

Varicella-zoster immune globulin (VZIG) is indicated for use in persons exposed to varicella who are in the following categories:

- High-risk children: immunocompromised children younger than 15 years of age, including HIV-infected children
- Unvaccinated children with leukemia or lymphoma
- Normal adults and adolescents who are nonimmune
- Pregnant women, particularly in the first and second trimester: subclinical infection is linked to fetal involvement; a "healthy" mother does not rule out congenital disease
- Newborns whose mothers experience the onset of varicella infection within 5 days before delivery or within 2 days postpartum
- Premature infants less than 28 weeks of gestation or less than 1000 g who have been exposed to varicella
- Premature infants older than 28 weeks of gestation (with a nonimmune mother) who have been exposed to varicella

When the NP is faced with a pregnant woman who has been exposed, consult with an obstetric specialist before recommending VZIG. Acyclovir may also be considered during pregnancy to decrease risk of complications of maternal infection (McCarter-Spaulding, 2001).

The dosage of VZIG is 125 U for each 10 kg, with 125 U as the minimum dose and 625 U as the maximum dose, given as soon as possible after exposure for up to 96 hours. It is not required for newborns over 3 days old who have mothers with maternal zoster infections (Palmer & Feldman, 2002). The product does not contain thimerosal.

INFECTIONS IN CHILDREN ATTENDING DAY CARE

Approximately 75% of infants, toddlers, and children in the United States spend significant "care time" in settings outside of their homes. This population is more immunologically susceptibility to illness, given their ages, habits, and close proximity to one another. The environment enhances easy exposure to many infectious agents, whether spread from diapers, airborne, or from play surfaces. Day care–related illnesses are primarily respiratory, gastrointestinal, and of communicable disease in origin. Children less than 24 months of age have a higher incidence of illness. Data reveal that they can exhibit over 60 days of illness and have at least six respiratory infections per year (Daiichi Pharmaceutical Corporation, 2001; Wald & Marcy, 2002). Infections typically spread in day care settings are listed in Table 24-10. With the increase in drug resistance, these infections are eliciting greater concern.

Nurse practitioners and other health care professionals play critical roles in educating parents and day care centers about ways to decrease the incidence and transmission of infectious diseases. Some general guidelines for exclusion are included in Box 24-2. Children should not be excluded simply for yellow or green nasal discharge, nonpurulent conjunctivitis, exanthem without fever or behavioral changes, erythema infectiosum (fifth disease), hepatitis B carrier status, or HIV infection. Postexposure measures may prevent or lessen the impact of any subsequent contracted disease. Exposure to invasive infection from *H. influenzae* type b, *N. meningitidis*, measles, hepatitis A, varicella, and pertussis may include the use of prophylaxis such as rifampin, IG, antibiotics, or specific vaccines within 72 to 120 hours of exposure (varicella, MMR, DTaP; Wald & Marcy, 2002). The NP can consult with the local public health agency for specific recommendations.

SPECIFIC INFECTIOUS DISEASES

Viral Diseases

Coxsackievirus

Etiology. Coxsackievirus is in the *Enterovirus* genus. It is related to both poliovirus and echovirus. These ribonucleic acid (RNA) viruses are divided into groups: A (23 serotypes) and B (six serotypes).

TABLE 24-10 *Pathogens and Modes of Transmission of Infection in Day Care*

Modes of Transmission	Bacteria	Viruses	Parasites, Fungi, Mites, and Lice
Respiratory	*Haemophilus influenzae* type b *Neisseria meningitidis* *Streptococcus pyogenes* *Streptococcus pneumoniae* *Bordetella pertussis* *Mycobacterium tuberculosis*	Adenovirus Coronavirus Influenza A and B Measles Mumps Rubella Varicella-zoster Parainfluenza Parvovirus B19 Respiratory syncytial virus Rhinovirus	
Fecal-oral	*Campylobacter jejuni* *Salmonella* species *Shigella* species *Clostridium difficile* *Yersinia enterocolitica* *Escherichia coli* O157:H7	Enteroviruses Hepatitis A virus Rotavirus Calicivirus Astrovirus Enteric adenovirus	*Cryptosporidium parvum* *Giardia lamblia* *Enterobius vermicularis*
Person to person via skin contact	*Streptococcus pyogenes* *Staphylococcus aureus*	Herpes simplex Varicella-zoster Molluscum contagiosum Human papillomavirus	*Pediculus capitis* *Sarcoptes scabiei* *Trichophyton* species *Microsporum* species
Contact with blood, urine, or saliva		Cytomegalovirus Hepatitis B Hepatitis C Herpes simplex Human immunodeficiency virus	

From Wald E, Marcy S: Infections in daycare environments. In Burg F et al, editors: *Gellis and Kagan's current pediatric therapy*, ed 17, Philadelphia, 2002, WB Saunders. Modified from American Academy of Pediatrics: *2000 red book: report of the Committee on Infectious Disease*, ed 25, Elk Grove Village, IL, 2000, American Academy of Pediatrics, p. 107.

BOX 24-2 *Recommendations for Excluding Children from Day Care*

- Illness prevents the child from participating in program activities.
- Illness results in greater care need than the child care staff can provide without compromising the health and safety of the other children.
- Child has fever, unusual lethargy, irritability, persistent crying, difficulty breathing, or other signs of possible severe illness.
- Diarrhea (defined as an increased number of stools in comparison to the child's normal pattern, with increased stool water or decreased form) that is not contained by diapers or toilet use.
- Vomiting more than two times in the previous 24 hours unless the vomiting is due to a noninfectious condition and the child is not dehydrated.
- Mouth sores associated with an inability to control drooling of saliva.
- Rash with fever or behavior changes, unless noninfectious.
- Purulent conjunctivitis, unless noninfectious.

Data from Wald E, Marcy SM: Infections in daycare environments. In Burg F et al, editors: *Gellis and Kagan's current pediatric therapy*, ed 17, Philadelphia, 2002, WB Saunders.

Epidemiology. Enteroviruses are spread by fecal-oral contamination, especially in diapered infants. They are also transmitted during parturition. Coxsackievirus has a worldwide distribution, with increased prevalence during the warm months of the year. Epidemics transpire from May to October.

Infection is most commonly reported in children from 1 to 4 years of age.

Incubation Period. Incubation period is 3 to 6 days. The virus is shed for several weeks after the infection begins and is viable on environmental surfaces for long periods of time.

Clinical Findings

Type A Infection

1. Acute respiratory infection: A mild upper respiratory infection (URI) is common and may include complaints of sore throat, fever, vomiting, diarrhea, and coryza. Cases of pneumonia have been described.
2. Nonspecific febrile illness: In young children, there is an undifferentiated febrile illness associated with myalgias and malaise.
3. Herpangina: There is a sudden onset of high fever lasting 1 to 4 days. Loss of appetite, sore throat, and dysphagia are common, with vomiting and abdominal pain in 25% of cases. Minute vesicles or ulcers appear on the anterior pillars of the fauces, tonsils, uvula, and pharynx and the edge of the soft palate. The vesicles are gray-white with red areolas. They are usually 1 to 2 mm in diameter. The lesions enlarge and evolve into 5 mm gray-yellow ulcers. The entire course usually lasts 3 to 6 days with complete recovery.
4. Acute lymphonodular pharyngitis: This manifests as an acute sore throat lasting approximately 1 week.
5. Hand-foot-mouth disease: This is a clinical entity evidenced by fever, vesicular eruption of the buccal mucosa of the mouth, and a maculopapular rash involving the hands and feet. The rash evolves to vesicles, especially on the dorsa of the hands and the soles of the feet, and lasts 1 to 2 weeks. See Color Fig. 1.
6. Aseptic meningitis: There are the usual signs of fever, stiff neck, and headache. Altered sensorium and seizures are common. Most cases appear in epidemics or as unique cases; most patients recover completely.
7. Paralytic disease: A Guillain-Barré–type syndrome has been described.
8. Childhood insulin-dependent disease: A causative link between this disorder and Type A infection has been proposed but not proven.

Type B Infection. Type B infections are similar to type A infections, but type B herpangina does not exist. Type B infections include the following:

1. Congenital or neonatal infection: Symptoms occur within 2 weeks of birth. Transplacental infection occurs, and serious disseminated disease affects the fetal liver, heart, meninges, and adrenal cortex. The neonatal infection often manifests as a sudden onset of vomiting, coughing, cyanosis, and dyspnea. It is often mistaken for pneumonia. There is pallor and tachycardia that progresses to myocarditis and congestive heart failure. No murmur is heard. Infants often go into cardiac collapse and die. For those who survive, the recovery can be rapid.
2. Pleurodynia (Bornholm disease or devil's grip): This condition usually occurs in epidemics, but some isolated cases can occur. It is most often caused by type B disease, but type A virus has been implicated. There is sudden severe chest pain, pleuritic in nature and aggravated by deep breathing, coughing, or sudden movements. The pain occurs in waves of spasms that last 15 to 30 minutes and is described by patients as feeling like being stabbed with a knife or being squeezed in a vise. It can be mistaken for coronary artery disease, pneumonia, or pleural inflammation. There may be a prodrome 1 to 10 days before the onset of chest pain ushered in by headache, malaise, anorexia, and myalgia. Fifty percent of patients have crampy abdominal pain. Low to high fever occurs, and a pleural friction rub often is heard. The disease lasts from 1 to 10 days (mean 3.5 days).
3. Orchitis: This type B infection is clinically similar to mumps.
4. Myocarditis or pericarditis: Type B infection can cause mild to severe acute and chronic heart disease, but middle-aged men are the most susceptible.

Diagnostic Studies. Viral cultures are obtained from throat, stool, and rectum. For best results, send specimens to the laboratory chilled to 39° F (4° C). Results are usually available in less than 1 week, and most viral diagnostic laboratories have the capability of recovering enteroviruses. Polymerase chain reaction (PCR) is highly sensitive for testing CSF but has limited availability. Serologic-specific titers 2 to 4 weeks apart can also confirm the diagnosis.

Differential Diagnosis. The differential diagnosis includes other causes of the aforementioned conditions (e.g., viral, bacterial [pneumonia, meningitis, sepsis], connective tissue diseases).

Management. There is no therapy available for treatment. IgG may be helpful in immunocompromised patients.

Prevention. Enteric precautions and good handwashing are the only efficient control measures.

Erythema Infectiosum

Etiology. Erythema infectiosum, or fifth disease, is caused by parvovirus B19. The virus is a member of the Parvoviridae family. It is called *fifth disease* because it was the fifth eruptive rash described. These rashes include the following:

- Scarlet fever
- Measles
- Rubella
- Dukes' disease (erythema subitum)
- Erythema infectiosum
- Roseola

Epidemiology. Humans are the only reservoir. Upper respiratory secretions and blood during the viremic stage are considered infectious. Distribution is worldwide. Erythema infectiosum is a disease of childhood, usually attacking 2- to 15-year-olds, but infants and adults are not immune. Secondary spread to household contacts is approximately 50%. The disease occurs most commonly in late winter and early spring; it is spread via vertical transmission from mother to fetus, by respiratory tract secretions and percutaneous exposure to blood or blood products.

Incubation Period. The incubation period is approximately 4 to 20 days. The rash erupts between 2 and 3 weeks after exposure. The period of communicability lasts until the rash appears. In patients with aplastic crisis (sickle cell) or chronic anemia, the period of communicability is extended 1 week.

Clinical Findings. The following two phases are seen in erythema infectiosum:

1. Prodrome: Consists of mild fever (15% to 30% of cases), myalgias, headache, and malaise.
2. Rash: Appears 7 to 10 days after the prodromal stage and occurs in three stages: It first appears on the face and is "slapped cheek" in nature. There is an intense red eruption on the cheeks with circumoral pallor that lasts 1 to 4 days. Next, a lacy maculopapular eruption appears on the trunk and then moves peripherally to the arms, thighs, and buttocks. Palms and soles are occasionally involved. This phase can last a month. Finally, the rash subsides. There may be periodic recurrences precipitated by trauma, heat, sunlight, or cold (see Color Fig. 1). In adolescents and adults, there may be mild URI and arthritis. If a rash is present, it will not be rubelliform or petechial in nature.

Diagnostic Studies. Laboratory testing is not indicated because serologic tests for parvovirus are limited in availability. Serum B19–specific immunoglobulin M (IgM) confirms the presence of infection. Serum B19–specific immunoglobulin G (IgG) confirms past infection and immunity. There are ELISA and radioimmunoassay tests for B19. The virus is difficult to grow.

Differential Diagnosis. This is not a difficult disease to diagnose. The differential diagnoses include rubella, enterovirus disease, lupus, atypical measles, and drug rashes.

Management. There is no specific treatment.

Complications. These are few and typically not significant. All previously healthy patients usually recover without sequelae. The most frequently reported complications are as follows:

- Arthritis: Symptoms begin 2 to 3 weeks after the onset of initial symptoms. Joint manifestations are transient and self-limited (Miller & Cassidy, 2000). Adolescents and adults are more prone to develop arthritis and arthralgia than are children.
- Hemolytic anemia: Most common in patients with immunodeficiency. Intravenous IG has been used.
- Aplastic crisis: Most common in patients with chronic hemolytic anemias, especially sickle cell anemia.
- Proven maternal infection during pregnancy can cause fetal hydrops and death (less than 10% probability of fetal death). There are no reports of congenital anomalies.
- Pneumonia.
- Thromobocytopenic purpura.
- Aseptic meningitis (rare).

Prevention. Women who are exposed to children with the disease either at home or at work are at increased risk for infection with parvovirus B19. Because B19 has a low risk for fetal infection and there is widespread inapparent infection in children and adults, all women are at some risk of exposure. Because avoidance can reduce but not eliminate the risk of exposure, routine exclusion of pregnant women from the workplace where B19 infection is present is not recommended. Serologic testing for IgG antibody to B19 and fetal ultrasonography can help assess exposure risks if a woman is concerned.

Pregnant health care workers should not care for aplastic B19 patients or immunocompromised patients with chronic parvovirus infection because they are highly contagious (AAP, 2003).

Children in the rash stage can attend school.

Intravenous IG has proven of some help for those with immunocompromised conditions.

Human Immunodeficiency Virus

Etiology. HIV is an RNA cytopathic human retrovirus with at least two serotypes: HIV-1 and HIV-2. They are in the lentivirus subgroup. Both serotypes cause clinically indistinguishable disease. There are some reports that HIV 2 could, in fact, be a milder form of infection, but deaths are reported. Mixed infections are also documented. Retroviruses integrate into the target cell's genome as proviruses, and the viral genome is copied during cell replication. HIV persists in infected individuals for life, and its protein envelope mutates frequently. This antigenic drift creates havoc with the body's immune system. The body's defense system recognizes only previously encountered immunogenic forms. Any information about HIV is subject to change, and the NP is cautioned to check with the CDC regarding any new changes in HIV or acquired immunodeficiency syndrome (AIDS) diagnosis or treatment.

Epidemiology. Although there are AIDS-like syndromes in other primates and felines, infection cannot be obtained from pets, animals, or insects. Humans are the only source of HIV. The mode of transmission is intimate sexual contact, sharing of contaminated needles for injection, transfusion of contaminated blood or blood products, perinatal exposure, and breastfeeding. HIV has been isolated from blood (lymphocytes, macrophages, and plasma), CSF, pleural fluid, cervical secretions, human milk, tears, saliva, and urine. However, only blood, semen, cervical secretions, and human milk are implicated in transmission. Without contact from these sources, transmission is rare in families, households, hospitals, clinics, schools, or child care settings (AAP, 2000).

Infectivity is low. The risk of sexual transmission from just one episode of intercourse with an infected person is low (penile-anal contact 0.1% to 3%; penile-vaginal contact 0.1% to 0.2%). Accidental needle sticks in occupational settings rarely account for seroconversion and have a low infectivity rate. Less than 0.3% of the documented cases occurred this way. Transmission from accidental needle sticks from nonoccupational sources has not been documented (AAP, 2003). The last comprehensive study of HIV transmission between women who had sex only with women confirmed no cases attributable to this mode of transmission (CDC, 1999b).

The incidence of AIDS in children and adolescents younger than 19 years old in the United States is approximately 2% of the total number of reported cases. In 2000 the CDC reported a decrease of 81% of reported AIDS diagnoses in children as compared with 1992 rates (AAP, 2003). Greater than 90% of children less than 13 years of age were infected perinatally. Less than 5% of cases have no immediately identifiable risk factor, but with further investigation most do fall into an identifiable risk category. The remaining cases acquired HIV from contaminated blood products (e.g., hemophiliac patients or those with other coagulation disorders). Adolescents obtained HIV in the adult manner. Persons less than 21 years of age account for 25% of HIV transmissions. The adolescent female incidence is now greater than that of males (AAP, 2003).

Transplacental infection is well documented. Most babies born to HIV-infected mothers are initially HIV positive owing to the placental transfer of maternal antibodies. If the mother has been infected with HIV during late pregnancy and has not had time to develop antibodies, both mother and child will be antibody negative. Risk of an untreated HIV-infected woman giving birth to an infected infant is 13% to 39%. In vaginal twin deliveries, the firstborn twin has a greater risk of developing HIV than the second. Premature rupture of membranes greater than 4 hours before delivery increases the risk of antiretroviral agent transmission to the newborn. Cesarean delivery appears to reduce the risk of fetal infection by 50%. This number increases to 87% if women are treated with prophylactic medications during the prenatal and intrapartum periods and the infant is treated neonatally (Yoger & Chadwick, 2000). The transmission of HIV appears to be greatest within 14 days before delivery (70% incidence) versus during labor (30% incidence) (AAP, 2000).

Infection through postpartum human milk transmission is documented (DeVange et al, 2002). An estimated one third to one half of HIV transmission worldwide occurs by this route (AAP, 2003). However, in developing countries where pediatric AIDS is pandemic, treatment regimens—out of nutritional necessity—include breastfeeding plus drug treatment for women and infants (John et al, 2001; Perinatal Transmission [PETRA] Study Team, 2002). Neonatal antiretroviral prophylaxis within 6 to 12 hours of birth for a duration of 6 weeks reduced the risk of perinatal HIV transmission by two thirds (AAP, 2003).

The AAP guidelines (AAP, 2003) for counseling HIV-infected pregnant women and mothers include the following:

- Women and their health care providers need to be aware of the potential risk of transmission of HIV infection to infants during pregnancy and in the postpartum period, as well as through human milk.
- Documented, routine HIV education and routine testing with consent of all women seeking prenatal care are strongly recommended so that each woman knows her HIV status and the methods available to prevent the acquisition and transmission of HIV and to document whether breastfeeding is appropriate.
- At the time of delivery, provision of education about HIV and testing with consent of all women whose HIV status is unknown are strongly recommended. Knowledge of the woman's HIV status assists in counseling on breastfeeding and helps each woman understand the benefits to herself and her infant of knowing her serostatus and the behaviors that decrease the likelihood of acquisition and transmission of HIV.
- In general, women who are known to be HIV seronegative should be encouraged to breastfeed. However, women who are HIV seronegative but at particular high risk of seroconversion (e.g., injection drug users) should be

educated about HIV with an individualized recommendation concerning the appropriateness of breastfeeding. In addition, during the perinatal period, information should be provided on the potential risk of transmitting HIV through human milk and about methods to reduce the risk of acquiring HIV infection.
- Each woman whose HIV status is unknown should be informed of the potential for an HIV-infected woman to transmit HIV during the peripartum period and through human milk and the potential benefits to her and her infant of knowing her HIV status and how HIV is acquired and transmitted. The health care provider needs to make an individualized recommendation to assist the woman in deciding whether to breastfeed.

Neonatal intensive care units should develop policies that are consistent with these recommendations for the use of expressed human milk for neonates. Current standards of the Occupational Safety and Health Administration (OSHA) do not require gloves for the routine handling of expressed human milk. However, gloves should be worn by health care workers in situations where exposure to breast milk might be frequent or prolonged, such as in milk banking.

Human milk banks should follow the guidelines developed by the FDA, CDC, and AAP. These guidelines stipulate that all donors be screened for HIV and assessed for risk factors that might indicate donor infection and that the milk be pasteurized and meet rigid storage requirements.

In addition, NPs need to be vigilant regarding maternal compliance with the recommended neonatal HIV prophylaxis. Such compliance has been shown to be lower in women with asymptomatic HIV and in those who have poor social networks (Demas et al, 2002).

Incubation Period. The incubation period is variable. Symptoms of HIV infection in infants untreated perinatally are usually evident by the median age of 12 to 18 months. The infection can have a long latency period (longer than 5 years), but 15% to 20% of these children die before 4 years of age (median age of death is 11 months) (AAP, 2003). Intrauterine transmission usually occurs by 10 weeks of gestation and is associated with early, severe disease in the newborn. Intrapartum transmission occurs more in premature infants born before 34 weeks of gestation, in low-birth-weight infants, and in mothers who use IV drugs during pregnancy.

Seroconversion usually occurs between 6 and 12 weeks after exposure, and 95% of HIV-infected persons seroconvert within 6 months. In transfusion-associated infection, the time between exposure and clinical disease is months to years, with a mean of 3.5 years. The incubation time of HIV in adolescents and young adults has a median range of 8 to 12 years.

Clinical Findings. The current diagnosis categories for children with HIV infection are based on guidelines established in 1994 by the CDC (Box 24-3). The complete pediatric clinical classication system is available from the CDC; this system outlines the signs, symptoms, and conditions associated with the four HIV infection clinical categories for children.

AIDS in pediatric patients exhibits variable symptoms. Infant examinations are usually normal or demonstrate subtle lymphadenopathy with hepatosplenomegaly, failure to thrive, diarrhea, pneumonia, or thrush. *Pneumocystis carinii* pneumonia (PCP) is the most common cause of death in infants under 1 year of age. Other opportunistic diseases are *Mycobacterium avium* infection, severe cytomegalovirus (CMV) after 6 months of age, disseminated herpes, disseminated histoplasmosis, RSV, measles (despite vaccination), and anemia. Children—other than infants—generally have more recurrent bacterial infections, parotid gland swelling, lymphoid interstitial pneumonitis (30% to 50% incidence), or neurologic deficiencies that progress to encephalopathy. *Streptococcus pneumoniae, H. influenzae* type b, *Staphylococcus aureus,* and *Salmonella* organisms are common infections in pediatric AIDS patients. Sinusitis, cellulitis, and purulent middle ear infections are common. Malignancies are uncommon in pediatric AIDS, but they do occur. Children can have lymphoma, non-Hodgkin's B-cell lymphoma (Burkitt type), and leiomyosarcoma. Kaposi sarcoma is rare in children (Yoger & Chadwick, 2000).

Diagnostic Tests. Infants born to HIV-infected, seropositive mothers also are seropositive at birth owing to passive transfer of maternal antibodies. Maternal HIV IgG can persist for as long as 15 to 18 months. HIV proviral DNA testing (polymerase chain reaction [PCR]) will identify HIV-infected newborns early in the neonatal period. Serial HIV testing can be performed to assess the origins of the antibodies present. Positive cultures of the virus from blood or body fluid, increased HIV antibody, clinical disease, or the development of a new antibody to a specific viral protein indicates infant infection. See Table 24-11 for recommended testing times.

Laboratory tests are nonspecific in that a number of immunodeficiency states can give similar findings. The diagnosis of infection is made serologically in children over 18 months by ELISA testing, which is generally highly sensitive and specific. The test is repeated, and, if positive, confirmation is made by Western blot or immunofluorescent antibody testing.

Viral culture is not widely available. Serum antibodies are present in all infected persons. Some AIDS patients become seronegative late in the disease because the weakened immune system cannot manufacture antibodies.

BOX 24-3 *Diagnosis of Human Immunodeficiency Virus (HIV) Infection in Children**

Diagnosis: HIV Infected

1. A child younger than 18 months of age who is known to be HIV seropositive or born to an HIV-infected mother *and*
   - Has positive results on two separate determinations (excluding cord blood) from one or more of the following HIV detection tests:
     - HIV culture
     - HIV polymerase chain reaction
     - HIV antigen

   Or
   - Meets criteria for acquired immunodeficiency syndrome (AIDS) diagnosis based on the 1987 AIDS surveillance case definition
2. A child 18 months of age or older born to an HIV-infected mother or any child infected by blood, blood products, or other known modes of transmission (e.g., sexual contact) who
   - Is HIV-antibody positive by repeatedly reactive enzyme immunoassay (EIA) and confirmatory test (e.g., Western blot or immunofluorescent assay [IFA])

   Or
   - Meets any of the criteria in number 1

Diagnosis: Perianatally Exposed (Prefix E)

A child who does not meet the criteria above who

- Is HIV seropositive by EIA and confirmatory test (e.g., Western blot or IFA) and is younger than 18 months of age at the time of the test

Or

- Has unknown antibody status but was born to a mother known to be infected with HIV

Diagnosis: Seroreverter (SR)

A child who is born to an HIV-infected mother and who

- Has been documented as HIV-antibody negative (i.e., two or more negative EIA tests performed at 6 to 18 months of age or one negative EIA test after 18 months of age)

And

- Has had no other laboratory evidence of infection (has not had two positive viral detection tests, if performed)

And

- Has not had an AIDS-defining condition

From Centers for Disease Control and Prevention: 1994 revised classification system for human immunodeficiency virus infection in children less than 13 years of age, *MMWR Recommendations Rep* 43(RR12):1-19, 1994.

*This definition of HIV infection replaces the definition published in the 1987 AIDS surveillance case definition.

TABLE 24-11 *Testing Schedule for Human Immunodeficiency Virus in the Exposed Infant*

Test	Time after Birth
First DNA PCR from peripheral blood (not cord blood); confirm if positive	Within 48 hr
Second DNA PCR; confirm if positive	1-2 mo
Third DNA PCR; confirm if positive	2-4 mo

Infection is confirmed if two separate, confirmed samples are positive; infection is excluded if two separate, confirmed assays are negative when performed at the above times.

Data from American Academy of Pediatrics: *2003 red book: report of the Committee on Infectious Diseases*, ed 26, Elk Grove Village, IL, 2003, American Academy of Pediatrics.

See text for definitions of abbreviations.

Lymphopenia occurs as the disease progresses. There are decreased circulating CD4 cells (T-suppressor, T-helper cells), and the helper-suppressor ratio is less than 1.

Differential Diagnosis. The differential diagnosis includes other causes of immunologic deficiency, such as recent therapy with an immunosuppressive agent, lymphoproliferative disease, congenital immunologic states, severe malnutrition, graft-versus-host reaction, congenital CMV, or toxoplasmosis.

Management. Current drug regimens include combination therapy with protease inhibitor and nucleoside analogue reverse transcriptase inhibitor (NRTI) agents. Protease inhibitor agents include nelfinavir or retonavir (RTV). The NRTI agents include zidovudine (ADV; formerly known as azidothymidine, or AZT), didanosine (ddl), lamivudine (3TC) and stavudine (d4T), zalcitabine (ddC), saquinavir (SQV), and indinavir (IDV). Efavirenz (Sustiva) is a newer nonnucleoside reverse transcriptase inhibitor and is used for children who can swallow capsules. Studies are ongoing regarding the use of other new classes of antiretroviral drugs (e.g., fusion inhibitors and ribonucleotide reductase inhibitors).

Treatment should only be undertaken in concert with pediatric HIV specialists, because drug regimens are constantly being revised. The CDC is also a good source for the latest information regarding treatment. Many centers have ongoing clinical trials for which patients may be eligible. Information about such trials is available from the AIDS Clinical Trials Information Service (see Resource Box).

Treatment of associated conditions with appropriate medical therapy is indicated.

An important role of the NP in HIV treatment is in helping to boost adherence rates. The treatment regimens are highly challenging for parents because of complex dosing schedules and unwillingness of children to take the required medications. Many preparations are not offered in liquid form, or the taste is not attractive to children. To enhance compliance, some clinicians employ several tools: improving information via computer-assisted age-dependent programs, using electronic pillboxes, routinely measuring drug levels, developing simpler drug protocols, studying possible social and economic factors that predict compliance, and offering more support networks to families (Van Rossum et al, 2002). In infants and children with poor virologic response to treatment, adherence to medication can be predictive (Van Dyke et al, 2002).

Adolescents can present a particular noncompliance risk because of denial and fear of their infection, misinformation, distrust of and inexperience with the medical system, self-esteem issues, unstable living situations, and lack of familial and social support systems (Working Group, 2001).

There are virologic, immunologic, and clinical considerations for changing antiretroviral therapy (Working Group, 2001). The practitioner should be attuned to the clinical indications for changing therapy that would prompt a referral to the specialist for further evaluation. These include the following:

- Impaired growth in head circumference, decline of cognitive function, and motor dysfunction
- Persistent decline in weight-growth velocity despite adequate nutrition
- Advancement from one clinical category to another

Complications. HIV becomes a multisystemic illness with multiorgan complications. Management becomes complicated. The mortality rate is extremely high.

Prevention of Complications and Transmission

Recommendations for Childhood Vaccinations. Specific immunization recommendations are as follows:

- Children with symptomatic HIV infection: As with other immunizations for children suffering from immunologic deficiencies, live viral vaccines (MMR excepted) and BCG should not be given. DTP, DTaP, IPV, HIB, HB, Prevnar, and MMR (unless severely immunocompromised) vaccines are administered according to the usual schedule. MMR may be repeated within 4 weeks after the first dose is given to achieve rapid seroconversion. Yearly influenza vaccine should be given when children are 6 months of age. Passive immunization must be given when symptomatic HIV-infected children are exposed to wild diseases (measles, tetanus, varicella) regardless of immunization status. Children with asymptomatic HIV infection should follow the same schedule.
- Children who live with a symptomatic HIV-infected person: The use of live vaccines is contraindicated with the exception of MMR. MMR can be given because these viruses do not shed. Yearly influenza vaccines should be given to household members who live with infected persons.
- There is no HIV-preventive vaccine.

Reduction of Perinatal Transmission of HIV. The use of combination therapy or monotherapy to reduce perinatal transmission of HIV is recommended. Current treatment regimens recommend using either zidovudine, nevirapine, or zidovudine plus lamivudine, depending on the country where treatment is occurring. Developing countries seek the most cost-effective, efficacious, simple, and tolerable regimen. The CDC, WHO, and United Nations AIDS agencies are useful resources for current treatment regimens.

Patient education remains the only method to reduce the risk of acquisition and transmission.

Control Measures. The following control measures should be taken:

- Work-related exposure: Health care workers with parenteral or mucosal membrane exposure to HIV should confirm that the exposure indeed came from an HIV-infected person. Serial HIV testing should be obtained after exposure. AIDS counseling should be provided. Use of antiretroviral chemoprophylaxis for postexposure prophylaxis (PEP) must balance the risk of transmission against the toxicity of the medications. The recommended HIV PEP for percutaneous injuries, mucous membrane exposures, and nonintact skin exposures is available from the CDC website (see Resource Box).
- Adolescent education: Adolescents must be counseled about the risk of HIV transmission (e.g., sexual transmission, sharing of needles or syringes) and the use of condoms.
- School attendance: Children with AIDS or HIV infection should go to school if they are healthy enough to do so. Factors that must be taken into account include the risk to the immunosuppressed child of "normal germs" from "healthy kids and school personnel." The benefit from attendance far outweighs the risks. Because casual transmission is unknown, there is no real risk to other children as long as the infected child can control body secretions. Children who display biting behavior or have oozing wounds should be cared for in a setting that minimizes risk to others. The child's primary care provider is the only person with an absolute need to know the child's primary diagnosis. If the family decides to inform the school, those informed should maintain confidentiality. If the family choses not to inform the school, parents should get assurance that the school will notify them of any communicable disease outbreaks (e.g., varicella, measles).

Routine screening of school-age children for HIV antibodies is not recommended (AAP, 2003).

Hepatitis A Virus

Etiology. Hepatitis A virus (HAV) is a picornavirus and causes a primary infection in the liver.

Epidemiology. HAV is a highly contagious infection spread through person-to-person contact and fecal-oral contamination of food and water. It accounts for 50% of all viral hepatitis in the United States. It is rarely transmitted by contaminated blood transfusion. Human infection from nonhuman primates is also reported. Transmission occurs readily in households and day care centers. Eighty percent of cases in infants younger than 2 years of age and 50% of infected children between 3 and 4 years of age have nonsymptomatic (anicteric hepatitis) or nonspecific illness. Adults tend to have more severe disease. Children 5 to 14 years of age have the highest rates, and those over 40 years of age have the lowest rates (AAP, 2003). The high anicteric disease incidence allows considerable spread of disease before the index case is identified. Infants are protected by maternal antibodies during the first few months of life. The infection is unequally distributed among states and communities and varies with socioeconomic and living conditions. There is increasing incidence of HAV in intravenous drug users. There is no seasonal variance. It is vaccine preventable.

Incubation Period. The period of contagion is as long as the patient sheds virus and usually lasts 1 to 3 weeks. The patient is most contagious from 1 to 2 weeks before the onset of illness until 1 week after the onset of jaundice. The incubation period is 15 to 50 days (average 25 to 30 days).

Clinical Findings. The following two phases may be seen:

1. Preicteric phase: This phase manifests as an acute febrile illness. Malaise, nausea, anorexia, vomiting, digestive complaints, and occasional abdominal complaints occur. This phase goes unnoticed in many children. There can be dull right upper quadrant pain during exercise.
2. Jaundiced phase: Jaundice appears shortly after the onset of symptoms (70% incidence in older children and adults). Urine darkens and stools become clay colored. Often these are the only apparent signs of the illness. Diarrhea is common in infants, whereas constipation is more common in older children and adults. Patients feel sick. Infants have poor weight gain during the icteric phase.

Fulminant disease is rare. There is no chronic disease. The icteric phase lasts from a few days to almost a month and may be subtle in children. Complete recovery can be expected within 1 month with occasional relapses lasting for up to 6 months (AAP, 2003).

Diagnostic Studies. Serologic testing is widely available. IgM-specific antibodies indicate recent infection. These are replaced by IgG-specific antibodies 2 to 4 months later and serve as indicators of past infection. Changes in liver enzymes indicate the degree of injury. There is elevation of serum transaminases (serum glutamic-oxaloacetic transaminase [SGOT], aspartate aminotransferase [AST], serum glutamate pyruvate transaminase [SGPT], alanine aminotransferase [ALT]). Prothrombin time can be elevated.

Differential Diagnosis. Any cause of jaundice is in the differential diagnosis of HAV.

- Infancy: physiologic jaundice, hemolytic disease, galactosemia, hypothyroidism, biliary metabolic disorders, biliary atresia, α_1-antitrypsin deficiency, and choledochal cysts. Hypervitaminosis A causes a yellow pigmentation of the skin often mistaken for jaundice in children. Infections such as toxoplasmosis, rubella, CMV, and herpes (TORCH) also cause hepatitis.

- Older infants, children, and adolescents: hemolytic-uremic syndrome, Reye syndrome, malaria, leptospirosis, brucellosis, chronic hemolytic diseases with gallstone development, Wilson disease, cystic fibrosis, Banti syndrome, collagen-vascular disease, infectious mononucleosis, CMV, coxsackievirus, toxoplasmosis, Weil disease, yellow fever, acute cholangitis, amebiasis, and hepatitis B, C, and D. Drugs and poisons such as pyrazinamide, isoniazid, zoxazolamine, gold, cinchophen, phenothiazines, and methyltestosterone are among others that also cause hepatitis.

Management. Therapy is supportive in nature. The use of gamma globulin within 2 weeks of exposure is discussed earlier in this chapter.

Complications. Although patients can become very ill, most cases of HAV heal completely. Fulminant hepatitis with liver failure is rare.

Hepatitis B Virus

Etiology. Hepatitis B virus (HBV) is a hepadnavirus. It is highly contagious and causes severe liver disease.

Epidemiology. The most common method of transmission is percutaneous or mucous membrane exposure to contaminated blood or sexual secretions, or both. Saliva has not been shown to be infectious. Fecal-oral transmission cannot be demonstrated experimentally. HBV survives in a dried state for almost 1 month. Prolonged percutaneous contact with contaminated fomites can be a source of infection. Surface and core antigens are useful markers for epidemiologic studies. Patients are infectious when they are hepatitis B surface antigen (HBsAg) positive or if they are chronic carriers of HBV. Hepatitis B e antigen (HBeAg) correlates with viral replication and indicates chronic carriage. Antibodies to core and surface antigen lessen infectivity.

The major reservoir for HBV is healthy chronic carriers and patients with acute disease. Populations living in China, the Pacific Islands, sub-Saharan Africa, and other high endemic areas have a high infection and carriage state. In the United States the highest rate is seen in Alaskan Eskimo populations (Snyder & Pickering, 2000.) Perinatal transmission from female carriers (HBsAg positive or HBeAg positive, or both) to their newborn children has a 70% to 90% infant infection rate unless intervention is undertaken. Adolescents and adults who abuse IV drugs or who engage in sexual activity with multiple partners, or both, have the greatest risk of acquiring HBV. There is also a higher incidence of infection in the gay community. Health care workers who are exposed to blood and blood products or who care for the developmentally disabled are also at a high risk, as are chronic renal dialysis patients. Tattooing or body piercing with contaminated instruments is another route of infection. Breastfeeding is not contraindicated.

Incubation Period. The incubation period is 45 to 160 days (average of 90 days).

Clinical Findings. HBV has a range of illness from asymptomatic seroconversion to fulminating disease and death. HBV usually has a gradual onset. Arthralgia and skin problems such as urticaria or other rashes can be the first apparent signs. Papular acrodermatitis has been described in infants. Acute hepatitis B infection is somewhat similar to the icteric phase of HAV, but it is usually more severe. Skin, mucous membranes, and sclerae are icteric. The liver is enlarged and tender. Ten percent of patients develop chronic disease.

Diagnostic Studies. Serologic tests include HBsAg, hepatitis B core antigen (HBcAg), HBeAg, and antibodies to these antigens; the results can be useful in determining the stage of infection (Table 24-12). Positive HBsAg and HBcAg assays indicate active infection. Changes in liver enzymes indicate the degree of injury. There is elevation of serum transaminases (SGOT, AST, SGPT, ALT). Prothrombin time can be elevated, especially in fulminating disease.

Differential Diagnosis. Any cause of jaundice is in the differential diagnosis of HBV. See the section on differential diagnosis of HAV.

Management. Therapy is supportive in nature. The use of active and passive vaccination has been discussed previously. Those over 18 years of age with chronic HBV and who have liver disease may benefit from interferon alfa-2b. This drug has also been used in children, but results have been erratic. Remissions have been long term without further therapy.

Complications. There are hepatic and extrahepatic complications.

Chronic Persistent Hepatitis. The older one is when HBV is acquired, the less risk of chronic disease (Snyder & Pickering, 2000). From 20% to 30% of chronic cases acquired the disease in childhood. Most patients with this diagnosis are asymptomatic. Some have minimal nonspecific constitutional complaints such as fever, nausea, and minimal hepatomegaly. The condition is benign in childhood, although there is inflammatory liver disease. Chronic persistent hepatitis can progress to cirrhosis, liver failure, or liver cancer in adults and is usually diagnosed by liver biopsy. Often the disease follows a mild anicteric hepatitis.

Chronic Active Hepatitis. This condition has increased likelihood of progressing to cirrhosis and liver failure. There is recurrent episodic jaundice, elevated liver enzymes, and increased prothrombin time. Evolution of portal hypertension and ascites can begin. Often the disease follows a mild anicteric hepatitis.

Fulminating Hepatitis. This is a progressive course that is distinguished by liver failure and can occur a few days to a month after acute hepatitis. Elevated bilirubin (greater

TABLE 24-12 *Interpretation of the Hepatitis B Serologic Panel*

HBsAg*	Anti-HBs	Anti-HBc IgM†	Anti-HBc IgG	Interpretation	Comments
+	–	–	–	Early acute infection	First indicator to appear as early as 1-2 wk after infection but before clinical symptoms. Usually persists throughout the illness. Ensure household and sexual contacts are vaccinated.
+	–	+	+	Acute infection	Highly infectious, active replication of virus. Ensure household and sexual contacts are vaccinated.
+	–	–	+	Chronic infection	Low replication of the virus, low infectivity, or HbsAg carrier.
–	–	+	–	"Window period" following acute infection	Patient probably not infectious.
–	–	–	+	Remote infection with loss of detectable anti-HbsAg; remote infection with possible low-level HbsAg; possible false-positive test	Patient not infectious to household, sexual, needle-stick exposures.
–	+	+/–	+	Resolved infection	Patient is immune, not infectious.
–	+	–	+/–	Healed infection	Patient is immune, not infectious.
–	+	–	–	Immune following vaccination; resolved infection with loss of detectable anti-HBc	Patient is immune, not infectious.

Adapted from State of Alaska Epidemiology Bulletin: Serologic test for viral hepatitis, part 2. Available at *www.epi.hss.state.ak.us* (accessed Feb 13, 2002); Centers for Disease Control and Prevention: Viral hepatitis B. Available at *www.cdc.gov* (accessed Feb 14, 2003).
*The presence of HBsAg alone is insufficient for a diagnosis of acute infection.
†Anti-HBc IgG may also be reported as simply anti-HBc (or HBcAb) and can persist indefinitely.
See text for definitions of abbreviations.

than 20 mg/dl), elevated ammonia levels, marked elevated transaminases, encephalopathy, bleeding, coma, ascites, and abnormal encephalograph (EEG) changes occur. There is a 30% mortality rate.

Hepatoma. Primary hepatocellular carcinoma is associated with chronic HBV infection.

Extrahepatic Manifestations. Polyarteritis nodosa, glomerulonephritis, mixed cryoglobinemia, a serum sickness–like prodrome, and polymyalgia rheumatica are associated with HBV.

Hepatitis C Virus

Etiology. Hepatitis C virus (HCV), a single-stranded RNA virus with seven genotypes in the Flaviviridae family, causes the chronic form of what used to be called non-A, non-B hepatitis.

Epidemiology. The risk factors associated with HCV are illicit IV or intranasal drug use (40%), imprisonment, occupational or sexual exposure (10%), and transfusions (10%). Ten percent of cases have unexplained risk factors. Children with hemophilia or those on chronic hemodialysis are at greatest risk for this type of hepatitis. Transmission of HCV from HIV-positive mothers to their infants is documented, but prenatal transmission is uncommon. Transmission from breastfeeding is thought to be rare. Eighty-five percent of cases become chronic (Snyder & Pickering, 2000). Incidence is 0.2% for children less than 12 years of age and 0.4% for those 12 to 19 years of age (AAP, 2003).

Incubation Period. HCV has an incubation period of 2 to 24 weeks (average 7 to 9 weeks).

Clinical Findings. Onset of symptoms is often insidious, and most children are asymptomatic. Flulike prodromal symptoms followed by jaundice occur in fewer than 20% of cases. Incidence of chronic hepatitis infection in children is less than 10%; less than 5% develop cirrhosis (AAP, 2003). Chronic hepatitis with cirrhosis (a late occurrence, often 20 to 30 years) is associated with hepatosplenomegaly, ascites, clubbing, palmar erythema, spider angiomas, and, uncommonly, hepatocellular cancer. Fulminant hepatitis C is uncommon.

Diagnostic Studies. Mild to moderate fluctuations in aminotransferase elevations can occur. Confirmation of anti-HCV by ELISA or radioimmunoblot assay or HCV RNA by PCR is diagnostic. A newborn can be anti-HCV positive from maternal transfer for up to 12 months, so testing should be done after that time. Liver biopsy is confirmatory.

Differential Diagnosis. Differential diagnoses include hepatitis A and B and other causes of chronic hepatitis.

Management. Treatment of acute hepatitis is supportive. Chronic HCV infections in children respond to therapy with interfereon alfa-2 therapy. Ribavirin (Rebetrol) was approved in 2003 for use in children 3 years of age and older (*Infect Dis Children* Editorial Staff, 2003). Hepatitis A and hepatitis B vaccines should be given to prevent further liver complications. Breastfeeding by an HCV-positive mother is not contraindicated unless she has cracked or bleeding nipples. Children with HCV infection need not be excluded from daycare facilities (AAP, 2003).

Prognosis. The course of HCV is generally mild even with cirrhosis. Liver transplantation is an option, although reinfection is common and gradually progressive. The outcome of chronic HCV disease in children is less known. It is important for patients to refrain from alcohol to prevent further liver injury.

Hepatitis D Virus

Hepatitis D virus infection is uncommon in children, but it must be considered in cases of fulminant hepatitis. It cannot cause infection unless the patient also is infected with HBV. Incubation is 2 to 8 weeks. It is diagnosed most commonly in drug users, hemophiliacs, and immigrants from southern Italy and parts of Eastern Europe, South America, Africa, and the Middle East. Mother to newborn transmission is uncommon (AAP, 2003).

Hepatitis E Virus. Hepatitis E virus is similar to the caliciviruses. It is passed via the fecal-oral route. Endemic areas include India, the Middle East, Southeast Asia, and Mexico. Most cases in the United States are found in immigrants or visitors from these locations. Laboratory studies include IgM and IgG assays. This infection carries a high morbidity rate for pregnant women. There is no treatment or vaccine. Chronic infection is not seen. Contaminated water is the most common reservoir (AAP, 2003).

Herpesvirus

Etiology. Herpes simplex virus (HSV) is among the most widely disseminated infectious agents in humans. HSV has two antigenic types. HSV-1 is associated chiefly with nongenital infections of the mouth, lips, eyes, and central nervous system. HSV-2 is most commonly associated with genital and neonatal infection. Type 1 strains can be found in the genital tract (autoinoculation or oral-genital contact). Type 2 lesions found in the mouth or pharynx usually result from oral sexual activity.

Epidemiology. Primary infection with type 1 virus usually occurs in infants and children between 1 and 4 years of age. Distribution is worldwide, but the infection is more frequent in crowded environments. It is spread by intimate, direct contact. The virus has been recovered from stool, urine, skin lesions, saliva, and respiratory secretions. The primary site of clinical infection is gingivostomatitis (12.1%), usually occurring in the second year of life. There is no seasonal variation, and adults are the chief source of infection. Type 2 infections usually occur as a result of sexual activity. Sexual molestation must always be ruled out when the infection is found in nonneonates.

Neonatal HSV infection is usually acquired from the mother during the birthing process. Direct exposure occurs as the fetus passes through the vaginal vault. Viral migration from the vault to the fetus is the most common method of infection. Occasionally, a scalp monitor probe becomes contaminated and is the source of infection. Although the majority of neonatal infections are caused by HSV-2, approximately 25% are HSV-1. Risk of infection for an infant born to a mother with a primary genital infection is 33% to 50%. The risk for infants born to mothers with recurrent HSV genital infection is less than 5%. The incidence is 1 in 3000 to 1 in 20,000 live births (AAP, 2000). Most infants with congenital HSV infection are born to women without a history or clinical findings of active infection during pregnancy. Postnatal transmission is described but is less common. Mothers can inoculate their babies from oral, breast, or skin lesions. Fathers also can inoculate infants with nongenital lesions. There can be lateral transmission from an infected baby in the nursery. Postnatal transmission from nursery personnel with fever blisters is extremely rare.

Incubation Period. Period of communicability for types 1 and 2 (when not in the neonatal period) is 2 days to 2 weeks (AAP, 2003). Some cases of congenital infection occur more than 6 weeks after birth. Infection can be transmitted during either primary or recurrent infections, whether children are clinically ill or asymptomatic.

Clinical Findings. Manifestations are determined by the port of entry of the host, age, state of health, and immune competence. Eczema alone or in combination with other manifestations is also a complicating factor. Specific clinical findings, diagnosis, and treatment of gingivostomatitis, neonatal herpetic infection, eczema herpeticum, herpes vulvovaginitis, and herpes keratoconjunctivitis are discussed in other chapters.

Traumatic Herpetic Infection. This is a localized infection that occurs in a susceptible child because of an abrasion, teething, laceration, or burn that is inoculated with herpesvirus by an orally infected parent who kisses the "booboo." Vesicles appear at the site of the lesion. There may be fever, constitutional symptoms, and regional lymph node involvement.

Acute Herpetic Meningoencephalitis. Primary central nervous system involvement is an unusual manifestation outside the neonatal period. HSV-1 causes a rapidly progressing infection with a 70% fatality rate. Encephalitis can be focal, mimicking a mass lesion. Diagnosis is made by brain biopsy. In contrast, HSV meningitis is usually a relatively benign disease most often caused by HSV-2.

Recurrent Infections. As with varicella, the body does not truly eradicate the virus, and recurrent infections are common. The usual manifestation of recurrent infections is herpes labialis, the common fever blister, and involvement of skin adjacent to the lips. Some incidence of recurrent aseptic meningitis can be attributed to HSV infection. Constitutional symptoms are rare except in immunocompromised patients.

Diagnostic Tests. Tests may include viral culture, cytology-Papanicolaou smears, Tzanck stains, ELISA, fluorescent techniques, glycoprotein G assay, blood or CSF PCR in neonates, or brain biopsy in cases of encephalitis. Cultures in neonates need to be taken from skin vesicles, mouth, nasopharynx, eyes, urine, blood, stool or rectum, and CSF. Serologic tests usually are not helpful for diagnosing acute infection. Antibodies are not useful because increases are only seen after the critical diagnostic period. If encephalitis is suspected, an EEG and MRI of the brain are performed (Kohl, 2000).

Differential Diagnosis. The diagnosis is usually not a problem if vesicles are present. Coxsackievirus can cause a vesicular stomatitis.

Management. Treatment is supportive in nature except in life-threatening illness (neonatal infection or immunocompromised patients).

Complications. Usually the infection is mild. Major problems have been discussed. Bacterial superinfection is always a problem. There is an increased incidence of cervical cancer in women with HSV-2 infections.

Prevention. The prevention of neonatal infection is directly tied to the monitoring of women during pregnancy and labor. All pregnant women must be asked about HSV infection in themselves and all sexual partners. Signs and symptoms of HSV should be carefully monitored throughout pregnancy. Again, during labor, all women must be requestioned about HSV. The mother must be carefully examined for signs and symptoms of infection. Cesarean delivery is indicated in women with apparent infection unless membranes are ruptured for more than 4 to 6 hours. Scalp monitoring should be avoided.

After birth, the infant must be carefully examined for vesicular lesions. Any lesions found should be cultured. The child should be started on acyclovir while awaiting culture results if HSV is strongly suspected. Infants born to mothers with a history of HSV but no signs of active disease follow the same protocol. Intrapartum cultures from mother and child should be obtained on the day of delivery (see Chapter 39).

Toddlers and infants with primary gingivostomatis who are drooling should be excluded from child care centers. Children with "fever blisters" may attend school as long as they have control over their saliva. Covering lesions with a bandage is appropriate for children with active nonmucosal involvement. Wrestlers should be excluded from competition until lesions have healed (AAP, 2003).

Infectious Mononucleosis

Etiology. Infectious mononucleosis is part of the Epstein-Barr family of herpesvirus.

Epidemiology. Infectious mononucleosis (IM) is worldwide in distribution. By 5 years of age, 70% to 90% of children in poor urban settings or developing countries are seropositive for Epstein-Barr virus. In these children, primary infection tends to produce only mild symptoms or is subclinical. In more affluent socioeconomic groups, seroconversion is apparent in 40% to 50% of children (Barone & Krilov, 2001). Most symptomatic cases of IM occur during adolescence and in young adults (incidence is 1 in 2500 students). The mode of transmission is close personal contact (e.g., kissing). Pharyngeal secretions are the main source of transmission; fomite contamination can be a problem. About 15% to 20% of healthy immune individuals secrete virus at any one time. Up to 50% of patients on immunosuppressive therapy, including those on steroids, shed virus.

Incubation Period. Because IM virus is found in the saliva and blood of both clinically ill and asymptomatic infected persons for many months, the period of communicability is difficult to assess. The period of incubation is thought to be from 2 to 6 weeks (average 20 to 30 days).

Clinical Findings. IM is the "great impostor" and can mimic any disease imaginable. It is a disease of the primary lymphoid tissue and peripheral blood. There is enlargement of lymphoid tissue: regional lymph nodes, tonsils, spleen, and liver. Atypical lymphocytes are seen in the peripheral blood. Almost all body organs are involved, including but not limited to the lungs, heart, kidneys, adrenals, central nervous system, and skin. Symptoms are variable and can last up to 2 to 3 weeks. Clinical presentation can include the following:

- Fever: Moderate to high fever (less than 103° F [39.5° C]) lasting 1 to 3 days is common.
- Sore throat: Usually begins a few days after the fever. The throat is very painful. There is marked tonsillar

enlargement, grayish-colored exudates, ulceration, and pseudomembrane formation. Petechiae are found on the palate.
- Lymphadenopathy: Both the anterior and especially the posterior cervical nodes are involved; any lymphoid tissue can be affected. Nodes are firm but usually non-tender, and they are discrete in nature.
- Splenomegaly: Occurs in 50% to 75% of cases. Rupture is rare.
- Hepatomegaly: Is common. Almost all patients have abnormal liver function tests; 5% to 25% have clinical hepatitis.
- Skin rash: Occurs in 20% of cases. Can be maculopapular, urticarial, scarlatiniform, hemorrhagic, or nodular. The rash occurs more frequently in patients taking ampicillin and probably represents a form of arteritis or vasculitis.
- Periorbital edema: Reported in 25% of cases.

Other systemic manifestations reported as primary disease and not complications include myalgia, arthralgia, chest pain, ocular pain, photophobia, conjunctivitis, gingivitis, abdominal pain, diarrhea, cough, pneumonia, rhinitis, epistaxis, bradycardia, aseptic meningitis, Guillain-Barré syndrome, Bell's palsy, Reye syndrome, and acute cerebellar ataxia.

Diagnostic Studies. The CBC has a classic picture of more than 10% atypical lymphocytes and 50% lymphocytosis. There are a number of serologic tests. Monospot and the serum heterophile test are positive in 80% to 90% of infected patients over 4 years of age. Children older than 4 years of age usually must be ill for approximately 2 weeks before seroconverting. Viral culture and Epstein-Barr–specific core and capsule antibody testing are usually used for diagnosis if the primary screening tests are negative and there is continued suspicion of IM. CMV must be considered in patients who have all the symptoms of IM but are negative on primary testing. It is often impossible to differentiate the two clinically, but CMV infection is seen more in adults (Jenson, 2000).

Differential Diagnosis. Infectious mononucleosis is in the differential diagnosis of almost every infectious disease. Conditions and infections typically associated with a mononucleosis-like syndrome are gram-positive alpha-beta hemolytic streptococcal pharyngitis, leukemia, lymphoreticular malignancies, adenoviruses, toxoplasmosis, CMV, rubella, HIV, hepatitis, systemic lupus erythematosus (SLE), drug reactions, and diphtheria (Barone & Krilov, 2001).

Management. Treatment is supportive, with adequate fluids and calories. Corticosteroids and acyclovir are not recommended for routine disease. Contact sports and strenuous exercise should be avoided if the patient has hepatosplenomegaly. Participation is acceptable after the splenomegaly has resolved.

Complications. Usually most clinically healthy patients experience few sequelae. Rare complications include splenic rupture, thrombocytopenia, agranulocytosis, hemolytic anemia, orchitis, myocarditis, and chronic IM. Fatal disseminated disease, or B-cell lymphoma, occurs in patients with congenital or acquired cellular immunity deficiencies. Burkitt B-cell lymphoma and nasopharyngeal carcinoma are also caused by Epstein-Barr virus; these conditions are more commonly found in central Africa and Southeast Asia. Death from IM occurs in approximately 1 out of 3000 cases (Barone & Krilov, 2001).

Prevention. Persons with a recent history of IM or an infectious mononucleosis–like disease should not donate blood.

Influenza

Etiology. This is the only remaining pandemic disease with no effective control. Influenza virus is an orthomyxovirus of three antigenic types, A, B, and C. Types A and B are still responsible for epidemic disease. Type A is further classified into two surface antigens—hemagglutinin (H) and neuraminidase (N). Three hemagglutinin subtypes and two neuraminidase types are known to cause disease in humans. Specific antibodies to the virus are important in immunity. Influenza A has major changes between subtypes that occur at 10-year intervals. This process is called *antigenic shift*. Minor variation within a specific subtype is referred to as *antigenic drift* and occurs with both type A and type B.

After the emergence of a newly shifted strain, the highest incidence of the illness occurs in infants and children 5 to 14 years old, with an attack rate of 30% to 50% (Wright, 2000a). Healthy children under 5 years and those with chronic diseases have excessively high rates of hospitalization (AAP, 2003).

Epidemiology. Influenza is a highly contagious disease and is spread person to person by direct contact, droplet contamination, and fomites recently contaminated with infected nasopharyngeal secretions. Viremia is a rare occurrence. In temperate climates, epidemics always occur in the winter months, last approximately 4 to 8 weeks, and peak 2 weeks after the index case. In recent years, some epidemics have lasted 3 months. Children shed the virus longer than adults and therefore are particularly good transmitters within a community.

Incubation Period. The incubation period is 1 to 3 days. Patients become infectious 24 hours before the onset of symptoms. Viral shedding usually ceases 7 days after the onset of illness.

Clinical Findings. Influenza patients are sick! There is a sudden onset of high fever, 102° to 106° F, headache, chills, coryza, vertigo, sore throat, pain in the back and extremities, and dry hacking cough that can resemble pertussis. Vomiting, diarrhea, and croup occur in young children. Infants can appear septic. Conjunctival injection, epistaxis, and myocarditis (evident by weak heart sounds and rapid, weak pulse) are common. In severe infection, there can be involvement of the lower respiratory tract with atelectasis or infiltrates. Severe myocardial involvement can cause distention of the right side of the heart and congestive heart failure.

Diagnostic Studies. Special viral cultures taken from the nasopharyngeal cavity by swab or aspiration within 72 hours of the onset of illness can isolate the virus in 2 to 6 days to confirm the diagnosis. With the exception of direct fluorescent antibody (DFA) tests, other diagnostic tests are of little help. DFA tests are hampered by false-positive and false-negative reactions. There are numerous serologic tests: viral agglutination, complement fixation, immunofluorescence testing, and ELISA. Results from the ELISA or immunofluorescence techniques are available within several hours. The CBC shows leukopenia.

Differential Diagnosis. The differential diagnosis includes other viral respiratory infections (common cold, parainfluenza, respiratory syncytial virus), allergic croup, epiglottitis, and bacterial upper respiratory infections.

Management. Treatment is supportive in nature (bed rest, fluids, antipyretics). Given its expense, antiviral therapy should be reserved for high-risk patients and those in institutions (AAP, 2003). Amantadine diminishes the severity of type A illness but has no effect on type B. It is FDA approved only for treatment in patients 1 year of age and older; rimantadine is used for treating those 13 years of age and older (AAP, 2003). See Appendix A for dosage. Both should be started within 48 hours of symptom onset and continued for 2 to 5 days until the patient is asymptomatic for 24 to 48 hours. The newest classification of drugs, the neuraminidase inhibitors, includes zanamivir (Relenza) and oseltamivir (Tamiflu) and treats both hepatitis A and B. These drugs decrease the release of virus from cells and relieve flu symptoms approximately 1 to 1.5 days sooner than in untreated control subjects. Zanamivir is FDA approved for patients 7 years of age and older and is administered with a breath-activated inhaler (twice daily for 5 days). Oseltamivir is an oral agent. Currently it is FDA approved for use in children 1 year of age or older (dosage: 1 tablet twice daily for 5 days). Both are used to treat disease and oseltamivir is approved as prophylaxis against familial spread of influenza A and influenza B in patients 13 years of age and older (AAP, 2003).

Complications. Complications include Reye syndrome and respiratory infections (acute otitis media [AOM], pneumonia, acute myositis, toxic shock, myocarditis, cystic fibrosis, and asthma exacerbations) followed by a bacterial superinfection, usually with *H. influenzae* (Wright, 2000a). Do not give aspirin to influenza sufferers!

Prevention. As previously discussed, influenza vaccine should be used. Amantadine, rimantadine, and oseltamivir are approved for use in children and adults for prophylaxis against specific types of influenza infections. The prophylactic doses are the same as for treatment.

Measles (Rubeola)

Etiology. Measles (rubeola) is a *Morbillivirus* in the Paramyxoviridae family and is similar to mumps and influenza. There is only one antigenic type. Measles is typlified by a rash, indicating viremia. It is a serious illness in children! The disease is associated with high mortality and morbidity rates worldwide.

Epidemiology. Humans and primates are the only known reservoir of infection. The source of the infection is respiratory secretions, blood, and urine of infected persons. Virus is transmitted through droplet contact, fomites, and, less likely, aerosol transmission. Peak incidence of infection in susceptible persons occurs during the winter and spring months. The failure rate after the first vaccine at 12 months is approximately 5%; after the second vaccine the failure rate is less than 1% (AAP, 2003).

Incubation Period. The incubation period is 8 to 12 days. A person is contagious 1 to 2 days before the onset of symptoms or 3 to 5 days before the rash to 4 days after the appearance of the rash (AAP, 2003). There is no carrier state; disease or two vaccinations usually confers lifelong immunity.

Clinical Findings. The clinical manifestations are divided into three stages:

1. Incubation period: There are no specific symptoms.
2. Prodromal period: This is the first sign of the illness and lasts 4 to 5 days. This stage consists of URI symptoms; low to moderate fever (greater than 101° F [38.3° C]); and cough, coryza, and conjunctivitis (the "three Cs" of measles). An enanthem can be found on the oral mucosa opposite the lower molars. These Koplik spots last 12 to 15 hours. They are small, irregular bluish-white granules on an erythematous background and are pathognomonic of measles infection.
3. Rash stage: The rash of unmodified measles usually appears on the third or fourth day of the illness. As the rash appears, temperature rises, often to 105° F. The rash first appears behind the ears and on the forehead. It is maculopapular in nature. Papules enlarge, coalesce, and move progressively downward, engulfing the face, neck, and arms over the next 24 hours. By the end of the second 24 hours, the rash has spread to the back, abdomen, and thighs. As the legs become more involved, the face begins to clear. The entire process takes approximately 3

days. Respiratory symptoms are most severe on day 3 of the rash. The more severe the rash, the more severe the illness. It can become hemorrhagic. This type of measles can be fatal because of disseminated intravascular coagulation (DIC). After the fourth day of the rash stage, the rash begins to fade. The disease peaks and defervesces. After the rash clears, a residual light pigmentation occurs, lasting approximately 1 week. This desquamates finely. Maternal antibody level and improperly given vaccine can alter the presentation and clinical course of measles.

Modified Measles. This most commonly appears in children who have been passively immunized with IG after exposure to the disease. It can occur in infants with partial maternal immunity. The incubation period can persist as long as 20 days. The illness is an abbreviated version of typical disease. The prodrome period can be as early as 1 to 2 days with normal to low-grade fever. URI symptoms are minimal to absent. Koplik spots usually do not appear. The rash is so mild that it is often missed. There are usually no complications.

Diagnostic Studies. Confirmation of disease can be made by viral isolation in tissue culture and serial antibody titers drawn 3 weeks apart. A single measles IgM level is useful if drawn after the rash appears but not later than 30 to 60 days after the onset of the rash. Measles is a reportable disease in the United States.

Differential Diagnosis. Any viral rash (e.g., roseola, rubella, echovirus, coxsackievirus, IM, adenovirus, and Epstein-Barr virus), toxoplasmosis, scarlet fever, Kawasaki syndrome, meningococcemia, Rocky Mountain spotted fever, drug rashes, and serum sickness are included in the differential diagnosis.

Management. Treatment is supportive in nature. Bacterial superinfections are treated with appropriate antibiotics.

Children living in countries where malnutrition is an issue are at greater risk for death with measles infection. These children, and those with severe measles, have low vitamin A levels. Therefore vitamin A supplementation is recommended in the following circumstances (AAP, 2000):

- All children diagnosed with measles in areas where vitamin A deficiency is a recognized problem
- Children between 6 months and 2 years of age who are hospitalized with severe measles, manifested by pneumonia, croup, or diarrhea
- Infants who are older than 6 months of age diagnosed with measles with the following risk criteria: immunodeficiency, ophthalmologic evidence of vitamin A deficiency or xerophthalmia, impaired intestinal absorption (e.g., cystic fibrosis, short bowel syndrome), moderate to severe malnutrition, and recent travel from an area where measles has a high mortality rate

Use of vitamin A in infants younger than 6 months of age has not been proven efficacious (AAP, 2003).

The dosage of vitamin A is a one-time dose of 100,000 International Units (IU) for children between 6 months and 1 year of age and 200,000 IU for children who are 1 year of age and older. Vitamin A is repeated the next day and 1 month later if there is ophthalmologic evidence of vitamin A deficiency.

Complications. Measles is a severe disease. The measles virus is responsible for a significant inflammatory reaction that extends from the nasopharynx to the bronchi. Death is generally due to respiratory and neurologic sequelae or to bacterial superinfection. One must carefully document complications before specific treatment is undertaken.

Bacterial Superinfection and Viral Complications. These usually manifest as a URI, obstructive laryngitis, otitis, mastoiditis, cervical adenitis, bronchitis, and pneumonia. The causative organism is usually the measles virus or group A β-hemolytic streptococci, pneumococci, *H. influenzae*, *S. aureus*, or an exacerbation of underlying TB.

Myocarditis. This is a rare but reported complication. Transient electrocardiograph changes are common.

Purpura Fulminans (Black Measles). This is a severe complication with multiorgan bleeding.

Disseminated Intravascular Coagulation. Activation of the coagulation system leads to intravascular fibrin deposit and platelet destruction.

Neurologic Complications. EEG changes are common, especially during the rash stage, but are usually not significant. However, 1 to 2 per 1000 cases suffers from an acute measles encephalitis that more often occurs after the second and fifth day of the onset of the rash (may also occur before the rash). The child seems to be either doing well or recovering from the disease. Then there can be a sudden onset of fever, headache, vomiting, drowsiness, convulsions, and possibly coma. Frequently, there are signs of meningeal irritation. The CSF demonstrates increased protein and lymphocytic pleocytosis. An acute demyelinating encephalomyelitis can develop that may be due to an immunologic reaction.

Subacute Sclerosing Panencephalitis. This is a rare condition that is considered a late complication of measles. The incidence increases if the measles disease occurs before 18 months of age. It usually occurs 7 to 12 or more years after infection and is considered a "slow virus." The incidence is less than 0.06% per million cases. The infection is slow, progressive, and evidenced by behavioral and intellectual deterioration and seizures, and it may be fatal, frequently within 1 month. In the United States, it occurs more in Hispanic immigrant children living in the west and New York City (Maldonado, 2000). It is diagnosed by EEG changes, marked elevation of CSF globulin (especially IgG), exceptionally high serum measles antibody titer, and measles antibodies in the CSF.

Care of Exposed Persons. This is done with active and passive immunization, as discussed previously.

Mumps

Etiology. Mumps is an acute generalized viral disease with painful enlargement of one or more salivary glands (usually parotid glands) as the apparent sign. Mumps is a paramyxovirus. Only one serotype is known. Humans are the only natural reservoir.

Epidemiology. The source of infection is the saliva of infected persons. The virus is spread by direct contact, aerosol transmission, fomites, and, possibly, urine from infected persons. Viremia exists, and the virus is found in blood, urine, CSF, saliva, and upper respiratory secretions. Before mumps vaccination, mumps was a disease of childhood in the United States; 85% of infections occurred in children 2 to 14 years of age. Now, infection is more often seen in young adults born from 1967 to 1977 who lack immunity (Maldonado, 2000). Death from this virus is rare but occurs in about 2% of those who suffer from the complication of meningoencephalomyelitis. Infection occurs during all seasons but is most common during late winter and spring. Mumps virus crosses the placenta, and infection during the first trimester increases the risk of spontaneous abortion. Fetal malformations after prenatal mumps infection have not been demonstrated (AAP, 2003).

Incubation Period. The incubation period is 12 to 25 days (mean of 17 days). The period of communicability is 1 to 2 days before glandular swelling to 5 days after the onset of parotid swelling. The virus has been isolated 7 days before to 9 days after the onset of parotid swelling. One third of patients are asymptomatic but infectious. One attack usually confers lifelong immunity. Transplacental antibodies to mumps are protective for 6 months (Maldonado, 2000). Neonatal infection reflects maternal disease just before delivery.

Clinical Findings. There are two clinical stages:

1. Prodromal stage: Rare in children but can cause fever, headache, anorexia, neck pain, and malaise.
2. Swelling stage: Approximately 24 hours after the prodromal stage, one (in 25% of patients) or both of the parotid glands begin to swell in a characteristic manner. The gland fills the space between the posterior border of the mandible and mastoid, pushing downward and forward to the zygoma. The ear is pushed forward and upward. This can take a few hours to a few days. The area becomes swollen and painful. The enlarged glands decrease in size and usually return to normal in 3 to 7 days. Occasionally, a maculopapular, pink, discrete rash is seen on the trunk (Iannone, 2001). Pain on the affected side can be elicited by having the patient eat something sour. This is known as the "pickle sign." Stensen's duct is red and swollen. Twenty percent of patients are afebrile during this time. Fever is usually moderate and rarely high, with 10% to 15% of cases involving only submandibular gland swelling. Little pain is associated with the submandibular infection. However, the redness subsides more slowly. Wharton's duct is frequently swollen. Sublingual salivary glands are not commonly involved. When they are involved, there is bilateral swelling in the submental region in the floor of the mouth. Edema caused by lymphatic obstruction of the manubrium and upper chest is reported.

Diagnostic Studies. These include viral isolation and culture, serologic tests (enzyme immunoassay for IgG and IgM antibodies and specific mumps antibody), and elevated serum amylase. Saliva, spinal fluid, urine, and brain samples may be indicated, depending on symptoms.

Differential Diagnosis. Cervical or preauricular lymphadenitis, CMV, enteroviruses, tumor, suppurative parotitis by either bacterial or viral (coxsackievirus, parainfluenza 3) infection, idiopathic recurrent parotitis, parotid ductal obstruction, Mikulicz syndrome, uveoparotid fever, and cancer (especially lymphosarcoma) are included in the differential diagnosis.

Management. Treatment is supportive.

Complications. Complications include meningoencephalitis (10% incidence of CNS infection); orchitis/epididymitis (14% to 35% incidence in adolescents and adults); oophoritis (7% incidence in postpubertal women); pancreatitis (rare); thyroiditis (uncommon in children); myocarditis (13% incidence in adults); deafness (1 in 15,000 cases—transient or permanent); ocular complications (complete recovery can be expected); arthritis (rare in children); thrombocytopenia and hemolytic anemia (usually self-limited); mastitis (rare); and glomerulonephritis (rare).

Prevention. School and day care students should be kept home until 9 days after the onset of parotid swelling. Active and passive immunization has been discussed previously.

Parainfluenza Virus

Etiology. Parainfluenza virus, a paramyxovirus, is similar to the influenza and mumps viruses. Parainfluenza is the major cause of croup. It also is an important cause of bronchitis, bronchiolitis, and pneumonia. There are four antigenic types, classified 1 to 4. Type 4 has two subtypes, A and B, but less is known about them. Type 1 is associated more with croup, and type 3 is associated more with lower respiratory infection.

Epidemiology. The disease is spread by direct contact through infected nasopharyngeal secretions. Transmission occurs by person-to-person contact, as well as fomite contamination. Infection occurs throughout the year depending on the type. Type 3 is a major cause of lower respiratory tract disease in children under 6 months of age. Types 1 and 2 usually strike children 2 to 6 years of age and are seen more in summer and fall; reinfections occur at any age. Type 4 infections usually are mild.

Incubation. The incubation period is 2 to 6 days. Normal children usually shed type 1 virus for 4 to 7 days with a range of up to 14 days. Type 3 virus generally sheds for 8 to 9 days with a range of up to 3 weeks.

Clinical Findings. Eighty percent of parainfluenza infections affect the upper airways. This virus accounts for 50% of hospital admissions for croup and 15% of admissions for bronchitis, bronchiolitis, and pneumonia (Wright, 2000b). Sore throat is a common complaint in older children. Fever is found in only 20% of cases and is inversely proportional to the age of the child. Discrete maculopapular rashes of short duration can be found if the patient is carefully examined. Types 1 and 3 also have been associated with acute parotitis, causing an illness clinically indistinguishable from mumps virus. Reye syndrome has occurred in association with parainfluenza viral infection. Parainfluenza viruses have been recovered from the spinal fluid of victims of sudden infant death syndrome (SIDS).

Diagnostic Studies. These do not need to be done routinely. DFA tests are hampered by false-positive and false-negative reactions. There are numerous serologic tests: viral agglutination, complement fixation, immunofluorescent testing, and ELISA. Parainfluenza virus infection may not always cause a rise in antibody titers. Cultures can isolate the virus in 4 to 7 days. Serologic results can be confusing because of cross-reaction among paramyxovirus.

Differential Diagnosis. The differential diagnosis includes other viral URIs, allergic croup, and bacterial URIs. The most important clinical differential diagnostic consideration is laryngotracheitis and other acute upper airway obstructive diseases, such as acute angioneurotic edema, epiglottitis, and foreign body aspiration.

Management. The treatment is supportive. Antiviral therapy is not available (AAP, 2003). Antibiotics in cases of severe upper airway infection are reasonable until definitive test results are available. Cefuroxime covers most of the usual opportunistic bacterial organisms. Oral dexamethasone can be used in outpatient settings for those with mild croup (see Chapter 32 for more treatment information). No vaccine is available. Good hand hygiene is important.

Complications. Complications are infrequent. Secondary bacterial infections, including otitis media and pneumonia, may occur. Immunocompromised hosts can have significant secondary infections such as bacterial tracheitis, bronchitis, and pneumonia.

Poliomyelitis Virus

Etiology. The agent is an enterovirus with three serotypes of poliovirus (types 1, 2, and 3). The disease ranges from an asymptomatic illness to lower motor neuron paralysis.

Epidemiology. Humans are the only documented source of infection. Transmission is through fecal-oral contact and oral-oral upper respiratory secretions. The last North American epidemic occurred in 1979. Since 1979, almost all cases have been associated with oral vaccine use, as discussed earlier.

Asymptomatic disease occurs in 95% of those infected (AAP, 2003). Communicability is greatest 1 week before the onset of clinical illness and shortly afterward, due to respiratory secretions and high fecal excretion. Contagion exists for approximately 1 week for mouth secretions and for several weeks to months from feces. Contagion after receiving the oral polio virus vaccine (OPV) is longer from both oral secretions and feces, especially from immunocompromised individuals. The incubation period is 3 to 6 days for abortive polio and 7 to 21 days for the paralytic form.

Clinical Findings. There are three clinical forms:

1. Nonspecific febrile illness (abortive polio): A mild and brief illness. There is an acute onset of fever to 103° F. Malaise, pharyngitis, headache, nausea, vomiting, abdominal pain, constipation, and anorexia are common findings. The entire illness lasts a few hours to a couple of days.
2. Nonparalytic polio: Manifests as aseptic meningitis in 1% to 5% of cases (AAP, 2003). The patient manifests abortive symptoms and becomes sicker. Pain and stiffness of the neck, trunk, back, and legs are common. Headache is intense; constipation is common. Hyperesthesia and paresthesia occur. There may be a fleeting bladder paralysis. Usually there is a 1- to 2-week symptom-free period between the abortive and the nonparalytic stages.
3. Paralytic disease: Produces nonparalytic findings plus weakness of one or more muscle groups. The incubation period for paralytic polio is from 4 to 21 days. This most likely coincides with the replication of the virus in the oropharyngeal and gastrointestinal tracts. There is asymmetric distribution of weakness. Cranial or skeletal muscle can be involved, with lower extremities more commonly affected. Bladder paralysis occurs in up to 20% of the cases with concomitant bowel atony. The muscle paralysis is a flaccid type, without sensory loss, with subsequent atrophy caused by denervation and disuse. Generally, the greater the paralytic symptoms the more severe the disability (Morag & Ogra, 2000). Two thirds of patients with acute motor neuron disease develop paralytic polio (AAP, 2003).

Diagnostic Studies. The diagnostic test of choice are viral cultures: two stool and two pharyngeal samples at least 24 hours apart within the first 2 weeks after the beginning of symptoms. If confirmatory, these should be sent to the CDC for further analysis.

Differential Diagnosis. Polio is rare. Differential diagnoses include other conditions causing muscular weakness: Guillain-Barré syndrome, peripheral neuritis, encephalitis, rabies, tetanus, botulism, demyelinating encephalomyelitis, tick-bite paralysis, spinal cord tumors, familial periodic paralysis, myasthenia gravis, and hysterical paralysis. Conditions that cause decreased limb movement or pseudoweakness are also differential diagnoses and include unrecognized trauma, toxic synovitis, acute osteomyelitis, acute rheumatic fever, scurvy, and congenital syphilitic osteomyelitis.

Management. There is no specific treatment. Patients with paralytic disease should be hospitalized.

Complications. The following may be seen:
- Gastrointestinal problems, including bleeding and acute gastric dilation
- Cardiopulmonary problems, consisting of mild hypertension and myocarditis
- Acute pulmonary edema
- Pulmonary embolism
- Metabolic problems (hypercalciuria and renal stones)

Postpolio syndrome can occur decades after initial wild-type infection and occurs in 30% to 40% of persons. Symptoms include muscle pain and weakness or paralysis. There is an increased risk in those who had residual infirmities and in women.

Prevention. Prevention is active and passive vaccination, as discussed previously.

Roseola Infantum (Exanthem Subitum)

Etiology. Roseola infantum is also known as exanthem subitum. The causative agent is human herpesvirus 6 (and, less commonly, herpesvirus 7). Herpesvirus 6 may be associated with multiple sclerosis (Leach, 2000).

Epidemiology. Humans are the only natural reservoir. The method of transmission is probably from oral, nasal, and conjunctival routes from other family members or caregivers (Leach, 2000). The disease is most common in children between 6 and 24 months of age. It is rare in children younger than 3 months or older than 3 years of age. Most children are seropositive by 2 years of age. This would indicate that there is asymptomatic illness or roseola without rash. Secondary cases are rare, and occasional outbreaks are reported. Cases occur all year long but tend to cluster in the spring and early summer.

Incubation Period. Incubation period has a mean of 9 to 10 days. The period of communicability is probably greatest during the fever phase before the rash erupts.

Clinical Findings. There is a sudden onset of fever from 101° to 106° F (39.9° to 40° C) for 3 to 5 days, but the child does not seem particularly ill. There may be signs of a URI (rhinitis, sore throat), gastrointestinal (GI) complaints (diarrhea, vomiting, abdominal pain), and, occasionally, a febrile convulsion (5% to 10% of cases). As the fever breaks, a diffuse, nonpruritic, discrete, rose-colored, maculopapular rash, 2 to 3 mm in diameter, appears. It fades on pressure and rarely coalesces. The roseola exanthema is similar to the rash of rubella. The rash lasts 1 to 2 days, begins on the trunk, and spreads centrifugally (Fig. 24-1).

Diagnostic Studies. Specific tests include serology, viral culture, antigen detection, and PCR, but no test is currently in use for ambulatory care. There may be initial leukocytosis with white blood cell counts as high as 20,000/mm^3 during the first 26 hours. Then classic viral leukopenia occurs.

Differential Diagnosis. Most viral rashes, scarlatina, and drug hypersensitivity are included in the differential diagnoses. However, the clinical course usually makes this illness easy to diagnose. A roseola-like illness is associated with parvovirus B19, echovirus 16, other enteroviruses, measles, and adenoviruses. Until the rash develops, fever without focus and bacterial sepsis are in the differential diagnosis. Continued high fever without a ready source usually leads to a septic workup for some of these children. If a febrile seizure occurs, meningitis is usually added to the differential diagnosis.

Management. There is no specific treatment.

Complications. Rare complications include febrile convulsions, encephalitis, hepatitis, and pneumonitis.

Rubella (German or 3-Day Measles)

Etiology. Rubella is an acute disease of childhood that occurs in two forms, postnatal and congenital. Rubella is an RNA virus of the genus *Rubivirus*, in the Togaviridae family.

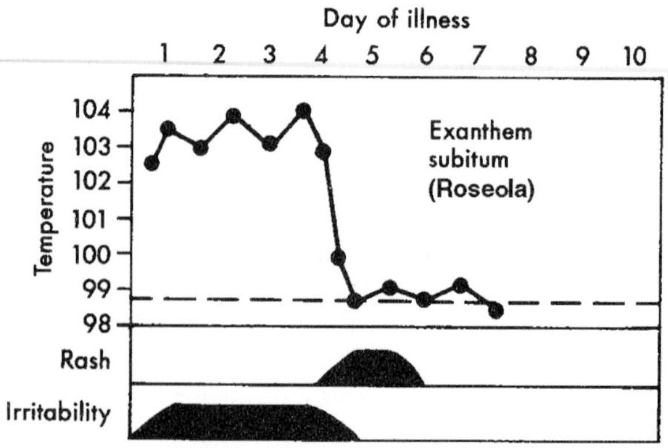

FIGURE 24-1 Schematic diagram illustrating the symptoms of roseola. (Adapted from Katz S, Gershon A, Hotez P: *Krugman's infectious diseases of children*, ed 10, Philadelphia, 1998, Mosby, pp 708-714.)

Epidemiology. Humans are the only reservoir. Infection is spread through nasopharyngeal secretions or transplacentally during either apparent or silent infections. It is worldwide in distribution. The virus has been isolated in blood, stool, and urine of infected individuals. It also has been isolated on fomites for as long as 24 hours. With the arrival of immunization, the numbers of epidemics declined. Most cases occur in unvaccinated children, teenagers, and young adults. In closed populations (boarding schools and the military), the attack rate is close to 100%. Males and females are equally affected. Approximately 25% to 60% of infections are subclinical. There is transplacental immunity for approximately 5 to 6 months if the mother is immune. There is probable lifelong immunity for naturally occurring disease. Verified second attacks are rare.

Incubation Period. The incubation period is 14 to 21 days. The period of maximum communicability is approximately 7 days before to 5 to 7 days after the onset of rash.

Clinical Findings. Postnatal disease is marked by three stages:

1. Prodrome: There are mild catarrhal symptoms. This stage is occasionally missed.
2. Lymphadenopathy: Usually begins within 24 hours, but can begin as early as 7 days, before the rash appears, and can last for more than 1 week. The postauricular, posterior cervical, and posterior occipital are the primary lymph nodes involved. There is generalized lymph node involvement, and at times splenomegaly is noted.
3. Rash: An enanthem can appear in 20% of cases just before the general rash. These Forschheimer spots, which consist of small rose-colored to reddish spots located on the soft palate, were first noted in 1898. They are not considered pathognomonic for rubella and are noted in scarlet fever and other URIs. The rubella rash can be the first obvious sign of illness. It begins on the face and can fade before it spreads to the chest during the next 24 hours. The rash is composed of discrete maculopapules that occasionally coalesce. It spreads caudally, lasting a mean of 3 days. There can be itching without a rash or a fine, branlike desquamation. A low-grade fever can occur during the eruption. There is no photophobia; anorexia, headache, and malaise are rare.

Diagnostic Studies. Viral cultures and serologic testing of acute and convalescent titers at least 2 weeks apart are done. Hemagglutination inhibition studies are the most widely used method but are being supplanted by latex agglutination enzyme and fluorescent immunoassay, among others. Rubella-specific IgM is an important test in the newborn.

Differential Diagnosis. The disease can be difficult to diagnose unless there is an epidemic. The rash can be confused with scarlet fever, mononucleosis, echovirus, roseola, rubeola, and drug eruptions.

Management. There is no specific therapy.

Complications. Complications in postnatal rubella are rare. They include arthritis (most common complication, affecting female adolescents more often than younger children); neuritis (pain/paresthesia of arms, wrists, hands, and popliteal area occurring 1 to 2 months after the infection); encephalitis (1 in 6000 cases during the eruptive stage with 20% fatality rate); and idiopathic thrombocytopenic purpura (rare occurrence).

Prevention. Children with postnatal rubella should be kept home from school or day care for approximately 1 week after the rash erupts. Active and passive immunization has been discussed previously.

Reinfection. There are conflicting studies. Because illness without rash exists, the actual numbers of reinfections are unknown. Rubella virus has many antigenic sites, causing the production of numerous antibodies. Their duration is unknown. In serologically immune persons, the reinfection rate from wild virus is 3% to 10%. The reinfection rate in those immunized is approximately 14% to 18%. Many of these reinfections are subclinical. Accidental vaccination of a pregnant woman should not be considered a reason for pregnancy termination, because there is little evidence that such an occurrence causes congenital rubella syndrome (Wharton, 2002).

Varicella

Etiology. Varicella is a common, highly contagious virus. It is a herpesvirus with only one antigenic strain, *Herpesvirus varicellae.* Chickenpox is the primary illness. Shingles (herpes zoster) is the reactivation infection (see Chapter 37). It derives its name not from chickens but from the propensity of the lesions to resemble chickpeas.

Epidemiology. Humans are the only reservoir of infection, and illness is spread by direct contact, droplets, and airborne transmission. Victims of shingles are also infectious for causing primary varicella illness. Immunity is usually life long. Symptomatic reinfection is rare, but asymptomatic reinfection occurs. Secondary attacks are usually mild. Asymptomatic primary infection is rare. Immunocompromised patients are at risk of developing generalized zoster. Ninety percent of varicella patients are younger than 10 years of age, and all but a few individuals contract the disease. There seems to be a shift in the epidemiology as adolescents and young adults contract the disease. Chickenpox is worldwide in distribution and endemic in most large cities. Epidemics occur but at irregular intervals. The incidence is greater in late autumn, winter, and spring. Primary varicella is associated with mortality rates of fewer than 2 per 100,000 cases; death is usually secondary to pneumonia. Those immunocompromised have a mortality rate of about 7% (Myers & Stanberry, 2000). Since the advent of the varicella vaccine before 1995, one study showed that there has been a steady decline in varicella disease (approximately 78% decrease) and hospitalizations due to complications (69% decrease) (Seward et al, 2002).

Incubation Period. The incubation period is 10 to 21 days, with a mean of 14 days. The period of communicability is 1 to 2 days before the rash erupts until all lesions are crusted over, which takes about 3 to 7 days. This can be prolonged to 28 days in VZIG recipients (AAP, 2003). Figure 24-2 shows differences in distribution of the maculopapular eruptions of scarlet fever, chickenpox, and smallpox and prodromal symptoms.

Clinical Findings. The following two phases are seen in varicella:

1. Prodrome: Not always present. It is composed of low-grade fever, listlessness, headache, backache, mild abdominal pain, and occasionally URI symptoms. These symptoms may occur 1 to 2 days before onset of the second phase.
2. Rash: Classic appearance. It is centripetal, beginning on the scalp, face, or trunk. Crops of pruritic lesions progress from spots to "teardrop vesicles" that cloud over and umbilicate in 24 to 48 hours. After a few days, all morphologic forms can be seen simultaneously. Scabs last from 5 to 20 days, depending on the depth of the lesions. There can be high fever, to 105° F. The more severe the rash, the higher the fever. Lesions can develop on all mucosal tissues, mouth, pharynx, larynx, trachea, vagina, and anus.

Diagnostic Studies. These are of little importance except in the case of exposure of pregnant women. The virus can be cultured. Tzanck smears of lesions demonstrate multinucleated giant cells containing intranuclear inclusion bodies that are diagnostic of herpesviruses (herpes zoster virus or herpes simplex virus). PCR of skin lesions is widely used.

Differential Diagnosis. The rash is classic; therefore the diagnosis is usually not a problem. See discussion later in this chapter on differentiating varicella from smallpox. Occasionally, impetigo, cigarette burns, and insect bites can cause some confusion in children with a mild rash.

Management. Chickenpox is usually a benign infection in normal children. Treatment is supportive in nature, including: management of itching with antihistamines or oatmeal baths; acetaminophen for fever; and antistaphylococcal penicillin or cephalosporins for bacterial superinfections until the bacterial agent has been identified. Children with fever for more than several days, or increasing temperatures 4 or more days after the appearance of the rash, should be evaluated closely for invasive disease (Annunziato & Gershon, 2002). Aspirin is contraindicated because of the possibility of Reye syndrome. Ibuprofen is not recommended because of a possible causal relationship with bacterial superinfections (Annunziato & Gershon, 2002). Intravenous acyclovir and vidarabine are effective in treating varicella in immunocompromised patients. VZIG can prevent or modify the course of the infection if given within 48 hours of rash onset or less than 72 hours after exposure. It is not effective after the disease has progressed. Oral acyclovir is expensive and is not routinely recommended for most children (AAP, 2003). When given to otherwise healthy children within 24 hours after eruption of the rash, there is a modest decrease in the symptoms and duration of the illness. Indications for the use of acyclovir include children older than 12 years with chronic pulmonary disorders, those receiving chronic salicylate therapy, or those receiving intermittent or short courses of oral or aerosolized corticosteroids. Dosing information can be found in Appendix A.

Complications. The following complications can occur: pyodermas (about a 5% incidence, causing serious invasive disease [AAP, 2000]); idiopathic thrombocytopenic purpura (1% to 2% incidence); pneumonia (rare in children, but with a 10% to 20% incidence in adolescents); CNS complications (encephalitis in 1 per 1000 cases, more commonly in children under 5 years and over 20 years; ataxia in 1 per 4000 cases, usually mild and resolves without residua); Reye syndrome (usually due to taking aspirin during the infection); and, rarely, glomerulonephritis, orchitis, hepatitis, toxic shock, osteomyelitis, necrotizing fasciitis, myositis, myocarditis, arthritis, and appendicitis.

Prevention. The following are recommended:

- Children exposed to chickenpox can attend school for about 1 week. If they begin to show signs of illness, they must be kept home for 1 week. If they do not break out in a rash, they can return to school. Children with active disease are to be kept home until all lesions are dry.
- Exposed patients: Use of VZIG has been previously discussed. VZIG is associated with asymptomatic infection. Varicella titers should be obtained 2 months after VZIG is given to assess immune status.
- Chickenpox vaccine has been previously discussed.

Congenital Varicella

Neonatal involvement is directly tied to the timing of the maternal infection. Infection early in pregnancy (at 8 to 20 weeks of gestation) can result in significant anomalies and scarring. Twenty percent of infants develop the disease in mothers who became infected prenatally, with 2% demonstrating embryopathy (Myers & Stanberry, 2000). Maternal infection occurring within 1 week from the estimated date of delivery to 1 week after delivery frequently results in

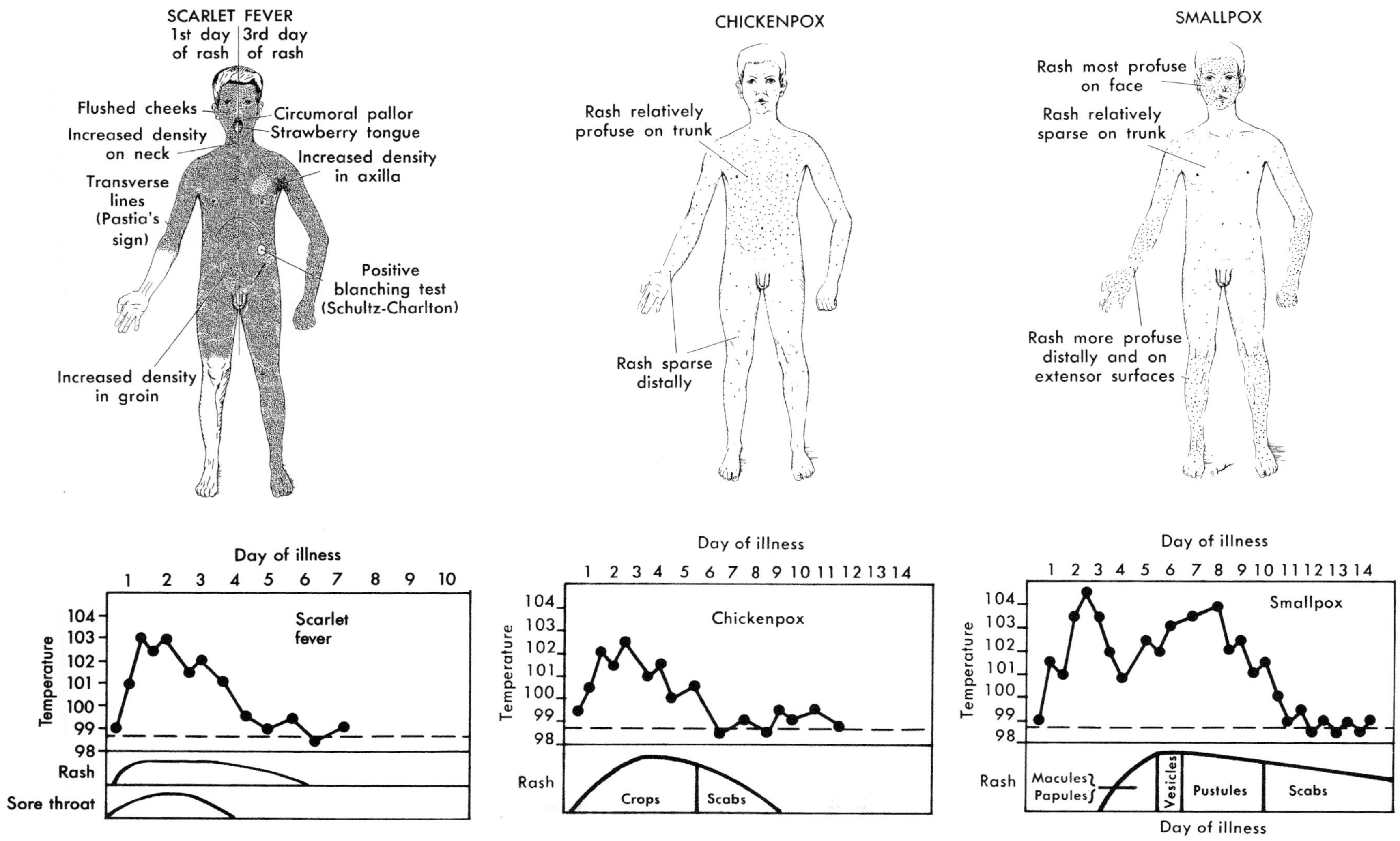

FIGURE. 24-2 Differences in distribution of the maculopapular eruptions of scarlet fever, chickenpox, and smallpox. (Adapted from Katz S, Gershon A, Hotez P: *Krugman's infectious diseases of children*, ed 10, Philadelphia, 1998, Mosby, pp. 708-714.)

neonatal varicella-zoster infection. There is no time for maternal antibodies to develop and cross the placenta. Infants should be given VZIG as soon as possible if their mothers develop varicella 5 days before the delivery or within 2 days postpartum. Despite VZIG, 50% of infants may develop mild varicella infection (Myers & Stanberry, 2000).

West Nile Virus

Etiology. West Nile Virus (WNV) is an arbovirus (family Flaviviridae). The virus is commonly found in Africa, West Asia, and the Middle East. Since 1999 it has been identified as occurring in most states of the United States. It recurs yearly when warmer weather occurs and mosquitoes begin breeding. Temperate weather and drought conditions are also believed to encourage mosquito-borne illnesses.

Epidemiology. It is mainly spread to people by bites from infected mosquitoes; however, evidence now points to uncommon human-to-human spread via organ transplantation, blood transfusions, and breastfeeding (CDC, 2001). Mosquitoes become infected by feeding on the blood of previously mosquito-infected birds and then transferring the virus via saliva to other birds, horses, humans, and other animals. The infection can be fatal to birds (especially crows, jays, and magpies). A hallmark of the presence of WNV in communities has been the discovery of dead birds. Bird-to-human transmission is not believed to occur.

Symptoms in humans develop 3 to 14 days after being bitten by an infected mosquito. Approximately 1 in 100 people who develop the infection will have the severe form of the disease (less than 1%). The disease causes the highest morbidity and mortality rates in older adults, those with preexisting chronic diseases, and those immunosuppressed. The mortality rate has been approximately 5% annually in the United States since 1999 (AAP, 2003).

Clinical Findings. Eighty percent of people bitten by an infected mosquito have minimal symptoms or are asymptomatic (Chettle, 2002). Symptoms of mild infection occur in approximately 20% of people and include fever (102° to 104° F); headache; muscle aches; eye pain; rash on neck, body, arms, or legs; lymphadenopathy; weakness; anorexia; nausea; and vomiting. Those with mild disease experience symptomatic relief within a week, with fatigue lingering longer.

Those with symptoms of severe infection may experience high fever; body and muscle weakness; rash on neck, body, arms, or legs; GI upset; and CNS symptoms (severe headache, change in mental status [disorientation], awkward gait/paralysis, stiff neck and nerve abnormalities, tremors/seizures, stupor/coma).

Laboratory Studies. IgM antibody capture enzyme-linked immunosorbent assay (MAC-ELISA) of serum or CSF is the test of choice and is collected within 8 days of illness onset. If positive, this test should be followed up by a more specific plaque reduction neutralization test to confirm WNV; CBC (normal or elevated white blood cells, low lymphocytes, anemia); and MRI or CT scan (or both) if patient has neurologic findings.

Management. For asymptomatic or mild cases, no treatment is necessary. Hospitalization is indicated for those with symptoms of meningitis or encephalitis. No virus-specific treatment is available for these patients; the FDA is testing interferon alfa-2b on these patients. The benefits of organ transplantation, transfusions, and breastfeeding far outweigh the risks of acquiring the disease and should not be curtailed (Zacharyczuk, 2002a).

Complications. With severe infection, complications include encephalitis, meningoencephalitis, meningitis, myocarditis, pancreatitis, and fulminant hepatitis.

Prevention. The goal of prevention is to avoid mosquito bites. No validated test is available to screen for WNV in donated blood. Mosquito abatement programs have been instituted in communities to reduce mosquito breeding grounds. NPs are encouraged to consider WNV in their differential diagnoses in any area where the virus has been identified and to counsel families about ways to minimize their exposure risk. Counseling should include the following:

- Stay indoors during the mosquitoes' most active times—dawn and dusk; if must be outdoors during these times, wear light-colored, long-sleeved shirts and long pants.
- Apply insect repellent with N,N-diethyl-meta-toluamide (DEET) to exposed skin and clothing except to children under 6 months of age.
- Children 6 months to 2 years: Apply DEET less than 10% once per day and only if in high-risk areas; do not apply to face or hands; use sparingly. Wash DEET off with soap and water when the child is inside.
- Children 3 to 12 years: Use DEET less than 10% sparingly and not more than three times daily; do not use on face or hands; wash off with soap and water when returned indoors.
- Older than 12 years: Use DEET less than 30% sparingly; do not spray directly on face but apply to hands first and then apply to face. Wash off with soap and water when returned indoors.
- Inventory outdoor areas for standing water that can serve as breeding areas for mosquitoes (e.g., old tires, pots/containers, bird bath [change once a week], pool or spa covers). Keep pools and spas clean and chlorinated.
- Use tight-fitting screens on all doors and windows.
- Report any dead birds, especially crows, jays, hawks, magpies, and owls, to local health department or pest control agency.

No vaccine is available for humans, birds, or horses. A vaccine is undergoing trials and is expected to be tested on humans in 2003. It is a modified yellow fever vaccine.

Hantavirus

Hantavirus is a Sin Nombre virus carried by deer mice, white-footed mice, cotton rats, and rice rats. It is spread by aerosolization of the rodent's saliva, urine, and feces excretions. These rodents are distributed equally throughout the United States; eradication of rodents is neither feasible nor desirable given their role in ecologic function (CDC, 2002d).

The illness from this viral infection, Hantavirus pulmonary syndrome (HPS), carries a mortality rate of about 37% (45% in those with cardiopulmonary disease); the elderly are at particular risk (CDC, 2002d). Human avoidance of infection is the goal in dealing with this disease. The virus is susceptible to common household disinfectants and chlorine.

To control outbreaks, the CDC recommends home and work environment modifications and the safe cleanup of rodent waste and nests (CDC, 2002d). The NP can make the following recommendations to patients if rodent infestation is suspected or discovered in their environments:

- Use rubber or latex gloves, goggles, or glasses for all cleanup activities.
- Disinfect areas of infestation with common household disinfectants and chlorine solutions.
- When cleaning out sheds, attics, basements, or other storage areas, aerate the areas first for at least 30 minutes to reduce exposure to aerosolized particulates.
- Avoid live or dead wild animals, especially rodents and rodent nesting sites.

New Viruses

As technology has become more sophisticated, researchers have been able to identify previously unidentified causative agents of infectious diseases. Other factors that have led to the more global emergence of pathogens include drug resistance, exotic travel (exotic diseases), and ownership of exotic pets (Zacharyczuk, 2002b). It is important for NPs to pay attention to the history of lifestyle habits of their patients in order to stay vigilant to the potential existence of new pathogens.

Metapneumovirus (human pneumovirus) is a respiratory pathogen of the Paramyxoviridae family. It may prove to be a significant cause of bronchiolitis in children (in addition to influenza and RSV). It resembles RSV in its symptomatology and epidemiology. Though not a new organism, technologic advances allowed it to be identified and monitored starting in 2001. One study revealed that approximately 25% of children 6 to 12 months of age and almost all 5-year-olds tested were seropositive for this agent. Seventy percent of children hospitalized for respiratory complications caused by this virus were found to harbor only this one virus during their illness. It was detected only between January and April. The role of antiviral agents in treating this virus is currently unknown (Brunell, 2002).

Enteroviruses E13 and E18 had previously been seen rarely in the United States until 2001. These enterovirus serotypes were identified in three or four large outbreaks of aseptic meningitis in 2001. Similar small viruses include poliovirus, coxsackieviruses A and B, and echoviruses. Always circulating in the population, the enteroviruses are the most common cause of aseptic meningitis. They are rarely tested for because there is no treatment (Kronemyer, 2002b). Antiviral agents currently in use have no benefit. The National Enterovirus Surveillance System (NESS) of the CDC has an ongoing surveillance system and encourages practitioners to test for enterovirus in patients diagnosed with aseptic meningitis. It is currently not a reportable disease in the United States.

Bacterial Infections

Cat-Scratch Disease

Etiology. *Bartonella henselae* is the organism thought to be responsible for cat-scratch disease (CSD). CSD is the most common cause of chronic persistent lymphadenopathy (Stechenberg, 2000). It is a slow-growing, gram-negative bacillus.

Epidemiology. CSD is believed to be a common infection (more than 24,000 cases per year), with most cases occurring in patients under 20 years of age. Infection occurs after direct, cutaneous contact with an infected animal. In 87% to 99% of the cases, a cat (usually a kitten) is involved. Other sources include dog scratches, monkey contact, wood splinters, and other inanimate objects. Most of the animals are healthy and are CSD skin test negative. Person-to-person contact has not been reported (AAP, 2003; Stechenberg, 2000). The CSD agent may be the cause of bacillary angiomatosis and peliosis hepatis. These infections have been reported in HIV-infected patients.

Incubation Period. The incubation period between injury and primary skin lesion is 7 to 12 days. The lymphadenopathy may take 5 to 50 days to develop but averages 12 days.

Clinical Findings. In approximately one third of cases, patients manifest systemic illness; the rest are not very sick. The illness appears in two stages:

1. Skin lesion: Cutaneous, 3 to 5 mm lesions arise approximately 1 week after inoculation and can persist for months. The nonpruritic lesions initially begin as vesicles or pustules and evolve into papules. They may be misdiagnosed as impetigo secondary to an insect bite. The cutaneous lesions heal completely without scarring. Up to 10% of patients may have the inoculation lesions present as nonsuppurative conjunctivitis or ocular granuloma (the affected eye is not painful, with little or no discharge, but may be red and swollen). Mucous membrane ulcers

have been found at the onset of the lymphadenopathy stage. Two weeks after the inoculation, the preauricular, submandibular, cervical, supraclavicular, axillary, epitrochlear, or inguinal nodes closest to the lesion begin to swell. There can be single or multiple nodes involved. Multiple node-site involvement usually indicates several different inoculation sites. The node may swell up to 5 cm. The area around the infected node is usually warm, tender, indurated, and erythematous during the first few weeks. Cellulitis is uncommon, but large nodes may suppurate. The lymphadenopathy usually lasts approximately 1 to 4 months and up to 1 year in some cases.
2. Systemic cat-scratch disease (SCSD): In one third of cases, patients manifest systemic illness. This can be associated with fever up to 106° F (41.2° C), malaise, fatigue, anorexia, emesis, headache, heptosplenomegaly, sore throat, exanthema, blindness, arthralgia, seizures, coma, and conjunctivitis.

Enlarged mediastinal or pancreatic nodes can cause pleurisy, obstructive phenomena, and splenic and hepatic abscesses. Significant weight loss has been reported.

Diagnostic Studies. A diagnostic test is available from the CDC. It is an indirect immunofluorescent assay (IFA) and is available only to state health departments. CT or ultrasonography may be useful in identifying hepatic or splenic abscesses and granulomas. The CBC may show leukocytosis and increased eosinophils. The erythrocyte sedimentation rate (ESR) may be elevated early in the disease process. Lymph node biopsy stained with Warthin-Starry silver stain also is diagnostic.

Differential Diagnosis. The differential diagnosis includes any cause of lymphadenopathy. The most common of these are bacterial and viral infections (e.g., streptococci [especially Group A β-hemolytic], staphylococci, anaerobic bacteria, atypical mycobacteria, tularemia, brucellosis, CMV, HIV, Epstein-Barr virus, systemic fungal infections, toxoplasmosis). Neck masses from other sources (e.g., cystic hygromas, bronchogenic cysts, tumors) are in the differential.

Management. Symptomatic treatment is usually sufficient in most cases. Antipyretics can be used if there is moderate fever. Painful nodes can be treated with moist wraps. Incision and drainage of suppurative lesions should be avoided because of the high risk of sinus tract formation. Needle aspiration can yield material for diagnostic testing. Biopsy may be required if neoplasm is in the differential. Systemic antibiotics may be used for SCSD. Oral azithromycin has shown some clinical success in reducing the initial lymph node volume in half the infected patients (500 mg in one dose the first day; 250 mg days 2 through 5; smaller children: 10 mg/kg per 24 hours on day 1; 5 mg/kg per 24 hours days 2 through 5) (Stechenberg, 2000).

Complications. Complications include Parinaud oculoglandular syndrome, encephalopathy (5% incidence), severe chronic systemic disease, erythema nodosa, neuroretinitis, thrombocytopenia purpura, hepatosplenomegaly, primary atypical pneumonia, breast tumor, angiomatoid papules, and osteomyelitis. Almost all of these problems resolve completely (Stechenberg, 2000).

Lyme Disease

Etiology. *Borrelia burgdorferi*, a spirochete, is the causative agent.

Epidemiology. Lyme disease is the most commonly reported vector-borne infection in the United States. In the United States, three clusters (the Northeast [Maryland to Massachusetts], the Midwest [Wisconsin and Minnesota], and the West [Northern California and Oregon]) have reported the most cases. In the East, the natural host to *B. burgdorferi* is the white-footed mouse. The eastern deer tick *(Ixodes scapularis)* becomes infected by feeding on the mouse and transmits the organism to humans. The western deer tick *(Ixodes pacificus)* feeds mostly on lizards, and they are not effective hosts for *B. burgdorferi.* Lyme disease has been reported in habitats that are inhospitable to the tick. The vector in these cases has not been identified. There is varied risk of transmission, depending on the percentage of ticks actually infected with *B. burgdorferi.* In the Northeast and Midwest, 14% to 20% of nymphal and 35% to 40% of adult ticks are infected. In endemic locations, up to 80% of adult ticks are infected. In the West, the rate of infected ticks is only 1% to 3%.

The risk of infection after a tick bite is directly related to how long the tick has fed. It takes hours for the tick to fully implant its mouth into the host's skin and days to become fully engorged. Nymphal ticks must feed for 36 to 48 hours and adult ticks for 48 to 72 hours before the risk of transmission of *B. burgdorferi* is significant. The disease is not regarded as being teratogenic to fetal development (Shapiro, 2000).

Incubation Period. The incubation period from the bite to the rash stage is approximately 1 to 2 weeks (range 3 to 31 days). Late manifestation of the disease may appear more than 1 year later.

Clinical Findings. Lyme disease is divided into three stages:

1. Stage 1 (early localized disease): Generally, within 1 to 2 weeks after the bite, a typical rash appears at the inoculation site (this time frame can range from 3 to 32 days). Erythema migrans begins as a red, annular macule or papule at the site of the tick bite and progresses into large annular erythematous lesions 5 to 15 cm in diameter. Erythema migrans can vary in morphology. The center of the lesion may be clear, vesicular, or necrotic. The lesion may be pruritic or painful. It

typically is located in the axillary, periumbilical, thigh, or groin areas. Organisms are present in the lesions. They may be cultured or seen in biopsy material. The rash remains for a few weeks and will fade even if untreated. The patient may experience fever, malaise, headache, arthralgia, and stiff neck during this phase. Without treatment these symptoms, including the rash, may become intermittent, lasting for weeks to months.

2. Stage 2 (early disseminated disease): Through spirochetemia, the organism disseminates through the skin causing multiple skin lesions. These are morphologically similar to, but smaller than, the local lesion. They develop several days to several weeks after the primary lesions. The other systemic manifestations noted in the local disease may return. Infections of eye, bone, heart, synovium, muscle, liver, spleen, and CNS occur because of the hematogenous and lymphatic spread of the organism. The patient may experience iritis, optic neuritis, conjunctivitis, osteomyelitis, pericarditis and myocarditis (though rare, this may be manifested by varying degrees of heart block), mild arthritis, hepatitis, lymphadenitis, aseptic meningitis, and cranial neuropathies (especially seventh nerve palsy in children). Stage 2 can last from weeks to 2 years without treatment. Most of the symptoms (including the rash) wax and wane during this time.
3. Stage 3 (late disease): Stage three usually begins with pauciarticular or monarticular arthritis. The knees are most commonly affected. They are red, hot, and swollen but not as painful as with other types of bacterial arthritis. Untreated, the arthritis initially resolves in a few weeks but becomes recurrent, migratory (but rarely to small joint), and chronic. Lyme arthritis can occur in patients without initial skin lesions. Rarely, adults suffer late CNS sequelae (progressive encephalopathy), radicular syndrome, or chronic leukoencephalitis.

Diagnostic Studies. Cultures from leading-edge biopsy are possible but time consuming, and detection rate is low. The organism is slow growing and may take up to 4 weeks to isolate. The organism, if found, can be stained with Warthin-Starry silver or immunohistochemical (with monoclonal or polyclonal antibodies). Because *B. burgdorferi* occurs in such low concentrations, it is often either missed or confused with normal skin structures. In patients without rash, manifesting late-stage signs and symptoms, the diagnosis of Lyme disease should be based on clinical findings, with serologic testing as an adjunct (AAP, 2000).

Serologic tests performed by reference laboratories are the most accurate means to diagnose Lyme disease. Positive results, however, may mean prior infection rather than present acute infection, because antibodies can remain elevated for years (Shapiro, 2000). IgM- and IgG-specific antibodies can be done via the ELISA testing method; any result needs to be followed up with the Western blot test. Because of the timing of antibody formation, serologic testing is useful in stage 2 or 3 only. The test kits available commercially are unreliable (Gerber & Shapiro, 2001). The antibodies persist for 6 to 8 weeks and then decline. IgG-specific antibodies appear 6 to 8 weeks after inoculation and peak at 4 to 6 months. They can remain elevated indefinitely. Note that early antimicrobial intervention may prevent the production of Lyme antibodies. There are many false-positive cross-reactions with other spirochetes, lupus, and varicella organisms. Children with typical symptoms of the disease do not need routine serologic testing (AAP, 2003).

B. burgdorferi has been successfully detected 80% of the time in joint fluid of untreated patients by using sensitive PCR testing. This test is in development.

Differential Diagnosis. The rash is characteristic but may not be present in all cases. It may suggest eczema, tinea, granuloma annulare, cellulitis, or an insect bite. Lyme disease should be included in the differential diagnosis of osteomyelitis, septic arthritis, infectious hepatitis, nonresponsive lymphadenopathy, meningitis, multiple sclerosis, amyotrophic lateral sclerosis, Alzheimer's disease, juvenile arthritis, and Bell's palsy.

Management. Clinical judgment is crucial in determining whether to treat a patient for Lyme disease. False-positive and false-negative test results are frequently reported. There are many clinically asymptomatic but serologically positive cases, and Lyme disease may not be the cause of a patient's multisystemic illness.

Early Localized Disease (Stage 1)

1. Amoxicillin (patients younger than 8 years of age), 50 mg/kg per day orally (PO; from the Latin, *per os*, by mouth) divided into three doses a day (maximum dose 500 mg) for 14 to 21 days
2. Doxycycline (patients age 8 years or older), 100 mg PO twice daily for 14 to 21 days
3. For patients unable to take amoxicillin or doxycycline either use erythromycin, 30 to 50 mg/kg per day PO (maximum 250 mg/dose), divided four times daily for 14 to 21 days, or cefuroxime, 30 mg/kg per day divided twice daily (maximum 500 mg/dose) for 14 to 21 days

Early Disseminated Disease without Focal Findings. Same as early focal disease.

Early Disseminated Disease with Focal Findings

1. Isolated facial palsy: Same as stage 1 but for 28 to 30 days. Do not use corticosteroids. The palsy will spontaneously resolve over 2 to 8 weeks in most cases. Antibiotic use prevents the late stage.
2. Arthritis: Treat for 28 to 30 days with either amoxicillin (younger than 8 years: 25 to 50 mg/kg per day divided

twice daily [maximum 2000 mg/day]) or doxycycline (older than 8 years: 100 mg twice daily). If symptoms fail to resolve after 8 weeks or there is joint inflammation, a second joint is inflamed, or there is evidence of extraarticular infection, repeat treatment either PO or use ceftriaxone, 75 to 100 mg/kg per day (maximum 2000 mg/day) every day IV or IM or penicillin, 300,000 IU/kg per day (maximum 20 million U/day) IV divided every 4 hours for 14 to 28 days.
3. Carditis or CNS disease: Same dosage of ceftriaxone or penicillin as for arthritis. Do not use corticosteroids.

Complications. Many of these have been previously discussed in the section on clinical findings. Gerber and Shapiro (2001) and Sigal (2002) take issue with the notion of a diagnosis of "chronic Lyme disease." Children may be more prone to initially have arthritis symptoms than adults. It is common for symptoms to persist for 2 to 3 weeks even after successful antibiotic treatment. Arthritis recurrences decrease over time. Children virtually always have specific physical findings (rash, Bell's palsy, swollen joints), but nonspecific symptoms persist after treatment (headache, fatigue, arthralgias). The authors postulate that these lingering symptoms indicate inadequate treatment. Treated appropriately, children recover irrespective of the stage of the disease at which they were treated. Parental concerns with chronic symptoms after adequate treatment need to be addressed carefully, and other behavioral or organic causes may need to be explored.

Prevention

1. Avoid tick-infested areas. Use tick skin repellent with DEET (less than 10% if 12 years of age or less; less than 30% in children over 12 years of age). Inspect skin carefully every day during the tick season. Spray permethrin on clothing and wear light-colored long pants (tucked into shoes), long sleeves, and a hat.
2. Infection risk is low. The risk in endemic areas is less than 2%. Chemoprophylaxis is not necessary.
3. Three doses of vaccine are necessary for persons 15 to 70 years of age in endemic areas; the need for booster doses has not been determined.
4. Post–tick bite prophylaxis with doxycycline (single 200 mg dose) can be effective in preventing the disease when given within 72 hours after a bite from *I. scapularis* (Nadelman et al, 2001). However, this prophylaxis should be given only to those who live in highly endemic areas and when the tick is a nymphal deer tick that is at least minimally engorged with blood (Gerber & Shapiro, 2001).

Meningococcal Disease

Etiology. *Neisseria meningitidis* is a gram-negative diplococcus. It is a common commensal organism in the human nasopharynx. It was first described in 1805. It has no animal or environmental reservoirs. There are 13 serotypes identified, and groups A, B, C, W-135, and Y are largely the causes of invasive disease. Groups B and C are the most common in the United States. Group B is a greater threat to younger children, with 50% of all meningococcal infection occurring in children younger than 2 years of age (25% to 33% of these are under 1 year of age) (Caserta, 2001).

Epidemiology. The organism is spread from person to person via respiratory tract secretions and in most cases causes asymptomatic colonization. This can persist for weeks to months. Carriage rates range from 2% to 30% in nonepidemic periods depending on the study (Estabrook, 2000). Carriage rate is higher in areas of crowding, especially in day care centers. During epidemics, the carriage rate can rise to 100% in a closed population. Disease occurs most often during winter and early spring in children who are younger than 5 years of age. The peak attack rate occurs in children 3 to 5 months of age. Epidemics occur in semi-closed communities (e.g., day care centers, schools, colleges, and military bases). Patients with functional or anatomic asplenia, terminal complement component (C_5-C_9) deficiency, C_3, or properdin deficiency are at increased risk of invasive or recurring meningococcal disease (AAP, 2003). In children, the risk increases in environments where there is tobacco smoke (Kriz, Bobak, & Kriz, 2000).

Incubation Period. The incubation period is 1 to 10 days. Patients are contagious until 24 hours after initiation of treatment.

Clinical Findings. Colonization can lead to invasive disease. Bacteremia and sepsis result and, depending on hematogenous spread, multiple patterns of illness can result, including bacteremia without sepsis, meningococcemic sepsis without meningitis, meningitis with or without meningococcemia, meningoencephalitis, and specific organ infection (Estabrook, 2000).

1. Occult bacteremia: This appears in a febrile child with URI or gastrointestinal-like symptoms. There may be a maculopapular rash. Often these children are treated as having a viral illness. Some have recovered without antimicrobial intervention, whereas others have developed meningococcal meningitis.
2. Acute meningococcemia: Abrupt fever (71%; less than 1% with hypothermia), chills, pharyngitis, headache, purulent conjunctivits, myalgias (30%), weakness, malaise, prostration, irritability (21%), emesis (34%), and a maculopapular rash may quickly progress into septic shock (42%) manifested by hypertension, DIC, acidosis, adrenal hemorrhage, renal failure, myocardial failure, and coma. Bacteremia can result in meningitis, purulent pericarditis, myocarditis, pneumonia, or septic arthritis. Seventy-one percent of patients manifest petechiae or purpura or both (49%) (Estabrook, 2000).

3. Chronic meningococcemia: This is rare. A nontoxic-appearing child has fever, headache, and rash. The rash consists of painful, discrete pinkish-red macules up to 20 mm in diameter that progress into lesions on an erythematous base. The rash usually spares the face and scalp but is concentrated on the extremities. The symptoms are recurrent, lasting 6 to 8 weeks. Bacteremia can occur, and without treatment, acute infection can result.

Diagnostic Studies. The diagnosis is confirmed with a positive culture from blood, CSF, or synovial fluid. Latex agglutination testing exists, but it does not detect group B meningococcus. It may be of some value in cases where oral antibiotics were given and organism growth has been suppressed. PCR testing exists but is used only in research laboratories. A CBC shows leukopenia (21%), decreased platelets (14%), and elevated ESR and C-reactive protein.

Differential Diagnosis. The list of differential diagnoses is long and includes septicemia caused by other invasive bacteria (e.g., pneumococcus or *H. influenzae*, viral meningitis, leptospirosis, syphilis). Collagen vascular diseases, primary hematology/oncology disease, erythema nodosa, erythema multiforme, Rocky Mountain spotted fever, mycoplasma, coxsackievirus, echovirus, rubella and rubeola infections, Henoch-Schönlein purpura, idiopathic thrombocytopenic purpura, viral exanthems, and Kawasaki syndrome are also in the differential diagnosis.

Management. Aqueous penicillin G (250,000 to 300,000 U/kg per day IV divided every 4 hours for 5 to 7 days) is the drug of choice. An alternative is cefotaxime (100 mg/kg per 24 hours) or ceftriaxone (100 mg/kg per 24 hours). The patient is kept in respiratory isolation until 24 hours after the induction of treatment. Some *N. meningitidis* strains studied by the CDC are resistant to penicillin. In these cases (after susceptibility testing) or if the patient is allergic to penicillin, cefotaxime, or ceftriaxone, chloramphenicol (75 to 100 mg/kg per 24 hours IV divided into four doses) may be substituted.

Control Measures. Exposed contacts must be carefully monitored. Household, school, or child contacts who develop a febrile illness must be evaluated for invasive disease promptly. If the child is suspected of having meningococcemia, IV antibiotics should be started pending culture results.

1. Chemoprophylaxis: Close contacts (household daycare, nursery school, those who shared oral secretions [kissing, shared utensils or toothbrushes]) of the index case 7 days before the onset of symptoms are at increased risk of invasive disease. Medical personnel are usually not considered at high risk unless they performed mouth-to-mouth resuscitation, intubation, or suctioning before antibiotic therapy was instituted (AAP, 2000). Rifampin, 10 mg/kg per dose (maximum dose 600 mg) PO twice daily for a total of four doses, is the prophylactic treatment of choice for those over 1 month of age. Infants younger than 1 month of age should be given 5 mg/kg per dose PO twice daily for a total of four doses. Ceftriaxone, 125 mg IM, in one dose is also useful and can be given to pregnant women and children 15 years of age and younger. The dose for those older than 15 years of age is 250 mg IM. Ciprofloxacin, 500 mg PO, in a single dose can be given to nonpregnant adults 18 years of age and older. IV antibiotic therapy does not eradicate carriage; therefore chemoprophylaxis is recommended for the index case before hospital discharge unless the child was treated with ceftriaxone or cefotaxime.
2. Vaccine: Vaccine, in conjunction with chemoprophylaxis, is advisable to prevent extended outbreaks only if the identified strain is contained in the vaccine.

Complications. Complications are caused by inflammation, intravascular hemorrhage and necrosis in multiple organ systems, and shock. Organ abscesses and infarcts cause necrosis of tissue and gangrene. Skeletal deformities and limb amputations are not infrequent. Meningitis can lead to ataxia, seizures, deafness (2% to 6%), arthritis and pericarditis (8% to 24%), and, more rarely, blindness, palsies, paralysis, developmental delays, and hydrocephalus. Immune-complex reactions are responsible for arthritis symptoms. Mortality rate is 10% to 15% in the United States (Caserta, 2001).

Streptococcal Disease

Etiology. Streptococci are gram-positive spherical cocci that are classified based on their ability to hemolyze red blood cells. Complete hemolysis is known as β-hemolytic. Partial hemolysis is α-hemolytic. Nonhemolysis is γ-hemolytic. Cell wall carbohydrate differences further subdivide the streptococci. These differences are identified as Lancefield antigen subgroups A–H and K–V. Subgroups A–H and K–O are associated with human disease.

Group A β-hemolytic Streptococci

EPIDEMIOLOGY. There are more than 100 M-protein types of group A β-hemolytic streptococci (GABHS). Transmission is through infected upper respiratory tract secretions. Fomites, especially unwashed hands, are a common source of indirect contact. Food-borne epidemics, especially via water, milk, ice cream, and eggs, are reported. Most commonly streptococcus microbes involve the respiratory tract, skin, soft tissues, and blood. Both streptococcus pharyngitis and impetigo are associated with crowding, whether at home, school, or other institution. Pharyngitis is rare in infancy, but the incidence rises with age until adolescence (commonly from 5 to 15 years of age). It is not common in adults unless there is an epidemic. URIs occur year round but are most common in the winter. Temperate climates have greater incidences of pharyngeal infection (especially in colder times of the year) than tropical climates. Carriage state is high, and 15% to 50% of asymptomatic children have GABHS cultured from their throats. By contrast, streptococcus skin infection (impetigo) is more common in toddlers and preschool-age children, and it occurs more often during summer, early fall in tropical areas, or in warmer weather in temperate climates. Those at increased risk for invasive GABHS are those with varicella infection, IV drug use, HIV, diabetes, or chronic heart or lung disease; the very young; and the elderly. Incidences of GABHS bacteremia, streptococcus toxic shock syndrome (TSS), and streptococcus necrotizing folliculitis have increased (AAP, 2003).

INCUBATION PERIOD. The incubation period is 2 to 5 days for pharyngitis and 7 to 10 days for skin acquisition to lesions of impetigo. The period of communicability is from the onset of symptoms up to a few months in untreated persons.

CLINICAL FINDINGS. The following may be seen in GABHS:

Respiratory tract infection. Pharyngitis and pneumonia are described in Chapter 32.

Scarlet fever. This is caused by erythrogenic toxin. It is uncommon in children younger than 3 years of age. The incubation period is approximately 3 days (range, 1 to 7 days). There is abrupt illness with sore throat, vomiting, headache, chills, and malaise. Fever can reach 104° F (40° C). Tonsils are erythematous, swollen, and usually covered in exudate. The pharynx also is inflamed and can be covered with a gray-white exudate. The palate and uvula are erythematous and reddened, and petechiae are present. The tongue is usually coated red. Desquamation of the coating leaves prominent papillae (strawberry tongue) (see Fig. 24-2).

The rash appears within 12 to 48 hours. The exanthema is red and finely papular and makes the skin feel coarse, akin to sandpaper. The rash begins in the axilla, groin, and neck, spreads centripetally, is generalized within 24 hours, and blanches on pressure (Schultz-Charlton sign). The face is usually spared. There is circumoral pallor, and the cheeks are flushed. There is increased rash density on the neck, axilla, and groin. Pastia's lines, transverse linear hyperpigmented areas with tiny petechiae, are seen in the folds of the joints. In severe disease, small vesicles (miliary sudamina) can be found on the hands, feet, and abdomen. Rash, sore throat, and constitutional symptoms resolve in approximately 5 to 7 days. The rash begins to desquamate shortly thereafter. Fine branlike flakes begin on the face and slowly spread to the trunk and extremities. This process takes up to 6 weeks (Todd, 2000).

Scarlet fever can occur after wound infection (surgical scarlet fever), burns, or streptococcus skin infection. The disease is similar to regular scarlet fever, but there is no pharyngeal or tonsillar involvement.

Skin infections. The characteristic lesion for streptococcal impetigo is a honey-colored scab on an erythematous base (see Color Fig. 14). Localized lymphadenopathy is common. A small, transient, vesicular lesion may precede the scab lesion. Deep soft tissue infection may develop after impetigo. Streptococcal soft tissue abscesses result from puncture wounds contaminated with GABHS. Infants having weepy eczema can have secondary GABHS skin infection. The eczema area develops the typical impetiginous lesions. Erysipelas is an acute cellulitis with lymphadenitis. The skin becomes red and indurated. It begins as a small lesion and spreads marginally for 4 to 6 days. The lesion's borders are firm, raised, and tender. Fever, chills, vomiting, irritability, and other constitutional symptoms are present. These subside when the rash stops spreading. Bacteremia, abscesses, metastatic foci, and death are reported.

Bacteremia. This can occur after respiratory (pharyngitis, tonsillitis, AOM) and localized skin infections. Some children have no obvious source of infection. Meningitis, osteomyelitis, septic arthritis, pyelonephritis, pneumonia, peritonitis, and bacterial endocarditis (acute rheumatic fever) are rare but can be associated with GABHS bacteremia.

Vaginitis. GABHS causes vaginitis in prepubertal females. Vulvar erythema, serous discharge, and irritation (especially with walking and urination) are common findings. Although the infection is usually the result of autoinoculation, it can be a symptom of sexual molestation if infected saliva is used as a sexual lubricant.

Perianal streptococcal cellulitis. This is uncommon and occurs in either sex. Manifestations include local itching, pain, blood-streaked stools, erythema, and proctitis. Although infection is usually the result of autoinoculation, it can be a symptom of sexual molestation if infected saliva is used as a sexual lubricant.

Necrotizing fasciitis. This occurs in children and often is associated with varicella.

Streptococcal toxic shock syndrome. Toxic shock syndrome caused by GABHS appears as an acute multiorgan disease similar to TSS caused by *S. aureus* (Box 24-4). It is more often caused by a nonmenstrual infection (from surgical and gynecologic procedures and invasive infections). The overall incidence of TSS is declining. Pain at the trauma or surgical site of infection (may look like cellulitis or necrotizing fasciitis) is the most common finding (Rifkin & Gusic, 2002). The pain is typically more severe than that suggested by the physical examination. Infection can also be characterized by symptoms suggestive of *S. aureus* TSS infection: fever, rash, severe diarrhea, severe myalgias, hypotension, respiratory distress, desquamation (palms and soles usually after 7 to 21 days), transient toxic cardiomyopathy, headaches, depressed mentation, and multiorgan dysfunction (especially renal). The rash is similar to that seen with Kawasaki syndrome and scarlet fever. The mortality rate can reach 50%. The *S. pyogenes* organism must be isolated to make the diagnosis (unlike that of *S. aureus* TSS infection). The infection can be transmitted by close contact; contact and droplet isolation is recommended.

Diagnostic studies. Culture of the organism is the most useful method of establishing the diagnosis. A positive throat culture confirms the diagnosis; however, a positive culture may identify a carrier state. Many rapid streptococcal identification tests are not as sensitive as a culture in picking up GABHS; therefore a negative rapid test must be followed up by a culture unless the rapid streptococcal identification test is highly sensitive. The specificity of most rapid tests is good (95%); therefore, if the rapid test is positive, the diagnosis of GABHS is confirmed. The STREP A OIA MAX (a trademarked optical immunoassay test marketed by Thermo BioStar) is reportedly a highly sensitive and specific test that has proven reliability and accuracy. Documentation of past GABHS infection is done by drawing a titer for antibodies to various streptococcal enzymes, such as antistreptolysin O (ASO).

DIFFERENTIAL DIAGNOSIS. A differential diagnosis is acute pharyngitis caused by viruses, especially adenoviruses and infectious mononucleosis. Other bacterial upper respiratory diseases in the differential diagnosis, though rare, include diphtheria, tularemia, toxoplasmosis, mycoplasma, tonsillar tuberculosis, salmonellosis, and brucellosis. Staphylococcal impetigo must be differentiated from GABHS pyoderma. Septicemia, meningitis, osteomyelitis, septic arthritis, pyelonephritis, and bacterial endocarditis can result from other bacteria causing similar infections. Cultures or serologic testing differentiate the offending organism.

MANAGEMENT. Antimicrobial therapy is the treatment of choice:

1. Potassium penicillin V PO is the drug of choice (250 mg two or three times daily for 10 days) for children less than 27 kg ($\geq$27 kg, 500 mg two to three times daily). If compliance is good, penicillin PO (500 mg/day in two divided doses for 10 days) can be given to adolescents and adults. Amoxicillin (40 mg/kg once daily for 10 days) has demonstrated effectiveness (AAP, 2003).
2. Benzathine penicillin G IM (600,000 U if child is less than 60 pounds, or 1.2 million U for larger children and adults). If given IM, allow mixture to warm to room temperature.
3. Erythromycin estolate (20 to 40 mg/kg per day divided into two or four doses) or erythromycin ethylsuccinate (40 mg/kg per day in two to four divided doses for 10 days), if allergic to penicillin. Clarithromycin for 10 days or azithromycin for 5 days (maximum 1 g per day),

BOX 24-4 *Centers for Disease Control and Prevention Case Definition of Streptococcal Toxic Shock Syndrome*

1. Isolation of group A streptococci
   A. From a normally sterile site (e.g., blood, CSF, peritoneal fluid, tissue biopsy, surgical wound)
   B. From a nonsterile site (e.g., throat, superficial skin lesion, etc.)
2. Clinical signs of severity
   A. Hypotension: systolic blood pressure 90 mm Hg or less in adults or below 5th percentile for age in children
   And
   B. Two or more of the following signs:
      - Renal impairment: creatinine 2 mg/dl or greater for adults or at least twice the upper limit of normal for age
      - Coagulopathy: platelets less than or equal to 100,000/mm^3 or DIC
      - Liver involvement: elevated SGPT, SGOT, or bilirubin concentration greater than or equal to twice the upper limits of normal
      - Adult respiratory distress syndrome
      - A generalized erythematous macular rash that may desquamate
      - Soft tissue necrosis, including necrotizing fasciitis, myositis, or gangrene

An illness fulfilling criteria 1A, 2A, and 2B can be defined as a definite case. An illness fulfilling criteria 1B, 2A, and 2B can be defined as a probable case if no other etiology can be found.

Modified from Centers for Disease Control and Prevention, Working Group on Severe Streptococcal Infection: Defining the group A streptococcal toxic shock syndrome: rationale and consensus definition, *JAMA* 269:390-391, 1993; American Academy of Pediatrics: *1997 red book: report of the committee on infectious diseases*, ed 25, Elk Grove Village, IL, 2000, American Academy of Pediatrics, p 578.

clindamycin, and oral cephalosporins (cephalexin, cephradine, cefadroxil, cefaclor, cefixime, cefuroxime) can also be used but are much more expensive.
4. Topical antibiotics may be used with simple uncomplicated impetigo (one to two single lesions). Mupirocin, bacitracin, and neosporin can be effective. For multiple or migrating lesions, a systemic antibiotic is indicated.
5. Asymptomatic carriers generally do not need treatment. If treatment is warranted, clindamycin (20 mg/kg per day divided into three doses; maximum 1.8 g/day) for 10 days is the drug of choice.

Supportive care. This includes antipyretics, fluids, and rest. If clinical relapse occurs, another culture should be done. If positive, a second course of penicillin is indicated, preferably benzathine penicillin IM. If recurrent infection is a problem, simultaneous culturing of the family for chronic carrier state is advised. Children can return to school as soon as they are afebrile and on antibiotics for at least 24 hours.

COMPLICATIONS. These are usually caused by spread of the disease from the localized infection and have already been discussed.

Group B β-hemolytic Streptococci. Group B β-hemolytic streptococci (GBBHS) are a leading cause of perinatal bacterial infection. There are nine serotypes (Ia, Ib, Ia/c, II, III, IV, V, VI, and VII) associated with human infection. Type III is the most frequent cause of neonatal meningitis. GBBHS colonizes the GI tract and vagina, with colonization rates in pregnant women and newborns that range from 15% to 40% (AAP, 2003). Infection occurs in approximately 1 to 4 per 1000 live births in infants whose mothers did not receive prenatal prophylaxis (AAP, 2003). Transmission occurs by direct contact, mother to child during parturition, and after birth by contact with colonized persons, usually through hand contamination. Early-onset disease is more common in high-risk deliveries or premature infants, small-for-gestational-age infants, infants born after prolonged rupture of membranes, and mothers with genital tract infections. It can cause disease in older persons with diabetes mellitus or immunologic disorders. Chapter 39 discusses this problem and the management of the disease in infants.

Non–Group A or B Streptococci. These organisms are associated with invasive disease. They may cause urinary tract infections (UTIs), endocarditis, respiratory disease, and meningitis in newborns, older children, and adults. The incubation period and communicability times are unknown. Culture is the best method of establishing the diagnosis. Groups C, F, and G are less susceptible to penicillin and cephalosporins. Therefore ampicillin or vancomycin with an aminoglycoside is the combination of choice for severe infection attributed to these three groups. The other groups are usually susceptible to penicillin.

Tuberculosis

Etiology. TB is caused by *Mycobacterium tuberculosis*, an aerobic, nonmotile, nonsporulating, pleomorphic rod; *M. tuberculosis* does not stain with the usual tests and is a very slow-growing organism, averaging approximately 21 days to culture. This organism is spread primarily by droplet contamination; fomite transmission is uncommon. Children who are foreign born account for more than 33% of pediatric cases (AAP, 2003).

Incubation Period. The incubation period is 2 to 10 weeks. Risk of disease is highest in the first 2 years after infection. Infection is defined as converting from a negative to a positive tuberculin skin test. The skin test will be reactive within 2 to 12 weeks after initial infection (median 3 to 4 weeks) (AAP, 2003). The majority of cases in the United States are found among the urban, low income (including homeless and correctional facility residents), and those who are of the nonwhite racial and ethnic groups from Asia, Africa, and Latin America.

Clinical Findings

Primary Pulmonary Tuberculosis. Most children ages 3 to 15 years are asymptomatic when first noted to have a positive TB skin test. Eighty percent of infected children who are older than 4 years of age and prepubertal do not progress to disease. Chest radiographs are usually negative for signs of pulmonary disease 1 to 6 months after initial infection. Symptoms may include fever, malaise, cough, decreased appetite, weight loss, night sweats, chills, erythema nodosum, and phlyctenular keratoconjunctivitis (a hypersensitivity reaction marked by elevated clear nodules with surrounding hyperemia near the limbus). In children under 12 years of age, there is usually minimal cough and little expulsion of bacilli; therefore there is less contagion from these children (AAP, 2003).

Enlarging lymph nodes can encroach on mediastinal structures, causing compression, obstruction, or erosion. Compression on the esophagus causes dysphagia or aspiration. Major arteries and veins can also be compressed by enlarging nodes with resulting edema. Superior vena cava syndrome can occur.

Fistulas can occur between the lymph node and the bronchial lumen and cause fibrosis, bronchiectasis, and pneumonia. Recurrent cough, stridor, and wheezing are signs of increasing pulmonary infection. Most children do not suffer significant pulmonary infection, and most reinfections resolve even without chemotherapy. However, progressive primary TB does occur in immunosuppressed children. Instead of resolving, the lesions continue to evolve, often involving an entire lobe. Older children and adolescents suffer from upper lobe infiltrates and cavitation. Calcification and lymphadenitis may be minimal.

Miliary Tuberculosis. Infants and children younger than 3 years of age frequently develop miliary TB. During early stages of the disease, bacilli reach the bloodstream directly from the initial focus or by way of the regional lymph nodes. Necrosis and caseation of multiple organs can occur. Lesions are the size of millet seeds; hence the name "miliary" TB. It is also common in very old and immunosuppressed patients, especially those with AIDS. The disease has a precipitous onset. Moderate to high fever is common. Malaise, decreased appetite, weight loss, and fatigue are constitutional symptoms at the outset. Lymphadenopathy, hepatomegaly, splenomegaly, tachypnea, dyspnea, rales, wheezes, and stridor are often found on physical examination. Other signs and symptoms are present, depending on which organs are involved.

Diagnostic Studies. Chest radiographs showing hilar adenopathy suggest TB, but culture of the organism is essential to establish the diagnosis. *M. tuberculosis* is a slow-growing organism. It often takes 2 to 10 weeks to isolate it in the bacteriology laboratory. Acid-fast bacilli stains can be helpful. DNA probes are useful but have limited availability. Histologic examination for acid-fast bacilli is helpful.

Tuberculin skin testing is based on the delayed hypersensitivity to *M. tuberculosis* antigens. The test usually becomes positive 2 to 12 weeks after infection with the bacilli. The preparation currently available for skin testing is PPD. The Mantoux test uses 0.1 ml of 5 tuberculin units (TU) PPD. It is injected intradermally into the volar surface of the forearm, producing a wheal.

Tuberculin skin tests (Mantoux) are read 48 to 72 hours later by experienced health care professionals. The induration is measured, not the erythema. Pediatric patients are considered at high risk for TB if they meet any of the following medical risk criteria:

- Contacts with adults who have active TB
- Born in or have parents from TB-prevalent parts of the world
- Have clinical signs suggestive of TB on chest radiograph or other clinical evidence
- HIV positive or have an immunosuppressive disorder
- Have other risk factors, including Hodgkin's disease, lymphoma, diabetes mellitus, chronic renal failure, or malnutrition
- Incarcerated adolescents
- Exposed to high-risk adults (e.g., those with HIV infection, the homeless, substance abusers, migrant farm workers)
- Residents of homeless shelters or some medically underserved, low-income populations, such as Asian, African, Middle Eastern, Latin American immigrants (AAP, 2003)

A Mantoux skin test is defined as positive if the following reactions occur:

- Induration (larger than 15 mm) in children 4 years of age or older without any risk factors
- Induration (larger than 10 mm) in children younger than 4 years of age or with medical risk factors as listed previously
- Induration (larger than 5 mm) in children who are household contacts of active or previously active TB cases suspected to have TB because of either a chest radiograph consistent with active or previously active TB or clinical findings of TB diagnosed with immunosuppressive disorders or HIV infection (AAP, 2003)

Skin testing is not always valid. Ten percent of children with positive cultures can have a negative skin test. This decreased reactivity can also occur in immunocompromised patients, infants younger than 6 months of age, BCG recipients, those with poor nutrition, and those with miliary TB or early TB infection, HIV, or concomitant infection (measles, varicella, influenza). Patients sensitized to nontuberculous mycobacteria can cross-react and have a less than 10 mm sized reaction to TB skin testing. BCG cross-reaction has been discussed previously. High-risk groups and patients living in areas where TB is endemic or on the rise should be skin tested yearly. Low-risk groups do not need to be routinely tested (AAP, 2003).

Differential Diagnosis. The NP should consider TB in patients with symptoms of basilar meningitis, hydrocephalus, cranial nerve palsy, or stroke. Permanent neurologic dysfunction can result and has a worse prognosis in infants than in toddlers and older children. The differential diagnosis includes mycotic infections, staphylococcal pneumonia, sarcoidosis, chronic pneumonia, and Hodgkin's lymphoma.

Management. The AAP (2003) recommends drugs and treatment regimens based on the disease state, as listed in Tables 24-13 and 24-14. Pyridoxine is not routinely recommended for children and adolescents. It is recommended for use in those individuals whose diets are either limited in meat or milk, in those with HIV, in breastfeeding infants and their mothers, and for pregnant adolescents (AAP, 2003).

Complications. The following complications can occur:

Chronic Reactivation Pulmonary Tuberculosis. This complication is a progression of the primary disease. It is most common in adolescents and in those who had their initial infection after 7 years of age. It can be highly contagious; complete recovery is expected with appropriate treatment.

Lymph Node Disease. This is an extrapulmonary form of TB affecting the superficial lymph nodes. It can be caused by drinking raw milk contaminated with *M. bovis* or after initial infection with *M. tuberculosis*. The nodes are firm (but not hard), fixed to underlying tissue, and nontender. The lymphadenopathy is usually unilateral at first and can progress to multinode involvement. Tuberculin skin testing

TABLE 24-13 Commonly Used Drugs for Tuberculosis

Drug	Daily Dose	Twice-Weekly Dose
Isoniazid (I)	10 mg/kg prevention (maximum, 300 mg); 10-15 mg/kg treatment (maximum, 300 mg); available as syrup or tablets; crushed tablets are more palatable than the syrup	20-30 mg/kg/dose (maximum, 900 mg)
Rifampin (R)	10-20 mg/kg (maximum, 600 mg); available as syrup or tablets	10-20 mg/kg/dose (maximum, 600 mg)
Pyrazinamide (Z)	20-40 mg/kg (maximum, 2000 mg); tablets only	50 mg/kg/dose (maximum, 2000 mg)
Streptomycin (S)	20-40 mg/kg (maximum 1000 mg); IM only	20-40 mg/kg/dose (maximum, 1000 mg)
Ethambutol (E)	15-25 mg/kg (maximum, 2500 mg); tablets only	50 mg/kg/dose (maximum, 2500 mg)

TABLE 24-14 Drug Treatment Regimens for Tuberculosis in Infants, Children, and Adolescents‡

Type of TB Illness	Isoniazid (I)	Rifampin (R)	Pyrazinamide (Z)	Streptomycin (S)
Prophylaxis				
• Isoniazid susceptible	Daily for 9 months†			
• Isoniazid resistant		Daily for 6 months		
• If resistant to both I and R, consult TB specialist				
Pulmonary and extrapulmonary disease (miliary, lymph node, bone, joint infection)‡	Daily for 2 months, then 2-3 times weekly for 4 months*	Daily for 2 months, then 2-3 times weekly for 4 months*	Daily for 2 months	
		OR		
	Daily for 6 months, then daily for 4 months	Daily for 6 months, then daily for 4 months	Daily for 6 months	
• Hilar adenopathy only	Daily for 6 months	Daily for 6 months		
Meningitis (treat for a total of 9-12 months)	Daily for 2 months, then once daily or twice weekly for 7-10 months	Daily for 2 months, then once daily or twice weekly for 7-10 months	Daily for 2 months	Daily for 2 months or Ethambutol

Data from American Academy of Pediatrics: *Red book: report of the Committee on Infectious Diseases, 2003*, ed 26, Elk Grove Village, IL, 2003, American Academy of Pediatrics, p 649; American Thoracic Society and CDC: Targeted tuberculin testing and treatment of latent Tb infection, *MMWR* 49(RR06):1-54, June, 2000; Ampofo KK, Saiman L: Tuberculosis. In Burg F et al, editors: *Gellis and Kagan's current pediatric therapy*, ed 17, Philadelphia, 2002, WB Saunders.

Boxes indicate that these drug regimens are given concurrently (no length of time indicated).

*Directly observed therapy (DOT) is desirable.

†DOT twice a week can be used for 9 months if daily therapy cannot be achieved.

‡Treatment recommendations are in constant flux; it is advised that NPs consult a pediatric Tb specialist before initiating treatment for any type of tuberculosis infection to ensure that the most current treatment is prescribed; different regimens will be used if child also has concurrent HIV infection.

is usually positive; a chest x-ray is normal 70% of the time. The diagnosis is made by culturing node tissue biopsies.

Pleural Effusion. This occurs in approximately 8% of children with primary disease. It is caused by an extension of the bacillus into the pleural space by subpleural foci or hematogenous spread, or both. It usually occurs 6 months to years after the primary infection. It is infrequent to rare in children under 6 years of age (Starke & Munoz, 2000).

Tuberculous Meningitis. This is the most serious complication of TB. It generally follows primary pulmonary disease in untreated infants and young children, usually developing within 6 months. Meningeal infection is also common in miliary TB. Bacilli migrate to the subarachnoid space. Caseous lesions can enlarge, encapsulate, and form a tuberculoma that can act just like any other CNS mass lesion. The incidence is 0.3% in those 6 months to 4 years of age. Tuberculin skin testing is negative in 50% of cases, with 20% to 50% of cases also having negative chest x-rays (Starke & Munoz, 2000). Diagnosis is via CSF culture. Symptoms include fever, malaise, irritability, drowsiness, decreased developmental milestones, nuchal rigidity, seizures, and other neurologic symptoms.

Skin Tuberculosis. This variant is rare in the United States and occurs in 1% to 2% of all TB cases. It occurs in two forms: (1) the TB chancre and (2) multiple skin lesions resulting from hematogenous spread. Those at high risk include those with HIV, those with poor hygiene, and those who are malnourished.

Ocular Tuberculosis. Bacilli usually reach the eye by hematogenous spread. Infected upper respiratory secretions can spread to the cornea, sclera, and conjunctiva by sneezing or by contaminated fingers. Yellow-gray nodules appear at the posterior pole or palpebral conjunctiva. Coalescence of the nodules can form small ulcers. Phlyctenular conjunctivitis, small jelly-like gray nodules seen on the conjunctiva, is the result of a hypersensitivity reaction.

Hematogenous Spread of Tuberculosis to Other Organs or Body Systems. Spread can be to endocrine and exocrine glands, urogenital tract, heart and pericardium, skeleton, abdomen, tonsils, adenoids, larynx, middle ear, and mastoids.

TEMPERATURE AND FEVER

Fever is defined as an abnormally elevated body temperature with a temperature of 100.4° F (38° C) or higher. Fever results from a resetting of the hypothalamic heat regulatory center or when heat production exceeds heat loss. Peripheral warm and cold neurons and the temperature of blood circulating in the hypothalamus act on the heat regulatory center to keep the human body at a preset core temperature of 98.6° F (37° C). Axillary temperature may be 1° F lower. Body temperature is lower in the morning and peaks in the late afternoon. In children over 2 years of age, normal temperature fluctuations can range from 1.4° to 2° F (0.8° to 1.2° C). Those under 2 years of age maintain fairly unwavering temperatures.

The human body generates heat by metabolic processes (increased cellular metabolism, muscle activity, and involuntary shivering). Heat conservation is maintained by vasoconstriction and heat preference behaviors. Heat loss occurs by sweating, evaporation, conduction, radiation, convection, vasodilation, and cold preference behaviors. These factor inputs are integrated by the thermoregulatory neurons (Powell, 2004a).

The normal hypothalamic setpoint is altered by many different agents. Febrile illnesses in neonates are usually the result of congenital infections, those acquired at delivery (late-onset group B streptococcal infection), those acquired in the nursery (especially premature infants), those acquired at home (pneumococcal or meningococcal infection), or those acquired as a result of anatomic or physiologic dysfunction (e.g., renal). Other causes for fever in children are related to bacterial and viral infections, vaccines, biologic agents, tissue damage, malignancy, drugs, collagen-vascular disorders, endocrine disorders, inflammatory disorders, and other disease states. Temperatures higher than 105.8° F (41° C) are rarely of infectious origin but are due to CNS dysfunction (e.g., malignant hyperthermia, drug fever, heat stroke). Fever-causing agents produce endogenous pyrogens that reset the hypothalamic center. This process takes approximately 90 minutes. Clinically, this means that blood cultures should be obtained before the fever spikes, because there would be a greater bacterial or fungal yield.

The incidence of fevers above 106° F (41.2° C) in emergency departments is 0.05%. A temperature of 107° F or higher is considered a harmful fever and has the potential complication of death or brain damage if not treated (Adam, 2001). The increased metabolic processes can exacerbate problems in children with chronic illness.

Fever is the most common presenting complaint in pediatric practice. There are two situations that are particularly worrisome for any NP: fever without a source or focus in infants and young children and fever of unknown origin. Each of these situations is discussed separately, and guidelines for their management are given.

Fever without Focus in Infants and Young Children

Managing fever without an identifiable source in infants and young children is a challenge. The assessment of the child who has an acute fever often involves a careful investigation for a source of infection. Children between birth and 24 months are at greatest risk for unsuspected bacteremia; it is less common in those over 36 months.

History

The following should be included in the history of the illness:

- Duration and degree of fever (fever documented at home by reliable caregiver should be considered accurate)
- Possible associated symptoms: vomiting, diarrhea, respiratory symptoms, rash (especially petechiae or purpura)
- Change in play activities
- Irritability, inconsolability

- Lethargy (level of consciousness characterized by poor or absent eye contact or failure to recognize parents or interact with persons or objects in the environment)
- Review of known exposures (family illness, contacts with other ill children, day care contacts)
- Recent vaccination
- Recent travel history
- Past medical history of malignancy, splenectomy, shunt, indwelling catheter, immunologic disorders, recurrent bacterial infections, serious bacterial infection
- Neonatal history of complications, prior antibiotics, prior surgeries, hyperbilirubinemia
- Chronic illness
- Current medications, including antipyretics and antibiotics

Risk Criteria

High Risk

- Any febrile infant younger than 1 month of age; any toxic-appearing child regardless of age
- Infant 1 to 3 months of age who is toxic appearing
- Infant 1 to 3 months of age with a fever of 102.2° F
- Infant 1 to 3 months of age with a chronic illness, with unreliable caretakers, who was premature, with white blood cell (WBC) count greater than 15,000 or stool greater than 5 WBCs per high-power field (hpf)

Low Risk

- Infant 1 to 3 months of age with a fever greater than 100.4° F rectally or infant or child 3 to 36 months of age with a fever greater than 102.2° F who is nontoxic appearing with a history of previously being healthy and has nonfocal bacterial infection. Continue with the workup even if an infant under 3 months of age has otitis media
- Infant 3 to 6 months of age with rectal temperature greater than 100.4° F but less than 102.2° F who is not ill appearing
- Infant or child 3 to 36 months of age who is mildly ill appearing with rectal temperature greater than 102.2° F (39.0° C) and fewer than 15,000 WBCs; stool fewer than 5 WBCs/hpf if diarrhea present; negative chest x-ray if cough present

Laboratory Studies

A negative, low-risk ambulatory workup is characterized by the following laboratory results:

- CBC with WBC count below 15,000/mm^3, fewer than 1500 bands/mm^3
- Blood culture—no growth in 48 hours (72 hours for those immunocompromised or if fungal infection suspected in the neonate; Steele, 2001b)
- Catheterized urinalysis (fewer than 5 WBCs/hpf, negative leukocytes and nitrites)
- When diarrhea is present, fewer than 5 WBCs/hpf in stool
- If cough is present, a negative chest x-ray

Differential Diagnosis

The differential diagnosis includes the following:

- Upper respiratory tract disease such as viral URI, otitis media, and sinusitis
- Lower respiratory tract disease such as bronchiolitis and pneumonia
- Gastrointestinal disease, primarily bacterial, or gastroenteritis
- Musculoskeletal infections such as cellulitis, septic arthritis, and osteomyelitis
- Urinary tract infection (especially *E. coli*)
- Bacteremia (pneumococci [incidence 75% before PCV-7 vaccine]), *H. influenzae* type B (15%), meningococci (5%), and group A and B streptococci, salmonella, and *S. aureus* (5%). Of infections caused by pneumococci, 60% have traditionally been vaccine serotypes and 15% nonvaccine serotypes. Since the advent of PCV-7 vaccine, most infections caused by pneumococci are expected to be nonvaccine serotypes (Klein, 2002).

Research studies and analysis of data have established practice guidelines for the outpatient management of infants and children from 0 to 36 months of age (Baraff et al, 1993; Children's Hospital and Health Center, 1998; Prober, 1999). The practice guidelines for the management of infants and children 0 to 36 months of age with fever without a focus include the following universal points:

- *Fever* is defined as a rectal temperature of 100.4° F (38.0° C) or greater in infants 0 to 90 days old; greater than 100.4° F (38.0° C) but less than 102.2° F (39° C) in infants 3 to 6 months old; or greater than 102.2° F (39° C) in infants and children 3 to 36 months old. Refer to the algorithm (Fig. 24-3) for management of these different fever thresholds.
- *Fever without focus* is an acute febrile illness in which the etiology of the fever is not apparent after careful history and physical examination.

Management

Some general practice guidelines include the following management strategies (see Fig. 24-3):

- Refer all toxic-appearing 0- to 36-month-old infants and children to an emergency department for lumbar puncture and possible parenteral antibiotic therapy after prompt laboratory workup.
- Febrile infants younger than 4 weeks of age, regardless of whether they meet the low-risk criteria identified

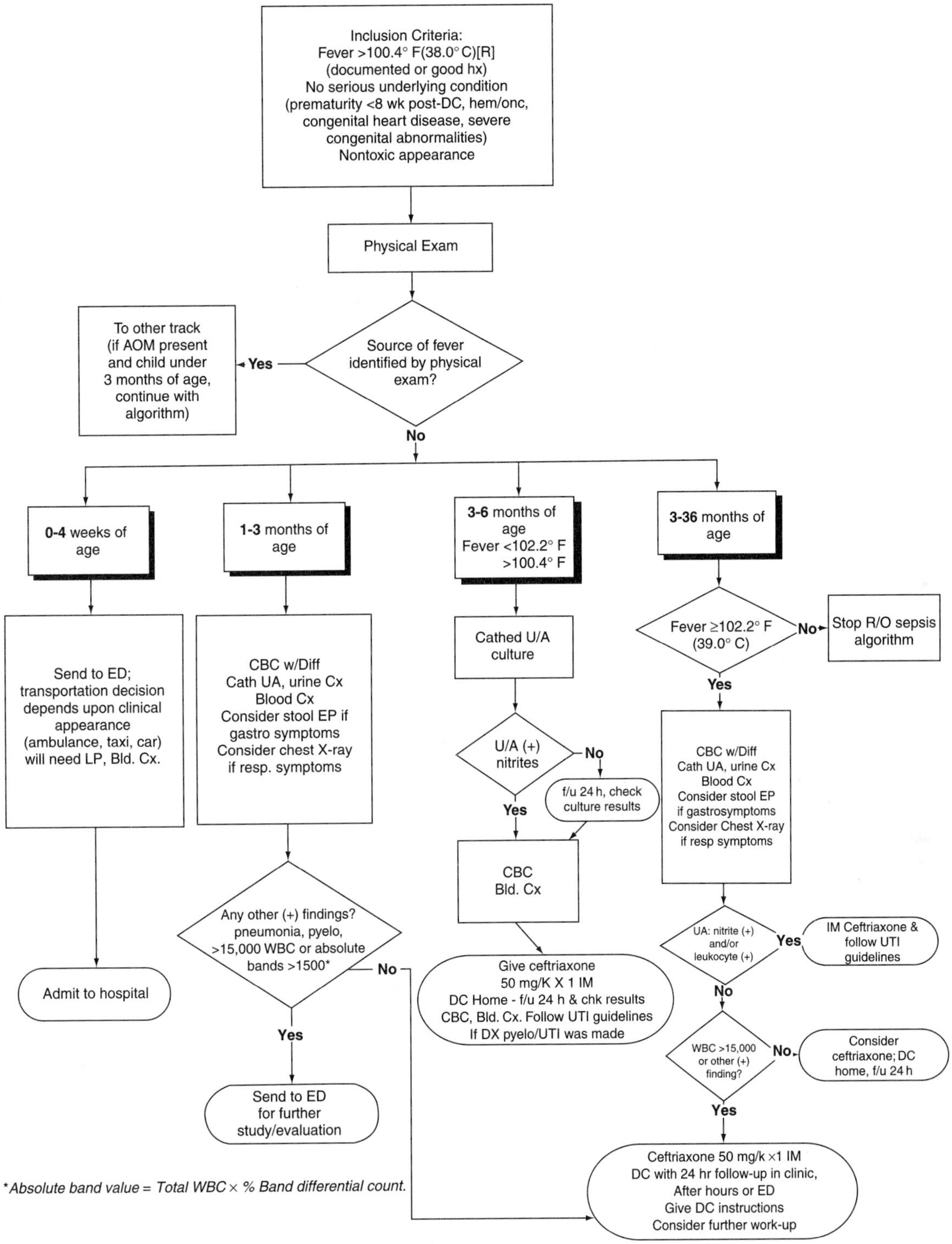

FIGURE 24-3 Fever without focus algorithm. *Hx*, History; *R*, rectal; *DC*, discharge; *AOM*, acute otitis media; *ED*, emergency department; *LP*, lumbar puncture; *Bld. Cx*, blood culture; *EP*, enteric pathogens (culture); *W/diff*, with differential; *Cx*, culture; *Pyelo*, pyelonephritis; *WBC*, white blood cell count; *Cathed*, catheterized; *U/A*, urinalysis; *f/u*, follow-up; *h*, hours; *IM*, intramuscularly; *Chk*, check; *UTI*, urinary tract infection; *Dx*, diagnosis; *Resp*, respiratory; *hem/onc*, hematologic/oncology issue. (Adapted from Children's Hospital and Health Center: *R/O sepsis algorithm*, San Diego, 1998, Children's Hospital and Health Center.)

previously, should have a sepsis evaluation (culture of CSF, blood, and catheterized or suprapubic urine specimen; a CBC and differential; and complete analysis of the CSF) and hospitalization for parenteral antibiotics.
- Infants 28 to 90 days old who are nontoxic appearing and meet the low-risk criteria listed previously can be managed as outpatients using the algorithm illustrated in Fig. 24-3. Febrile infants 28 to 90 days old who do not meet the laboratory low-risk criteria should be hospitalized.
- Infants between 3 and 6 months of age with fever greater than 100.4° F (38.0° C) but less than 102.2° F (39.0° C) and nontoxic appearing may be managed using the algorithm illustrated in Fig. 24-3.
- Refer all toxic-appearing children to the emergency department for further workup and treatment.

Children 3 to 36 months of age with rectal fevers greater than 102.2° F (39.0° C) and nontoxic appearing can be managed as outpatients using the aforementioned algorithm (Fig. 24-3). Return for visit appointment in 24 hours, if the fever persists longer than 48 hours, or the child is worse.

An important point to remember in treatment is that bacteremia can be an occult infection in young infants and children (i.e., nontoxic-appearing patient whose blood culture is positive for a pathogenic organism). A useful axiom to remember is that the higher the WBC count and the greater the absolute number of neutrophils or bands, the greater the risk of bacteremia in a febrile child. Remember that all toxic-appearing infants under 28 days old need immediate hospitalization. Others require further evaluation or hospitalization. Also remember that the younger the infant, the greater the uncertainty about the possibility of a serious bacterial infection, and the greater the need to rule out this possibility.

Parents of infants who are managed as outpatients need detailed instructions on signs and symptoms that indicate a worsening of their infants' illness. Instruct parents to bring their infant in immediately if any of these signs and symptoms appear: change in or new rash; duskiness, cyanosis, or mottling; coolness of extremities; poor feeding or vomiting; irritability; difficulty in comforting or arousing; seizure activity (eye rolling or jerking of extremities); or bulging anterior fontanel. Careful follow-up of such infants must be ensured (Powell, 2004b).

Fever of Unknown Origin

The classic definition of *fever of unknown origin* (FUO) is (1) a prolonged fever (rectal temperature greater than 101° F [38.3° C] or oral temperature greater than 100.0° F [37.8° C]) for at least 3 weeks or more without an etiology; and (2) no specific diagnosis after 3 to 7 days or after 3 days of outpatient visits, extensive studies, and continued fevers (Durack, 1997). A child with an FUO requires that the health care providers to frequently rethink and reevaluate historical, clinical, and laboratory data.

Many FUOs are atypical presentations of common disorders. Few are exotic. In the United States most FUOs are caused by salmonellosis, tuberculosis, rickettsial diseases, syphilis, Lyme disease, Kawasaki syndrome, cat-scratch disease, inflammatory bowel disease, rheumatic fever, infectious mononucleosis, CMV, hepatitis, coccidioidomycosis, histoplasmosis, malaria, and toxoplasmosis. Less common are tularemia, brucellosis, rat-bite fever, and leptospirosis (Powell, 2004b).

In children under 6 years of age, the most common causes of FUO are UTI/pyelonephritis, respiratory illnesses, localized infections (abscess, osteomyelitis), juvenile arthritis (JA), and, rarely, leukemia. In adolescents the most common causes include TB, inflammatory bowel disease, autoimmmune disorders, lymphoma, and the causes listed for children under 6 years of age.

The approach to evaluating a child with an FUO should include a detailed history, a thorough physical examination, and screening laboratory studies.

History

- Careful analysis of symptoms or signs, a meticulous review of systems, history of the fever pattern, and patient's age
- Past medical history of recurrent infections, surgery, transfusions, and contact with ill individuals or exposure to wild and domestic animals
- Medication use and family medical history, including autoimmune disease or inflammatory bowel disorder
- History of pica; history of travel with souvenirs of dirt, rocks, or artifacts

Physical Examination

- Skin findings (e.g., rashes, lesions), presence or absence of sweating
- Local or generalized lymphadenopathy or hepatosplenomegaly
- Joint examination and palpation of bones for tenderness, swelling
- Palpation of sinus and mastoid areas
- Eye examination looking for palpebral or bulbar conjunctivitis, conjunctival hemorrhages, and ophthalmologic examination if JA is suspected
- Pelvic examination in adolescent females
- Rectal examination and guaiac test
- Mouth and throat examination for exudates, erythema, absence of fungiform papillae

Laboratory Studies

- CBC with differential, ESR
- Blood and CSF
- Urinalysis plus blood and urine cultures
- PPD with controls
- Chest, sinus, mastoid, and GI tract radiographs
- Liver chemistries
- Serum protein analysis
- Heterophil antibody and antinuclear antibody titer in older children

Other tests may involve bone marrow, radionuclide scans, total body CT, MRI, or biopsies (Powell, 2004b).

Differential Diagnosis

Infectious diseases, collagen-vascular disease (JA, SLE), malignancies, drug fever (typically secondary to ingestion of phenothiazines, antidepressants, atropine, amphetamine, and other anticholinergic medications), nosocomial, HIV-associated illnesses, and Münchausen syndrome by proxy are included in the differential diagnosis of an FUO.

Management

Consider hospitalizing the child if there is evidence of systemic illness or failure to thrive, if the child is very young, or if the parent(s) anxiety is extreme. Otherwise, the child should be followed up with frequent visits, documented fever pattern, and other specialized tests if screening tests indicate the need or if other physical findings develop. Empirical use of antibiotics should be avoided unless the child has possible disseminated tuberculosis (Powell, 2004b).

HELMINTHIC ZOONOSES

Description

Domesticated dogs and cats and wild animals kept as pets can be infected with intestinal helminth parasites. Mild to severe illnesses can result when helminth are transmitted to children by fecal contamination. With a reported 59% of U.S. households having one or more pets (Kazacos, 2000), close contact is inevitable. Helminth zoonoses (transmitted from animal to a human host) are briefly presented, and the most common infections known to occur in children are discussed.

Transmission of zoonotic infections can occur by several routes:

- Direct infection by ingestion of eggs or the penetration of larvae into the body (infections such as tapeworms and roundworms are acquired from their eggs; hookworms penetrate the skin)
- Indirect infection by ingestion of larvae in food (e.g., fish, meat, snails, freshwater shrimp, land crabs)
- Exposure to an intermediary vector (e.g., mosquito, flies, fleas, ticks)

Helminth larvae can live for extended periods of time in human and animal organs and tissues, causing an inflammatory condition referred to as larva migrans (LM). Larva migrans can affect many organs and tissues within the body. When LM has been identified, the resulting clinical syndromes produced are classified as visceral, ocular, neural, cutaneous, or covert toxocariasis and asymptomatic or clinically inapparent infection (Kazacos, 2000).

The true incidence of LM is unknown, because it is not reportable in the United States. Some studies within the United States have shown an average prevalence rate of *Toxocara canis* (dog) or *T. cati* (cat) seropositivity of 3%. The rates vary, however, depending on location and socioeconomic factors.

Different species of roundworms and hookworms found in dogs, cats, and raccoons are common causes of LM in humans. Dogs carry the most common cause of zoonotic infection worldwide *(T. canis)*. Young puppies under 3 months have been known to carry this roundworm 90% to 100% of the time; however, dogs of any age can harbor the parasite (Kazacos, 2000). Another infection *(Baylisascaris procyonis)* is being increasingly seen in young children who are in contact with raccoons. The LM from this infestation can lead to a fatal or severe neurologic disease.

Prevention of zoonotic infections includes identifying possible sources of exposure, referral of pets to veterinarians for testing, decontamination of soiled environments, and prevention of further exposure. The latter intervention includes education about safe pet fecal cleanup, the regular deworming of pets, good handwashing, behavioral modification in cases of pica and geophagia, and covering sandboxes when not in use. Information should be provided to families with pets, especially puppies, kittens, and raccoons, about having them tested for helminth infestations. Communities should be encouraged to promote leash laws and responsible pet ownership (cleaning up pet fecal waste), to disallow dogs from playgrounds and parks where children play, and to restrict open access to sandboxes (Kazacos, 2000).

Toxocara canis

Etiology and Incidence

Infection with *T. canis* can cause zoonotic visceral LM (VLM), ocular LM (OLM), and, in severe cases, neural LM (NLM). Ingestion of eggs can occur from contact with contaminated soil (in sandboxes, parks, playgrounds, schoolyards, public places where dogs have visited), hands, food, and fomites such as toys. Once the eggs are ingested and hatched, the larvae can penetrate the intestines and migrate to the liver and lungs and other tissues of the body. With initial or mild infections, the larvae seem to be able to reach other locations, such as the brain and eye, more easily. Neural LM syndrome can result, which may be mild (subtle neurologic or behavior changes) to severe (CNS involvement). Children from 1 to 5 years old (average 2 years) are most commonly affected by VLM; OLM can occur in children and young adults.

History

Assess for history of pica or geophagia; exposure to dogs, cats, or environments where animals are known to frequent; and recent travel, fever, abdominal pain, hepatomegaly, or respiratory symptoms (cough, wheezing, asthma, pneumonia). In the case of OLM, there may be no history of pica or symptoms of VLM.

Physical Examination

- OLM: decreased vision, strabismus, or leukokoria; patient may be asymptomatic
- Covert toxocariasis
- Abdominal pain, hepatomegaly, anorexia, nausea, vomiting
- Lethargy; sleep and behavior changes
- Coughing, wheezing
- Fever
- Cervical adenitis
- Limb pain

Laboratory Studies

- CBC reveals leukocytosis, marked eosinophilia, hypergammaglobulinemia, elevated blood group isohemagglutinin titers.
- Elevated *T. canis* antibody titer (ELISA with confirmatory Western blot test) in OLM.
- CT and MRI may be used to detect granulomatous lesions in OLM.

Differential Diagnosis

Toxocariasis should be considered in any child with nonspecific symptoms, notably recurrent abdominal pain, reactive airway disease, or allergies of unknown cause. A normal eosinophilia count should not predispose the NP from ruling out this infection, if suspected. Infected patients do not pass eggs or larvae in their excreta.

Management

Management is based on controlling inflammatory reactions (corticosteroids and antihistamines) and trying appropriate anthelmintic therapy (rates of successful treatment with anthelmintics are mixed) (Kazacos, 2000). A pediatric infectious disease expert should be consulted for treatment recommendations. Family pets need evaluation by a veterinarian.

INFECTIOUS AGENTS USED IN BIOTERRORISM

Since September 2001, the United States has become more aware of a potential threat of infectious diseases acquired through biologic warfare. Most of these diseases have not been seen in clinical practice settings. The most anticipated of these agents are discussed.

Children are at particular risk for exposure to and absorption of biologic agents (e.g., anthrax and botulinum toxin). Factors that predispose them to such risk include being within closer proximity to the ground, having faster ventilation rates and thinner skins, having an increased risk of dehydration, and having greater undeveloped cognition.

Agents of biologic warfare are categorized by the CDC according to their potential for aerosol transmission, susceptibility of the population, degree of person-to-person transmission, expected high morbidity and mortality rates, the likelihood for delayed diagnosis, and the lack of effective and efficacious treatments (Unger, 2002). Agents at highest risk to the populace are known as category A weapons of bioterrorism. These include specific bacteria, viruses, botulinum toxin, *Bacillus anthracis* (anthrax), *Francisella tularensis* (tularemia), variola virus (smallpox), and viruses of hemorrhagic fever (Ebola, Marburg, Lassa fever).

Ensuring that NPs are knowledgeable in identifying infectious diseases, fevers without focus, and fevers of unknown origin can enhance the national bioterrorism surveillance network. NPs can help their communities in the early detection and prompt large-scale medical response by developing an awareness of syndromes and symptoms that might suggest a biologic warfare agent exposure (Bechtel, 2002d; Unger, 2002). NPs also can join other health care providers in developing pediatric readiness plans. These readiness plans should include triage, isolation and treatment/care facilities, transportation, communication, housing, and the establishment of vaccination clinics on a massive scale for children, especially in communities where emergency departments may not have the procedural skills to address a severely ill pediatric population. NPs can request health alerts by E-mail from the CDC (see Resources Box).

See Table 24-15 for a full discussion of each agent.

Anthrax

Anthrax is found naturally in soil, surviving as long as 40 years in that medium. It has traditionally been known as

TABLE 24-15 *Agents of Bioterrorism*

Disease	Signs and Symptoms	Incubation Time (Range)	Person-to-Person Transmission	Isolation	Diagnosis	Postexposure Prophylaxis for Children and Adolescents (see App. A for dosing)	Treatment in Children and Adolescents (see App. A for dosing)
Anthrax *(Bacillus anthracis)*							
Inhalation	Flulike symptoms (fever, fatigue, muscle aches, dyspnea, nonproductive cough, headache), chest pain; possible 1-2 day improvement then rapid respiratory failure and shock. Meningitis may develop.	1-6 days (up to 6 wk)	None	Standard precautions	Chest x-ray evidence of widening mediastinum; obtain sputum and blood culture. Sensitivity and specificity of nasal swabs unknown—do not rely on for diagnosis.	Prophylaxis for 60 days: Amoxicillin* Doxycycline Ciprofloxacin *Alternative:* Ofloxacin or levofloxacin or gatifloxacin	Penicillin G* Amoxicillin* Ciprofloxacin *Alternative:* Ofloxacin or levofloxacin or gatifloxacin
Cutaneous	Intense itching followed by painless papular lesions, then vesicular lesions, developing into eschar surrounded by edema.	1-12 days	Direct contact with skin lesions may result in cutaneous infection	Contact precautions	Peripheral blood smear may demonstrate gram-positive bacilli on unspun smear with sepsis.		
Gastrointestinal (GI)	Abdominal pain, nausea and vomiting, severe diarrhea, GI bleeding, and fever.	1-7 days	None	Standard precautions	Culture blood and stool.		
Botulism (botulinum toxin)	Afebrile, excess mucus in throat, dysphagia, dry mouth and throat, dizziness, then difficulty moving eyes, mild pupillary dilation and nystagmus, intermittent ptosis, indistinct speech, unsteady gait, extreme symmetric descending weakness, flaccid paralysis; generally normal mental status.	Inhalation: 12-80 hr Foodborne: 12-72 hr (2-8 days)	None	Standard precautions	Laboratory tests available from CDC or Public Health Department; obtain serum, stool, gastric aspirate, and suspect foods before administering antitoxin. Differential diagnosis includes polio, Guillain-Barré, myasthenia, tick paralysis, stroke, meningococcal meningitis.	Pentavalent toxoid (types A, B, C, D, E) may be available in the future One 10 ml vial trivalent botulism antitoxin IV	Botulism antitoxins Supportive care, ventilation **Avoid clindamycin and aminoglycosides**

Continued

TABLE 24-15 *Agents of Bioterrorism—cont'd*

Disease	Signs and Symptoms	Incubation Time (Range)	Person-to-Person Transmission	Isolation	Diagnosis	Postexposure Prophylaxis for Children and Adolescents (see App. A for dosing)	Treatment in Children and Adolescents (see App. A for dosing)
Pneumonic plague ***(Yersinia pestis)***	High fever, cough, hemoptysis, chest pain, nausea and vomiting, headache. Advanced disease: purpuric skin lesions, copious watery or purulent sputum production; respiratory failure in 1-6 days.	2-3 days (2-6 days)	Yes, droplet aerosols	Droplet precautions until 48 hr of effective antibiotic therapy	A presumptive diagnosis may be made by Gram, Wayson, or Wright stain of lymph node aspirates, sputum, or cerebrospinal fluid with gram-negative bacilli with bipolar (safety pin) staining.	Doxycycline Ciprofloxacin	Streptomycin Gentamycin *Alternatives:* Doxycycline Ciprofloxacin
Smallpox (variola virus)	Prodromal period: malaise, fever, rigors, vomiting, headache, and backache. After 2-4 days, skin lesions appear and progress uniformly from macules to papules to vesicles and pustules, mostly on face, neck, palms, soles, and subsequently progress to trunk.	12-14 days (7-17 days)	Yes, airborne droplet nuclei or direct contact with skin lesions or secretions until all scabs separate and fall off (3-4 wk)	Airborne (includes N95 mask) and contact precautions	Swab culture of vesicular fluid or scab, send to BL-4 (Biologic Level 4) laboratory. All lesions are similar in appearance and develop synchronously, opposed to chickenpox. Electron microscopy can differentiate variola virus from varicella.	Early vaccine within 4-5 days if available depending upon CDC guidelines	Supportive care, vaccinations within 72 hours of rash; possible use of cidofovir
Tularemia	Fever, headache, acute inflammation, pharyngitis	2-10 days (average 2-6)	No	Standard precautions	Respiratory secretions and blood: antibody titers (>four-fold increase). Light microscopy and fluourescent-labeled antibody. **Pneumonic**: x-ray findings of lobar/subsegmental infiltrates, hilar adenopathy, pleural effusion, atypical infiltrates.	Doxycycline Ciprofloxacin	Doxycycline Ciprofloxacin Vaccine currently available only for high-risk persons (laboratory workers)
• **Ulceroglandular:**	Skin papules, granulomatous lesions with necrotic, caseous areas.						
• **Oculoglandular:**	Edematous/inflamed conjunctiva with yellow nodules, ulcers or palpebral conjunctiva/sclera. Cervical/submaxillary/preauricular lymphadenopathy.						

• **Typhoidal:**	Fever >102° F (39.4° C), chills, headache, aches, vomiting photophobia, hepatosplenomegaly, exanthems on upper extremities (+/− face and neck), diarrhea.						
• **Pneumonic:**	Respiratory symptoms of pneumonia or pleuritis.						
Hemorrhagic fevers • Crimean-Congo • Dengue • Ebola and Marburg • Hanta pulmonary syndrome • Yellow fever • Lassa fever	Generally: fever, muscle aches, dizziness, malaise, weakness. exhaustion, +/− rash, +/− headache. With disease progression: ecchymosis, bleeding from orifices with GI symptoms, can lead to shock, delirium, seizures, renal failure.	Depends on agent Crimean: 2-10 days Ebola/Marburg: 3-9 days Dengue: 2-7 days Lassa: 6-17 days	Ebola and Lassa only via blood or body fluids	Mask, contact, and standard precautions, depending on agent; DEET for mosquito-bite resistance	Serology or specific virologic techniques.	Only Yellow fever vaccine available	Supportive: ribavirin therapy may be useful for some agents in certain cases

Adapted from North Carolina Statewide Program for Infection Control and Epidemiology (SPICE): Bioterrorist Agents, 2002. Available from University of North Carolina website: *www.unc.edn/depts/spice/bioterrorism* (accessed Nov 8, 2003); Cain, 2002a, 2002b; Reavis, 2002a, 2002b; Unger, 2002.

*If strains are sensitive.

woolsorters' disease due to inhaling the spore-forming gram-positive rod after exposure to hides, wool, or other animal products during processing. It has been largely eliminated in developed countries secondary to the anthrax vaccine for animals. Three forms have been identified: cutaneous, inhalation, and gastrointestinal.

If appropriate treatment is not started within 48 hours after the onset of symptoms, the mortality rate can reach 95%. Prophylaxis is effective if administered as soon as possible after exposure. Doxycycline, amoxicillin, penicillin (if the organism is sensitive), and ciprofloxacin are recommended agents. Amoxicillin is recommended for children younger than 12 years old. Currently all of the anthrax vaccine is held by the U.S. Department of Defense and cannot be obtained by the private sector. The CDC is studying other prophylaxis regimens that include antibiotics plus anthrax vaccination (Unger, 2002). Cephalosporins and trimethoprim-sulfamethoxazole are contraindicated because of known anthrax resistance.

Botulinum Toxin

The poison protein molecules that make up botulinum toxin are secreted by vegetative cells of *Clostridium botulinum* bacteria. These substances are the most toxic poison known to exist in a natural state. There are seven strains designated A through G. Each strain has its own exotoxin; any strain can prove deadly. This gram-positive, spore-forming bacillus occurs naturally in soil and is anaerobic. Infection is generally via a food-borne route. Food is heated high enough to drive off dissolved oxygen but not high enough to destroy all of the *C. botulinum* spores. Any surviving spores germinate and begin producing their exotoxins. Canned vegetables, fish, and marine mammals can serve as such vehicles. Other avenues of infection with *C. botulinum* include the GI tract (due to overgrowth), wound infections, and aerosol exposure from a laboratory accident or terrorism. It is not contagious or spread by person-to-person contact.

Botulinum toxin can be detected in serum, stool, gastric aspirate, and vomitus. Preventive prophylaxis after exposure and active treatment excludes the use of antibiotics but includes careful use of passive immunization with equine antitoxin for adults. Skin testing before the use of the sera is imperative. There is also an investigational pentavalent botulinum toxoid vaccine (with toxoids A through E) currently available from the CDC for military and laboratory personnel only. Commercial products are under development for potential mass immunization purposes (Cain, 2002a). Any known aerosolized exposure requires the immediate cleaning or disposal of clothes and thorough cleansing and rinsing of skin and hair.

Pneumonic Plague

Infection with the *Yersinia pestis* organism manifests in three forms: bubonic, pneumatic, and septicemic. In the fourteenth century, catastrophic epidemics caused by the bubonic form occurred in Europe. The scourge was referred to as the "black death" or "great pestilence." Today, small outbreaks occur around the world. Bubonic is the most common form and is acquired from infected fleas or rats. Pneumonic is acquired from aerosolized droplets, and septicemic plague results from direct contact with infected animals (hides or secretions) or people (secretions). The pneumonic form is an anticipated biologic warfare agent. The concern is that an antibiotic-resistant strain of pneumonic *Y. pestis* would be used (Reavis, 2002a). The pneumonic form is also the most invasive and pathogenic; the mortality rate can be greater than 50% in untreated cases.

Laboratory testing depends on isolating *Y. pestis* from cultures of blood, sputum, CSF, or aspirates from lymphadenopathy. Management depends on rapid diagnosis. Exposure to plague plus either a temperature of 101.2° F (38.5° C) or the new onset of a cough necessitates starting antibiotic therapy. Asymptomatic people with known exposure should also start antibiotic prophylaxis for 1 week. Unfortunately, the symptoms at the onset of pneumonic plague suggest a respiratory infection. Patients may not seek treatment until the more advanced symptoms of plague appear.

There is no vaccine for pneumonic plague. Standard and droplet precautions for 72 hours after starting antibiotic treatment are recommended. Bubonic plague can be successfully controlled with the use of health education and environmental treatment (sunlight and heat, rodenticides).

Smallpox

There are two forms of this viral disease, variola major and variola minor. Two other forms of the virus are known as hemorrhagic and malignant, and these are frequently fatal. The last known naturally acquired case in the world occurred in 1977. The virus is spread from person to person via virus-containing aerosolized droplets from saliva that are then inhaled by exposed persons. Such droplets can also remain viable for up to 1 week on bedding, clothing, and other surfaces. Those most at risk have been within 6 feet of an infected person.

Historically, unimmunized patients with smallpox suffered an average fatality rate of 30%. The disease is not transmittable before the appearance of the rash. The infected person is most contagious within the first week of having the rash. Those with pharyngeal and oral lesions are more contagious. However, until all of the scabs have fallen off, the virus has the potential to spread (Unger, 2002).

Smallpox is anticipated to be a formidable warfare agent because of the propensity for its rash to resemble that of chickenpox and to be dismissed as such. However, the astute NP will be able to distinguish the two diseases by the pattern of symptoms preceding the rash. See Fig. 24-2 for the distinguishing differences that aid diagnosis as compared with the features of scarlet fever and varicella.

Laboratory diagnosis can be made by DFA, electron microscopy, or PCR from fluid obtained from the lesions. Management involves interrupting the mode of transmission: isolation of those infected, as well as isolation and vaccination of contacts and those exposed to the contacts. This approach to epidemiologic control is referred to as "search and containment" or "ring" vaccination. Public health experts are still undecided whether to embrace this more selective ring approach or vaccinate on a mass level if an outbreak should occur. See the prior discussion regarding the smallpox vaccine.

There is no known, effective treatment for active smallpox infection. Antibiotics for secondary infections and supportive therapy are the mode of treatment. Antivirals may be attempted (although they are not known to be effective) and include cidofovir, adefovir dipivoxide, cyclic cidofovir, and ribovarin.

Tularemia

The etiologic agent in tularemia is *Francisella tularensis.* The organism is a small, aerobic, gram-negative bacterium without toxins. Tularemia is also known as "rabbit fever" and "deerfly fever" in the United States. Small amounts of the bacteria are highly virulent. Two strains have been identified: strain B, which is less virulent (currently found in Europe), and the more virulent strain A (found in the United States, Europe, and Japan). Without antibiotic treatment, strain A has been known to have a wide-ranging mortality rate (5% to 60%; Cain, 2002b).

F. tularensis is found in and on soil, water, and vegetation and can be endemic in wild mammals (rabbits, hares, squirrels, voles, mice, water rats). It is spread from animal to animal and animal to human by direct contact with an infected animal or its environment (e.g., nests or sharing an ecologic niche) or by a bite from an infected tick, mosquito, or deer fly that has bitten another infected animal. It is more commonly acquired by hunters and outdoorsmen; it is a particular concern of laboratory workers working with the agent.

The agent enters humans via the cutaneous or mucous membrane routes and invades phagocytes and macrophages. If used as a biologic warfare agent, it may be spread in aerosol form and may be absorbed by the eye or respiratory system. It can also be transmitted by contaminated food or water. Oculoglandular, oropharyngeal, typhoidal (systemic tularemia), gastrointestional, and pneumonic refer to the different forms of the infection.

Successful treatment will entail prompt diagnosis of this rare disease. Any suspicious atypical pharyngitis, atypical pneumonia, pleuritis, and hilar lymphadenopathy would be clues. The differential diagnosis for pulmonary tularemia includes psittacosis, legionellosis, Q fever, mycoplasma and *C. pneumoniae* infections, anthrax, and plague (Unger, 2002). Laboratory diagnosis is made from blood and respiratory secretions via fluorescent-labeled antibody. Should a mass outbreak occur, the treatment of choice is doxycycline and ciprofloxacin for both children and adults (Cain, 2002b). Beta-lactam antibiotics are ineffective. A current vaccine is available only to high-risk laboratory workers.

Viral Hemorrhagic Fevers

There are four categories of viral hemorrhagic fevers:

- Arenavirus—Lassa fever, Argentine hemorrhagic fever
- Bunyavirus—Crimean-Congo hemorrhagic fever, hantavirus, pulmonary syndrome, hemorrhagic fever with renal syndrome
- Filovirus—Ebola, Marburg
- Flavivirus—Yellow fever, dengue, Omsk hemorrhagic fever, Kyasanur Forest disease viruses

Most are spread from infected animal hosts or arthropod vectors (zoonotic); severity of illness ranges from mild to life threatening (23% to 100% mortality rate range). The animal host is often specific to individual viruses. Humans may contract the viruses where these hosts and vectors are found. Infection is usually from contact with the host or vector urine, saliva, or feces. Human-to-human contact can occur from contact with bodily fluids or fomites, such as infected needles. The hosts for Ebola and Marburg are unknown (Reavis, 2002b). If used as a biologic agent, it is expected to be distributed in an aerosol form to infect the human vascular system (Unger, 2002).

Prevention focuses on avoiding exposure to hosts and vectors via the following measures:

- Controlling rodent populations and discouraging their entry into living and work spaces
- Effectively and safely cleaning up rodent habitats and excreta
- Controlling mosquitoes
- Avoiding bites from ticks and mosquitoes in endemic areas (protective clothing, insect repellents, screens, mosquito netting)
- Obtaining prophylaxis if available
- Educating patients traveling to known areas of infectivity

RESOURCE BOX

Infectious Disease

AIDS INFORMATION

U.S. Department Health and Human Services
1-800-448-0440
www.hivatis.org

Association of State and Territorial Health Officials
1-601-576-7634
www.astho.org

AIDS Clinical Trials Information Service
www.actis.org

Biological Warfare Agent Health Alerts
Available by E-mail request from www.healthalerts@cdc.gov

Centers for Disease Control and Prevention
1-800-311-3435
www.cdc.gov

Vaccine Adverse Event Reporting System (VAERS)
1-800-822-7967
www.vaers.org

Food and Drug Administration
www.fda.gov/cber/vaers/vaears.htm

In the United States, the CDC is encouraging control of rodent populations, rapid diagnostic testing, and stockpiling vaccines and supportive treatment medications. Further information is available from the CDC in the guideline *Infection Control for Viral Hemorrhagic Fevers in the African Health Care Setting* (CDC, WHO, 1998). Diagnosis is anticipated to be from serologic testing or from virologic techniques. The only vaccine currently available is for yellow fever. Treatment will be supportive, though ribavarin is expected to be attempted in certain cases.

REFERENCES

Adam H: Management of fever. In Hoekelman R: *Primary pediatric care,* ed 4, St Louis, 2001, Mosby.

American Academy of Pediatrics: *2000 red book: report of the Committee on Infectious Diseases,* ed 25, Elk Grove Village, IL, 2000, American Academy of Pediatrics.

American Academy of Pediatrics: *2003 red book: report of the Committee on Infections Diseases,* ed 26, Elk Grove Village, IL, 2003, American Academy of Pediatrics.

American Journal of Nurse Practitioners Editorial Staff: CDC immunization recommendations, *Am J Nurse Pract* 6(3):9-12, 2002.

Annunziato P, Gershon A: Varicella-zoster virus infection. In Burg F et al, editors: *Gellis and Kagan's current pediatric therapy,* ed 17, Philadelphia, 2002, WB Saunders.

Baraff LJ et al: Practice guidelines for the management of infants and children 0 to 36 months of age with fever without source, *Pediatrics* 92:1-12, 1993.

Barone S, Krilov L: Infectious mononucleosis and other Epstein-Barr virus infections. In Hoekelman R: *Primary pediatric care,* ed 4, St Louis, 2001, Mosby.

Bechtel B: Efficacy of the PCV7 extends beyond invasive disease to OM and pneumonia prevention, *Infect Dis Children* 15(7):55-56, 2002a.

Bechtel B: Wild rotavirus infection may not cause intussusception, *Infect Dis Children* 15(5):20-21, 2002b.

Bechtel B: Aventis to donate smallpox vaccine, *Infect Dis Children* 15(5):17-18, 2002c.

Bechtel B: Why should pediatricians care about bioterrorism? Children are most at risk, *Infect Dis Children* 15(7):24-25, 2002d.

Bechtel B: Pediatric flu vaccine recommendation looks unlikely, according to ACIP, *Infect Dis Children* 15(11):16, 2002e.

Bechtel B: Intranasal influenza vaccine granted approval by FDA, *Infect Dis Children* 16(7):3, 2003.

Besser R: Antibiotic resistance, 2002. Available at *www.cdc.gov/drug-resistance/community* (accessed Sept 10, 2002).

Black S: Prevention of pneumococcal disease: efficacy trial, *Infect Dis Children Suppl,* June 2002, pp 4-6.

Brunell P: A new respiratory virus, *Infect Dis Children* 15(7):4-10, 2002.

Cain W: Botulism toxin, *Am J Nurse Pract* 6(4):25-27, 2002a.

Cain W: Tularemia, *Am J Nurse Pract* 6(5):24-26, 2002b.

Caserta M: Meningococcemia. In Hoekelman R: *Primary pediatric care,* ed 4, St Louis, 2001, Mosby.

Centers for Disease Control and Prevention: 1994 revised classification system for human immunodeficiency virus infection in children less than 13 years of age, *MMWR Morb Mortal Wkly Rep* 43(12):1-10, 1994.

Centers for Disease Control and Prevention: Prevention of pneumococcal disease: recommendations of the Advisory Committee on Immunization Practices, *MMWR Morb Mortal Wkly Rep* 46(RR-8):1-24, 1997.

Centers for Disease Control and Prevention: Measles-mumps-rubella vaccine use and strategies for elimination of measles-rubella and congenital rubella syndrome and control of mumps: recommendations of the Advisory Committee on Immunization Practices (ACIP), *MMWR Morb Mortal Wkly Rep* 47(RR-8):1-57, 1998.

Centers for Disease Control and Prevention, World Health Organization: Infection control for viral hemorrhagic fevers in the African health care setting, 1998. Available at *www.cdc.gov.*

Centers for Disease Control and Prevention: Prevention of hepatitis A through active or passive immunization: recommendations of the ACIP, *MMWR Morb Mortal Wkly Rep* 48(RR-12):1-37, 1999a.

Centers for Disease Control and Prevention, Division of HIV/AIDS Prevention: HIV/AIDS and US women who have sex with women (WSW), 1999b. Available at *www.cdc.gov/hib/pubs/facts/wsw* (accessed Aug 3, 2002).

Centers for Disease Control and Prevention: *Tuberculosis: what the clinician should know*, ed 4, 2000a. Available at *www.cdc.gov* (accessed Sept 15, 2002).

Centers for Disease Control and Prevention: Preventing pneumococcal disease among infants and young children, *MMWR Morb Mortal Wkly Rep* 49(RR-09):1-38, 2000b.

Centers for Disease Control and Prevention, Division of Vector-Borne Infectious Diseases: West Nile virus, 2001. Available at *www.cdc.gov* (accessed Feb 16, 2003).

Centers for Disease Control and Prevention: Recommended childhood immunization schedule—United States, 2002, *MMWR Morb Mortal Wkly Rep* 51:31-33, 2002a.

Centers for Disease Control and Prevention: Flu season 2002-2003, *Influenza Vaccine Bulletin* 3, 2002b.

Centers for Disease Control and Prevention, National Immunization Program: Varicella vaccine. Available at *www.cdc.gov/nip/vaccine/varicella* (accessed Sept 15, 2002.)

Centers for Disease Control and Prevention: Hanta virus pulmonary syndrome—United States: updated recommendations for risk reduction, *MMWR Morb Mortal Wkly Rep* 51(RR-9):1-16, 2002d.

Centers for Disease Control and Prevention: Viral hepatitis B. Available at *www.cdc.gov* (accessed Feb 14, 2003).

Centers for Disease Control and Prevention, National Immunization Program: Dosages and schedules for hepatitis A vaccines. Available at *www.cdc.gov.nip* (accessed Feb 16, 2003).

Chettle C: West Nile virus: spread of the mosquito borne illness, *Nurseweek*, Nov 2002, pp 22-23.

Children's Hospital and Health Center: *R/O sepsis algorithm*, San Diego, 1998, Children's Hospital and Health Center.

Daiichi Pharmaceutical Corporation: Sound advice: illness in children attending childcare, *Daiichi Pharm Corp Newslettor* 1(5):1-12, 2001.

Demas P et al: Maternal adherence to the zidovudine regimen for HIV-exposed infants to prevent HIV infection: a preliminary study, *Pediatrics* 110(3):e35, 2002.

DeVange P et al: Validation of performance on the gen-probe human immunodeficiency virus type 1 viral load assay with genital swabs and breast milk samples, *J Clin Microbiol* 40(11):3929-3937, 2002.

Dowell SR et al: Principles of judicious use of antimicrobial agents for pediatric upper respiratory tract infection, *Pediatrics* 101:163-165, 1998.

Durack D: Fever of unknown origin—reexamined and redefined. In Mackowiak P, editor: *Fever: basic mechanisms and management*, ed 2, Philadelphia, 1997, Lippincott-Raven.

Estabrook M: *Neisseria meningitidis*. In Behrman RE et al, editors: *Nelson textbook of pediatrics*, ed 16, Philadelphia, 2000, WB Saunders.

Gerber M, Shapiro E: Late lyme disease: clearing up confusion, *Contemp Pediatr* 18(7):46-56, 2001.

Iannone R: Contagious exanthematous diseases: mumps. In Hoekelman R: *Primary pediatric care*, ed 4, St Louis, 2001, Mosby.

Infectious Diseases in Children Editorial Staff: MMR and varicella vaccines safe and effective when given together, *Infect Dis Children* 15(8):28-29, 2002.

Infectious Diseases in Children Editorial Staff: FDA approves drug for use in pediatric hepatitis C, *Infect Dis Children* 16(10): 36-37, 2003.

Institute of Medicine: Immunization safety review: measles-mumps-rubella vaccine and autism, 2001a. Available at *www.iom.edu* (accessed Aug 26, 2002).

Institute of Medicine: Immunization Safety Committee report on thimerosal-containing vaccines and neurodevelopmental disorders, 2001b. Available at *www.iom.edu* (accessed Aug 26, 2002).

Institute of Medicine: Immunization safety review: multiple immunizations and immune dysfunction, 2002a. Available at *www.iom.edu* (accessed Aug 28, 2002).

Institute of Medicine: Hepatitis B and demyelinating neurological disorders, 2002b. Available at *www.iom.edu* (accessed Aug 28, 2002).

Jenson H: Epstein-Barr virus. In Behrman RE et al, editors: *Nelson textbook of pediatrics*, ed 16, Philadelphia, 2000, WB Saunders.

John G et al: Timing of breast milk HIV-1 transmission: a meta-analysis, *East Afr Med J* 78(2):75-79, 2001.

Kazacos K: Protecting children from helminthic zoonoses, *Contemp Pediatr Veterinary Med Suppl*, Mar 2000, pp 2-24.

Klein J: Management of the febrile child without a focus of infection in the era of universal pneumococcal vaccine, *Pediatr Infect Dis J* 21(6):584-588, 2002.

Kohl S: Herpes simplex virus. In Behrman RE et al, editors: *Nelson textbook of pediatrics*, ed 16, Philadelphia, 2000, WB Saunders.

Kriz P, Bobak M, Kriz B: Parental smoking, socioeconomic factors, and risk of invasive meningococcal disease in children: a population based case-control study, *Arch Dis Child* 83: 117-121, 2000.

Kronemyer B: *Haemophilus influenze* type b becomes rare disease in the US, *Infect Dis Children* 15(7):52, 2002a.

Kronemyer B: Two rarely detected viruses are now predominant enterovirus serotypes, *Infect Dis Children* 15(5):86-87, 2002b.

Leach C: Roseola (herpesvirus types 6 and 7). In Behrman RE et al, editors: *Nelson textbook of pediatrics*, ed 16, Philadelphia, 2000, WB Saunders.

Maldonado Y: Measles; subacute sclerosing panencephalitis; rubella; mumps. In Behrman RE et al, editors: *Nelson textbook of pediatrics*, ed 16, Philadelphia, 2000, WB Saunders.

McCarter-Spaulding D: Varicella infection in pregnancy, *J Obstet Gynecol Neonatal Nurs* 6:667-673, 2001.

Miller M, Cassidy J: Postinfectious arthritis and related conditions. In Behrman RE et al, editors: *Nelson textbook of pediatrics*, ed 16, Philadelphia, 2000, WB Saunders.

Mitchell M: Microbiologic diagnosis of infections. In Finberg L, Kleinman R: *Saunders manual of pediatric practice*, ed 2, Philadelphia, 2002, WB Saunders.

Morag A, Ogra P: Enteroviruses. In Behrman RE et al, editors: *Nelson textbook of pediatrics*, ed 16, Philadelphia, 2000, WB Saunders.

Myers M, Stanberry L: Varicella-zoster virus. In Behrman RE et al, editors: *Nelson textbook of pediatrics*, ed 16, Philadelphia, 2000, WB Saunders.

Nadelman R et al: Prophylaxis with a single-dose doxycycline for the prevention of Lyme disease after an *Ixodes scapularis* tick bite, *N Engl J Med* 345(2):79-84, 2001.

Nelson M: Update on management of RSV infection, *US Pharmacist* 27:7, 2002. Available at *www.uspharmacist.com* (accessed Oct 8, 2002).

New information for use of anthrax vaccine evolving, *Infect Dis Children* 15(5):22-23, 2002.

Oregon State Health Division: Smallpox: spread, control and counterintuition, *CDC Summary* 51(4):1-2, 2002.

Palmer S, Feldman S: Passive immunization for infectious diseases (excluding intravenous immune globulin). In Burg F et al, editors: *Gellis and Kagan's current pediatric therapy*, ed 17, Philadelphia, 2002, WB Saunders.

Perinatal Transmission (PETRA) Study Team: Efficacy of three short-course regimens of zidovudine and lamivudine in preventing early and late transmission of HIV-1 from mother to child in Tanzania, South Africa, and Uganda: a randomized, double-blind, placebo-controlled trial. Lancet 359:1178-1186, 2002.

Pharmacology Consult Staff: FluMist: the new intranasal influenza vaccine, *Infect Dis Children* 16(9):11-12, 2003.

Powell K: Fever. In Behrman RE et al, editors: *Nelson textbook of pediatrics*, ed 17, Philadelphia, 2004a, WB Saunders.

Powell K: Fever without focus. In Behrman RE et al, editors: *Nelson textbook of pediatrics*, ed 17, Philadelphia, 2004b, WB Saunders.

Prober CG: Managing the febrile infant: no rules are golden, *Contemp Pediatr* 16:48-55, 1999.

Reavis C: Plague, *Am J Nurse Pract* 6(2):19-21, 2002a.

Reavis C: Hemorrhagic fevers, *Am J Nurse Pract* 6(3):29-32, 2002b.

Rifkin B, Gusic M: Toxic shock syndrome in a post-op teenage girl, *J Infect Dis Children* 15(5):112-115, 2002.

Sagliocca L et al: Efficacy of hepatitis A vaccine in prevention of secondary hepatitis A infection: a randomized trial, *Lancet* 353:1136-1139, 1999.

Seward J et al: Varicella disease after introduction of varicella vaccine in the United States, 1995-2000, *JAMA* 287(5):606-611, 2002.

Shapiro E: Lyme disease. In Behrman RE et al, editors: *Nelson textbook of pediatrics*, ed 16, Philadelphia, 2000, WB Saunders.

Sigal L: Misconceptions about Lyme disease: confusions hiding behind ill-chosen terminology, *Ann Intern Med* 136(5): 413-419, 2002.

Snyder J, Pickering L: Viral hepatitis. In Behrman RE et al, editors: *Nelson textbook of pediatrics*, ed 16, Philadelphia, 2000, WB Saunders.

Starke J, Munoz I: Tuberculosis. In Behrman RE et al, editors: *Nelson textbook of pediatrics*, ed 16, Philadelphia, 2000, WB Saunders.

State of Alaska Epidemiology Bulletin: Serologic test for viral hepatitis, part 2. Available at *www.epi.hss.state.ak.us* (accessed Feb 13, 2002).

Stechenberg B: Bartonella: cat scratch disease. In Behrman RE et al, editors: *Nelson textbook of pediatrics*, ed 16, Philadelphia, 2000, WB Saunders.

Steele R: Acellular pertussis vaccine for older children. Pediatric infectious disease report given at the Pediatric Academic Societies' 2001 Annual Meeting. Baltimore, April 28-May 1, 2001a.

Steele R: Laboratory documentation of bacteremia. Pediatric infectious disease report given at the Pediatric Academic Societies 2001 Annual Meeting. Baltimore, April 28-May 1, 2001b.

Stephenson M: Unfamiliar with disease, parents are worried about vaccine safety, *Infect Dis Children* 15(7):48, 2002.

Todd J: Group A streptococcus. In Behrman RE et al, editors: *Nelson textbook of pediatrics*, ed 16, Philadelphia, 2000, WB Saunders.

Unger J, editor: Bioterrorism: what all primary care practitioners need to know, *Nursing Contact Hours for NPs* 2:41-52, 2002.

University of Wisconsin-Madison Department of Bacteriology: Bacteria 303—the bacterial flora of humans. Available at *http://bact.wisc.edu/Bact303* (accessed Dec 12, 2002).

Van Dyke R et al: Reported adherence as a determinant of response to highly active antiretroviral therapy in children who have human immunodeficiency virus infection, *Pediatrics* 109(4):e61, 2002.

Van Rossum A et al: Results of 2 years of treatment with protease inhibitor-containing antiretroviral therapy in Dutch children infected with human immunodeficiency virus type 1, *Clin Infect Dis* 34:1008-1016, 2002.

Wald E, Marcy S: Infections in daycare environments. In Burg F et al, editors: *Gellis and Kagan's current pediatric therapy*, ed 17, Philadelphia, 2002, WB Saunders.

Wharton M: Rubella. In Burg F et al, editors: *Gellis and Kagan's current pediatric therapy*, ed 17, Philadelphia, 2002, WB Saunders.

Woods C, Abramson J: Immunization practices. In Burg F et al, editors: *Gellis and Kagan's current pediatric therapy*, ed 17, Philadelphia, 2002, WB Saunders.

Working Group on Antiretroviral Therapy and Medical Management of HIV-infected Children (National Pediatric and Family Resource Center, Health Resources and Services Administration—National Institutes of Health): Guidelines for the use of antiretroviral agents in pediatric HIV infection, Dec 2001. Available at *www.nih.gov* (accessed Sept 15, 2002).

World Health Organization, Department of Vaccines and Biologicals: Supplementary information on vaccine safety. Part 2. Background rates of adverse events following immunizations. WHO/V&B/00.36, 2000. Available at *www.who.int/vaccines-documents/* (accessed Sept 15, 2002).

Wright P: Influenza viruses. In Behrman RE et al, editors: *Nelson textbook of pediatrics*, ed 16, Philadelphia, 2000a, WB Saunders.

Wright P: Parainfluenza viruses. In Behrman RE et al, editors: *Nelson textbook of pediatrics*, ed 16, Philadelphia, 2000b, WB Saunders.

Yoger R, Chadwick E: Acquired immunodeficiency syndrome (human immunodeficiency virus). In Behrman RE et al, editors: *Nelson textbook of pediatrics*, ed 16, Philadelphia, 2000, WB Saunders.

Zacharyczuk C: Blood transfusions, transplants and breast milk all linked to West Nile, *Infect Dis Children* 15(10):14, 2002a.

Zacharyczuk C: Emerging pathogens: always lurking around the bend, *Infect Dis Children* 15(7):28, 2002b.

25 Atopic Disorders and Rheumatic Diseases

Catherine J. Goodhue, Margaret A. Brady

Atopic disorders and rheumatic diseases of children share certain characteristics that lend to their combined discussion in this chapter. Inflammation, chronicity, and genetic predisposition are common to both groups of disorders. The triad of atopic disorders that may or may not coexist consists of atopic dermatitis, allergic rhinitis (or "hay fever"), and asthma.

The two most common childhood rheumatic diseases are juvenile arthritis (JA) and systemic lupus erythematosus (SLE). Both are collagen-vascular disorders that nurse practitioners (NPs) are likely to encounter in their practice. Fibromyalgia is a rheumatic disease that is gaining attention in the literature. Brief discussions of this disease, as well as chronic fatigue syndrome, are presented. Although the incidence of rheumatic fever has diminished significantly in the United States, it is still a disease that merits attention by NPs. Therefore review of its clinical presentation and treatment also is included. The immunopathogenesis and management of Henoch-Schönlein purpura, the most common vasculitis syndrome of childhood, also are discussed.

ANATOMY AND PHYSIOLOGY

Information related to the anatomy and physiology of the organ systems involved in atopic disorders and rheumatic diseases is contained in Chapters 31, 32, 37, and 38.

PATHOPHYSIOLOGY AND DEFENSE MECHANISMS

Atopic or Allergic Disorders

Allergy results as part of a specific acquired alteration in the body that has an immunologic basis. The union of antigen and antibody creates a cascade of events that culminates in biochemical reactions. There are four types of allergic reactions: I (anaphylactic reactions), II (cytotoxic reactions), III (Arthus-type reactions), and IV (delayed-type hypersensitivity). All four types of allergic reactions are mediated by circulating or cellular antibodies and generally can occur in any individual. In contrast, atopic disorders are forms of allergic reactivity that occur only in certain susceptible individuals with some unknown and probably genetic predisposition. Certain antigens (e.g., cat dander, ragweed) are problematic for atopic individuals but not for others. These atopic individuals become sensitized to the offending allergen, and an atopic disorder is the end result.

The development of an atopic disorder or allergic response involves a susceptible individual who is both exposed to an offending antigen and has a predisposition to selective synthesis of immunoglobulin E (IgE) when in contact with common environmental antigens. If these conditions are in place and contact with an offending antigen occurs, the following biochemical chain of cascading events unfolds:

- There is a brisk proliferation of T helper type 2 (Th2) cells that secrete cytokines: interleukin (IL)-3, IL-4, IL-5, IL-9, and IL-13.
- Cytokines are involved in IgE synthesis and activation of eosinophils.
- IgE binds to receptors on mast cells, basophils, and Langerhans cells.
- Chemical mediators that cause biochemical reactions and allergic-related injury to target organs (skin and respiratory tract) are released. Examples of chemical mediators include
  - Histamine
  - Prostaglandins
  - Leukotrienes
  - Eosinophil chemotactic factor of anaphylaxis

- High-molecular-weight neutrophil chemotactic factor
- Platelet-activating factor
- Arachidonic acid—cyclooxygenase and lipoxygenase products

The end result of this biochemical process is tissue injury of a target organ. Examples of tissue injury include inflammation and hyperresponsiveness, resulting in such symptoms as obstruction, increased mucus discharge, and pruritus.

Immediate allergic reactions can involve sneezing, hives, wheezing, vomiting, or anaphylaxis. Acute reactions can be followed by a late-phase response resulting from the release of toxic mediators by activated eosinophils and mononuclear cells recruited to the site of the acute allergic reaction (Boguniewicz & Leung, 2001).

The pathogenesis of atopic diseases involves a complex interrelationship of genetic, environmental, and immunologic factors. The main defense mechanism to protect against atopic disorders is the elimination of the offending substance to prevent IgE development and antigen-antibody interaction. For example, if there is a family history of atopic disorders, breastfeeding offers the protection of limited exposure to cow's milk protein and the benefit of maternal IgA and IgG antibodies. Once chemical mediators are released, the body's protective responses reduce inflammation and repair tissue damage. Pharmacologic therapy cannot cure atopic disorders but reduces symptoms and checks the allergic process. For example, drugs may be used to control inflammation (corticosteroids), compete with histamine for receptor sites on target tissues (antihistamines), and prevent mast cell degranulation and mediator release (cromolyn sodium).

Rheumatic Diseases

Juvenile arthritis is the term currently used in the United States to describe a group of conditions involving chronic inflammation of synovial joints in children younger than 16 years of age. The British use the term *chronic juvenile arthritis* (CJA) to describe these same conditions. Both JA and SLE are connective tissue disorders marked by inflammatory changes in connective tissues throughout various parts of the body. The exact cause of these collagen diseases is unknown; however, an autoimmune basis is postulated as a key factor in rheumatic disease.

There is no natural defense mechanism identified to prevent either of these diseases; however, periods of remission do occur in some children with SLE for unknown reasons, and many children with JA achieve complete remission with puberty. Because inflammation is a significant factor in these two rheumatic diseases of childhood, administration of corticosteroid preparations is a key therapy to control inflammation responsible for tissue injury and possible permanent tissue changes.

Considerations in the Pathogenesis of Juvenile Arthritis

The exact etiology of most forms of JA is unknown; however, there are two theories about its causation. Genetics is believed to be a predisposing factor to most forms of this disorder. JA, associated with clinical findings of iritis and the production of antinuclear antibodies, is found in children with histocompatibility complex antigens—human leukocyte antigen (HLA)–DR5. Children with seropositive, polyarticular disease are found to have HLA-DR4. Infectious agents also have been implicated in JA, including *Yersinia enterocolitica* and related enteric pathogens and *Klebsiella*.

The pathophysiology of JA is marked by proliferation of macrophage-like and fibroblastoid synoviocytes with subsequent infiltration of neutrophils and lymphocytes, evidence of autoimmunity, and cytokine production. The end result is nonsuppurative inflammation of the synovium that can lead to articular cartilage and joint structure erosion. Children with JA have no demonstrable immunodeficiency (Hollister, 2001; O'Neil, 2002a).

Considerations in the Pathogenesis of Systemic Lupus Erythematosus

Various immune phenomena are associated with SLE, including altered immunologic reactions in the T- and B-lymphocyte function. There is a strong link between a faulty immune mechanism and SLE. The disease is sometimes familial. Approximately 20% of children with SLE have a first-degree relative with the disease, and more than 50% of monozygotic twins are concordant for SLE. This familial pattern suggests altered cellular immunity in genetically predisposed individuals as a key factor in the pathogenesis of SLE.

There is an HLA and complement deficiency association with SLE. Other factors such as hormones (in patients older than 10 years, SLE is ninefold more common in females than males and is often precipitated by menarche, oral contraceptive use, or pregnancy), infectious agents (viral agents mostly), temperate climates, exposure to ultraviolet light, and certain drugs (e.g., hydralazine and procainamide) are thought to play a role in its pathogenesis. Characteristic pathologic findings include the production of numerous autoantibodies and impairment in the normal suppression of autoreactive B-cell clones. Immune complexes are abundant and their clearance may be impaired. In addition, the deposition of immune complexes causes inflammation of the endothelium of blood vessels leading to vasculitis in many organs that results in ischemic damage (O'Neil, 2002b).

Assessment

History. Additional key factors to consider in the history of a child who has an atopic disorder include the following:

- A family history or personal history of allergies, asthma, atopic dermatitis (eczema), or allergic rhinitis is frequently found.
- Pruritus is a significant finding in atopic dermatitis and allergic rhinitis.
- The rash of atopic dermatitis is characteristically found in certain locations of the body.
- Nighttime coughing and wheezing are characteristic of asthma.
- Signs and symptoms of allergic rhinitis and asthma may be associated with certain allergens or key triggering agents and may be seasonal.
- Coughing or shortness of breath with exercise or exertion is characteristic of asthma.

Additional key factors to consider in the history of a child who has a rheumatic disease include the following:

- History of a characteristic rash or joint involvement, or both, is common.
- The child can have other systemic manifestations of disease.

Physical Examination. The physical examination sections in Chapters 31, 32, 37, and 38 should be reviewed.

Diagnostic Studies. Various diagnostic studies or procedures can be used in the outpatient evaluation and management of children with either atopic disorders or rheumatic diseases.

Atopic Disorders. Routine chest radiographs are not indicated in most children with asthma. However, chest radiographs can be useful in selected cases of asthma or suspected asthma: in a child with atypical signs or symptoms; if a secondary infection does not clear with standard therapy; or if there are signs and symptoms of significant pulmonary involvement.

Pulmonary function tests, such as forced vital capacity, forced expiratory volume in 1 second, and forced expiratory flow, are important diagnostic tests in the diagnosis of asthma, especially in young children. Peak expiratory flow rate (PEFR) and pulse oximetry measurements can be easily and quickly done in most pediatric settings and provide additional information useful to the diagnosis and management of asthma.

Eosinophil count, determination of serum IgE concentration, radioallergosorbent test (RAST), ImmunoCAP, and prick test are not needed to confirm the diagnosis or to monitor treatment of the majority of children with an atopic disorder.

Rheumatic Diseases. Laboratory blood studies, including antinuclear antibodies (ANA), anti-DNA antibody, and determination of serum complement levels, are common tests ordered in children with SLE. Other related blood, serologic, and urine laboratory studies are indicated, depending on organ involvement (e.g., renal involvement is a frequent complication). A positive rheumatoid factor by latex fixation, ANA, or erythrocyte sedimentation rate (ESR) may be useful markers in JA.

Imaging studies are done to assess and manage joint pathology.

Management Strategies

The atopic disorders and rheumatoid diseases tend to be chronic conditions with exacerbation and remission of symptoms. Individual management strategies are based on the specific disease process and are discussed in each of their respective sections. However, certain key concepts apply to these conditions.

General Measures. The following general measures should be taken in the management of atopic disorders and rheumatic diseases:

- Encourage self-care and learning about one's disease
- Address issues of living with a chronic disease, such as
  - School, peer, and family dynamics
  - Body image
  - Adolescent adjustment
  - Patient-parent role in management of a long-term illness or chronic condition

Medications. The control of inflammation associated with atopic disorders and rheumatoid diseases is a key principle in the management of these illnesses. Corticosteroids, whether used topically on the skin, inhaled via the nostrils or throat, taken orally for systemic effect, or taken intramuscularly or intravenously for rapid systemic absorption, are a mainstay of treatment. Other pharmacologic agents commonly used are as follows:

- For atopic conditions:
  - Antipruritic agents—to control itching
  - Antihistamines—to control symptoms associated with the release of chemical mediators
  - Anticholinergics—to reduce vagal tone in the airways (may also decrease mucous gland secretion)
  - Bronchodilators—to control bronchospasm
  - Cromolyn sodium and nedocromil—to inhibit mast cell release of histamine

  - Leukotriene modifiers—to disrupt the synthesis or function of leukotrienes
  - Antibiotics—to treat secondary infections
  - Immunomodulators—to inhibit the inflammatory response
- For rheumatic diseases:
  - Analgesics (salicylates or nonsteroidal agents)—to relieve arthritis or joint pain; to relieve pain in general
  - Other therapeutic agents—to relieve signs and symptoms specific to the disease process and organ system involvement

Parent and Patient Education. Both patients and parents need to be instructed about the following:

- Signs and symptoms necessitating the immediate reevaluation of the child.
- Medications—clear instructions are needed on how much to give, when to give, side effects to watch for, how to administer, and how long medication should be taken. A written plan is highly recommended.
- Correct administration of inhaled medications. For example, when two puffs or sprays are ordered, the child should activate one puff or spray and then inhale followed in 1 to 2 minutes by a second puff or spray and second inhalation. A parent or child may think incorrectly that being told to take two puffs or two sprays means to activate two puffs or sprays and then inhale.
- Any other measures relevant to the treatment plan (e.g., bathing instructions, monitoring peak flow rate, avoidance of allergens, and environmental control).
- Parent support groups and professional organizations and resource groups.

SPECIFIC IMMUNOLOGIC PROBLEMS OF CHILDREN: COMMON ATOPIC DISORDERS

Asthma

Description

Asthma is a chronic respiratory disease and is characterized by the following features (Boguniewicz & Leung, 2001; National Heart, Lung, and Blood Institute [NHLBI], 1997):

- Immunohistopathologic responses produce
  - Shedding of airway epithelium and collagen deposition beneath the basement membrane
  - Edema
  - Mast cell activation
  - Inflammatory infiltration by eosinophils, lymphocytes (Th2-like cells), and neutrophils (especially in fatal asthma)
- Airway inflammation contributes to airflow limitations, including
  - Acute bronchoconstriction
  - Airway edema
  - Mucous plug formation
- Airflow obstruction is often reversible, either spontaneously or with treatment.
- Persistent inflammation can result in airway wall remodeling and irreversible changes.
- Airway inflammation also triggers hyperresponsiveness (to any of a variety of stimuli, such as physical, chemical, or pharmacologic agents, allergens, exercise, cold air) and is a factor in disease chronicity.

Asthma in children is classified as mild intermittent, mild persistent, moderate persistent, or severe persistent depending on symptoms, recurrences, need for specific medications, and pulmonary function measurements (Table 25-1). Children classified at any level of asthma can have episodes involving mild, moderate, or severe exacerbations. Exacerbations involve progressive worsening of shortness of breath, cough, wheezing, chest tightness, or any combination of these symptoms. The degree of airway hyperresponsiveness is usually related to the severity of asthma. Children younger than 5 years of age experience greater airway hyperresponsiveness than do older children.

Many children experience early- and late-phase responses to their asthma episode. The early asthmatic response (EAR) phase is characterized by activation of mast cells and their mediators, with bronchospasm being the key feature. EAR starts within 20 to 30 minutes of mast cell activation and resolves within approximately 1 hour if the individual is removed from the offending allergen. The late-phase asthmatic response is a prolonged inflammatory state that usually follows the EAR within a few hours, is often associated with respiratory symptoms more severe than the EAR presentation, and can last from hours to days (Moy, 2002).

Exercise-induced bronchospasm describes the phenomenon of airway narrowing during or minutes after the onset of vigorous activity. Most asthmatics exhibit airway hyperirritability after rigorous activity and display exercise-induced bronchospasm. However, for some children, exercise is the only stimulus that triggers their asthma. Although asthma is not always associated with an allergic disorder in children, many pediatric patients with chronic asthma have an allergic component. For this reason, asthma is discussed in this chapter.

Etiology and Incidence

It is not known for certain whether hyperresponsiveness of the airways is present at birth in genetically predisposed children or acquired. However, the genetic predisposition

TABLE 25-1 ***Classification of Asthma Severity in Children: Clinical Features before Treatment***

Classification and Step	Symptoms*	Nighttime Symptoms	Lung Function
Step 1: Mild intermittent	Symptoms ≤2 times per week Asymptomatic and normal PEF between exacerbations Exacerbations brief (few hours or days); varying intensity	≤2 times per month	FEV_1 or PEF ≥80% predicted PEF variability <20%
Step 2: Mild persistent	Symptoms >2 times per week but <1 time per day Exacerbations may affect activity	>2 times per month	FEV_1 or PEF ≥80% predicted PEF variability 20%-30%
Step 3: Moderate persistent	Daily symptoms Daily use of inhaled short-acting β_2-agonist Exacerbations affect activity, ≥2 times per week; may last days	>1 time per week	FEV_1 or PEF >60%; ≥80% predicted PEF variability >30%
Step 4: Severe persistent	Continual symptoms Limited physical activity Frequent exacerbations	Frequent	FEV_1 or PEF ≤60%predicted PEF variability >30%

Adapted from National Heart, Lung, and Blood Institute: *Highlights of the Expert Panel Report 2: guidelines for the diagnosis and management of asthma,* NIH pub no 97-4051A, Bethesda, MD, 1997, National Institutes of Health.
*Having at least one symptom in a particular step places the child in that particular classification.
FEV_1, forced expiratory volume in 1 second; *PEF,* peak expiratory flow.

for the development of an IgE-mediated response to common aeroallergens, known as atopy, remains the strongest identifiable predisposing risk factor for asthma.

The morbidity and mortality statistics of asthma in childhood demonstrate an alarming increase in the prevalence of asthma and its complications. Asthma has become a leading reason for pediatric hospital admissions and accounts for 5.8 million visits annually to pediatric settings (Centers for Disease Control and Prevention, 2002). Occupational or environmental exposure can cause airway inflammation associated with asthma. Factors known to precipitate or aggravate asthma in children include the following:

- Atopic individual response to allergens—inhaled, topical, ingested
- Viral infections
- Exposure to known irritants (paint fumes, smoke) and occupational chemicals
- Gastroesophageal reflux
- Exposure to tobacco smoke (for infants, especially smoking by mother)
- Environmental changes—rapid changes in barometric pressure, weather, especially cold air
- Exercise
- Psychologic factors (e.g., anxiety attack or panic disorder)
- Allergic rhinitis and sinusitis
- Emotional stress (both positive and negative emotions)
- Drugs (e.g., aspirin, β-blockers)
- Food additives (sulfites)
- Endocrine factors

Allergen-induced asthma results in hyperresponsive airways. The majority of children with asthma show evidence of sensitization to any of the following inhalant allergens:

- House dust mites, cockroaches, indoor molds
- Saliva and dander of cats and dogs
- Outdoor seasonal molds
- Airborne pollens—trees, grasses, and weeds

Food allergens (e.g., cow's milk protein) can cause asthma but are generally problematic only in infants (Boguniewicz & Leung, 2001). The mechanism by which allergens cause asthma is explained in the earlier section on pathophysiology and defense mechanisms.

Clinical Findings

History. The history of a patient being seen for asthma can include the following:

- Family history of asthma or other related allergic disorders (e.g., eczema or allergic rhinitis)
- Conditions associated with asthma (e.g., chronic sinusitis, nasal polyposis, gastroesophageal reflux, and chronic otitis media)

- Complaints of chest tightness or dyspnea
- Cough, particularly at night and in the early morning
- Cough or shortness of breath with exercise or exertion
- Seasonal, continuous, or episodic pattern of symptoms
- Episodes of recurrent "bronchitis" or pneumonia
- Precipitation of symptoms by known aggravating factors

Physical Examination. The following may be seen on physical examination:

- Wheezing (may be absent if severe obstruction) or coughing
- Prolonged expiratory phase, high-pitched rhonchi
- Diminished breath sounds
- Signs of respiratory distress, including tachypnea, retractions, nasal flaring, use of accessory muscles, increasing restlessness, apprehension, agitation, drowsiness to coma
- Tachycardia, hypertension or hypotension, pulsus paradoxus
- Cyanosis of lips and nail beds if underlying hypoxemia
- Other possible associated findings include sinusitis, flexural eczema, and rhinitis

Diagnostic Studies. Use of various laboratory and radiographic tests should be individualized to the child and based on symptoms, severity or chronology of the disease, response to therapy, and age. Tests to consider include the following:

- A complete blood count (CBC) if secondary infection or anemia is suspected (also check for elevated numbers of eosinophils).
- Chest radiograph only if secondary respiratory infection or other pulmonary disorders are suspected or if under 1 year of age with persistent wheezing.
- Sinus radiographs may be helpful if sinusitis is suspected; however, computed tomography (CT) scans are more sensitive and specific.
- Allergic workup, including skin testing, immunoglobulins, RAST, or ImmunoCAP.
- Sweat test if cystic fibrosis is a possibility.
- Oxygen saturation by pulse oximetry to assess severity of acute exacerbation. Pulse oximetry measures the oxygen saturation (SaO_2) of hemoglobin—the percent of total hemoglobin that is oxygenated—as follows:
  - Greater than 95%, mild
  - 90% to 95%, moderate
  - Less than 90%, severe lack of oxygen
- Pulmonary function tests:
  - Formal spirometry testing is the gold standard in children older than 5 years for diagnosing asthma.
  - Start with PEFR assessment in children 4 to 5 years of age or older; use to assess the severity of airflow obstruction and to monitor the effectiveness of β-agonist treatment (measurements before and after treatments).
  - Consider the use of more sophisticated pulmonary studies for the child with severe asthma.

Pulmonary monitoring and typical findings include the following:

- Can use PEFR in some children as young as 4 to 5 years. Use child's personal best value as a guideline to help detect possible changes in airway obstruction; can use predicted range for height and age if personal best rate is not available (Table 25-2 and Fig. 25-1).

TABLE 25-2 ***Predicted Average Peak Expiratory Flow for Normal Children and Adolescents***

Height (in)	Males and Females (L/min)
43	147
44	160
45	173
46	187
47	200
48	214
49	227
50	240
51	254
52	267
53	280
54	293
55	307
56	320
57	334
58	347
59	360
60	373
61	387
62	400
63	413
64	427
65	440
66	454
67	467

From National Heart, Lung, and Blood Institute: *Executive summary: guidelines for the diagnosis and management of asthma*, NIH pub no 94-3042A, Bethesda, MD, 1994, National Institutes of Health. Adapted from Polger G, Promedhar V: *Pulmonary function testing in children: techniques and standards*, Philadelphia, 1971, WB Saunders.

NOTE: It is recommended that peak expiratory flow rate (PEFR) objectives for therapy be based on each individual's "personal best," which is established after a period of PEFR monitoring while the individual is under effective treatment.

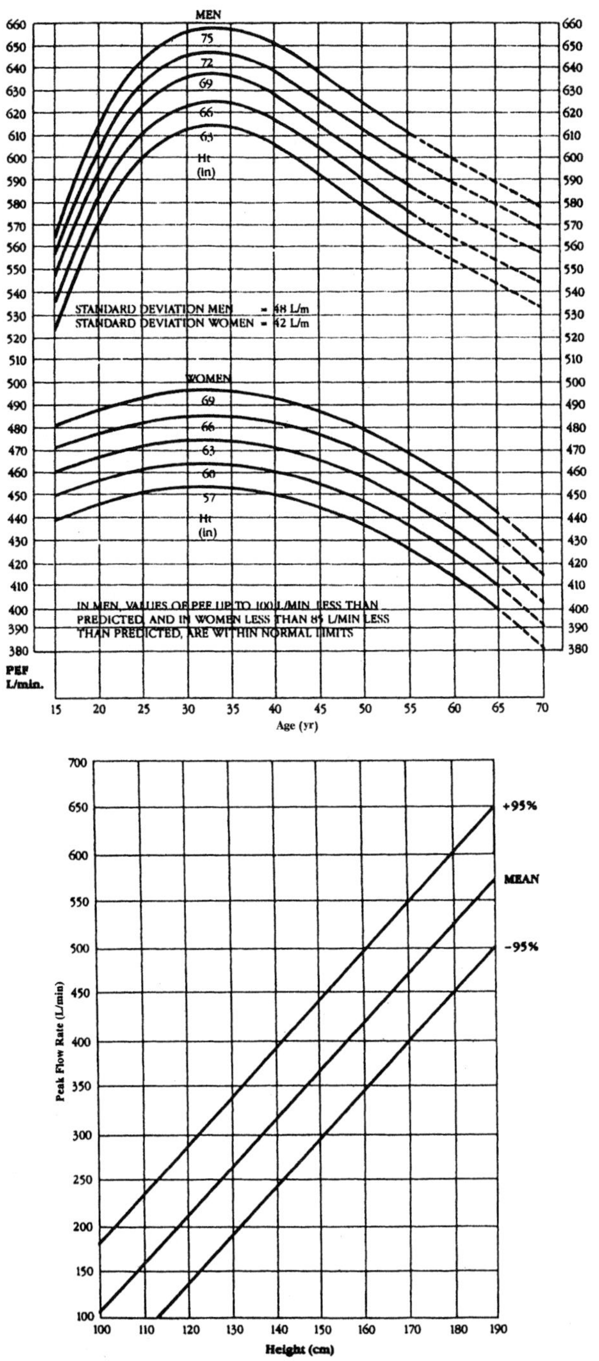

FIGURE 25-1 Sample peak expiratory flow rate nomogram. (From National Heart, Lung, and Blood Institute: *Executive summary: guidelines for the diagnosis and management of asthma*, pub no 94-3042A, Bethesda, MD, 1994, National Institutes of Health. *Top*, Adapted from Nunn AJ, Gregg I: New regression equations for predicting peak expiratory flow in adults, *BMJ* 298:1068-1070, 1989. *Bottom*, Adapted from Godfrey S, Kamburoff PL, Nairn JR: Spirometry, lung volumes and airway resistance in normal children aged 5 to 18 years, *Br J Dis Chest* 64:15-24, 1970.)

- Interpretation of PEFR reading (see Box 25-1 for use of peak flow meter and interpretation of results)—if PEFR is in the
  - Green zone: 80% to 100% of personal best signals good control.
  - Yellow zone: 50% to 80% of personal best signals caution.
  - Red zone: below 50% of personal best signals major airflow obstruction.
- Chest radiograph findings: hyperinflation of the lungs with flattening of the diaphragm on radiograph with or without patchy infiltrate or atelectasis (Boguniewicz & Leung, 2001; Moy, 2002).

Differential Diagnosis

Numerous conditions can cause airway obstruction and be incorrectly confused with asthma, especially in young children and infants. Examples include the following:

- Acute bronchiolitis, laryngotracheobronchitis, bronchopneumonia
- Bronchial foreign body aspiration
- Congenital malformations of the respiratory, cardiovascular, or gastrointestinal systems
- Cystic fibrosis

BOX 25-1 *Use of the Peak Flow Meter and Its Interpretation*

Steps to Follow in Using a Peak Flow Meter

1. Have child stand up.
2. Make sure that indicator is at the base of the numbered scale.
3. Ask child to take a deep breath.
4. Have the child place the peak flow meter in the mouth with the lips sealing the mouthpiece.
5. Tell the child to blow out as hard and fast as possible.
6. Record the rate.
7. Repeat steps 2 through 6 two more times.
8. Record the highest of the three values.

Peak Expiratory Flow Rate (PEFR)

The maximum flow rate that is produced during forced expiration with fully inflated lungs.

Personal Best Value

The highest value that an individual achieves in measuring PEFR is known as one's "personal best" value or rate. Using the personal best value is the most accurate gauge to use to interpret changes in peak flow measurements, because the child's own scores are used as the standard for comparison.

- Tracheal or foreign body compression (e.g., aortic ring, tumors)
- Chronic lower respiratory tract infections caused by immunodeficiency disorders
- Recurrent aspirations

Management

"Guidelines for the Diagnosis and Management of Asthma—Update on Selected Topics 2002" (NHLBI, 2002) and *Highlights of the Expert Panel Report 2: Guidelines for the Diagnosis and Management of Asthma* (NHLBI, 1997) are the most recent standards for the treatment of asthma in children. Management strategies are based on whether the child has mild intermittent, mild persistent, moderate persistent, or severe persistent asthma. A stepwise approach is recommended. If control of symptoms is not maintained at a particular step of classification and management, the health care provider first should reevaluate for compliance and administration factors. If these factors do not appear to be responsible for the lack of symptom control, the health care provider should go to the next higher step. Likewise, gradual stepdowns in treatment may be considered every 1 to 6 months.

In this chapter, the outpatient management of mild intermittent, mild persistent, moderate persistent, and severe asthma is discussed, as is the outpatient management of acute exacerbations. The practitioner should refer to other textbooks for management of severe asthma requiring hospitalization.

Chronic Asthma. Treatment of chronic asthma in children is based on general control measures and pharmacotherapy. General control measures include the following:

- Avoid exposure to known allergens or irritants.
- Administer yearly influenza vaccine.
- Control environment to eliminate or reduce offending allergen.
- Provide allergen immunotherapy.
- Treat rhinitis, sinusitis, or gastroesophageal reflux.
- See section on patient education for other measures.

The pharmacologic management of asthma in children is based on the classification of the severity of asthma and the child's age. A child's classification can change over time. Also, within any classification, a child may experience mild, moderate, or severe exacerbations. Table 25-1 lists the four classifications of asthma based on severity of clinical manifestations. A stepwise approach to treatment is based on severity of symptoms and the use of pharmacotherapy to control chronic symptoms, maintain normal activity, prevent recurrent exacerbations, minimize adverse side effects, and maintain nearly "normal" pulmonary function. Tables 25-3 and 25-4 show the management plan for children

TABLE 25-3 ***Stepwise Approach for Managing Infants and Young Children (5 Years of Age and Younger) with Acute or Chronic Asthma***

Classify Severity: Clinical Features Before Treatment or Adequate Control		Medications Required To Maintain Long-Term Control
	Symptoms/Day Symptoms/Night	Daily Medications
Step 4 **Severe Persistent**	Continual Frequent	▪ **Preferred treatment:** – **High-dose inhaled corticosteroids** **AND** – **Long-acting inhaled β_2-agonists** **AND**, if needed, – Corticosteroid tablets or syrup long term (2 mg/kg/day, generally do not exceed 60 mg per day). (Make repeat attempts to reduce systemic corticosteroids and maintain control with high-dose inhaled corticosteroids.)

TABLE 25-3 ***Stepwise Approach for Managing Infants and Young Children (5 Years of Age and Younger) with Acute or Chronic Asthma—cont'd***

Step 3 **Moderate Persistent**	Daily >1 night/wk	■ **Preferred treatments:** – **Low-dose inhaled corticosteroids and long-acting inhaled β_2-agonists** **OR** – **Medium-dose inhaled corticosteroids.** ■ Alternative treatment: – Low-dose inhaled corticosteroids and either leukotriene receptor antagonist or theophylline. If needed (particularly in patients with recurring severe exacerbations): ■ **Preferred treatment:** – **Medium-dose inhaled corticosteroids and long-acting β_2-agonists.** ■ Alternative treatment: – Medium-dose inhaled corticosteroids and either leukotriene receptor antagonist or theophylline.
Step 2 **Mild Persistent**	>2/wk but <1x/day >2 nights/mo	■ **Preferred treatment:** – **Low-dose inhaled corticosteroids (with nebulizer or MDI with holding chamber with or without face mask or DPI).** ■ Alternative treatment (listed alphabetically): – Cromolyn (nebulizer is preferred or MDI with holding chamber) OR leukotriene receptor antagonist.
Step 1 **Mild Intermittent**	≤2 days/wk ≤2 nights/mo	■ No daily medication needed.

Quick Relief
All Patients

- Bronchodilator as needed for symptoms. Intensity of treatment will depend on severity of exacerbation.
  - Preferred treatment: **Short-acting inhaled β_2-agonists** by nebulizer or face mask and space/holding chamber
  - Alternative treatment: Oral β_2-agonists
- With viral respiratory infection
  - Bronchodilator q4-6hr up to 24 hr (longer with physician consult); in general, repeat no more than once every 6 wk
  - Consider systemic corticosteroid if exacerbation is severe or patient has history of previous severe exacerbations
- Use of short-acting β_2-agonists >2 times a week in intermittent asthma (daily, or increasing use in persistent asthma) may indicate the need to initiate (increase) long-term-control therapy.

Step down
Review treatment every 1 to 6 mo; a gradual stepwise reduction in treatment may be possible.

Step up
If control is not maintained, consider step up. First, review patient medication technique, adherence, and environmental control.

Goals of Therapy: Asthma Control

- Minimal or no chronic symptoms day or night
- Minimal or no exacerbations
- No limitations on activities; no school/parent's work missed
- Minimal use of short-acting inhaled β_2-agonist
- Minimal or no adverse effects from medications

Note

- The stepwise approach is intended to assist, not replace, the clinical decisionmaking required to meet individual patient needs.
- Classify severity: assign patient to most severe step in which any feature occurs.
- There are very few studies on asthma therapy for infants.
- Gain control as quickly as possible (a course of short systemic corticosteroids may be required); then step down to the least medication necessary to maintain control.
- Minimize use of short-acting inhaled β_2-agonists. Over-reliance on short-acting inhaled β_2-agonists (e.g., use of short-acting inhaled β_2-agonist every day, increasing use or lack of expected effect, or use of approximately one canister a month even if not using it every day) indicates inadequate control of asthma and the need to initiate or intensify long-term-control therapy.
- Provide parent education on asthma management and controlling environmental factors that make asthma worse (e.g., allergies and irritants).
- Consultation with an asthma specialist is recommended for patients with moderate or severe persistent asthma. Consider consultation for patients with mild persistent asthma.

From Executive Summary of the NAEPP Expert Panel Report: *Guideline for the diagnosis and management of asthma*: update on selected topics, 2002, NIH pub no 02-5075, Bethesda, MD, June 2002, National Institutes of Health.
DPI, Dry powder inhaler; *MDI*, metered-dose inhaler.

TABLE 25-4 *Stepwise Approach for Managing Asthma in Adults and Children Older Than 5 Years of Age: Treatment*

Classify Severity: Clinical Features Before Treatment or Adequate Control			Medications Required To Maintain Long-Term Control
	Symptoms/Day **Symptoms/Night**	**PEF or FEV_1** **PEF Variability**	**Daily Medications**
Step 4 **Severe Persistent**	Continual Frequent	≤60% >30%	▪ **Preferred treatment:** – **High-dose inhaled corticosteroids** AND – **Long-acting inhaled β_2-agonists** AND, if needed, – Corticosteroid tablets or syrup long term (2 mg/kg/day, generally do not exceed 60 mg per day). (Make repeat attempts to reduce systemic corticosteroids and maintain control with high-dose inhaled corticosteroids.)
Step 3 **Moderate Persistent**	Daily >1 night/wk	>60%-<80% >30%	▪ **Preferred treatment:** – **Low-to-medium dose inhaled corticosteroids and long-acting inhaled β_2-agonists.** ▪ Alternative treatment (listed alphabetically): – Increase inhaled corticosteroids within medium-dose range OR – Low-to-medium dose inhaled corticosteroids and either leukotriene modifier or theophylline. If needed (particularly in patients with recurring severe exacerbations): ▪ **Preferred treatment:** – **Increase inhaled corticosteroids within medium-dose range and add long-acting inhaled β_2-agonists.** ▪ Alternative treatment: – Increase inhaled corticosteroids within medium-dose range and add either leukotriene modifier or theophylline.
Step 2 **Mild Persistent**	>2/week but <1x/day >2 nights/mo	≥80% 20-30%	▪ **Preferred treatment:** – **Low-dose inhaled corticosteroids.** ▪ Alternative treatment (listed alphabetically): cromolyn, leukotriene modifier, nedocromil, OR sustained release theophylline to serum concentration of 5-15 mcg/mL.
Step 1 **Mild Intermittent**	≤2 days/wk ≤2 nights/mo	≥80% <20%	▪ No daily medication needed. ▪ Severe exacerbations may occur, separated by long periods of normal lung function and no symptoms. A course of systemic corticosteroids is recommended.

Quick Relief
All Patients

- Short-acting bronchodilator: **2-4 puffs short-acting inhaled β_2-agonists** as needed for symptoms.
- Intensity of treatment will depend on severity of exacerbation; up to 3 treatments at 20-minute intervals or a single nebulizer treatment as needed. Course of systemic corticosteroids may be needed.
- Use of short-acting β_2-agonists >2 times a week in intermittent asthma (daily, or increasing use in persistent asthma) may indicate the need to initiate (increase) long-term-control therapy.

TABLE 25-4 *Stepwise Approach for Managing Asthma in Adults and Children Older Than 5 Years of Age: Treatment—cont'd*

Step down
Review treatment every 1 to 6 months; a gradual stepwise reduction in treatment may be possible.

Step up
If control is not maintained, consider step up. First, review patient medication technique, adherence, and environmental control.

Goals of Therapy: Asthma Control

- Minimal or no chronic symptoms day or night
- Minimal or no exacerbations
- No limitations on activities; no school/work missed
- Maintain (near) normal pulmonary function
- Minimal use of short-acting inhaled β_2-agonist
- Minimal or no adverse effects from medications

Note

- The stepwise approach is meant to assist, not replace, the clinical decisionmaking required to meet individual patient needs.
- Classify severity: assign patient to most severe step in which any feature occurs (PEF is % of personal best; FEV_1 is % predicted).
- Gain control as quickly as possible (consider a short course of systemic corticosteroids); then step down to the least medication necessary to maintain control.
- Minimize use of short-acting inhaled β_2-agonists. Over-reliance on short-acting inhaled β_2-agonists (e.g., use of short-acting inhaled β_2-agonist every day, increasing use or lack of expected effect, or use of approximately one canister a month even if not using it every day) indicates inadequate control of asthma and the need to initiate or intensify long-term-control therapy.
- Provide education on self-management and controlling environmental factors that make asthma worse (e.g., allergens and irritants).
- Refer to an asthma specialist if there are difficulties controlling asthma or if step 4 care is required. Referral may be considered if step 3 care is required.

From Executive Summary of the NAEPP Expert Panel Report: *Guidelines for the diagnosis and management of asthma: update on selected topics, 2002,* NIH pub no 02-5075, Bethesda, MD, June 2002, National Institutes of Health.
FEV_1, Forced expiratory volume in 1 second; *PEF*, peak expirate, flow.

5 years of age and younger and for children older than 5 years of age, respectively.

Important considerations to note in the pharmacologic treatment of asthma include the following:

- Control of asthma should be gained as quickly as possible by starting at the classification step most appropriate to the initial severity of the child's symptoms or at a higher level (e.g., a course of systemic corticosteroids or higher dose of inhaled corticosteroid). After control of symptoms, decrease treatment to the least amount of medication needed to maintain control.
- Systemic corticosteroids may be needed at any time and step if there is a major flare-up of symptoms.
- Children with intermittent asthma may have long periods in which they are symptom free; they can also have life-threatening exacerbations, often provoked by respiratory infection. In these situations, a short course of systemic corticosteroids should be used (NHLBI, 1997).
- Variations in asthma necessitate individualized treatment plans.
- The β_2-agonist can be given by nebulization with a compressor (e.g., Pulmo-Aide). Nebulization can be a more effective route than metered-dose inhaler (MDI) therapy for young infants (2 years of age or younger) or children who progress to moderate or severe airway obstruction.
- A spacer or holding chamber (Aerochamber or Inspirease) enhances the delivery of MDI medications to the lower airways of a child and is strongly recommended. Spacers eliminate the need to synchronize inhalation with activation of MDI.
- Dry powder inhalers (DPIs) such as Serevent Diskus, Pulmicort Turbuhaler, and Flovent Diskus do not need spacers or shaking before use. The child must rinse mouth with water and spit after inhalation. DPIs should not be used in children younger than 4 to 5 years.
- Different inhaled corticosteroids are not equal in potency to each other on a per puff or microgram basis. Table 25-5 compares the daily low, medium, and high doses of the various inhaled corticosteroids used for children. Combination inhaled corticoseroid/long-acting β_2-agonist can now be used in children age 12 years and older.
- For treatment of exercise-induced bronchospasm:
  - Use either an inhaled short-acting β_2-agonist or a mast cell stabilizer (cromolyn or nedocromil) or both. Combination of both types of drugs is the more effective therapy. A long-acting β_2-agonist can be used in older children.
  - Use two puffs of a β_2-agonist, cromolyn, or nedocromil 20 minutes before exercise.
  - An extended warming-up period may promote a refractory state and eliminate the need for repeat medications (Boguniewicz & Leung, 2001; Moy, 2002).

Table 25-6 identifies the usual dosages for long-term control medications (exclusive of inhaled corticosteroids)

TABLE 25-5 ***Estimated Comparative Daily Dosages for Inhaled Corticosteroids***

	Low Daily Dose		Medium Daily Dose		High Daily Dose	
Drug	**Child***	**Adult**	**Child***	**Adult**	**Child***	**Adult**
Beclomethasone CFC (42 or 84 μg/puff)	84-336 μg	168-504 μg	336-672 μg	504-840 μg	>672 μg	>840 μg
Beclomethasone HFA (40 or 80 μg/puff)	80-160 μg	80-240 μg	160-320 μg	240-480 μg	>320 μg	>480 μg
Budesonide DPI (200 μg/inhalation)	200-400 μg	200-600 μg	400-800 μg	600-1200 μg	>800 μg	>1200 μg
Inhalation suspension for nebulization (child dose)	0.5 mg		1.0 mg		2.0 mg	
Flunisolide (250 μg/puff)	500-750 μg	500-1000 μg	1000-1250 μg	1000-2000 μg	>1250 μg	>2000 μg
Fluticasone						
• MDI: 44, 110, or 220 μg/puff	88-176 μg	88-264 μg	176-440 μg	264-660 μg	>440 μg	>660 μg
• DPI: 50, 100, or 250 μg/inhalation	100-200 μg	100-300 μg	200-400 μg	300-600 μg	>400 μg	>600 μg
Triamcinolone acetonide 100 μg/puff	400-800 μg	400-1000 μg	800-1200 μg	1000-2000 μg	>1200 μg	>2000 μg

From Executive Summary of the NAEPP Expert Panel Report: *Guidelines for the diagnosis and management of asthma: update on selected topics, 2002,* NIH pub no 02-5075, Bethesda, MD, June 2002, National Institutes of Health.
DPI, Dry powder inhaler; *MDI,* metered-dose inhaler.
*≤12 years of age.

used to treat asthma in children. Quick-relief medications are listed in Table 25-7.

Practice parameters are guides and should not replace individualized treatment based on clinical judgment and unique differences in patients.

Acute Exacerbations of Asthma. The treatment of acute episodes of asthma is based on classification of the severity of the episode. Acute episodes are classified as mild, moderate, and severe (Table 25-8). Early recognition of warning signs and treatment should be stressed in both patient or parent education, or both.

Characteristics of a *mild acute episode* are

- Wheezing, usually end expiratory
- Increased respiratory rate

TABLE 25-6 ***Long-Term Control Medications for the Treatment of Asthma***

Medication	**Dosage Form**	**Child Dose**‡	**Adult Dose**	**Comments**
Inhaled Corticosteroids—See Table 25-5				
Systemic Corticosteroids ***(applies to all three corticosteroids)***				
Methylprednisolone	2, 4, 8, 16, 32 mg tablets	0.25-2 mg/kg daily in a single dose in AM or qod as needed for control	7.5-60 mg daily in a single dose in AM or qod as needed for control	For long-term treatment of severe persistent asthma, administer single dose in morning either daily or on alternate days (alternate-day therapy may produce less adrenal suppression). If daily doses are required, one study suggests improved efficacy and no increase in adrenal suppression when administered at 3:00 PM.
Prednisolone	5 mg tablets, 5 mg/5 ml, 15 mg/5 ml	Same as above	Same as above	

TABLE 25-6 ***Long-Term Control Medications for the Treatment of Asthma—cont'd***

Medication	Dosage Form	Child Dose[‡]	Adult Dose	Comments
Prednisone	1, 2.5, 5, 10, 20, 50 mg tablets; 5 mg/ml, 5 mg/5 ml	Short-course "burst": 1-2 g/kg/day, maximum 60 mg/day for 3-10 days	Short-course "burst" to achieve control: 40-60 mg per day as single or 2 divided doses for 3-10 days	Short courses or "bursts" are effective for establishing control when initiating therapy or during a period of gradual deterioration. The bursts should be continued until patient achieves 80% PEFR personal best or symptoms resolve. This usually requires 3-10 days but may require longer. There is no evidence that tapering the dose following improvement prevents relapse.
Cromolyn and Nedocromil				
Cromolyn	MDI 1 mg/puff nebulizer; 20 mg/ampule	1-2 puffs tid-qid 1 ampule tid-qid	2-4 puffs tid-qid 1 ampule tid-qid	One dose before exercise or allergen exposure provides effective prophylaxis for 1-2 hr.
Nedocromil	MDI 1.75 mg/puff	1-2 puffs bid-qid	2-4 puffs bid-qid	See cromolyn above.
Inhaled Long-Acting β_2-Agonists ***(should not be used for symptom relief or for exacerbations; use with inhaled corticosteroids)***				
Salmeterol	MDI 21 μg/puff DPI 50 μg/blister	1-2 puffs q12hr 1 blister q12hr	2 puffs q12hr 1 blister q12hr	May use one dose nightly for symptoms. Do not use as a rescue inhaler for symptom relief or for exacerbations.
Formoterol	DPI: 12 μg/single-use capsule	1 capsule q12hr	1 capsule q12hr	
Sustained-release albuterol	4 mg tablet* 8 mg tablet[†]	4 mg bid	4-8 mg bid	For children 6 yr and older.
Methylxanthines				
Theophylline (numerous manufacturers)	Liquids Sustained-release tablets and capsules	Starting dose 10 mg/kg per day; usual maximum dose: ≥1 yr of age: 16 mg/kg per day <1 yr of age: 0.2 (age in wk) + 5 = mg/kg per day	Starting dose 10 mg/kg per day up to 300 mg maximum; usual maximum 800 mg/day	Routine serum theophylline level monitoring is required (serum concentration 5-15 μg/ml); not commonly used with pediatric patients.
Leukotriene Modifiers				
Montelukast	4 or 5 mg chewable tablet, 10 mg tablet	4 mg qhs (2-5 yr) 5 mg qhs (6-14 yr) 10 mg qhs (>14 yr)	10 mg qhs	
Zafirlukast	10 or 20 mg tablet	20 mg daily (7-11 yr) (10 mg tablet bid)	40 mg daily (20 mg tablet bid)	Take zafirlukast at least 1 hr before or 2 hr after meals.
Zileuton	300 or 600 mg tablet		2400 mg daily (give tablets qid)	Monitor hepatic enzymes (ALT).
Combined Medication				
Fluticasone/salmeterol DPI	100, 250, or 500 μg/50 μg	1 inhalation bid; dose depends on severity of asthma	1 inhalation bid; dose depends on severity of asthma	

*Proventil and Repetabs come in 4 mg only.
[†]Volmax comes in 4 mg and 8 mg.
[‡]≤12 years of age.
ALT, Alanine aminotransferase; *DPI*, dry powder inhaler; *MDI*, metered-dose inhaler; *PEFR*, peak expiratory flow rate.

TABLE 25-7 *Quick-Relief Medications for the Treatment of Asthma*

Medication	Dosage Form	Child Dose*	Adult Dose	Comments
Short-Acting Inhaled β_2-Agonists				
Metered-Dose Inhalers				
Albuterol	90 μg/puff, 200 puffs	1-2 puffs 15-30 min before exercise	2 puffs 15-30 min before exercise	An increasing use or lack of expected effect indicates diminished control of asthma.
Albuterol HFA	90 μg/puff, 200 puffs	2 puffs tid-qid	2 puffs tid-qid	Not generally recommended for long-term treatment. Regular use on a daily basis indicates the need for additional long-term control therapy.
Bitolterol	370 μg/puff, 300 puffs		2 puffs q8hr maximum: 2 puffs q4hr	Differences in potency exist so that all products are essentially equipotent on a per puff basis.
Pirbuterol	200 μg/puff, 400 puffs		1-2 puffs q4-6hr	May double usual dose for mild exacerbations. **Nonselective agents (e.g., epinephrine, isoproterenol, metaproterenol) are not recommended because of their potential for excessive cardiac stimulation, especially at high doses.**
Dry Powder Inhalers				
Albuterol Rotahaler	200 μg/capsule	1 capsule q4-6hr as needed and before exercise	1-2 capsules q4-6hr as needed and before exercise	
Nebulizer Solution				
Albuterol	5 mg/ml (0.5%)	0.05 mg/kg (minimum 1.25 mg, maximum 2.5 mg) in 2-3 ml of saline q4-6hr	1.25-5 mg (0.25-1 ml) in 2-3 ml of saline q4-8hr	May mix with cromolyn or ipratropium nebulizer solutions; may double dose for mild exacerbations
Bitolterol	2 mg/ml (0.2%)	Not established	0.5-1.5 mg (0.25-0.75 ml) in 2-3 ml of saline q8hr	May not mix with other nebulizer solutions. Minimum 4 hr interval.
Levalbuterol	0.31 mg/3 ml 0.63 mg/3 ml 1.25 mg/3 ml	0.31 mg tid q6-8hr maximim: 0.63 mg tid	0.63 mg tid q6-8hr maximum: 1.25 mg tid	For children 6-11 yr
Anticholinergics				
Metered-Dose Inhalers				
Ipratropium	18 μg/puff, 200 puffs	1-2 puffs tid	2 puffs q6hr	Evidence is lacking for producing added benefit to β_2-agonists in long-term asthma therapy.
Nebulizer Solution				
Ipratropium	0.25 mg/ml (0.025%)	0.25 mg q6hr	0.25-0.5 mg q6hr	
Systemic Corticosteroids (Dosage applies to all three corticosteroids)				
Methylprednisolone	2, 4, 8, 16, 32 mg tablets	Short-course "burst": 1-2 mg/kg/day, maximum 60 mg/day, for 3-10 days	Short-course "burst" to achieve control: 40-60 mg per day as single or 2 divided doses for 3-10 days	Short courses or "bursts" are effective for establishing control when initiating therapy or during a period of gradual deterioration.

TABLE 25-7 *Quick-Relief Medications for the Treatment of Asthma—cont'd*

Medication	Dosage Form	Child Dose*	Adult Dose	Comments
Prednisolone	5 mg tablets, 5 mg/5 ml, 15 mg/5 ml			
Prednisone	1, 2.5, 5, 10, 20, 25 mg tablets: 5 mg/ml, 5 mg/5 ml			The burst should be continued until patient achieves 80% PEFR personal best or symptoms resolve; this usually requires 3-10 days but may require longer; there is no evidence that tapering the dose following improvement prevents relapse.

Adapted from the National Heart, Lung, and Blood Institute: *Highlights of the Expert Panel Report 2: guidelines for the diagnosis and management of asthma*, NIH pub no 97-4051A, Bethesda, MD, 1997, National Institutes of Health; and Taketomo CK, Hodding JH, Kraus DM: *Pediatric dosage handbook*, ed 9, Hudson, OH, 2002, Lexi-Comp.
PEFR, Peak expiratory flow rate.
*≤12 years of age.

TABLE 25-8 *Classifying Severity of Asthma Exacerbations**

	Mild	Moderate	Severe	Respiratory Arrest Imminent
Symptoms				
Breathless	While walking	While talking (infant—softer, shorter cry; difficulty feeding)	While at rest (infant—stops feeding)	
	Can lie down	Prefers sitting	Sits upright	
Talks in	Sentences	Phrases	Words	
Alertness	May be agitated	Usually agitated	Usually agitated	Drowsy or confused
Signs				
Respiratory rate	Increased	Increased	Often >30/min	
	Guide to rates of breathing in awake children:			
	Age	*Normal rate*		
	<2 mo	<60/min		
	2-12 mo	<50/min		
	1-5 yr	<40/min		
	6-8 yr	<30/min		
Use of accessory muscles; suprasternal retractions	Usually not	Commonly	Usually	Paradoxic thoracoabdominal movement
Wheeze	Moderate, often only end expiratory	Loud; throughout exhalation	Usually loud; throughout inhalation and exhalation	Absence of wheeze
Pulse/min	<100	100-120	>120	Bradycardia
	Guide to normal pulse rates in children:			
	Age	*Normal rate*		
	2-12 mo	<160/min		
	1-2 yr	<120/min		
	2-8 yr	<110/min		

Continued

TABLE 25-8 *Classifying Severity of Asthma Exacerbations—cont'd*

	Mild	Moderate	Severe	Respiratory Arrest Imminent
Pulsus paradoxus	Absent <10 mm Hg	May be present 10-25 mm Hg	Often present >25 mm Hg (adult), 20-40 mm Hg (child)	Absence suggests respiratory muscle fatigue
Functional Assessment				
PEFR % predicted or % personal best	80%	Approximately 50%-80%	<50% predicted or personal best, or response lasts <2 hr	
PaO_2 (on room air) and/or	Normal (test not usually necessary)	>60 mm Hg (test not usually necessary)	<60 mm Hg: possible cyanosis	
PCO_2	<42 mm Hg (test not usually necessary)	<42 mm Hg (test not usually necessary)	≥42 mm Hg: possible respiratory failure	
SaO_2% (on room air) at sea level	>95% (test not usually necessary)	91%-95%	<91%	
Hypercapnia (hypoventilation) develops more readily in young children than in adults and adolescents				

From National Heart, Lung, and Blood Institute: *Highlights of the Expert Panel Report 2: guidelines for the diagnosis and management of asthma*, NIH pub no 97-4051A, Bethesda, MD, 1997, National Institutes of Health.
*The presence of several parameters, but not necessarily all, indicates the general classification of the exacerbation. Many of these parameters have not been systematically studied, so they serve only as general guides.
PaO_2, Partial pressure of oxygen in arterial blood; *PCO_2*, partial pressure of carbon dioxide; *PEFR*, peak expiratory flow rate; *SaO_2*, oxygen saturation in arterial blood.

- No signs of respiratory distress, cyanosis, or activity restriction
- PEFR or forced expiratory volume (FEV) greater than 80% of expected value
- Ability to speak in normal sentences between breaths

Children with a *moderate acute episode* of asthma manifest the following:

- Audible wheeze
- Use of accessory muscles
- Increase in respiratory rate
- Unable to walk or utter more than three to five words between breaths

Manifestations of a *severe acute episode* of asthma in children include the following signs of severe respiratory distress:

- Cyanosis
- Use of accessory muscles plus lower rib and suprasternal retractions
- Agitation and the ability to say only single words between breaths
- Loud wheezing both on inhalation and expiration (NHLBI, 1997)

The *initial pharmacologic treatment* for acute asthma exacerbations is inhaled short-acting β_2-agonists, two to four puffs every 20 minutes for three treatments by way of MDI with or without a spacer, or a single nebulizer treatment (0.05 mg/kg; minimum 1.25 mg, maximum 2.5 mg of 0.5% solution of albuterol in 2 to 3 ml of normal saline).

If the initial treatment results in a good response (PEFR greater than 80% of patient's best), the inhaled short-acting β_2-agonists can be continued every 3 to 4 hours for 24 to 48 hours. If a child has been on corticosteroids, the dose should be doubled for 7 to 10 days.

An incomplete response (PEFR between 50% and 80% of personal best or symptoms recur within 4 hours of therapy) is treated by continuing β_2-agonists and adding an oral corticosteroid. The β_2-agonist can be given by nebulizer. Parents should contact their child's health care provider for additional instructions. If there is marked distress (severe acute symptoms) or a poor response (PEFR less than 50%) to treatment, the child should have the β_2-agonist repeated immediately and should be taken to the emergency department. Emergency medical rescue (911) transportation should be used if the distress is severe and nonresponsive.

Children who experience acute asthma exacerbations more than once every 4 to 6 weeks should be reevaluated as to their treatment plan (Boguniewicz & Leung, 2001; NHLBI, 1997, 2002).

Complications

Complications from asthma can range from mild secondary respiratory infections to respiratory arrest. Unresponsiveness to pharmacologic agents can lead to status asthmaticus and ultimately to death. Chronic high-dose steroid use leads to growth retardation and other related side effects.

Patient and Parent Education and Prevention

The practitioner needs to remember that day-to-day management of asthma is the responsibility of the child or parent. Education should be tailored to meet the patient's individual and family needs. Therefore the NP should provide instruction on the following:

- Factors responsible for asthma symptoms (i.e., inflammation, airway hyperresponsiveness, and obstruction)
- Environmental control of allergens or triggers such as smoking and dust
- Medication use (when to take, how often to take, side effects)
- Home PEFR monitoring
- How to use inhalers, spacer devices, or aerosol equipment (Box 25-2)
- Proper cleaning of aerosol equipment
- What to do if symptoms worsen (what medications to add or increase; how frequently to use inhaled medication; specific indications about when to seek additional medical treatment for worsening of symptoms); development of a written action plan with the child or parent to cover these issues (Fig. 25-2)
- Need to have an adequate supply of all medications (including oral corticosteroids) at home and medications readily accessible to the child at school or other settings where the child frequents
- Management of the child at school, camp, or other places away from home

The NP should stress that asthma is a chronic disease that can be controlled—the goal of therapy is to maintain normal activity. The child should wear a medical alert bracelet. Patients and parents should be acquainted with local asthma education programs and activities such as asthma camp. Also, written instructions and handouts should be provided for parents, child, and other significant individuals (e.g., school personnel).

Prognosis

Asthma is a chronic disease that, for most children, can be successfully managed with proper pharmacologic therapy, allergen and environmental control, and patient education. Mild asthma is more likely to disappear with increasing age than is moderate or severe asthma.

Allergic Rhinitis

Description

Allergic rhinitis (AR) is a disorder that results in nasal edema and other related local manifestations owing to the release of chemical mediators from the antigen-antibody reaction. Manifestations can be seasonal or perennial depending on exposure and subsequent sensitization to the offending allergen.

Etiology and Incidence

AR is second only to asthma as the most common atopic disorder. There is an increased incidence in families with an atopic history. Both genetic (the presence of an abnormal sensitivity that is associated with IgE production) and environmental factors are linked to its etiology. Many of the allergens that cause asthma produce allergic rhinitis in the same child. Food allergens can occasionally cause rhinitis.

The nasal mucosa is particularly vulnerable to inhaled allergens. The nasal mucosa of a susceptible individual comes in contact with an allergen that binds to a specific IgE antibody. Superficial mucosal mast cells and basophils then degranulate and release chemical mediators. This causes an early-phase reaction of edema, cellular recruitment, and increased vascular permeability with hyperemia and increased serous and mucoid secretions. A late-phase response can occur that results in additional release of chemical mediators and nasal obstruction (Hurwitz, 2000).

AR tends to be seasonal, perennial, or episodic. Seasonal allergic rhinitis (hay fever or seasonal pollenosis) is rarely observed in children younger than 4 or 5 years of age but can occur anytime after 2 years of age. Seasonal AR results from sensitization to airborne allergens, such as pollens of trees, grasses, weeds (ragweed and other weeds), and outdoor molds. There can be geographic variations in seasonal AR depending on climate and when the allergens are released into the environment.

Perennial allergic rhinitis has year-round signs and symptoms that may be more severe in the winter. Onset of

BOX 25-2 *How To Use a Metered-Dose Inhaler*

Using an inhaler seems simple, but most patients do not use it the right way.

Steps for Using an Inhaler for Children <5 Years

1. The use of a mask chamber, such as the InspirEase, with an MDI allows the delivery of inhaled medications even in an uncooperative child.
2. The child should be placed in the parent's lap and the mask placed around the child's mouth.
3. Press down on the MDI while firmly holding the mask around the child's mouth. The child will eventually take a deep breath and inhale the medication.

Steps for Using an Inhaler for Children ≥5 Years
Getting Ready

1. Take off the cap and shake the inhaler.
2. Breathe out all the way.
3. Hold the inhaler the way as shown in A, B, or C below.

Breathe in Slowly

4. Start breathing in slowly through mouth, then press down on the inhaler one time. (If a holding chamber is used, first press down on the inhaler. Within 5 seconds, begin to breathe in slowly.)
5. Keep breathing in slowly, as deeply as possible.

Hold Your Breath

6. Hold breath for a slow count to 10 if possible.
7. For inhaled quick-relief medicine (beta$_2$-agonists), wait about 1 minute between puffs. There is no need to wait between puffs for other medicines.

A. Hold inhaler 1 to 2 inches in front of mouth (about the width of two fingers).

B. Use a spacer/holding chamber. These come in many shapes and can be useful to any patient.

C. Put inhaler in mouth. Do not use for steroids.

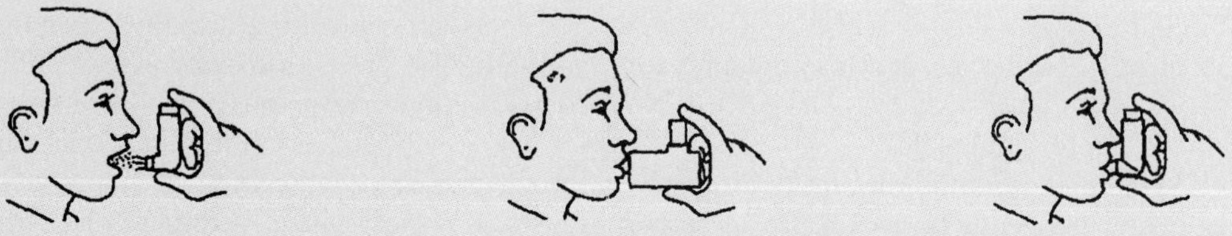

Step A or Step B is best, but Step C can be used if patient has trouble with Step A or Step B.

Clean Inhaler as Needed

Look at the hole where the medicine sprays out from your inhaler. If "powder" can be seen in or around the hole, clean the inhaler. Remove the metal canister from the L-shaped plastic mouthpiece. Rinse only the mouthpiece and cap in warm water. Let them dry overnight. In the morning, put the canister back inside. Put the cap on.

Know When To Replace Inhaler

For medicines taken each day (an example): a new canister has 200 puffs (number of puffs is listed on canister) and child is told to take 8 puffs per day: 8 puffs per day for 25 days equals 200 puffs in canister.

So this canister will last 25 days. If child started using this inhaler on May 1, replace it on or before May 25. Write the date on your canister. For quick-relief medicine, take as needed and count each puff. Do not put canisters in water to see if they are empty. This does not work.

Adapted from facts about controlling asthma. NIH pub no 97-2339, National Asthma Education and Prevention Program. National Heart, Lung, and Blood Institute. A reproducible handout.

The Pediatric Asthma Coalition of New Jersey

"Your Pathway to Asthma Control"

www.pacnj.org

Asthma Action Plan

(Press Firmly)

Name	Date of Birth	Effective Date / / to / /
Doctor/Nurse Practitioner		Parent/Guardian
Doctor's Office Phone Number		Parent's Phone
Emergency Contact After Parent		Contact Phone

The colors of a traffic light will help you use your asthma medicines.

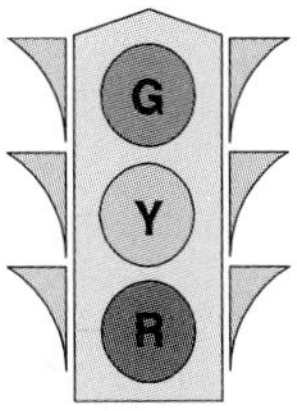

Green means **Go Zone!**
Use preventive medicine.

Yellow means **Caution Zone!**
Add prescribed yellow zone medicine.

Red means **Danger Zone!**
Get help from a doctor.

Pay Attention to Symptoms.

GO (Green)

You have *all* of these:
- Breathing is good
- No cough or wheeze
- Sleep through the night
- Can work and play

And/or Peak flow above ______

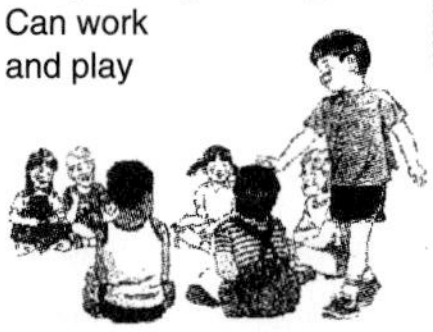

Use these medicines every day.

MEDICINE/DOSAGE	HOW MUCH TO TAKE	WHEN TO TAKE IT
COMMENTS:		

For asthma with exercise, take:

CAUTION (Yellow)

You have any of these:
- First sign of a cold
- Exposure to known trigger
- Cough
- Mild wheeze
- Tight chest
- Coughing at night

And/or Peak flow from ______ to ______

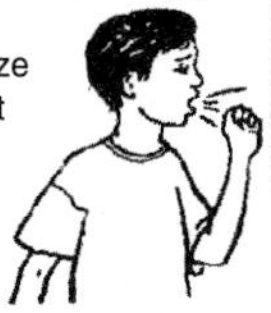

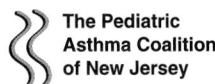

Continue with green zone medicine and ADD:

MEDICINE/DOSAGE	HOW MUCH TO TAKE	WHEN TO TAKE IT
FIRST ➡		
NEXT ➡		
COMMENTS:		

➡ **IF QUICK RELIEVER/YELLOW ZONE MEDICINE IS NEEDED MORE THAN 2-3 TIMES A WEEK THEN CALL YOUR DOCTOR.**

DANGER (Red)

Your asthma is getting worse fast:
- Medicine is not helping within 15-20 minutes
- Breathing is hard and fast
- Nose opens wide
- Ribs show
- Lips blue
- Fingernails blue
- Trouble walking and talking

And/or Peak flow below ______

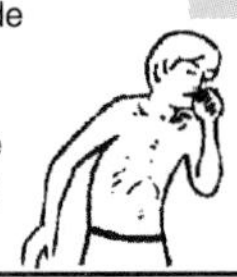

Take these medicines and call your doctor

EMERGENCY MEDICINE/DOSAGE	HOW MUCH TO TAKE	WHEN TO TAKE IT
COMMENTS:		

Get help from a doctor now! It's Important!

Asthma is a potentially life threatening illness. If you cannot contact your doctor, go directly to the emergency room. DO NOT WAIT. Make an appointment with your primary care provider within two days of an ER visit or hospitalization.

Check all items that trigger your asthma and things that could make your asthma worse:

- ❑ Chalk dust
- ❑ Cigarette smoke & second hand smoke
- ❑ Colds/Flu
- ❑ Dust mites, dust, stuffed animals, carpet
- ❑ Exercise
- ❑ Mold
- ❑ Ozone alert days
- ❑ Pests-rodents & cockroaches
- ❑ Pets-animal dander
- ❑ Plants, flowers, cut grass, pollen
- ❑ Strong odors, perfumes, cleaning products, scented products
- ❑ Sudden temperature change
- ❑ Wood smoke
- ❑ Foods: ______ ______ ______
- ❑ Other: ______ ______ ______ ______

☐ This student is capable and has been instructed in the proper method of self-administering the medications named above (or attached prescription).
☐ This student is not approved to self-medicate.

Check asthma severity: ❑ Mild Intermittent ❑ Mild Persistent ❑ Moderate Persistent ❑ Severe Persistent

PHYSICIAN/IPA/APN SIGNATURE______________________________

PHYSICIAN STAMP

WHITE - School Nurse Copy PINK- Patient Copy YELLOW- Doctor Copy

Approved by the New Jersey Thoracic Society, Medical Section of the American Lung Association of New Jersey.

Adapted from the NYC Childhood Asthma Initiative Adapted from the NHLBI

Funding provided by the New Jersey Department of Health and Senior Services

Printed 2002

Permission to Reproduce Blank Form

FIGURE 25-2 Sample Asthma Action Plan.

manifestations can occur before the second year of life, and offending substances tend to be indoor allergens, including the following:

- Dust mites
- Cockroaches
- Feathers
- Allergens or danders of household pets
- Indoor mold spores

Clinical Findings

Common nasal symptoms and findings on physical examination include the following:

- Reduced patency from chronic or recurrent bilateral nasal obstruction
- Mouth breathing, snoring, nasal speech
- Pale to purplish color and edema (bogginess) of nasal mucous membranes
- Clear, watery to seromucoid rhinorrhea
- Nasal crease—horizontal crease across the lower third of nose
- Itching and rubbing of nose or "allergic salute"
- Nasal stuffiness, postnasal drip, sneezing, congested cough
- Dennie-Morgan line or pleat—extra groove in lower eyelid

  Associated manifestations include the following:
  - Itching of palate, pharynx, or eyes
  - High arched palate
  - Redness of the conjunctiva, tearing, lid and periorbital edema, infraorbital cyanosis or allergic shiners
  - Enlarged tonsillar and adenoidal tissue
  - "Cobblestone" appearance of the pharynx or palpebral conjunctivae (or both) as a result of increased lymphoid tissue
  - Malocclusion if problem is chronic

Diagnostic Studies. Characteristic symptoms and clinical findings are the key to diagnosis. A history of atopy in the child or family member is helpful in making the diagnosis of AR. The presence of eosinophils on nasal smear can help substantiate the diagnosis but is a nonspecific, nonuniversal finding. Referrals for skin or serologic testing for IgE antibody to specific allergens should be reserved for the child with significant symptoms who does not respond to traditional management. The RAST or ImmunoCAP, in vitro tests, can be done for suspected allergens (Boguniewicz & Leung, 2001).

Differential Diagnosis

Conditions to include as differential diagnoses are the common cold, purulent rhinitis, sinusitis, adenoidal hypertrophy, foreign body obstruction, nasal polyposis of cystic fibrosis, nasopharyngeal tumors, choanal atresia or stenosis, and vasomotor rhinitis. Overuse of topical nasal decongestants can cause drug-induced rhinitis.

Management

There are three strategies for the management of AR: avoidance, pharmacology, and immunotherapy.

Avoidance Strategies. Avoiding exposure to the offending allergen or irritant as much as possible is essential. Allergens causing seasonal rhinitis are more difficult to avoid than are the indoor allergens such as molds because pollens are smaller and lighter and thus remain in the air longer.

Key avoidance measures for indoor allergens and irritants include the following:

- Control house dust, paying special attention to the child's bedroom.
  - Use dust mite–proof mattress and pillow covers.
  - Wash bed linens in hot water weekly.
  - Use vertical blinds instead of horizontal blinds or curtains.
  - Remove carpeting from bedroom.
  - Use plastic or wood furniture instead of cloth.
- Eliminate smoking from the child's environment; if household members still smoke despite education, stress that they should smoke outside the house.
- Keep pets outdoors; consider not having pets.
- Reduce mold; avoid damp basements.
- Use dehumidifiers, air conditioners with efficient filters, and air-cleaning devices with an electronic precipitator or with a high-efficiency particulate air (HEPA) filter.
- Eliminate milk, egg, or wheat for infants with perennial allergic rhinitis, if these prove to be offending substances.

Pharmacologic Therapy. Oral antihistamines, nasal cromolyn, nasal antihistamine, and nasal corticosteroids are part of the therapy for AR. Pharmacologic agents should be started 1 to 2 weeks before pollen season for children with seasonal AR. For perennial AR, start with maximum recommended dose and then taper to minimal dose needed to control symptoms. Some practitioners still occasionally use decongestants or combination decongestant and antihistamine preparations. Antibiotics need to be prescribed for secondary infections. Consult Appendix A for drugs and their administration.

Oral Antihistamines

- Oral antihistamines are especially helpful in seasonal allergic rhinitis.
- Oral antihistamines relieve symptoms of itching, sneezing, and rhinorrhea, but do little to relieve nasal obstruction.
- Oral antihistamines are divided into different classes (Table 25-9).

TABLE 25-9 Antihistamine Classes

Class	Name	Comments
Ethanolamines	Diphenhydramine (Benadryl)	Combination antihistamine and decongestant
	Clemastine (Tavist)	
	Carbinoxamine (Clistin, Rondec)	
Ethylenediamines	Pyrilamine (in Rynatan, Atrohist)	
	Tripelennamine	
Alkylamines	Chlorpheniramine (Chlor-Trimeton)	
	Brompheniramine (in Dimetane, Bromfed)	
Piperazines	Hydroxyzines (Atarax, Vistaril)	
Piperidines	Cyproheptadine (Periactin)	
Nonsedating antihistamines	Loratadine (Claritin)	Approved for children ≥2 yr old
	Cetirizine (Zyrtec)	Approved for children ≥2 yr old
	Fexofenadine (Allegra)	Approved for children ≥6 yr old

- Dosage of drug may need to be increased until relief of symptoms is obtained or side effects are experienced (see Appendix A).
- Patient can develop a tolerance to a particular antihistamine and may need to rotate drugs if tolerance develops.
- If side effects with one antihistamine are experienced, switch to another antihistamine in a different class or one in the same class but with different actions.
- Sedating antihistamines may interfere with daytime activities and negatively affect school performance.

Nasal Antihistamine

- Azelastine is a nasal antihistamine spray approved for use in seasonal AR in children 5 years of age and older.
- Azelastine acts by competing with histamine for H_1-receptor sites.

Decongestants

- Decongestants may help relieve nasal congestion.
- Decongestants may be used alone or in combination with an antihistamine.
- Topical decongestants can cause rebound rhinorrhea if used for more than 3 to 5 days; errors in administration can cause systemic absorption and side effects.

Nasal Cromolyn

- Nasal cromolyn can be used for both seasonal and perennial AR.
- Prophylaxis prevents the mast cell release of histamine and other chemical mediators.
- Best results occur when therapy is initiated before seasonal exposure.
- One to two sprays are administered in each nostril four times a day with tapering if symptoms are controlled (Boguniewicz & Leung, 2001).

Intranasal Corticosteroids

- Corticosteroids are effective agents to reduce inflammation and subsequent nasal obstruction. Have child clear nasal passages of mucus before their use.
- Corticosteroids are considered first-line therapy (Moy, 2002).
- Corticosteroids can be effective alone or together with antihistamines.
- Corticosteroids can take 1 week or more before clinical benefit is observed.
- Side effects can include local burning, irritation, soreness, or epistaxis.
- Table 25-10 lists usual dosages per nostril for intranasal corticosteroid preparations (Taketomo, Hodding, & Kraus, 2002).

Antibiotics

- Treat secondary infections (e.g., sinusitis and otitis media) with appropriate antibiotic coverage.

Immunotherapy. Allergen immunotherapy is indicated when symptoms are severe and have not improved with avoidance measures and pharmacologic therapy or when complications of chronic or recurrent sinusitis or otitis media and hearing loss are problematic. It should only be performed in a facility that has both the necessary equipment and health care professionals who are prepared to treat anaphylaxis.

Complications

Sinusitis may complicate allergic rhinitis owing to associated swelling of the mucosal lining of the sinuses with secondary infection. Likewise, eustachian tube dysfunction and its sequela, serous otitis media, are common complications.

TABLE 25-10 ***Intranasal Corticosteroid Preparations Used for Allergic Rhinitis: Usual Doses***

Drug	Dose	Number of Inhalations or Sprays and Daily Frequency	Age
Beclomethasone (Vancenase, Beconase inhaler)	42 μg/inhalation	1 tid	6-12 yr
		1 bid-qid or 2 bid	≥12 yr
Beclomethasone—aqueous inhalation (Beconase AQ)	42 μg/inhalation	1-2 bid	≥6 yr
(Vancenase AQ 84 μg)	84 μg/spray	1-2 once daily	≥6 yr
Budesonide* (Rhinocort Aqua)	32 μg/spray	2 sprays	≥6 yr
(Rhinocort)	50 μg/inhalation	2 sprays bid or 4 sprays daily	≥6 yr
Flunisolide (Nasalide, Nasarel)	25 μg/spray	1 spray tid or 2 sprays twice daily; maintenance dose is 1 spray daily	6-14 yr
		2 sprays bid; maintenance 1 spray daily	≥14 yr
Fluticasone (Flonase)	50 μg/spray	1 spray daily; 2 sprays daily if severe or poor response	≥4 yr
		2 sprays daily	>12 yr
Mometasone (Nasonex)	50 μg/spray	1 spray daily	3-11 yr
		2 sprays daily	>12 yr
Triamcinolone (Nasacort)	55 μg/spray	2 sprays daily	6-11 yr
		2 sprays daily; after 4-7 days may increase to 4 sprays daily or 2 sprays bid or 1 spray qid	≥12 yr
Triamcinolone AQ (Nasacort AQ)	55 μg/spray	2 sprays daily; maintenance dose 1 spray daily	>12 yr
(Tri-Nasal)	50 μg/inhalation	2 sprays daily; may increase to 4 sprays daily or 2 sprays bid	>12 yr

Adapted from Taketomo CK, Hodding JH, Kraus DM: *Pediatric dosage handbook*, ed 9, Hudson, OH, 2002, Lexi-Comp.
*Reduce slowly every 2-4 wk to smallest effective dose.

Malocclusion, the development of a high-arched palate, and the typical allergic facies can result from long-standing allergic rhinitis.

Patient and Parent Education and Prevention

Because allergic rhinitis is often a chronic problem, parents and children need to have specific information about control of this disorder.

- Instruct on environmental control. Handouts and a review of ways to individualize this information are essential.
- Review pharmacologic therapy, including the following:
  - Indications for and changes in medications
  - Frequency of use
  - Common side effects and contraindications
  - How to use intranasal sprays or inhalers if prescribed

Prognosis

Perennial allergic rhinitis can be a chronic problem unless offending allergens are identified and eliminated from the environment. If this is not possible, pharmacologic therapy is usually helpful in reducing symptoms. As the child grows and the nasal passages increase in size, symptoms may also lessen. Symptoms from seasonal allergic rhinitis often worsen from the adolescent years to mid-adulthood. Moving to a new environment often results in a short respite (1 to 3 years) from symptoms. However, the child frequently becomes sensitized to new airborne pollens, and symptoms of seasonal AR return.

Atopic Dermatitis

Description

Atopic dermatitis (AD) is a common skin disorder of childhood that is characterized by acute and chronic skin eruptions. The term *eczema* is sometimes used interchangeably with *atopic dermatitis.* Eczema means flaring up, which describes the acute symptom complex (erythema, scaling, vesicles, and crusts) seen with atopic dermatitis but does not adequately describe the chronic skin changes that can result from this disorder. Atopic dermatitis manifests a typical morphology and distribution of flexural lichenification or linearity in adults and facial and extensor involvement in infants and children. AD is frequently referred to as the "itch that rashes." With AD, the skin's ability to act as a protective barrier is impaired, resulting in dryness, cracking, and susceptibility to skin infection (see Color Fig. 13).

Etiology and Incidence

AD affects approximately 10% to 12% of the general population in the United States, with higher incidence in other countries. AD develops in 80% of cases by the first year of life and in another 10% by their second birthday. Asthma also develops in approximately 30% of those with AD, and AR develops in 30% of those with AD.

The exact etiology is unknown and may vary from individual to individual. Although many children have high IgE levels, an exact immune mechanism for this disorder is not evident. Abnormalities in histamine production (increased in the skin), chemotaxis, monocytes, and cytokines are associated with AD. The strongest predictor of AD is a positive family history of AD; a family history of asthma is also a predictor but less so than AD. Sweating increases itching in the atopic skin. A predisposition to development of pruritus is believed to be a key factor (Krafchik, 2002).

Clinical Findings

The following are seen in atopic dermatitis (Table 25-11):

- More than one third of cases begin before age 3 months. Dry skin is the only initial sign. These infants are generally not brought in for health care until pruritus and the itch-scratch-itch cycle develops, generally around 2 to 3 months of age.
- Acute manifestations (more common in infants) include the following:
  - Intense itching
  - Redness
  - Papules, vesicles, and edema
  - Serous discharge and crusts
  - Generalized dry skin (xerosis) with dry hair and scalp; diaper area usually spared
- Chronic manifestations (more common in children and adolescents) include the following:
  - Lichenification—thickened, leathery, hyperpigmented skin
  - Scratch marks
- Characteristics of infantile phase:
  - Begins at age 2 to 3 months; resolves around 2 to 3 years of age, with approximately one third of cases continuing into the childhood phase
  - Cheeks, forehead, scalp, extending to trunk as oval patches or to the extremities; lateral extensor surface of arms and legs
  - Tends to be acute
- Characteristics of childhood phase:
  - Beginning around age 18 to 24 months and lasting to adolescence; approximately one third of cases progress to adolescent AD
  - Wrists (hands), neck, ankles (feet), popliteal and antecubital fossae, buttock-thigh crease, flexural areas
  - Eyebrows can be thin and broken off
  - Tends to be chronic; possible lichenification
  - Involvement only of the feet in some children

TABLE 25-11 ***Assessment of Atopic Dermatitis***

Onset	Signs and Symptoms	Prognosis
Initial presentation		
• <3 mo old (one third of cases)	Dry skin first sign	Often not noticed
• 2-3 mo	Itch-scratch-itch cycle starts	
Infantile phase	Acute presentation—common in infants: intense itching; redness, papules, vesicles, edema; serous discharge and crusts; xerosis, dry hair, scalp; diaper area sparing; cheeks, forehead, scalp, extremities	Two thirds of cases resolve by 2-3 yr
Childhood phase (starts 18-24 mo of age)	Involves wrists, hands, popliteal and antecubital fossa; eyebrows thin and broken off; some only have feet involved; may have allergic/atopic facies and white dermatographism	One third continue into teenage years
Adolescent phase	Common in children and teenagers; thickened, leathery, hyperpigmented skin; scratch marks	New or recurrent problem

From Burns et al: *Pocket reference for pediatric primary care*, Philadelphia, 2001, WB Saunders.

- Characteristics of adolescent phase:
  - Often manifested by hand dermatitis only; can involve the popliteal and antecubital fossae, face, neck, upper arms and back, dorsa of hands, fingers, feet, and toes
  - May be new occurrence or recurrence of a chronic condition
  - Dry skin and lichenification are prominent findings
  - Erythema and scaling with less exudates
  - Postinflammatory hypopigmentation or hyperpigmentation that disappears
  - Continuing disease as adults in approximately 30% of children with AD
- Other key features of AD:
  - Tendency toward dry skin and a lowered threshold for itching (itch-scratch-itch cycle)
  - Tendency to worsen during dry winter months or with heat in the summer
  - Chronic AD often secondarily infected with *Staphylococcus aureus* (most commonly) or *Streptococcus pyogenes*
- Possible associated features:
  - Atopic pleats—extra groove in lower eyelid called Dennie-Morgan fold or pleat, nasal crease across top of nose
  - Accentuated palmar creases
  - Allergic shiners, mild facial pallor, or dry hair
  - Keratosis pilaris—follicular papules occurring on the extensor aspect of the arms, anterior thighs, and lateral aspects of the cheeks
  - Nummular eczema, dyshidrotic eczema, juvenile plantar dermatitis, nipple eczema, or ichthyosis vulgaris
  - White dermatographism—white line, flare and wheal reaction following stroking of the skin (Habif et al, 2001; Krafchik, 2002; Morelli & Weston, 2001; Sly, 2000)

Diagnostic Studies. Diagnosis of atopic dermatitis is based on characteristic historical and physical findings. A chronic or recurring rash that is pruritic and has a characteristic distribution and appearance, together with a family or personal history of atopy, is key in leading to the diagnosis of atopic dermatitis. Histologic examination of the skin is rarely needed and is reserved only for cases that are difficult to diagnose. Serum IgE concentration is elevated in many children with this problem; for the vast majority of children, immunologic testing (e.g., IgE, RAST, ImmunoCAP, or prick test) is not needed to confirm the diagnosis or to monitor treatment. Skin testing and desensitization are not recommended for children with atopic dermatitis only. If secondary fungal infection is suspected, collect scrapings and use potassium hydroxide (KOH) to look for fungal hyphae.

Differential Diagnosis

Other types of dermatitis, including seborrheic dermatitis, contact dermatitis, allergic contact dermatitis, nummular dermatitis, psoriasis, and scabies, are included in the differential diagnosis. A few genetic conditions are associated with similar skin eruptions (e.g., phenylketonuria, Wiskott-Aldrich syndrome, histiocytosis X, and acrodermatitis enteropathica). Pityriasis alba can also be a differential diagnosis.

Management

Treatment strategy is based on the following key concepts:

1. The itch-scratch-itch cycle must be interrupted.
2. Dryness of the skin must be corrected.
3. If there are known offending agents, they must be eliminated.
4. Secondary bacterial or viral infections must be treated.

Acute versus chronic care management is also a consideration. The following therapies are key factors in the control of atopic dermatitis:

- Antipruritic/sedative agents are essential to control pruritus (Taketomo, Hodding, & Kraus, 2002). These agents are essential to help control active exacerbations of AD and also are helpful as maintenance therapy.
  - Hydroxyzine (Atarax, Vistaril) has excellent antihistaminic and antipruritic qualities but can cause drowsiness and behavioral changes. If an antihistamine is needed throughout the day, the usual oral dose of Atarax in children is 2 mg/kg per day divided every 6 to 8 hours (Takemoto, Hodding, & Kraus, 2002). This dose may need to be increased.
  - Diphenhydramine hydrochloride (Benadryl) is also a useful antihistamine, especially if sedation is also needed. The usual oral dose of diphenhydramine hydrochloride in children is 5 mg/kg per day in divided doses every 6 to 8 hours, not to exceed 300 mg/day.
  - Nonsedating or low-sedating antihistamines may be considered (see Table 25-9 and Appendix A).
- Use wet compresses if there are weeping, oozing lesions and signs of acute skin inflammation. They also help rehydrate the skin.
  - Aluminum acetate (Burow solution in a 1:20 or 1:40 preparation). Solution should be lukewarm or body temperature.
  - Use a soft cloth that is moderately wet; remoisten as needed. Corticosteroid topical preparations can be applied either before or after application of compresses.
  - Can use up to 5 days; effective during the acute stage of atopic dermatitis.

- Aveeno or oatmeal baths help soothe acute episodes of pruritus, followed by application of a heavy cream emollient.
- Daily bath or shower, 10 to 15 minutes, to reduce skin dryness. Excessive soaking in the bathtub depletes the skin of natural moisturizers if not immediately followed with moisturizing topical agents. Use lukewarm, not hot, water. Immediately pat the child and quickly apply occlusive ointments. Some recommend two baths daily, each less than 5 minutes, immediately followed by lubricating oils or ointments as a way to restore water to the skin. Avoid bubble baths and oils.

Hydration is a key element in the treatment of atopic dermatitis. Children with severe atopic dermatitis may need soaking after baths to maintain skin hydration. This should be done at bedtime. Wet gauze and bandage wraps, wrung out to dampness, can be placed on the extremities with a dry dressing over them. Cotton pajamas or soaks can also be used with a wet, wrung-dry pajama or soak next to the skin and then covered with a corresponding dry pajama or sock. For some children with atopic dermatitis, frequent bathing may exacerbate their pruritus and thus aggravate their skin problems. Bathing must be limited in these patients. Instead, liberal application of water-in-oil moisturizers is the preferred treatment (Kristal & Klein, 2000).

- Immediately after bath or shower, gently pat dry within 3 minutes; no rubbing or scrubbing. Emolliate with a moisturizer. Lubricants maintain the skin's hydration, and emollients are the treatment of choice for dry skin.
  - An emollient (e.g., petrolatum [Vaseline, Aquaphor]) can be applied just before getting out of the bath water or just after getting out of the bath while still damp. This is also a good time to apply topical corticosteroid preparations, because absorption of the agent is more effective if the skin is hydrated.
  - Use mild soap such as Dove or Neutrogena for the axilla and groin. Do not use drying or deodorant soaps and no oils in bath water.
  - Cetaphil is a nondrying soap-free cleansing agent and can be substituted for bathing. Instruct parents to leave Cetaphil on the skin; it should not be wiped off after applying.
- Emollients can be applied three to four times a day as needed, such as fragrance-free Eucerin cream, Crisco (plain, not butter flavored), or petroleum jelly. If a child is sensitive to fragrances, scented creams such as Nivea should be avoided.
- Topical corticosteroid preparations are a mainstay of therapy. Do not apply topical steroids containing propylene glycol.
  - When applied over large areas of dermatitis or if occlusion (covering with plastic wrap) is used, the possibility of significant systemic absorption is greatly increased, especially in infants and young children.
  - Apply a thin layer of 1% hydrocortisone cream (acute stage) or ointment (chronic stage) to affected areas three or four times a day.
  - Use of fluorinated, topical corticosteroid preparations in children should only be done in consultation with a physician. Never use fluorinated, topical corticosteroid preparations on the face; instead, use 1% hydrocortisone ointment sparingly two to three times a day until symptoms improve and then withdraw. Do not use for an extended period of time because corticosteroids cause thinning of the skin. (See Appendix A for a listing of topical corticosteroids by potency rating.)
- Recently approved immunomodulators (tacrolimus 0.03% and 0.1% ointment and pimecrolimus 1% cream) can be used in children 2 years and older. These nonsteroidal antiinflammatory medications block calcineurin. This results in the inhibition of T-cell activation. The most common side effect is stinging or burning when applied. These preparations can be used on the face (Taketomo, Hodding, & Kraus, 2002).
- Systemic antibiotic agents are essential if secondary skin infection with *S. aureus* or *S. pyogenes* is suspected.
  - Oral erythromycin, first- or second-generation cephalosporins, or cloxacillin should be prescribed for 10 to 14 days depending on resistance of staphylococcus to a particular antibiotic.
  - If bacterial skin infections are recurrent or frequent, a 3-week course of oral antibiotics is recommended.
  - Topical antibiotic preparations are contraindicated, although the use of mupirocin has been demonstrated to reduce colony counts of *S. aureus.*
  - Topical antibacterial scrubs are contraindicated because they dry out the skin and cause irritation.
  - Topical antifungal medication is recommended if KOH positive for hyphae.
- Tar preparations may be added to help manage chronic and lichenified forms of dermatitis.
  - These are topical agents that have limited use.
  - Patients should be cautioned about photosensitivity.
- Systemic corticosteroid agents are rarely needed.
- Eliminate known or suspected offending agents.
  - Avoid nonbreathable fabrics—nylon or wool; wool is irritating whereas soft cotton clothing is not.
  - Avoid chlorine, turpentine, harsh soaps, fragrances, and bleach.

- Known atopic agents should be avoided (e.g., feather pillows, fuzzy toys, stuffed animals, pets).
- Dietary restrictions may include the elimination of cow's milk from the diet of infants predisposed to atopy. Eggs, fish, chocolate, nuts, and citrus fruits are generally not allowed until 12 months of age.
- Control of house dust to reduce mite exposure is encouraged. Careful attention to the child's bedroom is important.
- Commercial powders (e.g., benzyl benzoate [Acarosan, Capture]) may help control dust mites in carpets.

- Manipulate the environment. A decrease in environmental humidity and an increase in antigen presentation are key causative factors. Therefore increase environmental humidity and decrease exposure to antigens. Cool temperatures (air conditioning) help.
- Keep fingernails short.
- Refer to a dermatologist if child is unresponsive to traditional therapy or has an unusual manifestation (Krafchik, 2002; Morelli & Weston, 2001).

Complications

Secondary skin infections are a frequent complication of AD. *S. aureus* is the most frequent bacterial organism associated with skin infection. Treatment of secondary skin infection is imperative in the management of atopic dermatitis. Kaposi varicelliform eruption (eczema herpeticum) is a significant complication that can result in severe illness in children. Lichenification, a secondary skin change marked by thickening of the skin, is associated with chronic itching. Keratoconus is occasionally seen and is associated with chronic rubbing of the eyelids. Individuals with AD may be prone to molluscum contagiosum, tinea, and warts.

Patient and Parent Education and Prevention

Practitioners should provide patients and parents instruction in the following:

- Environmental control of allergens or triggers
- Medication use (when, how much, and how often to use; side effects; and proper application of topical preparations)
- What to do if symptoms worsen or signs of secondary skin infection appear and when to seek additional medical treatment for worsening of symptoms
- Precipitating factors:
  - Extreme temperatures/humidity
  - Excess sweat
  - Emotional stress
  - New clothes—wash with mild detergent (with no dyes or perfumes) before wearing them to remove formaldehyde and other chemicals
  - Harsh washing detergents—add second rinse cycle when washing clothes
  - Coarse clothes
  - Excess soap and water
  - Allergies
  - Cutaneous or systemic infection
- Keeping fingernails trimmed

The practitioner should stress that AD is often a recurrent disease that can be controlled. The goal of therapy is to prevent the itch-scratch-itch cycle and hydrate the skin. Specific written instructions and handouts should be provided to parents regarding bathing, skin care, and use of soaps and other skin cream or lotions.

Prognosis

With appropriate treatment, AD can generally be controlled. In most children, the symptoms of AD become quiescent by age 5 years; however, there is an adolescent and adult stage of the disease. Approximately 25% of children with atopic dermatitis go on to have persistence of symptoms throughout adulthood. Self-image problems may result if atopic dermatitis is severe.

DISEASES WITH AN AUTOIMMUNE BASIS

Juvenile Arthritis

Description

JA is a disease with an autoimmune basis and represents a group of conditions with onset of symptoms in children younger than 16 years of age that causes chronic inflammation of synovial joints for 6 weeks or more. There are various subtypes of JA disease in children that are categorized based on differences in their disease onset, severity, duration, and pattern of complications. The subtypes are systemic arthritis, polyarthritis–rheumatoid factor (RF) negative, polyarthritis-RF positive, oligoarthritis (inflammation of one to four joints), extended oligoarthritis, enthesitis-related arthritis (characterized by joint inflammation at the sites of insertion of fascia or tendons [enthesitis] and spine arthritis), and psoriatic arthritis (O'Neil, 2002a).

Etiology and Incidence

The exact etiology of JA is unknown. Genetics is believed to be a factor in most forms of JA. Certain histocompatibility complex antigens are more prevalent in the JA population. Infectious agents such as rubella, parvovirus, *Klebsiella*, *S. pyogenes*, and *Y. enterocolitica* also have been implicated in the etiology of JA. Cytokine production, proliferation of macrophage-like synoviocytes, infiltration with neutrophils and lymphocytes, and autoimmunity are thought to be the major pathologic processes causing chronic joint inflammation.

Prevalence estimates of JA in children are 1.1 in 1000 to 1 in 1500. The rate of JA in girls is significantly higher than in boys except for two subtypes: systemic arthritis and enthesitis-related arthritis. Oligoarthritis makes up approximately 50% to 60% of the cases of JA, and its peak age is early childhood. Systemic arthritis (representing 10% to 15% of JA cases) and polyarthritis-RF negative (representing 15% to 20% of JA cases) occur throughout childhood. Polyarthritis (RF positive) and enthesitis-related arthritis have a peak age of 8 years of age and older (O'Neil, 2002a).

Clinical Findings

History. The major complaints of the child with JA are

- Pain—generally a mild to moderate aching
- Joint stiffness—worse in the morning and after rest

Physical Examination. Typical manifestations of JA are

- Nonmigratory monoarticular or polyarticular involvement of large or proximal interphalangeal joints for more than 3 months
- Systemic manifestations—fever, erythematous rashes, leukocytosis, and nodules

Less commonly seen are ocular disease (e.g., iridocyclitis, iritis, or uveitis), pleuritis, pericarditis, anemia, fatigue, and growth failure.

Key physical findings are

- Swelling with effusion or thickening of synovial membrane, or both
- Heat over inflamed joint and tenderness along joint line
- Loss of joint range of motion and function; child typically holds the affected joints in slight flexion and may walk with limp

There are three major patterns of presentation:

1. *Acute febrile pattern* with an evanescent pale or salmon pink macular rash, arthritis, hepatosplenomegaly, leukocytosis, and polyserositis; this group does not develop iridocyclitis.
2. *Polyarticular (five or more synovial joints) pattern* of chronic pain and symmetric joint swelling; low-grade fever, fatigue, nodules, and anemia may be present but are not prominent as in acute form; iridocyclitis is an occasional feature in this group.
3. *Pauciarticular pattern* with involvement of few joints, typically the weight-bearing joints; synovitis may be mild and painless, joint involvement is asymmetric, and approximately 30% of these children have asymptomatic iridocyclitis.

Each of the seven subtypes of JA has a typical pattern of presentation. For more information on their specific presentation, the NP should consult other texts on this subject. Some children with JA may develop iridocyclitis, pleuritis, pericarditis, anemia, and fatigue in addition to their joint involvement (Hollister, 2001; O'Neil, 2002a).

Diagnostic Studies. Diagnosis is based on physical findings and history; there is no diagnostic laboratory test for rheumatoid arthritis (RA). A positive RF by latex fixation may be present, and ANA may be present in pauciarticular disease with iridocyclitis. Other laboratory findings that may be useful include ESR, leukocytosis, anemia, hyperglobulinemia, and hypoalbuminemia. Imaging studies (magnetic resonance imaging [MRI]) can help in managing joint pathology. Analysis of synovial fluid is not helpful in diagnosis of JA.

Differential Diagnosis

The various causes of monoarticular arthritis should be considered in the differential diagnosis. These include tumors, leukemia, cancer, bacterial infections, toxic synovitis, rheumatic fever, SLE, Lyme disease, inflammatory bowel disease, septic arthritis, and chondromalacia patellae.

Management

Children with severe involvement should be followed by a specialist in pediatric rheumatology. Other pediatric subspecialists, such as orthopedists, ophthalmologists, and cardiologists, may be consulted as needed. Therapy depends on the degree of local or systemic involvement.

Pharmacologic agents include the following (O'Neil, 2002a):

- Nonsteroidal antiinflammatory drugs (NSAIDs): Children with oligoarthritis generally respond well to NSAIDs.
    - Aspirin: 80 to 100 mg/kg/day (qid)
    - Ibuprofen: 30 to 40 mg/kg/day (tid to qid)
    - Tolmetin: 20 to 30 mg/kg/day (tid)
    - Naproxen: 10 to 20 mg/kg/day (bid)
    - Indomethacin 1 to 2 mg/kg/day (bid or qid)
- Oral or parenteral corticosteroids, sulfasalazine, etanercept (Enbrel) (a newly approved drug that soaks up tumor necrosis factor, an immune-system protein), or methotrexate is indicated in severe forms of JA.
- Intraarticular corticosteroid injections are used if there is severe joint involvement.
- Pharmacologic therapy for iridocyclitis is given as indicated by an ophthalmologist.
- Physical therapy—range of motion muscle-strengthening exercises and heat treatments—is used for joint involvement, and occupational therapy is beneficial. Rest and splinting are used if indicated.

Complications

Systemic involvement can include iridocyclitis, pleuritis, pericarditis, and hepatitis. Residual joint damage caused by granulation of tissue in the joint space can be a problem. Children most likely to develop permanent crippling disability are those with hip involvement, unremitting synovitis, or positive RF tests.

Patient and Parent Education and Prevention

The following education and preventive measures are taken:

- For children on aspirin therapy:
  - Educate parents about the risk of Reye syndrome and its signs and symptoms.
  - Recommend influenza vaccine.
- Offer chronic disease counseling as indicated in Chapter 23.
- Encourage normal play and recreation.
- Educate about side effects of medications, as well as about splinting, orthotics, and bracing requirements.
- Instruct about need to follow up with an ophthalmologist. Frequency of follow-up for uveitis screening is based on subtype of JA. Those with systemic arthritis, polyarthritis (both RF-negative and RF-positive subtypes), and enthesitis-related arthritis should be seen every 6 months. Those classified as oligoarthritis, extended arthritis, and psoriatic arthritis are seen every 3 months if ANA positive or every 4 months if ANA negative.
- Ensure that parent and child understand that physical therapy is a mainstay of treatment for chronic childhood arthritis and should be part of the child's daily routine. A daily plan that includes passive, active, and resistive exercises is important (Hudson-Barr & Lambert, 2002).
  - Water therapy and the use of heat or cold will reduce pain and stiffness. Swimming is an excellent activity for these children except those with severe anemia and cardiac disease.
  - Tricycle/bike riding and low-impact dance are other useful sport activities.
- Refer to the Arthritis Foundation, which has excellent resources for family members and children (see Resource Box).
- Instruct on the need to involve school personnel in the identification of needed school-related services through an individualized education plan (IEP).
- Discuss the challenge of pain management and its assessment in children with chronic arthritis, and encourage parents to advocate for effective pain control on behalf of their child.

Prognosis

The course of the disease is variable, and there is no curative treatment. After an initial episode, the child may never have another episode, or the disease may go into remission and recur months or years later. The disease process of JA wanes with age and subsides in 95% of children by puberty. Onset of JA in the teenage years is related to progression to adult rheumatoid disease.

Systemic Lupus Erythematosus

Description

SLE is a chronic systemic disease that can involve many organ systems. Autoantibody formation resulting from activation of B lymphocytes is a key characteristic of this immune complex disease. It is more acute and severe in children than in adults.

Etiology and Incidence

The exact cause is unknown, but SLE is believed to be a disease of altered immune regulation. In SLE, immune complexes are deposited in various tissues of the body and their clearance is impaired. Deposits of immune complexes trigger a generalized inflammatory response that can lead to tissue damage such as vasculitis and numerous organ system abnormalities (commonly the heart and renal system).

The mechanism triggering immune complex formation is unknown. Females are predominantly affected, frequently between ages 9 and 15 years. SLE is often precipitated by menarche, pregnancy, or use of oral contraceptives. Onset before age 3 years is rare; adult onset tends to occur at around 30 to 40 years of age. Altered cellular immunity in genetically predisposed individuals is postulated as a key factor in this disease. Approximately 20% of children with SLE have a first-degree relative with SLE (O'Neil, 2002b).

Clinical Findings

Clinical findings depend on organ involvement.

History. The history may include the following:

- Joint involvement
  - Most common initial finding
  - Nondeforming arthritis
  - Often symmetric joint involvement
- Arthralgia
- Systemic manifestations
- Fever—intermittent or sustained
- Fatigue
- Anorexia and loss of weight
- Malaise

Physical Examination. The following may be seen on physical examination (Hollister, 2001; O'Neil, 2002b):

- Malar or "butterfly" rash—scaly erythematous maculopapular rash covering malar areas extending over the bridge of the nose and cheeks; may spread down the face to the chest and extremities; "butterfly" rash and other lesions can be photosensitive
- Discoid rash with plugging of the follicles, hypopigmentation and hyperpigmentation, and scarring
- Lesions may also include small ulcerations in the skin and mucous membranes, indurations, purpura, and erythema nodosum
- Alopecia
- Mucous membrane manifestations
  - Gingivitis, mucosal hemorrhage, erosions, ulcerations
  - Silvery whitening of the vermilion border of the lips or thickening, redness, ulceration, or crusting of the lips
- Raynaud's phenomenon is present in some children
- Polyserositis—pleurisy, pericarditis, and peritonitis
- Hepatosplenomegaly and lymphadenopathy
- Signs and symptoms of central nervous system involvement, as well as cardiac and renal involvement (e.g., cardiac failure or renal failure)

Diagnostic Studies. Initial laboratory testing includes CBC, ANA, ESR, serum chemical analysis (metabolic and protein screen), and urinalysis. The ANA test is positive in 95% of children who have active, untreated SLE. A negative ANA excludes SLE from the diagnosis except for the rare false-negative test. A positive ANA test should be followed up with testing for disease-specific types of ANA. Elevated titers of anti-DNA antibody and depressed levels of serum complement are found in active disease involving the skin and central nervous and renal systems. Leukopenia, anemia, elevated sedimentation rate, and hypergammaglobulinemia are frequent laboratory findings. Other laboratory and radiographic studies depend on organ involvement (e.g., histopathologic studies, urine testing, and serologic testing).

Differential Diagnosis

Diseases that resemble SLE include rheumatic fever, RA, and viral infections. A temporary, drug-induced SLE can be caused by several pharmacologic agents, including hydantoin compounds, hydralazine, isoniazid (INH), procainamide, and sulfonamides.

Management

Children with SLE need to be followed up by a specialist in collagen-vascular disorders. Other pediatric subspecialists may be consulted. Therapy depends on the degree of local or systemic involvement. General measures include avoiding sun exposure and daylight fluorescent light, as well as applying sunscreen for ultraviolet A (UVA) and ultraviolet B (UVB) protection. The following measures also may be helpful:

- NSAIDs are used for relief of arthritis, serositis, or pain (if nephritis is present, use with caution).
- Oral steroids are prescribed if renal, cardiac, or central nervous system involvement is present. The dose is adjusted depending on clinical and laboratory findings.
- Antimalarial drugs may be used to treat cutaneous manifestations.
- Immunosuppressant agents may be added if the response to steroids is inadequate.

Use of other pharmacologic agents or therapies depends on the type and level of organ system involvement.

Complications

Currently, SLE is considered, for the most part, a controllable disease in children. The severity of the illness is variable. A diagnosis of SLE in childhood does not always mean a poor prognosis, especially if renal involvement is not present. Renal failure, central nervous system lupus, myocardial infarction, cardiac failure, and infection are the leading causes of death in children. Exposure to ultraviolet light may bring out or worsen skin lesions and can also result in exacerbation of systemic problems that can cause death. Side effects resulting from chronic use of high-dose corticosteroids can be a problem.

Patient and Parent Education

The practitioner should educate patients and parents as follows:

- About the effect of sun exposure and the need for sunscreen protection
- About the need to rest between activities, because fatigue is a frequent problem for children with SLE
- That SLE is a chronic disease that can have periods of remissions followed by exacerbations

Prognosis

SLE is a chronic disease with periods of exacerbations with waxing and waning of symptoms; however, complete remission can occur. Children with mild disease do well; patients with severe major organ involvement have a poor prognosis.

Fibromyalgia

Description

Fibromyalgia is a benign, intermittent, noninflammatory musculoskeletal pain syndrome. It is a complex syndrome that involves fatigue and generalized pain involving muscles, ligaments, and tendons. Symptoms are often vague and variable, with no major organ system abnormalities found. Its presentation can range from a generalized increased sensitivity to pain to a more classic pattern of specific symptoms. Fibromyalgia can occur as a primary condition or in conjunction with other rheumatologic disorders (secondary fibromyalgia). Fibromyalgia was first described in children in 1985.

Etiology and Incidence

The cause of fibromyalgia is unknown. It is considered a subset of musculoskeletal pain syndromes. Females are affected more often than males (Miller, 2002; Silver & Wallace, 2002).

Clinical Findings

History. The history may include the following common symptoms (Silver & Wallace, 2002; Yunus, 2002):

- Pain at multiple sites
- Fatigue
- Insomnia or prolonged night awakenings
- Tingling or numbness in limbs
- Complaints of swelling of hands and feet without objective findings
- Dizziness or weakness
- Associated conditions:
  - Chest pain or shortness of breath
  - Irritable bowel syndrome
  - Headaches
  - Chronic fatigue syndrome

Physical Examination. Local areas of tenderness or trigger points in muscles (usually at areas of tendon insertion) with pressure are characteristic physical findings. Pressure causes pain at the site and also in a circumferential or linear pattern surrounding the site.

Diagnostic Criteria. The criteria for the diagnosis of fibromyalgia established by the American College of Rheumatology are as follows:

- History of widespread pain that involves both sides of the body, is above and below the waist, and includes axial skeletal pain.
- Pain in 11 of 18 bilateral point sites on digital palpation using approximately 4 kg of pressure. Sites to evaluate are occiput, trapezius, supraspinatus, gluteal, greater trochanter, low cervical, second rib, lateral epicondyle, and knee (Yunus, 2002).

Diagnostic Studies. Laboratory studies are of little benefit. Blood count, liver functions, and muscle enzymes are normal. If secondary fibromyalgia, order appropriate tests to diagnose rheumatoid disorder.

Differential Diagnosis

In chronic fatigue syndrome, tiredness rather than pain is the major complaint. Fibromyalgia initially may be mistaken for other rheumatoid diseases but does not have the associated rashes, weight loss, fever (over 101° F), or joint swelling.

Management

Children and their parents need reassurance that they do not have a life-threatening disease but have a chronic condition that can be a lifelong problem. Treatment focuses on relieving symptoms and can include the following:

- Physical therapy for range-of-motion exercises, mild low-impact aerobic exercises (e.g., swimming, bicycling, and walking), and muscle strengthening.
- Amitriptyline (10 to 25 mg) taken before bedtime has been helpful in stabilizing abnormal sleep patterns and in reducing pain. Cyclobenzaprine (10 mg at bedtime) also has helped to stabilize sleep patterns but should be used for no longer than 2 to 3 weeks at a time.
- Psychotherapy to help cope with this condition and deal with stress.
- Analgesics and NSAIDs do not help relieve the pain and should not be prescribed.

Patient and Parent Education

The practitioner should educate patients and parents as follows:

- About fibromyalgia and that it is not a psychosomatic disorder
- About the possibility that this could be a chronic problem and they can have periods of remissions followed by exacerbations

Prognosis

The outcome of fibromyalgia in children is not clear (Hollister, 2001).

Chronic Fatigue Syndrome

The existence of or cause of chronic fatigue syndrome continues to be a debated topic. Criteria to assist in the classification of this syndrome have been developed by the Centers for Disease Control and Prevention (CDC). The presentation of chronic fatigue syndrome in children and adolescents is similar to that seen with adults. The key patient complaint is fatigue that must have a defined day of onset, is unexplained, and is persistent or relapsing. This fatigue is not relieved by rest or sleep and results in reduced activity. Other significant clinical findings include impaired memory or concentration, low-grade fever, sore throat, painful cervical or axillary lymph nodes, muscle pain, and neuropsychiatric problems. These clinical findings must have been present for 6 months or longer.

Epstein-Barr virus (EBV) infection has been implicated in the etiology of chronic fatigue syndrome. However, EBV does not explain all the symptoms. No single immunologic abnormality has been consistently identified as the causative factor. The etiology of chronic fatigue syndrome remains undetermined, and treatment is based on symptoms. Care must be taken in diagnosing this disorder in children, and other conditions (e.g., hypothyroidism, sleep apnea, hepatitis B or C, SLE, cancer, and major depressive and other psychiatric disorders) must first be ruled out (Craig & Kakumanu, 2002; Krilov & Fisher, 2002). For a definitive diagnosis of chronic fatigue syndrome once other conditions are ruled out, the child is best referred to a specialist in this area.

Acute Rheumatic Fever

Description

Acute rheumatic fever (ARF) is a nonsuppurative complication of a group A β-hemolytic streptococcus (GABHS) pharyngeal infection that results in an inflammatory process involving the joints, heart, central nervous system, and subcutaneous tissue. ARF is diagnosed based on a set of criteria called the Jones criteria (see Box 31-9) that were updated in 1992. Recurrent ARF can follow subsequent GABHS pharyngeal infections.

Etiology and Incidence

The exact pathologic mechanism that is responsible for the inflammatory changes in various organs and tissues is unknown. Abnormalities in the host immune response to streptococcal cell wall proteins are believed to be involved. Serotypes 1, 3, 5, 6, 18, and 24 are associated with ARF. There appears to be a genetic influence on susceptibility to GABHS infection. The risk of an initial attack of ARF following a GABHS pharyngeal infection is 0.2 to 2 per 100,000; the risk for recurrent ARF following subsequent episodes of GABHS pharyngitis (symptomatic or asymptomatic infection) is 50%. The most commonly affected group is 5- to 15-year-olds (Amin & Strong, 2002; Kaplan & Markowitz, 2002). See Chapter 31 for further discussion of ARF and cardiac involvement.

Clinical Findings

The diagnosis of an initial attack of ARF is based on the following:

- Evidence of documented (culture, rapid streptococcal antigen test, or antistreptolysin O [ASO] titer) GABHS pharyngeal infection
- Findings of two major manifestations or one major and two minor manifestations of ARF (Kaplan & Markowitz, 2002)

Major Manifestations

- Carditis (pancarditis)
- Polyarthritis (migratory and painful)
- Sydenham chorea
- Erythema marginatum
- Subcutaneous nodules

Minor Manifestations

Clinical Findings and History

- Fever, polyarthralgia, prior history of ARF

Diagnostic Studies

- Elevated acute-phase reactants (ESR, white blood cells, C-reactive protein)
- Prolonged PR interval on electrocardiogram

Children may be diagnosed with ARF without evidence of a preceding streptococcal infection in the following two situations: a child with Sydenham chorea or with acquired heart disease (commonly mitral valve regurgitation without a congenitally abnormal or prolapsed valve) that can only be linked to ARF.

Differential Diagnosis

No single diagnostic test exists for ARF, and many diseases are included in the differential diagnosis (e.g., JA, connective tissue diseases, infective endocarditis, and Lyme disease).

Management

The treatment of ARF includes the following:

- Antibiotic therapy to eradicate GABHS infection. Benzathine penicillin G is the drug of choice unless there is an allergic history; erythromycin is then the drug of choice. A patient with a history of ARF who has an upper respiratory infection should be treated for GABHS whether or not GABHS is recovered.
- Antiinflammatory therapy. Aspirin can be used for arthritis at 30 to 60 mg/kg per day in four divided doses for 2 to 6 weeks with a reduction in dosage as symptoms are relieved. Corticosteroids are indicated only with severe carditis and manifestations of heart failure (Sondheimer et al, 2001).
- Referral for treatment of congestive heart failure if needed. Medical management or valve replacement may be necessary.
- Bed rest is generally indicated only for children with congestive heart failure. Children with Sydenham chorea may need to be kept in bed to protect them until their choreiform movements are controlled (Kaplan & Markowitz, 2002; Sondheimer et al, 2001).

- Children with severe chorea may benefit from a trial of haloperidol (0.5 to 2 mg every 8 hours) (Amin & Strong, 2002).

The prevention of ARF includes the following:

- Treat GABHS pharyngeal infections with the appropriate antibiotics. Antibacterial prophylaxis for those with a prior history of ARF is required because of their greatly increased risk of recurrent ARF with subsequent inadequately treated GABHS infections. Intramuscular penicillin G every 21 to 28 days is more effective than daily penicillin V.
- Antibacterial prophylaxis is continued for 3 to 5 years of therapy or discontinued at adolescence for children with transient cardiac involvement. For those with persistent myocardial or valvular disease, treatment is lifelong (Sondheimer et al, 2001).
- Children with a history of ARF need bacterial endocarditis prophylaxis treatment for dental or surgical procedures in addition to their regular antibiotic prophylaxis (see Chapter 31).

Complications

Chronic congestive heart failure (CHF) can occur after an initial episode of ARF or follow recurrent episodes of ARF. Residual valvular damage is responsible for CHF.

VASCULITIS SYNDROME

Henoch-Schönlein Purpura

Description

Henoch-Schönlein purpura (HSP) is an overwhelming disease of childhood that is marked by acute vasculitis with associated inflammatory changes in various organ systems.

Etiology and Incidence

HSP is the most common vasculitis syndrome seen in children and can occur anytime from infancy (as early as 6 months) to adulthood. However, it is primarily a disease of childhood. Ninety percent of patients with HSP are less than 10 years of age. Immunoglobulin A (IgA) is involved in the immunopathogenesis of HSP. There is widespread leukocytoclastic vasculitis with IgA deposition in vessel walls. Patients with depositions of IgA in their renal mesangium have an associated nephritis. Although there are two subclasses of IgA, IgA1 and IgA2, only subclass IgA1 is involved in the pathogenesis of HSP (O'Neil, 2002c; Saulsbury, 2001).

Clinical Findings

Clinical findings can vary with age. Infants younger than 2 years of age tend to have milder disease and are less likely to have nephritis and abdominal complications. In adults, nephritis is generally severe and a more frequent associated finding. Approximately 10% of children develop nephritis. Symptoms of nephritis may not be manifested for 4 weeks to 3 months. HPS is more commonly seen in the fall and winter months. This condition often follows a respiratory infection. Cutaneous purpura concentrated on the legs and buttocks must be present to make the diagnosis (O'Neil, 2002c; Saulsbury, 2001).

History. A history of cutaneous purpura concentrated on the legs and buttocks is a key historical feature. In addition, the history may include the following:

- Urticarial or maculopapular rash may precede purpuric lesions
- Arthritis
  - Typically involves knees and ankles and is migratory
  - May precede the appearance of purpuric lesions
- Colicky abdominal pain
- Vomiting
- Hematuria (a hallmark of HSP nephritis)
- Gross or occult gastrointestinal (GI) bleeding

Physical Examination. The two most common manifestations of HSP are

- Skin vasculitis: cutaneous purpura—sine qua non for the diagnosis
  - Diameter: 0 to 2 mm
  - Concentrated on the legs and buttocks
  - Can involve trunk, face, and upper extremities
  - Typically lasts 3 days to 1 month
- Arthritis
  - Initially incapacitates but is self-limited and nondeforming
  - Commonly is periarthritis and involves the knees and ankles
  - Warmth, swelling, and erythema over the joints

Other common features that may be found include the following:

- Signs of GI obstruction (partial obstruction to intussusception) or bleeding
- Signs of nephritis (can occur within 3 months of disease onset)
  - Hypertension or azotemia
  - Hematuria and proteinuria (classic findings of nephritis)

Other, less common, physical findings are related to complications caused by vasculitis in other body organs (e.g., respiratory, cardiac, and central nervous systems).

Diagnostic Studies. The diagnosis of HSP is based on clinical findings. A urinalysis must be done to check for hematuria and proteinuria. Renal biopsy may be warranted if renal involvement is severe. Checking stools for blood is important in children complaining of abdominal pain. If GI obstruction is a consideration, abdominal radiographs should be ordered. Other diagnostic studies (e.g., chest radiographs, CT scans, or electroencephalographs) are ordered based on the signs and symptoms of complications such as shortness of breath, seizures, mental status changes, or hypertension. Such studies are useful to identify specific organ system involvement and the severity of the complication.

Differential Diagnosis

Diseases that cause a similar rash with renal abnormalities are part of the differential diagnosis and include poststreptococcal glomerulonephritis, hemolytic-uremic syndrome, and SLE. Other forms of vasculitis such as Wegener granulomatosis and polyarteritis nodosa are considerations (Bock, 2001).

RESOURCE BOX

National Organizations and Resources for Asthma and Atopic Dermatitis

Allergy and Asthma Network—Mothers of Asthmatics, Inc.
1-800-878-4403
1-703-641-9595
www.aanma.org
An excellent resource for parents

American Academy of Allergy, Asthma, and Immunology
1-800-822-2762
1-414-272-6071
www.aaaai.org

American Lung Association
1-800-586-4872
www.lungusa.org

Asthma and Allergy Foundation of America
1-800-727-8462
www.aafa.org

Asthma and Allergy Information Center and Hotline
1-800-727-5400

National Asthma Education Program Information Center
1-301-951-3260
Provides an excellent resource packet titled "Managing Asthma: A Guide for Schools and an Asthma Management Kit for Clinicians"

National Eczema Association for Science and Education
1-800-818-7546
Fax: 1-503-224-3363
E-mail: nease@teleport.com
www.nationaleczema.org

National Heart, Lung, and Blood Institute
National Asthma Education and Prevention Program
NHLBI Information Center
1-301-251-1222
www.nhlbi.nih.gov

National Jewish Center for Immunology and Respiratory Medicine
1-800-222-5864
www.njc.org
Some organizations have local branches listed in local telephone directories

What you need to know about asthma
www.asthma.about.com

U.S. Environmental Protection Agency
www.epa.gov/iaq/asthma
Information about indoor air quality and information for parents

NATIONAL ORGANIZATIONS AND RESOURCES FOR AUTOIMMUNE DISEASE IN CHILDHOOD (JUVENILE ARTHRITIS AND SYSTEMIC LUPUS ERYTHEMATOSUS)

American Autoimmune Related Diseases Association
1-800-598-4668 (information line)
1-313-371-8600
www.aarda.org

American Juvenile Arthritis Organization
1-404-872-7100 extension 6271
1-800-933-7023
www.arthritis.org/communities/juvenile_arthritis/about_ajao.asp

Lupus Foundation of America, Inc.
1-301-670-9292
1-800-558-0121
www.lupus.org

Management

Children with HSP need to be referred to a pediatrician and subspecialists depending on organ system involvement. Hospitalization is necessary with moderate to severe GI and renal system involvement or if pulmonary, cardiac, or central nervous system manifestations are present. Treatment is generally supportive, and careful attention is given to maintaining hydration and electrolyte balance. In addition, the following are key components of the management plan:

- Monitor for GI blood loss
- Monitor for hematuria and proteinuria
- Monitor and treat hypertension
- Prescribe analgesics and NSAIDs for arthritis
- Prescribe corticosteroids for arthritis and abdominal pain (shortens their duration)
- Treat complications

The skin lesions do not require special care and will resolve without treatment. Study data do not demonstrate that corticosteroids reduce either the duration of illness or the frequency of recurrences. Corticosteroid use has not been shown to be effective in treating established nephritis. Use of other pharmacologic agents or therapies depends on the type and level of organ system involvement. Follow-up includes urine checks weekly for 6 months and then monthly for 3 years (Gusic, 2000).

Complications

Many other infrequent complications of HSP are seen in children, such as myositis, orchitis, hemorrhagic cystitis, pancreatitis, cholecystitis, bowel infarction, perforation or stricture, seizures, ataxia, pulmonary hemorrhage, carditis, anterior uveitis, and episcleritis.

Patient and Parent Education

The practitioner should educate patients and parents as follows:

- About the illness, its complications, and the risk of recurrence
- About the need to closely monitor for nephritis for at least 3 months, including blood pressure and urinalysis testing

Prognosis

The rash and other symptoms can last anywhere from a few days to weeks, with 2 weeks to 3 months being the typical pattern. For the first year after onset of HSP, the recurrence rate in children is 10%. The presence of nephritis is a potentially serious complication with long-term sequelae, including end-stage renal disease (O'Neil, 2002c).

REFERENCES

Amin Z, Strong WB: Acute rheumatic fever. In Burg FD et al, editors: *Gellis and Kagan's current pediatric therapy*, ed 17, Philadelphia, 2002, WB Saunders.

Bock GH: Henoch-Schönlein purpura. In Hoekelman RA et al, editors: *Primary pediatric care*, ed 4, St Louis, 2001, Mosby.

Boguniewicz M, Leung YM: Allergic disorders. In Hay WW et al editors: *Current pediatric diagnosis and treatment*, ed 15, New York, 2001, McGraw-Hill.

Centers for Disease Control and Prevention: National Center for Health Statistics. Available at *www.cdc.gov/nchs/products/pubs/pubd/hestats/asthma/asthma.htm* (accessed Aug 5, 2002).

Craig T, Kakumanu S: Chronic fatigue syndrome: evaluation and treatment, *Am Fam Physician* 65(6):1083-1090, 2002.

Gusic BR: Henoch-Schönlein purpura. In Schwartz MW: *The 5-minute pediatric consult*, Philadelphia, 2000, Williams & Wilkins.

Habif TP et al: *Skin disease: diagnosis and treatment*, St Louis, 2001, Mosby.

Hollister JR: Rheumatic diseases. In Hay WW et al, editors: *Current pediatric diagnosis and treatment*, ed 15, New York, 2001, McGraw-Hill.

Hudson-Barr DC, Lambert SA: Juvenile idiopathic arthritis. In Hayman LL, Mahon MM, Turner JR, editors: *Chronic illness in children*, New York, 2002, Springer.

Hurwitz ME: Treatment of allergic rhinitis with antihistamines and decongestants and their effects on the lower airway, *Pediatr Ann* 29(7):411-420, 2000.

Kaplan EL, Markowitz M: Rheumatic fever. In Finberg L, Kleinman RE, editors: *Saunders manual of pediatric practice*, ed 2, Philadelphia, 2002, WB Saunders.

Krafchik BR: Atopic dermatitis. In Finberg L, Kleinman RE, editors: *Saunders manual of pediatric practice*, ed 2, Philadelphia, 2002, WB Saunders.

Krilov LR, Fisher M: Chronic fatigue syndrome in youth: maybe not so chronic after all, *Contemp Pediatr* 19(4):61-68, 2002.

Kristal L, Klein PA: Atopic dermatitis in infants and children: an update, *Pediatr Clin North Am* 47:877-895, 2000.

Miller ML: Musculoskeletal pain syndromes. In Behrman RE, Kliegman RM, Jenson HB, editors: *Nelson textbook of pediatrics*, ed 17, Philadelphia, 2002, WB Saunders.

Morelli JG, Weston WL: Skin. In Hay WW et al, editors: *Current pediatric diagnosis and treatment*, ed 15, New York, 2001, McGraw-Hill.

Moy JN: Asthma. In Finberg L, Kleinman RE, editors: *Saunders manual of pediatric practice*, ed 2, Philadelphia, 2002, WB Saunders.

National Heart, Lung, and Blood Institute: Guidelines for the diagnosis and management of asthma—update on selected topics 2002. Available at *www.nhlbi.nih.gov/guidelines/asthma/execsumm.pdf* (accessed June 28, 2002).

National Heart, Lung, and Blood Institute: *Highlights of the Expert Panel Report 2: guidelines for the diagnosis and management of asthma*, NIH pub no 97-4051A, Bethesda, MD, 1997, National Institutes of Health.

O'Neil KM: Juvenile arthritis. In Finberg L, Kleinman RE, editors: *Saunders manual of pediatric practice*, ed 2, Philadelphia, 2002a, WB Saunders.

O'Neil KM: Systemic lupus erythematosus. In Finberg L, Kleinman RE, editors: *Saunders manual of pediatric practice*, ed 2, Philadelphia, 2002b, WB Saunders.

O'Neil KM: Systemic vasculitis syndromes of childhood. In Finberg L, Kleinman RE, editors: *Saunders manual of pediatric practice*, ed 2, Philadelphia, 2002c, WB Saunders.

Saulsbury FT: Henoch-Schönlein purpura, *Curr Opin Rheumatol* 13:35-40, 2001.

Silver DS, Wallace DJ: The management of fibromyalgia-associated syndromes, *Rheum Dis Clin North Am* 28:405-417, 2002.

Sly M: Allergic disorders. In Behrman RE, Kliegman RM, Jenson HB, editors: *Nelson textbook of pediatrics*, Philadelphia, 2000, WB Saunders.

Sondheimer HM et al: Cardiovascular diseases. In Hay WW et al, editors: *Current pediatric diagnosis and treatment*, ed 15, New York, 2001, McGraw-Hill.

Taketomo CK, Hodding JH, Kraus DM: *Pediatric dosage handbook*, ed 9, Hudson, OH, 2002, Lexi-Comp.

Yunus MB: A comprehensive medical evaluation of patients with fibromyalgia syndrome, *Rheum Dis Clin North Am* 28:201-217, 2002.

26

Endocrine and Metabolic Diseases

Jean Betschart Roemer

The endocrine system is a secretory feedback system in which glands secrete circulating hormones that affect multiple organs and tissues. During the process of growth and sexual development, there is always the possibility of an abnormal secretion of a particular hormone or combination of hormones. Normal variations commonly occur in the timing and pattern of growth and sexual development. These can present a diagnostic challenge for the practitioner. In contrast, other symptoms and physical findings that the primary care nurse practitioner (NP) might note are clearly associated with specific endocrine disorders marked by either hyposecretion or hypersecretion of hormones. The primary care NP has responsibility to identify children with these disorders and refer them to an endocrinologist for additional diagnostic studies and treatment.

Diabetes mellitus is an endocrine disorder that involves alterations in glucose metabolism. In diabetes mellitus, the hormone insulin is diminished, absent, or ineffective, and glucose metabolism is adversely affected at the cellular level. Types 1 and 2 diabetes are common endocrine-metabolic disorders of childhood and adolescence.

Metabolic disorders generally affect multiple organs and tissues by altering metabolic processes to produce deleterious end products that result in the presence of abnormal substances. Early identification of metabolic disorders is imperative, because metabolic diseases can cause significant, irreversible changes in multiple organ systems and other problems, some of which are life threatening. Newborn screening programs can identify congenital hypothyroidism and a variety of inborn errors of metabolism that are treatable endocrine disorders. Early intervention can alter the outcomes for children born with these problems and may prevent mental retardation and other consequences associated with untreated metabolic and endocrine disorders.

STANDARDS FOR SCREENING

Screening for congenital hypothyroidism is recommended for all neonates during the first week of life. Otherwise, routine screening for thyroid disorders is not warranted in asymptomatic children or adults. Persons with a history of upper body irradiation may benefit from regular physical examination of the thyroid. Screening for phenylketonuria (PKU) is recommended for all newborns before discharge from the nursery. Infants who are tested before 24 hours of age should undergo a repeat screening test before the third week of life (U.S. Preventive Services Task Force, 1998). Routine prenatal screening for maternal PKU is not recommended. Table 26-1 lists available newborn screenings for common metabolic disorders.

ANATOMY AND PHYSIOLOGY

The endocrine system is a looped regulatory system that involves the hypothalamus, the pituitary gland, and other endocrine glands outside the central nervous system. The pituitary gland secretes various protein hormones that stimulate other endocrine glands or body cells. These in turn respond by secreting specific hormones that affect hormone production in the pituitary gland (Fig. 26-1).

Outline of the endocrine loop system:

1. The hypothalamus secretes hormones that regulate specific anterior pituitary cells:
   - Growth hormone–releasing hormone (GHRH) and somatostatin-regulated growth hormone (GH)
   - Prolactin-releasing factor (PRF)
   - Thyroid-stimulating hormone (TSH)–releasing hormone (thyrotropin-releasing hormone [TRH])
   - Corticotropin-releasing hormone (CRH)
   - Luteinizing hormone–releasing hormone (LHRH)

TABLE 26-1 *Newborn Screenings for Metabolic Disorders*

Screen	Description	States Mandating Screening	Severity	Test	Comments
Biotinidase deficiency	Autosomal recessive, multiple carboxylase deficiency	19 states, District of Columbia, and U.S. Virgin Islands	Neurologic signs including hearing loss and optic atrophy	Colorimetric assay for biotinidase using dried blood spot	Zero mortality rate with screening and treatment
Branched-chain ketoaciduria: maple syrup urine disease	Autosomal recessive, branched-chain ketoacid decarboxylation and high body fluid ketoacids	23 states, District of Columbia, and U.S. Virgin Islands	Lethal if unrecognized and untreated; irreversible retardation	Bacterial inhibition assay (BIA) for leucine using dried blood spot	Infants often have irreversible damage by the time they are identified
Congenital adrenal hyperplasia	Family of disorders; defects in enzymes required for biosynthesis of adrenal corticosteroids	11 states	Life-threatening adrenal crisis	Enzyme/radioimmunoassay for 17α-hydroxyprogesterone (17OHP) in 21-hydroxylase deficiency on dried blood spot	
Congenital hypothyroidism	Insufficient thyroid hormone	50 states, District of Columbia, Puerto Rico, and U.S. Virgin Islands	Mental retardation, poor growth	Radioimmunoassay for T_4, thyroid-stimulating hormone (TSH), or both	Mortality not expected but may be underestimated as a result of failure to diagnose
Galactosemia	Inherited disorder of galactose metabolism	44 states, District of Columbia, and U.S. Virgin Islands	Failure to thrive, vomiting, liver disease, mental retardation; fatal in most cases	Elevated blood galactose content	
Homocystinuria	Autosomal recessive defect in catabolism of sulfur-containing amino acids	20 states, District of Columbia, and U.S. Virgin Islands	50% mortality rate by 25 yr of age; developmental delay; marfanoid habitus	BIA for elevated levels of blood methione	Mortality not expected with screening and treatment
Phenylketonuria	Autosomal recessive disorder of phenylalanine hydroxylation	50 states, District of Columbia, Puerto Rico, and U.S. Virgin Islands	Developmental delay, severe mental retardation, seizures	Measurement of blood phenylalanine level by BIA using dried blood spot; automated fluorometric assay	Registries of affected females are being developed to track those at risk

Data from American Academy of Pediatrics Policy Statement: Newborn screening fact sheet (RE9632), *Pediatrics* 98:467-472, 1996.

2. The anterior pituitary responds to these hormones by releasing the following corresponding hormones:
   - GH
   - Prolactin
   - Thyrotropin (TSH)
   - Corticotropin (adrenocorticotropic hormone [ACTH])
   - Gonadotropic hormones: follicle-stimulating hormone (FSH) and luteinizing hormone (LH)
3. These anterior pituitary hormones affect the following target organs or endocrine glands:
   - Growth plate of bones
   - Breast tissue to maintain lactation

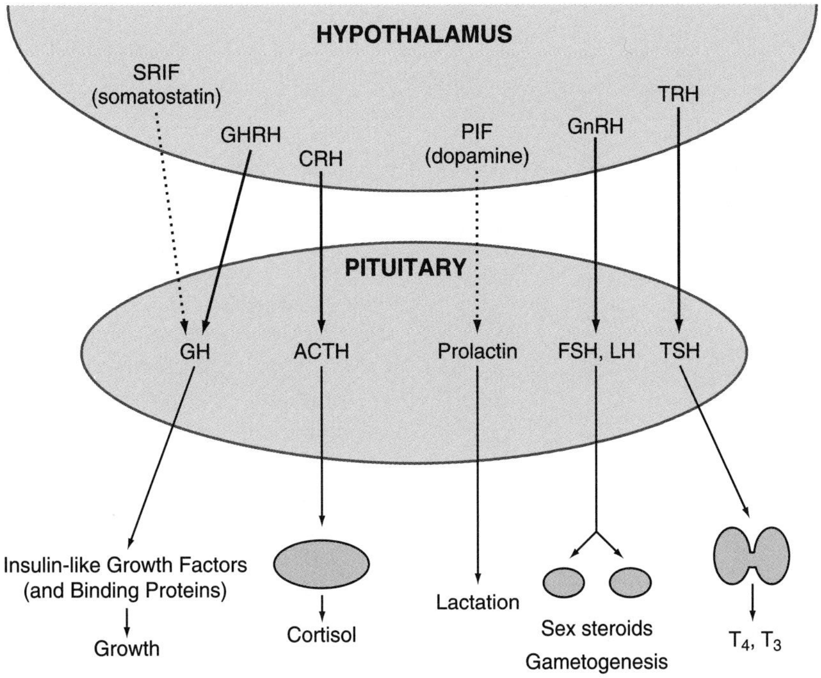

FIGURE 26-1 Hormonal influences of the hypothalamus and pituitary gland. *Solid line* represents stimulatory influence; *dotted line* represents inhibitory influence. *ACTH*, Adrenocorticotropin; *CRH*, corticotropin-releasing hormone; *FSH*, follicle-stimulating hormone; *GH*, growth hormone; *GHRH*, growth hormone-releasing hormone; *GnRH*, gonadotropin-releasing hormone; *LH*, luteinizing hormone; *PIF*, prolactin inhibitory factor; *SRIF*, somatotropin release-inhibiting factor; *T_3*, triiodothyronine; *T_4*, thyroxine; *TRH*, thyrotropin-releasing hormone; *TSH*, thyroid-stimulating hormone. (From Behrman RE, Kliegman RM: *Nelson essentials of pediatrics*, ed 3, Philadelphia, 1998, WB Saunders, p 649.)

- Thyroid gland
- Adrenal glands
- Gonads

4. The following endocrine glands secrete the identified hormone, which then influences hypothalamic hormone production:
   - Thyroid: T_3 (triiodothyronine) and T_4 (thyroxine)
   - Adrenals: corticosteroids
   - Gonads: LH stimulates synthesis of progesterone and androgens; FSH stimulates estradiol
5. The posterior pituitary is an extension of the ventral hypothalamus and secretes arginine vasopressin, the antidiuretic hormone, and oxytocin, a hormone significant in parturition and breastfeeding.

The metabolism of essential amino acids, carbohydrates, and lipids involves complex biochemical functions that transform these substances so they can be used at the cellular level. When metabolic pathways are altered, fundamental biochemical processes are adversely affected in multiple ways and with varying degrees of severity.

PATHOPHYSIOLOGY

Endocrine pathology occurs when there is an alteration in regulation of the normal feedback system that results in hyposecretion or hypersecretion of one or more hormones. Multiple factors cause alterations in hormone production. These include tumors, trauma, infection, systemic disease, genetic disorders, congenital malformation or agenesis of an endocrine gland, idiopathic causes, and iatrogenic causes (medications). The defect or problem can originate at the pituitary-hypothalamic level, in end-organ abnormalities, or for unknown reasons that lead to unresponsiveness to endogenous hormone. Hypothyroidism and hyperthyroidism are examples of disease entities in which the interrelationships of the hypothalamic-pituitary-thyroid axis are altered at any one of several possible sites (Fig. 26-2).

Many metabolic diseases are caused by inborn errors of metabolism. Alteration in genetic constitution results in disrupted biochemical functioning. In children with PKU (a deficiency of the enzyme phenylalanine hydroxylase or its cofactor tetrahydrobiopterin), there is a resulting excessive

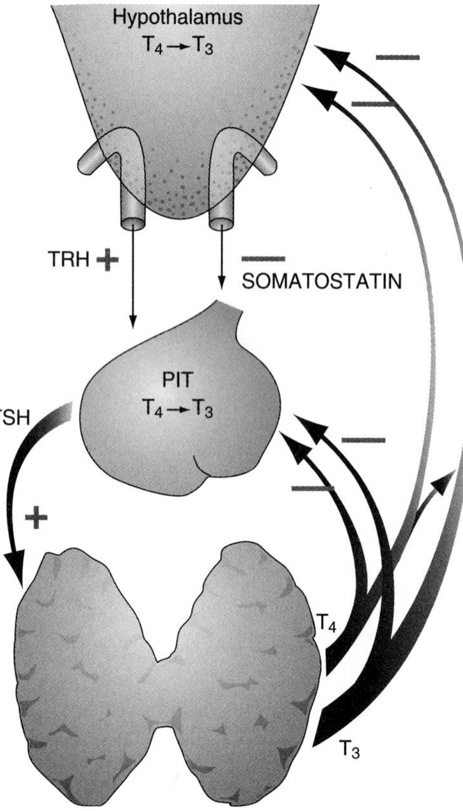

FIGURE 26-2 Interrelationships of the hypothalamic-pituitary-thyroid (HPT) axis. (From Wilson JD, Foster DW, editors: *Williams textbook of endocrinology*, ed 8, Philadelphia, 1992, WB Saunders, p 169.)

accumulation of phenylalanine, an essential amino acid. In galactosemia the defect involves deficiency of galactose 1-phosphate uridyltransferase and the resulting inability to metabolize galactose. Type 1 diabetes is an example of an acquired immune-mediated metabolic disease. In diabetes mellitus, a reduction in insulin production or deficiency of its action results in abnormal metabolism of carbohydrate, protein, and fat.

ASSESSMENT

Endocrine and metabolic disorders are manifest in various organs throughout the body and can alter numerous body functions. An assessment of the endocrine pathology most commonly seen in children is best approached by consideration of the following five areas:

1. Disturbance of growth and sexual development
2. Posterior pituitary gland dysfunction
3. Thyroid problems
4. Adrenal disorders
5. Primary and secondary gonad dysfunction

History

Endocrine disorders and metabolic diseases are either congenital or acquired. Symptoms might differ based on age of the patient at the time of manifestation of the disease. Key factors to consider in the history of a child who is suspected of having an endocrine or metabolic disorder are identified using the classification previously described under Assessment.

- Disturbance in growth and sexual development
  - Is the child growing less or more than 2 inches per year? Is the child still wearing last year's clothes?
  - What are the heights of mother, father, and other family members?
  - Is the child showing signs of sexual development (pubic hair, breast development, axillary or facial hair or both, menses, scrotal and testicular growth)? If yes, at what age did these occur?
  - Is the child taking any medications that affect growth (e.g., steroids)?
  - Are past measurements of stature available for review? Have the plots on standard growth curves crossed percentile lines?
- Posterior pituitary gland dysfunction
  - Are there symptoms of hypofunction, including polydipsia and polyuria?
- Thyroid problems
  - Are symptoms present of hypofunction or hyperfunction of this gland (as identified later under each of these problems)?
  - Does the child have another condition associated with secondary thyroid problems, such as trisomy 21, Turner syndrome, exposure to radiation, or type 1 diabetes mellitus?
  - Was there maternal exposure to radioiodine, goitrogens (e.g., thiourea or thiouracil), or iodine medication during pregnancy?
- Adrenal disorders
  - Are there symptoms of adrenal hypofunction that manifest as either acute adrenal crisis with vomiting, dehydration, and collapse or as a chronic form of disease with weakness, fatigue, and pallor?
  - Are there symptoms of adrenal hyperfunction in the newborn that manifest as alterations in sexual development or cause significant electrolyte and water disturbances?
  - Are there symptoms of acquired hyperfunction (Cushing syndrome) that cause classic symptoms such as

moon face, truncal adiposity, muscle wasting and weakness, lethargy, and hypertension?

- Primary and secondary gonad dysfunction
  - When did the child show signs of sexual development (pubic hair, breast development, axillary or beard/facial hair, menses, scrotal and testicular growth)? This is a key question in premature pubertal development.
  - How has the child been growing? Has growth accelerated? If delayed sexual development is suspected, questions regarding growth rate are important.
  - What is the child's diet and exercise history? Diet and exercise history is important if secondary amenorrhea resulting from anorexia or bulimia is suspected.
- Metabolic diseases
  - Are there classic signs and symptoms of diabetes mellitus, PKU, or galactosemia present as identified in this chapter under the specific disease entity?
  - Is there a positive family history of diabetes mellitus, PKU, or galactosemia? Type 1 diabetes mellitus is associated with certain markers found on chromosome 6 in specific human leukocyte antigen (HLA) regions; PKU and galactosemia are autosomal recessive diseases.

Physical Examination

Endocrine and metabolic disorders can affect numerous body systems. Attention to detail when performing a physical examination on a child with a suspected disorder is important. Review the following:

- Measure stature. Supine length is the preferred position for measuring children younger than 2 years of age. Use a stadiometer for children older than 2 or 3 years of age. Height and weight are plotted on a standardized growth chart. Serial measurements of growth to determine growth rate or velocity are essential to the assessment of growth problems.
- Check for proportionate appearance. Measure sitting and standing heights for upper to lower segment ratio, (see Chapter 33) check for height age, and measure growth velocity.
- Plot rate of weight gain and body mass index (BMI).
- Inspect the child's genitalia carefully. Look for signs of either normal or ambiguous genitalia.
- Identify the stage of sexual development using Tanner staging criteria (see Chapter 9).
- Note facial, axillary, and body hair for presence, distribution, and texture.
- Examine the skin for striae and acanthosis nigricans (see Color Fig. 11) of the neck, axilla, breast, knuckles, and skin folds.
- Palpate the neck carefully for enlargement of the thyroid gland.
- Perform a detailed physical examination of the newborn, observing for dysmorphic features.
- Acquired endocrine disorders are often due to either hyposecretion or hypersecretion of a specific hormone or combination of hormones. The child may appear sick. Signs of dehydration, exophthalmos, and tachycardia are physical findings associated with endocrine pathology. Newborns with PKU and galactosemia have normal newborn examinations, but physical symptoms develop as the deleterious effects of metabolic alterations become apparent. Other characteristic physical findings are identified later under the specific disease entity.

Diagnostic Tests

Laboratory studies measuring hormone levels are key diagnostic tools of endocrine disorders. Many of these studies are expensive. Accurate interpretation of data requires strict adherence to laboratory protocol for timing the collection of blood specimens.

Specific blood and urine studies that identify end products of abnormal metabolism or elevated or diminished levels of various substances, such as glucose, galactose, amino acids, calcium, or sodium, are important in the diagnosis of metabolic disorders.

Radiographic and imaging studies (e.g., bone age, skull radiographs, ultrasonography, radioactive isotopes, computed tomography [CT], and magnetic resonance imaging [MRI]) are also important diagnostic tools in evaluating certain endocrine disorders.

MANAGEMENT STRATEGIES

General Measures

Chronic disease issues and the effects of these diseases on lifestyle must be addressed:

- Family, school, peer, and emotional adjustment
- Body image, self-esteem, and social competence
- Disease understanding, acceptance, and self-care

Receiving encouragement in self-care and learning about one's disease and the patient-parent role in management of a long-term illness or chronic condition are essential for successful outcomes.

Genetic Counseling

Genetic counseling is necessary (see Chapter 41). There are significant implications for the family of a child with endocrine and metabolic disorders that are genetically linked.

Medications

Hormone replacement, whether temporary or lifelong, and therapy with other pharmacologic agents are often essential components of management of these disorders. Often, these need to be administered via injection, creating distress in both the child and caregiver. Short and clear instructions about medications are important: how much to give, when to give it, administration guidelines, possible side effects, and when to make adjustments in medication.

Dietary Considerations

Often, metabolic diseases require rigid adherence to dietary plans and restrictions. Parents and patients must be knowledgeable about dietary needs and restrictions and the effect of diet on the disease process.

Patient and Parent Education

Close supervision and frequent follow-up are necessary for children with metabolic and endocrine disorders. They are best evaluated initially and periodically by a multidisciplinary health care team of providers who have expertise in pediatric endocrinology. Parents and children must learn about the nature of the disorder, the treatment, possible complications, and the plan for long-term follow-up. A multidisciplinary care team can best provide the support and education required. The primary care provider, as part of the team, is in an ideal position to support and reinforce the plan of care. Additionally, it is essential that primary health care needs and anticipatory guidance are not overlooked.

SPECIFIC ENDOCRINE AND METABOLIC DISORDERS OF CHILDREN

Common Disorders Detected in the Newborn Period

Ambiguous Genitalia

Description. The diagnosis of ambiguous genitalia is made when a child is born with varied degrees of both male and female external genitalia. The term *true hermaphrodite* refers to a child who has both male and female gonadal structures. This is rare. It is more common to see either *female pseudohermaphroditism* (a female with ambiguous external genitalia and female gonads) or *male pseudohermaphroditism* (a male with ambiguous external genitalia and male gonads). When children are born with ambiguous genitalia, it should be treated as a medical emergency in order to ensure the correct assignment of sex as quickly as possible. There are many causes leading to abnormal sexual differentiation. A referral to a pediatric endocrinologist is necessary to determine the exact etiology as quickly as possible and to institute a treatment plan.

Congenital Adrenal Hyperplasia

Description. The most common etiology of ambiguous genitalia is congenital adrenal hyperplasia (CAH), which can be caused by a group of disorders of adrenal steroid biosynthesis. With CAH there is a deficiency of one of the several enzymes necessary for the adrenal cortex to produce cortisol and aldosterone; thus there are several forms of CAH. These disorders can disrupt adrenal or adrenal and gonadal steroidogenesis. The most frequent enzyme deficiency that results in CAH is 21-hydroxylase (95%). This enzyme deficiency involves overproduction of ACTH, leading to hyperplasia of the adrenal gland and excessive adrenal androgen secretion. When aldosterone and cortisol pathways are blocked or inhibited, excessive sodium is lost through the kidneys, resulting in an inability to maintain serum electrolyte balance. The androgen pathway is overstimulated, and virilization ensues. Patients with CAH fall into two categories: those who are salt losers and those who are not. About 75% of newborns with CAH detected with newborn screening are salt losers (Styne & Glaser, 2002). Genetic markers have been identified for CAH.

Clinical Findings

History. Parents may have experienced either the unexplained death of other infants or death of their own siblings with the same disorder.

Physical Examination. Patients with CAH who are not salt losers display varied features. There may be enlargement of the clitoris or penis, development of pubic hair, acne, and acceleration of growth. In affected females, diagnosis is usually made at birth because of ambiguous genitalia. There are normal internal genitalia with varying degrees of virilization of the external genitalia ranging from enlarged clitoris to complete fusion of the labial-scrotal folds, forming a penile urethra. Males often appear normal at birth. Signs of precocious sexual growth may appear in the child by 6 months of age or develop more gradually over the next 4 to 5 years.

Infants who are salt losers begin to have symptoms shortly after birth. Females are more easily identified because of the virilization of their external genitalia (although a female case might be missed if mild virilization is overlooked). Males have normal genitalia and appear normal. These males are often diagnosed at 7 to 14 days in adrenal crisis. Precocious sexual growth might appear by 6 months of age.

In the salt-losing variety of CAH, symptoms begin shortly after birth and manifest as

- Failure to regain birth weight
- Progressive weight loss
- Vomiting
- Lack of appetite
- Dehydration

Untreated symptoms of acute adrenal insufficiency include the following:

- Hyponatremia
- Hypochloremia
- Hyperkalemia
- Vascular collapse

If untreated, other symptoms include the following:

- Rapid somatic growth
- Advanced epiphyseal maturation leading to short stature as adults
- Progressive penile or clitoral enlargement
- Early appearance of facial, axillary, and pubic hair
- Acne

Diagnostic Tests. Laboratory findings include high plasma renin activity, low serum and urinary aldosterone levels, and elevated 17α-hydroxyprogesterone.

Management. The diagnosis and treatment of infants with suspected salt-losing CAH constitute a medical emergency, requiring immediate attention. Primary care should continue for well and sick visits between endocrinology appointments, and the provider should be familiar with the medical therapy involved. Surgical repair is required for those children with ambiguous genitalia.

Pharmacologic Management. Children with salt-losing CAH are given the following:

1. Hydrocortisone (Cortef). This replaces deficient cortisol and suppresses ACTH overproduction, thus inhibiting excessive production of androgen and further virilization. The administration of glucocorticoids suppresses ACTH secretion and produces atrophy of the adrenal cortex. The pituitary-adrenal axis may take 1 to 18 months to return to normal.

   Adjustments in the dosages of the glucocorticoids are based on periodic evaluation of plasma renin activity, 17α-hydroxyprogesterone, and serum androgens and on clinical assessment of growth and pubertal development. Hydrocortisone is the glucocorticoid most often used, with doses of 10 to 20 mg/m^2 per 24 hours administered orally in three divided doses. The morning dose is given as early as possible to blunt the body's normal early morning corticotropin increase. Individualizing dosage is important and is based on growth, bone age, and hormonal levels (American Academy of Pediatrics, 2000).

   All patients with classic forms of CAH must take glucocorticoids lifelong. When growth is completed, the child may be switched to prednisone, given once or twice daily, or dexamethasone, given as a single dose at bedtime, if adequate suppression of androgens can be maintained. Glucocorticoids should be increased during periods of stress (e.g., fever or surgery) in salt-losing and non–salt-losing patients (American Academy of Pediatrics, 2000).
2. Fludrocortisone (Florinef). This mineralocorticoid is administered to replace aldosterone at a dose of 0.05 to 0.2 mg daily given orally as a single dose or in two divided doses (Lee & Levitsky, 2002) and is required for children who are salt-losers and have elevated plasma rennin activity.
3. Sodium chloride. Sodium chloride supplements (5 ml of 10% NaCl given twice a day) is often needed in infancy and in hot weather (Lee & Levitsky, 2002).

The management of children with non–salt-losing and nonclassic 21-OH deficiency (American Academy of Pediatrics, 2000) involves the following:

1. Hydrocortisone therapy is used for children with non–salt-losing congenital adrenal hyperplasia. However, many of these children, especially boys, may not be diagnosed until 3 to 7 years of age. Administration of hydrocortisone therapy will slow growth and bone maturation to more normal rates for some children.
2. Patients with nonclassic 21-OH deficiency do not always require treatment. Many remain asymptomatic throughout their lives. For some, symptoms may develop during puberty, after puberty, or postpartum. They will also require glucocorticoid but in lower dosages than what is prescribed for patients with classic 21-OH deficiency. Advanced bone age, severe acne, hirsutism, menstrual irregularity, and infertility are indications for therapy.

Psychosocial Support. Assessment of the child's feelings about body changes and differences can be important. Children with ambiguous genitalia or precocious virilization are at risk for developing disturbances in self-concept and self-esteem. Precocious development can enhance feelings of being different. Play therapy can be a useful strategy to help children play out and cope with their differences. Understandably, parents also may have enormous concerns and grief over the diagnosis. Home health referral can be helpful for follow-up, support, and reinforcement to ensure that medications are taken properly and the child and family are adjusting.

Complications. The inability to fight infection, hypoglycemia, and hyponatremia can lead to vascular collapse and death. The child should be monitored for signs of cortisol and androgen excess, growth and weight gain, pubertal development, and osseous maturation. Psychosocial problems with self-esteem and feeling of being different are discussed under Psychosocial Support.

Patient and Parent Education. The primary care NP's role is to listen to parent and patient concerns and provide anticipatory guidance, make referrals, and reinforce the following:

- Children with CAH should wear medical identification bracelets. Patients or parents also need to carry medical information about the child's condition in case medical therapy is needed from an unfamiliar provider.
- Families must learn the need for lifelong medication therapy and medical follow-up.
- Caretakers must know the symptoms of acute adrenal insufficiency (vomiting, lethargy, dehydration) that require immediate medical attention.
- Education must also include when and whom to call for help in times of unusual stress. At these times there might be a need to triple the dose of hydrocortisone (e.g., illness with fever, pain, or vomiting). The parents should be prepared to give their child an intramuscular injection of hydrocortisone sodium succinate before transport to an emergency department if vomiting, lethargy, and dehydration are evident.

Phenylketonuria

Description. PKU is a disorder of amino acid metabolism in which phenylalanine cannot be converted to tyrosine because of a deficiency of the enzyme phenylalanine hydroxylase. As a result toxic levels of phenylalanine accumulate in the blood (hyperphenylalaninemia). If undetected and untreated, PKU causes progressive neurologic dysfunction with psychomotor retardation. Presently all 50 states mandate routine screening tests for all infants in the first few days of life after the initiation of feeding. Hyperphenylalaninemias can be classified as follows:

Disorder	Plasma phenylalanine level (mg/dl)	Level of mental retardation (if not treated)
Classic PKU	>20	Severe, profound
Atypical (variant) PKU	6-20	Mild to moderate
Benign persistent hyperphenylalaninemia	2-6	None (no treatment necessary)
Biopterin defects	4-40	None to severe

Etiology and Incidence. PKU most often occurs in Caucasians, with an incidence of 1:14,000 to 1:20,000 live births (Behrman, Kliegman, & Jenson, 2004). It is inherited as an autosomal recessive trait.

Clinical Findings. The neonate with PKU appears normal at birth. However, if the PKU is untreated, signs and symptoms develop, such as vomiting, irritability, and musty-smelling urine. On physical examination, the child with more advanced disease has a light complexion, eczematoid rash, hypertonicity with hyperactive deep tendon reflexes, seizures, and mental retardation.

Diagnostic Tests. Routine screening is done by the collection of blood from the heel of an infant, placed on filter paper. Patients with classic PKU who are on normal diets have serum concentrations of phenylalanine greater than 30 g/dl and a low concentration of tyrosine.

Management. Successful prevention of mental retardation caused by PKU is possible by limiting dietary phenylalanine intake to amounts that permit normal growth and development. Treatment involves the use of a low-phenylalanine, tyrosine-enriched diet with a low-phenylalanine milk substitute, such as Lofenalac. Previously, it was thought that phenylalanine restriction should be followed strictly until a child was 8 years of age, when it then could be relaxed. However, recent studies in older individuals who had stopped their low-phenylalanine diet have raised concerns of a possible link between a decline in intellectual performance and the discontinuation of dietary restriction. Therefore a diet low in phenylalanine may need to be lifelong because it is not clear whether the low-phenylalanine diet can ever be safely eliminated (Yudkoff, 2002). Adolescent females with PKU should be aware that strict dietary adherence must resume if they become pregnant and, ideally, should be started preconception.

Management of PKU should be done at a facility where blood levels of phenylalanine can be followed up and dietary adjustments made. Phenylalanine blood levels below 5 mg/dl are desired. Consultation with or referral to a dietitian is essential. Be sure to stress the need for mothers enrolled in the Women, Infants, and Children's (WIC) Nutritional Program to discuss their infant's need for special formula with the WIC dietitian.

Galactosemia

Description. Galactosemia is a disorder of galactose metabolism, with three possible inborn errors of galactose metabolism currently identified. A deficiency in one of the three enzymes results in the inability of the galactose to be converted to glucose 1-phosphate. Classic galactosemia, the most common form, is caused by a deficiency of galactose 1-phosphate uridyltransferase (GALT). Galactose is broken down from the disaccharide lactose, which is primarily found in milk. Without GALT, galactose metabolites accumulate in the tissues, leading to the clinical manifestations.

Etiology and Incidence. The incidence of galactosemia with complete or nearly complete GALT deficiency is about 1 in 40,000 to 60,000 live births; it is an autosomal recessive trait (Gibson, 2002).

Clinical Findings. The neonate born with galactosemia appears normal, with clinical manifestations beginning after milk feeding.

History. In galactosemia, there might be a history of vomiting, weight loss, diarrhea, and lethargy.

Physical Examination. If therapy is delayed or therapy is not yet effective, the following might be observed: jaundice, hepatomegaly, hypotonia, severe neonatal *Escherichia coli* infections, or cataracts. Death can occur.

Diagnostic Tests. Urine testing for glucose with a glucose oxidase method for reducing substance can be done for the initial workup. Confirmation of the diagnosis depends on assay of transferase activity in erythrocytes.

Management. A galactose-free formula is used for infants with galactosemia, and clinical manifestations subside after galactose intake is restricted. A galactose-restricted diet is the mainstay of therapy for a child. Foods that contain galactose (usually lactose, the disaccharide of glucose and galactose) are restricted. Strict avoidance of milk and all dairy products, as well as foods labeled as containing galactose or lactose, is recommended; fruits and vegetables that contain lower amounts of galactose should be eaten. Milk substitutes such as soybean and casein hydrolysate are used instead of milk. Lifelong dietary restrictions of galactose should continue, because there is no evidence that older children can more effectively metabolize galactose with maturation. Galactose intake of no more than 0.5 to 1 mg/kg/day is recommended for older patients with galactosemia (Gibson, 2002). Pregnant teenagers should be advised to continue the restricted diet throughout pregnancy.

Growth Hormone Disorders

Assessment of growth is an important component in the routine health care of children. Growth is an indicator of a child's mental and physical health and the quality of the environment. Differentiation of abnormal growth patterns from normal variants is integral to the practice of the NP. Recognition and referral of those children whose abnormal growth pattern is indicative of a pathologic process are extremely important. Children with poor growth should be carefully monitored to assess genetic, prenatal, endocrine, nutritional, metabolic, psychologic, or systemic chronic illness. Growth hormone deficiency (GHD) and GH excess are two endocrine disorders that require referral to a pediatric endocrinologist for appropriate treatment. Constitutional short stature (CSS) is a variation of normal growth. Table 26-2 differentiates GHD and CSS.

Constitutional Short Stature

Description. The most common cause of short stature is constitutionally delayed growth. In most cases, children with CSS do not have GH abnormalities or any other detectable alteration. Constitutional delay in growth is a variation of normal growth and is not a disease. By adulthood, the child's

TABLE 26-2 ***Short Stature: Characteristics of Growth Hormone Deficiency (GHD) and Constitutional Short Stature (CSS) in Children***

Condition	Etiology	Onset	Presentation	Endocrine/Metabolic Disturbance
GHD	Most cases are idiopathic; pituitary or hypothalamic disease; trauma; minor organic hypothalamic lesion; infection; radiation	Congenital or acquired	<4 cm of growth per year with normal birth weight; signs and symptoms of increased central nervous system pressure; microphallus; proportional short stature; delayed bone age	Deficiency or impairment in secretion of growth hormone–releasing hormone
CSS	Variation of normal growth; not a disease	First years of life impaired growth	Growth velocity is normal; delayed puberty and pubertal growth spurt; delayed bone age; positive family history	None—final height is appropriate for parents' height

final height is within the normal adult range. This entity needs to be differentiated from those of a pathologic nature.

Clinical Findings

History. The history may include the following:

- Typical growth pattern (Styne, 2002).
- Normal length and weight at birth with a slow decrease in height for age between birth and the second or third birthday. The height velocity decrease is gradual, with the child's percentiles of height for age falling during infancy.
- Growth resumes at a normal rate of 5 cm or more per year after age 2 to 3 years but is at or slightly below the 5th percentile for age.
- Delayed pubertal development.
- Family history of delayed growth and pubertal development.
- Determination of height velocity is the most critical factor in evaluating the growth of a child.

Physical Examination. The following may be seen on physical examination:

- Delayed bone age, but the rate of growth is normal for bone age.
- Final height is within the target range predicted for family height.

The neurologic examination is normal.

Diagnostic Test. The same screening tests are indicated as listed for GHD to rule out pathologic processes.

Management. Because it is difficult at times to differentiate CSS from that due to GHD, an endocrine referral may be necessary. Reassurance and support should be provided to the child regarding ultimate height and development. The use of growth hormone therapy (GHT) in these children is controversial.

Growth Hormone Deficiency

Description. GH is released in response to sleep, exercise, and hypoglycemia. It is responsible for the stimulation of growth in children, whose long bones are not fused. A deficiency is suspected when there are low levels of human growth hormone (hGH) in the serum or if the level fails to increase in response to sleep, exercise, and hypoglycemia.

Etiology and Incidence. The incidence of idiopathic GHD is approximately 1 in 3500 (Cuttler, 2002). GHD in children can be either congenital or acquired. The majority of the cases of GHD are idiopathic. It is suspected that either there is a deficiency or an impairment in the secretion of hGH-releasing hormone, or there is a minor organic hypothalamic lesion. Other causes of GHD include pituitary or hypothalamic disease, trauma, infection, embryologic defects, tumors, and irradiation.

Clinical Findings

History. A history of GHD can include the following:

- Poor growth rate (less than 4 cm per year) with history of normal birth weight
- Prolonged labor or breech delivery
- Headache, visual field disturbances, polyuria, polydipsia (if a tumor is present)
- Normal intelligence

Physical Examination. The following may be noted on physical examination:

- Proportional short stature
- Increased subcutaneous adiposity
- Hypoglycemia
- Microphallus in males
- Delayed bone age
- Childlike face with large, prominent forehead
- High-pitched voice

Diagnostic Tests. Diagnostic evaluation of a child with a suspected growth disorder is highly individualized and should be conducted in conjunction with a pediatric endocrinologist. Constitutional growth delay can be differentiated from genetic short stature by the level of skeletal maturation, which in the latter is consistent with chronologic age. Height velocity is the most critical factor in evaluation and might indicate pathology if decreased after the third year of age. Children with congenital GH deficiency often are diagnosed in the newborn period with hypoglycemia, prolonged hyperbilirubinemia, microphallus, or a combination of these three. In addition, with congenital GHD, linear growth commonly slows during the first 3 years of life (Cuttler, 2002; Vogiatzi & Copeland, 1998). In addition to a complete history, the diagnostic evaluation includes the following:

- Growth measurements and evaluation of growth charts
- Determination of midparental height (take the average of the mother's and father's heights; add 2.5 inches for boys and subtract 2.5 inches for girls)
- Complete blood count
- Sedimentation rate
- Urinalysis
- Stool for occult blood and ova and parasites
- Chemistry panel
- Thyroid function tests
- Bone age
- Karyotype (short girls)
- Growth hormone levels (IGF-1 and IGFBP-3)

A diagnosis of GHD is made when serum hGH is low and hGH levels fail to increase after specific stimulation tests.

Management. A child with GHD is best managed by a pediatric endocrinologist. Primary care providers should be aware of the type of therapy being used, including expected response and possible adverse reactions. The treatment of GHD has expanded because of the increased availability of synthetic GH. The recommended dose of GH for GHD is 0.18 to 0.3 mg/kg per week divided into daily subcutaneous doses. Adolescents can receive higher doses of 0.7 mg/kg per week. The dose for females with Turner syndrome and children with chronic renal failure is 0.35 to 0.375 mg/kg per week, divided into daily subcutaneous injections (Cuttler, 2002). The younger the child is when GH therapy is initiated, the greater the effect. If begun early enough, adult height can be within the same range as the child's peers without GHD. Reported side effects of GH include insulin resistance, pseudotumor cerebri, edema, growth of nevi, and carpal tunnel syndrome (Cuttler, 2002).

The average annual cost of GHT is based on a weight-dependent dose. For a 30 kg child, GHT is approximately $19,000, which may or may not be covered by health insurance. Therefore cost might place a burden on the family. Some states offer assistance through programs for children with special health care needs. The manufacturers of growth hormone also offer a program for financial assistance.

Excessive Growth Syndrome: Pituitary Gigantism

Description. Pituitary gigantism is a result of hypersecretion of GH, usually caused by a pituitary adenoma. The adenoma also can interfere with the functioning of other pituitary hormones. Hyposecretion of gonadal hormones can lead to pubertal delay or menstrual disturbances.

Clinical Findings

History. If the tumor occurs before the fusion of the epiphyses, the child will be extremely tall with a history of sudden growth. If the tumor occurs after closure of the epiphyses, the child will show signs of acromegaly. Complaints of impaired vision from compression of the optic nerve and symptoms of increased intracranial pressure occur.

Physical Examination. Signs of acromegaly that occur after fusion of the epiphyses include coarse facial features, protruding jaw, rapid increase in height, large hands and feet, and thickened skin.

Diagnostic Tests. The definitive laboratory result for the diagnosis of acromegaly is failure of serum GH level to decrease to less than 2 μg/L after ingestion of glucose (Fisher, 2000). In children, an increase in blood glucose suppresses GH secretion. The presence of a tumor is confirmed with skull films and CT or MRI.

Differential Diagnosis. Other conditions associated with excessive growth include

- Precocious puberty
- Hyperthyroidism
- Constitutional tall stature
- Klinefelter syndrome
- Syndromes of XYY, XXYY
- Marfan syndrome
- Soto syndrome

Management. The patient should be referred to a pediatric endocrinologist. The goal of therapy is to eliminate excessive GH secretion. In those with a pituitary lesion, the treatment regimen includes surgery, radiation, or pharmacologic therapy.

Diabetes Mellitus

Diabetes mellitus is a group of metabolic diseases causing hyperglycemia. Diabetes is a chronic disease that affects more than 17 million people in the United States (U.S. Department of Health and Human Services, 2002). The prevalence has increased because of a number of factors, primarily related to the increased incidence of obesity. Diabetes is the leading cause of adult blindness, kidney failure, and nontraumatic amputations and a major cause of heart disease and stroke. Chronic hyperglycemia is associated with complications of diabetes such as cardiovascular damage and dysfunction of the eyes, kidneys, and nerves. There are two major forms of diabetes, which have been termed *type 1 diabetes* (insulin-dependent diabetes mellitus [IDDM]; juvenile-onset diabetes) and *type 2 diabetes* (non–insulin-dependent diabetes mellitus [NIDDM]; adult- or maturity-onset diabetes). There are also other specific types of diabetes, including gestational diabetes and impaired glucose tolerance. Classification is not always clear because there may be considerable heterogenicity between various forms of the disorder (American Diabetes Association, 2002a).

Onset of type 1 diabetes is rapid, the illness is acute, ketones are present in blood and urine, and blood glucose levels can be very high. Type 2 diabetes is being diagnosed at an alarming rate in obese children with a strong family history. The diagnostic classification is not always clear on diagnosis. Verification through use of autoantibodies substantiates type 1 diabetes but is not universally recommended because of cost issues. Glycohemoglobin (Hgb) A_{1c} measurements are not currently recommended for the diagnosis of diabetes (American Diabetes Association, 2002a).

Type 1 Diabetes

Etiology and Incidence. Type 1 diabetes results from defects in insulin secretion, insulin action, or both. It is immune mediated, and thus there is beta cell destruction in the pancreas leading to absolute insulin deficiency. It occurs at a rate of 12 to 14 per 100,000, with a higher incidence in white American children than in other racial groups of children and adolescents. However, type 1 diabetes can occur at any age. The peak incidence related to age-group is adolescence. A seasonal pattern is noted, with diagnosis peaking in fall and winter months (Capriles & Levitsky, 2002). Markers of the immune destruction include islet cell antibodies (ICAs), insulin autoantibodies (IAAs), autoantibodies to glutamic acid decarboxylase (GAD65), and autoantibodies to the tyrosine phosphates. Also, this disease has strong histocompatibility antigen (HLA) associations (American Diabetes Association, 2002a).

Clinical Findings

HISTORY. Children may become ill quite suddenly. Onset is usually acute, appearing over a period of weeks or days. Typically, a child may have had a viral illness, cold, or flu, and parents notice increased urination and thirst during the recovery period. Weight loss can be significant. Often the diagnosis is not made until symptoms of ketoacidosis arise and the child appears ill. Acute symptoms such as vomiting, weight loss, and dehydration are flulike, sometimes delaying the diagnosis. Ketonuria and ketonemia occur. Table 26-3 identifies key clinical findings associated with type 1 diabetes mellitus.

The symptoms of patients with hyperglycemia may include

- Polydipsia
- Polyphagia
- Nocturia
- Blurred vision
- Weight loss
- Fatigue

Signs and symptoms of ketoacidosis include

- Dehydration
- Fruity-smelling breath
- Abdominal pain or vomiting
- Kussmaul breathing
- Flushed cheeks and face
- Mental confusion
- Lethargy
- Obtunded responses

PHYSICAL EXAMINATION. Note the degree of dehydration and look for signs of ketoacidosis (ketonuria or ketonemia). Other findings can include the following:

- Weight loss or slow rate of growth
- Muscle wasting
- Tachycardia
- Vaginal yeast, thrush, or other infection
- Glycosuria or ketononuria (or both)

DIAGNOSTIC TESTS

- Symptoms of diabetes together with a random plasma glucose concentration greater than or equal to 200 mg/dl (11.1 mmol/L)
- Fasting plasma glucose greater than or equal to 126 mg/dl (7.0 mmol/L)
- A 2-hour after-meal plasma glucose greater than or equal to 200 mg/dl (11.1 mmol/L) during an oral glucose tolerance test (OGTT) (American Diabetes Association, 2002a)

Management. The general goals of therapy for children with type 1 diabetes include achieving normal growth and development, optimal glycemic control, minimal acute or chronic complications, and a positive psychosocial adjustment to diabetes. Goals must be individualized for each child based on age, ability to recognize hypoglycemia, and self-care skills. Target ranges for blood glucose levels in children and teens vary depending on the judgment of the provider and individual goals set with the child and his or her parents.

TABLE 26-3 ***Type 1 Diabetes Mellitus: Key Clinical Findings***

History	Polydipsia, polyphagia, polyuria, nocturia, blurred vision, weight loss, fatigue
Onset	Usually acute, ketones in blood and urine, high blood glucose level
Laboratory findings	Ketonuria or ketonemia
Physical findings	Signs of ketoacidosis: dehydration; slow, labored breathing or air column; flushed cheeks and face; mental confusion; lethargy; fruity odor (acetone) on breath
Diagnostic tests	Random plasma glucose concentration ≥200 mg/dl (11.1 mmol/L)
	Fasting plasma glucose ≥126 mg/dl (7.0 mmol/L)
	Two hours after meal, plasma glucose ≥200 mg/dl (11.1 mmol/L) during an oral glucose tolerance test
Other tests	Verification of autoantibodies substantiates type 1 diabetes but is not universally recommended
	Glycosylated hemoglobin (Hgb A_{1c}) measurements are not currently recommended for the diagnosis of diabetes; useful for follow-up monitoring

From Burns CE et al: *Pocket reference for pediatric primary care*, Philadelphia, 2001, WB Saunders.

The guidelines for target fasting and before-meal glucose and for Hgb A_{1c} levels are age based (Wolfsdorf & Weinstein, 2002):

- Children younger than 5 years of age: 100 to 200 mg/dl and less than 9% Hgb A_{1c}
- Children between 5 and 11 years of age: 70 to 180 mg/dl and less than 8% Hgb A_{1c}
- Children 12 years of age and older: 70 to 150 mg/dl and less than 7% Hgb A_{1c}

The classic Diabetes Control and Complications Trial revealed that those who kept blood glucose levels as close to normal as possible had a 60% reduction in the risk, development, and progression of eye, kidney, and nervous system complications (American Diabetes Association, 2002c). This study included only adolescents and adults. Although it cannot be generalized, most practitioners feel strongly that the effects of hyperglycemia are common to all people with diabetes.

Assessment of the quality of diabetes control is determined by Hgb A_{1c} levels, a daily log of metered glucose values, and clinical symptoms. Hgb A_{1c} levels indicate an approximate level of glycemic control over the past 60 days. Acceptable control for children younger than 7 years is a value of approximately 8.0%, and for older children and teens, levels less than 8.0% are desirable. A target level that approaches normal is desirable only if it can be reached without severe or frequent episodes of hypoglycemia. This value must be used together with consideration of metered serum glucose values. If the Hgb A_{1c} level is acceptable but daily values have wide excursions (e.g., moving between 40 and 400 mg/dl), diabetes is not well controlled. Clinical symptoms would include the frequency and severity of hypoglycemia, ketonuria, or weight loss.

Hypoglycemia is the most immediate reason for making adjustments in insulin doses; however, the presence of ketonuria is also an indication for prompt action. Box 26-1 identifies key points to consider for insulin adjustment.

The usual diabetes regimen includes medical nutritional therapy and some form of insulin therapy. Insulin therapy can vary from two or more injections daily to insulin pump therapy. Blood glucose is monitored before meals, at bedtime, when there are symptoms of high or low blood glucose, and occasionally during the night. After initial stabilization at diagnosis, frequent follow-up visits at a minimum of 3-month intervals are essential. At first, the family may be in contact with the health care provider on a daily basis as blood glucose levels normalize. At each visit the management plan is reviewed with the child and family and modified based on the physical and psychosocial needs of the patient and family. Follow-up visits may focus on obtaining information regarding hypoglycemic episodes or ketonuria, results of blood glucose self-monitoring, insulin dose adjustments, and social or emotional issues. Traditional multidisciplinary team approaches are one way to manage a newly diagnosed case in a child, especially when the child is ill and hospitalized at the time of diagnosis. However, when the child is not ill, many centers are successfully managing their patients and providing education on an outpatient basis. The goals are to educate the child and family about diabetes management and to stabilize blood glucose levels.

BOX 26-1 *Considerations for Insulin Adjustments*

Hypoglycemia

- Is there a known reason for the hypoglycemia?
  - Insufficient food; delayed meal?
  - Exercise?
  - Extra insulin taken?
  - Illness?
- Was hypoglycemia severe? Easily treated by mouth?
- Is there a long period of time between meals and snacks?
- Which insulin is most likely to be peaking at the time of hypoglycemia?

Hyperglycemia

- Is there a known reason for hyperglycemia?
  - Too much food; sweets?
  - Meals/snacks too close together?
  - Insufficient exercise?
  - Insulin omission?
  - "Bad" pump site?
  - Illness?
- Are ketones present in the urine?
- Which insulin is most likely to be peaking at the time of hyperglycemia?
- Does the high blood glucose follow hypoglycemia?

The management team includes the child, parents, primary care provider, pediatric endocrinologist, nurse educator, dietitian, and social worker. All members are essential for the physical and psychologic well-being of the child. Diabetes management must integrate education and support for insulin, medical nutrition therapy, and exercise into daily life.

The physical examination should include assessment of the following:

- Adequate physical growth and sexual development (children in poor control may not grow normally)
- Blood pressure measurement
- Fundus and vision evaluation

- Laboratory studies should include the following:
  - Glycosylated hemoglobin every 3 months
  - Total urinary protein excretion measured once yearly in children who have had diabetes for more than 5 years (American Diabetes Association, 2002b)
  - Lipid profile done on children older than 2 years of age at time of diagnosis and when glucose control is established, and every 3 years thereafter if levels are not elevated (American Diabetes Association, 2002b)
  - Yearly thyroid screen

INSULIN THERAPY. The insulin regimen selected must be based on a number of individual factors such as age of the child, tolerance to injections, ability of caregivers to administer insulin, amount of flexibility required in the daily schedule, level of exercise, and motivation of the child and parents. At diagnosis, most children are started on an injection regimen of NPH insulin along with lispro (Humalog) or aspart (Novolog) three times per day. Insulin glargine (Lantus) is an option for providing basal insulin and is usually given once a day with injections of lispro or aspart when the child eats. It cannot be mixed with other insulins, thus requiring an additional injection. Commercially prepared premixed insulins generally do not allow for flexibility of daily dosage adjustment based on blood glucose values and exercise levels, although these insulins may be useful for those who do not require multiple daily insulin therapy or who cannot accurately mix their doses. Total insulin dosage is 1 U/kg per day unless the child is stable. A range of 0.5 to 1.5 U/kg per day is acceptable and allows for individual differences such as age, activity, eating habits, and metabolic requirements. Typically, an adolescent will require about 1.4 U/kg. The type and schedule of insulin delivery is highly variable and depends on a number of factors, such as the child's routine schedule and the need for flexibility in daily routine. A multiple daily insulin regimen (four injections per day) or an insulin pump can provide the ability to be more flexible in the daily regimen. (See Table 26-4 for a description of commercially available insulin preparations.) Many children use a "pen," an insulin delivery device that may be disposable and looks like a pen. It can conveniently provide insulin for active children.

Another type of insulin delivery is continuous subcutaneous insulin infusion (CSII), better known as insulin pump therapy. A fast-acting insulin, such as Novolog, is infused at an hourly rate, known as a basal rate, through a small, flexible, subcutaneous soft cannula. The cannula is replaced in a new site by the wearer every 2 days. A bolus of

TABLE 26-4 *Commercially Available Insulin*

Product	Manufacturer	Onset (hr)	Peak (hr)	Duration (hr)	Origin
Rapid Acting					
Lispro (Humalog)	Lilly	0.25	1-2	3-4	Human analog
Humulin R	Lilly	0.75	2	6	Human
Novolin R	Novo Nordisk	0.5	2-5	8	Human
Aspart (Novolog)	Novo Nordisk	0.16	1-2	3-5	DNA origin
Velosulin BR (buffered regular for insulin pump therapy)	Novo Nordisk	0.5	1-3	8	Human
Intermediate Acting					
Humulin N	Lilly	3	6-7	13	Human
Novolin N	Novo Nordisk	1.5	4-12	24	Human
Iletin II (NPH)	Lilly	1-3	6-12	18-24	Pork
Humulin L	Lilly	1-3	6-12	12-28	Human
Novolin L	Novo Nordisk	2.5	7-15	12	Human
Iletin II (Lente)	Lilly	1-3	6-12	12-28	Pork
Long Acting					
Humulin U	Lilly	4-6	14-24	36	Human
Mixtures					
Glargine (Lantus)	Aventis	1.0	1-24	24-32	DNA origin
Humalog 75/25	Lilly	0.25	1-6	13	Human
Humulin 50/50	Lilly	0.5-1	6-12	24	Human
Humulin 70/30	Lilly	0.5-1	6-12	24	Human
Novolin 70/30	Novo Nordisk	1.5	4-12	24	Human

insulin is programmed by the user to cover the amount of carbohydrates consumed. Insulin pump therapy provides the mechanism for children or their parents to control blood glucose levels based on food consumed and activity. It is becoming an increasingly popular way for children and adolescents with diabetes to receive insulin. Close parental supervision is required, and parents must be willing to test blood glucose levels as needed during the day and night. It can provide a better quality of life and may improve glycemic control in a motivated child or family.

Generally, adjustments of the insulin dose are based on the patterns of the blood glucose over several days. In general, it is wise to decrease insulin doses if there is any unexplained or severe hypoglycemic event. However, in raising insulin doses, it is most acceptable to look for patterns of control over a 3- to 4-day period. However, most often, parents are given a scale or algorithm of regular, lispro, or aspart insulin doses based on before-meal blood glucose. Insulin doses are often based on the amount of carbohydrate eaten.

Parents and teens are taught to make adjustments in insulin based on patterns of control. They are helped to adjust insulin to avoid hypoglycemia and hyperglycemia. Usually, a 10% adjustment in insulin can be made safely by parents. However, for young children dose adjustments are best made in one-half unit increments, or even smaller units on an insulin pump.

The usual sites for insulin injection are the legs, arms, and upper outer quadrant of the buttocks. School-age children and adolescents can be encouraged to use their abdomen as a regular injection site. However, young children with minimal subcutaneous abdominal fat have difficulty with this site. Rotation of injection sites is necessary to avoid lipohypertrophy and to prevent poor absorption of insulin.

MEDICAL NUTRITION THERAPY. The principles of medical nutritional therapy (MNT) for children and adolescents differ from those for adults, primarily because children and teens have unique caloric requirements and do not usually require weight reduction. Children need sufficient calories and protein for growth and development. General goals for youth with type 1 diabetes are to

- Provide adequate energy to ensure normal growth and development
- Integrate insulin regimens into usual eating and physical activity habits (American Diabetes Association, 2002d)

Nutrition recommendations for children and teens are based on a nutrition assessment. The distribution of calories from fat and carbohydrate can vary and can be individualized based on the nutrition assessment and treatment program (i.e., insulin regimen). Additional goals focus on preventing excessive glycemic excursions, hypoglycemia, and hyperlipidemia; controlling blood pressure; and preventing future complications of diabetes (Betschart, 2001). Generally, calories are spread among three meals and two to three snacks daily. Caloric intake is based on body size and surface area and can be calculated from a standard recommended dietary allowance (RDA) table, with the division of calories being approximately 60% to 70% carbohydrate, less than 30% fat, and 15% to 20% protein (American Diabetes Association, 2002d). Various approaches to nutrition therapy currently are being used for children and teens. Counting grams of carbohydrates is one approach that allows for a total number of grams of carbohydrate for each meal and snacks, which can then be covered by a fast-acting insulin. MNT for children and adolescents includes the following:

- Taking in recommended nutrients and vitamins
- Maintaining a consistent day-to-day intake of food
- Carefully monitoring carbohydrate intake
- Avoiding overtreatment of hypoglycemia
- Decreasing cholesterol, total fat, and saturated fat intake
- Maintaining ideal body weight

Reevaluation of the nutritional program should be done at least annually in consideration of the growth and development of the infant, child, or adolescent. Consultation and ongoing relationship with a dietitian should be encouraged.

EXERCISE. Exercise may not result in improved glycemic control in children with type 1 diabetes but is encouraged to promote cardiovascular fitness and long-term weight control and to enhance social interaction and self-esteem through team play (American Diabetes Association, 2002e). Exercise improves glucose utilization, leading to an increased uptake of glucose, and thereby lowers blood glucose levels. Therefore additional carbohydrates with protein or fat can be eaten before exercise. Because there is commonly a prolonged hypoglycemic effect from exercise, there exists a possibility of nocturnal hypoglycemia on active days. To replenish glycogen stores depleted during high-intensity exercise, a child or teen with diabetes may require additional food at bedtime and may need to test his or her blood glucose at 3:00 to 4:00 AM (American Diabetes Association, 2002e).

Complications. The acute complications of diabetes include ketoacidosis, severe or prolonged hypoglycemia, vaginal yeast infections or thrush, and cellulitis resulting from infection or injury. Chronic complications include microvascular disease such as retinopathy, nephropathy, neuropathy, eating disorders, depression, and cognitive defects, as well as macrovascular diseases such as arterial obstruction with gangrene of extremities and ischemic heart disease.

Type 2 Diabetes

Etiology and Incidence. Type 2 diabetes includes disorders that range from predominantly insulin resistance with relative insulin deficiency to predominantly an insulin secretory defect with insulin resistance. Type 2 diabetes is most commonly associated with the obese, the sedentary, and those with strong genetic predisposition. Although type 2 diabetes is found primarily in adults, increasing numbers of youths have been diagnosed with this form of diabetes (Glaser, 2002b; Rosenbloom et al, 1999).

Type 2 diabetes is more common than type 1. The prevalence of type 2 diabetes ranges from 8% to 46% of North American children, with African American, Hispanic, and American Indian ethnicity most at risk (American Diabetes Association, 2000). Because obesity in North America continues to increase, the incidence of type 2 diabetes in youths has also increased proportionately.

There are probably many different causes of this form of diabetes. Although the specific etiologies of type 2 diabetes are not known, autoimmune destruction of beta cells does not occur. Most patients with this form of diabetes are obese, and obesity itself causes some degree of insulin resistance (American Diabetes Association, 2002a).

Clinical Findings

History. The history of patients with diabetes may include

- Polydipsia
- Polyphagia
- Polyuria
- Nocturia
- Blurred vision
- Weight loss
- Fatigue
- Family history of type 2 diabetes

The onset of symptoms is often insidious. Most often patients are not acutely ill on diagnosis, but occasionally ketonuria and ketonemia may occur even in non–immune-mediated diabetes (American Diabetes Association, 2002a).

Polycystic ovarian syndrome (PCOS), a reproductive disorder characterized by hyperandrogenism and chronic anovulation with insulin resistance and obesity, is also common in youths with type 2 diabetes. Hypertension and disorders of lipid metabolism are also associated with type 2 diabetes.

Physical Examination. The following may be found on physical examination:

- Dehydration
- Obesity (greater than 85th percentile BMI for age and sex)
- Weight loss
- Acanthosis nigricans, noted especially in the axilla, base of the neck, groin, knuckles, and other skin folds (see Color Fig. 11)
- Glycosuria, ketonuria
- Vaginal yeast, thrush, or other infection
- PCOS symptoms (acne, hirsutism)

Diagnostic Tests. In asymptomatic, at-risk children, a fasting plasma glucose should be drawn at age 10 or puberty, whichever comes first, and should be repeated at 2-year intervals. Children who have the following characteristics should be tested (American Diabetes Association, 2003):

- BMI greater than 85th percentile for age and sex
- Weight for height greater than 85th percentile
- Weight greater than 120% of ideal for height
- Plus any two of the following risk factors:
  - Family history of type 2 diabetes in first- or second-degree relative
  - Race/ethnicity of Native American, African American, Hispanic American, Asian American, Pacific Islander
  - Signs of insulin resistance or conditions associated with insulin resistance (e.g., acanthosis nigricans)

In a symptomatic child, diagnosis is made if the following exist:

- Symptoms of diabetes plus a random plasma glucose concentration greater than or equal to 200 mg/dl (11.1 mmol/L)
- Fasting plasma glucose greater than or equal to 126 mg/dl (7.0 mmol/L)
- A 2-hour after-meal plasma glucose greater than or equal to 200 mg/dl (11.1 mmol/L) during an OGTT (American Diabetes Association, 2000, 2002a)

Management

Healthy Lifestyle. The goal of treatment for type 2 diabetes is the normalization of blood glucose values and Hgb A_{1c}. Successful control of the associated complications, such as hypertension and hyperlipidemia, is important. As is true for type 1 diabetes, the treatment plan must be individualized. Because the spectrum of disease is broad, ranging from ketoacidosis and hyperosmolar nonketotic states to apparent lack of symptoms, each case must be decided individually.

Lifestyle changes must be comprehensive. Self-management skills and education must include self-monitoring of blood glucose (SMBG), as well as MNT. Most often MNT requires that the whole family change food shopping and eating habits. Children with type 2 diabetes must learn healthy eating and be strongly encouraged to engage in daily sports or exercise. Referral to a dietitian is essential. Hgb A_{1c} levels can drop or even normalize with significant weight loss.

Pharmacotherapy. If dietary intervention and exercise are not successful, pharmaceutical therapy is warranted.

However, efficacy and safety data are not available for oral agents for use by children. In adolescents, metformin can be effective, especially in girls with PCOS if there is no renal impairment. When optimal glycemic control is not otherwise achieved, insulin therapy may be added. If MNT, exercise, and a weight loss program fail to control blood glucose levels, insulin remains the treatment of choice for children. Insulin regimens are similar to those for type 1 diabetes. Insulin pumps and insulins, such as insulin glargine (Lantus), provide a helpful means of providing round-the-clock basal insulin. Lispro (Humalog) and aspart (Novolog) prevent postprandial hyperglycemia.

EXERCISE. Sports and regular exercise are strongly encouraged in children and teens with diabetes as part of a healthy lifestyle program. Making exercise part of the daily regimen is a family goal. Often, children with type 2 diabetes are sedentary by nature and come from inactive families. Regular vigorous exercise (30 minutes a day) becomes a goal of treatment to reduce insulin resistance and promote insulin sensitivity (American Diabetes Association, 2002d).

Patient and Parent Education for Type 1 and Type 2 Diabetes. The cornerstone of treatment for diabetes has been and continues to be education regarding diabetes issues and management for the child and family. Diabetes is a relentless illness in that it affects every facet of daily life. Therefore it is crucial for parents to have a sound understanding in order to fit diabetes tasks into the activities of daily living. Education of the child, family, and caregivers should include insulin therapy, self-monitoring of glucose, nutrition and meal planning, exercise, managing sick days, school issues, coping skills, and prevention of complications. Those with diabetes should always wear a form of medical identification. School personnel must be informed of the plan of care and must implement an individualized care plan for the child. The American Association of Diabetes Educators provides excellent resources (see Resource Box).

Thyroid Disorders

Thyroid disorders arise from inadequate or excessive production of thyroid hormone resulting from congenital anomaly or biosynthetic alteration. The thyroid gland, located below the larynx in the anterior middle portion of the neck, is necessary for growth and development in children, including mental development, sexual maturity, and metabolism.

Congenital Hypothroidism

Hypothyroidism is a deficiency in thyroid hormone that can be either congenital or acquired (juvenile hypothyroidism).

Description. Congenital hypothyroidism (CH) results from an inadequate production of thyroid hormone that is due to different etiologies. CH is the most common cause of preventable mental retardation. Untreated hypothyroidism leads to irreversible brain damage and variable degrees of growth failure, deafness, and neurologic abnormalities.

Etiology and Incidence. CH has an overall incidence of 1 in 4000 births (Fisher, 2002). More female than male infants are affected (2:1). The majority of cases of CH are due to partial or complete failure of the thyroid gland to develop, most likely the result of an autosomal recessive genetic condition. Enzymatic deficiencies are rarely known to cause CH. Thyroid dysgenesis is more prevalent in children with Down syndrome.

Clinical Findings. Often the signs and symptoms of CH are difficult to assess, because most newborns with CH look normal. Normal newborn thyroid test results might decrease vigilance for clinically symptomatic patients because of false-negative results. The most common neonatal signs are prolonged jaundice, constipation, and umbilical hernia.

History. The patient's history may include the following:

- Family history of CH
- Prolonged gestation
- Increased birth weight
- Lag in first stooling
- Feeding or sucking difficulties
- Constipation
- Lethargy

Physical Examination. The following may be seen on physical examination:

- Respiratory distress
- Large posterior fontanel, delayed closure
- Abdominal distention with umbilical hernia
- Hypotonia, hypoactivity
- Macroglossia
- Poor peripheral circulation
- Peripheral cyanosis
- Hypothermia
- Jaundice (prolonged)
- Dry, cool, scaly skin
- Delayed mental responsiveness
- Delayed osseous development

Diagnostic Tests. Clinically, symptoms of hypothyroidism can go unrecognized during the first month of life. Newborn screening is performed in all 50 states, the District of Columbia, Puerto Rico, and the U.S. Virgin Islands. Screening tests use T_4 measurements of blood collected on filter paper before hospital discharge. If the T_4 result is low, a TSH level is obtained on this blood. If the TSH level is elevated, the newborn screen is reported as abnormal. The practitioner may repeat the thyroid screen to determine whether laboratory values are still abnormal before referral. When the TSH level is 20 mU/L or higher, a pediatric endocrinology workup is necessary (Nejad, 2002). During the first weeks of life, hypothyroidism can develop in neonates with normal T_4 and TSH levels on newborn screening. Infants with the symptoms of hypothyroidism should always be retested. Subsequent testing of serum is imperative in infants and should be done in a timely manner if there are suspicions of congenital hypothyroidism. Because infants with Down syndrome have an increased risk of acquired thyroid disease, repeat screening at 6 and 12 months and then annually (American Academy of Pediatrics, 2001).

Management. The American Thyroid Association Committee on Neonatal Screening recommends a starting dose of levothyroxine sodium (Synthroid) of 10 to 15 μg/kg per day to maintain serum T_4 levels within a 10 to 15 μg/dl range (American Academy of Pediatrics, American Thyroid Association, 1993; Styne & Glaser, 2002). Improvement is usually noted within 7 to 21 days. Linear growth and skeletal maturation respond dramatically. Intellectual capacity improves with early treatment. Two key points need to be followed throughout the treatment:

1. Thyroid tests (T_4, free T_4, and TSH levels) need to be done every month for the first 6 months; every other month between 6 and 12 months; and every 3 months thereafter.
2. Bone age needs to be determined at the start of therapy and at 1 year of age.

Differential Diagnosis. Thyroid failure secondary to hypothalamic or pituitary insufficiency must be differentiated from primary hypothyroidism resulting from a defect in the thyroid gland.

Prevention. Neonatal screening programs are the mainstay of prevention. However, remember to be vigilant because infants with thyroid problems may be missed.

Acquired Hypothyroidism

Etiology. The majority of the cases of juvenile hypothyroidism are due to autoimmune chronic lymphocytic thyroiditis, or Hashimoto thyroiditis. Other causes include thyroidectomy, ingestion of a goitrogenic substance (propylthiouracil), iodine deficiency, and irradiation of the thyroid tissue.

Clinical Findings. Manifestations of juvenile hypothyroidism are even more subtle than manifestations of CH.

History. A child's chief complaint may be only delayed growth. The following are other symptoms:

- Decreased appetite
- Lethargy
- Poor school performance
- Cold intolerance
- Delayed puberty

Physical Examination. The following may be noted on physical examination:

- Goiter
- Tenderness of the anterior neck
- Weakness
- Delayed dentition
- Cool, dry, carotenemic skin
- Reflexes diminished or absent

Diagnostic Tests. If acquired hypothyroidism is suspected, a referral to a pediatric endocrinologist is suggested to determine the cause of the disease. Initial laboratory tests that may be ordered before referral include the following:

- Serum T_4, free T_4, and TSH assays
- Serum thyroid antibody measurement

Management. The drug of choice in children and adolescents with acquired hypothyroidism is levothyroxine sodium. Dosage must be individualized based on age and ranges from 8 to 10 μg/kg per day for newborns to 100 to 200 μg/kg per day for adults. In follow-up serum TSH should be monitored 2 to 3 months after a change in dosage and with symptoms of hypothyroidism or hyperthyroidism (McGhee et al, 2001).

Hyperthyroidism

Description. Hyperthyroidism is present when there are excessive levels of circulating thyroid hormone.

Etiology and Incidence. Hyperthyroidism in children and adolescents is uncommon and is usually caused by Graves' disease or, less frequently, autoimmune thyroiditis. Graves' disease occurs five times more often in girls than in boys with an increased frequency of occurrence during the adolescent years (Glaser, 2002a; Nejad, 2002). Chronic thyroiditis, tumors of the thyroid, and exogenous thyroid hormone excess also can cause hyperthyroidism.

Clinical Findings. Symptoms most often occur in children between 10 and 14 years of age and usually develop over several months.

History. The history may include the following:

- Emotional instability
- Increased sweating
- Weight loss
- Insomnia
- Tremors
- Behavioral problems, difficulty concentrating, or deterioration in school performance

Physical Examination. The following may be noted on physical examination:

- Goiter
- Eyelid lag (exophthalmos)
- Tachycardia and palpitations
- Systolic hypertension
- Thyroid bruit

Diagnostic Tests. Total thyroxine (T_4), free T_4, triiodothyronine T_3, and TSH concentrations should be ordered before referral. Laboratory findings include the following:

- Elevated total thyroxine (T_4) free T_4, and triiodothyronine T_3
- Suppressed and often nondetectable TSH concentrations
- Rarely, elevated T_3 with normal or slightly elevated T_4 (Glaser, 2002a)

Differential Diagnosis. Diseases that are associated with hypermetabolism, such as leukemia, severe anemia, and chronic infections, need to be ruled out using appropriate diagnostic tests.

Management. The patient should be referred to an endocrinologist. In mild cases, therapy may not be necessary. Treatment includes the use of propylthiouracil, which blocks the formation of T_4 and T_3. Propranolol may be added to control nervousness and tachycardia. Alternative therapy includes radiation and surgical removal of the thyroid gland.

Pubertal Disorders

Precocious Puberty

Description. *Precocious puberty* has classically been defined as pubertal development occurring before age 8 years in girls and 9 years in boys. Because African American females begin puberty about 2 years earlier than Caucasian females, some now suggest setting the age cutoff at before 7 years in white girls and before 6 years in African American girls as premature puberty (Misra & Park-Bennett, 2002). True precocious puberty refers to a premature maturation of the hypothalamic-pituitary axis, which initiates sexual development, as opposed to pseudoprecocious puberty, which refers to autonomous secretion of sex steroids as a result of an adrenal or gonadal tumor or exogenous hormones. Girls are more apt to have precocious puberty with no underlying pathology. On the other hand, boys with symptoms of true precocious puberty are found to have central nervous system pathology such as hamartomas, astrocytomas, or gliomas. See Table 26-5 for age guidelines and key points associated with precocious puberty.

Etiology. Causes of precocious puberty are numerous. The etiology can be idiopathic or due to central nervous system disorders, trauma, postinflammation and postsurgical damage, hypothalamic hamartomas, tumors and space-occupying lesions, CAH, gonadal tumors, and variants of normal development such as premature thelarche and premature adrenarche (Misra & Park-Bennett, 2002).

Clinical Findings. Clinical manifestations often associated with precocious puberty may be seen on the history and physical examination. It is crucial to elicit information as to the rate of progression of sexual development.

History. The history may include the following:

- Breast development
- Pubic hair growth
- Axillary hair and odor
- Menstruation
- Behavioral changes

TABLE 26-5 ***Precocious and Delayed Puberty: Age Guidelines***

	Age		
	Female	**Male**	**Key Points**
Precocious puberty	<8 yr*	<9 yr	Girls often have no underlying pathology; boys often have central nervous system pathology
Delayed puberty	13 yr or 5 yr since fist sign of puberty and menarche	14 yr or 5 yr since first sign of puberty and completion of genital growth	No signs of puberty by these ages or failure to complete puberty

From Burns CE et al: *Pocket reference for pediatric primary care*, Philadelphia, 2002, WB Saunders.
*Misra and Parke-Bennet (2002) suggest using 7 years as the age cutoff in white girls and 6 years in African American girls.

Physical Examination. Findings on physical examination include the following:

- Accelerated linear growth
- Advanced bone age
- Genital maturation
- Acne

Neurologic symptoms suggest central nervous system pathology.

Diagnostic Tests. Referral to a pediatric endocrinologist is necessary because of the large number of possible causes and treatments. Laboratory tests that might be ordered before referral include the following (Misra & Park-Bennett, 2002):

- Blood
  - Testosterone (boys)
  - Estradiol (girls)
  - Thyroid function test
  - Basal and gonadotropin-releasing hormone (GnRH)–stimulated levels of LH and FSH
  - Dehydroepiandrosterone sulfate (DHEAS) and human chorionic gonadotropin in boys
- Radiologic
  - Pelvic ultrasonography (girls)
  - Testicular ultrasonography (boys)
  - Skeletal age determination
  - CT or MRI (if cranial lesion is suspected)

Differential Diagnosis. Benign conditions such as premature thelarche and premature adrenarche must be ruled out.

Management. Treatment of precocious puberty is aimed at eliminating the cause. Radiation, surgery, or chemotherapy is indicated in the case of central nervous system tumors. When a definitive diagnosis is not found, as is usually the case in girls, the treatment of choice is administration of a long-acting GnRH agonist to decrease the circulating gonadotropin and return the sex steroids to the prepubertal levels. It is important to treat precocious puberty in order to increase final adult height.

Delayed Puberty

Description. Puberty is considered delayed in a female if any of the following is present (Misra & Park-Bennett, 2002):

- No initial changes of puberty seen by age 13
- No menarche by 15 years of age plus no thelarche or pubarche
- No menarche by 16 years of age with breast budding and pubic hair development

Puberty is considered delayed in a male if the following is present:

- No initial changes of puberty (testicular enlargement or pubic hair development) seen by age 14

See Table 26-5 for age guidelines for delayed puberty.

Etiology. Multiple causes can delay the onset or progression of puberty. Some causes include the following:

- Chromosomal abnormalities such as Klinefelter, Noonan, and Turner syndromes
- Acquired disease, infection
- Chemotherapy
- Head trauma, radiation, surgery
- Constitutional delay in puberty
- Temporary conditions such as chronic illness, stress, malnutrition, or anorexia nervosa
- Permanent deficiencies such as hypothalamic or pituitary gonadotropin deficiency or tumors

Clinical Findings

History. The history might also include cryptorchidism or amenorrhea.

Physical Examination. Underdeveloped genitalia, short stature, and immature body proportions may be seen on physical examination.

Diagnostic Tests. Initially, bone age determination and hormonal evaluations, including testosterone, estradiol (ultrasensitive assays), plasma LH, and FSH level assays, should be ordered. Additional tests might include the following:

- GnRH stimulation testing
- Thyroid function tests
- Blood and urinary pH
- Urine specific gravity
- Complete blood count and sedimentation rate (to rule out chronic infection)
- Karyotype
- Radiologic examinations—pelvic ultrasonography, MRI, or CT (to rule out cranial pathology)

Management. Because there are various causes of delayed puberty, a pediatric endocrinology referral is necessary. Once the underlying cause is identified, hormonal replacement or hormonal stimulation therapy is the treatment of choice for hypogonadism or low gonadotropin levels.

Hypercholesterolemia and Hyperlipidemia

Description. Cholesterol levels should be less than 170 mg/dl (low-density lipoprotein [LDL] less than 110 mg/dl). Borderline acceptable results are 170 to 190 mg/dl (LDL 110 to 129 mg/dl). High results are greater than 200 mg/dl (LDL 130 mg/dl or greater). For a number of years attention has been focused on the control and prevention of coronary artery disease (CAD). Because of the relationship between dietary factors (fat and cholesterol) and atherosclerotic disease, it is important to identify children at risk in early childhood. However, the prediction of adult cholesterol levels based on multiple childhood screenings of serum cholesterol levels does not provide an accurate classification of all individuals (Schieken, 1999).

Etiology and Incidence. Atherosclerosis begins in childhood and is related to elevated blood levels of cholesterol. Children with elevated serum cholesterol, particularly LDL cholesterol levels, frequently have a family history of CAD. This is often a result of blood cholesterol elevation tendency, which leads to early CAD and premature death. Aortic fatty streaks are seen in children as young as the second decade of life, and fibrous plaques have been noted in autopsies of teens. Genetic disorders for familial hypercholesterolemia, familial combined hyperlipidemia, and familial hypertriglyceridemia are found in a small percent of the population. Familial hypercholesterolemia, the best understood of this group of disorders, is an autosomal dominant disease that results from alternation in either the number of or function of LDL cholesterol receptors with a resultant disorder of lipoprotein metabolism and transport (Rocchini, 2002).

The risk factors that indicate the need to screen children for hypercholesterolemia are as follows:

- Family history of heart disease—if parent or grandparent has/had a history of premature atherosclerotic disease defined as clinical manifestations of atherosclerosis in men younger than 50 years or in women younger than 60 years (Rocchini, 2002); if a parent or grandparent at age 55 years or younger underwent coronary angioplasty for coronary atherosclerosis, angioplasty, or coronary bypass surgery or had a documented myocardial infarction, angina pectoris, peripheral vascular disease, cerebrovascular accident, or sudden cardiac death (Schieken, 1999)
- Either parent has a known total cholesterol level of 240 mg/dl or higher (Schieken, 1999)

Children with incomplete or unknown family histories or with other risk factors should be screened at the discretion of the provider (Tershakovec & Stallings, 2002). The National Institutes of Health (NIH) has published a childhood risk assessment and screening algorithm that includes the classification, education, and follow-up of patients based on LDL cholesterol levels (Figs. 26-3 and 26-4).

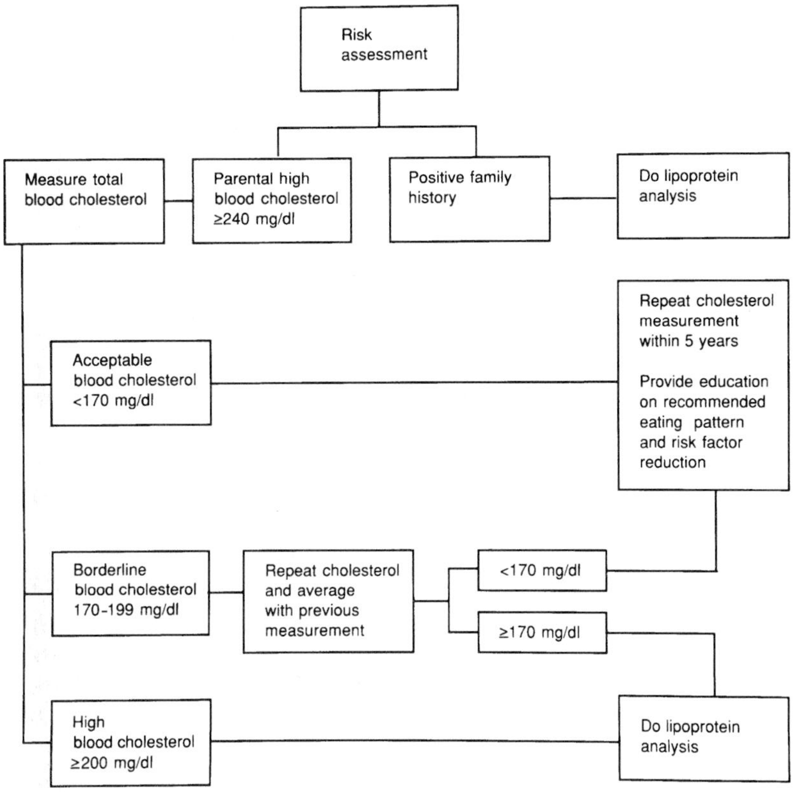

FIGURE 26-3 Risk assessment of children based on high parental blood cholesterol or a positive family history of premature atherosclerotic disease. (Reprinted from National Cholesterol Education Program: Report of the Expert Panel on Blood Cholesterol Levels in Children and Adolescents, National Heart, Lung, and Blood Institute, US Department of Health and Human Services, PHS NIH Publication No. 91-2732, Washington, DC, 1991, US Government Printing Office.)

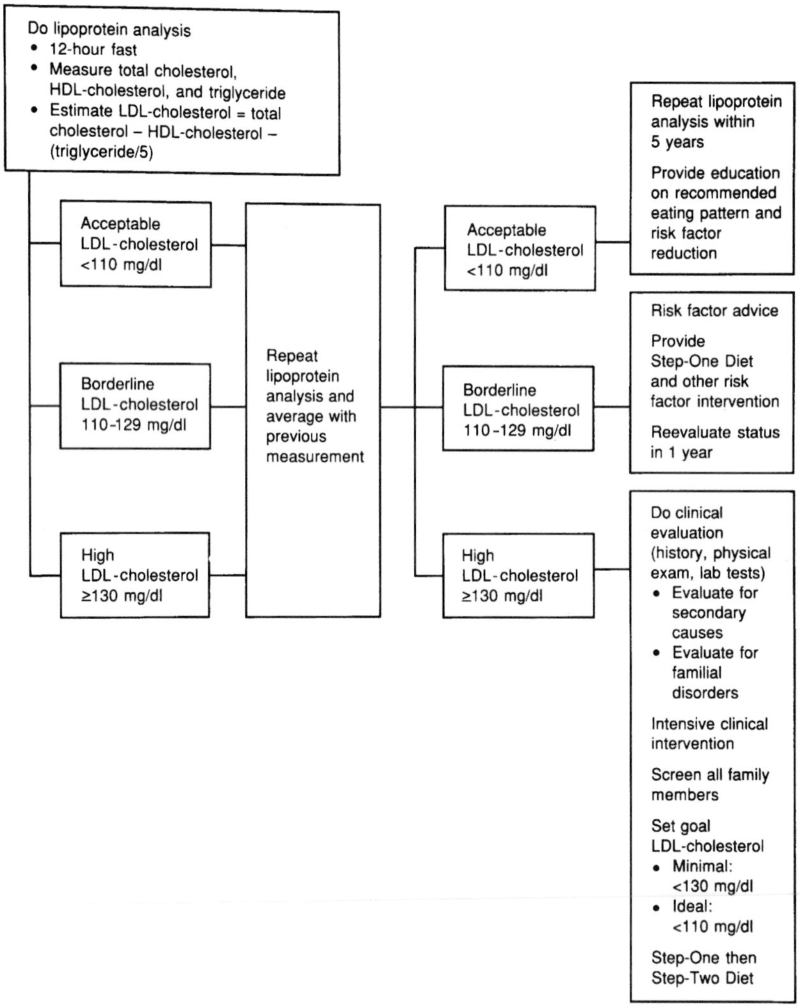

FIGURE 26-4 Classification, education, and follow-up of patients based on low-density lipoprotein (LDL) cholesterol level. (Reprinted from National Cholesterol Education Program: Report of the Expert Panel on Blood Cholesterol Levels in Children and Adolescents, National Heart, Lung, and Blood Institute, US Department of Health and Human Services, PHS NIH Publication No. 91-2732, Washington, DC, 1991, US Government Printing Office.)

Clinical Findings

History. Risk factors for hyperlipidemia and hypercholesterolemia are as follows:

- Family history of heart disease as identified earlier
- High-cholesterol, high-fat diet
- Obesity
- Lack of exercise, physical inactivity
- Smoking
- Hypertension
- Physical inactivity
- Diabetes mellitus

Diagnostic Tests. See Fig. 26-4. The initial lipoprotein analysis should be repeated and the two averaged to obtain an average LDL cholesterol level.

Differential Diagnosis. Differential diagnoses include the following:

1. Secondary hyperlipidemia
   - Exogenous factors such as drugs (e.g., corticosteroids, isotretinoin, thiazides, anticonvulsants, anabolic steroids, certain oral contraceptives), alcohol, obesity
   - Endocrine and metabolic disorders (e.g., hypothyroidism, diabetes mellitus, lipodystrophy, pregnancy)
   - Storage diseases (e.g., glycogen storage disease)
   - Obstructive liver disease (e.g., biliary atresia, cirrhosis)
   - Other causes such as anorexia nervosa, collagen disease, or Klinefelter syndrome
2. Homozygous familial hypercholesterolemia (rare)
   - Plasma cholesterol levels of 600 mg/dl or higher

- Cutaneous xanthomas (during the first 6 years of life)
- Atherosclerosis (onset before 10 years of age)
- Most affected persons die of complications of myocardial infarction before age 30 years (Tershakovec & Stallings, 2002)

3. Heterozygous familial hypercholesterolemia (1 in 500 in the general population)
   - Affected children's total cholesterol levels greater than 250 mg/dl with LDL cholesterol greater than 200 mg/dl
   - Tendon xanthomas seen in teenagers
   - Xanthomas seen in adults (Tershakovec & Stallings, 2002)

Management. The following plan of action should be taken:

1. Rule out secondary causes of hypercholesterolemia before a treatment regimen is begun.
2. Perform hyperlipidemia screening if family risk factors are identified or if history cannot be ascertained.
3. Manage other risk factors, including a history of smoking, low high-density lipoprotein (HDL) cholesterol concentration (less than 35 mg/dl), hypertension, severe obesity, or diabetes mellitus. These risk factors may contribute to earlier onset of coronary heart disease. Counsel about their link to cardiovascular disease as adults and the need for lifestyle changes beginning in childhood or adolescence to promote and prevent future cardiovascular disease.
4. Manage blood cholesterol (see Fig. 26-3).
5. Manage blood LDL cholesterol (see Fig. 26-4).
6. Provide nutritional management: See Table 26-6 for step-one and step-two diets and see Table 26-7 for dietary interventions based on total and LDL cholesterol levels.
7. Drug therapy is recommended for children age 10 years or older under the following conditions:
   - If, after a trial of dietary intervention for 6 months, LDL cholesterol is greater than or equal to 190 mg/dl and cholesterol is greater than 160 mg/dl in a child with a positive family history of premature cardiovascular disease.
   - Two or more other risk factors (see 3) are still present after concerted efforts to control them. Most lipid specialists do not recommend lipid-lowering drugs unless dietary means are unable to reduce the total cholesterol to below 250 mg/dl and LDL cholesterol to below 175 mg/dl (Rocchini, 2002).
8. Recommended drugs include bile acid sequestrants (such as cholestyramine and colestipol). However, compliance is frequently problematic, and most specialists in this field have switched to 3-hydroxy-3-methylglutaryl coenzyme A (HMG-CoA) reductase inhibitors, such as lovastatin and atorvastatin. HMG-CoA reductase inhibitors (statins), nicotinic acid, and other cholesterol-lowering drugs must be used with caution in children, and referral to a specialist in this area is best (Rocchini, 2002).

Prevention. Although the genetic component is fixed in disorders of lipoprotein metabolism and transport, the environmental components that are associated with adult

TABLE 26-6 *Characteristics of Step-One and Step-Two Diets for Lowering Blood Cholesterol*

	Recommended Intake	
Nutrient	**Step-One Diet**	**Step-Two Diet**
Total fat	Average of no more than 30% of total calories	Same
Saturated fatty acids	Less than 10% of total calories	Less than 7% of total calories
Polyunsaturated fatty acids	Up to 10% of total calories	Same
Monounsaturated fatty acids	Remaining total fat calories	Same
Cholesterol	Less than 300 mg/day	Less than 200 mg/day
Carbohydrates	About 55% of total calories	Same
Protein	About 15%-20% of total calories	Same
Calories	To promote normal growth and development and to reach or maintain desirable body weight	Same

From National Cholesterol Education Program: *Report of the Expert Panel on Blood Cholesterol Levels in Children and Adolescents,* NIH pub no 91-2732, Washington, DC, 1991, National Heart, Lung, and Blood Institute, US Department of Health and Human Services, Public Health Service, US Government Printing Office.

TABLE 26-7 ***Cutoff Points of Total and Low-Density Lipoprotein (LDL) Cholesterol for Dietary Intervention in Children and Adolescents with a Family History of Hypercholesterolemia or Premature Cardiovascular Disease***

Category	Total Cholesterol (mg/dl)	LDL Cholesterol (mg/dl)	Dietary Intervention
Acceptable	<170	<110	Recommended population eating pattern: normal diet with reduced cholesterol intake
Borderline	170-199	110-129	Step-one diet prescribed, other risk-factor intervention
High	≥200	≥130	Step-one diet prescribed, then step-two diet if necessary

From National Cholesterol Education Program: *Report of the Expert Panel on Blood Cholesterol Levels in Children and Adolescents*, NIH pub no 91-2732, Washington, DC, 1991, National Heart, Lung, and Blood Institute, US Department of Health and Human Services, Public Health Service, US Government Printing Office.

CAD are subject to intervention. Promotion of a healthy lifestyle should begin in childhood.

1. Risk reduction is essential. Health education that emphasizes exercise, weight control, prudent diet (including breastfeeding, late introduction of appropriate solids, control of salt intake, and reduced saturated fat intake), and stress management is the best preventive approach.
2. The American Academy of Pediatrics (1998) nutritional recommendations relative to lowering cholesterol levels in healthy children (2 to 18 years of age) are as follows:
   - Saturated fatty acids should be less than 10% of total calories.
   - Total fat over several days should be no more than 30% of total calories and no less than 20% of total calories.
   - Dietary cholesterol should be less than 300 mg per day.

   It is further recommended that a range of appropriate values of cholesterol be averaged over several days for a child or adolescent.
3. Early and sustained management of hypertension and diabetes is essential.
4. Smokers (patient or family members) should be counseled and referred to effective intervention programs. The effect on children's personal health and the negative impact of passive smoking should be emphasized.

RESOURCE BOX

National Organizations and Resources for Problems of Endocrine and Metabolic Disease

American Association of Diabetes Educators (AADE)
1-312-424-2426 or 1-800-338-3633
www.aadenet.org

American Diabetes Association
1-800-DIABETES
www.diabetes.org

American Dietetic Association
www.eatright.org

Barbara Davis Center for Childhood Diabetes
1-303-315-8796

Children's Diabetes Foundation at Denver
1-303-863-1200
www.childrendiabetesfdn.com

Children with Diabetes
1-513-755-0186
www.childrenwithdiabetes.com

Books, video, and compact disc for kids with diabetes:
www.diabetes.fyi.net

Endocrine Society
1-888-ENDOCRINE
www.endo-society.org

Human Growth Foundation (HGF)
1-800-451-6434
www.hgfound.org

RESOURCE BOX

National Organizations and Resources for Problems of Endocrine and Metabolic Disease—cont'd

Juvenile Diabetes Foundation (JDF)
1-800-JDF-CURE
www.jdfcure.com

Little People of America
Little People of America, Inc.
PO Box 65030
Lubbock, TX 79464-5030
1-888-LPA-2001 (English and Spanish)
E-mail: LPADatabase@juno.com
www.lpaonline.org

Magic Foundation for Children's Growth
1327 N. Harlem Ave.
Oak Park, IL 60302
1-708-383-0808
www.magicfoundation.org

Medic Alert Foundation
1-800-432-5378
www.medicalert.org

Pediatric Endocrinology Nursing Society (PENS)
PO Box 2933
Gaithersburg, MD 20886
www.pens.org

Pituitary Network Association
PO Box 1958
Thousand Oaks, CA 91358
1-805-499-9973
www.pituitary.com

Short Stature Foundation
17200 Jamboree Rd, Suite J
Irvine, CA 92714-5828
1-800-243-9273

Thyroid Foundation of America
410 Stuart Street
Boston, MA 02116
1-800-832-8321
www.allthyroid.org
www.tsh.org

REFERENCES

American Academy of Pediatrics: Cholesterol in childhood (RE9805), *Pediatrics* 101(1):141-147, 1998.

American Academy of Pediatrics: Health supervision for children with Down syndrome (RE0016), *Pediatrics* 107(2):442-449, 2001.

American Academy of Pediatrics: Technical report: congenital adrenal hyperplasia (RE0027), *Pediatrics* 106(6):1511-1518, 2000.

American Academy of Pediatrics, Section on Endocrinology and Committee on Genetics, and American Thyroid Association, Committee on Public Health: Newborn screening for congenital hypothyroidism: recommended guideline, *Pediatrics* 91:1203-1209, 1993.

American Diabetes Association: Clinical practice recommendations 2002: report of the Expert Committee on the Diagnosis and Classification of Diabetes Mellitus, *Diabetes Care* 25(suppl 1): S5-S20, 2002a.

American Diabetes Association: Clinical practice recommendations: standards of medical care for patients with diabetes mellitus, *Diabetes Care* 25(suppl 1):S33-S49, 2002b.

American Diabetes Association: Clinical practice recommendations: implications of the Diabetes Control and Complications Trial, *Diabetes Care* 25(suppl 1):S25-S27, 2002c.

American Diabetes Association: Clinical practice recommendations: evidence-based nutrition principles and recommendations for the treatment and prevention of diabetes and related complications, *Diabetes Care* 25(suppl 1):S61-S63, 2002d.

American Diabetes Association: Clinical practice recommendations: diabetes mellitus and exercise, *Diabetes Care* 25(suppl 1): S64-S68, 2002e.

American Diabetes Association: Position paper: type 2 diabetes in children and adolescents, *Diabetes Care* 23(3):381-389, 2000.

American Diabetes Association: Standards of medical care for patients with diabetes mellitus, *Diabetes Care* 26(1):S33-S50, 2003.

Behrman RE, Kliegman RM, Jenson HB: *Nelson textbook of pediatrics*, ed 17, Philadelphia, 2004, WB Saunders.

Betschart J: Diabetes during childhood and adolescence. In Franz JM, editor: *A core curriculum for diabetes education*, ed 4, Chicago, 2001, American Association of Diabetes Educators.

Capriles CC, Levitsky LL: Type 1 diabetes mellitus. In Finberg L, Kleinman RE, editors: *Saunders manual of pediatric practice*, ed 2, Philadelphia, 2002, WB Saunders.

Cuttler L: Growth hormone treatment. In Finberg L, Kleinman RE, editors: *Saunders manual of pediatric practice*, ed 2, Philadelphia, 2002, WB Saunders.

Fisher DA: Congenital hypothyroidism. In Finberg L, Kleinman RE, editors: *Saunders manual of pediatric practice*, ed 2, Philadelphia, 2002, WB Saunders.

Fisher DA, editor: *Pediatric endocrinology*, San Juan Capistrano, 2000, Quest Diagnostics Inc.

Gibson JB: Disorders of carbohydrate metabolism. In Finberg L, Kleinman RE, editors: *Saunders manual of pediatric practice*, ed 2, Philadelphia, 2002, WB Saunders.

Glaser N: Hyperthyroidism. In Finberg L, Kleinman RE, editors: *Saunders manual of pediatric practice*, ed 2, Philadelphia, 2002a, WB Saunders.

Glaser N: Type 2 diabetes mellitus. In Finberg L, Kleinman RE, editors: *Saunders manual of pediatric practice*, ed 2, Philadelphia, 2002b, WB Saunders.

Lee M, Levitsky LL: Disorders of the adrenal gland. In Burg FD et al, editors: *Gellis and Kagan's current pediatric therapy*, ed 17, Philadelphia, 2002, WB Saunders.

McGhee B et al: *Pediatric drug therapy handbook and formulary 2002-2003*, Department of Pharmacy, Children's Hospital of Pittsburgh, Cleveland, 2001, Lexi-Comp.

Misra M, Park-Bennett S: Disorders of puberty. In Burg FD et al, editors: *Gellis and Kagan's current pediatric therapy*, ed 17, Philadelphia, 2002, WB Saunders.

Nejad AS: Thyroid disorders. In Burg FD et al, editors: *Gellis and Kagan's current pediatric therapy*, ed 17, Philadelphia, 2002, WB Saunders.

Rocchini AP: The child at risk for cardiovascular disease. In Burg FD, Ingelfinger JR, Polin RA, et al, editors: *Gellis and Kagan's current pediatric therapy*, ed 17, Philadelphia, 2002, WB Saunders.

Rosenbloom A et al: Emerging epidemic of type 2 diabetes in youth, *Diabetes Care* 22:345-354, 1999.

Schieken RM: The child at risk for coronary heart disease as an adult. In Burg FD et al, editors: *Gellis and Kagan's current pediatric therapy*, ed 16, Philadelphia, 1999, WB Saunders.

Styne DM: Constitutional delay in growth and adolescence. In Finberg L, Kleinman RE, editors: *Saunders manual of pediatric practice*, ed 2, Philadelphia, 2002, WB Saunders.

Styne DM, Glaser NS: Endocrinology. In Behrman RE, Kliegman RM, Arvin A, editors: *Nelson essentials of pediatrics*, ed 4, Philadelphia, 2002, WB Saunders.

Tershakovec AM, Stallings VA: Disorders of lipoprotein metabolism and transport. In Behrman RE, Kliegman RM, Arvin A, editors: *Nelson essentials of pediatrics*, ed 4, Philadelphia, 2002, WB Saunders.

US Department of Health and Human Services: Fact sheet 2002.05:24; targets efforts on diabetes mellitus. Available at *www.hhs/gov/news* (accessed Sept 21, 2002).

US Preventive Services Task Force: *Guide to clinical preventive services: an assessment of 169 interventions*, Baltimore, 1998, Williams & Wilkins.

Vogiatzi MG, Copeland KC: The short child, *Pediatr Rev* 19(3):92-99, 1998.

Wolfsdorf JI, Weinstein DA: Diabetes mellitus in children and adolescents. In Burg FD et al, editors: *Gellis and Kagan's current pediatric therapy*, ed 17, Philadelphia, 2002, WB Saunders.

Yudkoff M: Disorders of amino acid metabolism. In Finberg L, Kleinman RE, editors: *Saunders manual of pediatric practice*, ed 2, Philadelphia, 2002, WB Saunders.

27

Hematologic Diseases

Martha K. Swartz

Blood is a major homeostatic force of the body. Essential body functions carried out by blood include the transfer of respiratory gases, hemostasis, phagocytosis, and the provision of cellular and humoral agents to fight infection. Abnormalities of blood cells are seen in various disease states and alterations in nutrition. Therefore diagnostic hematologic studies are essential parts of pediatric practice. For the pediatric provider, the types of hematologic diseases encountered in the clinical setting range from common nutritional deficiencies in which treatment is straightforward to those rare disorders with a genetic or chronic component that necessitate extensive referral and a multidisciplinary approach. In pediatrics, particularly, early diagnosis of blood disorders is important to ensure the best possible prognosis.

ANATOMY AND PHYSIOLOGY

Blood is made up of a cellular component with specialized functions and a fluid component called plasma. The cellular component consists of red blood cells (RBCs), or erythrocytes; white blood cells (WBCs), or leukocytes; and platelets, or thrombocytes. Leukocytes are further differentiated into granulocytes, monocytes, and lymphocytes. Plasma is a clear yellow fluid in which proteins (primarily albumins, globulins, and fibrinogen) are the major solutes. These plasma proteins maintain intravascular volume, contribute to the coagulation of blood, and are important in acid-base balance.

Blood formation in the human embryo initially takes place in the yolk sac during the first several weeks of gestation. In the second trimester, blood is formed primarily in the liver, spleen, and lymph nodes. During the last half of gestation, hematopoiesis shifts from the fetal liver and spleen to the bone marrow where, by birth, most blood formation takes place. Bone marrow produces erythrocytes, granulocytes, monocytes, and platelets and provides lymphocytes and lymphocytic precursors to the spleen, lymph nodes, and other lymphatic tissues.

Erythrocytes

Production of RBCs is regulated by the specific hormone erythropoietin, produced primarily by renal glomerular epithelial cells. In response to a decrease in the number of circulating RBCs or a decrease in the PaO_2 of arterial blood, erythropoietin stimulates the bone marrow to convert certain stem cells to proerythroblasts. Substances essential for RBC formation include iron, vitamin B_{12}, folic acid, amino acids, and other nutrients. The RBC matures through the following stages: proerythroblast, erythroblast, normoblast, reticulocyte, and erythrocyte.

As cellular differentiation occurs, the nucleus present in the early forms of the cell is extruded and replaced by hemoglobin (Hgb). The RBC assumes its characteristic nonnucleated biconcave disk shape, which is easily distorted, thereby enabling it to pass through small capillaries and sinuses without being destroyed. The large surface-to-volume ratio also facilitates rapid gas exchange.

The youngest red cells are the reticulocytes; after release from the bone marrow, they stay in circulation for about 1 day before becoming mature RBCs. The reticulocyte count is about 4% to 6% for the first 3 days of life, which reflects the relatively greater amount of erythropoiesis that occurs in the fetus. This increased reticulocyte count is followed by a sudden drop to the normal range of 0.5% to 1.5% (see Appendix C). A mature RBC lasts about 120 days before it is destroyed through phagocytosis in the spleen, liver, or bone marrow.

Hemoglobin

Hemoglobin is the oxygen-carrying protein molecule in the RBC. Each hemoglobin molecule is made up of two pairs of polypeptide chains (the globin portion) attached to heme groups, which are large disks containing iron and porphyrin, a nitrogen-containing organic compound. Various forms of hemoglobin are found in the embryo, fetus, and adult, depending on changes in globin chain synthesis. At birth, approximately 70% of hemoglobin is made up of fetal hemoglobin (Hgb F). By 12 months of age, 95% of hemoglobin consists of the normal adult hemoglobin molecules (Hgb A), which are composed of two α- and two β-polypeptide chains attached to four heme groups. Hgb F remains present at levels of less than 2%. Hgb A_2, another type of normal hemoglobin composed of two α- and two β-globin chains, makes up about 2.5% of the total hemoglobin.

Each of the four iron atoms in the hemoglobin molecule combines reversibly with an atom of oxygen to form oxyhemoglobin. This reaction occurs when the oxygen concentration is relatively high, as in the lungs, where oxygen crosses the alveolocapillary membrane and saturates about 96% of the hemoglobin. This percentage is the arterial oxygen saturation (SaO_2), and it is measured through pulse oximetry or arterial blood gas determination. When the oxygen concentration is lower, as in the tissues, oxygen is released to meet cellular needs.

The level of hemoglobin in a newborn ranges from 15 to 22 g/dl and then drops to its lowest point at 3 to 6 months, which is a physiologic anemia caused by the shortened survival of fetal RBCs and the rapid expansion of blood volume during this period. A decrease in hemoglobin can also develop secondary to a decrease in RBC production, blood loss, or increased RBC destruction. Because of these processes, transport of oxygen to the tissues is adversely affected, and the individual can become clinically anemic.

Antigenic Properties of Red Blood Cells

Red cells are classified into different types according to the presence of antigens on the cell membrane. The most common antigens are A, B, and Rh. A person inherits either A or B antigen (type A or B blood), both antigens (type AB blood, which is the universal recipient), or neither antigen (type O blood, which is the universal donor). Of the six types of Rh factors, the most common is D, which accounts for the Rh designation. In the United States, 85% of whites and 95% of blacks are Rh+ (Guyton & Hall, 2001). Clinically, these distinctions become important when blood transfusions are necessary or in assessment for maternal-fetal blood incompatibilities.

Leukocytes

Leukocytes, or WBCs, are larger and fewer in number than erythrocytes. Normally, about 5000 to 10,000 leukocytes are contained in a microliter of blood. The primary function of WBCs is protection of the body from invasion by foreign organisms and distribution of antibodies and other factors of the immune response.

Five distinct types of WBCs can be grouped into two broad classifications: granulocytes (also known as polymorphonuclear leukocytes [PMNs], or "polys") and agranulocytes (Table 27-1). Granulocytes contain large granules and horseshoe-shaped nuclei that become segmented and are connected by thin strands (Table 27-2). With Wright's stain, the cytoplasm stains blue or pink. Granulocytes are further divided into neutrophils; eosinophils, which absorb the acid dye eosin; and basophils, which absorb a basic dye. The agranulocytes include lymphocytes (also known as immunocytes) and monocytes.

Granular Leukocytes

In children, granulocytes make up 30% to 60% of all WBCs. They mature in the bone marrow through the following stages: stem cells, myeloblasts, promyelocytes, myelocytes, metamyelocytes, band forms, and mature segmented neutrophils. This maturational process takes approximately 6 to 11 days. Once a neutrophil is released into the bloodstream, it circulates for about 6 to 9 hours before entering the tissues, where the major function of PMNs is phagocytosis of harmful particles and cells, particularly bacterial organisms.

A frequency distribution of the types of WBCs is obtained by the differential count, and quantitative alterations within the categories are important diagnostically (see Table 27-1). A relative increase in the number of band (or other immature) cells is often called a "shift to the left," a term derived from how the differential count used to be tabulated on written forms. This phenomenon is indicative of the body's immunologic response to an infectious process.

Basophils and eosinophils are also important in the body's inflammatory and allergic responses. Basophils, which account for less than 1% of circulating leukocytes, release heparin and histamine into the bloodstream during systemic allergic reactions. They contain receptor sites for immunoglobulin E (IgE), levels of which are elevated in people with allergies; they also prevent clot formation in the microcirculation. Eosinophils are found in the mucosa of the gastrointestinal tract and in the lungs. They are weakly phagocytic. Eosinophilia is also associated with allergic reactions, as well as parasitic infections and drug reactions.

Monocytes

Monocytes, which contain a large lobulated nucleus, are relatively immature cells that circulate for about 8 hours before migrating to tissues, where they assume their mature form as macrophages. Like granulocytes, which are the first line of defense against microbe invasion, their primary function is phagocytosis of bacteria and cellular debris. Fixed and mobile macrophages are located primarily in the liver, spleen, lymph nodes, and gastrointestinal tract and make up

TABLE 27-1 *Hematologic Values and Normal Leukocyte Differential Count during Infancy and Childhood*

Hematologic Values

	Hemoglobin (g/dl)		Hematocrit (%)		Reticulo-cytes (%)	MCV (fl)	Leukocytes (WBC/mm^3)		Neutrophils (%)		Lympho-cytes (%)	Eosino-phils (%)
Age	**Mean**	**Range**	**Mean**	**Range**	**Mean**	**Lowest**	**Mean**	**Range**	**Mean**	**Range**	**Mean***	**Mean**
Cord blood	16.8	13.7-20.1	55	45-65	5.0	110	18,000	(9,000-30,000)	61	(40-80)	31	2
2 wk	16.5	13.0-20.0	50	42-66	1.0		12,000	(5,000-21,000)	40		63	3
3 mo	12.0	9.5-14.5	36	31-41	1.0		12,000	(6,000-18,000)	30		48	2
6 mo-6 yr	12.0	10.5-14.0	37	33-42	1.0	70-74	10,000	(6,000-18,000)	45		48	2
7-12 yr	13.0	11.0-16.0	38	34-40	1.0	76-80	8,000	(4,500-13,500)	55		38	2
Adult												
Female	14.0	12.0-16.0	42	37-47	1.6	80	7,500	(5,000-10,000)	55	(35-70)	35	3
Male	16.0	14.0-18.0	47	42-52		80						

*Relatively wide range.
fl, Femtoliters; *MCV*, mean corpuscular volume; *WBC*, white blood cell.

Normal Leukocyte Differential Count

	Granulocytes				Agranulocytes	
Age	**Segmented Neutrophils (%)**	**Band Neutrophils (%)**	**Eosinophils (%)**	**Basophils (%)**	**Lymphocytes (%)**	**Monocytes (%)**
Birth	47 ± 15	14.1 ± 4	2.2	0.6	31 ± 5	5.8
6 mo	23	8.8	2.5	0.4	61	4.8
12 mo	23	8.1	2.6	0.4	61	4.8
2 yr	25	8.0	2.6	0.5	59	5.0
4 yr	34 ± 11	8.0 ± 3	2.8	0.6	50 ± 15	5.0
6 yr	43	8.0	2.7	0.6	42	4.7
8 yr	45	8.0	2.4	0.6	39	4.2
10 yr	46 ± 15	8.0 ± 3	2.4	0.5	38 ± 10	4.3
12 yr	47	8.0	2.5	0.5	38	4.4

Absolute neutrophil count (ANC) = WBC × (% Seg + Band)

Data from Behrman R et al: *Nelson textbook of pediatrics*, ed 17, Philadelphia, 2004, WB Saunders, p 1605; Wallach J: Interpretation of diagnostic tests, ed 6, Boston, 1996, Little, Brown.

the mononuclear phagocyte system, formerly known as the reticuloendothelial system (Bullock & Henze, 2000).

Lymphocytes

Lymphocytes (or immunocytes), although not phagocytic, protect the body against specific antigens. They originate in the bone marrow but differentiate in lymphoid tissues such as the spleen, liver, thymus, lymph nodes, and intestines. Thymus-dependent lymphocytes, or T cells, are part of the cell-mediated immune response in which cytotoxic agents and macrophages are synthesized. B-cell lymphocytes are precursors of the humoral immune response whereby the cells are transformed into plasma cells that release immunoglobulins or antibodies into the bloodstream.

Platelet Cells and Coagulation Factors

The smallest cellular components in blood are the platelets, or thrombocytes, which are essential to hemostasis and clot formation. Circulating platelets are fragments of megakaryocytes, which are precursor cells that form in the bone marrow. The normal platelet count ranges from 150,000 to 300,000 cells/mm^3.

TABLE 27-2 *Overview of Leukocytes*

Cell Type	Characteristics	Diagram
Granulocytes (Polymorphonuclear Leukocytes, Polys)		
Neutrophils	Have small, fine, [illegible] ink or lilac [illegible]hilic granules [illegible]ained and a [illegible]gmented, irregularly lobed, purple nucleus.	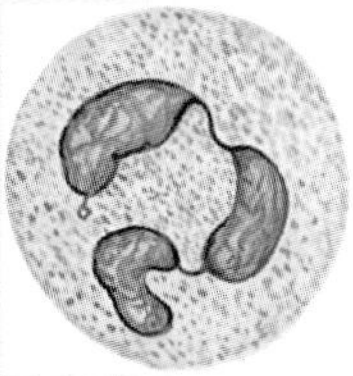
Eosinophils	Have large round granules that contain red-staining basic mucopolysaccharides and multilobed purple-blue nuclei.	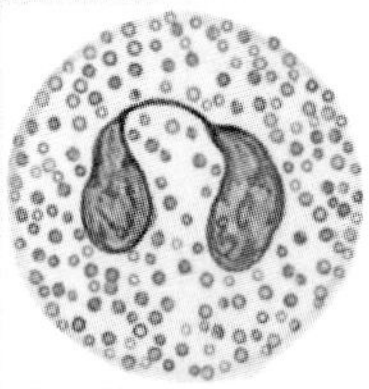
Basophils	Coarse blue granules conceal the segmented nucleus. Granules contain histamine, heparin, and acid mucopolysaccharides.	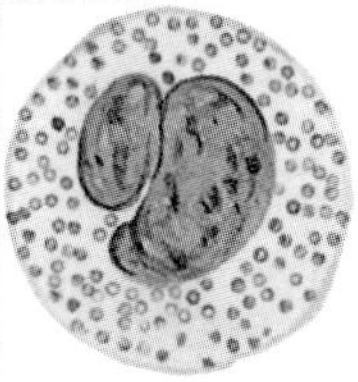
Agranulocytes		
Lymphocytes	Small cell with a large, round, deep-staining, single-lobed nucleus and very little cytoplasm. The cytoplasm is slightly basophilic and stains pale blue.	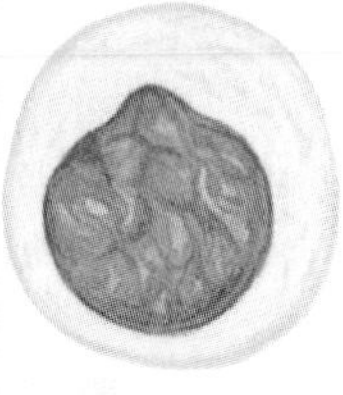
Monocytes	Large cell with a prominent, multi-shaped nucleus that sometimes is kidney shaped. Chromatin in the nucleus looks like lace, with small particles linked together like strands. The gray-blue cytoplasm is filled with many fine lysozymes that stain pink with Wright's stain.	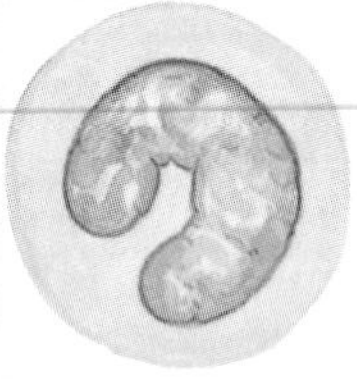

From Bullock B, Henze R: Hematology: adaptations and alterations in function. In Bullock B, editor: *Focus on pathophysiology*, Philadelphia, 2000, Lippincott Williams & Wilkins, p 359; McCance K, Huether S: *Pathophysiology: the biologic basis for disease in adults and children*, ed 4, St Louis, 2002, Mosby.

When a blood vessel is injured (or in the presence of intrinsic damage to the blood), platelets adhere to the inner surface of the vessel and form a hemostatic plug. As the platelets are degraded, a series of at least 13 clotting factors or proteolytic enzymes are released that bring about the clotting process in a cascading sequence of successive reactions (Fig. 27-1).

The basic reactions that occur in the sequential process of blood coagulation are as follows: As factor X is activated, prothrombin (factor II) is converted to thrombin, which then catalyzes the conversion of fibrinogen (factor I) to fibrin (Table 27-3). Fibrin provides the matrix in which blood cells aggregate to form a clot. A deficiency of any of the proteins in the pathway leads to a clotting disorder. In particular, if factor VIII is deficient (as in classic hemophilia A) or the number of platelets is inadequate (thrombocytopenia), activation of factor X is impaired.

PATHOPHYSIOLOGY

Hematologic problems are generally classified as disorders of RBC function, WBC function, and platelet and coagulation function. These three broad categories are further divided into disorders of blood cell production, maturation, or destruction. Knowledge of these pathophysiologic classifications gives the provider a rationale for routine screening and useful algorithms to guide further clinical investigation.

Classification of the Anemias

Anemia is generally defined as a reduction in blood hemoglobin concentration or a decrease in red cell mass below the normal range. The reduction in the amount of circulating hemoglobin also causes a decrease in the oxygen-carrying potential of the RBC. Morphologically (according to RBC size, shape, and color), anemias are described as hypochromic, microcytic; as macrocytic; or as normochromic, normocytic. This approach is a useful method for ruling out particular causes of anemia when trying to determine the underlying etiology (Table 27-4). In toddlers and young children, approximately 90% of cases of anemia are accounted for by iron deficiency, lead poisoning, infections, or hemoglobinopathy.

Anemias that are caused by inadequate production include acquired and constitutional aplastic anemia, red cell aplasia, and transient erythroblastosis of childhood (TEC). Maturational anemias are caused by nutritional disturbances such as iron deficiency, lead poisoning, and deficiencies in folic acid and vitamin B_{12}. Anemias are also a common occurrence in chronic illnesses in which either

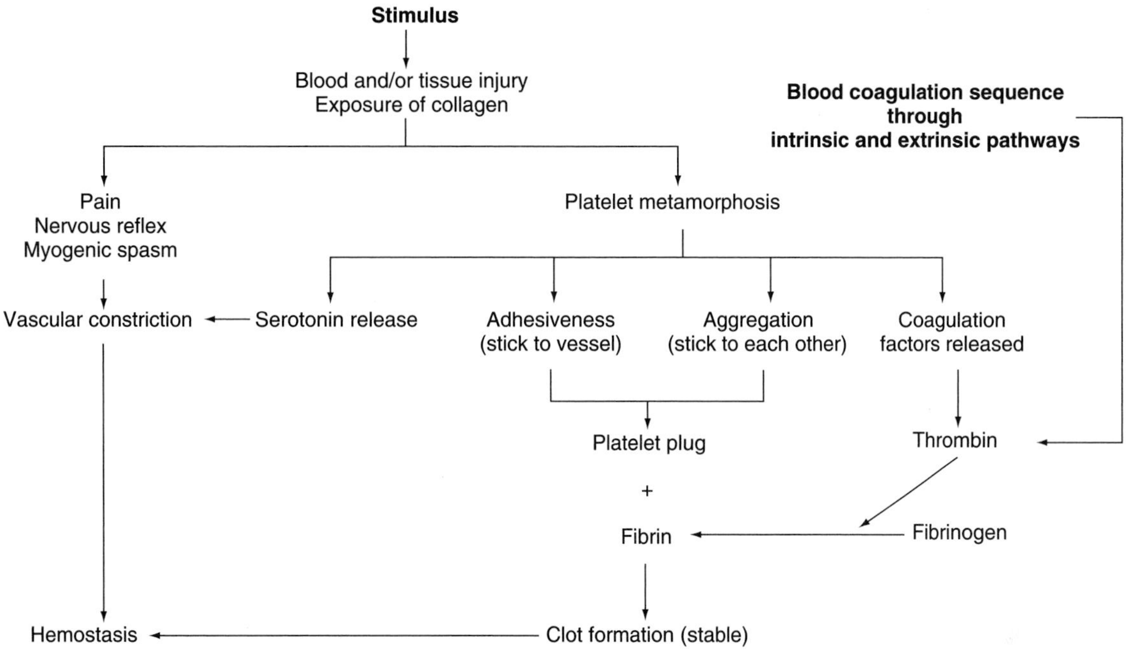

FIGURE 27-1 Hemostatic mechanisms. (From Bullock B, Henze R: Hematology: adaptations and alterations in function. In Bullock B, editor: *Focus on pathophysiology*, Philadelphia, 2000, Lippincott Williams & Wilkins.)

TABLE 27-3 ***Blood Coagulation Factors***

Factor (International Nomenclature)	Common Synonyms
I	Fibrinogen
II	Prothrombin
III	Tissue thromboplastin, thrombokinase
IV	Calcium
V	Proaccelerin, labile factor, accelerator globulin
(VI)	Obsolete term
VII	Proconvertin, stable factor
VIII	Antihemophilic globulin (AHG), antihemophilic factor (AHF), antihemophilic factor A
IX	Plasma thromboplastin component (PTC), Christmas factor, antihemophilic factor B
X	Stuart-Prower factor, Stuart factor
XI	Plasma thromboplastin antecedent (PTA), antihemophilic factor C
XII	Hageman factor, contact factor, antihemophilic factor
XIII	Fibrin-stabilizing factor (FSF), plasma transglutaminase

red cell survival time is decreased or the bone marrow response or transport of iron is impaired. Such conditions include chronic inflammatory illnesses, chronic infections, renal and liver disease, endocrine disorders, and malignant neoplastic diseases.

Anemias that result from increased cell destruction are hemolytic anemias and are caused by defects in the red cell membrane, hereditary hemoglobinopathies (as in sickle cell anemia), and congenital enzyme defects. These syndromes also include hereditary spherocytosis (HS) and glucose-6-phosphate dehydrogenase (G6PD) deficiency.

White Blood Cell Dysfunction

The WBC count and differential are useful diagnostic guides in the management of a variety of childhood illnesses. The normal range of granulocyte and lymphocyte counts varies throughout childhood (see Table 27-1). Neutrophilic leukocytosis (absolute neutrophil count [ANC] less than 7500 cells/μl) occurs in pathologic conditions such as acute infections, cancer, hemorrhage, hemolysis, tissue necrosis, or toxic exposure. A relative increase in the number of circulating immature band neutrophils (i.e., a shift to the left) is also indicative of an inflammatory process or acute bacterial infection.

TABLE 27-4 *Acute Anemia in Childhood and Adolescence*

Classification	History	Physical Findings	Screening Tests	Diagnostic Tests	Treatment
I. Microcytic					
Iron-deficiency anemia	Infant and toddler Excessive cow's milk ingestion Poor solid food intake	Waxy, sallow appearance of skin	Hgb: <7 g/dl MCV: <60 fl Retic: ↓ to sl ↑	Serum Fe: ↓ TIBC: ↑ % Saturation: ↓	Ferrous sulfate, 6 mg/kg/day of elemental iron Discontinue cow's milk Limit formula to <24 oz/day and encourage solid food
Homozygous thalassemia (Cooley's anemia)	Infant and toddler Growth failure Ethnic background consistent	Hepatosplenomegaly Frontal bossing	Hgb: var ↓ MCV: 50-60 fl		
II. Macrocytic					
Diamond-Blackfan anemia	*See III. Normocytic*				
Megaloblastic anemia	Variable, depending on etiology	Variable, depending on etiology	Hgb: var ↓ MCV: ↑ Retic: ↓ Platelets and WBC: ↓ Hypersegmented polys	Bone marrow: megaloblastic Vitamin B_{12} level: nl to ↓ Folate Others	Variable, depending on etiology (e.g., folic acid, vitamin B_{12} transfusion)
III. Normocytic					
A. Production Defect					
Diamond-Backfan anemia	Age: 65% <6 mo; 90% <1 yr Insidious onset	25% with physical abnormalities	Hgb: 2-3 g/dl MCV: ↑ in 30% (100% after treatment) Retic: <1%	Bone marrow: erythroid hypoplasia and lymphocytosis Hgb F: ↓ RBCi antigen: ↑	Prednisone: 2 mg/kg/day in 3-4 doses until Hgb >10 g/dl
Transient erythroblastopenia of childhood	1 to 3 yr of age Viral illness in preceding 3 mo	None	Hgb: 3-9 g/dl MCV: normal Retic: <1%	Bone marrow: erythroid hypoplasia	Supportive
Aplastic crisis of hemolytic anemia	Underlying hemolytic anemia Viral syndrome in preceding 1 to 3 wk Sudden exacerbation of pallor	Splenomegaly	Hgb: <7 g/dl Retic: <1% Smear: abnormalities of chronic anemia	Bone marrow: erythroid hypoplasia	Supportive
Marrow infiltration	Variable, depending on etiology Bleeding Infection	Petechiae, purpura Infection Hepatosplenomegaly	Hgb: var ↓ Retic: ↓ to nl Platelets: ↓ WBC: ↓ or ↑ Smear: variable	Bone marrow: infiltration by nonhematopoietic cells	Variable, depending on etiology (e.g., leukemia, neuroblastoma)
Aplastic anemia	Bleeding Infection	Petechiae, purpura Infection Multiple anomalies possible with Fanconi's anemia	Hgb: var ↓ MCV: ↑ in Fanconi anemia Retic: ↓ Platelets and WBC: ↓	Bone marrow: hypoplasia of all hematopoietic elements	Variable

TABLE 27-4 Acute Anemia in Childhood and Adolescence—cont'd

Classification	History	Physical Findings	Screening Tests	Diagnostic Tests	Treatment
B. Hemolytic					
Autoimmune hemolytic anemia	Jaundice Gastrointestinal symptoms Dark/red urine	Icterus Hepatosplenomegaly	Hgb: var ↓ Retic: ↑ (occ ↓) Smear: microspherocytes	Direct Coombs' test: positive	Corticosteroids: prednisone or intravenous equivalent: 2-6 mg/kg/day Transfusion indicated
Hemolytic-uremic syndrome	Infant and toddler Viral prodrome Gastrointestinal bleeding in 20% Sudden pallor, purpura Central nervous system symptoms	Purpura Hypotension Central nervous system abnormalities	Hgb: 7-8 g/dl Retic: ↑ Platelets: ↓ Smear: microangiopathy	None Renal tests: failure	Supportive: early dialysis ? Plasma infusion/exchange ? Antiplatelet drugs
C. Blood Loss					
Splenic sequestration crisis of sickle cell (SS) disease (internal blood loss)	SS disease: 5 mo to 2 yr of age Hgb SC or S-thalassemia: all ages Sudden weakness, dyspnea, abdominal distention Shock	Hypotension Massive splenomegaly	Hgb: <4 g/dl Retic: ↑ Smear: sickle cells	None	Plasma expanders: whole or reconstituted blood

Adapted from Green M, Haggerty R: *Ambulatory pediatrics IV*, Philadelphia, 1990, WB Saunders, pp 378-379.
Fe, Iron; *Hgb*, hemoglobin; *MCV*, mean corpuscular volume; *nl*, normal; *occ*, occasionally; *polys*, polymorphonuclear leukocytes; *RBCi*, red blood cell i antigen; *Retic*, reticulocytes; *sl*, slightly; *TIBC*, total iron-binding capacity; *var*, variably; *WBC*, white blood cell count.

Alterations of Granulocytes

Neutropenia (ANC less than 1500 cells/μl) results from decreased cellular production (as in various hematologic diseases, infections, drug-induced states, and nutritional deficiencies), increased peripheral destruction (as in autoimmune disorders), or peripheral pooling (as in bacterial infections, hemodialysis, and cardiopulmonary bypass). Most cases of neutropenia are discovered during evaluation of the WBC count in a child with an acute febrile illness. Neutropenia is classified as mild (ANC of 1000 to 1500 cells/μl), moderate (ANC of 500 to 1000 cells/μl), or severe (ANC less than 500 cells/μl). In an otherwise healthy child who is not taking any medication (typically antibiotics), the neutropenia should be monitored at least twice weekly. If it does not resolve over a 6-week period, the child should be managed in consultation with a hematologist and an immunologist (Platt, 1999; Yang, 2002). In rare cases when the ANC is less than 500 cells/μl, the child should be hospitalized for extensive culturing and coverage with broad-spectrum antibiotics.

Qualitative abnormalities of granulocytes are usually related to defects in the function of phagocytosis. These defects occur with collagen-vascular disorders and bacterial infections. The ingestion of certain drugs such as aspirin or corticosteroids leads to dysfunction of the phagocyte (Bullock & Henze, 2000). Granulomatous diseases are relatively rare disorders of granulocytes, particularly neutrophils, in which the enzymes necessary for bactericidal activity are lacking. Such diseases result in severe, recurrent infections of the skin, lymph nodes, lungs, liver, and bone.

Lymphocytic Disorders

Lymphocytosis is produced by viral illnesses, including mumps, measles, rubella, rubeola, varicella, and hepatitis. Pertussis and chronic lymphocytic leukemia also elevate the lymphocyte count. An increase in the number of atypical lymphocytes is evident in infectious mononucleosis, cytomegalic inclusion disease, and toxoplasmosis.

Malignant White Blood Cell Disorders

Leukemia refers to a group of malignant diseases with qualitative and quantitative changes in circulating leukocytes. Leukemia is characterized by diffuse, abnormal growth of leukocytic precursors in the bone marrow. Such an uncontrolled increase in immature WBCs leads to anemia and thrombocytopenia. Life-threatening infections occur because of a decrease in the function of circulating WBCs. Leukemias are further classified according to the course of the illness and the types of cells and tissues involved.

Malignant lymphomas, as in Hodgkin's disease, are solid neoplasms that are lymphocytic in origin. Lymphocytes are the only WBCs involved, with the malignant process occurring during their maturation or storage in bone marrow. They are associated with lymphadenopathy and tumor development in the liver, spleen, thymus, bone marrow, and submucosa of the gastrointestinal and respiratory tracts. Lymphomas are classified as Hodgkin's or non-Hodgkin's lymphomas and according to the type of cell involved (B cells or T cells). As the cell becomes more undifferentiated, the tumor becomes more aggressive (Bullock & Henze, 2000). As in leukemia, immune deficiencies develop and are followed by infection.

Platelet and Coagulation Disorders

In pediatrics, the most common cause of thrombocytopenia (platelet count less than 100,000/μl) is immune or idiopathic thrombocytopenic purpura (ITP). It is associated with destruction of circulating platelets brought about by an immune-mediated process.

When thrombocytopenia occurs, it is critical to rule out acute lymphocytic leukemia (ALL). If the child is febrile, meningococcemia and overwhelming sepsis should be considered (Hagani & Bussel, 2002a; Platt, 1999). Secondary thrombocytopenia results from drug hypersensitivity, viral infections, and autoimmune conditions. Thrombocytosis, or an elevation in the platelet count, is associated with certain malignancies or with polycythemia vera.

Disorders of coagulation can be brought about by deficiencies of any of the clotting factors. Single-coagulation-factor deficiencies are usually hereditary. The most common are deficiencies in factor VIII (classic hemophilia A), factor IX (hemophilia B or Christmas disease), and factor XI (hemophilia C or Rosenthal syndrome).

ASSESSMENT

History

A comprehensive, focused history and physical assessment are important aspects of the evaluation of a child with anemia or other suspected hematologic disorder. Many hematologic processes are inherited. Therefore the family history, nationality, and geographic origins are aids to diagnosis. For example, thalassemia occurs most often among patients of Mediterranean or Asian descent; G6PD deficiency is found in these ethnic groups and is also common among blacks. The nurse practitioner (NP) should obtain information about family members with a history of any of following:

- Anemia
- Jaundice
- Splenomegaly
- Gallbladder disease
- Sickle cell or thalassemia disease or trait
- Bleeding tendencies
- Drug and toxin exposure
- Bone marrow failure
- Chronic illnesses
- Lead exposure

The child's medical history and a review of systems are important, with particular attention paid to the following:

- Episodes of jaundice (including in the newborn period)
- Extremity pain
- Abdominal pain
- Blood loss (particularly from mucous membranes)
- Weight loss
- Recent infections
- Drug exposure
- Travel
- Behavioral changes
- Pallor
- Petechiae, ecchymoses
- Adenopathy
- Gastrointestinal and genitourinary disorders
- Changes in stool characteristics indicating gastrointestinal bleeding (i.e., black, tarry stools)

The nutritional history of the child (and of the breast-feeding mother) should include the following:

- Dietary intake of iron sources, vitamins, milk, and meat
- A 24-hour dietary recall
- Any history of pica (particularly when iron deficiency or plumbism is suspected)

Physical Examination

The physical examination of the child should be comprehensive, and vital signs and growth parameters should be documented. The following positive signs are particularly important to identify:

- Pallor (especially of the conjunctivae and palmar creases)
- Jaundice
- Petechiae
- Fundal hemorrhages
- Excessive bruising
- Bleeding from mucous membranes
- Lymphadenopathy
- Frontal bossing
- Joint or extremity pain
- Heart murmurs and signs of congestive heart failure
- Hepatomegaly or splenomegaly
- Congenital anomalies that are associated with hematologic disorders

Screening

In many states, routine screening is done on the cord blood of newborns to detect sickle cell disease, sickle cell trait, and other hemoglobinopathies. Routine hemoglobin screening should be done (American Academy of Pediatrics, Committee on Practice and Ambulatory Medicine, 2000)

- At 9 to 12 months of age, when fetal stores are depleted
- In menstruating adolescents

Lead screening should also be an integral part of pediatric primary care (see Chapter 42). A child considered to be at risk for exposure should have blood drawn to determine the level of lead at 9 to 12 months of age (American Academy of Pediatrics, Committee on Practice and Ambulatory Medicine, 2000). If the initial blood lead level is 10 μg/dl or greater, the child should be retested more frequently and may need individual case management.

Workup of Anemia

Anemia may be suspected on the basis of clinical judgment and the established norms of hematocrit (i.e., the percentage of blood volume occupied by RBCs) and hemoglobin values. The initial laboratory approach is to obtain the following:

- Complete blood count (CBC)
- Reticulocyte count
- Peripheral smear to examine the morphologic characteristics and staining properties of the RBC

In the description of the smear, *anisocytosis* refers to cells of unequal size, *poikilocytosis* denotes cells of abnormal shape, and *hypochromic* describes cells that are paler than usual.

The results of the RBC indices obtained in the CBC are useful in classification of the anemia, first according to the size of the RBC and then based on the pathophysiology (see Table 27-4):

- Mean corpuscular volume (MCV) is a measure of the average volume or size of the RBC and is calculated by dividing the hematocrit by the total number of RBCs. The calculated value of the MCV is expressed in cubic micrometers. A decrease in the MCV is seen in iron deficiency or thalassemia when the RBC is microcytic or smaller than usual. The MCV is increased in the megaloblastic anemias (such as folic acid anemia or juvenile pernicious anemia) when the RBC is abnormally large.
- Mean corpuscular hemoglobin (MCH) represents the average amount of hemoglobin in an RBC and is computed by dividing the hemoglobin concentration by the number of RBCs.
- Mean corpuscular hemoglobin concentration (MCHC) is the average percentage of hemoglobin in an RBC and is obtained by dividing the hemoglobin by the hematocrit.

In addition to the aforementioned screening tests, further diagnostic studies may be indicated to identify the type of acute anemia seen in childhood (Fig. 27-2). These measures include the following:

- Free erythrocyte protoporphyrin (FEP), which is a measure of the porphyrin precursors that have not been converted into heme.
- Serum iron (SI or Fe), which indicates iron concentration levels in plasma.
- Total iron-binding capacity (TIBC), which denotes the number of binding sites available for iron (the ratio SI/TIBC expresses the saturation).
- Serum ferritin (SF) concentration, which indicates the level of iron stores in the liver, spleen, and bone marrow. A decrease in this level is one of the earliest markers of iron deficiency.
- Red cell distribution width (RDW), which is the coefficient of variation of the MCV (or the standard deviation of the measured MCVs divided by their mean MCV times 100). It is a measure of variation in size of RBCs. A larger RDW indicates greater diversity in cell size. An increased RDW is seen with iron deficiency. The most common use of RDW is to differentiate thalassemia minor (in which the RDW is elevated) from iron deficiency.
- Hemoglobin electrophoresis, which identifies the percentages of different types of hemoglobin and is useful

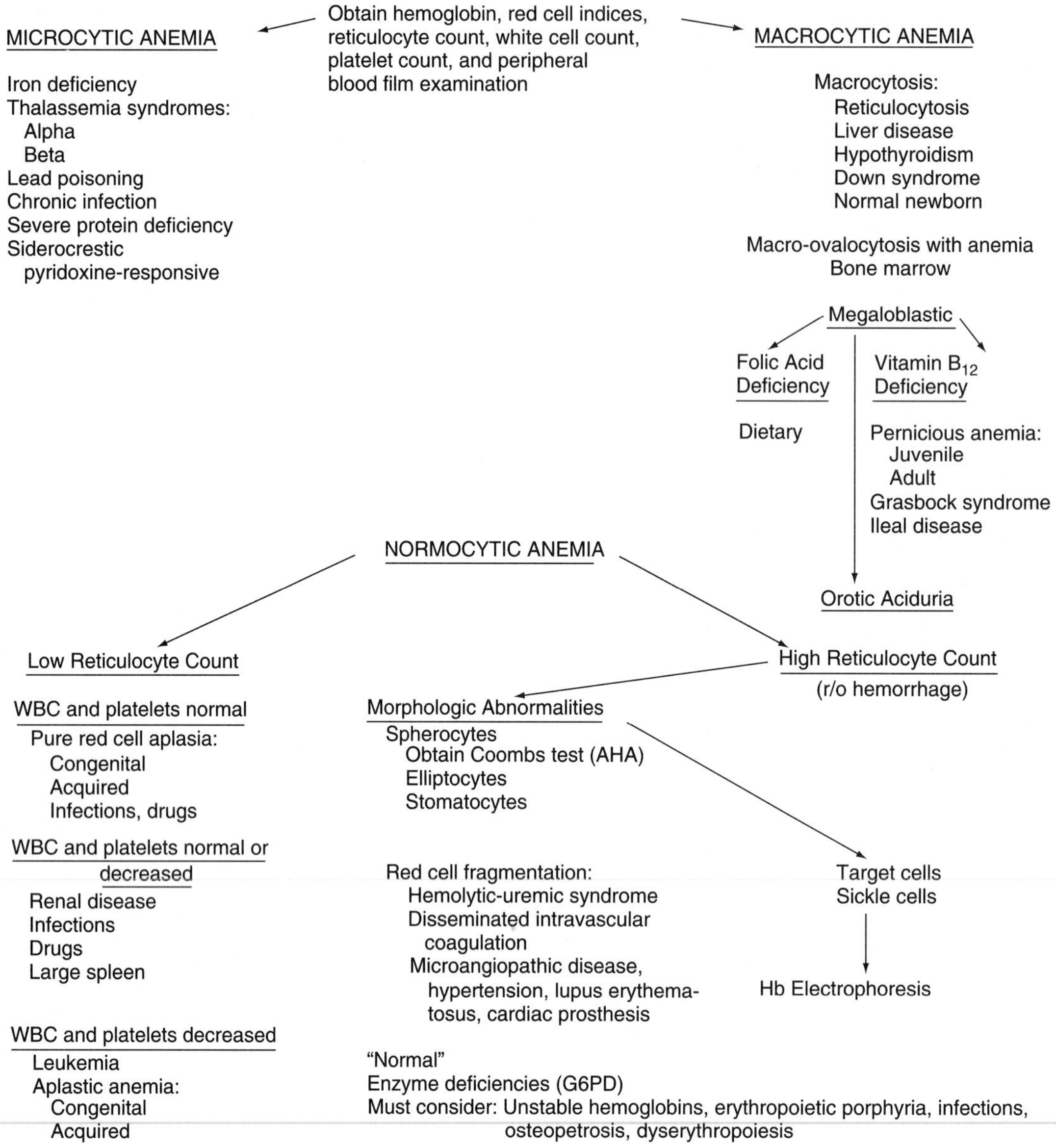

FIGURE 27-2 A diagnostic approach to anemia. *AHA*, Antihuman globulin antibody; *G6PD*, glucose-6-phosphate dehydrogenase; *Hb*, hemoglobin; *WBC*, white blood cell count. (From Nathan D, Oski FA: *Hematology of infancy and childhood*, ed 4, Philadelphia, 1993, WB Saunders, p 352.)

in the diagnosis of sickle cell anemia, thalassemia, and other hemoglobinopathies.

- Bone marrow aspiration, which examines for the presence of precursors of all the hematologic lines: erythroid elements, myeloid elements, and platelets/megakaryocytes. This procedure is necessary for the diagnosis of aplastic anemia (complete bone marrow failure), leukemia, and other malignancies.

White Blood Cell Count

The WBC count and differential are obtained on a smear of blood one cell layer thick, usually with a Wright stain procedure that contains both basic and acidic dyes.

The ANC is calculated from the results of the differential: if WBCs = 3600, percentage of segmented neutrophils = 20, band neutrophils = 5, lymphocytes = 60, monocytes = 10, and eosinophils = 5, then

$$\begin{aligned} \text{ANC} &= \text{WBC} \times (\%\ \text{Seg} + \text{Band}) \\ &= 3600 \times 0.25 \\ &= 900 \end{aligned}$$

Tests for Coagulation Disorders

- Platelet count (normal range is 150,000 to 300,000/mm^3).
- Platelet function tests such as platelet function analyzer (PFA).
- Prothrombin time (PT) (normal range is 11.5 to 14 seconds).
- Activated partial thromboplastin time (APTT) is the current method used to determine partial thromboplastin time (PTT) and is commonly still referred to as the PTT (normal range is 25 to 40 seconds).
- Specific coagulation factor assays determine which clotting factors are absent.

The PT and PTT measure all of the clotting factors except factor XIII. If the PT and APTT are elevated in association with thrombocytopenia, the probable diagnosis is disseminated intravascular coagulation. If the platelet count is normal, the PTT or PT is prolonged, or both, a coagulation factor deficiency is possible (Kaufman & Rao, 2002a; Platt, 1999). The typical laboratory findings of hemophilia are normal PT and PFA and an abnormal APTT (Hagani & Bussel, 2002b).

Bone Marrow Aspiration

Bone marrow aspiration or biopsy may be necessary to evaluate the specific types of cells present, including any foreign or malignant cells and maturation of the blood cell lines. In infants, the usual sites of aspiration are the proximal end of the tibia and posterior aspect of the iliac crest. In older children, the posterior part of the iliac crest or sternum can be used.

MANAGEMENT STRATEGIES

The types of management strategies used to treat children with hematologic problems are as varied as the disorders themselves. Most commonly, the plan of care focuses on provision of adequate nutrition and iron supplementation. Changes may be needed in the child's environment because of lead exposure. For some problems, management centers on teaching the family ways to prevent symptom exacerbation. For other rarer disorders, the focus is on helping the child and family cope with a chronic or potentially fatal condition and on collaborating with pediatric hematologists and oncologists in the delivery of care. Effective patterns of communication and referral among all the interdisciplinary providers, including laboratory personnel, are crucial.

Improvements in technology have brought about positive changes in the clinical management of children with hematologic disorders. The recognition of blood group antigens and infectious agents makes red cell transfusion a relatively safe procedure. Advances in pediatric hematology have led to an understanding of coagulation proteins and have dramatically improved the clinical course of children with coagulopathies. Unparalleled progress in the treatment of malignant hematologic diseases is likely to continue, and future breakthroughs will be possible as a result of gene replacement therapy.

Despite these many improvements, the family coping with having a child with chronic hematologic illness may experience numerous psychologic ramifications, often in the context of limited resources (Carroll, 2000). In cases of sickle cell disease or bleeding disorders, the family may experience overwhelming guilt and responsibility associated with the knowledge that the disease is genetically transmitted. Families of a child with leukemia may have difficulty coping with chronic uncertainty and with the needs of other siblings. Clinical issues such as pain management and problems with venous access may need to be addressed. Parents may be fearful that the therapeutic effects of narcotics and blood products may be outweighed by the potentially deleterious side effects. Reimbursement and financial health care coverage may become an area of real concern as children reach the maximum lifetime amount of insurance reimbursement. Families may also be hesitant to join organized support networks for fear of stigma. NPs and other health care providers need to be aware of these many issues that families of a chronically ill child may face while also keeping in mind the effects of culture and ethnicity on family management styles. The Resource Box at the end of this chapter identifies some Internet sites that may be of help to families and providers caring for a child with a chronic hematologic illness.

SPECIFIC HEMATOLOGIC PROBLEMS

Erythrocyte Disorders

Anemias are classified on the basis of two overall functional disturbances: anemias caused by nutritional deficiencies or inadequate production of RBCs and anemias brought about by increased destruction (hemolysis) of RBCs. Anemias occurring in the neonatal period are generally secondary to blood loss, isoimmunization, or congenital hemolytic anemias.

Anemias Caused by Inadequate Production of Red Blood Cells

Iron Deficiency Anemia

Description. Iron deficiency anemia is a common childhood anemia that is caused by inadequate availability of iron to sustain bone marrow erythropoiesis. Anemia caused by iron deficiency is the most common hematologic disease of infancy and childhood. Mild to moderate iron deficiency anemia is characterized by hemoglobin levels of 7 to 10 g/dl (Recht & Pearson, 1999). Hematologic markers are important in identifying various states of iron deficiency that range from iron depletion, to iron deficiency with anemia, to iron deficiency anemia.

Etiology and Incidence. Iron deficiency anemia is seen in approximately 9% of children age 1 to 2 years and 9% to 11% of adolescent girls. It usually occurs between ages 9 and 24 months and earlier in preterm infants (Tender & Cheng, 2002). Two factors that account for this relatively high rate of anemia are the rapid increase in body size and blood volume during the first 2 years of life and insufficient iron in the diet. Typically, the young child has a history of a diet low in iron-containing foods and a high intake of milk (more than 1 qt/day). Milk impairs iron absorption and can cause gastrointestinal irritation leading to occult blood loss, which compounds the problem. Iron deficiency is also common among girls in the adolescent years after menarche, when iron intake is often inadequate.

Clinical Findings

HISTORY. Clinical findings are noted as follows; however, children with mild to severe anemia may be asymptomatic:

- Irritability and restlessness are often noticed in infants and toddlers only in retrospect, after treatment, and associated with hemoglobin below 8 g/dl.
- Pica may be present in unusual circumstances.
- Anorexia has been reported with hemoglobin levels below 8 g/dl.
- Developmental delays (mental and motor areas) and behavioral disturbances that may be irreversible have been reported in infants and young children (Wu, Lesperance, & Bernstein, 2002).

PHYSICAL EXAMINATION. In mild to moderate iron deficiency, few symptoms are seen (Recht & Pearson, 1999). The child may appear normal, or pallor may be present. Rarely, in anemias that develop slowly, the physical examination may reveal tachycardia, or systolic murmurs and signs of congestive heart failure.

DIAGNOSTIC TESTS. The following may be seen:

- A microcytic, hypochromic anemia on CBC
- Low reticulocyte count
- RDW increased
- Low ferritin
- Elevated FEP (40 to 160 μg/dl) (Tender & Cheng, 2002)

Reticulocyte hemoglobin content (CHr) is a new test being studied to diagnose iron deficiency before anemia is present. Although controversial, the two most commonly used screening tests for iron deficiency anemia are hemoglobin and hematocrit, with hemoglobin being the more direct and sensitive marker of anemia compared with hematocrit measurements (Wu, Lesperance, & Bernstein, 2002). Iron deficiency anemia is frequently identified in routine screenings of hemoglobin level via finger-stick sampling. If there is a low hemoglobin level for age (in the range of 8 to 11 g/dl), a history of low iron intake, and no concern about other possible causes for the anemia or the possibility of another hemoglobinopathy, this is suggestive of iron deficiency anemia. A practical approach that many clinicians use to diagnose this form of anemia is to initially begin a trial of iron supplementation without further diagnostic testing and then follow the child's hemoglobin levels. They typically see the child again in 4 weeks. If there is a response to treatment with supplemental iron, a diagnosis of iron deficiency anemia is made (Wu, Lesperance, & Bernstein, 2002). Figure 27-3 presents a diagnostic approach to anemia based on mean corpuscular volume.

If there is no response to iron therapy, other studies, such as those identified in this section, are ordered to confirm iron deficiency or differentiate another etiology. Other causes of anemia, such as blood loss with occult rectal bleeding, should be considered in children with a low hemoglobin level on screening who eat a normal diet with adequate servings of iron-rich foods. Table 27-5 identifies age- and gender-specific laboratory cutoff values for childhood anemia.

Differential Diagnosis. If resistant to treatment, iron deficiency should be differentiated from other microcytic, hypochromic anemias such as lead poisoning, thalassemia minor, anemia of chronic disease, and hereditary sideroblastic anemia (see Fig. 27-3). In lead poisoning, the FEP may be above 200 μg/dl, and basophilic stippling may be seen on the RBCs in the peripheral smear. β-Thalassemia is indicated by elevations in Hgb A_2.

Management. Responses to treatment with iron supplementation are important diagnostically as well as therapeutically. For a child whose laboratory data reveal a microcytic, hypochromic anemia and an elevated FEP panel and whose history and physical examination are consistent with iron deficiency, a trial of iron is started (4 to 6 mg/kg per day of elemental iron in three divided doses) (Recht & Pearson, 1999). Peripheral reticulocytosis may be seen after the first 4 days of treatment, and hemoglobin should return to a normal level within 4 to 6 weeks. At the least, the hemoglobin should be rechecked 1 month after treatment. If a therapeutic response is observed (hemoglobin increase of greater than 1 g/dl or greater than 3% increase in hematocrit), iron supplementation should continue for 2 to 3 months to ensure adequate stores. Otherwise, compliance issues and alternative diagnoses should be

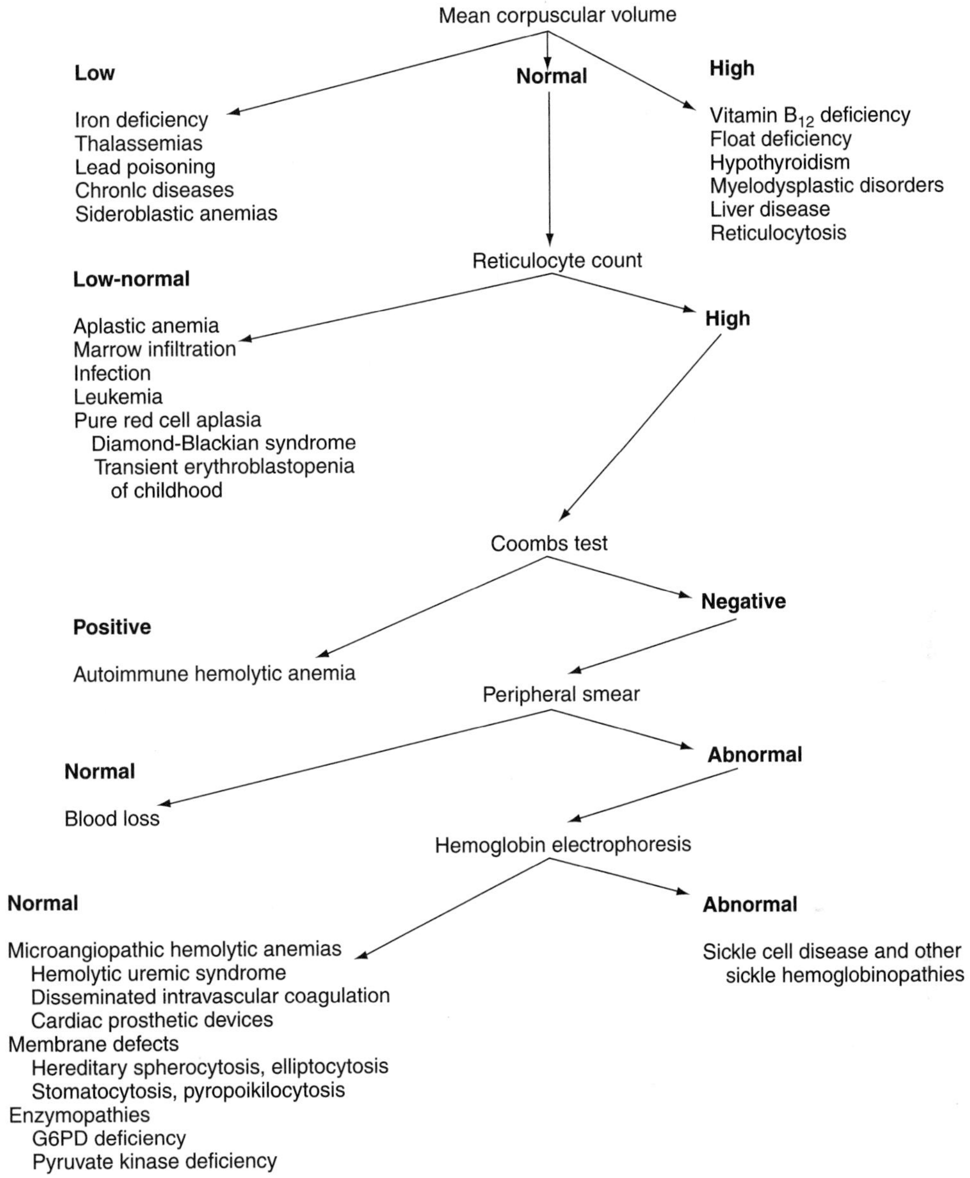

FIGURE 27-3 Diagnostic approach to anemia in the child, based on the mean corpuscular volume. (From Green M, Haggerty R, Weitzman M: *Ambulatory pediatrics*, ed 5, Philadelphia, 1999, WB Saunders, p 351.)

explored. Dietary counseling is critical and levels should be rechecked 6 months after iron supplements are stopped (Tender & Cheng, 2002; Wu, Lesperance, & Bernstein, 2002).

Complications. The lack of a therapeutic response may be due to poor compliance, inadequate dosage, the presence of unrecognized blood loss, or an alternate diagnosis. A more extensive determination of the child's iron status is obtained by measuring serum iron, iron-binding capacity, and the venous lead level. Stool guaiac should be checked for occult blood loss.

Children with extremely low hemoglobin (less than 7 g/dl), hypotension, or signs of congestive heart failure should be referred and may need to be hospitalized. Laboratory results that also indicate referral are neutropenia, thrombocytopenia, nucleated RBCs, or immature myeloid elements (Tender & Cheng, 2002; Platt, 1999). When disorders of erythrocytes, platelets, and leukocytes are all found, a bone marrow disorder is probable.

Education and Prevention. Parents or caretakers should be counseled about the adequacy of the child's diet. Whole cow's milk should be avoided in infants younger

TABLE 27-5 Age- and Gender-Specific Laboratory Cutoff Values for Anemia

Age (yr)	Hemoglobin Concentration (g/dl)	Hematocrit (%)	MCV (fl)
1 to <2	<11.0	32.9	<77
2 to <5	<11.1	33.0	<79
5 to <8	<11.5	33.5	<80
8 to <12	<11.9	35.4	<80
12 to <15, male	<12.5	37.3	<85
15 to <18, male	<13.3	39.7	<85
12 to <15, female	<11.8	35.7	<85
15 to <18, female	<12.0	35.9	<85

From Burg F et al, editors: *Gellis and Kagan's current pediatric therapy*, ed 17, Philadelphia, 2002, WB Saunders.
MCV, Mean corpuscular volume.

than 12 months. For full-term infants, dietary iron supplementation (as in iron-enriched infant cereal) should begin at 4 to 6 months of age. For preterm infants, supplementation with oral iron drops should begin as early as 2 months. If the child is treated therapeutically with oral iron supplements, parents should be advised to avoid giving the iron with meals, that vitamin C juice enhances absorption, and that the child's stools will probably turn black. Parents should also be cautioned to keep the medication safely out of reach to avoid accidental ingestion.

Megaloblastic Anemias

Description. Megaloblastic anemias are characterized by oval macrocytes and hypersegmented PMNs in the peripheral blood and megaloblasts in the bone marrow.

Etiology. The relatively rare megaloblastic anemias are due primarily to a lack of folic acid, vitamin B_{12}, or both. These two substances function as coenzymes in the synthesis of nuclear protein. Megaloblastic anemias may develop if the diet lacks these two substances or if the gastric intrinsic factor necessary for the absorption of vitamin B_{12} is absent.

Clinical Findings

HISTORY. Patients with megaloblastic anemia may include

- Young infants who are being fed powdered milk products or goat's milk, which are deficient in folic acid and vitamin B_{12}
- Older children who are exclusively vegetarian or who have severe nutritional deficiencies, absorption problems, or tapeworm infestations

PHYSICAL EXAMINATION. The following may be seen:

- Weakness, pallor
- Beefy-red, smooth, sore tongue

DIAGNOSTIC TESTS. The following results may be seen:

- Elevated MCV (greater than 95 fl) and MCHC
- Blood smear showing macro-ovalocytes with anisocytosis and poikilocytosis
- Normal white cell count and platelet count, but possibly decreased in more severe cases
- Large and hypersegmented neutrophils

Management. In general, management of folic acid deficiency and juvenile pernicious anemia (caused by a lack of vitamin B_{12}) is best done in consultation with a pediatric hematologist. Treatment is through dietary supplementation and correction of the underlying disorder (e.g., infection) if possible.

In folic acid deficiency confirmed by measurement of the RBC folate level, folic acid may be administered in a dose of 0.5 to 1 mg/24 hr and continued for 3 to 4 weeks. Prolonged use of folic acid should be avoided (Glader, 2004).

In vitamin B_{12} deficiency, a prompt hematologic response is usually seen after parenteral administration of vitamin B_{12}. If neurologic involvement is present, 1 mg should be given intramuscularly daily for at least 2 weeks. A maintenance dose of a 1 mg intramuscular injection of vitamin B_{12} is administered monthly throughout the patient's life (Glader, 2004).

Transient Erythroblastopenia of Childhood

Description. Idiopathic erythroblastopenia of childhood, or transient erythroblastosis of childhood (TEC), is a benign disorder of unknown cause that occurs in children during the first few years of life, usually after age 1 year. It is characterized by anemia, reticulocytopenia, and erythroid hypoplasia of the bone marrow. The cause of this acquired decrease in red cell production is not clear, although it frequently follows a viral infection (Glader, 2004; Segel, Hirsh, & Feig, 2002b).

Etiology. TEC is associated with temporary failure of erythropoiesis caused by probable viral suppression or as a result of an IgG-mediated autoimmune response.

Clinical Findings

HISTORY. TEC occurs mainly in previously healthy children between 6 months and 3 years of age. The child may have a history of a preceding infection.

PHYSICAL EXAMINATION. Patients have symptoms of anemia, including pallor.

DIAGNOSTIC TESTS. The following are seen in TEC:

- Anemia (in which the hemoglobin content may be as low as 2.5 g/dl or only slightly decreased)

- Markedly low reticulocyte count
- WBC count usually normal
- Platelets normal or elevated
- High serum iron level reflecting decreased utilization
- Bone marrow aspiration results indicating erythyroid hypoplasia

Differential Diagnosis. The syndrome can be differentiated from congenital hypoplastic anemia (Diamond-Blackfan syndrome) by the normal size of the RBCs (MCV less than 80 fl). Approximately 25% of children with Diamond-Blackfan syndrome have dysmorphic features (e.g., short stature, congenital heart disease, and mental retardation), whereas children with TEC have a normal physical examination (Segel, Hirsh, & Feig, 2002b).

Management. TEC is self-limited, with recovery taking place 1 to 2 months after diagnosis. No specific treatment is indicated, although transfusions may be required for severe anemia. The NP should consult with a physician; a referral to a hematologist may be needed.

Hemolytic Anemias

Hemolytic anemias can be classified as either hereditary or acquired. In particular, the hereditary and congenital anemias are manifested in infancy and early childhood. They may be due to a variety of hemoglobinopathies or to defects in the red cell membrane.

Sickle Cell Anemia and Trait

Etiology. Sickle cell disease describes a group of complex, chronic disorders that are characterized by hemolysis, unpredictable acute complications that may become life threatening, and the possible development of chronic organ damage (American Academy of Pediatrics, Committee on Genetics, 2002). Children who have sickle cell anemia or disease do not form the normal Hgb A molecule but rather synthesize hemoglobin S (Hgb S), which carries the amino acid valine instead of glutamic acid. Because of this change, Hgb S tends to polymerize or come out of solution at low PaO_2, low pH, low temperature, and low osmolality. This process damages the RBC by giving it a "sickled" appearance and causes a chronic hemolytic anemia with associated ischemia and vaso-occlusive problems.

Incidence. Sickle cell disease has an autosomal recessive inheritance pattern. It is found most often in people of African descent but is also detected among ethnic groups from the Mediterranean, the Caribbean, and India. In the United States, sickle cell disease occurs in about 1 of every 400 black infants (Lane, Nuss, & Ambruso, 2003). This incidence exceeds that of most other serious genetic disorders in children, including cystic fibrosis and hemophilia (American Academy of Pediatrics [AAP], 2002).

Children with sickle cell trait who are heterozygous for the gene essentially have a benign clinical course. Their RBCs contain only 30% to 40% Hgb S, and sickling does not occur under most conditions. It is only in rare instances of hypoxia, such as in shock, while flying in unpressurized aircraft, or traveling to high elevations, that signs of vaso-occlusion can occur.

Clinical Findings. Most infants with sickle cell disease born in the United States are now identified by routine neonatal screening. In those states that have not yet implemented universal screening, neonatal screening for sickle cell disease should be requested for those infants considered to be high risk, including those of African, Mediterranean, Middle Eastern, Indian, Caribbean, and Central and South American ancestry (AAP, 2002). A careful family medical history is also important.

PHYSICAL EXAMINATION. Symptoms begin to emerge in the second 6 months of life as the amount of Hgb S increases and Hgb F declines. Subsequently, painful, vaso-occlusive crises occur. The following may be noted:

- Pale and slightly jaundiced appearance with splenomegaly
- Painful swelling of the hands and feet (hand-foot syndrome) caused by infarction in the small bones
- Low-grade fever
- Leukocytosis
- Painful involvement of the larger bones (in older patients)
- Priaprism
- Diffuse abdominal pain
- Chest pain
- Sequestration crisis, which occurs when large amounts of blood are pooled in the abdominal organs and the spleen becomes enlarged

After age 5, splenomegaly usually disappears because of autoinfarction. Rates of height and weight gain are usually slowed after 7 years, and puberty may be delayed 3 to 4 years.

DIAGNOSTIC TESTS. The following laboratory results are seen in sickle cell disease (Platt, 1999; Segel, Hirsh, & Feig, 2002b):

- Hematocrit of 20% to 29% with sickled cells, nucleated RBCs, and Howell-Jolly bodies on the peripheral smear
- Hemoglobin 6 to 10 g/dl (severe sickle syndromes)
- MCV greater than 80
- Reticulocyte count of 20% to 29%
- Increased WBC and platelet count
- Hemoglobin electrophoresis (after infancy) showing a predominance of Hgb S and no Hgb A
- Blood film shows irreversibly sickled cells or chronic elliptocytes

Differential Diagnosis. Chronic hemolytic anemia should be included in the differential diagnosis. Other syndromes characterized by hemolytic anemia and vaso-occlusion are hemoglobin SC disease and a combination of Hgb S with α- or β-thalassemia. These diseases may be differentiated through electrophoresis and family testing if necessary.

Management. The following measures are instituted:

- Baseline laboratory data (CBC, reticulocyte count) are monitored every few months.
- Seven-valent pneumococcal conjugate and 23-valent pneumococcal polysaccharide vaccines are administered.
- Penicillin V prophylaxis (125 mg orally, twice daily) is initiated by 2 months of age. At age 3 years, the dose is increased to 250 mg orally, twice a day, and continued at least until the fifth birthday (AAP, 2002).
- Yearly influenza immunization is administered.
- Meningococcal vaccine is administered for children older than 2 years of age (Segel, Hirsh, & Feig, 2002b).
- Folic acid supplementation may be indicated if the diet is low in green leafy vegetables. Oral folic acid is administered, if needed, to prevent folic acid deficiency: 0.5 mg/day for children less than 5 years of age; 1 mg/day after age 5 years (Segel, Hirsh, & Feig, 2002b).
- Aggressive treatment of infections and maintenance of hydration and body temperature are used to prevent hypoxia and acidosis; volume replacement may be necessary to prevent circulatory collapse.

Children with sickle cell disease are usually comanaged by specialists in hematology and their primary care provider. Emergency admission or referral is necessary in the presence of the following:

- Fever (to rule out sepsis) greater than 101° F
- Pneumonia
- Sequestration crisis (splenomegaly with decreased hemoglobin or hematocrit)
- Aplastic crisis (decreased hematocrit and reticulocyte count)
- Severe painful crisis
- Unusual headache, visual disturbances
- Priapism

Consultation is also necessary for the chronic sequelae of persistent bone pain or leg ulcers, as well as issues of pregnancy and contraception.

Complications. Because of functional asplenia, the greatest concern is febrile illness indicating infection. In view of the serious threat of pneumococcal sepsis in children younger than 5 years, all complaints of fever, poor feeding, lethargy, and irritability should be evaluated in person rather than by telephone (Platt, 1999). The consequences of hemolysis may include chronic anemia, jaundice, cholelithiasis, and delayed growth and sexual maturation. Vaso-occlusion and tissue ischemia may result in acute and chronic injury to virtually every organ system (AAP, 2002).

Patient and Family Education. The parents of children with sickle cell anemia need a great deal of support in raising a child with a genetically transmitted chronic disease. Clear patterns of communication should be established between the family and the provider. Initial education includes the genetics and pathophysiology of the disease and the importance of regular health maintenance visits. Parents should be counseled about the need for early evaluation and treatment of febrile illness, acute splenic sequestration, aplastic crisis, and acute chest syndrome. As the child grows, the family should be educated in other potential clinical complications such as stroke, enuresis, priapism, cholelithiasis, delayed puberty, retinopathy, avascular necrosis of the hip and shoulder, and leg ulcers (AAP, 2002).

Preventive Care. Preventive measures for infants and children include the following:

- Timely administration of routine immunizations, including pneumococcal and meningococcal vaccines, as well as yearly influenza vaccine
- Prophylactic antibiotics
- Genetic counseling
- Support groups

Thalassemias. The thalassemias are a group of hereditary, hypochromic anemias that are associated with the absence or decreased synthesis of the normal hemoglobin polypeptide chains—usually the α- and β-chains (Quirolo & Vichinsky, 2004). They occur primarily in people of Mediterranean and Southeast Asian descent.

β-Thalassemias cover a broad clinical spectrum of disorders that are classified according to patterns of inheritance and the severity of the anemia. The heterozygous states are thalassemia minor and thalassemia minima, which are essentially silent carrier states. Homozygous forms are thalassemia intermedia and thalassemia major, or Cooley's anemia.

β-Thalassemia Minor

DESCRIPTION. β-Thalassemia minor disease or trait is associated with a mild, hypochromic, microcytic anemia in which hemoglobin levels are 2 to 3 g/dl below normal and the MCV averages 65 fl (Quirolo & Vichinsky, 2004). It may be confused with iron deficiency or lead poisoning and can be differentiated by measuring serum iron or lead levels, transferrin saturation, or serum ferritin levels (Table 27-6). Thus it is particularly important to avoid long-term unnecessary administration of iron supplements that could result in iron overload. In thalassemia minor, the RDW coefficient is elevated. The primary diagnostic feature is increased Hgb A_2 (greater than 3.5%) on electrophoresis.

CLINICAL FINDINGS. Clinically, most individuals with thalassemia trait are asymptomatic, although mild pallor and splenomegaly may be found. A hemoglobin of 9.5 to 11 g/dl

TABLE 27-6 *Red Blood Cell (RBC) Disorders Associated with Anemia in Infants and Children*

	Clinical Presentation			
Disease	**History**	**Physical Findings**	**Laboratory Diagnosis**	**Treatment**
Iron deficiency	Fatigue Irritability Excess milk intake	Pallor or none	RBC hypochromic, microcytic Mean cell volume (MCV) ↓ Serum iron ↓ Total iron-binding capacity ↑ % Saturation ↓ Ferritin ↓ Blood in stool or urine Ratio of MCV/RBC >13	Correct diet Eliminate source of bleeding Ferrous SO_4 6 mg/kg per day of elemental iron
α- and β- thalessemia trait	None Pallor Family history	None Pallor	RBC hypochromic, microcytic MCV ↓↓ Basophilic stippling (β-thalassemia trait) ↑ Hemoglobin (Hgb) A_2 (β-thalassemia trait) Ratio of MCV/RBC <13	None for child Test both parents Genetic counseling Avoid iron therapy
Hereditary spherocytosis	None Family history History of neonatal jaundice	Pallor, jaundice Splenomegaly	Spherocytosis Coombs' test negative Reticulocyte % ↑ Osmotic fragility increased Mean corpuscular hemoglobin concentration ↑	No splenomectomy if Hgb >10 g/dl (100 g/L) and reticulocyte <10% Folic acid (0.5 mg qd <5 yr of age; 1.0 mg qd >5 yr of age) Splenomectomy and immunizations to pneumococcus, *Haemophilus influenzae*, and meningococcus and penicillin prophylaxis
Chronic inflammation	Depends on the cause of the inflammation and the severity of anemia (fatigue to symptoms of congestive heart failure)	Depends on the cause of the inflammation and the severity of anemia (pallor to signs of congestive heart failure)	Nonspecific tests: erythrocyte sedimentation rate Acute-phase reactants: C-reactive protein, fibrinogen, haptoglobin Serum ferritin Serum iron and total iron-binding capacity % iron saturation Bone marrow iron stores Bone marrow sideroblasts	Treat underlying disease or condition Treat anemia
Lead intoxication	Pica—ingestion of lead-containing substances Neurobehavioral problems (e.g., irritability, poor appetite, inattention, hyperactivity) Neurodevelopmental delay (e.g., learning problems to severe cognitive dysfunction)	Poor speech Visual-motor integration problems Encephalopathy, neuropathy, cerebral edema if severe poisoning	Basophilic stippling Erythrocyte protoporphyrin blood lead	Eliminate source of lead in the child's environment Diet rich in iron and calcium Iron supplementation, 3-6 mg/kg/day to reduce further absorption of lead Chelation therapy based on lead levels and symptoms (use Centers for Disease Control and Prevention guidelines)

Adapted from Segel G, Hirsh M, Feig S: Managing anemia in a pediatric office practice: part 1, *Pediatr Rev* 23:75-83, 2002.

and an MCV of less than 80 fl/cell is commonly seen in prepubertal children. The MCV/RBC count per milliliter is less than 13 (the Mentzer index). In contrast, the Mentzer index of iron deficiency is usually greater than 13 for iron deficiency (Segel, Hirsh, & Feig, 2002a). The degree of anemia may be exacerbated in concurrent illness or pregnancy.

MANAGEMENT. No specific treatment is known for β-thalassemia minor. Primary emphasis should be on education of all family members and genetic testing, and counseling should be offered.

β-Thalassemia Major

DESCRIPTION. Homozygous β-thalassemia major (or Cooley's anemia) is associated with severe anemia resulting from decreased or absent production of Hgb A and hemolysis caused by the precipitation of excess α-chains in the RBCs.

CLINICAL FINDINGS. Affected infants usually become symptomatic in the first year of life and have pallor, failure to thrive, hepatosplenomegaly, and a severe anemia with an average hemoglobin of 6 g/dl and low MCV (60 to 70 fl). RBC morphology reveals significant microcytosis, poikilocytosis, hypochromia, target cells, and nucleated RBCs. Hgb A and Hgb F levels are elevated.

MANAGEMENT. Proper management of the child requires collaboration with a pediatric hematologist. Exchange transfusions are usually necessary every 4 to 5 weeks with a post-transfusion level of 9.5 g/dl as the goal. Iron chelation therapy is indicated. Splenectomy and bone marrow transplants may be indicated as well (Quirolo & Vichinsky, 2004).

COMPLICATIONS. If the condition is left untreated, the characteristic facies of frontal bossing and maxillary overgrowth will develop as a result of bone marrow expansion.

Hereditary Spherocytosis

Description. Hereditary spherocytosis (HS) is a hemolytic anemia characterized by a deficiency or abnormality of the RBC membrane protein spectrin, which reduces the RBC surface area. The RBC membranes assume a more spherical shape. Hence, RBCs are more likely to be sequestered and prematurely destroyed in the spleen (Segel, Hirsh, & Feig, 2002a). The disease process of HS can range from low-grade chronic hemolysis to severe transfusion-dependent anemia (Altman, 2002).

Incidence. HS occurs in 1 in 5000 persons of predominantly northern European ancestry.

Clinical Findings

PHYSICAL EXAMINATION. Jaundice usually appears in the newborn period, and it may be difficult to differentiate HS from hyperbilirubinemia caused by ABO incompatibility. After age 2, splenomegaly is usually present. Chronic fatigue, malaise, and abdominal pain may also be noted.

DIAGNOSTIC TESTS. Laboratory findings in HS include the following:

- Chronic anemia (hemoglobin is 6 to 10 g/dl).
- Reticulocyte count ranges from 5% to 20%.
- On peripheral smear, a small proportion of the RBCs are spherocytic and smaller than normal and lack the central pallor of the usual biconcave disk-shaped cell.
- Osmotic fragility of the cells is increased, as is the rate of autohemolysis of incubated blood.

Management. The treatment of choice is splenectomy, which usually produces a clinical cure. Except in severe cases, it should be deferred until 5 or 6 years of age because of the increased risk of infection before that age. Pneumococcal vaccine should be given before splenectomy.

After splenectomy, prophylactic penicillin therapy (age less than 5 years: 125 mg orally twice a day; age greater than 5 years: 250 mg orally twice a day) is recommended. Because of increased hemolysis, children with HS and active hemolysis should receive 1 mg of folic acid daily until splenectomy. There is remission of the disease after splenectomy (Segel, 2004).

Complications. Aplastic crises (which can be indicated by fever, fatigue, abdominal pain, and jaundice) associated with parvovirus infections are the most serious complications during childhood. Febrile illnesses should be vigorously treated. A splenectomized child with a temperature over 101.5° F and without an obvious source of infection should be hospitalized and treated with intravenous antibiotics until blood cultures prove to be negative (Altman, 2002).

Glucose-6-Phosphate Dehydrogenase Syndrome

Description. G6PD syndrome is a drug-induced hemolytic anemia caused by genetic deficiency of the G6PD enzyme in the RBC. Symptoms are generally associated with infections or exposure to oxidant metabolites of certain drugs that cause precipitation of hemoglobin, injury to the red cells, and rapid hemolysis.

Etiology and Incidence. G6PD syndrome is transmitted as an X-linked recessive trait. In the United States, about 10% of black males and 1% to 2% of black females are affected. It may also occur in a more severe form in Greeks, Italians, Arabs, Southeast Asians, and Chinese.

Clinical Findings

HISTORY. Patients generally have a history of recent infection (particularly hepatitis) or oxidant drug ingestion—specifically, aspirin-containing antipyretics, sulfonamides, antimalarials, naphthaquinolones, and the fava bean. The degree of hemolysis is dependent on the amount of the drug ingested and the extent of enzyme deficiency.

PHYSICAL EXAMINATION. The patient may have pallor and jaundice, if there is chronic hemolysis, or jaundice, pallor, lethargy, headache, and red or dark clear urine after drug ingestion.

DIAGNOSTIC TESTS. Several dye reduction tests provide the diagnosis. Screening tests available to measure a deficiency of G6PD should be used in high-risk groups. These tests measure G6PD enzyme activity in the red blood cell. After a hemolytic crisis, however, screening may produce a false-negative result because the younger blood cells that remain after hemolysis may show normal enzymatic activity. A more representative enzyme assay can be obtained 2 to 3 months after the episode (Segel, Hirsh, & Feig, 2002b).

Management. No specific treatment is available for this syndrome. Red cell transfusion and supportive therapy may be indicated in cases in which the anemia is severe.

Education. Patients and families should be taught to avoid the offending drugs—the most common being aspirin, sulfonamide antibiotics, and antimalarials.

Platelet and Blood Coagulation Disorders

Platelet disorders should be ruled out in a child before undergoing extensive surgery. Platelet disorders should also be considered in a child with petechiae, frequent nosebleeds, mucous membrane bleeding, and excessive bleeding from minor trauma. Evaluation of these complaints includes a family history of bleeding or platelet disorders and a history of drug or toxin exposure. Initial laboratory studies should include a CBC, platelet count, PT, and APTT. Among the diagnoses that may be differentiated with these tests are ITP, hemophilia, von Willebrand's disease, and leukemia.

Immune or Idiopathic Thrombocytopenic Purpura

Description. Immune or idiopathic thrombocytopenic purpura (ITP) is the most common of the thrombocytopenic purpuras in childhood and is believed to be an autoimmune response in which circulating platelets are destroyed. It usually occurs after viral illnesses (Scott, 2002).

Incidence. Most cases occur between ages 2 and 5 years, and the incidence is increased in fair-skinned children.

Clinical Findings. ITP is essentially a clinical diagnosis and does not rest on any one diagnostic test. It is characterized by the following:

- Acute onset of petechiae, purpura, and bleeding in an otherwise healthy child; the bruising or bleeding may be most prominent over the legs.
- A viral illness 1 to 4 weeks before onset in 70% of cases.
- Hemorrhage of the mucous membranes, particularly the gums and lips.
- Nosebleeds that can be severe and difficult to control.
- The liver, spleen, and lymph nodes are not generally enlarged.

Diagnostic Tests. Laboratory findings in ITP include

- Low platelet count (less than 150,000/mm^3) with an otherwise normal CBC
- Normal PT and PTT
- Megathrombocytes on the peripheral smear (Platt, 1999)

Differential Diagnosis. If the smear shows fragmented RBCs, blood urea nitrogen and creatinine levels should be measured to rule out hemolytic-uremic syndrome. If the PT and PTT are elevated with thrombocytopenia, disseminated intravascular coagulation is a possibility, and cultures should be taken to identify sources of infection. A prolonged PT and APTT with a normal platelet count suggest a coagulation factor deficiency. If the syndrome is complicated by prolonged thrombocytopenia, neutropenia, anemia, bone pain, or congenital anomalies, the child should be referred to a hematologist for possible bone marrow aspiration to rule out ALL and other disorders (Platt, 1999). In a sick, febrile child with isolated thrombocytopenia, petechiae, or purpura, the major diagnosis to consider first is meningococcemia. Such children should also be referred, hospitalized, and treated for presumed sepsis.

Management. The prognosis for children with ITP is excellent, with spontaneous recovery in 75% of cases in the first 3 months (Scott, 2002). Most cases of ITP can be managed on an outpatient basis without any specific therapy. If the platelet count is greater than 50,000/mm^3 and no bleeding is observed, children and parents should be taught to avoid contact sports, aspirin ingestion, and any other herbal or pharmacologic agents that interfere with platelet function and to notify the practitioner of any bleeding. Epistaxis can be treated with local measures. In severe cases (platelets less than 50,000/mm^3) in which the diagnosis of leukemia is ruled out, a short course of corticosteroid therapy may reduce severity in the initial phases. A suggested dosage schedule for prednisone is 2 mg/kg per day for 10 days and then tapered over a period of 10 days (Platt, 1999). Intravenous immune globulin (IVIG) is also given to children with active severe bleeding and who have contraindications for steroid use (Neufeld, 2002).

Complications. The most serious complication is intracranial hemorrhage, which occurs in less than 1% of cases (Scott, 2002).

Hemophilia

Description. Inherited deficiencies are known for each of the coagulation factors, with most of them resulting in abnormal bleeding. Hemophilia refers to a deficiency of factor VIII (hemophilia A) or factor IX (hemophilia B). In hemophilia A and B, absence or deficiency of the coagulation factor results in prolonged bleeding either spontaneously from small vessels or as a result of trauma.

In plasma, factor VIII is complexed with von Willebrand factor (vWf), which is a specific circulatory protein and acts as a carrier protein. von Willebrand's disease (also known as vascular hemophilia) is a heterogeneous group of hereditary bleeding disorders caused by a quantitative or qualitative abnormality of vWf protein, which also results in a bleeding disorder (Table 27-7).

Etiology and Incidence. Because the genes for the coagulation factors are sex linked (carried on the X chromosome) and recessive, the disease affects primarily males. Females are generally only carriers of the disorder. About 1 in 5000 males is affected with hemophilia A, which is five times more common than hemophilia B (Scott, 2002). von Willebrand's disease is seen in both sexes.

Clinical Findings. The following are seen in hemophilia:
- A positive family history in the vast majority of cases
- Excessive bruising
- Prolonged bleeding from mucous membranes after minor lacerations
- Hemarthroses characterized by pain and swelling in the elbows, knees, and ankles
- A greatly prolonged APTT

A specific assay for factor VIII or IX activity confirms the diagnosis.

Clinical findings associated with von Willebrand's disease include the following:
- Mucous membrane bleeding (epistaxis, menorrhagia), easy bruising, and excessive posttraumatic or postsurgical bleeding
- History of ecchymosis of trunk, upper arms, and thighs
- Factor VIII clotting activity usually decreased
- vWF antigen usually decreased
- Decreased vWF
- Bleeding time generally prolonged but may be normal (Kaufman & Rao, 2002b)

Management. Treatment consists of prevention of trauma and replacement therapy to increase factor VIII activity in plasma. Several products are available for replacement, including human plasma fraction concentrates (antihemolytic factors), cryoprecipitate, and desmopressin (DDAVP). Local measures include the application of cold and pressure to affected, painful joints. As with all bleeding disorders, aspirin should be avoided (Scott, 2002).

Ideally, most children with hemophilia should be enrolled in a local hemophilia treatment center to facilitate a collaborative, interdisciplinary approach to management. The primary provider should remain central to the care of the child. All immunizations should be given subcutaneously with a 26-gauge needle, followed by firm pressure at the site for several minutes. Iron replacement may also be necessary in children with severe bleeding disorders.

TABLE 27-7 ***Comparisons of Hemophilia A, Hemophilia B, and von Willebrand's Disease***

	Hemophilia A	Hemophilia B	von Willebrand's Disease
Inheritance	X-linked	X-linked	Autosoma dominant
Factor deficiency	Factor VIII	Factor IX	von Willebrand factor and VIIIC
Bleeding site(s)	Muscle, joint, surgical	Muscle, joint, surgical	Mucous membranes, skin, surgical, menstrual
Prothrombin time (PT)	Normal	Normal	Normal
Activated partial thromboplastin time (APTT)	Prolonged	Prolonged	Prolonged or normal
Bleeding time	Normal	Normal	Prolonged or normal
Factor VIII coagulant activity (VIIIC)	Low	Normal	Low or normal
von Willebrand factor antigen (vWF: Ag)	Normal	Normal	Low
von Willebrand factor activity (vWF: Act)	Normal	Normal	Low
Factor IX	Normal	Low	Normal
Ristocetin-induced	Normal	Normal	Normal, low, or increased at low-dose ristocetin
Platelet agression	Normal	Normal	Normal
Treatment	DDAVP* or recombinant VIII	Recombinant IX	DDAVP* or vWF concentrate

From Behrman R, Kliegman R: *Nelson essentials of pediatrics*, ed 4, Philadelphia, 2002, WB Saunders, p 639.
*Desmopressin (DDAVP) for mild to moderate hemophilia A or type I von Willebrand's disease.

von Willebrand's disease is treated depending on the type and severity of the bleeding. DDAVP, plasma-derived von Willebrand factor, platelet transfusion (if platelet type disease is present), and local measures to control bleeding may be part of the treatment plan (Kaufman & Rao, 2002b).

A written treatment plan stating the dosage of the replacement product for the location of the bleed should be in the chart and given to the parents to carry with them. The child should wear a medical alert bracelet or necklace.

Complications. Without factor replacement, bleeding persists, particularly in closed areas such as the joints. Brain hemorrhage can be a serious consequence of head trauma. Continued hemorrhage results in anemia and eventually hypovolemic shock.

The use of therapeutic replacement materials derived from blood carries some inherent risk. Hepatitis infection was a problem in the past. Infection with human immunodeficiency virus (HIV) unfortunately was frequently seen in patients who were exposed to multiple donors before the revision of blood donor screening tests and the use of heat-treated concentrates.

Cancer

Leukemias

Description. The leukemias represent a group of malignant hematologic diseases in which normal bone marrow elements are replaced by abnormal, poorly differentiated lymphocytes known as blast cells. Leukemias are classified according to cell type involvement (i.e., lymphocytic or nonlymphocytic) and by cellular differentiation. Acute lymphoblastic leukemia (ALL) is characterized by predominantly undifferentiated WBCs.

Incidence. The leukemias are the most common form of childhood cancer and account for about one third of pediatric malignancies. ALL accounts for about 77% of cases, with a peak incidence between 2 and 6 years of age. Acute myeloid leukemia (AML) accounts for about 11% of all cases. Most of the other leukemias are of the chronic myeloid form (Tubergen & Bleyer, 2004).

Etiology. As with all types of malignancy, the exact cause of leukemia is unknown. Several factors associated with increased risk have been identified, including infection, radiation, chemical and drug exposure, and genetic factors.

Clinical Findings. Most of the clinical signs and symptoms of leukemia are related to leukemic replacement of the bone marrow and the absence of blood cell precursors. The child may be anemic, pale, listless, irritable, or chronically tired and have the following:

- A history of repeated infections
- Bleeding episodes characterized by epistaxis, petechiae, and hematomas
- Lymphadenopathy and hepatosplenomegaly
- Bone and joint pain

All these symptoms may be vague or nonspecific, in which case it is important for the provider to have a high index of suspicion for cancer.

Diagnostic Tests. The following are used to diagnose leukemia:

- CBC with differential WBC, platelet, and reticulocyte counts. Thrombocytopenia is present in up to 85% of cases, and anemia is also usually present. WBC count may be elevated, normal, or low with varying levels of neutropenia.
- Peripheral smear, which may demonstrate malignant cells.
- Bone marrow examination, which shows an infiltration of blast cells replacing normal elements of the marrow.

Further classification regarding cell type, morphologic characteristics, and cell surface markers is generally made at the cancer treatment center to which the child is referred.

Management. The treatment program for most types of acute leukemia involves an induction phase (usually with vincristine, prednisone, and L-asparaginase), prophylactic central nervous system therapy, and a maintenance phase of therapy. Approximately 75% to 80% of children diagnosed with ALL are now thought to be curable. Key genetic features are now identifiable. Treatment decisions and risk categorizations are based on genetic classification schemes (Friedman & Weinstein, 2002). The role of the primary care provider is crucial to facilitate proper referrals and effective interdisciplinary communication and to assist the family in their coping and adaptation processes.

Long-term sequelae of cancer therapy for ALL have been identified in research studies and include effects on cognition and neuropsychologic functioning. Central nervous system irradiation has been linked to learning disabilities and impaired IQ, especially in children younger than 5 years who also received intrathecal therapy. As a result, cranial radiation dosages have been reduced and earlier neuropsychologic testing is recommended. Other documented potential late effects of treatment include the following:

- Short stature, muscle wasting, and avascular necrosis of the bone caused by high-dose steroid therapy—more pronounced in young children.
- Obesity and gonadal dysfunction resulting from a neuroendocrine effect.

- Potential alterations in pubertal development and gonadal function if given high-dose alkylating agents, especially if given in puberty and to girls.
- Cardiomyopathy if given anthracyclines. Children given these drugs are at risk for this problem. They need to be educated just before their teen years about avoiding alcohol, which increases the likelihood of cardiotoxicity, and cautioned about cigarette smoking.
- Malignant glioma associated with cranial irradiation.
- Second leukemias (usually AML) again associated with therapy with alkylating agents.
- Infertility with alkylator therapy.
- Cystitis or bladder dysfunction with cyclophosphamide.
- Delayed recovery of normal immune function (may need readministration of immunization).
- Psychosocial effects associated with chronic illness.
- Relapse of ALL.
- Possibility of hepatitis C virus infection if the child had a blood transfusion before 1992.

Risk-directed treatment based on high-risk features at diagnosis, response to chemotherapy, and transplantation options has drastically improved cure rates in the past two decades. It is hoped that the incidence and severity of late-term effects will likewise diminish (Wolfe & Marson, 2002).

Lymphomas

Non-Hodgkin's Lymphoma

Description. The non-Hodgkin's lymphomas (NHLs) are a diverse group of solid tumors of the lymphatic tissues that form from malignant profileration of T cells, B cells, or indeterminate lymphocyte cells. Different classification systems have been used. In pediatrics, the common types of NHL are small noncleaved cell lymphoma (Burkitt's and non-Burkitt's subtypes, B-cell origin), lymphoblastic lymphoma, and large cell lymphoma (Gilchrist, 2004).

Incidence. The incidence rate in children younger than 20 years of age is 10.5 per 1 million white children compared with 7.3 per 1 million black children (Gilchrist, 2004). In children, the incidence of NHL peaks at 5 to 7 years of age and again at 12 to 14 years of age (Wollner & Finlay, 2002).

Clinical Findings. The most common site of origin is in the lymphoid structures of the intestinal tract. The most common manifestations in children are (1) acute abdomen, including abdominal pain, distention, fullness, and constipation, and (2) nontender lymph node enlargement.

DIAGNOSTIC TESTS. Diagnostic studies are ordered depending on the location of the lymphoma and symptoms. They include computed tomography (CT) of the area in question, gallium scan, bone marrow aspirates and biopsies, lumbar puncture with central nervous system fluid analysis, CBC, lactate dehydrogenase and electrolyte levels, and 8-hour creatinine clearance if indicated (Wollner & Finlay, 2002).

Management. The diagnosis is confirmed by surgical biopsy, and the extent of the disease process can be determined by scans, bone marrow aspiration, and lumbar puncture. Because of rapid developments in treatment and the importance of careful histologic evaluation, these children should be referred to a major pediatric cancer center for care.

Lymphomas are sensitive to chemotherapy. Cranial irradiation or intrathecal chemotherapy is part of the treatment plan if central nervous system involvement is present. Maintenance therapy may be continued for 6 months to 2 years. The prognosis has improved dramatically over the past few years. For early-stage disease in which the disease is localized, 90% of patients can expect long-term disease-free survival. Patients with more extensive disease may have a 70% to 80% failure-free survival rate (Albano et al, 2003).

Hodgkin's Disease

Description. Like the NHLs, Hodgkin's disease is a malignancy of the lymph nodes. It usually originates in a cervical lymph node and spreads to other lymph node regions and, if left untreated, to organ systems, including liver, spleen, bone, bone marrow, and brain. Unlike in NHL, involvement of the bone marrow and central nervous system is rare (Gilchrist, 2004). Clinical and pathologic staging of the disease is usually done by specialists according to what is known as the Ann Arbor staging criteria.

Incidence. Hodgkin's disease represents 50% of the lymphomas of childhood. It is rare in children younger than 5 years. Sixty percent of children with Hodgkin's disease are between 10 and 16 years old (Albano et al, 2003).

Clinical Findings. The most common manifestations of Hodgkin's disease include the following:

- Painless enlargement of the lymph nodes, usually in the cervical area; the nodes may feel firm, are often matted together, and are nontender to palpation.
- Chronic cough if the trachea is compressed by a large mediastinal mass.
- Fever, decreased appetite, weight loss, and night sweats.

DIAGNOSTIC TESTS. Hematologic findings are often normal but may include the following:

- Anemia
- Elevated or depressed leukocytes or platelets

RESOURCE BOX

Hematologic Disorders

Cooley's Anemia Foundation
129-09 26th Avenue, #203
Flushing, NY 11354
1-718-321-CURE (2873)
1-800-522-7222
www.cooleysanemia.org

Leukemia and Lymphoma Society
1311 Mamaroneck Ave.
White Plains, NY 10605
1-914-949-5213
www.leukemia.org

National Hemophilia Foundation
116 West 32nd Street, 11th Floor
New York, NY 10001
1-212-328-3700
www.hemophilia.org

Sickle Cell Disease Association of America, Inc.
200 Corporate Pointe, Suite 495
Culver City, CA 90230-8727
1-800-421-8453
www.sicklecelldisease.org

- Elevated sedimentation rate and serum copper level
- Abnormal liver function test results

Management. The diagnosis is confirmed by histologic examination of an excised lymph node, followed by bone marrow studies and gallium scans to determine the extent of the disease. The child should receive treatment at a pediatric oncology center in collaboration with the primary provider. Optimum results are obtained through irradiation and chemotherapy with numerous agents. Children with Hodgkin's disease have a better response to treatment than do adults, with a 75% overall survival rate at more than 20 years follow-up (Albano et al, 2003).

REFERENCES

Albano E et al: Neoplastic disease. In Hay W et al, editors: *Current pediatric diagnosis and treatment*, ed 16, New York, 2003, Lange Medical Books/McGraw-Hill.

Altman A: Hemolytic anemias. In Burg F et al, editors: *Gellis and Kagan's current pediatric therapy*, ed 17, Philadelphia, 2002, WB Saunders.

American Academy of Pediatrics, Committee on Genetics: Health supervision for children with sickle cell disease, *Pediatrics* 109:526-535, 2002.

American Academy of Pediatrics, Committee on Practice and Ambulatory Medicine: Recommendations for preventative pediatric health care, *Pediatrics* 105:645, 2000.

Bullock B, Henze R: Hematology: adaptations and alterations in function. In Bullock B, editor: *Focus on pathophysiology*, Philadelphia, 2000, Lippincott Williams & Wilkins.

Carroll B: Sickle cell disease. In Jackson P, Vessey J, editors: *Primary care of the child with a chronic condition*, ed 3, St Louis, 2000, Mosby.

Friedman A, Weinstein H: Acute leukemia. In Burg F et al, editors: *Gellis and Kagan's current pediatric therapy*, ed 17, Philadelphia, 2002, WB Saunders.

Gilchrist GS: Lymphoma. In Behrman R, Kliegman R, Jenson H, editors: *Nelson textbook of pediatrics*, ed 16, Philadelphia, 2004, WB Saunders.

Glader B: Anemias of inadequate production. In Behrman R, Kliegman R, Jenson H, editors: *Nelson textbook of pediatrics*, ed 17, Philadelphia, 2004, WB Saunders.

Guyton A, Hall J: *Textbook of medical physiology*, ed 10, Philadelphia, 2001, WB Saunders.

Hagani A, Bussel J: Platelet disorders (thrombocytopenia and thrombocytopathy). In Finberg L, Kleinman R, editors: *Saunders manual of pediatric practice*, ed 2, Philadelphia, 2002a, WB Saunders.

Hagani A, Bussel J: Hemophilia. In Finberg L, Kleinman R, editors: *Saunders manual of pediatric practice*, ed 2, Philadelphia, 2002b, WB Saunders.

Kaufman M, Rao S: Disseminated intravascular coagulation. In Finberg L, Kleinman R, editors: *Saunders manual of pediatric practice*, ed 2, Philadelphia, 2002a, WB Saunders.

Kaufman M, Rao S: von Willebrand disease. In Finberg L, Kleinman R, editors: *Saunders manual of pediatric practice*, ed 2, Philadelphia, 2002b, WB Saunders.

Lane P, Nuss R, Ambruso D: Hematologic disorders. In Hay W et al, editors: *Current pediatric diagnosis and treatment*, ed 15, New York, 2003, McGraw-Hill.

Neufeld E: Disorders of platelet number and function. In Burg F et al, editors: *Gellis and Kagan's current pediatric therapy*, ed 17, Philadelphia, 2002, WB Saunders.

Platt O: Hematologic problems. In Dershewitz RA, editor: *Ambulatory pediatric care,* ed 3, Philadelphia, 1999, Lippincott-Raven.

Quirolo K, Vichinsky E: Hemoglobin disorders. In Behrman R, Kliegman R, Jenson H, editors: *Nelson textbook of pediatrics,* ed 17, Philadelphia, 2004, WB Saunders.

Recht M, Pearson H: Nutritional anemias. In McMillan J et al, editors: *Oski's pediatrics: principles and practice,* ed 3, Philadelphia, 1999, Lippincott Williams & Wilkins.

Scott J: Hematology. In Behrman R, Kliegman R, editors: *Nelson essentials of pediatrics,* ed 4, Philadelphia, 2002, WB Saunders.

Segel G: Hereditary spherocytosis. In Behrman R, Kliegman R, Jenson H, editors: *Nelson textbook of pediatrics,* ed 16, Philadelphia, 2004, WB Saunders.

Segel G, Hirsh M, Feig S: Managing anemia in a pediatric office practice: part 1, *Pediatr Rev* 23:75-83, 2002a.

Segel G, Hirsh M, Feig S: Managing anemia in a pediatric office practice: part 2, *Pediatr Rev* 23:111-121, 2002b.

Tender J, Cheng T: Iron deficiency anemia. In Burg F et al, editors: *Gellis and Kagan's current pediatric therapy,* ed 17, Philadelphia, 2002, WB Saunders.

Tubergen DG, Bleyer A: The leukemias. In Behrman R, Kliegman R, Jenson H, editors: *Nelson textbook of pediatrics,* ed 17, Philadelphia, 2004, WB Saunders.

Wolfe L, Marson K: The child cured of cancer. In Burg F et al, editors: *Gellis and Kagan's current pediatric therapy,* ed 17, Philadelphia, 2002, WB Saunders.

Wollner N, Finlay J: Non-Hodgkin lymphoma. In Finberg L, Kleinman R, editors: *Saunders manual of pediatric practice,* ed 2, Philadelphia, 2002, WB Saunders.

Wu A, Lesperance L, Bernstein H: Screening for iron deficiency, *Pediatr Rev* 23:171-177, 2002.

Yang Y: Neutropenia and lymphopenia. In Burg F et al, editors: *Gellis and Kagan's current pediatric therapy,* ed 17, Philadelphia, 2002, WB Saunders.

28 Neurologic Disorders

Catherine G. Blosser, Catherine E. Burns

Neurologic disorders in children are difficult for primary care providers to assess and manage. Central nervous system (CNS) problems can affect many systems, be manifested in many ways, and have profound effects on the lives of children and their families. No other body system has as much influence on development. The problems may be subtle or overwhelming. The nurse practitioner's (NP's) work is important: screening and identifying neurologic problems, referring to the appropriate health care resources, monitoring general health, serving as a case manager and patient advocate as school and long-term care issues arise, and supporting families as they deal with grief and caregiving issues.

ANATOMY AND PHYSIOLOGY

Anatomy

Any NP interested in the functional neurologic capabilities of patients is well served by understanding neurologic anatomy and physiology. The nervous system is divided into two parts: the CNS and the peripheral nervous system (PNS). The CNS consists of the brain and spinal cord. The PNS is made up of a network of afferent nerves and sense organs, which send information to the brain, and the efferent nerves, which send information out to the body for responses. Descending tracts from the brain to the gray matter of the spinal cord include the extrapyramidal tract, which conveys information from the cerebellum to the motor cells of the anterior column, and the pyramidal tract, which is the main motor pathway from the cerebral cortex to the spinal nerves and carries messages for voluntary movement. Most pyramidal tract fibers cross in the medulla, so the left half of the brain controls the right side of the body and vice versa. The anatomic units of the brain and their functions are listed in Table 28-1 and shown in Figs. 28-1 and 28-2.

Autonomic Nervous System

The autonomic nervous system (ANS) also involves CNS and PNS components. However, the sensory neurons and the efferent fibers that supply the organs, smooth muscles, and glands are sufficiently different to merit a separate classification. The ANS consists of the parasympathetic and sympathetic systems. The sympathetic system begins in the thoracolumbar area of the spinal cord and extends distally, whereas the parasympathetic system begins in the medulla and midbrain with relays to the thalamus and higher centers. The principal sympathetic system neurotransmitters are epinephrine and norepinephrine. The parasympathetic fibers produce acetylcholine. The two systems function in balance: one excites whereas the other inhibits (Box 28-1).

Physiology

Nerve impulses are transmitted along a nerve fiber through changes in polarization of the membrane, during which electrical activity is produced. Certain chemicals diffuse across the synapses between nerves and end organs. The primary transmitter is acetylcholine; however, other transmitters, including norepinephrine and dopamine, are also important.

PATHOPHYSIOLOGY AND DEFENSE MECHANISMS

Pathophysiology

The nervous system is so intimately related to functioning of the entire body that problems in any system can have neurologic implications. For example, seizures result from uncontrolled firing of cerebral neurons. Coma results from the inability of cerebral neurons to fire or the inability of the CNS to process stimuli and

TABLE 28-1 ***Anatomic Units of the Nervous System and Functions***

Anatomic Unit	Functions
I. Central nervous system	
A. Brain	
1. Forebrain—cerebrum	
a. Cortex (gray matter)	Posterior—motor skills
1) Frontal area	Anterior—decision making, emotions, memory, judgment, ethics, abstract thinking Broca's area—speech
2) Parietal area	Sensory integration, language, reading, writing, pattern recognition
3) Temporal area	Memory storage, auditory processing, olfaction, limbic system in deep temporal lobe—arousal
4) Occipital area	Visual processing
b. Diencephalon	
1) Thalamus	Receives and sorts sensory input, modulates motor impulses from cortex
2) Hypothalamus	Integrates autonomic functions
2. Midbrain	Connects brain with cerebellum, pons, medulla
3. Hindbrain	
a. Pons	Bridges cerebellum, medulla, midbrain; cranial nerves V, VI, VIII arise here
b. Medulla	Proximal end of spinal cord; contains reticular system—arousal; cranial nerves IX-XII arise here
c. Cerebellum	Coordination and movement; balance; smooth movements
B. Cranial nerves	Sensory and motor components; olfaction; vision; hearing; facial, tongue, pharyngeal, eye, shoulder movements
II. Spinal cord	
A. Dorsal roots	Afferent sensory fibers
B. Ventral roots	Efferent motor fibers
III. Protective layers	
A. Meninges	Protection of delicate nervous tissues
B. Ventricles	
C. Cerebrospinal fluid	

respond accordingly. Paralysis occurs when the peripheral nerves are unable to respond or do not receive signals through the pyramidal system of afferent and efferent nerves. Of course, more specific problems occur when special areas of the nervous system or individual nerves are damaged. Broad incapacity occurs with neurotransmitter problems.

Systemic Problems

The brain is extremely sensitive to changes in physiology anywhere in the body. Thus any metabolic change, whether from external or internal factors, affects the CNS. Examples include delirium from toxins and diabetic coma.

Genetic Problems

All chromosomal defects are associated with some neurologic effects because they are disorders involving many genes. Some of the single-gene defects may have direct neurologic effects (such as neurofibromatosis), whereas others, typically inborn errors of metabolism, can have indirect effects via the abnormal metabolites released (e.g., phenylketonuria).

Congenital Defects

Because the CNS is structurally complex, there are many opportunities for defects to occur during fetal development. Hydrocephaly, spina bifida, and other problems can result.

Injuries

Head and spinal cord injuries are common and can have long-term serious consequences for the child, especially because such complex neurologic tissue has relatively little ability to heal.

Defense Mechanisms

Peripheral nerves can regenerate somewhat if conditions are right. In the spinal cord, the axons of injured neurons cannot regrow within the cord, but they can grow in

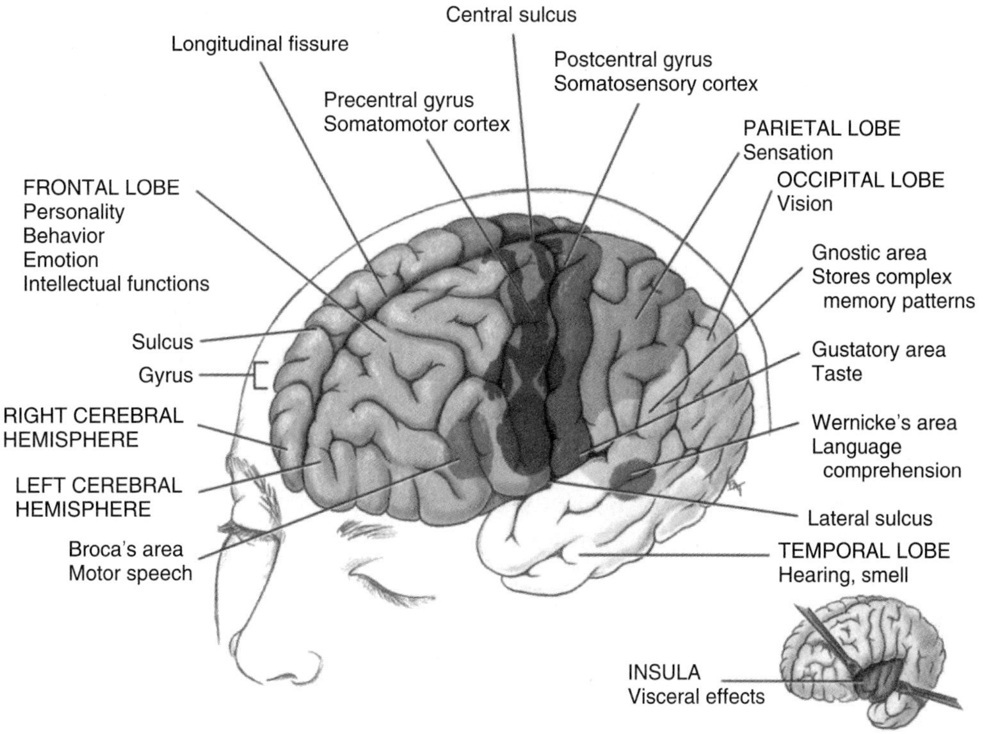

FIGURE 28-1 Lobes and functional areas of the cerebrum. (From Polaski AL: *Luckmann's core principles and practice of medical-surgical nursing*, Philadelphia, 1996, WB Saunders, p 245.)

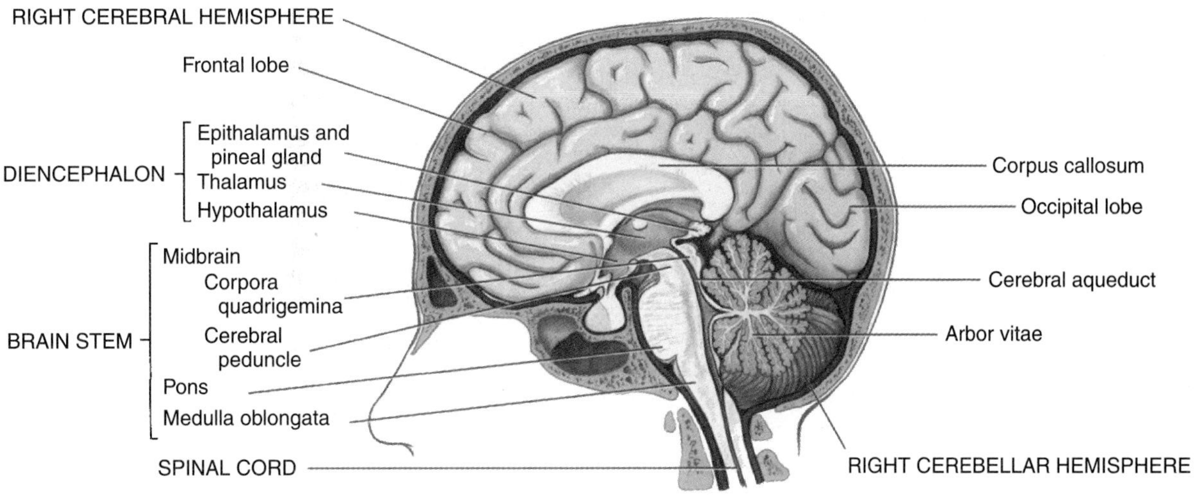

FIGURE 28-2 Midsagittal section of the brain showing the major portions of the diencephalons, brainstem, and cerebellum. (From Polaski AL: *Luckmann's core principles and practice of medical-surgical nursing*, Philadelphia, 1996, WB Saunders, p 245.)

BOX 28-1 *Autonomic Nervous System: Parasympathetic and Sympathetic Functions*

Parasympathetic System

Pupil constriction
Increased saliva
Lacrimal gland vasodilation
Coronary vessel vasoconstriction
Bronchial muscle constriction
Stomach peristalsis
Colon peristalsis
Genitalia vasodilation
Urinary bladder constriction
Skin vessel dilation

Sympathetic System

Pupil dilation
Decreased saliva
Coronary vessel vasodilation
Bronchial muscle relaxation
Stomach constriction
Adrenaline secretion
Colon relaxation
Sphincter relaxation
Sphincter constriction
Genitalia vasoconstriction
Urinary bladder relaxation
Skin vessel constriction

Data from Anderson P: *Basic human anatomy and physiology*, Monterey, CA, 1984, Wadsworth.

peripheral nerves outside the cord. In this case, if the cut ends are reconnected with special attention to the myelin sheath, regeneration of the injured nerve begins at the proximal end of the neuron soon after injury. The growth rate is approximately 2.5 to 3.0 mm per day (Menkes & Sarnat, 2000).

ASSESSMENT OF THE NERVOUS SYSTEM

Assessment of the nervous system requires a careful history and detailed physical examination. The examiner needs to determine (1) if a neurologic disorder exists, (2) where the disorder is located, and (3) the process that most likely produces the symptoms and affects the suspected location of the dysfunction (Menkes & Sarnat, 2000). For children with complex or severe neurologic problems, social, environmental, developmental, and family issues need thorough exploration. Historical information from patients over 3 years of age and from one or more family members is most likely to provide the most accurate picture of the issues. Imaging or laboratory studies may be required. See Chapter 2 for information regarding disease assessment, daily living, and developmental history.

History

Neurologic Disease History

- History of present illness:
  - Onset. When did the first symptoms appear? Was the onset insidious or sudden? Was it associated with any injury or strain? If yes, describe the trauma. Was the onset accompanied by any constitutional symptoms? How has the disorder evolved?
  - Pain and headache. Location and character, path of radiation, severity, extent of disability produced, effect of various activities or stimuli (including light sensitivity), relief measures, changes from day to night, effects of previous treatment, presence of pain or discomfort in other parts of the body.
  - Sensory deficits. Changes in hearing, vision, taste, loss of pain sensation, vertigo, dizziness.
  - Injury. How, when (time and date), why, where, mechanism or manner in which the injury was produced. Immediate treatment provided.
  - Reflexive responses. Vomiting, coughing, primitive reflexes, tics.
  - Behavioral changes. Irritability, stupor, changes in appetite, lack of attention, random activity, emotional lability, changes in school performance.
  - Motor and balance changes. Ataxia, spasticity, increased or decreased tone.
- Medical history:
  - Prenatal history: Maternal and paternal ages, alcohol, drug ingestion, radiation exposure, nutrition, prenatal care, injuries, hyperthermia, smoking, human immunodeficiency virus (HIV) exposure, maternal illness, bleeding, toxemia, diabetes, previous abortions and stillbirths.
  - Birth history and neonatal course: Complications, labor and delivery, resuscitation, trauma, congenital anomalies, feeding history (reflux, colic, frequent formula changes), jaundice, convulsions, infection, gestational age, sleeping habits.
  - Injuries or infections. Meningitis, encephalitis, head injuries, seizures—types, frequency, medications; frequent musculoskeletal injuries (can suggest coordination or impulsive behavior).
  - Cardiovascular or respiratory disorders.

- Environmental or drug exposure. Consider lead exposure.
- Metabolic disorders. Diabetes mellitus, thyroid disease. Hypoglycemia causes confusion, convulsion, loss of consciousness. Hyperglycemia causes lethargy, coma. Hyperthyroidism causes tremor. Hypothyroidism causes weakness, coma.
- Past neurologic disease and tests. Tics, hydrocephaly.
- Psychiatric disorders. Hallucinations.
- Drug ingestion.
- Urinary tract disease. Uremic syndrome manifests with confusion, convulsions, coma.
- Physical growth.

- Family disease history:
  - Family members with similar symptoms or genetic disorders.
  - Consanguinity.
  - Migraine history.
  - Mental functioning of family members.
- Review of systems:
  - Growth pattern, including height, weight, body mass index (BMI), and head circumference.
  - Review *all* systems. Allergies, medications, immunizations, hearing, vision, dental, skin integrity, behavior, nutritional status, and eating disorders are all important areas to assess.

Developmental History

Achievement of all developmental milestones—language, gross motor, fine motor, social, and cognitive—and school performance should be reviewed. Inquire about developmental changes, loss of skills, and lack of progression.

Functional Health

Inquire about the effects of symptoms on all areas of health promotion and safety, nutrition, elimination, activity, communication, role relationships, values and beliefs, sexuality, sleep, coping (management style) and stress tolerance, temperament, and self-concept. The "management style" of family members is crucial for the NP to assess, because it suggests how different family members may react over time to any chronic illness of their child (Jackson Allen & Vessey, 2004). Management styles and "chronic sorrow" are discussed more fully in Chapter 11.

Social Context

Because neurologic problems can have such profound, chronic consequences on the child and family, it is important to understand the social context of the child and family. Learn about the family composition, home environment, stressors, strengths, resources, financial issues, identified social supports (e.g., family, friends, health professionals), and community agencies involved with the family and child (Menkes & Sarnat, 2000). Race and ethnicity need to be explored since they can influence family perceptions and attitudes towards social support networks (Jackson Allen & Vessey, 2004).

Physical Examination

A complete physical examination is always important. The following should be noted:

- Abnormalities of the skin (café au lait lesions, angiomas, other pigmentation changes)
- Anomalies
- Low-set ears
- Cardiovascular system (including blood pressure)
- Musculoskeletal system
- Hearing
- Vision; eye problems, including cataract, corneal clouding, cherry-red spot
- Head circumference, growth measurements
- Tanner stage
- Hepatomegaly

Neurologic Examination

The provider conducting the neurologic examination moves from the highest level of functioning to the lowest. Cerebral function is tested first; then cranial nerves, motor function, and sensory function; and finally reflexes. In infants and children, watching them carefully while collecting the history and actively playing with them provides a great deal of neurologic information. Useful tools include a tennis ball, some small toys (especially a small car), a bell, and something that attracts attention (e.g., pinwheel) (Menkes & Sarnat, 2000).

Behavior and Mental Status. Test the following cortical functions through evaluation of behavior and mental status:

- Responsiveness
- Judgment
- Language and speech (receptive, expressive, written)
- Memory
- General knowledge
- Ability to relate to others
- Mood and affect

The level of consciousness is also a CNS function and includes speech flow, voice quality, and organization of thoughts.

Cranial Nerves. Cranial nerves I through XII are tested.

Motor Examination. When conducting the motor examination, look for symmetry and quality of movement.

Gait, posture, coordination, balance, strength, and tone are all aspects of this examination.

- Muscle strength and size. Look at muscle size and contour. Look for symmetry. Have the child stand from a lying position. Look for Gowers' sign (i.e., a child using the arms to push off from bent knees and gradually climbing the body and straightening up, which is common in children with muscular dystrophy). Ask the child to move extremities against resistance and to grip your fingers hard.
- Muscle tone. Muscle tone might be considered the resting strength of the muscle. Is the trunk or are the extremities floppy, rigid, or somewhat stiff when the child is resting? How difficult is it to move body parts passively? Tone may be increased or decreased all over or differ between the legs and the trunk and arms.
- Fine motor coordination. Fine motor coordination is tested by having the child pick up small pellets, write, stack blocks, cut with scissors, turn book pages, or do other hand activities.
- Involuntary movements. Tremors are fine involuntary movements. Chorea or choreiform movements are large, irregular jerking and writhing movements. Athetoid movements are slow writhing movements, especially of the hands and feet. Dystonia is an uncontrolled change in tone with movement and a tendency to hyperextend the joints.
- The reflexes involve a combination of motor functioning and transmission of nerve impulses from various parts of the body to the spine and brain and back again. When a reflex is abnormal, the question is why. Did the impulse not go through, or did the child have a problem in the ability to move responsively because of either efferent signals or problems of muscle tissue contractility? The reflexes and their testing are described later.

Sensory Examination. Examine for pain sensation and stereognosis. This part of the examination is always limited in infants and young children. Use a light pinprick to check for mild pain sensation.

Reflexes. The types of reflexes tested include deep tendon, superficial, and primitive reflexes.

- Deep tendon reflexes include the biceps, brachioradialis, triceps, patellar, and Achilles.
- Superficial reflexes include the upper abdominal, lower abdominal, cremasteric, gluteal, and plantar.
- Primitive reflexes include sucking, rooting, asymmetric tonic neck, grasp, trunk incurvation, stepping, and others found in Table 28-2.

Cranium Examination. The neurologic examination should always include measurement of head circumference and inspection of the skull for symmetry and shape. Auscultation over the skull or above the eyes can reveal a cranial bruit. Percussion of the skull can give a sound resembling a cracked pot when the sutures are separated, as with increased intracranial pressure. The skull of the infant can be transilluminated to look for the absence of cortical tissue with a flashlight outfitted with a rubber adaptor. The anterior fontanel should normally be slightly depressed with very faintly perceived pulsations.

Autonomic Nervous System. Alterations in blood pressure, sweating, or body temperature can be indicators of ANS problems.

Meningeal Signs. Signs of meningeal irritation such as with meningitis include Kernig and Brudzinski signs. Kernig sign is resistance and pain elicited on extension of the leg at the knee with the patient in the supine position and the hips flexed perpendicular to the trunk. Brudzinski sign consists of spontaneous flexion of the knee and hip provoked by passive flexion of the neck.

Neurologic Examination of the Infant. The neonate's neurologic functioning is largely subcortical. Therefore the examination is more limited than in an older infant or child. The cranium can be measured and transilluminated to look for structural or brain development problems. Assessing posture and muscle tone is fundamental. The primitive reflexes are all tested, although they can be absent or decreased in a satiated or sleepy infant. Tendon reflexes can be tested as in an older child. Babinski sign is not helpful in an infant. In older children and adults, its presence is an important sign of upper motor neuron disease.

Motor testing should include observation for symmetry of movements, consistent fisting of the hands, opisthotonos, scissoring, abnormal tone, and tremors. The infant's cry can be an indicator of several diseases; for example, it is high pitched with increased intracranial pressure, resembles mewing in cri du chat syndrome, and is hoarse with hypothyroidism.

Cranial nerves can be tested. Vision (cranial nerve II) is indicated by blinking in response to a bright light. Cranial nerves III, IV, and VI can be tested by assessing the neonate's ability to track through the visual fields. Facial grimaces test for cranial nerves V and VII. Hearing (cranial nerve VIII) can be tested with a small bell. The gag reflex tests cranial nerves IX and X. The olfactory nerve (cranial nerve I) is not functional until 5 to 7 months of age, but inhaled irritants (e.g., ammonia, vinegar) will produce a reaction in cranial nerve V in newborns (Menkes & Sarnat, 2000).

Diagnostic Studies

Radiographs have relatively little diagnostic value for the neurologic system since the advent of computed tomography (CT) and magnetic resonance imaging (MRI). CT

TABLE 28-2 *Primitive Reflexes*

Reflex	Age Appears	Age Disappears	How to Elicit	Response	Notes
Newborn Reflexes					
Rooting	Birth	3-4 mo	Head midline, stroke perioral area	Infant opens mouth and turns head to stimulated side	Absence indicates severe CNS disease or depressed infant; sleeping infant may not respond
Sucking	Birth	3-4 mo	Place nipple or finger 3-4 cm into mouth	Suck should be strong: push finger up and back; note rate	Absence indicates CNS depression; satiated or sleeping baby may not respond well
Asymmetric tonic neck (ATNR)	Birth	4-6 mo	With baby supine, rotate head to one side; hold 15 sec	Arm and leg extend on facial side; arm and leg on other side flex	Obligatory response when child cannot get out of position is abnormal; persistence beyond 4-6 mo indicates CNS lesion (e.g., CP)
Palmar grasp	Birth	3-6 mo	Place finger into infant's palm and press against palm	Infant flexes all fingers around examiner's finger	Grasp should be strong and symmetric
Trunk incurvation (Galant)	Birth	2 mo	Suspend baby prone; stroke 2-3 cm from spine with fingernail	Baby flexes toward stimulus	Asymmetry is significant; tests for spinal cord lesions; should not persist after 6 mo
Stepping	Birth	6-8 wk	Infant is held as though weight bearing with feet on surface	Infant steps along, raising one foot at a time	Tests brainstem, spinal column; absence indicates paralysis or depressed baby
Moro	Birth	4 mo	Present loud noise or allow infant's head to drop slightly	Arms spread and fingers extend and then flex; then arms come toward each other; cry is possible	Asymmetry indicates paralysis or fractured clavicle, absence indicates brainstem problem, usually severe; persistence also abnormal
Crossed extension	0-4 mo		Passively extend one leg and press knee to table; prick sole of that foot with pin	Other leg should slightly extend and adduct	
Plantar grasp	Birth	8-10 mo	Place finger firmly against base of toes	Toes should curl down	Tests S1-S2 spinal nerves; lessens by 8 mo, suspect asymmetry
Later Reflexes					
Landau	3 mo	15 mo-2 yr	Suspend infant prone by supporting abdomen	Infant should lift both head and legs	Abnormal if arm tone increased with internal rotation, arm held at side, or arm does not lift as noted
Neck righting	6 mo	2 yr	With infant supine, turn head to one side	Infant's trunk rotates in direction of head	Absent or decreased can indicate spasticity; can also rotate trunk and then look for head to follow; tests midbrain
Parachute	6-8 mo	Never	Suspend infant prone and lower quickly toward table	Infant should extend arms, hands, fingers	Response should be symmetric as well as "protective"

CNS, Central nervous system; *CP*, cerebral palsy.

scans display differences in density of the intracranial tissues and structures. An MRI can provide additional information related to aneurysms (e.g., hemorrhages, calcifications, abscesses), brain structure, and the cellular activity of various parts of the neurologic system (e.g., tumors, CNS, and spinal cord and malformations).

- Laboratory studies can provide indicators of systemic disease, infection, or inflammation. Laboratory studies are especially important for children receiving medication for seizures. Drug levels, liver function, and blood studies may be monitored routinely.
- Lumbar puncture provides a specimen of cerebrospinal fluid (CSF). The fluid provides information about metabolism, infections, and trauma within the CNS.
- The electroencephalogram (EEG) provides information about the electrical activity of the CNS, which is important in assessing the function, not the structure, of the system.
- Ultrasonography can be useful in infants to evaluate brain tissue.
- Other studies can include polysomnography (helps assess narcolepsy, apnea of infancy, certain movement disorders, and nocturnal seizures); electromyography (tests muscle activity); nerve conduction studies; evoked responses (brainstem-auditory, somatosensory, and visual); electronystagmography (measures eye movements to assess vertigo and postconcussion syndrome); and cerebral arteriography (visualizes cerebral blood vessels to evaluate vascular anomalies and tumors).

MANAGEMENT STRATEGIES

Counseling

Counseling for neurologic problems involves several components. The family should understand the pathology, including possible etiologies, and the treatment plan. Parents also need information about the prognosis with and without treatment, as well as any genetic implications of the diagnosis. The latter can best be communicated through formal genetics counseling. Family members should have time to ask questions about all these issues.

Counseling also involves helping families cope with the diagnosis and its implications for the patient and family, both short term and long term. Congenital problems are often identified at birth or shortly thereafter. Families need to receive diagnoses truthfully, humanely, and promptly. Issues of etiology need to be addressed to relieve the guilt that some parents feel about causing the problem. A plan of care needs to be mutually agreed on by the family and care provider before the infant or child is discharged from the hospital or clinic.

Using sensitive, acceptable terminology when discussing any physical limitation is crucial. The NP is encouraged to use the following terms appropriately (Miller & Bachrach, 1998). Correct language can influence not only how parents relate to their child's condition but also communicate to others a more accurate reflection of the child's abilities (e.g., schools, employers).

- *Impairment*: existence of a deviation from normal movement or an inability to control an involuntary movement (one can be impaired without being disabled)
- *Disability*: a restriction in an ability to execute a normal activity of daily living that someone of similar age could execute (all people with disabilities are impaired)
- *Handicap*: existence of a disability that prevents the person from achieving a normal role in society that someone of a similar age is expected to achieve (all people with handicaps have disabilities)

Anticipatory Guidance

Neurologic Development

Families are sometimes concerned about problems that providers believe are within normal limits. In these situations, no neurology referral is necessary. The family needs to understand the predicted neurologic development and be provided with time lines and markers that they can use to monitor their child's development. Misperceptions about the implications of minor variations need to be dealt with, and the family should always be given the opportunity to return for further assessment or discussion if concerns remain. The temperament of the child and the child's learned social behavior versus pathologic symptoms may need to be addressed (e.g., breath-holding vs. seizures).

Educational Needs

Many neurologic problems in children affect learning, although neurologic problems are not synonymous with mental retardation. Sensory problems affect the child's ability to receive the input necessary for learning. Motor problems can affect both the child's ability to interact with the environment and the child's ability to communicate or indicate understanding. Management should always consider the educational needs of the child. Special infant or preschool educational programs can assist the child to learn by using the most appropriate learning modalities. Teachers often need assistance in understanding the limitations and strengths of the child.

Genetics Counseling

Many neurologic conditions are genetic in origin. See Chapter 41 for a discussion of genetics assessment and management, including counseling.

Physical, Occupational, and Speech Therapy

Physical therapy can be useful to help restore or maintain function or to teach new motor skills. The physical therapist should be accustomed to dealing with children. Occupational and speech therapy may also be essential to promote maximal development. Early intervention programs offer such assistance in many states and are generally free to qualifying patients.

Social Services

Children with multiple handicapping conditions and their families frequently have ongoing issues of coping, as well as identification and management of medical and financial resources. Medical social workers can be a great help to these families.

Medications

A variety of medications are used to control the effects of neurologic problems. Most require time for the effects to become apparent, need dose adjustments, and are affected by the metabolism of the individual child. Thus blood levels are often needed. Side effects of medications need to be weighed against their beneficial effects. Many require tapering of dosages when treatment with the medication is to be discontinued. A variety of anticonvulsant medications are described in Table 28-5.

SPECIFIC NEUROLOGIC PROBLEMS OF CHILDREN

Degenerative Disorders

Degenerative disorders consist of a group of neurodegenerative disorders whose etiologies affect either the gray matter or white matter of the brain. The diagnosis is based on age of onset, clinical features, genetic transmission, and chemical and chromosomal studies. Gray matter diseases involve neurons, and their onset is heralded by seizures, decrease in cognitive functioning, and visual changes. White matter diseases usually lead to demyelination and are evidenced by decreasing motor skills, ataxia, and spasticity (Swaiman & Ashwal, 1999). Gray matter disorders include Menkes syndrome (also called kinky-hair syndrome), progressive infantile poliodystrophy, neuronal ceroid-lipofuscinoses, and Rett syndrome. White matter disorders include Schilder's disease, acute disseminating encephalomyelitis, acute hemorrhagic leukoencephalitis, and multiple sclerosis. Only Rett syndrome and multiple sclerosis are discussed in this chapter.

Degenerative disorders are believed to be the result of biochemical or metabolic dysfunctions (in turn caused by genetic, immune-mediated demyelination or by unknown causes) that lead to anatomic or functional insults to major portions of the brain. These insults usually affect the basal ganglia, cerebellum, brainstem, spinal cord, peripheral and cranial nerves, or cerebrum. Such insults can also follow infections or an altered immune state.

Rett Syndrome

A mutation in the X-linked, methyl-CpG-binding protein 2 gene (MECP2) has been identified in 80% of females with classic Rett syndrome features (Milunsky et al, 2001). This neurodevelopmental disorder was previously thought to affect only females and be lethal to males. However, there has been some recently reported variation to the X-linked Rett syndrome gene that occurs in males but is not lethal and results in mental retardation and neurologic impairment (Dotti et al, 2002). Defects in MECP2 have also been demonstrated in patients with autism, schizophrenia, learning disabilities, and neonatal encephalopathy (International Rett Syndrome Association, 2002). MECP2 is abundant in the brain. When not disabled by mutation, it silences certain genes that control motion and emotion.

Rather than cause brain degeneration, Rett syndrome arrests maturation of certain areas of the brain. Typically, the patient is female, with onset at 5 to 18 months. Affected girls cease to gain developmental milestones. CNS irritability and withdrawal develop, and then these girls begin to lose skills, including speech and hand skills. Stereotypic hand movements, slowed head growth leading to microcephaly, autistic-like behavior, dementia, and disorganized breathing and apnea followed by hyperpnea occur. Seizures, scoliosis, and spastic paraparesis and quadriparesis are late developments in the syndrome.

Physical therapy, occupational therapy, speech therapy, and seizure management are important to preserve functional abilities. As with all neurodevelopmental problems, families need significant support and social services. Life expectancy varies. Differential diagnoses include cerebral palsy, autism, psychosis, and other neurodegenerative diseases.

Multiple Sclerosis

There is a 3% to 5% incidence of multiple sclerosis (MS) in children under 6 years of age; 80% of cases occur between ages 10 and 15 years (juvenile-onset MS). Twice as many females than males are affected. The etiology is not clear, but proposals include environmental, infectious, toxic, immunologic, or genetic causes. No specific virus has been isolated. Nonviral organisms can cause demyelination and include *Campylobacter, Hartmanella*, mycobacterium, diphtheria, and tetanus toxins. High amounts of animal fat, protein, vitamin D, and meat have correlated as risk factors (Swaiman & Ashwal, 1999).

Repeated attacks of demyelination occur in the CNS, including the optic nerve. The initial symptoms include ataxia and fever followed by encephalopathy, hemiparesis, seizures, and optic neuritis. These episodes of focal neurologic dysfunction can last weeks or months and be followed by partial or complete recovery. Repeated episodes are frequently preceded by fever, nausea/vomiting, and lethargy and may occur within months or years of each other.

MS may be in a clinician's differential diagnosis during the initial episode of neurologic dysfunction, but the final diagnosis is usually not clear until after a second episode when a pattern of disability and recovery is established. Long-term outcome is not predictable.

The laboratory workup includes a lumbar puncture, an MRI, and visual-evoked responses. The MRI will show characteristic plaque formation and demyelination. Treatment involves exercises—resistance, aerobic, and stretching—and routines that promote agility and speed. The use of corticosteroids during exacerbations is traditional therapy (Fenichel, 2001). New research is underway to find drugs that will prevent and treat relapses, alter the progression of the disease, and be neuroprotective and restorative (Joy & Johnston, 2001).

Nondegenerative Disorders

Cerebral Palsy

Description. Cerebral palsy (CP) is a chronic, nonprogressive disorder that impairs control of movement by damaging motor areas in the brain. Symptoms appear within the first few years of life. Depending on the area affected and the extent of damage, children with CP can also have mental impairment (up to 66%); seizures (up to 50%); a lag in growth and development; neurosensory disorders affecting touch, pain, and continence; perceptual disorders; impaired vision and hearing; speech/swallowing/chewing difficulties; and other learning or emotional difficulties. It is important to note that the degree of disability can vary from person to person and that the degree of impairment is not necessarily profound (National Institute of Neurological Disorders and Stroke [NINDS], 2001).

Cerebral palsy is categorized by the type of movement: spastic, athetoid (or dyskinetic), ataxic, and mixed (usually involves a combination of spastic and athetoid). These types are further described by the body parts involved: diplegic, hemiplegic, or quadriplegic (sometimes called "tetraplegic") and by specific impairment to muscle movement or function (Table 28-3). Children may exhibit varying degrees of involvement and severity; capabilities may improve over time depending on the degree of involvement

TABLE 28-3 ***Terms Used to Describe Cerebral Palsy***

Movement Type	Description	Associated Impairments
Spastic	Inability of a muscle to relax	Often evident after 4-6 mo; retarded speech; convergent strabismus; toe-walking; flexed elbows
Athetoid	Inability to control muscle movement (continuous, writhing movements)	
Ataxic	Problems with balance and coordination	
Body Part Involved		
Diplegic	Affects both legs more than both arms	
Hemiplegic	Affects one side of the body (upper extremity is usually affected more than the lower extremity)	Often not detected at birth; right side often more affected than left; 50% develop seizures; growth arrest on affected limb(s)
Quadriplegic	Affects all four extremities	Affects upper extremities more than lower; 50% with grand mal seizures; IQ impairment can be severe
Specific Problems with Movement or Function		
Dystonia	Muscle tone problems	
Choreic	Disorganized tone	
Tremor	Involuntary, rhythmic movements of opposing muscles	
Ballismus	Violent, jerky movements	
Rigidity	Stiffness	

Adapted from Menkes J, Sarnat H: *Child neurology*, ed 6, Philadelphia, 2000, Lippincott Williams & Wilkins.

and treatment. The clinician is encouraged to maintain an approach that is optimistic yet realistic.

Etiology. The term *cerebral palsy* refers to chronic impairment of motor function as a result of some damage to or anomaly in the brain hemisphere(s). Once believed to be caused only by birth complications (neonatal or perinatal asphyxia or trauma), only 6% of CP cases are now believed to be caused by such occurrences (NINDS, 2001). Current research suggests additional possibilities. These include prenatal factors, prematurity or low birth weight, trauma to the brain, and congenital cerebral malformations. The condition is neither hereditary nor contagious. In approximately 25% to 50% of cases, the etiology cannot be determined (Berkowitz, 2000). Small for gestational age, low birth weight (less than 2500 g), preterm babies (less than 37 weeks of gestation), and multiple births are at greater risk for CP. Complicated labor and delivery, breech presentation, Apgar score of less than 3 at 10 minutes or more, traumatic delivery, microcephaly, maternal vaginal bleeding (between sixth and ninth months of pregnancy), severe proteinuria late in pregnancy, maternal hyperthyroidism/mental retardation/seizures, intracranial hemorrhage, toxemia, preeclampsia, antepartal hemorrhage, postmaturity, fetal distress, maternal stroke, coagulation in the fetus or newborn, and neonatal seizures are all considered risk factors (Menkes & Sarnat, 2000; NINDS, 2001). Other etiologies may include intrauterine drug exposure (e.g., alcohol, cocaine, tobacco, crack), intrauterine infections (e.g., cytomegalovirus, toxoplasmosis, rubella), and congenital brain malformations. In the United States it is estimated that children who acquire CP postnatally account for 10% to 20% of those with the disorder (NINDS, 2001). In such cases, the cause can be attributed to meningitis, encephalitis, head trauma (e.g., secondary to shaken baby syndrome or other abuse, car accidents, falls), and kernicterus (Berkowitz, 2000; Fenichel, 2001; Menkes & Sarnat, 2000).

Incidence. Approximately 500,000 Americans have CP (NINDS, 2001). The prevalence is 1 to 3 per 1000 live births across many studies. The incidence has not declined in many years and may be slowly increasing in the very low birth weight population because more of these babies are now surviving (Menkes & Sarnat, 2000). Children who are immobile, who are profoundly retarded, or who need special feeding have a decreased life expectancy. Otherwise, affected children are expected to reach adulthood (Fenichel, 2001).

Clinical Findings

History. The history that should be obtained from a patient with CP in terms of pathology, development, and functional health patterns follows.

PATHOLOGY

- Prenatal/natal history of risk factors as listed previously
- Seizures
- Hearing and vision or ocular problems such as strabismus, nystagmus, optic atrophy
- Growth parameters, especially decreased head circumference
- Early head injury or meningitis
- Muscle tone (can be hypotonic before 6 months, but then become hypertonic; unusual posture or favor one side)

Generalized, prolonged, and cramped synchronized movements in preterm infants were more often seen in those more likely to be diagnosed with CP (Ferrari et al, 2002).

DEVELOPMENT. Milestones may be delayed but should still be attained; persistent primitive reflexes are common (e.g., Moro and tonic neck). Hand preference before 1 year is highly suspect.

FUNCTIONAL HEALTH PATTERNS. Assess the following:

- Feeding history of regurgitating through the nose, inability to coordinate suck and swallow, inability to advance the diet to textured foods—in short, oral-motor coordination problems
- Irritability or depressed affect (including unusual sleepiness) as a neonate
- Difficulty with movement, cuddliness, grasp and release, self-feeding, and head control to look around; inability to change position per developmental level
- Persistent primitive reflexes
- Communication problems, either language or speech proficiency

Physical Examination

- Skin. Dermatologic signs of syndromes, such as neurofibromatosis, may be present.
- Orthopedic examination. Scoliosis, contractures, and dislocated hip may be present.
- Neurologic examination. The following may be seen on the neurologic examination:
  - Deep tendon reflexes are increased.
  - Tone is increased, although occasionally decreased; hypotonia before 6 months of age is common. Tone may also be mixed.
  - Minimal muscle atrophy.
  - No fasciculations.
  - Persistent primitive reflexes (e.g., tonic neck and Moro after 6 months).
  - Delayed reflexes (e.g., parachute reflex remains absent after 9 to 10 months; side-protective reflexes remain absent after 5 months).
  - Asymmetric movements.
  - Preferred handedness before 1 to 2 years of age.

  - Structural defects, such as hydrocephaly or microcephaly.
- Vision and hearing. Visual refractive errors occur in 50% of children, and strabismus is found in 33%. Hearing problems may have resulted from the initial brain insult.
- Development. Assessment of motor, fine motor, language, and personal social skills is needed. The Denver Developmental Screening Test II (Denver II) can be used for initial screening. Look also at the quality of movements (e.g., smoothness of gait, grasping, clarity of speech). In children with CP, motor milestones are commonly delayed.
- Feeding assessment. A patient with CP can have a reversed swallow wave; uncoordinated suck and swallow; decreased tone of the lips, tongue, and cheeks; increased gag reflex; involuntary tongue and lip movements; increased sensitivity to food stimuli; poor occlusion; and delayed inhibition of the suck reflex. Evaluate the diet, height, weight, and body mass index for adequate nutrition.

Diagnostic Studies

- Imaging studies. A CT scan can be obtained to identify brain malformations. Structures and abnormalities that are nearer to bony structures can be more clearly visualized with an MRI.
- Chromosomal and metabolic studies. These studies can be done to identify genetic disorders, especially single-gene defects.

Differential Diagnosis. The first and main requirement is to differentiate central from peripheral disorders. CP is always central and is characterized by brisk deep tendon reflexes. Many other conditions can have CP/motor involvement features. These conditions include intrauterine infections, fetal alcohol syndrome, hydrocephalus, tumors, agenesis of the corpus callosum or other brain malformations, Tay-Sachs disease, phenylketonuria, Lesch-Nyhan syndrome, spinal cord injury, hypothyroidism, muscle diseases, seizures, and many genetic and metabolic disorders. Also, mental retardation results in delayed milestones but should not include increased reflexes. Neuromuscular disorders are associated with signs of weakness, muscle atrophy, and decreased deep tendon reflexes. A condition that is characterized by the deterioration of once-acquired motor skills is not CP.

Management. The management of children with CP described here can serve as a model for the management of children with a variety of neurologic problems.

Referral of Suspected Cases. Children with CP should be evaluated and cared for at centers that provide interdisciplinary caregivers, including developmental pediatricians, orthopedists, neurologists, nurses, speech pathologists, physical and occupational therapists, education consultants and psychologists, and social workers. The care of children with CP may also involve an ophthalmologist, feeding clinic and nutritionist services, and genetics counseling.

Family Education about the Diagnosis. Families need to understand the diagnosis and its nonprogressive but incurable characteristics. They need to understand that the extent of brain damage is not always related to the extent of disability. Thus no one can predict what the future for a given child will be. It is known that children who receive special services, such as physical therapy, speech therapy, and other interventions, have better outcomes than do children who are left to develop on their own. United Cerebral Palsy has educational materials and a variety of services available for affected children and their families (see Resource Box).

Family Support. Generally, families grieve when given the diagnosis of CP and need support during this time. Support groups or opportunities to meet other families with affected children are often helpful. The emotional needs of siblings must not be overlooked either. The social worker can be very helpful to families trying to cope with complex health problems.

CP services are long term and expensive. Many children will be eligible for Supplemental Security Income or state program benefits for the severely handicapped. Respite care can be a benefit that is available to families. The Individuals with Disabilities Education Act of 1997 (IDEA) requires children with disabilities to be assessed for and instructed in the use of assistance devices. Again, social workers can be very helpful in connecting families to appropriate services; NPs can play an important role in the multidisciplinary team involved with ensuring that services are received.

Nutrition. Children with CP often have inadequate nutrition because of their problems with biting, sucking, chewing, swallowing, and self-feeding. Additionally, children with athetosis may need as much as 50% to 100% more calories to support their increased caloric needs because of their constant writhing movements. Children with spasticity, on the other hand, may need fewer calories because of their decreased movements. Occasionally, the problems are so severe that a gastrostomy is needed, sometimes with fundoplication to prevent reflux and aspiration. Special positioning, feeding therapy by a speech pathologist, and special feeding devices can help. High nutrient density is a key to providing a nutritious diet (i.e., getting more nutrients into the same volume of food). Feeding clinics are often helpful to plan management of nutrition.

Elimination. Constipation is common because of lack of exercise, inadequate fluid and fiber intake, medications, poor positioning, low abdominal muscle tone, and other factors. Stool softeners such as docusate sodium may help. Laxatives such as senna concentrate (Senokot) or milk of magnesia may be useful.

Bladder control and urinary retention are also problems for children with CP. Most achieve bladder control between 3 and 10 years of age. Mental retardation makes toilet training difficult for some. Children with CP are three times more likely to suffer urinary tract infections (Jackson Allen & Vessey, 2004).

Dentistry. Orofacial muscle tone can contribute to malocclusion, and problems with oral mobility make daily dental hygiene difficult. These children have more gum disease (often secondary to the use of antiepileptic drugs) and caries (Hoekelman, 2001; Jackson Allen & Vessey, 2004). A careful dental care program is necessary.

Drooling. Inability to manage oral secretions results in drooling. Social isolation, wet clothing, skin excoriation, malodorous breath, discomfort, choking, gagging, and aspiration can make these oral secretions a serious problem. Glycopyrrolate, 0.05 to 1.0 mg by mouth, twice or three times daily, may help, but side effects may also be problematic (e.g., constipation, difficulty urinating, restlessness). Surgical intervention is a last resort and commonly involves removing the submandibular gland or nerves, or cutting/rerouting the salivary duct. Newer studies are proving the efficacy of botulinum toxin A (Botox) injections (Suskind & Tilton, 2002).

Pulmonary. Positioning problems, an increase in gastroesophageal reflux, and difficulty in clearing secretions place children with CP at higher risk for respiratory problems, notably pneumonias (especially from aspiration; Hoekelman, 2001). The duration of respiratory symptoms with upper respiratory infections (URIs) also is increased in these children (Jackson Allen & Vessey, 2004).

Skin. The skin is more likely to break down and cause decubiti secondary to positioning problems. There is an increased incidence of skin latex allergies with CP (Jackson Allen & Vessey, 2004).

Movement and Mobility. Positioning and seating, standing, transportation, bathing, dressing, mobility for play and getting to school, and oral hygiene are important to assess and manage. Occupational and physical therapists are essential to these aspects of care. Families need help incorporating various strategies into their homes and lifestyles. The goals of therapy are to improve physical conditioning and gain maximum independence in mobility, fine motor activities, self-care, and communication. Therapists try to promote efficient movement patterns, inhibit primitive reflexes, and achieve isolated extremity movements. Bracing, adaptive devices, and early intervention programs beginning in infancy are important. Children need to experience different environments for developmental growth. Wheelchairs and motorized wheelchairs can be beneficial in helping children explore their environment more efficiently. Furthermore, although the condition is not progressive in terms of the brain lesion, contractures, scoliosis, dislocated hips, and other deformities can develop if the child is allowed to maintain abnormal positions for long periods. Thus therapy for range of motion is a long-term need for many of these children. Orthopedic care may be necessary.

Communication. With the combined problems of lack of oral-motor control and the high incidence of mental retardation, communication can be a real problem for children with CP. Speech therapy is important to achieve oral speech when possible or to use augmentative devices such as computers with voices to allow language development and communication of needs even without oral speech. Hearing deficits need to be identified and managed by an audiologist. Computers with specially outfitted input devices have greatly increased the ability of those with speech and movement disabilities to communicate with others.

Advocacy. Families often need help accessing services through schools because children with CP may have special education needs. Some insurance companies try to avoid the costs of long-term care and therapy. The primary care provider is important to families as an advocate and resource.

Special Education. Early intervention programs and specialized educational programs through school systems are often beneficial.

Other Treatments. Drugs are sometimes used to alter muscle tone or abnormal movements. These include botulinum toxin A (Botox), anticholinergics (e.g., trihexyphenidyl, benztropine, procyclidine hydrochloride), alcohol or phenol injections into muscles, oral diazepam (Valium), baclofen (Lioresal), tizanidine (Zanaflex), and dantrolene (Dantrium). Surgery is used to release contractures or to sever overactivated nerves (called a *selective dorsal root rhizotomy*) (Finberg & Kleinman, 2002). Selective dorsal rhizotomy (of spinal nerves) plus intrathecal baclofen decrease spasticity and increase range of motion of affected limbs. Although functional spasticity can be helped with these last two procedures, the selective motor, balance, and weakness problems are not improved. Strength training can help with balance and weakness (Hoekelman, 2001).

Experimental surgery is ongoing and includes the implantation of electrodes into the cerebellum (to stimulate selected nerves, leading to improved coordination of movement) and cutting parts of the thalamus (to alter messages from the muscles and sensory organs) (NINDS, 2000).

Complications. Children who receive no intervention have poorer functional abilities; they make less progress developmentally and are at risk for unnecessary contractures and deformities. Box 28-2 lists associated problems seen in CP.

Prevention and Screening. The incidence of CP can be decreased to some extent through good prenatal care. Recent research compared the blood of newborns who later developed CP with the blood of newborns who did not. Results revealed some interesting elevations in interferons or other inflammatory cytokines. It is postulated that these substances are the result of maternal infection and caused indirect fetal damage (Mast, 2002). Other studies are focusing on preterm infants with histologic chorioamnionitis as a red flag. It is anticipated that continued research into new areas will eventually lead to further preventive interventions.

BOX 28-2 *Problems Associated with Cerebral Palsy*

Cognitive

Learning disabilities
Mental retardation

Seizure Disorders

Language and Speech Disorders

Articulation
Vocal strength and quality
Language processing

Vision

Refractive errors
Strabismus
Amblyopia
Cataracts
Retinopathy of prematurity
Cortical blindness
Homonymous hemianopsia (hemiplegia)

Hearing

Conductive
Sensorineural

Other Sensory

Tactile hypersensitivity or hyposensitivity
Dsypraxia
Balance and movement problems
Proprioception difficulties
Stereognosis

Motor

Prolonged primitive reflexes
Absence of protective reflexes
Delayed motor milestones
Hip subluxation and dislocation
Scoliosis
Contractures

Feeding and Eating Problems

Chewing, sucking, and swallowing deficits
Drooling
Hypoxemia
Fatigue
Underweight and overweight
Gastroesophageal reflux
Aspiration

Bowel

Constipation
Encopresis

Urinary

Bladder control
Urinary retention
Urinary tract infections

Dental

Malocclusions
Enamel deficits and caries
Gum hyperplasia (with phenytoin)

Pulmonary

Respiratory infections
Pneumonia

Skin

Decubitus
Latex allergy

Behavioral and Emotional

Behavioral disorders
Attention-deficit disorder, with and without hyperactivity
Self-injurious behaviors
Depression
Autism
Growth failure
Other

From Jackson Allen P, Vessey J: *Primary care of the child with a chronic condition*, ed 4, St Louis, 2004, Mosby.

Until that time, early identification and intervention can significantly improve the outlook for affected children and their families.

Bell Palsy

Description. Bell palsy is an acute unilateral paralysis or weakening of any facet of the facial nerve. The patient may initially experience localized pain or tingling in one ear, and then typically be seen in the clinic with sagging on one side of the face with the eyelid completely or partially closed. There may be a hypersensitivity to loud noises, loss of taste on the anterior two thirds of the tongue, and changes in lacrimation and salivation. The history usually reveals a recent URI or exposure to cold temperature. Onset is rapid and can progress to maximum intensity within hours. Symptoms may last for 1 to 9 weeks (average 2 to 4 weeks) with spontaneous remission and recovery. The younger the child, the more complete the remission (Menkes & Sarnat, 2000).

Etiology. There is edema of cranial nerve VII and venous congestion in areas of the nerve canal. Infectious agents have been implicated, including Epstein-Barr, mumps, herpes simplex and herpes zoster, and Lyme disease and other spirochetes. There may be a genetic predisposition that involves trigeminal and auditory nerve pathways (Menkes & Sarnat, 2000).

Clinical Findings

Physical Examination. A neurologic assessment of all facial nerve functions may be difficult in children and is not critical to making an accurate diagnosis (Fenichel, 2001). The NP should note the following:

- Unilateral motor changes in forehead, cheek, and perioral area; face muscles pull to the normal side when the child makes facial expressions.
- Normal blood pressure.
- Dribbling liquids from the weak side when offered fluids.
- Eating and drinking are more difficult.
- Eyelid fails to close on the affected side, and complete blinking may be absent.
- Taste (50% of patients), lacrimation, and salivation may be impaired.
- No limb weakness.
- No skin lesions to suggest herpes near the ear on the affected side of the face.

Diagnostic Studies. None are indicated unless the patient fails to improve within 4 weeks or other concurrent neurologic symptoms evolve (Fenichel, 2001).

Differential Diagnosis. Guillain-Barré syndrome (usually includes an additional symptom of absent tendon reflexes of limbs), hypertension, infection, trauma, Melkersson syndrome (involves recurrent facial palsies with swollen lips, tongue, cheeks, or eyelids), acute otitis media, polymyelitis, histiocytosis X, varicella, and post-DTP (diphtheria-tetanus-pertussis) vaccine reaction.

Management. If lid closure is incomplete, prescribe artificial tears to the affected eye several times daily and patch the eye if the child plays outdoors, during active play, and when sleeping. Steroids are not indicated in children (Fenichel, 2001). Eighty percent will recover but have some partial palsy; others may experience recovery within 6 weeks to 6 months but experience incomplete nerve recovery. Recurrence rates are approximately 7% in children (Menkes & Sarnat, 2000).

Complications. If recovery is incomplete, lack of salivating in response to food, facial contractures, tics, and lacrimation may occur.

Epilepsy and Seizure Disorders

Description. Approximately 25,000 to 40,000 children in the United States experience their first nonfebrile seizure every year (Hirtz et al, 2000). Seizures are due to the misfiring of the cortical neurons of the brain. Convulsive seizures occur when misfiring causes attacks of involuntary contraction of voluntary muscles (see Table 28-4 for types of seizures). When seizures are recurrent and unrelated to fever, the disorder is called *epilepsy.* Seizures represent either brain dysfunction or significant underlying disorders. A patient may demonstrate characteristics of more than one type of seizure. The peak incidence is during three distinct periods: neonatal, between 5 and 10 years (absence and benign focal), and during adolescence (partial complex) (Finberg & Kleinman, 2002).

Etiology. Different kinds of seizures arise from disorders in diverse parts of the brain. Seizures can result from a variety of genetic (25%), symptomatic (50%; e.g., electrolyte problems, metabolic dysfunction related to acute and chronic illnesses, head trauma, tumors, toxins), or idiopathic conditions (Finberg & Kleinman, 2002). More than 30,000 genes are expressed in the brain, and an increasing number of brain malfunctions are being traced to chromosomal changes (Menkes & Sarnat, 2000). Approximately one third of children who have a prior history of cognitive or motor impairments will have a recurrent unprovoked seizure within 1 year. In contrast, two thirds of those with such histories will experience a recurrence. Ninety percent to 95% of the recurrences happen within 2 years (Children's Hospital Medical Center, 1999; Fenichel, 2001).

Clinical Findings

History. The history of a patient with seizures should include the following:

- Description of the seizure: focal or generalized, loss of consciousness, aura, length of postictal sleep or confusion, duration of the episode, and associated illness

TABLE 28-4 *Classification of Seizures*

Seizure Type	Age	Pattern	Comments
I. Partial or focal seizures		Begin locally	Affect one hemisphere
A. Simple partial		Consciousness not impaired	Last 10-20 sec
1. With motor symptoms	Any age	Any part of body: includes jacksonian seizures	Due to birth trauma, inflammation, stroke, tumors (if new onset of tumor with progressive neurologic symptoms)
2. With sensory or somatosensory symptoms	Any age	"Pins and needles," numb; auras include lights, tastes, sounds	
3. With autonomic symptoms	Any age	Recurrent abdominal pain, headache, sweat, laugh, cry, tachycardia, dilated pupils	May have migraine quality; family history of migraine or seizures
4. Compound forms	Any age		
B. Complex partial	Any age; may behard to recognize in young child	Consciousness impaired; clonic activity, forced head/eye deviation, focal tonic posturing, automatisms—purposeless motor activities (e.g., lip smacking, repetitious swallowing/chewing, finger/hand fidgeting, tics)	Last 1-2 min
1. Impaired consciousness only		Staring spell	
2. With cognitive symptoms		May have confusion	
3. With affective symptoms		Aura of fear	
4. With "psychosensory" symptoms		May have odd smell/taste; visual or auditory hallucination	
5. With "psychomotor" symptoms		Automatisms	
6. Compound forms			
C. Partial seizures, secondary generalized		Seizure begins in one part of body but then generalizes	Aura can let person seek safe position
II. Idiopathic localization-related seizures			
A. Benign focal (or rolandic)	4-13 yr		Resolve by adolescence; treatment may not be needed
1. Diurnal		Alert; unilateral twitching, drooling, paresthesia of face, gums, tongue, buccal mucosa; may progress into hemiclonic or hemitonic movements	With or without postictal weakness of affected side
2. Nocturnal		Advances to generalization	
III. Generalized seizures			Usually no aura
A. Absence	4-12 yr	Petit mal; 5-30 sec; lapses of consciousness (short staring "spells"); can have associated movements; no falling; no aura	Hyperventilation for 3-4 min can trigger seizure; blinking lights can also trigger
B. Myoclonic (infantile spasms)	Infancy	Head drops or sudden flexing; may suddenly cry out; older children exhibit trunk or extremity flexion	Hypsarrhythmia on EEG with no normal background activity; difficult to treat
C. Clonic		Rhythmic jerking	
D. Tonic		Intense muscle contractions	
E. Tonic-clonic	Any age; most common type of seizure	Grand mal; begins with loss of consciousness; stiffening, violent jerking; postictal phase of sleep and confusion; 15% incontinent	Aura in some; may have abdominal pain or headache; life threatening if continues, producing hypercarbia, respiratory acidosis, lactic acidosis; some occur in sleep
F. Atonic		Similar to myoclonic	Child often falls

EEG, Electroencephalogram.

- Any underlying medical diagnosis (e.g., diabetes, renal disease, cardiovascular disorder)
- Previous CNS infection or birth trauma
- Intrauterine infection, trauma, bleeding
- Toxic exposure or drug use
- Anticonvulsant medication stopped abruptly
- Recent head injury
- Family history of seizures

Physical Examination. The following should be determined on physical examination:

- Focal abnormalities, weakness
- Presence of seizure activity during the examination
- Hypertension (for renal disease)
- Systemic disease
- Cardiovascular disorder
- Neurocutaneous disease, café au lait spots of neurofibromatosis, ash leaf spots or adenoma sebaceum of tuberous sclerosis, facial hemangioma of Sturge-Weber syndrome
- Signs of head trauma
- Transillumination of the skull in infants

Diagnostic Studies. The most current recommendations for laboratory/imaging evaluation include the following (Hirtz et al, 2000; Reuter & Brownstein, 2002; Ryan, 2002):

- Complete blood count (CBC) (including platelets, liver function tests [LFTs])—useful for diagnostic purposes or as a baseline before anticonvulsant therapy is started.
- Metabolic screen—only if child is younger than 6 months, if a metabolic problem is suspected because of history, or if concurrent vomiting, diarrhea, or dehydration exists or patient fails to return to baseline alertness after seizure.
- Blood glucose—standard in all patients.
- Urine/serum toxicology—only if illicit drug exposure suspected.
- Lumbar puncture—only if child is younger than 6 months; any age patient with persistent changes in mental status or failure to return to baseline functioning; patients with meningeal signs.
- EEG—standard in all children after first nonfebrile seizure. An abnormal EEG supports the seizure diagnosis. However, a normal EEG when the child is not seizing does not rule out a seizure disorder.
- MRI—imaging studies are not routinely indicated if the initial seizure is followed by a normal neurologic examination and return to baseline mental status. Imaging is recommended (1) if the patient demonstrates cognitive changes after several hours and postictal focal dysfunction (signs of increased intracranial pressure, such as found with tumors, abscesses, strokes, or vascular malformations); (2) if the seizure lasted more than 15 minutes; (3) in infants younger than 6 months old; and (4) if any new onset of focal neurologic deficit has occurred. An MRI is now the preferred imaging study over CT scans because of its increased sensitivity.
- CT scan—used only in cases of marked cognitive, motor, or neurologic dysfunction of unknown etiology (e.g., head injury, brain infection or tumor, abscesses); abnormal EEGs; or focal seizure symptoms that may or may not evolve into a generalized seizure.
- Polysomnography (simultaneous EEG, electromyogram, electrocardiogram [ECG], and electrooculogram) can be useful to assess nocturnal seizures.

Differential Diagnosis. Consider breath-holding, syncope, migraine headaches, gastroesophageal reflux, night terrors, metabolic problems, tumors or other CNS problems, or a cardiovascular problem. Vertigo has been confused with epilepsy. Tics (involuntary, spasmodic, nonrhythmic, repetitive movements) are stereotypic but not associated with impaired consciousness and at times can be suppressed by the patient.

Pseudoseizures. Pseudoseizures, or "hysterical seizures," may be difficult to distinguish from true seizures, even after direct observation. The NP is more likely to suspect such pseudoseizures in a patient with seizures who has gained more recent control of a seizure disorder. In such cases, the pseudoseizures serve as attention-getting behaviors for the child who misses the attention gained before control. Pseudoseizures also may be seen in adolescents, more often in girls than in boys (3:1). Incest or sexual abuse must be addressed in these girls (Fenichel, 2001). The seizures should be regarded as real and not a consequence of a severe psychologic problem. Distinguishing characteristics of pseudoseizures include the following:

- Unilaterally or bilaterally coordinated motor activity more like thrashing and jerking rather than tonic-clonic; no aura or complaints of malaise, heart palpitations, feeling like choking before seizure onset
- Discomfort, distress expressed; sometimes ataxia, fumbling, or consciousness impaired but not absent
- No incontinence; patient does not hurt self or bite tongue
- No postictal stage
- Occur at home
- No EEG changes, even during episodes

Treatment for pseudoseizures involves developing alternative gains to seizure behavior. Most children stop after the diagnosis is made and interventions are in place. Sometimes a referral for counseling may be indicated, depending on the etiology. No anticonvulsants are used in the case of children who do not have an underlying seizure disorder.

Management

Referral. A child with suspected seizures should be referred to a neurologist for diagnosis and initiation of treatment. Anticonvulsant drugs are usually prescribed, especially after a second seizure. Delaying treatment does not affect ultimate control. There is a 90% recurrence rate after a second generalized type of seizure; less if it is a partial seizure (Fenichel, 2001).

Management of Stable Patients with Diagnosed Seizure Disorders. NPs monitor stable children with seizures. Such activity includes prescribing anticonvulsants, monitoring drug levels, and performing case management. Any change in status requires consultation with or referral to the neurologist.

Drug Monitoring. All NPs working with patients receiving anticonvulsants should be familiar with the common drugs (Table 28-5) and their major side effects (see also Appendix A). Helping with compliance issues is also a component of the monitoring role. Start with one drug. Fenichel (2001) offers some general comments about antiepileptic drug (AED) therapy:

- Patients can be controlled with subtherapeutic blood levels.
- Patients can be free of side effects at levels beyond the therapeutic range.
- Phenytoin (Dilantin) saturates the enzyme system; therefore even a small increase in dosage can cause a marked increase in blood levels.
- Half-lives are longer with the introduction to a new drug; steady concentrations (and elimination) of the drug are achieved at 5 half-lives.
- Half-lives vary by patient and other drugs being taken (e.g., antibiotics, anticonvulsants, antipyretics).

TABLE 28-5 ***Antiepileptic Drug Therapy for Children****

Seizure Type	Drug	Blood Levels (g/ml)	Laboratory Monitoring
Partial, generalized tonic-clonic in children >2 yr; contraindicated for absence and myoclonic	Carbamazepine (Tegretol)	4-12	CBC; baseline, at 6-12 wk, then annually; drug blood levels
Partial, generalized, status epilepticus	Phenytoin (Dilantin)	10-30	Drug blood levels
Simple partial, tonic-clonic	Phenobarbital (Luminal)	10-45	None
Absence	Ethosuximide (Zarontin)	40-120	None
First-line generalized seizures if >10 yr, myoclonic, absence	Valproic acid (Depakene)	50-120	Baseline (and after 1 mo) LFTs, ammonia, prothrombin, partial thromboplastin
Partial, tonic-clonic, myoclonic	Primidone (Mysoline)	8-12	None
Partial, myoclonic, infantile spasms	Vigabatrin (not approved in United States)	1.4-14	
Partial, generalized, Lennox-Gastaut syndrome	Felbamate (Felbatol)†	Not monitored	LFTs, CBC with diff., platelets, retic ct. monthly (requires close monitoring)
Refractory partial-onset, rolandic	Gabapentin (Neurontin)— an adjunct drug with other AEDs used for partial seizures	5-15	Depends on other AED used
Partial, Lennox-Gastaut syndrome, absence, atonic, juvenile myoclonic	Lamotrigine (Lamictal)—an adjunct drug only with valproic acid	2-20	
Partial, generalized	Topiramate (Topomax)	2-25	None
Partial	Oxcarbazepine (Trileptal—similar to Tegretol)	5-50	None
Partial, generalized	Zonisamide (Zonegran)	10-40	None
Partial	Levetiracetam (Kepra)	20-60	None
Partial, generalized	Tigabine (Gabatril)— adjunct drug only	5-70	None

Data from Burg F et al, editors: *Gellis and Kagan's current pediatric therapy*, ed 17, Philadelphia, 2002, WB Saunders; Fenichel G: *Clinical pediatric neurology: a signs and symptoms approach*, ed 4, Philadelphia, 2001, WB Saunders.
*See Appendix A for dosing information.
†Drug not approved by Food and Drug Administration for pediatric use; consult before using.
AEDs, Antiepileptic drugs; *CBC*, complete blood count; *LFTs*, liver function tests; *retic ct.*, reticulocyte count; *diff.*, differential.

- If gastrointestinal side effects occur, decreasing the dosage and increasing the frequency of administration may help; try changing to an enteric-coated pill or taking the drug after eating.
- Administer drug twice daily or daily for better compliance.
- The first signs of toxicity usually include sedation, changes in behavior, and changes in cognition; other drug toxicities may cause decreases in memory and attention span or interpersonal relationship difficulties. It is important to note that some patients may exhibit these changes and have drug levels within the normal range.
- Metabolites of the drugs can cause hypersensitivity side effects.
- Do routine drug level monitoring based on the clinical picture.

Antiepileptic Drug Withdrawal. After 2 years or longer without seizures, consideration may be given to gradually withdrawing anticonvulsant therapy. Waiting is particularly efficacious in patients with an abnormal EEG and partial seizures. Whether or not to withdraw medication in children with generalized seizures is still under debate (Sirven, Sperling, & Wingerchuk, 2001). Those with seizure onset after 5 years of age who have normal mentation are excellent candidates. Some evidence indicates that spike-and-wave paroxysmal features on the EEG are a contraindication to drug withdrawal. Children with mental retardation, CP, focal motor deficits, age of onset younger than 2 years, symptomatic seizures, and abnormal EEGs are not good weaning candidates. Weaning is supervised closely and occurs over 6 weeks to 4 to 6 months, with one drug removed at a time. Of children who have been seizure free for 2 years and have no risk factors, 70% to 75% remain seizure free without drugs. If seizures do recur, 50% do so within the first 6 months of weaning and 60% to 80% within 2 years. Three fourths of recurrences occur during weaning or within the first year (Bouma, Peters, & Brouwer, 2002; Hoekelman, 2001). If the onset of seizures occurred during a time of anoxia, head injury, meningitis, or encephalitis, AED treatment can be stopped after recovery from the condition is complete. The patient can always be restarted should there be a recurrence (Fenichel, 2001).

Ketogenic Diet. The ketogenic diet is useful in young children with all types of seizures, particularly in those with myoclonic forms, infantile spasms, atonic/kinetic types, and with the mixed seizures of Lennox-Gastaut syndrome (Fenichel, 2001). The diet is considered when the side effects of AEDs are intolerable or when allergies to AEDs preclude administration. The ideal child is between 2 and 5 years old because the desired steady state of ketosis is easier to maintain. The diet is stringent and requires utmost vigilance to the ratios of calories, protein, fat, carbohydrate, vitamins, and minerals. It is best managed under very tight control with medical and dietitian leadership. Side effects usually involve abdominal pain and diarrhea. A prescreening process, including psychologic testing to determine the child's and family's emotional functioning, coping, and problem-solving abilities, is recommended. A dietitian should screen the child for nutrition and growth status. A nurse should interview the family for understanding of and education about the protocol. The diet is started while the child is admitted to the hospital, where metabolic and neurologic states can be monitored. One study in 1996 demonstrated that for carefully selected and monitored children, 10% will achieve a seizure-free state within 1 year, and 23% will have a reduction in seizures (Hoekelman, 2001).

Surgery. Surgery has been successful in helping some children with complex partial seizures. However, as with the ketogenic diet, selection of appropriate children is done with great care. Focal resection surgery is currently used only in children with well-localized related epilepsy whose seizures are well documented, who have failed to respond to AEDs, and whose development has been assessed over time. Seizure-free rates after resection have been documented to reach 90%, with minimal loss of neurologic function (Finberg & Kleinman, 2002). Hemispherectomy or interhemispherectomy can be curative. Side effects of the surgery include hemiparesis, incontinences, stuttering, and poor hand coordination. Temporal lobotomies are an option for treating intractable partial complex seizures localized to the temporal area; side effects are aphasia and superior quadrant visual loss. Slightly more than 50% of candidates achieve freedom from seizures. Callosotomy and vagus nerve stimulation, as palliative surgeries, are options for children with multiple regions of hemispheric involvement that result in intractable seizures. In vagus nerve stimulation, a programmed stimulation generator is implanted in the anterior chest wall. The left vagus nerve is stimulated. How stimulation works is not completely known, but there are resultant changes in the central spinal fluid amino acids and an activation of the noradrenergic system. Side effects include neck pain, voice changes and hoarseness, and possible infection (Fenichel, 2001; Hoekelman, 2001). Both children and adults are good candidates.

Counseling. Older children need to understand the seizures they are experiencing and their significance. They also need to know about the anticonvulsant medications they are taking. Teenagers want to drive. Laws vary from state to state, but generally a teenager who has been seizure free for 2 years and has demonstrated good drug compliance should be allowed to drive. Parents need to understand the diagnosis, treatment, and necessary follow-up. They also need to understand the implications of seizure disorders and long-term prognoses. Negative attitudes continue to surround epilepsy and may need to be addressed. Epilepsy is not synonymous with mental retardation.

Children with epilepsy may experience social stigmas and problems with self-esteem. Other mental health problems may also occur in these children as they try to cope with a chronic disease. Parents are encouraged to treat children as normally as possible (Hoekelman, 2001).

Safety. Uncontrolled seizures can present safety hazards for an unsupervised child. The child and family need to consider the situations that the child will be in and be sure that someone knows what to do if a seizure occurs. School personnel need to be informed and prepared. Safety helmets worn at all times are sometimes warranted if falls and head injury occur frequently. Swimming alone is never recommended, but swimming, contact sports, and climbing are to be allowed if the child is well controlled. Scuba diving is contraindicated. A recent study revealed that fatal car crashes attributed to seizures were rare (0.6%) versus those due to other medical conditions (84%). The authors of the study summarized their findings by noting that "seizure-related car crashes do not pose any substantial risk to safety," but they recognized the need to adhere to state laws and to keep one's seizures well controlled (Scherer & Krauss, 2001).

Immunizations. The decision to give pertussis vaccine to children with neurologic seizures or other neurologic conditions needs to be made on an individual basis. If used, diphtheria-tetanus-acellular pertussis (DTaP) is recommended. Children who will be in child care centers, special clinics, or residential care centers should be immunized if possible. Progressive neurologic conditions with developmental delays are reason for deferral of pertussis vaccine. Infants and children with a personal history of seizures have been noted to have a sevenfold increase in post–diphtheria-pertussis-tetanus (DPT) immunization seizures. Thus DTaP and acetaminophen at the time of administration and every 4 hours for the first 24 hours is recommended. Other neurologic conditions that predispose to seizures or neurologic deterioration or a seizure history in an infant should result in consideration of deferral of pertussis immunization (American Academy of Pediatrics Committee on Infectious Diseases, 2003).

Complications. *Status epilepticus* is defined as a prolonged single seizure lasting more than 20 to 30 minutes or recurrent seizures without an interictal stage. A child who has generalized tonic-clonic seizures and who is in status epilepticus is at risk for brain damage and intellectual deficits (Fenichel, 2001). Lack of oxygenation, decreased cerebral perfusion, metabolic acidosis, hypoglycemia, hyperkalemia, lactic acidosis, increased temperature, and increased intracranial pressure can all result in significant risk of morbidity and mortality. Such an occurrence needs to be handled as a medical emergency. Mortality rate in children is estimated at less than 6%, and most deaths are attributed to the illness that preceded the seizure (Hoekelman, 2001). Status epilepticus can be triggered by an acute brain infection, progressive neurologic disease, AED failure, or, rarely, a febrile seizure in an otherwise healthy child without other risk factors. However, most cases of status epilepticus occur in children with underlying neurologic deficits. It is difficult to diagnose status epilepticus in children with absence or complex partial seizures, because the children may just appear confused (Fenichel, 2001). Adverse outcomes can include behavioral problems, mental retardation, and focal motor deficits. Diazepam rectal gel (Diastat) is recommended for use by health care providers, parents, and caregivers (including school personnel) in children over 2 years of age who have a seizure lasting more than 5 minutes. It is administered once and takes effect in 5 to 15 minutes. Its use has decreased emergency department visits by 67%, and it is safe at higher than recommended doses, with less than 1% incidence of respiratory depression. The most common side effect is somnolence. It is available in a premeasured portable packet and dosed according to age and weight (Francis, 2003).

Prevention and Screening. Epilepsy cannot be prevented, but early diagnosis and intervention can often reduce the disabilities and risks associated with the condition.

Febrile Seizures

Description. Febrile seizures are the most common type of seizures in children. They are brief, generalized, clonic or tonic-clonic in nature and can be either simple or complex. Fever develops in most children at the time of the attack, and temperatures can be as low as 100.1° to 101.4° F (37.8° to 38.5° C). Little postictal confusion is associated with febrile seizures. Simple febrile seizures last less than 15 minutes and do not recur within a 24-hour period; complex febrile seizures last longer than 30 minutes, can recur on the same day, and can have focal attributes (Menkes & Sarnat, 2000).

Etiology and Incidence. The etiology of febrile seizures is unclear and by definition excludes seizures that are caused by intracranial illness or are related to an underlying CNS problem. There is some confusion as to whether the seizures are triggered by the height of the temperature or by the action of the temperature rising. Current research slightly favors the former interpretation (Menkes & Sarnat, 2000). There is believed to be a familial predisposition (24%) that inherently leaves the child with a more temperature-sensitive immature neuronal membrane (Menkes & Sarnat, 2000). Research is ongoing to identify specific genes that might play a role in this familial predisposition. So far, four chromosomal areas have been identified that warrant further study. It is hoped that by gaining a better understanding of febrile seizures, better treatments can be found (Ryther, 2001).

Febrile seizures generally occur in children between 3 months and 5 years of age; the median age is 18 to 22 months (93% are between 6 months and 3 years). Boys are affected more than girls. Two percent to 4% of all children have febrile seizures. The risk for subsequent febrile seizures is 30% to 50% (Hoekelman, 2001; Menkes & Sarnat, 2000).

Clinical Findings

History. The history of a patient with febrile seizures involves the following:

- Description of seizure duration, type (generalized or focal), frequency in 24 hours
- Relationship of the seizure to the febrile episode
- Abnormal neurologic status before the seizure, which is not consistent with a febrile seizure
- Family history of afebrile seizures
- Maternal smoking in the perinatal period
- Prematurity or neonatal hospitalizations for more than 28 days
- Parents' impression of slow development

Physical Examination. The physical examination is the same as that described earlier for seizures.

Diagnostic Studies. Diagnostic studies include the following (Behrman, Kliegman, & Jenson, 2004):

- Lumbar puncture in infants younger than 2 months of age
- Blood glucose in all children (CBC, calcium, electrolytes, urinalysis *not* indicated in an otherwise fully recovered child—need to individualize assessment)
- EEG if neurologic signs are present or seizure was atypical
- MRI with atypical febrile seizure features

Differential Diagnosis. Consider sepsis, meningitis, metabolic or toxic encephalopathies, hypoglycemia, anoxia, trauma, tumor, and hemorrhage. Febrile delirium and febrile shivering can be confused with seizures. Breath-holding spells can mimic febrile seizures; however, the former are always related to crying or tantrums. Febrile seizures come at unpredictable times during sleep, eating, play, or other generally calm times and are related to the onset of an illness. Epileptic seizures occur without concurrent illness and at unpredictable times.

Management. The following steps should be taken in the management of a febrile seizure:

- Protect the airway, breathing, and circulation if the seizure is still occurring. Place the child in a side-lying position to prevent aspiration or airway obstruction.
- Do not put anything in the child's mouth.
- Time the duration of the seizure, and observe whether it is focal or generalized.
- Reduce the fever with acetaminophen or ibuprofen, although the use of antipyretics will not necessarily prevent another febrile seizure.
- The child should be seen shortly after the seizure. Advise transport to an emergency center if the seizure lasts more than 10 minutes.
- Anticonvulsants are not recommended for febrile seizures but may be considered in any of the following situations (Menkes & Sarnat, 2000):
  - The child has abnormal neurologic findings or developmental delays.
  - The initial seizure was complex febrile *and* there is a family history of afebrile seizures.
  - The child has recurrent, prolonged simple febrile seizures.

Prophylaxis. If prophylaxis is indicated, diazepam by mouth 0.33 mg/kg every 8 hours is given during a febrile illness (usually for 2 to 3 days). Side effects of diazepam include transient ataxis, lethargy, and irritability (Fenichel, 2001). An alternative to diazepam if transient ataxis or lethargy exists is continuous daily phenobarbital to achieve a blood level of 15 μg/ml. Phenobarbital, however, has behavioral side effects that are often intolerable to the family.

Education. The family should receive information about febrile seizures, their risks, and their management. Education should include information explaining the febrile seizure, reassurance that no long-term consequences are associated with febrile seizures, information that febrile seizures recur in some children and that nothing can be done to prevent the seizures, and first-aid information in case another seizure occurs at some time. The decision to use prophylaxis must be individualized to meet parents' values and needs (Gordon et al, 2001). A follow-up phone call to the parents after 1 week is often helpful.

Complications. Death or persisting motor deficits do not occur in patients with febrile seizures. No indication has been found that intellect or learning is impaired. An affected child has an increased risk for the development of epilepsy (less than 5%) if the seizure is prolonged and focal; if the child has repeated seizures with the same febrile episode; or if the child has had a prior neurologic deficit, a family history of epilepsy, or both. Two thirds of patients who have had one simple febrile seizure will not have any more. The younger the age at onset (less than 18 months) of the first febrile seizure, the lower the temperature threshold needed to cause the child to seize and the more likely the child is to have a recurrence.

Headaches

Description. Headaches in children fall into two classifications—acute and chronic. Table 28-6 lists the more common types found in these classifications. Rosenblum and Fisher (2001) note studies that found that by the time children are 7 years old, 40% will have experienced

TABLE 28-6 *Most Common Types of Headaches*

Characteristics	Vascular (Migraine)	Cluster	Chronic, Low Grade	Tension
Prevalence	2.5% occurrence in children <7 yr; 5% occurrence prepuberty; 5% occurrence postpuberty if male	Uncommon in children Occur mostly in females, over 10 yr of age	Most common type of chronic headaches in all ages	All ages, both sexes
History	10% occurrence postpuberty if female Female:male = 3:2 Positive family history (90% of patients have both parents with history; 80% have one parent with history); 50% have history of motion sickness	No family history Unilateral headache recurring daily over 4-8 wk with 1-2 yr between occurrences Typically occurs in fall or spring Pain occurs in burst lasting 30-90 min and repeated several times a day	Use of caffeine (including caffeinated drinks) or nonprescription analgesics Throbbing pain, anxiety, malaise if does not take the above routinely	Positive family history with childhood onset; fatigue, stress, depression, exertion
Pattern	Recurrent pattern May be aura Transitory neurologic changes (nausea/vomiting, malaise, personality changes, photophobia, phonophobia) Appears sick Periodic "ice-pick" pain on top of head described by adolescents Resolves after sleeping Pain lasts 2-4 hr in younger children; 48-72 hr in adolescents	Hurts to lie down, pain intense (constant or throbbing), scalp tender, conjunctiva injected, tearing No nausea/vomiting	Generalized pain, low intensity, dull ache, does not interfere with most activities, but may decrease them	Bilateral, diffuse (site may shift), dull, aching pain ("tight band around head"), located in neck and back of head May appear on awakening and continue all day; does not increase with activity No nausea, vomiting, photophobia, phonophobia, or neurologic changes; negative neurologic examination Lasts 30 minutes, all day, or for several days Can occur at same time as more classic migraine headache
Triggers	Stress, exercise, head trauma, menstrual cycle, hunger, noise, travel, cold weather	None	Withdrawal from caffeine or analgesics	May be stress, musculoskeletal dysfunction

Differential diagnosis	Benign occipital epilepsy of childhood (same visual changes as migraine but are followed by either unilateral or clonic-tonic, complex partial seizure pattern, then headache and nausea—occurs usually as child falls asleep)	Chronic paroxysmal one-sided head pain (hemicrania)		
Diagnostic tests	None (EEG if suspect benign occipital epilepsy)	None	None	None
Treatment (see Appendix A for dosing)	*Acute*: acetaminophen, ibuprofen, naproxen, sumatriptan (Imitrex), rizatriptan benzoate (Maxalt), ergot; promethazine for nausea/vomiting; cold frontal compresses *Prophylaxis*: propranolol (Inderal), amitriptyline (Elavil), cyproheptadine (Periactin) *Others*: biofeedback/relaxation	*Supression*: prednisone 1 mg/kg/day for 5 days, then taper for 2 wk *Acute attack*: sumatriptan, oxygen, lithium	*Acute only*: acetaminophen, ibuprofen, naproxen, or other nonsteroidal antiinflammatory drugs	*Acute*: analgesics, nonsteroidal antiinflammatory drugs, amitriptyline, tizanidine *Other*: massage, relaxation techniques, cold, alternating with warm compresses to occipital area

Adapted from Fenichel G: *Clinical pediatric neurology: a signs and symptoms approach*, ed 4, Philadelphia, 2001, WB Saunders, pp 77-89; Rosenblum R, Fisher P: A guide to children with acute and chronic headaches, *J Pediatr Health Care* 15(5):229-235, 2001; Burg F et al, editors: *Gellis and Kagan's current pediatric therapy*, ed 17, Philadelphia, 2002, WB Saunders; Hershey A et al: Effectiveness of nasal sumatriptan in 5-12 year old children, *Headache* 41(7):693-697, 2001.

headaches. By mid-adolescence this number rises to 75%. A person may experience different types of headaches.

Characteristics of *classic migraine* include nausea, abdominal pain, vomiting, unilateral pain, pulsating pain, relief with sleep, an aura, visual changes such as dark or blind spots, and a family history of headache. Infants and toddlers may be seen with irritability, sleepiness, and pallor. In preadolescents, common migraine symptoms are more likely. Nausea and vomiting might not occur, and the pain can be more frontal. Lethargy and sleep can follow. Visual changes are rare, and the pain quality is variable. Times between headaches are pain free. Abdominal migraine is rare; symptoms include pain, nausea, and vomiting with minimal or no headache. Such symptoms can also be suggestive of complex partial seizures (Finberg & Kleinman, 2002).

Muscle contraction or *tension headaches* are also common. There is no prodrome, and the pain is dull and bifrontal or occipital, with nausea and vomiting occurring only rarely. Tension headaches can last for days or weeks but do not interfere with activities. In children it can be difficult to differentiate migraine and muscle contraction headaches. Psychosocial stress seems to be a major factor in tension headaches in both children and adolescents.

Traction or *inflammatory headaches* are much more rare, occurring when a mass is causing inflammation or traction on the brain. They have many similar symptoms as those of headaches caused by brain tumors. The key point for these headaches is increasing severity, often with accompanying neurologic signs.

Ninety-seven percent to 99% of brain tumors in children cause symptoms of intracranial pressure, including the following:

- Pain that is worse in the mornings on awakening and standing up
- Pain that wakens child from sleep
- Involve vomiting but not nausea
- Headache is accompanied by diplopia
- Increased pain with straining, sneezing, coughing, defecation, or changes in position
- Occipital and neck pain
- Edema of the optic disc
- Mental changes

All of these symptoms point toward a significant structural headache needing prompt referral (Fenichel, 2001) (Box 28-3).

BOX 28-3 *Signs and Symptoms Suggestive of Increased Intracranial Pressure*

Infants

Full anterior fontanel
Open metopic and coronal sutures
Poor growth
Impaired upward gaze
Abnormal head growth
Shrill cry
Lethargy
Vomiting

Children

Persistent unilateral headache
Papilledema
Abnormal eye movements (or one or both eyes suddenly turn in)
Ataxia
Hemiparesis
Abnormal deep tendon reflexes
Severe, excruciating headache of recent onset, unlike any previously experienced; no normal period of functioning between episodes of headache
Cranial bruits

Etiology and Incidence. Pain fibers line the walls of the large intracranial blood vessels; the meninges and periosteum; the muscles around the head, neck, scalp, eyes, and jaw area; and the sinuses. The pain-sensitive blood vessels can be stimulated by inflammation and vasodilation. Intracranial pressure can cause pain as a result of traction and displacement of intracranial arteries. Low serotonin levels and temporary increases in dopamine levels are theorized as possibly contributing to the initiation of headache symptomatology (Rosenblum & Fisher, 2001).

Double-blind studies have implicated food allergies as triggering some headaches, but results have been inconsistent. The suspect foods include cow's milk, eggs, chocolate, wheat, benzoic acid, cheese, tomatoes, and rye (Menkes & Sarnat, 2000). The NP may choose to try an elimination diet as part of the treatment regimen.

Clinical Findings. Children less than 10 years of age often have a poor sense of time and may not serve as the best historians. The most important questions to ask patient and parent(s) regard frequency, location, and associated symptoms.

History. The following factors are assessed in the history of a child with headache:

- Duration. Recent severe onset is worrisome.
- Frequency and triggers. Children with recurrent, low-intensity headaches, with no neurologic changes, and who recover completely between episodes are unlikely to have serious intracranial etiology (Fenichel, 2001).
- Location. Occipital or consistently localized headaches can indicate underlying pathology. Facial pain might be

sinusitis. Ocular motor imbalance can produce a dull periorbital discomfort, whereas temporomandibular joint pain tends to localize around the periauricular or temporal areas.

- Quality and severity of pain. Sharp, throbbing, or pounding pain is probably vascular (migraine). Dull and constant pain may be tension or organic. Severity can be assessed by asking about limitations to activities and missed school days. How many "different kinds of headaches" are experienced?
- Presence of an aura or other premonitory symptoms.
- Age of onset, progression of the headaches over time, and longest period of time without symptoms.
- Home management and medications used.
- Self-coping activities.
- Associated symptoms. Nausea, vomiting, visual changes, dizziness, paresthesia, confusion, ataxia, pallor, photophobia, and phonophobia can occur with migraine. Changes in gait, personality, mentation, or behavior that do not occur at the same time as the headache are worrisome and merit further evaluation with medical referral.
- Head trauma. If associated with headache, head trauma can represent a subdural hematoma or postconcussive syndrome.
- Psychologic symptoms. Evaluate for the presence of depression, school stressors, or concerns about family functioning (Rosenblum & Fisher, 2001).
- Family history. Most children with headache, especially migraine, have a family history of headaches.

Physical Examination. The physical examination is usually normal. The following areas must be assessed:

- Blood pressure
- Neurologic examination
- Optic fundi
- Height and weight
- Head circumference (infants up to 24 months)
- Pericranial muscles for tenderness
- Sinuses (frontal and maxillary)
- Teeth
- Temporomandibular joints (mouth and jaw)
- Thyroid gland
- Cranial bruits (over temples and orbits)

Diagnostic Studies. Imaging studies are rarely indicated unless the history suggests symptoms of increased intracranial pressure (see Box 28-3) or when a complaint of "dizziness" fits the criteria listed in Table 28-7. Parents seek medical attention for pain relief for their child, as well as for reassurance that there are no intracranial processes occurring (brain tumors). Recent behavioral changes; reduced visual acuity; abnormalities on neurologic examination; pain on awakening, coughing, or straining that leads to a need to change positions; and persistent wakening at night with a headache are additional indications for neuroimaging studies (Evans & Lewis, 2001; Rosenblum & Fisher, 2001). In most cases a good history and physical examination can help the clinician distinguish the harmful from the merely painful headache. A CT scan without contrast is usually adequate to determine the presence of a brain tumor. If abnormal, an MRI should be done. An EEG should be obtained if the history and physical examination suggest a seizure process; cervical and spinal x-rays are indicated following a history of a motor vehicle accident or neck/cervical injury (Rosenblum & Fisher, 2001).

TABLE 28-7 *How to Proceed When the Complaint Is "Dizziness"*

Complaint of "Dizziness"	Studies Indicated
Light-headed	None
Double vision (posterior fossa location)	MRI
Sensation of whirling motion of oneself or of room/objects (vertigo)	MRI
Confusion	MRI, EEG, comprehensive metabolic screen

EEG, Electroencephalogram; *MRI,* magnetic resonance imaging.

Differential Diagnosis. The differential diagnosis consists of sinusitis, an intracranial mass, pseudotumor cerebri, sleep disorder, hyperthyroidism, hypertension, and temporomandibular joint dysfunction. Visual acuity is rarely a cause of headaches. These and other causes of headaches in children are outlined in Table 28-8.

Management. Treatment can include general pain management, abortive therapy to interrupt migraine headaches, and prophylactic medications to prevent or reduce the frequency and severity of acute attacks (see Table 28-6).

Prophylactic therapy is considered when headaches cause a child to miss school more than once monthly. Anticonvulsants are also used, especially if the child has a seizure disorder. Calcium channel blockers have not been studied in large, controlled trials, but as a group they can be used in children with normal cardiovascular systems (Fenichel, 2001).

Refer all patients with organic (structural) headaches. Patients with refractory headaches (after more than three classic prophylactic regimens have failed) should be referred for adjunct counseling, relaxation, and other coping techniques (e.g., biofeedback, yoga).

TABLE 28-8 ***Other Causes of Headaches in Children***

Cause	Characteristics
Drugs	
Cocaine	Migraine-like pain in patient with no history of migraine headaches
Marijuana	Frontal, mild
Analgesics and cardiovascular agents	Pain follows administration (of drug) or withdrawal (typical of analgesics)
Food additives (nitrites, monosodium glutamate common)	Pain occurs only in individual genetically sensitive; pain is diffuse, throbbing after ingestion
Physiologic	
Vasculitis	Uncommon in children; can occur as part of a collagen vascular disease, such as systemic lupus erythematosus
Chronic hypertension	Low-grade, occipital pain on awakening or frontal during day
Eyestrain	Dull, aching pain behind eyes relieved when eyes are closed; caused by muscular fatigue during prolonged ocular convergence—not a refractive error
Temporomandibular joint syndrome (TMJ)	>8 yr old; pain on one side of face and vertex of TMJ; may be a history of jaw injury
Whiplash and neck injury	Pain dull, aching in neck, shoulders, upper arms with poor neck rotation; no nausea or vomiting; caused by muscles contracted to "splint" area of dysfunction in cervical joint areas or soft tissue
Following partial or generalized seizure	Diffuse pain
Infectious illness	Uncommon
Dental disease	Uncommon
Malfunctioning shunt	History of ventriculoperitoneal, ventriculopleural, or ventriculoatrial shunt

Adapted from Fenichel G: *Clinical pediatric neurology: a signs and symptoms approach*, ed 4, Philadelphia, 2001, WB Saunders, pp 85-89.

Counseling. For nonorganic headaches (e.g., no tumor, aneurysm, or metabolic or structural cause), reassure the parents and patient. The patient should be taught pain and stress management techniques. School attendance should be mandatory, although a quiet rest period may be allowed at school if needed. School nurses can be helpful in developing a plan for school attendance. If the child remains home, activities should be restricted to bed and only homework done. The child should be returned to school if the pain improves during the school day. Minimize attention to the headache. Relaxation exercises or biofeedback training can be helpful. Trigger factors should be avoided.

Complications. Brain tumors, abscesses, hematomas, and arteriovenous malformations in children are generally associated with ataxia, papilledema, intellectual changes, or behavioral changes. These processes crowd out other intracranial structures, precipitating edema and interfering with the normal actions of CSF and vessels. Infants may initially accommodate well to the increase in intracranial pressure because of the ability of their cranial sutures to expand. Serious pathology is also indicated with headaches that interrupt sleep, increase in frequency and severity over a period of only a few weeks, occur on rising and then fade, are exacerbated by changes in position or with straining, persist at the occiput, or are related to personality, ataxic, or behavioral changes. If a headache is symptomatic of a brain tumor, 95% will have reported the headaches for under 4 months (Menkes & Sarnat, 2000).

Head Injury

Description. Head trauma involves tissue damage to the brain and its surrounding structures, and injury can range from mild to severe. Head injuries can be either open or closed. Open head injuries produce more focal injuries. Closed head injuries cause more multifocal or diffuse damage. Primary effects are from the initial injury and are related to mechanical forces that tear connections within the brain and cause contusions where the brain hits the skull surfaces (e.g., shaken baby syndrome). Axons to distant areas, fibers in the corpus callosum connecting the two hemispheres, or both can be torn. Contusions and hemorrhage can occur. Secondary effects of the trauma, such as hypoxia, ischemia, hypotension, brain swelling, hemorrhage, contusion, and status epilepticus, can affect recovery. Brain injury is the leading cause of death in those under 35 years of age. Half of all deaths due to such injuries occur in children under 15 years, with males being victims twice as much as females. Children in special education and those with a diagnosis of attention-deficit hyperactivity disorder (ADHD) often suffer recurrent episodes of head trauma (Semrud-Clikeman, 2001).

Clinical Findings and Management. Immediate assessment and care of a head-injured patient is outside the scope of this chapter. More information is found in Chapter 40, including the Glascow Coma Scale (GCS), which has been traditionally used to measure the severity of head injury. The reliability of the GCS has been recently questioned as to the value of its accuracy in predicting outcome. Schaan, Jaksche, and Boszczyk (2002) noted the difficulties of the requisite site-of-accident GCS score and difficulty "scaling" patients because of sedation and intubation. New scales that combine CT scans and clinical parameters (pupil dilation, hemiparesis, and brainstem signs) to predict outcome are being researched. It is acknowledged by Schaan, Jaksche, and Boszczyk (2002) that predictive scales of outcome alone should not be used to modify patient management (Table 28-9).

The NP is likely to encounter posttrauma patients. Seizures occur in 3% to 5% of children after head trauma, usually within the first 24 hours. The impact of mild to moderate head injury on school performance and adjustment can be significant. Eighty percent of children with a history of severe head injury require special education. Both clinicians and school personnel should be alert to a lack of progress and deterioration of skills. There is a strong association between development before and after head injury and behavioral problems (Semrud-Clikeman, 2001). Children (2 to 6 years) are usually more impaired than adolescents, secondary to immature brain development and general vulnerability. The longer the coma, the poorer the outcome; the greater the CNS damage, the greater the number of psychologic disorders that result. A neuropsychologic evaluation may be helpful to plan appropriate educational and behavioral management.

The most common causes of head trauma differ according to age. Infants and toddlers are more likely to obtain head trauma from falls, physical abuse, and motor vehicle accidents. Young children suffer head trauma from pedestrian and bicycle accidents, and adolescents suffer head trauma from motor vehicle accidents in which they are the driver (Semrud-Clikeman, 2001). Concussions are commonly related to sports injuries. See Chapter 15 for information

TABLE 28-9 ***Head Injury Acuity***

Characteristics	Mild	Moderate	Severe
Length of time patient was unconscious or had posttraumatic amnesia	<1 hr	1-24 hr	>24 hr
Glasgow Coma Scale score	13-15	9-12	3-8
Symptoms	Usually alert in the emergency department with headache, lethargy, irritability, withdrawn, may or not be labile	Occasional brain swelling and hematomas. Headache, concentration/problem solving and memory problems; symptoms can last for several months.	Approximately 50% mortality rate; impaired memory, concentration, and organizational skill problems.
Sequelae	Repeated "minor" damage (e.g., head trauma with sports) can result in changes in neuropsychology (attention, arousal and information processing). ADHD, decreased attention span, emotional changes, sleep disturbances, memory problems, headache, language deficits can result.	Same as for "mild."	Seizures, hemaparesis, aphasia, cognitive problems, behavior changes. Anxiety, attention problems (similar to ADHD).

Adapted from Semrud-Clikeman M: *Traumatic brain injury in children and adolescents: assessment and intervention,* New York, 2001, Guilford Press.
ADHD, Attention-deficit hyperactivity disorder.

on posttrauma management of head injuries related to sports.

Prevention. Wearing helmets by children using bicycles, skateboards, scooters, motorcycles, and in-line skates prevents many head injuries. Protection of children from falls in the home or from playground equipment is also important in reduction of head injuries. School-age children and adolescents should have properly fitting headgear appropriate for their sports participation. Adequate seat restraints can reduce the incidence of head injuries from motor vehicle accidents.

Prevention of secondary brain trauma from hemorrhage, edema, and other factors can be maximized by the prompt management of head trauma events.

Disturbances of Head Growth

Macrocephaly. *Macrocephaly* is defined as a head circumference more than 2 standard deviations (SD) above the mean for age and sex or one that increases too rapidly. "Large" heads may be genetic and only of statistical significance; the NP's initial evaluation should be to measure both parents' head circumferences. Macrocephaly can also be attributed to hydrocephaly, megalencephaly (enlarged brain), subdural hematoma, tumor, thickening of the skull, or other problems. Benign familial macrocephaly occurs as or can be related to a genetic syndrome (anatomic or metabolic), such as Sotos syndrome (cerebral gigantism). At birth, infants with anatomic megalencephaly will have macrocephaly at birth, but those with a metabolic etiology will be normocephalic at birth. In cases of excessive volumes of CSF, the fluid may be located within the brain (in the ventricular cavities) or outside the brain, in the subarachnoid spaces.

A CT scan can be diagnostic with consultation or referral if abnormal. A CT finding of "benign enlargement of the subarachnoid spaces" is transient in nature. The subarachnoid enlargement resolves by school age, though the macrocephaly will remain (Piatt, 2000).

Hydrocephaly. Hydrocephaly is a condition in which an increased volume of CSF causes progressive ventricular dilation. The etiology includes a wide variety of disorders, such as infection, tumor, hemorrhage, and congenital malformation. The patient can have a large head, an excessive rate of head growth, irritability, vomiting, loss of appetite, impaired upgaze and other extraocular movements, hypertonia, and hyperreflexia. Papilledema may not be present in an infant, whereas it does appear in older children with closed cranial sutures. In a neonate, the head can sometimes be transilluminated. Prompt referral and surgical treatment are necessary.

Microcephaly. *Microcephaly* is defined as a head circumference 2 SD below the mean for age and sex or one that is increasing slower than normal. Different ethnic groups have different standards of head circumferences. On examination, the skull will appear to be normally shaped; palpation may reveal some overlapping bones along the suture lines. This disorder can result from conditions in which the brain never formed correctly because of genetic or chromosomal abnormalities. Disease processes that interfere with normal brain growth can also be causative (these infants will be born with normal head circumferences at birth). Brain damage that occurs prenatally will not be evidenced initially, but a decreasing head circumference curve will start to occur after the infant reaches 3 to 6 months of age. A head circumference less than 3 SD below the mean for age and sex can indicate later mental retardation (Fenichel, 2001).

Commonly, microcephalic children have delayed developmental milestones and neurologic problems. Management of microcephaly is supportive and directed toward management of the resulting deficits. Protein-calorie malnutrition, craniosynostosis, and hypopituitarism are treatable causes of microcephaly. Referral to a pediatrician or neurologist should be made for diagnosis. Development of an interdisciplinary management plan may be useful.

Craniosynostosis. The NP needs to be able to distinguish between primary and secondary skull malformations. Congenital (or "true" or "primary") craniosynostosis involves early closure or absence of skull sutures. More than one suture can be involved, although this phenomenon is more often found when there is an associated syndrome (Rohan, Golombek, & Rosenthal, 1999). Growth along the remaining open suture lines produces progressive skull deformity in one or more directions. The skull is flat over the closed suture(s). Increased intracranial pressure can result as the brain tries to grow within the confined space. Primary craniosynostosis occurs in 1 to 2.5 per 1000 births, is ethnically neutral, and can vary in type and prominence between genders (Berkowitz, 2000). Craniosynostosis can be found in over 60 genetic syndromes—Crouzon, Apert, Carpenter, Chotzen, Pfeiffer, and others. The sagittal suture is most commonly fused. In young infants the frontal metopic suture may normally be prominent, but this is not clinically significant and does not require intervention (Menkes & Sarnat, 2000).

An initial skull radiograph is indicated should craniosynostosis be suspected. A follow-up CT scan may be needed, as indicated by the x-ray results. However, often the most expedient action for the NP to take is to refer the patient to an experienced pediatric neurosurgeon or craniofacial plastic surgeon first. Treatment is often surgical. If the condition is genetic, management will need to be planned according to the problems associated with the syndrome. Genetic counseling is important.

Secondary synostosis results when outside forces put pressure on the growing cranium, causing the skull to become misshapen (referred to as *deformational plagiocephaly*). This is most commonly seen with premature infants (termed *deformational scaphocephaly*), after shunting in an infant with hydrocephaly (termed *sagittal synostosis*), in children who have microcephaly and aberrant positioning in utero, during birth, or perinatally because of torticollis or positioning traditions. The success of the Back to Sleep campaign has resulted in infants with secondary (or pressure-related) occipital flattening but without the compensatory growth along other suture lines seen with primary synostosis. Most cases of deformational plagiocephaly are self-correcting through positional changes; sometimes physical therapy is indicated in recalcitrant cases (e.g., with torticollis). Figure 28-3 illustrates the different descriptions for the deformities of primary craniosynostosis.

Central Nervous System Infections

Description. All the infections of the CNS have similar symptoms. These infections can be manifested acutely (over 1 to 24 hours) or chronically (over 1 to 7 days or more).

Etiology. Bacteria, viruses, fungi, spirochetes, protozoa, and parasites can all cause CNS infection. The meninges, superficial cortical structures, blood vessels, and brain parenchyma can be involved. The most common microbes are as follows (Fenichel, 2001):

- Newborn: group B streptococci, *Escherichia coli, Listeria monocytogenes*, and other enterobacteria
- Infancy and preschool age: bacterial infections most common—*Haemophilus influenzae* type B, *Neisseria meningitidis, Streptococcus pneumoniae, Mycobacterium tuberculosis*
- School age: *N. meningitidis, S. pneumoniae, M. tuberculosis*

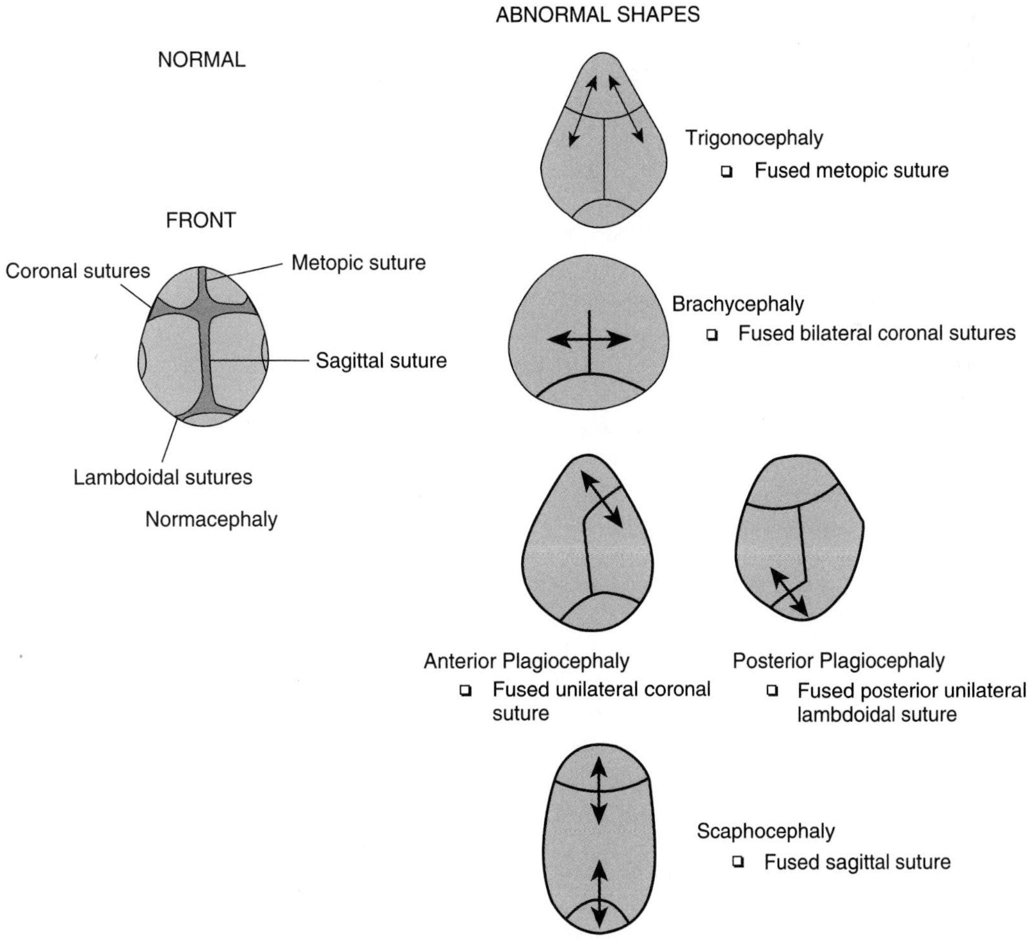

FIGURE 28-3 Characteristics of skull deformities seen with craniosynostosis. (Adapted from Cohen MM: Craniosynostosis update 1987, *Am J Med Genet Suppl* 4:99-148, 1988.)

Clinical Findings

History. The following may be noted from the history:

- Recent head injury or neurosurgical procedure
- Immunodeficiency diseases
- Infections of the sinuses or other structures of the head

Physical Examination. Findings on physical examination include the following:

- Systemic signs, including fever; malaise; impaired heart, lung, or kidney function
- CNS signs, including headache; stiff neck and spine; nausea and vomiting; fever or hypothermia; changes in mental status, ranging from irritability to lethargy or coma; seizures; and focal or sensory deficits in cranial nerves, notably III, IV, and VI
- Presence of Kernig or Brudzinski sign of meningeal irritation (may be absent in a young infant)
- Bulging fontanel and increasing head circumference in a young infant
- Papilledema late in the course in older children or adolescents
- Cranial nerve palsies

By age, the most common findings are as follows:

- From 0 to 3 months: fever, hypothermia, lethargy, irritability, poor feeding, apnea, focal seizures, enteric or respiratory symptoms; nuchal rigidity and a bulging fontanel (infrequent)
- From 3 months to 5 years: petechial rash, localized CNS signs as described earlier
- From 6 to 18 years: petechial rash, cranial nerve VII palsy (Lyme disease), sinusitis symptoms, localized CNS signs

Diagnostic Studies. Blood cultures, CBC with differential, urinalysis, chemistry panel, and lumbar puncture for CSF studies are done. Enterovirus meningitis and herpes simplex virus rapid tests are available. EEGs, CT or MRI scan, and brain biopsy may be needed.

Management and Complications. The NP needs to refer all children with potential CNS infection as rapidly as possible. Hypovolemia, hypoglycemia, hyponatremia, acidosis, septic shock, increased intracranial pressure, seizures, and other complications can occur quickly and need aggressive management. Hearing loss can occur in all forms of meningitis. Blindness, hydrocephaly, cerebral palsy, seizures, and developmental delays can also occur depending on the type of organism involved. Outcomes depend on the following four factors (Menkes & Sarnat, 2000):

- Type of infectious agent and severity of initial infection
- Age of patient (the younger, the worse the outcome)
- Length of symptoms before the diagnosis and initiation of treatment
- Antibiotic used and amount

The Floppy Infant

A floppy infant should arouse suspicion. The otherwise alert baby has hypotonia and depressed spontaneous movements. Other symptoms seen in a range of known causes include seizures, failure to react to pain, muscle wasting, absent reflexes, tongue fasciculation, and unilateral muscular movement deficits (Finberg & Kleinman, 2002). Etiologies usually focus on a metabolic or CNS dysfunction or a systemic illness. Most conditions involving the CNS are serious and lasting; others may be transitory, such as a brachial plexus nerve palsy after birth or congenital myasthenia gravis. Hypotonic infants can increase their tone over the first year of life and then demonstrate spastic CP. A baby can have low tone but still not lack strength when actively moving. The infant may also be weak, which means that its maximum effort lacks strength. Babies with Werdnig-Hoffmann disease (infantile spinal muscular atrophy) are weak. Floppy infants with brisk reflexes almost certainly have a CNS disorder. Acquired floppy infant syndrome has been known to occur in breastfed infants whose mothers were vegetarian; these infants were found to be deficient in cobalamin intake (Renault et al, 1999). Prenatal use of benzodiazepines has resulted in neonatal hypotonia (Gonzalez de Dios, Moya-Benavent, & Carratala-Marco, 1999). All these babies need to be referred to specialists, including a geneticist. The diagnostic tool of choice is the MRI; sometimes muscle biopsies or various neurophysiologic studies are employed. Many conditions of floppy infant syndrome do not respond well to treatment; rehabilitation can help maximize function (Finberg & Kleinman, 2002).

Reye Syndrome

Description and Etiology. Reye syndrome is an encephalopathy that is decreasing in incidence. It is a systemic disorder of mitochondrial function occurring during or after a viral infection and, more often, with the use of salicylates during such viral illnesses (Fenichel, 2001). Inborn metabolic disorders are also frequently associated with symptoms suggestive of Reye syndrome (Burg et al, 2002). Infrequent cases are seen with varicella or nonspecific respiratory infections, notably *H. influenzae* type B. The decline has been associated with the decreased use of salicylates in younger children.

Clinical Findings. Unless treated, the clinical course in Reye syndrome proceeds in five predictable stages. After the initial prodromal symptoms of the illness, severe vomiting then progresses to irrational behavior; to stupor and coma; to apnea, fixed pupils, and decorticate posturing with increasing brain edema; and then to death.

Management. Immediate referral with admission to a hospital setting for supportive care is essential. About 70% of patients survive, some with severe neurologic sequelae. Infants are more severely affected than older children.

Tethered Cord

The spinal cord is attached to the base of the brain and free at the caudal end, allowing for freedom of movement during growth, activities, and skeletal changes (including such abnormalities as scoliotic curves). With a tethered cord, however, the caudal end is fixed, causing abnormal stretching and damage to nerve cells, fibers, and blood vessels. Eventually symptoms of neurologic deterioration occur (Tarcan et al, 2001). It is often associated with a congenital spinal anomaly, such as spina bifida (90%), but tethering can also result from bony protrusions, tough membranous bands, lipomas, tumors, cysts, scarring, and trauma in the caudal equina area.

Not all tethering leads to clinical symptoms. If symptoms do occur, they manifest as functional deficits to nerves that emanate from the caudal equina area. Common findings or complaints include leg weakness, incontinence of bladder and bowel (or worsening of such), back or leg pain (especially with flexion/extension), groin or genitorectal pain, loss of reflexes and sensation in the legs, scoliosis, or deformity of the legs or hips (Royal Australian College of General Practitioner spinal bifida continence management guideline, 2002). Though not necessarily abnormal, the following skin changes are often seen in individuals later diagnosed with tethered cord and should be noted for reference: midline dimples, hair tufts, fatty deposits, birthmarks, and sacral sinuses or tracts. Symptoms are not necessarily evident in infancy but can be manifested in early childhood to adulthood (Fenichel, 2001).

Imaging methods of the entire spinal cord are used for diagnostic purposes (MRI). A referral to a pediatric neurosurgeon is indicated for suspect tethered cord. Surgery is usually the treatment of choice and can reverse or stabilize the neurologic functions. If a child has reached full skeletal height with minimal symptoms, monitoring is all that is often done. In children who have had surgery for tethered cord, the NP is encouraged to be watchful for retethering, which can occur as the child gets older. In a child with a history of repaired spina bifida, the NP needs to be vigilant for early symptoms of tethered cord.

Arnold-Chiari Malformation

Arnold-Chiari malformations consist of two types of uncommon congenital spinal cord anomalies whose sequelae are usually not evident until late childhood or into adulthood. Type I malformation involves the herniation of the caudal end of the cerebellar vermis through the foramen magnum. Type II malformation is present in 50% of children with lumbar meningomyelocele. The herniation can lead to brainstem and upper cervical cord compression that may ultimately cause necrosis of both structures. Etiology is believed to be secondary to embryonic segmentation disorders of the neural tube (Finberg & Kleinman, 2002).

The symptoms of a malformation may not be readily apparent. Type I malformation can cause headache, neck pain, atrophy and decreased reflexes in the lower extremities, sensory losses, and scoliosis. Any child with meningomyelocele should be suspected of having type II malformation. Type II malformation involves the same herniation as type I plus an alteration in the shape and development of the medulla. Further symptoms of type II may include hydrocephaly, respiratory distress, syncope, poor feeding, vomiting, dysphagia, tongue paralysis, and cardiopulmonary failure (Fenichel, 2001). Epilepsy is not related. Diagnosis is made by MRI and may inadvertently be found at the time of an MRI for a possibly unrelated reason (e.g., headache). Management strategies are not always successful; surgery to relieve the compression or a ventriculoperitoneal shunt may be tried in symptomatic cases. Older children may benefit from a cervical laminectomy to relieve compression as the child grows.

Meningomyelocele

Description. Failure of the vertebrae, skull, meninges, brain, or spinal cord to be encapsulated by the lamina of the vertebrae along the dorsal midline of the body is referred to as a *dysraphic defect.* Meningomyelocele refers to the protrusion of both the spinal cord nerve roots (myelo) and the three layers of membranes (meninges) that cover the spinal cord and brain through this spinal defect. The protruding dural sac may contain only the meninges (10% to 20% of cases) or both meninges and nerve roots (the remaining cases). The term *spina bifida cystica* is often used interchangeably with *meningomyelocele.* When the vertebral arches fail to close, but there is no subsequent herniation of cord or meninges, the term *spina bifida occulta* is used. Most cases of spina bifida cystica occur in the thoracolumbar area (90%). Meningoceles may also protrude through the skull and may or may not be covered with skin. Such a cranial meningocele consists only of a CSF-filled meningeal sac; no nerve roots are involved, and therefore no neurologic deficits exist. However, there may be brain malformation under the mass that does have neurologic consequences. Encephaloceles or cephaloceles refer to cranial lesions that contain a meningocele sac plus cerebral cortex, cerebellum, or portions of brainstem that protrude from fissures in the occipital (most common), frontal, or nasal cavity areas of the skull.

Functional mobility depends on the level and degree of the defect. At birth a child with a meningomyelocele in the lumbosacral area would demonstrate flaccid paralysis of the legs, sensory deficits below the spinal defect, neurogenic bladder, deformities of the ankles and feet, atrophied muscles, and possibly apnea if hydrocephaly is present. Long-term dysfunction would include flaccid paraplegia, continued sensory deficits, neurogenic bladder and bowel, and recurrent urinary tract infections (UTIs).

Etiology and Incidence. Closure of the neural tube usually occurs during the third and fourth weeks of gestation. Genetic and environmental factors are both believed to play a causative role in the failure of the closure to occur. A woman who has had a previous child born with dysraphia has about a 2% recurrence rate with future pregnancies. A lack of sufficient levels of folic acid and vitamin A increases the incidence of neural tube defects. All women of childbearing age are now encouraged to take 0.4 mg/day of folic acid. A woman wishing to conceive should take 4 mg/day for 4 weeks before conception and through the first trimester (Fenichel, 2001). Intake of other drugs and toxins is associated with neural tube defects; such drugs and toxins include retinoic acid derivatives (e.g., vitamin A, a paradox given that insufficient levels also cause the defect), valproic acid, and alcohol. Diabetes mellitus (including gestational diabetes), maternal hyperthermia during the first month of pregnancy, trisomy 18 and 13, and Meckel syndrome are also risk factors (Burg et al, 2002; Finberg & Kleinman, 2002).

The incidence in the United States is approximately 0.4 to 1 per 1000 live births; this rate is decreasing. African Americans have a lower incidence (Burg et al, 2002).

Clinical Findings. Diagnosis is made prenatally with the use of a maternal serum test to look for an increase in the concentration of α-fetoprotein; if elevated, an ultrasound and amniocentesis are done. α-Fetoprotein is the primary plasma protein that exists within the fetus and amniotic fluid. The concentration of the protein is elevated should there be a defect in the skin of the fetus. If the prenatal screen indicates that the fetus has possible spina bifida cystica, a fetal ultrasound will confirm the diagnosis. Cranial ultrasounds will be done to look for hydrocephaly (and in turn the Arnold-Chiari type II malformation). In the neonatal period, serial cranial ultrasounds are done to watch for the development of hydrocephaly, if this condition has not shown up prenatally. Other physical anomalies that can accompany meningomyelocele include cleft lip and palate, omphalocele, diaphragmatic hernia, tracheoesophageal fistula, congenital heart disease, bladder exstrophy, and imperforate anus (Burg et al, 2002). It is preferable that these infants be delivered by cesarean section.

Management and Complications. Management of a myelomeningocele entails surgical resection of the involved neural tube structures and closure within a week after birth. If surgery is not done during that time, death may result in the first year from meningitis or sepsis. Intrauterine surgery has also been successfully done to close the defect and prevent exposure of the neural tube to amniotic fluid and possible postnatal infection. If the defect occurs in a high spinal region or there is clinical hydrocephalus at birth, survival is also compromised. Despite early treatment, mental retardation is common in those with recalcitrant hydrocephaly, shunt problems, and ventriculitis; about 30% of those without such medical problems suffer cognitive deficits.

The NP's role in the care of a child with dysraphia involves delivering well-child care, assessing and treating acute illnesses (especially UTIs and constipation), monitoring shunt function, and communicating and often coordinating services with the myriad of specialists that will be involved (e.g., orthopedists, ophthalmologists [strabismus is common], neurologists, nephrologists, physical therapists, social workers, geneticists). In addition, the NP needs to be alert to the onset of symptoms indicative of Arnold-Chiari type II malformation and tethered cord, and watch for seizures (15% incidence), learning difficulties, and ADHD.

Tic Disorders

Tics, or habit spasms, are found in children and adults. Boys are two to three times more likely to be affected than girls. The most common time for onset is age 7 to 11 years (range is from 2 to 15 years). Four types of tic disorders are recognized: Tourette syndrome, transient tic disorder, chronic motor or vocal tic disorder, and unspecified type. Some tics can be suppressed with effort and are not a part of voluntary movements. Other forms of tics come and go spontaneously and tend to decrease when the child is out of school. Duration of affliction can be lifelong; half of the children with tics outgrow them in late adolescence. Others many experience this resolution only to see them recur in middle age.

Tourette syndrome is the most complex of the tic disorders. It is chronic, hereditary (autosomal dominant with varying levels of penetrance, which is gender related), and characterized by tics that vary in severity over time. Boys with Tourette syndrome frequently have concomitant ADHD, whereas girls are more likely to experience obsessive-compulsive disorder (OCD). One half of children are diagnosed with ADHD and one third with OCD (Fenichel, 2001). If the onset of tics is associated with the initiation of a drug, such as one for ADHD, the relationship is generally regarded now as less causative and more of an indication of a predisposition toward Tourette syndrome (Fenichel, 2001).

RESOURCE BOX

Neurologic Diseases

Brain Injury Association of America
1-800-444-6443
www.biausa.org/

International Rett Syndrome Association (IRSA)
1-800-818-RETT
www.rettsyndrome.org

National Headache Foundation
1-800-NHF-5552
www.headaches.org

National Spinal Cord Injury Association
1-800-962-9629
www.spinalcord.org

Spina Bifida Association of American
1-800-621-3141
www.sbaa.org

Tourette Syndrome Association, Inc.
1-718-224-2999
http://tsa-usa.org

United Cerebral Palsy
1-800-872-5827
www.ucpa.org

To meet the diagnostic criteria for Tourette syndrome, the tics must

- Be a combination of motor and verbal tics
- Be repeated many times every day for more than a year with no tic-free periods of longer than 3 months
- Cause marked distress or impairment socially, occupationally, or otherwise
- Begin before age 18 years
- Not be related to some other medical condition or substance use (American Psychiatric Association, 1995)

Simple motor tics usually affect the head, eyes, or face (eye blinks, eyebrow raising, nose flaring, grimacing, lip smacking); head or arm jerking, kicking, toe curling, and shoulder shrugging can also occur. More complex motor tics include head shaking, touching, hitting, jumping, smelling objects, repeating movements, self-mutilating activities such as lip biting, and other behavior. Initial vocal tics include sniffing, grunting or snorting, throat clearing, and coughing. Hissing and barking can occur, but swearing is rare in children. If swearing (or coprolalia) is repressed by the patient, it usually results in barking or coughing noises (Fenichel, 2001).

Differential Diagnosis. Consider hyperkinesis, choreiform (harder to suppress and occurs during voluntary movements) or dystonic movements, genetic disorder such as Huntington's or Wilson's disease, OCD, structural lesion in the brain, and pharmacologic side effect. Tics are not associated with degenerative diseases.

Management. Parents should be encouraged to ignore tics, given their tendency to wax and wane. The decision to treat with medicine depends on how much the tics bother the child rather than the parents (Fenichel, 2001). Pharmacologic management of motor or vocal tics may include haloperidol (Haldol), pimozide (Orap), fluphenazine (Prolixin), thiothixene (Navane), clonazepam (Klonopin), and clonidine (Catapres). Fluoxetine (Prozac) and other drugs have also been used. Drugs may need to be rotated to maintain effectiveness over time. Because of the comorbidity with ADHD and OCD, management strategies must also involve the family, educational measures, and other supportive measures, including medication.

REFERENCES

American Academy of Pediatrics Committee on Infectious Diseases: *2003 redbook: report of the Committee on Infectious Diseases*, ed 26, Elk Grove Village, IL, 2003, American Academy of Pediatrics.

American Psychiatric Association: *Diagnostic and statistical manual of mental disorders*, ed 4, Washington, DC, 1995, The Association.

Anderson P: *Basic human anatomy and physiology: clinical implications for the health professions*, Monterey, CA, 1984, Wadsworth.

Behrman R, Kliegman R, Jenson J: *Nelson textbook of pediatrics*, ed 16, Philadelphia, 2004, WB Saunders.

Berkowitz C: *Pediatrics: a primary care approach*, ed 2, Philadelphia, 2000, WB Saunders.

Bouma P, Peters A, Brouwer O: Long term course of childhood epilepsy following relapse after antiepileptic drug withdrawal, *J Neurol Neurosurg Psychiatry* 72(4):507-510, 2002.

Burg F et al, editors: *Gellis and Kagan's current pediatric therapy*, ed 17, Philadelphia, 2002, WB Saunders.

Children's Hospital Medical Center: *Evidence-based clinical practice guideline for medical management of first unprovoked seizure in children 2 to 18 years of age*, Cincinnati, 1999, Children's Hospital Medical Center.

Dotti M et al: A Rett syndrome MECP2 mutation that causes mental retardation in men, *Neurology* 58(2):226-230, 2002.

Evans R, Lewis D: Is an MRI scan indicated in a child with new-onset daily headache? *Headache* 41(9):905-906, 2001.

Fenichel GM: *Clinical pediatric neurology: a signs and symptoms approach*, ed 4, Philadelphia, 2001, WB Saunders.

Ferrari F et al: Cramped synchronized general movements in preterm infants as an early marker for cerebral palsy, *Arch Pediatr Adolesc Med* 156:422-423, 2002.

Finberg L, Kleinman R: *Saunders manual of pediatric practice*, ed 2, Philadelphia, 2002, WB Saunders.

Francis A: Diastat, an at-home treatment for adults and children makes patients feel empowered, *Advance for Nurses Online.* Available at *www.advancefornurses.com* (accessed Jan 29, 2003).

Gonzalez de Dios J, Moya-Benavent M, Carratala-Marco F: "Floppy infant" syndrome in twins secondary to the use of benzodiazepines during pregnancy, *Rev Neurol* 29(2):121-123, 1999.

Gordon K et al: Treatment of febrile seizures: the influence of treatment efficacy and side-effect profile on value to parents, *Pediatrics* 108(5):1080-1088, 2001.

Hershey A et al: Effectiveness of nasal sumatriptan in 5-12 year old children, *Headache* 41(7):693-697, 2001.

Hirtz D et al: Practice parameter: evaluating a first nonfebrile seizure in children. Report of the Quality Standards Subcommittee of the American Academy of Neurology, the Child Neurology Society, and the American Epilepsy Society, *Neurology* 55(5):616-623, 2000.

Hoekelman R: *Primary pediatric care*, ed 4, St Louis, 2001, Mosby.

International Rett Syndrome Association: Rett syndrome: rosetta stone of neurologic diseases. Available at *www.rettsyndrome.org* (accessed June 19, 2002).

Jackson Allen P, Vessey J: *Primary care of the child with a chronic condition*, ed 4, St Louis, 2004, Mosby.

Joy J, Johnston R, editors: *Multiple sclerosis: current status and strategies for the future*, Washington, DC, 2001, National Academies Press, pp 277-324.

Mast J: Cerebral palsy. In Burg F et al, editors: *Gellis and Kagan's current pediatric therapy*, ed 17, Philadelphia, 2002, WB Saunders.

Menkes J, Sarnat H: *Child neurology*, ed 6, Philadelphia, 2000, Lippincott Williams & Wilkins.

Miller F, Bachrach S: *Cerebral palsy: a complete guide for caregiving*, Baltimore, 1998, Johns Hopkins Press Health Book.

Milunsky J et al: Mutation analysis in Rett syndrome, *Genet Test* 5(4):321-325, 2001.

National Institute of Neurological Disorders and Stroke: *Cerebral palsy: hope through research*, Bethesda, MD, 2001, National Institutes of Health.

Piatt JH Jr: Infants heads: too big? Too small? Misshapen? For the primary physician, *Doernbecher J* 6(2):25-29, 2000.

Polaski A: *Luckmann's core principles and practice of medical-surgical nursing*, Philadelphia, 1996, WB Saunders.

Renault F et al: Neuropathy in two cobalamin-deficient breast-fed infants of vegetarian mothers, *Muscle Nerve* 22(2):252-254, 1999.

Reuter D, Brownstein D: Common emergent pediatric neurologic problems, *Emerg Med Clin North Am* 20(1):155-176, 2002.

Rohan A, Golombek S, Rosenthal A: Infants with misshapen skulls: when to worry, *Contemp Pediatr* 16(2):47-73, 1999.

Rosenblum R, Fisher P: A guide to children with acute and chronic headaches, *J Pediatr Health Care* 15(5):229-235, 2001.

Royal Australian College of General Practitioner spina bifida continence management guideline: spinal cord tethering, *Aust Fam Physican* 31(1):80-83, 2002.

Ryan M: Evaluating a first nonfebrile seizure in children, *Clin Adv* 5(3):76, 2002.

Ryther R: The genetics of febrile seizures, *Seizure Genetics Newsletter*, Vanderbilt University Epilepsy Genetics Research Group, Winter 2001. Available at *www.phg.mc.vanderbilt.edu/epilepsynews/epnews* (accessed July 7, 2002).

Schaan M, Jaksche H, Boszczyk B: Predictors of outcome in head injury: proposal of a new scaling system, *J Trauma* 52(4):667-674, 2002.

Scherer P, Krauss G: Seizure-related car crashes are uncommon, *Epilepsia* 42(suppl 7):215-216, 2001.

Semrud-Clikeman M: *Traumatic brain injury in children and adolescents: assessment and intervention*, New York, 2001, Guilford Press.

Sirven J, Sperling M, Wingerchuk D: Early versus late antiepileptic drug withdrawal for people with epilepsy in remission, *Cochrane Database Systems Review* 3:CD001902, 2001.

Suskind D, Tilton A: Clinical study of botulinum-A toxin in the treatment of sialorrhea in children with cerebral palsy, *Laryngoscope* 12(1):73-81, 2002.

Swaiman K, Ashwal S: *Pediatric neurology: principles and practice*, ed 3, St Louis, 1999, Mosby.

Tarcan T et al: Long-term followup of newborns with myelodysplasia and normal urodynamic findings: is followup necessary? *J Urol* 165(2):564-567, 2001.

29 Eye Problems

Catherine G. Blosser, Margaret A. MacDonald, Nancy Barber Starr

Ophthalmic diseases occur more often in the very young or elderly, with the exception of eye trauma, refractive errors, and some other disorders. Infants and children are particularly susceptible to permanent central visual loss (amblyopia), opacities (congenital cataracts), refractive errors, strabismus, and other conditions that interfere with visual acuity. With detection and correction, these conditions will not lead to permanent loss in the mature central visual system of the older child or adult (American Academy of Ophthalmology, 2002). Priorities of the nurse practitioner (NP) in caring for children with eye problems or concerns include promoting optimal growth and development of the ocular structures and maximizing visual acuity. To this end, NPs seek to maintain good vision and health, detect abnormalities, treat those conditions that fall within their scope of practice, refer patients with conditions requiring physician expertise, and provide education and reassurance to parents and children. In some cases, consultation with a pediatrician or family practice physician suffices to ensure optimal care. Other cases warrant direct referral to an ophthalmologist.

Care of blind or visually impaired children is discussed in Chapter 17 because there is a significant effect on development and learning.

STANDARDS FOR VISUAL SCREENING AND CARE

The objective related to vision in the *Healthy People 2010* objectives (U.S. Department of Health and Human Services, 2000) is to

- Increase the proportion of primary care providers who routinely refer or screen infants and children for impairments of vision, hearing, speech, and language and who assess other developmental milestones as part of well-child care.

The *Guide to Clinical Preventive Services* (U.S. Preventive Services Task Force, 1996) clinical intervention states the following:

- Vision screening to detect amblyopia and strabismus is recommended once for all children before entering school, preferably between ages 3 and 4. Clinicians should be alert for signs of ocular misalignment when examining infants and children. Stereoacuity testing may be more effective than visual acuity testing in detecting these conditions. Evidence is insufficient to recommend for or against routine screening for diminished visual acuity among asymptomatic schoolchildren. Recommendations against such screening may be made on other grounds, including the inconvenience and cost of routine screening and the fact that refractive errors can be readily corrected when they produce symptoms.

Put Prevention into Practice: The Clinician's Handbook of Preventive Services (U.S. Public Health Service, 1997) outlines recommendations from major authorities, including the following:

- The American Academy of Pediatrics (AAP) and Bright Futures: All children from birth to 2 years of age need their external eye structures assessed at each well-child examination. Visual acuity testing should first be performed at 3 years of age. If the child is uncooperative, retesting should occur 6 months later. Subsequent testing should occur at 4, 5, 10, 12, 15, and 18 years of age. Subjective assessment by history should occur during visits at all other ages. All infants should be examined by 6 months of age to evaluate fixation preference, alignment, and the presence of any eye disease. Children should again be medically evaluated for these problems by 3 to 4 years of age. Children who are difficult to screen (infants, toddlers, children with developmental delays) should undergo photoscreening techniques to detect amblyopia, media opacities, and treatable ocular disease processes (AAP, 2002).

- The American Academy of Ophthalmology (AAO), the American Association for Pediatric Ophthalmology and Strabismus (AAPOS), and the American Optometric Association (AOA): Eye and vision screening should be performed at birth and approximately 6 months, 3 years, and 5 years of age. The AAO has published recommendations regarding screening methods and indications for referral to be used by primary care clinicians in screening preschool children (see Tables 29-3 and 29-4). Screening after 5 years of age should occur every 2 years throughout the school years and may be performed during routine health care visits, in preschool and day care settings, at schools, or at public screenings.

For high-risk children, the AAO recommends that asymptomatic children have a comprehensive examination by an ophthalmologist if they are at high risk because of health and developmental problems that make screening by the primary care clinician difficult or inaccurate (e.g., retinopathy of prematurity [ROP] or diagnostic evaluation of a complex disease with ophthalmologic manifestations); a family history of conditions that cause or are associated with eye or vision problems (e.g., retinoblastoma, significant hyperopia, strabismus [particularly accommodative esotropia], amblyopia, congenital cataract, or glaucoma); or multiple health problems, systemic disease, or the use of medications that are known to be associated with eye disease and vision abnormalities (e.g., neurodegenerative disease, juvenile rheumatoid arthritis, systemic steroid therapy, systemic syndromes with ocular manifestations, or developmental delay with visual system manifestations).

DEVELOPMENT AND PHYSIOLOGY OF THE EYE

Development of the Ocular Structures

At 21 days of gestation the human embryo is one fifth of an inch in length, and the first recognizable ocular tissue is visible on each side of the head. Within 10 days the eyes become much more prominent and, by the end of the eighth week, have moved medially toward the front of the face. The eyelids are completely formed, and the edges of the upper and lower lids fuse and seal the eye while it develops. At 16 weeks of gestation the eyes are fully anterior, and over the ensuing weeks they continue to move closer to the bridge of the nose. By the seventh month of pregnancy the fetus can open its eyes.

Development of the eye as a visual organ is not complete at birth, yet newborns have the ability to fix their gaze, follow an object to midline, and react to a change in the intensity of light. Over the first 2 to 3 months of extrauterine life, the ability to focus at any range develops as the eyes become coordinated horizontally and vertically. By 3 months of age, infants can follow moving objects, and by 4 months, they can indicate visual recognition of familiar objects. The shape and contour of the eyeball change, and visual acuity and binocularity gradually increase with age. The size of the orbits doubles by the time the child is 1 year of age and doubles again by 6 years of age. When eye growth is completed at 10 to 12 years of age, the diameter of the eyeball is about 2.5 cm.

During early childhood, the visual pathways are developing that will ensure central vision. The brain must receive equally clear, bilaterally focused images, at the same time, for this development to occur. The visual pathways are amenable to corrective influences (e.g., adequate treatment of amblyopia) until age 10 years (AAO, 2002).

Anatomy and Physiology of the Eye

The eyeball consists of three layers of tissue: the fibrous tunic, the vascular tunic, and the inner tunic or retina (Fig. 29-1). The fibrous tunic consists of the sclera and the cornea. The vascular tunic, the middle layer, is composed of the choroid, the ciliary body, and the iris. All the structures of the eye are dedicated to accurate and efficient functioning of the innermost layer of the eyeball, the retina. The optic disc consists only of nerve fibers (no rods or cones), so no visual images are formed here. Thus it is referred to as the blind spot.

The inside of the eyeball consists of the anterior and posterior cavities. The anterior cavity is divided into anterior and posterior chambers. The anterior chamber lies between the cornea and the iris. The posterior chamber lies between the iris and the suspensory ligament. Aqueous humor circulates throughout these chambers to maintain intraocular pressure and link the circulatory system with the avascular lens and cornea. The other cavity within the eyeball, the posterior cavity, lies between the lens and the retina. The gelatinous vitreous humor found in this cavity contributes to the maintenance of intraocular pressure and holds the retina in place. The lens, which separates the cavities, hangs by the suspensory ligament. Six muscles guide movement of the globe. Four rectus muscles (superior, inferior, lateral, and medial) move the eyeball up, down, in, and out, respectively. Two oblique muscles (superior and inferior) rotate the eyeball on its axis. Cranial nerves III (oculomotor), IV (trochlear), and VI (abducens) innervate these muscles.

The focusing of light rays involves four basic processes: refraction of light rays, accommodation of the lens, constriction of the pupil, and convergence of the eyes. *Refraction* is the bending of light rays as they pass from one

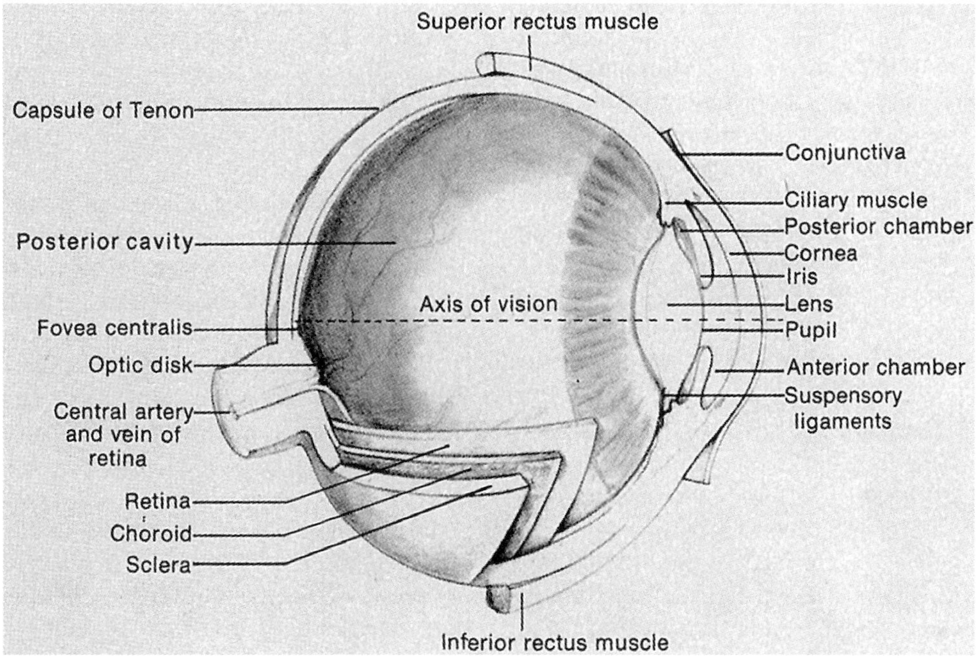

FIGURE 29-1 Structure of the eye, transverse section. (From Anderson PD: *Basic human anatomy and physiology: clinical implications for the health professions*, Sudbury, MA, 1984, Jones & Bartlett. Copyright ©1984, Jones & Bartlett Publishers, *www.jbpub.com*. Reprinted with permission.)

transparent medium (air) to another (cornea or lens). The lens modifies the degree of refraction to create the sharpest image on the retina. *Accommodation* is the ability of the lens to focus on close objects by increasing its curvature. The normal eye refracts light rays from an object 20 feet away to focus a clear image onto the retina; hence the fraction 20/20 is used to denote the accepted standard of normal vision. The circular muscle fibers of the iris, which contract in response to light, cause constriction of the pupil. Regulating the light entering the eye can also facilitate production of a precise image. To maintain single binocular vision, close objects require the eyes to rotate medially so that the light rays from the object hit the same points on both retinas. This rotation is called *convergence.* A normal neonate demonstrates disconjugate fixation, but convergence and accommodation normally develop by 3 to 4 months of age, with parallel alignment by 5 to 6 months of age without nystagmus or strabismus.

After an image is formed on the retina, light impulses are converted into nerve impulses and transmitted to the visual centers located in the occipital lobes of the cerebral cortex. Lesions in various places along the neural tracts from the eye to the cortex cause different types of loss of visual fields (Fig. 29-2).

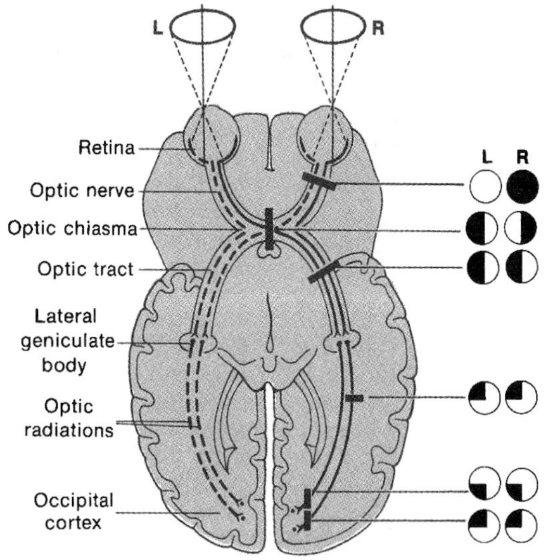

FIGURE 29-2 Visual pathway. On the right are diagrams of the visual fields with areas of blindness darkened to show the effects of injuries in various locations. (From Anderson PD: *Basic human anatomy and physiology: clinical implications for the health professions*, Sudbury, MA, 1984, Jones & Bartlett. Copyright ©1984, Jones & Bartlett Publishers, *www.jbpub.com*. Reprinted with permission.)

PATHOPHYSIOLOGY OF THE EYES

Potential problems with the eyes or visual system can take the form of specific disorders, infections, or injuries to the eye. The most common disorders of the eye interfering with vision are refractive errors (myopia, hyperopia, astigmatism, and anisometropia). Less common disorders include strabismus, amblyopia, ptosis, nystagmus, cataracts, glaucoma, ROP, and retinoblastoma. Infections and injuries may be relatively minor and superficial or be critical and involve deep tissues of the eye. Certain systemic diseases (e.g., juvenile rheumatoid arthritis) and medications (e.g., steroids) can also affect the eyes and warrant extra assessment measures.

ASSESSMENT

Assessment of the eye, as with all body systems, requires a thoughtful history and careful physical examination, as well as certain specialized screening tests.

History

The history should include the following:

- Medical history
  - Systemic history: birth weight; pertinent prenatal, perinatal, postnatal factors (e.g., prematurity, infections); past hospitalizations and surgery, general health and development
  - Ocular history, including date (and results) of the last vision screening and prior eye problems or diseases, including diagnoses and treatments
  - If history of eye injury: unilateral or bilateral injury? Were there visual changes or photophobia?
  - Family medical history of ocular problems (including eye surgeries) such as glaucoma, blindness, poor vision, difficulty walking in dim light, photophobia, use of thick glasses, lazy eye, strabismus, nystagmus, leukokoria, retinoblastoma, congenital cataracts
  - History of chronic systemic disease in patient or family (e.g., inflammatory bowel disease, connective tissue disorders, cardiac defects of Marfan syndrome, midfacial hypoplasia; abnormalities of teeth, umbilical cord, or urinary tract; neurologic or skin anomalies, developmental delay, mental retardation, diabetes, sickle cell hemoglobinopathies, Tay-Sachs disease, tuberculosis)
  - Presence of allergies and to what substances
  - Current medications (e.g., steroids); past or present substance abuse
  - Prescription and use of eyeglasses or contact lenses (Does the child have glasses that were prescribed? Are they used? If not, why?); use of sunglasses with ultraviolet (UV) protection or protective glasses
- Present symptoms of eye dysfunction or disease
  - Visual loss or change in vision such as blurring, diplopia, spots, and halos in older children; problems with fixing, tracking, squinting, head tilt, eye-hand coordination, grasp, gait, balance, behavior, and changes in the ability to maintain eye contact in younger children
  - Pain or sensitivity to light (photophobia) resulting in irritability and shielding or rubbing of the eyes
  - Swollen eyelids, pruritus, excessive tearing or discharge, erythema, burning, eye fatigue, strabismus
  - Constant blinking, chronic bulbar conjunctival injection

Physical Examination

The physical examination can be challenging, depending on the child's age. The components need to be done quickly to accommodate the child's short attention span. Knowledge of visual developmental norms is essential in assessing a child's visual capabilities (Table 29-1). The examination should include the following:

- Gross inspection should be made of the external structures (lids, bulbar conjunctiva, lacrimal structures, and the size, symmetry, and reactivity of the pupils), orbits, eye muscle balance, and mobility.
- The red reflex is tested in all ages. It needs to be assessed for color, intensity, and clarity (opacities or white spots).
- In older children, funduscopic examination allows for visualization of the retina, choroid, fovea, macula, optic disc and cup, and entry and exit of the vessels and nerves.

TABLE 29-1 *Normal Visual Developmental Milestones*

Birth-2 wk:	Infant sees and responds to change in illumination; refuses to reopen eyes after exposure to bright light; increasing alertness to objects; fixes on contrasts (e.g., black and white).
2-4 wk:	Infant fixes on an object.
By 1 mo:	Infant fixes on and follows an object.
By 3-4 mo:	Infant recognizes parent's smile; looks from near to far and focuses close again; beginning development of depth perception; follows 180-degree arc; reaches toward toy.
By 4 mo:	Color vision near that of an adult; tears are present.
By 6-10 mo:	Infant fixes on and follows toy in all directions.
By 12 mo:	Vision is close to fully developed.

- Examination of the eye is sometimes facilitated by using a cotton-tipped applicator to evert the eyelid. Eyelid eversion is accomplished by having the patient look down while the examiner grasps the lashes with the thumb and index finger, places the applicator in the middle of the lid, pulls the eyelid down and out, and everts it over the applicator. Irrigation of the eye with normal saline is another technique useful in situations where removal of a foreign body or irritating substance is desired.
- Growth parameters (especially head growth and shape) and the head and neck or other structures should be examined if a systemic condition is suspected.
- A rule of thumb is that if the examiner cannot see into the eye (e.g., absent red light reflex), the patient cannot see out.

Screening Tests

Conducting Screening Tests

Fatigue, hunger, anxiety, and environmental distractions can interfere with vision testing. Testing should always precede the administration of immunizations or any procedure that might cause discomfort. While testing, observe children for behavior indicating that they are having difficulty, such as straining, squinting, excessive blinking, head tilting or shaking, and thrusting of the trunk and head forward. The tendency to peek out from behind the eye shield may or may not reflect difficulty; the child may do so out of a desire to be successful and please the tester. The examiner should also resist the tendency to correct a mistake or give the child nonverbal clues that can influence the results. Children who have difficulty performing any of the vision tests in the primary care provider's office should be tested again at another time.

Red Light Reflex

Performing an adequate red light reflex test (Bruchner test) will allow the NP to detect the presence of asymmetric refractive errors, strabismic deviations, and abnormalities in the ocular media (e.g., cataracts, corneal abnormalities, retinoblastoma). Disease processes involving the cornea, lens, vitreous, or retina will block the light from entering or exiting the pupil and result in an abnormal red light reflex. The recommended technique follows:

- Darken the examination room (a lighted room will cause the pupils to constrict, causing a poor red reflex). The darker the room, the easier it is to detect more subtle asymmetries between the red reflexes.
- Stand 2 to 3 feet away from the infant/child and use the ophthalmoscope light set at 0 or +1 to illuminate the face.
- Look at both pupils simultaneously and separately; observe the red reflexes for symmetry. Examining the red reflex slightly off-axis to the center of the pupil enhances the color (ask a child to look to one side or use a distraction; infants can be approached from the side).
- The red reflexes should be symmetric; any dark spots, opacities, or leukokoria requires prompt referral to an ophthalmologist.
- Dilation of the pupils with 1% tropicamide and 2.5% phenylephrine ophthalmic drops (allow 30 minutes for them to take effect) enhances the examination in questionable situations where asymmetric reflexes have been detected. Infants with a positive family history of retinoblastoma should have a dilated red reflex test done at 1 to 2 weeks of age and every 2 months (Lin & Edmond, 2003; Retinoblastoma International, 2000).
- The red light reflex can also be documented by taking a Polaroid shot of the patient's face in a darkened room from a distance of 3 to 5 feet.
- In children with fair skin pigmentation, the red reflex will be a bright red-orange color; in those with darker pigmentation, the red reflex will be a dark red-brown color.

Visual Acuity Testing

Visual acuity testing (Tables 29-2 and 29-3), for both near and distance vision, should be performed on all children every time they come for a routine checkup, when problems with visual acuity are suspected, and when eye trauma occurs. If the child wears eyeglasses or contact lenses, visual acuity measurement must be obtained with correction.

Color Vision Testing

The human retina contains 6 million red and green cones and approximately 1 million blue cones. Alterations in color vision occur when the normal photopigments in the photoreceptor cones are replaced with different ones. Color ranges are then interpreted or perceived differently.

TABLE 29-2 ***Visual Acuity Norms***

Age	Visual Acuity	Visual Range (Degrees)
Birth	20/100	45
6 wk	20/100	90
4 mo	20/80	180
1 yr	20/40	180
3-4 yr	20/30	180
6 yr	20/25 or 20/20	180

TABLE 29-3 Recommended Ages and Methods for Pediatric Eye Evaluation Screening

Recommended Age	Method	Indications for Referral to an Ophthalmologist
Newborn-3 mo	Red reflex	Abnormal or asymmetric
	Inspection	Structural abnormality
3-6 mo (approximately)	Fix and follow	Failure to fix and follow in a cooperative infant
	Red reflex	Abnormal or asymmetric
	Inspection	Structural abnormality
6-12 mo and until child is able to cooperate for verbal visual acuity	Fix and follow with each eye	Failure to fix and follow
	Alternate occlusion	Failure to object equally to covering each eye
	Corneal light reflex	Asymmetric
	Red reflex	Abnormal or asymmetric
	Inspection	Structural abnormality
3 yr (approximately)	Visual acuity* (monocular)	20/50 or worse, or 2 lines of difference between the eyes
	Corneal light reflex/cover-uncover reflex	Asymmetric/ocular refixation movements
	Red reflex	Abnormal or asymmetric
	Inspection	Structural abnormality
5 yr (approximately)	Visual acuity* (monocular)	20/40 or worse, or 2 lines of difference between the eyes
	Corneal light reflex/cover-uncover reflex	Asymmetric/ocular refixation movements
	Red reflex	Abnormal or asymmetric
	Inspection	Structural abnormality
Every 1-2 yr after age 5 yr	Visual acuity* (monocular)	20/30 or worse, or 2 lines of difference between the eyes
	Corneal light reflex/cover-uncover reflex	Asymmetric/ocular refixation movements
	Red reflex	Abnormal or asymmetric
	Inspection	Structural abnormality

From American Academy of Ophthalmology, Pediatric Ophthalmology Panel; *Preferred practice guidelines: pediatric eye evaluations*, San Francisco, 2002, American Academy of Ophthalmology.

NOTES: These recommendations are based on panel consensus. Although the child may be retested if screening is inconclusive or unsatisfactory, undue delays should be avoided; if inconclusive on retesting, referral for comprehensive pediatric medical eye evaluation is indicated.

Use of medication for papillary dilation facilitates evaluation of the red reflex. For infants, a combined weak solution of phenylephrine hydrochloride and cyclopentolate (Cyclomydril Ophthalmic [Alcon, Ft. Worth, TX]) is associated with fewer side effects. (Isenberg S, Everett S, Parelhoff E: A comparison of mydriatic eye drops in low-weight infants, *Ophthalmology* 92:278-279, 1984.)

*Figures, letter, "tumbling E" or optotypes, LEA symbols, vision-testing machines.

Red/green color deficiency is an X-linked inherited disorder. Inherited color deficiencies are more common in males and affect about 6% of males of European ancestry (females 0.26%); 3.1% of black, Native American, or Hispanic males (females 0.7%); and 4.9% of Asian males (females 0.64%) (Reichel, 2000).

Color vision deficiency may also be acquired. A patient with acquired deficiency may have had normal color vision and then experienced color changes and losses. Diabetes, infections, optic neuritis, and toxins are systemic conditions that can lead to such losses. Blue/yellow deficiency is the most common type of acquired color discrepancy.

Significant color blindness can affect school performance; can have safety implications, in that the child may be unable to distinguish traffic or vehicle brake lights; and can affect career choices. Color vision is tested by using the Hardy-Rand-Rittler test (for preschoolers) or Ishihara's plates (for school-age children).

Peripheral Vision Testing

Examination of peripheral visual fields provides information with regard to retinal function, the neuronal visual pathway to the brain, and the function of cranial nerve II (optic nerve). In an infant, assessment is limited to a rough estimate of peripheral visual fields by watching the child's response to a familiar object (e.g., bottle, toy) or a threatening gesture as it is brought into each of the four quadrants. In children mature enough to cooperate, peripheral visual fields can be measured by confrontation or by finger counting. Peripheral visual fields should be approximately

50 degrees upward, 70 degrees downward, 60 degrees medially (toward the nose), and 90 degrees laterally.

Testing for Ocular Mobility and Alignment

The Hirschberg test (also called the corneal light reflex) evaluates extraocular muscle function by projecting a small light source onto the cornea of the eye with the child looking straight ahead. A normal test reveals the reflected light as a small white dot symmetrically located in the same position of each eye (often slightly nasal of center). The cover-uncover test and the alternating cover test should be performed with the child fixating straight ahead, first on a near point and then on a far point about 20 feet away (Fig. 29-3). The process is sometimes aided by asking the child questions

CORNEAL LIGHT REFLEX

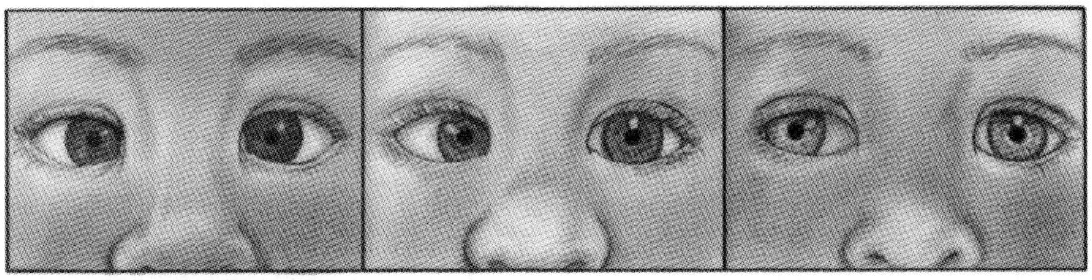

A Pseudostrabismus **B R Esotropia** **C R Exotropia**

Symmetric Corneal Light Reflex

A. *Pseudostrabismus* has the appearance of strabismus due to epicanthal fold but is normal for a young child.

Asymmetric Corneal Light Reflex

Strabismus is true disparity of the eye axes. This constant malalignment is also termed tropia and is likely to cause amblyopia.

B. Esotropia—inward turn of the eye.

C. Exotropia—outward turn of the eye.

COVER TEST

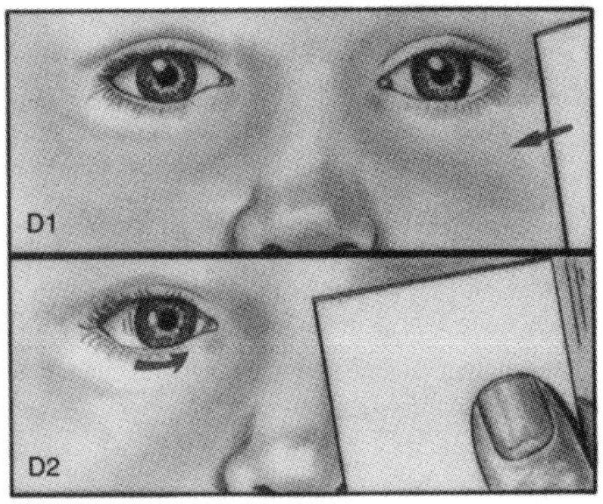

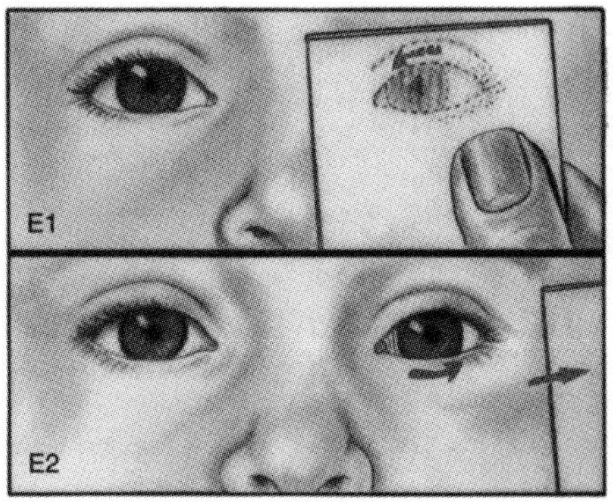

D Right, uncovered eye is weaker

D. Uncovered eye—if it jumps to fixate on designated point, it was out of alignment before (i.e., when you cover the stronger eye, the weaker eye now tries to fixate).

Phoria—mild weakness, apparent only with the cover test and less likely to cause amblyopia than a tropia but still possible.

E Left, covered eye is weaker

E. Covered eye—if this is the weaker eye, once macular image is suppressed it will drift to relaxed position.

As eye is uncovered—if it jumps to re-establish fixation, weakness exists.

Esophoria—nasal (inward) drift.

Exophoria—temporal (outward) drift.

FIGURE 29-3 Extraocular muscle function testing (corneal light reflex and cover test). (From Jarvis C: *Physical examination and health assessment*, ed 2, Philadelphia, 1996, WB Saunders, p 340.)

about the object (e.g., "How many cows do you see?"). During the alternating cover test the examiner rapidly covers and uncovers the eye while shifting between the two eyes. Any movement is an indication of misalignment.

Assessment of Visual Loss

If significant visual disturbance is suspected, the following functional vision assessments should be performed, the results documented, and the child referred immediately to an ophthalmologist:

- Shine a penlight into the eye from a lateral position and turn the light off and on several times to assess light perception. If the child can identify when the light is on or off, vision is described as "LP" (light perception).
- If hand movements can be seen 12 inches from the child's face, it is documented as "H/M at 1 ft." Indication of search and recognition should be seen as the hand is slowly moved back and forth with periodic cessation.
- Ask the child to count the number of fingers seen when one, two, or three fingers are held up 12 inches from the child's face. If the child is correct, document the vision as "C/F 1 ft."

Diagnostic Studies

Laboratory Studies

Studies such as a complete blood count (CBC), cultures, and Gram stain are done if identification of infection or particular organisms would be helpful in guiding management.

Ultrasound or radiographic studies such as computed tomography (CT) or magnetic resonance imaging (MRI) are sometimes useful in determining a diagnosis of orbital cellulitis, trauma, or tumor or in substantiating a concern about the central nervous system (CNS).

Fluorescein Staining

Fluorescein staining may be used to determine the extent of damage to the corneal epithelium as a result of trauma, infection, or exposure to a foreign body. Moisten a small strip of fluorescein tape and place it in the lower conjunctival cul-de-sac. Allow the fluorescein to mix with tears. Examine the cornea with a cobalt blue filter light; any injury will take up the fluorescein stain and appear as a greenish area.

Other Visual Testing Tools

Visual evoked cortical potentials testing involves delivering a stimulation to the CNS by displaying a specific checkerboard or striped grating of different special frequencies in front of the infant or child. An electrical response in the CNS is evoked. This test is used by ophthalmologists to estimate visual acuity in infants and children who are preverbal (McKeown, 2000). Preferential looking, or forced choice preferential looking, testing can be done in an ambulatory care setting. This requires use of special black-and-white and gray-striped cards to provide the spatial frequencies. Photoscreening systems screen for amblyogenic risk factors (strabismus, media opacities, major refractive errors) in infants, toddlers, and those with developmental delays. A camera or video system may be used to take images of the papillary and red reflexes. This system is undergoing more thorough study at the current time as to its applicability and practicability (AAP, 2002).

MANAGEMENT STRATEGIES

Referral for Ophthalmologic and Specialty Management

Many eye problems require referral to ophthalmologists or optometrists for management. See Table 29-4 for referral points. Although any child with eye pathology should be referred to an ophthalmologist, optometrists can be a valuable resource in caring for children with refractive errors or certain common eye conditions (e.g., corneal abrasions, foreign bodies). It is recommended that NPs acquaint themselves with the statutory guidelines for scope of practice and prescription privileges as designated by the state boards of optometry within their state in order to optimize referral possibilities.

Ophthalmologic or optometric management of potential or present central vision deficiencies may include the following:

Occlusion

Patching one eye or using pharmacologic penalization to occlude the vision in one eye are techniques used to treat strabismus and improve or prevent amblyopia.

Corrective Lenses

In children, eyeglasses are used to correct refractive errors. Contact lenses are occasionally recommended for older children (and frequently for adolescents) (Box 29-1). Keratorefractive (Lasik) surgery is undergoing research in the United States and other countries for its application in children; however, its use is controversial. It is currently contraindicated in children under 18 years old (Francesconi, Azar, & Talamo, 2000).

General guidelines for glasses and contact lenses can be found in Box 29-1. Glasses must be changed frequently in children because of head growth. Because the child may be reluctant to wear eyeglasses that hurt or pinch, parents

TABLE 29-4 *Indications for a Comprehensive Pediatric Medical Eye Evaluation*

Indication	Specific Examples
Abnormalities in the screening evaluations (see Table 29-3)	Detection of a red reflex abnormality or asymmetry
	Detection of a structural eye abnormality
	Detection of an ocular alignment or motility abnormality
	Unable to perform vision screening at age 3-3 $^1/_2$ or older
	Visual acuity 20/50 or worse, or a 2-line difference in a 3-year-old
	Visual acuity 20/40 or worse, or a 2-line difference in a 5-year-old
	Visual acuity 20/30 or worse, or a 2-line difference in a 6-year-old or older child
Signs or symptoms of eye problems by history or observations by family members*	Defective ocular fixation or visual interactions
	Abnormal light reflex (including both the corneal light reflections and the "red" fundus reflection)
	Ocular alignment or movement abnormality
	Nystagmus (shaking of eyes)
	Persistent tearing
	Persistent ocular discharge
	Persistent redness
	Persistent light sensitivity
	Squinting
	Eye closure
	Head tilt
	Learning disabilities
Risk factors (general health problems, systemic disease, or use of medications that are known to be associated with eye disease and visual abnormalities)	Prematurity
	Perinatal complications (evaluation at birth and at 6 mo)
	Neurologic disorders or neurodevelopmental delay (on diagnosis)
	Juvenile rheumatoid arthritis (on diagnosis)
	Diabetes mellitus (5 yr after onset, yearly thereafter)†
	Systemic conditions with ocular manifestations (at 6 mo or on diagnosis)
	Chronic systemic steroid therapy or other medications (e.g., hydroxychloroquine) known to cause eye disease
A family history of conditions that cause or are associated with eye or vision problems	Retinoblastoma
	Childhood cataract
	Childhood glaucoma
	Retinal dystrophy/degeneration
	Strabismus
	Amblyopia
	Glasses in early childhood
	Sickle cell disease
	Systemic syndromes with ocular manifestations

From American Academy of Ophthalmology Pediatric Ophthalmology Panel: *Pediatric eye evaluations*, San Francisco, 2002, American Academy of Ophthalmology.

NOTES: These recommendations are based on panel consensus except where noted.

*"Headache" is not included because it is rarely caused by eye problems in children. This complaint should first be evaluated by the primary care physician.

†Klien R et al: The Wisconsin epidemiologic study of diabetic retinopathy. II. Prevalence and risk of diabetic retinopathy when age at diagnosis is less than 30 years, *Arch Ophthalmol* 102:520-526, 1984.

should assess the fit of the eyeglasses on a monthly basis and watch for behavior that indicates discomfort in a preverbal child (e.g., constantly removing glasses, rubbing at the frames or face).

Contact lenses, in addition to the cosmetic benefit, provide better refractive error correction than eyeglasses do and thereby enhance visual acuity and the total corrected field of vision. The NP can promote eye health by reinforcing instructions regarding proper contact lens care and reminding the patient that contact lenses should not be worn when the eye is inflamed or topical ophthalmic medications are being used.

BOX 29-1 *Recommendations for Use of Corrective Lenses*

Eyeglasses

Polycarbonate lenses are lightweight, strong, and shatterproof; scratch-resistant coating is recommended.

Silicone nose pads with nonskid surfaces prevent glasses from slipping.

Comfort cables secure frames by wrapping around the child's ears and are available for children 1 to 4 years old. Straps are recommended for infants under 1 year of age and allow them to roll and lie down.

Flexible hinges allow outward bending for easy removal by the child.

Match the frame to the child's facial shape and features to encourage compliance; if old enough allow the child to choose the frames.

To encourage compliance with infants and children, do not fight them when they remove glasses; be persistent, replace the glasses, and provide distraction. Parents may need to set the glasses aside for a few hours before trying again. Seek counsel from the prescribing provider for further help.

Tinted lenses can be used for photosensitivity; ultraviolet light filters are helpful with aphakia (absence of lens), congenital absence of iris, and albinism.

Do not place the glasses down with lenses in contact with surfaces.

Clean glasses daily with liquid soap and a soft cloth (do not use paper products).

Contact Lenses

Contact lenses are appropriate for children 13 years and older or in children who can demonstrate ability to manage lens hygiene, including insertion and removal.

Contact lenses are helpful for an aphakic child who would otherwise need very thick glasses that distort images.

Wear protective outer eyewear for sports.

Do not wear contact lenses if one or both eyes are inflamed or when using topical ophthalmic medications. Those with recurrent conjunctival or corneal infections, inadequate tears, severe allergies, or excessive exposure to dust or smoke should not wear contact lenses.

Adapted from American Academy of Ophthalmology: Eyeglasses for infants and children. Medem Medical Library website. Available at *www.medem.com* (accessed Jan 16, 2003).

Ophthalmic Medications

Caution and precision must be exercised when administering ocular medications to children because their smaller body mass and faster metabolism may potentiate the action of the drugs and result in adverse ocular and systemic side effects.

Topical ophthalmic medications such as antibiotics, mydriatics, and corticosteroids are frequently found in ointment or solution vehicles. These topical agents are primarily used for treating disorders affecting the anterior segment of the eye. Solubility is one of several factors that influence the absorption of topical ophthalmic medications. Those that are water soluble (e.g., anesthetics, steroids, and alkaloids) penetrate the corneal epithelium easily. Fat-soluble preparations (e.g., most antibiotics) do not penetrate the epithelium of the cornea unless it is inflamed.

Topical Antibiotics

Prescription of topical antibiotics is ideally based on empirical evidence that infection exists. The best choice of a topical antibiotic is one that is not often prescribed for problems in other body systems. Topical ophthalmologic preparations such as 10% sodium sulfacetamide, 4% sulfisoxazole, and broad-spectrum antibiotics are effective and rarely produce a hypersensitivity reaction. Topical penicillins, on the other hand, are to be avoided. Ophthalmic ointments are generally preferred over solutions for use in children because they last longer, do not sting, do not need to be given as often, and are less likely to be absorbed into the lacrimal passage. Ointments interfere with vision because they coat the eye, and they are more likely to cause contact dermatitis. Special care must be taken to ensure that the tip of the tube or dropper is not contaminated. Ophthalmic ointment should be transferred from the tube to moistened cotton swabs (one for each eye) and then rolled into the lower portion of each conjunctival sac (see Appendix A for ophthalmic drugs).

Ophthalmic Corticosteroids

Although ophthalmic corticosteroids are effective in the treatment of ocular inflammation (excluding ocular allergy), a patient with a condition severe enough to warrant consideration of corticosteroid use should be referred to an ophthalmologist. Steroids are associated with numerous complications, such as an increased incidence of herpes simplex keratitis and corneal ulcers, corneal perforation and intraocular sepsis, glaucoma, slowed healing of corneal abrasions and wounds, increased intraocular pressure, and cataract formation. They should never be used for suspected eye infections, for red eye of unknown origin, in immunocompromised children, or in any eye trauma that involved plants or soils (Trobe, 2001). A child receiving long-term ophthalmologic steroids should be assessed frequently for signs of adrenal suppression or other side effects. Encourage parents to keep scheduled tonometry appointments at 2- to 3-month intervals.

Other Topical Preparations

Decongestants or antihistamines or a combination of the two, mast cell stabilizers, and nonsteroidal antiinflammatory drugs are agents used in treating various ophthalmologic conditions, such as allergic conjunctivitis. Over-the-counter vasoconstrictors or vasoconstrictor-antihistamine preparations should be tried first for mild allergic conjunctivitis (Trobe, 2001). Cycloplegic agents are used for iritis.

Systemic Medications

In ocular infections involving the posterior segment and the orbit, systemic antibiotic preparations are necessary. A combination of topical and systemic antibiotics can also be used. In general, these conditions warrant referral to an ophthalmologist. Systemic drugs may also cause damage to the eyes (Table 29-5).

Eye Injury Prevention

Ocular trauma accounts for one third of all cases of acquired blindness in children. Male-to-female trauma incidence ratio is 4:1, with males 11 to 15 years old outnumbering all other age-groups. Most of the injuries could be prevented. The majority of the injuries are the result of sports-related accidents, toy darts, sticks, stones, fireworks, BB shot, paintball sports, other projectiles, and alpine skiing (Andley, Liang, & Lou, 2000). Parental supervision and education of children regarding prevention of eye injury are essential to minimize these injuries. Prevention includes such fundamental concepts as the following:

- Children need to be instructed to
  - Not run with or throw sharp objects
  - Use protective eyewear when hammering, using power tools, or participating in a sport where there is a high

TABLE 29-5 ***Systemic Drugs Causing Ocular Side Effects***

Drug	Ocular Side Effects	Intervention
Corticosteroids (prednisone at dosage of 15 mg/day for ≥1 yr)	Cataracts (25% incidence)	Monitor with ophthalmologic examinations.
Digoxin at moderately toxic ranges	Snowy, flickering, yellow vision	Resolves when drug is administered in correct range.
Isoniazid in greater than recommended dosages	Loss in color vision, ↓ visual acuity, and visual field changes	Effects are reversible only if discovered early. Ophthalmologic examination can be done before treatment and every 6 mo; any changes warrant stopping isoniazid and referring to an ophthalmologist.
Isotretinoin	Pseudotumor cerebri (after initiating treatment) with resultant blurred vision, visual field loss, and varying visual acuity changes	Monitor for symptoms.
Minocycline hydrochloride	Pseudotumor cerebri and orthostatic blackouts, evidenced by blurred vision, visual field loss, varying visual acuity changes, diplopia	Monitor for symptoms.
Phenytoin and carbamazepine	Blood levels in moderately toxic ranges can produce diplopia, blurred vision, nystagmus	Resolve when therapeutic doses are within normal ranges.

Adapted from Trobe J: *The physician's guide to eye care,* San Francisco, 2001, The Foundation of the American Academy of Ophthalmology.

ocular risk (e.g., hockey, badminton, racquetball, lacrosse, basketball, baseball) (Vinger, 2000)
  - Use orthodontic headwear that breaks away if force is applied
  - Not shine laser pointers in eyes
  - Use eye wash fountains when indicated
- Parents further need to be instructed to
  - Store harmful chemicals and sharp objects out of the reach of small children
  - Limit and supervise the use of BB guns, air rifles, darts, and fireworks

Sunglasses

Ultraviolet (UV) A and UVB radiation from the sun can damage the lens and retina of the eye and cause cataracts and other conditions harmful to vision later in life. Sunglasses should be used to minimize such damage by absorbing these light wavelengths, even if wearing UV-treated contact lenses (Andley, Liang, & Lou, 2000; School of Public Health, 2002). It is never too early to start wearing sunglasses. Wearing a hat with a wide (3-inch) brim cuts the radiation exposure in half.

Sunglasses that have large-framed, wraparound lenses with side shields provide the best protection. The lens and frame should be constructed of nonbreakable plastic or polycarbonate. The protection comes from the chemical coating on top of, or incorporated into, the lenses. Gray, brown, and green colors are sufficient for general purposes and lead to minimal color distortion. Darker colors or polarized lenses alone do not offer the protection that is needed. Lenses should only be purchased if they carry the American National Standards Institute (ANSI) label or American Optometry Association (AOA) notation. ANSI communicates their standards by labeling their lenses Z80.3 and "general purpose," "special purpose" (for snow and water sports), and "cosmetic use" (lowest protection). AOA sets higher UV radiation standards (School of Public Health, 2002).

Sports Protection

Protective glasses or goggles are mandatory for all functionally one-eyed individuals (with best corrected vision less than 20/40 in the poorer-seeing eye) or for any athlete who has had eye surgery or trauma or whose ophthalmologist recommends eye protection (Vinger, 2000). Additionally, these children or adolescents should not participate in boxing or full-contact martial arts. Wrestling has a low rate of reported injury, but specific protective eyewear is available; however, there are no standards for eyewear in this sport. Eye protection is recommended for any child or adolescent participating in sports that have a high eye injury rate. The greatest number of injuries occurs in basketball and baseball or softball. However, eye protection is also recommended for pool activities, racquet sports, football, soccer, hockey, lacrosse, and squash. Eye protection also should be used in shop class or labs or when working with high-velocity projectiles (e.g., hammer on metal, power tools, or lawn mowers).

Protective glasses or goggles should be properly fitted with lenses made from CR-39 or 2 to 3 mm plastic-blend polycarbonate set deeply in a grooved frame with padding or rubber bridges around the nose. A headband or wraparound earpieces should be used to secure the glasses. Parents should only buy the protective eyewear certified by American Society for Testing and Materials (ASTM) or National Operating Committee on Standards for Athletic Equipment (NOCSAE) for use in the particular sport (see Resource Box).

Laser Pointers

The Food and Drug Administration (FDA) released a warning in 1997 about the misuse of laser pointers. Although harmless when used as intended by lecturers, reports of eye injury have appeared when the pointers are used as toys. The light energy from the laser aimed at the eye can be more damaging than staring directly into the sun and results in retinal scarring (De La Paz & D'Amico, 2000).

Vision Therapy, Lenses, and Prisms

Vision therapy, lenses, and prisms are controversial methods of treatment claimed by some to be effective therapy for learning disabilities and dyslexia. The latest joint organizational policy of the AOA and the American Academy of Optometry (1997, p. 2) states that "vision therapy does not directly treat learning disabilities or dyslexia . . . but is a treatment to improve visual efficacy and visual processing." These interventions consist of (1) visual training, including muscle exercises, ocular pursuit, tracking exercises, or "training" glasses (with or without bifocals or prisms); (2) neurologic organizational training (laterality training, crawling, balance board, perceptual training); and (3) wearing of colored lenses (AAP, 1998).

The most recent AAP, American Academy of Ophthalmology, and AAPOS joint statement, "Learning Disabilities, Dyslexia, and Vision: A Subject Review," states that "vision problems are rarely responsible for learning difficulties. No scientific evidence exists for the efficacy of eye exercises ('vision therapy') or the use of special tinted lenses in the remediation of these complex pediatric developmental and neurological conditions. . . . Avoid remedies involving eye exercises, filters, tinted lenses, or other optical devices that have no known scientific proof of efficacy" (AAP, 1998, p. 1). Indeed, current research has shown that dyslexia is a language-based disorder—not a visual-perceptual problem—caused by neurobiologic and genetic factors (International Dyslexia Association, 2002).

When counseling parents who inquire about vision therapy, the NP should be aware of the pressure that parents may be under from optometrists advocating vision therapy for learning disabilities and the divergent opinions held by educators and the ophthalmologic community about this modality of treatment. Managing a child with academic difficulties requires a multidisciplinary approach involving education, as well as psychologic and other medical specialists. Screening for ocular defects early is a routine part of the NP practice, and defects should be referred to the appropriate specialist.

COMMON EYE DISORDERS

Visual Disorders

Refractive Errors and Amblyopia

Description. Alterations in the refractive power of the eye include myopia, hyperopia, astigmatism, compound refractive errors, and anisometropia (DeRespinis, 2001). In a normal eye, light from a distant object focuses directly on the retina. When variations in axial length of the eyeball or curvature of the cornea or lens exist, light focuses in front of or behind the retina. This abnormal focusing produces an alteration in the refractive power of the eye that results in a visual acuity deficit (see Box 29-2 for further definitions).

Amblyopia is a usually unilateral deficit in which there is defective development of the visual pathways—due to a lack of clear focused images reaching the brain—needed to attain central vision. This results in reduced or permanent loss of vision that is not correctable once visual maturity is complete (by approximately 10 years of age) (AAO, 2002). Amblyopia is labeled (or typed) according to the structural or refractive problem that is causing the poor visual image to reach the brain: deprivational, or obstruction of vision (e.g., due to ptosis, cataract, nystagmus); strabismic (due to strabismus or lazy eye); or refractive (myopia, hyperopia, astigmatism, anisometropia).

Etiology and Incidence. Refractive errors are the most common visual disorder seen in children (Hoekelman, 2001). Approximately 20% of children have significant refractive errors by their teen years. Myopia may be present at birth, but it is more likely to develop during the middle school years (6 to 12 years of age). The incidence is 25% among 12- to 17-year-olds. Mild hyperopia is normal in a young child but should resolve spontaneously by school age. Amblyopia affects approximately 2% of children under 6 years of age (AAO, 2002).

Clinical Findings. The following may be noted:

- Squinting
- Fatigue
- Headaches
- Pain in or around eyes
- Dizziness
- Mild nausea
- Developmental delay
- Tendency to cover or close one eye when concentrating
- Family history of refractive errors, strabismus, or amblyopia

Management. Detection of visual problems in children at an early age is essential to prevent the development of otherwise avoidable permanent visual loss. The following steps are involved:

- Refer to an ophthalmologist or optometrist for prescription corrective lenses.
- Older children should have an annual refraction and eyeglass evaluation.
- Unilateral visual occlusion may be necessary and, occasionally, surgery may be necessary.
- Extended-wear contact lenses may be prescribed in unilateral aphakia, severe anisometropia, corneal scarring with irregular astigmatism, and keratoconus.

BOX 29-2 *Descriptive Terms for Refractive Errors*

Myopia, or nearsightedness, exists when the axial length of the eye is increased in relation to the eye's optical power. As a result, light from a distant object is focused in front of the retina rather than directly on it. A myopic child sees close objects clearly, but distant objects are blurry.

Hyperopia, or farsightedness, exists when the visual image is focused behind the retina. As a result, distant objects are seen clearly but close objects are blurry.

Astigmatism exists when the curvature of the cornea or the lens is uneven; thus the retina cannot appropriately focus light from an object regardless of the distance, which makes vision blurry close up and far away. Rarely, astigmatism can be caused by an alteration in the corneal sphere caused by a soft tissue mass on the inner aspect of the eyelid, such as a chalazion or hemangioma.

Anisometropia is a different refractive error in each eye. It may consist of any combination of refractive errors discussed above, or it may occur with aphakia.

- Support and reassurance according to the child's developmental level are needed during the period of adjustment to contact lenses or eyeglasses.
  - Infants and toddlers need distraction, with replacement of glasses if removed.
  - Verbal children may be aided by the use of positive reinforcement such as sticker charts.
  - School-age children and teenagers should participate in the selection of frames. If desired, contacts may be considered.
- Claims of certain diets or exercises as means of correcting or preventing refractive errors have not been substantiated by research efforts. (See the discussion in Management Strategies earlier in the chapter.)

Complications. Untreated or insufficiently treated amblyopia in young childhood will result in irreversible and lifelong visual loss.

Strabismus

Description. Strabismus is a defect in the position of the eyes in relation to each other, commonly called a "lazy eye." In strabismus, the visual axes are not parallel because the muscles of the eyes are not coordinated; when one eye is directed straight ahead, the other deviates. As a result, one or both eyes appear crossed. In children, strabismus may be manifested as a phoria or a tropia (Box 29-3). Pseudostrabismus is present when the sclera between the cornea and the inner canthus is obscured by closely placed eyes, a flat nasal bridge, or prominent epicanthal folds (see Fig. 29-3). Upper eyelid ptosis may accompany strabismus in some cases (Zwaan, 1999).

Etiology and Incidence. Affecting approximately 4% of children, nonparalytic strabismus usually develops before 5 years of age. Esodeviations are the most common type of strabismus, account for more than 50% of deviations, and are visible when the child is looking at a near object. Early-onset (infantile) esotropia is evident before 6 months of age and requires surgical correction. Accommodative esotropia becomes evident later, usually at 2 to 3 years of age. Exodeviations occur 25% of the time and are usually intermittent and more visible when the child is looking far away. Infantile exotropia is more rare and is more often associated with intracranial pathology. Intermittent exotropia is seen in approximately 70% of infants before 3 months (McManaway & Frankel, 2001). Both types of strabismus may be hereditary or the result of various eye diseases (e.g., neuroblastoma), trauma, systemic or neurologic dysfunction that paralyzes the extraocular muscles, uncorrected hyperopia, and accommodation and accommodative convergence (McManaway & Frankel, 2001; Rubin, 2001).

BOX 29-3 *Descriptive Terms for Strabismus*

A **phoria** is an intermittent deviation in ocular alignment that is held latent by sensory fusion. The child can maintain alignment on an object.

A **tropia** is a consistent or intermittent deviation in ocular alignment. A child with a tropia is unable to maintain alignment on an object of fixation.

Phorias and tropias are classified according to the pattern of deviation seen:

- **Hyper** (up) and **hypo** (down) are used to classify vertical strabismus.
- **Exo** (away from the nose) and **eso** (toward the nose) describe horizontal deviations.
- **Cyclo** describes a rotational or torsional deviation.

Clinical Findings. Clinical findings can involve the following:

- Intermittent exotropia may be seen in normal children 6 months to 4 years old who are ill or tired or when they are exposed to bright light or with sudden changes from close to distant vision. It is more often seen when the child is looking with distant fixation (Robb, 2000).
- When only one eye is affected, the child always fixates with the unaffected eye.
- When both eyes are affected, the eye that looks straight at any given time is the fixating eye.
- The angle of deviation may be inconsistent in all fields of gaze, actually changing in some forms of strabismus.
- Persistent squinting, head tilting, face turning, overpointing, awkwardness, or marked decreased visual acuity in one eye may be seen.
- Cataracts, retinoblastoma, anisometropia, and severe refractive errors are found infrequently.

Diagnostic Testing. The corneal light reflection technique and the cover-uncover and alternating cover tests are assessments used to screen for strabismus. Asymmetry of light reflection on the cornea is indicative of a deviation in ocular alignment. The cover-uncover test is used to detect tropias, whereas the alternating cover test detects phorias (see Fig. 29-3). The photoscreener can also be used to detect strabismus.

Management. Management steps include the following:

- Any ocular misalignment seen after 4 months of age is considered suspicious, and the child should be referred (Miller & Apt, 2002). Hypertropia or hypotropia, exotropia, acquired esotropia or exotropia, cyclovertical deviation, or any fixed deviation is an indication for referral as soon as it is first observed. Patients who

acquire esotropia under 3 years of age usually develop strabismic amblyopia if not treated after the onset of the deviation (Pratt-Johnson & Tillson, 2001).
- The unaffected eye is occluded, which forces the child to use the deviating eye. Occlusion has traditionally been accomplished by patching the "good" eye. Recent research has demonstrated that "pharmacologic penalization" with the daily instillation of 1% atropine sulfate was equally effective for moderate amblyopia at 6 months (Kushner, 2002; Pediatric Eye Disease Investigational Group, 2002).
- Surgical alignment of the eyes may be necessary. It is ideally done before 2 years of age and usually between 6 and 18 months of age (Pratt-Johnson & Tillson, 2001).
- Orthoptic exercises as a treatment modality are indicated only in certain forms of intermittent strabismus or when the visual axes are nearly aligned.
- Corrective lenses may or may not be indicated, depending on the presence of refractive errors.
- Annual follow-up with an ophthalmologist is needed for monitoring of visual acuity, refraction, alignment, and mobility if surgery was performed.
- Assessment for amblyopia should be done at every visit, even after straightening the eyes, because changes in alignment can occur through the fifth year.
- The ocular status of an affected child's siblings is monitored.
- Local botulinum toxin injection may also be used with certain deviations (Jockin, 2002).

Complications. Amblyopia (secondary visual loss) occurs in 30% to 50% of children with strabismus (Behrman, Kliegman, & Jenson, 2004). Uncorrected strabismus can have a negative effect on self-esteem.

Blepharoptosis

Description and Etiology. Blepharoptosis or ptosis is drooping of the upper eyelids affecting one or both eyes. It can be congenital or acquired, secondary to trauma or inflammation. Congenital ptosis caused by an abnormality in development of the levator muscles or cranial nerve III may be an autosomal dominant trait. Other possible etiologies include trauma to cranial nerve III during the birthing process, trauma to the eyelid or neck, chronic inflammation (particularly of the anterior segment of the eye), or a neurologic disorder. The more recent the onset of the ptosis, the more urgent the referral (Trobe, 2001).

Management. Management involves the following steps:
- Correct any underlying systemic disease.
- Evaluate for anisometropia (unequal refractive errors in each eye), anisocoria, and decrease in pupillary light reflex.
- Refer to an ophthalmologist. If vision is compromised, surgery is performed in an effort to prevent amblyopia and developmental delay. If vision is not compromised, correction is usually delayed until the child is at least 3 years old.

Nystagmus

Description. Nystagmus is the presence of involuntary, rhythmic movements that may be pendular oscillations or jerky drifts of one or both eyes. Movement is horizontal, vertical, rotary, or mixed.

Etiology. Nystagmus occurs in association with albinism, high refractive errors, CNS abnormalities, and various diseases of the inner ear and the retina and middle ear trauma.

Clinical Findings. Oscillation in the newborn's eyes is common and exists for a short time during the neonatal period. Involuntary oscillation that persists or occurs beyond the initial weeks of life indicates pathology. The movements may be constant or varied, depending on the direction of gaze. Rhythmic head movements sometimes manifest as nystagmus (Behrman, Kliegman, & Jenson, 2000). The NP should note the field(s) of gaze within which the nystagmus is evident (e.g., field of gaze straight ahead, left, or up) (Trobe, 2001).

Management. Management consists of treating any underlying systemic disorder and referring the patient to an ophthalmologist. Any acquired nystagmus is most worrisome and should alert the NP to refer for prompt evaluation.

Cataracts

Description. *Cataract,* a partial or complete opacity of the lens affecting one or both eyes, is the most common cause of an abnormal pupillary reflex. Some cataracts are considered clinically significant, others insignificant.

Etiology. Cataracts may be congenital or a result of infection (e.g., congenital rubella, cytomegalovirus [CMV], toxoplasmosis), trauma to the eye, metabolic disease (e.g., galactosemia), long-term use of systemic corticosteroids or ocular corticosteroid drops, CNS anomalies (e.g., craniosynostosis, cranial defects), genetic defects (e.g., Down syndrome, albinism), and demyelinating sclerosis and ataxia-telangiectasia. They may also be seen in children who have other ocular abnormalities, such as strabismus or pendular nystagmus, and in children with diabetes mellitus, atopic dermatitis, or Marfan syndrome. Prematurity is also associated with cataracts.

Clinical Findings. The following history and physical examination findings are present:
- A history of maternal prenatal infection, drug exposure, or hypocalcemia is usually elicited.
- Cataract appears as a black dot or line surrounded by a red reflex, usually bilateral.

- Visual acuity deficits may vary.
- A pale red reflex in people of color should not be confused with a cataract.

Management. Surgical removal of the lens optically clears the visual axis. The resultant aphakic refractive error is corrected with lenses. Any sensory deprivation amblyopia is corrected.

Complications. Visual developmental delay (amblyopia), especially in neonates with bilateral congenital cataracts that are dense, has been reported.

Prognosis. The success of treatment depends on the cataract type. Visual outcomes tend to be better with unilateral than bilateral cataracts. Good results are more likely if cataracts are removed before 3 months of age.

Glaucoma

Description. Glaucoma is a disturbance in the circulation of aqueous fluid that results in an increase in intraocular pressure and subsequent damage to the optic nerve. It is classified according to age at the time of its appearance and other associated conditions.

Etiology and Incidence. Infantile glaucoma, which occurs in the first 3 years of life—usually before 6 months of age—is a congenital abnormality of the structures that drain the aqueous humor. It is an anomaly of the drainage apparatus over 50% of the time. The incidence is approximately 1 in 10,000 live births and occurs more in males (Quinn, 2002). It is also seen in association with other developmental anomalies, such as neurofibromatosis; diffuse facial nevus flammeus (port-wine stain); or Sturge-Weber, Marfan, Hurler, or Pierre Robin syndromes. Secondary or juvenile glaucoma occurs between 3 and 30 years of age, when the drainage network for aqueous humor becomes obstructed after ocular infection, trauma, neoplasm, or long-term corticosteroid use.

Clinical Findings. Symptoms of infantile glaucoma (unilateral or bilateral) include the following:

- "Classic triad" of tearing, photophobia, and excessive blinking or blepharospasm (only one third of patients manifest this triad [Behrman, Kliegman, & Jenson, 2004]) caused by irritation
- Edematous, hazy corneas
- Palpable orbital globe, bulbar conjunctival erythema, and visual impairment

Symptoms of secondary glaucoma include the following:

- Extreme pain
- Blurred vision
- Tunnel vision
- Pupillary dilation
- Erythema (often in only one eye)
- Change in configuration of optic nerve cupping, with asymmetry between the eyes and loss of vision over time

Management. Early diagnosis is important. The goal is normalization of intraocular pressure and prevention of optic nerve damage along with correction of associated refractive errors and prevention of amblyopia.

- Refer to an ophthalmologist. Primary treatment is surgery as early as possible (often multiple surgeries are required). Medications may include topical β-blockers and carbonic anhydrase inhibitors.
- Parent and patient education must emphasize the importance of medication compliance and discourage excessive physical or emotional stress and straining at stool.
- A medical identification tag is worn at all times.
- Routine tonometry and an ophthalmoscopic examination are needed for every member of the family every 2 years.

Complications. Stretching of the cornea and sclera and blindness can occur.

Retinopathy of Prematurity

Description. ROP is a developmental, vascular disorder. It involves the abnormal growth of the retinal vessels in incompletely vascularized retinas of premature infants. Previously, ROP was called *retrolental fibroplasia.* An international classification of ROP has been identified and is important both for understanding the disease and for predicting outcome. The classification system describes ROP according to the distance to which the vascularization has reached away from the optic nerve (zone I, II, or III), severity of inflammatory changes (stage), and duration (clock hours) (Phelps, 2002). ROP is important because of the increasing incidence, the critical window of time for treatment, and the need for monitoring for late complications.

Etiology and Incidence. ROP is a multifactorial retinal vasculopathologic disease primarily caused by early gestational age and low birth weight. It occurs primarily in premature infants born at less than 30 to 32 weeks of gestation or weighing less than 1500 g. Infants weighing less than 1251 g have an incidence of 66%. Those with gestational ages less than 26 weeks have a 90% incidence; the incidence drops to 70% at 26 to 28 weeks and less than 45% after 29 weeks (Phelps, 2002).

Abnormal vasculopathology affects the normal progression of growth of the retinal vessels from the optic nerve outward. Exposure to supplemental oxygen for greater than 30 days is an additional risk (not causative) factor, causing vaso-obliteration (Palmer, 2000). The incidence of ROP is increasing because of survival of the very smallest babies who require prolonged oxygen and ventilation.

Other neonatal factors increase the risk of ROP (e.g., history of maternal bleeding, anemia, intraventricular hemorrhage, sepsis, hypotension, necrotizing enterocolitis [Paysse, 2002]). An increased incidence of the disease is noted in whites, with multiple births, and in infants with longer neonatal transport times after delivery to specialty neonatal intensive care units. There are no gender differences (Phelps, 2002).

Clinical Findings. ROP is initially diagnosed by a pediatric ophthalmologist while the infant is in the nursery. Once the baby is discharged, the following may be seen:

- Leukokoria (white fibrovascular tissue in the retrolental space), glaucoma, cataracts
- Vitreous haziness, hemorrhage
- Retinal and iris changes
- Pallor of optic nerve
- Strabismus
- Cataracts
- Detached retinas (often with secondary glaucoma, entropion, and eye infections)

An infant (especially if full or near term) not previously diagnosed with ROP who has detached retinas or leukokoria needs an opthalmologic evaluation to rule out genetic disorders (e.g., Norris syndrome, familial exudative vitreoretinopathy [X-linked recessive]).

Management. Retinopathy of prematurity progresses at variable rates; the worst prognosis is seen when the vascularization at birth was in zone I (closest to the optic nerve). Zone II onset or slower progression can lead to complete resolution; zone III is associated with full recovery (Phelps, 2002). The NP's role in managing ROP is to ensure that all premature infants receive initial and follow-up examinations as indicated by their gestational maturity and size. Examinations should be performed by a pediatric ophthalmologist experienced in examining preterm infants. Initial ophthalmologic examinations should be done on all infants born at less than 29 weeks of gestation or weighing 1500 g or less or those born at 29 to 34 weeks with an unstable course during hospitalization. They should occur at 4 to 6 weeks of chronologic age or 31 to 32 weeks of postconceptual age; cicatricial fundus (scarring) changes need to be followed throughout life (AAO, 2002; Paysse, 2002; Phelps, 2002). The NP further needs to do the following:

- Discuss with parents the implications of their child's disease.
- Monitor for late sequelae or ROP progression (e.g., strabismus, pseudostrabismus, amblyopia, myopia, anisometropia, leukokoria, cataracts).
- Assist children who have sequelae to maximize their potential by referring to early intervention services for low-vision children.
- Follow up all children yearly (even if ROP has resolved completely) if ROP needed any treatment; less frequent follow-up is needed if no treatment was needed (Paysse, 2002).

Cryosurgery or laser therapy is employed to arrest the progression of abnormally growing blood vessels. It can lead to the reduction of poor outcomes in those with moderate or severe ROP (Palmer, 2000; Phelps, 2002).

Complications. Retinal detachment, amblyopia, serious myopia, strabismus, glaucoma, and cicatrix (residual retinal scars) leading to later vision loss are possible complications. Any cicatricial formation is complete at about 8 months. Less than 10% of infants have any significant retinal sequelae or visual impairment (Behrman, Kliegman, & Jenson, 2004). Educational problems, including low IQ, poor social development, perceptual interpretation of the environment, motor skill development, and language acquisition; stereotypic behavior such as rocking or moving the head; and behavioral problems are possible (Wheeler et al, 1997).

Prevention. Minimizing or preventing ROP can be accomplished by decreasing the occurrence of premature births and minimizing the oxygen needed. Using vitamin E to maintain physiologic serum levels and reducing exposure to high ambient and supplemental lighting has not been fruitful in reducing ROP (Palmer, 2000; Phelps, 2002).

Retinoblastoma

Description. Retinoblastoma is a rare malignant tumor of the retina but is the most common tumor affecting the neonatal eye. Tumors usually manifest by 2 years of age (Murphree & Christensen, 2000).

Etiology and Incidence. Retinoblastoma is the most common childhood ocular malignancy. It may be found as a single tumor in one eye or as multiple tumors in one or both eyes. Both hereditary and nonhereditary forms may occur (Gupta, Hamming, & Miller, 2002; Murphree & Christensen, 2000). Bilateral disease occurs one third of the time, usually develops at an earlier age (by 15 months), and is the heritable form of the disease. Unilateral disease occurs two thirds of the time, is due to genetic mutation, and is commonly recognized by 25 months. The overall incidence is approximately 1 in 20,000 live births, without race or sex preference.

Clinical Findings. The following may be seen:

- Positive family history
- Strabismus—either the first (Gupta, Hamming, & Miller, 2002) or second (Murphree & Christensen, 2000) most common finding
- White pupil (leukokoria)—50% of cases detected by this symptom alone by the primary care provider or parents

(Phelps, 2002); either the first (Murphree & Christensen, 2000) or second (Gupta, Hamming, & Miller, 2002) most common finding
- Decreased visual acuity
- Possible inflammation and photophobia (causes pain), orbital cellulitis, hyphema, abnormal red reflex, nystagmus, glaucoma, hypopyon (pus in anterior chamber of eye), or signs of global rupture

Diagnosis is made via CT scan, ultrasound, or MRI.

Management. Refer the patient to an ophthalmologist for diagnosis and management by a multidisciplinary team. Irradiation, systemic plaque radiotherapy, thermotherapy, photocoagulation, chemotherapy, and cryotherapy are therapeutic modalities. Surgical removal of the affected eye is sometimes necessary if the tumor is large or intraocular. An ocular prosthesis for enucleation can be fitted 3 to 4 weeks after surgery. Siblings and parents should receive fundi examinations.

Frequent follow-up (every 3 months until 6 or 7 years of age), to assess treatment and to monitor for recurrence, is important. An ophthalmologist, a pediatric oncologist, a radiation oncologist, a social worker, and a genetic counselor need to be involved.

Complications. Metastasis is possible if the diagnosis is delayed. Those who survive are at high risk for a secondary nonocular malignancy (often pinealoblastoma or sarcoma of the head or orbit), cataracts, radiation retinopathy, optic neuropathy, or bone marrow suppression; metastasis is usually fatal.

Prognosis. The size and extent of the tumor determine the prognosis. If the orbit or optic nerve is involved, the prognosis is poor. Five-year survival rates with prompt diagnosis and treatment are 95% (Gupta, Hamming, & Miller, 2002). In those with a hereditary etiology, secondary malignancies can occur (e.g., osteogenic sarcoma).

Infections

Conjunctivitis

Conjunctivitis is an inflammation of the palpebral conjunctiva (the lining of the upper and lower eyelids) and occasionally the bulbar conjunctiva (layer of conjunctival tissue over the sclera). It is the most frequently seen ocular disorder in pediatric practice. Bacteria (most commonly *Haemophilus influenzae*) are responsible for the infection 60% to 70% of the time in children; both gram-negative and gram-positive organisms are implicated. *Staphylococcus aureus* is now regarded as not, or minimally, contributory (*Contemporary Pediatrics*, 2000). Conjunctivitis also occurs as a viral (less than 20% incidence) or fungal infection, or as a response to allergens or chemical irritants (*Contemporary Pediatrics*, 2000). Bacterial conjunctivitis is often unilateral whereas viral conjunctivitis is most often bilateral. Unilateral disease can also suggest a toxic, chemical, mechanical, or lacrimal cause. A major indicator of etiology is also age of the patient (Table 29-6).

Blockage of the tear drainage system, injury, foreign body, abrasion or ulcers, keratitis, iritis, herpes simplex virus, and infantile glaucoma are all in the differential diagnosis.

Conjunctivitis in the Newborn (Ophthalmia Neonatorum)

Description. Conjunctivitis in the newborn, also known as ophthalmia neonatorum or neonatal blennorrhea, is a form of conjunctivitis that occurs in the first month of life. In most states, conjunctivitis of the newborn is a reportable infectious disease.

Etiology and Incidence. Conjunctivitis occurs in 0.3% to 11% of newborns and is of aseptic (chemical) or septic origin. The most common cause is chemical conjunctivitis from the prophylactic instillation of silver nitrate at birth. *Chlamydia* is the most common infectious or septic cause. *Staphylococcus, Streptococcus, Pseudomonas, Haemophilus, Neisseria gonorrhoeae*, and herpes simplex virus (HSV) are also implicated (Kapur, Yoder, & Polin, 2002).

Clinical Findings

- Chemical conjunctivitis usually occurs in the first 24 to 72 hours of life.
- Septic conjunctivitis caused by
  - *C. trachomatis* usually begins in the first 2 weeks of life (Neu, 2002; Schaffer, 2002).
  - *Neisseria gonorrhoeae* usually appears in the first 2 to 5 days of life (up to 28 days).
  - HSV occurs at birth or in the first weeks of life.
- Symptoms most commonly seen include the following:
  - Chemical-induced conjunctivitis frequently manifests as nonpurulent discharge and edematous bulbar and palpebral conjunctiva.
  - *C. trachomatis* specifically causes moderate eyelid swelling and bulbar conjunctival infection.
  - *Neisseria gonorrhoeae* specifically causes acute conjunctival inflammation, erythema, and excessive, purulent discharge.
  - HSV specifically causes conjunctivitis and corneal opacity, often unilateral.

There may be a maternal history of vaginal infection during pregnancy or current sexually transmitted disease (STD).

LABORATORY STUDIES. Giemsa staining and direct immunofluorescent monoclonal antibody staining, cultures, and antigen detection tests can be used. Gonorrhea should also be tested for in any infant younger than 2 weeks. A culture for gonorrhea (on chocolate agar or Thayer-Martin medium) or aggressive scraping for a

TABLE 29-6 *Types of Conjunctivitis*

Type	Incidence/Etiology	Clinical Findings	Diagnosis	Management
Ophthalmia neonatorum	Neonates: *C. trachomatis, Neisseria gonorrhoeae* (GC), herpes simplex virus (HSV) Silver nitrate reaction occurs in 10% of neonates	Erythema, chemosis, purulent exudates with GC; clear to mucoid d/c with *Chlamydia*	Culture (DFA, EIA) Gram stain R/O GC, chlamydia	Saline irrigation to eyes until clear followed by erythromycin ointment GC: IM or IV ceftriaxone or cephotaxime (AAP, 2003) Chlamydia: PO EES HSV: IV or PO antivirals
Bacterial conjunctivitis	Preschoolers and sexually active teens: *Haemophilus influenzae* (nontypeable), *Streptococcus pneumoniae, GC*	Erythema, chemosis, itching, burning, mucopurulent d/c, matter in eyelashes; ↑ in winter	Cultures (optional) Gram stain (optional) Chocolate agar (for GC) R/O pharyngitis, GC, AOM, URI, seborrhea	Sulfacetamide sodium 10% ophthalmic solution OR Ofloxacin 0.3% solution OR Erythromycin 0.5% ophthalmic ointment Amoxicillin or Augmentin oral suspension if concurrent acute otitis media Warm soaks to eyes tid until clear No sharing towels, pillows No school until treatment begins
Chronic bacterial conjunctivitis	School-age children and teens: Bacteria, viruses, *C. trachomatis*, review compliance and prior drug choices of conjunctivitis treatment	Same as above; foreign body sensation	Cultures Gram stain R/O dacryostenosis, blepharitis, corneal ulcers	Gentamicin 0.3% ophthalmic solution/ointment OR Erythromycin 0.5% ophthalmic ointment Lacrimal duct massage tid-qid 10 strokes Refer to ophthalmologist if no improvement in 3 days
Inclusion conjunctivitis	Neonates and sexually active teens: *C. trachomatis*	Erythema, chemosis, clear or mucoid d/c, palpebral follicles	Cultures (DFA, EIA) R/O sexual activity	Erythromycin PO for 2-3 wk Tetracycline PO (adolescents only)
Viral conjunctivitis	Adenovirus 3, 4, 7, HSV, herpes zoster, varicella	Erythema, chemosis, tearing (bilateral); HSV and herpes zoster: unilateral with photophobia, fever; zoster: nose lesion; ↑ spring and fall	Cultures R/O corneal infiltration	Refer to ophthalmologist if herpes lesions or photophobia present Cool compresses tid-qid
Allergic and vernal conjunctivitis	Atopy sufferers, seasonal	Stringy, mucoid d/c, swollen eyelids and conjunctivae, itching, tearing, palpebral follicles, headache, rhinitis	Eosinophilia in conjunctival scrapings	Vasocon 0.1%, 0.012%, 0.03% ophthalmic solution; refer to allergists if needed

AOM, Acute otitis media; *d/c*, discharge; *DFA*, DNA fluorescent antibody test; *EIA*, enzyme immunoassay; *EES*, erythromycin ethylsuccinate; *IM*, intramuscular; *IV*, intravenous; *PO*, oral; *qid*, four times a day; *R/O*, rule out; *tid*, three times a day; *URI*, upper respiratory tract infection.

Gram stain are used for diagnosis (do not just sample the purulent discharge) (Schaffer, 2002). *Chlamydia* should also be tested for if gonorrhea is suspected, due to the comorbidity of these organisms.

Management

- Irrigate the eyes with sterile normal saline until clear of exudate.
- Gonococcal conjunctivitis: Infants should receive a 7- to 14-day course of intravenous or intramuscular ceftriaxone or cefotaxime. Ocular morbidity can result in missed infections.
- Nongonococcal conjunctivitis: A topical ophthalmic antibiotic preparation such as erythromycin 0.5% ointment (0.25- to 0.5-inch strip to each eye) is applied two to four times a day. The eyes should be cleansed with water or saline on cotton balls before instillation of the ointment into the lower conjunctival sac.
- Herpes simplex conjunctivitis: Hospitalization and topical and systemic antivirals are needed.
- Chemical-induced conjunctivitis resolves spontaneously within 3 to 4 days without specific treatment.

Prevention. Prophylactic administration of silver nitrate 1% ophthalmic solution (2 drops to each eye) or an ophthalmic antibiotic ointment such as 1% tetracycline or 0.5% erythromycin (0.25- to 0.5-inch strip into each eye within 1 hour of delivery) is common practice for prophylaxis after birth. It is required by law in most states and territories to prevent gonococcal conjunctivitis in the newborn. It should be determined at the time of the first visit whether infants born at home have received this prophylaxis.

Inclusion Conjunctivitis (Chlamydia)

Etiology. Inclusion conjunctivitis is usually caused by one of eight known strains of *Chlamydia trachomatis* and is most often seen in a neonate or sexually active adolescent. Neonates will usually demonstrate symptoms within the first 4 to 12 days of life (to 6 weeks), whereas *N. gonorrhoeae* symptoms are usually detected earlier.

Clinical Findings

- Maternal history of an STD or a history of a sexual partner with an STD
- Conjunctival erythema and mild to severe mucopurulent to bloody discharge, usually bilateral
- Follicular reaction (large, round elevations) in the conjunctiva of the lower eyelids
- Associated cervicitis or urethritis
- Infants may have symptoms suggestive of pneumonia (due to *Chlamydia*)

LABORATORY STUDIES. Conjunctival scrapings for Giemsa staining are indicated. A rapid screen of certain antigens can also be done using direct fluorescent antibody (Microtrak) or electroimmunoassay (Chlamydiazyme) testing kits. A specimen should also be gathered appropriately to test for gonorrhea, because of the comorbidity of these two organisms. Ocular morbidity can result if gonorrhea is missed.

Management. The following treatment is recommended:

- A 2-week course of systemic erythromycin ethylsuccinate (EES) (50 mg/kg per day in three to four divided doses or 500 mg twice a day for 10 to 14 days in infants or children younger than 9 years). A second course is sometimes required. The Centers for Disease Control and Prevention (CDC) issued a cautionary warning about an increased incidence of pyloric stenosis in infants following systemic EES for pertussis. More recent research has confirmed this possible connection after systemic treatment for *C. trachomatis* in newborns in the first 2 weeks of life (CDC, 1999; Mahon, Rosenman, & Kleinman, 2001). This was not the case with erythromycin ophthalmic ointment. Practitioners are encouraged to use systemic EES with caution; if no other alternatives are viable they need to have a high index of suspicion for the development of pyloric stenosis. Trimethoprim-sulfamethoxazole (0.5 ml/kg per day in two divided doses for 14 days) is an alternative systemic treatment after the neonatal period (Schaffer, 2002).
- Doxycycline (100 mg twice a day for 10 to 14 days), erythromycin base (250 mg four times daily for 14 days), or azithromycin (1 g orally in a single dose) can be used in young adults.
- Topical treatment, as well as oral, is often recommended.
- Mothers of infants with *C. trachomatis* conjunctivitis, partners of such mothers, and partners of sexually active adolescents also need examinations and treatment (CDC, 2002).

Complications include chlamydial pneumonia or gastroenteritis in infants. Complications may occur 6 to 8 weeks following the conjunctivitis.

Bacterial Conjunctivitis

Description. Acute bacterial conjunctivitis is commonly called *pinkeye*.

Etiology and Incidence. Bacterial conjunctivitis is predominantly caused by nontypeable *H. influenzae*, *Streptococcus pneumoniae*, and adenovirus. It is most common in the winter and in preschoolers. It is infrequently caused by *Staphylococcus* (*Contemporary Pediatrics*, 2001).

Clinical Findings. The following may be noted:

- Erythema of one or both eyes (key finding)
- Burning, stinging, or itching of the eyes and a feeling of a foreign body
- Photophobia
- Petechiae on bulbar conjunctiva
- Yellow-green purulent discharge

- Encrusted and matted eyelashes on awakening
- Symptoms of upper respiratory infection, otitis media, or acute pharyngitis

LABORATORY STUDIES. Routine culture testing is not necessary. Gram stain and culture can be done if the conjunctivitis is chronic, recurrent, or difficult to treat.

Differential Diagnosis. Chronic bacterial conjunctivitis that is resistant to treatment requires consideration of nasolacrimal duct obstruction in infants, poor compliance (conjunctivitis needs to be treated for 7 days), or wrong choice of drug. Cultures or scrapings are appropriate at that point. Leukemia can cause chronic conjunctivitis (*Contemporary Pediatrics*, 2001).

Management. Bacterial conjunctivitis is considered a self-limited disease (unless caused by gonorrhea or chlamydia) and usually resolves within 7 to 10 days. However, because both gram-negative and gram-positive organisms have been implicated, children who receive topical antibiotics demonstrate faster clinical improvement, can return to day care or school faster, and cause less parental work loss (*Contemporary Pediatrics*, 2001). Older children and teens are ideally managed without antibiotic treatment to avoid the overuse of antibiotics and because of the self-limited nature of this disease (Kane & Ellis, 2002).

The NP will want to choose broad-spectrum coverage and start treatment before any laboratory results would be available. The use of topical antibiotics leads to little resistance and little systemic absorption because of the high concentrations and short time use. Parents can be instructed to put pressure over the lacrimal duct when instilling the medication to prevent drainage into the nasolacrimal system. The recent introduction of the *S. pneumoniae* (Prevnar) vaccine is expected to decrease the incidence of conjunctivitis caused by that organism (*Contemporary Pediatrics*, 2001).

UNCOMPLICATED CONJUNCTIVITIS. The drugs of choice include the following:

- Ofloxacin as a first-line drug provides excellent penetration, pH, tolerability, and compliance.
- Sodium sulfacetamide 10% ophthalmic solution or ointment can be used.
- Trimethoprim sulfate plus polymixin B sulfate ophthalmic solution (Polytrim) is less irritating to the eye but is less bactericidal than ofloxacin. There is an increase in resistance to *S. pneumoniae* in some areas of the country.
- Erythromycin 0.5% ophthalmic ointment is recommended for patients with sulfa allergy.

Neomycin is to be avoided because of possible sensitization. Chloramphenicol 1% can increase the chance of aplastic anemia, though rarely; the aminoglycosides (gentamycin and tobramycin) are demonstrating poor *S. pneumoniae* coverage and have been implicated in corneal toxicity (*Contemporary Pediatrics*, 2001).

CONJUNCTIVITIS-OTITIS SYNDROME. This syndrome is usually caused by *H. influenzae*. Treatment requires amoxicillin or amoxicillin with clavulanic acid (Augmentin) at 80 mg/kg of amoxicillin per 24 hours in children younger than 24 months or another appropriate antibiotic for 10 days. Concurrent use of a topical antibiotic is not necessary (*Contemporary Pediatrics*, 2001).

Patient Education. If only one eye is involved, it is likely that the infection will spread within a day or two to involve both eyes. The patient (or parent) is instructed to do the following:

- Cleanse the eyelashes several times a day with a weak solution of no-tears shampoo and warm water. The importance of wiping from the inner canthus outward and using a different cloth or cotton ball for each eye should be emphasized.
- Use warm soaks three to four times a day to relieve itching and burning.
- Instill prescription ophthalmic solutions or ointments into the lower conjunctival sac. A moistened cotton swab may be used to facilitate instillation of ointments.
- Wash hands frequently and avoid shared linens to limit spread of the infection.
- Also treat seborrheic dermatitis on the scalp and face if present. Refer to Chapter 37 for treatment recommendations.

Some day care centers exclude children with conjunctivitis until they have completed 1 to 2 days of treatment. Improvement in the child's condition should be seen within 48 hours. If medication compliance is not in question and improvement is not seen within 72 hours of administration, the parent should be instructed to return so that a smear of the exudate can be taken for culture and sensitivity testing.

Complications. If vision is blurred or ophthalmoscopic examination reveals a bulging iris and a contracted, fixed pupil, suspect more serious inflammation of the uveal tract (iritis, cyclitis, or choroiditis) and refer immediately to an ophthalmologist because severe ocular morbidity can result.

Viral Conjunctivitis

Etiology and Incidence. Usually caused by an adenovirus, viral conjunctivitis can also be caused by herpes simplex, herpes zoster, or varicella virus. It is more common in children older than 6 years of age and in the spring and fall (*Contemporary Pediatrics*, 2001).

Clinical Findings. The following may be noted:

- Pharyngitis with enlarged preauricular nodes
- Itchy, red, and swollen conjunctiva
- Hyperemia and swollen eyelids

- Tearing and profuse clear, watery discharge
- Fever, headache, anorexia, malaise, upper respiratory symptoms (pharyngitis-conjunctivitis-fever triad with adenovirus)
- Photophobia with measles or varicella rashes
- Herpetic vesicles on the eyelid margins and eyelashes (marginal blepharitis) or on the conjunctiva and cornea (keratoconjunctivitis)
- Vesicles with superficial painful ulcerations, particularly on the tip of the nose (may be associated with herpes)

Management

- Good hygiene is essential. Viral conjunctivitis is self-limited and should resolve in 7 to 14 days. Conjunctivitis is often difficult to distinguish from keratitis. If the NP has any question, referral for ophthalmologic care is recommended.
- Warm or cold compresses and artificial tears can be used.
- Sodium sulfacetamide 10% ophthalmic solution or ointment (1 to 2 drops or 0.5 inch into the lower conjunctival sac four times daily) or broad-spectrum antibiotic preparations may be used to prevent secondary bacterial infection, but there is no consensus on this treatment (*Contemporary Pediatrics*, 2001).
- Antihistamine or vasoconstrictive ophthalmic solutions may be used for symptomatic relief.
- With HSV infection, immediate referral to an ophthalmologist should occur because of potential complications. Vidarabine or trifluridine (Viroptic) may be used in treatment. Topical corticosteroids should be avoided because they may worsen the course.
- Molluscum on the eyelid margins requires referral for excision.

Complications. Involvement of deeper layers of the cornea (keratitis) can occur and must be differentiated from conjunctivitis. Scarring of the cornea resulting in blindness is a significant complication of HSV infection.

Allergic Conjunctivitis

Description. Allergic conjunctivitis usually occurs in childhood but can occur after adolescence. The incidence is 15% of the general population (Friedlander, 2002). Four types of allergic conjunctivitis have been identified: (1) hay fever–associated conjunctivitis is characterized by mild injection and swelling; (2) vernal conjunctivitis is more severe, is more common in 3- to 12-year-olds, and has an increased prevalence in warm weather; (3) atopic keratoconjunctivitis occurs with atopic dermatitis and is notable for significant itching; and (4) giant papillary conjunctivitis occurs most often in contact lens wearers allergic to the thimerosal in contact lens solutions. Individuals with atopic conjunctivitis have an increased susceptibility to herpes simplex infection (blepharitis or keratitis) (Raizman, 1998).

Etiology. Seasonal allergens, often unidentified, cause these types of conjunctivitis. Rhinitis, eczema, and asthma may be associated conditions (Collum & Kilmartin, 2001).

Clinical Findings. The following may be noted:

- Family history of atopy or seasonal allergies
- Rhinitis, eczema, asthma
- Acute attacks precipitated by allergens (e.g., pollen, animals, molds, dust, dust mites, occasionally food)
- Severe itching and tearing
- Redness and swelling of the conjunctiva or eyelid (or both)
- Follicular reaction of the conjunctiva
- Stringy, mucoid discharge
- Bilateral involvement most common
- Cobblestone papillary hypertrophy in the tarsal conjunctiva

LABORATORY STUDIES. Conjunctival or nasal smears reveal numerous eosinophils.

Management. The following steps are taken when approaching treatment:

- Prevention is best; avoid allergens (leads to a 30% improvement [Finegold, 1998]).
- For mild cases, saline solution or artificial tears are administered along with cool compresses. Refrigerated eyedrops are more soothing.
- The next step is decongestants and antihistamines—given topically or systemically (can cause ocular dryness). Prescribed agents can provide quicker, more long-term relief with fewer side effects than over-the-counter agents (Paradis & Granet, 2002). Topical decongestants such as naphazoline hydrochloride (Naphcon or Vasocon) ophthalmic solution (1 to 2 drops every 3 to 4 hours) or combination (Naphcon-A or Vasocon-A) opthalmic solution (1 to 2 drops four times a day) can be used sparingly to reduce ocular congestion, irritation, and itching. Vasoconstrictors (e.g., Visine) should be avoided because of rebound congestion; these drugs should not be used for more than 3 days or more frequently than recommended.
- Topical mast cell stabilizers may be helpful for maintenance therapy or vernal conjunctivitis.
    - Cromolyn sodium 4% (Opticrom, Crolom), 1 to 2 drops four times a day for children older than 4 years on a regular basis.
    - Alocril 2% or lodoxamine tromethamine (Alomide) 0.1%, 1 to 2 drops four times a day for children older than 2 years.
    - Olopatadine (Patanol) is a mast cell stabilizer combined with an antihistamine for children older than 3 years (1 drop twice daily). Olopatadine will cover all of the symptoms of itching, redness, swelling, and discharge (Paradis & Granet, 2002).

- Nonsteroidal antiinflammatory drugs can be used for late-phase treatment of itching and burning.
  - Ketorolac tromethamine (Acular) 0.5%, 1 drop four times a day up to 1 week in children older than 12 years.
- Topical steroids are sometimes used in severe cases of allergy, but they must be used with caution because of possible side effects (increased intraocular pressure, potential for viral infection, contraindication with herpes, potential to cause cataracts, and poor corneal healing). At maximum they should be used for 1 week. If additional therapy is required, referral for ophthalmologic care is necessary.
- Refer to an allergist or ophthalmologist if unresponsive to treatment or if the following present: corneal abrasions, impaired vision, need for corticosteroids, severe keratoconjunctivitis, or atypical manifestations.
- Maintain a high threshold of suspicion for herpes-induced blepharitis or keratitis.

Blepharitis

Description. Blepharitis is an acute or chronic inflammation of the eyelash follicles or meibomian sebaceous glands of the eyelids (or both) (Table 29-7). It is usually bilateral. There may be a history of contact lens wear or a contact with another symptomatic person (Paysse, 2002).

Etiology. Blepharitis is commonly caused by contaminated makeup or contact lens solution. Poor hygiene, tear deficiency, rosacea, and seborrheic dermatitis of the scalp and face are also possible etiologic factors. The ulcerative form of blepharitis is usually caused by *S. aureus.* Nonulcerative blepharitis is occasionally seen in children with psoriasis, seborrhea, eczema, allergies, or lice infestation and in children with trisomy 21.

Clinical Findings. The following can be seen in blepharitis:

- Swelling and erythema of the eyelid margins and palpebral conjunctiva
- Flaky, scaly debris over eyelid margins on awakening; presence of lice
- Gritty, burning feeling in eyes
- Mild bulbar conjunctival injection
- Ulcerative form: hard scales at the base of the lashes (if the crust is removed, ulceration is seen at the hair follicles, the lashes fall out, and an associated conjunctivitis is present)

TABLE 29-7 ***Common Eye Infections***

Condition	Clinical Findings	Management	Prevention
Blepharitis	Swelling, erythema of eyelid margins and palpebral conjunctiva, pruritus, flaking	Cleanse eyes, warm compresses, antibiotic drops or ointment	New eye makeup, clean contacts and glasses, hygiene
Hordeolum	Tender, red, swollen furuncle at eyelid margin	Warm compresses, remove eyelash, antibiotic drops or ointment	Hygiene
Chalazion	Initially, mild erythema and slight swelling; later, slow-growing, round painless mass	As for hordeolum plus treat cellulitis if present	Hygiene
Nasolacrimal duct obstruction (dacryostenosis)	Tearing or mucus, continuous or intermittent, blepharitis; express thin mucopurulent discharge from punctum	Daily massage, antibiotic ointment with inflammation or infection, normal saline for nasal congestion	Massage duct, minimize nasal congestion (see Fig. 29-4)
Nasolacrimal duct infection (dacryocystitis)	Tenderness and swelling over lacrimal duct, edema and erythema of tear sac, excoriation of skin; express purulent discharge from punctum	Warm compresses, massage, oral antibiotic	As above
Periorbital cellulitis	Acute onset, pain, swelling and erythema; temperature >39° C, systemic symptoms	Outpatient systemic antibiotic therapy with close follow-up or hospitalization if moderate to severe infection, nonresponsive, or younger than 1 yr	HIB vaccine, hygiene, thorough cleansing of any skin disruption around eye, prompt treatment of sinusitis

HIB, Haemophilus influenzae type b.

Management. Explain to the patient that this may be chronic or relapsing. The patient is instructed to perform the following procedures:

- Scrub the eyelashes and eyelids with a cotton-tipped applicator containing a weak (50%) solution of no-tears shampoo to maintain proper hygiene and debride the scales.
- Use warm compresses twice daily for 5 to 10 minutes and wipe away lid debris.
- Apply sodium sulfacetamide 10% ophthalmic solution (1 to 2 drops into each eye twice a day) or erythromycin 0.5% ophthalmic ointment (0.25 to 0.5 inch into each eye twice daily) until symptoms subside and for at least 1 week thereafter. Ointment is preferable to eyedrops because of increased duration of contact with the ocular tissue.
- Chronic staphylococcal blepharitis and meibomian keratoconjunctivitis respond to tetracycline or erythromycin (250 mg daily for maintenance). Doxycycline (50 to 100 mg twice daily) can be used chronically in children older than 12 years (Steinemann, 2000).
- Treat associated seborrhea, psoriasis, eczema, or allergies as indicated.
- Remove contact lenses and wear eyeglasses for the duration of the treatment period. Sterilize or clean lenses before reinserting.
- Purchase new eye makeup.
- Use artificial tears for patients with inadequate tear pools.

Hordeolum

Description. Commonly called a stye, hordeolum is an infection of the sebaceous glands of the eyelids (external hordeolum) or meibomian glands of the eyelid (internal hordeolum). It can be caused by bacterial infection of the Zeis or Moll's glands (Fraunfelder, 2000).

Etiology. The causative organism is *S. aureus* or, rarely, *Pseudomonas aeruginosa.* It is common in those with chronic eyelid or skin disease or diabetes mellitus (Fraunfelder, 2000).

Clinical Findings. A tender, swollen, red furuncle is seen along the eyelid margin. The patient complains of a foreign body sensation. A hordeolum on the palpebral conjunctiva can be inspected by rolling back the eyelid.

Differential Diagnosis. If the hordeolum does not resolve, consider preseptal cellulitis, sebaceous cell cancer, or pyogenic granuloma (Fraunfelder, 2000).

Management

- Rupture often occurs spontaneously when the furuncle becomes large and a point develops. Removal of an eyelash near the furuncle frequently promotes rupture.
- Warm, moist compresses three to four times daily, 15 minutes each time, facilitate the process of rupturing. Hygiene for the eye can be maintained by scrubbing the eyelashes and eyelids with a cotton-tipped applicator containing a weak (50%) solution of no-tears shampoo once or twice a day.
- Sodium sulfacetamide 10% solution or ointment (1 to 2 drops or 0.25 to 0.5 inch into each eye four times a day) or an antibiotic ophthalmic ointment (e.g., erythromycin, 0.25 to 0.5 inch into each eye four times a day) until 2 to 3 days after resolution is effective treatment.
- Steroids are not indicated.
- Refer for incision and drainage if the hordeolum does not rupture on its own after coming to a point.
- Multiple or recurrent hordeolum: erythromycin 250 mg four times daily for 14 days; dicloxacillin 125 to 250 mg four times daily or cloxacillin 500 mg four times daily for 14 days. Prophylaxis: tetracycline 250 mg daily or doxycycline 50 to 100 mg daily.

Chalazion

Description. Chalazion is a chronic, sterile inflammation of the eyelid resulting from a lipogranuloma of the meibomian glands that line the posterior margins of the eyelids. It is deeper in the eyelid tissue than a hordeolum and may result from an internal hordeolum or retained lipid granular secretions.

Clinical Findings. Initially, mild erythema and slight swelling of the involved eyelid are seen. After a few days the inflammation resolves, and a slow growing, round, nonpigmented, painless (key finding) mass remains. It may persist for long periods of time. It is more commonly seen in adults.

Management. The following steps are taken:

- Warm compresses are used three to four times a day for 15 minutes for 2 to 3 days. Massage the eyelid and tarsal plate 40 times with the flattened finger. Hygiene for the eye can be maintained by scrubbing the eyelashes and eyelids with a cotton-tipped applicator containing a weak (50%) solution of no-tears shampoo once or twice a day (Wessels, 2000).
- Erythromycin ophthalmic ointment 0.5% (0.25 to 0.5 inch into each eye four times a day) or sodium sulfacetamide 10% (1 to 2 drops or 0.25 to 0.5 inch of ointment into each eye four times a day) can be used if a hordeolum is present.
- If cellulitis is present, erythromycin (30 to 50 mg/kg per 24 hours in divided doses every 6 to 8 hours) or cephalexin (20 to 40 mg/kg per 24 hours in divided doses every 8 hours) can be used.

- Referral to an ophthalmologist for surgical incision or corticosteroid injections is made if the condition is unresolved after medical treatment.

Complications. Fragile, vascular granulation tissue called pyogenic granuloma that enlarges and bleeds rapidly can occur if a chalazion breaks through the conjunctival surface.

Nasolacrimal Duct Obstruction: Dacryostenosis and Dacryocystitis

Description. Nasolacrimal duct obstruction, or dacryostenosis, is an abnormal stricture of the nasolacrimal duct or tear sac, usually at the nasal end. Dacryocystitis is an inflammation of the involved nasolacrimal duct.

Etiology. Nasolacrimal duct obstruction is fairly common in neonates (2% to 6% of live births [Milder, 2000]). It is thought to be due to congenital failure of the duct to canalize, but it may also occur secondary to infection or trauma. Congenital failure of the duct to canalize may be unilateral or bilateral, and clinical signs appear 3 to 12 weeks after birth. When inflammation is seen, it is most commonly caused by *S. aureus* and is often unilateral.

Clinical Findings. The following are seen:

- Continuous or intermittent tearing and mucoid discharge at the inner canthus that can become purulent
- Blepharitis in lids and lashes
- Occasional nasal obstruction and drainage
- Expression of thin mucopurulent exudate from the punctum lacrimale

The following additional symptoms may be noted if infection is present:

- Tenderness and swelling over the lacrimal duct
- Edema and erythema of the tear sac
- Excoriation of the surrounding skin
- Fever
- Expression of purulent material

Laboratory Studies. A white blood cell (WBC) count (elevated) and cultures are obtained if the inflammation is severe.

Differential Diagnosis. Punctual or canalicular atresia, conjunctivitis, foreign body, and nasal mucosal edema are differential diagnoses.

Management. Treatment of dacryostenosis or chronic dacryocystitis in infancy is as follows:

- Duct blockage usually resolves spontaneously in the first 6 months and in more than 90% of infants by 12 months of age (Milder, 2000). Treatment consists of minimizing stagnation in the tear duct and avoiding infection.
- Daily massage of the lacrimal sac may be performed to facilitate canalization of the duct. The technique involves placing a clean finger over the medial canthus and pressing in a posterior direction until the fingertip enters the space behind the inferior bony orbital ridge. Gentle pressure applied in a downward and medial direction transmits hydrostatic force through the nasolacrimal duct to the obstruction (Ballard, 2000) (Fig. 29-4). This technique should be performed about 10 times, three to four times a day.
- A topical ophthalmic ointment such as 0.5% erythromycin may be prescribed (0.25 to 0.5 inch into each eye four times a day) for 5 days and at the first sign of infection.
- Saline drops into the nose, followed by aspiration before feeding and at bedtime, helps relieve any concurrent nasal congestion.
- Refer children with persistent nasolacrimal duct obstruction to an ophthalmologist for evaluation and possible duct probing. If this is a recurring problem in older children, probing is usually always necessary. Some ophthalmologists may probe the duct as early as 4 months of age, whereas others wait until 9 to 12 months.

If dacryocystitis occurs, the following actions are indicated:

- Warm compresses four times a day
- Continued lacrimal sac massage as described previously
- Topical antibiotics with the addition of an oral antistaphylococcal antibiotic that treats for β-lactamase resistance (mild cases: Augmentin 20 to 40 mg/kg three times daily for 10 days; severe cases: cefuroxime 50 to 100 mg/kg three times daily for three days followed by Augmentin for 7 days [Trobe, 2001])

Complications. Periorbital or orbital cellulitis is a complication of dacryocystitis.

Periorbital Cellulitis

Description. Periorbital cellulitis, or inflammation of the tissues surrounding the involved eye, is often associated with trauma or focal infection near the eye, bacteremia, or sinusitis. It is predominantly an infection in children, spread from the upper respiratory tract or middle ear.

Etiology. Periorbital cellulitis is most commonly seen in children 6 months to 2 years of age. It can also occur with infected lacerations, abrasions, insect stings or bites, impetigo, or a foreign body where the infection is spread via venous or lymphatic channels (Fraioli, 2000). It may also be secondary to paranasal sinusitis. The etiology is often unknown, but the bacteria most commonly responsible for periorbital cellulitis are streptococcal organisms, *S. aureus*, and, until the introduction of the HIB vaccine, *H. influenzae* type b (Duboraw, Stasior, & Krohel, 2000).

Clinical Findings. The following may be noted:

- Acute febrile illness (temperature higher than 39° C if associated with bacteremia)

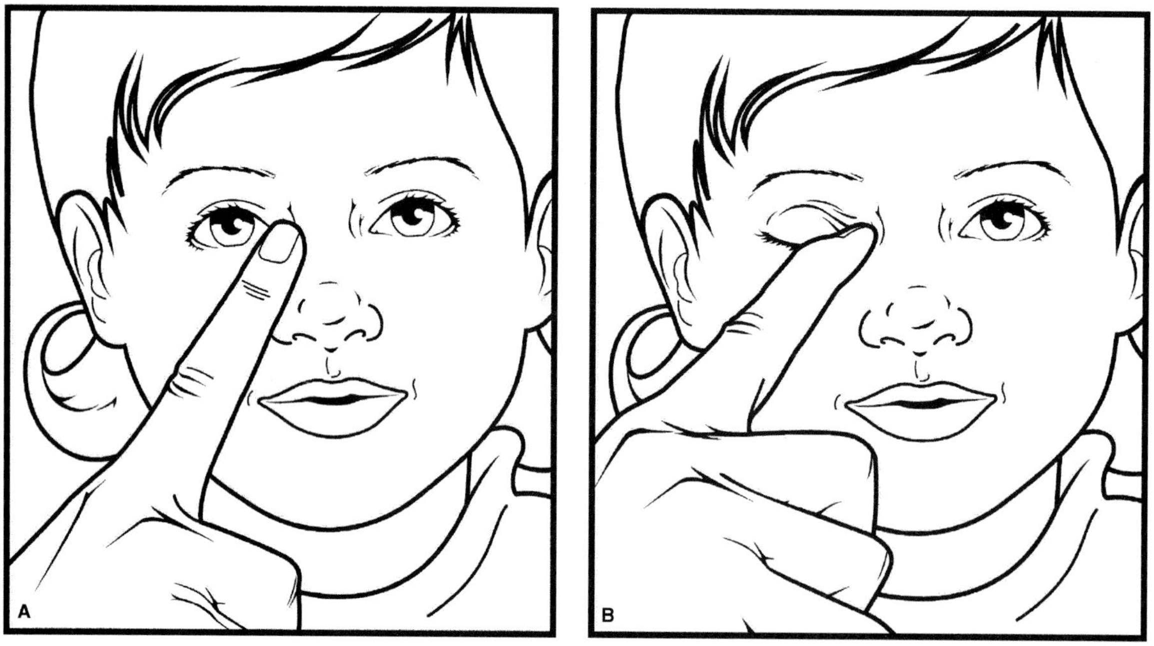

FIGURE 29-4 Technique to clear nasolacrimal duct Obstruction. **A,** Incorrect technique. **B,** Correct technique. The finger is pushing behind the bone, "in and up." Note that the finger tip is not visible in the proper technique.

- Swelling and erythema of tissues surrounding the eye
- Orbital discomfort/pain
- Deep red color of the eyelid (color is purple-blue with *H. influenzae* infection)
- Symptoms of bacteremia or sinusitis
- Paralysis of extraocular muscles

Laboratory Studies. Depending on the severity of the cellulitis, the following can be useful:

- CBC with differential (WBC count usually greater than 15,000 if bacteremic)
- Blood cultures and culture of purulent wounds near the eye
- Lumbar puncture (infants younger than 1 year)
- CT scan to rule out sinusitis, orbital cellulitis, or subperiosteal abscess
- Visual acuity, extraocular movement, and pupillary reaction testing

Differential Diagnosis. Conjunctivitis (bilateral conjunctival inflammation), cavernous sinus thrombosis, and orbital cellulitis (proptosis, limited extraocular movement, and reduced visual acuity) are the differential diagnoses in children; in neonates consider conjunctivitis, dacryocystitis, and ruptured dacryocystocele (Fraioli, 2000).

Management. The child may be managed as an outpatient if the cellulitis is mild, the orbit is not involved (full eye movements are present, no pain with eye movement, visual changes, or ptosis), the child exhibits no symptoms of systemic bacterial sepsis, and the child is over 1 year of age. However, management must be made on a case-by-case basis. Consultation is needed when proptosis, ophthalmoplegia, or changes in visual acuity occur; these conditions are suggestive of more extensive infection involving the orbit.

- Outpatient management begins with ceftriaxone (50 to 75 mg/kg [up to a maximum of 1 g] intramuscularly divided every 12 hours). The child is monitored daily until blood cultures are negative for 48 hours or clinical improvement is seen. Oral antibiotics may then be used to complete a 7- to 14-day course. Cloxacillin, amoxicillin with clavulanic acid, and cefixime are first-line choices for treatment (Fraioli, 2000). If a rapid clinical response is not seen, further evaluation and treatment should be done. Warm soaks to the periorbital area every 2 to 4 hours for 15 minutes may provide comfort and speed healing. The parent is advised to call immediately if there is any change in condition.
- Hospitalization and intravenous administration of nafcillin, or a combination of oxacillin and cefuroxime (chloramphenicol is used as an alternative), followed by a 10-day course of oral antibiotics, are required for any of the following:
  - Moderate to severe cases of cellulitis
  - A poor response to outpatient management

  - A purulent wound near the eyelid
  - Children younger than 1 year
  - Children with suspected sepsis

Complications. Complications include orbital cellulitis or extension of the infection into the orbit, subperiosteal or orbital abscess, optic neuritis, retinal vein thrombosis, panophthalmitis, meningitis, epidural and subdural abscesses, and cavernous sinus thrombosis.

Keratitis and Corneal Ulcers

Description. Keratitis, or inflammation of the cornea, can cause a dramatic alteration in visual acuity and can progress to corneal ulceration and blindness. A corneal ulcer begins as a well-defined infiltration at the center or edge of the cornea and subsequently suppurates and forms an ulcer that may penetrate deep into the corneal tissue or spread to involve the width of the cornea. Involvement is usually unilateral.

Etiology and Incidence. Causes of keratitis include HSV-1, although other viruses, as well as bacteria, fungi, and amebae, may be responsible. Bacterial causes progress rapidly and can destroy the cornea within 24 to 48 hours. The most common risk factor for keratitis is trauma; less common causes include an allergic reaction, conjunctivitis, a systemic infection, toxic chemicals, and the use of corticosteroids (Coster & Badenoch, 2000). The FDA has recently issued a warning against the use of improperly fitted (or purchased OTC from outlets) decorative contact lenses popular with teenagers (Clinician News Staff, 2003).

Clinical Findings. Symptoms vary in intensity according to the depth and extent of ulceration. The following are reported or seen:

- Exposure to an infected individual
- History of illness, eye trauma, foreign body, or the use of antibiotics
- Vesicles on the skin or eyelids and herpes lesions elsewhere on the body
- Severe pain, sensation of a foreign body, and photophobia
- Tearing, erythema, and spasms of the eyelid
- Blurred vision
- Gritty sensation in eye
- Occasional corneal opacification
- Area staining green with a fluorescein strip (if herpes, a dendritic ulcer is seen)

Management. When a corneal ulcer is suspected, the child should be referred immediately. Delay can result in loss of vision in the eye. Do not attempt to treat. A patch is never placed over an eye thought to have an infection (Trobe, 2001).

- Steroids should never be used.
- Treatment with antivirals such as trifluridine or vidarabine may be used to speed healing in herpes simplex infections.

Complications. Corneal opacification, scarring, and loss of vision can occur if treatment is delayed.

Inflammation of the Uveal Tract

Description. Inflammation of the uveal tract and other ocular structures is often called *uveitis.* The inflammation may be anterior (affecting the iris, ciliary body, or both) or posterior (affecting the choroid). Adjacent ocular structures can also be involved, including the retina, vitreous, sclera, lens, and optic nerve.

Etiology. Many processes have been implicated. Known etiologies include viral or bacterial infections, ocular trauma, and infection elsewhere in the eye, as well as allergy, malignancy, and systemic diseases such as juvenile rheumatoid arthritis, inflammatory bowel, Kawasaki syndrome, herpes simplex, tuberculosis, Lyme disease, CMV, toxoplasmosis, syphilis, acquired immunodeficiency syndrome, ulcerative colitis, and Steven-Johnson syndrome (Behrman, Kliegman, & Jenson, 2004; Power, 2000; Rosenbaum & George, 2000). The inflammation may be acute or chronic.

Clinical Findings. The following may be noted:

- Acute onset of pain (key finding)
- Photophobia and blurred or decreased vision (key findings)
- Excessive tearing and eyelid edema
- Conjunctival erythema
- Circumcorneal injection
- Hypopyon (pus layer in the bottom of the anterior chamber)
- Cloudy appearance of the eye with a bulging iris and a contracted, irregular, or fixed pupil

If chronic, there may be no ocular pain, photophobia, redness, or tearing.

Differential Diagnosis. Conjunctivitis is the differential diagnosis.

Management. Evaluate and treat any underlying systemic disease. Refer the patient to an ophthalmologist. A definitive diagnosis is made by slit-lamp examination. The prognosis is improved with early treatment, and delay may result in scarring of the pupil with cataract formation or the development of glaucoma. Cycloplegics and topical corticosteroids (depending on the cause of the inflammation) are often used in treatment. Mydriatics are used regularly to prevent posterior synechiae. Nonsteroidal antiinflammatory agents are used as an adjunct to treatment.

Complications. Anterior and posterior synechiae (adhesions of iris to lens and cornea), changes in intraocular pressure, corneal edema, various degrees of visual impairment, retinal detachment, glaucoma, enucleation, and cataracts are possible complications (Behrman, Kliegman, & Jenson, 2004; Rosenbaum & George, 2000).

Trachoma

Description. A chronic infectious disease of the eye, trachoma is characterized by follicular keratoconjunctivitis with neovascularization of the cornea. It is the second leading cause of blindness from any cause in the world and is preventable (Taylor & Taylor, 2000).

Etiology and Incidence. Trachoma is a chronic keratoconjunctivitis caused by *Chlamydia trachomatis* and is endemic in hot, dry, dusty, poverty-stricken areas with poor personal and community hygiene. It is rare in the United States but is endemic among Navaho Indians in the southwestern United States (Hammerschlag, 2004).

Clinical Findings. The following are noted:

- Inflammation
- Pain
- Photophobia
- Excessive tearing
- Granulation follicles on the upper eyelids and eventual invasion of the cornea causing blindness

Management. Consult with an ophthalmologist because treatment is difficult and recommendations vary. Treatment consists of adequate doses of oral tetracycline (doxycycline, azithromycin), erythromycin, and a topical antibiotic ointment to rapidly reduce inflammation to prevent scar formation. Steroids are contraindicated.

Reinforce the need for frequent handwashing and careful cleansing of the eyes. Discourage sharing of towels and handkerchiefs.

THE INJURED EYE

Corneal Injury

Description

Damage to or loss of the epithelial cells of the cornea in the form of a corneal abrasion (Table 29-8) or tear is relatively common. Scratches from paper, brushes, fingernails,

TABLE 29-8 *Common Eye Injuries*

Injury	Clinical Findings	Treatment
Corneal injury (abrasion)	Sensation or evidence of foreign body, pain, photophobia, tearing, blepharospasm, ↓ vision, + fluorescein staining	Rest, topical antibiotics, oral analgesics, follow-up in 24 hr; refer for any severe injury
Foreign body	Vertical striation on cornea, pain, tearing, sensation of foreign body, irregular or peaked pupil, perforating wound	Do not remove intraocular foreign body; if extraocular, irrigate eye to remove; topical antibiotic and patch; follow-up in 24 hr
Burns Chemical Thermal UV radiation	Pale, necrotic appearance to skin and eyelids, opaque cornea, visual impairment, photophobia, tearing, pain with UV injury only	Chemical and thermal: emergency; continuous irrigation for 20-30 min; to ophthalmologist with ongoing irrigation UV: topical antibiotic, patch, analgesics, heals in 1-2 days
Hyphema	Pain, tearing, photophobia; blood in anterior chamber, hazy iris, or inability to detect red reflex, change in visual acuity	Refer to ophthalmologist; restrict intake, place eye shield; increased risk if child has sickle cell trait or disease or other hematologic disorder
Lacerations	Pain, visual disturbance, uveal prolapse	Apply eye shield and refer immediately to ophthalmologist
Retinal detachment	Impaired vision, visual field impairment, "flashing light" sensation	Refer immediately to ophthalmologist
Hematoma/contusion of orbit	Retinal clouding, visual changes, bruised eyelid; symptoms of retinal detachment	Refer immediately to ophthalmologist to rule out closed head injury; CT scan, MRI, ultrasound radiography
Orbital fracture	Pain, diplopia, ↓ infraorbital nerve root sensation, facial bruising, globe displacement, swelling, corneal laceration, irregular pupil, hyphema or absent red light reflex	Plain film radiography, CT scan; refer immediately to an ophthalmologist; may need surgery

CT, Computed tomography; ↓, decrease; *MRI*, magnetic resonance imaging; +, positive; *UV*, ultraviolet.

contact lens overuse, improperly fitted cosmetic contact lenses, plants, or a foreign body in the conjunctival sac are often responsible.

Clinical Findings

The following may be noted:

- Evidence and sensation of a foreign body
- Severe pain and photophobia
- Tearing and blepharospasm
- Decreased vision
- Conjunctival erythema

Other Studies. Fluorescein staining with superficial uptake is indicative of a minor corneal abrasion. If the fluorescein staining goes deep into the cornea, subepithelial corneal damage (e.g., corneal ulceration or corneal tear) is possible. Vertical striations on the cornea suggest a foreign body embedded under the eyelid.

Management

The following steps are taken:

- Refer severe corneal injuries or possible subepithelial damage to an ophthalmologist.
- Patching is no longer indicated (Scoper, 2000).
- Use elbow restraints for the infant to ensure that the eye is not rubbed or further irritated.
- If no symptoms of corneal infection, use topical antibiotics (0.5% erythromycin or Polysporin ointment twice daily for 5 days); use a broader-spectrum topical antibiotic if early infection is suspected (Wilson, 2002).
- Repeated instillation of local anesthetic is not recommended because it interferes with reepithelialization of the cornea.
- Oral analgesics may be used to ease the discomfort.
- Advise the patient to return daily for follow-up evaluation or refer for slit-lamp examination within 24 to 36 hours. If no improvement is seen after 24 to 48 hours or if symptoms worsen, refer to an ophthalmologist.

Foreign Body

Description

A superficial foreign body in the eye is usually lodged on the surface of the eye or superficially in the cornea. It rarely results in serious trauma. Foreign objects may penetrate the globe (intraocular) with more serious consequences.

Etiology

Foreign bodies commonly occur in younger children during play and in older children during sports. Foreign bodies can include dirt particles, BB gun pellets, and debris thrown up by a lawn mower or in shop class.

Clinical Findings

The following may be noted via direct ophthalmoscope set at +10 to +12:

- Pain and foreign body sensation
- Foreign body in conjunctival sac
- Tearing
- Inflammation
- Irregular or peaked pupil
- Photophobia
- Opaque lens
- Perforating wound to the cornea or iris

Other Studies. Fluorescein staining may be useful if no foreign body is visualized. Ultrasonography or CT scan may be needed, depending on the foreign body and its location. An MRI is contraindicated. Refer any suspected intraocular penetration by a metal object or fragment (ask if patient had been engaged in a metal-on-metal activity [Johnson & Ellis, 2000]).

Management

Recommendations include the following:

- Never remove an intraocular foreign body, and never remove a foreign body if the history indicates that a projectile object was possibly involved in the injury. Refer immediately to an ophthalmologist.
- View the upper bulbar conjunctiva by having the patient look down while the upper lid is pulled away from the globe and illuminating the upper recess. Evert the eyelid to visualize the superior tarsal conjunctiva.
- Use of a topical anesthetic (proparacaine 0.5% or tetracaine 0.5%; 1 drop) facilitates patient cooperation.
- Remove an extraocular foreign body via irrigation with sterile saline or Dacriose. A moistened cotton swab may be used. Cautiously and gently roll it across the cornea to remove the extraocular foreign body, but only in cooperative patients; this maneuver might cause considerable additional damage to the epithelial surface (Eisenbaum, 2003; Trobe, 2001).
- If any difficulty is encountered when removing a foreign body from the eye, stop all efforts, patch the eye, and refer the patient immediately to an ophthalmologist.
- After removing any extraocular object, instill fluorescein stain and inspect the cornea with cobalt-blue light to look for green staining or lines. Instill an ophthalmic antibiotic solution (e.g., sulfacetamide or gentamicin with cycloplegic [Cyclopentolate 1%]) and patch the eye.
- Reschedule the patient in 24 hours or refer to an ophthalmologist for follow-up (Trobe, 2001).

Complications

Sympathetic ophthalmia, chronic siderosis, or a uveitis of the uninjured eye can occur any time from 10 days to years after a penetrating injury of the globe.

Burns

Etiology

Burns to the eyes and surrounding tissues can be thermal (caused by exposure to steam, flame, intense heat, cinders, or cigarettes), chemical (e.g., cleaning agents, fertilizers, pesticides, battery fluid, or laboratory products), or induced by UV light (e.g., from bright snow, laser pointers, or a sunlamp). The amount of damage to the eye is directly related to the length of exposure and the nature of the source of the burn. Chemical burns are true emergencies because of the progressive damage that can occur. Burns on the eyelids are classified and treated the same as burns elsewhere on the body.

Clinical Findings

The following may be noted:

- Pale or necrosed appearance of the surrounding skin and eyelids
- Opacity of corneal tissue
- Visual impairment (decreased acuity)
- Initial exquisite pain or delayed complaints of pain (e.g., in UV burns, pain emerges about 6 hours after exposure)
- Photophobia
- Tearing within 12 hours of exposure
- Swollen corneas
- Fluorescein stain revealing pinpoint uptake

Management

The following steps are taken:

- Instill a topical anesthetic if available.
- Chemical burns require immediate, ongoing irrigation. With the eyelids held apart, instill a steady, gentle solution of tepid water, saline, or Ringer's irrigation for 20 to 30 minutes or until the pH of the tear film is 7.3 to 7.7. Refer to an ophthalmologist after irrigation to determine the extent of the damage. Do not patch the eye; allow tearing to continue to cleanse the eye. Cool compresses applied to the surrounding skin may be comforting. Hospitalization may be needed for sedation and analgesia.
- Thermal burns may be treated the same way as acid or alkaline chemical burns, as discussed previously (Wander, 2000).
- UV burns are treated by using topical antibiotic prophylaxis, patches, and analgesics. Healing should occur in 1 to 2 days.

Lacerations

Description

Lacerations from injuries cause perforation of the cornea and lead to uveal prolapse. Twenty-eight percent of lacerations occur in the home, and causes include accidents (77%), assaults (22%), recreational activities (11%), and self-infliction (1%) (Scoper, 2000).

Management

Apply an eye shield to protect the eye. Refer the patient immediately to an ophthalmologist to rule out damage to the globe and surrounding structures.

Traumatic Hyphema

Description

A hyphema is an accumulation of visible blood or blood products in the anterior chamber of the eye.

Etiology and Incidence

A hyphema is the result of blunt trauma to the globe without penetration or perforation. This condition is most often caused by balls, fists or fingers, elbows, rocks, exploding airbags, and sticks. It may also occur in infants with birth trauma or in patients with retinoblastoma, juvenile xanthogranuloma of the iris, or abnormal hematologic profiles such as sickle cell trait or disease (Behrman, Kliegman, & Jenson, 2004; Romano, 2000). Hyphema is the most common contusion injury to the eye seen in children. It is responsible for more hospitalizations than any other ophthalmologic condition.

Clinical Findings

Vision, pupil motility, the lids and adnexa, the cornea and anterior segment, and the red reflex should all be assessed. The following may be noted:

- History of traumatic eye injury
- Somnolence (often associated with intracranial trauma)
- Blood appearing as a dark red fluid level between the cornea and iris on gross examination or as a hazy-appearing iris
- Inability to detect a bilateral red light reflex
- Pain, photophobia, and tearing
- Visual acuity changes and impaired vision (light perception and hand motion perception)

- Abnormal pupillary reflex
- Need for slit-lamp examination

Management

The goals of treatment include resolving the hyphema, making the patient comfortable, and preventing complications; however, no consensus has been reached on how to best accomplish such treatment (e.g., hospitalization or not, systemic medication or not, which medications). There is a risk of recurrent bleeding regardless of the size of the original bleed (Romano, 2000). However, the following steps should be taken:

- Refer the patient immediately to an ophthalmologist.
- Restrict oral intake until the child has been seen by an ophthalmologist.
- Place a perforated eye shield (not a patch) over the eye—avoid pressure to prevent reinjury.
- If a hematologic disorder is detected, ensure quick intervention and close follow-up.

The following steps are commonly recognized for treatment of traumatic hyphemas:

- Hospitalize all children and limit activity (may have bathroom privileges). Elevate the head of the bed to 30 to 45 degrees. Encourage the child to sleep in a supine position. Discourage reading or close eye work during this period.
- No atropine drops, antibiotics, tonometry, topical anesthetics, antiglaucoma agents, steroids, or topical dilating agents should be used (Romano, 2000).
- Acetaminophen (Tylenol) is the analgesic of choice; avoid aspirin and nonsteroidal antiinflammatory agents because they may add to the risk of a rebleed. Sedatives may be necessary in pediatric patients.
- Surgery may be necessary to remove the trapped blood from the chamber if it is causing an increase in intraocular pressure, in sickle cell patients, or if greater than 50% of the hyphema remains without some clearing in the first 4 days (Romano, 2000).
- Hospital discharge is usually after a week. The child should be followed closely by an ophthalmologist, because long-term monitoring is necessary to detect possible traumatic cataract, retinal detachment, or glaucoma.

Complications

A second hemorrhage can occur within 3 to 5 days of the first, leading to glaucoma, amblyopia, or corneal blood staining that can result in permanent visual loss. Patients with abnormal hematologic profiles (e.g., sickle cell disease or trait) are more likely to rebleed and are more likely to have visual loss because of glaucoma (Behrman, Kliegman, & Jenson, 2004; Romano, 2000).

Retinal Detachment

Description

Retinal detachment is detachment of the neurosensory retina from its retinal pigment epithelium base within the globe. Frequently associated with severe ocular trauma or child abuse, retinal detachment also occurs as a congenital abnormality or with pronounced myopia, aphakia, cataracts, ROP, Marfan syndrome, viral retinitis, penetrating trauma, retinoblastoma, or various retinopathies. There may be concurrent ocular disease or a family history of retinal detachment (Kirsch, 2000).

Clinical Findings

The following may be noted:

- Blurry vision that becomes progressively worse
- Dark cloud in one visual field, flashing lights, or a "shower of floaters"
- Darkening of retinal vessels on funduscopic examination
- Gray elevation at the site of detachment

Management

Instruct the patient not to eat, and refer the patient to an ophthalmologist for surgery to reattach the retina.

Orbital Hematoma/Contusion of the Globe

Etiology

This condition is usually the result of a blow to the globe. The degree of damage depends on the energy of the object hitting the globe. Such injuries commonly occur as a result of sports activities, motor vehicle accidents, assault, or BB gun accidents (Wilson & Edwards, 2000).

Clinical Findings

The following may be seen:

- Milky white appearance of the retina
- Visual acuity changes
- Severe bruising of the eyelids and periorbital tissues
- Lens dislocation
- Retinal detachment or edema
- Vitreous, retinal, or choroid hemorrhage
- Rupture of the eyeball

Management

Refer the patient immediately to an ophthalmologist. A closed head injury, damage to the skull, and facial bone fractures will need to be ruled out via CT scan, MRI, or ultrasound radiography. Occasionally cryopexy or laser photocoagulation surgery is needed for contusions of the globe.

Complications

Possible complications include permanent visual loss, retinal necrosis, subretinal hemorrhage, and retinal or macular holes.

Orbital Fractures

Description

An orbital fracture is a fracture of the walls of the orbit secondary to blunt trauma to the face or eye(s). The orbital floor is more commonly fractured. The inferior rectus muscle may become caught in the fracture site.

Etiology

The usual cause of an orbital fracture is a blow or blunt trauma to the orbit (e.g., ball, fist, motor vehicle accident [hitting the dashboard], fall).

Clinical Findings

The following may be noted:

- Pain, diplopia
- Loss of sensation along the path of the infraorbital nerve (upper lip and ipsilateral cheek)
- Ecchymosis of the lids, nosebleed, trouble chewing
- Limited ocular movement (especially upward) and weakness in downward movement
- Globe displacement with a sunken-eye appearance or a protruding eye
- Bony discontinuity or "step-off"
- Subcutaneous emphysema in surrounding tissues and edema
- Enophthalmos
- Corneal laceration
- Irregular pupil
- Hyphema or absent red light reflex (Trobe, 2001)

Diagnostic Studies. Plain film radiography and CT scan are the best imaging modalities.

Management

- An orbital fracture is an ophthalmologic emergency requiring immediate intervention and referral. Diagnostic studies are performed to rule out injury to the skull and cranial contents. Open reduction may be necessary if any of the orbital bones are displaced or to rule out displacement of the globe or enophthalmos.
- Icing the injury for 24 hours, followed by heat for 2 to 3 days, allows the swelling to subside before surgical repair. Surgery is often best done within 2 weeks of the injury.
- Antibiotics and nasal decongestant may also be used.

Pterygium

A pterygium is a fibrovascular mass of thickened bulbar conjunctiva that extends beyond the limbus onto the cornea. Elastic and hyaline degenerative changes occur. The lesion is usually triangular and commonly found on the nasal side of the orbit—less often on the temporal side (Behrman, Kliegman, & Jenson, 2004; Rich, 2000). It is caused by irritation of the bulbar conjunctiva from sunlight, wind, dust, fumes, or airborne allergens; it can also be hereditary. Growth rates of the lesions vary. A pinguecula may precede the pterygium, which will occur as a yellow-white, slightly raised mass on the bulbar conjunctiva. The lesion is usually painless, may itch, and may be accompanied by occasional complaints of blurred vision if the lesion enlarges. It can be confused with melanoma, squamous cell carcinoma, intraepithelial epithelioma, or a dermoid cyst. Treatment involves protecting against irritants (wear goggles or sunglasses, use topical lubricants such as artificial tears) and using mild vasoconstrictors or short-term steroids for inflammation. Surgical removal may be needed if the pterygium impedes vision. Complications include visual impairment to blindness (occurrence 40% to 50%), recurrence after surgical removal, restricted ocular mobility (especially with abduction), and diplopia.

Subconjunctival Hemorrhage

Subconjunctival hemorrhage is splotchy bulbar conjunctival redness that spontaneously occurs or is secondary to intrathoracic pressure (from coughing, sneezing, or straining) that results in the bursting of conjunctival vessels. It is commonly found in neonates as a benign occurrence to a vaginal delivery. The hemorrhages usually spontaneously resolve within 1 week. No treatment is indicated (Trobe, 2001).

Entropion

Entropion is a condition in which the eyelids invert so that the cilia or epithelium rubs against the corneal surface, causing abrasion or irritation. Both the upper and lower eyelids may be involved. There is a rare congenital form. On examination, there is evidence of lid laxity. Pain or irritation and photophobia are typical symptoms. Complications include corneal scarring and corneal infections (Dailey, 2000). Management involves surgical intervention.

Ectropion

Ectropion is a condition in which the eyelid margins evert, resulting in the overflow of tears down the cheeks. It may be seen in patients with Down syndrome. Management

RESOURCE BOX

Eye Problems

Blind Children's Center
1-800-222-3566
www.blindcntr.org

National Federation of the Blind: National Organization of Parents of Blind Children
1-410-659-9314
www.nfb.org/nopbc.htm

Prevent Blindness America
1-800-331-2020
www.preventblindness.org

Protective Eyewear Certification Council
c/o Paul Vinger, M.D.
297 Heath's Bridge Rd.
Concord, MA 01742
www.protecteyes.org

Vision World Wide
1-800-431-1739
www.visionww.org/bookstore.htm

involves lubrication for mild cases; surgery is indicated for chronic or symptomatic cases.

REFERENCES

American Academy of Ophthalmology, Pediatric Ophthalmology Panel: *Preferred practice guidelines: pediatric eye evaluations*, San Francisco, 2002, American Academy of Ophthalmology.

American Academy of Ophthalmology: Eyeglasses for infants and children. Medem Medical Library website. Available at *www.medem.com* (accessed Jan 16, 2003).

American Academy of Optometry, American Optometric Association: Vision, learning and dyslexia, *J Am Optom Assoc* 68:284-286, 1997.

American Academy of Pediatrics: Learning disabilities, dyslexia, and vision: a subject review, *Pediatrics* 102:1217-1219, 1998.

American Academy of Pediatrics: *2003 red book: report of the Committee on Infectious Diseases*, ed 26, Elk Grove Village, IL, 2003, American Academy of Pediatrics.

American Academy of Pediatrics: Use of photoscreening for children's vision screening, *Pediatrics* 109(3):524-525, 2002.

Anderson PD: *Basic human anatomy and physiology: clinical implications for the health professions*, Boston, 1984, Jones & Bartlett.

Andley U, Liang J, Lou M: Biochemical mechanisms of age-related cataract. In Albert D et al, editors: *Principles and practice of ophthalmology*, ed 2, Philadelphia, 2000, WB Saunders.

Ballard E: Excessive tearing in infancy and early childhood: the role and treatment of congenital lacrimal duct obstruction, *Postgrad Med Online* 107(6), 2000.

Behrman RE, Kliegman R, Jenson H, editors: *Nelson textbook of pediatrics*, ed 16, Philadelphia, 2000, WB Saunders.

Centers for Disease Control and Prevention: Hypertrophic pyloric stenosis in infants following pertussis prophylaxis with erythromycin—Knoxville, Tennessee, 1999, *MMWR Morb Mortal Wkly Rep* 48(49):1117-1120, 1999.

Centers for Disease Control and Prevention: Guidelines for the treatment of sexually transmitted diseases 2002, *MMWR Morb Mortal Wkly Rep* 2002:51(RR-6):2002.

Clinician News staff: Improper use of cosmetic lenses a disturbing national trend, *Clinician News* 7(2), March 2003, p 6.

Collum L, Kilmartin D: Acute allergic conjunctivitis. In Abelson M, editor: *Allergic diseases of the eye*, Philadelphia, 2001, WB Saunders.

Contemporary Pediatrics editorial staff: Management of conjunctivitis: diagnosis and treatment of bacterial disease, *Contemp Pediatr Suppl* 2000.

Contemporary Pediatrics editorial staff: Management of conjunctivitis: mimics and non-bacterial disease, *Contemp Pediatr: Suppl* 2001.

Coster D, Badenoch P: Bacterial corneal ulcers. In Fraunfelder F, Roy F, editors: *Current ocular therapy*, ed 5, Philadelphia, 2000, WB Saunders.

Dailey R: Entropion. In Fraunfelder F, Roy F, editors: *Current ocular therapy*, ed 5, Philadelphia, 2000, WB Saunders.

De La Paz M, D'Amico D: Photic retinopathy. In Albert D et al, editors: *Principles and practice of ophthalmology*, ed 2, Philadelphia, 2000, WB Saunders.

DeRespinis PA: Eyeglasses: why and when do children need them? *Pediatr Ann* 30(8):455-461, 2001.

Duboraw C, Stasior G, Krohel G: Orbital cellulitis and abscess. In Fraunfelder F, Roy F, editors: *Current ocular therapy*, ed 5, Philadelphia, 2000, WB Saunders.

Eisenbaum A: Eye. In Hay WW et al, editors: *Current pediatric diagnosis and treatment*, ed 16, New York, 2003, McGraw-Hill.

Finegold I: Successful management of ocular allergy with atopic diseases. Presented at the American College of Allergy, Asthma, and Immunology meeting, Philadelphia, Nov 6-11, 1998.

Food and Drug Administration: FDA issues warning on misuse of laser pointers. Press release P97-45, Dec 18, 1997. Available at *www.fda.gov/bbs/topics* (accessed Dec 19, 1998).

Fraioli A: Conjunctivitis and orbital cellulitis in childhood. In Albert D et al, editors: *Principles and practice of ophthalmology*, ed 2, Philadelphia, 2000, WB Saunders.

Francesconi C, Azar D, Talamo J: Incisional refractive surgery. In Albert D et al, editors: *Principles and practice of ophthalmology*, ed 2, Philadelphia, 2000, WB Saunders.

Fraunfelder F: Hordeolum. In Fraunfelder F, Roy F, editors: *Current ocular therapy*, ed 5, Philadelphia, 2000, WB Saunders.

Friedlander M: Allergic conjunctivitis. In Fanaroff A, Martin F, editors: *Neonatal-perinatal medicine*, vol 2, *Diseases of the fetus and infant*, ed 7, St Louis, 2002, Mosby.

Gupta B, Hamming N, Miller M: Neonatal eye disease: retinoblastoma. In Fanaroff A, Martin F, editors: *Neonatal-perinatal medicine*, vol 2, *Diseases of the fetus and infant*, ed 7, St Louis, 2002, Mosby.

Hammerschlag M: *Chlamydia trachomatis*. In Behrman RE, Kliegman R, Jenson H, editors: *Nelson textbook of pediatrics*, ed 17, Philadelphia, 2004, WB Saunders.

Hoekelman R: *Primary pediatric care*, ed 4, St Louis, 2001, Mosby.

International Dyslexia Association: Website. Available at *www.interdys.org* (accessed Oct 15, 2002).

Jockin Y: Strabismus and amblyopia. In Burg F et al, editors: *Gellis and Kagan's current pediatric therapy*, ed 17, Philadelphia, 2002, WB Saunders.

Johnson D, Ellis P: Intraocular foreign body: steel or iron. In Fraunfelder F, Roy F, editors: *Current ocular therapy*, ed 5, Philadelphia, 2000, WB Saunders.

Kane K, Ellis M: When should acute non-venereal conjunctivitis be treated with topical antibiotics? *J Fam Pract* 51(4):312, 2002.

Kapur R, Yoder M, Polin R: The immune system: development and disorders of organ systems. In Fanaroff A, Martin F, editors: *Neonatal-perinatal medicine*, vol 2, *Diseases of the fetus and infant*, ed 7, St Louis, 2002, Mosby.

Kirsch L: Retinal detachment. In Fraunfelder F, Roy F, editors: *Current ocular therapy*, ed 5, Philadelphia, 2000, WB Saunders.

Kushner B: Atropine vs. patching for treatment of amblyopia in children, *JAMA* 287(16):2145-2146, 2002.

Lin J, Edmond J: Leukocoria. American Association for Pediatric Ophthalmology and Strabismus website. Available at *http://med-aapos.bu.edu/aapos/pediintro* (accessed Jan 20, 2003).

Mahon B, Rosenman M, Kleinman M: Maternal and infant use of erythromycin and other macrolide antibiotics as risk factors for infantile hypertrophic pyloric stenosis, *J Pediatr* 139(3):380-384, 2001.

McKeown C: The pediatric eye exam. In Albert D et al, editors: *Principles and practice of ophthalmology*, ed 2, Philadelphia, 2000, WB Saunders.

McManaway J, Frankel C: Strabismus. In Hoekelman R, editor: *Primary pediatric care*, ed 4, St Louis, 2001, Mosby.

Milder B: Dacryocystitis and dacryolith. In Fraunfelder F, Roy F, editors: *Current ocular therapy*, ed 5, Philadelphia, 2000, WB Saunders.

Miller K, Apt L: Strabismus. In Rudolph A, Rudolph C, editors: *Rudolph's pediatrics*, ed 21, New York, 2002, McGraw-Hill Medical Publishing Division.

Murphree A, Christensen L: Retinoblastoma. In Fraunfelder F, Roy F, editors: *Current ocular therapy*, ed 5, Philadelphia, 2000, WB Saunders.

Neu N: Chlamydial diseases. In Burg F et al, editors: *Gellis and Kagan's current pediatric therapy*, ed 17, Philadelphia, 2002, WB Saunders.

Palmer E: Retinopathy of prematurity. In Fraunfelder F, Roy F, editors: *Current ocular therapy*, ed 5, Philadelphia, 2000, WB Saunders.

Paradis A, Granet D: Don't let children rub their eyes! *Infect Dis Child* 15(5):66-67, 2002.

Paysse E: Retinopathy of prematurity. In Singh K, Smiddy W, Lee A, editors: *Ophthalmology review*, New York, 2002, Thieme.

Pediatric Eye Disease Investigational Group: A randomized trial of atropine vs. patching for treatment of moderate amblyopia in children, *Arch Ophthalmol* 120(3):268-278, 2002.

Phelps DL: Retinopathy of prematurity. In Fanaroff A, Martin F, editors: *Neonatal-perinatal medicine*, vol 2, *Diseases of the fetus and infant*, ed 7, St Louis, 2002, Mosby.

Power W: Introduction to uveitis. In Albert D et al, editors: *Principles and practice of ophthalmology*, ed 2, Philadelphia, 2000, WB Saunders.

Pratt-Johnson J, Tillson G: *Management of strabismus and amblyopia: a practical guide*, ed 2, New York, 2001, Thieme.

Quinn G: Introduction: ocular disorders and the primary care practitioner. In Burg F et al, editors: *Gellis and Kagan's current pediatric therapy*, ed 17, Philadelphia, 2002, WB Saunders.

Raizman M: Pathophysiology and differential diagnosis of ocular allergy. Presented at the American College of Allergy, Asthma, and Immunology meeting, Philadelphia, Nov 6-11, 1998.

Reichel E: Hereditary gene dysfunction syndromes. In Albert D et al, editors: *Principles and practice of ophthalmology*, ed 2, Philadelphia, 2000, WB Saunders.

Retinoblastoma International: Presenting signs and symptoms of leukocoria, 2000. Available at *www.kidseyecancer.org* (accessed Jan 20, 2003).

Rich L: Pterygium and pseudopterygium. In Fraunfelder F, Roy F, editors: *Current ocular therapy*, ed 5, Philadelphia, 2000, WB Saunders.

Robb R: Strabismus in childhood. In Albert D et al, editors: *Principles and practice of ophthalmology*, ed 2, Philadelphia, 2000, WB Saunders.

Romano P: Traumatic hyphema. In Fraunfelder F, Roy F, editors: *Current ocular therapy*, ed 5, Philadelphia, 2000, WB Saunders.

Rosenbaum J, George R: Uveitis. In Fraunfelder F, Roy F, editors: *Current ocular therapy*, ed 5, Philadelphia, 2000, WB Saunders.

Rubin S: Management of strabismus in the first year of life, *Pediatr Ann* 30(8):474-480, 2001.

Schaffer D: Conjunctiva. In Burg F et al, editors: *Gellis and Kagan's current pediatric therapy*, ed 17, Philadelphia, 2002, WB Saunders.

School of Public Health, University of California-Berkeley: The best pair of shades, *Wellness Letter* 18(10):4, 2002.

Scoper S: Corneal abrasion, contusions, lacerations and perforations. In Fraunfelder F, Roy F, editors: *Current ocular therapy*, ed 5, Philadelphia, 2000, WB Saunders.

Steinemann T: Staphylococcus. In Fraunfelder F, Roy F, editors: *Current ocular therapy*, ed 5, Philadelphia, 2000, WB Saunders.

Taylor K, Taylor J: Trachoma. In Fraunfelder F, Roy F, editors: *Current ocular therapy*, ed 5, Philadelphia, 2000, WB Saunders.

Trobe J: *The physician's guide to eye care*, San Francisco, 2001, Foundation of the American Academy of Ophthalmology.

US Department of Health and Human Services: *Healthy people 2010*, vol 1, *Child and adolescent focused objectives*, Washington, DC, 2000, US Department of Health and Human Services.

US Preventive Services Task Force: *Guide to clinical preventive services*, ed 2, Baltimore, 1996, Williams & Wilkins.

US Public Health Service: *Put prevention into practice: the clinician's handbook of preventive services*, ed 2, Germantown, MD, 1997, International Medical Publishing.

Vinger P: A practical guide for sports eye protection, *Physician Sportsmed* 28(6):49-66, 2000.

Wander A: Thermal burns. In Fraunfelder F, Roy F, editors: *Current ocular therapy*, ed 5, Philadelphia, 2000, WB Saunders.

Wessels I: Chalazion. In Fraunfelder F, Roy F, editors: *Current ocular therapy*, ed 5, Philadelphia, 2000, WB Saunders.

Wheeler L et al: Educational intervention strategies for children with visual impairment with emphasis on retinopathy of prematurity, *J Pediatr Health Care* 11(6):275-279, 1997.

Wilson D, Edwards A: Chorioretinal concussions and lacerations. In Fraunfelder F, Roy F, editors: *Current ocular therapy*, ed 5, Philadelphia, 2000, WB Saunders.

Wilson M: Cornea. In Burg F et al, editors: *Gellis and Kagan's current pediatric therapy*, ed 17, Philadelphia, 2002, WB Saunders.

Zwann J, editor: Eye problems. In Dershewitz RA, editor: *Ambulatory pediatric care*, ed 3, Philadelphia, 1999, Lippincott-Raven.

30 Ear Disorders

Ann Marie Petersen-Smith

The ear provides the body with the ability to hear and maintain equilibrium. Appropriate functioning of the ear is essential for hearing, acquisition of speech, and the ability to maintain an upright position. The ear extends from the external to the inner ear structures. Malfunction of any of the structures of the ear can have an impact on both the ear and surrounding tissue. Additionally, ear dysfunction can cause systemic problems that can have a lifelong impact. Adequate hearing is important for learning, socialization, and language development. Caring for children with ear problems is an important role of the nurse practitioner (NP), and understanding of ear anatomy, physiology, and disorders allows the NP to thoughtfully assess the system and its functions.

STANDARDS FOR HEARING SCREENING

Universal detection of hearing loss before 3 months of age is endorsed by the Joint Committee on Infant Hearing (2000a, 2000b), the *Healthy Hearing 2010* objectives for the nation's hearing health (U.S. Department of Health and Human Services, 2000), and the National Institutes of Health (NIH) (1993). These recommendations also include follow-up by 3 months of age and appropriate family-centered intervention by 6 months of age. Screening of newborns or infants can be done by using evoked otoacoustical emission testing or the auditory brainstem response. However, the U.S. Preventive Services Task Force (USPSTF) (2001) maintains that there is insufficient evidence to recommend for or against routine screening of asymptomatic newborns. The USPSTF does agree with the need for predischarge screening of newborns with one or more neonatal risk factors and screening for hearing loss in children 1 month to 3 years of age with certain risk factors.

During childhood, routine screening of asymptomatic children older than 3 years is debated. The USPSTF (2001) does not recommend screening beyond 3 years of age or in adolescence. However, the Joint Committee on Infant Hearing, the American Academy of Pediatrics (AAP), and Bright Futures Guidelines all recommend pure-tone audiometry at 3, 4, 5, 10, 12, 15, and 18 years of age, with subjective assessment at other ages (U.S. Public Health Service, 1997). The American Speech-Language-Hearing Association recommends annual pure-tone audiometry from age 3 to grade 3 (U.S. Public Health Service, 1997). Screening of high-risk children, including those with frequently recurring otitis media (OM), middle ear effusion, or both, or those with chronic exposure to loud noises, should include annual audiologic screening and monitoring the development of communication skills.

DEVELOPMENT, ANATOMY, AND PHYSIOLOGY

Development

Development of the ear begins during the third week of gestation and is complete by the third month of embryonic life. Insult to the fetus during this time can cause irreparable damage to the ear. Ear development occurs at the same time as kidney development, so malformation or dysfunction in one system should alert the practitioner to problems in the other.

Anatomy and Physiology

The external ear is responsible for transmission of sound waves from outside the ear to the middle ear and for clearance of debris. The canal contains glands that secrete sweat, sebum, and cerumen, which help lubricate the hair follicles and aid in the removal of debris. Patency of the ear canal is imperative for proper functioning.

The tympanic cavity constitutes the middle ear. The tympanic membrane is at the proximal end of the external auditory canal and separates the external ear from the middle ear. The middle ear is a small chamber in the temporal bone that contains the ossicles—the malleus, incus, and stapes—which function to transmit sound waves from the external auditory canal to the inner ear. The malleus lies against the tympanic membrane, which vibrates when sound waves hit it. The stapes rests against the oval window, and its vibration causes the oval window to stimulate the fluids of the inner ear.

The eustachian tube has three physiologic functions with respect to the middle ear: (1) ventilation of the middle ear to equalize air pressure in the middle ear with atmospheric pressure and to replace oxygen that has been absorbed; (2) protection from nasopharyngeal sound, pressure, and secretions; and (3) drainage of secretions from the middle ear into the nasopharynx.

The inner ear functions to transmit sound and aid in balance. Vibrations of the tympanic membrane, ossicles, and oval window set the inner ear fluids in motion. The fluid sound waves reach the cochlea, wherein lies the organ of Corti, which contains the hearing receptor hair cells. The hair cells transmit impulses to the auditory nerve (cranial nerve VIII), which transmits stimuli to the auditory cortex of the temporal lobe in the brain. The equilibrium receptors lie in the semicircular canals and vestibule of the inner ear. The semicircular canals respond to changes in direction of movement. The vestibule contains receptors essential to the maintenance of equilibrium (Fig. 30-1).

PATHOPHYSIOLOGY AND DEFENSE MECHANISMS

Pathophysiology

The processes that negatively affect the ear are usually localized; however, ear pathology can be related to systemic dysfunction or disorders. Common localized pathology includes disruption of defense mechanisms; viral, bacterial, or fungal infections in the inner, middle, and outer ear; foreign bodies in the ear; and trauma. Neurologic dysfunction, poor immunologic competence, and congenital anomalies are common systemic disorders that can affect the ear and its functions. External influences such as excessive noise in the environment can cause irreparable damage to the ear's hearing function.

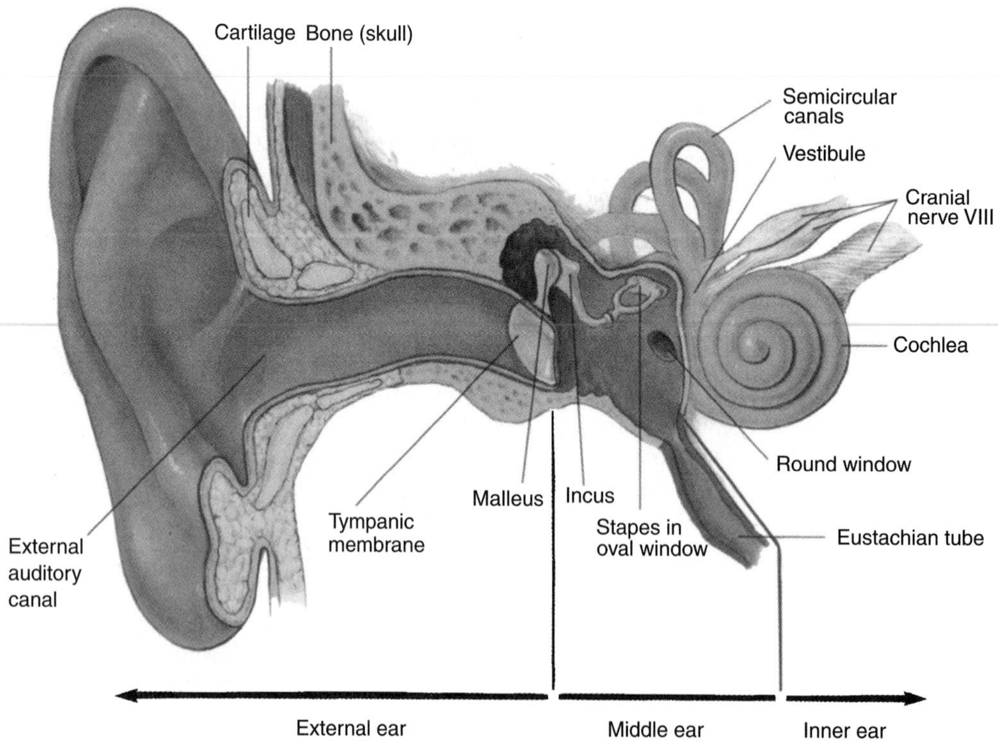

FIGURE 30-1 Anatomy of the ear. (From Jarvis C: *Physical examination and health assessment,* ed 2, Philadelphia, 1996, WB Saunders, p 365.)

Defense Mechanisms

Debris formed by keratinizing cells in the ear is lubricated and extruded by the cilia in the external auditory canal. Maintenance of an acidic pH in the ear canal prevents the growth of pathogenic bacteria. Additionally, the surface lining of the external ear is water resistant and has ample blood and lymph supply. These characteristics, as well as the antibacterial properties of cerumen, help protect against invading microorganisms. In comparison to the distal end of the external auditory canal, the proximal end has fewer hair fibers, a thinner epithelial layer, and more nerve fibers that cause great discomfort when touched. This sensitivity to pain serves a protective function by deterring the insertion of foreign bodies into the ear, thus avoiding damage to the middle ear.

The inner ear is also well protected inasmuch as the structures for both hearing and equilibrium are set deep within the skull.

ASSESSMENT

History

The history of a patient with an ear disorder should include the following:

- Previous medical history significant for craniofacial abnormalities or syndromes associated with craniofacial anomalies
- Pain (onset, location, quality, duration, alleviating or aggravating factors)
- Associated symptoms such as fever, vomiting and diarrhea, nasal congestion, or other symptoms of upper respiratory infection
- Itching or discharge
- Tinnitus or hearing loss
- Past medical history pertinent to the ear
- Family history of ear dysfunction
- Craniofacial abnormality (cleft lip/palate) or syndrome associated with craniofacial abnormality (Down syndrome, Treacher Collins syndrome)
- Prematurity
- Exposure to risk factors: environmental tobacco smoke (ETS), bottle propping, day care, noise, swimming
- Family history of or presence of kidney malformation
- Diabetes mellitus

Physical Examination

The physical examination includes the following:

- Inspection of the external structures of the ear for symmetry, skin abnormalities, discharge, or lesions. The inner and outer canthi of the eye should form a straight line with the superior portion of the pinna. If the pinna inserts below this line, the ear is said to be low set.
- Observation for developmental milestones related to hearing (Box 30-1).
- Palpation and rotation of the external ear for tenderness and inflammation; push on the tragus and apply pressure to the mastoid process.
- An otoscopic examination, which can be better accomplished in a young child at the end of the physical examination with the child on an examining table or seated on the parent's lap. Pulling the ear downward, outward, and backward can enhance visualization of the external auditory canal in infants and small children. In older children and adolescents, the external auditory canal is lifted upward and backward, slightly away from the head.

BOX 30-1 *Developmental Milestones Used to Assess Hearing*

Birth to 3 Months

Startles (Moro reflex) to loud noise
Awakens to sounds
Blinks or widens eyes to noises

Age 3 to 6 Months

Quiets to parent's voice
Stops activity to listen to new sound
Looks for source of sound
Reciprocates vocally and initiates sounds

Age 6 to 12 Months

Coos and gurgles with inflection
Responds to simple phrases
Turns to localize sound in any plane
Responds to own name

Age 12 to 18 Months

Points to unexpected sound or familiar objects when asked
Follows simple direction without cues
Imitates some sounds, first words by 12 to 15 months

Age 18 to 24 Months

Points to body parts when asked
Has expressive vocabulary of 20 to 50 words
50% of speech intelligible to strangers

Adapted from Northern J, Downs M: *Hearing in children*, ed 4, Baltimore, 1991, Williams & Wilkins.

- Decreased tympanic membrane mobility secondary to effusion is noted through pneumatic otoscopy, tympanometry, or acoustic reflectometry.
- Examination of the canal for redness, edema, or discharge. Assess all 360 degrees of the tympanic membrane, the bony processes, and the cone of light (see Color Fig. 3). Use pneumatic otoscopy to note the position, color, gloss, and movement of the eardrum. Look for air-fluid level or bubbles behind the tympanic membrane. Note any retraction or perforation.

Common Diagnostic Studies

- *Evoked otoacoustic emission testing* (EOAE) is the method of hearing screening being used for universal newborn screening. Dr. Kemp first described the phenomenon of otoacoustic emissions in 1978. The normal-hearing ear emits detectable 20 dB sounds called *spontaneous otoacoustic emissions.* The normal ear also emits these sounds when given a stimulus. EOAE is highly sensitive and easy to perform. It can be completed in less than 10 minutes. EOAE does not quantify hearing deficit but identifies whether the cochlea is functioning. It does have an approximately 10% false-positive result and may not identify a child with auditory nerve damage (Finitzo, Albright, & O'Neal, 1998; Mason & Hermann, 1998).
- *Auditory brainstem response* (ABR) measures the initiation of sound-induced electrical signals in the cochlea. The ABR is useful in identifying hearing loss in a young infant or in children unable to cooperate with audiometry. Automated ABR is now available as a screening device. It takes 10 to 15 minutes to perform, has a 5% false-positive rate, and can be administered in a noisy nursery.
- *Audiometry,* useful in assessing hearing loss in children, measures hearing threshold via bone or air conduction, or both, in decibels at varying frequencies (Tables 30-1 and 30-2). Twenty decibels is about as loud as a whisper, 90 dB produces pain, and 40 dB is normal speaking loudness. The frequencies of normal speaking range from 250 to 4000 Hz. Hearing loss, especially in the higher frequencies (2000 to 6000 Hz), can cause significant problems in understanding speech. A screening audiogram that tests each ear at 20 dB and frequencies of 500, 1000, 2000, and 4000 Hz is a useful assessment tool in office pediatrics. If a more detailed audiogram is needed, a qualified audiologist should perform it.
- *Pneumatic otoscopy* helps assess tympanic membrane mobility. A good seal with the speculum and otoscope is required before insufflation of air into the ear canal. Brisk movement of the membrane should be seen; altered mobility suggests middle ear effusion or possible perforation.
- *Tympanometry* assesses movement of tympanic membranes by applying from -400 to $+100$ mm H_2O pressure to the ear canal. Movement of the tympanic membrane is translated into a graph called a *tympanogram* (Fig. 30-2). The type A tympanogram has a compliance peak between ±100 mm H_2O and reflects a normal tympanic membrane. The type B tympanogram generally has no peak or a flattened wave and suggests effusion, perforation, or the presence of a pressure-equalizing tube. The type C tympanogram has a sharp peak between -100 and -200 mm H_2O and reflects negative ear pressure. (See Fig. 30-3 for types of tympanograms.) Tympanograms are helpful when otitis media with effusion is persistent or a question remains regarding the results of physical examination of the eardrum. Tympanograms are of little use in children younger than 7 months because their ear canals are hypercompliant in response to pressure from the tympanometer.
- *Acoustic reflectometry* is a newer sonar technology that can be used in the primary care setting. The handheld instrument, which consists of an acoustic transducer that has 44 different frequencies at 80 dB, can be used to detect the presence of middle ear effusion. A microphone records sound reflection back from the eardrum. A microprocessor measures the difference in frequency of the sound emitted and the sound returned. A fluid-filled middle ear space restricts vibration of the eardrum, so sound is intensified when returning to the device. The result is a spectral gradient angle that is displayed on a panel on the device. The angle size correlates with the likelihood of middle ear disease. It is a painless procedure, does not require an airtight seal, and does not pressurize the canal.
- *Tympanocentesis* with aspiration of middle ear fluid is helpful for the relief of pain and identification of persistent infecting organisms. It is rarely used in clinical pediatrics and is generally considered outside the scope of practice of the NP.
- Laboratory tests of blood and urine are rarely indicated unless questions remain regarding perinatal infection, systemic illness, or concomitant kidney dysfunction.

TABLE 30-1 *Audiologic Tests for Infants and Young Children*

Test	Characteristics	Age Range	Advantages	Disadvantages
Behavioral observation audiometry (BOA)	Behavioral test: responses to noisemakers or calibrated sounds are observed	0-5 mo	Low cost	Insensitive to unilateral or less than severe hearing loss; highly subject to observer bias; child tires rapidly when subjected to repeated stimuli
Visual reinforced audiometry (VRA)	Behavioral test: child is given an animated toy for turning to sounds	5-24 mo	Low cost; child responds at softer levels and for longer periods compared with BOA	Insensitive to unilateral loss (unless earphones used); need two examiners to reduce bias
Play audiometry	Behavioral test: child is trained to respond to tones by playing game	2-5 yr	Low cost; can detect unilateral and mild hearing loss	Requires cooperation of child
Screening audiometry	Behavioral test: child raises hand or responds verbally to tones at fixed levels (20-25 dB)	4 yr and older	Can be performed by trained paraprofessional in most children age 4 yr and older; can detect unilateral and mild hearing loss	Further tests required if failed
Otoacoustic emissions (OAE)	Physiologic test: response of inner ear to brief clicks or tones is measured with specialized instrument	Any	Child's response not needed; takes fewer than 2 min if child is quiet; can be performed by a trained paraprofessional; low cost; can detect unilateral and mild hearing loss	Cannot tell type or degree of loss; further tests required if failed
Auditory brainstem response (ABR) audiometry	Physiologic test: averaged number of response or brainstem to brief tones or clicks	Any	Child's response not needed; can detect unilateral and mild loss; can determine degree and slope of loss (with tone bursts and bone conduction testing)	Requires audiologist and equipment to administer and interpret; expensive; requires sedation beyond about 6 mo of age

From Daly KA, Hunter LL, Giebink GS: Chronic otitis media with effusion, *Pediatr Rev* 20(3):85-93, 1999.

TABLE 30-2 *Evaluation of Audiometric Results*

Average Threshhold at 500-2000 Hz (dB)	Description	Significance
−10 to +15	Normal	
16-25	Slight loss	Difficulty hearing faint speech, slight verbal deficit
26-40	Mild loss	Auditory learning dysfunction, language or speech problems
41-55	Moderate loss	Trouble hearing conversational speech, may miss 50% of class discussion
56-70	Moderately severe loss	
71-90	Severe loss	Educational retardation, learning disability, limited vocabulary
90	Profound loss	

A normal tympanogram is depicted below. Four features of the tympanogram can be used to evaluate the ear under test:

❶ **Static admittance (Peak Ya)** is a measure of the height of the tympanometric peak. Given appropriate norms, static admittance is a useful indicator of middle ear disease.

❷ **Equivalent ear canal volume (+200 Vea)** is the admittance value determined with an ear canal air pressure of +200 daPa (dekapascals). An abnormally high equivalent ear canal volume suggests the presence of a tympanic membrane perforation, or a patent tympanostomy tube.

❸ **Tympanometric peak pressure (TPP)** is the position of the tympanometric peak on the pressure axis. TPP is an imprecise measure of the middle ear pressure. By itself, TPP is not an accurate indicator of middle ear disease.

❹ **Tympanometric gradient (GR) or tympanometric width** is a measure of the width of the tympanometric peak. Defined as the pressure interval required for a 50% reduction of peak eardrum admittance, tympanometric width is a good indicator of the presence of **middle ear effusion**.

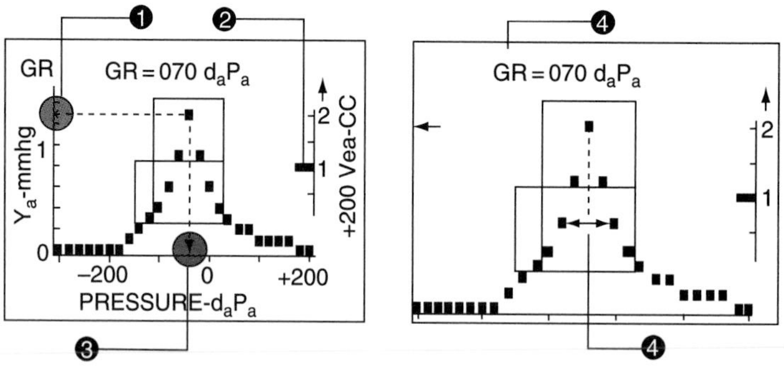

FIGURE 30-2 A normal tympanogran. (From WelchAllyn: MicroTymp Portable Tympanometric Instrument operating instructions. Available at *www.welchallyn.com*, Skaneateles Falls, NY.)

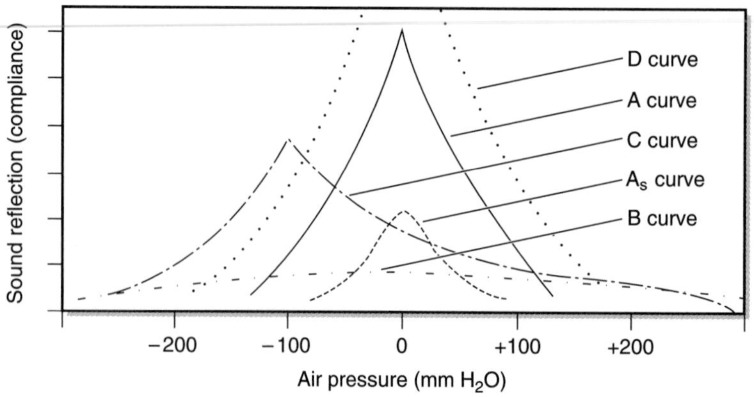

FIGURE 30-3 Tympanogram. Five types of tympanogram curves. Generally, an *A* curve indicates a normal tympanic membrane, a *B* curve is abnormal, a *C* curve may be abnormal, and a *D* curve indicates hypermobility. An A_s curve may be normal in infants. (From Harrison CJ, Belhorn TH: Acute otitis media: management and prophylaxis, *Clin Rev*, Apr 1992, p 55.)

MANAGEMENT STRATEGIES

Medications

Medications are used only when indicated. Antibiotics and antifungals are necessary when infection is present. The following practice guidelines regarding the judicious use of antimicrobial agents in pediatric patients have been developed by the AAP (Dowell et al, 1998).

- Otitis media should be classified as acute otitis media (AOM) or otitis media with effusion (OME). AOM is diagnosed when there is fluid present in the middle ear with signs of acute local or systemic illness such as otalgia, otorrhea, or fever. With OME, fluid is present in the middle ear without signs or symptoms of acute infection.
- Antimicrobials are indicated to treat AOM if there is documented middle ear effusion and signs or symptoms of acute local or systemic infection. Pneumatic otoscopy can be used to assess the tympanic membrane for color, position, translucency, and mobility. Tympanometry and acoustic reflectometry also can be used to validate effusion. Fever without other findings, such as ear pain or red or bulging tympanic membrane, may be unrelated to middle ear effusion.
- A short course of antimicrobials (5 to 7 days) is acceptable for treating uncomplicated AOM in certain patients. Data support short-course therapy in older children (older than 2 years of age) with mild AOM.
- Antimicrobial agents are not indicated for the initial treatment of OME. Antibiotic therapy or bilateral myringotomy with insertion of typanotomy tubes is recommended in children with documented bilateral effusion that persists for 3 months and significant hearing loss.
- Persistent middle ear effusion after treatment of AOM does not require antimicrobial therapy.
- The use of antimicrobial prophylaxis is appropriate treatment for the use of recurrent AOM with the following criteria: three or more distinct and well-documented episodes of AOM in a 6-month time frame or four or more episodes in 12 months.

The NP should be familiar with these recommendations and be aware of their role in the prevention of superinfections caused by the indiscriminate use of antibiotics. Systemic corticosteroids are not recommended for the treatment of AOM or persisitent OME (Bluestone & Klein, 1999). The use of topical nasal steroids in the treatment of AOM or persistent OME is controversial; however, they have been shown to decrease inflammation in the eustachian tubes and upper respiratory tract (Williams, 1999) (see further discussion under OME). Antipyretics and analgesics are useful in treating fever and discomfort. Use of ceruminolytics or removal of the impaction is essential when excessive cerumen impedes examination of the ear or alters hearing. Acidic eardrops help maintain an environment in the external auditory canal that prevents the growth of fungi and bacteria. Ototopical preparations must be administered appropriately to help ensure successful treatment. The bottle of ototopic should be warmed before instilling the drops, the tragus should be pumped a few times after instillation of the drops, and the affected ear should remain up for at least 2 to 3 minutes after the procedure is complete (Carlson, 2002).

Education and Counseling

Education and counseling of the patient and family regarding both the prevention of additional problems and the treatment course are important in the treatment of ear problems. Areas of particular importance include avoiding passive smoke exposure, avoiding bottle propping, minimizing exposure to other children with minor acute illnesses, and decreasing exposure to loud noises.

Prevention of Noise-Induced Hearing Loss

Firecrackers (especially Chinese ones), toy cap pistols, firearms, loud pop music, squeaking toys, snowmobiles, farm equipment, lawn mowers, and ill-fitted hearing aids have all been shown to cause some degree of hearing loss (Nash et al, 1997). The NP should actively educate patients and parents to avoid damaging sources of sound and use protective devices. Three types of protective devices are readily available at pharmacies or hardware stores: earmuffs, form-fitting foam earplugs, and premolded earplugs. Maintaining an awareness of risk factors should lead the NP to early detection of cochlear damage and hearing loss.

Removal of Cerumen

Cerumen in the ear canal can be removed with the use of a cerumen scoop (curettage) or by gently irrigating the ear or both. Before irrigation, 2 to 3 drops of docusate sodium (Colace), triethanloamine (Cerumenex), mineral oil, or other warm oil may be instilled to help soften the obstructive wax (Singer, Sauris, & Viccelio, 2000). Baking soda mixed with water is also effective. Mix one-half teaspoon of baking soda with 2 ounces of water and instill a few drops in the affected ear two times daily for 1 week. After 1 week the solution should be discarded. Tap water irrigation alone is also as effective as using a softener before irrigation. For dry, hardened wax, softeners may decrease the amount of irrigant required (Spiro, 1997). Irrigation is then accomplished by using a bulb syringe or "water pick" (on low setting). The irrigation solution can be warm water or hydrogen peroxide diluted 1:1 with warm water. Irrigation should not be attempted if the tympanic membrane is possibly perforated or tympanostomy tubes are in place.

Curretage requires skill, but it is less messy than and may be as effective as irrigation. Blunt plastic ear curettes may be less traumatic than the metal variety. Always carefully explain the procedure to parents and inform them that the ear canal is extremely sensitive and fragile and bleeds easily when touched. This may avoid an adverse parent reaction when there is blood on the curette or in the ear canal.

Follow-up and Referral

Close follow-up of infection and assessment for hearing loss are necessary in order to detect changes in hearing and monitor recurrence of illness. An otolaryngology referral is indicated for unusual ear conditions, congenital malformation of the head and neck structures, craniofacial anomalies, sensory dysfunction involving hearing or speech, when appropriate therapy for OM has failed, or if ongoing effusion or infection persists (American Academy of Pediatrics Policy Statement, 2002). Myringotomy or placement of pressure-equalization tubes (PETs) can help relieve discomfort and prevent further infection. Audiologic referral is necessary if ear pathology is prolonged or when the child's ability to hear is questioned. Speech and language evaluations are imperative to resolve questions about whether the child's verbal development is delayed because of persistent or recurring ear problems. Chapter 32 addresses criteria for tonsillectomy and adenoidectomy.

Pressure-Equalizing Tubes

Indications for tympanostomy and the insertion of PETs are listed in Box 30-2. Every child with recurrent or persistent AOM or chronic OME must be considered on an individual basis for the placement of PETs. Otolaryngologists may wait until the fall or winter months to insert PETs because the tubes take more care during the summer and most ear disease wanes in the summer months.

Paradise and colleagues (2001) reported that the immediate placement of PETs in children less than 3 years of age with persistent OME did not have a significant improvement in developmental outcomes, including speech and language acquisition. The authors concluded that waiting to insert PETs had no detrimental effect on development. Rovers and colleagues (2001) demonstrated that the insertion of PETs in young children did not significantly improve their quality of life for up to 1-year follow-up.

BOX 30-2 *Indications for Tympanostomy and the Insertion of Pressure-Equalizing Tubes*

Children between ages 1 and 4 years, children with craniofacial anomalies, and other children at high risk for acute and recurrent AOM benefit the most from PETs in terms of resolution of otitis media and child development.

- Otitis media with effusion lasting more than 3 months or with language delay, hearing loss, severe retraction pocket, vertigo, tinnitus, or frequent superimposed acute otitis media
- Recurrent otitis media (if the child has two or more infections despite prophylaxis; if avoidance of prophylaxis or long-term antibiotics is desired; if language delay, hearing loss, or multiple drug allergies)
- Severe eustachian tube dysfunction (persistent ear popping, pain, vertigo, tinnitus, or fluctuating hearing loss)
- Complications of otitis media present or suspected (mastoiditis, facial nerve paralysis, brain abscess, labyrinthitis)

Adapted from DeRosa J, Grundfast KM: Surgical management of otitis media, *Pediatr Ann* 31(12):814-820, 2002; Pizzuto MP, Volk MS, Kingston LM: Common topics in pediatric otolaryngology, *Pediatr Clin North Am* 45:973-991, 1998.
AOM, Acute otitis media; *PETs*, pressure-equalizing tubes.

Insertion of PETs in a child with recurrent OM or prolonged middle ear effusion results in less discomfort with AOM, appropriate ventilation of the middle ear space, and improved hearing. Additionally, the use of PETs may decrease the incidence of AOM in some children. Baseline hearing status should be established in any child having PETs inserted. Children with persistent hearing loss after PETs are placed should be further evaluated (AAP Section on Otolaryngology and Bronchoesophagology, 2002). The procedure takes less than 15 minutes and is usually done using general anesthesia. The child is usually discharged after about an hour and is treated with otic drops for several days.

The examiner can establish that the tube is functioning properly if the tube spans the eardrum, the lumen is unobstructed, and no middle ear effusion is present. If appropriate functioning of the tube cannot be established, pneumatic otoscopy or tympanometry may be useful. A flat (type B) tympanogram with large volume measurements confirms appropriate function of the PET. A normal (type A) tympanogram suggests a clogged or extruded tube.

Using ototopical drops for 5 to 7 days can occasionally clear clogged PETs. Otic suspensions, such as Pediotic, that are mildly acidic should be used because they are less irritating to middle ear mucosa. Water and ceruminolytics are contraindicated. If the child can taste the drops or complains of stinging, the drops are most likely reaching the middle ear space and indicate a functioning tube.

Generalized water precautions for children with PETs are controversial. Water does not enter the middle ear space via the PET during bathing, showering, or surface swimming. Diving and head dunking may allow water into the middle ear space; however, chlorinated pools have few bacteria and earplugs are probably unnecessary. However, lakes, ponds, rivers, and bath water may have increased bacterial counts, so earplugs are recommended if head dunking may occur.

Viral myringitis or early AOM without otorrhea in a child with PETs will most likely resolve spontaneously because of increased middle ear ventilation. Antibiotics are not indicated. Tympanostomy tube otorrhea (TTO) occurs usually when a child with PETs has an upper respiratory infection and has drainage coming from the tubes. TTO occurs in about 20% of all children with PETs, most of which are self-limited episodes (Hannley, Denneny, & Holzer, 2000). TTO usually involves the same bacterial pathogens seen in AOM. Ofloxacin otic drops have been approved for use as monotherapy for TTO by instilling 5 to 10 drops (5 drops if age 5 years or younger) into the affected ear twice daily for 10 days (Bluestone, 2001). Other ototopical medications are listed in Table 30-3. If the otorrhea has not improved after 5 to 7 days of topical

TABLE 30-3 ***Commonly Used Topical Preparations for Ear Disease***

Product Name (Manufacturer)	Antibiotic	Antiinflammatory	Acid	Comments
Auralgan (Wyeth-Ayerst)				Benzocaine in a glycerin and propylene base; used for anesthesia in cases of severe AOM; **do NOT use in presence of TM perforation**
Cipro HC Otic (Alcon Labs)	Ciprofloxacin	Hydrocortisone	Glacial acetic acid	FDA approval for otitis externa only; however, based on clinical studies on the safety of ciprofloxacin by Force et al (1995) this preparation is used clinically with an open TM
Ciloxan Ophthalmic (Alcon Labs)	Ciprofloxacin	None	Acetic	Sterile ophthalmic preparation (Force et al, 1995); demonstrated safety and efficacy for use with open TM
Floxin Otic (Daiichi Pharmaceuticals)	Ofloxacin	None	Hydrochloric	Only FDA-approved product for (a) acutely infected tympanostomy tubes in children 1 yr and older and (b) chronic suppurative otitis media in children 12 yr and older
Cortisporin Otic Solution (Monarch Pharmaceuticals)	Polymyxin B and neomycin	Hydrocortisone	Hydrochloric	May be painful on instillation; demonstrated to be ototoxic in animal models by Rohn et al (1993); human studies have demonstrated no ototoxicity in children or adults with courses of up to 2 wk (Merifield et al,1993; Welling et al, 1995)
Cortisporin Otic Suspension	Polymyxin B and neomycin	Hydrocortisone	None	May be used when solution is poorly tolerated
Cortisporin Ophthalmic	Polymyxin B and neomycin	Hydrocortisone	Sulfuric	May be used when this combination is desired and both otic solution and suspension are poorly tolerated
Debrox Otic Solution (SmithKline Beecham)	None	None	Citric	Excellent choice for cleansing of the EAC; also contains carbamide peroxide as an added ceruminolytic
Domeboro Otic (Bayer Pharmaceutical Division)	None	None	Acetic and boric	Excellent antimicrobial and antifungal activity; may be used in conjunction with other topicals

Continued

TABLE 30-3 Commonly Used Topical Preparations for Ear Disease—cont'd

Product Name (Manufacturer)	Antibiotic	Antiinflammatory	Acid	Comments
Gentamicin Ophthalmic	Gentamicin	None	Hydrochloric	May be used by some otolaryngologists as a first-line agent in patients with a sulfa allergy; demonstrated ototoxicity in animal models; Gyde (1976) reported no ototoxicity when used in adults
Inflamase Mild (1/8%), Inflamase Foret (1%) (Ciba Vision Ophthalmics)	None	Prednisolone	None	Excellent choice for inflammatory conditions such as granular myringitis
Pediotoic (King Pharmaceuticals)	Polymyxin B and neomycin	Hydrocortisone	None	Usage has declined dramatically with introduction of Floxin
TobraDex Ophthalmic (Alcon Labs)	Tobramycin dexamethasone		Sulfuric	No documented ototoxicity with either agent; excellent broad-spectrum coverage
Vasocidin Ophthalmic (Ciba Vision Ophthalmics)	Sulfacetamide prednisolone		Hydrochloric	Used by many otolaryngologists as a first-line agent and as a prophylactic agent (Garcia et al, 1994)

Data from *Physician's Desk Reference* (2001). From Ramsey AM: Diagnosis and treatment of the child with a draining ear, *J Pediatr Health Care* 16(4):166-167, 2002.

AOM, Acute otitis media; *EAC,* external auditory canal; *FDA,* Food and Drug Administration; *TM,* tympanic membrane.

therapy, treatment with oral antibiotics is appropriate. If the otorrhea is resistant to oral and ototopical agents, referral to an otolaryngologist is recommended.

Many PETs fall out well before their usefulness has been expended, and 20% to 50% of children require a second set (Pizzuto, Volk, & Kingston, 1998). Once the PET has been extruded from the tympanic membrane, follow-up every 6 to 12 months is suggested until the tube falls out of the external canal. For the rare set of PETs that remain in situ, surgical removal is suggested after 2 years (AAP Section on Otolaryngology and Bronchoesophagology, 2002). Complications of PETs include otorrhea, otitis externa, granuloma, cholesteatoma, PET obstruction, tympanic membrane perforation, and tympanosclerosis.

SPECIFIC EAR PROBLEMS IN CHILDREN

Otitis Externa

Description

Otitis externa (OE) is an inflammatory reaction of the external auditory canal. Inflammation is evidenced as (1) simple infection with edema, discharge, and erythema; (2) furuncles or small abscesses that form in hair follicles; or (3) impetigo or infection of the superficial layers of the epidermis. OE can also be classified as mycotic OE, caused by fungus, or as chronic external otitis, a diffuse low-grade infection of the external auditory canal. Severe infection or systemic infection can be seen in patients with diabetes who are immunocompromised or who have received head and neck irradiation (Hannley, Denneny, & Holzer, 2000).

Etiology

OE is most frequently caused by retained moisture in the external ear canal, which changes the acidic environment of the external ear canal to a neutral or basic environment, thereby promoting bacterial or fungal growth. Chlorine in swimming pools adds to the problem because it kills the normal ear flora and allows the growth of pathogens. The most common pathogens in "swimmer's ear" are *Pseudomonas aeruginosa* and *Staphylococcus aureus* (Hughes & Lee, 2001).

Purulent otorrhea from a perforated tympanic membrane secondary to AOM can cause OE. Furunculosis of the external canal is generally caused by *S. aureus* and *Streptococcus pyogenes* carried by dirty fingers. Otomycosis is usually caused by *Aspergillus* or *Candida* and is caused by recent use of systemic or topical antibiotics or steroids. Otomycosis is also more common in children with diabetes or immune dysfunction (Hughes & Lee, 2001). Foreign bodies that disrupt the lining of the ear canal can also lead to OE.

Clinical Findings

History. The following can be found:

- Itching and irritation progressing to severe pain
- Pressure and fullness in ear and occasionally hearing loss that can be conductive or sensorineural
- Rare systemic complaints and symptoms
- Rare hearing loss and otorrhea

Physical Examination. Findings on physical examination can include the following:

- Pain, often quite severe, with movement of the tragus or on attempts to examine the ear with an otoscope
- Swollen external auditory canal with debris, making visualization of the tympanic membrane difficult
- Rare otorrhea
- Occasional regional lymphadenopathy
- Tragal tenderness with a red, raised area of induration that can be deep and diffuse or superficial and pointing, which is characteristic of furunculosis
- Red crusty or pustular spreading lesions
- Black spots over the tympanic membrane, indicative of mycotic infection
- Dry-appearing canal with some atrophy or thinning of the canal and virtually no cerumen visible with chronic OE

Laboratory Studies. Culturing the discharge from the ear is not customary but can be done if clinical improvement is not seen during or after treatment, or if chronic OE is suspected. Culturing requires a swab premoistened with sterile nonbacteriostatic saline or water.

Differential Diagnosis

AOM with perforation, TTO, chronic suppurative otitis media (CSOM), necrotizing OE, cholesteatoma, mastoiditis, posterior auricular lymphadenopathy, dental infection, and eczema are all in the differential diagnoses.

Management (Box 30-3)

The following steps are taken:

- Remove any foreign body (see the next section).
- Meticulous and repeated clearing of the canal is the cornerstone of effective treatment (Hannley, Denneny, & Holzer, 2000). If no perforation of the tympanic membrane exists, irrigate the canal with saline or Burow's solution. Burow's solution is soothing, decreases edema, and kills *Pseudomonas.*
- Antibiotic eardrops are the mainstay of therapy for OE (see Table 30-3). The fluoroquinolone ototopical products (ciprofloxacin and ofloxacin) are effective against *Pseudomonas, S. aureus,* and *Streptococcus pneumoniae,* which may be a factor if the OE is a complication of AOM. Neomycin is effective against *S. aureus* but has no activity against *Pseudomonas* (Capoot et al, 2002). Medications containing neomycin cause an allergic contact dermatitis in approximately 5% of recipients (Hughes & Lee, 2001). Polymixin, which is often found in combination with neomycin, also has good *S. aureus* and *Pseudomonas* coverage. Eardrops that contain steroids may help relieve swelling and pain faster than antibiotic alone (Pistorius et al, 1998).
- If significant swelling is present, insert a wick soaked with the antibiotic eardrop solution. A foam (Pope), cotton, hydrogel polymer (Merocel XL) (Capoot et al, 2002) or gauze (0.25 inch) wick usually works well (Walsh, 2002). The tip of the wick is lubricated with water-based lubricant just before insertion into the ear. Once in place, the wick should be impregnated with antiobiotic for as long as it remains in the auditory canal. This may require reapplication of drops every 2 to 3 hours (Capoot et al, 2002). Wicks are usually removed after several days if they have not fallen out on their own. The wick falls out when the swelling has subsided, and treatment with direct application of drops to the ear canal should continue for the duration of treatment.
- Oral or parenteral antibiotics are generally not needed except for systemic illness or failed topical treatment.
- Avoid cleaning, manipulating, and getting water into the ear. Swimming is prohibited during acute infection.

BOX 30-3 ***Management of Otitis Externa***

Treatment Guidelines

- Administer analgesics as needed
- Remove any foreign body
- Lance any furuncles
- Irrigate with saline or Burow's solution
- Instill antibiotic drops
- If impetigo: cleanse with antiseptic acid and apply antibiotic ointment
- If mycotic: cleanse with 5% boric acid in ethanol solution, followed by antifungal solution

Prevention

- Avoid water in ears
- Use acetic or boric acid and alcohol solutions in ear after swimming
- Avoid scratching, cleaning, and prolonged use of ceruminolytics

- Administer analgesics for pain, as needed. Narcotic analgesics may be necessary for severe pain and are indicated for short-term use.
- Lance a furuncle that is superficial and pointed with a 14-gauge needle. If it is deep and diffuse, a heating pad or warm oil-based drops can speed resolution.
- If impetigo is present, clear the canal by using half-strength hydrogen peroxide or other antiseptic solutions, followed by a warm-water rinse. Apply an antibiotic ointment (mupirocin) once or twice a day for 5 to 7 days. The child should avoid touching the ear. Fingernails should be short and hands cleansed with antibacterial soap. Systemic antibiotics are generally unnecessary.
- A dermatology consultation is indicated if no improvement in symptoms is seen within 1 week.
- Mycotic OE is treated with a solution of 5% boric acid in ethanol, which is antiseptic and promotes drying. Clotrimazole-miconazole solution can be used alone or with a topical antibiotic corticosteroid solution for 5 to 7 days.
- A follow-up visit may be necessary after 1 to 2 weeks for reevaluation of the OE and removal of debris.

Complications

Infection of surrounding tissues with impetigo, irritated furunculosis, and malignant OE with progression and necrosis caused by *Pseudomonas* infection are possible complications.

Prevention

The patient should be instructed to do the following:

- Avoid water in the ear canals.
- Use well-fitting earplugs for swimming if susceptible.
- Use acidic drops (diluted vinegar or diluted alcohol, 3 to 5 drops) daily, especially after swimming, to prevent the recurrence of OE. Over-the-counter drugs such as VoSol Otic eardrops can be used (5 drops in each ear after swimming).
- Avoid persistent scratching or cleaning of the external canal.
- Avoid prolonged use of ceruminolytic agents.

Foreign Body in the Ear Canal

Description

A foreign body in the external ear canal is a problem frequently seen in pediatric patients.

Etiology

Foreign bodies are usually placed in the ear canal by the child. Insects can also be found in the canal.

Clinical Findings

History. The history can include the following:

- Child reports putting something into the ear
- Complaints of buzzing, fullness, or an object in the ear
- Ear pain or otorrhea

Physical Examination. A foreign body is visible with the naked eye or by otoscopic examination.

Management

The following steps are taken:

- Straighten the ear canal by pulling on the pinna, and gently shake the patient's head.
- Bayonet forceps can be used to grasp the object, especially if it is irregularly shaped.
- If the object is metal, try using a magnet to retrieve it.
- Kill insects by instilling 70% alcohol in the ear canal before flushing.
- Irrigate the ear canal with water; if vegetable matter, use 70% alcohol.
- Refer the patient to an otolaryngologist if you are unable to extract the object without causing discomfort or trauma to the canal wall.

Complications

Infection, perforation of the tympanic membrane, and damage to the ossicles are possible if the object is not removed.

Prevention

Educate children and their parents not to put objects in the ear.

Acute Otitis Media

Description

AOM is an infection of the middle ear that can be of several types (see Color Fig. 4). Table 30-4 defines characteristics of different types of AOM.

Etiology

AOM often follows eustachian tube dysfunction. When the eustachian tube is obstructed, negative pressure develops as air is absorbed in the middle ear (see Color Fig. 5). The negative pressure pulls fluid from the mucosal lining and causes an accumulation of sterile fluid. Viruses are associated with up to 90% of cases of AOM; however, viruses are the sole pathogen in only 5% to 6% of episodes (Heikkinen, 2000). At least one otopathogen has been found in 87% to 95% of cases of AOM (Rodriguez & Schwartz, 1999). Bacteria pulled in from the eustachian tube lead to the accumulation of purulent fluid. *Streptococcus pneumoniae* (40% to 50%), *Haemophilus influenzae* (20% to 30%), and *Moraxella*

TABLE 30-4 Types of Acute Otitis Media

Type	Characteristics
AOM	Suppurative effusion of the middle ear
Bullous myringitis	AOM in which bullae form between the inner and middle layers of the tympanic membrane and bulge outward
Persistent otitis media	AOM that has not resolved when antibiotic therapy has been completed or AOM recurs within days of treatment
Recurrent otitis media	Three separate bouts of AOM within a 6 mo period or six within a 12 mo period; often a positive family history of OM and other ENT disease in father of child

AOM, Acute otitis media; *ENT*, ear, nose, throat.

catarrhalis (10% to 15%) are the most common infecting organisms (Dowell et al, 1999; Hoberman et al, 2002). *Streptococcus pneumoniae* causes the most cases of AOM, is the least likely bacterium to resolve without treatment, and is responsible for the increasing treatment failures because of the emergence of multiple drug resistance (drug-resistant *S. pneumoniae* [DRSP]) (Dowell et al, 1999). Currently, nearly 50% of strains of *S. pneumoniae* are penicillin nonsusceptible. Approximately 30% to 35% of *H. influenzae* strains, and virtually all strains of *M. catarrhalis*, are β-lactamase-producing bacteria (Hoberman et al, 2002).

Young children have shorter, more horizontal, and more flaccid eustachian tubes that are easily disrupted by viruses, which predisposes them to AOM. Other predisposing factors include upper respiratory infection, allergies, Down syndrome, cleft palate, bottle propping during feedings, day care attendance, and passive cigarette smoke. Cigarette smoking leads to functional eustachian tube obstruction and decreases the protective ciliary action in the eustachian tube.

Incidence

Most episodes of AOM occur in the first 24 months of life, and 94% of children suffer at least one episode by age 2 (Block, 2002). It is the most common indication for antibiotic prescriptions in the United States (Kozyrskyj et al, 1998). The incidence of AOM is greater in males, white children, and Native Americans, including Eskimos. Approximately 20% of children have recurrent AOM (Eden, Fireman, & Stool, 1996).

Clinical Findings

History. The following can be noted:

- Previous medical history significant for craniofacial anomalies or congenital syndromes associated with craniofacial anomalies, prematurity, or exposure to risk factors (eustachian tube dysfunction, bottle propping, and day care)
- Ear pain, manifesting in an infant or a young child as irritability, inability to sleep, or ear pulling; severe ear pain with bullous myringitis
- Lethargy, dizziness, tinnitus, and unsteady gait
- Diarrhea and vomiting
- Fever
- Sudden hearing loss
- Stuffy nose, rhinorrhea, and sneezing
- Rare facial palsy and ataxia

Physical Examination. The following can be apparent on physical examination:

- Tympanic membrane showing increased vascularity, erythema, bulging, and obscured or absent landmarks (see Color Fig. 4).
- Tympanic membrane that is red, yellow, or purple. Redness alone should not be used to diagnose AOM, especially in a crying child.
- Thin-walled, sagging bullae filled with straw-colored fluid are seen with bullous myringitis.
- Decreased tympanic membrane mobility secondary to effusion (see Color Fig. 8) is noted with pneumatic otoscopy, tympanometry, or acoustic reflectometry.

Laboratory Findings. Tympanometry reflects effusion (type B pattern). Tympanocentesis to identify the infecting organism is helpful in the treatment of infants younger than 2 months. In older infants and children, tympanocentesis is rarely done and is useful only if the patient is in a toxic state or immunocompromised or in the presence of resistant infection or acute pain from bullous myringitis (Barkin & Rosen, 1999). If a tympanocentesis is warranted, refer the patient to an otolaryngologist for this procedure.

Differential Diagnosis

Otitis media with effusion (OME), mastoiditis, dental abscess, sinusitis, lymphadenitis, parotitis, peritonsillar abscess, trauma, eustachian tube dysfunction, impacted teeth, temporomandibular joint dysfunction, and immune deficiency are differential diagnoses. Any infant 2 months of age or younger with an AOM should be evaluated for fever without focus and not just treated for an ear infection.

Management

The following are issues to be considered when treating AOM (Fig. 30-4):

- Currently, much controversy surrounds the use of antibiotics in the treatment of AOM. The main reason for the ongoing discussion is the increasing rate of antibiotic-resistant bacteria related to the injudicious use of antibiotics (see the earlier section on judicious use of antibiotics). Ample evidence has also been presented that as many as 70% to 90% of cases of AOM resolve without antibiotics (Takata et al, 2001), usually those caused by *H. influenzae* or *M. catarrhalis* (Dowell et al, 1999). Little and colleagues (2002) suggested that antibiotic use be delayed for 2 to 3 days to observe for spontaneous resolution of symptoms. They also identified predictors of poor outcome when immediate antibiotics were not prescribed, such as the presence of ear drainage, three or more previous courses of antibiotics compared with none, fever, vomiting, and cough.
- There seems to be some agreement that antibiotic treatment of a carefully diagnosed and documented AOM is appropriate. Diagnosis is made with pneumatic otoscopy, which can assess position, color, translucency, and mobility. Treatment is also recommended if the AOM is accompanied by clear local signs (bulging membrane with cloudy or yellow fluid, very red membrane, or otorrhea), if systemic signs (fever) are present, if more than three attacks of AOM have occurred in the past 18 months, or if the patient has a history of OME or PET use (Dowell et al, 1998; Pelton & Barnett, 1998).
- Ten days of antibiotic therapy is suggested for AOM with perforation, in children with an underlying medical condition, or in children younger than 24 months. The risk of treatment failure is higher in younger children. Amoxicillin is still the first-line drug choice for AOM. Children with AOM who have high fever most likely have *S. pneumoniae* in the middle ear fluid and might benefit from high-dose amoxicillin therapy (80 to 90 mg/kg per day) (Dowell et al, 1999; Hoberman et al, 2002). Children at low risk for DRSP (no antimicrobial exposure in the previous month, no day care attendance, older than 2 years) are still appropriate for the 40 to 45 mg/kg per day dosage (Dowell et al, 1999; Hoberman et al, 2002). Recommendations from the DRSP Therapeutic Working Group (Dowell et al, 1999) suggest amoxicillin-clavulanate (70 to 90 mg/kg per day divided in two doses, given twice daily, with the clavulanate component at 10 mg/kg per day); cefuroxime axetil and intramuscular ceftriaxone (50 mg/kg daily as a single dose or three doses over a 3- to 5-day period) are useful alternative agents for clinical treatment failure. A recent study has shown that the 3-day ceftriaxone regimen is significantly superior to the 1-day regimen in eradicating *S. pneumoniae* from the nasopharynx (Haiman et al, 2002). Clindamycin should be reserved for use only after all other medication options have failed or after a tympanocentesis has been performed and susceptible bacteria identified (Hoberman et al, 2002). Treatment failure is defined as "lack of clinical improvement in signs and symptoms such as ear pain, fever and tympanic membrane findings of redness, bulging or otorrhea after 3 days of therapy" (Dowell et al, 1999). The NP is cautioned to keep current on updated recommendations for the treatment of AOM because of the rapid changes in resistance patterns and newly developed treatments. Table 30-5 lists the current antibiotics approved by the Food and Drug Administration for the treatment of AOM. A high bacteriologic and clinical failure rate has been identified when AOM is treated with trimethoprim-sulfamethoxazole; consequently, it should no longer be considered as appropriate empiric therapy for AOM (Leiberman et al, 2002).
- Five- to 7-day treatment regimens may be appropriate for other groups of children not heretofore mentioned (e.g., children older than 2 to 6 years, with a mild episode and few previous infections) (Kozyrskyj et al, 1998; Pelton & Barnett, 1998; Pichichero, 2000).
- Persistent OM occurs when antibiotic therapy has been completed and evidence of AOM is still present or AOM recurs within days of treatment. Re-treatment with a broader-spectrum antibiotic is suggested. OME should not be considered treatment failure and should be expected in up to 70% of cases (Dowell et al, 1999).
- Recurrent AOM (being "otitis prone") is present when more than three bouts of AOM have occurred in 6 months or six in 12 months. Children with recurrent AOM are more likely to have a family history of AOM in the father and have other ear, nose, and throat (ENT) diseases. The use of prophylactic antibiotics in the treatment of recurrent AOM is a highly debated issue. Antibiotic-resistant bacteria are the key concern. Prophylaxis should be reserved for children who suffer frequent, severe bouts of AOM (three or more episodes within a 6-month period or four or more episodes within 12 months) (Dowell et al, 1998); children less than 2 years of age; and Native Americans. Block and colleagues (2001) suggest that a highly restricted use of chemoprophylaxis for recurrent AOM appears to have minimal adverse consequences in the community. When used, prophylaxis is thought to

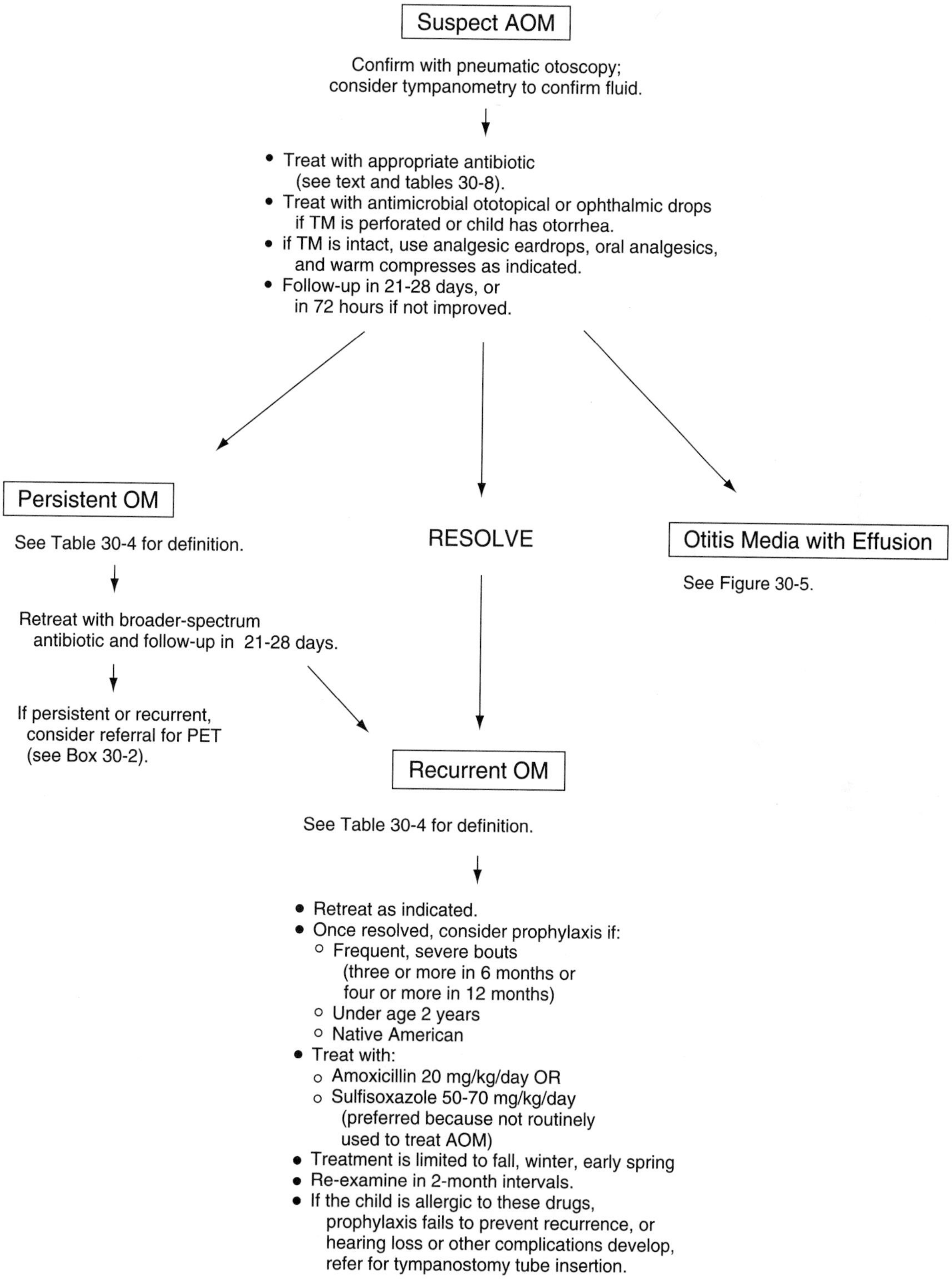

Suspect AOM
Confirm with pneumatic otoscopy;
consider tympanometry to confirm fluid.
• Treat with appropriate antibiotic
(see text and tables 30-8).
• Treat with antimicrobial ototopical or ophthalmic drops
if TM is perforated or child has otorrhea.
• if TM is intact, use analgesic eardrops, oral analgesics,
and warm compresses as indicated.
• Follow-up in 21-28 days, or
in 72 hours if not improved.
Persistent OM
See Table 30-4 for definition.
Retreat with broader-spectrum
antibiotic and follow-up in 21-28 days.
If persistent or recurrent,
consider referral for PET
(see Box 30-2).
RESOLVE
Otitis Media with Effusion
See Figure 30-5.
Recurrent OM
See Table 30-4 for definition.
• Retreat as indicated.
• Once resolved, consider prophylaxis if:
○ Frequent, severe bouts
(three or more in 6 months or
four or more in 12 months)
○ Under age 2 years
○ Native American
• Treat with:
○ Amoxicillin 20 mg/kg/day OR
○ Sulfisoxazole 50-70 mg/kg/day
(preferred because not routinely
used to treat AOM)
• Treatment is limited to fall, winter, early spring
• Re-examine in 2-month intervals.
• If the child is allergic to these drugs,
prophylaxis fails to prevent recurrence, or
hearing loss or other complications develop,
refer for tympanostomy tube insertion.

FIGURE 30-4 Management of acute otitis media. See Tables 30-3 and 30-5 for medications.

TABLE 30-5 ***Medications Approved by the Food and Drug Administration to Treat Acute Otitis Media as of 2003***

Drug	Dose	Comments
Amoxicillin	40-90 mg/kg per day given bid	First choice unless contraindicated
Amoxicillin-clavulanate (Augmentin)	40-90 mg/kg per day given bid with clavulanate <10 mg/kg per day	Good β-lactamase coverage; costly and more likely to cause diarrhea
Amoxicillin-clavulanate (Augmentin 600ES)	90/6.4 mg/kg per day bid	Higher amoxicillin per tsp than Augmentin; less diarrhea than with Augmentin
Azithromycin (Zithromax)	10 mg/kg per day on day 1 (max dose 500 mg/day) then 5 mg/kg per day on days 2-5 given qd (max dose 250 mg/day)	Children older than 6 mo, 5-day treatment course
Cefdinir (Omnicef)	14 mg/kg per day qd or bid	Broad-spectrum third-generation cephalosporin
Cefpodoxime (Vantin)	10 mg/kg per day given bid	Broad spectrum of coverage, costly; third generation
Cefprozil (Cefzil)	30 mg/kg per day given bid	Broad spectrum of coverage, cost similar to that of other cephalosporins; second generation
Ceftibuten (Cedax)	9 mg/kg per day given q.d.	Children older than 6 mo; active against β-lactamase; third generation
Ceftriaxone (Rocephin)	50 mg/kg per day IM in 1-3 doses over 5 days	Costly; third generation
Cefuroxime (Ceftin)	30 mg/kg per day given bid 125 mg bid if younger than 2 yr 250 mg bid if 2-12 yr old 250-500 mg bid if older than 12 yr	Broad spectrum of coverage, costly; second generation
Clarithromycin (Biaxin)	15 mg/kg per day given bid	Children older than 6 mo
Loracarbef (Lorabid)	30 mg/kg per day given bid	Broad spectrum of coverage, costly; second generation

IM, Intramuscularly.

decrease recurrent infection, which can lead to chronic OME and potential hearing loss and have a detrimental effect on language and cognition. Treatment has traditionally been once daily with amoxicillin (20 mg/kg per day) or sulfisoxazole (50 to 75 mg/kg per day; preferable because it is no longer routinely used to treat AOM), with treatment limited to fall, winter, and early spring (Blumer, 1998; Pizzuto, Volk, & Kingston, 1998). Cephalosporins and trimethoprim-sulfamethoxazole are not recommended for prophylaxis (Ahuja & Thompson, 1998). Children who are treated should be reexamined at 2-month intervals. The NP needs to watch community resistance patterns and treat breakthrough infections.

- Decongestants and antihistamines are not helpful in the treatment of AOM.
- Antimicrobial ototopical drops (oflaxacin or Cortisporin) or ophthalmic drops (tobramycin or gentamicin) are indicated if the tympanic membrane is perforated and the child has otorrhea.
- Analgesic eardrops (Auralgan Otic) are helpful for pain relief in the absence of perforation or PET.
- Oral antipyretics and analgesics should be given as needed: acetaminophen (10 to 15 mg/kg every 4 to 6 hours) or children's ibuprofen (5 to 10 mg/kg every 6 to 8 hours).
- Warm compresses may be helpful.
- A follow-up appointment needs to be scheduled if symptoms are not significantly improved in 48 to 72 hours, and a follow-up appointment should be scheduled 21 to 28 days after the initial diagnosis.

Complications

Persistent AOM, persistent OME, tympanic membrane perforation (see Color Fig. 6), OE, mastoiditis, cholesteatoma, tympanosclerosis (see Color Fig. 7), hearing loss of 25 to 30 dB for several months, ossicle necrosis, pseudotumor cerebri, cerebral thrombophlebitis, and facial paralysis are possible complications.

Prevention and Education

Patients and parents should be instructed regarding the following:

- *H. influenzae* type b vaccine is not helpful because the *H. influenzae* responsible for AOM is usually nontypable. Pneumococcal seven-valent conjugate vaccine (Prevnar) may help decrease the incidence of pneumococcal AOM (Pelton, 2002; Sagraves, 2002).
- Annual influenza vaccine may help prevent otitis media. Influenza viruses are among the common viruses associated with AOM (Heikkinen, Thint, & Chonmaitree, 1999). Use of influenza vaccine, especially in high-risk children who attend day care centers, has proven effective in reducing the incidence of OM. Early treatment of influenza with the antiviral oseltamivir can help reduce OM (Chonmaitree, 2002; Whitley et al, 2001).
- Xylitol, a sugar found in fruits and the bark of birch trees, has bacteriostatic effects against *S. pneumoniae* and interferes with bacterial adhesion to mucous membranes (Kemper, 2002). Unfortunately, to be beneficial it has to be chewed five times a day and causes excessive gas and diarrhea.
- Bottle propping, feeding infants lying down, and passive smoke exposure should be avoided.
- Avoid the use of pacifiers. Although the relationship cannot be fully explained, multiple studies have shown that pacifier use increases the incidence of AOM (Jackson & Mourino, 1999; Niemela et al, 2000; Warren et al, 2001).
- Breastfeeding until at least 4 months of age is protective against single and recurrent episodes of AOM (Duncan et al, 1993).
- The importance of keeping follow-up appointments should be stressed.
- Educate regarding the problem of drug-resistant bacteria and the need to avoid the use of antibiotics unless absolutely necessary.
- If antibiotics are used, the child needs to complete the entire course of the prescription.
- If the child is in day care, another, less populated, day care environment may need to be considered.

Otitis Media with Effusion

Description

OME, also referred to as middle ear effusion, secretory, nonsuppurative, or serous OM, is characterized by an accumulation of fluid in the middle ear and a decrease in mobility of the tympanic membrane with pneumatic otoscopy (see Color Fig. 8). Chronic OME is defined as middle ear effusion (MEE) persisting longer than 3 months.

Etiology and Incidence

OME usually begins with eustachian tube dysfunction (ETD) caused by viral illness, anatomic abnormalities, barotrauma, allergies, or a combination of these conditions. ETD changes the middle ear mucosa in the following sequence: (1) the mucosa becomes secretory with increased mucus production; (2) the mucus becomes viscous as the mucosa absorbs water; and (3) fluid becomes stuck behind the tympanic membrane (Williams, 1999).

In another process, ETD causes OME, which then becomes AOM. OME is a natural consequence of both treated and untreated AOM. MEE resolves in 65% of untreated children within 30 days and in 60% of antibiotic-treated children within 30 days (Daly, Hunter, & Giebink, 1999). Approximately 90% of effusions of less than 2 to 3 months' duration resolve without treatment within a few months. OME that lasts longer than 2 to 3 months has only a 15% to 30% resolution rate even when monitored for 30 months (Rosenfeld, 1996).

Thirty percent of children with OME have bacteria (nontypable *H. influenzae, M. catarrhalis,* and *S. pneumoniae*) in their middle ear effusions (Daly, Hunter, & Giebink, 1999). OME is the most common cause of hearing loss in children. Risk factors for chronic OME are listed in Box 30-4.

BOX 30-4 ***Risk Factors for Chronic OME or Longer Duration of OME***

Environmental

- Group child care
- Number of hours in child care
- Exposure to children at home or in child care
- Number of smokers and cigarettes smoked in household
- Feeding in supine position
- Shorter duration of breastfeeding
- Autumn season

Characteristics of Child or Specific Disease History

- Early onset of otitis media
- Several prior episodes
- Bilateral OME
- Male gender
- Lower socioeconomic status
- Having a sibling with a history of otitis media

Data from Daly KA, Hunter LL, Giebink GS: Chronic otitis media with effusion, *Pediatr Rev* 20(3):85-93, 1999.
NOTE: Many of these are also implicated in the increased risk of acute otitis media and recurrent otitis media.
OME, Otitis media with effusion.

Clinical Findings

History. The following features may be noted in the affected child:

- Often asymptomatic, afebrile, and without complaints of otalgia
- Fullness in the ear or the feeling of "talking in a barrel"
- Complaint of hearing loss in older children
- Dizziness or impaired balance
- Chronic vomiting with failure to thrive, which can be related to chronic OME

Physical Examination. An abnormal-appearing tympanic membrane, often described as dull, varying from bulging and opaque with no visible landmarks to retracted and translucent with visible landmarks and an air-fluid level, may be seen (see Color Fig. 9). Pneumatic otoscopy reveals decreased tympanic membrane mobility. Head and neck structures should be examined for abnormalities.

Laboratory Findings. The tympanogram is flat—type B. The audiogram can show hearing loss of 15 to 31 dB.

Differential Diagnosis

Differential diagnoses include all causes of hearing loss and anatomic abnormalities, including AOM; unilateral OME can indicate nasopharyngeal carcinoma.

Management

Treatment of OME is controversial and varied. The Agency for Health Care Policy and Research issued guidelines for the treatment of OME in 1994 (Fig. 30-5), which have not been revised to date.

- Current treatment guidelines suggest that OME does not need treatment with antibiotics. For OME lasting longer than 3 months, a hearing evaluation might prove useful. PET should be considered if OME is bilateral for more than 4 months and hearing loss has been documented. PET would also be considered for OME that is unilateral and lasts longer than 6 months.
- Evaluate relevant risk factors and recurrence.
- Follow up every 4 to 8 weeks. For persistent OME, following a period of watchful waiting, one or two courses of antibiotics spaced 4 to 6 weeks apart might be helpful (Roddey & Hoover, 2000).
- Oral corticosteroids in combination with antimicrobials have been used in selected patients with OME and found to be effective, but only for short periods of time and not to any significant statistical degree. These reports are therefore not currently of sufficient strength to recommend the use of steroids routinely to treat OME in a child of any age because the evidence of possible adverse effects outweighs the evidence for possible benefits (Cincinnati Children's Hospital Medical Center, 1999). A referral to an otolaryngologist is recommended before the use of oral corticosteroids.
- Antihistamines and decongestants are not helpful unless the child has nasal allergies (see Chapter 25).
- Nasal corticosteroids can be helpful in conjunction with antibiotics if nasal congestion or allergy symptoms are present (Williams, 1999). However, nasal steroids given to children during an upper respiratory infection may actually hasten the onset of AOM (Ruohola et al, 2000).
- Recommend that the child be given preferential seating in school and be spoken to face to face.
- After 3 months of persistent OME, refer to an otolaryngologist for evaluation. If persistent hearing loss or speech delay is apparent, refer to an audiologist and speech therapist for evaluation and treatment. Box 30-5 lists risk factors for hearing loss.

Complications

Complications include recurrent AOM and hearing loss that may be temporary conductive or, over time, permanent high-frequency sensorineural hearing loss. It is debated how much of an effect chronic OME has on cognitive ability, language, and learning, including attention and behavior. Studies are underway to examine this further (Berman, 2001; Minter et al, 2001).

Prevention and Education

- Stress the importance of follow-up until the tympanic membrane and hearing are normal.
- Advise parents of the length of time (weeks to months) required for resolution of OME.
- Encourage parents to decrease background noise, speak louder than usual, and focus on the child's face when speaking because of the mild, transient hearing loss.
- Remind parents of their important role in language development of their child. Conversation and parent interaction through reading and play, along with affirmative sounds and gestures, are the most important factors in language development and school readiness (Berman, 2001).

Cholesteatoma

Description

Cholesteatoma is an epidermal inclusion cyst of the middle ear or mastoid consisting of desquamated debris from the keratinizing, squamous epithelial lining of the middle ear (see Color Fig. 10).

Etiology and Incidence

Cholesteatomas can be congenital or acquired. Varied theories explaining their formation include the following: an inflammatory process, perforation of the tympanic membrane, and failure of desquamated tissue to clear from the middle ear. The incidence rate is unknown.

Clinical Findings

History. The history can include

- Chronic OM with malodorous purulent otorrhea
- Vertigo and hearing loss

Physical Examination. A pearly white lesion is present on or behind the tympanic membrane. Aural polyps are considered cholesteatomas unless proven otherwise. Congenital cholesteatomas are often in the most anterior, inferior position of the tympanic membrane (Thompson, 1999).

Differential Diagnosis

Tympanosclerosis, debris from chronic OME, malignant rhabdomyosarcoma, and aural polyps are some of the differential diagnoses.

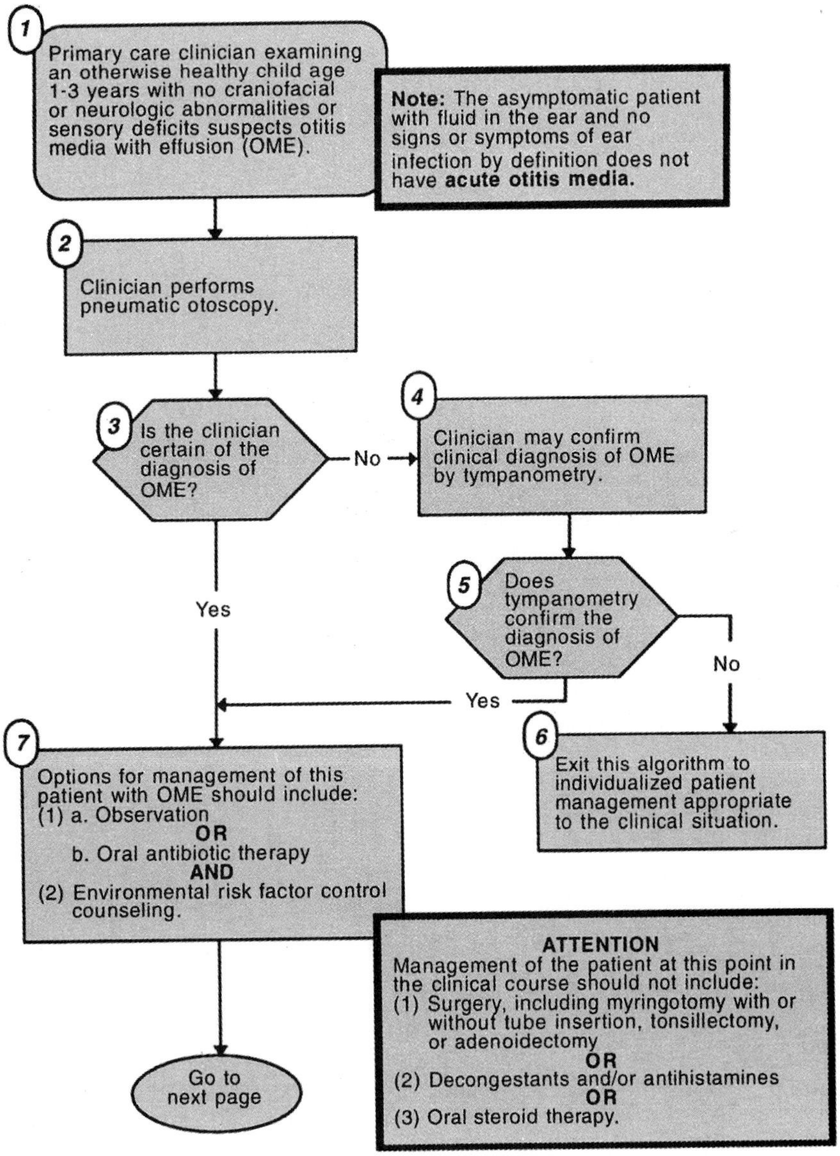

FIGURE 30-5 Management of otitis media with effusion. (From Agency for Health Care Policy and Research: *Quick reference guide for clinicians: managing otitis media with effusion in young children*, AHCPR pub no 94-0623, Rockville, MD, 1994, Agency for Health Care Policy and Research.)

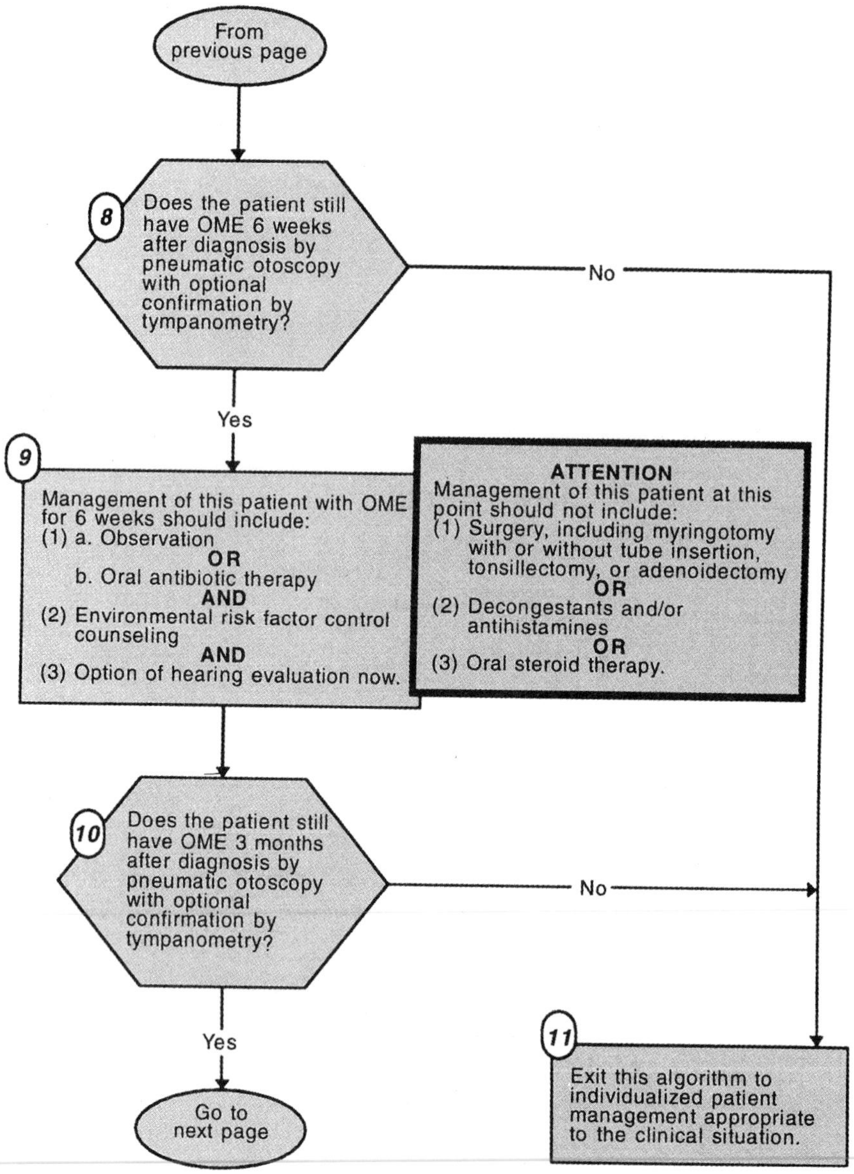

FIGURE 30-5 cont'd

Management

Accurate diagnosis and immediate otolaryngologic referral for surgical excision are needed.

Complications

Complications include irreversible structural damage, permanent bone damage, facial nerve palsy, hearing loss, and intracranial infection, especially in untreated cases. Recurrence is 50%, with a 50% cure rate at best (Thompson, 1999).

Mastoiditis

Description

Mastoiditis is a suppurative infection of the mastoid cells.

Etiology

Mastoiditis may accompany OM. The mucoperiosteal lining of the mastoid air cells becomes inflamed, with subsequent progressive swelling and obstruction of drainage from the mastoid. Common organisms identified include *S. pyogenes, S. aureus,* coagulase-negative staphylococcus, *S. pneumoniae,*

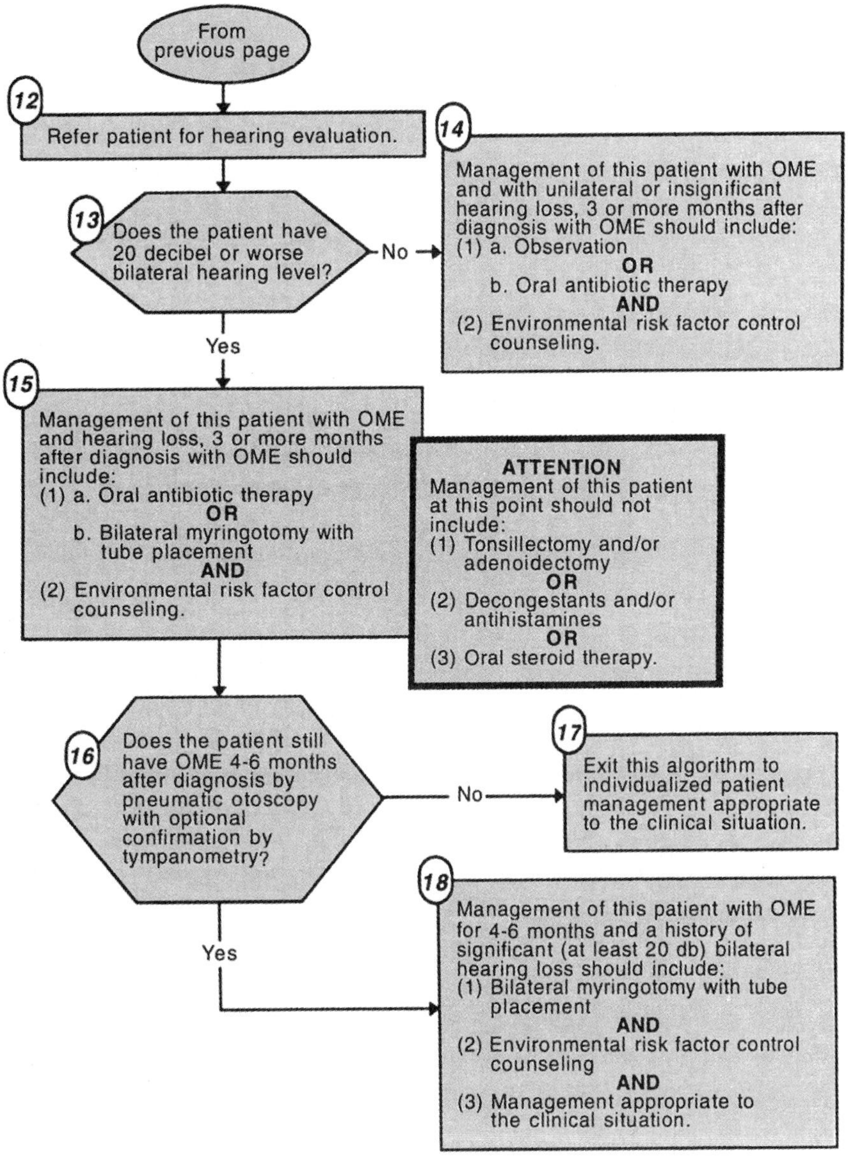

FIGURE 30-5 cont'd

H. influenzae, and *Mycobacterium tuberculosis* (rare). Antibiotic treatment for AOM does not safeguard against and may actually mask mastoiditis with a normal tympanic membrane (Luntz et al, 2001). Intracranial complications of mastoiditis are not rare and may develop despite treatment.

Incidence

Mastoiditis is uncommon but potentially life threatening. A multicenter study of pneumococcal mastoiditis (stated to be the most common causative organism) found that over 50% of cases occurred in children less than 12 months of age, with many children not having a history of recurrent AOM. Male to female ratio was 2:1 (Kaplan et al, 2000).

Clinical Findings

- Concurrent or recurrent AOM
- Fever and otalgia
- Persistent OM unresponsive to antibiotic therapy
- Postauricular swelling

BOX 30-5 *Risk Factors for Hearing Loss Caused by OME**

- Bilateral OME for 3 months or longer
- If two or more present:
  - OME present for longer than 8 weeks
  - Speech development slower than peers
  - Speech less clear than previously
  - Child decreases amount of talking
  - Child less responsive to name and other familiar sounds
  - Child says "Huh?" or "What?" frequently
  - Child sits close to TV or wants volume louder
  - Child has difficulty learning (reading, spelling)
  - Child is hyperactive or overly inattentive

From Daly KA, Hunter LL, Giebink GS: Chronic otitis media with effusion, *Pediatr Rev* 20(3):89, 1999.
*Child should be tested audiologically if one or two of the above are present.
OME, Otitis media with effusion.

Infants may have swelling above the ear, displacing the pinna inferiorly or laterally. In older children, the swelling pushes the earlobe superiorly and laterally.

Laboratory Studies

- Radiography (may show coalescence of mastoid air cells and loss of bony trabeculation)
- Computed tomography (CT) can provide definitive anatomic information
- Tympanocentesis (culture and Gram stain help identify offending organism) (Barkin & Rosen, 1999)

Management

Urgent ENT referral is imperative. Hospitalization and intravenous antibiotics are usually required. Antibiotic coverage should include an antistaphylococcal agent (Luntz et al, 2001).

Prevention

The pneumococcal conjugate vaccine may reduce the incidence of mastoiditis caused by *S. pneumoniae.*

Sensorineural and Conductive Hearing Loss

Description

Hearing loss is defined as bilateral pure-tone hearing loss of 40 dB or more at frequencies of 500, 1000, and 2000 Hz in the better ear. Three types of hearing loss are recognized—sensorineural, conductive, and central—although there may also be a combined type. Either or both ears may be involved. The average age at detection of hearing loss is somewhere between 14 and 24 months if profound and up to 48 months for lesser degrees (AAP Joint Committee on Infant Hearing, 2000; Bachmann & Arvedson, 1998).

Sensorineural hearing loss (SNHL) occurs because of damage to the cochlear structure of the inner ear or to fibers of the auditory nerve. SNHL may be mild or severe, is permanent, and is not usually treatable. Noise-induced hearing loss (NIHL) is a preventable type of SNHL that is permanent and incurable and affects cognitive, social, emotional, and psychologic functioning (Nash et al, 1997).

Conductive hearing loss results from blocked transmission of sound waves from the external auditory canal to the inner ear (e.g., AOM, OME). Bone conduction is usually normal with decreased air conduction. Conductive hearing loss is usually in the range of 15 to 40 dB (mild to moderate) and is not permanent. Middle ear effusions result in an average hearing loss of 27 to 31 dB.

Etiology

SNHL and conductive hearing loss can be associated with craniofacial anomalies (e.g., aural atresia, cleft lip/cleft palate, external ear deformity without atresia, dysmorphic facies without external ear deformity), genetic aberrations/congenital deformities (e.g., white forelock, café au lait spots, family history of SNHL, metabolic abnormalities), or environmental exposure (e.g., ototoxic drugs, bacterial or viral meningitis, loud noises, head trauma). SNHL occurs when hair cells in the cochlea are injured by exposure to excessive noise over a variable period. SNHL can also come from prenatal and perinatal exposure (e.g., intrauterine infections, toxic chemicals, erythroblastosis fetalis). Conductive hearing loss can also be caused by AOM and OME with or without perforation, tumors, cerumen impaction, or idiopathic causes (e.g., otosclerosis).

Incidence

SNHL occurs in 1 to 3 per 1000 infants in well-baby nurseries and in 2 to 4 per 1000 infants in the intensive care unit (Sokol & Hyde, 2002). Fifty percent of cases are genetically linked, 20% to 25% are from environmental factors, and 25% to 30% are from an uncertain cause. Hereditary SNHL accounts for 20% to 50% of all cases of severe to profound SNHL. SNHL occurs in 10.3% of children following meningitis (Bachmann & Arvedson, 1998; Williams, 1999). One study reported that of all cases of hearing loss, 90% were sensorineural, with the highest rate among black male children. Thirty percent of all children with hearing loss had another neurodevelopmental condition (Van Naarden, Decoufle, & Caldwell, 1999).

Conductive hearing loss occurs in 15% of school-age children (Williams, 1999). Congenital deformities causing conductive hearing loss occur in 1 in 10,000 to 20,000 live births (Stewart & Downs, 1993).

Clinical Findings

History. Hearing loss is often a "silent disease" (Williams, 1999). Careful consideration and attention to identified risk factors are essential in identifying hearing loss in children (Williams, 1999; Joint Committee on Infant Hearing, 2000a, 2000b).

The risk factors for SNHL in newborns include the following:

- Neonatal intensive care unit admission for 2 days or longer
- Usher syndrome, Waardenburg syndrome, or findings associated with other syndromes known to include hearing loss
- Family history of hereditary childhood sensorineural hearing loss
- Congenital infections such as toxoplasmosis, bacterial meningitis, syphilis, rubella, cytomegalovirus, and herpes
- Craniofacial anomalies, including morphologic abnormalities of the pinna and ear canal
- Ototoxic drug exposure
- Birth weight less than 1500 g
- Hyperbilirubinemia requiring exchange transfusion or causing kernicterus
- Severe depression at birth (e.g., Apgar score of 0 to 3 at 5 minutes, failure to initiate a response by 10 minutes, or hypotonia at up to 2 hours of age)
- Prolonged mechanical ventilation for greater than 10 days

The risk factors for hearing loss in children 1 month to 3 years of age include the following (Joint Committee on Infant Hearing, 2000a, 2000b):

- Kidney malformation
- Parental or caregiver concern regarding hearing, speech, language, or developmental delay; parents tend to be about 12 months ahead of care providers in identifying hearing loss in children (Bachman & Arvedson, 1998)
- Family history of permanent childhood hearing loss
- Stigmata or other findings associated with a syndrome known to include SNHL, conductive hearing loss, or eustachian tube dysfunction
- Syndromes associated with progressive hearing loss such as neurofibromatosis and osteopetrosis
- Neurodegenerative disorders, such as Hunter syndrome, or sensorimotor neuropathies, such as Friedreich's ataxia and Charcot-Marie-Tooth disease
- Head trauma
- Recurrent or persistent OME for at least 3 months

Other risk factors or indicators for hearing loss include the following:

- Failure to learn to speak at the appropriate age or failure to respond to auditory stimuli; speech that sounds like baby talk or is monotone and difficult to understand; avoidance of speaking
- Failed school screening audiogram; decreased note taking; seeming to misunderstand, ignore, confuse, or miss what is being said
- Increased volume of TV
- Aggression, increased physical complaints, difficulty in school and social situations
- Environmental exposure to firecrackers, toy cap pistols, firearms, loud music, squeaking toys, and machines (e.g., snowmobiles, farm equipment, lawn mowers)

Physical Examination. The following may be found in children with SNHL and conductive hearing loss:

- Presence of craniofacial anomalies (see Etiology).
- Presence of genetic stigmata associated with SNHL (see Etiology).
- Abnormal hearing screening during routine well-child care visits or other office visits. For children younger than 6 months, an ABR test is recommended. Behavioral testing using a conditioned response or an ABR is appropriate for children older than 6 months.
- A complete physical examination with special attention to the eyes, skin, and skeletal and nervous systems is needed.
- Ears—preauricular pits, auricular malformation or appendage, abnormal tympanic membrane integrity, or impaired mobility with pneumatic otoscopy.
- Eyes—cataracts, corneal opacities, coloboma, blindness, nystagmus, exophthalmos, night blindness, heterochromia iridis, or blue sclerae (associated with genetic disorders that can cause SNHL).

Diagnostic Tests. Audiometry is often the first testing performed. In younger children, an ABR or EOAE may be ordered. For SNHL, tests are ordered as indicated by the history and physical findings:

- Urinalysis, serum blood urea nitrogen, and creatinine to rule out renal disease.
- Complete blood count, TORCH (toxoplasmosis, rubella, cytomegalovirus, herpes simplex) screen, sickle cell screen.
- CT as indicated to rule out inner ear malformation.
- For conductive hearing loss, a tympanogram can show decreased mobility of the tympanic membrane.
- Tympanometry is used as the confirmatory test after suspected decreased mobility is noted with pneumatic otoscopy.

RESOURCE BOX

AHQR National Guideline Clearinghouse
www.guideline.gov

American Academy of Audiology
www.audiology.org

American Academy of Family Physicians
www.aafp.org

American Academy of Pediatrics Virtual Classroom
Online case studies and pneumatic otoscopy course
www.aap.org/otitismedia

Bright Futures
www.brightfutures.org

Centers for Disease Control and Prevention
www.cdc.gov

Clinical Education Series
Intermountain HealthCare
Introduction to Otitis Media
36 State Street
Salt Lake City, UT 84111
1-801-442-2000

Contemporary Pediatrics
www.contemporarypediatrics.com

Johns Hopkins University School of Medicine
A View Through the Otoscope:
Distinguishing Acute Otitis Media with Effusion

University of Michigan
www.med.umich.edu/1libr/topics

University of Iowa Virtual Hospital
www.vh.org

Differential Diagnosis

Mixed SNHL with conductive hearing loss is included in the differential diagnosis.

Management

The following should occur for any child with suspected hearing loss:

- Refer any child with suspected hearing loss to an audiologist and otolaryngologist for full evaluation as soon as possible. In the referral, include information about the patient's symptoms, history or physical findings, and any known diagnosis associated with hearing loss.
- Encourage the use of amplification devices as appropriate. They may be personal (e.g., hearing aids) or group (e.g., teacher microphone). Cochlear implants with an external speech processor are sometimes used for profound SNHL.
- Recommend special school and teaching strategies such as front-of-room placement and facing the child when speaking.
- Evaluate and treat AOM and OME if present (see the AOM and OME sections).
- Screen for hearing loss if bilateral middle ear effusion is present for 3 months or longer.
- Ensure a family-centered approach in making decisions regarding interventions for the child (e.g., Public Law 99-457, Individuals with Disabilities Education Act [IDEA]).
- Refer to Chapter 17 for discussion of children who are deaf.

Complications

Significant hearing loss impedes speech, language, cognitive development, and social interaction skills.

Prevention

- Recommend avoidance of environmental factors associated with hearing loss.
- Avoid ototoxic drug use.
- Immunize against mumps, rubella, varicella, *H. influenzae* type b, *S. pneumoniae*, influenza, and other diseases that can cause SNHL through central nervous system damage.
- Treat prenatal and perinatal infections promptly.
- Provide Rh_0(D) immune globulin to prevent erythroblastosis fetalis in susceptible women.

REFERENCES

Ahuja G, Thompson J: What role for antibiotics in otitis media and sinusitis, *Postgrad Med* 104(3):93-99, 1998.

American Academy of Pediatrics Joint Committee on Infant Hearing: Year 2000 position statement: principals and guidelines for early hearing detection and intervention programs, *Pediatrics* 106(4):798-817, 2000.

American Academy of Pediatrics Policy Statement: Guidelines for referral to pediatric surgical specialists, *Pediatrics* 110(1): 187-191, 2002.

American Academy of Pediatrics Section on Otolaryngology and Bronchoesophagology: Follow-up management of children with tympanostomy tubes, *Pediatrics* 109(2):328-329, 2002.

Bachmann KR, Arvedson JC: Early identification and intervention for children who are hearing impaired, *Pediatr Rev* 19(5):155-165, 1998.

Barkin R, Rosen P, editors: *Emergency pediatrics: a guide to ambulatory care*, ed 5, St Louis, 1999, Mosby.

Berman S: Management of otitis media and functional outcomes related to language, behavior, and attention: is it time to change our approach? *Pediatrics* 107(5):1175-1177, 2001.

Block SL: Therapeutic nihilists: lend me your ears or the witches cauldron of acute otitis media, *Pediatr Ann* 31(12):784-791, 2002.

Block SL et al: Restricted use of antibiotic prophylaxis for recurrent acute otitis media in the era of penicillin non-susceptible Streptococcus pneumoniae, *Int J Otorhinolaryngol* 61:47-60, 2001.

Bluestone C: Efficacy of ofloxacin and other ototopical preparations for chronic suppurative otitis media in children, *Pediatr Infect Dis J* 20:111-115, 2001.

Bluestone C, Klein J: Chronic suppurative otitis media, *Pediatr Rev* 20(8):277-279, 1999.

Blumer J: Traditional management of acute otitis media. In *Otitis media: management strategies for the 21st century*, Bala Cynwyd, PA, 1998, Meniscus Educational Institute.

Capoot GD et al: The child with otitis externa: current and comprehensive management, *Contemp Pediatr* (suppl):4-18, 2002.

Carlson L: Update on otitis media, *Am J Nurse Pract*, Oct 2002, pp 9-14.

Chonmaitree T: Does influenza vaccination prevent acute otitis media? *Inside Influenza* 2(3):1-11, 2002.

Cincinnati Children's Hospital Medical Center: Evidence based clinical practice guidelines for medical management of otitis media in children 2 months to 6 years of age, 1999. Available at *www.guideline.gov* (accessed Jan 15, 2003).

Daly KA, Hunter LL, Giebink GS: Chronic otitis media with effusion, *Pediatr Rev* 20(3):85-93, 1999.

DeRosa J, Grundfast KM: Surgical management of otitis media, *Pediatr Ann* 31(12):814-820, 2002.

Dowell S et al: Otitis media—principles of judicious use of antimicrobial agents, *Pediatrics* 101:165-171, 1998.

Dowell SF et al, and the Drug-Resistant *Streptococcus pneumoniae* Therapeutic Working Group: Acute otitis media: management and surveillance in an era of pneumococcal resistance—a report from the Drug-Resistant *Streptococcus pneumoniae* Therapeutic Working Group, *Pediatr Infect Dis J* 18:1-9, 1999 [published erratum appears in *Pediatr Infect Dis J* 18(4):341, Apr 1999].

Duncan B et al: Exclusive breast-feeding for at least 4 months protects against otitis media, *Pediatrics* 91:867-872, 1993.

Finitzo T, Albright K, O'Neal J: The newborn with hearing loss: detection in the nursery, *Pediatrics* 102:1452-1460, 1998.

Force RW et al: Topical ciprofloxacin for otorrhea after tympanostomy tube placement, *Arch Otolaryngol Head Neck Surg* 121(8): 880-884, 1995.

Gyde MC: When the weeping stopped: an otologist views otorrhea and gentamicin, *Arch Otolaryngol* 102(9): 542-546, 1976.

Haiman T et al: Dynamics of pneumococcal nasopharyngeal carriage in children with nonresponsive acute otitis media treated with two regimens of intramuscular ceftriaxone, *Pediatr Infect Dis J* 21:642-647, 2002.

Hannley M, Denneny J, Holzer S: Use of ototopical antibiotics in treating 3 common ear diseases, *Otolaryngol Head Neck Surg* 122:934-940, 2000.

Harrison CJ, Belhorn TH: Acute otitis media: management and prophylaxis, *Clin Rev*, April 1992, p 55.

Heikkinen T: Role of viruses in the pathogenesis of AOM, *Pediatr Infect Dis J* 19(suppl 5):517-523, 2000.

Heikkinen T, Thint M, Chonmaitree T: Prevalence of various respiratory viruses in the middle ear during acute otitis media, *N Engl J Med* 340:260-264, 1999.

Hoberman A et al: Treatment of otitis media consensus recommendations, *Clin Pediatr*, July/Aug 2002, pp 373-390.

Hughes E, Lee J: Otitis externa, *Pediatr Rev* 22:191-198, 2001.

Jarvis C: *Physical examination and health assessment*, ed 2, Philadelphia, 1996, WB Saunders, p. 365.

Joint Committee on Infant Hearing: Joint Committee on Infant Hearing 2000 position statement, *Pediatrics* 106:798-817, 2000a.

Joint Committee on Infant Hearing: Joint Committee on Infant Hearing 2000 position statement: principles and guidelines for early hearing detection and intervention programs, *Am J Audiol* 9:9-29, 2000b.

Kaplan SL et al: Pneumococcal mastoiditis in children, *Pediatrics* 106(4):695-699, 2000.

Kemper K: Otitis media: when parents don't want antibiotics or tubes, *Contemp Pediatr* 19:47-58, 2002.

Kozyrskyj A et al: Treatment of acute otitis media with a shortened course of antibiotics, *JAMA* 279:1736-1742, 1998.

Leiberman A et al: Bacteriologic and clinical efficacy of trimethoprim/sulfamethoxazole for treatment of acute otitis media, *Pediatr Infect Dis J* 20:260-264, 2002.

Little P et al: Predictors of poor outcome and benefits from antibiotics in children with acute otitis media: pragmatic randomized trial, *BMJ* 325:22-25, 2002.

Luntz M et al: Acute mastoiditis—the antibiotic era: a multicenter study, *Int J Otorhinolaryngol* 57:1-9, 2001.

Mason J, Hermann K: Universal hearing screening by automated brainstem response measurement, *Pediatrics* 101:221-228, 1998.

Merifield DO, Parker NJ, Nicholson NC: Therapeutic management of chronic suppurative otitis media with otic drops, *Otolaryngol Head Neck Surg* 109(1):77-82, 1993.

Minter KR et al: Early childhood otitis media in relation to children's attention-related behavior in the first six years of life, *Pediatrics* 107(5):1037-1042, 2001.

Nash D et al: When loud noises hurt, *Contemp Pediatr* 14(6):97-109, 1997.

National Institutes of Health: Early identification of hearing impairment in infants and young children, *NIH Consens Statement* 11(1):1-24, 1993.

Niemela M et al: Pacifier as a risk factor for acute otitis media: a randomized, controlled trial of parental counseling, *Pediatrics* 106:483-488, 2000.

Paradise JL et al: Effect of early or delayed insertion of tympanostomy tubes for persons with persistent otitis media on developmental outcomes at the age of three years, *N Engl J Med* 344:1179-1187, 2001.

Pelton S, Barnett ED: New strategies for the treatment of AOM. In *Otitis media: management strategies for the 21st century*, Bala Cynwyd, PA, 1998, Meniscus Educational Institute.

Pelton SI: Vaccination for the prevention of acute otitis media: proof of concepts and current challenges, *Pediatr Ann* 31(12):804-809, 2002.

Physician's Desk Reference, ed 55, Montvale, NJ, 2001, Medical Economics.

Pichichero M: Short course of antibiotic therapy for respiratory infections: a review of the evidence, *Pediatr Infect Dis J* 19:929-937, 2000.

Pistorius G et al: Prospective randomized, comparative trial of ciprofloxacin otic drops, with or without hydrocortisone, vs. polymyxin B-neomycin-hydrocortisone otic suspension in the treatment of acute otitis externa, *Infectious Diseases in Clinical Practice* 8:387, 1998.

Pizzuto MP, Volk MS, Kingston LM: Common topics in pediatric otolaryngology, *Pediatr Clin North Am* 45:973-991, 1998.

Ramsey AM: Diagnosis and treatment of the child with a draining ear, *J Pediatr Health Care* 16(4):161-169, 2002.

Roddey O, Hoover H: Otitis media with effusion in children: a pediatric office perspective, *Pediatr Ann* 29:623-629, 2000.

Rodriguez WJ, Schwartz RH: *Streptococcus pneumoniae* causes otitis media with higher fever and more redness of tympanic membranes than *Haemophilus influenzae* or *Moraxella catarrhalis, Pediatr Infect Dis J* 18(10):942-944, 1999.

Rohn GN, Meyerhoff WL, Wright CG: Ototoxicity of topical agents, *Otolaryngol Clin North Am* 26(5):747-758, 1993.

Rosenfeld R: How can meta-analysis help in treatment of otitis media? Presented at the Sixth International Symposium on Recent Advances in Otitis Media, 1996.

Rovers MM et al: Randomized controlled trial of the effect of ventilation tubes (Grommets) on quality of life at age 1-2 years, *Arch Dis Child* 84:45-49, 2001.

Ruohola A et al: Intranasal fluticasone propionate does not prevent acute otitis media during viral upper respiratory infection in children, *J Allergy Clin Immunol* 106:467-471, 2000.

Sagraves SR: Increasing antibiotic resistance: its effect on the therapy for otitis media, *J Pediatr Health Care* 16(2):79-85, 2002.

Singer A, Sauris E, Viccelio A: Ceruminolytic effects of docusate sodium: a randomized, controlled trial, *Ann Emerg Med* 36:228-232, 2000.

Sokol J, Hyde M: Hearing screening, *Pediatr Rev* 23(5):155-161, 2002.

Spiro S: A cost effectiveness analysis of ear wax softeners, *Nurse Pract* 22(8):28-32, 1997.

Stewart J, Downs M: Congenital conductive hearing loss: the need for early identification and intervention, *Pediatrics* 91:355-359, 1993.

Takata G et al: Evidence assessment of management of acute otitis media: the role of antibiotics in treatment of uncomplicated acute otitis media, *Pediatrics* 108:239-243, 2001.

Thompson JW: Cholesteatomas, *Pediatr Rev* 20(4):134-136, 1999.

US Department of Health and Human Services: *Healthy people 2010.* Objectives: draft for public comment: child and adolescent focused objectives, 2000. Available at *http://web.health.gov/healthypeople* (accessed Oct 21, 2002).

US Preventive Services Task Force: Recommendations and rationale for newborn hearing screening, 2001. Available at *www.ahqr.gov/news/press/pr2001/newbornpr.htm* (accessed Oct 21, 2002).

US Public Health Service: *Put prevention into practice: the clinician's handbook of preventive services*, ed 2, Germantown, MD, 1997, International Medical Publishing.

Van Naarden KV, Decoufle P, Caldwell K: Prevalence and characteristics of children with serious hearing impairment in metropolitan Atlanta 1991-1993, *Pediatrics* 103(3):570-575, 1999.

Walsh M: Otitis externa, 2002. Available at *www.emedicine.com/emerg/topics350.htm* (accessed Feb 2, 2003).

Warren J et al: Pacifier use and the occurrence of otitis media in the first year of life, *Pediatric Dentistry* 23:103-107, 2001.

Welling DB, Forrest LA, Goll F III: Safety of ototopical antibiotics, *Laryngoscope* 105(5 Pt 1):472-474, 1995.

Whitley R et al: Oral oseltamivir treatment of influenzae in children, *Pediatr Infect Dis J* 20:127-133, 2001.

Williams MA: Hearing loss. In Dershewitz RA, editor: *Ambulatory pediatric care*, ed 3, Philadelphia, 1999, Lippincott-Raven.

31 Cardiovascular Disorders

Catherine G. Blosser, Jan Freitas-Nichols

Most cardiovascular problems in the pediatric population are due to congenital heart disease (CHD), which occurs in 0.5% to 0.8% of all live births and 22% of stillborns. CHD is the leading cause of early death from all congenital anomalies (Hoffman, 2002). Incidence rates vary depending on diagnostic techniques used and the inclusion/exclusion criteria of studies. Changes in growth can produce dramatic changes in the severity of congenital cardiovascular malformations (CCVMs). By 1 week of age, 40% to 50% of infants with CHD have been detected (50% to 60% by 1 month of age) (Bernstein, 2004). Defects such as small ventricular septal defects (VSDs) or a bicuspid aortic valve cause little or no disability to an infant or child, although the diagnosis itself can cause great concern for parents and caregivers. Three categories of risk factors for CHD have been identified: familial, maternal, and fetal entities.

In almost every instance of CHD an accurate diagnosis can be made through noninvasive procedures. Evaluation and diagnosis can occur as early as 16 to 18 weeks of gestation with fetal echocardiography and as early as 10 weeks of gestation with the newer high-frequency transvaginal echocardiography. In addition to cardiac malformations, fetal echocardiography is used to diagnose arrhythmias and hemodynamic changes (Allen, Phillips, & Chan, 2001). Early detection of CHD decreases the morbidity and mortality rates associated with undiagnosed, complex problems of the heart.

The incidence of the type of CCVM has been found to vary by gender. Transposition of the great vessels and aortic stenosis are more common in males; atrial and ventricular septal defects and patent ductus arteriosus (PDA) occur more in females. Race is thought to play some role, but the connection is not clear (Allen, Phillips, & Chan, 2001). The lack of early prenatal care (before 12 weeks) has not been implicated in CCVM rates.

The nurse practitioner (NP) must maintain a high index of suspicion regarding any signs or symptoms of cardiovascular disease. Such suspicion allows early identification and referral of infants and children with potential cardiovascular problems. Additional roles that the NP offers include provision of support to families and children once a diagnosis is made and education of families about prevention of acquired heart disease. This chapter presents information on both congenital and acquired heart disease in the pediatric population that should assist the NP in assessment, management, family support, and referral.

STANDARDS OF CARE

The *Guide to Clinical Preventive Services* (U.S. Preventive Services Task Force, 1996) recommendations related to cardiovascular health are as follows:

- Measurement of blood pressure (BP) during office visits is recommended for children and adolescents. This recommendation is based on proven benefits from the early detection of treatable causes of secondary hypertension; evidence is insufficient to recommend for or against routine periodic BP measurement to detect essential (primary) hypertension in this age-group. Sphygmomanometry should be performed in accordance with the recommended technique for children, and hypertension should only be diagnosed on the basis of readings at each of three separate visits. Criteria defining hypertension vary with age. Age-, sex-, and height-specific BP nomograms for U.S. children and adolescents have been published.
- Routine counseling to promote physical activity and a healthy diet for the primary prevention of hypertension is recommended.

The American Academy of Pediatrics (AAP) recommends measuring BP in children every year beginning at 3 years of age (AAP, 2000).

The National Institutes of Health National High Blood Pressure Education Program (NIH NHBPEP) on BP control in children and adolescents recommends measuring BP annually beginning at 3 years of age (NIH NHBPEP, 1996).

ANATOMY AND PHYSIOLOGY

Fetal Circulation

Knowledge of the fetal circulation is essential for understanding the circulatory changes that occur in the newborn at delivery (Fig. 31-1). Fetal circulation has four unique features that differ from postnatal circulation:

- Oxygenation of the blood occurs in the placenta, not the lungs.
- Fetal pulmonary vascular resistance is high and systemic vascular resistance is low (high pressure on the right side of the heart, low pressure on the left side).
- The foramen ovale, the opening in the septum between the two atria, permits a portion of the blood to flow from the right atrium directly to the left atrium.
- A PDA provides a connection between the pulmonary artery and the aorta that allows blood to flow from the pulmonary artery to the aorta and bypass the fetal lungs.

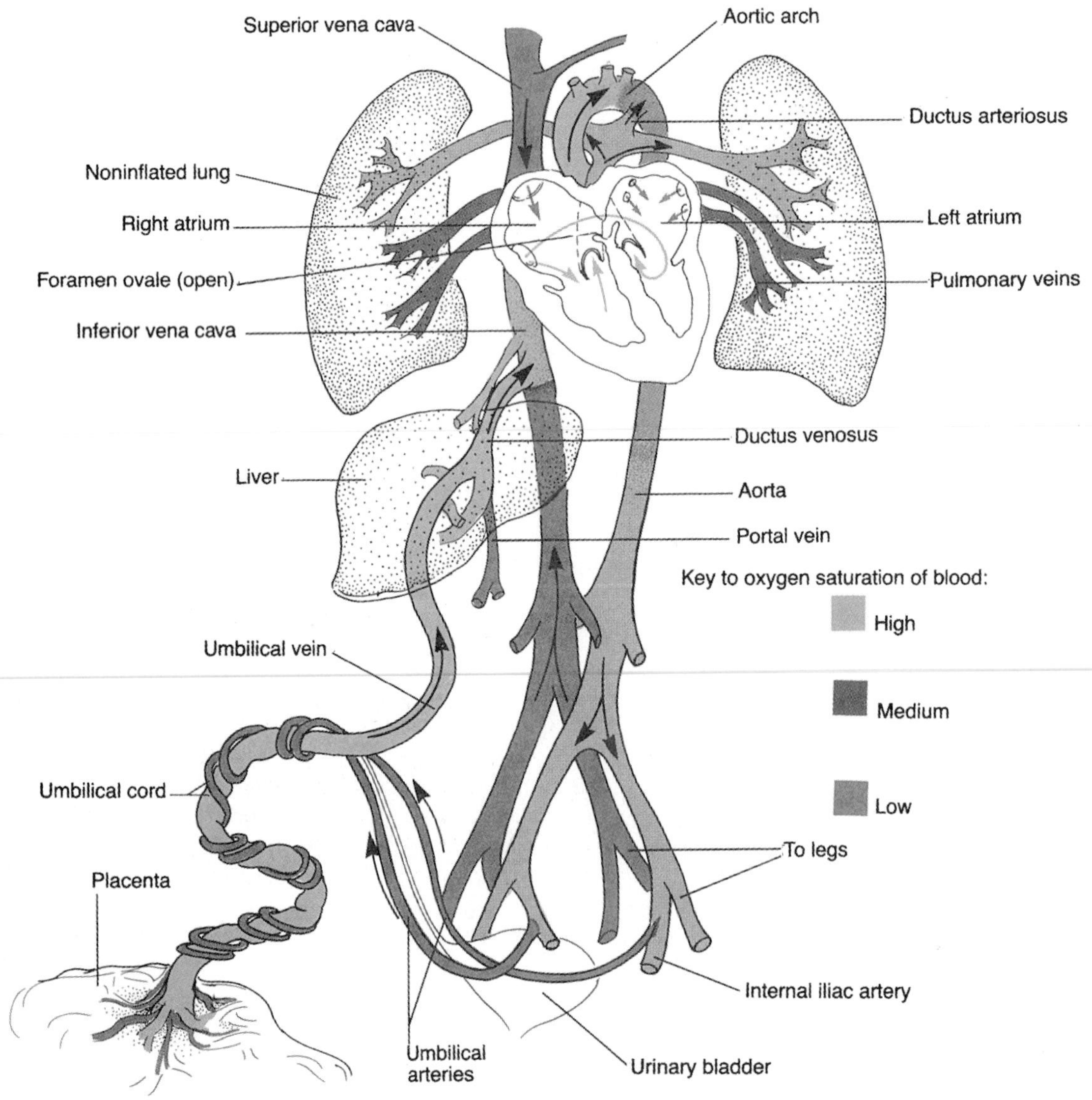

FIGURE 31-1 Fetal circulation. (From Gorrie TM, McKinney ES, Murray SS: *Foundations of maternal-newborn nursing*, Philadelphia, 1994, WB Saunders.)

Oxygen is diffused into the fetal circulation from the maternal uterine arteries in the placenta. From the placenta, oxygenated blood flows through the umbilical vein and is diverted through the liver to the inferior vena cava by the ductus venosus. When this well-oxygenated blood reaches the right atrium, it flows preferentially toward the atrial septum, through the foramen ovale, and into the left atrium. Oxygenated blood then flows into the left ventricle and out the aorta. Approximately two thirds of the blood from the aorta flows toward the head and neck to ensure that the fetal brain constantly receives well-oxygenated blood.

Venous blood returns from the head and upper extremities through the superior vena cava to the right atrium. This blood preferentially flows toward the tricuspid valve into the right ventricle. From the right ventricle, the blood enters the pulmonary artery. Because pulmonary vascular resistance is high and systemic resistance is low, most blood in the pulmonary artery flows through the ductus arteriosus into the descending aorta to supply oxygen and nutrients to the trunk and lower extremities. Only a small amount of blood flows into the pulmonary circuit to perfuse the lungs.

The fetal circulation is best described as two parallel circuits, with the left ventricle supplying blood to the upper extremities and the right ventricle serving the lower extremities and the placenta. At the time of transition to extrauterine life, these separate blood flows become a serial circuit.

Neonatal Circulation

A number of complex events occur at birth that rapidly shift the fetal circulation toward a neonatal circulation. Clamping the umbilical cord with subsequent removal of the placenta as the oxygenating organ causes an immediate circulatory change in which the lungs become the new source of oxygenation. This change causes an increase in systemic vascular resistance (systemic BP). With the first breath, mechanical inflation of the lungs and an increase in oxygen saturation bring about a dramatic fall in pulmonary vascular resistance and, consequently, increased pulmonary blood flow. This activity leads to beginning constriction of the ductus arteriosus. As the pressures within the heart become relatively higher on the left side and lower on the right, the foramen ovale closes. Functional closure of the ductus arteriosus and foramen ovale usually occurs within the first hours to days of life, and a serial circuit forms out of the once-parallel pulmonary and systemic circulation.

The transition toward complete anatomic closure, or obliteration of fetal structures by tissue growth or constriction, is more gradual. Pulmonary vascular resistance drops gradually over the first 6 to 8 weeks of life, which may protect the pulmonary circulation against volume overload in some congenital heart anomalies. Shunt murmurs or symptoms of congestive heart failure (CHF) gradually become apparent as the infant approaches 8 weeks of age. At this time, resistance to flow is less, and shunting to the pulmonary bed increases.

Conditions that cause persistence of fetal shunts, thus allowing unoxygenated blood to flow from the right side of the heart to the left, may cause cyanosis. Any murmur or cyanosis in a newborn should be carefully monitored and evaluated to detect cardiac abnormalities.

Normal Cardiac Structure and Function

The heart is a muscular, four-chambered organ located in the mediastinum, the space in the chest between the lungs. The four chambers are divided into two larger muscular pumping chambers, the ventricles, and two smaller receiving chambers, the atria. The right side of the heart receives blood low in oxygen returning from the systemic circulation by way of the inferior and superior venae cavae. The blood enters the right atrium and passes through the tricuspid valve to the right ventricle. It is then pumped through the pulmonic valve into the pulmonary artery and from there to the lungs, where it is oxygenated. Blood returning from the lungs enters the left atrium by way of the pulmonary veins and then passes through the mitral valve into the left ventricle. It is next pumped through the aortic valve into the aorta to provide oxygenated blood for the systemic circulation.

The heart valves are one-way valves that open and close because of pressure changes within the heart, controlling the flow of blood from chamber to chamber. The tricuspid valve has three cusps held in place by the chordae tendineae. The pulmonary valve directs blood flow from the right ventricle into the pulmonary artery, which bifurcates into right and left arteries to allow flow into both lungs. The pulmonary veins entering the left atrium contain no valves, so blood can flow freely from the lungs into the atrium. The mitral valve controls flow from the left atrium into the left ventricle. The aortic valve controls flow from the high-pressure left ventricle out to the body.

Conduction System

Myocardial contraction is stimulated by electrical depolarization along the conduction tract within the heart. Depolarization begins at the sinoatrial node, which is high in the wall of the atrium. This node acts as the pacemaker of the heart by regularly beginning the depolarizing impulses of each heartbeat. The wave of depolarization travels from the sinoatrial node throughout the atria and produces contraction of the atrial muscle. The impulses reach the atrioventricular (AV) node, which is located in the lower portion of the right atrium at the junction of the atrium and ventricle. From the AV node, the depolarization wave passes through the bundle of His, the fibers extending from the AV node along the intraventricular septum. Depolarization spreads through the left and right branches of the bundle of His and through the Purkinje fibers extending into the ventricular muscle. Impulses then spread throughout the ventricles and cause contraction. The electrocardiogram (ECG) can demonstrate this pattern of changing electrical impulses.

Heart Sounds

Heart sounds are a reflection of the heart's functioning, although the intensity varies with age, thickness of the chest wall, and cardiac output. At the time of ventricular contraction, the beginning of systole, the mitral and tricuspid valves close and produce the first heart sound (S_1). S_1 is the "lubb" of lubb-dupp. Although the left side of the heart reacts slightly before the right side, closure of the mitral and tricuspid valves occurs so closely together that S_1 appears as a single sound. S_1 is best heard at the apex of the heart and is synchronous with the apical and carotid pulses.

After the blood has been ejected, the heart relaxes, the mitral and tricuspid valves open, and the aortic and pulmonary valves close to keep the blood from rushing back into the ventricles. This closure results in the second heart sound (S_2). S_2 reflects the onset of diastole and is the "dupp" of lubb-dupp.

PATHOPHYSIOLOGY

The term *congenital heart disease* (CHD) implies only that a cardiovascular malformation is present at birth. It does not indicate the etiology or cause of the malformation. When CHD is diagnosed in an infant or child, parents may

TABLE 31-1 ***Congenital Malformation Syndromes Associated with Congenital Heart Disease***

Syndrome	Resultant Heart Defect(s)
Chromosomal Disorders	
Trisomy 21 (Down syndrome)	Endocardial cushion defect, VSD, ASD, PDA, TOF
Trisomy 18	VSD, ASD, PDA, coarctation of aorta, bicuspid aortic or pulmonary valve
Trisomy 13	Same as trisomy 18
XO (Turner syndrome)	Bicuspid aortic valve, coarctation of aorta
Fragile X syndrome	Mitral valve prolapse, aortic root dilation
Teratogenic Agents	
Congenital rubella	PDA, peripheral pulmonic stenosis
Fetal hydantoin syndrome	VSD, ASD, coarctation of aorta, PDA
Fetal alcohol syndrome	ASD, VSD
Fetal valproate effects	Coarctation of aorta, hypoplastic left side of the heart, aortic stenosis, pulmonary atresia, VSD
Maternal phenylketonuria	VSD, ASD, PDA, coarctation of aorta
Retinoic acid embryopathy	*Conotruncal anomalies
Others	
Apert syndrome	VSD
Crouzon's disease	PDA, coarctation of aorta
DiGeorge syndrome	Interrupted aortic arch, ASD, truncus arteriosus, TOF
Infant of a diabetic mother	Hypertrophic cardiomyopathy, VSD, conotruncal anomalies*
Marfan syndrome	Aortic stenosis, mitral valve stenosis, total anomalous pulmonary venous return, aortic aneurysm, mitral valve prolapse
Neurofibromatosis	Pulmonary stenosis
Noonan syndrome	Pulmonic stenosis, ASD, cardiomyopathy
Treacher Collins syndrome	VSD, ASD, PDA
Williams syndrome	Supravalvular aortic stenosis, peripheral pulmonic stenosis

Adapted from Behrman R, Kliegman R, Jenson H, editors: *Nelson textbook of pediatrics*, ed 16, Philadelphia, 2000, WB Saunders, p 1345.

*Conotruncal anomalies: TOF, pulmonary atresia, truncus arteriosus, transposition of the great arteries.

ASD, Atrial septal defect; *PDA*, patent ductus arteriosus; *TOF*, tetralogy of Fallot; *VSD*, ventricular septal defect.

incorrectly assume that they are somehow responsible for the child's defect. Health care professionals must be clear about what is and what is not known about CHD to spare parents needless worry and guilt.

Most CHD is due to a complex interaction of genetic and environmental or intrauterine factors, a pattern called *multifactorial inheritance*. The heart is essentially formed by 6 weeks of fetal life, a time when the fetus is most susceptible to infectious or teratogenic exposure or to predisposing genetic or chromosomal factors (Moore & Persaud, 1998). Up to 25% of children with CHD also have noncardiac abnormalities (Behrman, Kliegman, & Jenson, 2000).

Genetic risk factors are most significant for children who have a family history of CHD. The incidence is between 2% and 30% and depends on the type of defect, familial relationship, and whether more than one first-degree relative is affected (Bernstein, 2004). The single greatest risk factor is a parent or sibling with a congenital heart abnormality. The risk is highest when the defect occurs in the mother or full sibling and lowest when the defect is in the father or half sibling (Allen, Phillips, & Chan, 2001). Certain chromosomal abnormalities or syndromes are associated with CHD (e.g., infants with Down syndrome [trisomy 21] have a 50% incidence of CHD) (Table 31-1).

Two to four percent of CHD is caused by well-documented teratogens and maternal conditions or environmental influences. Teratogens include maternal thalidomide, diazepam, lithium, warfarin, corticosteroids, phenothiazine, alcohol, gastrointestinal drugs, and retinoic acid. Paternal use of cocaine is frequently implicated in cases of CHD (Allen, Phillips, & Chan, 2001; Bernstein, 2004) (Box 31-1).

BOX 31-1 *Risk Factors Suggestive of Congenital Heart Disease*

Perinatal Risk Factors

- Maternal infections and exposures (CMV, rubella, other viral syndromes)
- Maternal use of tobacco, alcohol, street drugs, or prescription drugs
- Maternal health disease (CHD, lupus, diabetes)
- Maternal age at child's birth (increase in chromosomal abnormalities after 40 years of age)
- Maternal pregnancy history (excessive weight gain, gestational diabetes)

Neonatal Risk Factors

- Fetal or newborn distress (aspiration, hypoxia, cyanosis)
- Prematurity (increased incidence of CHD in premature infants)
- Presence of associated anomalies (genetic or chromosomal abnormalities or syndromes)
- Neonatal infections (GABHS)
- Birth weight (term infants, less than 2500 g; SGA, less than 2 standard deviations from the mean for gestational age)

Newborn Risk Factors

- Murmur at birth or early infancy
- Hypertension (at birth or beyond)
- Feeding difficulty (SOB, easily fatigued, diaphoresis, poor intake)
- Cyanosis (increase with crying, feeding, exertion)
- Tachypnea (persistent, with crying, feeding)

Toddler, School-age, and Teenage Risk Factors

- Deviation from normal growth and development (normal milestone development, following own growth curve)
- Deviation from activity level appropriate for chronologic age (keeps up with peers; able to run, ride bike)
- Frequent respiratory tract infections (pneumonia, URIs that last longer than normal)
- Prior murmurs, blue spells
- Documented GABHS infection
- Hypertension (documented on a minimum of three separate visits)
- Chest pain with exertion
- SOB with exertion (beyond normal peers)
- Syncope or dizziness (especially associated with noted heart rate change)
- Tachycardia or bradycardia (fluttering in chest, racing heart)

Family History Risk Factors

- CHD (especially siblings, parents, first-degree relatives)
- Sudden death or premature myocardial infarction (before age 50)
- Hypertension
- Rheumatic fever
- Genetic syndromes
- Hypercholesterolemia

CHD, Congenital heart disease; *CMV*, cytomegalovirus; *GABHS*, group A β-hemolytic streptococcus; *SGA*, small for gestational age; *SOB*, shortness of breath; *URIs*, upper respiratory infections.

CHD has been associated with infectious exposure in the first 8 weeks of gestation, especially to cytomegalovirus, mumps, or rubella. A woman who contracts rubella during this phase of pregnancy has a 50% risk of having a baby with congenital rubella syndrome. Infants born to mothers with insulin-dependent diabetes have a threefold risk of having CHD (Allen, Phillips, & Chan, 2001).

ASSESSMENT OF THE CARDIOVASCULAR SYSTEM

Cardiac assessment includes a comprehensive history, a thorough physical assessment, and a variety of diagnostic tests.

History

Review of the family, maternal, fetal, neonatal, and infant medical history, as well as growth and development, is helpful in the cardiac evaluation of a newborn or child with a suspected cardiac abnormality (see Box 31-1 for risk factors).

Physical Examination

Physical assessment in a child with suspected CHD should be adapted to the age of the child (Box 31-2). It is not always possible to follow the same pattern of assessment with each child evaluated. Be flexible, yet thorough, in any evaluation and include all aspects of the physical examination in an order that best suits the comfort and needs of the infant or child. Emphasis should be on a developmental approach to cardiac assessment.

Vital Signs

Heart rate, respiratory rate, and BP vary considerably throughout childhood. Measurements of vital signs must be obtained on each visit with the child at rest because crying and exercise affect results. The normal ranges for various age-groups and gender are available for comparison.

- *Heart rate* (Table 31-2). Heart rates should always be obtained by auscultation of the heart in children younger

BOX 31-2 *Developmental Approach to Cardiac Assessment*

Infants

Complete the assessment with the infant in the parent's arms to keep the infant quiet and cooperative.
Perform uncomfortable aspects of the examination after auscultation to ensure a quiet listen.
Keep the infant covered and warm to minimize discomfort and physiologic changes associated with chilling.
Observe color, respiratory effort, and general effort level while the baby is quiet.

Toddlers

Approach the child quietly, calmly, and slowly. A loud, boisterous greeting may frighten the toddler.
Complete the assessment wherever the child is most comfortable—sitting on the floor, in the parent's lap, on the examination table.
Allow the child to handle a stethoscope while the history is being taken.
Have a toy or distraction item available during the examination.
Consider "listening" to the parent first to improve comfort with the examination.

School Age

Clearly explain the plan and expectations before the examination.
Answer the child's questions honestly.
Talk about topics of interest (school, sports) during the examination.
School-age children may be modest and prefer to keep a gown on during most of the examination.
School-age children may be helpful in discussion of symptoms and events surrounding current concerns.

Adolescents

Questions should be directed at the adolescent and parent.
Communicate in a manner that conveys honesty, professionalism, and interest in their concerns.
Ensure privacy related to both the physical examination and information sharing.
Provide a choice of having a parent present for any or all aspects of the history and examination.
Adolescents are very "body aware" and need reassurance that their concerns are valid, even when the symptom is within normal limits.

TABLE 31-2 ***Normal Heart Rates (Beats per Minute) in Infants and Children***

Age	Resting (Awake)	Resting (Asleep)	Exercise/ Fever
Newborn	100-180	80-160	Up to 220
1 wk-3 mo	100-220	80-200	Up to 220
3 mo-2 yr	80-150	70-120	Up to 220
2-10 yr	70-100	60-90	Up to 220
10 yr-adult	55-90	50-90	Up to 220

than 10 years. Assessment should include rate and rhythm variations. An increased heart rate can be caused by excitement, anxiety, hyperthyroidism, heart disease, anemia, or fever. Rhythm is assessed for regularity.

- *Pulses.* Pulses should be checked in the upper and lower extremities and evaluated for character (strength) and variation between the different sites. A bounding pulse may indicate PDA. Weak or thready pulses indicate CHF or an obstructive lesion such as severe aortic stenosis. Good brachial pulses in conjunction with weak, "thready," or absent femoral pulses indicate coarctation of the aorta.
- *BP.* Assessment should begin at 3 years of age or younger if heart disease is suspected. It is important to always use a BP cuff that is appropriate for the child's size. For arm pressure, the width of the cuff should be two thirds the length of the upper arm measured from the axilla to the antecubital space. A cuff that is too narrow or does not fit around a chubby arm may cause an erroneously high reading. Initial evaluation should compare the pressure in all four extremities. Pressure in all extremities should be equal, with pressure in the legs being slightly higher (10 to 20 mm Hg) in a child who walks. In a child 2 to 10 years of age, the average systolic blood pressure is determined by a simple equation: $90 + (2 \times \text{age in years})$.
  - The pulse pressure (difference between systolic and diastolic pressure) is normally 20 to 50 mm Hg throughout childhood. A wide pulse pressure caused by an unusually high systolic reading can be due to an increased heart rate. If it is due to an abnormally low diastolic pressure, it may be an indication of PDA, aortic regurgitation, or other cardiac pathology.
- *Respiratory rate.* Evaluation of the respiratory system includes the respiratory rate, assessment of effort, and breath sounds in all five lobes of the lungs. It is important to evaluate the respiratory rate in a quiet infant or child. A stethoscope should be used to listen for breath sounds while counting the rate. A respiratory rate above 40 in a young child or 60 in a newborn who is quiet, resting, and afebrile warrants further evaluation. Ease or difficulty of respiratory effort and adventitious sounds such as rales, rhonchi, or wheezing should be assessed. An infant with cyanotic CHD may be happily tachypneic and not show significant signs of grunting or dyspnea; the use of accessory muscles for breathing results in intercostal retractions, nasal flaring, or tracheal pulling. An infant or child with CHF demonstrates significant tachypnea, as well as dyspnea.

General Appearance

- Observation of an infant is best accomplished before any other part of the physical examination occurs so that the observer can get a true picture of the appearance, general nutritional state, respiratory effort, color, physical abnormalities, and distress or discomfort level before the child has been disturbed. It is important to validate with the caregiver the child's comfort level to assess any variation from normal.
- During this observation period one should notice unusual facial characteristics (e.g., malformed ears, wide-spaced eyes, noticeable anomalies) or extracardiac anomalies (e.g., cleft lip or palate, polydactyly, microcephaly) that may be associated with a syndrome or chromosomal abnormalities. Children may have obvious stigmata such as those seen with Down syndrome, Marfan syndrome (unusually tall with an arm span wider than the head-to-toe height), Turner syndrome (webbed neck, pixie-like facies), or fetal alcohol syndrome (microcephaly and pinched facies), all of which are associated with CHD.
- Overall skin color should be assessed for signs of mottling or central cyanosis while the infant is at rest. Cyanosis caused by heart disease is recognized as a pale blue or ruddy red color of the mucous membranes (lips, tongue, nail beds). The tongue is the best indicator because it lacks pigmentation and is richly served by the vascular system. Peripheral cyanosis or acrocyanosis, a blueness or pallor noted around the mouth and on the hands or feet, can be a normal variant, especially if it intensifies when the child is cold or crying. Clubbing of the fingers and toes may be seen in children with long-standing cyanosis.
- Note any wheezing, nasal flaring, retractions, prominent neck veins, or head bobbing with respirations (Allen, Phillips, & Chan, 2001).
- Signs of peripheral or periorbital edema should be noted. Edema or puffiness around the eyes may be evident in an infant with CHF even in the absence of peripheral edema

of the hands or feet. True pitting edema of the feet is an unusual finding in an infant with CHF.

- Diligent measurement of height and weight, accurate plotting on standardized charts, and continued analysis of growth and development are important tools that should be included at each assessment. Although many children with CHD fall within the normal ranges of height, weight, and development, a large number of infants and children with heart disease experience poor weight gain, less than normal linear growth, and delays in achieving developmental milestones.

Palpation

- Palpation of the chest should include assessment of all five areas, including the aortic, pulmonic, tricuspid, and mitral areas and Erb's point (Fig. 31-2). Chest palpation is best accomplished by using the open palm of the hand near the base of the fingers. The hand should be gently moved from location to location across the chest to assess abnormal precordial activity, including pulsations, lifts, heaves, or thrills, and to determine the location of the apical impulse. The apical impulse is used to determine the size of the heart and is the most lateral point at which cardiac activity can be palpated. In infants and children, the impulse is normally palpated at the apex of the heart in the fourth intercostal space just to the left of the midclavicular line. At approximately 7 years of age the point shifts to the fifth intercostal space. In the presence of cardiomegaly, the apical impulse is shifted laterally or downward.

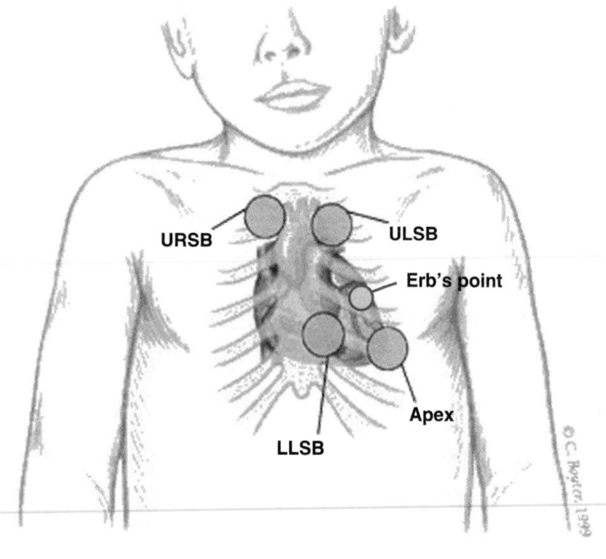

Upper right sternal border (URSB; aortic listening area)
- aortic valve clicks of aortic stenosis, venous hum

Upper left sternal border (ULSB; pulmonic listening area)
- pulmonary valve clicks of pulmonary stenosis, pulmonary flow murmurs, atrial septal defect, PDA, venous hum

Lower left sternal border (LLSB; tricuspid area)
- ventricular septal defects, Still's murmur, tricuspid value regurgitation, hypertrophic cardiomyopathy, subaortic stenosis

Apex (mitral area)
- aortic or mitral valve clicks, mitral valve regurgitation

Erb's point
- aortic ejection click of aortic stenosis, or dilated aortic root

FIGURE 31-2 Traditional auscultatory areas for clicks and murmurs. (Adapted from McConnell M, Adkins S, Hannon D: Heart murmurs in pediatric patients: when do you refer? *Am Fam Pract* 60[2]:558-565, 1999. © C. Boyter, 1999.)

- Thrills are characterized by a palpable vibration caused by turbulent blood flow through abnormal structures or defects in the heart. The turbulent flow may be due to valvular narrowing or stenosis or defects such as VSD.
- Peripheral pulses (radial, brachial, carotid, dorsalis pedis, and posterior tibial) should be assessed for amplitude and intensity. Symmetry between the upper and lower extremity pulses is important for assessment of obstructed blood flow as in coarctation of the aorta. A fast pulse rate may indicate arrhythmia or CHF (Allen, Phillips, & Chan, 2001).
- The liver and spleen should be assessed for enlargement. A liver more than 1 cm below the right costal margin may indicate hepatomegaly and is an important finding in the assessment of a child with suspected heart disease. Infants may have a palpable liver edge as a normal finding.
- The back should be examined for scoliosis, a finding associated with enlarged hearts (Allen, Phillips, & Chan, 2001).

Auscultation of Heart Sounds

- Auscultation of the heart should be approached in the same manner for every child. The practitioner can start either at the top of the heart and move downward toward the apex or mitral area or move in reverse as long as the same method is followed each time. It is important to try to assess heart sounds in a quiet environment with a cooperative child to ensure a thorough and accurate assessment.
- Determination of heart rate and rhythm followed by identification of heart sounds and detection of murmurs should occur in each of five previously noted areas of the heart (see Fig. 31-2).
- Heart sounds represent various events in the cardiac cycle. Four individual heart sounds can be heard: S_1, S_2, S_3, and S_4. S_1 and S_2 represent normal heart sounds, whereas the presence of S_3 or S_4 may indicate cardiac enlargement or volume overload. At each area of examination, the NP should accurately identify the first (S_1) and second (S_2) heart sounds.

- S_1 has the following characteristics:
  - It is characteristically heard in the beginning of systole; it indicates closure of atrioventricular valves (mitral and tricuspid).
  - Typically, it is a single heart sound—the "lubb" of the lubb-dupp.
  - It may be differentiated from early systolic clicks by the low frequency of the sound (clicks have a higher frequency).
  - It is usually best heard at apex.
- S_2 has the following characteristics:
  - It is characteristically heard at the end of systole; it indicates closure of the aortic and pulmonic valves.
  - It is normally split (aortic valve closes slightly ahead of the pulmonic valve).
  - It is the "dupp" of the lubb-dupp.
  - It widens with inspiration and narrows or becomes singular with expiration.
  - It is best assessed at the upper left sternal border in the pulmonic area.
  - Pulmonary hypertension causes early closure and accentuation of S_2, which may sound like a loud single second heart sound.
  - Wide splitting of S_2 without becoming single sound on expiration may indicate increased pulmonary flow (typical of ASD).
- S_3 and S_4 have the following characteristics:
  - S_3 is associated with rapid ventricular filling; it may be heard in a quiet infant or child with a rapid heart rate.
  - S_3 "gallop" is best heard at the apex with the bell of the stethoscope during early diastole. When combined with S_1 and S_2, it gives an impression of the word "Kentucky."
  - S_4 is always pathologic; it represents increased force of atrial contraction and ventricular distention.
  - S_4 "gallop" sounds like the word "Tennessee." It is best heard in late diastole just before S_1.
  - S_4 is low pitched and is best heard at the apex with the bell of the stethoscope.
- Clicks: Ejection and nonejection clicks may be appreciated as extra heart sounds. Ejection clicks are evident early in systole, immediately after S_1, and give the impression of a split first heart sound. Pulmonic ejection clicks are high in frequency, vary with respiration, and disappear with inspiration. An aortic ejection click, heard best at Erb's point, is constant in intensity with a sound of a "snap" or a "click." Nonejection clicks are heard best in midsystole, or midway between S_1 and S_2 in the cardiac cycle at the apex. These clicks are best heard in upright or standing patients, vary with respirations, and are due to mitral valve prolapse. See Fig. 31-2 for a description of cardiac conditions associated with each of these clicks.

Murmurs

A murmur is an extra sound that may be detected during examination of the heart. Up to 80% of children may have a murmur, especially at approximately 3 to 4 years of age (Allen, Phillips, & Chan, 2001; Noonan, 1999). Less than 5% of murmurs denote pathology. A murmur alone is not a diagnosis. It may be caused by normal blood flow through normal cardiac structures (innocent or physiologic murmur) or by turbulent blood flow caused by a defect or abnormal cardiac structures. Murmurs may also be due to normal transitional physiologic processes and may be intensified by anything that increases cardiac output (e.g., anemia, fever, exercise).

Innocent or Functional Murmurs. Functional or innocent cardiac murmurs are common in children and can be evident in newborns. These murmurs are asymptomatic and are usually classic in quality (Box 31-3). Innocent or functional murmurs are not caused by abnormal cardiac structures but are due to transitional flow or mildly turbulent flow through a normal heart. Table 31-3 describes common innocent murmurs.

BOX 31-3 *Characteristics of Innocent Murmurs*

- Usually grade I-II/VI in intensity and localized
- Changes with position (sitting to lying)
- May vary in loudness or presence from visit to visit
- May increase in loudness (intensity) with fever, anemia, exercise, or anxiety
- Musical or vibratory in quality
- Systolic in timing except for venous hum, which is continuous
- Duration is short
- Best heard in LLSB or pulmonic area (except for venous hum)
- Rarely transmitted
- May disappear with Valsalva maneuver, position, or gentle jugular pressure
- Vital signs: normal
- ECG: normal
- General health status: good

ECG, Electrocardiogram; *LLSB*, left lower sternal border.

TABLE 31-3 *Common Innocent Murmurs*

	Stills	Pulmonary Flow Murmur of Childhood	Pulmonary Flow Murmur of Infancy	Venous Hum
Other names	Innocent Vibratory Functional Physiologic Head start murmur	Flow murmur	Peripheral pulmonary stenosis	
Description	Midsystolic, louder in supine position or with inspiration	Early systolic to midsystolic; decreases or disappears with standing; increases with cardiac output or in supine position	Short, midsystolic ejection murmur	Constant swishing sound, disappears with head turning, compression of jugular vein(s), or supine position; varies with respirations
Age	Any age, but most common between 2-6 yr	Any age, but more commonly heard in thin-chested adolescents between 8-14 yr	Common during newborn period, especially in preterm infants	Any
Best heard	Midpoint, left midsternal border to apex	Pulmonary outflow area; radiates to lung fields	Murmur radiates from left upper sternal border to both axilla and back, usually gone by age 6 mo	In upright position, left and right upper chest
Quality	Short, vibratory, musical, "twangy string"	Soft, blowing with normally split S_2; no click or thrill	Soft with middle to high pitch	Soft, high pitch; does not radiate
Intensity	Grade II-III	Grade I-III	Grade I-II	Grade II-III
Differential diagnosis	Small VSD, IHSS	ASD, PS	Supravalvular PS or AS	PDA

Adapted from Allen H, Phillips J, Chan D: History and physical examination. In Allen H et al: *Moss and Adams' heart disease in infants, children, and adolescents: including the fetus and young adult*, ed 6, Philadelphia, 2001, Lippincott Williams & Wilkins; Asprey D: Innocent heart murmur. In Burg F et al: *Gellis and Kagan's current pediatric therapy*, Philadelphia, 2002, WB Saunders.

NOTE: Innocent murmurs typically increase with cardiac output (excitement, fever, anemia).

AS, Aortic stenosis; *ASD*, atrial septal defect; *IHSS*, idiopathic hypertrophic subaortic stenosis; *PDA*, patent ductus arteriosus; *PS*, pulmonic stenosis; *VSD*, ventricular septal defect.

Families and older children should be reassured that nothing is wrong with the heart. They should be told that this murmur may come and go and may be louder at times of fever, anxiety, pain, or exercise but in no way represents cardiac pathology. Families should be reminded that activities need not be limited and that special precautions are not necessary.

Criteria for Describing a Heart Murmur. All cardiac murmurs should be thoroughly evaluated to determine an accurate diagnosis. Every murmur is assessed according to the criteria listed in Table 31-4. These are further illustrated and discussed in Fig. 31-3. Characteristics of pathologic murmurs needing referral are listed in Box 31-4. It is important to note that the presence of a murmur causes great anxiety for a family waiting for a diagnosis.

All murmurs should have a second opinion from a pediatric colleague or pediatric cardiologist if the diagnosis is uncertain or there is a suspicion of heart disease (Noonan, 1999). Interestingly, the percentage of referrals for murmurs to pediatric cardiologists has increased. One study revealed that 51% to 73% of such referrals resulted in a diagnosis of Still's murmur (innocent murmur). This increase in referrals is believed to be related to primary care providers' discomfort with evaluating pediatric murmurs, as well as the increasingly litigious nature of health care (Noonan, 1999). The NP is encouraged to consult with peers and develop confidence with diagnosing innocent murmurs instead of referring all murmurs to cardiologists.

Common Diagnostic Studies. If the NP fully intends to refer for a cardiology consult, performing any of the following routine diagnostic studies is not cost-effective (Noonan, 1999).

- *Chest radiograph.* Radiography provides the following information: cardiac size and size of specific chambers and great vessels, cardiac contour, status of pulmonary blood flow, and status of the lungs and other surrounding tissue (Fig. 31-4).
- *ECG.* ECG monitors the electrical activity of the heart from different locations and in different planes of the body.
- *Echocardiogram.* Echocardiography uses reflected sound waves to identify intracardiac structures and their motion. The types of recordings include two-dimensional, M-mode, contrast, and Doppler studies (Fig. 31-5).
- *Complete blood count (CBC).* CBC rules out severe anemia or polycythemia as a cause of a murmur.
- *Arterial blood gases.* Determination of arterial blood gas content assesses blood levels of oxygen and carbon dioxide. Respiratory acidosis occurs with pulmonary disease, and metabolic acidosis occurs with cardiac disease.

Other diagnostic tests may include the following:

- *Cardiac catheterization.* An opaque catheter is introduced into the heart chambers via the large peripheral vessels. The dye introduced through the catheter is observed via fluoroscopy and provides information about cardiac output, vascular resistance, and the response of the heart to exercise and medications.
- *Hyperoxia test.* Supplementation of 100% oxygen results in "pinking" and increased arterial oxygen saturation when the disease is primarily pulmonary; minimal or no color improvement indicates that the disease is cardiac.
- *Magnetic resonance imaging.* This technique uses a strong magnetic field to cause movement of nuclei to yield an image of the heart structures.
- *Electron beam computed tomography (EBCT) and radionuclide studies.* These studies are used to more clearly evaluate anomalies.
- *Exercise testing.* A graded treadmill or bicycle ergometer is used to determine cardiac output (myocardial blood flow and rhythm) response to exercise for endurance and capacity measurement.

TABLE 31-4 ***Describing a Heart Murmur***

Grade or intensity: • Does not necessarily indicate severity of the problem • May be altered with positional change from supine to sitting	Grade I: Barely audible; heard faintly after a period of attentive listening Grade II: Soft but easily audible Grade III: Moderately loud, no thrill Grade IV: Loud, thrill present Grade V: Loud, audible with stethoscope barely on the chest
Timing with cardiac cycle	Systolic Diastolic Continuous
Location on chest where murmur is loudest	Aortic Pulmonic
Radiations or transmission to other locations	To back To apex To carotids
Quality	Musical Harsh blowing
Duration	Point of onset and length of time systole and diastole murmurs last (e.g., "early systole, heard throughout cardiac cycle")
Pitch	Low Middle High

SYSTOLIC MURMURS

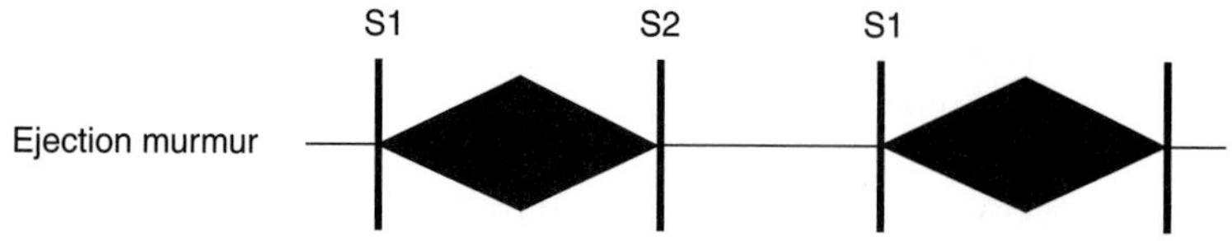

- Comprise most murmurs heard and occur between S1 and S2.
- Are either regurgitation murmurs (e.g., the holosystolic murmur of a VSD that begins with S1 and continues throughout systole) or ejection murmur caused by flow of blood through narrowed or stenotic areas (e.g., AS).
- Best heard at second left or right intercostal space (ICS)
- Begin after S1 and end before S2.
- Include all innocent and physiologic murmurs

DIASTOLIC MURMURS

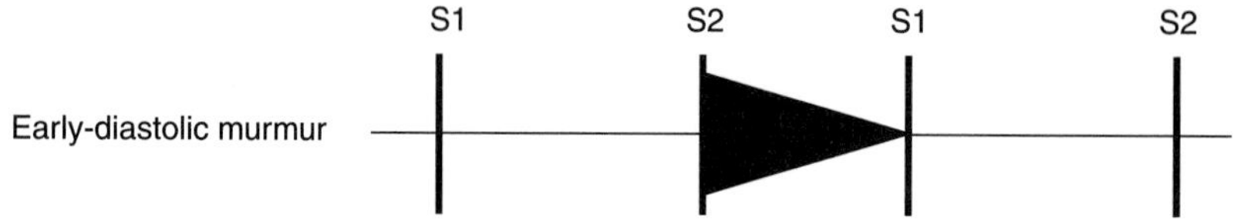

- Occur between S2 and the return to S2.
- Always indicate cardiac pathology.
- Murmur that starts with S2 and has a decrescendo quality is most commonly due to aortic or pulmonic regurgitation.
- Mid-diastolic "rumble," a short low-pitched rumble heard best at the apex, is commonly due to atrioventricular valve stenosis or increased flow across a nonstenotic valve, such as seen with a large VSD or PDA.

CONTINUOUS MURMURS

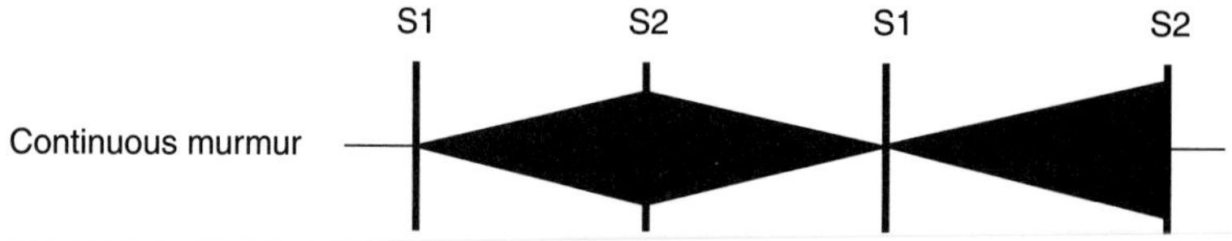

- Start at S1 and go completely through systole and diastole.
- Most common cause is PDA.
- These murmurs need to be differentiated from the coexistence of separate systolic and diastolic murmurs and venous hums.

AS, Aortic stenosis; PDA, Patent ductus arteriosus; VSD, Ventricular septal defect.

FIGURE 31-3 Types of heart murmurs. (Adapted from Allen H et al: *Moss and Adams' heart disease in infants, children, and adolescents, including the fetus and young adult*, ed 6, Philadelphia, 2001, Lippincott Williams & Wilkins, p 150.)

BOX 31-4 *Auscultatory Findings That Suggest a Need for Referral*

- A murmur in a patient with a syndrome known to have a high incidence of congenital heart disease (e.g., trisomy 21)
- Any diastolic murmur
- Any systolic murmur that is associated with a thrill
- Pansystolic murmurs
- Continuous murmurs that cannot be suppressed
- Systolic clicks
- Opening snaps
- Fixed splitting of the second heart sound not associated with bundle branch block
- An accentuated S_2
- S_4 gallops

From Asprey D: Innocent heart murmur. In Burg F et al: *Gellis and Kagan's current pediatric therapy*, Philadelphia, 2002, WB Saunders.

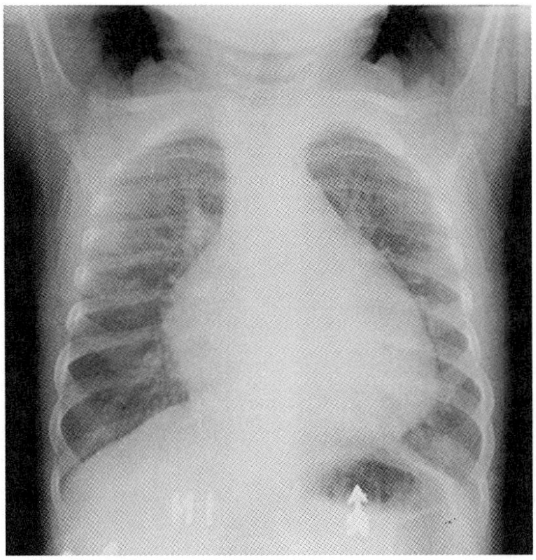

FIGURE 31-4 Chest radiogram of a 3-month-old with ventricular septal defect and congestive heart failure. Cardiomegaly with increased pulmonary vascular markings from pulmonary venous congestion is visible.

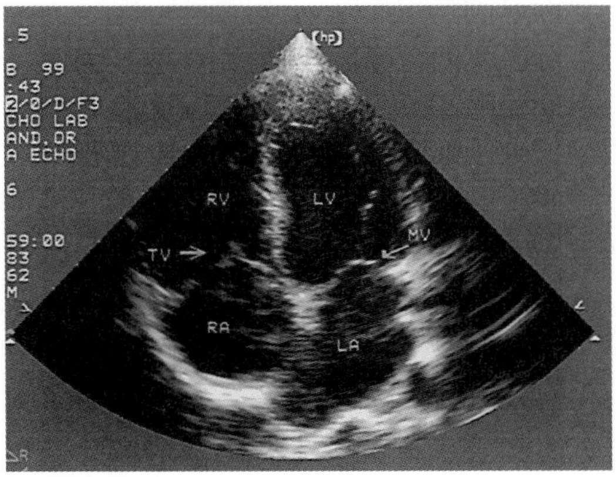

FIGURE 31-5 Echocardiogram of a 2-year-old with atrial septal defect.

MANAGEMENT STRATEGIES

Referral

Practitioners in primary care settings are likely to identify infants, children, and adolescents with suspected cardiac disease. Early detection and prompt referral with appropriate follow-up early in life can greatly reduce the morbidity and mortality rates associated with CHD. Pediatric cardiologists are the recommended specialists to whom to refer, because they can best determine the extent of workup necessary to confirm or eliminate a diagnosis (Bernstein, 2004).

Findings suggestive of cardiac disease are the presence of cyanosis, symptoms of CHF, a nonfunctional murmur, or a difficult to differentiate murmur in the presence of poor growth and development. A murmur alone in a child who is otherwise doing well should be referred to a pediatric cardiologist for further evaluation in a timely but not urgent time frame (2 to 4 weeks). An infant with suspected disease who has a murmur, symptoms of CHF, cyanosis, or poor feeding should be evaluated as soon as possible by a pediatric cardiologist. Newborns should be evaluated within 1 or 2 days of noticeable signs. An older child with dizziness, chest pain with exertion, dysrhythmia, dyspnea, syncope, signs of CHF, or abnormal vital signs should also be referred as soon as possible.

It is important for the practitioner to establish a relationship with a pediatric cardiologist who has diagnostic capabilities immediately available and can proceed with intervention should it prove necessary.

Family Support

Families with infants or children in whom a cardiac problem has been diagnosed may feel fearful, confused, and even guilty. The severity of the cardiac illness or disorder, the type of treatment needed, and the prognosis of the child dictate the kind of support that a family requires. Families need the support of their primary care provider to help them understand the diagnosis, to cope with the short- and long-term consequences, and to advocate for them within the referral center, which may be an overwhelming experience.

Parents and their designated support people should clearly understand the diagnosis and have diagrams of the defect and general information to take away with them for future reference. Should medication be necessary, parents should understand the reason for the treatment, as well as the regimen for administration and side effects. They should have a good understanding of the signs and symptoms of deterioration (e.g., CHF) and clear information regarding how to proceed should symptoms develop. Infant and child cardiopulmonary resuscitation certification is critical for anyone caring for a child with a heart condition.

Support of a family with a new diagnosis or a critical diagnosis is time consuming but necessary. When an infant or child must be seen frequently in a tertiary care center, routine primary care with well-child information and normal counseling may be neglected. It is important to encourage families to schedule and keep regular visits with the primary care provider for routine health supervision and maintenance care. The family needs to understand the importance of additional ongoing subspecialty care with the pediatric cardiologist.

Every opportunity to connect with a family and provide reassuring information is usually welcomed and helpful. The NP helps the family understand the diagnosis and treatment plan, provides an opportunity for family members to express their feelings and concerns, and coordinates necessary community-based interventions.

Primary Health Care for Children with Cardiovascular Diseases

The goals of primary health care for a child with cardiovascular disease include the following (Koot & Wallander, 2001):

- Adequate nutritional intake and optimal growth
- Optimal psychosocial development and functioning, especially concerning anxiety, vulnerability, independence, and acceptance of physical limitation(s)
- Enhancement of self-esteem, social support, and coping
- Provision of comprehensive health care
- Promotion of compliance with treatment regimens
- Prevention or identification of cardiac complications
- Anticipatory guidance regarding ongoing preventive care and health maintenance, emphasizing normal aspects of the child's growth and development to enhance the family's coping

Specific areas that may need additional attention at various ages are listed in Box 31-5. Providing more detailed information regarding the following areas may be helpful to these families:

- *Lifestyle and stress management.* Discuss with the family the need to treat the child as normally as possible. Encourage the family members to contact health care providers when they have questions or need reassurance. Direct parents to support groups that provide informational and emotional support for families. Discuss lifestyle changes regarding dietary practices, exercise patterns, and stress management for the patient and the family. Prevention of respiratory infections through good handwashing should be emphasized. All caregivers must understand that respiratory infections require prompt evaluation and treatment.
- *Exercise and sports participation.* Reassure the parents that the child generally "self-limits" activity according to ability. Exercise tolerance studies should be completed before entrance into sports or any activities that require strenuous physical exertion. Parameters for sports participation for children with carditis, hypertension, CHD, dysrhythmias, mitral valve prolapse, and heart murmurs are available in Chapter 15.
- *Diet and nutrition.* Depending on the child's condition, the family may need help in modifying the diet to provide maximum calories or limit various types of foods. Nutritional referral may at times prove helpful (see Chapter 12 for more detailed information).

BOX 31-5 *Key Areas of Primary Health Care for Children with Cardiovascular Disease*

Infancy (Birth to 2 Years)

Growth and development
Nutrition
Immunizations
Attention to siblings

Preschool Years

Development
Discipline
Dental care
Endocarditis prophylaxis

School Age (6 to 12 Years)

School program
Activity recommendations and sports
Endocarditis prophylaxis

Adolescence

Sexuality concerns, contraception, and pregnancy
Delayed puberty
Genetic counseling
Athletics/exercise
Vocational counseling
Endocarditis counseling

Adapted from Uzark K: Recognition and management of congenital heart disease in the neonate. Presented at the National Association of Pediatric Nurse Associates and Practitioners 17th Annual Conference, San Diego, CA, 1996.

Prevention of Bacterial Endocarditis

Although uncommon in children, bacterial endocarditis (also called subacute bacterial endocarditis [SBE] or infectious endocarditis) has a high morbidity and mortality rate (see later) and warrants primary prevention whenever indicated. The incidence in children is less than that of adults, which is 1.7 to 3.8 per 100,000. Children with underlying CHD or rheumatic heart disease are the most susceptible (Thornton, 2000). The initial symptoms are a high fever with the sudden onset of a murmur and peripheral emboli. The most common pathogens are *Staphylococcus aureus*, the streptococcus family, and *Neisseria gonorrhoeae*.

The standard for prophylaxis against SBE was established in 1997 by the American Heart Association. These recommendations identify how the practitioner can (1) stratify risk categories into high, moderate, or negligible; (2) identify procedures for which prophylaxis is and is not recommended; and (3) simplify treatment regimens (Box 31-6 and Tables 31-5 and 31-6). Prophylaxis is initiated shortly before the procedure and given perioperatively. A high index of suspicion for bacterial endocarditis should be maintained if any unusual clinical findings (e.g., petechiae, fever) are present after any procedure.

Primary Prevention

Immunization schedules should be maintained into and throughout adulthood to prevent potential complications from preventable diseases. Genetics counseling is recommended for parents with significant family histories of CHD (Allen, Phillips, & Chan, 2001; Bernstein, 2004). Early prenatal care and education are essential, and women should be counseled regarding the avoidance of teratogens during pregnancy.

BOX 31-6 *Relative Risk of Endocarditis for Various Cardiovascular and Underlying Conditions*

High Risk

Prosthetic valves
Previous episode of endocarditis
Complex cyanotic congenital heart disease (e.g., single-ventricle states, transposition of the great vessels, tetralogy of Fallot)
Surgically constructed systemic artery–to–pulmonary artery shunts
Intravenous drug use
Indwelling central catheters

Moderate Risk

Uncorrected patent ductus arteriosus
Uncorrected ventricular septal defect
Uncorrected atrial septal defect (other than secundum)
Bicuspid aortic valve
Mitral valve prolapse with regurgitations
Rheumatic mitral or aortic valve disease
Other acquired valvular diseases
Hypertrophic cardiomyopathy

From Dajani A, Taubert K: Infective endocarditis. In Allen H et al: *Moss and Adams' heart disease in infants, children, and adolescents: including the fetus and young adult*, ed 6, Philadelphia, 2001, Lippincott Williams & Wilkins.

CONGENITAL HEART DISEASES

An infant or child with heart disease may have a variety of disease manifestations. Signs and symptoms in infants with CHD depend on the type of cardiac defect, the timing of PDA closure, and the fall in the pulmonary vascular resistance. Cyanosis and CHF are more obvious signs. Some infants and older children may simply have a murmur without symptoms. In older children, chest pain with exertion or syncope is often the chief complaint. The NP must be open to all diagnostic possibilities.

Congestive Heart Failure

CHF is the most common emergency in children with heart disease. It is the major reason, other than elective procedures, for hospitalization of these children. Those under 6 months old usually have an underlying intracardiac left-to-right shunt (e.g., VSD), whereas those older than 4 years of age succumb to CHF from acquired heart diseases (e.g., Kawasaki disease, rheumatic heart disease [RHD], myocarditis, or endocarditis) (Allen, Phillips, & Chan, 2001).

CHF refers to a set of clinical signs and symptoms that indicate myocardial dysfunction. This dysfunction results in cardiac output that is inadequate to provide blood and oxygen to body tissues. Compensatory mechanics in the body respond by affecting fluid homeostasis. Electrolyte and hormonal imbalances and water retention result, further complicating pulmonary and peripheral congestion (Anderson et al, 2002). VSD and PDA are examples of conditions that lead to increased myocardial workload caused by excessive volume secondary to shunting of blood. Structural or valvular abnormalities (e.g., coarctation or aortic stenosis) impede the normal flow of blood through cardiac structures and thereby increase the pressure load on the heart. Any condition that decreases the effectiveness of myocardial function (e.g., myocarditis, anemia, dysrhythmia) can also result in failure of the heart to maintain adequate cardiac output (Table 31-7).

Alterations in cardiac function occur because the cardiac muscle is overtaxed and compensation mechanisms are activated in an attempt to maintain adequate cardiac output. Ventricular dilation and hypertrophy are early indicators of the heart's reaction to increased workload. Tachycardia is an adaptive mechanism to increase cardiac

TABLE 31-5 ***Procedures for Which Endocarditis Prophylaxis Is or Is Not Recommended***

	Prophylaxis Recommended	Prophylaxis NOT Recommended
Dental	Dental extractions Periodontal procedures Dental implant placement and reimplantation of avulsed teeth Root canal instrumentation Initial placement of orthodontic bands but not brackets Intraligamentary local anesthetic injections Teeth or implant cleaning where bleeding is expected	Restorative dentistry Nonintraligamentary local anesthetic injections Intracanal endodontic treatment; postplacement and buildup Rubber dam placement Postoperative suture removal Placement of removable prosthodontic or orthodontic appliances Taking oral impressions Fluoride treatments Taking oral radiographs Orthodontic appliance adjustment Shedding of primary teeth
Respiratory tract	Tonsillectomy or adenoidectomy Surgery involving respiratory mucosa Rigid bronchoscopy Flexible bronchoscopy with biopsy	Endotracheal intubation Flexible bronchoscopy without biopsy Pressure tympanostomy tube insertion/removal
Gastrointestinal tract	Sclerotherapy for esophageal varices Esophageal stricture dilation Biliary tract surgery Operations involving intestinal mucosa	Gastrointestinal endoscopy without biopsy Transesophageal echocardiography
Genitourinary tract	Cystoscopy Urethral dilation Urethral catheterization with infection	Vaginal delivery Cesarean section Urethral catheterization without infection Therapeutic abortion Circumcision
Other procedures		Cardiac catheterization, including device placement and pacemakers Skin biopsy

Adapted from Dajani A et al: Prevention of bacterial endocarditis: recommendations by the American Heart Association, *JAMA* 277:1794-1801, 1997; Dreyer W: Infective endocarditis. In Burg F et al, editors: *Gellis and Kagan's current pediatric therapy*, ed 17, Philadelphia, 2002, WB Saunders.

output and promote delivery of oxygen to the heart and body. If demands on the heart are increased past the point of maximal effectiveness, the result is decreased cardiac output, pulmonary and systemic congestion, and associated clinical symptoms (Box 31-7).

Acyanotic Congenital Heart Disease (Left-to-Right Shunts)

Acyanotic lesions have a communication between the two sides of the heart through which extra blood shunts from the high-pressure, oxygenated, left side of the heart to the low-pressure, unoxygenated, right side of the heart. The result is an increase in pulmonary blood flow (Fig. 31-6).

Atrial Septal Defect

Description. An atrial septal defect (ASD) is a defect or hole in the atrial septum. Of the three types of ASD, the most common involves the midseptum in the area of the foramen ovale and is called an ostium secundum–type defect (Fig. 31-7). Defects of the sinus venosus type are high in the atrial septum, near the entry of the superior vena cava, and are frequently associated with anomalous pulmonary venous return. A primum ASD is in the lower portion of the septum and may be seen in children with Down syndrome.

Incidence. ASD is one of the most commonly recognized congenital cardiac anomalies in adults. ASD of the ostium secundum variety is twice as common in females and accounts for 7% to 10% of CCVMs (Anderson et al, 2002; Bernstein, 2004).

TABLE 31-6 Prophylactic Regimens for Dental, Oral, Respiratory Tract, or Esophageal Procedures

	Agent	Regimen
Standard general prophylaxis	Amoxicillin	50 mg/kg p.o. (maximum 2 g) 1 h before procedure
Unable to take oral medications	Ampicillin	50 mg/kg i.m. or i.v. (maximum 2 g) within 30 min before procedure
Penicillin allergic	Clindamycin	20 mg/kg p.o. (maximum 600 mg) 1 h before procedure
	or	
	Cephalexin or cefadroxil	50 mg/kg p.o. (maximum 2 g) 1 h before procedure
	or	
	Azithromycin or clarithromycin	15 mg/kg p.o. (maximum 500 mg) 1 h before procedure
Penicillin allergic and unable to take oral medications	Clindamycin	20 mg/kg i.v. (maximum 600 mg) within 30 min of procedure
	or	
	Cefazolin	25 mg/kg i.m. or i.v. (maximum 1 g) within 30 min before procedure

Dajani A, Taubert K: *Infective endocarditis.* In Allen H et al: *Moss & Adams' heart disease in infants, children, and adolescents, including the fetus and young adult,* ed 6, Philadelphia, 2001, Lippincott Williams & Wilkins, p 1307.
IM, Intramuscularly; *IV,* intravenously; *PO,* orally.
For patients in the high-risk category for endocarditis, half the dose may be repeated 6 hours after the initial dose (except for azithromycin—a second dose is not necessary).

- Cephalosporins should not be used in individuals with immediate-type hypersensitivity reaction (urticaria, angioedema, or anaphylaxis) to penicillins.
- If the child is also being treated for an acute infection with an antibiotic, the drug chosen should be from a different class for the prophylaxis.

TABLE 31-7 Conditions That Can Lead to Congestive Heart Failure in Children

Age	Condition
Premature infant	Patent ductus arteriosus
Birth-1 wk	Hypoplastic left heart syndrome
	Coarctation of the aorta
	Critical aortic stenosis
	Interrupted aortic arch
	Arteriovenous malformations
	Tachycardia
	Cardiomyopathy
1 wk-3 mo	Ventricular septal defect
	Truncus arteriosus
	Atrioventricular canal (endocardial cushion defect)
	Total anomalous pulmonary venous return
	Coarctation
	Tachycardia
	Patent ductus arteriosus
	Aortic stenosis
	Tricuspid atresia
Over 1 yr	Bacterial endocarditis
	Rheumatic fever
	Myocarditis

Clinical Findings

History

- Often completely asymptomatic
- May fatigue easily or have exertional dyspnea
- May be somewhat underdeveloped physically
- May have a history of frequent upper respiratory tract infections or pneumonia

Physical Examination

- Typically, a murmur may not be noticed until the child is 2 to 3 years of age, when examination of a quiet child can be performed.
- Mild left precardial bulge or palpable lift at the left sternal border may be seen.
- S_1 is normal or split, with accentuation of the tricuspid valve closure sound.
- S_2 is split widely and is relatively fixed in relation to respiration in patients with normal pulmonary pressure.
- A grade I–III/VI, widely radiating, medium-pitched, not harsh systolic ejection murmur is heard best at the pulmonic area. If the shunt is large, increased blood flow across the tricuspid valve is responsible for a middiastolic, rumbling murmur at the left lower sternal border (LLSB).
- There is seldom a thrill.
- Arterial pulses are normal and equal.

BOX 31-7 *Signs and Symptoms of Congestive Heart Failure*

Infants

Tachypnea
Tachycardia
Rales/wheezing
Cardiomegaly and hepatomegaly
Periorbital edema
Poor feeding
Poor weight gain
Diaphoresis

Children

Tachypnea
Tachycardia
Rales/wheezing
Cardiomegaly and hepatomegaly
Orthopnea
Shortness of breath or dyspnea with exertion
Peripheral edema
Poor growth and development

- In older patients (teenage or older), the pulmonic and the tricuspid murmurs decrease in intensity and the second heart sound may be single and accentuated. A diastolic murmur of pulmonic incompetence can appear.

Diagnostic Tests

- Chest radiography reveals cardiac enlargement. The main pulmonary artery may be dilated and the pulmonary vascular markings increased.
- The ECG shows right axis deviation with right atrial enlargement.
- The echocardiogram identifies the specific location of the defect in the atrial septum and shows chamber enlargement.
- Cardiac catheterization is rarely necessary unless the diagnosis is in doubt, shunt size is indeterminable, or pulmonary vascular disease is suspected (Bernstein, 2004).

Management. Management of ASD includes the following:

- Small defects found in infancy may close on their own.
- Larger defects require surgical intervention, usually after 1 year and before school entry or when the defect is identified in an older child. Such intervention can be planned electively to prepare the infant's or child's family for surgery. Surgical closure may involve a patch placed over the defect or primary suture closure for smaller defects. Surgical mortality rate is less than 1%. Technology is advancing rapidly in the area of nonsurgical repair of ASDs, allowing the defect to be closed by a device in the cardiac catheterization laboratory.
- An ECG every 3 to 5 years is necessary to rule out any late-occurring conduction abnormalities.
- No SBE prophylaxis precautions are necessary if the defect is small and isolated (see Table 31-6).
- Long-term outcome is excellent for patients after ASD repair.

Ventricular Septal Defect

Description. The ventricular septum is made up of four components: the membranous septum, the inlet septum, the trabecular septum, and the outlet or infundibular septum. A VSD is a hole or defect in one of these areas of the ventricular septum. Most commonly, defects occur in the region of the membranous septum and are referred to as perimembranous defects because

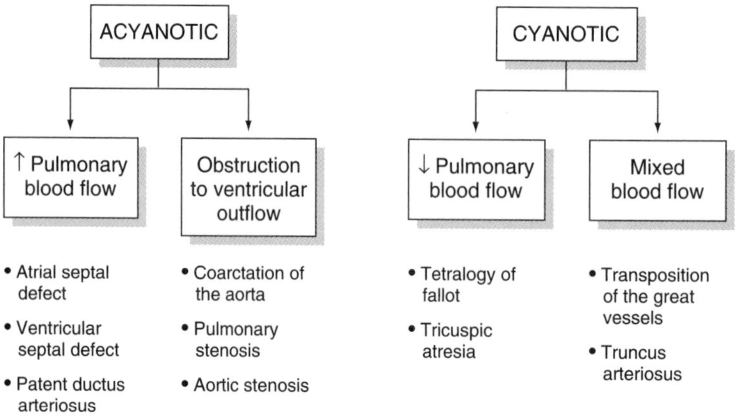

FIGURE 31-6 Classification of congenital heart disease.

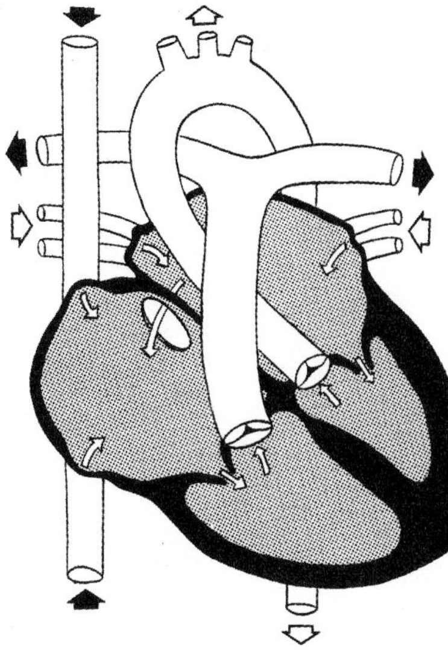

FIGURE 31-7 Atrial septal defect. (Used with permission of Ross Products Division, Abbott Laboratories, Columbus, OH 43216. From *Clinical education aid no. 7*. Copyright 1970 Ross Products Division, Abbott Laboratories.)

they are larger than the membranous septum itself. Other defects occur in the trabecular or muscular portion of the septum (Fig. 31-8).

Incidence. VSD is the most common childhood cardiac defect with an incidence of 25% and is slightly more common in females. Defects result from a deficiency in fetal

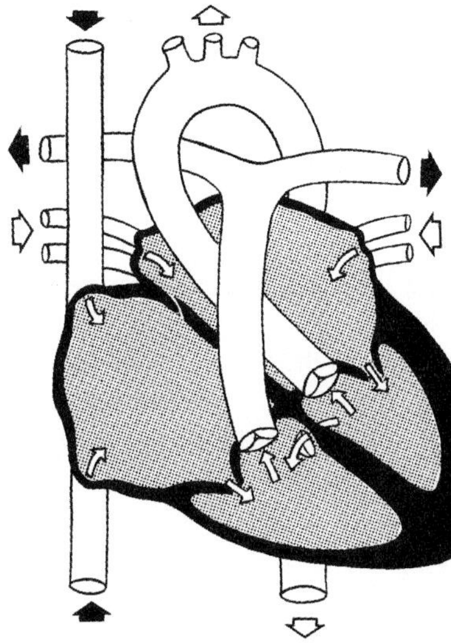

FIGURE 31-8 Ventricular septal defect. (Used with permission of Ross Products Division, Abbott Laboratories, Columbus, OH 43216. From *Clinical education aid no. 7*. Copyright 1970 Ross Products Division, Abbott Laboratories.)

growth or a failure of alignment or fusion of component parts. It is associated with chromosomal syndromes such as Down, but 95% of cases have no chromosomal anomaly. Approximately 30% to 50% of VSDs are small; the vast majority close by 4 years of age (Bernstein, 2004; Emblad et al, 2001).

Clinical Findings

History

- A murmur that may not have been evident at birth is noticed at 2 to 6 weeks of life as pulmonary vascular resistance falls.
- Signs of CHF may be present (e.g., pale skin color, poor weight gain, feeding difficulty, effort intolerance and fatigue, diaphoresis with crying or feeding).
- Small defects may be completely asymptomatic.

Physical Examination

- Small VSD
  - Harsh, high-pitched, grade II–IV/VI holosystolic murmur at LLSB
  - All other findings within normal limits
- Large VSD
  - Low-pitched, grade II–V/VI holosystolic murmur at LLSB
  - VSD murmur that becomes higher pitched over time indicates that the defect is becoming smaller
  - Diastolic rumble at the apex
  - "Thrill" along the left sternal border
  - Signs of progressing CHF after the first weeks of life
  - S_3 or S_4 gallop if CHF is present

Diagnostic Tests

- Chest radiography findings vary depending on the size of the shunt. Patients with small shunts have normal heart size and pulmonary vascular markings that are just beyond the upper limits of normal. Patients with large shunts have cardiac enlargement involving both the left and right ventricles and a left atrium with pulmonary vascular markings that are significantly increased. (See Fig. 31-4.)
- The ECG is normal in patients with small defects and may show cardiac enlargement and left ventricular hypertrophy (LVH) with large shunts.
- Echocardiography (two-dimensional, Doppler, or transesophageal) provides visualization of defects and pinpoints the exact anatomic location. In "pinhole" VSDs, a murmur may be present; however, a defect may not be visualized on the echocardiogram.
- Cardiac catheterization may be necessary to provide a clear anatomic picture if surgery is being considered. Surgery is required in infancy for those with uncontrolled CHF, including failure to thrive or recurrent respiratory infections (McDaniel & Gutgesell, 2001).

Management

- Infants with small defects and no symptoms of CHF are monitored every 1 to 2 months throughout the first year of life and then biannually to assess for closure of the defect. These newborns may exhibit localized, softly blowing systolic murmurs located at the LLSB (Stockman & Lohr, 2001). Some defects may never close but cause no difficulty. SBE prophylaxis is needed at the time of high-risk surgical or dental procedures.
- Larger defects with signs of CHF are managed as follows:
  - Digoxin or diuretics (or both) may be helpful.
  - Adequate caloric intake to enhance growth must be ensured.
  - Families must be taught the signs and symptoms of developing or progressing CHF.
- If no improvement is seen over weeks or months, surgery is indicated before 6 months.
  - Surgical repair consists of closure of the defect with a Dacron patch.
  - ECG is necessary every 3 to 5 years to rule out any late-occurring conduction abnormalities.
  - SBE prophylaxis precautions are necessary until 6 months after repair (Dajani & Taubert, 2001).

Long-term outcome is excellent after VSD repair.

Patent Ductus Arteriosus

Description. In the normal newborn, the first stage of ductus arteriosis functional closure should occur in the first 12 to 72 hours with the second stage of fibrous, permanent sealing by 2 to 3 weeks (Moore, Brook, & Heymann, 2001). The ductus arteriosus may remain patent in some infants and leave a connection between the aorta and the pulmonary artery. As pulmonary vascular resistance falls, aortic blood is shunted back into the pulmonary artery and recirculates through the lungs (Fig. 31-9).

Incidence. PDA accounts for 5% to 10% of all cases of CHD. The incidence in females outnumbers that in males 2:1. In intensive care nurseries with premature infants weighing less than 1750 g, the frequency of PDA is as high as 45% to 80% (Moore, Brook, & Heymann, 2001). In utero exposure to rubella in the first trimester is associated with PDA.

Clinical Findings

History

- The patient may be asymptomatic if the PDA is small.
- Increasing signs of CHF may appear in the first weeks of life.

Physical Examination

- In the immediate postnatal period, the murmur is soft, systolic, and heard along the left sternal border, under the left clavicle, and in the back.

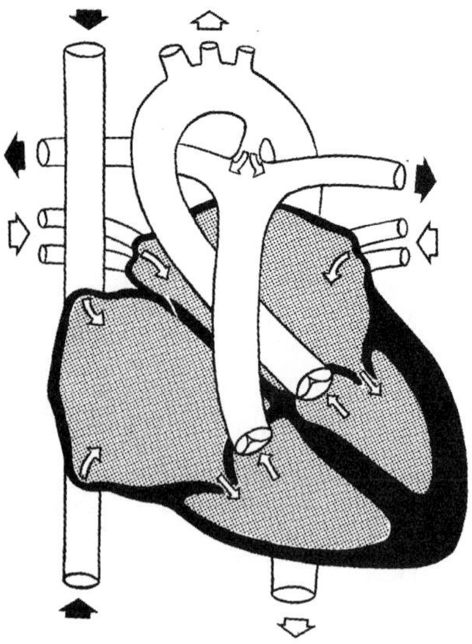

FIGURE 31-9 Patent ductus arteriosus. (Used with permission of Ross Products Division, Abbott Laboratories, Columbus, OH 43216. From *Clinical education aid no. 7.* Copyright 1970 Ross Products Division, Abbott Laboratories.)

- After the first weeks of life, a typical grade II–V/VI, harsh, rumbling, continuous "machinery murmur" is heard in the left infraclavicular fossa and pulmonic area with a thrill at the base.
- Physical findings of CHF (e.g., hepatomegaly, rales, fatigability, tachypnea, failure to thrive) may be present with a large shunt.

Diagnostic Tests

- Chest radiography findings include the following:
  - With a small to moderate shunt, the heart is not enlarged.
  - If the shunt is large, evidence of both left atrial and ventricular enlargement is apparent.

In both cases, the aorta is prominent, as is the main pulmonary artery segment. Pulmonary vascular markings may be increased.

- ECG reveals left ventricular hypertrophy with large shunts.
- Echocardiograms show enlargement of the left atrium. This clue is important for detecting the presence of CHF and is especially useful in diagnosing PDA in a premature infant. The echocardiogram also shows directional shunting through the ductus.
- Cardiac catheterization, two-dimensional echocardiology, and Doppler echocardiology are used if medical management is not successful and surgical closure is contemplated (Moore, Brook, & Heymann, 2001).

Differential Diagnosis. See Table 31-8.

TABLE 31-8 *Congenital Heart Disease: Differential Diagnosis of Cardiac Defects*

Feature	Atrial Septal Defect	Ventricular Septal Defect	Patent Ductus Arteriosus	Transposition of the Great Vessels	Tetralogy of Fallot	Tricuspid Atresia	Aortic Stenosis	Pulmonic Stenosis	Coarctation of the Aorta
Incidence of total CHD	10%, 2:1 female to male	20%	10%	5%, 3:1 male to female	8%	2%	5%, 4:1 male to female	8%	5%
Age at initial presentation	Variable; may be asymptomatic into adulthood	Variable depending on size; large by 4-8 wk; small by 6 mo	Neonate to 3 mo	Immediately at birth	Usually by 6 mo	Usually newborn	Depends on severity; critical in newborn	Depends on severity; newborn to school-age children	First weeks of life or 3-5 yr
Clinical findings	Murmur on preschool examination	CHF or murmur	CHF or murmur	Cyanosis	Cyanosis	Cyanosis	Murmur CHF; older child, chest pain	Cyanosis or murmur	CHF in newborn; hypertension in preschooler
Auscultation	Midsystolic murmur at ULSB with wide-split second heart sound	Holosystolic murmur at LLSB	Continuous murmur under left clavicle, referred to back	Usually no murmur	Early systolic ejection murmur at second left intercostal space; holosystolic murmur at LLSB	ASD murmur may be associated with PDA	Systolic ejection murmur at URSB, constant systolic click at apex with bicuspid valve	Late systolic ejection murmur at ULSB, intermittent systolic ejection click	Systolic ejection murmur in left intraclavicular region with transmission to back
Radiologic findings	May have mild cardiomegaly	Normal or cardiomegaly	Cardiomegaly	Egg-shaped heart	Boot-shaped heart	Cardiomegaly	Normal	Normal	Rib notching

Continued

TABLE 31-8 Congenital Heart Disease: Differential Diagnosis of Cardiac Defects—cont'd

Feature	Atrial Septal Defect	Ventricular Septal Defect	Patent Ductus Arteriosus	Transposition of the Great Vessels	Tetralogy of Fallot	Tricuspid Atresia	Aortic Stenosis	Pulmonic Stenosis	Coarctation of the Aorta
Pulmonary vasculature	Normal to slightly increased	Normal or increased	Increased markings	May have increased markings or be normal	Decreased pulmonary vascularity	Decreased pulmonary markings	Normal	Decreased in severity	Normal
ECG	May have RsR_I in V_I, right atrial enlargement	Combined ventricular hypertrophy	Combined ventricular hypertrophy	RV hypertrophy	RV hypertrophy	Right atrial enlargement, absent RV voltage	Left ventricular hypertrophy	RV hypertrophy	RV hypertrophy
Associations	Holt-Oram syndrome, Down syndrome in PAPVR, mitral valve prolapse	Associated with many defects	Associated with many defects	VSD, PDA, coronary artery anomalies	Down syndrome	VSD, PDA, ASD	Marfan syndrome, Turner syndrome, Williams syndrome	Turner syndrome, Williams syndrome, neurofibromatosis	Turner syndrome, neurofibromatosis, PDA
Treatments	Surgical closure	Observation, digoxin and/or diuretics; if large, surgical closure	Surgical closure if large	Newborn PGE, septostomy, arterial switch (Jatene)	Tetralogy repair, BT shunt	Shunt and surgical repair	Catheter valvulotomy or surgical repair	Catheter valvuloplasty or surgery	Surgical repair or balloon dilation

ASD, atrial septal defect; *BT*, Blalock-Taussig; *CHF*, congenital heart failure; *ECG*, electrocardiogram; *LLSB*, left lower sternal border; *PAPVR*, partial anomalous pulmonary venous return; *PDA*, patent ductus arteriosus; *PGE*, prostaglandin E; *RV*, right ventricular; *ULSB*, upper left sternal border; *URSB*, upper right sternal border; *VSD*, ventricular septal defect.

Management

- Pharmacologic management of a preterm infant with PDA depends on the magnitude of the shunt. Indomethacin, a prostaglandin inhibitor that constricts and closes the ductus, may be given to preterm infants to effect closure.
- Surgical intervention in an asymptomatic infant with a small left-to-right shunt is unnecessary because a small PDA usually undergoes spontaneous closure by age 2 years. Patients with large shunts or infants with pulmonary hypertension should have their PDA surgically closed within the first few months of life to prevent the development of progressive pulmonary vascular obstruction. Surgical ligation of the ductus is a low-risk procedure because cardiopulmonary bypass is not necessary. Cardiac catheterization techniques are commonly used to close the shunt. PDA is one of the few defects that is effectively "cured" by surgical intervention.
- Families should be reassured that their child will live an active, normal life.
- SBE prophylaxis precautions are recommended 6 months after the repair (Dajani & Taubert, 2001).

Cyanotic Congenital Heart Disease (Right-to-Left Shunts)

Cyanotic CHD (see Fig. 31-6) represents 10% to 18% of all congenital heart lesions (Moller & Hoffman, 2000). Cardiac cyanosis is due to obstruction of pulmonary blood flow or mixing of oxygenated and unoxygenated blood. Visible cyanosis occurs when greater than 3 to 5 g/dl of desaturated hemoglobin is present in arterial blood. Cyanosis, given a constant hemoglobin oxygen saturation, is more readily apparent with polycythemia and less readily apparent with anemia or the presence of fetal hemoglobin, which shifts the oxygen-hemoglobin saturation curve. With cyanotic heart defects, desaturated blood enters the systemic arterial circulation, regardless of whether cyanosis is clinically evident. Polycythemia is a compensatory mechanism to increase the oxygen-carrying capacity but puts the patient at risk for cerebral thromboses (Bernstein, 2004). Common heart conditions causing cyanosis in the immediate newborn period include transposition of the great arteries (TGA), tetralogy of Fallot (TOF), truncus arteriosus, and tricuspid atresia.

Transposition of the Great Arteries

Description. TGA is the result of incomplete septation and migration of the truncus arteriosus during fetal development. In TGA, the aorta arises from the right ventricle and the pulmonary artery arises from the left ventricle. The aorta receives the unoxygenated systemic venous blood and returns it to the systemic arterial circuit. The pulmonary artery receives oxygenated pulmonary venous blood and returns it to the pulmonary circulation (Fig. 31-10). There may be a number of other CCVMs.

Incidence. TGA accounts for 5% to 7% of all cases of CHD and occurs 60% to 70% more frequently in males (Wernovsky, 2001). Without treatment, there is a 30% mortality rate in the first week of life, 50% in the first month, 70% in the first 6 months, and 90% by the first year. With treatment, 90% survive. The incidence is 20 to 30.5 per 100,000 live births (Wernovsky, 2001).

Clinical Findings

History

- Cyanosis is immediately evident by 1 hour of birth (52%) or within the first day after birth (92%).
- There may be symptoms of CHF.
- Affected infants are often large for gestational age with retardation of growth and development after the neonatal period.

Physical Examination

- Infants may have no murmur at birth or may have a murmur characteristic of associated lesions such as VSD, ASD, or PDA.
- S_2 is loud and single.

Diagnostic Tests

- Chest radiography and ECG findings may be normal in the early newborn period, or the heart may appear egg shaped.
- ECG findings show right axis deviation and right ventricular hypertrophy.

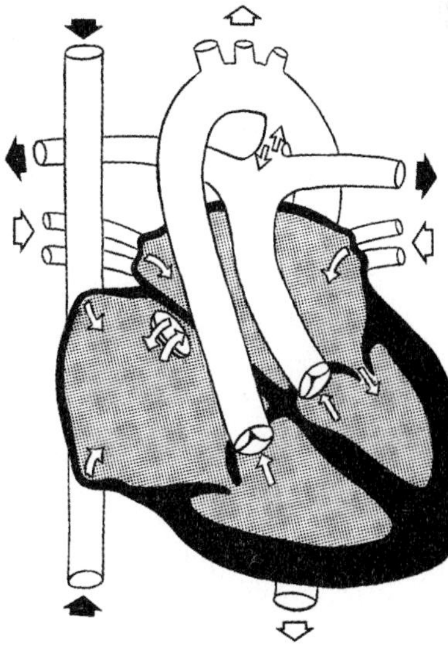

FIGURE 31-10 Complete transposition of the great vessels. (Used with permission of Ross Products Division, Abbott Laboratories, Columbus, OH 43216. From *Clinical education aid no. 7.* Copyright 1970 Ross Products Division, Abbott Laboratories.)

- Usually two-dimensional and Doppler echocardiography is obtained for diagnosis. Results show the pulmonary artery arising from the left ventricle and the aorta arising from the right (Wernovsky, 2001).

Management

- Immediate referral and transfer to a pediatric cardiac center are necessary. Correction of electrolyte and acid-base imbalance may be necessary.
- Pharmacologic management (in addition to oxygen administration) may include intravenous prostaglandin E_1 (PGE_1) to delay closure of the ductus arteriosus.
- A balloon atrial septostomy may be performed in the catheterization laboratory to promote mixing of oxygenated and unoxygenated blood in the atria.
- The current surgical repair is the arterial switch (Jatene procedure) and is usually performed in the first few days of life. Neoaortic (i.e., new) regurgitation is a common finding after such a procedure.
- These patients are monitored closely throughout life with annual echocardiogram follow-up. Families require information and support as their child develops.
- SBE prophylaxis precautions are indicated.

Prognosis. Some institutions have realized 5-year survival rates of up to 98% with the Jatene procedure (Wernovsky, 2001). However, long-term patency and inadequate growth of the coronary arteries warrant close monitoring. The NP should refer any patient with such a repair to a pediatric cardiologist, especially with a history of palpitations, syncope, and shortness of breath with exertion.

Tetralogy of Fallot

Description. The tetralogy of Fallot (TOF), also referred to as TET (short for tetralogy), is a combination of four anatomic cardiac defects resulting in right ventricular outflow tract obstruction: (1) pulmonary valve stenosis, (2) right ventricular hypertrophy, (3) VSD, and (4) an aorta that overrides the ventricular septum (Fig. 31-11). A child may not display signs of cyanosis if the valvular stenosis is mild. In contrast, when the right-to-left shunting increases across the VSD because of increased right-sided pressure secondary to constriction of the right ventricular outflow tract, the child will appear cyanotic.

Incidence. TOF, the most common cyanotic lesion, accounts for 3.5% to 9% of all cases of CHD. There is no racial bias; the defect occurs up to 56.4% more frequently in males (Siwik, Patel, & Zahka, 2001).

Clinical Findings

History

- Infants are likely to have a history of maternal diabetes, maternal phenylketonuria, or maternal trimethadione or retinoic acid use (Siwik, Patel, & Zahka, 2001).

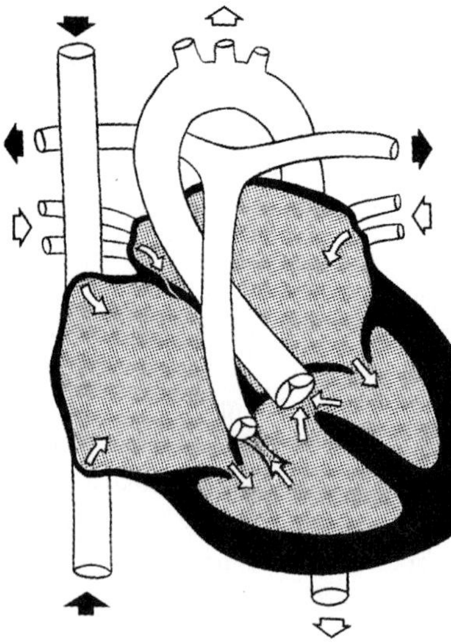

FIGURE 31-11 Tetralogy of Fallot. (Used with permission of Ross Products Division, Abbott Laboratories, Columbus, OH 43216. From *Clinical education aid no. 7*. Copyright 1970 Ross Products Division, Abbott Laboratories.)

- The severity of symptoms depends on the degree of right ventricular outflow obstruction.
  - With mild obstruction, the cyanosis may be so slight that it is not initially evident. These infants have a VSD murmur and possibly a pulmonary stenosis murmur.
  - Severe obstruction results in cyanosis at birth.
- Most affected infants are cyanotic by 4 months of age, fatigue easily with crying or feeding, and demonstrate dyspnea.
- Hypercyanotic episodes, or TET spells (the infant becomes intensely cyanotic, is extremely dyspneic, and appears to be unable to get air), are induced by crying, defecating, or feeding and occur during the first 2 to 3 months of life.
- Poor weight gain is common.
- Older children can have dyspnea on exertion, squatting episodes, poor appetite, clubbing, poor growth, increasing cyanosis, and alterations in consciousness from irritability to syncope.

Physical Examination

- Cyanosis of the mucous membranes and dyspnea may be evident.
- A grade III–V/VI, harsh systolic ejection murmur is heard at the left mid to upper sternal border with a palpable thrill and a holosystolic murmur at the LLSB.
- Observable sternal lift secondary to right ventricular hypertrophy may be present.
- Usually no diastolic murmur is heard.
- A loud aortic closure can be heard at the left sternal border.

Diagnostic Tests
- Chest radiography shows a boot-shaped heart with decreased pulmonary vascular markings.
- ECG shows right ventricular hypertrophy and may show a conduction delay in V_1.
- Two-dimensional echocardiography is diagnostic when it shows the extent of the pulmonary obstruction and demonstrates the anatomy of the overriding aorta and VSD.
- Pulse oximetry desaturation to 85% occurs, with resultant increase in hemoglobin/hematocrit values.
- Cardiac catheterization may be done before surgery.

Management
- In neonates with severe pulmonary obstruction, patency of the ductus arteriosus is critical and can be accomplished with PGE_1 as described in management of TGA.
- For hypercyanotic episodes, or TET spells, the child should be cradled in a knee-chest position until the spell subsides. This maneuver increases systemic resistance, decreases right-to-left shunting, and increases pulmonary blood flow, thus alleviating symptoms. Immediate intervention is required for infants who are "spelling."
- Open heart surgical repair is performed in infancy.
- These children are routinely monitored for life because they may develop an outflow tract obstruction or a late arrhythmia may develop many years after the initial repair. Sports participation is usually unrestricted if there are no residual defects after surgery. The NP should seek a cardiology consult before clearing for sports participation (Stockman & Lohr, 2001).
- SBE prophylaxis precautions are indicated.

Tricuspid Atresia

Description and Incidence. Pulmonary atresia results in the absence of communication between the right ventricle and the pulmonary artery. The degree of the obstruction can be variable. The atresia can be at the level of the main pulmonary artery or the pulmonary valve. Atresia of the pulmonary valve is the most common type (Fig. 31-12). The right ventricle may be hypoplastic with ventricular hypertrophy. Survival depends on having a concurrent PDA, ASD, or patent foramen ovale to allow mixing of blood. Less than 3% of all children with CHD have tricuspid atresia. Up to 20% have multiple cardiac abnormalities. The etiology of this condition is unknown (Epstein, 2001).

Clinical Findings

History
- Cyanosis in the first week of life with dyspnea on exertion
- Fatigue with the effort of crying or feeding
- Occasional hypoxic episodes

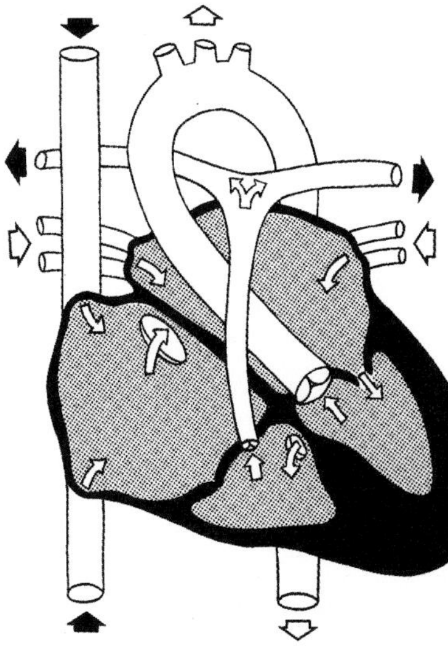

FIGURE 31-12 Tricuspid atresia. (Used with permission of Ross Products Division, Abbott Laboratories, Columbus, OH 43216. From *Clinical education aid no. 7*. Copyright 1970 Ross Products Division, Abbott Laboratories.)

- Failure to thrive (poor weight gain)
- CHF (develops over time)
- Hepatomegaly (may or may not be present)

Physical Examination
- Grade III–V/VI, harsh pansystolic murmur along the middle left sternal border
- Usually a single S_2
- May or may not be a thrill

Diagnostic Tests
- Chest radiography is generally normal initially, with x-ray changes occurring as the degree of cardiomegaly and obstruction of the pulmonary blood flow progresses.
- ECG shows LVH with small or absent right ventricular voltage.
- Two-dimensional echocardiography is diagnostic and shows the specifics of the atresia (Allen, Phillips, & Chan, 2001).

Management
- Intravenous PGE_1 before shunting may be indicated in newborns. Shunts and eventual total surgical repair, usually with a Fontan procedure (multiple surgical interventions), are required.
- Families require support throughout the child's life. Frequent surgeries and hospitalizations can interfere with normal social development. Early recognition and intervention for developmental delays are important to the child's future.
- SBE prophylaxis precautions are indicated.

Complications. Complications include development of collateral arterial and venous vessels and protein-losing enteropathy. A decrease in exercise tolerance throughout life can be expected, as well as left ventricular dysfunction. Complications may be fewer as surgical correction becomes more common at earlier ages. For patients with long-term complications, heart transplantation can be an option (Epstein, 2001).

Obstructive Cardiac Lesions

Aortic Stenosis

Description. Normally, the aortic valve opens to allow oxygenated blood to flow from the left ventricle to the aorta. Stenosis may be valvular, subvalvular, or supravalvular, with valvular being the most common. Valvular stenosis is usually characterized by a bicuspid valve. Stenosis causes increased pressure load on the left ventricle leading to LVH and, ultimately, ventricular failure. Obstruction of the aortic valve may cause a decrease in coronary artery blood flow. Unless severe, congenital aortic stenosis is often not diagnosed until early adulthood (Fig. 31-13).

Incidence. Aortic stenosis (AS) accounts for 3% to 5% of all cases of CHD and is four times more common in males. Twenty percent of patients with AS have associated cardiac abnormalities (Freed, 2001).

Clinical Findings

History

- The patient may be asymptomatic, depending on the severity of the defect.

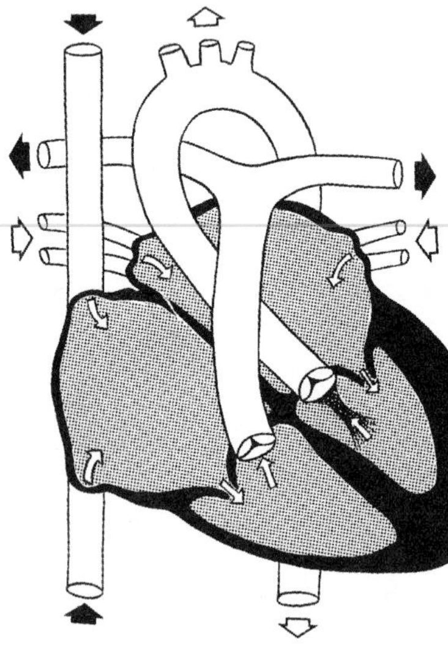

FIGURE 31-13 Subaortic stenosis. (Used with permission of Ross Products Division, Abbott Laboratories, Columbus, OH 43216. From *Clinical education aid no. 7.* Copyright 1970 Ross Products Division, Abbott Laboratories.)

- Growth and development may be normal.
- Activity intolerance, fatigue, chest pain (angina pectoris), or syncope can develop or increase with age.
- CHF may be evident in 10% of newborns with AS (Freed, 2001).

Physical Examination

- BP may reveal a narrow pulse pressure or a high systolic pressure in the right arm.
- A grade III–IV/VI, loud, harsh systolic ejection murmur is best heard at the upper right sternal border or atypically at the base with radiation to the LLSB and apex.
- With a valvular lesion, a faint, early diastolic murmur may be heard.
- In the most severe lesions, S_2 is single or closely split.
- S_3 or S_4 heart sounds may also be heard.
- A thrill may be present at the suprasternal notch.

Diagnostic Tests

- Chest radiographs are usually normal or may show left ventricular hypertrophy.
- ECG can be normal or reveal LVH and inverted T waves.
- Two-dimensional and Doppler echocardiograms are the diagnostic examinations of choice (Freed, 2001).
- Exercise testing may be done.

Management

- The timing of treatment depends on the severity of the obstruction. Treatment is usually not necessary unless the stenosis is moderate to severe. However, aortic stenosis and symptoms of obstruction tend to progress with age.
- Balloon valvuloplasty of the stenotic valve is now the initial treatment of AS. Aortic valvulotomy may be used if valvuloplasty is not successful. Both techniques are used in infancy, with similar mortality rates (10% to 20%) (Freed, 2001).
- Avoidance of high-risk sports is often recommended because of the risk of sudden death. Families should be counseled to encourage their children to avoid competitive athletics. Following exercise testing, the child should be directed to participate in light activities, such as recreational swimming, bicycling, or golf (Koot & Wallander, 2001).
- Aortic stenosis has the highest complication rate for bacterial endocarditis; therefore SBE prophylaxis is always necessary (Freed, 2001).

Pulmonic Stenosis

Description. Normally, the pulmonary valve opens to allow the flow of blood from the right ventricle into the pulmonary artery. Pulmonic stenosis is characterized by narrowing or noncompliance of the pulmonic valve as blood is ejected through it. Right-sided pressure is increased as the ventricle pumps against the obstruction. Right ventricular hypertrophy occurs as a result of this increased load. Pulmonary stenosis can also occur in the pulmonary arterial system and cause mild to severe obstruction to pulmonary blood flow. Mild pulmonic stenosis is usually identified on routine examination.

Incidence. Isolated pulmonic stenosis makes up approximately 8% to 10% of all cases of CHD. Approximately 1% to 2% may have other cardiac defects (Latson & Prieto, 2001).

Clinical Findings

History

- The patient is usually asymptomatic, with a murmur noted on routine physical examination.
- Exertional dyspnea and fatigue are noticeable as stenosis progresses.
- Cyanosis from obstruction to pulmonary blood flow may be evident with severe pulmonic stenosis in infancy.
- Growth and development are usually normal.

Physical Examination

- A grade II–IV/VI, harsh, mid-to-late systolic ejection murmur is heard at the upper left sternal border over the pulmonic region, with transmission along the left sternal border, neck, and back and into both lung fields.
- An intermittent systolic ejection click may be evident in the pulmonic area that decreases with inspiration and increases with expiration (Latson & Prieto, 2001).
- Cyanosis and symptoms of right-sided CHF can occur in severe cases.
- S_2 may be fixed as stenosis progresses.

Diagnostic Tests

- Chest radiographs may be within normal limits in infants or show prominent main pulmonary artery segments in 80% to 90% of cases. Right-sided cardiac enlargement and decreased peripheral pulmonary vascular markings may be evident if heart failure develops (Latson & Prieto, 2001).
- ECG may be normal with mild stenosis, abnormal in 80% of cases with moderate stenosis, and 100% abnormal with severe stenosis (abnormal = right atrial and ventricular hypertrophy).
- The two-dimensional and Doppler echocardiograms are helpful in confirming the diagnosis, identifying the gradient, and monitoring progression of the stenosis (Latson & Prieto, 2001).
- Angiocardiography may be used to provide information about the location and severity of the stenosis.

Management

- Balloon valvuloplasty is indicated and has proven successful in neonates. If unsuccessful, valvulotomy is indicated.
- With mild stenosis, families need to be encouraged to treat their children normally and not limit their activity. In those with moderate stenosis, the stenosis can progress to severe narrowing during periods of rapid growth, such as during infancy or adolescence (Latson & Prieto, 2001).
- SBE prophylaxis is necessary in those with moderate to severe stenosis.

Coarctation of the Aorta

Description. Coarctation of the aorta is a narrowing of a small or long segment of the aorta (Fig. 31-14). Coarctatation may occur as a single defect caused by a disturbance in the development of the aorta or may be secondary to constriction of the ductus arteriosus. The severity of the coarctation, its location, and the degree of obstruction determine the effect of the coarctation. A preductal coarctation may go unnoticed until the ductus begins to close and causes obstruction of blood flow to the lower part of the body. Systolic and diastolic hypertension exists in vessels above the area of narrowing. Hypotension is present in vessels below the area of narrowing. One study showed that the average age at diagnosis was 10 years (Beckman, 2001).

Incidence. Coarctation of the aorta is not always apparent until the ductus closes after birth. After this closure, though, rapid CHF and shock may occur. It accounts for 6% to 8% of cases of CHD and occurs twice as often in males. Patients with Turner syndrome have close to a 35% incidence of coarctation (Beckman, 2001).

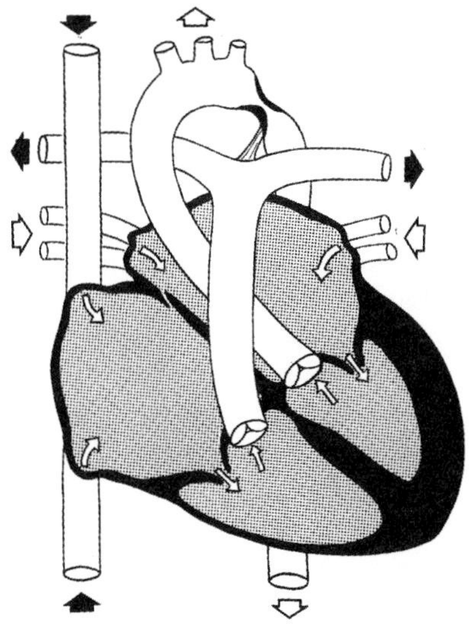

FIGURE 31-14 Coarctation of the aorta. (Used with permission of Ross Products Division, Abbott Laboratories, Columbus, OH 43216. From *Clinical education aid no. 7.* Copyright 1970 Ross Products Division, Abbott Laboratories.)

Clinical Findings

History. In older children, coarctation may go unnoticed until the BP is checked and mild hypertension is noted in the upper extremities, or a murmur is detected. Retrospectively, children with coarctation may have had complaints of leg pain with exercise or headaches.

Physical Examination

- Upper extremity hypertension with lower extremity hypotension is present, although milder cases may cause only a minimal discrepancy between upper and lower extremity blood pressures. In severe cases, poor lower extremity perfusion may be noticed with lower body mottling or pallor.
- Delayed timing and absent or weak arterial femoral and other distal pulses may occur.
- Bounding brachial, radial, and carotid pulses may occur.
- Signs of CHF may be evident.
- A systolic ejection murmur may be detected in the left infraclavicular region with transmission to the back.
- Ventricular heaving at the apex may occur.
- The patient may or may not have a systolic thrill at the suprasternal notch.
- Gallup rhythm may occur in infants with CHF.

Diagnostic Tests

- Chest radiography may reveal a normal or slightly enlarged heart.
- ECG findings depend on the severity of the lesion and the age of the patient. In infants, right ventricular hypertrophy may be seen; in older children, left ventricular changes are found secondary to hypertension.
- Two-dimensional or Doppler echocardiography is helpful in confirming the diagnosis and locating the constricted aortic segment. It may also show associated cardiac abnormalities.
- Magnetic resonance imaging can define the location, severity, and anatomy of the aortic arch.

Management

- In critical or severe coarctation, initial management is aimed at maintaining the ductus arteriosus to keep blood flowing to the lower part of the body. PGE_1 may be used.
- Surgical repair is completed either as an emergency during the neonatal period or electively at 2 to 3 years of age if upper extremity hypertension is not severe. The most common surgical intervention involves resection of the constricted area with an end-to-end anastomosis of the upper and lower portions of the aorta. Restenosis is more likely to occur if repair was done before 1 year of age (Beckman, 2001). Balloon dilation of the coarcted area may be performed in recoarctation or in the case of isolated mild coarctation. Other procedures, including bypass grafting, may be necessary with unusually long coarcted segments. Surgical mortality is rare. Recent advances in stenting are being explored to see if this will prevent later restenosis (Beckman, 2001).
- Monitoring of hypertension postoperatively is imperative. In older children with long-standing hypertension, antihypertensive medication may be required for several months after repair. Long-term prognosis is excellent unless there are associated intracardiac defects.
- Competitive sports should be restricted only if they involve high-impact activities where there is an increased chance of chest impact or heavy isometric exercise (Beckman, 2001). Any hypertension needs to be under control.
- SBE prophylaxis precautions are necessary.

ACQUIRED HEART DISEASE

Chest Pain

Description

Chest pain in the pediatric population is a common complaint and does not usually represent a serious cardiovascular problem. However, chest pain of any kind can cause great anxiety for children, adolescents, and their parents. It is important to thoroughly evaluate the complaint, with a careful history (especially a family history of sudden death or early cardiac disease) and thorough physical examination. ECG and other laboratory tests may be indicated if findings are present. Reassurance is of the utmost importance.

Etiology and Incidence

The most frequent cause of chest pain is musculoskeletal, originating in the chest wall or chest cage. Costochondritis, Tietze syndrome, idiopathic chest pain, precordial catch syndrome, slipping-rib syndrome, hypersensitive xiphoid syndrome, trauma, and muscle strain are diagnoses assigned to specific types of chest pain; all are of musculoskeletal origin, benign, and rarely require any treatment. The pain is often related to sports or casual athletic activity. Chest pain secondary to a pulmonary problem (asthma, pneumonia, embolism, pneumothorax) or gastrointestinal problem (reflux esophagitis, esophageal foreign body), herpes zoster, or sickle cell disease should be included in the differential diagnosis. Chest wall pain, particularly with exercise, may indicate exercise-induced asthma but rarely indicates cardiac disease. Chronic chest pain that is vague and occurs over many months in a variety of circumstances, particularly around stressful events, may be psychogenic (anxiety or hyperventilation). Pain associated with syncope, exertional dyspnea, or irregularities in heart rhythm needs careful evaluation for a cardiac cause.

Usually, children or adolescents who have pain of cardiac origin describe a specific history with details that are consistent from event to event. Most pediatric patients with chest pain do not have cardiac pathology.

The incidence of chest pain is approximately 0.288%, and it occurs slightly more often in males. The mean age at initial evaluation is 12 to 14 years. Most cases resolve spontaneously (Driscoll, 2001).

Clinical Findings

History. To determine the etiology of the chest pain, the NP should elicit the following historical information:

- Past medical history or family history for sudden death, heart disease or condition, asthma, eczema, Marfan syndrome, sickle cell disease
- Past and present casual or more intense sports activities, including any resultant trauma or muscle strains
- Characteristics of the chest pain
  - Relationship of pain to exercise; any syncope or exertional dyspnea
  - Any burning, substernal pain that worsens with reclining or with spicy foods (gastrointestinal etiology)
  - Pain that is sharp or stabbing, lasting several seconds to minutes, located over the midsternum or infranipple area, and occurring with nonexertion or deep inspirations (more likely musculoskeletal in origin)
  - Pain that awakens the patient (more likely organic)
- Any other associated symptoms such as fever, nausea, vomiting, headaches, choking episodes
- Any recent, major stressful events
- Medication, tobacco, or other drug use, including oral contraceptives (embolism)

Physical Examination. A complete chest (lungs and heart) and abdominal examination should be performed. Key findings to focus on include the presence of the following:

- Cardiac murmur, rubs, or clicks
- Point tenderness of one or more costochondral joints exaggerated with physical activity or deep inspirations (costochondritis or Tietze syndrome [if associated with warmth, swelling, or tenderness over costochondral junction])
- Irregular heart rhythm (cardiac disease)
- Shortness of breath, coughing, wheezing, chest pain with exercise
- Rales, wheezing, tachypnea, decreased breath sounds (pulmonary disease)

Diagnostic Tests. In most cases, only the history and physical are necessary to make the diagnosis; other tests are not indicated unless the following problems are suspected:

- Febrile, cardiac, or pulmonary condition: chest radiograph
- Exercise-induced asthma: pulmonary function testing with exercise
- Cardiac disease: 24-hour Holter monitor or stress test (or both)
- Signs of CHD, pericarditis, or myocarditis: ECG

Musculoskeletal, respiratory, psychogenic, and gastrointestinal disorders, as discussed earlier, as well as miscellaneous entities such as sickle cell crisis, aortic abdominal aneurysm (Marfan syndrome), pleural effusion (collagen-vascular disorders), and shingles, are in the differential diagnosis.

Management

- When chest pain has no clear-cut cause, the child appears well, and all aspects of the evaluation are normal, reassurance may be the most important treatment. Frequently, when reassured that the pain has no organic cause, the pain subsides or becomes less of an issue for the child.
  - Costochondritis and Tietze syndrome are usually responsive to nonsteroidal antiinflammatory treatment and rest.
  - Antacids may be tried if esophagitis is suspected; see Chapter 33.
  - See management of foreign body ingestion in Chapter 33.
  - See Chapters 25 and 32 for management of asthma and respiratory diseases.
- In cases in which pulmonary, gastrointestinal, or cardiac disease is a concern, treatment, referral, or evaluation is necessary.
- Follow-up is indicated to ensure that no new findings have emerged, to ensure that the child is participating in normal activities, and to monitor potential psychoemotional problems.

Hypertension

Definition

Hypertension is defined as a systolic or diastolic (or both) BP in the 95th or higher percentile for age, sex, and height on at least three consecutive occasions. *High-normal BP* is defined as average systolic or diastolic BP in the 90th percentile or higher but less than the 95th percentile. *Normal BP* is defined as systolic and diastolic BP below the 90th percentile for age, sex, and height (NIH NHBPEP, 1996).

Etiology and Incidence

Hypertension is a significant problem in children and young adults and results from the interaction of genetic and environmental factors. Increasingly, children are found to have high BP associated with obesity, sedentary lifestyles, and stress. It is estimated that hypertension occurs in 1% of children; the etiology is genetic in 60% of cases (Schieken, 2001). The believed differences in blood pressure between the sexes and some races have not stood up to findings of more recent research that corrected for body size and maturity (Schieken, 2001). Primary hypertension is most common in children with mild hypertension; blood pressure measurements show considerable variability over time. Secondary hypertension is more commonly seen in children under age 6 years with significant or severe hypertension (Kay, Sinaiko, & Daniels, 2001). The primary cause of secondary severe hypertension is renovascular or parenchymal renal diseases. Other causes include cardiovascular, endocrine, metabolic and drug-induced, and central nervous system conditions (Anderson et al, 2002). The onset of primary hypertension is more likely to occur after age 10 years. Neonates with hypertension are severely ill with neurologic and cardiac symptoms.

An elevation in systolic blood pressure is more common in children. An increase in left ventricular myopathy is seen more with mild to moderate systolic BP elevation than with diastolic BP elevation. Systolic blood pressure hypertension in children should be a primary prognostic finding (Sorof, 2002).

The NP plays an important role in the early recognition and treatment of hypertension. Interventions should strive to normalize systolic BP hypertension, even if the diastolic BP is within normal limits for age.

Clinical Findings

History

- Neonatal history of prolonged mechanical ventilation, umbilical catheterization
- Diet, activities, and other habits (e.g., smoking, drinking)
- Medications taken, including oral contraceptives, cold medications, steroids, and diet aids
- Chronic illness, especially renal disease, past history of urinary tract infections, diabetes, or seizures
- Headache, chest pain, dyspnea, muscle weakness, palpitations, abdominal pain, facial palsy, decreased vision, excessive sweating
- Family history of a first-degree relative with myocardial infarction (especially before 50 years of age), stroke, hypertension, diabetes, hyperlipidemia, sudden cardiac death, polycystic kidney disease, neurofibromatosis, pheochromocytoma, or obesity

Physical Examination

- Body habitus, especially obesity (per body mass index); poor growth (height, weight)
- Dysmorphic features
- Edema, pallor, flushing, skin lesions (suggestive of tuberous sclerosis or systemic lupus erythematosus [SLE])
- Absent, diminished, or pounding pulses in all extremities
- Fundi, thyroid gland, abdominal mass, flank bruit; decreased visual acuity, facial palsy
- Elevated BP

Accurate BP measurement is essential. An appropriately sized cuff must be used with the cubital fossa supported at the heart level. The right arm is preferred for comparison with normative charts, but right thigh measurement is also recommended if elevated pressure is suspected. The child or adolescent should be seated and have been resting in that position for 3 to 5 minutes. Deflation should be controlled at 2 to 3 mm Hg per second. Systolic pressure is recorded at the onset of tapping sounds; diastolic pressure is recorded at the disappearance (not the muffling) of sounds. Some authorities recommend recording the pressure twice on each occasion and using an average of each to record.

Management

See Fig. 31-15 for an algorithm to identify children with high BP. Early identification and prompt evaluation of these children are critical.

- BP measurements should be done annually on all children 3 years and older, with baseline and serial measurements documented carefully in the child's record. Standardized measurements are available (Tables 31-9 and 31-10).

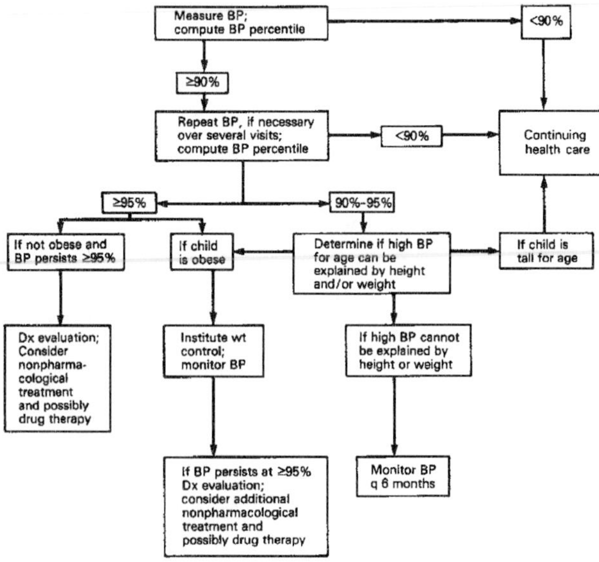

FIGURE 31-15 Algorithm for identifying children with high blood pressure *(BP)*. NOTE: Whenever BP measurement is stipulated, the average of at least two measurements should be used. (From American Academy of Pediatrics: Algorithm for identifying children with high blood pressure, *Pediatrics* 79:7, 1987. Reproduced by permission of *Pediatrics*, vol 79, p 7, copyright 1987.)

TABLE 31-9 ***Blood Pressure Levels for the 90th and 95th Percentiles of Blood Pressure for Girls Age 1 to 17 Years by Percentiles of Height***

		Systolic BP (mm Hg)							Diastolic BP (mm Hg)						
Age	**Height Percentiles* BP† ↓**	**→5%**	**10%**	**25%**	**50%**	**75%**	**90%**	**95%**	**5%**	**10%**	**25%**	**50%**	**75%**	**90%**	**95%**
1	**90th**	97	98	99	100	102	103	104	53	53	53	54	55	56	56
	95th	101	102	103	104	105	107	107	57	57	57	58	59	60	60
2	**90th**	99	99	100	102	103	104	105	57	57	58	58	59	60	61
	95th	102	103	104	105	107	108	109	61	61	62	62	63	64	65
3	**90th**	100	100	102	103	104	105	106	61	61	61	62	63	63	64
	95th	104	104	105	107	108	109	110	65	65	65	66	67	67	68
4	**90th**	101	102	103	104	106	107	108	63	63	64	65	65	66	67
	95th	105	106	107	108	109	111	111	67	67	68	69	69	70	71
5	**90th**	103	103	104	106	107	108	109	65	66	66	67	68	68	69
	95th	107	107	108	110	111	112	113	69	70	70	71	72	72	73
6	**90th**	104	105	106	107	109	110	111	67	67	68	69	69	70	71
	95th	108	109	110	111	112	114	114	71	71	72	73	73	74	75
7	**90th**	106	107	108	109	110	112	112	69	69	69	70	71	72	72
	95th	110	110	112	113	114	115	116	73	73	73	74	75	76	76
8	**90th**	108	109	110	111	112	113	114	70	70	71	71	72	73	74
	95th	112	112	113	115	116	117	118	74	74	75	75	76	77	78
9	**90th**	110	110	112	113	114	115	116	71	72	72	73	74	74	75
	95th	114	114	115	117	118	119	120	75	76	76	77	78	78	79
10	**90th**	112	112	114	115	116	117	118	73	73	73	74	75	76	76
	95th	116	116	117	119	120	121	122	77	77	77	78	79	80	80
11	**90th**	114	114	116	117	118	119	120	74	74	75	75	76	77	77
	95th	118	118	119	121	122	123	124	78	78	79	79	80	81	81
12	**90th**	116	116	118	119	120	121	122	75	75	76	76	77	78	78
	95th	120	120	121	123	124	125	126	79	79	80	80	81	82	82
13	**90th**	118	118	119	121	122	123	124	76	76	77	78	78	79	80
	95th	121	122	123	125	126	127	128	80	80	81	82	82	83	84
14	**90th**	119	120	121	122	124	125	126	77	77	78	79	79	80	81
	95th	123	124	125	126	128	129	130	81	81	82	83	83	84	85
15	**90th**	121	121	122	124	125	126	127	78	78	79	79	80	81	82
	95th	124	125	126	128	129	130	131	82	82	83	83	84	85	86
16	**90th**	122	122	123	125	126	127	128	79	79	79	80	81	82	82
	95th	125	126	127	128	130	131	132	83	83	83	84	85	86	86
17	**90th**	122	123	124	125	126	128	128	79	79	79	80	81	82	82
	95th	126	126	127	129	130	131	132	83	83	83	84	85	86	86

From National Institutes of Health, National High Blood Pressure Education Program: *Update on the Task Force Report (1987) on high blood pressure in children and adolescents*, NIH pub no 96-3790, September 1996. Available at *www.nhlbi.gov* (accessed Jan 20, 2003).

*Height percentile determined by standard growth curves.

†Blood pressure percentile determined by a single measurement.

TABLE 31-10 *Blood Pressure Levels for the 90th and 95th Percentiles of Blood Pressure for Boys Age 1 to 17 Years by Percentiles of Height*

Age	Height Percentiles* → / BP† ↓	Systolic BP (mm Hg)							Diastolic BP (mm Hg)						
		5%	10%	25%	50%	75%	90%	95%	5%	10%	25%	50%	75%	90%	95%
1	**90th**	94	95	97	98	100	102	102	50	51	52	53	54	54	55
	95th	98	99	101	102	104	106	106	55	55	56	57	58	59	59
2	**90th**	98	99	100	102	104	105	106	55	55	56	57	58	59	59
	95th	101	102	104	106	108	109	110	59	59	60	61	62	63	63
3	**90th**	100	101	103	105	107	108	109	59	59	60	61	62	63	63
	95th	104	105	107	109	111	112	113	63	63	64	65	66	67	67
4	**90th**	102	103	105	107	109	110	111	62	62	63	64	65	66	66
	95th	106	107	109	111	113	114	115	66	67	67	68	69	70	71
5	**90th**	104	105	106	108	110	112	112	65	65	66	67	68	69	69
	95th	108	109	110	112	114	115	116	69	70	70	71	72	73	74
6	**90th**	105	106	108	110	111	113	114	67	68	69	70	70	71	72
	95th	109	110	112	114	115	117	117	72	72	73	74	75	76	76
7	**90th**	106	107	109	111	113	114	115	69	70	71	72	72	73	74
	95th	110	111	113	115	116	118	119	74	74	75	76	77	78	78
8	**90th**	107	108	110	112	114	115	116	71	71	72	73	74	75	75
	95th	111	112	114	116	118	119	120	75	76	76	77	78	79	80
9	**90th**	109	110	112	113	115	117	117	72	73	73	74	75	76	77
	95th	113	114	116	117	119	121	121	76	77	78	79	80	80	81
10	**90th**	110	112	113	115	117	118	119	73	74	74	75	76	77	78
	95th	114	115	117	119	121	122	123	77	78	79	80	80	81	82
11	**90th**	112	113	115	117	119	120	121	74	74	75	76	77	78	78
	95th	116	117	119	121	123	124	125	78	79	79	80	81	82	83
12	**90th**	115	116	117	119	121	123	123	75	75	76	77	78	78	79
	95th	119	120	121	123	125	126	127	79	79	80	81	82	83	83
13	**90th**	117	118	120	122	124	125	126	75	76	76	77	78	79	80
	95th	121	122	124	126	128	129	130	79	80	81	82	83	83	84
14	**90th**	120	121	123	125	126	128	128	76	76	77	78	79	80	80
	95th	124	125	127	128	130	132	132	80	81	81	82	83	84	85
15	**90th**	123	124	125	127	129	131	131	77	77	78	79	80	81	81
	95th	127	128	129	131	133	134	135	81	82	83	83	84	85	86
16	**90th**	125	126	128	130	132	133	134	79	79	80	81	82	82	83
	95th	129	130	132	134	136	137	138	83	83	84	85	86	87	87
17	**90th**	128	129	131	133	134	136	136	81	81	82	83	84	85	85
	95th	132	133	135	136	138	140	140	85	85	86	87	88	89	89

From National Institutes of Health, National High Blood Pressure Education Program: *Update on the Task Force Report (1987) on high blood pressure in children and adolescents*, NIH pub no 96-3790, September 1996. Available at *www.nhlbi.gov* (accessed Jan 20, 2003).

*Height percentile determined by standard growth curves.

†Blood pressure percentile determined by a single measurement.

- High-normal BP: At least two follow-up BP measurements should be taken within 1 to 2 months of the initial reading to determine whether this high reading is a single, isolated event. If subsequent readings fall below the 95th percentile, the child should continue with routine BP checks during annual visits.
- Sustained elevated BP: If the BP is significantly elevated, laboratory evaluation includes a CBC, erythrocyte sedimentation rate (ESR), fasting serum lipids, urinalysis and culture, electrolytes, blood urea nitrogen, creatinine, and glucose. Additional organ assessments would include echocardiography (better than ECG and chest x-ray), a thorough ophthalmologic examination, and renal ultrasound (Falkner & Sadowski, 2000).
- Hypertension secondary to obesity can be as serious as hypertension secondary to other organic disease and should be treated as such. For those with high-normal blood pressure without any indication of end-organ involvement, treatment should consist of nonpharmacologic intervention: diet, exercise, and weight management. Caloric restriction with exercise is more effective than caloric restriction alone when using the nonpharmologic approach initially (Falkner & Sadowski, 2000). Recommendations should include the following:
  - Dietary intervention to control/reduce obesity includes ingestion of a low-fat, high-fiber diet with lots of fresh fruits and vegetables; elimination of foods high in sodium and salt added to foods; adequate calcium (1200 mg/day); and adequate potassium from fruits and beans.
  - Increased physical exercise and sports participation balanced with relaxation techniques. Aerobic exercise is recommended, not static or isometric exercise. Other techniques that are helpful are pairing with family or friends for exercise and maintaining a diary or log of exercise.
  - Avoid smoking, caffeine consumption, drinking, and drug consumption.
- Drug therapy (in conjunction with appropriate referrals) is considered if no change is seen after 6 to 12 months of diet and exercise therapy or if the patient is symptomatic, has severe hypertension, or has end-organ damage (Falkner & Sadowski, 2000). The patient should be referred to a specialist who has experience using pharmacologic agents in children. The goal is to reduce systolic or diastolic BP below the 90th percentile. Studies are lacking regarding drug efficacy and pharmacokinetics, recommendations regarding antihypertensive drugs, and age-appropriate preparations for children (Flynn, 2002). None of the antihypertensive drugs has been approved by the Food and Drug Administration for use in children. Table 31-11 lists the most current

TABLE 31-11 ***Manufacturers' Pediatric Dosing Recommendations for Antihypertensive Medications***

Class	Drugs	Manufacturer's Recommendations (Dose or Other Comments)
ACE inhibitors	Captopril	Suggested dosage comparable to or less than that used in adults
	Enalapril	Initial dose: 0.08 mg/kg/day (up to 5 mg); maximum dose: 0.58 mg/kg/day (up to 40 mg)
Beta-adrenergic antagonist	Propranolol	Initial dose: 1 mg/kg/day divided bid; usual dose 2-4 mg/kg/day; maximum dose: 16 mg/kg/day
Central-adrenergic agonists	Methyldopa	Initial dose: 10 mg/kg/day, divided bid-qid; maximum dose: 65 mg/kg/day, up to 3 g/day
Direct vasodilators	Diazoxide	Per-kilogram doses same as for adults
	Hydralazine	Initial dose: 0.75 mg/kg/day, divided qid; maximum dose 7.5 mg/kg/day up to 200 mg/day
	Minoxidil	Initial dose: 0.2 mg/kg/dose once daily; effective range: 0.25-1.0 mg/kg/day up to 50 mg/day
Diuretics	Chlorothiazide	10-20 mg/kg/day divided bid up to 1 g/day; up to 30 mg/kg/day in infants <6 mo
	Furosemide	2 mg/kg/day once daily; increase up to 6 mg/kg/day
	Hydrochlorothiazide	1 mg/lb/day, divided bid, maximum 50 mg/day for hypertension; 1.5 mg/lb/day in infants <6 mo
	Spironolactone	1.5 mg/lb/day (3.3 mg/kg/day)

From Flynn JT: Pharmacologic management of childhood hypertension: current status, future challenges, *Am J Hypertens* 15(2, pt 2):31S-33S, 2002.
ACE, Angiotensin-converting enzyme.

recommendations for treating childhood hypertension. Factors that influence drug choice include age, lifestyle, cause of the hypertension, blood pressure, drug side effects, and other existing medical problems.

Periodic echocardiograms may be recommended to evaluate LVH.

Complications

Increases in blood pressure in children and adolescents can lead to adverse effects. These include increases in left ventricular mass, increases in carotid intimal medial thickness, and coronary artery calcification, especially if combined with obesity, lipid and lipoprotein abnormalities, and tobacco use (Daniels, 2002).

Prevention

- Because much of hypertension is genetic in origin, prevention through optimal health promotion and maintenance is essential. Regular health maintenance, including evaluation of BP and health education regarding risk factors, is critical. Counseling should emphasize both behavioral modification and parental involvement. Decreasing body mass index and increasing aerobic fitness have been shown to reduce elevations in age-related blood pressure. Specific preventive measures include the following:
  - Healthful nutrition
  - Prevention of obesity
  - Decrease in dietary fat and sodium
  - Aerobic exercise every other day for a period of at least 20 minutes
  - Stress management
  - Avoidance of caffeine and tobacco use and prescription or over-the-counter medications that can exacerbate high BP (e.g., cold medications with ephedrine or phenylephrine, steroids)
  - Monitoring of BP if oral contraceptives are used
- Children and adolescents with systemic hypertension may have significant rise in BP during exercise. Athletes with significant hypertension should have their BP measured regularly (every 2 months) to monitor the impact of exercise on BP. The AAP recommends the following (AAP, 1997):
  - Youths with severe hypertension need to be restricted from competitive sports and highly static (isometric) activities until their hypertension is under adequate control and there is no evidence of target organ damage. Power lifting should be discouraged because the Valsalva maneuver and other improper breathing maneuvers can cause BP elevations (Falkner & Sadowski, 2000). Because cardiovascular conditioning may be less strenuous than competitive athletics, complete restriction of exercise may not be necessary for those with severe hypertension.
  - When hypertension and other cardiovascular diseases coexist, eligibility for participation in competitive athletics is usually based on the type and severity of the other cardiovascular disease.
  - A young athlete with hypertension, regardless of degree of severity, should be strongly encouraged to adopt healthy lifestyle behaviors, including avoidance of exogenous androgens, growth hormone, drugs of abuse (especially cocaine, ethanol, and anabolic steroids), use of tobacco (by all routes), and high sodium intake. Advise that the use of diuretic drugs and β-blockers has been prohibited by some athletic governing bodies. In these instances, other types of medication may need to be considered.

Kawasaki Disease

Description

Kawasaki disease (also known as mucocutaneous lymph node syndrome or infantile polyarteritis) is characterized by an acute generalized systemic microvasculitis occurring throughout the body in the first 10 days of the disease. During this initial stage, inflammation of the arterioles, venules, and capillaries of the heart can occur and later progress to the formation of a coronary artery aneurysm in some children. It is self-limited and is the most common cause of acquired heart disease in children in Japan and the United States (Burno, 2001).

Etiology and Incidence

Although the etiology of Kawasaki disease remains unconfirmed, clinical evidence supports an infectious cause. It exhibits geographic and seasonal outbreaks, predominantly reported in the late winter and early spring. Person-to-person spread is low, but it occurs with greater frequency in siblings (1%). Between 4 and 18.8 per 100,000 children contract Kawasaki disease each year in the United States (Burno, 2001). Although children of all racial groups are susceptible, the incidence is proportionately higher in Asian American children and exhibits a 1.5:1 male-to-female ratio. More than 85% of cases occur in children younger than 5 years, with an average age of 2 to 3 years old (Burno, 2001). Recurrence rates are approximately 2% (Takahashi, 2001).

Clinical Findings

Diagnostic criteria are listed in Box 31-8. Children younger than 6 to 12 months may have atypical findings. There are four stages in which changes in cardiovascular pathology

BOX 31-8 *Diagnostic Criteria for Kawasaki Disease*

The child must exhibit fever plus four of the other five criteria *or,* if fewer than four criteria, coronary vessel involvement:

1. Fever for 5 days or longer
2. Bilateral conjunctival injection without exudate
3. Polymorphous rash that may be urticarial or pruritic
4. Inflammatory changes in the lips and oral cavity
5. Changes in the extremities such as peripheral edema, erythema of the palms and soles, or desquamation of the hands and feet (convalescent period)
6. Cervical lymphadenopathy that is often unilateral, anterior cervical

occur, depending on the length of time since the onset of symptoms.

Stage 1. The acute phase (days 0 to 14) begins with an abrupt onset of high fever (greater than 39.0° C) that is unresponsive to antipyretics or antibiotics. Typically, significant irritability, bilateral conjunctival inflammation, erythema of the oropharynx, dryness and fissuring of the lips, "strawberry tongue," cervical lymphadenopathy, a polymorphous rash, erythema of the urethral meatus, tachycardia, and edema of the extremities are noted.

- Laboratory findings: an elevated ESR and platelet count (as high as 700,000/mm^3), positive C-reactive protein, leukocytosis with left shift, slight decreases in red blood cells and hemoglobin, hypoalbuminemia, increased α_2-globulin, and sterile pyuria

Stage 2. The subacute phase (2 to 4 weeks after illness onset) begins with resolution of the fever and lasts until all other clinical signs have disappeared.

- Irritability may be prolonged throughout this phase.
- Desquamation of the fingers (at the junction of nail tip and digit) occurs first, followed by the toes.
- Transient jaundice, abnormal liver function tests, arthralgia or arthritis, transient diarrhea, orchitis, facial palsy, and sensorineural hearing loss may occur.
- The risk for development of a coronary artery aneurysm is greatest in this period.

Stage 3. During the convalescent phase, all clinical signs of Kawasaki disease have resolved, but laboratory values may not have returned to normal. This phase is complete when all blood values are normal (6 to 8 weeks from onset).

Stage 4. The chronic phase (40 days to 4 years after illness onset) of coronary complications can persist into adulthood. Although the child may exhibit a normal echocardiogram, some studies suggest that there may be long-term coronary arteritis (Burno, 2001). Children may develop dyslipidemia as evidenced by mild to moderate low-density lipoproteins or lower high-density lipoproteins (Takahashi, 2001).

Diagnostic Tests

- CBC with differential, ESR, platelet count, C-reactive protein, liver transaminases, γ-glutamyltransferase (GGT), and urinalysis are done.
- Blood, urine, cerebrospinal fluid, and group A β-hemolytic streptococcus (GABHS) pharyngeal cultures may be indicated given the patient's symptomatology.
- Two-dimensional echocardiography; if abnormal, a cardioangiography is obtained.

Differential Diagnosis

Measles, other adenoviruses, scarlet fever, drug reactions, Stevens-Johnson syndrome, erythema multiforme, mononucleosis, juvenile arthritis, leptospirosis, inflammatory bowel disease, sarcoidosis, SLE, rickettsial infection, and toxic shock are differential diagnoses for the triad of red eyes, prolonged fever, and rash (Burno, 2001; Kato, 2000).

Management

Early diagnosis is essential to prevent aneurysms in the coronary arteries and extraparenchymal muscular arteries. Goals of treatment include (1) evoking a rapid antiinflammatory response, (2) preventing coronary thrombosis by inhibiting platelet aggregation, and (3) minimizing long-term coronary risk factors by exercise, diet, and smoking prevention.

- Treatment includes the following:
  - Intravenous gamma globulin therapy (a single dose of 2 g/kg over a period of 10 to 12 hours in the first 10 days of the illness) is effective in reducing the incidence of coronary artery abnormalities (Takahashi, 2001). The use of immunoglobulin after the tenth day must be individualized (Pichichero, 2001).
  - High-dose aspirin is given for its antiinflammatory properties (80 to 100 mg/kg per day in four divided doses every 6 hours initially). Once the fever resolves, aspirin is continued at an antiplatelet dose (3 to 5 mg/kg per day) in patients without ECG evidence of coronary artery changes until the ESR and platelet count have returned to normal (6 to 8 weeks). If coronary artery abnormalities develop, aspirin or dipyridamole therapy is used indefinitely, otherwise, it can be stopped. Warfarin (Coumadin) is sometimes added in patients with evidence of turbulent flow through the affected vessel sections.

- A two-dimensional echocardiogram is useful to diagnose and monitor the progression of coronary artery abnormalities. An echocardiogram should be obtained as soon as the diagnosis is established as a baseline study, with subsequent studies done in the subacute and convalescent phases. Cardiac catheterization and angiography are done if large or multiple aneurysms appear.
- If varicella or influenza develops, aspirin treatment should be stopped for 1 to 2 weeks and another antiplatelet drug substituted to minimize the risk of Reye syndrome (Takahashi, 2001).
- Live virus vaccines should be delayed until 9 to 12 months after administration of intravenous gamma globulin (Pichichero, 2001).
- Patients with no coronary or cardiac changes on echocardiography at any stage should be followed by a cardiologist throughout the first year. Afterward, the NP may follow the patient; no activity restrictions are required at that point (Pichichero, 2001).
- Patients with any range of transient coronary artery dilation (including giant aneurysms) should be followed by a cardiologist for years. Physical activities depend on degree of cardiac abnormality; some modification is justified (Pichichero, 2001).

Complications

The acute disease is self-limited; however, if left untreated, significant cardiac sequelae will develop in 15% to 25% of cases (Pichichero, 2001). The process of aneurysm formation and subsequent thrombosis or scarring of the coronary artery may occur as late as 6 months after the initial illness. Possible complications include recurrence (less than 2%); coronary aneurysm (less than 20%); CHF or massive myocardial infarction (death is more likely in the first year); myocarditis or pericarditis, or both (30%); and pericardial effusion, mitral valve insufficiency, and coronary vessel stenosis (Kato, 2000; Takahashi, 2001).

Prognosis

There is a 0.3% mortality rate. The risk of coronary aneurysm is reduced to 3% in patients older than 1 year if intravenous immunoglobulin is given within 10 days of the illness. Aneurysm regression occurs in half of all patients, commonly by 1 year after the illness (80% resolve within 5 years), but vessels do not dilate normally in response to increased oxygen demand by the myocardium. Patients with coronary artery abnormalities are at risk for myocardial infarction, sudden death, and myocardial ischemia for years after the illness. Prompt treatment of chest pain, dyspnea, extreme lethargy, or syncope is always warranted. Surgical revascularization and transcatheter revascularization are used for some coronary sequelae of Kawasaki disease (Takahashi, 2001).

Acute Rheumatic Fever

Description

Acute rheumatic fever (ARF) is a systemic connective tissue disease. In its acute stage, it results in inflammation of the heart, joints, central nervous system, and cutaneous and subcutaneous tissues. The most significant sequela of ARF is rheumatic heart disease, which can cause significant damage and scarring of the mitral valve (see Chapter 25 for more information).

Etiology and Incidence

In the 1950s and early 1960s, ARF and its major complication, valvular heart disease, were significant problems worldwide. During the late 1960s and 1970s, the disease almost disappeared in the United States and Western Europe, only to resurge in the mid-1980s. It remains a common childhood illness in underdeveloped countries and is the leading cause of acquired heart disease in children worldwide (Ayoub, 2001). It occurs most commonly in school-age children 5 to 15 years old.

The relationship between pharyngitis caused by GABHS infection and the subsequent immune response of ARF is well established. This disease classically occurs after a latent period of 10 to 20 days following streptococcal pharyngitis or tonsillitis. Progression of symptoms is evident within 3 to 5 weeks of a streptococcal infection that has usually been untreated or only partially treated.

ARF occurs as a sporadic infection in approximately 0.2% to 0.3% of patients whose GABHS infections were not treated. With each subsequent GABHS reinfection, further cardiac damage can be expected (Ayoub, 2001). Treatment with antibiotic prophylaxis to prevent recurrences has decreased the prominence of this disease in developed countries.

Clinical Findings

The diagnosis of ARF is based on a set of guidelines known as the Jones criteria (Dajani et al, 1992) (Box 31-9). The presence of two major or one major and two minor criteria with evidence of a preceding GABHS infection indicates a high probability of ARF. Children with fewer manifestations can also have ARF. The incidence of manifestations include the following: arthritis of large joints (65%), carditis (50%), chorea (15% to 30%), cutaneous nodules (5%), and subcutaneous nodules (less than 5% to 7%).

BOX 31-9 *Jones Criteria for Rheumatic Fever**

Evidence of Preceding GABHS Infection

Positive throat culture or rapid streptococcal antigen test result
Elevated or rising streptococcal antibody titer

Minor Manifestations

Arthralgia
Fever
Elevated acute-phase reactants
Elevated erythrocyte sedimentation rate
Elevated C-reactive protein

Major Manifestations

Carditis
- Tachycardia out of proportion to degree of fever
- Cardiomegaly
- New murmurs or change in preexisting murmurs
- Muffled heart sounds
- Precordial friction rub
- Precordial pain
- Changes in electrocardiogram (especially prolonged PR interval)

Polyarthritis
- Swollen, hot, red, painful joint(s)
- After 1 to 2 days, affects different joints (migratory)
- Favors large joints—knees, elbows, hips, shoulders, wrists

Erythema marginatum
- Erythematous macules with clear center and wavy, well-demarcated border
- Transitory
- Nonpruritic
- Primarily affects trunk and extremities (inner surfaces)

Chorea
- Sudden, aimless, irregular movements of extremities
- Involuntary facial grimaces
- Speech disturbances or emotional lability
- Muscle weakness (can be profound)
- Muscle movements exaggerated by anxiety and attempt at fine motor activity; relieved by rest

Subcutaneous nodes
- Nontender swelling
- Located over bony prominence
- May persist for some time and then gradually resolve

From Dajani AS et al: Guidelines for the diagnosis of rheumatic fever: Jones criteria, updated 1992, *Circulation* 87:302-307, 1993.

*The presence of two major or one major and two or more minor criteria with evidence of preceding group A β-hemolytic streptococcal (GABHS) infection indicates a high probability of rheumatic fever.

Diagnostic Tests

- Rapid streptococcal antigen screening or streptococcal culture is done during the acute illness in children over 2 years of age. Up to two thirds of children with ARF may have negative cultures as a result of the body having eliminated the bacteria during the latent period of the infection.
- Other tests include antistreptolysin O titer (ASO), CBC, ESR, and C-reactive protein (see Chapter 25 for further information).

Management

See Chapter 25 for further discussion of ARF.

- Treatment and prevention of GABHS infection are essential.
- Use antiinflammatory agents to control clinical manifestations of the disease (salicylates or steroids, depending on the degree of carditis).
- Maintain supportive therapy, including treatment of CHF and choreiform movements.
- Compliance with drug regimens, including ongoing antibiotic prophylaxis, is essential. Compliance may require monthly penicillin injection in a patient who is unable to comply with the twice-a-day oral regimen.
- Prevention of recurrence can be achieved with prompt identification and treatment of future GABHS infections. In approximately 70% to 80% of patients, valvular disease will resolve if they are compliant in taking antibiotic prophylaxis (Ayoub, 2001).

Infective Endocarditis

Description

Infective or bacterial endocarditis, formerly referred to as subacute bacterial endocarditis, is a condition in which a bacterial or fungal (less common) infection invades traumatized endocardial (endothelial) surfaces of the heart, most commonly the cardiac valves. Infective endocarditis (IE) usually occurs in children or adults with underlying structural cardiac abnormalities (CHD, ARF), but it does rarely occur in those without structural heart disease. The incidence of IE has increased as more children with CHD are surviving, due to aggressive treatments. Half of the cases occur in children over 10 years of age, but infection can occur in any age-group. Premature neonates may acquire it secondary to umbilical arterial catheters or central venous lines. Infection carries high morbidity and mortality rates and can lead to destruction of heart valves or disseminated sepsis. The importance of prevention in patients who are at risk, as well as the importance of early diagnosis and treatment, cannot be overemphasized (Dajani & Taubert, 2001).

Etiology

The disease is thought to involve the introduction of pathogens into the bloodstream. The most common portal of entry is orally, from the release of bacteria during dental work or oral surgery, or with other surgical procedures (e.g., cardiac catheterization or surgery requiring indwelling catheters, or in those who are at risk because of structural abnormalities of the heart). *Streptococcus viridans* is the most common causative organism, followed by *S. aureus.* Together, these two groups account for 80% of IE cases. The microorganisms that are released into the bloodstream at the time of mild or severe bacteremia grow on the endocardium and form vegetation, fibrin deposits, and platelet thrombi. The lesion may invade surrounding tissues, such as heart valves, or may break off and embolize in other organs such as the lungs, kidney, spleen, or brain.

Clinical Findings

- Exposure within 2 weeks before onset of symptoms
- Acute manifestations: short duration of illness, high fever (greater than 39° C), myalgias, night sweats, arthralgias, headache, general malaise, decreased appetite, increase in intensity of preexisting murmur or new onset of murmur
- Embolization symptoms: hematuria, acute onset of respiratory distress, splenomegaly, neurologic changes (stroke, brain abscesses, hemorrhage, meningitis), petechiae (in conjunctiva, buccal mucosa, palatal area, nail beds, palms, and soles)

Diagnostic Tests

- The diagnosis is based on clinical findings and results of blood cultures. A persistent low-grade fever in a patient with known cardiac abnormalities should be evaluated immediately with three sets of blood cultures over 24 hours from different sites (detects 97% of cases of IE) before the administration of empirical antibiotic therapy. Three cultures over 1 to 2 hours are sufficient in patients who are severely ill. When three cultures are positive for the same organism, IE must be considered and treatment instituted.
- The ESR and white blood cell count are elevated in the acute stage; anemia may be evidenced.
- Two-dimensional echocardiography is helpful in detecting vegetation, new valvular insufficiency, or obvious damage to a valve (Dajani & Taubert, 2001). The use of transesophageal echocardiography to diagnose IE in children is yet to be fully studied.

Management

- Treatment should begin as soon as IE is suspected in order to decrease the subsequent morbidity and mortality associated with untreated bacteremia.
- High doses of appropriate antibiotics are given intravenously for 4 to 6 weeks.

Prevention

IE in those at risk because of structural heart disease is prevented by administering prophylactic antibiotic therapy before procedures known to increase the risk of IE. Such procedures include dental work and manipulation of the respiratory, genitourinary, or gastrointestinal tract (see the management strategies section on prevention of bacterial endocarditis and Tables 31-5 and 31-6).

Myocarditis

Myocarditis refers to active inflammation of the myocardium, the muscular walls of the heart. It may go unrecognized in many children whose infective illness resolves spontaneously, or it may lead to fulminant disease with rapid progression resulting in chronic cardiomyopathy. Although rare, myocarditis is often caused by viral infections, most commonly enteroviruses, coxsackievirus A and B, echoviruses, and poliovirus. Influenza, cytomegalovirus (CMV), varicella, mumps, human immunodeficiency virus, respiratory syncytial virus, and rubella are other viral causes. Nonviral infections (fungal, bacterial, protozoan, rickettsial), various medications, autoimmune or inflammatory disorders (e.g., ARF, SLE), and toxic reactions to infectious agents or other disorders (e.g., Kawasaki disease) may also be etiologic agents; however, the etiology is often unknown. Myocarditis may occur in epidemics, usually in infants in association with coxsackievirus B (Towbin, 2001).

Clinical Findings

History. Symptoms of myocarditis, which are secondary to reduced myocardial function, are caused by interstitial inflammation or damage. As a result, muscle function decreases and causes enlargement of the heart with decreased contractility. As this process progresses, cardiac function decreases and symptoms of CHF become evident. The following history is characteristic:

- Infants
  - Fever, irritability or listlessness, episodes of pallor, diaphoresis
  - Tachypnea or respiratory distress
  - Poor appetite and vomiting
- Children and adolescents
  - Recent flulike or gastrointestinal viral illness (10 to 14 days previously)
  - Lethargy, low-grade fever, pallor
  - Decreased appetite and abdominal pain
  - Exercise intolerance, malaise, rashes, palpitations, respiratory distress (late finding), decreased pulse oximetry reading

Physical Examination

- Pallor, mild cyanosis, skin cool and mottled with poor perfusion (in infants)
- Rapid laborious respirations, grunting, decreased pulse oximetry reading
- Tachycardia, gallop rhythm, muffled heart sounds, apical systolic murmur, weak pulses
- Hepatomegaly

Diagnostic Tests. The NP should refer patients with symptoms suggestive of myocarditis to pediatric cardiologists. Diagnostic testing will usually involve chest radiography, ECG, two-dimensional echocardiography, CBC, ESR, cardiac and liver enzymes, viral titers, blood cultures, metabolic studies (e.g., thyroid and carnitine), and viral cultures from the myocardium.

Differential Diagnosis

Sepsis, asthma, recurrent vomiting, and chronic viral illness are in the differential.

Management

Treatment is supportive with bed rest and medications, such as digitalis, diuretics, and angiotensin-converting enzyme blockers. Occasionally, anticoagulation and antiarrhythmia medications may be used. Many experimental therapies are under study, including the use of intravenous gamma globulin and vaccines for enteroviruses (Towbin, 2001). Severe cases may require hospitalization for mechanical ventilation and inotropic support. Recovery often takes 2 to 3 months; follow-up is indefinite. Pericardial effusion and pericarditis can occur concurrently. Scarring of the myocardium may occur and cause persistent heart failure and ventricular arrhythmias.

Prognosis

Cardiomyopathies may result in a need for cardiac transplantation. Up to 75% of neonates die; mortality rates in older infants and children range from 10% to 25%. Fifty percent of children and adolescents show full recovery; 25% continue to have abnormal ECGs and chest x-rays, although they remain clinically asymptomatic (Towbin, 2001).

Pericarditis

Pericarditis refers to an inflammation or other abnormality of the pericardium, the sac that surrounds the heart. Excess fluid accumulates in the pericardial space and causes the normally compliant pericardium to distend. As intrapericardial pressure increases, the heart becomes compressed and its ability to fill is limited. Pericarditis may be seen in individuals without a prior history of cardiac disease. Viral infection (usually coxsackievirus or adenovirus) is the most common cause of pericarditis in children (40% to 75% of cases). Other etiologic agents include infections (tuberculosis, other bacteria), trauma, hypersensitivity to medication (INH, hydralazine), collagen-vascular and connective tissue diseases (ARF, juvenile rheumatoid arthritis, SLE), Kawasaki disease, postsurgical complications, and complications of systemic infection. Pericarditis is most common in children younger than 2 years and demonstrates equal sex distribution (Nowlen & Bricker, 2000). It is a serious illness that may have rapidly fatal consequences if not diagnosed and treated in a timely manner. The following findings should alert the NP to refer the patient to a pediatric cardiologist:

- History of precordial or substernal chest pain altered by respiration, coughing, or position (may not be found in small children); lethargy, loss of appetite, abdominal pain; fever, irritability; tachycardia; viral illness 10 to 14 days before onset of symptoms
- Physical examination findings: distended neck veins; tachycardia, pericardial friction rub (an early sign heard best along the left sternal border with the patient leaning forward), or muffled heart sounds (if the effusion is large); Kussmaul sign (slow, deep respirations); pulsus paradoxus—decrease in BP of greater than 10 mm Hg during inspiration with patient in a supine position (normal fluctuation is 4 to 6 mm Hg); hepatomegaly

Myocarditis is the main differential diagnosis. Management consists of pericardiocentesis if tamponade becomes evident, nonsteroidal antiinflammatory and analgesic medications, or, rarely, sternotomy/thoracotomy to control any intrapericardial bleeding. Cardiac tamponade can occur with large or rapid effusions. There is a relapse rate of 15% if the causative agent was viral. Most children recover fully within a 3- to 4-week period.

HEART CONDUCTION DISTURBANCES

Cardiac Arrhythmias

Description

Abnormal heart rates (see Table 31-2) or rhythms, also called arrhythmias or dysrhythmias, result from abnormal impulse formation or conduction. They can manifest as a primary disorder or as a consequence of cardiac or other systemic disorders (Fish & Benson, 2001; Vetter, 2000). The NP should be familiar with the following descriptions of arrhythmias:

- Sinus arrhythmias—variable heart rate that increases with inspiration and decreases with expiration
- Bradycardia or slow heart rate (less than 60 beats per minute in newborns, 40 beats per minute in children)
  - Sinus bradycardia
  - Complete atrioventricular (AV) block
- Tachycardia, or a rate that exceeds the upper limits of normal (220 beats per minute in newborns, 190 beats per minute in older children)
- Conduction disturbances
- AV block (first-, second-, and third-degree block)
- Premature atrial contractions—depolarization may or may not be conducted through the AV node
- Premature ventricular contractions—premature QRS complex with a prolonged duration or morphologic difference from the preceding QRS

Etiology and Incidence

Most abnormal heart rhythms in children with entirely normal hearts are benign, but an arrhythmia in a child with a cardiac abnormality can be lethal. Any patient who has an arrhythmia or syncope with exertion requires an evaluation for underlying cardiac disease. There are known familial or genetic linkages associated with arrhythmias, although specific genes have not been identified (Fish & Benson, 2001).

The most commonly seen bradycardia in an otherwise normal child is a sinus bradycardia. This arrhythmia may be caused by hypoxia, acidosis, increased intracranial pressure, abdominal distention, hypothermia, or hypoglycemia. It may also be caused by drugs such as β-blockers or digoxin. Mild slowing may be due to increased vagal tone or cardiac conditioning (e.g., athletes) (Fish & Benson, 2001). A complete AV block (complete heart block) can either be congenital, as seen in infants of mothers with an autoimmune disease such as SLE, or may be acquired after cardiac surgery. This conduction abnormality is also seen postoperatively in patients who have had surgery in the area of the septum (ASD, VSD) or the AV (tricuspid or mitral) valves (Fish & Benson, 2001). The hemodynamic effect of a slow heart rate depends on how different it is from the patient's usual heart rate.

Sinus tachycardia can be caused by predisposing factors that increase cardiac output, including fever, anxiety, infection, drug exposure, CHD, Wolff-Parkinson-White syndrome, dehydration, pain, or anemia. It also can be a symptom of hyperthyroidism. The most common pathologic tachycardia is supraventricular tachycardia (SVT), which occurs most often in males younger than 4 months of age. SVT can also occur in young children, as well as young adults (Vetter, 2000).

Premature contractions can be seen in an infant or child with an otherwise normal heart. It is not unusual to see multiple premature atrial contractions on the ECG of a newborn. Occasional premature ventricular contractions are also seen in otherwise normal infants. Premature ventricular contractions that are uniform in appearance, which means that they have the same QRS complex appearance every time, are usually of no consequence.

Clinical Findings

History

- Bradycardia with a sudden decrease in heart rate can cause syncope or severe dizziness.
- SVT can be of sudden onset and variable duration.
  - Infants tolerate several hours of SVT with rates up to 250 beats per minute before demonstrating evidence of poor feeding, irritability, or pallor that can eventually lead to CHF if not converted.
  - Older children may feel quite ill after a few minutes and have complaints of "butterflies" in the chest, dizziness, palpitations, pain in the neck, abdominal pain with nausea and vomiting, and syncope

Physical Examination

- Slow or fast heart rate; rhythm—regular, irregular, or regularly irregular

Diagnostic Tests. Tests include ECG (the basic screening tool) and 24-hour Holter monitor or event monitor if symptoms are sporadic and the ECG is normal.

Differential Diagnosis

Heart rates that are elevated or slowed because of exercise, physical conditioning, or other physiologic reasons are included in the differential diagnosis.

Management

Identification of an arrhythmia can be challenging. A sinus arrhythmia requires no treatment. Refer all other rhythm abnormalities to a pediatric cardiologist for evaluation. Other findings that require a referral include the following:

- Abnormal ECG
- History of unusual heart rhythm

- History of syncope or dizziness on exertion with palpitations
- History of cardiac abnormality, heart surgery, or Wolff-Parkinson-White syndrome

Complications

Death can occur with some arrhythmias if untreated.

Education/Prognosis

- Recurrent SVT—the child or parent may be taught to monitor the heart rate and use vagal maneuvers to break the spell.
- Most arrhythmias in children with normal hearts are benign. Such is not the case for children with an abnormal heart. Arrhythmia in a child with a cardiac abnormality can be lethal.

Wolff-Parkinson-White Syndrome

Wolff-Parkinson-White syndrome (WPWS) is the most common type of electrophysiologic abnormality in which cardiac excitation occurs along accessory conduction routes between atria and ventricles. This results in early activation of the ventricles, leading to tachycardia (Vetter, 2000).

The condition is more likely to be discerned in infants with other cardiac anomalies who are younger than 1 month of age. These infants demonstrate SVT. However, there is an asymptomatic form seen more in adults and young children. In children between 6 and 8 years of age, asymptomatic cases often manifest with ventricular fibrillation and cardiac arrest (3% to 4%). In children (and adults) over 10 years of age, atrial fibrillation may be the initial indicator that may then precipitate ventricular fibrillation (Vetter, 2000).

The cause of WPWS is unknown. The syndrome is associated with other CHDs, hypertrophic cardiomegaly, and tuberous sclerosis. Approximately 0.1% to 0.3% of the general population is affected, but the incidence increases to 0.27% to 0.86% in patients with CHD. There is a genetic association in 3% of cases.

The ECG typically shows a short PR interval for age, and the QRS complex is "slurring." Management usually involves prophylaxis with antiarrythmic medications or catheter ablation.

RESOURCE BOX

Cardiovascular Disorders

American Heart Association
1-800-242-8721
www.amhrt.org

Mended Hearts
1-888-432-7899
www.mendedhearts.org

National Heart, Lung, and Blood Institute
1-301-592-8573
www.nhlbi.nih.gov

REFERENCES

Allen H, Phillips J, Chan D: History and physical examination. In Allen H et al: *Moss and Adams' heart disease in infants, children, and adolescents: including the fetus and young adult,* ed 6, Philadelphia, 2001, Lippincott Williams & Wilkins.

American Academy of Pediatrics: Algorithm for identifying children with high blood pressure, *Pediatrics* 79:7, 1987.

American Academy of Pediatrics: Recommendations for preventive pediatric health care (RE 9939), *Pediatrics* 105(3):645, 2000.

American Heart Association Committee on Rheumatic Fever, Endocarditis, and Kawasaki Disease of the Council on Cardiovascular Disease in the Young: guidelines for long-term management of patients with Kawasaki disease, *Circulation* 89(2):916-922, 1994.

Anderson R et al: *Paediatric cardiology,* ed 2, New York, 2002, Churchill Livingstone.

Asprey D: Innocent heart murmur. In Burg F et al: *Gellis and Kagan's current pediatric therapy,* Philadelphia, 2002, WB Saunders.

Ayoub E: Acute rheumatic fever. In Allen H et al: *Moss and Adams' heart disease in infants, children, and adolescents: including the fetus and young adult,* ed 6, Philadelphia, 2001, Lippincott Williams & Wilkins.

Beckman R: Coarctation of the aorta. In Allen H et al: *Moss and Adams' heart disease in infants, children, and adolescents: including the fetus and young adult,* ed 6, Philadelphia, 2001, Lippincott Williams & Wilkins.

Behrman R, Kliegman R, Jenson H, editors: *Nelson textbook of pediatrics,* ed 16, Philadelphia, 2000, WB Saunders.

Bernstein D: The cardiovascular system. In Behrman RE, Kliegman RM, editors: *Nelson essentials of pediatrics,* ed 17, Philadelphia, 2004, WB Saunders.

Burno J: Kawasaki disease, *Adv Pediatr* 48:157-177, 2001.

Dajani AS et al: Guidelines for the diagnosis of rheumatic fever: Jones criteria 1992 update, *JAMA* 268(15):2069-2073, 1992.

Dajani A, Taubert K: Infective endocarditis. In Allen H et al: *Moss and Adams' heart disease in infants, children, and adolescents: including the fetus and young adult,* ed 6, Philadelphia, 2001, Lippincott Williams & Wilkins.

Dajani A et al: Prevention of bacterial endocarditis: recommendations by the American Heart Association, *JAMA* 277:1794-1801, 1997.

Daniels S: Cardiovascular sequelae of childhood hypertension, *Am J Hypertens* 15(2, pt 2):61S-63S, 2002.

Driscoll D: Chest pain in children and adolescents. In Allen H et al: *Moss and Adams' heart disease in infants, children, and adolescents: including the fetus and young adult,* ed 6, Philadelphia, 2001, Lippincott Williams & Wilkins.

Emblad P et al: *Pediatric pearls of wisdom,* ed 2, Lincoln, 2001, Boston Medical Publishing.

Epstein M: Tricuspid atresia. In Allen H et al: *Moss and Adams' heart disease in infants, children, and adolescents: including the fetus and young adult,* ed 6, Philadelphia, 2001, Lippincott Williams & Wilkins.

Falkner B, Sadowski R: Hypertension in children and adolescents. In Moller J, Hoffman J: *Pediatric cardiovascular medicine,* New York, 2000, Churchill Livingstone.

Fish F, Benson D: Disorders of cardiac rhythm and conduction. In Allen H et al: *Moss and Adams' heart disease in infants, children, and adolescents: including the fetus and young adult,* ed 6, Philadelphia, 2001, Lippincott Williams & Wilkins.

Flynn J: Pharmacologic management of childhood hypertension: current status, future challenges, *Am J Hypertens* 15(2, pt 2): 30S-33S, 2002.

Freed M: Aortic stenosis. In Allen H et al: *Moss and Adams' heart disease in infants, children, and adolescents: including the fetus and young adult,* ed 6, Philadelphia, 2001, Lippincott Williams & Wilkins.

Gorrie T, McKinney E, Murray S: Fetal circulation. In *Foundations of maternal-newborn nursing,* Philadelphia, 1994, WB Saunders.

Hoffman J: Incidence, mortality and natural history. In Anderson R et al: *Paediatric cardiology,* ed 2, New York, 2002, Churchill Livingstone.

Kato H: Kawasaki disease. In Moller J, Hoffman J: *Pediatric cardiovascular medicine,* New York, 2000, Churchill Livingstone.

Kay J, Sinaiko A, Daniels S: Pediatric hypertension, *Am Heart J* 142(3):422-432, 2001.

Koot H, Wallander J: *Quality of life in child and adolescent illness: concepts, methods, and findings,* New York, 2001, Brunner-Routledge-Taylor & Francis.

Latson L, Prieto L: Pulmonary stenosis. In Allen H et al: *Moss and Adams' heart disease in infants, children, and adolescents: including the fetus and young adult,* ed 6, Philadelphia, 2001, Lippincott Williams & Wilkins.

McConnell M, Adkins S, Hannon D: Heart murmurs in pediatric patients: when do you refer? *Am Fam Pract* 60(2):558-565, 1999.

McDaniel N, Gutgesell H: Ventricular septal defects. In Allen H et al: *Moss and Adams' heart disease in infants, children, and adolescents: including the fetus and young adult,* ed 6, Philadelphia, 2001, Lippincott Williams & Wilkins.

Moller J, Hoffman J: *Pediatric cardiovascular medicine,* New York, 2000, Churchill Livingstone.

Moore K, Persaud TVN: *The developing humans,* ed 6, Philadelphia, 1998, WB Saunders.

Moore P, Brook M, Heymann M: Patent ductus arteriosus. In Allen H et al: *Moss and Adams' heart disease in infants, children, and adolescents: including the fetus and young adult,* ed 6, Philadelphia, 2001, Lippincott Williams & Wilkins.

National Institutes of Health National High Blood Pressure Education Program: *Update on the Task force report (1987) on high blood pressure in children and adolescents,* NIH pub no 96-3790, Sept 1996. Available at *www.nhlbi.gov* (accessed Jan 20, 2003).

Noonan J: Innocent murmurs and the pediatrician, *Clin Pediatr* 38(9):519-520, 1999.

Nowlen T, Bricker J: Pericardial diseases. In Moller J, Hoffman J: *Pediatric cardiovascular medicine,* New York, 2000, Churchill Livingstone.

Pichichero M: Kawasaki disease. In Hoekelman R: *Primary pediatric care,* ed 4, St Louis, 2001, Mosby.

Ross Products Division, Abbott Laboratories: *Clinical education aid no. 7,* Columbus, OH, 1970, Ross Products Division, Abbott Laboratories.

Schieken R: Systemic hypertension. In Allen H et al: *Moss and Adams' heart disease in infants, children, and adolescents: including the fetus and young adult,* ed 6, Philadelphia, 2001, Lippincott Williams & Wilkins.

Siwik E, Patel C, Zahka K: Tetralogy of Fallot. In Allen H et al: *Moss and Adams' heart disease in infants, children, and adolescents: including the fetus and young adult,* ed 6, Philadelphia, 2001, Lippincott Williams & Wilkins.

Sorof J: Prevalence and consequences of systolic hypertension in children, *Am J Hypertens* 15(2, pt 2): 57S-60S, 2002.

Stockman J, Lohr J: *Essence of office pediatrics,* Philadelphia, 2001, WB Saunders.

Takahashi J: Kawasaki syndrome (mucocutaneous lymph node syndrome). In Allen H et al: *Moss and Adams' heart disease in infants, children, and adolescents: including the fetus and young adult,* ed 6, Philadelphia, 2001, Lippincott Williams & Wilkins.

Thornton S: Differential diagnosis of infective endocarditis, *J Am Acad Nurse Pract* 12 (5):177-183, 2000.

Towbin J: Myocarditis. In Allen H et al: *Moss and Adams' heart disease in infants, children, and adolescents: including the fetus and young adult,* ed 6, Philadelphia, 2001, Lippincott Williams & Wilkins.

US Preventive Services Task Force: *Guide to clinical preventive services,* ed 2, Baltimore, 1996, Williams & Wilkins.

Uzark K: Recognition and management of congenital heart disease in the neonate. Presented at the National Association of Pediatric Nurse Associates and Practitioners 17th Annual Conference, San Diego, CA, 1996.

Vetter V: Arrhythmias. In Moller J, Hoffman J: *Pediatric cardiovascular medicine,* New York, 2000, Churchill Livingstone.

Wernovsky G: Transposition of the great vessels. In Allen H et al: *Moss and Adams' heart disease in infants, children, and adolescents: including the fetus and young adult,* ed 6, Philadelphia, 2001, Lippincott Williams & Wilkins.

32 Respiratory Disorders

Catherine J. Goodhue, Margaret A. Brady

Respiratory problems are a leading cause of illness in children and a major reason for health care visits. Viral upper respiratory tract infections (URIs) and otitis media are common diagnoses seen every day by practitioners. Guiding parents in the appropriate management of upper respiratory disorders is often a challenge for health care providers seeking to treat such problems as the common cold, otitis media, rhinitis, tonsillopharyngitis, and sinusitis. Parents seeking to relieve their child's upper respiratory tract symptoms are often tempted to use a variety of over-the-counter medications readily available to them or to pressure the nurse practitioner (NP) to prescribe needless antibiotics. In contrast, a child with a lower respiratory tract disorder such as asthma or bacterial pneumonia can experience a potentially life-threatening illness that demands prompt attention. NPs who ask key questions about the history of the respiratory symptoms; do a systematic and complete examination of the upper and lower airways, including the sinuses; and, if indicated, order specific laboratory tests and radiographic examinations can determine an accurate diagnosis and develop a successful treatment plan in most cases. When children have complicated problems, they can be referred with baseline information to the appropriate medical specialist for additional studies and treatment.

ANATOMY AND PHYSIOLOGY

Upper Respiratory Tract

The upper respiratory tract includes the nostrils, nasopharynx, larynx, upper part of the trachea, eustachian tubes, and sinuses. Air is warmed and humidified as it travels through the nasal passages, and particles are filtered out by coarse nasal hairs. A blanket of mucus covers the surface epithelium of the nasal mucosa. Nasal secretions contain lysozymes and secretory immunoglobulin A (IgA) to defend against microbial invasion. Similarly, the paranasal sinuses are lined with ciliated, mucus-secreting epithelium. The maxillary and ethmoid sinuses are the earliest sinuses to develop and can be visualized on plain radiographs by 1 to 2 years of age. The sphenoid and frontal sinuses become visible on radiographs at approximately 5 to 6 years of age. The sinuses become clinically significant sites of infection as follows:

- Maxillary and ethmoid sinuses as early as infancy
- Sphenoid sinuses around the third and fourth year of life
- Frontal sinuses around the sixth to tenth year of life

The sinuses continue to grow through adolescence.

Lower Respiratory Tract

The right lung has three lobes, upper, middle, and lower, with the upper and middle being separated by a minor fissure. The left lung has two lobes, upper and lower, separated by a major fissure. The upper left lobe has an area called the *lingula* that corresponds to the right middle lobe. The right main stem bronchus is shorter and wider than the left bronchus. It forms a smaller angle away from the trachea than the left bronchus does. This anatomic variation explains why foreign bodies usually end in the right main stem bronchus. Although the body surface and the number of respiratory airways and alveoli increase tenfold from birth to adult life, the tissue available for gas exchange increases approximately twentyfold. The newborn's chest is cylindrically shaped and has relatively horizontal ribs, which limits the infant's ability to expand his or her chest. The shape of the chest changes during the first few years of life because of greater transverse growth of the lower part of the chest wall. This differential growth results in the ribs being positioned lower anteriorly than posteriorly. The change in positioning of the ribs adds rigidity to the thorax of older children.

The diaphragm is the main muscle of respiration, and the intercostal, sternocleidomastoid, spinal, neck, and abdominal muscles are accessory muscles that can be used to increase effort. Normal exhalation occurs from elastic recoil of the lung.

Primitive airways appear at approximately the fourth week of gestation. At approximately the sixteenth week of gestation, the number of bronchial branches equals that in adults. Subsequent growth continues by increasing the length of the respiratory tract. During the sixteenth to twenty-sixth weeks of gestation, vascularization of the future respiratory portion of the lung occurs. Cartilage, glands, and muscles of the airways and type II alveolar cells are formed by the twenty-eighth week. Type II cells allow the fetus to produce surfactant. The airways continue to grow, and terminal sac formation occurs. at approximately the thirty-sixth week, the terminal sacs divide and alveoli are formed. Approximately 50 million primitive alveoli are present at birth.

After birth, the alveolar ducts branch off the third respiratory bronchioles. Alveoli continue to form and number 100 to 200 million in older children and 200 to 600 million in adolescents. The alveolar sacs continue to increase in size. The adult lung contains approximately 300 million alveoli.

Other structures important for gas exchange and pulmonary function are present at birth and include cartilage, mucous glands, goblet cells, and ciliated cells of the conducting airways. Smooth muscle is also present; therefore even very young infants can have bronchospasm.

Airway resistance is higher in newborns and young children than in adults. The airways of young infants and children are easily obstructed by inflammation, foreign bodies, or mucus secretion. The maximal inspiratory pressure generated by an infant is equal to that of an adult. However, the chest wall and supporting structures are softer and more flexible, so chest wall retraction is greatest in young infants. The chest wall of a newborn is highly compliant (Behrman, Kliegman, & Jenson, 2004).

PATHOPHYSIOLOGY INVOLVED IN AIRWAY DISEASE

All lung disorders eventually result in some form of airway obstruction. Narrowing of the lumen of the airway results from one or more of the following:

- Presence of intraluminal material (e.g., secretions, tumors, or foreign matter)
- Mural thickening (e.g., edema or hypertrophy of the glands or mucosa)
- Contraction of smooth muscle (e.g., spasm)
- Extrinsic compression

These factors rarely occur in isolation. They cause pulmonary malfunction by impairing tracheobronchial hygiene and impeding normal airflow. Even small blockages in an infant's or a young child's airway can lead to severe airway obstruction related to the proportional size of the infant's or young child's airways.

The two major types of airway obstruction are complete and partial. In complete obstruction, neither airflow nor drainage of secretions occurs. Such occlusion leads to lobar atelectasis after the residual gas diffuses into the pulmonary circulation. In partial obstruction, flow of air and drainage of secretions occur but are impaired. Partial obstruction can be further divided into the following two separate classifications:

The first consists of a bypass valve obstruction caused by narrowing of the lumen; a wheeze may be produced. Although resistance to flow is increased, air can still flow in during inspiration and out during expiration.

The second is a check-valve or ball-valve obstruction; air entry is possible, but during expiration the lumen is completely occluded so that escape of air is impossible. Bronchial foreign bodies and emphysema are associated with bypass, check-valve, or ball-valve obstructions that result in overinflation of lung airways.

High airway obstruction occurs above the level of the secondary bronchi and generally interferes more with inspiration than expiration. If the obstruction is complete and above the bifurcation of the trachea, asphyxia and death can result. Partial obstruction may result in severe dyspnea, stridor (a harsh, high-pitched inspiratory sound), and subcostal retractions. Coughing is the mechanism to remove nonfixed, high airway obstruction. Poor inspiratory airflow limits the effectiveness of coughing. The sound produced by coughing can help detect the level of obstruction and assists in making a diagnosis. Obstructions next to the larynx produce a cough that sounds croupy or barking; obstructions in the trachea or major bronchi produce a brassy sound.

Lower airway obstructions are caused by peripheral lesions that are usually diffuse in location and involve bronchioles smaller than 3 mm. The usual mechanism of narrowing is spasm, accumulation of secretions, edema of the mucous membrane, extrinsic compression, or any combination of these factors.

Complete obstruction causes atelectasis. A large percentage of the lung volume needs to be involved before symptoms become apparent; small atelectatic changes do not produce obvious clinical manifestations.

The primary clinical manifestation of lower airway obstruction is expiratory-phase symptoms. Wheezing is the principal sound patients make if the obstruction allows enough air to pass through the narrowed lumen. Chest excursion is diminished, and the expiratory phase is prolonged. Increased airway resistance during exhalation results in overinflation of the lungs, which in turn eventually increases the anteroposterior diameter of the chest. Chronic overinflation results in the "barrel chest" typical of a patient with chronic lung disease such as cystic fibrosis or emphysema. The accumulation of fluids and inflammation in the lower airways usually result in a repetitive hacking, ineffectual cough. On physical examination, percussing an overinflated chest elicits hyperresonance.

The more marked the obstruction, the more symptoms induced. The body attempts to compensate by using accessory muscles to assist in breathing. Dyspnea can result, often in association with orthopnea and exercise intolerance. Cyanosis is an ominous sign that can suggest impending death.

Fine crackles or rales also indicate respiratory pathology and are short crackling sounds heard during inspiration. These sounds are not cleared by coughing and are caused by airways suddenly opening after having been previously closed. The gas pressure between the compartments equalizes and creates the crackling sound.

DEFENSE SYSTEMS

The respiratory defense system includes both mechanical and biologic processes. Mechanical defenses include

- Filtering of particles
- Warming and humidifying of inspired air
- Clearing of airway through mucociliary and coughing actions
- Spasm and breathing changes

Approximately 75% of inspired air is warmed as it passes through the nose, paranasal sinuses, pharynx, larynx, and upper portion of the trachea. Final warming and humidifying of the airstream take place in the trachea and large bronchi. Heat and moisture are removed during the expiratory phase of respiration. The nose has a large surface area on which particles larger than 5 mm are impacted and filtered to prevent them from entering the lower airways. The trachea and bronchioles are lined with various defensive cells and mucous glands. Goblet cells secrete the mucous layer that lies on the tip of cilia. Particles entering the conducting airway are quickly cleared by the mucociliary defenses. Coughing can propel particles, but in young infants and children, coughing is often unproductive in expectorating mucus.

The temporary cessation of breathing, reflex shallow breathing, laryngospasm, and even bronchospasm are compensatory efforts aimed at stopping foreign matter from further entry into the lower respiratory tract. However, these respiratory efforts offer limited protection and have significant drawbacks.

Biologic processes that protect the respiratory system include

- Phagocytosis
- Absorption of noxious gases in the vasculature of the upper airway
- Absorption of particles by the lymph system

Phagocytosis, aided by the secretory immunoglobulins IgA, plus interferon, lysozyme, and lactoferrin, is the principal antimicrobial defense. Particles reaching the alveoli can be phagocytized by alveolar macrophages, cleared from the lung by the mucociliary system, or carried by lymphocytes into regional nodes or the blood. These particles can take days to months to clear.

The respiratory defense system is at risk for compromise from numerous environmental factors. Damage to epithelial cells is caused by a variety of substances and gases such as sulfur, nitrogen dioxide, ozone, chlorine, ammonia, and cigarette smoke. Hypothermia, hyperthermia, morphine, codeine, and hypothyroidism can adversely alter mucociliary defenses. Dry air from mouth breathing during periods of nasal obstruction, tracheostomy placement, or inadequately humidified oxygen therapy results in dryness of the mucous membrane and slowing of the cilia beat. Cold air is also irritating to the lower airways.

Phagocytic ability is also reduced by many substances, including ethanol ingestion and cigarette smoke. Hypoxemia, starvation, chilling, corticosteroids, increased oxygen, narcotics, and some anesthetic gases also impair phagocytosis. Recent acute viral infections can reduce antibacterial killing capacity. Damage from infection and chemical irritants may or may not be reversible (Behrman, Kliegman, & Jenson, 2004).

ASSESSMENT OF THE RESPIRATORY SYSTEM

History

1. History of the present illness:
   - Onset. Was the onset acute or insidious or preceded by the common cold (or both)?
   - Key signs and symptoms. Has the child had symptoms or signs of a daytime or nighttime cough, fever, rhinorrhea, sore throat, lesions in the mouth, retractions, cyanosis, dyspnea, or increased respiratory effort? See Table 32-1 for key characteristic and causes of cough.
   - Progression. Are the respiratory signs or symptoms increasing in severity, lessening, or about the same? Is the child easily fatigued, less active, or having trouble sleeping?

TABLE 32-1 ***Key Characteristics of Cough, Common Causes, and Questions to Ask in a Pediatric History***

Purpose	A cough is a protective reflex to ensure airway patency
Characteristics	
Age factor	Infants have a weak, nonproductive cough
Quality	Staccato-like, brassy, barking (LTB), whooping (pertussis), weak, honky (psychogenic)
Duration	Acute (most causes are infectious), recurrent (associated with allergies and asthma), or chronic (e.g., cystic fibrosis); continuous or intermittent; a *chronic cough* is defined as coughing that lasts more than 2 to 4 wk
Productive	Mucus producing or nonproductive
Timing	During the day, night (associated with asthma), or both
Associated symptoms	Fever—may indicate bacterial infection Rhinorrhea, sneezing, wheezing, atopic dermatitis—associated with asthma and allergic rhinitis Malaise, sneezing, watery nasal discharge, mild sore throat, no or low fever, not ill appearing—typical of URI Tachypnea—pneumonia or bronchiolitis in infants (infants may not have a cough)
Causes	
Congenital anomalies	Tracheoesophageal fistula, laryngeal cleft, vocal cord paralysis, pulmonary malformations, tracheobronchomalacia, congenital heart disease, congestive heart failure
Infectious agents	Viral (respiratory syncytial virus, adenovirus, parainfluenza), bacterial (tuberculosis, pertussis, *S. pneumoniae*), fungal, and others (*Chlamydia* and *Mycoplasma*)
Allergic conditions	Allergic rhinitis, asthma
Other	Foreign body aspiration, gastroesophageal reflux, psychogenic cough, environmental triggers (air pollution, tobacco smoke, wood smoke, glue sniffing, volatile chemicals), cystic fibrosis, drug induced, HIV, tumor

Adapted from Noble JE: Cough. In Berkowitz C, editor: *Pediatrics: a primary care approach*, ed 2, Philadelphia, 2000, WB Saunders, pp 271-274; McNamara M: Cough. In Schwartz MW, editor: *The 5-minute pediatric consult*, ed 2, Philadelphia, 2000, Lippincott Williams & Wilkins, pp 20-21.
HIV, Human immunodeficiency virus; *LTB*, laryngotracheobronchitis; *URI*, upper respiratory infection.

- Associated symptoms. Has there been a decrease in appetite or feeding? Any rashes, headache, or abdominal pain?
- Contacts. Are any family members or close contacts (day care, school) ill with similar signs and symptoms?
- Similar illnesses in the past. Does the child have a history of respiratory tract infections, allergies, or asthma? How many similar past infections has the child had (e.g., croup, pneumonia, sinusitis, streptococcal tonsillopharyngitis, frequent colds)?
- Treatment. Have any over-the-counter or prescription drugs been used? Have any other treatment modalities been used, including folk cures, complementary therapies, or home remedies?

2. Family history:
   - Do others in the family have a history of allergies or asthma? Is there any family history of ear-nose-throat or respiratory problems that could be familial or genetic diseases such as cystic fibrosis (CF)?
3. Review of systems:
   - Note any infections, constitutional diseases, or congenital problems that might have a respiratory component.
4. Environment:
   - Does anyone in the family or in the day care setting smoke? Does the child live or attend school in an urban or industrial area subject to air pollution (e.g., near a major highway or industrial plant)?

Physical Examination

Chapter 2 covers physical examination of the respiratory system. Additional information pertinent to the physical examination of a child with suspected respiratory disease includes the following:

- Measurement of vital signs and observation of general appearance:
  - A normal respiratory rate is age dependent and, if elevated, is a key indicator of lower respiratory involvement.
  - The level of anxiety, nasal flaring, and position of comfort are useful indicators of respiratory distress.
- Inspection of
  - The nose for rhinorrhea—clear, mucoid, mucopurulent; foreign bodies, erosion, polyps, lesions, bleeding; and color of the mucous membrane.
  - The throat, pharynx, and tonsillar areas for lesions, vesicles, exudate, enlargement of any structure, or other abnormalities. If epiglottitis is a consideration, do not inspect the mouth.
  - The chest for the depth, ease, symmetry, and rhythm of respiration. These elements are key indicators of lower respiratory tract involvement. The use of accessory muscles and the presence of retractions should be noted. A prolonged expiratory phase is associated with respiratory obstruction in the lower airways.
- Palpation or percussion (or both) of
  - The paranasal and frontal areas to check for signs of sinus tenderness.
  - The chest for signs of dullness or hyperresonance caused by consolidation, fluid, or air trapping.
- Auscultation of the chest:
  - Upper tract involvement frequently causes rhonchi or referred breath sounds.
  - Lower tract involvement is suggested by fine crackles or rales (interrupted abnormal breath sounds) or by wheezing.
- Determination of respiratory distress is based on physical findings—consider the anxiety level, respiratory rate and rhythm, use of accessory muscles, color, breath sounds, and pulse oximetry.

Diagnostic Procedures

Diagnostic procedures used to evaluate respiratory illness in children managed as outpatients include the following:

- Monitoring oxygenation by pulse oximetry and blood gases:
  - Pulse oximetry can be used to continuously measure peripheral oxygen saturation. Results generally correlate well with simultaneous arterial saturation (SaO_2). The equation to determine the partial pressure of O_2 (PaO_2) is $PaO_2 = FiO_2$ $(Ba - PH_2O) - 1.2$ $PaCO_2$. FiO_2 is the fractional oxygen concentraion (FiO_2) of the inspired gas. The partial pressure of H_2O is constant at 47 and that of CO_2 is usually 45. This dependence on barometric pressure (Ba) is the limiting factor: The higher the altitude at which one lives, the more hypoxic one becomes (e.g., the PaO_2 of room air at sea level $= 0.21\ [760 - 47] - 1.2 \cdot 45 = 95.73$). If Ba falls 50 mm Hg, the resultant PaO_2 of room air changes drastically (e.g., $PaO_2 = 0.21[710 - 47] - 1.2 \cdot 45 = 85$). People living in higher altitudes suffer from chronic hypoxia (Maggi, 1998). When first arriving at a high elevation, many individuals experience a transient mountain sickness with symptoms that include headache, insomnia, irritability, breathlessness, nausea, and vomiting. This phenomenon can last approximately 1 week before acclimatization begins to occur. The affected person begins to increase production of red blood cells. Changes in hemoglobin result in decreased O_2 affinity, which makes more O_2 available to the cells. Finally, a functional nonpathologic right ventricular hypertrophy takes place. These effects last as long as the person remains at high altitude.
- Blood gas studies can help the NP in assessing possible respiratory collapse. A rising $PaCO_2$ is an ominous sign. Box 32-1 lists normal values for blood gases at sea level.
- Radiographic imaging, including radiographs, ultrasonography, magnetic resonance imaging (MRI), and computed tomography (CT) of the sinuses, soft tissues of the neck, and chest. Fluoroscopy is useful in the evaluation of stridor and abnormal movement of the diaphragm. Contrast studies are useful for patients with recurrent pneumonia, persistent cough, or suspected fistulas.
- Pulmonary function tests are discussed in Chapter 25 in the section on asthma.
- Other specialized tests, including cultures and blood work, are addressed under the specific illness.

BOX 32-1 *Normal Blood Gas Values at Sea Level*

- Normal PaO_2: 90 to 100 mm Hg
- Normal $PaCO_2$: 38 to 42 mm Hg
- Capillary PO_2: roughly one half arterial PO_2
- Capillary PCO_2: same as arterial PCO_2
- Hypoventilation: $PaCO_2$ greater than 45 mm Hg; as $PaCO_2$ rises, the risk of respiratory failure increases
- Hyperventilation: $PaCO_2$ less than 35 mm Hg (usually need a respiratory rate greater than 60 breaths per minute)

- Other imaging studies that might be needed to assess these children include bronchograms (useful in delineating the smaller airways), pulmonary arteriograms (evaluation of the pulmonary vasculature), and radionuclide studies (evaluation of the pulmonary capillary bed). Endoscopy, bronchoscopy, percutaneous tap, lung biopsy, sweat testing, and microbiology studies are other helpful diagnostic procedures if used appropriately. Children who are significantly ill or have unusual signs and symptoms that require such procedures should be referred to medical specialists.

BASIC RESPIRATORY MANAGEMENT STRATEGIES

General Measures

General management measures include the following:

- Fluid. Hydration is important to keep mucous membranes and secretions moist. Intake of fluids should be encouraged and parents of young children given guidelines regarding the amount of fluids that their child should take and the frequency of feedings.
- Humidification. For a child with laryngotracheobronchitis (LTB), taking the child out into the cold night air, opening a freezer door, or turning on the shower at home is often beneficial. A cold-mist vaporizer helps provide moisture to the nares and oropharynx; the vaporizer must be cleaned daily so that it will not become a source of infection. To prevent the growth of organisms, nebulizers and humidifiers should be cleaned first with soapy water, rinsed thoroughly, soaked for one-half hour in a solution of 1 part vinegar to 2 or 3 parts distilled water, and then air-dried. Control 3 is a commercial product that can be substituted for vinegar. However, it is expensive.
- Bulb syringe. Because infants are obligate nose breathers, parents should be instructed in use of the bulb syringe to relieve obstruction of the infant's nares with mucus. Use the bulb syringe gently and intermittently because improper use can cause irritation, inflammation, and respiratory obstruction from tissue damage. Be sure to obstruct one nostril while suctioning the other.
- Normal saline nose drops or spray. Use before feedings and when mucus is thick or crusted. Follow by suctioning the nares with a bulb syringe; remember that the naris not being suctioned must be occluded.

Children who are significantly ill or have unusual manifestations need referral to or consultation with a pediatrician or pediatric subspecialist.

Medications

The following pharmacologic agents may be needed to treat various respiratory illnesses:

- Antibiotics. Specific agents are discussed in the section on individual illnesses. If an antibiotic is prescribed, the drug should be taken until completed.
- Analgesics and antipyretics. Acetaminophen and ibuprofen may be prescribed for relief of pain or fever.
- Decongestants and antihistamines. The use of decongestants and antihistamines is controversial. Often they do not shorten the course of a disease but can provide relief of nasal symptoms. Use these agents with caution, especially in children younger than 9 months to 1 year.
- Expectorants. Water is one of the most effective expectorants. Over-the-counter agents provide some symptomatic relief but do not shorten the course of respiratory illnesses. Use with care in children younger than 1 year.
- Cough medication. Cough suppressant medications should be prescribed judiciously because coughing is a protective mechanism to clear secretions. Prescribing a cough suppressant at bedtime can help the child and parent sleep. Use very carefully in infants younger than 1 year.

The American Academy of Pediatrics (AAP) has guidelines for the judicious use of antimicrobial agents in pediatric patients with common respiratory illnesses such as otitis media, pharyngitis, sinusitis, and cough/bronchitis. The NP should be familiar with the recommendations. All health care providers must be cognizant of their role in the prevention of superinfections caused by the indiscriminate use of antibiotics.

Patient and Parent Education

Parents should be educated about assessment and management of changes in the child's condition (Box 32-2). Include the following:

- Indications for immediate reevaluation of the child
  - Signs and symptoms of respiratory distress
  - Other indicators of worsening of the illness (e.g., toxic appearance, malaise, feeding difficulty)
- Information on when to expect improvement in the child's symptoms and, if symptoms do not improve as expected, what to do next
- Clear instructions about medications—how much to give, when to give, side effects to watch for, how long to give, and the necessity of completing the course of antibiotics

BOX 32-2 *Parental Education for At-Home Care of the Child with a Respiratory Tract Infection: Issues to Discuss*

Fluid: Give guidelines on amount and frequency of fluids child should take.
Humidification: For laryngotracheobronchitis, take the child out into the cold night air, open a freezer door, or turn on the shower at home. In dry climates, humidifiers help in respiratory illnesses; instruct about cleaning of nebulizers and humidifiers.
Bulb syringe: Instruct to use the bulb syringe gently and intermittently and to obstruct one nostril while suctioning the other.
Normal saline nose drops or spray: Use before feedings and when mucus is thick or crusted. Follow by suctioning nares with bulb syringe.
Other educational issues to cover:
- Indications for immediate reevaluation of child:
  - Signs and symptoms of respiratory distress
  - Other indicators of worsening of illness (e.g., toxic appearance, malaise, feeding difficulty)
- Information on when to expect improvement in the child's symptoms and, if symptoms do not improve as expected, what to do next
- Clear instructions about medications—how much to give, when to give, side effects to watch for, how long to give, and to complete the course of antibiotics
- Infection control information if needed
- Instructions on next return visit

From Burns C et al: *Pocket reference for pediatric primary care,* Philadelphia, 2001, WB Saunders.

- Infection control information if needed
- Instructions on the next return visit

INDICATIONS FOR TONSILLECTOMY AND ADENOIDECTOMY

The only two absolute indications for tonsillectomy are suspicion of tumor and severe aerodigestive tract obstruction. For any other indication, the risk-benefit ratio of the procedure must be weighed. Significant morbidity and mortality rates are associated with this procedure. Complications, including anesthesia problems, hemorrhage, and infection, occur in approximately 10% of cases. Many indications for adenoidectomy exist and include the following: chronic persistent upper airway problems manifested by obstructive sleep apnea, chronic persistent otitis media, unresponsive chronic sinus infections, persistent mouth breathing, nasal speech, adenoid facies (narrow high arched palate and elongated mandible), and persistent or chronic nasopharyngitis (if related to chronic hypertrophied infected adenoid tissue). The morbidity and mortality rates connected with this procedure are not as high as with tonsillectomy. This procedure may often be accompanied by tonsillectomy (Wetmore, 2004).

UPPER RESPIRATORY TRACT DISORDERS

Nasopharyngitis (Common Cold or Upper Respiratory Tract Infection) and Tonsillopharyngitis

Description

Nasopharyngitis and tonsillopharyngitis are frequent problems seen in pediatric practice. Young children have, on average, six to seven URIs, or colds, per year. (See Table 32-2 for a differential diagnosis of URI from sinusitis and purulent rhinitis.) When tonsillar involvement is significant, the term *tonsillopharyngitis* or *tonsillitis* is used; when tonsillar involvement is minor, the term *nasopharyngitis* is used. Nasopharyngitis is most often caused by a viral agent (Turner & Hayden, 2004).

Management

Only supportive care is needed for a URI as addressed in the sections entitled General Measures and Patient Education under Basic Respiratory Management Strategies. Antibiotics are not appropriate treatment. The use of antipyretics, analgesics, decongestants, antihistamines, and cough medication is controversial but can help alleviate the distress caused by URI symptoms if used cautiously.

TABLE 32-2 ***Differentiation of Common Upper Respiratory Infections in Children***

Site of Infection	Symptoms	Duration of Symptoms (days)	Etiologic Agent	Management	Duration of Treatment	Comments
The common cold (viral URI)	Malaise, sneezing, watery nasal discharge, mild sore throat, may have a fever, not ill appearing	0-10	Rhinoviruses (cause 40% of URIs), RSV, parainfluenza, enteroviruses, adenoviruses	No antibiotics; symptomatic Rx, e.g., saline nose drops, increased fluids; for infants, bulb-syringe the nose before meals and bedtime; for older children, cough suppression at night if unable to sleep; humidifier		If lasts longer than 10-14 days, consider other diagnosis (e.g., sinusitis)
Acute purulent rhinorrhea	Thick, yellow nasal discharge (often associated with URI)	>3	Part of the natural history of URI; superinfection by *Streptococcus pneumoniae, Haemophilus influenzae,* β-hemolytic streptococci	Symptomatic care; a wait-and-see approach for antibiotics: if >10- to 14-day duration, treat with amoxicillin or dicloxacillin if staphylococci suspected	Best approach, wait and see	Avoid indiscriminate and frequent use of antibiotics (development of antibiotic resistance)
Acute purulent sinusitis	Persistent nasal symptoms for more than 10 days with URI, nasal drainage, cough, recalcitrant asthma	10-30	*S. pneumoniae, Moraxella catarrhalis,* nontypable *H. influenzae*	Amoxicillin, erythromycin-sulfamethoxazole, or amoxicillin-clavulanate	10-14 days	By 7 days should be asymptomatic; change antibiotics 48-72 hr after start of treatment if no response
Subacute sinusitis	Same as above but persistent for at least 30 days	30-120	Same as above; may be β-lactamase producing	Amoxicillin-clavulanate		Initial acute infection did not clear, need to switch antibiotics
Chronic/ recurrent sinusitis	Malaise, easy fatigability, unilateral or bilateral nasal discharge, postnasal discharge, nasal obstruction if middle turbinate significantly obstructed	>120	Same as above plus α-hemolytic streptococci and *Staphylococcus aureus*	Amoxicillin-clavulanate, azithromycin, cefixime	3-6 wk	May need endoscopic sinus surgery if chronic sinusitis does not respond to prolonged medical management; investigate differential diagnoses

RSV, Respiratory syncytial virus; *Rx,* medication; *URI,* upper respiratory infection.

Acute Viral Pharyngitis and Tonsillitis

Etiology. Viral infection is the leading cause of nasopharyngitis and tonsillopharyngitis. Adenovirus is the most common cause of viral pharyngitis and tonsillitis. The enteroviruses (coxsackievirus, echovirus), herpesvirus, and Epstein-Barr virus are also common. Although not a virus, *Mycoplasma pneumoniae* is a frequent cause of pharyngitis and tonsillitis in school-age children. Viral infections occur year-round, and it is helpful to know what agents are currently infecting children in the community. It can be difficult to differentiate viral from bacterial infections because of overlapping symptoms. However, hoarseness, cough, coryza, and conjunctivitis are classic features of a viral infection (Gaebler, 2002).

Clinical Findings

History. The following may be reported:

- Gradual onset
- Prominent nasal symptoms of rhinorrhea (key finding)
- Sore throat and dysphagia
- Mild cough
- Low-grade fever

Physical Examination. Virus-specific findings include the following:

- Epstein-Barr virus can produce exudate on the tonsils, soft palate petechiae, and diffuse adenopathy.
- Adenovirus can produce exudate on the tonsils and cervical adenopathy.
- Enteroviruses can produce vesicles or ulcers on the tonsillar pillars and posterior fauces; coryza, vomiting, or diarrhea may be present.
- Herpesvirus produces ulcers anteriorly and marked adenopathy.

Diagnostic Tests. If a diagnosis of viral infection is in doubt, a culture should be done. Cultures are useful in differentiating viral infection from group A β-hemolytic streptococci (GABHS) infection. If infectious mononucleosis is suspected, a heterophil antibody test and complete blood count (CBC) can be helpful in confirming the diagnosis.

Management. For viral infection, only supportive care is needed, including fever and sore throat pain relief with acetaminophen or ibuprofen. Fluid intake should be encouraged (Gaebler, 2002).

Acute Bacterial Pharyngitis and Tonsillitis

Etiology. The three most common bacterial causes of pharyngitis and tonsillitis in children and adolescents are GABHS, *Neisseria gonorrhoeae*, and *Corynebacterium diphtheriae*. GABHS accounts for less than 10% of infections in children with sore throat and fever. *N. gonorrhoeae* pharyngitis is a sexually transmitted disease that can mimic GABHS pharyngitis or can run a subclinical course. *C. diphtheriae* causes diphtheria and is discussed later in this chapter. The latter two organisms are rare causes of tonsillopharyngitis.

Clinical Findings

History. The following characterize GABHS infection:

- Less commonly seen in children younger than 2 years; most commonly found in 5- to 11-year-old children
- Abrupt onset without nasal symptoms
- Fever, malaise, sore throat, dysphagia
- Nausea, abdominal discomfort, vomiting, headache

Physical Examination. The following may be seen:

- Petechiae, beefy-red uvula, red tonsillopharyngeal tissue
- Tonsillopharyngeal exudate (frequently)
- Tender anterior cervical lymph nodes
- Scarlatiniform rash

Diagnostic Tests. A positive throat culture confirms the diagnosis and is still the test of choice; however, a positive culture can also identify a carrier state. Some rapid streptococcal identification tests are not as sensitive as culture in detecting GABHS; therefore a negative rapid test must be followed by culture. The specificity of the rapid streptococcal test is very good (95%); therefore if the rapid test is positive, the diagnosis of GABHS is confirmed. The Strep A Optical Immuno Assay (rapid streptococcal test) reportedly has a sensitivity better than routine throat culture does. Documentation of past GABHS infection is obtained by antibody titer to various streptococcal enzymes such as antistreptolysin O (ASO).

Management. The goal of antibiotic therapy is to prevent the development of rheumatic fever, the spread of illness to others, and the development of suppurative complications. Antibiotics also shorten the course of the illness and the severity of symptoms. The management plan includes the following:

- Antimicrobial therapy (based on clinical need)—one of the following (AAP Committee on Infectious Diseases, 2003):
  - Benzathine penicillin G intramuscularly (600,000 U if less than 60 lb; 1.2 million U for larger children and adults).
  - Potassium penicillin V orally (250 mg two to three times a day for 10 days in children less than 27 kg; 500 mg two to three times a day for 10 days in children greater than 27 kg and adolescents).
  - Erythromycin estolate (20 to 40 mg/kg per day in two to four divided doses for 10 days) or erythromycin ethylsuccinate (40 mg/kg per day in two to four divided doses) if allergic to penicillin. Resistance to erythromycin has been reported in Finland and Japan but is not yet a significant problem in the United States.

  - A 10-day course of a narrow-spectrum (first-generation), orally administered cephalosporin is now acceptable, particularly if the child is allergic to penicillin. However, about 15% of patients allergic to penicillin also are allergic to the cephalosporins (AAP Committee on Infectious Diseases, 2003).
  - If evidence of penicillin resistance is present, a β-lactamase–resistant antibiotic can be used such as amoxicillin-clavulanate or dicloxacillin.
- Supportive care—antipyretics, fluids, rest.
- Reculture is not generally needed except in situations in which it is necessary to ensure eradication of the organism.
- If the child continues to have symptoms of streptococcal pharyngitis and a positive culture for streptococcus, this child may represent an actual treatment failure or have a new infection with a different serologic type of streptococcus.
- Noncompliance with pharmacologic therapy can explain treatment failure, and in these instances an injection of benzathine penicillin is recommended.
- For a compliant patient with recurrence soon after completion of antimicrobial therapy, treat with any of the following drugs: the same antimicrobial agent, amoxicillin-clavulanate, clindamycin, narrow-spectrum cephalosporin, erythromycin, or another macrolide (AAP Committee on Infectious Diseases, 2003).
- If clinical relapse occurs, a second course of antibiotic is indicated, as discussed earlier. If recurrent infection is a problem, culturing of the family for the chronic carrier state is advised. Toothbrushes or orthodontic devices may harbor GABHS and should be cleaned or discarded.
- Children can return to school when they are afebrile and have been taking antibiotics for at least 24 hours.

Complications. Major late complications caused by GABHS are rheumatic fever and acute glomerulonephritis. Suppurative complications include cervical adenitis, sinusitis, otitis media, pneumonia, and retropharyngeal or peritonsillar abscess. Recurrent GABHS tonsillopharyngitis can also be a problem. Syndenham chorea is linked to GABHS infection.

Acute Purulent Rhinitis

Description

Acute purulent rhinitis often represents a superinfection of a common cold or purulent sinusitis. Remember that thick, yellow discharge is a common sequela of an uncomplicated URI.

Etiology

Likely organisms involved in the superinfection are pneumococci, *Haemophilus influenzae*, β-hemolytic streptococci, and *Staphylococcus aureus*.

Clinical Findings

History. Complaints of URI with characteristic symptoms and a profuse and continuous, purulent, yellow to green nasal discharge for more than 3 days are reported.

Physical Examination. A yellow to green nasal discharge is seen.

Differential Diagnosis

A nasal foreign body and sinusitis are the differential diagnoses. The mucopurulent discharge associated with the common cold (acute viral rhinitis) is intermittent and worse in the early morning on awakening. Allergic rhinitis is discussed in Chapter 25.

Management

Controversy surrounds the appropriateness of early intervention with antibiotic therapy if the only major symptom is a purulent nasal discharge. The following approaches may be considered:

- Take a wait-and-see plan. Advise symptomatic treatment because the discharge may be only a symptom of an uncomplicated URI.
- Removal of purulent material—may need to instill saline into the nares and use a bulb syringe or do saline washes.
- Family education—tell to return should symptoms persist for more than 10 to 14 days or if worsening.

Sinusitis

Description

Inflammation and secondary infection of the paranasal sinuses can be either an acute or a chronic problem. Sinusitis is a complication of approximately 5% to 10% of URIs in children. Persistence of URI symptoms for longer than 10 days without improvement separates a simple URI from sinusitis. The maxillary and ethmoid sinuses are most frequently involved. Inflammation and edema of the mucous membranes lining the sinuses cause obstruction and set up an ideal situation for bacteria to invade the sinus cavities. Certain conditions predispose children to chronic sinus infections, including allergies, nasal deformities, CF, nasal polyps, and human immunodeficiency virus (HIV) infection.

Differentiation of acute from chronic sinusitis is based on the duration of respiratory symptoms. In acute sinusitis, respiratory symptoms last more than 10 days but less than 30 days. When respiratory symptoms persist more than 30 days and do not improve, a diagnosis of subacute sinusitis is made. If symptoms last more than 120 days, a diagnosis of chronic sinusitis is appropriate. Remember that sinus inflammation is part of the natural history of a cold or allergic rhinitis. Thick, yellow discharge is a common and normal finding with a URI. Therefore the NP must be cautious to not overdiagnose sinusitis and subsequently indiscriminately use antibiotics (Nash & Wald, 2001).

Etiology

The common bacterial organisms responsible for superinfections are *Streptococcus pneumoniae, H. influenzae, Moraxella catarrhalis,* and GABHS. The role of viruses in sinusitis is not clear. Anaerobic and staphylococcal agents are implicated in chronic sinusitis. The various sinuses develop, aerate, and become clinically important at different times during childhood. Ethmoiditis can occur after 6 months of age, in contrast to frontal sinusitis, which is first seen around 10 years of age. Cases of recurrent and chronic sinusitis are often caused by recurrent viral URI associated with day care attendance, smoking in the home, older siblings at home who reinfect the child, or certain predisposing conditions such as allergies, immunodeficiency disorders, or CF.

Clinical Findings in Acute Sinusitis

History. The following may be reported:

- URI more severe or prolonged than usual
- Coughing during the day, often worse at night, and rhinorrhea lasting more than 10 days
- Fever—low grade or temperature higher than 39° C
- Clear or mucopurulent rhinorrhea or postnasal drip
- Facial pain
- Sore throat, bad breath, headache (Nash & Wald, 2001; Rahbar & McGill, 2002)

Physical Examination. The nasal mucosa is often reddened or swollen, and sometimes periorbital edema is apparent.

Clinical Findings in Chronic Sinusitis

History. The following may be reported:

- Protracted respiratory symptoms (more than 30 days)
- Nasal congestion and discharge (more than 90 days)
- Cough (day and night)
- Malaise, fatigue, anorexia
- Fever (rare but can be low grade)
- Sore throat (frequent complaint)

Physical Examination. The following are frequently seen (Behrman, Kliegman, & Jenson, 2000):

- Nasal discharge, either unilateral or bilateral, that varies from day to day
- Postnasal discharge
- Swelling of the middle turbinates, which can result in nasal obstruction
- Allergic rhinitis manifestations (e.g., boggy pale turbinates)

Diagnostic Tests. If the clinical findings suggest sinusitis, radiographs are not needed. Facial swelling, acute sinusitis unresponsive to 48 hours of antibiotics, and a child with a toxic appearance, chronic or recurrent sinusitis, and chronic asthma are indications for imaging studies, including either sinus radiographs, ultrasonograms, or CT scanning. A Waters view is usually sufficient to demonstrate sinusitis on a radiograph. Nasal cultures are not useful.

Differential Diagnosis

Viral upper respiratory tract illness, allergic rhinitis, and other causes of headache are the differential diagnoses.

Management

Antimicrobial therapy should be prescribed for a course of 10 days in sinusitis or, if the child is responding slowly but not symptom free, an additional 7 days. Most children show dramatic improvement in 3 to 4 days (Berman et al, 2001). Failure to improve in 48 hours suggests a resistant organism or complications. The course of therapy may be up to 21 days in acute sinusitis and up to 6 weeks in chronic sinusitis.

In uncomplicated sinusitis in children:

- Amoxicillin (40 mg/kg per day in three divided doses) is the desirable therapy (Ditmar, 2002). Other sources treat with amoxicillin at 80 to 90 mg/kg per day divided into three doses. If the child is allergic to penicillin:
  - Erythromycin-sulfamethoxazole (based on erythromycin, 10 mg/kg per dose three to four times a day).
- If a β-lactamase–positive organism is suspected (e.g., failure to improve with treatment or residence in a geographic area that has a high prevalence of β-lactamase–producing *H. influenzae*) or for chronic sinusitis:
  - Amoxicillin-clavulanate 45 mg (amoxicillin component) per kilogram per day divided every 12 hours.
  - Cefuroxime axetil, cefpodoxime, a newer macrolide, or erythromycin plus sulfamethoxazole.

Additional management considerations include the following:

- The use of decongestants, antihistamines, or both in the treatment of acute sinusitis is controversial and has not proved effective (Nash & Wald, 2001). They can be useful in recurrent or chronic sinusitis, especially if allergic manifestations are present (see the management section for allergic rhinitis). See Chapter 25 for information on the use of decongestants and antihistamines.
- Children with complications or signs of invasive infection should be referred to the appropriate medical specialist. Surgical drainage by an otolaryngologist, treatment of allergies and control of allergic rhinitis by an allergist, or both may be necessary.

- Comfort measures include the use of acetaminophen, ibuprofen, or codeine for severe pain. A humidifier helps relieve the drying of mucous membranes associated with mouth breathing. Increase oral fluid intake; saline irrigation of the nostrils is recommended by some allergists.
- Diving is contraindicated with sinusitis.

Complications

Chronic or recurrent sinusitis can become a problem often requiring referral to an otolaryngologist or allergist. Orbital cellulitis secondary to ethmoiditis, manifested by swelling and erythema of the eyelids, proptosis, decreased extraocular movements, and altered vision, is a serious, life-threatening complication that is a medical emergency. Intracranial complications such as cavernous sinus thrombosis, subdural empyema, and brain abscess can also occur. Chronic sinusitis is also associated with intractable wheezing in children with asthma (Behrman, Kliegman, & Jenson, 2004; Nash & Wald, 2001).

Diphtheria

Description

Diphtheria occurs as an acute infection of the upper respiratory tract, the trachea, or both. Diphtheria can cause membranous obstruction of the upper airway. It also produces a neurotoxin. Although only about five cases of diphtheria are reported annually in the United States, it remains an important and dangerous disease.

Etiology

Corynebacterium diphtheriae is a gram-positive rod with three strains that can be either toxigenic or nontoxigenic. Transmission results from intimate contact with an infected person or carrier. Discharge from the nose, throat, eye, and skin lesions can produce infection. Although rare, fomites can act as a vehicle of transmission, and food-borne outbreaks have been reported. The incubation period averages from 2 to 5 days; communicability lasts for 2 weeks or less in untreated cases. Chronic carriage can occur even with antimicrobial therapy.

Clinical Findings

Characteristic signs and symptoms follow.

Primary Infection

- Low-grade fever
- Grayish, adherent pseudomembrane found in either the nasopharynx, pharynx, or trachea
- Sore throat, serosanguineous nasal discharge, hoarseness
- Cutaneous lesions infected with diphtheria (less often seen)

Toxin Production

- The ability of a strain of *C. diphtheriae* to produce toxin is related to bacteriophage infection of the bacterium, not to colony type.
- Toxin production is more lethal than the primary infection and can induce the following:
  - Myocarditis
  - Motor paralysis
  - Guillain-Barré–type paralysis

Diagnostic Tests. A confirmatory diagnosis is based on a positive culture of *C. diphtheriae*. Specimens should be obtained from the nose, throat, any skin lesions, and either beneath the membrane or from a portion of the membrane. A special culture medium is needed, and toxigenicity tests are performed if *C. diphtheriae* is confirmed. Culture results take 8 to 48 hours; treatment begins when diphtheria is suspected. Do not wait for laboratory confirmation. Results of the CBC may be normal or show a slight leukocytosis and thrombocytopenia.

Differential Diagnosis

Acute streptococcal pharyngitis and infectious mononucleosis are included in the differential diagnosis of pharyngeal diphtheria. A nasal foreign body or purulent sinusitis can resemble nasal diphtheria; epiglottitis and viral croup can also cause obstruction, as does laryngeal diphtheria.

Management

Children with diphtheria require hospitalization. Treatment consists of the following:

- Antitoxin administration and antimicrobial therapy with erythromycin or penicillin G
- Supportive care for respiratory, cardiac, and neurologic complications as appropriate
- Immunization of the child after recovery because disease does not necessarily confer immunity

Prevention

Universal immunization against diphtheria with regular booster injections is the only effective method of control. Infection can occur in immunized or partially immunized children, but the severity of the disease is greatly diminished. Disease generally occurs in nonimmunized children; the frequency of severe life-threatening complications in this group is high. Care of a child exposed to diphtheria is individualized and based on immunization status, likelihood of follow-up, and compliance with antimicrobial therapy. The AAP Committee on Infectious Diseases (2003) lists specific guidelines that should be followed for the care of exposed children.

Pertussis

Description

Pertussis is commonly known as whooping cough because of the high-pitched inspiratory whoop that is characteristic of this illness in young children. It is an acute, highly communicable infection that produces a toxin responsible for the severe symptoms associated with pertussis. If this disease occurs in unvaccinated infants younger than 1 year, it is often associated with pneumonia, seizures, and encephalopathy. Pertussis in older children and vaccinated children produces a milder respiratory illness (Behrman, Kliegman, & Jenson, 2004). Outbreaks of pertussis still occur despite the availability of an effective vaccine. Older children and adults can be the vector of pertussis because their symptoms are not severe.

Etiology

Pertussis is caused by *Bordetella pertussis, Bordetella parapertussis*, and *Bordetella bronchiseptica.* Transmission of these gram-negative pleomorphic bacilli is via aerosol droplets from close contact with infected individuals, who generally have mild or atypical illness that is not recognized as pertussis. The incubation period is between 6 and 21 days; the period of communicability is greatest during the catarrhal stage until before or during the early paroxysmal stage of coughing. Cases of pertussis occur in adults, who constitute a reservoir for the disease. The highest incidence of mortality occurs under 1 month of age (1.3%) (AAP Committee on Infectious Diseases, 2003).

Clinical Findings

Manifestations of this disease vary by age-group, stage of disease, and whether the child has received any immunization against pertussis.

Characteristics of the disease in infants and young children include the following:

- Catarrhal stage—1 to 3 weeks
    - Mild cough, coryza, sneezing, and fever to 101° F
- Paroxysmal stage—2 to 4 weeks
    - Persistent staccato, paroxysmal cough ending with an inspiratory whoop
    - Vomiting at the end of paroxysmal coughing and whoop
    - Cyanosis, sweating, prostration, and exhaustion after coughing
- Convalescent stage—2 to 3 weeks
    - Waning of paroxysmal coughing episodes

Specific findings in infants younger than 6 months are

- Apnea (common)
- No inspiratory whoop

Findings in older children include

- Persistent irritating cough but no inspiratory whoop
- Low-grade fever

Diagnostic Tests. Culturing for *B. pertussis* requires special media and takes 7 days for incubation. The organism is found most frequently during the catarrhal or early paroxysmal stage. A positive culture from the nasopharynx is diagnostic; however, false-negative results do occur. Leukocytosis (20,000 to 30,000/mm^3) with 70% to 80% lymphocytes is a common finding in young children and appears around the end of the catarrhal stage.

Management

The following steps are involved:

- Young infants and children with severe respiratory symptoms require hospitalization.
- Erythromycin (40 to 50 mg/kg per day [maximum, 2 g/day] in four divided doses for 14 days) can improve symptoms if given in the catarrhal stage.
- Antimicrobial therapy given in the paroxysmal stage does not alter the course of pertussis per se, but administration of erythromycin limits spreading of the organism.
- Corticosteroids should not be used. Albuterol may modestly reduce symptoms, but the associated fussing from the treatment may trigger paroxysms (Behrman, Kliegman, & Jenson, 2004).

Care of Exposed Children. The AAP Committee on Infectious Diseases (2003) lists specific guidelines for the care of exposed children and adults, including the following:

- Immunization coverage with diphtheria-tetanus-acellular pertussis (DTaP)
- Chemoprophylaxis with erythromycin (40 to 50 mg/kg per day [maximum, 2 g/day] orally in four divided doses for 14 days) for all household and close contacts, including children in day care, irrespective of their immunization status
- Close monitoring of respiratory symptoms for 20 days after last contact with an infected individual

Complications

Secondary bacterial pneumonia, seizures, epistaxis, subconjunctival hemorrhage, encephalopathy, and death can occur. Activation of tuberculosis is associated with pertussis infection.

Prevention

Active immunity follows natural pertussis; reinfections are mild and may not be noticed. Young infants are at greatest risk for pertussis. The recommended guidelines for giving the initial series of DTaP vaccines and booster doses should be followed. Remember that just one DTaP immunization can reduce the severity of symptoms in an infant infected with pertussis. Universal immunization of children younger than 7 years is crucial to control of this disease.

Only children with valid contraindications to receiving pertussis vaccine, as identified in Chapter 24, should be excluded from receiving the vaccine. Immunity from pertussis immunization wanes over time, and the vaccine does not confer active immunity. Pertussis in older children, adolescents, and adults is a mild, often unrecognized disease that, if transmitted to an unimmunized infant, can result in life-threatening illness.

Recurrent Epistaxis

Etiology and Incidence

Recurrent epistaxis is commonly seen in children living in dry climates or during the winter months when artificial heating is used. The cause is often benign and due to mechanical trauma to the area (e.g., nose picking). Other factors that can also cause mucosal irritation that results in bleeding include allergies, neoplasms (e.g., polyps, hemangiomas), chronic rhinitis, chronic use of nasal sprays or drying agents such as decongestants, and viral or bacterial infections of nasal tissue. In adolescents, the use of recreational drugs such as cocaine causes local mucosal irritation. The anterior portion of the nasal septum, Kiesselbach area, is the usual site of involvement (Edelstein & Khabie, 2001; Inkelis, 2000).

Clinical Findings

History. The following may be reported:

- Tarry stools
- Frequent nose bleeds
- Recent URI
- Allergic rhinitis

Physical Examination. Bleeding from the nares can often be seen, and the anterior aspect of the nares is red and raw with or without fresh clots or old crusts. The nasal mucosa may be dry or cracked.

Diagnostic Tests. A baseline hematocrit may be indicated in severe or chronic epistaxis. It can reveal iron deficiency anemia secondary to the bleeding.

Differential Diagnosis

A bleeding disorder or nasal tumor is characterized by epistaxis that is severe, prolonged, and recurrent. Be suspicious of epistaxis in a child younger than 2 years of age, evidence of bleeding at other sites, and bleeding that lasts longer than 20 minutes. If these abnormalities occur and a coagulopathy is suspected, order a CBC, platelet count, prothrombin time (PT), and activated partial thromboplastin time (PTT).

Management

The following steps are taken:

- Have the child sit upright and lean forward to avoid swallowing the blood.
- Apply pressure to the nose (pinch the nares at the bony structure) for 10 minutes.
- Packing and topical vasoconstrictor drugs are occasionally needed.
- Use a bedside humidifier to moisten the air in dry climates or in winter with forced air heating.
- Apply topical cortisone or topical antibiotic to the area for 5 to 7 days to keep moist and assist healing.

Prevention

Use of a vaporizer and normal saline nose drops and application of petroleum jelly (Vaseline) or a topical antibiotic (Neosporin) to the inside of the nares are preventive measures.

Nasal Foreign Body

Description

It is not uncommon for young children to insert all types of foreign bodies into any body orifice. Nasal foreign bodies can be noted immediately by the parent or lie undetected until symptoms appear.

Clinical Findings

History. A persistent or recurrent unilateral purulent nasal discharge is reported.

Physical Examination. A foreign body may be seen with a purulent, foul-smelling nasal discharge.

Differential Diagnosis

Nasal polyps, purulent rhinitis, adenoiditis, sinusitis, and nasal tumors are conditions that are also associated with either bilateral or unilateral discharge.

Management

Management involves the following:

- Detection of a foreign body in the nasal cavity, which secures the diagnosis
  - Use of alligator forceps, suction with narrow tips, cotton-tipped applicators with collodion, and topical vasoconstrictor drugs if needed to remove the object, depending on its size and consistency
  - Good lighting (essential)
- Removal of the nasal foreign body, depending on its location, its composition, and the skill of the practitioner

- Referral to an otolaryngologist for young children who cannot cooperate or when the foreign body is extremely difficult or dangerous to remove, such as paper clips or staples (Dolitsky & Ward, 2001; Haddad, 2002)

EXTRATHORACIC AIRWAY DISORDERS

Laryngotracheobronchitis—Infectious Croup

Description

Laryngotracheobronchitis (LTB) is a rapid, acute, upper airway obstruction at the larynx characterized by a harsh, barking cough and inspiratory stridor.

Etiology

Viral agents are responsible for most cases of croup, with the parainfluenza viruses being the leading viral organisms, followed by the adenoviruses, respiratory syncytial virus (RSV), and rubeola. *M. pneumoniae* has been implicated in a small percentage of croup illnesses (Malhotra & Krilov, 2001). Other bacterial agents include *H. influenzae* type b, GABHS, pneumococcus, and staphylococcus. These organisms are infrequent causes of croup but cause very serious illness. Viral croup is common in children between 3 months and 5 years of age and occurs most often in the cold season of the year. Males are affected more often than females. Recurrent croup and recurrent laryngitis can develop in children until 6 years of age. A positive family history has been noted in 15% of children in whom croup develops.

Clinical Findings

Clinical manifestations depend on the type of infectious agent responsible for the croup and the area of the upper airway affected.

History. The history includes the following:

- URI symptoms of rhinitis, conjunctivitis, or both are sometimes present before stridor.
- Intermittent stridor occurs—mild to moderate.
- Gradual onset of symptoms occurs (1 to 2 days).
- Symptoms are worse at night.
- Most children with viral croup improve within a few days.

Physical Examination. The following can be seen:

- Slight dyspnea, retractions
- Mild, brassy, or barking cough
- Temperature elevated to 104° F
- Decreased breath sounds bilaterally with rhonchi and crackles

Diagnostic Tests. Usually the diagnosis is evident clinically. Radiography of the soft tissues of the neck and chest displays a classic pattern of subglottic narrowing but is usually not done unless there is a question about the diagnosis. Microbiology cultures can be helpful in selected cases.

Differential Diagnosis

The differential diagnoses include acute epiglottitis; acute spasmodic croup (no signs of infection); aspiration of a foreign body; retropharyngeal abscess; extrinsic compression from tumors, trauma, or congenital malformations; angioedema (anaphylaxis) or early asthmatic attack; infectious mononucleosis; and psychogenic stridor.

Table 32-3 differentiates acute infectious LTB from other common causes of stridor.

Management

Therapy depends on the cause, severity, and location of the disease. The aim of therapy is to provide adequate respiratory exchange.

- If bacterial infection is present, treat with an antibiotic that is likely to eradicate the suspected organisms, which are *S. aureus* and *H. influenzae.*
- Symptomatic relief of mild croup can be provided with the judicious use of steam from a hot shower or bath or "cold" steam from a humidifier. These measures usually terminate the laryngeal spasm. Often a ride in a car at night with the windows down accomplishes the same result. Occasionally, vomiting also relieves the spasm.
- Cough and cold medicines sometimes help, especially if the child has URI symptoms.
- If bronchospasm is also suspected, the use of bronchodilators in the usual doses prescribed for relief of asthma as discussed in Chapter 25 may be advantageous.
- Corticosteroids as part of the management of LTB are beneficial in decreasing the edema of the laryngeal mucosa. Corticosteroids reduce inflammatory edema and prevent destruction of ciliated epithelium (Behrman, Kliegman, & Jenson, 2004). A one-time dose of dexamethasone 0.6 mg/kg can be given as part of outpatient management. Antibiotics are not indicated.

Indications for Hospitalization. Children in distress with respiratory rates between 70 and 90 breaths per minute should be hospitalized. A child with a temperature higher than 102.2° F should be carefully evaluated; hospitalization may be necessary if other worrisome symptoms are also present. Racemic epinephrine by aerosol (a 2.25% solution diluted 1:8 with water in doses of 2 to 4 ml/15 min) may help. Corticosteroids are used and intravenous hydration may be necessary (Finberg & Bergelson, 2002).

TABLE 32-3 ***Differentiating Common Respiratory Diseases That Can Cause Stridor or Similar Signs***

Characteristic	LTB	Epiglottitis	Bacterial Tracheitis	Diphtheria	Foreign Body
Peak age	3-60 mo	2-7 yr	Most <3 yr	Any age/ unimmunized	Toddlers
Onset	Gradual, acute onset at night	Rapid	Acute	Gradual onset	Acute symptoms or gradual onset
Common findings	URI, seal-bark cough, mild-moderate dyspnea, symptoms worse at night	Sore throat, drooling, aphonia, looks toxic, dysphagia, tripod position	URI, may have cough, looks toxic, purulent sputum	Pharyngeal membrane, sore throat, nasal discharge, hoarseness	Coughing/choking episode, dyspnea, wheezing, cyanosis, signs and symptoms of secondary infection
Respiratory efforts	Rate generally <50	Marked distress	Marked distress	Minor to significant signs and symptoms of obstruction	Minor to significant distress
Fever	Common—low grade	High (39° C)	High (39° C)	Low grade	Normal to low grade
CBC	Generally normal	High, left shift	High, left shift	Normal to slight leukocytosis, decreased thrombocyte count	Normal unless secondary infection
Organism(s)	Usually viral: parainfluenza, adenovirus, RSV	Usually *Haemophilus influenzae* type b (HIB)	Usually *Staphylococcus aureus*	*Corynebacterium diphtheriae*	
Specific laboratory tests	None	None	None	Positive culture	None
Radiographic view/findings	Lateral or AP of neck/subglottic narrowing	Lateral of neck/thumb sign	Lateral of neck/subglottic narrowing	Signs of obstruction in severe cases	May see localized hyperinflation, mediastinal shift, atelectasis
Treatment	Humidification, corticosteroids in selected cases	Hospitalization, cefuroxime, corticosteroids	Hospitalization, *Staphylococcus* coverage	Hospitalization, erythromycin/ penicillin, antitoxin	Removal of foreign body, treatment of secondary infection/ bronchospasm
Intubation	Rare	Usually necessary	Frequently necessary	May be necessary	Endoscopy to remove foreign body
Prevention	None	Immunization—HIB	None	Immunization—DTaP	Education on child proofing home and monitoring child

AP, Anteroposterior; *CBC*, complete blood count; *LTB*, laryngotracheobronchitis; *RSV*, respiratory syncytial virus; *URI*, upper respiratory tract infection.

Complications

Increasing obstruction of the airways causes continuous stridor, nasal flaring, and suprasternal, infrasternal, and intercostal retractions. With further obstruction, air hunger and restlessness occur and are quickly followed by hypoxia, weakness, decreased air exchange, decreased stridor, increased pulse rate, and eventual death from hypoventilation. Anything that taxes the child's respiratory efforts such as crying or feeding causes more respiratory distress. Examination of the nasopharynx with a tongue depressor may result in sudden respiratory compromise. Severely ill children should be evaluated for acute epiglottitis.

Acute Spasmodic Croup

Description

Some children are prone to recurrent episodes of acute LTB. The term *acute spasmodic croup* is used to describe this condition. Recurrent croup may be related to airway hypersensitivity or allergy. The clinical manifestations and treatment plan are the same as indicated for acute LTB. The causes of spasmodic croup cannot be differentiated from the usual causes of croup; most likely a viral agent triggers the airway reaction.

Epiglottitis

Etiology

Epiglottitis occurs in children between 2 and 7 years of age. *H. influenzae* type b is usually the cause of this illness. Use of *H. influenzae* type b vaccine beginning at 2 months of age has resulted in a drastic decline in the number of children with invasive infections caused by this organism. Group A streptococcus is a rare cause of epiglottitis (Finberg & Bergelson, 2002).

Clinical Findings

History. An affected child has a sudden escalating course of fever, sore throat, and dyspnea and looks sick.

Physical Examination. Findings include the following:

- Inspiratory and sometimes expiratory stridor
- Drooling, aphonia, and high fever
- Rapidly progressive respiratory obstruction and prostration
- Flaring of the alae nasi and retraction of the supraclavicular, intercostal, and subcostal spaces
- Child assuming a position of hyperextension of the neck
- In older children, one may find
  - Complaints of sore throat and dysphagia
  - Stridor, brassy cough (uncommon), irritability, and restlessness
  - Child assuming a "tripod" position with mouth open and tongue hanging out

A rare, unusual finding is that of just a hoarse cough and a cherry-red epiglottis. No attempt should be made to examine the posterior pharynx because stimulation of the area can induce spasm and obstruction of the epiglottis and lead to respiratory arrest.

Diagnostic Tests. Blood cultures should be ordered. If the possibility of epiglottitis is thought to be remote in a patient with croup, a lateral neck radiograph may be obtained before the physical examination is undertaken. Absence of the "thumb" sign on the radiograph rules out the condition. A health care professional capable of supporting the airway and skilled in intubation must accompany the child to the radiology department and back.

Management

The time from the onset of symptoms until death may be only a matter of hours. Acute epiglottitis is a pediatric emergency! If epiglottitis is suspected, do not examine the throat. The child should not be placed in the supine position and should be immediately transported to the hospital. The child should be examined in the operating room by someone who can do an emergency tracheostomy. An airway must be established, either a nasotracheal airway or a tracheostomy. The diagnosis is confirmed in the operating room by depressing the tongue to view the swollen cherry-red epiglottis. Such children have a risk of reflex laryngospasm and acute and complete airway obstruction.

Begin the following treatments:

- Administer intravenous antibiotics that cover β-lactamase–producing *H. influenzae* in a septic dose schedule. Ceftriaxone sodium, 150 mg/kg per day in two divided doses, or an equivalent cephalosporin is given (Larsen et al, 2001).
- Administer oxygen.

The acute infection rarely lasts more than 48 to 72 hours. As improvement occurs, the child can be extubated, but antibiotic therapy should be continued for 10 days. Patients heal completely. Untreated or undertreated patients have a significant mortality rate. Remember that the time from the onset of symptoms to death can be a matter of hours. If *H. influenzae* is identified as the causative agent, rifampin prophylaxis (20 mg/kg in a single dose [maximum, 600 mg] for 4 days) should be given to all family contacts with children younger than 4 years and all child contacts younger than 4 years.

Prevention

Routine immunization against *H. influenzae* type b, the leading cause of epiglottitis, is the primary means of prevention.

Bacterial Tracheitis

Etiology

Bacterial tracheitis is an acute, potentially dangerous bacterial infection of the upper airway that does not involve the epiglottis. This condition occurs in younger children, usually younger than 3 years. *S. aureus* is the most common organism cultured. *H. influenzae* and *M. catarrhalis* have also been implicated as causative agents. Bacterial tracheitis usually follows a viral respiratory infection (generally parainfluenza virus type 1). No gender differentiation has been noted in the incidence or severity of symptoms (Behrman, Kliegman, & Jenson, 2004).

Clinical Findings

History. A brassy cough as part of a "typical viral LTB or URI" and a high fever may be reported.

Physical Examination. Copious purulent sputum is seen in older children. Inspiratory stridor develops and the child begins to look "toxic."

Diagnostic Tests. The diagnosis is based on confirming a bacterial upper airway infection. The white blood cell count will be elevated. Bacterial tracheitis can be differentiated from epiglottitis by its slower clinical course and a normal-appearing epiglottis on examination. The "classic" features of acute epiglottitis are absent (e.g., no thumb sign on a lateral neck film).

Management

Management issues include the following:

- The usual treatments for croup are ineffective, and hospitalization is necessary.
- Intubation or tracheostomy is usually necessary to bypass the swelling that develops at the level of the cricoid cartilage and to manage the copious purulent secretions.
- Antibiotics that cover staphylococcus are administered.
- Oxygen administration and airway support are necessary.
- Most patients become afebrile in 48 to 72 hours; the child is weaned from the artificial airway and usually does well.

INTRATHORACIC AIRWAY DISORDERS

Foreign Body Aspiration

Description

The symptoms and physical findings associated with aspiration of a foreign body depend on the nature of the material aspirated plus the location and degree of the obstruction. The cough reflex protects the lower airways, and most aspirated material is immediately expelled with coughing. Onset of a sudden episode of coughing without a prodrome or signs of respiratory infection should make the provider suspicious of foreign body aspiration.

Etiology

Objects that are either too large to be eliminated by the mucociliary system or cannot be expelled by coughing eventually lead to some form of respiratory symptomatology. Obviously, a large foreign body occluding the upper airway can cause suffocation. A small object in the lower respiratory tree may not produce symptoms for days to weeks. Obstruction results from either the foreign body itself or edema associated with its presence. Hot dogs are one of the most common causes of fatal aspiration.

Laryngeal Foreign Body

Clinical Findings

History. A rapid onset of hoarseness and the development of a croupy cough with aphonia are reported.

Physical Examination. The child can also have hemoptysis, dyspnea, wheezing, and cyanosis.

Diagnostic Tests. Because most foreign objects are not radiopaque, radiographs may not be useful in the diagnosis. If the history suggests foreign body aspiration, bronchoscopy must be undertaken. Direct laryngoscopy might reveal the presence of foreign matter.

Tracheal Foreign Body

Clinically, the child has a history of cough, hoarseness, dyspnea, and possibly cyanosis. The most characteristic signs of tracheal foreign body aspiration are the asthmatic wheeze and the audible slap and palpable thud sound produced by the momentary expiratory impact of the foreign body at the subglottic level.

Bronchial Foreign Body

The initial clinical findings are similar to those seen in either tracheal or laryngeal foreign body aspiration. Blood-streaked sputum may be expectorated. Children aspirating a metallic object often complain of a "metallic taste" in their mouths. If the object is nonobstructive and nonirritating, few or no initial symptoms may be seen. A small object can act as a bypass valve, and wheezes can be heard; emphysema or atelectasis can develop as the result of a large obstruction caused by a bronchial foreign body. The child may have limited chest expansion, decreased vocal fremitus, atelectasis, or emphysema-like changes with resulting hyporesonant or hyperresonant changes. Diminished breath sounds are often found. Crackles, rhonchi, and wheezes can be present if air movement is adequate. Most objects are aspirated into the right lung. A careful medical history may reveal a forgotten episode of choking.

Clinical Findings

History. An initial episode of coughing, gagging, and choking is described. Some objects are inhaled with no choking (e.g., a spear of grass). Hemoptysis rarely occurs as an early symptom but, on rare occasion, does occur as an initial symptom months or years after the aspiration event took place.

Physical Examination. If the acute episode is missed or not appreciated, a latent period of mild "wheezing" or cough may be seen. Lobar pneumonia, intractable wheezing, and status asthmaticus can develop.

Diagnostic Tests. Clinical suspicion is the clue to this diagnosis! Inspiratory and forced expiratory chest radiographs and chest fluoroscopy are useful in identifying radiolucent foreign bodies (Fig. 32-1).

Management. If the object is removed via bronchoscopy before permanent damage occurs, recovery is usually complete. Secondary lung infections and bronchospasms should be treated as suggested in the section on management of pneumonia and asthma.

Complications. If the foreign body is vegetable matter, vegetal or arachidic bronchitis can occur. This severe condition can be characterized by sepsis-like fever, dyspnea, and cough. If the material has been there for a long time, suppuration can occur.

Bronchitis

Description

The diagnosis of bronchitis is often made by practitioners and can be classified as acute or chronic. Acute bronchitis is usually caused by a viral agent resulting in inflammation of the tracheal and major bronchial mucosa. Chronic bronchitis, which is characterized by a productive cough lasting for more than 3 months, is usually a symptom of another chronic disorder (e.g., allergies, CF, cigarette smoking). It probably does not exist as a single pathologic entity in children (Leickley, 2002).

Etiology

This condition is usually preceded by a viral URI. Although a virus is the most common cause of true bronchitis, weakened tissue can succumb to a secondary bacterial infection. *S. pneumoniae, M. catarrhalis,* and *H. influenzae* are the most commonly cultured bacterial organisms.

Clinical Findings

History. The following are reported:

- A dry, hacking, unproductive cough begins a few days after the onset of rhinitis.
- The patient complains of low substernal discomfort or burning chest pain aggravated by coughing.
- The cough becomes productive after a few days, and shortness of breath can occur.

Physical Examination. Findings can vary and include the following:

- Low-grade or no fever
- Signs of nasopharyngeal infection, conjunctivitis, and rhinitis (common)
- Coarse breath sounds and coarse to fine moist rales
- The presence of rhonchi, which can be high pitched and resemble wheezes (sibilant)

Differential Diagnosis

Children with recurrent acute bronchitis must be evaluated for underlying pathology. Respiratory tract anomalies, foreign body aspiration, bronchiectasis, immunodeficiency, allergy, sinusitis, tonsillitis, exposure to air pollutants, adenoiditis, and CF must be considered in the

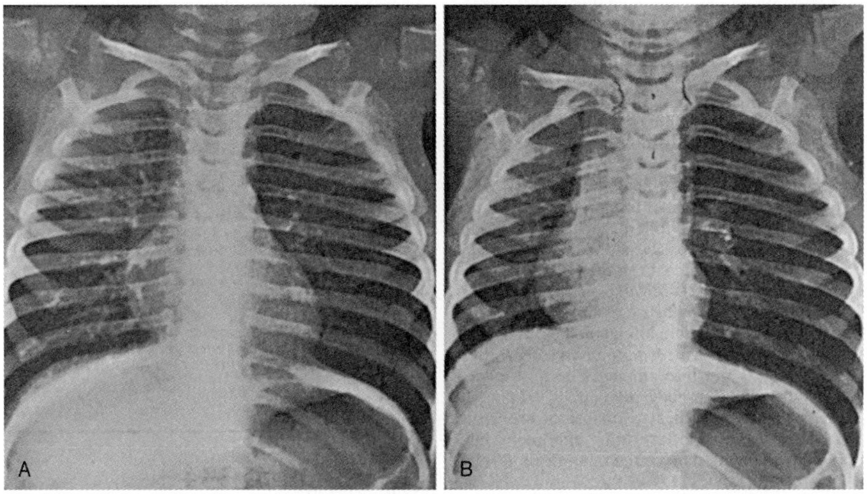

FIGURE 32-1 Obstructive overinflation caused by a peanut fragment in the left main stem bronchus. **A,** Inspiration. **B,** Expiration. (From Orenstein D: Foreign bodies in the larynx, trachea, and bronchi. In Behrman R, Kliegman RM, Jenson HB, editors: *Nelson textbook of pediatrics,* ed 16, Philadelphia, 2000, WB Saunders, p 1281.)

differential diagnosis. Check for tobacco or marijuana use in teenagers.

Management

No specific therapy is known, and most patients require none. Care is primarily supportive. Postural drainage and the use of a humidifier can be helpful. Cough suppressants should be prescribed judiciously. Antihistamines should not be used because of their excessive drying effect; these drugs tend to prolong the symptoms. If evidence of a bacterial infection such as high fever and crackles is observed, antibiotics may be considered. Mucus generally thins in 5 to 10 days, and the cough decreases.

Complications

In normal, healthy children, the condition is not serious; however, malaise continues for another week or so after the cough lessens. In undernourished or chronically ill children, otitis, sinusitis, and pneumonia are common.

Bronchiolitis

Description

Bronchiolitis is a common disease of the lower respiratory tract that causes inflammation leading to obstruction of the small respiratory airways. In mild cases, symptoms can last for 1 to 3 days. In severe cases, cyanosis, air hunger, retractions, and nasal flaring with symptoms of severe respiratory distress within a few hours may be seen.

Etiology

Bronchiolitis is a viral illness, with RSV responsible for more than 50% of cases. Parainfluenza virus (type 3), mycoplasma, or adenoviruses generally cause the remainder of cases. Adenovirus and RSV can cause long-term complications. Bronchiolitis commonly occurs in young children from infancy to 2 years of age. The source of infection is an older family member with a "mild" URI. Older children and adults have larger airways and tolerate the swelling associated with this infection better than infants do.

Clinical Findings

History. The following are reported:

- URI symptoms lasting for several days
- Moderate fever to 102° F
- Decrease in appetite
- Gradual development of respiratory distress

Physical Examination. Findings include the following:

- Paroxysmal wheezing
- High respiratory rate (approximately 60 to 80 breaths per minute)
- Varying signs of respiratory distress and pulmonary involvement (e.g., nasal flaring, retractions, cyanosis, prolonged expiration)
- Palpable liver and spleen because of their being pushed down by hyperinflated lungs

Diagnostic Tests. A chest radiograph displays hyperinflation of the lungs and increased anterior-posterior diameter. Some infants may have scattered areas of consolidation caused by atelectasis or inflammation of the alveoli. Early bacterial pneumonia can be difficult to detect and cannot be ruled out by radiographs. Immunofluorescence analysis of nasal washings is needed to detect RSV.

Differential Diagnosis

Making the diagnosis is not usually a problem. In mild afebrile cases, bronchial asthma can be confused with bronchiolitis. A successful challenge with bronchodilators favors the diagnosis of asthma. Less than 5% of cases of recurrent bronchiolitis have a virus as their cause. Other, rarer conditions to be ruled out include congestive heart failure, tracheal foreign body aspiration, organophosphate poisoning, CF, and bronchopneumonia with generalized obstructive emphysema.

Management

Most infants with mild signs of respiratory distress can be treated as outpatients.

- Supportive care consists of adequate hydration and use of antipyretics.
- Careful instructions must be given to parents regarding the following:
  - Management of rhinitis (use of saline drops)
  - Signs of increasing respiratory distress or dehydration that call for hospitalization
  - Indications for the use of antipyretics
  - Guidelines for feeding an infant with signs of mild respiratory distress (amount of fluid needed per 24 hours; smaller, more frequent feedings; monitoring of the respiratory rate; and guarding against vomiting)

Infants younger than 2 months and older infants with signs of severe respiratory distress should be hospitalized. Signs that suggest increasing respiratory distress include the following:

- Progressive stridor
- Stridor at rest
- Increasing respiratory rate
- Restlessness
- Hypoxia (recorded by either blood gas or pulse oximetry)
- Rising PCO_2 (recorded by blood gas)
- Pallor

- Cyanosis
- Depressed sensorium

In-hospital management focuses on supportive care and includes oxygen and elevation of the child to a sitting position at a 30- to 40-degree angle. The infant's neck should be extended to 30 to 40 degrees. Intravenous fluids are frequently needed because respiratory distress interferes with nursing or bottle feeding. Ribavirin (Virazole) can be considered in documented RSV infection in very ill infants with underlying diseases such as congenital heart lesions and immunodeficiencies. Ribavirin is expensive and a known teratogen in rats. Bronchodilators can be tried but are effective in only a small percentage of patients. Racemic epinephrine may be considered in infants with significant crackles. The use of corticosteroids is not effective (Weist, 2002).

Both LTB and bronchiolitis can cause significant respiratory tract damage. Occasionally, a hospitalized child may not be quickly weaned back to room air. Home management of these patients is extremely difficult and should be undertaken only by someone with excellent pulmonary skills and in consultation with a pediatrician or pediatric pulmonologist. The child should have an O_2 saturation study before discharge to help determine the O_2 requirements at rest, feeding, play, and sleep. A pneumogram to rule out apnea may also be indicated. Strict outpatient follow-up is mandatory for as long as the child is receiving home O_2.

Complications

The first 48 to 72 hours after the onset of cough is the most critical. Apneic spells are common in an infant. The child can be desperately ill but gradually improves. The fatality rate associated with bronchiolitis is less than 1%. Prolonged apnea, uncompensated respiratory acidosis, and profound dehydration secondary to loss of water from tachypnea and an inability to drink are the factors leading to death in young infants with bronchiolitis. A significant number of children in whom bronchiolitis developed during infancy suffer from reactive airway disease later in life.

Prevention

RSV immune globulin is used to protect high-risk infants from RSV. Palivizumab (Synagis) is an RSV-specific monoclonal antibody used for high-risk infants (see Chapter 25) (Bergelson & Finberg, 2002).

Pneumonia

Description

Pneumonia is a disease marked by inflammation of the parenchyma of the lung. Several subclassifications of pneumonia are recognized: bacterial, viral, other infectious agents, mycotic, aspiration, and a few other rare syndromes. It can also be characterized as lobar or interstitial pneumonia. Lobar pneumonia involves depositions in the alveolar space; in interstitial pneumonia, cellular infiltrates attack the walls of the alveoli and interstitial septae, with sparing of the alveolar space. Lobar and interstitial pneumonia, as well as bronchiolar and bronchial inflammation, can coexist in a child (Gaston, 2002). Table 32-4 differentiates the various forms of pneumonia commonly found in infants, children, and adolescents.

Bacterial Pneumonia

Description. Primary bacterial infection is less common in childhood than secondary bacterial infection after a viral infection. Viral infection affects the lung defenses by altering normal secretions, inhibiting phagocytosis, modifying the normal bacterial flora, and disrupting the epithelial layer. Thus the many childhood viruses set the stage for secondary bacterial infection. Children with immunologic problems or chronic illnesses are prone to primary bacterial pneumonia and experience recurrent pneumonias or fail to clear the initial infection completely. Differentiating bacterial from viral pneumonia is particularly important in infants younger than 6 months of age.

Etiology. The usual cause of bacterial pneumonia is *S. pneumoniae.* It causes more than 90% of cases of childhood bacterial pneumonia. Pneumococcal pneumonia occurs most commonly in the late winter and early spring, after the cycle of viral URIs. Asymptomatic carriers play a more important role in dissemination of disease than do sick contacts. Children younger than 4 years suffer the highest attack rate. Less common organisms include the following:

- GABHS is seen most frequently in children 3 to 5 years old.
- Group B β-hemolytic streptococcus causes pneumonia in neonates and infants.
- *Escherichia coli* and group B β-hemolytic streptococcus cause pneumonia in neonates; group B β-hemolytic streptococcus causes pneumonia in infants.
- *S. aureus,* a very serious infection, is more common in infants than in older children.
- Gram-negative organisms cause a small percentage of childhood pneumonias. These bacteria include *H. influenzae* (type b), *Klebsiella pneumoniae,* and *Pseudomonas aeruginosa.* They usually have significant morbidity and mortality rates. Altered host resistance is often associated with some of these infections.

Clinical Findings in Infants and Young Children

History. The following may be reported (Gaston, 2002):

- History of a mild URI for a few days and then an abrupt high fever to temperatures above 103.3° F (38.5° C)

TABLE 32-4 *Differentiating Various Forms of Pneumonia in Infants, Young Children, and Adolescents*

Characteristic	Bacterial	Viral	Mycoplasmal	Chlamydial
Common age	All ages	All ages	>5 y	3-19 wk
Onset	Acute; gradual	Acute; gradual	Slow	Gradual
Clinical findings	Depend on age; starts with URI, cough, dyspnea, tachypnea, rales, decreased breath sounds, grunting, retractions, toxic look	Depend on age; cough, coryza, hoarseness, crackles, wheezing	Persistent cough, malaise, headache	Tachypnea, staccato cough, crackles, wheezing rare, 50% have signs or history of conjunctivitis
Fever	Acute onset of fever (≥39° C)	Present	>39° C	Afebrile
CBC	WBCs often elevated >15,000/μl	Normal/slight elevation	Normal	Eosinophilia in 75% of cases
Organism(s)	90% caused by *Streptococcus pneumoniae*	RSV, parainfluenza, influenza (types A and B)	*Mycoplasma pneumoniae*	*Chlamydia trachomatis*
Radiographic findings	Lobar consolidation	Transient lobar infiltrates	Varies, interstitial infiltrates	Hyperinflation, infiltrates
Treatment	Depends on bacteria; penicillin, methicillin, cefuroxime, gentamicin, vancomycin	Supportive care	Erythromycin/clarithromycin	Erythromycin

CBC, Complete blood count; *RSV*, respiratory syncytial virus; *URI*, upper respiratory infection: *WBCs*, white blood cells.

- Cough, usually not severe
- Restlessness, shaking chills, apprehension

Physical Examination. Findings include the following:

- Nasal flaring, grunting, retractions
- Tachypnea generally greater than 50 breaths per minute in infants or greater than 40 breaths per minute at rest in a preschool child (may be the only clue), tachycardia, air hunger, cyanosis
- Fine crackles, dullness, diminished breath sounds
- Presence of a pleural effusion and signs of congestive heart failure
- Abdominal distention, downward displacement of the liver or spleen
- Nuchal rigidity without meningeal infection resulting from involvement of the right upper lobe
- Decreased peripheral perfusion and capillary refill
- Lethargy

Clinical Findings in Children and Adolescents

History. The patient can have

- Sudden onset of shaking chills, followed by a high fever, cough, chest pain
- Intermittent periods of drowsiness, restlessness, rapid respiration
- Dry, hacking, productive cough (with rust-colored or bloody sputum if expectorated)

Physical Examination. The following may be seen:

- Retractions, decreased tactile and vocal fremitus, and diminished breath sounds
- Dullness plus fine and crackling rales on the affected side
- Splinting of the affected side to minimize pleuritic pain or lying on the side in a fetal position—helps compensate for decreased air exchange and improves ventilation
- Progression to delirium, circumoral cyanosis, and posturing

Diagnostic Tests. Usual findings in a bacterial infection include the following:

- The white blood cell count is elevated with a left shift, and arterial blood gases are consistent with hypoxia.
- The organism may be found by culture of nasopharyngeal scrapings, tracheal aspirates, blood (only 30% of cases are positive), or lung tap fluid.
- Counterimmunoelectrophoresis results are positive.

- Radiographs are consistent with lobar or segmental consolidation. Staphylococcal pneumonia involves the right lobe 65% of the time. Pneumatoceles are common in staphylococcal pneumonia (Behrman, Kliegman, & Jenson, 2004; Bergelson & Finberg, 2002). Blood, urine, and cerebrospinal fluid cultures should also be obtained in infants younger than 3 months of age as part of a septic workup.

Differential Diagnosis. Other types of pneumonia, bronchiolitis, allergic bronchitis, congestive heart failure, acute bronchiectasis, aspiration of a foreign body, pulmonary abscess, and endotracheal tuberculosis are included in the differential diagnosis. Also, right lower lobe pneumonia can be confused with appendicitis. Right upper lobe pneumonia can often closely resemble meningitis.

Management. Management consists of appropriate antibiotic coverage, adequate fluid intake, and respiratory therapy (humidified oxygen) if needed. Older children with pneumococcal pneumonia can usually be treated safely at home if not in severe respiratory distress. Most children who are moderately ill and can be treated at home respond to amoxicillin. Common pharmacologic therapy is based on the infecting organism as outlined:

1. *S. pneumoniae* and β-hemolytic streptococcus:
   - Penicillin G (100,000 U/kg per 24 hours)—usually given as one 600,000 U intramuscular injection followed by oral penicillin.
   - Erythromycin and trimethoprim-sulfamethoxazole can be used in children with mild to moderate disease who are allergic to penicillin.
   - Third-generation cephalosporins are also used.
2. *S. aureus* (Behrman, Kliegman, & Jenson, 2004; Bergelson & Finberg, 2002):
   - Semisynthetic penicillinase-resistant penicillin (nafcillin, oxacillin, clindamycin, or vancomycin) should be used.
   - A chest tube may be needed if significant empyema is present.
3. *H. influenzae* (Nelson & Howenstine, 2002):
   - Mild—amoxicillin, amoxicillin-clavulanate, cephalosporin, erythromycin, clarithromycin, or azithromycin
   - Moderate to severe—cefuroxime or other second-generation cephalosporin, nafcillin, and gentamicin
4. *K. pneumoniae* and *P. aeruginosa*:
   - A third-generation cephalosporin and an aminoglycoside at the appropriate doses may be administered.

Pharmacologic management is often also based on age and the common organisms that are found in a particular age-group. Guidelines for treatment of pneumonia by age are as follows (Gaston, 2002):

- Infants and preschoolers:
  - Ampicillin/sulbactam at 200 mg/kg per day, divided every 6 hours; cefuroxime 150 mg/kg per day, divided every 8 hours; or ceftriaxone 75 mg/kg per day, divided every 12 to 24 hours.
  - For ill-appearing infants with lobar pneumonia, consider *S. aureus* (5% to 10% prevalence) as the infecting organism.
  - Remember that *Chlamydia trachomatis, Ureaplasma urealyticum*, and CMV can be acquired perinatally but not cause illness until later. See Chapter 24 for their management.
  - The infant who is clinically stable can be switched to ampicillin/clavulanic acid for a 10-day course of therapy. A 10-day course of ampicillin/clavulanic acid at 40 mg/kg per day divided every 8 hours can be used for a preschooler who is clinically stable, is not hypoxemic, is not in respiratory distress, and has reliable caretakers.
- School-age children and adolescents:
  - Ampicillin at 100 mg/kg per day, divided every 6 hours, or intravenous penicillin G at 150,000 U/kg per day, divided every 6 hours, can be used for the hypoxic hospitalized patient. For resistant pneumococcus, ceftriaxone at 80 mg/kg per day, once daily or divided twice daily, or a macrolide can be used. If sputum Gram stain suggests *H. influenzae* or *S. aureus*, parenteral ampicillin/sulbactam or cefuroxime or oral ampicillin/clavulanic acid can be used (Gaston, 2002).

Complications. By the second to third day, auscultation reveals a change in respiratory sounds as the infection begins to consolidate. Increased fremitus, tubular breath sounds, and the disappearance of crackles may be noted. As resolution occurs around the seventh day (the day of crisis in untreated cases involving children and adolescents), crackles can recur. Empyema is common in staphylococcal and GABHS infections.

Viral Pneumonia

Description. Viral pneumonia often involves both the conducting airways and the alveoli. This type of pneumonia is a common problem in young children and can result in serious illness in a young infant.

Etiology. Viruses commonly causing pneumonia in children, particularly infants, are RSV, adenoviruses, parainfluenza virus (types 1, 2, and 3), and enterovirus. Influenza virus, rhinovirus, and herpes simplex virus are less likely causative agents.

Clinical Findings

History. The onset of illness caused by viral pneumonia is similar to that caused by bacterial pneumonia—history of an initial URI. However, the progression of respiratory symptoms is slower in viral illnesses than in bacterial pneumonia.

Physical Examination. Findings may include the following:
- Tachypnea, cough, retractions
- Rales, wheezing, decreased breath sounds, cyanosis
- Other symptoms specific to the individual viral organism

Diagnostic Tests. The typical radiograph shows patchy (diffuse infiltrates) bronchopneumonia. Hyperinflation (hyperexpansion of the lungs) is a common radiographic finding (Fig. 32-2).

Management. Management of children with viral pneumonia is similar to that of children with bacterial pneumonia. Most children are managed as outpatients with
- General supportive measures consisting of hydration and antipyretics
- Antibiotics only if secondary bacterial infection is diagnosed
- Humidified oxygen, vigorous pulmonary therapy, and intubation (may be necessary for children in severe distress; such children require hospitalization)

Complications. Secondary bacterial pneumonia can be a frequent problem. Premature and young infants with chronic diseases and severe cases of pneumonia caused by RSV often require hospitalization (Behrman, Kliegman, & Jenson, 2004; Larsen et al, 2001).

Mycoplasmal Pneumonia

Description. Mycoplasmal pneumonia, or primary atypical pneumonia, is the most common cause of pneumonia in children older than 5 years through the young adult years. This disease is usually mild and self-limited.

Etiology. *M. pneumoniae*, an organism without a cell wall, is responsible for this form of pneumonia. It is transmitted from one symptomatic patient to another by droplet spread. The incubation period is 2 to 3 weeks, and asymptomatic carriage after infection can last for weeks.

Clinical Findings

History. Upper respiratory tract symptoms, low-grade fever (temperature greater than 39° C), and dry cough with scant sputum, often associated with a prodrome of chills, headache, sore throat, gastrointestinal symptoms, and malaise, are frequently reported. Rhinorrhea is not common (Gaston, 2002).

Physical Examination. Minimal changes or harsh breath sounds and rhonchi may be heard on auscultation.

Diagnostic Tests. Chest radiograph findings are nonspecific and reveal bronchovascular markings with areas of atelectasis.

Management. Erythromycin is the drug of choice for children younger than 9 years at 20 to 50 mg/kg per day in divided doses, two to four times per day. Azithromycin at 500 mg on day 1 is followed by 250 mg/day for the next 4 days. Tetracycline can be used in children 9 years of age or older (Gaston, 2002).

Complications. Most children have an uneventful recovery, but it is important to inform parents that their child's cough can last for several weeks. These children commonly have moderate dyspnea on exertion for 2 to 3 months. *M. pneumoniae* can spread to the blood, central nervous system, heart, skin, or joints. A child with sickle cell disease and mycoplasmal pneumonia has more severe pulmonary disease than the average child does.

Chlamydial Pneumonia of Infancy

Description. This type of pneumonia is transmitted from the infected genital tract of the mother to the infant. It does not become apparent until 2 to 19 weeks of age.

Etiology. *Chlamydia trachomatis* is an organism that has many subtypes within the species. Approximately 50% of infants born to infected mothers acquire this infection,

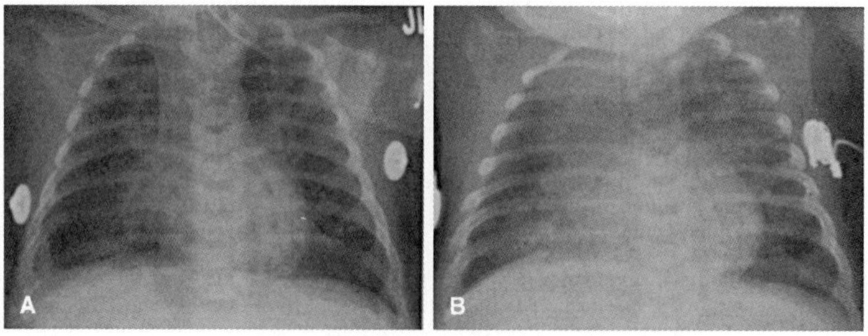

FIGURE 32-2 Six-month-old infant with rapid respirations and fever. An anteroposterior radiograph of the chest shows hyperexpansion of the lungs with bilateral fine air space disease and streaks of density, indicating the presence of both pneumonia and atelectasis. (From Prober CG: Pneumonia. In Behrman R, Kliegman RM, Jenson HB, editors: *Nelson textbook of pediatrics*, ed 16, Philadelphia, 2000, WB Saunders, p 761.)

but only 5% to 20% are at risk for chlamydial pneumonia. The incidence of this disease is increasing; the disease in untreated infants can linger and recur (AAP Committee on Infectious Diseases, 2003).

Clinical Findings

History. The infant is afebrile. A prior, concurrent, or no history of inclusion conjunctivitis is reported.

Physical Examination. Findings include

- Repetitive, staccato cough with tachypnea
- Cervical adenopathy
- Crackles and tachypnea, rarely wheezing

Diagnostic Tests. The diagnosis is often based on clinical signs and symptoms, as well as chest radiographic findings of hyperinflation and bilateral diffuse infiltrates. An eosinophil count of 300 to 400/mm^3 or greater and elevated serum IgG and IgM concentrations are indirect evidence of infection. An elevated serum titer of *Chlamydia*-specific IgM is diagnostic of the disease, but this test is not available in all laboratories. The organism may be cultured.

Differential Diagnosis. Other forms of bacterial, viral, or parasitic pneumonias or pertussis are included in the differential diagnosis.

Management. Most infants can be treated as outpatients; those with severe respiratory distress need hospitalization. Oral erythromycin (50 mg/kg per day in four divided doses for 14 days) is the treatment of choice (AAP Committee on Infectious Diseases, 2003). Some sources recommend a 10-day course of oral erythromycin at 50 mg/kg per day divided in four doses for 10 days (Gaston, 2002). Alternative therapies that are being studied for efficacy are azithromycin (10 mg/kg per day divided every 12 hours for 10 days) and clarithromycin (15 mg/kg per day divided every 12 hours for 10 days). However, these therapies have not been thoroughly investigated (Gaston, 2002).

Prevention. Identification and treatment of pregnant women with *C. trachomatis* in their genital tract are necessary for prevention.

Guidelines for Radiographic Follow-up after a Pneumonia

A follow-up chest radiograph should be obtained if there is no trend toward improvement; if there is persistent cough, dyspnea, or other physical findings; or if there is a worsening or recurrence of symptoms or physical findings. Patients who have had lobar pneumonia, mycoplasmal pneumonia, and *Chlamydia pneumoniae* tend to have a cough for weeks and moderate dyspnea on exertion for 2 to 3 months as part of a normal course in recovery. Children with recurrent pneumonias should be referral for further pulmonary evaluation.

Tuberculosis

Tuberculosis is discussed in Chapter 24.

Cystic Fibrosis

Description

CF is a multisystemic congenital disorder manifested by chronic obstructive pulmonary disease (COPD), gastrointestinal disturbances, and exocrine dysfunction.

Etiology and Incidence

CF is an autosomal recessive genetic disorder. It occurs in approximately 1 in 3500 white births. Although not common, it does occur in 1 in 17,000 black births and 1 in 90,000 Asian births. The basic insult is an inability to clear mucoid secretions and inadequate salt and water secretion on the cellular level. The endobronchial spaces are not cleared of their mucoid secretions, which leads to colonization by bacteria with resulting chronic inflammation and infection. Inadequate water secretion also causes desiccation of mucoid and proteinaceous secretions and, consequently, pulmonary and exocrine duct obstruction and tissue damage (Behrman, Kliegman, & Jenson, 2004).

Clinical Findings

CF is a multisystemic illness. Clinical manifestations include the following (Behrman, Kliegman, & Jenson, 2004):

- *Pulmonary.* CF is a major cause of severe chronic lung disease in children. The pulmonary system manifestations run the clinical spectrum from dry, frequent cough to COPD. Bronchitis, bronchiolitis, bronchiolectasis, and pneumonia are frequent. Bronchospasm resembling acute or chronic asthma may be present. The airways become colonized with *S. aureus, H. influenzae,* and, finally, *P. aeruginosa. Burkholderia cepacia* is a slower-growing organism found in children with CF. Pulmonary disease usually becomes progressive and leads to COPD, cor pulmonale, respiratory failure, and death. Other respiratory problems associated with CF include recurrent acute sinusitis and nasal polyps.
- *Gastrointestinal tract.* Meconium ileus develops in up to 15% of newborns born with CF. A meconium ileus syndrome equivalent can also develop in older patients, with desiccated fecal material causing gastrointestinal obstruction. Eighty-five percent of affected children have failure to thrive because of pancreatic enzyme insufficiency. These children have thick, fat-laden stools, poor muscle mass, and delayed maturation. Infants with CF who are fed soy-based formulas do very poorly, and severe hypoproteinemia and anasarca quickly result.

Other gastrointestinal problems associated with CF include intussusception, duodenal inflammation, gastroesophageal reflux, bile reflux, rectal prolapse, and vitamin E and K deficiencies with resulting bleeding diathesis or bleeding disorders.
- *Hepatobiliary tract.* Biliary cirrhosis occurs in 2% to 3% of children with CF and is characterized by jaundice, ascites, hematemesis from esophageal varices, and splenomegaly. Adolescent patients experience biliary colic and cholelithiasis.
- *Pancreas.* Recurrent acute pancreatitis is not uncommon. Diabetes mellitus develops in 8% of such patients, usually in the second decade of life.
- *Genitourinary tract.* Affected children have delayed sexual development. Ninety-five percent of males have fertility problems. The incidence of inguinal hernia, hydrocele, and undescended testes is higher. Females experience secondary amenorrhea, cervicitis, and decreased fertility. A pregnancy is usually carried to term if pulmonary function is not severely compromised.
- *Sweat glands.* Excessive salt loss can lead to hypochloremic alkalosis, especially in warm weather or after gastroenteritis. Children with CF often taste salty because of elevated amounts of NaCl lost in endogenous sweat.

Diagnostic Tests. The diagnosis of CF is based on an abnormal sweat test. Sweat tests should be done at a laboratory that regularly deals with children and routinely does these tests. Fifty to 100 mg of sweat should be collected to ensure accuracy and precision of the sweat test. A result of greater than 60 mEq/L of chloride is considered diagnostic of CF. Forty to 60 mEq/L is suggestive of CF, and less than 40 mEq/L is negative. Children with hypoproteinemia may elicit false-negative sweat test results.

Pancreatic function tests include 3-day stool collection to measure fat balance (a cumbersome test) and quantification of trypsin and chymotrypsin activity in a fresh stool sample (patients with CF have decreased stool trypsin and chymotrypsin activity). Glycosylated hemoglobin levels may be elevated in older children because of impaired pancreatic functioning (Behrman, Kliegman, & Jenson, 2004).

Pulmonary function tests are used to follow the clinical course.

Prenatal diagnosis has a 90% sensitivity for detecting a CF gene mutation on the long arm of chromosome 7. Newborn screening for immunoreactive trypsinogen is positive in 95% of cases. Routine screening of all newborns is not recommended.

Treatment

Children with CF have complicated treatment regimens and should be monitored by a multidisciplinary team. Pulmonary, nutritional, physical, and pharmacologic (antibiotic and antiinflammatory) therapy and psychologic counseling must be individualized for each child at each stage of the illness.

Syncope

A child with a syncopal episode requires a thoughtful approach. Many possible etiologies can produce syncopal episodes, including cardiovascular (neurally mediated, dysrhythmia, structural disease), neurologic (headache, seizure, transient ischemic attack), psychiatric (depression, panic attack, conversion reaction), and systemic or metabolic (drugs, carbon monoxide, electrolyte imbalance) (Johnsrude, 2000).

A detailed history and careful physical examination should be performed on all children with syncope. If warranted, the NP may order some initial screening diagnostic tests. Appropriate referral to pediatric specialists for further evaluation and diagnostic testing is suggested for children whose history, physical examination, or diagnostic tests suggest a potential pathologic problem that is outside the range of practice for the NP. See Chapter 31 for discussion about cardiac etiologies.

The initial approach to the assessment and management of syncope includes a thorough history and analysis of the symptom, a physical examination, and selected screening tests if indicated.

History

Important information to obtain about the syncopal incident includes whether the child had
- A triggering factor such as exercise, pain, or an emotional event
- A prior incident or incidents of syncope or fainting
- An associated injury, clonic-tonic movements, or vertigo
- Associated chest pain or palpitations
- A family history of sudden death
- The possibility of pregnancy or the use of drugs
- A history of exercise-induced reactive airway disease or respiratory distress
- A known psychologic stress or stressors at home or school or in social environments

Physical Examination

A detailed neurologic examination is needed if the syncopal episode suggests a seizure disorder. Careful evaluation of the head, eyes, ears, nose, and throat is done if vestibular disease is likely. A cardiovascular examination is always important.

Diagnostic Screening Tests

For possible cardiac causes of syncope, a 12-lead electrocardiogram (ECG) is performed and a 24-hour ambulatory monitor is used (if concerned with intermittent cardiac arrhythmia). If a seizure disorder is suspected, appropriate neurologic evaluation is done as outlined in Chapter 28. Note that a CBC, random glucose test, and glucose tolerance test have low yields and are not recommended as routine tests for a syncopal episode.

Pectus Excavatum

Description

Pectus excavatum, or funnel chest, is an abnormality of the skeleton and chest wall. Midline narrowing of the thoracic cavity and restriction in chest wall movement are characteristic.

Etiology and Incidence

Children with upper airway obstruction have a higher incidence, but about 86% of children with this defect are identified at birth or within the first year of life. The cause of pectus excavatum in these instances is often unknown. About 79% of cases occur in males, and a positive family history of chest wall deformity is found in about 37% of cases.

Clinical Findings

History. The parent may note a depression in the chest wall. A positive family history of chest wall deformity may be elicited.

Physical Examination. Findings include posterior depression of the sternum and costal cartilage.

Diagnostic Tests. Diagnostic tests include

- Chest radiography
- Exercise testing if substantial pectus deformity is present
- Other cardiac (echocardiogram) and pulmonary function studies as suggested by the degree of deformity and symptomatology

Management

If the deformity is the result of a pulmonary disease, early treatment of the underlying pulmonary problem occasionally resolves the skeletal deformity. Surgical repair depends on the severity of the defect, demonstration of a decrease in pulmonary function, progression of the defect on serial radiographs, or sometimes the patient's and parents' wish for cosmetic repair. If the patient is male with an associated scoliosis or has a severe defect, evaluate for Marfan syndrome.

> **RESOURCE BOX**
>
> ***Respiratory Disorders***
>
> **Cystic Fibrosis Foundation**
> 1-800-344-4823
> www.cff.org
>
> See Chapter 25 for resources related to respiratory conditions.

Complications

Pectus excavatum can also affect cardiac and pulmonary function.

REFERENCES

American Academy of Pediatrics Committee on Infectious Diseases: *2003 red book: report of the Committee on Infectious Diseases*, ed 26, Elk Grove Village, IL, 2003, American Academy of Pediatrics.

Behrman RE, Kliegman RM, Jenson HB, editors: *Nelson textbook of pediatrics*, ed 17, Philadelphia, 2004, WB Saunders.

Bergelson J, Finberg R: Lower respiratory infections. In Finberg L, Kleinman RE, editors: *Saunders manual of pediatric practice*, ed 2, Philadelphia, 2002, WB Saunders.

Berman S et al: Ear, nose and throat. In Hay WW et al, editors: *Current pediatric diagnosis and treatment*, ed 15, New York, 2001, McGraw-Hill.

Ditmar MK: Rhinitis and acute sinusitis. In Burg FD et al, editors: *Gellis and Kagan's current pediatric therapy*, ed 17, Philadelphia, 2002, WB Saunders.

Dolitsky JN, Ward RF: Foreign bodies of the ear, nose, airway and esophagus. In Hoekelman RA et al, editors: *Primary pediatric care*, ed 4, St Louis, 2001, Mosby.

Edelstein DR, Khabie N: Epistaxis. In Hoekelman RA et al, editors: *Primary pediatric care*, ed 4, St Louis, 2001, Mosby.

Finberg R, Bergelson J: Upper respiratory infections. In Finberg L, Kleinman RE, editors: *Saunders manual of pediatric practice*, ed 2, Philadelphia, 2002, WB Saunders.

Gaebler J: Pharyngitis and tonsillitis. In Finberg L, Kleinman RE, editors: *Saunders manual of pediatric practice*, ed 2, Philadelphia, 2002, WB Saunders.

Gaston B: Pneumonia, *Pediatr Rev* 23:132-140, 2002.

Haddad J: Foreign bodies in the ear, nose, and pharynx. In Burg FD editors: *Gellis and Kagan's current pediatric therapy*, ed 17, Philadelphia, 2002, WB Saunders.

Inkelis SH: Nosebleeds. In Berkowitz CD, editor: *Pediatrics: a primary care approach*, Philadelphia, 2000, WB Saunders.

Johnsrude CL: Current approach to pediatric syncope, *Pediatr Cardiol* 21:522-531, 2000.

Larsen GL et al: Respiratory tract and mediastinum. In Hay WW et al, editors: *Current pediatric diagnosis and treatment*, ed 15, New York, 2001, McGraw-Hill.

Leickley F: Bronchitis. In Finberg L, Kleinman RE, editors: *Saunders manual of pediatric practice*, ed 2, Philadelphia, 2002, WB Saunders.

Maggi C, Director, Critical Care and Pulmonary Medicine, Miller Children's Hospital, Long Beach, CA: Private correspondence, 1998.

Malhotra A, Krilov LR: Viral croup, *Pediatr Rev* 22(1):5-11, 2001.

McNamara M: Cough. In Schwartz MW, editor: *The 5-minute pediatric consult*, ed 2, Philadelphia, 2000, Lippincott Williams & Wilkins.

Nash D, Wald E: Sinusitis, *Pediatr Rev* 22(4):111-116, 2001.

Nelson RP, Howenstine MS: Pneumonia. In Finberg L, Kleinman RE, editors: *Saunders manual of pediatric practice*, ed 2, Philadelphia, 2002, WB Saunders.

Noble JE: Cough. In Berkowitz CD, editor: *Pediatrics: a primary care approach*, ed 2, Philadelphia, 2000, WB Saunders.

Rahbar R, McGill TJ: Rhinosinusitis. In Finberg L, Kleinman RE, editors: *Saunders manual of pediatric practice*, ed 2, Philadelphia, 2002, WB Saunders.

Turner RB, Hayden GF: The common cold. In Behrman J, Kliegman RM, Jenson HB, editors: *Nelson textbook of pediatrics*, ed 17, Philadelphia, 2004, WB Saunders.

Weist A: Bronchiolitis. In Finberg L, Kleinman RE, editors: *Saunders manual of pediatric practice*, ed 2, Philadelphia, 2002, WB Saunders.

Wetmore RF: Tonsils and adenoids. In Behrman J, Kliegman RM, Jenson HB, editors: *Nelson textbook of pediatrics*, ed 17, Philadelphia, 2004, WB Saunders.

33

Gastrointestinal Disorders

Ann M. Petersen-Smith

The gastrointestinal (GI) system functions to ingest and absorb nutrients and discard waste products. Appropriate functioning of the system is essential for normal growth and development and maintenance of other organ systems.

The nurse practitioner (NP) plays an integral role in the care of children with GI dysfunction. An understanding of the anatomy, physiology, and common disorders of the GI system allows NPs to thoughtfully assess and treat problems. This chapter focuses on GI disorders that involve organic pathology. Functional problems of the GI system such as obesity, anorexia, bulimia, encopresis, and constipation are discussed in Chapters 12 and 14.

ANATOMY AND PHYSIOLOGY

The GI system begins to develop during the third week of gestation. The primitive gut is initially formed and then divides into the foregut, midgut, and hindgut. The structures further develop in an intricate and complex fashion to become the digestive tract and accessory organs.

The GI tract extends from the mouth to the anus. It includes the organs of digestion and accessory organs such as the liver, pancreas, and gallbladder. The system provides the following functions:

- Ingestion of food
- Movement of food from the mouth toward the rectum
- Mechanical dissolution of food
- Chemical dissolution of food
- Absorption of nutrients
- Expulsion of waste products

The mouth serves as the site for ingestion, chewing, and mixing of food with saliva. The tongue senses the texture and taste of foods, which initiates salivation and release of gastric juices in the stomach. The esophagus transports food from the mouth to the stomach by *peristalsis*, the sequential contraction and relaxation of the musculature in the esophagus. The upper esophageal sphincter prevents air from being swallowed while breathing. The lower esophageal sphincter (LES) prevents food from being regurgitated from the stomach, which is important because intraabdominal pressure exceeds intrathoracic and atmospheric pressures. The stomach serves as a reservoir for ingested foods. It secretes digestive juices, mixes food with the gastric fluids, and propels the liquid material into the small intestine. The small intestine's primary function is absorption of nutrients (carbohydrates, fats, proteins, minerals, and vitamins) into the systemic circulation. Absorption occurs through villi, which cover the mucosal folds and serve as the functional unit of the intestine. Each villus contains an artery, a vein, and a lymph vessel, which serve to transport nutrients from the intestine into the systemic circulation. The villi are covered with enterocytes, whose major role is the digestion of carbohydrates and proteins. Enterocytes secrete proteins and enzymes known as brush border enzymes, which assist in digestion.

Carbohydrates must be converted to monosaccharides before their absorption is possible. This process begins in the mouth, where the salivary enzyme amylase breaks down complex starches into disaccharides. The brush border enzymes in the small intestine convert disaccharides into monosaccharides (sucrose to glucose and fructose, lactose to glucose and galactose, and maltose to glucose). When this process is hindered, disaccharides remain osmotically active and can cause diarrhea.

Fat absorption, which occurs mainly in the jejunum, is accomplished through the addition of lipases secreted by the pancreas. Lipases break down fats into particles that are easily absorbed by the villi. Fats then rely on the lymphatic system for absorption.

Proteins are converted to amino acids by pancreatic enzymes. The resulting amino acids are further divided into smaller amino acid particles that are absorbed via the brush border into the systemic circulation. After appropriate absorption of nutrients, the small intestine is left with the initial fecal liquid. This liquid is then propelled by peristalsis into the large intestine. The large intestine removes water from the fecal liquid and allows for short-term storage. The fecal mass, which consists of waste products, bacteria, intestinal secretions, and shed cells, is pushed into the sigmoid colon.

Entry of feces into the rectum stimulates the defecation reflex. This reflex stretches the rectal wall, relaxes the internal anal sphincter, and thereby creates the need to defecate. If this urge is ignored, further fluid resorption occurs as the stool is retained, gets larger, and becomes very dry. Excessive stretching of the colon from the hard, dry stool bolus can lead to decreased peristalsis, further complicating the retention of stool.

PATHOPHYSIOLOGY

The GI tract can be affected by illness, injury, or generalized problems that prevent it from functioning normally. Dysfunction can be localized or systemic. Categories of dysfunction include the following:

- Disorders of motility
- Infection
- Malabsorption syndromes
- Impairment of digestion, absorption, and nutrition
- Congenital malformations
- Genetic syndromes
- Metabolic disorders
- Behavioral problems
- Injuries and trauma

ASSESSMENT

History

The history assesses the following:

- Family history of gallbladder disease, ulcers, or allergy to any food product
- Past medical history related to the GI system (e.g., illnesses, surgeries, anatomic problems such as cleft lip/palate, esophageal atresia)
- Presence of pain (onset, location, type, quality, and aggravating and alleviating factors)
- Bowel habits (frequency, times per week, consistency, associated pain, aids such as medications or enemas)
- Constipation and diarrhea (patient's definition of each, how often they occur, treatment tried thus far)
- Changes in appetite
- Thirst level (increased or decreased)
- Food intolerance or allergy (what foods, symptoms, treatment)
- Belching and flatulence
- Vomiting
- Heartburn
- Feeding habits and nutrition history or current diet (what, when, how often, what tolerated)
- Apnea may be seen in infants with gastroesophageal reflux (GER)

Physical Examination

When assessing a suspected GI problem, a head-to-toe physical examination is frequently indicated.

- Plot growth parameters, including weight for height, to establish proportionality of the patient and exclude certain growth aberrations from the diagnosis.
- Determine body mass index (BMI). The BMI is a number that evaluates the child's weight status in relation to height to determine if a child is underweight or overweight. It is considered one of the first indicators used to assess body fat and a common method of tracking weight problems and obesity.
- Determine the patient's hydration status (skin turgor, mucous membranes, peripheral pulses, tears).
- Inspect the abdomen for visible peristalsis, rashes, lesions, asymmetry, masses, enlarged organs, and pulsations.
- Auscultate for frequency of bowel sounds (normal is 5 to 20 per minute).
- Percuss for density and to measure organs.
- Palpate both lightly and deeply.
- Assess peritoneal irritation:
    - Have the patient walk standing straight up or cough.
    - Have the patient stand on tiptoes and fall onto the heels.
    - Palpate for rebound tenderness.
    - Check for the obturator sign: A supine patient flexes the right thigh at the hip with the knee bent and internally rotates the hip. The sign is positive when it induces abdominal pain.
    - Check for the psoas sign: The patient lies on the left side and extends and then flexes the right leg at the hip. A positive sign is one that induces abdominal pain.
- Perform a rectal examination when intraabdominal, pelvic, or perirectal disease is suspected. This examination includes external inspection and internal palpation for masses, stool, or irregularities. The index finger should be used because of its increased sensitivity; however, in infants and young children use the fifth finger. Insert a gloved, lubricated finger into the rectum. Place the other hand on the abdomen for a bimanual examination. Young

pediatric patients should be supine with their feet held together and knees and hips flexed, putting their legs over their abdomen. Adolescent males can be lying on their side or standing with the hips flexed and the upper part of the body on the examination table. Adolescent females can be lying on their side or, if a concurrent pelvic examination is to be done, in the lithotomy position.
- Perform a gynecologic examination if pelvic pathology is suspected (see Chapter 36).

Common Diagnostic Studies

Laboratory tests are performed as indicated by the history, initial symptoms, and physical examination and include the following:
- Urinalysis (UA) and urine culture
- Complete blood count (CBC) with differential
- Serum chemistry screen, liver profile, lipid profile, erythrocyte sedimentation rate (ESR), C-reactive protein (CRP), thyroid function
- Pregnancy test
- Stool examination for ova and parasites, culture, blood, white blood cells, pH, Clinitest for reducing substances
- Fecal fat collection for 72 hours to rule out fat malabsorption
- Radiologic examination, including abdominal radiographs, abdominal and pelvic ultrasonography (US), chest radiographs (referred pain with pneumonia), upper and lower GI series, and radionuclide studies with scintiscan, depending on the suspected pathology
- Bone age to assess suspected growth abnormalities
- Papanicolaou smear and vaginal cultures and smears if pelvic pathology is suspected

Additional, more specialized tests can be ordered after consultation with a physician:
- Duodenal aspirate to identify existing infection
- Esophageal pH probe to establish GER, with a pH of less than 4 representing a reflux episode
- Breath hydrogen test if lactose intolerance is suspected
- Sweat chloride test if cystic fibrosis is suspected

MANAGEMENT STRATEGIES

Medications

Many common medications are used to treat various GI disorders:
- Antibiotics or antifungals may be necessary for bacterial or fungal infection.
- Antiemetics can be used to treat nausea or vomiting.
- Antidiarrheals are occasionally appropriate for persistent diarrhea or diarrhea associated with chronic disease, but they are never appropriate with acute diarrheal diseases because toxins need to be excreted from the body.
- Stool softeners, laxatives, and cathartics are useful in the acute treatment and long-term management of constipation and encopresis.
- Medications that alter GI motility or tone can be used to treat GER.
- Oral steroids, parenteral steroids, and other immunosuppressants may be indicated in the treatment of inflammatory bowel disease.
- Pain medication and antispasmodics may occasionally be used in selected acute and chronic GI conditions.
- Medications that alter gastric acidity can be used to treat GER and ulcer disease.
- Iron supplementation may be needed as supportive therapy for chronic disease.

Probiotics

Probiotics can be used as nutritional supplements. Probiotics are live microorganisms that, when ingested and colonized in the bowel, can have a therapeutic or preventive health benefit. Their effects have been most extensively studied in diarrheal disease and inflammatory bowel disease. Probiotics may be antagonistic to *Helicobacter pylori*, reduce symptoms of atopic disease, and be helpful in infant immunity (Markowitz & Bengmark, 2002; Vanderhoof & Young, 2002). See Chapter 43 for further information.

Nutrition

Normal nutrition that meets the recommended daily needs should be encouraged to promote normal GI function, growth, and development. Intake of fluids to ensure hydration is equally important. Dysfunction of the GI tract can be either short or long term and can require alterations in dietary intake. Consultation with a registered dietitian is important in designing an adequate diet for a child with a long-term GI problem. See Chapter 12 for more detail.

Activity

Age-appropriate activity should be encouraged on a regular basis to help maintain normal GI function. Some GI maladies require short-term rest, but generally the system functions better when activity is regular and consistent.

Counseling and Education

It is important to spend time assessing and planning for the unique needs of a child with GI dysfunction. Helping the family understand the disease or disorder and its course, prognosis, and management is essential. Planning for specific needs related to medication, diet, and activity assists the family to normalize life for the child.

UPPER GASTROINTESTINAL TRACT DISORDERS

Dysphagia

Description

In dysphagia, younger children are unable to swallow and older children can have an awareness that something is wrong with their swallowing ability.

Etiology

True dysphagia is never psychogenic, and patients with swallowing difficulties must be evaluated. Pharyngeal, laryngeal, and esophageal lesions, foreign bodies, anatomic malformations, physiologic dysfunction, neurologic dysfunction, and tumors can be responsible for symptoms.

Clinical Findings

History. The following may be reported:

- Progressive dysfunction
- Symptoms such as discomfort with swallowing or a sense of food getting stuck
- Picky eating, for example, a child preferring liquids to solids and refusing feedings

Physical Examination. Observe a feeding and the child's ability to swallow. Look for choking, vomiting, or regurgitation. Carefully palpate the neck to feel for masses.

Diagnostic Tests. Diagnostic tests include

- Lateral neck films
- Barium swallow
- Fluoroscopy

Differential Diagnosis

Obstructive and compressive lesions usually cause trouble only with solids. Physiologic dysfunction is usually associated with systemic disease, and the patient has trouble with both liquids and solids.

Management

Referral and treatment of the cause are needed.

Vomiting and Dehydration

Description

Vomiting is the forceful emptying of gastric contents. The type of emesis may assist in determining the cause (Murray & Christie, 1998, 2000). Nonbilious vomit is generally caused by infection, inflammation, metabolic, neurologic, or psychologic problems. An obstructive lesion generally causes bilious vomiting. Bloody vomit accompanies active bleeding in the GI tract.

Dehydration is the loss of water and extracellular fluid. Depending on the cause of dehydration, water and salts (primarily sodium chloride) may be lost in physiologic proportion or lost disparately, each producing a different clinical picture (Finberg, 2002). There are three types of dehydration: isonatremic (isotonic), hypernatremic (hypertonic), and hyponatremic (hypotonic). When dehydration is caused by simple diarrhea, homeostatic mechanisms can usually maintain sodium concentrations in the serum, resulting in isonatremia. When vomiting occurs with diarrhea and water intake is less, there is greater water loss than salt loss, potentially resulting in hypernatremic dehydration. When there is massive stool loss of water and salt, and only water is ingested, there is a large salt loss, potentially resulting in hyponatremia (Finberg, 2002).

Etiology and Incidence

Vomiting is one of the most common symptoms in childhood. Following is a list of the causes of vomiting by site of origin (Acker, 2002; Murray & Christie, 2000):

- Oropharynx: cleft palate and laryngopharyngeal cleft
- Upper GI: congenital stricture, foreign body, gastritis/esophagitis, gastric web pyloric stenosis, tracheoesophageal fistula, vascular ring, peptic ulcer disease
- Small intestine: annular pancreas, choledochal cyst, intestinal atresias and stenoses, intestinal malrotation with volvulus, intestinal pseudoobstruction
- Colon: Hirschsprung disease, intussusception, meconium ileus, necrotizing enterocolitis, fecal impaction
- Hepatobiliary or pancreatic dysfunction
- Infections: bacterial enteritis, otitis media, sepsis, urinary tract infection, viral gastroenteritis (VGE), hepatitis
- Neurologic: congenital anatomic malformation, gray and white matter degenerative disorders, hydrocephalus, kernicterus, brain tumors, migraine headache, head trauma
- Other: cow milk protein allergy, inborn errors of metabolism, maternal drug exposure/withdrawal, toxic ingestions, appendicitis, cyclic vomiting, pneumonia, drug/alcohol ingestion, eating disorders, pregnancy

Clinical Findings

History. The history should assess the following:

- Past history of illnesses, surgeries, or hospitalizations
- Medications currently being taken (including over-the-counter, herbal, cultural, and homeopathic remedies)
- Recent exposure to illness, injury, or stress
- Family history of GI disease or fetal or neonatal deaths

- Onset and duration of vomiting, quality and quantity, presence of blood or bile, odor, precipitating event
- Relationship of vomiting to meals, time of day, or activities
- Vomiting early in the morning
- Presence of associated symptoms: diarrhea, fever, ear pain, urinary tract infection (UTI) symptoms, vision changes, headache, seizures, high-pitched cry, polydipsia, polyuria, polyphagia, anorexia
- Symptoms of dehydration (Table 33-1)

Physical Examination. The following are needed:

- Assessment of dehydration (see Table 33-1). One of the most useful clinical signs of hydration is capillary refill time (CRT). Normal CRT is less than 2 seconds. Research has shown that a CRT of 2 to 2.9 seconds corresponds to a 50 to 90 ml/kg loss, 3.0 to 3.5 seconds corresponds to a 90 to 110 ml/kg loss, 3.5 to 3.9 corresponds to a 110 to 120 ml/kg loss, and more than 4 seconds corresponds to a 150 ml/kg loss (Finberg, 2002).
- Growth parameters and vital signs.
- Neurologic examination: nuchal rigidity, level of consciousness, and behavioral changes, which can include irritability or lethargy. Sensorium remains intact until there is greater than 6% of weight loss as a result of dehydration. Hypotension is a late manifestation of dehydration (Finberg, 2002).
- Abdominal examination: Inspect for distention, visible peristaltic waves; auscultate bowel sounds (i.e., increased with gastroenteritis, decreased with obstruction, absent with ileus or peritonitis); assess liver and spleen size, masses; perform a rectal examination as indicated.
- Respiratory examination: tachypnea, decreased oxygen saturation.
- Perform a pelvic examination as indicated.

Diagnostic Tests. Diagnostic studies are performed as indicated by the probable diagnosis (Acker, 2002):

- CBC with differential, blood culture, liver function tests, glucose, ammonia, electrolytes, CRP, ESR
- UA and urine culture

TABLE 33-1 ***Estimation of Dehydration***

	Extent of Dehydration			
Characteristic	**Mild**	**Moderate**	**Severe**	**Shock**
Weight loss—infants (%)	3-5	5-10	10-15	>15
Weight loss—children (%)	3-4	6-8	10	
Pulse	Normal	Slightly increased	Very increased	Rapid and weak
Blood pressure	Normal	Normal to orthostatic, >10 mm Hg change	Orthostatic to shock	
Behavior	Normal	Irritable, more thirsty	Hyperirritable to lethargic	Difficult to awaken/ unresponsive; too weak to stand; very dizzy
Thirst	Slight	Moderate	Intense	
Mucous membranes*	Normal	Dry	Parched	
Tears	Present	Decreased	Absent; sunken eyes	
Anterior fontanel	Normal	Normal to sunken	Sunken	
External jugular vein	Visible when supine	Not visible except with supraclavicular pressure	Not visible even with supraclavicular pressure	
Skin* (signs and symptoms less useful in children >2 yr of age)	Capillary refill >2 sec	Slowed capillary refill, 2-4 sec (decreased turgor)	Very delayed capillary refill (>4 sec) and tenting; skin cool, acrocyanotic, or mottled*	Capillary refill time >4 sec; cold/ acrocyanotic
Urine production	Slight decrease	Infants: no urine for >8 hr Children: no urine for >12 hr	Very decreased or absent	Anuria
Urine specific gravity	>1.020	>1.020; oliguria	Oliguria or anuria	

From Jospe N, Forbes G: Fluids and electrolytes: clinical aspects, *Pediatr Rev* 17:395-403, 1996.
*These signs are less prominent in patients who have hypernatremia.

- Toxicology screen
- Stool for culture and occult blood, leukocytes, parasites, fat, pH as indicated
- Rapid strep test/throat culture
- Pregnancy test
- Abdominal radiograph (obstructions, organomegaly, foreign body, ingestion, and some masses)
- Ultrasound (abscesses, masses, stenoses, cysts, appendicitis, pyloric stenosis)
- Barium swallow/enema (malrotation, pyloric stenosis, GER, masses)
- Endoscopy (obstruction, hemorrhage, infection; collect biopsies)
- Esophageal pH probe analysis
- Computed tomography (CT) scan or magnetic resonance imaging (MRI) looking for masses, inflammation, herniations, perforations, and obstructions
- Electroencephalogram (EEG)

Differential Diagnosis

The differential diagnosis includes all other causes of vomiting, including organic lesions, chronic problems, and eating disorders (weight loss); overfeeding (weight gain); esophageal disorders, achalasia, and stricture (undigested food in the vomitus); metabolic disease and increased intracranial pressure (early-morning vomiting); psychogenic or peptic ulcer disease (PUD) (vomiting after meals); hepatobiliary or pancreatic dysfunction (if vomiting does not relieve pain); obstruction (bilious vomiting); volvulus and malrotation (intermittent vomiting); and gastroenteritis (concurrent diarrhea).

Management

The following steps are taken:

- Determine the degree of dehydration and treat the cause.
- Provide for an initial period of bowel rest.
- Rehydrate (Box 33-1). After 1 to 2 hours with nothing by mouth, introduce an appropriate rehydration solution. Avoid plain water, apple juice, soda, milk, and sports drinks because none of these liquids provides appropriate replacement of sugars and electrolytes (Table 33-2). Begin with small amounts (as little as 5 to 10 ml) of clear liquids offered frequently. Breastfed infants should continue to breastfeed more frequently for shorter periods.
- Resume maintenance fluid levels (see Box 33-1).
- Avoid solids for 4 to 6 hours, and then reintroduce age-appropriate bland solids slowly as tolerated. Bland solids might include complex carbohydrates, bananas, applesauce, pretzels, and rice or rice cereal.
- Prescribe antiemetics cautiously (promethazine [Phenergan], 0.5 to 1 mg/kg per dose per rectum every 6 hours) if vomiting is excessive, dehydration imminent, and GI pathology excluded.
- Monitor urine output.

BOX 33-1 *Treatment of Dehydration*

Rehydration (with Increased Sodium Concentration)

Mild	ORS	40-50 ml/kg over 4 hr (10 ml/kg per hr)
Moderate	ORS	60-100 ml/kg over 4-6 hr (20 ml/kg per hr)
Severe	IV fluids	Ringer's lactate or normal saline, 20 ml/kg bolus over 1 hr; may repeat bolus if needed (until pulse, perfusion, mental status are normal)
		Follow with 5% dextrose with NaCl and KCl added (once the child has voided) for maintenance fluids and abnormal loss replacement (see later); if severe dehydration, give one half amount over 8 hr, the other one half over the next 16 hr; include bolus amounts in the 24 hr total
		Begin ORS as soon as possible

Maintenance

Total water volume	0-10 kg	100 ml/kg per 24 hr
	10-20 kg	1000 ml + 50 ml/kg for each kg over 10 kg/24 hr
	>20 kg	1500 ml + 20 ml/kg for each kg over 20 kg/24 hr

May give up to 150 ml/kg in first 24 hr

Replacement of Fluid Losses (If Continued, Heavy Losses)

10 ml/kg or 4-8 oz of ORS for each diarrhea stool (1 to 1.5 times the amount of stool)

BOX 33-1 *Treatment of Dehydration—cont'd*

Refeeding

Reintroduce age-appropriate diet within 24 hr. Avoid fatty foods and foods high in simple sugars.
Encourage complex carbohydrates, lean meats, yogurt, bananas, and applesauce.
Formula-fed infants should have full-strength formula. If that is not tolerated, use lactose-free or soy formula.
Breastfeeding infants should continue to breastfeed with shorter duration and more frequent feedings.
Use regular milk for older children.

Data from Lasche J, Duggan C: Managing acute diarrhea, *Contemp Pediatr* 16(2):74-83, 1999; Jospe N, Forbes G: Fluids and electrolytes: clinical aspects, *Pediatr Rev* 17(11):395-403, 1996; Northrup RS, Flanagan TP: Gastroenteritis, *Pediatr Rev* 15(12):461-472, 1994.
IV, Intravenous; *ORS*, oral rehydration solution.

TABLE 33-2 *Rehydration Solutions*

				Base		Carbohydrate		
	Sodium*	Chlorine*	Potassium*	Type	Concentration*	Type	Concentration (g/L)	Osmolality
Stool								
Pediatric diarrheal stool	50-100	75-90	25-35	HCO_3	25-40	—	—	250-300
Oral Rehydration Solutions								
Recommended:								
WHO ORS[II]	90	80	20	Citrate	30	Glucose	20	<300
WHO recommendations for ORS solutions	60-90	50-80	20-30	Citrate	25-35	Glucose	20	<300
Pedialyte (Ross)	45	35	20	Citrate	30	Glucose	25	<264
Rehydralyte (Ross)	75	65	20	Citrate	30	Glucose	25	<327
Cereal-based ORS	60-90	—[†]	—[†]	—[†]	—[†]	Starch[‡]	50	200-225
Infalyte (Mead-Johnson)	50	45	25	Citrate	34	Rice syrup solids	30	
Home sugar-salt solution	30-60	30-60	—	—	—	Sucrose	40	170-230
Other solutions:								
Soft drinks, cola, etc.	2	(—)[§]	0.1	HCO_3	13	F/G	50-150	<550
Apple juice	3	(—)[§]	32	—	0	F/G/S	63	<700
Chicken broth	250	(—)[§]	5	—	0	—	0	<450
Gatorade	20	(—)[§]	3	HCO_3	3	G/others	45	<330
Intravenous Solutions								
Recommended:								
Ringer's lactate	135	90	4	Lactate	49	—	—	<278
Normal saline	135	135	0	—	0	—	—	<270
5% dextrose in saline	135	135	0	—	0	Glucose	50	<545
Not recommended:								
5% dextrose in water	0	0	0	—	0	Glucose	50	<275

From Northrup RS, Flanigan TP: Gastroenteritis, *Pediatr Rev* 15(12):461-472, 1994.
*In millimoles or milliequivalents per liter.
[†]Variable.
[‡]From various cereals: rice, wheat, sorghum, etc.
[§]Value not reported.
[II]Not available in the United States but used worldwide.
F, Fructose; *G*, glucose; *ORS*, oral rehydration solution; *S*, sucrose; *WHO*, World Health Organization.

8. Treat fever.
9. Refer if the child has a toxic appearance or moderate to severe dehydration, projectile vomiting, abnormal examination, vomiting for greater than 12 hours, or vomiting of blood, bile, or fecal matter.

Cyclic Vomiting Syndrome

Description

Cyclic vomiting syndrome (CVS) is characterized by recurrent stereotypical spells of vomiting, between which the child is completely well (Li & Howard, 2002). The International Scientific Symposium on Cyclic Vomiting Syndrome (Li, 1995) identified the following diagnostic criteria:

- *Essential criteria* include recurrent severe, discrete episodes of vomiting; varying intervals of normal health between episodes; duration of vomiting lasts hours to days; and there is no apparent cause of vomiting (negative laboratory, radiographic, and endoscopic testing).
- *Supportive criteria* include a pattern that is stereotypical (each episode is similar as to onset, intensity, duration, frequency, associated symptoms, and signs within individuals) and self-limited (episodes resolve spontaneously if left untreated).
- *Associated symptoms* include nausea, abdominal pain, headache, motion sickness, photophobia, and lethargy.
- *Associated signs* include fever, pallor, diarrhea, dehydration, excess salivation, and social withdrawl.

Although the typical child with CVS is well up to 90% of the time, there is substantial morbidity and medical costs when the episodes occur (e.g., 20 missed days of school per child, high rate of intravenous rehydration, laboratory costs, imaging studies, endoscopic procedures, emergency department visits, and missed work by parent) (Li & Balint, 2000).

Etiology and Incidence

The prevalence of CVS is unknown. It causes one third of recurrent vomiting in children (Li & Howard, 2002). The female-to-male ratio is 5:4. CVS occurs in all races, and average age of onset is 5.3 years old. It generally takes 2.6 years to make the diagnosis, and the condition lasts an average of 3.4 years. Most children appear to outgrow CVS before or during the preteen years; however, approximately 28% of children with CVS suffer migraine headaches as adolescents and adults (Li & Balint, 2000).

Clinical Findings

History

- Very careful listening is important! This diagnosis is made mostly on history alone.
- Recurrent episodes. Episodes usually last 24 to 48 hours; they occur at regular intervals, usually every 2 to 4 weeks, although many children have unpredictable episodes.
- The child may have a prodromal period (some combination of pallor, anorexia, nausea, abdominal pain, or lethargy) or a recovery period (from ill to playing again) that is brief.
- Episodes more likely to occur at night (2:00 to 4:00 AM) or early in the morning (6:00 to 7:00 AM).
- Episodes generally begin and end abruptly.
- There may be a precipitating event (infection, positive or negative psychologic stress, diet changes, menstruation) (Li & Balint, 2000).
- Vomiting may occur as frequently as every 5 to 10 minutes, unmatched in any other disorder (Pfau et al, 1996).
- Bilious vomiting and hematemesis occur 76% and 32% of the time, respectively.
- Abdominal pain, retching, anorexia, nausea, or diarrhea may occur.
- Headache, photophobia, phonophobia, or vertigo may occur.
- Family history is positive for migraine headache.

Physical Examination

- The child appears ill. Children with CVS appear substantially more ill than children with VGE.
- The child appears pale, as if in shock.
- The child is often locked into a fetal position by unrelenting pain and nausea.
- Even before the child is dehydrated, the child may become so listless that he or she cannot walk or talk (Li, 2001).

Diagnostic Tests. Three questions are essential to make the diagnosis of CVS (Li & Howard, 2002):

- Has the child had at least three episodes? (One hundred percent respond "Yes.")
- Is the child completely asymptomatic between episodes? (One hundred percent respond "Yes.")
- Are the episodes stereotypical? (Ninety-eight percent respond "Yes.")

"Red flags" to be aware of and to guide further evaluation include severe headache, GI bleeding, unilateral abdominal pain, weight loss, failure to respond to any treatment, progressive worsening, prolonged episodes requiring repeat hospitalizations, and a change in pattern or symptoms (Li & Howard, 2002).

Laboratory testing is needed to exclude other diagnoses (approximately 12% of children with CVS-like history have a specific underlying disorder and may require guidance from a gastroenterologist) (Li & Howard, 2002; Ravelli, 2001).

- CBC with differential
- Electrolytes, glucose

- Liver function tests (LFTs), metabolic screening during an episode (lactate, ammonia, amino acids, and porphobilinogen)
- UA and urine culture, urine organic acids
- Radiology: small bowel radiography, abdominal US, MRI or CT of head or sinuses (or both), and endoscopy as indicated

Differential Diagnosis

The differential diagnosis includes any other cause of vomiting or abdominal pain.

Management

Supportive measures include the following (Li & Balint, 2000):

- Quiet, dark room
- Intravenous fluids to replace losses
- Antiemetics (diphenhydramine, lorazepam, promethazine)
- Sedation to reduce nausea (diphenhydramine, lorazepam)
- Analgesics as needed (meperidine, diphenhydramine)
- Abortive measures (administered at the onset of symptoms or if child has less than one episode per month)
- Antiemetics (granisetron, ondansetron)
- Migraine relief
    - Acute (ketorolac, sumatriptan)
    - Prophylactic—if more than one episode per month (amitriptyline, cyproheptadine, phenobarbital, propranolol)
    - Menstrual relief (leostrin)
- Prokinetic (erythromycin, which accelerates gastric emptying)

Referral to a gastroenterologist is recommended when further testing is needed (endoscopy), when atypical or "red flag" symptoms occur, or if the child fails to respond to treatment.

Gastroesophageal Reflux

Description

GER refers to the passage of gastric contents into the esophagus from the stomach through the LES. It can be a normal phenomenon. Three classifications of GER are recognized:

- Physiologic: infrequent, episodic vomiting
- Functional: painless, effortless vomiting with no physical sequelae
- Pathologic: frequent vomiting with alteration in physical functioning (e.g., esophagitis, failure to thrive [FTT], aspiration pneumonia)

Etiology and Incidence

The etiology is unclear and probably multifactorial. The LES usually is influenced by intraabdominal pressure, hormones, neurologic control, and age. LES tone is normal in infants and children with GER. Inappropriate relaxation of the LES may be responsible for many instances of GER. Animal studies suggest that newborn and infant gastric musculature may function differently from the gastric musculature of adults. Young infants have increased intraabdominal pressure because of their inability to sit upright.

Alterations in swallowing, pharyngeal coordination, and esophageal motility and delayed gastric emptying are also potential factors related to GER. Children with neurodevelopmental disability commonly have GER. Increased muscle tone, chronic supine positioning, and altered GI motility exacerbate GER.

Up to 70% of infants less than 1700 g have pathologic GER. Forty percent have symptomatic improvement by 4 months of age, and 85% are symptom free by 12 months (Orenstein, 1999; Sondheimer, 2003).

Clinical Findings

History. Important historical information to elicit includes the following:

- Careful birth, medical, and social history
- Concerns about feeding difficulty, pulling from the bottle or breast, refusing to eat, crying, choking, coughing, wheezing, apnea, weight loss, irritability, continuous unexplained crying, recurrent respiratory infections, pneumonia, and bloody emesis in younger children
- FTT
- Acute life-threatening event (ALTE) (Cadranel, 2001)
- Sandifer syndrome, abnormal behavior and posturing with tilting of the head to one side and bizarre contortions of the trunk
- Heartburn, painful belching, headache, dyspnea, abdominal pain, stool pattern changes, dental caries, or recurrent pneumonia
- A 24-hour diet history and discussion of feeding circumstances

Physical Examination. Findings can include the following:

- Signs of FTT
- Torticollis
- Hoarseness
- Anemia
- Tooth erosion resulting from destruction of enamel by gastric acids caused by frequent vomiting
- Rash, recurrent diarrhea, persistent vomiting, or early-morning vomiting (symptoms of other primary disease with GER as a secondary problem)

Diagnostic Tests. In most infants with vomiting and in older children with regurgitation and heartburn, a history and physical examination are sufficient to reliably diagnose GER, recognize complications, and initiate treatment

(North American Society for Pediatric Gastroenterology and Nutrition [NASPGN], 2001). The following tests may be obtained. Special studies should be ordered as indicated following consultation with a physician or a pediatric gastroenterologist.

- CBC with differential to rule out anemia and infection
- UA and urine culture
- Stool for occult blood
- Abdominal US to rule out pyloric stenosis if age appropriate
- Upper GI series (test is neither sensitive nor specific for the diagnosis of GER but is useful for the evaluation of anatomic abnormalities such as pyloric stenosis or malrotation) (NASPGN, 2001)
- Endoscopy to rule out esophagitis and other pathology if deemed necessary
- Esophageal pH monitoring (test is a reliable way to diagnose GER, with a pH lower than 4 indicating reflux; however, esophageal pH may be normal in some patients with GER, especially those with respiratory complications) (NASPGN, 2001)
- Intraluminal electric impedance measures episodes of GER independent of the pH of the fluid (especially useful for diagnosis in children with respiratory events related to GER because it can measure multiple indices such as heart rate, oxygenation, sleep state, and apnea episodes) (Wenzl et al, 1999)
- Radionucleotide scan with scintiscan if deemed necessary

Differential Diagnosis

Included in the differential diagnosis are anatomic obstruction, antral or esophageal webs, masses, malrotation, otitis media, UTI, gastroenteritis, formula intolerance, inborn errors of metabolism, brain tumors, increased intracranial pressure, Reye syndrome, obstructive uropathy, pancreatitis, and hepatobiliary problems (Chang, 1999).

Management

- See Figs. 33-1 and 33-2.
- A period of empiric therapy may be useful in determining if GER is causing a specific symptom.
- Breastfed infants should continue to breastfeed.
- Formula-fed infants: There is evidence that a 1- to 2-week trial of a hypoallergenic formula in formula-fed infants is helpful. Use smaller, more frequent feedings and frequent burping during feedings. Milk-thickening agents may decrease the number of episodes of vomiting but may not change the pH probe monitoring results (NASPGN, 2001).
- Prone positioning is the most beneficial for infants with GER; however, the risk of sudden infant death syndrome (SIDS) outweighs the benefits associated with lying prone. The supine position is preferred in all infants, including those with GER. In children older than 1 year of age, there is benefit to left-side positioning during sleep with the head of the bed elevated (Ewer, James, & Tobin, 1999; NASPGN, 2001).
- For older children, avoid chocolate, caffeine, high-fat foods, spicy foods, alcohol, and bedtime snacks. For children who are obese, weight loss is recommended.
- See Table 12-10 for feeding strategies in patients with GER.
- Medications can be helpful when the aforementioned measures have failed to give relief (Table 33-3). Chronic antacid therapy is generally not recommended.
- Close follow-up of growth parameters to ensure adequate weight gain is important.
- Refer for Nissen fundoplication or similar surgical procedures if the GER is severe, not well managed medically, or causing significant secondary morbidity.

Complications

Complications include FTT, aspiration, recurrent pneumonia, apnea, wheezing, esophagitis with pain, bleeding and formation of strictures, weight loss, irritability, malnutrition, and developmental delays. GER has been implicated in SIDS.

Patient Education

- Assure parents of infants that GER is usually self-limited and that symptoms improve as the child grows.
- Remind parents that GER may temporarily worsen during illness.
- Review medication information, including dosages and side effects.

Peptic Ulcer Disease

Description

PUD consists of a group of gastric and duodenal disorders. With duodenal ulcers, mucosal defects penetrate the duodenal mucosa and submucosa. Gastric ulcers result from gastric mucosal defects that penetrate the mucosa and submucosa.

Etiology and Incidence

Primary ulcers tend to be duodenal, have no underlying cause, and tend to be chronic with granulation tissue and fibrosis (Hassall, 2001). Secondary ulcers are more often gastric, generally more acute, and associated with known ulcerogenic events (Sondheimer, 2003). Ulceration in children is commonly associated with stressful situations, medications, and critical illness. A strong familial predisposition for PUD has been noted. There is no evidence that

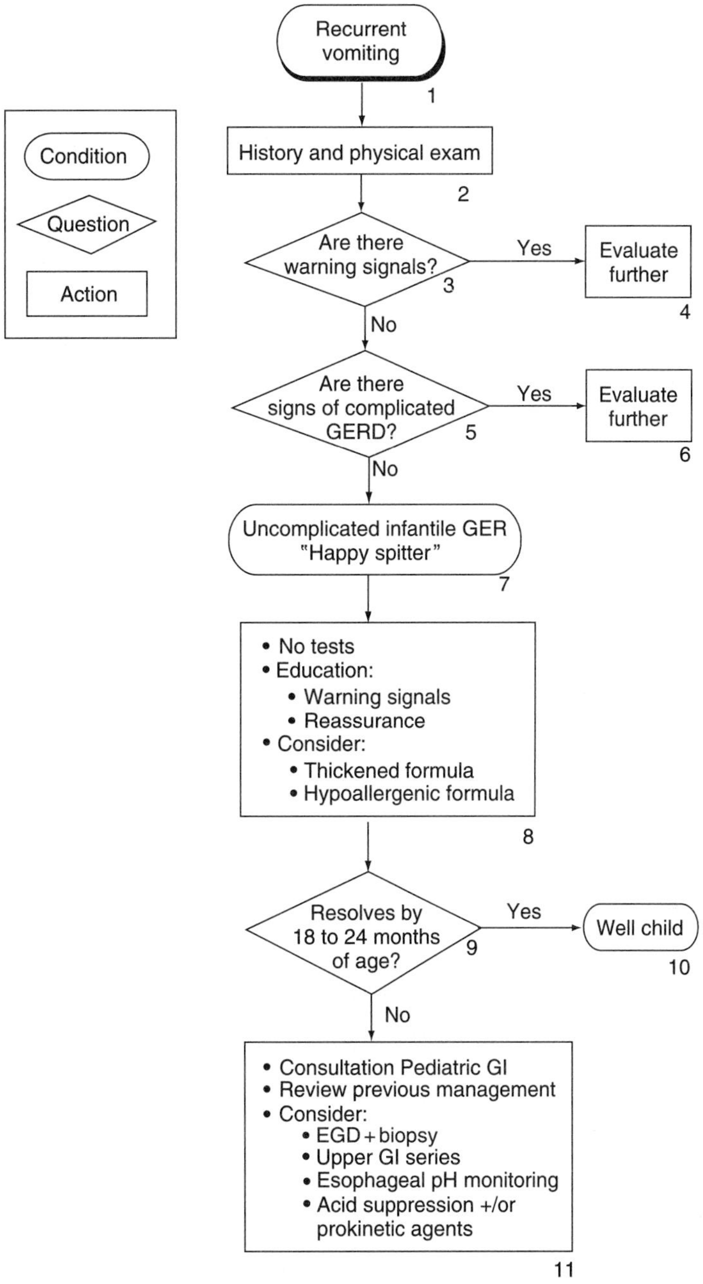

FIGURE 33-1 An algorithm for the management of an infant with uncomplicated GER (the "happy spitter"). *Pediatric GI*, Pediatric gastroenterologist; *EGD*, esophagogastroduodenoscopy; *UGI*, upper gastrointestinal series radiography. (From Rudolph CD et al: Guidelines for evaluation and treatment of gastroesophageal reflux in infants and children: recommendations of the North American Society for Pediatric Gastroenterology and Nutrition, *J Pediatr Gastroenterol Nutr* 32[suppl 2]:S14, 2001.)

diet plays a role in the formation of ulcers. Chronic aspirin therapy and nonsteroidal antiinflammatory drugs (NSAIDs) cause gastric mucosal damage but are not associated with ulcer formation. Smoking can cause duodenal ulcers and slows the rate of healing.

Primary gastric ulcers are about seven times less likely than duodenal ulcers to occur in children. Cytomegalovirus (CMV) and *H. pylori* are associated with PUD in children. The incidence of *H. pylori* infection is 10% in children with PUD. Colonization rates have been suggested

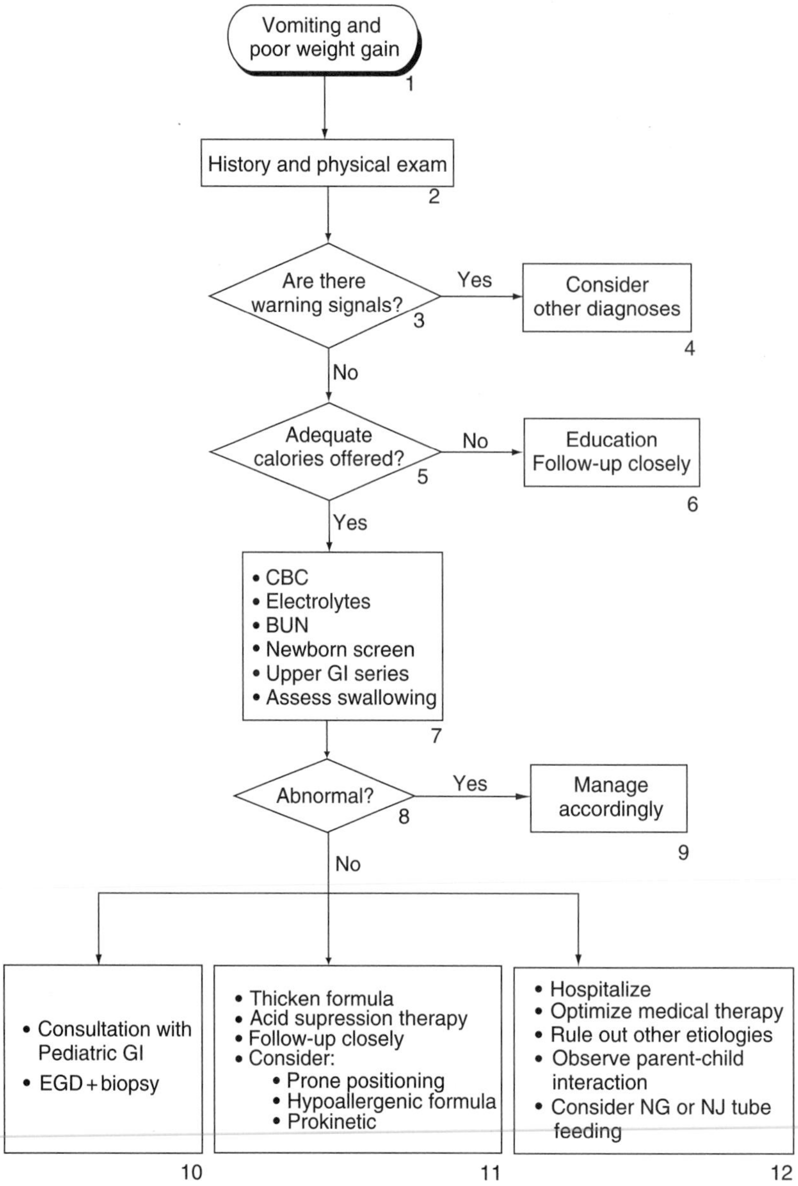

FIGURE 33-2 An algorithm for the management of an infant with vomiting and poor weight gain. *BUN*, blood urea nitrogen; *CBC*, complete blood count; *NG*, nasogastric; *NJ*, nasojejunal. (From Rudolph CD et al: Guidelines for evaluation and treatment of gastroesophageal reflux in infants and children: recommendations of the North American Society for Pediatric Gastroenterology and Nutrition, *J Pediatr Gastroenterol Nutr* 32[suppl 2]:S14, 2001.)

to be 8% to 63%. *H. pylori* is transmitted person to person (most likely by fecal-oral contamination) or by contaminated water sources and induces a chronic inflammation in the stomach and duodenal mucosa that destroys the protective mucosal layer. No correlation between *H. pylori* infection and recurrent abdominal pain has been found in children.

PUD is most common between ages 12 and 18 years, with boys being affected more frequently. It is more common among children of low socioeconomic status; blacks and Hispanics; and children living in crowded, unsanitary conditions who share a bed (Bechtel, 2002). The male-to-female ratio is about 2:1 to 3:1. Most children with duodenal ulcers have a positive family medical history, a key finding.

TABLE 33-3 ***Drugs Demonstrated to Be Effective in Gastroesophageal Reflux Disease***

Type of Medication	Recommended Oral Dosage	Adverse Effects/Precautions
Histamine$_2$-Receptor Antagonists		
Cimetidine	40 mg/kg/day divided tid or qid (adult dose: 800-1200 mg/dose bid or tid)	Rash, bradycardia, dizziness, nausea, vomiting, hypotension, gynecomastia, reduces hepatic metabolism of theophylline and other medications, neutropenia, thrombocytopenia, agranulocytosis, doses should be decreased with renal insufficiency
Nizatidine	10 mg/kg/day divided bid (adult dose: 150 mg bid or 300 mg hs)	Headaches, dizziness, constipation, diarrhea, nausea, anemia, urticaria, doses should be decreased with renal insufficiency
Ranitidine	5 to 10 mg/kg/day divided tid (adult dose: 300 mg bid)	Headache, dizziness, fatigue, irritability, rash, constipation, diarrhea, thrombocytopenia, elevated transaminases, doses should be decreased with renal insufficiency
Famotidine	1 mg/kg/day divided bid (adult dose: 20 mg bid)	Headache, dizziness, constipation, diarrhea, nausea, doses should be decreased with renal insufficiency
Proton Pump Inhibitors		
Omeprazole	1 mg/kg/day divided qd or bid (adult dose: 20 mg qd)	Headache, diarrhea, abdominal pain, nausea, rash, constipation, vitamin B_{12} deficiency
Lansoprazole	No pediatric dose available (adult dose: 15-30 mg qd)	Headache, diarrhea, abdominal pain, nausea, elevated transaminases, proteinuria, angina, hypotension
Pantoprazole	No pediatric dose available (adult dose: 40 mg qd)	Headache, diarrhea, abdominal pain, nausea
Rabeprazole	No pediatric dose available (adult dose: 20 mg qd)	Headache, diarrhea, abdominal pain, nausea
Prokinetic		
Cisapride	0.8 mg/kg/day divided qid (adult dose: 10-20 mg qid)	Rare cases of serious cardiac arrhythmia (FDA recommends ECG before administration) Beware of drug interactions Do not use in patients with liver, cardiac, or electrolyte abnormalities (FDA recommends K^+, Ca^{++}, Mg^{++}, and creatinine before administration)

From Rudolph CD et al: Guidelines for evaluation and treatment of gastroesophageal reflux in infants and children: recommendations of the North American Society for Pediatric Gastroenterology and Nutrition, *J Pediatr Gastroenterol Nutr* 32(suppl 2):S9, 2001.

bid, Twice a day; *ECG*, electrocardiogram; *FDA*, Food and Drug Administration; *hs*, at bedtime; *qd*, every day; *qid*, four times daily; *tid*, three times daily.

Clinical Findings

History

- Positive family history
- Can be asymptomatic
- Symptoms can wax and wane
- Recurrent epigastric abdominal pain
- Pain (onset, location, duration, severity) with eating, awakens from sleep (key finding)
- Vomiting and hematemesis
- Weight loss
- Bloody stool
- Infants: poor feeding, GI bleeding, vomiting, intestinal perforation
- Toddlers/preschoolers: poorly localized abdominal pain, vomiting, GI bleeding
- School-age children and adolescents: poorly localized epigastric or right lower quadrant (RLQ) pain, postprandial pain, dyspepsia
- Predisposing factors: alcohol, smoking, aspirin, NSAIDs, or corticosteroids

Box 33-2 delineates major and minor criteria for the diagnosis of dyspepsia.

BOX 33-2 *Major and Minor Criteria for the Diagnosis of Dyspepsia*

Major Criteria

Epigastric abdominal pain
Recurrent vomiting (at least three times per month)

Minor Criteria

Symptoms associated with eating (anorexia/weight loss)
Pain awakening the child at night
Heartburn
Oral regurgitation
Chronic nausea
Excessive belching/hiccuping
Early satiety
Periumbilical abdominal pain
Family history of peptic ulcer disease, dyspepsia, or irritable bowel syndrome

Adapted from Chelimsky G, Czinn S: Peptic ulcer disease in children, *Pediatr Rev* 22(10):349-355, 2001.

Physical Examination. A careful physical examination should be performed; however, there may be no physical findings. The physical examination should include the following (Chelimsky & Czinn, 2001):

- Height, weight, head circumference, BMI, and percentiles
- Funduscopic examination
- Careful mouth inspection looking for ulcers (associated with Crohn's disease), dental enamel erosion (associated with GER)
- Lung examination for wheezing (associated with GER)
- Abdominal examination for tenderness and hepatosplenomegaly
- Rectal examination to assess perirectal disease

Diagnostic Tests

- Diagnostic tests include CBC with differential, ESR, LFTs, and electrolytes; stool for blood, culture, ova, and parasites; and UA and urine culture.
- Upper GI series or endoscopy is indicated for GI bleeding, for persistent unexplained vomiting, and to diagnose ulcer disease.
- Test for *H. pylori* infection if the child has been endoscopically or radiologically diagnosed with a gastric or duodenal ulcer, has mucosa-associated lymphoid tissue (MALT) lymphoma, and occasionally to determine if the infection has been eradicated. Testing for *H. pylori* infection is *not* recommended for children with recurrent abdominal pain who do not have ulcer disease, asymptomatic children at increased risk of acquiring *H. pylori* infection, or children with positive family history (Gold et al, 2000). Tests for *H. pylori* include the following (Gold et al, 2000):
  - GI endoscopy with multiple biopsy sites is the most reliable way to diagnose infection with *H. pylori.* Rapid urease testing of biopsy tissue has poor positive predictive value in children.
  - Polymerase chain reaction (PCR) from tissue biopsy for *H. pylori* is expensive, difficult to do, easily compromised by contamination, and not widely available outside the research laboratory.
  - Determine serum gastrin level (especially if considering Zollinger-Ellison syndrome).
  - Determine serum IgG antibody titer for *H. pylori* (level greater than 500 U [normal 0 to 200]). This test should not be the sole basis for starting therapy.
  - Urea breath test: There is insufficient evidence that the urea breath test can be used to reliably diagnose or exclude *H. pylori*-associated disease (Gold et al, 2000).

Differential Diagnosis

All other causes of abdominal pain (see Table 33-6), GER, and GI bleeding are included in the differential diagnosis.

Management

- For PUD not related to *H. pylori*, the following treatment may be helpful:
  - Antacids: any liquid preparation, 0.5 ml/kg, given between 1 and 3 hours after eating and before bed.
- See Table 33-4 for medications used for PUD.
- Empirical therapy for suspected *H. pylori* is not recommended.
- For PUD related to *H. pylori* infection in association with symptomatic GI disease, eradication treatment is necessary. See Table 33-5 for treatment guidelines. Compliance with the treatment regimen is the single most important determinant of eradication (Huang & Hunt, 1999).

Complications

Recurrence, hemorrhage, perforation, gastric outlet obstruction, and gastric malignancy are possible complications.

Patient Education/Prevention/Prognosis

Treatment success depends on the child completing the drug regimen and the avoidance of spicy foods, caffeine, and chocolate. This area of pediatric primary care is being actively studied, and NPs must be aware of ongoing changes in recommendations for therapy.

TABLE 33-4 *Medications Used in the Treatment of Acid-Peptic Disease*

Medication	Pediatric Dose	How Supplied
Histamine$_2$-Receptor Antagonists		
Cimetidine	20-40 mg/kg/day up to 400 mg twice daily	Syrup: 300 mg/5 ml; tablets: 200, 300, 400, and 800 mg
Famotidine	1-1.2 mg/kg/day up to 20 mg twice daily*	Syrup: 40 mg/5 ml; tablets: 20 and 40 mg
Ranitidine	2-4 mg/kg/day up to 150 mg twice daily	Syrup: 75 mg/5 ml; tablets: 150 and 300 mg
Proton Pump Inhibitors		
Lansoprazole	0.8 mg/kg/day	Capsules: 15 and 30 mg
Omeprazole	0.8 mg/kg/day; effective dosage range of 0.3-3.3 mg/kg per 24 hr has been reported†	Capsules: 10 and 20 mg
Cytoprotective Agents		
Sucralfate	40-80 mg/kg/day up to 1 g four times per day‡	Suspension: 1 g/5 ml; tablets: 1 g

Adapted from Chelimsky G, Czinn S: Peptic ulcer disease in children, *Pediatr Rev* 22(10):353, 2001.
*40 mg/day in one dose for young adults.
†20 mg/day in one dose for young adults.
‡1 g four times daily for young adults.

TABLE 33-5 *Recommended Eradication Therapies for* H. pylori *Disease in Children*

Options	Medications	Dosage
First-line Options		
1	Amoxicillin	50 mg/kg/day up to 1 g bid
	Clarithromycin	15 mg/kg/day up to 500 mg bid
	Proton pump inhibitor (PPI): omeprazole (or comparable acid inhibitory doses of another PPI)	1 mg/kg/day up to 20 mg bid
2	OR Amoxicillin	50 mg/kg/day up to 1 g bid
	Metronidazole	20 mg/kg/day up to 500 mg bid
	Proton pump inhibitor: omeprazole (or comparable acid inhibitory doses of another PPI)	1 mg/kg/day up to 20 mg bid
3	OR Clarithromycin	15 mg/kg/day up to 500 mg bid
	Metronidazole	20 mg/kg/day up to 500 mg bid
	Proton pump inhibitor: omeprazole (or comparable acid inhibitory doses of another PPI)	1 mg/kg/day up to 20 mg bid
Second-line Options		
4	Bismuth subsalicylate	1 tablet (262 mg) qid *or* 15 ml (17.6 mg/ml qid)
	Metronidazole	20 mg/kg/day up to 500 mg bid
	Proton pump inhibitor: omeprazole (or comparable acid inhibitory doses of another PPI) *plus* an additional antibiotic:	1 mg/kg/day up to 20 mg bid
	amoxicillin	50 mg/kg/day up to 1 g bid
	or tetracycline*	50 mg/kg/day up to 1 g bid
	or clarithromycin	15 mg/kg/day up to 500 mg bid
5	OR Ranitidine bismuth-citrate	1 tablet qid
	Clarithromycin	15 mg/kg/day up to 500 mg bid
	Metronidazole	20 mg/kg/day up to 500 mg bid

From Gold BD et al: Medical Position Statement: the North American Society for Pediatric Gastroenterology and Nutrition. *Helicobacter pylori* infection in children: recommendations for diagnosis and treatment, *J Pediatr Gastroenterol Nutr* 31(5):496, 2000.
Initial treatment should be provided in a twice-daily regimen (to enhance compliance) for 7 to 14 days.
*Only for children 12 years of age or older.
bid, Twice daily; *qid*, four times daily.

LOWER GASTROINTESTINAL TRACT DISORDERS

Infantile Colic

Description

Infantile colic is characterized by persistent crying in infants younger than 3 months. The average infant cries for 2 to 3 hours per day. In contrast, an infant with colic usually cries for more than 4 hours per day. One definition of colic is the rule of threes: a healthy infant who cries for more than 3 hours per day, more than 3 days per week, for more than 3 weeks (Goldstein, Hagerman, & Reynolds, 2003).

Etiology and Incidence

No specific cause of colic has been identified, although both physical and psychosocial factors may play a role. Certain physical factors have been implicated and include sensitivity to diet (e.g., cow's milk), excessive gas, swallowed air during feeding, inadequate burping, hypermotile bowel, and cigarette smoke in the infant's environment. Psychosocial factors can include the perception of a stressful pregnancy, negative childbirth experience, unsatisfying interactions among family members, and overstimulation. The parents' inability to accurately interpret and respond to the infant's cries may contribute to colic. The infant may become overstimulated, underfed, or overfed. The stress created by a crying baby contributes to ineffective parental interventions and can exacerbate the problem. Carey's classic study on colic (1972) revealed that colicky babies have a low sensory threshold. More recent studies look at colic as a possible manifestation of a child with "difficult temperament" or just a manifestation of typical behavioral development (Barr, 2002).

Colic has been estimated to occur in anywhere from 5% to 28% of all infants (Clifford et al, 2002), although the incidence varies greatly depending on the definition used (Reijneveld, Brugman, & Hirasing, 2001). Using the Wessel definition, anywhere from 15% of infants (Clifford et al, 2002) to 30% to 40% of infants (Goldstein, Hagerman, & Reynolds, 2003) continue with colic symptoms past 3 months of life.

Clinical Findings

History. Parents or caregivers report that the infant is less than 3 months old and cries 3 hours or more a day for 3 days or more per week (Goldstein, Hagerman, & Reynolds, 2003). Additional findings include the following:

- Demands frequent feeding and is often fussy while feeding
- Has excessive gas
- Is inconsolable or is comforted for short periods only
- Is "tense" or "tight" and keeps legs stiff and fists clenched tightly

Physical Examination. If possible, see the family during a crying time. A thorough examination must be completed to rule out other pathology and should include the following:

- Evaluation of growth parameters
- Abdominal examination for masses, tenderness, and bowel sounds
- Stool for blood or mucus

Differential Diagnosis

All other causes of abdominal pain are in the differential diagnosis (see Table 33-6), as well as undetected corneal abrasion, UTI, other infection, or traumatic injury. Persistent mother-infant distress syndrome (increased crying and colicky behaviors that persist beyond 3 months of age) and latent distress (no colicky behavior at 6 weeks of age, but present at 3 months) are newer subcategories of colic being researched (Barr, 2002; Clifford et al, 2002).

Management

- No cure is known for infantile colic. The goal of treatment is to manage the situation until the colic resolves itself. Parents and providers who are flexible, creative, and persistent in seeking solutions are most likely to be successful. See Box 33-3 for management strategies.
- Medications (e.g., simethicone) are ineffective in treating colic. It may give the parents "something to do," but it can actually potentiate the myth of a physical cause. Sedation for either the parent or the child is sometimes indicated in extreme cases (Behrman, Kliegman, & Jenson, 2004).
- An extensively hydrolyzed whey formula was effective in diminishing crying in one study done in the Netherlands (Lucassen et al, 2000).

Complications

Stress created by a crying baby can contribute to parental feelings of hostility, anger, and guilt, ultimately leading to poor parent-child interaction. Parents may respond by unintentionally physically or emotionally abusing their infant.

Patient Education/Prevention/Prognosis

The National Center for Shaken Baby Syndrome "period of PURPLE crying" campaign has materials to educate parents about properties of early (first 3 months of life) crying. P stands for peak, U for unpredictability of crying bouts, R for resistance to soothing, P for painlike expression, L for long crying bouts, and E for evening clustering. See the Resource Box at the end of this chapter for contact information.

BOX 33-3 Management Strategies for Infantile Colic

- Acknowledge the importance of the concern.
- Provide support for the parents.
- Affirm the baby's good health.
- Help parents distinguish infant cries and understand infant state.
- Remind the parents that colic is temporary.
- Reinforce parents' efforts to comfort their infant.
- Encourage parents to take time off from child care by finding assistance from family or friends.
- Inform parents that the stress they feel is sensed by the infant, which may cause more crying.
- Allow parents to express feelings of anger, guilt, and frustration.
- Inform parents of equipment sold to soothe babies (vibrating infant seats and cribs).
- Share anecdotal reports of using noise from hair dryers or vacuum cleaners or a ride in the car to calm the infant.
- Implement strategies to calm the infant (decrease in environmental stimulation, swaddling the infant, carrying the infant, firm and gentle pressure to the abdomen, rocking, swinging).
- Ensure proper feeding (e.g., correct latch-on, frequent burping, avoidance of early addition of solids, change in diet if lactose intolerance or milk allergy is a problem).
- Have the parents keep a diary of the baby's crying for analysis by the health care provider; a diary may assist in identifying patterns that can lead to interventions.

Data from Dihigo S: New strategies for the treatment of colic: modifying the parent/infant interaction, *J Pediatr Health Care* 12(5):256-262, 1998; Fleisher D: Coping with colic, *Contemp Pediatr* 15(6):144-156, 1998; Goldstein E, Hagerman J, Reynolds A: Colic. In Hay et al: *Current pediatric diagnosis and treatment.*

Colic is resolved by 3 months of age in somewhere between 60% (Goldstein, Hagerman, & Reynolds, 2003) and 85% (Clifford et al, 2002) of infants.

Acute Abdominal Pain

Description

The location and character of abdominal pain can be helpful in identifying the disease process. Visceral pain is generally dull and diffuse. Visceral pain fibers are located in the muscular wall of hollow viscera and the capsule of solid viscera. Visceral nerves are stimulated by tension and stretching. Parietal pain is usually sharp, localized, and stimulated by inflammation in the parietal peritoneum. The shared innervation of many abdominal organs leads to poor localization of pain.

- *Epigastric* pain usually indicates pain from the liver, pancreas, biliary tree, stomach, and upper part of the small bowel.
- *Periumbilical* pain is generated from the distal end of the small intestine, cecum, appendix, and ascending colon.
- *Suprapubic* discomfort indicates distal intestine, urinary tract, and pelvic organ dysfunction.
- *Referred* pain is usually sharp, localized pain felt in remote areas innervated by the same nerves as the affected organ. When visceral pain is overwhelming, referred pain occurs.
- *Acute,* continuous pain is more indicative of an acute process.

Etiology

Primary GI causes of abdominal pain in children include appendicitis, viral and bacterial enteritis, inflammatory bowel disease, intussusception, pancreatitis, cholecystitis, and liver dysfunction.

Primary extra-GI causes of abdominal pain include ovarian cyst, salpingitis, sexually transmitted diseases, otitis media, pneumonia, pharyngitis, UTI, Henoch-Schönlein purpura, rheumatic fever, sickle cell disease, pleurisy, kidney pain, rectal or uterine disease, and hernia. Referred pain in the shoulder can be generated from pneumonia, subphrenic abscess, pleurisy, pancreatitis, and the spleen, gallbladder, and liver. Testicular pain occurs with kidney disease and appendicitis. Back pain can also accompany retroperitoneal hematoma, pancreatitis, and rectal or uterine disease (Barkin & Rosen, 1999).

Clinical Findings

History. The history should assess the following:

- Family history of gallbladder disease, hernia, kidney or liver disease, and other incidences of abdominal pain
- Past medical history of illnesses or surgeries
- History of trauma or abuse
- Pain: onset, location, duration, distribution, quality, radiation, changes in location, awakes child from sleep
- Activity level
- Appetite and food intake
- History of recent infection
- Fever (high fever is usually not associated with acute abdomen)
- Nausea, vomiting, diarrhea, or constipation
- Aggravating and alleviating factors
- Hematuria, dysuria, frequency, incontinence
- Menstrual history and last period, vaginal discharge, sexual activity, birth control, and penile discharge

Physical Examination. Adolescents should be examined with parents out of the room (for privacy and to elicit a complete history). The following are needed for all children:

- Complete physical examination
- Weight, BMI, and vital signs (temperature, heart rate, respiratory rate, and blood pressure)
- Abdominal examination, including rectal examination, psoas and obturator signs, rebound tenderness, decreased bowel sounds
- Pelvic examination as indicated
- Repeated examinations as necessary to observe for changes

See Differential Diagnosis for specific findings; also see sections on appendicitis and intussusception.

Diagnostic Tests. The following are performed as indicated:

- CBC with differential, serum electrolytes, ESR, amylase, pregnancy test (as indicated by the history and examination)
- UA and urine culture
- Stool for occult blood
- Pelvic examination—gonococcal or chlamydial culture (or both), Papanicolaou smear, vaginal smears
- Abdominal radiograph
- Chest radiograph (anteroposterior and lateral as indicated) to rule out pneumonia
- Abdominal or pelvic (or both) ultrasonography

Differential Diagnosis

See Table 33-6 and Fig. 33-3.

Management

Treatment involves the following:

- Consultation and referral, including surgery as indicated
- No sedatives or pain medication until the diagnosis is made
- Intravenous rehydration and gastric decompression as necessary
- Treatment of the cause

Complications

Complications include ruptured viscera, intraabdominal bleeding, strangulation leading to ischemia of the gut, and shock leading to death.

Appendicitis

Description

Appendicitis is inflammation of the appendix. Although a classic presentation is easy to discern, appendicitis can mimic many other intraabdominal conditions, making diagnosis tricky.

Etiology and Incidence

Following obstruction of the appendiceal lumen by a fecalith, lymphoid tissue, tumor, parasite, foreign body, or inspissated cystic fibrosis secretions, the appendix becomes distended and subject to ischemia and necrosis. Peritoneal inflammation around the infected appendix causes the characteristic symptoms. There is about a 36-hour window from the onset of pain to the rupture of the appendix, with 80% of children perforating by 48 hours (Pena, Taylor, & Lund, 1999).

Appendicitis is the most common reason for emergency abdominal surgery in childhood (Ashcraft, 2000). Frequency increases with age, but the average age of appendicitis in children is 10 years, with boys and girls equally affected. Children younger than 8 years have twice the perforation rate of those older than 8 years (Irish et al, 1998). Approximately one third of children have a perforated appendix by the time they seek treatment from a health care provider (Pena, Taylor, & Lund, 1999).

Clinical Findings

- The most reliable information is gained from the sequence of symptoms (Pena, Taylor, & Lund, 1999):
  - Periumbilical pain is felt (earliest sign).
  - Child awakens with pain that peaks in 4 hours, then subsides and migrates to RLQ (classic sign).
  - After a few hours, vomiting may occur (this follows periumbilical pain; in gastroenteritis, vomiting precedes the pain).
  - Anorexia occurs (although up to 50% of children state that they are hungry).
  - Stool is low volume and mucusy (gastroenteritis has high-volume, watery stools).
  - Low-grade fever (1 to 2° F) is often a late sign, but it is not reliable.
- The process evolves over 12 hours, with the potential for infants and young children to become sick much more quickly.
- Following perforation, symptoms lessen, with less vomiting, fever greater than 101° F, and the most comfortable position being on the side with the legs flexed.
- Infants demonstrate irritability, pain with movement, and flexed hips.
- The child may become quiet because crying and movement hurt.

Physical Examination. A complete physical examination is necessary. Reexamination may be needed in 4 to 6 hours. The following can be found:

- Presence of involuntary guarding, rebound tenderness, maximal pain over McBurney's point (1.5 to 2 inches in from the right anterior superior iliac crest on a line

TABLE 33-6 *Differential Diagnosis of Gastrointestinal Causes of Abdominal Pain in Children*

Disease	Major Symptoms	Signs	Excreta	Tests	Age of Onset
Anal fissure	Constipation, crying with defecation, bright red blood on stool or in diaper	Small tears in anal mucosa	Constipation with bloody streaks	Stool occult blood	Any
Appendicitis	Fever, anorexia, vomiting; process evolves over 12 hr	Diffuse, then localized to right-sided (RLQ) tenderness, guarding, maximal pain over McBurney's point	Constipation or diarrhea, rare blood and pus	CBC: increased neutrophils UA: pyuria Abdominal radiograph: may show fecalith Ultrasonography: may be abnormal	Frequency increases with age, peaking between 15-30 yr
Colic	Persistent crying in infant	Duration of crying >3 hr/day for 3 or more days/wk	Normal	Stool: r/o blood, mucus	<3 mo
Constipation	Poor appetite, soiling, straining with stools	Possible tenderness over colon and small bowel, rectal fissures, encopresis, fewer than three stools per week	Hard or soft, may have blood on outer surface of stool	Abdominal radiograph Barium enema if unresponsive to intervention	Peaks between 2-4 yr
Foreign body	Children may be asymptomatic *or* Coughing, choking, gagging, pain in throat or chest, anorexia, pain with swallowing	*May* have increased salivation, refusal to swallow, respiratory symptoms Normal abdominal examination	May see passage of FB	Chest radiograph if respiratory symptoms Abdominal radiograph if FB not seen to pass in stool or signs of abdominal pain/obstruction present	Highest incidence between 14 mo-6 yr
Gastroenteritis, viral or bacterial	Vomiting, diarrhea	General abdominal tenderness	Watery, bilious (green) vomitus, may or may not have blood in stool	Stool: may show bacteria, WBCs, blood, mucus	Any
Gastroesophageal reflux	Regurgitation, vomiting, irritability, recurrent pain after bedtime	Infants: gastric distention, effortless regurgitation during or after feedings; FTT, stridor, apnea, recurrent pneumonia, bronchospasm Older children: vomiting, sour taste in mouth, abdominal pain, burning sensation in substernal area; chronic nocturnal cough, wheezing, pneumonia; dysphagia, nausea, FTT	Rare hematemesis	Barium swallow with fluoroscopy; 24 hr esophageal pH probe study Esophageal manometry Endoscopy for esophageal biopsy	Commonly 0-24 mo with 60%-80% spontaneous resolution; can occur in specific disease disorders and in older children and adolescents

Continued

TABLE 33-6 *Differential Diagnosis of Gastrointestinal Causes of Abdominal Pain in Children—cont'd*

Disease	Major Symptoms	Signs	Excreta	Tests	Age of Onset
Hepatitis	Nausea, anorexia	Tender liver with or without spenomegaly, jaundice	Pale stools, diarrhea	Elevated ALT and AST Mild elevations of LDH and alkaline phosphatase Elevated bilirubin (direct and indirect) May have mild lymphocytosis Hepatitis panel may show active or carrier status	Any—dependent on type of hepatitis
Hernia (strangulated)	Vomiting, crying	Distention, bulge in inguinal area	Fecal vomitus	None—refer for immediate surgical evaluation	70% occur in first year
Hirschsprung's disease	Failure to pass stool within 24 hr in an infant or rectal stimulation required to pass stools; history of constipation since infancy in children	FTT, abdominal distention, palpable stool throughout abdomen but empty rectal ampulla	May have diarrhea, bilious (green) vomiting	Abdominal radiograph Barium enema Rectal examination: absence of stool in rectal ampulla Electrolytes, CBC	Infancy to adult
Inflammatory Bowel Diseases					
Crohn's disease	Umbilical or RLQ pain, diarrhea, weight loss, anorexia	Short stature, tender abdominal mass, fever, arthralgias or arthritis, perianal lesions	Loose and usually nonbloody stools unless anal fissures present	CBC, total protein, albumin, ESR, CRP Stool for blood and WBCs Bone age Refer for endoscopy	Childhood and adolescence with peak at 20-30 yr
Ulcerative colitis	Weight loss, abdominal pain	Tender colon	Bloody stools	Same as above	Peak incidence at 16-20 yr
Intestinal obstruction	Vomiting, abdominal distention; failure to pass feces in newborn after 24 hr; acute or gradual onset of periumbilical or lower abdominal pain	Alternating crampy and quiescent periods of periumbilical to lower abdominal pain, increased bowel sounds, obstipation	Bilious (green) emesis	Abdominal radiograph (flat, upright views)	Neonates; if occurs after 2 mo, usually due to intussusception or other causes
Intussusception	Episodic, cyclic abdominal pain with vomiting alternating with calm periods	Tender, sausage-shaped mass in RUQ, distention, legs drawn up at time of pain followed by periods of lethargy, absence of bowel sounds in RLQ; these "classic" symptoms occur in <50% of cases	Blood-tinged mucus ("currant jelly" stool); this occurs as a late sign	Abdominal ultrasound 100% reliable (abdominal radiography misses diagnosis in 33%-55% of cases) Barium enema	70% <2 yr old with peak incidence at 5 mo and 3 yr; as age of onset increases, further pathology is often present

TABLE 33-6 ***Differential Diagnosis of Gastrointestinal Causes of Abdominal Pain in Children—cont'd***

Disease	Major Symptoms	Signs	Excreta	Tests	Age of Onset
Irritable bowel syndrome	Recurrent, intermittent, dull, crampy abdominal pain, diarrhea, or constipation	Intense thirst, fluctuating abdominal distention, increased bowel sounds; history of others in family with recurrent abdominal pain especially with social stimulation, travel, holidays, trauma; healthy appearance; borborygmus and flatus in school-age and older children; vague tenderness in RLQ, LLQ, and epigastrium; pain usually not related to eating or defecation; occasional pallor and nausea	Watery, malodorous stools; first stool of day may be formed, followed by three or more watery stools through the day	CBC, ESR, UA, stools for O&P and occult blood Abdominal ultrasonography Upper GI series with small bowel follow-through	5-15 yr
Lactose intolerance	Bloating, gaseousness, crampy abdominal pain	Pain and diarrhea within hours of lactose ingestion; may have history of recent severe viral gastroenteritis In infants: vomiting, distention, abdominal pain after lactose-containing formula or bovine milk ingestion by breastfeeding mother	Acidic diarrhea	Breath hydrogen test after lactose challenge Reducing substances in stool Lack of normal increase in blood glucose after ingestion of lactose	5-15 yr rare in infancy; prominent in some ethnic groups
Mesenteric lymphadenitis	Fever, vomiting	Right-sided (RLQ often) or diffuse tenderness		Abdominal ultrasonography may show mesenteric adenitis	
Meckel diverticulum	Painless rectal bleeding	Anemia, periumbilical or lower abdominal pain may be manifested similar to appendicitis or volvulus	Bloody stools	CBC Stools for occult blood Refer for surgical consultation	65% incidence in children <5 yr old with peak at 2 yr

Continued

TABLE 33-6 *Differential Diagnosis of Gastrointestinal Causes of Abdominal Pain in Children—cont'd*

Disease	Major Symptoms	Signs	Excreta	Tests	Age of Onset
Necrotizing enterocolitis	Feeding intolerance; abdomen distended, tense, and tender	Possible palpable abdominal mass and cellulitis of abdominal wall, GI bleeding, shock		CBC, chemistry panel Abdominal radiograph/ultrasound	Premature and term infants
Parasites	Parasite dependent: possibly diarrhea, bloating, distention, flatulence	Parasite dependent: rectal itching, weight loss, malaise, cough, hepatomegaly, vague abdominal pain, anemia	May or may not have diarrhea, which may be bloody, greasy, or foul smelling; visible worms in stool or vomitus	Stools for O&P CBC: may show increased eosinophils	Any
Peptic ulcer disease	Poor appetite, weakness, epigastric pain with or without nausea	Vague abdominal pain or RLQ localization; epigastric tenderness, which can occur at night; vomiting	Black stools or coffee-ground vomitus	CBC Stool for occult blood Upper GI series Serum IgG antibody for *Helicobacter pylori* Urea breath test	Any, usually above 8 yr
Recurrent abdominal pain	At least three episodes of abdominal pain over 3 mo period	Periumbilical to generalized abdominal pain, sometimes sharp or dull and lasting 1-3 hr; occasional nausea/vomiting	Normal	CBC, ESR, chemistry screen UA and urine culture Stool O&P, culture, pH, reducing substances	Usually between 6 and 19 yr with peak at 9 yr
Volvulus or malrotation	Bilious (green) vomiting	Abdominal distention, GI bleeding, palpable epigastric mass, dehydration, lethargy, shock	May be bloody	CBC Abdominal radiograph Barium enema Upper GI series Refer immediately for surgical consultation	First month of life

Table developed by Catherine Blosser with information from Burg et al (2002); Teitelbaum, Leichtner, & Tunnessen (1999); Behrman & Kliegman (1998); Finberg & Kleinman (2002); Irish et al (1998).

ALT, Alanine aminotransferase; *AST*, aspartate aminotransferase; *CBC*, complete blood count; *CRP*, C-reactive protein; *ESR*, erythrocyte sedimentation rate; *FB*, foreign body; *FTT*, failure to thrive; *GI*, gastrointestinal; *LDH*, lactate dehydrogenase; *LLQ*, left lower quadrant; *O&P*, ova and parasites; *RLQ*, right lower quadrant; *r/o*, rule out; *RUQ*, right upper quadrant; *UA*, urinalysis; *WBCs*, white blood cells.

toward the umbilicus) on abdominal examination (most reliable finding); percussion is best method for eliciting rebound tenderness (Ashcraft, 2000)

- Heel-drop jarring test (on toes for 15 seconds, drops on heels); inability to stand straight or climb stairs; winces when getting off examination table or riding in a car over bumps
- Positive psoas sign or obturator sign (or both)
- Rovsing sign (pressure deep in left lower quadrant with sudden release elicits RLQ pain)
- Tenderness and possibly a mass on the right side on rectal examination

Scoring systems are available, and although they do not "substantially improve the diagnostic accuracy of an experienced examiner," they do help "focus attention on key aspects" of the diagnosis (Burd & Whalen, 2001).

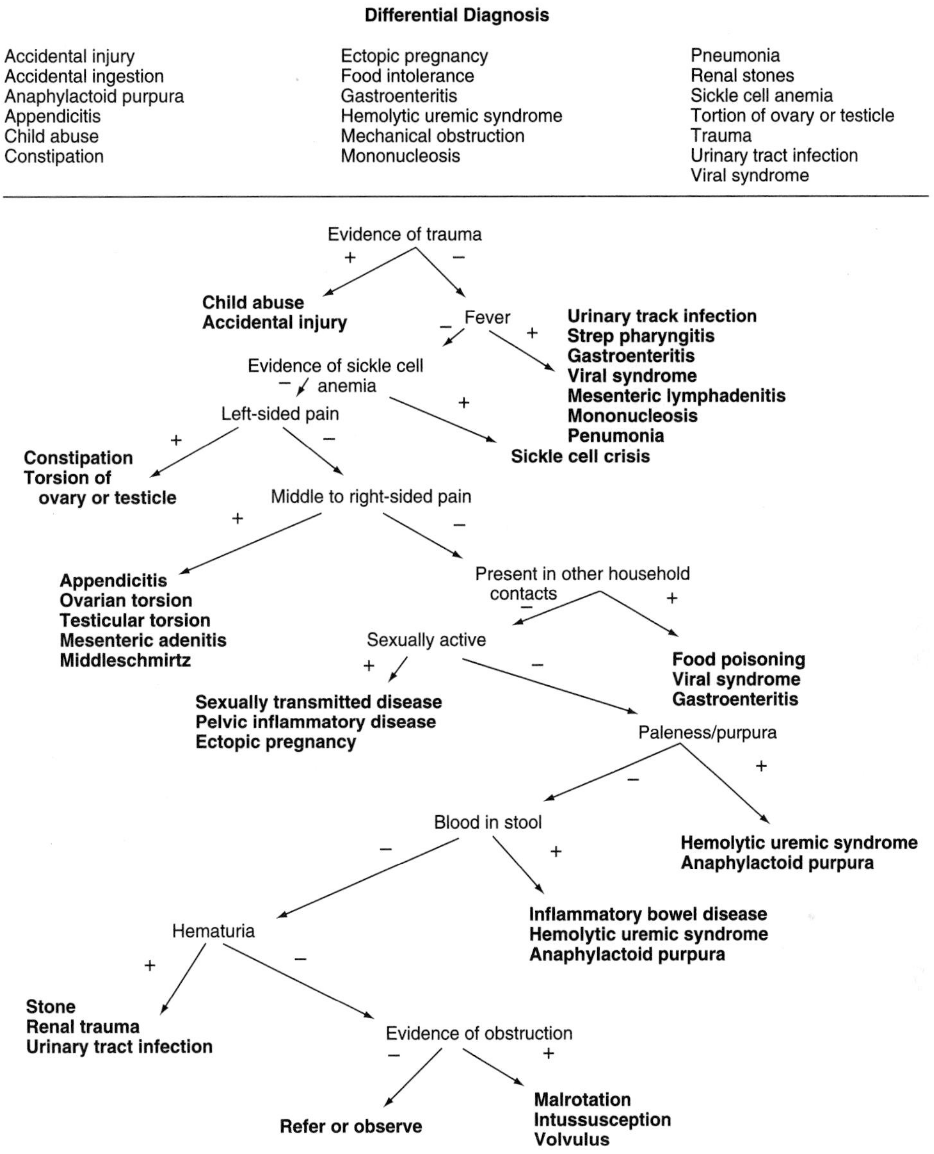

FIGURE 33-3 Decision tree for differential diagnosis of acute abdominal pain. (From Schwartz MW et al, editors: *Pediatric primary care: a problem-oriented approach*, ed 3, St Louis, 1997, Mosby.)

Diagnostic Tests. The following may be noted with appendicitis:

- CBC with differential shows increased neutrophils (greater than 10,000/mm^3 or greater than 75%).
- UA can show pyuria.
- CRP may be elevated if symptoms have been present for longer than 12 hours (low specificity).
- Examination of stool may demonstrate blood and pus (rare finding).
- Abdominal radiographs can show a fecalith, especially if rupture has occurred.
- Ultrasonography demonstrates thickened, noncompressible, larger than 6 mm mass (not as helpful if appendix is perforated).
- CT with contrast has highest accuracy, especially in equivocal cases (Pena et al, 2000).

Differential Diagnosis

The differential diagnosis includes viral gastroenteritis (fever and crampy abdominal pain with vomiting, diarrhea, or both), constipation, UTI (fever, chills, and urinary symptoms), pelvic inflammatory disease or organ pathology, pneumonia, duodenal ulcer (gnawing and burning), intestinal obstruction (crampy pain), peritonitis (worse pain when jumping or coughing), and intussusception (child younger than 2 years with a right upper quadrant [RUQ] mass).

Management

- A surgical consultation for an appendectomy is needed.
- Intravenous and preoperative antibiotics are given if perforation is suspected.
- Patients should be seen in follow-up 2 to 4 weeks after surgery. If appetite, bowel function, energy, and activity level are normal, no pain or fever is present, findings on physical examination are normal, and the wound is well healed, the child can resume unrestricted activity. If at the 2- to 4-week follow-up the child has signs of delayed infection, abnormal bowel function, or unexplained weight loss, refer back to the surgeon.

Complications

Perforation, peritonitis, pelvic abscess, ileus, obstruction, sepsis, shock, and death can occur.

Intussusception

Description

The invagination of bowel begins proximal to the ileocecal valve and is usually ileocolic, but it can be ileoileal or colocolic.

Etiology and Incidence

The cause is not generally apparent. Polyps, Meckel's diverticulum, Henoch-Schönlein purpura, constipation, lymphomas, lipomas, parasites, rotavirus, adenovirus, and foreign bodies can be predisposing factors. Intussusception may be a complication of cystic fibrosis. Intussusception is the most common cause of intestinal obstruction in the first 2 years of life, with males predominating by a 2:1 ratio. The peak incidence is between 3 and 12 months of age. The incidence is increased in the summer and the middle of winter (Orenstein, 2000).

Clinical Findings

History. The following can be reported:

- The classic triad for intussusception, present in just 20% of cases (Orenstein, 2000):
  - Paroxysmal, episodic abdominal pain with vomiting every 5 to 30 minutes
  - Screaming with drawing up of the legs with periods of calm, sleeping, or lethargy between episodes
  - Stool, possibly diarrhea in nature, with blood ("currant jelly"); approximately 40% have occult blood and 40% have gross blood
- Fever present in 1 of 10 cases (Orenstein, 2000)
- May follow an uncomplicated gastroenteritis or upper respiratory infection (Ashcraft, 2000; Orenstein, 2000)
- Possible severe prostration

Physical Examination

- Observe the baby's appearance and behavior over a period of time.
- A sausage-like mass may be felt in the RUQ of the abdomen (Danca's sign).
- The abdomen is often distended and tender to palpation.

Diagnostic Tests

- An abdominal flat-plate radiograph can appear normal, especially early in the course (Fig. 33-4).
- Abdominal ultrasonography establishes the diagnosis in 90% of the cases (Orenstein, 2000).
- An air or barium enema is diagnostic and frequently therapeutic.

Differential Diagnosis

The differential diagnosis includes incarcerated hernia, testicular torsion, acute gastroenteritis, appendicitis, colic, and intestinal obstruction.

Management

The following steps are taken:

- Emergency management and consultation with a pediatric radiologist and a pediatric surgeon.
- Rehydration and stabilization of fluid status.
- Radiologic reduction using an air or barium enema under fluoroscopy is the gold standard, but ultrasound-guided saline reduction has been shown to be as effective and is widely used in Europe (Orenstein, 2000).
- Surgery if perforation is suspected or radiologic reduction fails.
- Intravenous antibiotics are often administered to cover potential intestinal perforation.
- A period of observation following radiologic reduction is recommended; clear discharge instructions to return with any recurrence of symptoms are required, and close phone follow-up for up to 72 hours is prudent.

Complications

Swelling, hemorrhage, incarceration, and necrosis of the bowel requiring bowel resection may occur (Irish et al, 1998). Perforation, sepsis, shock, and reintussusception (5% to 10%, usually within 24 hours of radiologic reduction) can all occur (Orenstein, 2000).

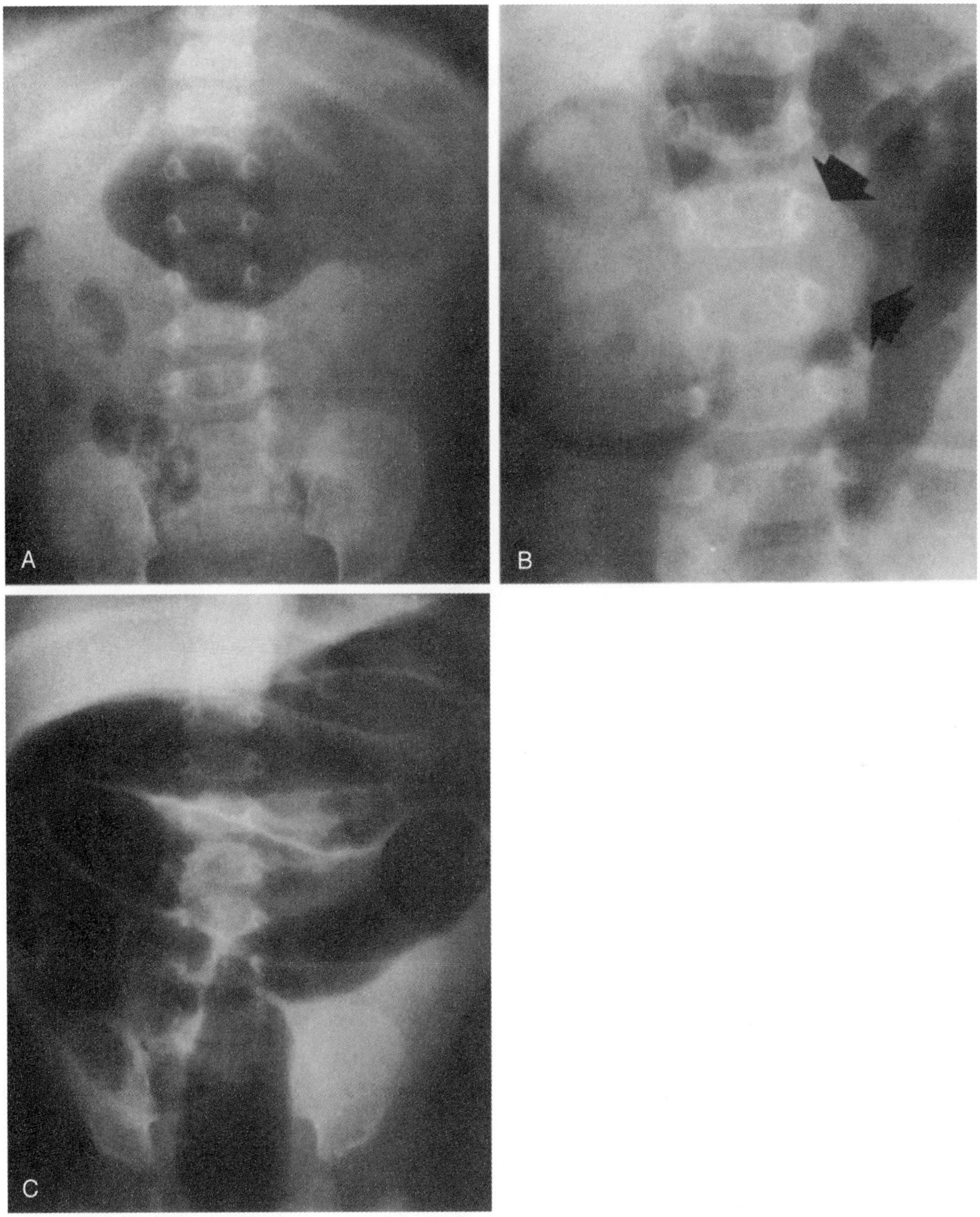

FIGURE 33-4 Intussusception. **A**, Plain abdominal radiograph demonstrating a gas-filled stomach and relatively little gas in the distal end of the bowel. This baby had typical clinical features of intussusception and a palpable upper abdominal mass. Therefore an enema with air was performed. **B**, The intussusception *(arrows)* is outlined by air. **C**, Reduction is proved by air refluxing into loops of small bowel. (From Burg FD et al, editors: *Gellis and Kagan's current pediatric therapy*, ed 15, Philadelphia, 1999, WB Saunders.)

Recurrent Abdominal Pain

Description

Recurrent abdominal pain (RAP) is defined as a minimum of three episodes of abdominal pain occurring over a 3-month period that interfere with normal activity. It is differentiated from chronic abdominal pain in that each episode of RAP is distinct and separated by periods of wellness. There are three classifications of RAP. With the first, there is a clear organic cause for the pain; second, there is a clear psychogenic etiology for the pain; and third, the one described here, neither a clear organic nor a psychogenic cause can be identified (Thiessen, 2002).

Etiology and Incidence

The cause of the pain remains unclear, but the pain is genuine. A localized increase in intraluminal pressure may cause stretching of the intestinal wall leading to functional abdominal pain. Intestinal dysmotility can prevent normal movement of intestinal contents and cause local distention, which is perceived as pain. The term *biopsychosocial dysfunctional pain* has been applied to children with RAP.

Affected children have an involuntary predisposition for the development of physiologic pain (e.g., a family history of RAP). Temperament and personality can make the child more vulnerable to environmental stressors (often minor) that precipitate the sensation of pain. Children who are perfectionists, are dependent, or have low self-esteem may be more likely to experience RAP. Maternal depression, overprotectiveness, and poor conflict resolution in the household are also contributing factors. However, some studies have shown that children with RAP have similar scores on measures of psychologic distress as children with an organic cause for their pain (Thiessen, 2002). Occasionally a precipitating event occurs, but commonly none is found. Positive and negative reinforcement of the pain can modify the RAP (Nurko, 1999b).

RAP occurs in 10% to 15% of children between ages 4 and 16 years. Males and females are affected equally until age 9; between 9 and 12 years of age, the female-to-male ratio is 1.5:1; and the incidence peaks at 10 to 12 years of age. Approximately 10% to 15% of children with RAP have an organic etiology (Theissen, 2002).

Clinical Findings

History. The NP should perform a complete review of systems, as well as a careful psychosocial history (home, school, parents, friends). Findings on history can include the following:

- Periumbilical, generalized, sharp or dull, constant or intermittent pain reported
- Pain occurring on a daily basis and lasting 1 to 3 hours with complete recovery between episodes, lasting at least 3 months
- Episodes described as vague and paroxysmal
- Nighttime pain rare
- Pain often accompanied by a dramatic reaction (clutching abdomen, doubling over, or throwing self to ground)
- School avoidance
- Slight or no fever, nausea, and vomiting
- Bowel habits rarely affected
- Complex rituals—hot pads, repositioning, gentle rubbing by parent—the only providers of relief (Nurko, 1999b)
- Parental history of recurrent abdominal pain
- Pain medications do not alleviate pain
- Illicit drug use
- Sexual activity or abuse and possibility of pregnancy
- Functional or autonomic symptoms (nausea, vomiting, pallor, perspiration, flushing, palpitations, headache)

See Box 33-4 for "red flags" for RAP.

BOX 33-4 *"Red Flags" for Recurrent Abdominal Pain*

Red Flags on History

Localization of the pain away from the umbilicus
Pain associated with a change in bowel habits, particularly diarrhea, constipation, or nocturnal bowel movements
Pain associated with night wakening
Repetitive emesis, especially if bilious
Constitutional symptoms, such as recurrent fever, loss of appetite or energy
Recurrent abdominal pain occurring in a child younger than 4 years of age

Red Flags on Physical Examination

Loss of weight or decline in height velocity
Organomegaly
Localized abdominal tenderness, particularly removed from the umbilicus
Perirectal abnormalities (e.g., fissures, ulceration, or skin tags)
Joint swelling, redness, or heat
Ventral hernias of the abdominal wall

From Thiessen P: Recurrent abdominal pain, *Pediatr Rev* 23(2):43, 2002.

Physical Examination. The physical examination is usually normal but should include the following:

- Abdominal examination: presence of pain, rebound tenderness, masses
- Perianal and rectal examination
- Weight and height plotted on growth curves
- Vital signs (temperature, heart rate, respiratory rate, blood pressure)
- Complete neurologic examination
- Pelvic examination as indicated
- Examination of skin and joints for lesions, swelling, discoloration
- Reexamination during an acute episode
- Complete reexamination with each subsequent visit
- Red flags on physical examination (see Box 33-4)

Diagnostic Tests. Laboratory tests are usually normal, but the following are ordered as indicated:

- CBC with differential, ESR, albumin, and liver and renal function tests if question of organic cause or systemic illness
- UA and urine culture to rule out infection
- Stool for occult blood, pH, reducing substances, culture, and ova and parasites
- Breath hydrogen testing if concerned about carbohydrate malabsorption (lactose intolerance)

Differential Diagnosis

See Fig. 33-5. The following are included in the differential diagnosis:

- All organic causes of abdominal pain, including urinary tract, GI tract, and extraabdominal causes
- Lactose intolerance (usually involving diarrhea, belching, flatulence, and bloating)
- Abdominal pain associated with depression (usually includes social isolation, decreased activity and attention span, difficulty sleeping, and irritability)
- School avoidance (usually associated with severe pain and anxiety on weekday mornings only)
- Irritable bowel syndrome (usually has onset of pain after age 14)

Management

Functional disorders and organic diseases are managed as follows:

For a functional disorder:

- Suggest that the pain can be functional (inorganic) early in the visit. Assure the patient and family that the symptoms are real and that they will not be ignored.
- Reassure the patient and family that no organic cause is present, which is good, and that the child is in no physical danger.
- Discuss how stressful events and emotional issues might affect the pain.
- Encourage return to school, normalization of lifestyle, and limiting attention given for pain episodes.
- Recommend increased dietary fiber (total dosage in milligrams equals the child's age plus 5); restrict caffeine and products with sorbitol (Zeiter & Hyams, 2001).
- Inform parents and child that GI medications generally do not help; however, anticholinergics, antidepressants, and serotonin receptor antagonists have been used (Zeiter & Hyams, 2001).
- Refer for psychologic dysfunction (maladaptive behavior, conversion reaction, depression, anxiety).
- Use psychologic management strategies for the pain (Zeltzer & Bursch, 2001):
  - Relaxation to promote self-regulation through reduction of tension and anxiety. This allows the child to take control of self.
  - Distraction to shift attention from abdominal pain and onto other activities. Attending school is a good distraction.
  - Hypnotherapy to focus attention away from ailing abdomen.
  - Biofeedback to provide evidence to the child that he or she can change muscle tension, skin temperature, and relaxation.
  - Psychotherapy.
  - Family therapy.
- Discuss "red flags" (Box 33-4) so that the parents/child can identify changes in status and illness.

If there is organic disease:

- Refer for organic problem or breath hydrogen testing.
- Establish regular follow-up.

Malabsorption Syndromes

Description

The inability to digest or absorb dietary nutrients leads to malabsorption syndromes. Children can be nearly asymptomatic or suffer from severe malnutrition and FTT.

Etiology and Incidence

Malabsorption syndromes are manifestations of other problems, not disease entities themselves. Improperly absorbed carbohydrates act as osmotic laxatives that pull fluid and electrolytes into the intestine. Carbohydrates are fermented in the bowel and produce abdominal distention and excessive flatus. Fats and proteins can also be malabsorbed and cause symptoms. Lactose malabsorption is the most common malabsorption syndrome.

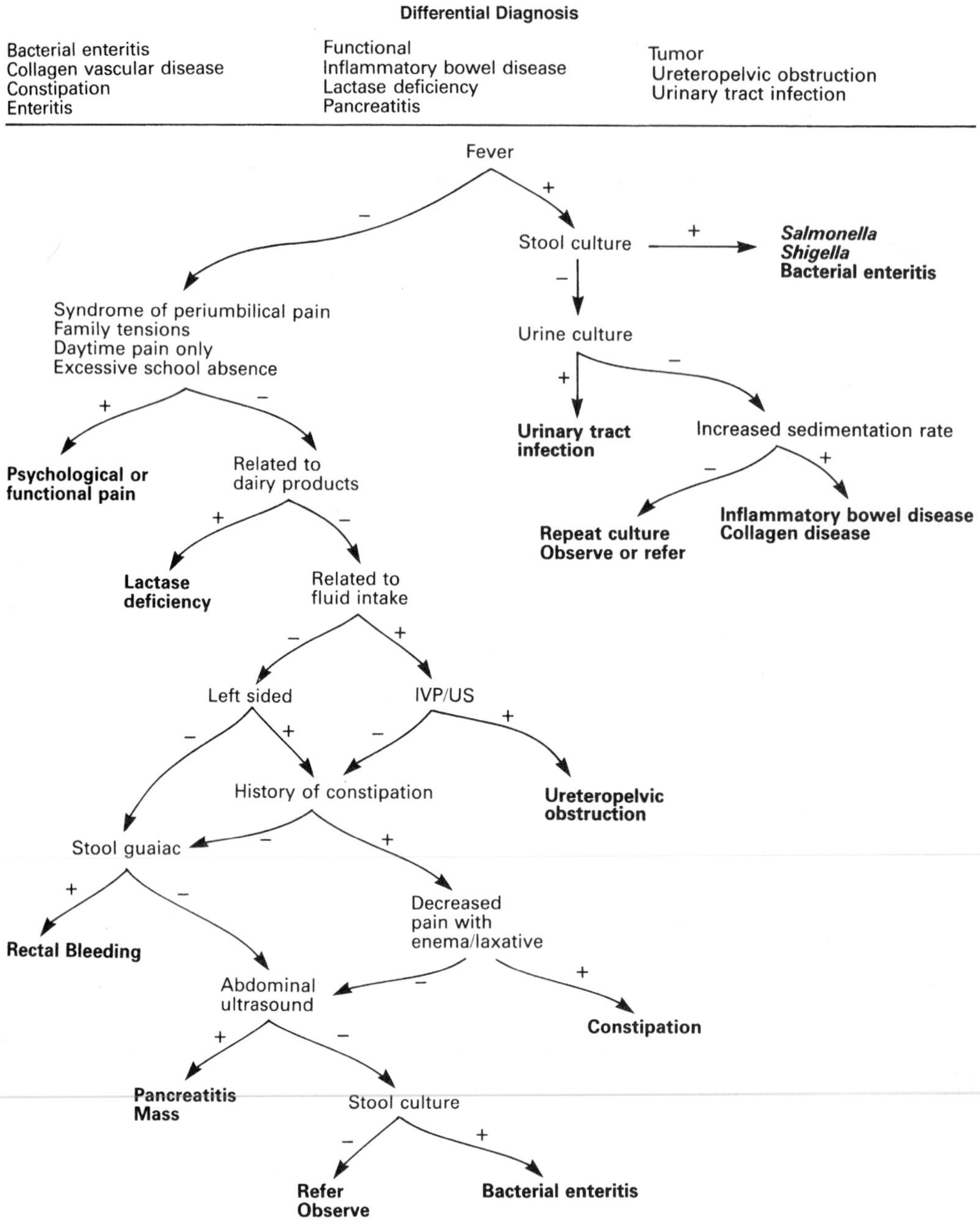

FIGURE 33-5 Decision tree for the differential diagnosis of chronic abdominal pain. (From Schwartz MW et al, editors: *Pediatric primary care: a problem-oriented approach*, ed 3, St Louis, 1997, Mosby.)

Malabsorption secondary to infection may occur. Postinfectious diarrhea is most common in children. Continued infection or damage to the intestinal mucosa from the infecting organism may prolong the diarrhea for weeks. The damaged intestine is unable to absorb nutrients appropriately, which causes an osmotic pull of fluid into the intestine, decreased reabsorption of bile acids, and fermentation leading to diarrhea (Lencer & Wolf, 1999).

Clinical Findings

History. The history can include the following:

- Symptoms that vary by cause
- Chronic diarrhea with frequent, large, foul-smelling, pale stools
- May not have diarrhea
- Excessive flatus with abdominal distention
- Increased appetite

- Growth failure (a common symptom of nutritional deficiency and malabsorption)
- Pallor, fatigue, hair and dermatologic abnormalities, dizziness, cheilosis, glossitis, peripheral neuropathy (symptoms of vitamin deficiency seen with malabsorption)

A complete dietary history is needed to distinguish between undernutrition and malabsorption. Aversions occur to foods that precipitate symptoms. Note that delayed puberty can coexist with malabsorption. Past surgical and trauma history is needed.

Physical Examination. The following should be included:

- Growth parameters and percentiles (weight, height, BMI, head circumference)
- Skinfold thickness and lean body mass
- Tanner stage
- Examination for delayed growth and puberty

Diagnostic Tests. The following are ordered as indicated:

- Stool assessment for occult blood, ova and parasites, white blood cells, and culture; liquid stool for pH and reducing substances; 72-hour fecal fat collection or Sudan stain for stool fat
- CBC with differential, serum calcium, phosphorus, alkaline phosphatase, total protein, ferritin, folate, and liver function tests
- Lactose and sucrose breath hydrogen testing
- Bone age

Differential Diagnosis

FTT, short stature, chronic diarrhea, cystic fibrosis, immune deficiency, hepatic disease, inflammatory bowel disease, and celiac disease are included in the differential diagnosis.

Management

- Treat persistent enteric infection.
- Identify and avoid offending foods. If malabsorption is a primary problem, lifelong food avoidance may be necessary. If it is a secondary problem, retrial of the food at intervals can be attempted.

Polyps

Description

Most children who have colonic juvenile polyps have only a few that are either hamartomatous without adenomatous dysplasia or adenomatous with malignant potential (Hoffenberg et al, 1999). It is imperative to identify if there are only isolated juvenile polyps (JPs) or if a juvenile polyposis coli (JPC) exists. Seventy-five percent to 90% of children with polyps have JP, which is usually found in the rectosigmoid colon. Occasionally, a few other polyps may grow after the diagnosis has been made. A JP is usually pedunculated and on histologic examination has well-differentiated mature epithelial cells. JPC usually involves 5 to 10 or more juvenile polyps that are limited to the colon. JPC can be associated with a protein-losing enteropathy and anemia, and it represents a high risk for malignancy.

Etiology and Incidence

The pathogenesis of juvenile polyps remains poorly understood (Hoffenberg et al, 1999). Recently two genes have been linked to JPC.

Clinical Findings

History. Rectal bleeding is the most common initial symptom in any age. Usually the blood coats or is mixed in with the stool. Bleeding can be daily, intermittent, or infrequent. Large volume loss is extremely rare (Hoffenberg, 2001).

- Most commonly diagnosed at age 4 years
- A visible prolapsed polyp
- Unexplained anemia
- Family history of colon polyps

Physical Examination. The following should be included (Hoffenberg, 2001):

- Anorectal examination to find polyp or other source of rectal bleeding
- Examination for lumps in muscle and bone suggestive of soft tissue tumors (familial adenomatous polyposis)
- Visual examination for mucocutaneous pigmentation, freckling (Peutz-Jeghers syndrome)
- Ophthalmologic examination for congenital hypertrophy of retinal pigment (familial adenomatous polyposis)

Diagnostic Tests

- Colonoscopy has replaced barium enema as the diagnostic test of choice
- Fecal occult blood test, even if blood appears to be present
- Stool culture for bacterial pathogens and parasites
- CBC with differential and ESR
- Prothrombin time and partial thromboplastin time

Management

- All polyps should be removed.
- Children with one to four JPs at diagnosis usually need no further follow-up unless there are recurrent symptoms. If there are five or more JPs, there is a family history of colon polyps, or the biopsied polyps are unusual, follow-up is recommended in 6 to 12 months.
- In JPC, all of the polyps must be removed and close follow-up maintained. Follow-up includes a colonoscopy 1 year after initial diagnosis and then, if no new polyps are noted, every 2 to 3 years. It is imperative to prevent complications from the JPC. Children who have JPC must be followed closely into adulthood to observe for signs of familial adenomatous polyposis syndrome,

which is associated with a number of malignant cancers in adulthood (located in the colon, ampulla of Vater, thyroid gland, stomach, pancreas, liver, or brain).

Anal Fissure

Description

Anal fissures are small tears in the anal mucosa.

Etiology and Incidence

The usual cause of an anal fissure is passage of frequent or hard stools. Anal stenosis and other trauma can also be causative factors. Anal fissures are the most common cause of rectal bleeding in all pediatric groups.

Clinical Findings

History. The following can be reported:

- Crying with bowel movement
- Bright red streaks of blood in the stool or diaper
- Withholding of stool

Physical Examination. With the patient in the knee-chest position and the anus slightly everted, small tears in the anal mucosa can be visible. An otoscope with a large speculum is needed if the external fissures are not readily visible. A digital anal examination with the fifth finger rules out anal stenosis.

Differential Diagnosis

Other sources of lower intestinal hemorrhage such as infection, formula intolerance, necrotizing enterocolitis, intussusception, juvenile polyps, hemolytic-uremic syndrome, Henoch-Schönlein purpura, irritable bowel disease, and vascular lesions are included in the differential diagnosis. Sexual abuse should be considered in children with large, irregular, or multiple fissures.

Management

- Treat the cause.
- Local wound care should include sitz baths twice a day and application of 0.5% hydrocortisone cream or K-Y jelly to the anus.

Complications

Recurrence of fissures is common (e.g., constipation causes a fissure, which leads to a retention-constipation cycle) (Sondheimer, 2003).

Prevention

Preventive measures include the following:

- Avoid constipation
- Encourage regular toileting habits
- Avoid the use of laxative medications and enemas

INFLAMMATORY BOWEL DISEASE

"Inflammatory bowel disease (IBD) is thought to result from inappropriate and ongoing activation of the mucosal immune system driven by normal luminal flora. There are likely defects in both the barrier function of the intestinal epithelium and the mucosal immune system" (Podolsky, 2002). More than 25% of children with IBD are diagnosed before age 20, with about one third having at least one extraintestinal manifestation (Oliva-Hemker, 1999). See Table 33-7 for extraintestinal manifestations and Table 33-8

TABLE 33-7 ***Extraintestinal Manifestations of Inflammatory Bowel Disease***

Site	Manifestation
Skin	Erythema nodosum, pyoderma gangrenosum
Liver	Fatty infiltration, sclerosing cholangitis, chronic hepatitis, cholelithiasis, Budd-Chiari syndrome
Bone	Osteopenia, aseptic necrosis
Joints	Arthralgia, arthritis, ankylosing spondylitis, sacroiliitis
Eye	Uveitis, episcleritis, keratitis
Renal/urologic	Nephrolithiasis, obstructive hydronephrosis, enterovesical fistula, immune complex glomerulonephritis
Hematologic	Anemia (iron, folate, vitamin B_{12} deficiency), thrombocytosis, thrombocytopenia
Vascular	Thrombophlebitis, vasculitis, portal vein thrombosis
Pancreas	Pancreatitis
Other	Growth delay, pubertal delay, possibly lymphoma, possibly acute myelocytic leukemia

From Hyams JS: Inflammatory bowel disease, *Pediatr Rev* 21(9):292, 2000.

TABLE 33-8 *Features of Crohn's Disease and Ulcerative Colitis*

Feature	Crohn's Disease	Ulcerative Colitis
Age at onset	10-20 yr	10-20 yr
Area of bowel affected	Oropharynx, esophagus, and stomach, rare; small bowel only, 25%-30%; colon and anus only, 25%; ileocolitis, 40%; diffuse disease, 5%	Total colon, 90%; proctitis, 10%
Distribution	Segmental; disease-free skip areas common	Continuous distal to proximal
Pathology	Full-thickness, acute, and chronic inflammation; noncaseating granulomas (50%), extraintestinal fistulas, abscesses, stricture, and fibrosis may be present	Superficial, acute inflammation of mucosa with microscopic crypt abscess
X-ray findings	Segmental lesions; thickened, circular folds, cobblestone appearance of bowel wall secondary to longitudinal ulcers and transverse fissures; fixation and separation of loops; narrowed lumen, "string sign"; fistulas	Superficial colitis; loss of haustra; shortened colon and pseudopolyps (islands of normal tissue surrounded by denuded mucosa) are late findings
Intestinal symptoms	Abdominal pain, diarrhea (usually loose with blood if colon involved), perianal disease, enteroenteric or enterocutaneous fistula, abscess, anorexia	Abdominal pain, bloody diarrhea, urgency, and tenesmus
Extraintestinal symptoms		
Arthritis/arthralgia	15%	9%
Fever	40%-50%	40%-50%
Stomatitis	9%	2%
Weight loss	90% (mean 5.7 kg)	68% (mean 4.1 kg)
Delayed growth and sexual development	30%	5%-10%
Uveitis, conjunctivitis	15% (in Crohn's colitis)	4%
Sclerosing cholangitis	—	4%
Renal stones	6% (oxalate)	6% (urate)
Pyoderma gangrenosum	1%-3%	5%
Erythema nodosum	8%-15%	4%
Laboratory findings	High erythrocyte sedimentation rate; microcytic anemia, low serum iron and total iron-binding capacity; increased fecal protein loss; low serum albumin; antineutrophil cytoplasmic antibodies present in 10%-20%; *Saccaromyces cerevisiae* antibodies positive in 60%	High erythrocyte sedimentation rate, microcytic anemia; high white blood cell count with left shift; antineutrophil cytoplasmic antibodies present in 80%

From Kirschner BS: Inflammatory bowel disease in children, *Pediatr Clin North Am* 35:189, 1989. Cited in Sundheimer J: Gastrointestinal tract. In Hay WW et al, editors: *Current pediatric diagnosis and treatment*, ed 16, New York, 2003, Lange Medical Books.

for features of Crohn's disease in contrast with ulcerative colitis (UC).

Crohn's Disease

Description

Crohn's disease is a chronic inflammatory disease with exacerbations and remissions involving any portion of the intestinal tract. Areas of intestine that are unaffected are called skip areas.

Etiology and Incidence

The cause is largely unknown. Susceptibility to Crohn's disease is most likely inherited (Podolsky, 2002). The disease is most likely a genetically determined response that is immunologically mediated. Crohn's disease has a multifactorial basis (heredity, diet, immunologic aberrations, and ineffective mucosal integrity) that is probably influenced by environmental factors (Israel, 1999). The disease occurs in 16 of every 100,000 individuals, affects males and females equally, and is more common in white people.

Twenty-five percent to 40% of cases are diagnosed in childhood and adolescence. Siblings are 17 to 35 times more likely to get Crohn's disease than is the general population (Hyams, 2000).

Clinical Findings

History. The following can be reported:

- Fever
- Weight loss (average of 5 to 7 kg)
- Delayed growth
- Arthralgias/arthritis in large joints, occasional joint destruction
- Obstructive symptoms associated with meals
- Pain in the umbilical region and RLQ; may awaken at night
- Anorexia
- Malabsorption and lactose intolerance
- Bloody diarrhea and pain with stooling
- Mouth sores, especially during exacerbations of the illness
- Use of NSAIDs, use of tobacco (Podolsky, 2002)

Physical Examination

- A complete physical examination is required.
- Carefully measure growth parameters (height, weight, and BMI).
- An abdominal examination is performed while observing for RLQ tenderness and a mass.
- Perianal skin tags, deep anal fissures, and perianal fistulas strongly suggest Crohn's disease.
- Clubbing of digits may be present.
- Erythema nodosum is common.

Diagnostic Tests. The following are ordered as needed:

- CBC, total protein, albumin, ESR, CRP
- Stool for culture, ova, parasites, and *Clostridium difficile* (with recent antibiotic use)
- Stool for blood and white blood cells
- Bone age (usually delayed by 2 years)

Differential Diagnosis

Rheumatoid arthritis, systemic lupus erythematosus, hypopituitarism, acute appendicitis, peptic ulcer, intestinal obstruction, intestinal lymphoma, anorexia, and growth failure are included in the differential diagnosis (Sondheimer, 2003).

Management

The goals of therapy are to (1) control the disease and induce a lasting remission; (2) prevent relapses; and (3) achieve normal nutrition, growth, and lifestyle. Treatment is pharmacologic, nutritional, surgical, and psychosocial. The following management steps are taken:

- Refer for endoscopy, definitive diagnosis, consultation, and follow-up care.
- Medications:
  - Antidiarrheals will not help inflammation but will help make the symptoms manageable.
  - Corticosteroids are used orally, rectally, or intravenously for acute exacerbations. They are not intended for use in remission.
  - Aminosalicylates (sulfasalazine, olsalazine, and mesalamine) are given topically (enema) or orally.
  - Immunomodulatory agents may be used (azathioprine, 6-mercaptopurine, methotrexate, and cyclosporine).
  - Antibiotics are used for acute exacerbation (ampicillin, gentamicin, clindamycin, or metronidazole).
  - Metronidazole (Flagyl) prophylaxis (15 mg/kg per day) is used for perianal disease until the patient has mild to no disease symptoms. The use of ciprofloxacin and clarithromycin is currently under investigation.
  - Anti–tumor necrosis factor (anti-TNF) agents such as Infliximab may be used.
  - The administration of healthy bacteria (probiotics) is also under investigation (Podolsky, 2002).
- Severe disease can require hospitalization, total parenteral nutrition, a nasogastric tube for decompression, and surgery. Seventy percent of patients eventually (10 to 20 years following diagnosis) require surgery (Hyams, 2000; Sondheimer, 2003).
- Monitor growth.
- If the small bowel is involved, an ophthalmologic examination is needed to rule out underlying ophthalmologic manifestations of the disease.
- Refer for nutritional therapy to help induce remission, prevent or correct malnutrition, and maintain and promote growth. See Box 12-9 for specific nutritional recommendations.
- Refer for psychosocial therapy as indicated. Depressive disorders are common.

Complications

Growth failure, fistula and abscess formation, intestinal obstruction, and malnutrition can occur. Perforation and hemorrhage are rare (Sondheimer, 2003). Cholelithiasis, nephrolithiasis, pancreatitis, pericarditis, and peripheral neuropathy are other complications of Crohn's disease (Winesett, 1997). There is also an increased risk of colon cancer.

Prevention/Prognosis

Follow recommended therapy to avoid sequelae. Crohn's disease is usually progressive. Over 50% experience symptoms affecting quality of life, 20% have severe disability, and 20% describe themselves as healthy (Sondheimer, 2003). Only 1% do not have at least one relapse after diagnosis and therapy (Hyams, 2000).

Ulcerative Colitis

Description

Ulcerative colitis is characterized by recurring bloody diarrhea with acute and chronic inflammation limited to the colon. Patients with ulcerative colitis have significant weight loss secondary to chronic caloric insufficiency.

Etiology and Incidence

The cause is largely unknown but is probably a genetically determined response that is immunologically mediated. It is thought to be an altered immunologic response in the intestinal mucosa. The disease has a multifactorial basis (heredity, diet, immunologic aberrations, and ineffective mucosal integrity) influenced by environmental factors (Israel, 1999). The overall incidence is 2 cases per 100,000, with the peak onset occurring among 16- to 20-year-olds. Approximately 20% occur in children younger than 20 years (Snyder, 2002).

Clinical Findings

History. The following can be reported:

- Fever
- Weight loss (average of 4 kg)
- Delayed growth and sexual maturation
- Arthritis/arthralgias of the large joints
- Anorexia
- Diarrhea
- Lower abdominal cramping, left lower quadrant pain
- Pain increased before stooling and passing flatus
- Stool with bright red blood and mucus
- Oral ulcers possible with active disease
- Skin lesions (erythema nodosum, pyoderma gangrenosum, and diffuse papulonecrotic eruptions)

Physical Examination

- Perform a complete physical examination.
- Carefully measure growth parameters (weight, height, and BMI).
- Abdominal examination can reveal rebound tenderness if the disease is severe.

Diagnostic Tests. The following are ordered as needed:

- CBC with differential, iron-binding capacity, total protein, albumin, ESR, CRP, platelet count
- Stool for white blood cells, blood, and culture
- Bone age (usually delayed up to 2 years)

Differential Diagnosis

Shigella, Salmonella, Yersinia, Campylobacter, Escherichia coli, C. difficile, irritable bowel syndrome, and Crohn's disease are the differential diagnoses (Sondheimer, 2003).

Management

The goals of therapy are to (1) control the disease and induce a lasting remission; (2) prevent relapses; and (3) achieve normal nutrition, growth, and lifestyle. Treatment is pharmacologic, nutritional, surgical, and psychosocial. Management involves the following:

1. Refer for endoscopy, definitive diagnosis, consultation, and close follow-up care.
2. Medications:
   - Aminosalicylates (sulfasalazine, mesalamine) orally or rectally
   - Parenteral or oral steroids for moderate to severe disease, tapered doses for remission
   - Immunomodulatory agents (azathioprine or 6-mercaptopurine) to wean off steroids
   - Hydrocortisone rectal preparation for tenesmus
   - Antispasmodics before meals
   - Iron supplementation to correct anemia
3. Nutrition (see Box 12-9 for nutritional recommendations):
   - Diet: high in protein and carbohydrate, normal amount of fat, and decreased roughage.
   - Lactose is poorly tolerated (Sondheimer, 2003).
   - Vitamin and iron supplementation is recommended.
   - Parenteral/enteral nutritional supplements (60 to 70 cal/kg per day) may be used.
   - Refer for nutritional therapy to prevent/correct malnutrition and maintain and promote growth.
4. Monitor growth.
5. Refer for surgery as indicated (can be curative).
6. Refer for ophthalmologic examination to rule out ophthalmologic manifestations of the disease.
7. Refer for psychosocial therapy as indicated. Depressive disorders are common.

Complications

Complications can include growth failure, toxic megacolon, intestinal perforation, liver disease, sepsis, colitis (children with pancolitis experience a much more severe course), cancer of the colon (can be a long-term sequela—1% to 2% per year after 10 years of disease), arthritis, uveitis, and malnutrition (Sondheimer, 2003).

Prevention/Prognosis

Follow the recommended therapy to avoid complications. Prognosis is good. Seventy percent will go into remission within 3 months of diagnosis, following initiation of therapy. Fifty percent will remain in remission. Up to 26% with severe disease require colectomy, whereas only 10% with mild disease do (Hyams, 2000).

Foreign Bodies in the Gastrointestinal Tract

Description

Most swallowed foreign bodies pass through the GI tract without difficulty. Some objects get lodged at points of narrowing (cricopharyngeal muscle, the carina, Schatzki ring, cardioesophageal junction, pylorus, ligament of Treitz). Anything 3 to 5 cm or larger might have trouble passing the ligament of Treitz. The need for surgical intervention for a GI foreign body is about 1% (Chen & Beierle, 2001).

Etiology and Incidence

The cause is a swallowed foreign body, with the highest incidence occurring between 6 months and 3 years of age (Chen & Beierle, 2001). Foreign body ingestion occurs equally in boys and girls, with developmentally delayed children at higher risk. Common items include coins (most commonly pennies), food, toys, marbles, buttons, and batteries. Bezoars are foreign bodies that have accumulated over time in the alimentary tract (Chen & Beierle, 2001). Bezoars are most often caused by plant or vegetable matter (phytobezoar), hair (trichobezoar), and persimmons (disopyrobezoar). Bezoars eventually cause obstructive symptoms because of increasing size.

Clinical Findings

History

- Often there is no history of swallowing a foreign body.
- Initially the child might have experienced a coughing, choking, or gagging episode (although this episode might not have been observed by the parents). Persistent wheezing that is unresponsive to bronchodilators may indicate a foreign body in the esophagus (Chen & Beierle, 2001).
- Subsequent symptoms can include discomfort in the throat or chest, refusal to eat, increased salivation, vomiting, pain with swallowing, and respiratory difficulty (Karjoo, 1998).

Physical Examination

- Most children are asymptomatic.
- GI examination is normal.
- Respiratory symptoms may be found if the foreign body is lodged in the esophagus and pressing on the trachea.

Diagnostic Tests

- If symptoms of obstruction persist, radiographic studies are ordered to rule out a foreign body. A dime is 17 mm, a penny 18 mm, a nickel 20 mm, and a quarter 23 mm in size. The radiographic studies should include the neck, the chest, and the upper abdomen (Chen & Bierle, 2001). Abdominal radiographs can be ordered if an object has not been seen in the stool and symptoms of distress or obstruction are present.
- A contrast study (barium esophogram) or forced expiratory film is needed if a foreign body is suspected but is not radiopaque.
- An alternative to radiography is a handheld metal detector.

Management

If asymptomatic or if the foreign body is in the stomach or intestine, no intervention is necessary and the family can be reassured. Smooth objects, buttons, and most coins can remain in the intestines for months without symptoms. The exception is new, mostly zinc pennies, which can cause a chemical reaction and poisoning. Watch for fecal passage and report any new associated symptoms. Follow-up radiography is indicated after 2 weeks if a coin has not been identified in stool. Emergent endoscopic removal of all batteries should be done because burns and injury can occur within 4 hours of ingestion.

If symptomatic or if the object is sharp or very large, give the child nothing by mouth until a decision is made. Consult with a physician and pediatric surgeon. Generally, foreign bodies that remain in the esophagus longer than 3 hours or in the small intestine longer than 5 days need to be removed. Removal is often accomplished via a Foley catheter technique or by gastroesophagoscopy. Sharp objects (e.g., open safety pins, wooden toothpicks, and fish bones) and small batteries also need to be removed; this is generally accomplished by endoscopy (Chen & Beierle, 2001). When it is unclear how long a foreign body has been in the esophagus or if it has been there more than 48 hours, it should be retrieved with an endoscope. Foreign bodies can erode into esophageal tissue and ultimately cause catastrophic perforation (Chen & Beierle, 2001).

Complications

Perforation or stricture formation can occur in up to 10% of children.

Prevention

Parent education, anticipatory counseling, and careful supervision of children are needed. Avoid ear piercing in children younger than 2 years because earrings are easily ingested.

FAILURE TO THRIVE (ORGANIC)

Description

Failure to thrive (FTT), also called growth deficiency (Brayden, Daley, & Brown, 2003), is described as inadequate weight gain as determined by standardized growth charts. The diagnosis is based on a child's weight being below the

3rd to 5th percentile or falling more than two major percentile groups or becoming flat. Weight almost always falls before height and head circumference do. Organic FTT is also referred to as undernutrition due to major organ system disease (Brayden, Daley, & Brown, 2003).

Etiology and Incidence

FTT can be associated with multiple medical conditions (Table 33-9) and psychologic factors (see Chapter 19). The purpose of this section is to discuss the assessment, laboratory findings, and differential diagnosis related to medical/organic causes of FTT; however, it is necessary to consider all physical and psychologic factors concurrently when evaluating FTT. Eight percent to 10% of children seen for primary care have signs of growth failure, with the number rising to 15% to 30% in inner-city emergency departments (Brayden, Daley, & Brown, 2003).

Clinical Findings

A thoughtful approach to the history, physical examination, and laboratory evaluation of children with FTT includes the following (Brayden, Daley, & Brown, 2003; Schwartz, 2000):

History

- Three-day diet history
- Careful family history of weight, height, BMI, growth patterns, and chronic health conditions
- Prenatal factors: drug, alcohol, and tobacco exposure; length of gestation; illnesses; weight gain; nutrition; TORCHES (toxoplasmosis, rubella, cytomegalovirus, herpes, syphilis); and human immunodeficiency virus (HIV) exposure
- Perinatal factors: birth weight, Apgar scores, complications, length of stay in the hospital, congenital anomalies, neurologic insults, newborn screening results
- Collection and interpretation of growth data for the child's measurements, percentiles, BMI, height for weight over time
- General parental concerns about the child's weight and growth
- General health history: hospitalizations, medications, surgeries, accidents, illnesses
- Developmental history
- Nutrition history: caloric intake; feeding behavior; feeding cues; cues to hunger and satiety; ability to suck, swallow, chew; progression to solids; frequency of feedings; amount taken per feeding; preparation of formula (overdilution), family eating patterns (meals and child feeding)
- Stooling and voiding history: diarrhea, constipation, vomiting, poor urine stream
- Social and family factors: family composition, caregiving environment, day care, family support, finances, parent-child relationship, parenting attitudes, typical day
- Careful review of systems

Physical Examination

- Weight, height, BMI, and head circumference (in those younger than 2 years) plotted on standardized growth curves and percentiles, including weight for height graphs
- Skinfold measurements

TABLE 33-9 ***Major Organic Causes of Failure to Thrive***

System	Cause
Gastrointestinal	Gastroesophageal reflux, celiac disease, pyloric stenosis, cleft palate/cleft lip, lactose intolerance, Hirschsprung's disease, milk protein intolerance, hepatitis, cirrhosis, pancreatic insufficiency, biliary disease, inflammatory bowel disease, malabsorption
Renal	Urinary tract infection, renal tubular acidosis, diabetes insipidus, chronic renal insufficiency
Cardiopulmonary	Cardiac diseases leading to congestive heart failure, asthma, bronchopulmonary dysplasia, cystic fibrosis, anatomic abnormalities of the upper airway
Endocrine	Hypothyroidism, diabetes mellitus, adrenal insufficiency or excess, parathyroid disorders, pituitary disorders, growth hormone deficiency
Neurologic	Mental retardation, cerebral hemorrhage, degenerative disorders
Infectious	Parasitic or bacterial infections of the gastrointestinal tract, tuberculosis, human immunodeficiency virus disease
Metabolic	Inborn errors of metabolism
Congenital	Chromosomal abnormalities, congenital syndromes (e.g., fetal alcohol syndrome), perinatal infections
Miscellaneous	Lead poisoning, malignancy, collagen-vascular disease, recurrently infected adenoids and tonsils

From Behrman RE, Kliegman R, Jenson HR, editors: *Nelson textbook of pediatrics*, ed 16, Philadelphia, 2000, WB Saunders, p 120.

- Vital signs (temperature, pulse, respiratory rate, blood pressure)
- Evidence of abuse or neglect
- Presence of dysmorphic features
- Upper and lower segment measurements (Fig. 33-6) to rule out dwarfism
- Skin, hair, nails, and mucous membranes
  - Scaling skin seen with zinc deficiency
  - Rough or hard skin with hypothyroidism
  - Edema with protein deficiency
  - Alopecia with hypervitaminosis or syphilis
  - Spoon-shaped nails with iron deficiency or GI diseases
  - Cyanosis with heart disease
  - Labial fissures with vitamin deficiency

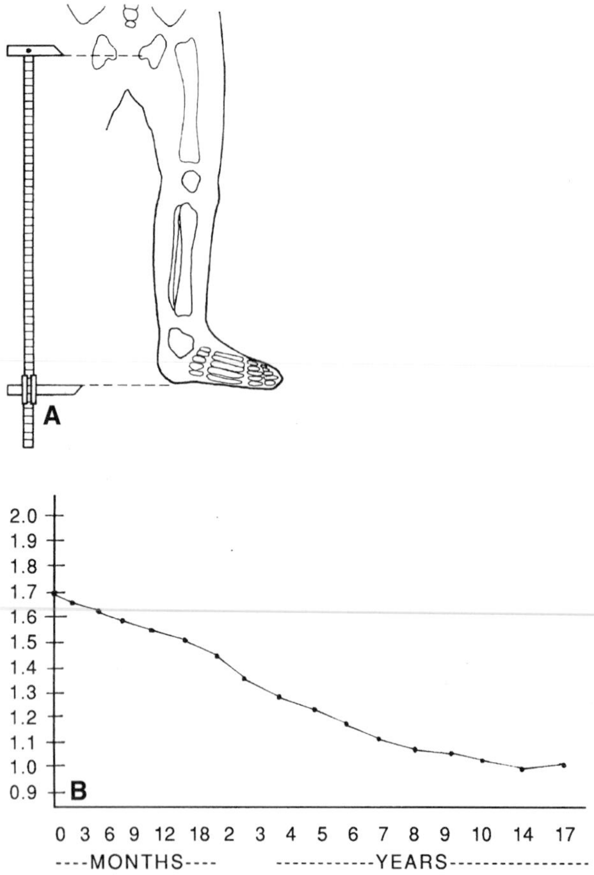

FIGURE 33-6 Upper:lower (U:L) segment ratios. **A**, To calculate U:L segment ratios use the following formula: (height − lower segment)/ lower segment. **B**, Normal U:L segment ratios. 1.7 at birth, 1.3 at 3 years of age, 1.0 at 14 years of age. High U:L ratios are characteristic of short limb dwarfism or bone disorders such as rickets. (From Behrman RE, Kliegman R, Jenson HB: *Nelson textbook of pediatrics*, ed 17, Philadelphia, 2004, WB Saunders; Siberry GK, Iannone R, editors: *The Harriet Lane handbook*, ed 15, St Louis, 2000, Mosby, p 278.)

- Oral findings: dental caries, tonsillar hypertrophy, submucous cleft palate or tongue enlargement
- Lymphadenopathy and splenomegaly with malignancy and immune deficiency
- Endocrine: thyroid enlargement, precocious or ambiguous sexual development
- Neuromuscular tone and strength
- Disproportionate somatic growth (dwarfism)

Diagnostic Tests

Appropriate use of laboratory tests is indicated by the history and physical examination.

- UA and urine culture
- CBC, differential and platelets, ESR
- Serum electrolytes (make sure to get total CO_2)
- Lead level
- Purified protein derivative (PPD) with *Candida* control
- HIV screening
- Serum protein, albumin, alkaline phosphatase, blood urea nitrogen (BUN), and creatinine
- Thyroid function and growth hormone (expensive, often done later in workup)
- Stool studies for fat, reducing substances, ova and parasites, and culture
- Sweat test
- Bone age
- Chest radiograph
- Renal ultrasonography and voiding cystourethrography
- Developmental testing

Differential Diagnosis

See Table 33-9.

Management

- Manage treatable causes.
- Provide nutritional support: vitamin supplementation with iron, zinc, and minerals; calorically enriched formula and foods (up to 150 cal/kg per day). See Box 12-4 for further information related to FTT.
- Provide parent education and support.
- Make referrals as needed.
- Provide close follow-up, initially every 1 to 2 weeks. Day care may provide structure for eating, as well as other activities.
- Acceptable weight gain by age (Brayden, Daley, & Brown, 2003):
  - Birth to 3 months: 20 to 30 g/day
  - Age 3 to 6 months: 15 to 20 g/day
  - Age 6 to 9 months: 10 to 15 g/day
  - Age 9 to 12 months: 6 to 11 g/day

- Age 12 to 18 months: 5 to 8 g/day
- Age 18 to 24 months: 3 to 7 g/day

LOWER GASTROINTESTINAL TRACT INFECTIONS

Acute Diarrhea

Description

Acute diarrhea is excessive loss of fluid and electrolytes in the stool. Significant stool losses are defined as greater than 10 g/kg per day in infants and greater than 200 g/day in children (Nurko, 1999a; Vanderhoof, 1998).

Etiology and Incidence

Four kinds of diarrhea are recognized (Nurko, 1999a; Vanderhoof, 1998):

1. Osmotic diarrhea results when osmotically active particles in the intestine draw excess fluid into the stool; this condition occurs with dumping syndrome, lactase deficiency, overfeeding, malabsorption syndromes, and excess ingestion of hypertonic juices.
2. Secretory diarrhea occurs in the presence of inhibition of ion absorption or stimulation of ion excretion, as seen in the presence of bacterial endotoxins.
3. Motility disorders cause diarrhea but not malabsorption. Bile salt and pancreatic enzyme deficiency can cause diarrhea by deletion or inhibition of the normal absorption process.
4. Inflammatory processes such as bacterial invasion, celiac sprue, and irritable bowel syndrome or surgical procedures can change the anatomy and functional ability of the intestine. Abnormal peristalsis for any reason can result in acute diarrhea.

Diarrhea can be caused by various viral and bacterial agents, including the following:

- *Campylobacter jejuni* is a gram-negative rod found in contaminated food and water. It is usually acquired by toddlers and children from household pets, which serve as reservoirs. *C. jejuni* is less common after age 7 to 8 years, although neonates are susceptible. It is most common in the summer months.
- *Clostridium difficile* is a gram-positive anaerobic bacillus. Asymptomatic carriers of *C. difficile* who take antibiotics (usually ampicillin, clindamycin, and cephalosporins) experience increased growth of the organism. *C. difficile* intestinal colonization rates in healthy neonates and young infants can be as high as 50% but are usually less than 5% in children older than 2 years and adults (American Academy of Pediatrics [AAP], 2003).
- *Yersinia enterocolitica* is a gram-negative rod found in contaminated food (uncooked pork and unpasteurized milk) and water. It produces an enterotoxin that causes secretion of fluid and electrolytes into the bowel. *Y. enterocolitica* causes diarrhea in children of all ages.
- *Salmonella* is a gram-negative rod found in contaminated, improperly cooked poultry, eggs, dairy products, and sausage. It is spread by human-to-human contact. *Salmonella* is most common in children younger than 4 years of age. The peak incidence is in the first months of life (AAP, 2003). Invasive disease is more common in children with underlying chronic illness (AAP, 2000).
- *Shigella* is a gram-negative rod found in contaminated food and water. Humans are the host and reservoir, and the organism is spread by the fecal-oral route. The organism multiplies and releases cytotoxin, which causes epithelial damage and ulceration. *Shigella* is most common in children 6 months to 3 years of age.
- Enterohemorrhagic *E. coli* strains are associated with diarrhea, hemorrhagic colitis, hemolytic-uremic syndrome, and postdiarrheal idiopathic thrombocytopenic purpura. *E. coli* O157:H7 is the prototype and can cause mild to severe, profuse, and bloody diarrhea. The disease can be transmitted from infected persons, carriers, or food and water contaminated by human feces. *E. coli* O157:H7 has been found in undercooked ground beef, raw fruit and vegetables, and unpasteurized fruit juices. Incubation is from 10 hours to 6 days; *E. coli* O157:H7 infection usually lasts 3 to 4 days and can be fatal.
- Viruses (human rotavirus, adenovirus, Norwalk-like virus, and small round viruses) invade the intestinal mucosa and leave a decreased surface area and decreased absorptive capacity. This type of diarrhea is the most common (Spitzer, 2002).

Acute diarrhea accounts for approximately 20% of acute care visits in children younger than 2 years. It is the cause of 8 in 1000 hospitalizations in children younger than 1 year and is the reason for 10% of preventable deaths in the United States. Acute diarrhea is responsible for 500 deaths per year in the United States among children 1 to 4 years of age. Poor access to care and poverty are correlated with increased mortality rates from diarrhea (Behrman, Kliegman, & Jenson, 2004).

Clinical Findings

History. The following should be included (Table 33-10):

- Pattern of diarrhea: when diarrhea began, number of stools, frequency, quality of stools
- Signs and symptoms associated with infectious diarrhea: bloody stool, abdominal pain, vomiting, or fever
- Number of wet diapers in the past 24 hours and approximate time of last voiding

- Dietary record, changes in diet that might correlate with increased stooling
- Family members with similar illness or other GI diseases
- Day care or school illness patterns and contacts
- Travel history
- Previous growth pattern

Physical Examination. Assess the following (see Table 33-10):

- Vital signs
- Hydration status (see Table 33-1)
- Weight and height
- State of alertness
- Anterior fontanel if still open

Diagnostic Tests. The following are ordered as indicated:

- Stool examination (color, consistency, blood, mucus, pus, odor, volume)
- Stool pH, Clinitest, and heme test
- Stool for ova and parasites, white blood cells, and culture
- Specific laboratory findings (Table 33-11)

Differential Diagnosis

Numerous causes, including infection (bacterial or viral), medication ingestion, parasitic infestations, anatomic abnormalities, dietary intolerances, and appendicitis, may be responsible for acute diarrhea.

Management

The following steps are taken:

- Restore and maintain hydration. Oral rehydration with an oral electrolyte solution should be attempted. Appropriate rehydration solutions include Pedialyte and Infalyte. It is inappropriate to use fruit juices, Kool-Aid, sports drinks, or soda. If the child is not vomiting, oral rehydration can be accomplished quickly (less than 4 hours) (see Table 33-2 and Box 33-1). For formula-fed infants, returning to full-strength formula as quickly as possible is recommended. If the child is unable to tolerate full-strength formula, a diluted formula (one fourth to half strength) can be used for a short time (4 to 6 hours) as tolerated. The child's regular formula can be used initially as long as it is tolerated. If not tolerated, use soy or hydrolysate formula. Breastfed infants should continue to breastfeed more frequently for shorter periods.
- For children who are taking solids, it is important to introduce bland, soft foods within the first 24 to 48 hours of rehydration. An age-appropriate diet with avoidance of fatty foods and foods high in simple sugars is recommended. Complex carbohydrates, lean meat, yogurt, fruit, and vegetables are well tolerated and assist in firming up the stool (AAP Provisional Committee on Quality Improvement, Subcommittee on Acute Gastroenteritis, 1996).
- Prescribe medications as indicated (see Table 33-10).
- Antidiarrheals are not generally recommended because the offending organism must be excreted. If diarrhea persists beyond the initial infection, cautious use of these agents in older children is acceptable. There is evidence that *Lactobacillus* given early in a diarrheal illness can shorten the duration of the diarrhea and lessen the number of stools per day (Van Niel et al, 2002). *Lactobacillus* is most effective above a threshold dose (10 billion colony-forming units) during the first 24 to 48 hours of diarrhea. This dose results in colonization of the intestine and inhibition of attachment by pathogens (Saxelin, Salminen, & Vapaatalo, 1991).
- Studies looking at the efficacy of zinc given to children with acute diarrhea show a decrease in the duration of illness. Further studies are needed to evaluate adverse effects and dosing (Strand et al, 2002).
- Administer parenteral hydration if necessary for the following:
  - Impaired circulation and possible shock
  - Weight less than 4 to 5 kg or a child younger than 3 months
  - Intractable diarrhea, lethargy, anatomic anomalies
  - Failure to gain weight or continued weight loss despite oral fluids
- Use telephone follow-up as indicated.

Complications

Chronic diarrhea or dehydration leads to acidosis, causing cardiovascular collapse and possible death.

- *C. jejuni* can lead to hemorrhagic necrosis of the jejunum, reactive arthritis, seizures, pseudotumor in the mesenteric lymph nodes, and hemolytic-uremic syndrome.
- *C. difficile* can cause pseudomembranous colitis, toxic megacolon, colonic perforation, relapse, intractable proctitis, and death in debilitated children.
- *Y. enterocolitica* can result in septicemia and acute ileitis syndrome.
- *Salmonella* can cause bacteremia, focal infection, and a carrier state.
- *Shigella* can lead to toxic megacolon, cholestatic hepatitis, hemolytic-uremic syndrome, Reiter syndrome, and bacteremia.
- *E. coli* O157:H7 can cause hemolytic-uremic syndrome.

Prevention

Preventive measures include the following:

- Good handwashing by the child and care providers. Liquid soap and paper towels are recommended at day care centers.

TABLE 33-10 ***Infectious Diarrhea: Signs, Symptoms, and Treatment***

Cause	Diarrhea	Bloody Stool	Abdominal Pain	Vomiting	Fever	Other	Treatment
Campylobacter jejuni	+++ Foul smelling		+	+	+		Erythromycin, 40 mg/kg per day in 3 divided doses for 5-7 days decreases fecal excretion in 24-48 hr; illness lasts 7-12 days
Clostridium difficile	++	+	+				Discontinue offending antibiotic (see text) Metronidazole, 30 mg/kg per day in 4 divided doses for 7-10 days *or* Vancomycin, 40 mg/kg per day in 4 divided doses for 7-10 days Cholestyramine helps bind the toxin and decrease diarrhea
Yersinia entercolitica	+ Green/ malodorous	+	+ RLQ pain		+		Usually resolves spontaneously in 3-4 days; if septic, TMP-SMZ, 8 mg TMP/kg per day in 2 divided doses for 7-10 days, *or* Chloramphenicol, 50-75 mg/kg per day in 4 divided doses for 7-10 days, *or* Tetracycline, 25-50 mg/kg per day in 4 divided doses for 7-10 days (older teens only)
Salmonella	++	+	+ Rebound tenderness	+	+	Sepsis Bacteremia	No treatment if uncomplicated Usually resolves spontaneously Antibiotics can prolong the carrier state Antibiotics indicated for children younger than 1 yr who are at risk for bacteremia and for patients who are immunosuppressed or have cardiac or valvular disease, lymphoproliferative diseases, sickle cell disease, or hemolytic anemias If indicated, use amoxicillin, 40 mg/kg per day in 3 divided doses for 7-10 days *or* TMP-SMZ, 8 mg TMP/kg per day for 7-10 days in 2 divided doses, *or* Chloramphenicol, 50-75 mg/kg per day in 4 divided doses for 7-10 days Steroids and prostaglandins may be necessary for severe illness
Shigella	+++ (initially) + (after 1-3 days)	+	+		+	Irritability Listlessness Patulous rectum	Need susceptibility information Resistance is common TMP-SMZ, 8 mg TMP/kg per day in 2 divided doses for 5 days *or*
Escherichia coli	++	+	+ Cramps and abdominal pain	−/+	+	Hemolytic-uremic syndrome	TMP-SMZ, 8 mg TMP/kg per day in 2 divided doses for 7-10 days if diarrhea is moderate to severe Do CBC, platelets, and kidney function tests
Virus	+++ Watery		+ Cramps	+	+		Symptomatic treatment and maintenance of fluids

CBC, Complete blood count; *RLQ*, right lower quadrant; *TMP-SMZ*, trimethoprim-sulfamethoxazole.

TABLE 33-11 *Laboratory Findings Associated with Infectious Diarrhea*

Cause	Bloody Stool	WBCs in Stool	Stool Culture	CBC	Other
Campylobacter jejuni	+ Gross	+	+	↑ WBCs	Darting and motility on microscopy
Clostridium difficile	+ Gross	+	+ For toxin	Slightly ↑ WBCs ESR nl	
Yersinia enterocolitica	+ Gross or occult	+	+		
Salmonella	+ Gross	+	+	↓, nl, or slightly ↑ WBCs with left shift	
Shigella	+ Gross	+	+	nl or slightly ↑ WBCs with left shift	
Escherichia coli	+ Gross	—	+		Hemolytic-uremic syndrome as a complication
Virus	—	—	±*		

*If virus is suspected, consider studying stool for reducing substances, Clinitest, heme test, and pH. Can test stool using enzyme-linked immunosorbent assay (ELISA) and latex agglutination assay for rotavirus.
CBC, Complete blood count; *ESR*, erythrocyte sedimentation rate; *nl*, normal; *WBCs*, white blood cells; +, present; −, not a clinical finding ±, may or may not be present; ↑, increased; ↓, decreased.

- Good sanitation and appropriate removal of soiled clothing and diapers. The diapering area should be cleaned after changing each baby at day care centers.
- Avoiding contaminated sources; meat should be properly cooked.
- With *Shigella*, culture all symptomatic contacts and treat those with positive stool cultures.

Chronic Diarrhea

Description

Chronic diarrhea is defined as one or more liquid to semiliquid stools passed per day for 14 days or longer.

Etiology

Causes include the following:

- Iatrogenic causes: excessive fluids (greater than 150 ml/kg per day) (including ingestion of large amounts of fruit juices) and a diet in which less than 25% of the total calories is from fat
- Infants: formula protein intolerance (50% crossover between cow's milk and soy formulas)
- Toddlers: chronic nonspecific diarrhea—usually appears in 6- to 30-month-old children and resolves by 5 years of age (Huffman, 1999; Liacouris & Baldassano, 1998; Vanderhoof, 1998)
- Children/adolescents: acquired lactose intolerance, short-bowel syndrome, Crohn's disease, ulcerative colitis, intestinal lymphangiectasia, secretory tumors, irritable bowel
- Viral or bacterial agent
- Overfeeding, malabsorption (disaccharide intolerance)
- Carbohydrate intolerance (sorbitol, fructose, etc.)
- Intractable diarrhea of infancy
- Radiation therapy
- Severe combined immunodeficiency syndrome

Clinical Findings

History. The following should be assessed:

- Occurrence of more than one liquid stool per day for 2 or more consecutive weeks
- Dietary history (including amount of fruit juices ingested per day)
- Stool consistency, blood, mucus, pus, particles of food
- Stool incontinence
- Day care exposure
- Teething
- Treatment by parents (any dietary manipulation, drug or home treatments)
- Recent travel

Physical Examination. Look for physical findings associated with the underlying pathology (see Differential Diagnosis). The physical examination includes

- Hydration status
- Weight and height measurements, skinfold thickness
- Skin and hair condition, color of skin and conjunctivae
- Vital signs (heart rate and blood pressure)
- Palpation of the thyroid
- Abdominal examination

Diagnostic Tests. The following are ordered as indicated:

- Stool for culture, ova and parasites, pH, Clinitest (for reducing substances), heme test, fat stain
- CBC with differential, ESR, and serum electrolytes and albumin
- Sweat chloride test
- Lactose tolerance test
- Urinalysis and urine culture

Differential Diagnosis

The differential diagnosis includes allergy (the patient usually has other systemic symptoms), hyperthyroidism (enlarged thyroid, increased heart rate), malabsorption (weight loss and growth retardation), cystic fibrosis (clubbing, respiratory symptoms), celiac disease, Crohn's disease, and nonacute UTI.

Management

The following steps are taken:

- Treat the underlying cause.
- Provide enteral or parenteral support if the patient is unable to maintain adequate intake orally.
- Treat toddler's diarrhea (chronic nonspecific diarrhea) as follows:
    - Normalize the diet.
    - Decrease excess intake of juice or fluids (100 ml/kg per day).
    - Give half of fluid as milk (whole or 2%).
    - Increase fat in the diet to a total of 4 g/kg per day.
    - Increase fiber.
- Refer the following patients to a gastroenterologist:
    - Newborns with diarrhea in first hours of life
    - Patients with abnormal growth delay/failure or abnormal physical findings (anorexia, abdominal pain, chronic bloating, vomiting, or weakness)
    - Those with severe illness

Complications

Malnutrition and growth failure can occur.

Intestinal Parasites

Description

Multiple organisms cause parasitic infestation in the GI tract. *Giardia lamblia, Enterobius vermicularis* (pinworm), *Ascaris lumbricoides* (roundworm), and *Taenia* (tapeworm) are some of the most common intestinal parasites that affect pediatric patients.

Etiology and Incidence

Giardia lamblia. *G. lamblia* is a flagellate protozoan generally found in contaminated mountain water sources, municipal water supplies, and food. It is the most common GI parasitic infection in the United States (Nash, 2001). Person-to-person spread is via the fecal-oral route, often in day care and industrial settings. The organism resides in the small intestine, and encystation occurs as feces dehydrate in transit. Cysts can be excreted for months or years and are resistant to chlorine (AAP, 2003). An increased incidence is seen in homosexuals and children. Seventy-six percent of infected individuals are asymptomatic.

Enterobius vermicularis. Pinworms are 1 cm long, white, and threadlike and live in the colon and rectum. The female lays eggs in the perianal area and dies. The eggs come from contaminated fomites and the anus, fingers, and mouth. They survive in bedding, clothing, and house dust for 2 weeks. The eggs are ingested, hatch, and become larvae in the small intestine; once mature, they migrate to the rectum. Eggs are easily transmitted within families, day care settings, and institutions.

Ascaris lumbricoides. Roundworm comes from fecal contamination of soil and contaminated vegetables. Ingested eggs hatch, and the larvae penetrate the wall of the small intestine and enter the pulmonary system via the circulatory system. They break out of blood vessels into the lungs, are coughed up and then swallowed, and become adult worms in the small intestine. The process takes 2 months. The worms can grow to 30 cm in length and survive cold, drying, and chemicals. They can penetrate the liver or perforate the intestine. Found in the rural southern part of the United States, they are most common in children younger than 10 years. A 50% prevalence has been noted in some tropical areas.

Taenia. Tapeworm, also known as "beef" or "pork" tapeworm, comes from the consumption of raw or undercooked beef or pork with encysted parasites. The larval form of pork tapeworm causes cysticercosis, with space-occupying lesions in the viscera, brain, and muscle. The incidence is unknown.

Clinical Findings

See Tables 33-12 and 33-13.

TABLE 33-12 *Intestinal Parasite Infestation: Signs, Symptoms, and Treatment*

Parasite	Gastrointestinal Symptoms	Diarrhea	Weight Loss	Other	Treatment
Giardia lamblia	+ Abdominal cramps, flatulence, bloating; may be protracted, intermittent illness	++ Rarely bloody, watery, greasy, foul smelling	+		Treat all positive stool cultures with the following: Furazolidone, 5-8 mg/kg per day in 4 divided doses for 7-10 days *or* Metronidazole, 40 mg/kg per day in 3 divided doses for 7-10 days Can repeat either if treatment fails
Enterobius vermicularis (pinworms)	—	—	—	Perirectal/ vaginal itching	Mebendazole, 100 mg tablet for 1 dose, then repeat in 2 wk, *or* Pyrantel pamoate, 11 mg/kg (max, 1 g) for 1 dose, then repeat in 2 wk Simultaneously treat family members Vaginitis is self-limiting
Ascaris lumbricoides (roundworm)	Worms in stool or vomit Bowel or biliary obstruction	—	+ Malnutrition		Pyrantel pamoate, 11 mg/kg for 1 dose (max, 1 g), *or* Mebendazole, 100 mg tablet per day for 3 days If intestinal obstruction present, piperazine citrate, 75 mg/kg per day (max, 3.5 g) for 2 days; makes worms flaccid and easier to pass
Taenia (tapeworm)	Worms in stool, abdominal pain, excessive appetite	—	—		Praziquantel, 20 mg/kg per day in 4 divided doses for 1 day

+, Present; ++, present to a greater degree; −, not present.

TABLE 33-13 *Laboratory Findings Associated with Intestinal Parasite Infestation*

Parasite	Stool Findings	Stool for Ova and Parasites	Stool Culture	CBC	Duodenal Aspirate	Other
Giardia lamblia		—	+ Three cultures over 1 wk		± May be necessary	EIA for *Giardia*
Enterobius vermicularis (pinworm)						Transparent tape test during night
Ascaris lumbricoides (roundworm)	Worms in stool	+	—	Marked eosinophilia		
Taenia (tapeworm)		+ Ova in stool				

CBC, Complete blood count; *EIA*, enzyme immunoassay; +, present; −, negative; ±, may or may not be present.

RESOURCE BOX

Gastrointestinal Disorders

American Pseudo-Obstruction and Hirschsprung's Disease Society
1-800-394-2747
1-508-685-4477
www.tiac.net/users/aphs
Newsletter, informational materials (including Spanish), networking, referrals to local resources, local chapters, advocacy, fund research, maintain research registry

CCFA: Crohn's and Colitis Foundation of America
1-800-932-2423 or 1-800-343-3637
1-212-685-3440
ccfa.org
Newsletter, informational materials (including Spanish), referrals to local resources, local chapters, advocacy, fund research

Cyclic Vomiting Syndrome Association
1-414-784-6842
beaker.iupui.edu/cvsa
Newsletter, informational materials, networking, referrals to local resources, local chapters, fund research, maintain research registry

International Foundation for Functional Gastrointestinal Disorders (IFFGD)
1-414-964-1799
www.execpc.com/iffgd
Newsletter, informational materials, referrals to local resources, advocacy

National Digestive Diseases Information Clearinghouse
1-301-654-3810
digestive.niddk.nih.gov

National Institute of Diabetes and Digestive and Kidney Diseases
1-301-496-3583
www.niddk.nih.gov

Purple Crying Campaign
www.dontshake.com
Materials for the prevention of shaking in relation to crying and colic.

Differential Diagnosis

The differential diagnosis includes all other causes of infectious and noninfectious diarrhea; pinworms, in particular, can be associated with "pinworm neurosis" after successful therapy or as a fantasy infestation in unaffected contacts (Lerman, 1999).

Management

See Table 33-12.

Complications

The following can occur:

- *G. lamblia* can lead to malabsorption, weight loss, and FTT.
- *E. vermicularis*, even untreated, is self-limited.
- *A. lumbricoides* can lead to Löffler syndrome (fever, respiratory symptoms, pulmonary infiltrates, excessive serum eosinophilia) caused by an allergic response as the larvae migrate to the lungs.
- *Taenia* can cause systemic cysticercosis.

Prevention

Most parasitic infestations can be prevented by good handwashing and good sanitation. The following parasites can be avoided or eliminated:

- *G. lamblia*: Treat questionable water with iodine or boiling for 20 minutes. Exclude symptomatic children from school/day care until asymptomatic.
- *E. vermicularis*: Avoid scratching. Wash sheets and clothing in hot water and detergent.
- *A. lumbricoides*: Appropriate food preparation is necessary to prevent infection.
- *Taenia*: Avoid raw or undercooked beef or pork.

REFERENCES

Acker M: Vomiting in children, *Adv Nurse Pract* 10:51-56, 2002.

American Academy of Pediatrics: *Report of the Committee on Infectious Diseases*, ed 26, Elk Grove Village, IL, 2003, American Academy of Pediatrics.

American Academy of Pediatrics Provisional Committee on Quality Improvement, Subcommittee on Acute Gastroenteritis: Practice parameter: the management of acute gastroenteritis in young children, *Pediatrics* 97:424-436, 1996.

Ashcraft KW: Consultation with the specialist: acute abdominal pain, *Pediatr Rev* 21(11):363-366, 2000.

Barkin R, Rosen P: *Emergency pediatrics: an approach to ambulatory care*, ed 4, St Louis, 1999, Mosby.

Barr RG: Changing our understanding of infant colic, *Arch Pediatr Adolesc Med* 156:1172-1174, 2002.

Bechtel B: Treating *H. pylori* in childhood may stave off cancer in adulthood, *Infect Dis Child* 15:59, 2002.

Behrman RE, Kliegman RM: *Nelson essentials of pediatrics*, ed 3, Philadelphia, 1998, WB Saunders.

Behrman RE, Kliegman R, Jenson HB, editors: *Nelson textbook of pediatrics*, ed 17, Philadelphia, 2004, WB Saunders.

Brayden RM, Daley MF, Brown JM: Growth deficiency. In Hay WW et al, editors: *Current pediatric diagnosis and treatment*, ed 16, New York, 2003, Lange Medical Books.

Burd RS, Whalen TV: Evaluation of the child with suspected appendicitis, *Pediatr Ann* 30(12):720-725, 2001.

Burg F et al, editors: *Gellis and Kagan's current pediatric therapy*, ed 15, Philadelphia, 1999, WB Saunders.

Cadranel S: Medical and surgical therapies for GERD, *J Pediatr Gastroenterol Nutr* 32:S19-S20, 2001.

Carey WB: Clinical applications of infant temperament measurements, *J Pediatr* 81:823-828, 1972.

Chang T: Gastroesophageal reflux. In Dershewitz RA, editor: *Ambulatory pediatric care*, ed 3, Philadelphia, 1999, JB Lippincott.

Chelimsky G, Czinn S: Peptic ulcer disease in children, *Pediatr Rev* 22:349-355, 2001.

Chen M, Beierle E: Gastrointestinal foreign bodies, *Pediatr Ann* 30:736-742, 2001.

Clifford TJ et al: Sequelae of infant colic: evidence of transient infant distress and absence of lasting effects on maternal mental health, *Arch Pediatr Adolesc Med* 156:1183-1188, 2002.

Dihigo S: New strategies for the treatment of colic: modifying the parent/infant interaction, *J Pediatr Health Care* 12(5):256-262, 1998.

Ewer A, James M, Tobin J: Prone and left lateral positioning reduce gastroesophageal reflux in preterm infants, *Arch Dis Child Fetal Neonatal Educ* S1:F201-F205, 1999.

Finberg L: Dehydration in infancy and childhood, *Pediatr Rev* 23:277-281, 2002.

Finberg L, Kleinman RE: *Saunders manual of pediatric practice*, ed 2, Philadelphia, 2002, WB Saunders.

Fleisher D: Coping with colic, *Contemp Pediatr* 15(6):144-156, 1998.

Gold B et al: Medical position statement: the North American Society for Pediatric Gastroenterology and Nutrition. *Helicobacter pylori* infection in children: recommendations for diagnosis and treatment, *J Pediatr Gastroenterol Nutr* 31:490-497, 2000.

Goldstein E, Hagerman RJ, Reynolds A: Child development and behavior. In Hay WW et al, editors: *Current pediatric diagnosis and treatment*, ed 16, New York, 2003, Lange Medical Books.

Hassall E: Peptic ulcer disease and current approaches to *H. pylori*, *J Pediatr* 138:462-468, 2001.

Hoffenberg E: Colonic polyps in children: from benign to worse, *Contemp Pediatr* 18: 118-134, 2001.

Hoffenberg E et al: Symptomatic colonic polyps in childhood: not so benign, *J Pediatr Gastroenterol Nutr* 28:175-181, 1999.

Huang H, Hunt R: Treatment after failure: the problem of non-responders, *Gut* 45:140-145, 1999.

Huffman S: Toddler diarrhea, *J Pediatr Health Care* 13(1):32-33, 1999.

Hyams JS: Inflammatory bowel disease, *Pediatr Rev* 21(9):291-295, 2000.

Irish MS et al: The approach to common abdominal diagnoses in infants and children, *Pediatr Clin North Am* 45:729-772, 1998.

Israel E: Inflammatory bowel disease. In Dershewitz RA, editor: *Ambulatory pediatric care*, ed 3, Philadelphia, 1999, JB Lippincott.

Jospe N, Forbes G: Fluids and electrolytes: clinical aspects, *Pediatr Rev* 17(11):395-403, 1996.

Karjoo M: Caustic ingestion and foreign bodies in the gastrointestinal system, *Curr Opin Pediatr* 10:516-522, 1998.

Kirschner BS: Inflammatory bowel disease in children, *Pediatr Clin North Am* 35:189, 1988.

Lasche J, Duggan C: Managing acute diarrhea, *Contemp Pediatr* 16(2):74-83, 1999.

Lencer W, Wolf AA: Malabsorption syndrome and chronic diarrhea. In Dershewitz RA, editor: *Ambulatory pediatric care*, ed 3, Philadelphia, 1999, JB Lippincott.

Lerman S: Common intestinal parasites. In Dershewitz RA, editor: *Ambulatory pediatric care*, ed 3, Philadelphia, 1999, JB Lippincott.

Li BU, editor: Proceedings of the International Symposium on Cyclic Vomiting Syndrome, *J Pediatr Gastroenterol Nutr* 21:S1, 1995.

Li BU: Cyclic vomiting syndrome: age-old syndrome and new insights, *Semin Pediatr Neurol* 8:13-21, 2001.

Li BU, Balint J: Cyclic vomiting syndrome: evolution in our understanding of a brain-gut disorder, *Adv Pediatr* 47:117-161, 2000.

Li BU, Howard J: New hope for children with cyclic vomiting syndrome, *Contemp Pediatr* 19:121-130, 2002.

Liacouras CA, Baldassano RN: Is it toddler's diarrhea? *Contemp Pediatr* 15(9):131-144, 1998.

Lucassen PL et al: Infantile colic: crying time reduction with a whey hydrolysate: a double-blind randomized placebo-controlled trial, *Pediatrics* 106(6):1349-1354, 2000.

Markowitz JE, Bengmark S: Probiotics in health and disease in the pediatric patient, *Pediatr Clin North Am* 49(1):127-141, 2002.

Murray K, Christie D: Vomiting in infancy: when to worry, *Contemp Pediatr* 17:81-174, 2000.

Murray KF, Christie DL: Vomiting, *Pediatr Rev* 19(10):337-341, 1998.

Nash T: Treatment of *Giardia lamblia* infections, *Pediatr Infect Dis J* 20:193-196, 2001.

North American Society for Pediatric Gastroenterology and Nutrition: Pediatric GE reflux guidelines, *J Pediatr Gastroenterol Nutr* 32:S1-S31, 2001.

Northrup RS, Flanigan TP: Gastroenteritis, *Pediatr Rev* 15(12):461-472, 1994.

Nurko S: Acute diarrhea. In Dershewitz RA, editor: *Ambulatory pediatric care*, ed 3, Philadelphia, 1999a, JB Lippincott.

Nurko S: Recurrent abdominal pain. In Dershewitz RA, editor: *Ambulatory pediatric care*, ed 3, Philadelphia, 1999b, JB Lippincott.

Oliva-Hemker M: More than a gut reaction: extraintestinal complications of IBD, *Contemp Pediatr* 16(10):45-64, 1999.

Orenstein J: Update on intussusception, *Contemp Pediatr* 17(3):180-191, 2000.
Orenstein SR: Gastroesophageal reflux, *Pediatr Rev* 20(1):24-28, 1999.
Pena BMG et al: Costs and effectiveness of ultrasonography and limited computed tomography for diagnosing appendicitis in children, *Pediatrics* 106(4):672-675, 2000.
Pena BMG, Taylor GA, Lund DP: Appendicitis revisited: new insights into an age-old problem, *Contemp Pediatr* 16(9):122-131, 1999.
Pfau B et al: Differentiating cyclic from chronic vomiting patterns in children: qualitative criteria and diagnostic implications, *Pediatrics* 97:364-368, 1996.
Podolsky D: Inflammatory bowel disease, *N Engl J Med* 347:417-429, 2002.
Ravelli A: Cyclic vomiting syndrome, *J Pediatr Gastroenterol Nutr* 32:S14-S15, 2001.
Reijneveld SA, Brugman E, Hirasing RA: Excessive infant crying: the impact of varying definitions, *Pediatrics* 108(4):893-897, 2001.
Rudolph CD et al: Guidelines for evaluation and treatment of gastroesophageal reflux in infants and children: recommendations of the North American Society for Pediatric Gastroenterology and Nutrition, *J Pediatr Gastroenterol Nutr* 32(suppl 2):S14, 2001.
Saxelin M, Salminen E, Vapaatalo M: Dose response colonization of feces after oral administration of *Lactobacillus casei* strain GG, *Microbiology Ecology of Health and Disease* 4:1-8, 1991.
Schwartz ID: Failure to thrive: an old nemesis in the new millennium, *Pediatr Rev* 21(8):257-264, 2000.
Schwartz MW et al, editors: *Pediatric primary care: a problem oriented approach*, ed 3, St Louis, 1997, Mosby.
Siberry GK, Iannone R, editors: *The Harriet Lane handbook*, ed 15, St Louis, 2000, Mosby.
Snyder JP: Inflammatory bowel disease: Ulcerative colitis and Crohn disease. In Finberg L, Kleinman RE, editors: *Saunders manual of pediatric practice*, ed 2, Philadelphia, 2002, WB Saunders.
Sondheimer J: Gastrointestinal tract. In Hay WW et al, editors: *Current pediatric diagnosis and treatment*, ed 16, New York, 2003, Lange Medical Books.
Spitzer MD: Viral causes of diarrhea, *Pediatr Rev* 23(7):257-258, 2002.
Strand TA et al: Effectiveness and efficacy of zinc for the treatment of acute diarrhea in young children, *Pediatrics* 109(5):898-903, 2002.
Teitelbaum SJ, Leichtner AM, Tunnessen WW: "Read my lips": abdominal pain in a 14 year old, *Contemp Pediatr* 16(3):31-41, 1999.
Thiessen P: Recurrent abdominal pain, *Pediatr Rev* 23:39-46, 2002.
Vanderhoof JA: Chronic diarrhea, *Pediatr Rev* 19(12):418-422, 1998.
Vanderhoof JA, Young RJ: Probiotics in pediatrics, *Pediatrics* 109(5):956-957, 2002.
Van Niel C et al: *Lactobacillus* therapy for acute diarrhea in children: a meta-analysis, *Pediatrics* 109:678-684, 2002.
Wenzl T et al: Gastroesophageal reflux and respiratory phenomena in infants: status of the intraluminal impedance technique, *J Pediatr Gastroenterol Nutr* 28:423-428, 1999.
Winesett M: Inflammatory bowel disease in children and adolescents, *Pediatr Ann* 26(4):227-234, 1997.
Zeiter DK, Hyams JS: Clinical aspects of recurrent abdominal pain, *Pediatr Ann* 30(1):17-21, 2001.
Zeltzer L, Bursch B: Psychological management strategies for functional disorders, *J Gastroenterol Nutr* 32:S40-S41, 2001.

34 Dental and Oral Diseases*

Charles Poland III, Kevin J. Hale

The focus of ambulatory care in the pediatric setting is directed toward keeping the child well and minimizing the impact of disease, developmental problems, and disturbances in behavior. This concept of care places a major emphasis on prevention, early intervention, and anticipatory guidance to minimize the effects of developmental, psychologic, and chronic disease in children.

Pediatric dentists use these same strategies to achieve their successes. The primary focus of pediatric dentistry is to establish preventive dental health habits that successfully guide the child and parent through childhood into adulthood free of dental disease. Dental caries, periodontal disease, and malocclusions are the primary oral diseases. The caries process that leads to dental cavities is most often initiated early in the life of a child, whereas periodontal disease is primarily a disease of adults. Both diseases are entirely preventable with modern preventive dental strategies and intervention in the disease process. Most malocclusions are genetically induced or result from premature tooth loss or digit/pacifier habits. Implementation of preventive measures, as well as definitive treatment of malocclusion, enhances the child's physical and psychosocial growth and development.

Oral Health in America: A Report of the Surgeon General (U.S. Department of Health and Human Services, 2000a) emphasized the following points:

- Optimal oral health is an integral part of total health.
- Oral diseases may be associated with other health problems.
- The mouth reflects the general health and well-being of the individual.

The report also pointed out that tooth decay, unfortunately, is the most prevalent chronic disease of childhood and represents the greatest unmet health care need, particularly in poor and minority populations. More than 40% of children in the United States have tooth decay by the time they reach kindergarten (Pierce, Rozier, & Vann, 2002), and once the caries process is initiated dental decay prevalence increases at an alarming rate through the adolescent years (Fig. 34-1). Tooth decay is a significant problem for nearly 18 million children, with 25% experiencing disease levels or related pain severe enough to interfere with routine daily activities (Crall, 2002). The incidence rates of caries and periodontal disease in the underserved and minority adult populations are similar and illustrate health care inadequacies for these social groups.

Incorporating oral health strategies into the nurse practitioner's (NP's) list of objectives provides hope that the onset of oral disease in children can be prevented or, at the very least, delayed, and that the incidence and severity of disease can be minimized. Because of the unique trust that parents have in their child's primary care provider, the NP can have a profound impact on the outcome of children's oral health. The dental profession alone cannot eliminate the prevalence of caries in young children by drilling and filling dental cavitations. Only in partnership with primary medical providers will prevention and earlier interception of the caries process dramatically reduce levels of childhood caries.

STANDARDS OF CARE

The projected goals for *Healthy People 2010,* found in Appendix D, are ambitious (U.S. Department of Health and Human Services, 2000b). These goals reflect the need to reduce the incidence of oral disease, particularly in children, and provide improved access to oral health care for all Americans. New and different strategies need to be implemented that involve the entire health care team, not just dentistry.

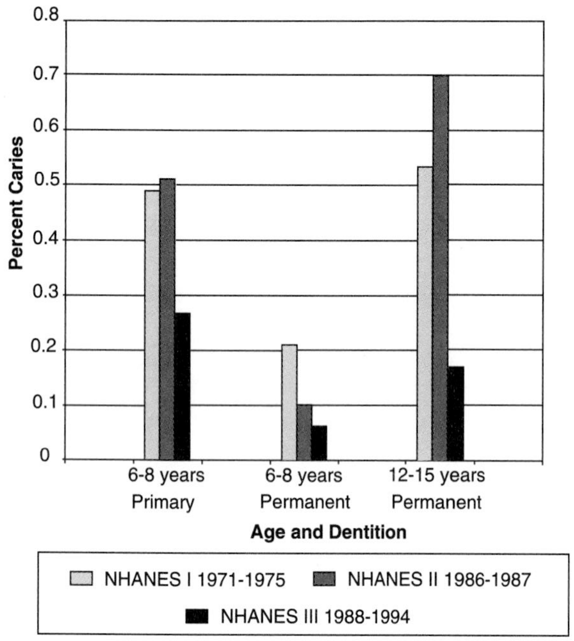

FIGURE 34-1 Untreated caries in primary and permanent teeth. (Data from the First National Health and Nutrition Examination Survey [NHANES I] 1971-1975, the Second National Health and Nutrition Examination Survey [NHANES II] 1986-1987, and the Third National Health and Nutrition Examination Survey [NHANES III] 1988-1994, National Institute of Dental and Craniofacial Research: Oral Health U.S., 2002.)

A child's first dental visit should occur no later than 1 year of age, and the dentist should then determine the frequency of subsequent visits (U.S. Preventive Services Task Force, 1996; U.S. Public Health Service, 1997).

The Bright Futures program has several publications that detail standards of dental care and oral health anticipatory guidance guidelines for each health supervision visit from infancy through adolescence (Casamassimo, 1996, 1997). The American Academy of Pediatric Dentistry (AAPD) outlines oral health policies, periodicity for prevention, and guidelines for pediatric dental care. The guideline emphasizes the need to start professional dental care at 12 months of age, when the caries process begins. It also provides the best reference for dental and nondental professionals seeking guidance about oral and dental health care for children (AAPD, 2002). Table 34-1 lists recommendations for preventive pediatric dental care.

New standards of care for primary medical providers include screening for oral health problems, conducting a preliminary oral risk assessment at 6 months of age, and providing sound advice on fluoride use and other preventive habits. Preventive strategies should promote toothbrushing with a fluoride dentifrice starting at age 12 months, restriction of sugary drinks and snacks, application of fluoride varnish by trained and appropriate health professionals, and referral to a "dental home" for a detailed risk assessment and an individualized oral health preventive program (AAP, 2003; Ismail & Sohn, 2002).

Dental Development

The oral cavity consists of the gingiva (gums), mucosa, tongue, hard and soft palate, and teeth. Tooth development is described in four stages: initiation, calcification, eruption, and shedding. *Initiation* refers to the initial development of the tooth follicle, which occurs in the first trimester in utero. *Calcification* refers to the deposition of inorganic mineral crystals of enamel and dentin on the teeth and affects the color, texture, and thickness of the tooth. This process ensures a hardened tooth structure before eruption. All 20 primary teeth begin hard tissue formation by 4 to 6 months of gestation. The first permanent molars and lower incisors are the first permanent teeth to develop and begin to calcify just before or soon after birth.

Teeth begin to erupt at about 6 to 7 months of age, and all 20 teeth are usually present by the end of the third year. This is referred to as the *primary dentition stage.* Permanent teeth begin erupting at around 6 years of age (the *transitional dentition stage*), and all 32 teeth, except the third molars, are in place by 13 to 14 years of age (the *early permanent dentition stage*). Dentists frequently refer to these three stages of dental development to describe the timing for interceptive or comprehensive orthodontic treatment. The timings of tooth eruption given in Table 34-2 are estimates and may vary by as much as 6 months or more. It is not unusual to see the mandibular lateral incisors delayed in their eruption until the mandibular cuspids erupt. The clinician should not be overly concerned about delayed eruption of teeth as long as the child is achieving other normal growth parameters. The clinician should, however, be concerned with contralateral asymmetric eruption patterns that persist for longer than 3 to 4 weeks and should refer the child to a pediatric dentist for evaluation. Several multiple congenital disorders and syndromes are associated with delayed eruption and missing teeth. These issues are normally secondary and can be dealt with when the "dental home" is established. The eruption of teeth in a premature infant is as variable as in a full-term infant; there is no need to adjust for age when anticipating tooth eruption.

TABLE 34-1 ***Recommendations for Preventive Pediatric Dental Care***

Age[1]	Infancy, 6-12 mo	Late Infancy, 12-24 mo	Preschool, 2-6 yr	School Age, 6-12 yr	Adolescence, 12-18 yr
Oral hygiene counseling[2]	Parents/ Guardians/ Caregivers	Parents/ Guardians/ Caregivers	Child/Parent/ Guardians/ Caregivers	Child/Parent/ Guardians/ Caregivers	Patient
Injury prevention counseling[3]	•	•	•	•	•
Dietary counseling[4]	•	•	•	•	•
Counseling for nonnutritive habits[5]	•	•	•	•	•
Fluoride supplementation[6,7]	•	•	•	•	•
Assess oral growth and development[8]	•	•	•	•	•
Clinical oral examination	•	•	•	•	•
Prophylaxis and topical fluoride treatment[9]		•	•	•	•
Radiographic assessment[10]			•	•	•
Pit and fissure sealants			If indicated on primary molars	First permanent molars as soon as possible after eruption	Second permanent molars and appropriate premolars as soon as possible after eruption
Treatment of Dental Disease/Injury	•	•	•	•	•
Assessment and treatment of developing malocclusion			•	•	•
Substance abuse counseling				•	•
Assessment and possible removal of third molars					•
Referral for regular and periodic dental care					•
Anticipatory guidance[11]	•	•	•	•	•

From American Academy of Pediatric Dentistry: *Guideline on periodicity of examination, preventive services, anticipatory guidance and oral treatment for children*, Chicago, 1992, AAPD.

[1]First examination at the erupton of the first tooth and no later than 12 months.

[2]Initially, responsibility of parent; as child develops, jointly with parents; then, when indicated, only child.

[3]Initially play objects, pacifiers, car seats; then when learning to walk; and finally sports and routine playing.

[4]At every appointment discuss the role of refined carbohydrates; frequency of snacking.

[5]At first discuss the need for additional sucking; digits vs. pacifiers; then the need to wean from the habit before the eruption of the first permanent front teeth. For school-age children and adolescent patients, counsel regarding any existing habits such as fingernail biting, clenching, or bruxism.

[6]As per AAP/ADA guidelines and the water source.

[7]Up to at least 16 years.

[8]By clinical examination.

[9]Especially for children at high risk for caries and periodontal disease.

[10]As per AAPD radiographic guidelines.

[11]Appropriate discussion and counseling should be an integral part of each visit for care.

Disruption in Development, Eruption, or Shedding of Teeth

Enamel Hypoplasia

Genetic defects, infection, malnutrition, trauma, and fluorosis are the most common causes of abnormal tooth development. Enamel hypoplasia is caused by a disturbance in the formation of the enamel matrix and is the most common defect. Enamel hypoplasia can appear as a simple opacity, severe discoloration of the enamel, or a misshapen tooth devoid of much of its enamel (Fig. 34-2). Treatment of malformed or discolored teeth usually requires crowning or placing a tooth-colored restoration on or in the affected tooth.

TABLE 34-2 Eruption Sequence

Primary Dentition	Age at Eruption (Months)
Maxillary	
Central incisor	7.5
Lateral incisor	9
Cuspid	18
First molar	14
Second molar	24
Mandibular	
Central incisor	6
Lateral incisor	7
Cuspid	16
First molar	12
Second molar	20
Permanent Dentition	**Age at Eruption (Years)**
Maxillary	
Central incisor	7-8
Lateral incisor	8-9
Cuspid	11-12
First bicuspid	10-11
Second bicuspid	10-12
First molar	6-7
Second molar	12-13
Mandibular	
Central incisor	6-7
Lateral incisor	7-8
Cuspid	9-10
First bicuspid	10-12
Second bicuspid	11-12
First molar	6-7
Second molar	11-13

Adapted from Logan WHG, Kronfeld R: The chronology of human dentition, *J Am Dent Assoc* 20, 1933.

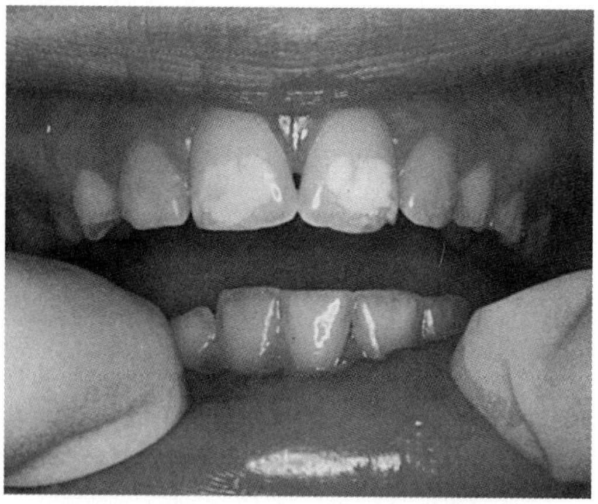

FIGURE 34-2 Enamel hypoplasia of the two central incisors. Note that fluorosis or a febrile illness would have affected other teeth during time of similar development.

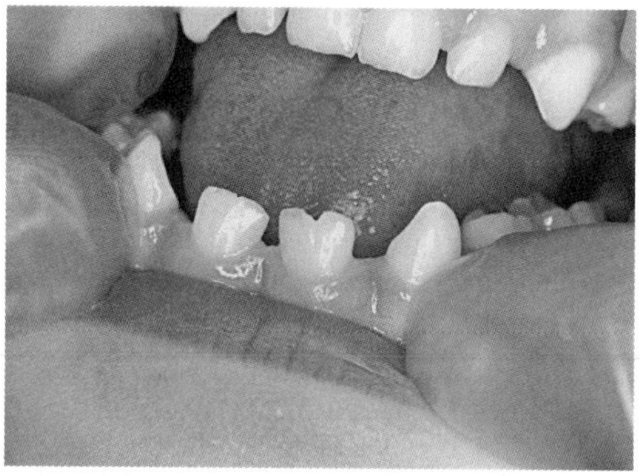

FIGURE 34-3 Fusion of deciduous incisors.

Hypocalcification

Hypocalcification defects of enamel are rare and are usually associated with metabolic diseases, such as rickets and parathyroid deficiency. Alterations in the size and shape of teeth include microdont (small tooth) and macrodont (large tooth). Fusion is a single enlarged tooth or joined "double" tooth in which the tooth count reveals a missing tooth when the anomalous tooth is counted as one (Fig. 34-3).

Hypodontia

Hypodontia refers to the absence of one or more teeth and is common in the permanent dentition. The third molars, second bicuspids, and maxillary lateral incisors are the most frequently missing teeth in the permanent dentition. Congenitally missing teeth in the deciduous dentition are much more rare but do occur, with the lateral incisors and cuspids most frequently missing. When this occurs, the permanent successor teeth are also frequently missing. Missing teeth require replacement with either a dental implant or a fixed or removable dental bridge.

Hyperdontia

Hyperdontia, the presence of supernumerary teeth, can occur in any location within the dental-alveolar areas, but is most commonly found in the anterior maxilla. Such teeth need to be identified, and the tooth may need to be removed to prevent asymmetric or delayed eruption of the permanent maxillary incisors.

Exfoliation

Exfoliation, or shedding, of deciduous teeth occurs as the permanent successor erupts into the mouth. The timing of this event is as variable as the eruption of deciduous teeth. Eruption of the permanent tooth normally stimulates the deciduous tooth root to be resorbed. When the deciduous tooth root is not resorbed properly, the permanent tooth can be diverted from its normal eruption path and forced into an abnormal position requiring orthodontic repositioning. Most pediatric dentists observe an overretained deciduous tooth for a period of 2 to 3 weeks in the hope that the tooth will exfoliate naturally before putting the child through an extraction procedure. When not associated with dental infection, premature loss of deciduous teeth should alert the clinician to other growth disturbances or inborn errors of metabolism.

DENTAL CARIES

Process of Caries Formation

Role of Infection

Dental caries have long been recognized as an infectious and transmissible disease that arises from an overgrowth of specific, normally occurring human dental flora (Keyes, 1960; Loesche, 1979). *Streptococcus mutans* (SM) and lactobacilli species are considered to be principle indicator organisms of a group of aciduric bacteria responsible for dental cavitation. The vertical inoculation of SM from the mother or close caregiver to the infant is well documented (Berkowitz & Jones, 1985; Davey & Rogers, 1984). In fact, genotypes of SM in infants appear to be identical to those present in mothers in approximately 71% of mother-infant pairs (Li & Caufield, 1995). Human dental flora is highly site specific and exhibits discrete windows of colonization. The eruption of teeth signals the time that SM can be introduced and begin colonizing. An infant can therefore be inoculated at 6 through 30 months of life (Berkowitz, Jordan, & White, 1975; Stiles et al, 1976). The average age of SM acquisition is approximately 2 years of age (Caufield, Cutter, & Dasanayake, 1993). Once this occurs, the caries process proceeds as a back-and-forth process of demineralization and remineralization of enamel.

Demineralization-Remineralization

Dental enamel is a permeable structure composed of an organic matrix and an inorganic hydroxyapatite crystal. The organic matrix permits exchange of the basic composition of the hydroxyapatite crystal with salivary calcium, phosphates, fluorides, and other dietary minerals. When the pH or ion concentration in the oral environment is altered, demineralization or remineralization occurs.

When carbohydrate substrate is introduced into the mouth, the oral plaque pH will fall within 2 to 3 minutes. When the pH falls below 5.5, the colonized cariogenic bacteria in the mouth metabolize this substrate and produce acid that begins the demineralization process. A single carbohydrate exposure creates an acid pH for up to an hour (Berg, 2002). Over the next 25 to 30 minutes, saliva will neutralize and buffer the plaque pH and support the remineralization process.

Tooth cavitation results from the cycle of demineralization-remineralization of subsurface enamel. In dynamic equilibrium, the caries process continues without destruction of enamel, but when the process reaches disequilibrium, enamel structure weakens to a point that cavitation occurs. Early subsurface lesions are not visible but may be present on most tooth surfaces (Fig. 34-4; see Color Fig. 11). Cavitation starts in this subsurface enamel before progressing through an intact layer of enamel. The advanced subsurface lesions may appear as white chalky lesions commonly found along the gingival margin of deciduous anterior teeth (see Color Fig. 12). Figure 34-5 illustrates the dynamic nature of the caries process and control strategies.

When in contact with the enamel surface, the element fluoride hastens the remineralization process, reducing the solubility of enamel crystal, enhancing the nucleation of calcium phosphate in the enamel crystal, and accelerating maturation of the enamel surface.

Modifiers of the Cavitation Process

Nutritional Modifiers. The uncontrolled frequent ingestion of natural and refined sugars, as well as cooked starches, maintains low plaque pH over a sustained time interval, promoting the demineralization process. The more times carbohydrates are ingested, the longer the mouth is predisposed to a constant acidic state. A child's eating habits will have a more significant influence on the caries process than will restricting any one food or snack. Therefore children who are "nibblers and sippers" have a higher risk for caries than do children who eat the same foods but are "wolfers and gobblers." Uncontrolled snacking on "sticky

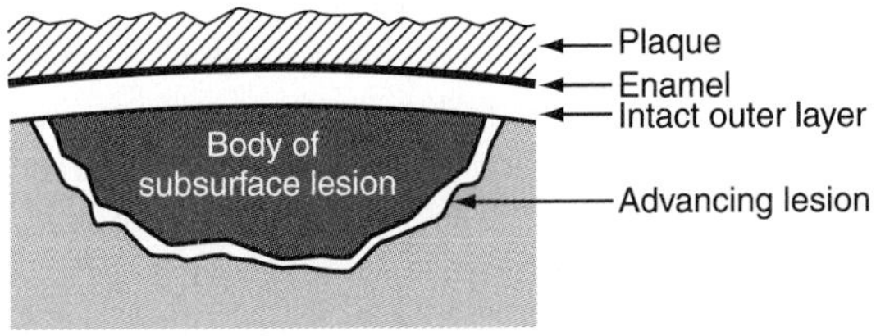

FIGURE 34-4 Caries process proceeds as a subsurface lesion beneath an intact layer of enamel.

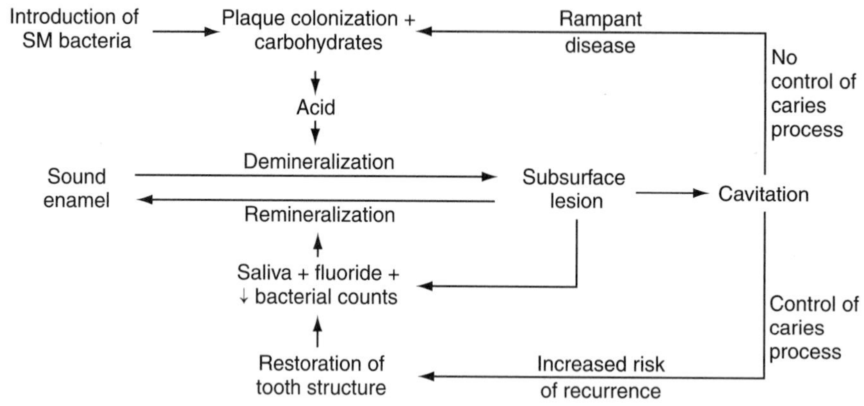

FIGURE 34-5 The dynamic process of caries formation and control. *SM, Streptococcus mutans.*

carbohydrates" (e.g., cookies, candy, potato chips, pretzels) or using a "sippy" cup containing milk or fruit juice throughout the day encourages the demineralization process.

Improper Bottle Feeding and Nursing. The most significant demineralization modifier of the caries process in young children is the milk bottle in bed or when used as a pacifier (i.e., behavior purposes, not nutritional). Uncontrolled day breastfeeding or sleeping with the breast nipple in the mouth once tooth eruption has commenced also produces the same prolonged acidic state. These inappropriate feeding/behavior practices may leave children at high risk for early childhood caries (ECC).

Bottle and nursing habits have been the focus of caries control in young children. While acknowledging that the bottle or improper nursing habit is a major modifier of the disease, the clinician should recognize that the bacterial component transmitted from a caregiver is the basic etiology of the caries process in young children. This is key in making an accurate caries risk assessment. This point was affirmed in a study of Head Start children: 86% of children with caries were reported to have taken the bottle to bed, whereas 69% of children with no caries also reported similar use of the bottle in bed (Tinanoff & O'Sullivan, 1997).

Impact and Incidence of Caries. Many health professionals have been misled into believing that dental caries is no longer a major health issue for children. However, nearly 20% of children ages 2 to 5 years have untreated caries, and in poor children 80% of these will remain untreated (Vargas, Crall, & Schneider, 1998). Approximately 336 hours of school time per 100 school-age children are lost annually because of dental problems or dental visits. Between 12 and 15 years of age, 17% of children have untreated caries (CDC, 2002).

Newly erupted teeth, particularly deciduous teeth, are highly susceptible to the caries process. The transmission of cariogenic bacteria, or "window of infectivity," is most critical between 6 and 31 months of age (Berg, 2002). Infants who are of low socioeconomic status, whose mothers have a low education level, who consume sugary foods, or who have high levels of cariogenic bacteria are 32 times more likely to have caries at age 3.5 years than children in whom those risk factors are not present (Nowak, 2000). Those with the least access to care demonstrate the highest prevalence of disease and SM salivary titers (Kaste et al, 1996). Over twice as many children (36%) are without dental insurance as compared to those with medical insurance (Vargas, Crall, & Schneider, 1998).

Clinical Findings

History

An adequate assessment of a child's oral health should begin by 6 months of age. The assessment should include a dental history and an examination of the child's mouth to screen for abnormalities and gross dental disease. The dental history should include the following:

- Parental dental history for risk assessment (Box 34-1)
- Assessment of risk factors for early childhood caries (Box 34-2 and Table 34-3)
- Family history of caries, craniofacial deformities, malocclusion, or periodontal disease
- Pattern of tooth eruption
- Fluoride content of the primary water supply
- Fluoride supplementation
- Use of toothbrush, toothpaste, and floss
- Age at the first dental visit and periodicity of subsequent preventive dental visits

BOX 34-1 *Parental Dental History for Risk Assessment*

- When was the last time you had a cavity filled?
- Do you have any untreated cavities or broken fillings in your mouth?
- When was the last time you visited a dentist?
- Do you see your dentist on a regular one- or two-times-a-year schedule for preventive dental services?

BOX 34-2 *Risk Factors for Early Childhood Caries*

- Active caries in the mother or close caregiver
- High SM counts in the mother
- High SM counts in the child
- Visible decalcified lesions
- Inappropriate bottle use
- Frequent snacks
- Physical handicaps
- Poverty
- Frequent use of medicines containing sucrose
- Complicated pregnancy
- History of poor family oral health
- Previous ECC
- Inadequate systemic fluoride
- High sugar intake
- Poor oral hygiene
- Oral dysfunction
- Children in free or reduced lunch programs
- Children with special health care needs
- Cultural customs

ECC, Early childhood caries; *SM*, *Streptococcus mutans*.

- Whether a "dental home" has been established
- Dental or mouth injuries
- Nutritional and eating behaviors
  - Infants and toddlers up to 3 years of age: feeding/behavioral habits, including the frequency and types of feedings/meals/snacks (e.g., nibblers and sippers) and the use of breast, bottle, or cup for behavioral purposes, not just nutrition
  - Preschool children 3 to 5 years of age: oral habits—finger sucking, pacifier use, parental involvement with toothbrushing and the use of dental floss
  - School-age children and adolescents: oral habits, orthodontic and facial orthopedic corrections, sports participation, and changes in nutritional practices that include an increase in the consumption of carbonated beverages and sugar-fortified juices and drinks
- Need for antibiotic prophylaxis with some dental procedures in children with an increased susceptibility to surgically induced bacteremias (e.g., children with cardiac defects)

Many dental procedures are not as traumatic to gingival tissue as daily toothbrushing and may not require antibiotic prophylaxis. Advising a patient or parent to take an antibiotic before having any "dental work" oversimplifies the variety of dental procedures available that a patient may require and leads to overuse of antibiotics and the risk of acquiring resistant bacteria. See Chapter 31 for specific information regarding situations where dental prophylaxis is indicated.

Oral Examination

The infant's mouth is best examined with the child's head lying on the lap of the parent or examiner or on an examination table with the hands and arms held above the baby's head by the parent. This position stabilizes the head and enables the examiner to look into the mouth with only overhead illumination. Talking throughout the examination eases the anxiety of both the parent and the child.

Examination of a toddler's mouth is accomplished with the toddler lying with legs around the parent's waist and head in the examiner's lap and the parent holding the child's hands and lower torso. Alternatively, the child stands between the examiner's legs, facing the same direction as the examiner, opens the mouth and tilts the head back. The examiner's crossed legs help hold the child and enable both the parent and the examiner to view the child's mouth. This method is also excellent for parents to use when brushing and flossing the child's teeth. Examining an older child's mouth can be performed with the child in the standing, sitting, or prone position (with a tongue blade and good lighting).

During the oral examination, the NP should note the following:

- Facial symmetry, jaw size
- Mouth—moistness, color, odor, lesions, frenulum
- Lips—cracking, scaling, maceration, lesions
- Gums—color, texture, bleeding, lesions, overgrowth, plaque
- Mucosa—color, lesions, hydration
- Tongue—color, texture, fissured, geographic, coated

TABLE 34-3 *AAPD Caries-risk Assessment Tool (CAT)*

Caries-risk Indicators	Low Risk	Moderate Risk	High Risk
Clinical Conditions			
	No carious teeth in past 24 mo	Carious teeth in the past 24 mo	Carious teeth in the past 12 mo
	No enamel demineralization (enamel caries "white-spot lesions")	One area of enamel demineralization (enamel caries "white-spot lesions")	More than one area of enamel demineralization (enamel caries "white-spot lesions")
	No visible plaque; no gingivitis	Gingivitis[a]	Visible plaque on anterior (front) teeth Radiographic enamel caries High titers of mutans streptococci Wearing dental or orthodontic appliances[b] Enamel hypoplasia[c]
Environmental Characteristics			
	Optimal systemic and topical fluoride exposure[d]	Suboptimal systemic fluoride exposure with optimal topical exposure[d]	Suboptimal topical fluoride exposure[d]
	Consumption of simple sugars or foods strongly associated with caries initiation primarily at mealtimes[e]	Occasional (i.e., one or two) between-meal exposures to simple sugars or foods strongly associated with caries	Frequent (i.e., three or more) between-meal exposures to simple sugars or foods strongly associated with caries
	High caregiver socioeconomic status[f]	Midlevel caregiver socioeconomic status (i.e., eligible for school lunch program or SCHIP)	Low-level caregiver socioeconomic status (i.e., eligible for Medicaid)
	Regular use of dental care in an established "dental home"	Irregular use of dental services	No usual source of dental care
General Health Conditions			
			Active caries present in the mother Children with special health care needs[g] Conditions impairing saliva composition/flow[h]

From American Academy of Pediatric Dentistry: *Reference manual 2002-2003: policy on the use of a caries-risk assessment tool (CAT) for infants, children and adolescents*, Chicago, 2002, AAPD, p 17.

[a]Although microbial organisms responsible for gingivitis may be different from those primarily implicated in dental caries, the presence of gingivitis is an indicator of poor or infrequent oral hygiene practices and has been associated with caries progression.

[b]Orthodontic appliances include both fixed and removable appliances, space maintainers, and other devices that remain in the mouth continuously or for prolonged time intervals and that may trap food and plaque, prevent oral hygiene, compromise access of tooth surfaces to fluoride, or otherwise create an environment supporting dental caries initiation.

[c]Tooth anatomy and hypoplastic defects such as poorly formed enamel, developmental pits, and deep pits may predispose a child to develop dental caries.

[d]Optimal systemic and topical fluoride exposure is based on the American Dental Association/American Academy of Pediatrics guidelines for exposure from fluoride drinking water or supplementation and use of a fluoride dentifrice.

[e]Examples of sources of simple sugars include carbonated beverages, cookies, cake, candy, cereal, potato chips, french fries, corn chips, pretzels, breads, juices, and fruits. Clinicians using caries-risk assessment should investigate individual exposures to sugars known to be involved in caries initiation.

[f]National surveys have demonstrated that children in low-income and moderate-income households are more likely to have dental caries and more decayed or filled primary teeth than children from more affluent households. Also, within income levels, minority children are more likely to have caries. Thus sociodemographic status should be viewed as an initial indicator of risk that may be offset by the absence of other risk indicators.

[g]Children with special health care needs are those who have or are at increased risk for a chronic physical, developmental, behavioral, or emotional condition and who also require health and related services of a type or amount beyond that required by children generally.

[h]Alteration in salivary flow can be the result of congenital or acquired conditions, surgery, radiation, medication, or age-related changes in salivary function. Any condition, treatment, or process known or reported to alter saliva flow should be considered an indication of risk unless proven otherwise.

- Hard and soft palate—intact, cleft, bifid uvula
- Teeth—number, size, shape, color, crowding, pits, fissures, caries, enamel hypoplasia and staining, and intraarch occlusion (best examined with the child's mouth closed and "lifting the lips" with a tongue blade; this is an effective technique to demonstrate to parents for brushing and monitoring for signs of early ECC)

Management Strategies

As a primary care provider, the NP has the opportunity to intercept the epidemic of dental disease and provide valuable and timely oral health prevention and education. Historically, many primary medical care providers waited until a child was 3 or 4 years of age before suggesting that the parents seek professional dental care. Often, parents were told to wait until all of the "baby teeth erupt" or until the child could cooperate with the dentist. Referral to a pediatric dentist was made only if decay was identified. This erroneous concept of pediatric oral health management ignored much of what is known about prevention of dental caries. Specifically, it failed to apply knowledge about the following:

- The role of bacterial reservoirs as a cause of dental caries. These reservoirs are found in families and passed from mother to child from generation to generation.
- The use of topical fluoride during early tooth eruption to increase host resistance to the caries process.
- The limited role of fluoridation of water: fluoridated water is only one part of the solution.

As a result, delay of treatment occurred to the extent that surgical or restorative dentistry became necessary. In some cases, this rehabilitative therapy was extensive. Out of fear of causing enamel fluorosis, primary care providers failed to advise parents to use fluoride toothpaste on an infant's newly erupted teeth. Parents should be instructed to use less than one fourth of the size of a pea of toothpaste to brush the teeth and then wipe the toothpaste off with a cloth.

Fluoride supplementation and pit and fissure sealants are two successful and readily available management strategies. Additionally, all children ought to have a "dental home" where comprehensive, continuous, accessible and affordable care is available, delivered, or supervised by qualified pediatric or family dentists.

Oral Checklist

It is no longer "best practice" to delay the timing of the first dental visit until after the caries process has begun or a cavity is detected. Pediatric dentists advise that a risk-based assessment of the child's liability to the caries process be completed before bacterial colonization has begun. The NP can develop and use a quick oral health checklist that would include the following:

- Completing an initial or follow-up risk assessment for caries (see Table 34-3).
- Reviewing relevant portions of the initial assessment with the parent to determine if continuous management of the child's dental care is being provided within a "dental home." It is not unusual for families to get off track with regular dental checkups, and a reminder from their primary care provider can be a powerful incentive to reinstitute the preventive dental program.
- Referring to a "dental home" based on the risk assessment, if one has not been established.
- Providing oral hygiene counseling for caries and periodontal disease prevention.
- Providing nutritional counseling for caries prevention.
- Determining the fluoride content of the primary water supply.
- Instituting systemic fluoride therapy when appropriate.
- Applying fluoride varnish to children under 2 years of age if (1) the risk assessment is high and the primary health care provider is trained in the identification of early childhood caries, and (2) the NP has been educated in the appropriate use, application, and limitations of fluoride varnish. There is scant evidence that application of fluoride varnish independent of other individualized preventive dental programs, outside the "dental home," provides caries protection. The other recommended measures described in this chapter have been shown to be extremely effective.

Referral to the "Dental Home"

Any abnormalities or questionable conditions should initiate a dental referral to the child's "dental home." The NP should be familiar with dental offices or networks within the community that provide appropriate "dental homes" for young children. At-risk children need to be referred earlier than 12 months of age; low-risk children should be seen by at least 18 months of age. However, the "gold standard" is to refer children for their first dental visit at 12 months of age.

The "dental home" should be expected to provide the following:

- An accurate risk assessment for dental diseases
- An individualized preventive dental health program based on the risk assessment
- Anticipatory guidance about growth and development issues (e.g., teething, digit or pacifier habits)
- A plan for emergency dental trauma
- Information about proper care of the child's teeth and gingiva
- Information about proper nutritional practices

- Pit and fissure sealants
- Restorative and surgical dental care when necessary that meets the parents' and child's psychologic needs
- Interceptive orthodontic and facial orthopedic care for children with developing malocclusions
- A special place for the child and parent to establish a positive attitude about dental health without acquiring the classic dental phobias that are still common in many adults
- Referrals to other dental specialists such as endodontists, periodontists, oral surgeons, and orthodontists when care cannot be directly provided within the "dental home"
- Comprehensive dental care in accordance with accepted guidelines and periodicity schedules for pediatric dental health (see Table 34-1)

Best practice dictates that the following infants should establish a "dental home" by 12 months of age or earlier:

- Children with special health care needs (e.g., those with oral dysfunction, those on seizure medications, those with mental retardation, those with Down syndrome, or those with cerebral palsy)
- Children with demonstrable caries, plaque, demineralization, or staining
- Children who sleep with a bottle or breastfeed all night
- Later-order siblings of a child or parent with mildly to moderately high caries rate
- Children of families of low socioeconomic status
- Any child who has one or more findings in the "high risk" category listed on Table 34-3

Dental care for most children is provided in a quiet, nonthreatening environment, particularly when professional dental care is started early in a child's life and the child becomes familiar with the dental surroundings. Family and pediatric dentists provide care to children. Pediatric dentists in particular have considerable training in child psychology and view themselves as teachers. They endeavor to guide and mold the child's attitude and behavior related to dental care and the dental office environment. Frequently, the child is separated from the parent during dental visits. At other times, the dentist may request that the parent help manage the child, particularly if the child is very young or noncommunicative. Very young children who require considerable treatment, children with overt-resistive behavior, or children with developmental delay may require sedation, general anesthesia, or physical stabilization (restraints).

Fluoride

When applied topically during the immediate posteruptive period, a small amount of fluoride toothpaste reduces enamel solubility, promotes the remineralization process, and enhances the enamel maturation process. These susceptible young teeth are then afforded the opportunity to resist demineralization and enhance remineralization.

Systemic fluoride reduces dental decay by at least 40% and is considered to be a significant part of successful preventive dental strategies (Berg, 2002). Children who live in communities with fluoridated water have shown rates of 50% to 70% fewer cavities (Consultant, 2001). Systemic fluoride supplementation is indicated for

- All children 6 months to 16 years of age who are living in areas without optimally fluoridated community water
- Breastfed infants older than 6 months
- Children who drink only fluoride-free bottled or osmotically purified water as their primary water source

The incidence of mild and moderate dental fluorosis is increasing (Fig. 34-6). Most commercially prepared fruit juices and sodas are reconstituted or made with fluoridated water. This practice is reported to be partially responsible for the increase in the ambient level of fluoride in a child's diet. Other sources of excessive ingestion of fluoride include young children swallowing too much fluoride toothpaste and fluoride supplementation when the primary water source contains optimal or high levels of fluoride. The NP should encourage the family to have an analysis of the fluoride content of the child's primary water source. If the water comes from a known community fluoride source, the NP should be aware of the inherent fluoride concentration. Approximately 66% of the water systems in the United States are now fluoridated (CDC, 2002). Review the child's ECC risk assessment before prescribing fluoride supplements. Recommended supplemental fluoride doses are listed in Table 34-4.

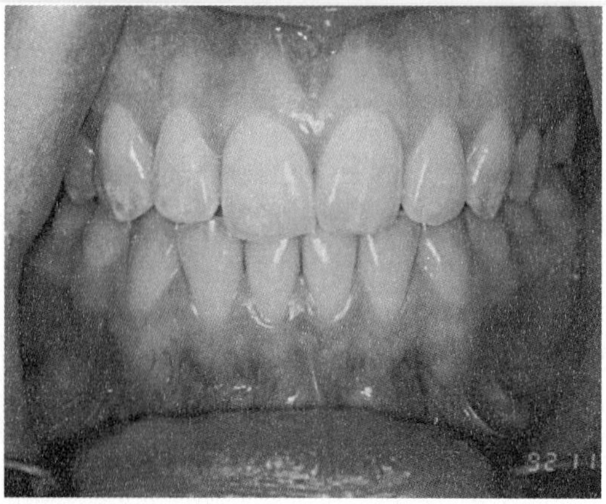

FIGURE 34-6 Mild dental fluorosis.

TABLE 34-4 ***Flouride Supplementation Regimen***

	Dose of Fluoride Administered		
Age	If <0.3 ppm of Fluoride in Drinking Water	If 0.3-0.6 ppm of Fluoride in Drinking Water	If >0.6 ppm of Fluoride in Drinking Water
Birth-6 mo	0	0	0
6 mo-3 yr	0.25 mg/day	0	0
3-6 yr	0.5 mg/day	0.25 mg/day	0
6-16 yr	1.0 mg/day	0.50 mg/day	0

Adapted from Mueller W: Oral medicine and dentistry. In Hay W, editor: *Current pediatric diagnosis and treatment*, ed 16, New York, 2003, McGraw-Hill.
ppm, Parts per million.

Sealants

Pit and fissure sealants provide one of the most beneficial and cost-effective preventive treatments available and are applied by dentists. Sealants involve the application of protective resin coatings that bond to the biting (occlusal) surfaces of molars and premolars (Fig. 34-7). Most molars and premolars are susceptible to decay in the poorly formed grooves on the biting surface. Some of the pits, fissures, or grooves are so deep and narrow that even the bristle of the toothbrush cannot effectively remove plaque and food debris. This inaccessibility allows caries to occur even in the presence of impeccable oral hygiene. Children with deep grooves on their posterior teeth should have sealants placed soon after eruption.

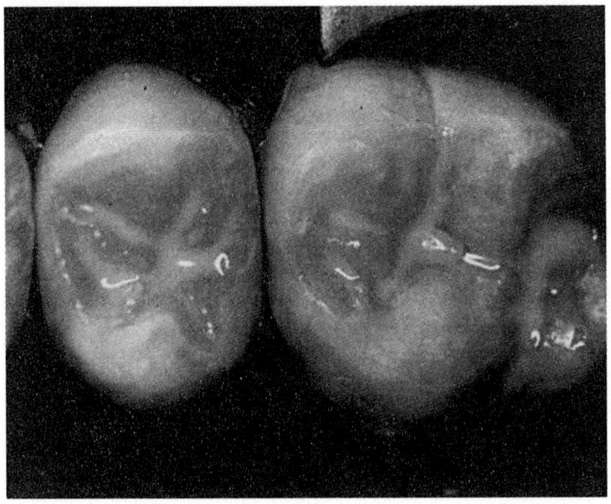

FIGURE 34-7 Sealants. Pit and fissure sealants are the most under-used preventive regimen in dentistry. They can prevent carious lesions from forming in the occlusal (biting) surfaces of most teeth with susceptible deep grooves. (Photo courtesy of Berg and Jones.)

Prevention

Compliance with keeping the recommended periodic well-child visits is generally high (Crall, 2002). The NP, then, is in a unique position to intercept the transmission of dental disease. When the infectious nature of the caries process for young children becomes a primary focus, there is an opportunity to break the cycle of infectivity by identifying high-risk children and their caregiver "infectors" through a risk-base assessment. The strategy to prevent dental decay in primary pediatrics is a three-tiered approach. The rationale for the second and third tiers is based on the timing of infectivity and the mechanism of demineralization-remineralization. These interventions facilitate the non-restorative repair of subsurface lesions before cavitation occurs.

First Tier: A Caries-risk Assessment of the Primary Care Provider (Usually the Mother) and the Infant

- The Caries-risk Assessment Tool (CAT) (see Table 34-3), the mother's dental history (see Box 34-1), and visual examination of the mother's dentition can provide a sufficient caries-risk assessment. Mothers with active decay or multiple fillings in multiple quadrants of the mouth are at higher risk than those who have never experienced decay.

Second Tier: Education to Delay Colonization and Benign Floral Enhancement of the Mother and Infant

Over 40% of adults ages 55 to 75 years have active root caries and high levels of cariogenic organisms (Shay, 1996). Because an infant cannot be colonized with dental flora until the eruption of the primary dentition, benign floral enhancement (BFE) offers important caries prevention (Berkowitz, Jordan, & White, 1975). Delaying this colonization, by modifying the mother's flora (lowering SM levels) before and during the colonization process, can significantly and favorably affect the child's caries index (Brambilla et al, 1998; Kohler, Andreen, & Jonsson, 1984). BFE can be accomplished in the parent by the following methods:

- Cautioning the parent to avoid bacterial inoculation practices (e.g., sharing utensils, cleaning pacifier with saliva)
- Removal of the parent's caries by a dentist
- Administration of meticulous oral hygiene (brushing twice daily and flossing once daily)

- Judicious administration of fluorides (toothpastes and rinses)
- Avoidance of simple sugars between meals in a protracted fashion (fruit juices and carbonated beverages); all of the child's caregivers should follow this recommendation
- Use of chlorhexidine (0.12%) mouth rinses to reduce the high titers of oral flora
- Use of xylitol gum or mints to reduce plaque and remineralize teeth (Isokangas et al, 2000)

Xylitol gum can be found in most drugstores. Orbit, Trident, and Carefree have several flavors available. Even if parents cannot access dental care, this gum can be somewhat helpful in BFE endeavors. See Appendix A for dosing information.

Third Tier: Promoting Initial Benign Floral Acquisition by the Infant

After BFE has been achieved, the goal is to develop a stable oral flora in the child that is not pathogenic. This is achieved by thorough daily oral hygiene procedures, provided by an adult. Ongoing management and prevention of dental caries requires continued reinforcement of the BFE program. The ultimate goal is to minimize the virulence of the parent's (caregiver's) and, potentially, the infant's dental flora.

In addition, the NP should be aware of the frequency and timing of carbohydrate ingestion and provide proper nutritional counseling, demonstrate proper brushing techniques ("lift the lip"), ensure that there is a "dental home," and ensure adequate topical and systemic fluoride intake.

Complications

Evidence shows a relationship of ECC to the systemic health of the child. One study demonstrated that children with ECC weighed significantly less than children without ECC. It concluded that the progression of ECC may affect growth adversely (Acs et al, 1992). Other studies have provided evidence that pregnant women with moderate to severe periodontal disease are more likely to deliver low-birth-weight infants (Offenbacher et al, 2001). Other complications include periodontal disease, local or diffuse abscesses, cellulitis, bone loss, tooth mobility, premature loss of teeth, and orthodontic complications (Sayany, 2002a, 2002b).

OTHER DENTAL DISEASES AND DENTAL PROBLEMS

Gingivitis and Periodontal Disease

Description, Etiology, and Incidence

Gingivitis is an inflammation of the marginal (margin of the gum or the gum line) and the interdental papillary portion of the periodontium. Gingivitis is the most prevalent lesion of the oral soft tissues in young children, with estimates varying from 80% to 90% of children (Carranza & Newman, 1996). Gingivitis results from retention of bacterial plaque in the soft tissue crevice around the neck of the tooth. Poor oral hygiene is the most common cause. Chronic gingivitis leads to periodontitis if the condition remains untreated over a long period of time.

Periodontal disease (periodontitis) is a bacterial inflammatory disease of the gingival and supporting alveolar bony structures; gingival bacterium penetrate deep into the periodontium, resulting in a permanent loss of alveolar bone and supporting structures. Prolonged poor oral hygiene is the precipitating etiologic factor. Inadequate nutrition may contribute to this disease, as well as Down syndrome and any systemic disease that alters the body's defense mechanisms to infection (e.g., juvenile diabetes and various forms of immunosuppression). Periodontitis it is not common in adolescent children without accompanying systemic disease.

Clinical Findings

Oral Examination. The examination findings of periodontitis include the following (Fig. 34-8; also see Table 34-7):

- Bleeding gums (even with light touch), fetid breath, and pain in gingival tissue
- Tooth mobility even when the gingiva appears normal or without severe marginal inflammation
- Severely stained teeth, cavitation of teeth, obvious signs of intraoral neglect

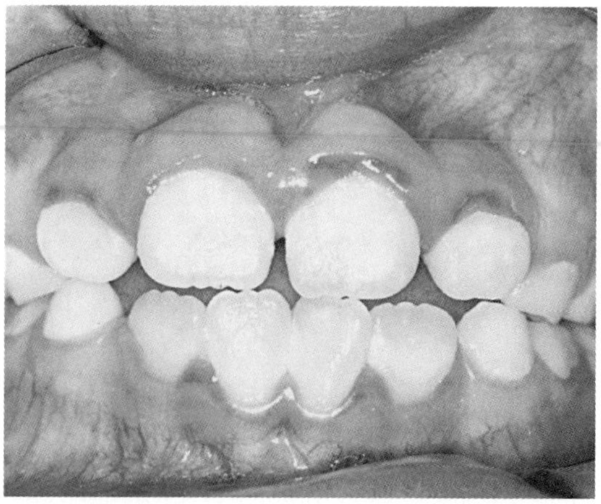

FIGURE 34-8 Gingivitis. Gingival inflammation is caused and perpetuated by plaque accumulation under the gingival crevice. Proper oral hygiene can correct this common condition. (Photo courtesy of Berg and Jones.)

- Erythema to considerable inflammation especially noticeable around first permanent molars and lower incisors
- Lateral gingival abcesses with a purulent discharge

Diagnostic Studies. Dental radiographs are needed to evaluate periodontal bone loss.

Management

The successful long-term treatment of periodontitis is difficult. Often, there is underlying systemic disease that will compromise the prognosis. In addition, poor oral hygiene habits that contributed to the etiology are difficult to change given the long history of neglect by the patient that initiated the disease. The resultant bony defects that are common with severe alveolar bone loss contribute to the difficulty of bacterial plaque removal. Tooth loss is often the resultant outcome without intense professional treatment and home care. Referral to a dentist for definitive diagnosis, treatment, and follow-up care is necessary.

Prevention

Prevention of these periodontal diseases requires using correct and thorough oral hygiene practices. For young children who lack the fine motor skills adequate enough to write their name in cursive or to tie their shoes, brushing and flossing is required by parents.

Dental Malocclusions

Description

Dental malocclusions are best defined as crowded, irregular, or protruding teeth that interfere with dental-oral function, affect dental-facial aesthetics, or increase the likelihood of injury to the teeth. Severe malocclusions may produce a functional disturbance that interferes with mastication, swallowing, speech, and normal function of the temporomandibular joint. Less severe malocclusions often require some physiologic compensation for the anatomic deformity to allow for adequate function.

Etiology

If the developmental sequence from primary dentition through transitional (or mixed dentition) to permanent dentition occurs in an orderly, symmetric, and timely fashion, a functional, aesthetic, and stable occlusion results. When this sequence is disrupted, final occlusion of the permanent dentition is affected. The most common factors initiating abnormal development of occlusion are as follows:

- Genetic control of the size, shape, and position of the maxilla and mandible within the facial structure and the direction of growth of both bones.
- Genetic control of tooth size, shape, development, and eruption.
- Abnormal oral musculature, tongue, and swallowing habits. Abnormal tongue position and deviation from the so-called normal movement of the tongue during swallowing have long been associated with anterior open bite, protrusion of the maxillary incisors, and, in some cases, lisping. Normal infants position the tongue anteriorly in the mouth at rest and during swallowing. A mature swallow pattern is characterized by relaxation of the lips, placement of the tongue behind the maxillary incisors, and elevation of the mandible until posterior teeth contact; this sequence is not usually observed before a child is 4 or 5 years of age.
- Digit/pacifier habits, seen in nonnutritional sucking. Thumb/finger sucking and pacifier use are common practices that should not be allowed to complicate or interfere with normal growth and development of the oral-facial structures. Nonnutritive sucking is a normal activity in most children younger than 2 years old, with many parents encouraging this habit for behavioral control. Any attempts to change this habit before age 24 to 30 months usually proves difficult and unnecessary. However, if continued beyond this age (depending on the frequency, duration, and intensity of the habit), the position of the teeth, as well as growth and function of the mandible, can be altered.
- Premature loss of deciduous teeth, particularly the second deciduous molar. When a primary or permanent tooth is lost prematurely, the forces that hold that tooth in space three-dimensionally are no longer in equilibrium. It is not unusual for the teeth anterior and posterior to the lost tooth to tip into the newly opened space.
- Overretained deciduous teeth.
- Bruxism. Bruxism is nonfunctional grinding or gnashing of teeth and occurs in approximately 15% of adult and child patients. The habit usually occurs at night and, if continued over a prolonged period, can result in abrasion of the permanent teeth. In adolescents, the habit is usually associated with stress and may lead to temporomandibular joint disturbances. Childhood night grinding has been shown to have association with chronic middle ear congestion but is not related to stress or emotional disturbances.

Incidence

The reported incidence of dental-facial malocclusion varies with the defining criteria used by different investigators. Using Grainger's Treatment Priority Index, approximately 25% of children age 6 to 11 years have nearly ideal occlusion, but by 12 to 17 years of age only 12% have nearly ideal occlusion. Crowding and misaligned teeth account for 40% of malocclusions in 6- to 11-year-old children and 85% of malocclusions in children 12 to 17 years old (Grainger, 1967).

Clinical Findings

Oral Examination. Evaluation of the child's developing occlusion is the first step in preventing and treating malocclusion. The Angle orthodontic classification system (Angle, 1900) uses the maxillary and mandibular permanent first molars and their relationship with each other to describe the anterior-posterior relationship of the dentition. It is essential that class I or normal occlusion be established for proper overjet and overbite to occur. This requires that the maxillary first permanent molar interdigitate into the mandibular first permanent molar. When the crown and root angulations of these molar teeth are in proper alignment, as well as being in a class I relationship, the premolars and canines of the dentition can fully interdigitate with each other. Classes I, II, and III malocclusion are illustrated and defined in Fig. 34-9.

This classification system has been expanded to describe not only the specific tooth-to-tooth relationships of the dental arches but also the skeletal relationship of the maxilla and mandible that forms the bite (Box 34-3; Figs. 34-10 and 34-11). In the examination the NP may find the following:

- The teeth are severely crowded.
- There is an excessive overjet or anterior reverse bite (class III).
- There is inadequate alignment for chewing function or normal speech.
- Deciduous posterior teeth are missing without space maintenance.
- There is flaring of the maxillary incisors (bucked teeth), development of an anterior open bite, or development of a posterior crossbite with a functional shift of the mandible.
- The child voices embarrassment over the appearance of his or her teeth.

Management

When such disruptions do occur, appropriate corrective measures are needed to restore normal occlusal development. Such corrective procedures may require some type of passive space maintenance, active tooth guidance, or a combination of both. The child should be referred between 3 and 8 years of age. A comprehensive evaluation in the primary or early mixed dentition stages identifies abnormalities that, if addressed early in a child's dental development, often prevent major orthodontic treatment later. Space maintenance and control of oral habits are the two main orthodontic treatments that prevent the oral neuromuscular complex from developing into an abnormal physical relationship (malocclusion).

Space Maintenance. By placing a space maintainer, three-dimensional forces are held in balance, and adequate room is saved for the unerupted developing permanent tooth. Space maintainers are either fixed (unilateral or bilateral) or removable. Unilateral fixed spacers are the most common (Fig. 34-12).

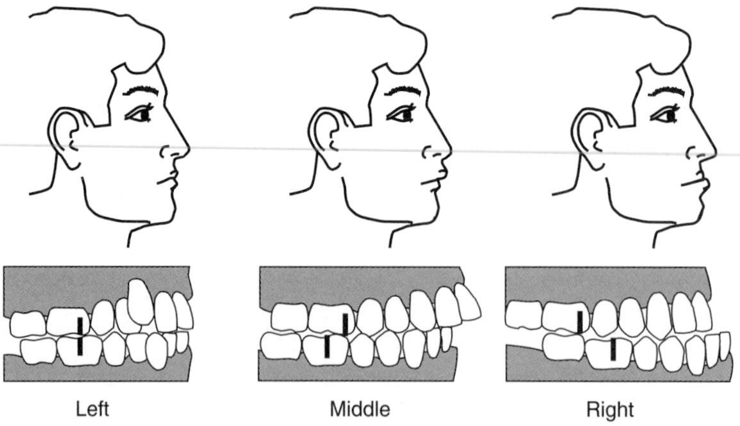

FIGURE 34-9 Orthodontic classification system. *Left*, Class I facial relationship and dental malocclusion: The molar relationship is the same as in normal occlusion; however, some other problem with alignment of the teeth exists, such as crowding in one section or throughout the entire dental arch. *Middle*, Class II facial relationship and dental malocclusion: This classification refers to any positioning of the maxillary molars more anterior to the class I position, the mandibular molars more posterior to the class I position, or a combination of the two. *Right*, Class III facial relationship and dental malocclusion: This classification is the opposite of class II, the class III classification being any positioning of the maxillary molars more posterior to the class I position, the mandibular molars more anterior to the class I position, or a combination of the two.

BOX 34-3 *Skeletal Relationships of the Maxilla and Mandible*

Overbite: Overbite is the amount of overlap of the maxillary incisors over the mandibular incisors. It is measured from the incisal edge of the maxillary teeth to the incisal edge of the mandibular teeth. It can also describe a negative overbite, which is an open bite in which the anterior teeth or incisors do not overlap each other (Ngan & Fields, 1997).

Overjet: Overjet is an anterior-posterior relationship description. It describes how far the maxillary incisors are in front of or behind the mandibular incisors. Parents often refer to an excessive overjet as a "bad overbite" when describing their child's occlusion. These two terms should not be confused because they have different treatment consequences.

Crossbite: In normal occlusion, the maxillary dentition occludes a half-tooth outside or lateral to the posterior mandibular teeth and in front of the mandibular incisor teeth. In an *anterior crossbite,* the maxillary anterior teeth are behind (lingual) the mandibular anterior teeth. Anterior crossbite of one or more of the permanent incisors (see Figs. 34-10 and 34-11) may be evidence of a localized discrepancy, which in most cases should be referred promptly to avoid serious complications. In a *posterior crossbite* the maxillary posterior teeth are either inside or outside their normal position relative to the mandibular posterior teeth; more rarely, the maxillary teeth are lateral to their mandibular counterpart, and the entire maxillary tooth is not in contact with the biting surface of the lower tooth. Such crossbite patterns result from skeletal structural problems of the maxilla or mandible, faulty eruption patterns of the posterior teeth, primary dentition crossbites, or the mandible shifting into an abnormal position.

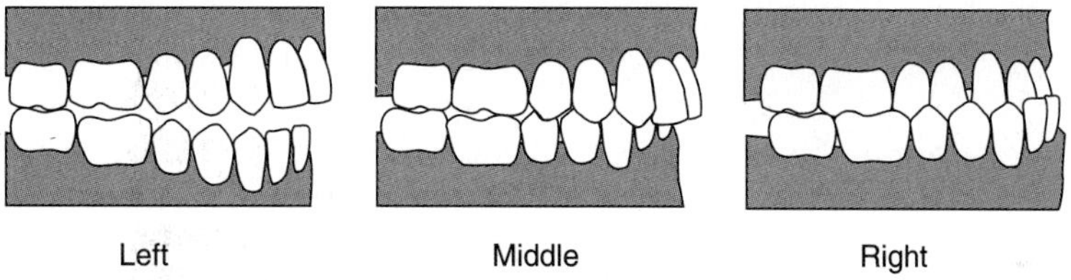

FIGURE 34-10 Classifications of relationships of the maxilla and mandible: dental bite relationships. *Left,* Anterior openbite (also called negative overbite). *Middle,* Anterior deepbite (overbite). *Right,* Posterior and anterior crossbite.

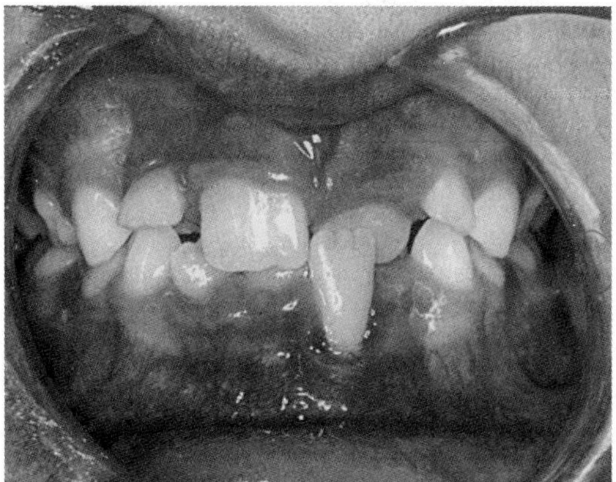

FIGURE 34-11 Anterior crossbite involving maxillary left central incisor and mandibular left central incisor. Note stripping of gingiva from facial of lower incisor as a result of this traumatic occlusion.

Bruxism. The treatment of choice for adolescents with bruxism is a nighttime mouth guard to prevent wear of the teeth and encourage oral-facial muscle relaxation. Younger children rarely continue to grind their teeth on a consistent enough basis to abrade their teeth or produce temporomandibular joint disturbances. The disorder is self-limited and rarely of any consequence, but it should be addressed by the "dental home" provider.

Nonnutritive Sucking. Flaring of the maxillary decidous incisors and persistence of a small open bite will have no abnormal effect on the position of the permanent incisors if the habit is stopped before the appearance of the erupting permanent incisors. Severe flaring of the deciduous maxillary incisors or a large anterior open bite, particularly when combined with a retrognathic mandible, can interfere with speech development and mastication and should receive attention. The presence of a posterior crossbite (maxillary

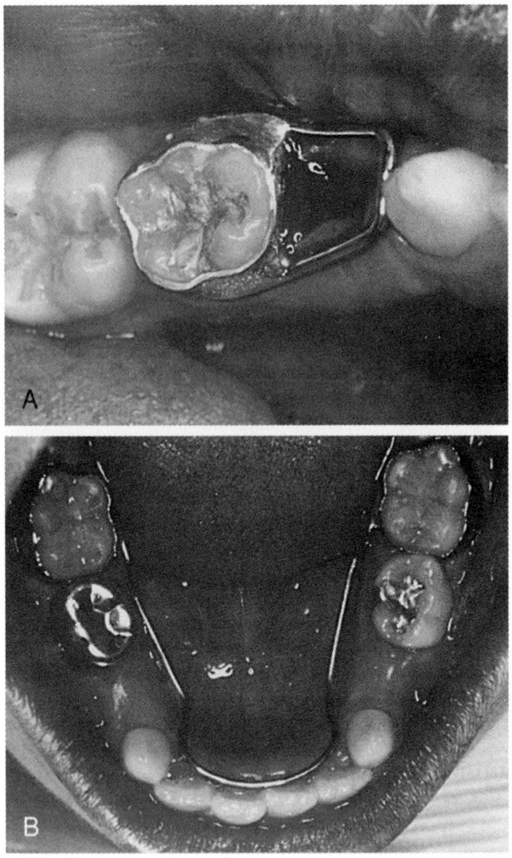

FIGURE 34-12 Fixed space maintainers. **A**, Unilateral. **B**, Bilateral.

canines or molars inside the mandibular teeth) accompanied by a shift of the mandible laterally when the child bites the teeth together signals a potentially serious developmental disturbance. These functional shifts of the mandible should be referred and treated as early as possible (between 3 and 4 years of age) to prevent asymmetric growth of the temporomandibular joint and excessive unilateral growth of the mandible causing lower facial asymmetry.

Many children suck their thumbs or fingers for short periods during infancy or early childhood. Although the habit may be considered normal during the first 2 years of life, many children never have a digit-sucking habit. Parents should be advised to observe the child, and if the sucking gradually diminishes, it is probable that the child will stop without intervention. However, if the child shows no inclination to stop the habit, it becomes a problem that should be addressed.

Corrective appliances for oral habits are indicated when the child reaches 4 to 5 years of age and when the child wants to discontinue the habit and needs only a reminder to accomplish the task. If an appliance is used, it should not be painful; it should not be used as a punishment; and it should not interfere with occlusal function, eating, speaking, or socialization. Instead, it should merely be a reminder. A retainer with a series of smooth loops placed lingual to the incisors has proved successful in helping children overcome maladaptive oral habits.

The parents' role in the correction of an oral habit is important. Parents are often overanxious about the habit and its possible effects and may be tempted to use negative reinforcement, which is rarely effective. This anxiety may result in nagging or punishment, and it often creates greater tension and intensifies the habit. Painting the child's thumb or fingers with a noxious-tasting substance is also ineffective.

Tongue and Swallowing Habits. Myofunctional therapy for tongue thrusting or a deviated swallow is sometimes considered for children in the normal transitional stages of swallow maturation, but this procedure should be seriously questioned. Some preschool children with a forward tongue position have not yet learned to follow the adult pattern, and with time will correct the problem. Dental open bite and abnormal tooth position are more likely caused by the influence of the resting position of the tongue rather than thrusting of the tongue while swallowing. Malocclusions that are caused from the resting posture of the tongue or lips are extremely challenging to treat and should be dealt with orthodontically, and then reevaluated after the child has completed all facial growth. Surgical correction may ultimately be recommended.

Interceptive and Comprehensive Orthodontic Treatment. Interceptive orthodontic treatment is designed to enhance the child's occlusal function and aesthetics at an early age and to minimize occlusal abnormalities that worsen with growth and as permanent teeth erupt. Typically, it involves correction of transverse (arch width) abnormalities, arch development to prevent dental crowding, anterior-posterior skeletal and dental relationships, and alignment of the eight incisors. This is accomplished by using either fixed or removable orthodontic appliances.

Comprehensive orthodontics may involve some combination of preventive or interceptive orthodontics, but more commonly refers to orthodontic treatment provided when the child is in the early permanent dentition stage or later when the second molar teeth are fully erupted. Such treatment can be instituted at any age into adulthood but is more efficiently provided during the early teen growth years, and depends on the specific facial or dental malocclusion. Severe skeletal-dental malocclusions may require orthodontic-surgical treatment and are usually treated after facial growth has subsided.

Complications

Impaired dental-facial aesthetics can have a profound effect on a child's psychosocial development and if extreme, should be considered a social handicap. Different cultures, families, and individuals have different views on dental-facial aesthetics, and these individual views should be respected. However, dental-facial aesthetics is a factor in how children feel about themselves, as well as how others view them.

Protruding incisor teeth have twice the chance of receiving some sort of trauma resulting in dental fractures or devitalization of the pulp (Andreasen, 1994). Minimizing the risk of dental trauma to anterior teeth through interceptive or definitive orthodontic treatment is considered a part of comprehensive preventive dental care.

Traumatic Injuries to the Face and Teeth

Description and Etiology

Traumatic injuries to a child's mouth and teeth are common as normal motor development and coordination evolve. Children with poor coordination or a lack of protective reflexes are particularly at risk. These injuries are not usually severe but require attention. All children are at risk while riding in a motor vehicle and must be placed in properly fitting child-restraint seats. The repeated vomiting that occurs in bulimia demineralizes tooth enamel and causes a unique type of trauma.

Injuries about the head, neck, and face occur in over half of all child abuse cases (U.S. Department of Health and Human Services, 2000a). Many of these children also have accompanying dental involvement, so this diagnosis must be kept in mind when evaluating injury to the mouth and oral cavity.

Falls account for most dental trauma in children 1 to 5 years old, peaking at 2 to 3 years when coordination is developing (AAPD, 2001). It is extremely important to identify nonvital dark deciduous teeth (Fig. 34-13). Deciduous teeth that appear dark have been subjected to enough trauma that the dental pulp tissues have undergone necrosis and lost their vitality.

Males have twice the injury rate of females. In children 6 to 17 years old, bicycle accidents, sports, and being struck by an object account for most injuries. Additionally, 8-year-olds experience a high number of orofacial injuries as they begin to develop athletic skills and growth spurts. Injuries are more numerous in those participating in team sports, but the injuries are more severe in individual sports (AAPD, 2001; Oral Health Program, Rhode Island Department of Health, 2001). Fights, sports, and vehicle accidents

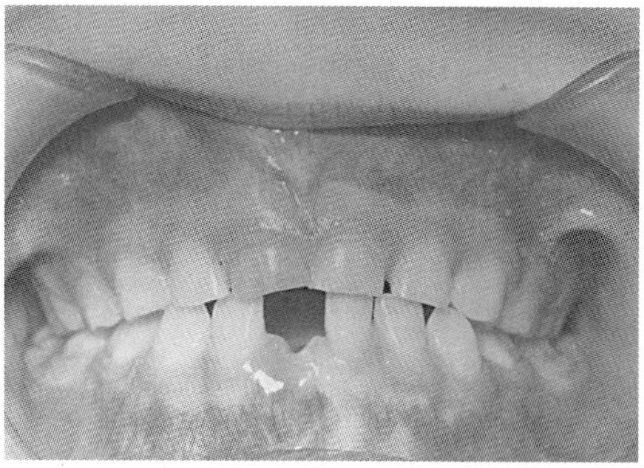

FIGURE 34-13 Dark, nonvital tooth indicating necrotic pulp.

account for most dental injuries in young adults. Motor vehicle accidents are responsible for oral trauma at all ages. At least one quarter of children visit the emergency department for craniofacial injuries before they reach 15 years of age; children with protrusion of the front teeth have twice the risk for anterior dental trauma (Nguyen et al, 1999).

Clinical Findings

History. When the child arrives at the office, it is most important to take a careful history to ensure that the child has no special health care needs that would alter routine dental care (e.g., cerebral palsy, cleft lip and palate, mental retardation, congenital heart disease). Recording when, where, and how the injury took place helps identify any suspicions of child abuse.

Oral and Facial Examination

Many pediatric health care providers have received little training in the detection of dental injuries, particularly those that are due to oral abuse. Collaboration with a pediatric dentist or a dentist with training in forensic oral pathology should be sought when oral abuse is suspected.

Examining a child with an oral/dental injury can be a challenge if the child is crying or agitated. Nevertheless, the examination must be thorough in order to identify injuries that require immediate treatment. The clinician needs to examine for the following:

- Facial asymmetry, bruising, and a full range of motion of the mandible
- Any injury to the lips, frenula, tongue, soft palate, gingiva, and other mucosal surfaces
- Soft tissue injury such as puncture wounds, foreign bodies, torn tissue that exposes underlying bone, or lacerations over 2 mm long that would require suturing
- Alignment of the teeth within the dental arch and alignment with the opposing dental arch

- Mobility in both a labial and palatal (lingual) direction while noting any teeth that exhibit more than 2 mm of movement
- Fractured teeth, with the extent of the fracture into dentin noted and whether any pulp tissue is exposed
- Findings suggestive of child abuse

Blunt trauma injuries are most commonly inflicted with an instrument, eating utensils, hands, or fingers. Contusions; lacerations; punctures; fractured, displaced, or avulsed teeth; and petechial hemorrhages on the palate are the common physical injuries of the oral cavity. The oral cavity is a frequent site of sexual abuse, and the clinician should be alert for the oral signs of gonorrhea or syphilis discussed later in this chapter. When bite marks are observed, the intercuspid distance should be measured to identify whether a child or an adult is responsible for the bite. Bite marks with an intercuspid distance of 3.0 cm or more are most likely caused by an adult. The physical findings should be photographed for later documentation. A pediatric dentist or forensic oral pathologist can often record bite marks with either photography or dental impressions of the bite marks.

Diagnostic Studies. When a missing tooth or tooth fragment cannot be found and identified, lateral soft tissue, neck, and thoracoabdominal radiographs for foreign bodies (teeth or tooth fragments) are indicated to ensure a patent airway free of tooth fragments.

Culture the child's mouth for gonorrhea or chlamydia (blood test for syphilis) if child abuse is suspected as the etiology of the clinical findings.

Management

When faced with providing the initial management of a traumatic dental-facial injury, the NP needs to be prepared to recognize severe trauma to the head, neck, or airway and separate out those injuries confined to the teeth and gingiva. Immediate management of dental trauma seeks to prevent the aesthetic disfigurement of tooth loss, future pain, infection, or expensive dental treatment. Table 34-5 identifies

TABLE 34-5 ***Traumatic Dental Injuries That Require Immediate Attention by a Dental Professional***

Injury	Clinical Features	Treatment Action
Fractured jaw	Facial asymmetry, swelling, pain, limitation of movement	Radiographic diagnosis, immobilization
Dental alveolar bone fracture	Mobility of segments of teeth rather than individual teeth	Radiographic diagnosis, intraarch stabilization
Dental crown fractures involving exposure of pulpal tissue	Pulp tissue visible in the tooth fracture site	Pulp capping and coverage of the fracture to prevent bacterial infection of pulp, dental abscess, and endodontics
Root fractures	Mobility of one or more teeth more than 2 mm in any direction	Radiographic diagnosis, intraarch stabilization
Intruded tooth	Tooth completely or partially intruded or jammed into its socket	Radiographic diagnosis Primary tooth—allowed to reerupt, followed by pulpotomy Permanent tooth—requires orthodontic repositioning and endodontics
Partial avulsions (extrusions)	Tooth dislodged from its socket and will not remain stable or has >2 mm mobility	Radiographic diagnosis to rule out root fracture Primary teeth—extract if severely mobile or intraarch stabilization and pulpotomy Permanent tooth—intraarch stabilization and endodontics
Complete avulsion	Entire tooth displaced from the dental socket intact	Radiographic confirmation Primary tooth (if found)—stop bleeding; do not reimplant Permanent tooth—gently clean root surface, reimplant immediately, intraarch stabilization; transport the tooth in saline, milk, or cold water to the dental office if necessary
Toothache accompanied by swelling	Cellulitis or localized facial erythema Broken or carious tooth	Confer with a pediatric dentist about antibiotic choice Start antibiotic therapy

dental injuries that require immediate dental intervention and referral. Table 34-6 identifies dental injuries that are of concern but can be dealt with by a dental professional within 1 to 3 days. The need for a tetanus booster should be considered and the patient's immunization record reviewed.

If the injury to the dentition appears to be minor, a follow-up appointment within 1 week with a pediatric dentist should be recommended to ensure that the child has no detrimental effects of pulp necrosis, subsequent infection, or peripheral root resorption from the injury. Giving advice over the telephone is often requested by a concerned parent but should be avoided, other than recommending a dental referral or office visit for evaluation.

Prevention

During the early years of life, a focus on injury prevention facilitates protection of the mouth and oral cavity. Preventive measures include the use of gates at the top and bottom of stairs, avoidance of walkers, use of safety seats and seat belts when in motor vehicles, and use of bike helmets.

Mouth Guards. As children become older and more involved in organized sports, the incidence and severity of oral/dental trauma increase. Fortunately, many of these injuries can be prevented through the use of dental mouth guards. During health supervision visits or sports physical examinations, the NP should stress the importance of mouth guard protection.

Although "boil and bite" mouth guards are available from retail stores, they are bulky and uncomfortable. Custom-fitted mouth guards afford the best protection and allow for better speech, breathing, and retention. Because they are more comfortable, compliance is rarely a problem. Mouth guards were first developed in the 1950s to prevent chronic brain concussion in football players before the use of facemasks was made mandatory. Although prevention of concussion continues to be the primary objective of mouth guards, they also protect the lips, gingiva, and teeth by:

- Keeping the lips away from the teeth and preventing lip lacerations
- Preventing violent contact of the upper and lower teeth that might result in tooth and jaw fracture
- Holding the jaws apart, acting as a shock absorber to minimize energy transfer through the maxilla and condylar fossa to the cranial bones, and thereby preventing concussion
- Spreading the forces of the blow throughout the dentition rather than being directed at any one tooth or segment of bone to prevent tooth fractures and avulsions

Mouth guards should be recommended for all sports that involve powerful physical contact with another player or with an object (e.g., a hardball or softball). Most football and hockey organizations mandate the use of mouth guards, and few oral injuries are seen in these sports. However, soccer, basketball, wrestling, baseball, and softball are the sports that the dental community now associates with oral/dental sports injuries. Mouth guards are also beneficial in activities such as skateboarding and in-line skating. The NP should advocate the use of mouth guards in such sports.

Dental Neglect

The AAPD defines *dental neglect* as the willful failure of a parent or guardian to seek and follow through with treatment necessary to ensure a level of oral health essential for adequate function and free from pain and infection (AAPD, 1999). Many factors influence a family to not seek

TABLE 34-6 ***Traumatic Dental Injuries That Require Attention by a Dental Professional within 1 to 3 Days***

Injury	Clinical Features	Treatment Action
Bumped deciduous incisors	Dark discolored anterior deciduous or permanent tooth	Radiographic diagnosis, pulpectomy, endodontics
Toothache not accompanied by swelling	Painful carious or fractured tooth often accompanied by mobility or a draining fistula	Start antibiotics/analgesics, insist on professional dental follow-up
Simple crown fractures	Fractures of enamel or dentin (or both) that do not expose the pulp	Restore the tooth to function and aesthetics as convenient
Broken braces, wires, dental appliances	Dental appliances loose or irritating to the child	Dental appointment as soon as possible; remove the appliance
Minor bumps	Teeth slightly loosened in their sockets with <2 mm mobility and stable in the dental arch	Insist on professional dental follow-up

dental care for the family's children. Ignorance, cultural values, lack of perceived health value, lack of finances, and geographic isolation are the most common reasons. Indicators of dental neglect include the following:

- Untreated rampant caries easily detected by a layperson
- Untreated pain, infection, bleeding, or trauma affecting the oral-facial region

The NP should first be certain that the parent or guardian thoroughly understands the significance of dental pathology and the potential for life-threatening infections if left untreated. Once such understanding is established, a place for the child to receive dental care should be identified. If the parent continues to be negligent after financial ability to support care has been determined, a referral to social services for investigation of child abuse by neglect is warranted.

Complications

Nonvital deciduous teeth have the potential to develop peripheral root resorption, chronic apical granulomas, and infection that can damage the permanent tooth bud or spread to other tissues, reducing the chance for retention of the tooth until it exfoliates at the normal age. Prompt endodontic treatment is needed.

Oral Problems of Infants

Natal and Neonatal Teeth

Natal teeth are present at birth, and neonatal teeth erupt within the first 30 days of life (Fig. 34-14). They are usually in the mandibular incisor area, and a large majority are primary incisors. Only a small percentage are supernumerary teeth. Natal teeth occur in 1 in 2000 to 3000 births. A 14.5% familial occurrence has been noted (Children's Health at Doernbecher, 2003). Natal teeth are also associated with several syndromes, such as Jadassohn-Lewansky and cleft palate and lip, endocrine disturbances, nutritional deficiencies, congenital syphilis, and fever of the mother during pregnancy (Pereira, 1998).

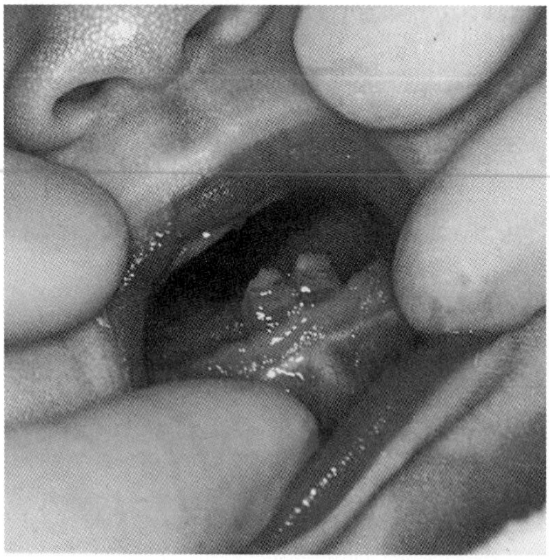

FIGURE 34-14 Natal teeth. Natal teeth are distinguished from neonatal teeth in that they are present at birth. These teeth are extracted if they present a risk of aspiration. (Photo courtesy of Berg and Jones.)

If the tooth is extremely loose, it should be extracted before the infant is discharged from the nursery to prevent aspiration. If the tooth is not excessively loose, it should be evaluated by a pediatric dentist before the child leaves the hospital or within the first few days of life.

Extracting a neonatal tooth on the basis that the tooth will interfere with breastfeeding is not warranted because children routinely breastfeed after tooth eruption. A lactation nurse should be consulted if the mother has discomfort adjusting to the infant's suckling; use of a breast pump and bottling of mother's milk can be considered.

Aspiration of the tooth, pain, refusal to feed, and maternal discomfort with breastfeeding can occur.

Teething Discomfort

The inflammation and sensitivity that can be present in gingival tissue as deciduous teeth erupt is commonly referred to as *teething*. The following may be noted:

- Actively erupting deciduous teeth
- Irritability and fussiness
- Gingival inflammation
- Eruption hematoma or eruption cysts
- Bacterial plaque accumulation

The following measures may help in managing the discomfort:

- Daily toothbrushing of the erupting deciduous teeth should be done to prevent the gingival inflammation and infection that occur with dental bacterial plaque accumulation.
- A cold liquid–filled teething ring provides an object that slightly anesthetizes the gums and allows the baby to chew and apply pressure to the gums. A hard rubber ring or beads also help without running the risk of aspirated fluid from a ruptured ring.
- A non–aspirin-containing analgesic can help.
- Topical creams or oil of clove should not be used. If the parents report that the child has a fever, look for other systemic infections because tooth eruption does not cause a fever. Fever speeds up selected metabolic processes and may stimulate accelerated tooth eruption.

Eruption Hematoma (Eruption Cyst)

An eruption hematoma is a bluish lesion on the gums preceding eruption of a tooth. These lesions are not true cysts but result from bleeding into the dental follicular space of the erupting tooth as it emerges through the alveolar bone beneath the alveolar mucosa. The 5 to 10 mm lesion is a well-circumscribed, dome-shaped, fluctuant, bluish swelling located over an erupting tooth.

The enlargement ruptures spontaneously and the tooth erupts. Rarely does an eruption hematoma cause the child discomfort requiring analgesics. If the gum appears to be infected, refer the patient to a pediatric dentist for excision of the overlying gingival tissue.

Oral Candidiasis

Pseudomembranous candidiasis (thrush) is commonly manifested as adherent white plaques that resemble curdled milk and is sometimes mistaken for formula remaining in the mouth (Fig. 34-15).

Candida albicans (a common inhabitant of the oral cavity) may be present in the normal oral flora in approximately 45% of the population (Dock & Creedon, 2002). Other forms of candidiasis (e.g., atrophic or chronic hyperplastic candidiasis) are rare in children but may be seen as red macules or red areas with white patches in those immunocompromised. The organisms multiply rapidly when host resistance is lowered, after exposure to broad-spectrum antibiotics, or in association with immunosuppression or systemic disease. Neonatal candidiasis is contracted during passage through the vagina and appears during the first 2 weeks of life. Other sources include digits (from sucking), the breast, the bottle nipple, or ingestion of antibiotics.

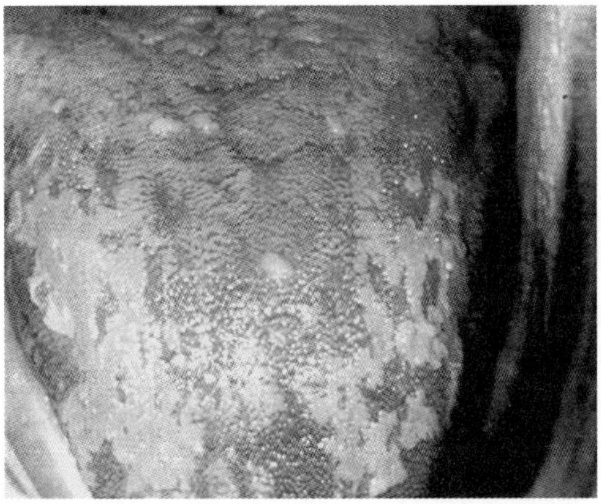

FIGURE 34-15 Oral candidiasis. White patches on the intraoral soft tissues that rub off, exposing an underlying bleeding tissue, are often *Candida* lesions. (Photo courtesy of Berg and Jones.)

The history may reveal a decrease in feeding. The oral examination commonly shows mild lymphadenopathy and raised, furry, white patches or red lesions combined with white patches on the buccal mucosa, tongue, and palate that may bleed when scraped with a tongue blade.

Oral candidiasis is often self-limited. Medication treatment typically involves using a topical antifungal suspension or gentian violet (see Chapter 37 for specific management regimens). If recurrent, look for other causes such as conditions associated with immunosuppression. Systemic antifungal agents are not recommended for children unless associated with immunosuppression or multiorgan involvement.

Oral Problems of Toddlers

Hyperplastic Maxillary Frenum

The wedge-shaped tissue connecting the upper lip to the area of the gum between the two central incisor teeth is called the *maxillary frenulum* or *frenum.* Many parents are concerned with an abnormally large frenum causing a diastema (spacing) between the teeth. No etiology is known for this condition.

A hyperplastic maxillary frenum is considered an aspect of normal variation. Ideally, primary teeth have wide spacing to allow room for the permanent teeth. As the primary teeth are exfoliated, the maxilla grows downward and forward; the maxillary frenum does not grow with the rest of the maxilla and becomes smaller in comparison.

If a space is still present between the two front teeth after all six of the permanent upper incisor teeth have erupted (at around 12 years of age), the frenum may need to be excised in conjunction with orthodontic treatment for either occlusion or cosmetic purposes. Early excision can result in scar tissue that is more dense and fibrous than the original tissue.

Mandibular Labial Frenum

The wedge-shaped tissue connecting the lower lip to the area of the gum in front of the two central incisor teeth is called the *mandibular labial frenulum* or *frenum.* On occasion, the mandibular labial frenum attaches into the marginal gingiva instead of the fixed gingival tissues and causes gingival recession on the labial surface of one or both incisors.

Premature or asymmetric gingival recession on the labial surface of the lower incisors will be evident. If present, refer to a pediatric dentist for evaluation and treatment. A gingival autograft surgical procedure is often necessary to prevent alveolar bone resorption and advanced periodontal disease in the area of gingival recession. Without surgical intervention, periodontal disease and tooth loss will occur.

Mandibular Lingual Frenum (Tongue-Tie)

A short fibrous strand of connective tissue that originates along the anterior ventral surface and tip of the tongue to the lingual mandibular gingiva is known as a *mandibular lingual frenum*, or *tongue-tie*. No etiology is known. A mandibular lingual frenum is considered to be a normal variation.

The NP should determine the ability to produce normal articulation sounds. Most speech pathologists believe that children will have no problem making normal speech sounds if the child can extend the tongue over the lower incisor teeth and touch the lower lip.

Refer to a speech pathologist and pediatric dentist for evaluation of any restriction of tongue movement, or if the NP or parent is concerned. Historically, lingual frenectomies were common and many times unnecessary. Consequently, many pediatric dentists do not approve of any surgical intervention or even evaluation of the condition. Stripping or recession of the lingual gingiva may accelerate periodontal disease and tooth loss. Surgical scarring and damage to Wharton ducts can occur as a result of surgical intervention.

Herpes Simplex Virus

Primary infection with herpes simplex virus type 1 (HSV-1) usually occurs as acute gingivostomatitis. The virus then becomes dormant in certain nerve cells until reactivated by triggering factors such as stress, menses, illness, and fatigue. Recurrent infection occurs as herpes labialis infection, commonly called cold sores or fever blisters. Table 34-7 differentiates oral herpes simplex infection, gingivitis, and aphthous ulcers. See Chapters 24 and 37 for more information.

Clinical findings include the following:

- Gingivostomatitis evidenced by
  - Erythema of the soft mucosa of the mouth
  - Yellow or white liquid-filled vesicles that rupture and form painful oral ulcers that are 1 to 3 mm in diameter and are covered with a whitish-gray membrane
  - Cervical lymphadenopathy
  - Friable gingiva that bleeds easily
  - Fever, irritability, headache
  - Weight loss and dehydration
- Herpes labialis
  - Cluster of small, clear vesicles with an erythematous base that become weepy and ulcerated and progress to crustiness, usually only on one side of the mouth

Management

Lesions heal spontaneously in 1 to 2 weeks. The following steps can be taken:

- Oral hygiene is performed with a soft toothbrush, cotton-tipped applicator, or cloth.

TABLE 34-7 ***Differentiating Oral Herpes Simplex Infection, Gingivitis, and Aphthous Ulcers***

	Etiology and Age	Clinical Findings	Treatment
Herpes simplex virus (HSV)	HSV type 1 primary infection is gingivostomatitis, which usually occurs before 5 yr of age; recurrent infection is herpes labialis and occurs at any age	Gingivostomatitis—erythematous soft mucosa of the mouth with vesicles that ulcerate and form white plaques on mucous membranes Herpes labialis—burning, itching cluster of small clear vesicles with an erythematous base that become crusty, usually near the mouth	Lesions heal spontaneously. Encourage fluids. Oral analgesics, oral anesthetics in older children. Occasional use of acyclovir (Zovirax) in severely ill children. Exclude from day care if drooling.
Gingivitis	Retention of bacterial plaque in the soft tissue of the neck of the tooth; most prevalent in young children because of poor hygiene	Early—mild erythema and inflammation at the margins of gum tissue Moderate—red, glazed bleeding gums Severe—spontaneously bleeding gums, fetid breath, enlarged gums	Antibacterial mouth rinses with chlorhexidine 0.12% if the child can expectorate. Improved oral hygiene. Refer to a dentist if severe.
Aphthous ulcers	Idiopathic in origin, precipitated by trauma, stress, sun, allergies, and certain chronic disorders; most common in adolescents	Tingle or burn before lesion occurs, pain with the lesion Single or multiple small circular lesions with an erythematous halo and pale center on the alveolar and buccal mucosa, tongue, soft palate, and floor of the mouth	Resolves spontaneously. Oral analgesics, topical anesthetics, antibacterial rinse as above. Topical steroids if severe (e.g., Kenalog in Orabase). Refer to a dentist if duration >14 days.

- Encourage fluids, especially cold ones, and a soft diet.
- Oral analgesics (acetaminophen or ibuprofen) may be used for control of pain.
- An equal mixture of diphenhydramine and Maalox applied topically provides symptomatic relief.
- Some clinicians recommend acyclovir (Zovirax), 20 to 40 mg/kg per day given in five doses for up to 5 days for children older than 1 year with severe gingivostomatitis, especially if at risk for dehydration.

Small children who cannot control their secretions should be excluded from day care during the initial course. It is not uncommon to have herpetic whitlow (see Chapters 24 and 37 for further discussions). Contact with the mouth and sharing of food and utensils should be avoided until the lesions have resolved.

Oral Problems in Preschoolers, School-Age Children, and Adolescents

Geographic Tongue (Glossitis Areata Migrans, Benign Migratory Glossitis)

A geographic tongue manifests as an irregular circular lesion on the dorsal surface of the tongue with a red, smooth, erythematous central area surrounded by a thin, yellowish-white line or band (Fig. 34-16).

The etiology of this anomaly is unknown. It has been linked to stress, alcohol, tobacco, spicy foods, citrus fruits or other local irritants, and heredity. Desquamation of the filiform papillae on the dorsum of the tongue is responsible for the appearance of the lesion, which characteristically changes shape with time before it spontaneously resolves. Reassure the concerned parent that the condition is commonly seen in children (1% to 3% prevalence; Dock & Creedon, 2002), is self-limiting, requires no treatment (other than elimination of any offending irritant), and may recur.

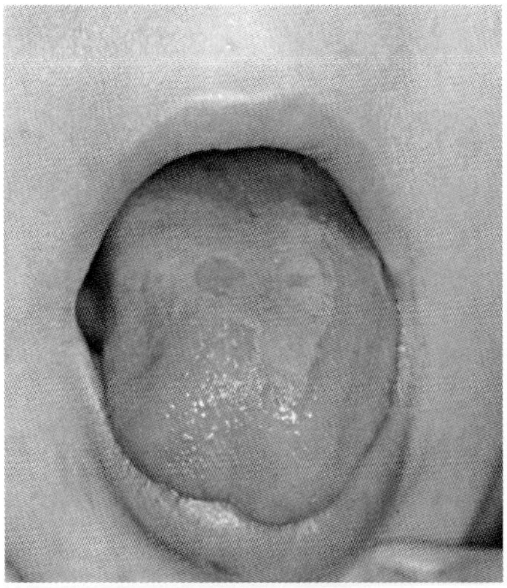

FIGURE 34-16 Geographic tongue in an 18-month-old child.

Parulis (Gum Boil)

A parulis is a chronic mass of granulation tissue localized on the gingiva that is the external portion of a draining apical dental abscess. Extensive decay or pulpal necrosis from a traumatic injury may produce such an abscess that can then lead to the formation of a parulis.

Facial pain, gingival swelling, erythema, fistula, granuloma (localized infection), lymphadenopathy, and fever (cellulitis) may be symptoms. Management involves referring the patient for tooth extraction, pulpectomy, or endodontics. If infection is localized, antibiotic therapy is not usually indicated. If cellulitis is present, antibiotic therapy is given before or along with endodontic therapy or extraction (penicillin VK or erythromycin). Referral to a pediatric dentist for follow-up care is necessary.

Smokeless Tobacco Use

Tobacco use in the form of either smoke or spit (chewing tobacco or snuff) damages oral soft tissue and predisposes the user to oral cancer. Approximately 28% to 30% of high school students and 11% of middle school students smoke. This represents about a 22% decrease from 1997 to 2001 (American Lung Association, 2002; CDC, 2002). Smokeless tobacco is chewed, held between the cheek and gum, or sniffed through the nose. Adolescents who use chewing tobacco or snuff have blood nicotine levels equal to those of smokers. Adolescent males, especially those participating in recreational team sports, are at greatest risk. The incidence is greater in whites. An estimated 12% to 29% of adolescent males use smokeless tobacco (Centers for Disease Control and Prevention, National Institutes of Health, 2001).

The oral examination will reveal erythema of isolated intraoral soft tissue areas; white patches (leukoplakia) or oral ulceration on the gingiva or buccal mucosa may also be detected. Management involves periodic oral cancer screening examinations by a dentist, preventive dental care, referral to a dentist for biopsy of any changes in the oral mucosa, education and counseling regarding smokeless tobacco use and its health implications (see Resource Box), and medication support or referral to tobacco cessation groups.

Smokeless tobacco use is associated with dental caries, discolored teeth, gingivitis, localized gum recession, soft tissue changes, and elevated cholesterol levels, blood pressure, and heart rate. Users have an increased risk of oral cancer, including epithelial dysplasia, carcinoma in situ, and squamous cell carcinoma.

Recurrent Aphthous Ulcers

Description. Recurrent aphthous ulcers are commonly called *canker sores* (Fig. 34-17). They recur frequently and are sometimes confused with herpetic lesions (see Table 34-7).

Etiology and Incidence. An aphthous ulcer is considered idiopathic in origin but can be precipitated by trauma, stress, sun, allergies, and endocrine or hematologic disorders. Onset may be in childhood but often occurs in adolescence with a prevalence rate of about 20% (Neville et al, 1995). Occasionally, these patients have underlying iron, vitamin B_{12}, or folate deficiency, or celiac disease.

Clinical Findings. The patient may report tingling or burning preceding the appearance of the oral lesions. The following can be seen on the oral examination:

- Single or multiple small, circular to oval lesions with an erythematous halo and a pale to yellow center
- Lesion(s) located on alveolar mucosa, ventral surface of the tongue, soft palate, buccal mucosa, or floor of the mouth
- Lesions are generally painful
- Lack of systemic symptoms

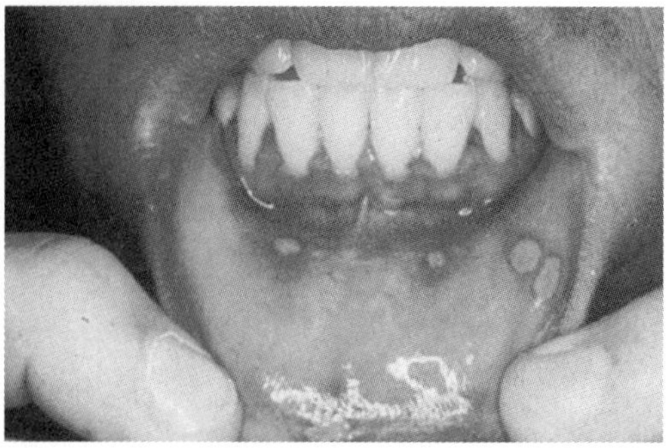

FIGURE 34-17 Apthous ulcers, also called *canker sores*, are vesicles at first; they become small round ulcers with a white base surrounded by a red halo.

Differential Diagnosis. The differential diagnosis includes herpes simplex or herpes zoster lesions, herpangina (coxsackievirus A), trauma, hand-foot-and-mouth disease, and

RESOURCE BOX

Dental Disorders

Academy of Sports Dentistry
c/o Dr. Dave Kumamoto
1-312-792-1354

American Academy of Pediatric Dentistry
1-312-337-2169
www.aapd.org

American Dental Association
1-800-947-4746
1-312-440-2500
www.ada.org

American Dental Hygienists' Association
1-312-440-8900
www.adha.org

American Society of Dentistry for Children
1-312-943-1244
E-mail: asdckids@aol.com

Bright Futures in Practice: Oral Health and Quick Reference Guidelines
National Center for Education in Maternal and Child Health
1-703-524-7802
www.brightfutures.org

Federation of Special Care Organizations
Academy of Dentistry for Persons with Disabilities
1-312-440-2661

National Cancer Institute Smokeless Tobacco Educational Program
Office of Cancer Communication
National Institute of Dental and Craniofacial Research
1-301-496-4261
www.nidcr.nih.gov

National Foundation of Dentistry for the Handicapped
1-303-298-9650

National Institute of Dental Research
1-301-496-4261
www.nidr.nih.gov

National Oral Health Information Clearinghouse
1-301-402-7364
www.aerie.com/nohicweb/ohurap.html
Produces and distributes patient and professional educational materials, including fact sheets, brochures, and information packets for patients with special oral health needs

Prevent Abuse and Neglect through Dental Awareness (PANDA)
Lynn Douglas Mouden, DDS, MPH
1-314-751-6247

chemical burns. Severe persistent lesions are associated with juvenile diabetes and inflammatory bowel syndrome.

Management. Aphthous ulcers spontaneously resolve in 1 to 2 weeks. The following comfort steps can be recommended:

- Palliative treatment with oral analgesics, topical anesthetics, diphenhydramine (Benadryl) elixir, and Maalox (can also use attapulgite [Kaopectate]) in a 50/50 mixture, or a viscous lidocaine (Xylocaine) solution for children older than 12 years. Children should not swallow solutions.
- Antibacterial rinses to mitigate secondary bacterial infection. Tetracycline elixir applied topically or used as a 2-minute rinse shortens the disease course.
- Topical steroid rinses or triamcinolone acetonide (Kenalog in Orabase) can provide some relief for severe ulcerations.
- Silver nitrate cauterization has been used to provide pain relief but delays healing.
- See Chapter 43 for complementary medicine suggestions.

Refer to an oral surgeon or a pediatric dentist for biopsy if the condition lasts more than 14 days.

Mucoceles

When a blockage or traumatic severance of a minor salivary gland duct occurs, a submucosal retention of saliva results. This retention cyst is called a *mucocele.* Mucoceles are most often seen on the inside of the lower lip, rarely on the upper lip, palate, or floor of the mouth; they can fluctuate in size and last for weeks or months. If they spontaneously rupture, recurrence is likely. Referral to a pediatric dentist or an oral surgeon is indicated for surgical removal of the mucocele and relevant minor salivary gland.

Sexually Transmitted Diseases Occurring in the Oral Cavity

Palatal petechia, focal ulcerations, and mucosal erythema may identify sexually active adolescents engaging in oral sex. A careful history to determine possible exposure is warranted, should the NP observe these findings. The patient should be referred for a physical examination to diagnose and treat any sexually transmitted diseases (e.g., *Candida, Trichomonas,* herpes, *Chlamydia, Neisseria gonorrhoeae,* and human immunodeficiency virus [Neville et al, 1995]). See Chapters 24 and 36 for more information. Refer to an oral surgeon or a pediatric dentist for any unusual lesions that do not resolve within 2 weeks.

REFERENCES

Acs G et al: Effect of nursing caries on body weight in a pediatric population, *Pediatr Dent* 14(55):302-305, 1992.

American Academy of Pediatric Dentistry: *Reference manual 1999-2000,* Chicago, 1999, AAPD.

American Academy of Pediatric Dentistry: *Reference manual 2001-2002,* Chicago, 2001, AAPD.

American Academy of Pediatric Dentistry: *Special issue: reference manual 2002-2003,* Chicago, 2002, AAPD.

American Academy of Pediatrics: Oral health risk assessment: timing and establishment of the dental home, *Pediatrics* 11(5):1113-1116, 2003.

American Lung Association: Fact sheet: teenage tobacco use, 2002. Available at *www.stateoftheair.org* (accessed Feb 5, 2003).

Andreasen JO: *Textbook and color atlas of traumatic injuries to the teeth,* ed 3, St Louis, 1994, Mosby.

Angle EH: *Treatment of malocclusion of the teeth and fractures of the maxillae, Angle's system,* ed 6, Philadelphia, 1900, SS White Dental Manufacturing Company.

Berg J: Prevention in dentistry. In Burg F et al, editors: *Gellis and Kagan's current pediatric therapy,* ed 17, Philadelphia, 2002, WB Saunders.

Berkowitz RJ, Jones P: Mouth-to-mouth transmission of the bacterium *Streptococcus mutans* between mother and child, *Arch Oral Biol* 30:377-379, 1985.

Berkowitz RJ, Jordan HV, White G: The early establishment of *Streptococcus mutans* in the mouths of infants, *Arch Oral Biol* 20:171-174, 1975.

Brambilla E et al: Caries prevention during pregnancy: results of a 30 month study, *J Am Dent Assoc* 129:871-877, 1998.

Carranza FA, Newman MG: *Clinical periodontology,* ed 8, Philadelphia, 1996, WB Saunders.

Casamassimo P: *Bright Futures in practice: oral health,* Arlington, 1996, National Center for Education in Maternal and Child Health.

Casamassimo P: *Bright Futures in practice: oral health quick reference cards,* Arlington, 1997, National Center for Education in Maternal and Child Health.

Caufield PW, Cutter GR, Dasanayake AP: Initial acquisition of mutans streptococci by infants: evidence for a discrete window of infectivity, *J Dent Res* 72:37-45, 1993.

Children's Health at Doernbecher: Natal teeth. University of Oregon Health Sciences Center website. Available at *www.ohsu.edu* (accessed Feb 3, 2003).

Centers for Disease Control and Prevention, National Institute of Dental and Craniofacial Research, National Institutes of Health: Oral health US, 2002. Available at *www.drc.nidcr.nih.gov* (accessed Feb 6, 2003).

Centers for Disease Control and Prevention, National Institutes of Health: Youth tobacco surveillance—US 2000, *Morb Mortal Wkly Rep* 50(SS-4):1-84, 2001.

Consultant: 20th century fluoridation takes a bite out of tooth decay, *Consultation Primary Care,* March 2001, p 472.

Crall JJ: *Pediatric oral health interfaces: financing and delivery system issues.* Commissioned by the American Academy of Pediatric Dentistry for its Filling the Gaps Interfaces Project, supported by the HRSA/Maternal and Child Health Bureau. The Interfaces Project, 2002.

Davey AL, Rogers AH: Multiple types of the bacterium *Streptococcus mutans* in the human mouth and their intra-family transmission, *Arch Oral Biol* 29:453-460, 1984.

Dock M, Creedon R: The teeth and oral cavity: oral pathology in children. In Rudolph A, Rudolph C, editors: *Rudolph's pediatrics*, ed 21, New York, 2002, McGraw-Hill.

Grainger RM: *Orthodontic treatment priority index*, PHS pub no 1000, series 2, no 25, Washington, DC, 1967, National Center for Health Statistics.

Ismail AI, Sohn W: *Oral health knowledge and practices of family physicians and pediatricians in the U.S.* Paper presented at the IADR/AADR/CADR 80th General Session, San Diego, March 6-9, 2002.

Isokangas P et al: Occurrence of dental decay in children after maternal consumption of xylitol chewing gum, a follow-up from 0 to 5 years of age, *J Dent Res* 79(11):1885-1889, 2000.

Kaste LM et al: Coronal caries in the primary and permanent dentition of children and adolescents 1-17 years of age: United States, 1988-1989, *J Dent Res* 75(spec iss):631-636, 1996.

Keyes PH: The infectious and transmissible nature of experimental dental caries, *Arch Oral Biol* 1:304-320, 1960.

Kohler B, Andreen I, Jonsson B: The effects of caries-preventive measures in mothers on dental caries and the presence of the bacteria *Streptococcus mutans* and *Lactobacillus* on their children, *Arch Oral Biol* 11:879-883, 1984.

Li Y, Caufield PW: The fidelity of initial acquisition of mutans streptococcus by infants from their mothers, *J Dent Res* 74:681-685, 1995.

Loesche WJ: Clinical and microbiological aspects of chemotherapeutic agents used according to the specific plaque hypothesis, *J Dent Res* 58:2404-2412, 1979.

Logan WHG, Kronfeld R: The chronology of human dentition, *J Am Dent Assoc* 20:379-427, 1933.

Mueller W: Oral medicine and dentistry. In May W, editor: *Current pediatric diagnosis and treatment*, ed 16, New York, 2003, McGraw-Hill.

Neville BW et al: *Oral and maxillofacial pathology*, Philadelphia, 1995, WB Saunders.

Ngan P, Fields HW: Open bite: a review of etiology and management, *Pediatr Dent* 19:91-98, 1997.

Nguyen Q et al: A systematic review of the overjet size and traumatic dental injuries, *Eur J Orthod* 21(5):503-515, 1999.

Nowak AJ, Warren JJ: Infants' oral health and oral habits, *Pediatr Clin North Am* 47:1043-1066, 2000.

Offenbacher S et al: Maternal periodontitis and prematurity. Part I. Obstetric outcome of prematurity and growth restriction, *Ann Periodontol* 6(1):164-174, 2001.

Oral Health Program, Rhode Island Department of Health: *Position paper: sports related oro-facial injuries*, 2001. Available at *www.health.ri.gov/disease/primarycare/oralhealth* (accessed Mar 18, 2003).

Pereira A: Natal teeth: a review of the literature and report of an unusual case, *Braz Dent J* 9(1):53-56, 1998.

Pierce K, Rozier R, Vann W Jr: Accuracy of pediatric primary care providers' screening and referral for early childhood caries, *Pediatrics* 109(5):E82, 2002.

Sayany Z: Dental caries and periodontal disease. In Burg F et al, editors: *Gellis and Kagan's current pediatric therapy*, ed 17, Philadelphia, 2002a, WB Saunders.

Sayany Z: Pediatric dental emergencies. In Burg F et al, editors: *Gellis and Kagan's current pediatric therapy*, ed 17, Philadelphia, 2002b, WB Saunders.

Shay K: Root caries in the elderly, an update for the next century, *J Indiana Dent Assoc* 96(4):37-43, 1996.

Stiles HM et al: Occurrence of *Streptococcus mutans* and *Streptococcus sanguis* in the oral cavity and feces of young children. In Stiles M, Loesche W, O'Brien T, editors: *Microbial aspects of dental caries*, Washington, DC, 1976, Information Retrieval.

Tinanoff N, O'Sullivan DM: Early childhood caries: overview and recent findings, *Pediatr Dent* 19:12-16, 1997.

US Department of Health and Human Services, Public Health Service: *Oral health in America: a report of the Surgeon General*, July 2000a. Available at *www.nidcr.nih.gov/sgr/oralhealth* (accessed Mar 3, 2003).

US Department of Health and Human Services: *Healthy people 2010*, Washington, DC, 2000b. Available at *www.healthypeople.gov* (accessed Mar 3, 2003).

US Preventive Services Task Force: *Guide to clinical preventive services*, ed 2, Baltimore, 1996, Williams & Wilkins.

US Public Health Service: *Put prevention into practice: the clinician's handbook of preventive services*, ed 2, Germantown, MD, 1997, International Medical Publishing.

Vargas C, Crall J, Schneider D: Sociodemographic distribution of pediatric dental caries. NHANES III, 1988-1994, *J Am Dent Assoc* 129:1229-1239, 1998.

35 Genitourinary Disorders

Nan Gaylord, Nancy Barber Starr

The genitourinary system is responsible for maintaining an optimal environment for metabolism, including regulation of water and electrolytes (sodium, potassium, chloride, calcium, phosphate, and magnesium), excretion of waste products (urea, creatinine, poisons, and drugs), acid-base regulation, and hormonal secretion (vitamin D, renin, erythropoietin, and prostaglandins). The male system has both reproductive and excretory functions. Genitourinary problems in children and adolescents range from commonly occurring, easily treated diseases to significant congenital or acquired conditions. Pediatric primary care providers play a significant role in working with children, adolescents, and families to identify problems, manage disorders, maintain optimal function, and provide education and support related to genitourinary function. Referral to and collaboration with pediatric urologists and nephrologists are also important components of patient management. However, first-line assessment and management, as well as provision of continuity of care, are important responsibilities of the nurse practitioner (NP).

Discussion of related functional health problems—enuresis and dysfunctional voiding—is included in Chapter 14.

STANDARDS OF CARE

The *Guide to Clinical Preventive Services* (U.S. Preventive Health Services Task Force, 2003) does not recommend any urine screening for asymptomatic bacteriuria in any child of any age. *Put Prevention into Practice: The Clinician's Handbook of Preventive Services* (U.S. Public Health Services, 2003) concurs with this recommendation. The American Academy of Pediatrics, Committee on Practice and Ambulatory Care (2000), recommends that a urinalysis (UA) be performed between ages 9 and 12 months and again at 5 years of age. Also, dipstick leukocyte esterase testing is recommended yearly by all of the aforementioned authorities and *Bright Futures* (2002) to screen for sexually transmitted diseases (STDs) in sexually active adolescents.

Blood pressure (BP) screening is recommended by the American Academy of Pediatrics, Committee on Practice and Ambulatory Care (2000), and *Bright Futures* (2002) at every recommended preventive health care visit beginning at 3 years of age. The other authorities previously listed suggest BP screening for children periodically, but no specific times are suggested. Although hypertension is frequently renal in origin in children, the management and treatment of the disorder are discussed in Chapter 31.

ANATOMY AND PHYSIOLOGY

The renal system is composed of two kidneys, two ureters, a bladder, and a urethra. The kidneys are positioned posteriorly on the abdominal wall. The main features of the kidney are the cortex, the medulla, and the collecting system. The renal medulla and nephrons are present at birth, but the peripheral tubules are small and immature. By adolescence, the kidneys are of adult size and weight. The ureters are muscular tubes that convey urine from the kidneys to the bladder by peristaltic contractions. The bladder is a muscular reservoir to collect the urine. It lies close to the anterior abdominal wall in early childhood. With growth, it descends into the pelvis and changes shape from cylindrical to pyramidal. As the bladder nears its capacity, nerve signals are transmitted to the brain to indicate that urination is required. When urination occurs, the sphincter between the bladder and urethra opens and contractions of the bladder create pressure that forces the urine out the urinary meatus. The male urethra is significantly longer than the female's as it leaves the bladder in the lower pelvis, passes through the prostate with openings for the release of bulbourethral gland fluids and semen with sexual activity, and extends the full length of the penile shaft. The urethral meatus is located on the tip of the glans in the male. In the female the urethra descends from the bladder and exits the body inside the labia minora, midline, just posterior to the clitoris.

Physiologically, the kidneys serve to filter, clear, reabsorb, and secrete substances essential to the body's metabolism. The urinary system begins forming and excreting urine at 3 months of gestational age. Glomerular filtration and renal blood flow begin to increase at birth and become stable by 1 to 2 years of age. In infants, total extracellular fluid volume is significantly greater than that of adults, and fluid composition tends to have a lower bicarbonate concentration. Normal urine excretion is 1.5 to 3 ml/kg per hour. Because the kidneys are still maturing throughout infancy and early childhood, urine is also more dilute than in adulthood. Concentrating capacity reaches adult values at 6 to 12 months.

PATHOPHYSIOLOGY AND DEFENSE MECHANISMS

Pathophysiology

Problems in the urinary system can occur at any point in the system from the kidneys to the urethral meatus. If the kidneys and ureters are involved, the disease is considered to be in the upper tract; if the problem is in the bladder, urethra, or meatus, it is considered a disease of the lower urinary tract. These differentiations can be difficult because frequently disease in one part of the system affects the entire system. Additionally, disease can be relatively silent in clinical presentation and physical appearance or noticeably problematic at any age. The main mechanisms can be classified as follows:

- Infection
- Inflammatory response
- Congenital malformation or condition
- Abnormalities acquired from injury, infection, or malfunction within the system

Defense Mechanisms

The urinary tract is normally a sterile system. The mucosal lining of the bladder serves as the first line of defense and provides inhibition of bacterial growth and adherence. The acid pH of the urine also protects the urinary system by inhibiting bacterial growth. Finally, actual flow of urine out of the bladder provides mechanical defense by its flushing action. If these defenses are compromised, the body initiates an inflammatory response.

ASSESSMENT OF THE GENITOURINARY SYSTEM

History

The following information should be obtained:

- History of the present illness
  - Onset and pattern of symptoms
  - Fever, abdominal pain, or both
  - Preceding injury or illness, especially streptococcal infection
  - Vomiting
  - Voiding pattern—stream force and direction, any dribbling or discharge
  - Color, odor, frequency, and volume of urine, dysuria, urgency; enuresis or incontinence
  - Diarrhea
  - Sexual activity or abuse
- Family history
  - Any familial history of renal disease, deafness, high BP, structural abnormalities, or syndromes involving the genitourinary system
- Past history of urinary tract infection (UTI), hematuria, proteinuria, or any other related finding

Physical Examination

Pertinent findings can include the following:

- Growth parameters—failure to thrive (FTT) can be associated with UTI in infants; increased weight can be associated with nephrotic syndrome
- BP—often elevated with nephritis and nephrotic syndrome
- Edema, pallor, dehydration
- Ear position and formation—if low set or abnormal, may have concurrent renal involvement
- Abdominal masses, ascites, flank or suprapubic tenderness
- Costovertebral tenderness
- External genitalia abnormalities

Diagnostic Studies

Diagnostic studies are ordered as indicated. The proper collection, transport, and storage of urine are essential to obtain accurate results. Most tests on urine, unless otherwise indicated, are best done on a first morning void. A second morning void, collected before the ingestion of large amounts of fluid, is recommended for microscopic examination. This practice collects fresh urine and increases the likelihood of seeing cellular casts, which can dissolve within 10 to 30 minutes. Urine should be evaluated within 30 minutes and, if stored, kept below 4° C but not overnight unless in a special preservative (e.g., boric acid). The efficacy and cost efficiency of routine UA is much debated.

The following should be noted on UA.

- Physical characteristics. Color, clarity, odor, specific gravity, and osmolality are noted.
- Chemical characteristics. Urine dipsticks are available and widely used to determine pH, specific gravity, glucose, ketones, protein, bile pigments, hemoglobin, nitrites, and leukocyte esterase. For correct results, strips must remain in their original containers and not be exposed to moisture, light, cold, or heat until used. Urine must be fresh, warmed if refrigerated, and read at correct time intervals for each test strip (Table 35-1).
  - Urine pH can vary from 4.6 to 8 and is diet dependent. Specific gravity is a measure of hydration and renal concentration ability and varies from 1.003 to 1.030. A random first-voided urine specimen specific gravity of 1.023 or more indicates intact renal concentrating ability. Urine with a specific gravity greater than 1.020 is considered concentrated.
  - A dipstick positive for blood indicates the presence of hemoglobin. Intact erythrocytes cause spotty changes on the dipstick, whereas free hemoglobin or myoglobin causes uniform changes of color.
  - The nitrite test is an indirect measure of bacteria in the urine. Common urinary pathogens contain enzymes that reduce nitrate in urine to nitrite. However, the urine should have been in the bladder at least 4 hours to show accurate results. Urine culture should be done on any urine sample positive for nitrites for confirmation of infection.

TABLE 35-1 ***Chemical Characteristics of Urine***

Constituent	Positives Indicate	False Positives Caused By	False Negatives Caused By
Glucose	Metabolic problem (e.g., diabetes), recent high glucose intake, galactosemia	Antibiotics, delay in reading, myoglobin, oxidizing contaminants	Ascorbic acid intake, ketones, high specific gravity
Ketones	Dehydration, starvation, strenuous exercise, stress, fever, metabolic problems (e.g., diabetes)		If urine left standing, acetone evaporates
Protein	Renal disease, orthostatic proteinuria	Exercise, fever, dehydration, alkaline or concentrated urine (specific gravity >1.020), semisynthetic penicillin, oxidizing, cleansing agents	Dilute or acidic urine
Blood (hemoglobin)	If concurrent microscopic examination is negative for RBCs: Free hemoglobin secondary to chemicals, illness, or drugs; myoglobin secondary to burns, muscle trauma, physical child abuse, myostitis, strenuous exercise If concurrent microscopic examination is positive for RBCs: Renal problems	Menses, oxidizing cleansing agents, dilute urine	Ascorbic acid
Nitrite	Bacteria causing urinary tract infection	Rare	Common; urine should be in bladder at least 4 hr
Leukocyte esterase	Pyuria (WBCs in urine); inflammation from irritation or infection of vulva, vagina, or urethra; inflammation of bladder or kidneys with or without infection	Oxidizing agents	Immunocompromised
Urobilinogen	Hemolytic disease; hepatic disease	Rare	Rare
Bilirubin	Hepatic disease; biliary obstruction	Rare	Rare

RBCs, Red blood cells; *WBCs*, white blood cells.

- Microscopic examination of urine. Urine can be spun by centrifuge and the sediment examined, or it can be examined unspun. When evaluating results, consideration must be given to which method was used, and repeated examination is recommended. Urine should be examined under the microscope for red blood cells (RBCs), white blood cells (WBCs), bacteria, casts, and crystals. Microscopic examination of a fresh specimen is essential if blood or protein is found on the dipstick or urinary tract symptoms are present (see earlier comments).
  - RBCs—The number of RBCs per high-power field (hpf) that are thought to be abnormal varies, but in general, more than 2 to 5/hpf (×40) in unspun urine or more than 2 to 10/hpf in spun urine is thought to be abnormal (Finberg & Kleinman, 2002; Liao & Churchill, 2001; Opas, 1999) (Fig. 35-1). If cells are dysmorphic, the origin of the blood is most likely the kidney.
  - WBCs—Fewer than 2 WBCs/hpf should be seen. More than 10 WBCs often indicates a symptomatic infection. If between 2 and 10 WBCs/hpf are seen, urine culture or other workup should be performed (Fig. 35-2).
  - Bacteria and leukocytes seen in an unspun sample are associated with colony counts on culture of 100,000 (Fig. 35-3).
  - Casts—RBC, hyaline, waxy, epithelial, leukocyte, or fatty casts are seen in various disease states (Fig. 35-4).
  - Crystals, if amorphous, are not unusual. Calcium oxalate, cystine, tyrosine, leucine, cholesterol, or sulfa crystals are abnormal.

Depending on the results of the UA and/or clinical symptoms, other tests may be indicated, including:

- Gram stain. A Gram stain of the urine can be helpful in identifying organisms.
- Urine culture and sensitivities. The method of collection of urine is an important factor to note when interpreting culture results. Bag collection is considered reliable only if the results are negative. Sterile catheterization or suprapubic bladder tap is recommended if a culture is indicated on children less than 24 months and those others unable to provide a midstream clean-catch urine (Al-Orifi et al, 2000).
  - Urine culture is easily done by standard culture methods or with a dipslide incubated overnight at room temperature. Urine should be cultured immediately but may be refrigerated for up to 24 hours before plating if kept in boric acid. Doubling of pathogens occurs in as little as 20 minutes at room temperature (Woodhead, 1999). Bacterial identification and sensitivities need only be performed in complicated or nonresponsive cases.
- Urethral swabs. Either urethral swabs (insertion of the specified sterile swab 1 to 2 cm into the urethral opening with a slow gentle twisting action on removal) or vaginal swabs are accurate methods of culture acquisition for diagnosis of *Neisseria gonorrhoeae* and *Chlamydia trachomatis* and are the only diagnostic methods available in some areas of practice. The culture media are specific for each of those organisms. This method of specimen collection for culture, however, is slowly being replaced with a urine nucleic acid amplification test for detection of these

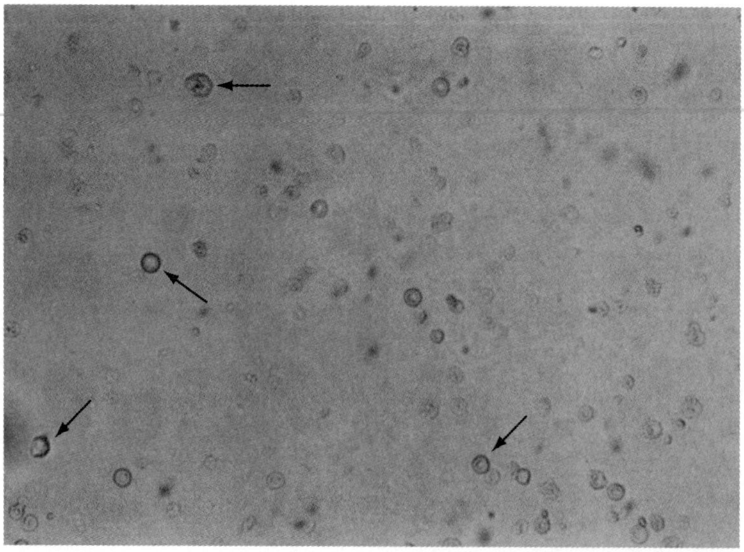

FIGURE 35-1 Red blood cells (RBCs) may originate from any part of the renal system. The presence of large numbers of RBCs suggests pathology. (From Graff SL: *A handbook of routine urinalysis*, Philadelphia, 1983, JB Lippincott.)

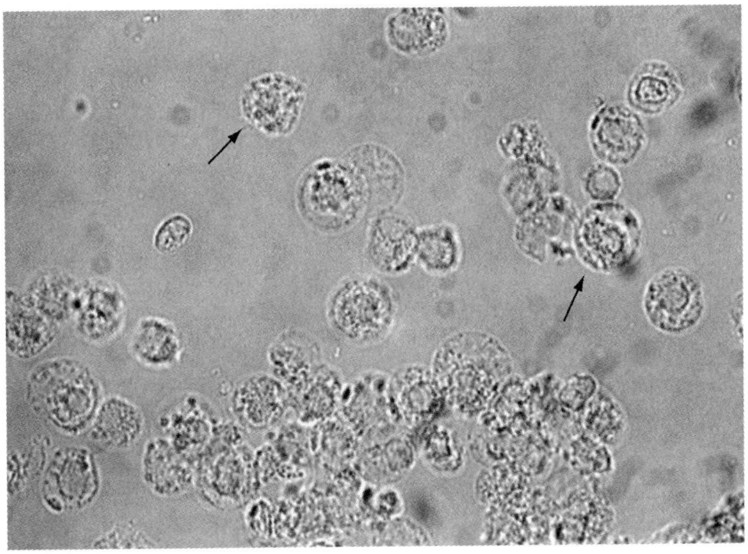

FIGURE 35-2 White blood cells (WBCs) in the urine (pyuria) may originate from any part of the renal system. The presence of more than 5 WBCs per high-power field (hpf) suggests pathology. (From Graff SL: *A handbook of routine urinalysis*, Philadelphia, 1983, JB Lippincott.)

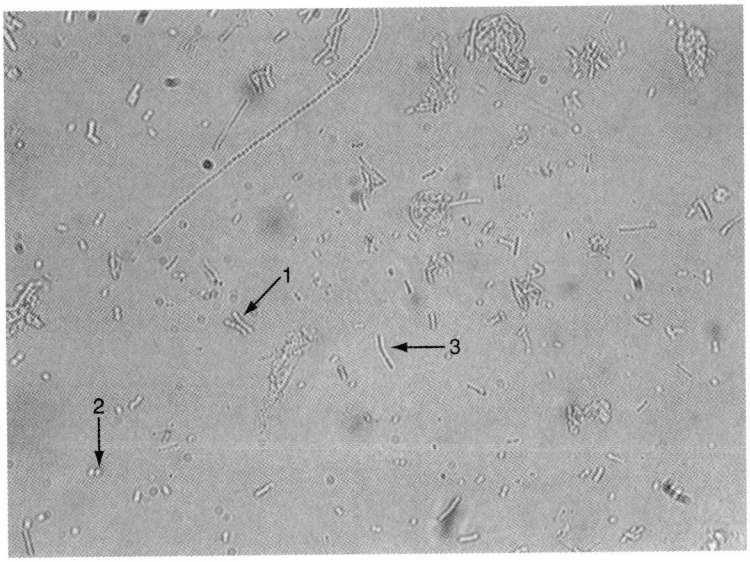

FIGURE 35-3 Bacteria (rods *[1]*, cocci *[2]*, and chains *[3]*) (500×). (From Graff SL: *A handbook of routine urinalysis*, Philadelphia, 1983, JB Lippincott.)

organisms (Sugunendran et al, 2001). If the urine test for these organisms is available, the specimen should only be between 10 and 20 ml of the first-catch urine with no cleansing of the perineum or penis. The *Trichomonas* nucleic acid amplification test is in the development process (Blake & Woods, 2001).

- A 24-hour urine collection. Collecting a 24-hour sample of urine is done to determine calcium excretion, the calcium-creatinine ratio, and quantification of protein.
- Blood work.
  - Serum or blood urea nitrogen (BUN) estimates the urea concentration in serum or blood and is a measure of toxic metabolites that can cause uremic syndrome.
  - Serum creatinine in combination with creatinine clearance is used to estimate the glomerular filtration rate (GFR) or kidney function.
  - Serum electrolytes and acid-base status can detect renal tubular abnormalities.

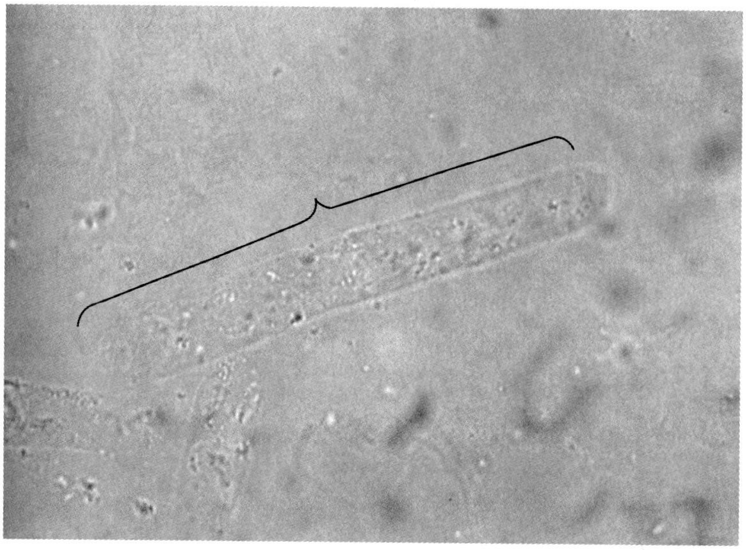

FIGURE 35-4 Hyaline casts. Viewed with an 80A filter (400×). (From Graff SL: *A handbook of routine urinalysis*, Philadelphia, 1983, JB Lippincott.)

- Ultrasonography. Ultrasonography of the renal system provides noninvasive structural information and is useful as a first-line evaluation of the renal system.
- Voiding cystourethrogram (VCUG). A VCUG is the most accurate test to evaluate reflux of urine from the bladder back into the ureters and kidneys.
- Intravenous pyelogram (IVP). IVPs are readily available and provide structural and functional information about the renal system.
- Nuclear imaging scans. These scans provide less structural and functional detail than an IVP but involve less radiation exposure. Nuclear scans are especially helpful in the early identification of pyelonephritis and parenchymal scarring and in monitoring reflux.

MANAGEMENT STRATEGIES

Education and Counseling

Education and counseling are essential components in the management of genitourinary tract disorders. Parents and children must be informed about the pathology, etiology, treatment, and prognosis with and without treatment. A plan of care that the family, as well as the care provider, is comfortable with must be decided on and initiated. Urinary problems can occur as early as the newborn period or anytime throughout childhood or adolescence. They vary in severity and chronicity. The NP must modify appropriate strategies for each individual situation.

Medication, Diet, and Activity

Depending on the diagnosis, medications can include antibiotics and steroids (see discussion of specifics later). Diet and activity may need to be modified in some chronic renal conditions. These modifications are usually carried out in consultation with appropriate specialists.

Referral

Referral to a pediatric urologist, nephrologist, or surgeon may be required. When a referral is made, the primary care provider retains the essential role of serving as case manager for the child and providing continuity of care over time. The primary care provider is often the one whom the family best knows and is most comfortable with in discussing concerns, potential plans, and longer-term management.

UPPER GENITOURINARY TRACT DISORDERS

Hematuria

Description

Hematuria refers to blood in the urine that may be persistent, recurrent, or transient. It is detected by dipstick, by microscopic examination, or with the naked eye (macroscopic) and can arise from any point in the urinary system. Hematuria is a symptom of disease or injury to the urinary system, although a few RBCs can be normal in a pediatric patient. The number of RBCs/hpf considered to be abnormal varies and ranges from any to more than 5/hpf in unspun urine to more than 5 to 10/hpf in spun urine (Finberg & Kleinman, 2002; Friedman, 2002; Patel, 2001; Ruley, 2001a). For management purposes, *hematuria* in this text is defined as more than 2/hpf in unspun or 5/hpf in spun urine.

Etiology and Incidence

Contributors to hematuria can be discovered from outside of the urinary meatus and throughout the urinary system to the kidneys. The term *gross hematuria* is related to the concentration of RBCs rather than to the location or significance of the disorder. The causes of macroscopic hematuria are as follows: UTI, 49%; trauma/irritation, 25%; glomerulonephritis (GN), 9%; coagulopathy/hemoglobinopathy, 3%; stones, 2%; and unknown, less than 9%. Hydronephrosis, tumor, cystitis cystica, or epididymitis are characterized by macrohematuria less than 1% of the time (Opas, 1999). Brownish, tea-colored urine with casts or protein is usually glomerular in origin; clots and red to pink urine with isomorphic RBCs but no protein usually originate from the lower tract. The incidence of hematuria is 0.5% to 2% when confirmed with repeat UA (Bender & Swinford, 2002; Finberg & Kleinman, 2002; Langman, 1999).

Clinical Findings

History. The following information is obtained:

- Previous medical history of cystic kidney disease, sickle cell, lupus, malignancy
- Family or previous history of hematuria, nephrolithiasis, cystic kidney, hemoglobinopathy, sickle cell disease or trait, systemic lupus erythematosus (SLE), hypertension, congestive heart disease, malignancy, deafness, renal failure
- Preceding illness—viral or streptococcal pharyngitis or impetigo
- Onset, duration, pattern, and timing of episodes
- Color of urine
- Dysuria, urgency, or frequency
- Presence of pain—back, abdominal, or flank, with voiding
- Straining or squatting with urination (tumor)
- Strenuous exercise or trauma (including bladder catheterization)
- Enuresis
- Trauma, foreign body, or sexual activity or abuse
- Current menstruation or medication
- Edema, rash, pallor, or arthralgias
- Drug ingestion, especially nonsteroidal antiinflammatory drugs (NSAIDs), aspirin, or antibiotics
- Symptoms related to chronic renal disease (Box 35-1)

BOX 35-1 *Seven "Red Flags" for Chronic Renal Failure*

1. Failure to thrive (poor growth, fatigue, anorexia, nausea, gastroesophageal reflux, vomiting)
2. Chronic anemia (normochromic, normocytic, nonresponsive to medication)
3. Complicated enuresis (daytime frequency, urgency, incontinence, chronic constipation, encopresis, infrequent voiding, straining to void, recurrent urinary tract infection)
4. Prolonged, unexplained vomiting or nausea (especially in the morning), anorexia, weight loss without diarrhea
5. Hypotension
6. Unusual bone disease (rickets, valgus deformity, fracture with minor trauma)
7. Poor school performance (headache, fatigue, inattention, withdrawal from family activity)

Adapted from Vogt BA: Identifying renal disease: simple steps can make a difference, *Contemp Pediatr* 14(3):115-117, 1997.

Physical Examination. Findings include

- FTT or falling growth curves (chronic renal insufficiency or long-standing acidosis)
- Malformed ears (congenital renal disease)
- Oliguria/anuria, edema, hypertension, and proteinuria, which are suggestive of glomerular disease
- Flank pain, which is suggestive of a lower tract disorder
- Abdominal or flank mass, which suggests an obstruction such as Wilms' tumor, cystic disease, or posterior valves
- External genitalia—excoriation, bleeding, foreign body, abuse

Laboratory Studies. The following studies are essential:

- Urinalysis (dipstick):
  - Color—a tea or smoky color indicates a nephrologic disorder; red indicates a urologic disorder.
  - If greater than 1+ hematuria by dipstick (which equals 3 RBCs/hpf or 0.02 mg/dl hemoglobin) for blood, microscopic examination for RBCs is needed to differentiate hemoglobin or myoglobin from RBCs.
  - If protein is present, refer to the section on proteinuria and nephritis for further workup. Note: The most significant differentiating factor is the presence of proteinuria. If present, rapid evaluation and early referral to a nephrologist are essential.
- Microscopic examination for RBCs, including size and shape, casts, crystals, and WBCs:
  - A few RBCs/hpf can be normal in a pediatric patient (see description of hematuria).

- Distorted, misshapen RBCs of different size suggest glomerular disease.
- A negative microscopic examination occurs in dilute urine because RBCs undergo lysis as a result of the hypotonicity of urine.

- Urine culture (approximately 33% are positive).
- For persistent hematuria:
  - UA on first-degree relatives.
  - Consider a complete blood count (CBC) with platelets, electrolytes, BUN, creatinine, sickle cell screen, tuberculin PPD (purified protein derivative), complement components C3 and C4, antinuclear antibody (ANA), antistreptolysin O titers, immunoglobulins, hepatitis serologies, and human immunodeficiency virus (HIV) (Sparrow, 2002).
  - Renal ultrasonography is performed if any concerns remain along with other indicated radiologic studies.
- If results show isolated, transient hematuria, monitor every year with UA, growth performance, and BP.

Differential Diagnosis

Five patterns of hematuria have been identified and may be helpful when considering the differential diagnosis of hematuria (Boineau & Lewy, 1989):

Type 1—microscopic and persistent
Type 2—microscopic and intermittent
Type 3—persistent macroscopic
Type 4—intermittent or recurrent macroscopic
Type 5—intermittent or recurrent macroscopic with persistent microscopic

Types 1 and 2 account for most cases of hematuria in pediatrics. Type 3 is common in urologic and nephrologic disorders such as UTI, GN, hemoglobinopathies, renal stones, and trauma. Types 4 and 5 occur with immunoglobulin A (IgA) nephropathy, hypercalciuria, and benign recurrent hematuria.

Other differential diagnoses to consider include the following:

- *Pseudohematuria* occurs when a false-positive dipstick reading is noted but no RBCs are found on the microscopic examination. The two most common causes are myoglobinuria and hemoglobinuria (see Table 35-1).
- *Extrarenal hematuria* is common with systemic bleeding disorders and is evidenced by macroscopic and microscopic hematuria.
- The presence of RBC casts, proteinuria, or both is a manifestation of *glomerular hematuria,* such as acute or chronic GN.

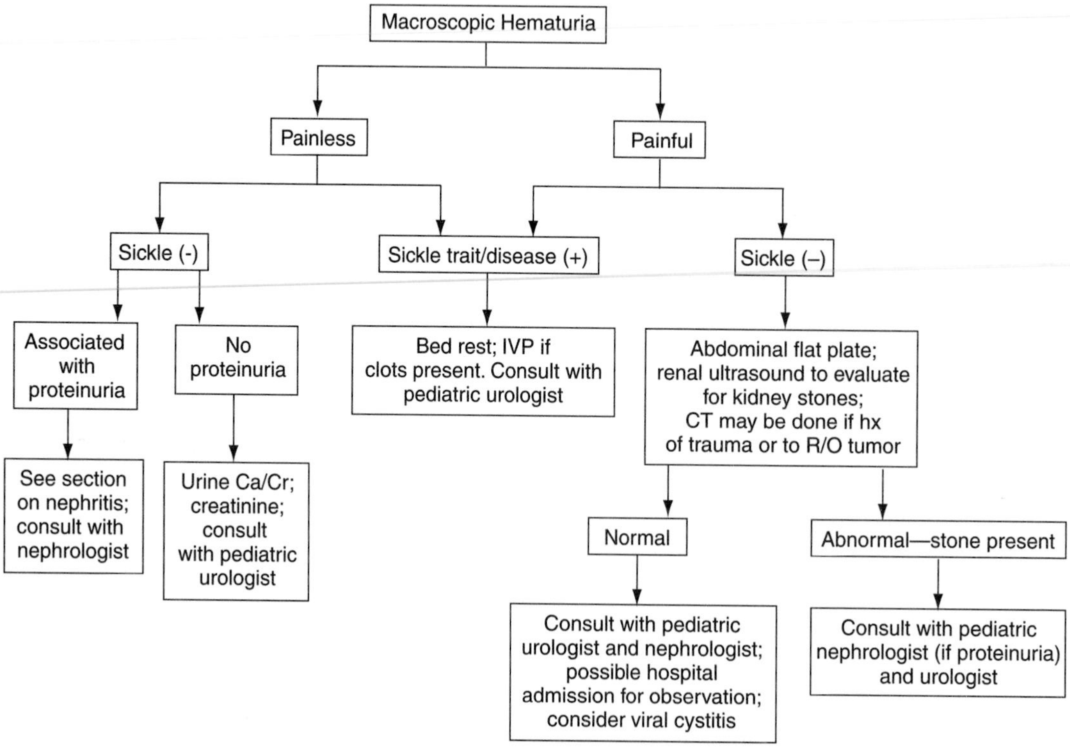

FIGURE 35-5 Management of macroscopic hematuria. *Ca/Cr,* Calcium/creatinine ratio; *CT,* computed tomography; *hx,* history; *IVP,* intravenous pyelogram; *R/O,* rule out. (Adapted from Dershewitz RA, editor: *Ambulatory pediatric care,* ed 3, Philadelphia, 1999, JB Lippincott-Raven.)

- *Idiopathic hypercalciuria* is an inherited tubulointerstitial disorder with excessive urinary calcium excretion in the presence of macroscopic and microscopic hematuria. It represents the most frequently seen isolated cases of hematuria in children and occurs more commonly in the southeastern United States and southern Canada. It occurs in 5% of healthy white children and accounts for 30% of cases of hematuria (Gallo, Schmeissing, & Langman, 1999). The diagnosis is made by laboratory examination of urine. The spot calcium-creatinine ratio done on the first morning specimen is elevated (greater than 0.21 mg/dl). Elevated 24-hour calcium excretion (greater than 3.5 mg/kg per 24 hours) confirms the diagnosis. Idiopathic hypercalciuria and Berger disease (see the section on nephritis) are responsible for 50% or more of cases of isolated hematuria in children.

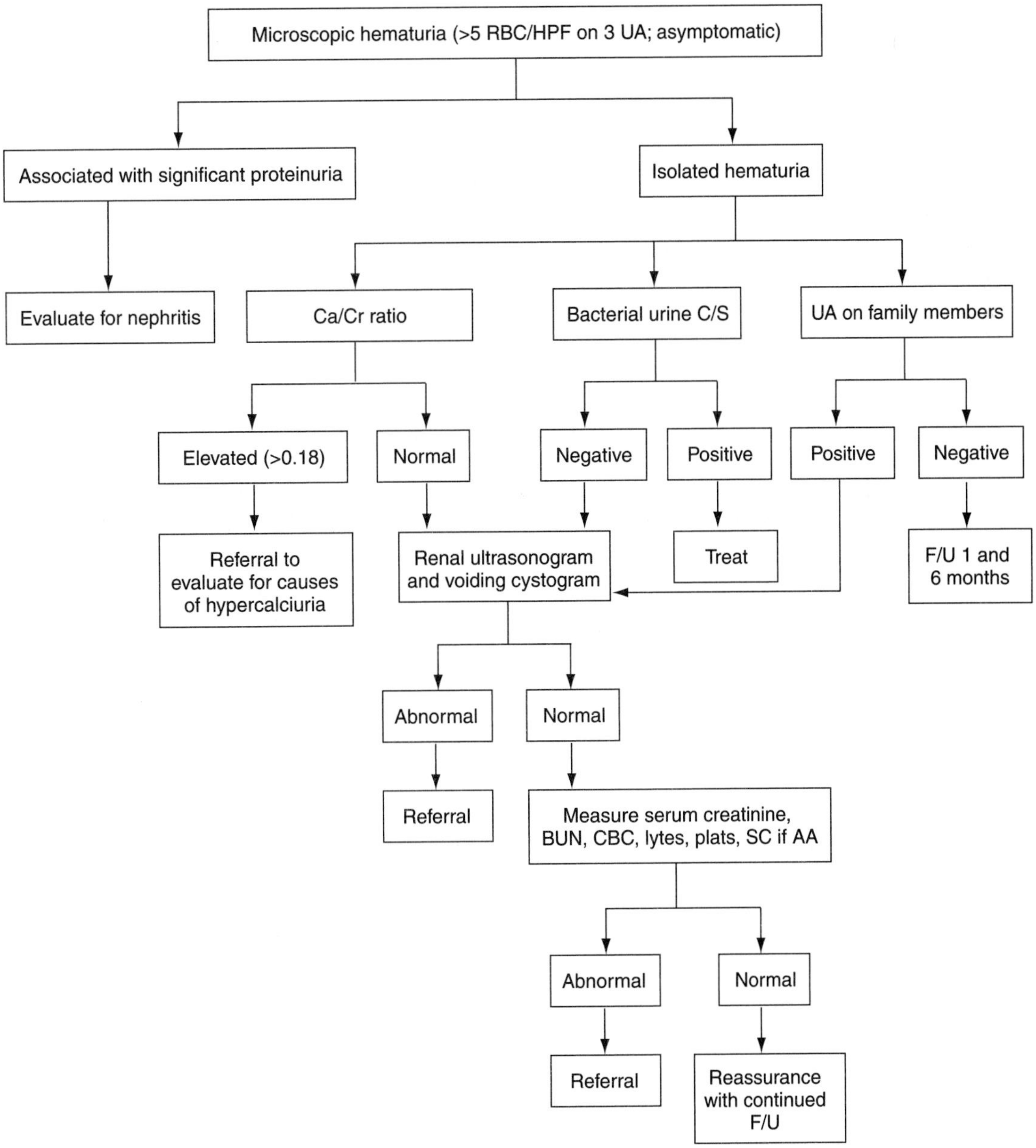

FIGURE 35-6 Management of asymptomatic microscopic hematuria. *AA*, African American; *BUN*, blood urea nitrogen; *CBC*, complete blood count; *Ca/Cr*, calcium/creatinine ratio; *C/S*, culture/sensitivity; *F/U*, follow-up; *lytes*, electrolytes; *plats*, platelets; *RBC/HPF*, red blood cells per high-power field; *SC*, sickle cell; *UA*, urinalysis. (Adapted from Dershewitz RA, editor: *Ambulatory pediatric care*, ed 3, Philadelphia, 1999, JB Lippincott-Raven.)

- Although rare, *renal stones (nephrolithiasis)* or *calcification (nephrocalcinosis)* can occur. If suspected, a renal ultrasonogram can be included as part of the workup.
- *Exercise-induced hematuria* occurs when hematuria is present after vigorous exercise, but not at other times.
- Hematuria caused by *viral* or *bacterial illnesses* is not uncommon, with adenovirus known to cause hemorrhagic cystitis (Sparrow, 2002). Though rare in children, renal tuberculosis may need to be considered in the work-up.
- Hematuria caused by external irritation of the urinary meatus will resolve with healing and removal of the offending irritant (e.g., soaps, bubble bath, lotions) or avoidance of the offending behavior (e.g., scratching, masturbation, sexual activity).

Management

A progressive approach to evaluating hematuria should be undertaken with the goal of not overlooking serious, treatable progressive conditions while avoiding unnecessary studies.

1. Macroscopic hematuria without proteinuria or casts (Fig. 35-5).
   - Urine culture is done initially to rule out UTI.
   - Ultrasonography may be done to evaluate for renal stones, an obstructive lesion, or tumor; IVP or VCUG is performed as indicated.
   - Type 4 or 5 hematuria may need an immunologic workup—antistreptolysin O (ASO), C3, ANA, anti-DNA, BUN, creatinine.
   - Consultation or referral to a nephrologist or urologist may be necessary, depending on the findings.
2. Microscopic hematuria. Initially, three first morning urine samples should be examined within 7 to 14 days to confirm the presence of hematuria (Fig. 35-6).
   - If exercise-induced hematuria is suspected, recheck the urine after refraining from exercise for 72 hours.
   - If repeated urine specimens are negative, recheck the urine in 1 month and again in 6 months.
   - If protein or casts are found in the urine (a red flag), suspect glomerular hematuria and see the section on nephritis.
   - If urine culture is positive, see the section on UTI.
   - If the calcium-creatinine ratio is greater than 0.18 to 0.21, suspect idiopathic hypercalciuria.
     - Increase fluid to dilute the calcium concentration.
     - Refer to a nephrologist.
     - Perform ultrasonography if nephrolithiasis is suspected.
     - Monitor BP.
   - If asymptomatic microscopic hematuria is suspected:
     - Perform microscopic examination of family members' urine.
     - Consultation with or referral to a nephrologist may be warranted.
     - Monitor UA, BP, and growth every 6 to 12 months.
3. Refer to a nephrologist for persistent microhematuria, recurrent gross hematuria, proteinuria, RBC or other casts detected by UA, family history, or any signs of renal failure.

Prognosis

Microscopic hematuria is a transient benign finding in the vast majority of patients but is a finding deserving of further evaluation (Lum, 2003; Ruley, 2001a).

Proteinuria

Description

Protein in the urine is commonly detected by dipstick tests. It may be transient, recurrent, or fixed. Proteinuria can be a symptom of disease, or it can reflect a benign, self-limited condition. The quantity of protein and the timing of its presence determine its significance. Qualitative protein in urine, as tested by dipstick, is considered positive if it registers 1+ (30 mg/dl) or more in urine with a specific gravity of less than 1.015. Quantitative protein is tested by measuring a timed urine. A level of less than 4 mg/m^2 per hour is considered normal, 4 to 40 mg/m^2 per hour is abnormal, and greater than 40 mg/m^2 per hour is nephrotic.

Four groups of proteinuria exist: isolated, transient or functional, glomerular, and tubulointerstitial.

- Orthostatic proteinuria and persistent asymptomatic proteinuria, which are members of the first group, termed *isolated proteinuria*, are the most common.
  - *Orthostatic proteinuria* accounts for up to 60% (75% in adolescents) of cases of proteinuria (Finberg & Kleinman, 2002; Opas, 1999). In this condition, the child excretes abnormal amounts of protein when upright but normal amounts when lying down. Orthostatic proteinuria is demonstrated by collecting urine as described in laboratory studies section.
  - *Persistent asymptomatic proteinuria* is a common, transient phenomenon in which an otherwise healthy child, with normal clinical and laboratory workup, has an abnormally high level of protein in the urine.
- The second group of proteinuria is transient or functional proteinuria and is caused by some type of stress.
  - *Exercised-induced proteinuria* is documented by collecting a urine sample, having the patient exercise vigorously for several minutes, and then collecting another sample. The postexercise sample is usually strongly positive.

- *Fever-induced proteinuria* can accompany any febrile state and usually subsides with resolution of the fever. Other stress-related causes include cold exposure, infection, congestive heart failure, and seizures. This type of proteinuria usually resolves in 1 to 2 weeks and does not require any workup.
- The third and fourth groups, *glomerular proteinuria*, which is typified by GN, and *tubulointerstitial proteinuria*, are least common and are characterized by high levels of proteinuria. Some authorities believe that persistent proteinuria in childhood, even at low levels, should be placed in these groups with a high index of suspicion for an underlying, progressive renal disorder.

Etiology and Incidence

Proteinuria originates from problems with glomerular filtration, tubular reabsorption or secretion, or both. The child is often asymptomatic. If proteinuria is significant enough to cause hypoproteinemia, edema is present.

The incidence of proteinuria is cited at 5% to 15% in school-age children. It drops to 2% if a criterion of 1+ is used and to 0.1% if greater than 2+ is used. It persists, however, in only 0.1% when four consecutive urine specimens are tested. Its peak incidence (2%) occurs in adolescence (16 years for boys, 13 for girls) (Finberg & Kleinman, 2002; Hogg et al, 2000; Langman, 1999; Ruley, 2001b).

Clinical Findings

History

- Family history of deafness, visual problems, and renal disease
- Recent strenuous exercise or febrile illness
- Polydipsia or polyuria
- Vague symptoms such as malaise, fatigue, or pallor
- Symptoms related to chronic renal disease (see Box 35-1)

Physical Examination

- BP (hypertension), pulse, respiratory rate
- Growth and development parameters (poor weight gain or FTT with chronic disease; weight gain with nephrotic syndrome)
- Edema, especially periorbital edema, or symptoms of fluid retention
- Abdominal examination for a mass, enlarged kidney, fluid, tenderness

Laboratory Studies. The following are done as indicated:

- UA (repeated three times over 1 to 2 weeks), preferably done on a first-voided specimen:
  - A 1+ protein (30 mg) is significant if the specific gravity is less than 1.015; 2+ protein (100 mg) is significant if the specific gravity is greater than 1.015.
  - False-positive results occur in highly concentrated or alkaline (pH greater than 5.5) urine. False-negative results occur in dilute or acidic urine.
  - At least 75% of asymptomatic patients with proteinuria in a single urine specimen have normal urine on repeated testing.
- A urine sample collected immediately after arising in the morning can be compared with a specimen collected after several hours of activity to rule out orthostatic etiology. The child must have voided before sleep to obtain accurate results. A typical result yields negative to trace amounts on overnight specimens but 1+ or greater on daytime specimens. If the result is equivocal, back-to-back urine samples (from arising to bedtime and bedtime to arising) can be evaluated for quantitative protein.
- Microscopic urine:
  - RBCs or WBCs (or both), casts, bacteria, oval fat bodies, or other abnormalities are present in most pathologic conditions.
- The protein-to-creatinine ratio on a random daytime urine sample is elevated. Normal values are less than 0.5 for a child 6 months to 2 years of age, less than 0.2 to 0.25 for a child older than 2 years, and less than 0.1 to 0.2 mg/dl for an adult; greater than 2 mg/dl is considered nephrotic (Hogg et al, 2000).
- A 12- or 24-hour timed urine collection for creatinine (normal, 10 to 15 mg/kg per 24 hours) and protein excretion (normal, less than 4 mg/m^2 per hour) is elevated. A back-to-back collection (e.g., bedtime to arising, arising to bedtime) is done to compare active or upright and resting levels.
- If protein in urine is greater than 4 mg/m^2 per hour, check the CBC, electrolytes, BUN, creatinine, albumin/total protein, C3, C4, cholesterol, liver function tests, and urine culture. Perform an ultrasonogram, VCUG, and radionuclide scans as indicated. Evaluate for systemic disease as indicated (e.g., ANA, ASO, Streptozyme, hepatitis B, HIV, tuberculosis).

Differential Diagnosis

Pseudoproteinuria can be caused by semisynthetic penicillins or benzalkonium chloride.

Management

The persistence, quantity, and presence of other abnormalities (e.g., hematuria) are key to evaluating proteinuria.

1. If protein by dipstick is trace or 1+ and specific gravity is greater than 1.015:

- Offer reassurance.
- Do monthly recheck of urine for 4 to 6 months.
- If protein is persistent, refer the patient to a nephrologist.

2. If protein by dipstick is greater than 1+, see Fig. 35-7. Evaluate the child for orthostatic proteinuria.
3. If morning's urine protein is 1+ or 2+, perform either:
- A quantitative 12- to 24-hour urine protein excretion test:
  - If less than 4 mg/m^2 per hour, reassure.
  - If greater than 4 mg/m^2 per hour, proceed as in Fig. 35-7.

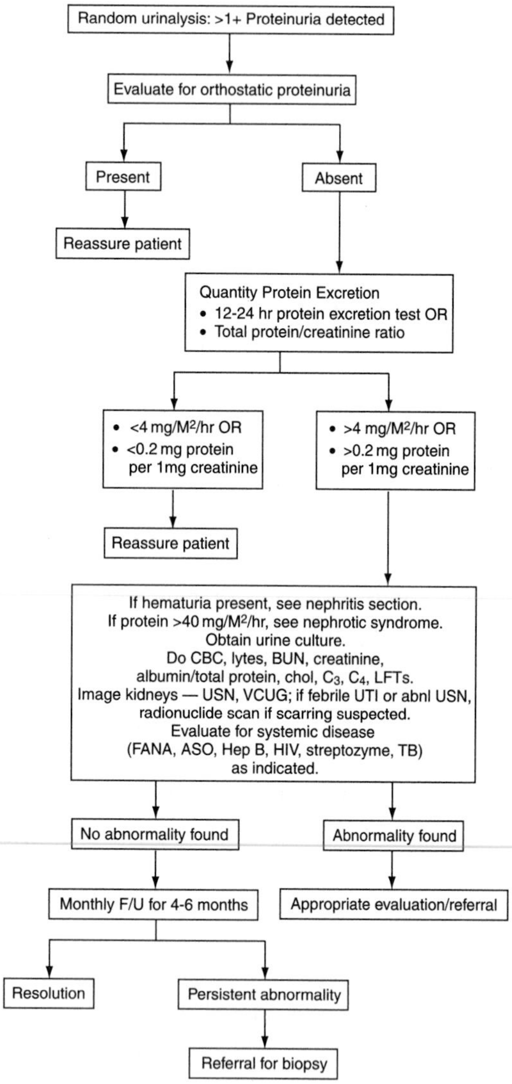

FIGURE 35-7 Evaluation of proteinuria. *abnl*, Abnormal; *alb/TP*, albumin/total protein; *ANA*, antinuclear antibody; *ASO*, antistreptolysin O; *BUN*, blood urea nitrogen; *C3*, complement 3; *C4*, complement 4; *CBC*, complete blood count; *chol*, cholesterol; *Cr*, creatinine; *FANA*, fluorescent antinuclear antibody; *F/U*, follow-up; *Hep B*, hepatitis B; *HIV*, human immunodeficiency virus; *LFTs*, liver function tests; *lytes*, electrolytes; *USN*, ultrasound; *VCUG*, voiding cystourethrogram. (Adapted from Dershewitz RA, editor: *Ambulatory pediatric care*, ed 3, Philadelphia, 1999, JB Lippincott-Raven.)

- A random urine total protein/creatinine ratio and UA with microscopic:
  - If UA is normal and there is less than 0.2 mg of protein/1 mg of creatinine, reassure as normal.
  - If protein/creatinine ratio is greater than 0.2 mg of protein/1 mg of creatinine, proceed as in Fig. 35-7.

4. If protein by dipstick is greater than 2+, evaluate for nephrotic syndrome (see later section).
5. If hematuria is present, evaluate for nephritis (see later section).
6. Follow-up is important to monitor for any change in status.
7. Refer the following to a nephrologist: persistent unexplained nonorthostatic proteinuria, any hematuria or RBC or WBC casts, polyuria or oliguria, nephrotic levels of protein, elevated BUN or creatinine, elevated BP, or a child with a family history of renal failure, GN, sensorineural hearing loss, kidney transplantation, or systemic complaints (joint pain, rashes, or arthralgias).

Prognosis

Orthostatic proteinuria with a 10-year follow-up showed resolution in 50% and the remainder with a normal GFR.

Nephrotic Syndrome

Description

Nephrotic syndrome is due to excessive excretion of protein in urine. The classic definition of nephrotic syndrome is massive proteinuria (greater than 40 mg/m^2 per hour and a protein-creatinine ratio on spot urine of greater than 1.0), hypoalbuminemia (less than 2.5 g/dl), edema, and hyperlipidemia. The latter two findings may not be present in all cases or at all times. The main mechanism of the massive protein loss is increased glomerular permeability. The loss can be selective (albumin only) or nonselective (including most serum proteins), and such selectivity is an important distinction in diagnosis. With protein loss, the liver increases its synthesis of protein and thereby causes concurrent hyperlipidemia and lipiduria.

The classification of nephrotic syndrome as described by the International Collaborative Study of Kidney Diseases in Children (Warshaw, 1994) is as follows:

- Primary nephrotic syndrome, unrelated to systemic disease, is also called minimal change nephrotic syndrome (MCNS) or idiopathic nephrotic syndrome, lipoid nephrosis, or nil disease. Minimal change disease is characterized by the child's age (1 to 7 years), normal vascular volume despite edema (normal BP and normal heart size), absence of gross hematuria or urinary casts, and absent or transient microhematuria with normal

serum creatinine, complement components, and ANA. Histopathologic examination shows glomerular lesions without inflammation and mild to no morphologic abnormality. This type occurs in 80% to 90% of cases and is usually characterized by resolution of symptoms in response to steroids.
- Secondary nephrotic syndrome occurs in association with or secondary to systemic disorders (e.g., SLE, Henoch-Schönlein purpura [HSP]), infectious processes (e.g., syphilis, hepatitis B, HIV, or malaria), drug toxicities (e.g., NSAIDs, mephenytoin), allergens, or other renal disorders (e.g., IgA or congenital nephritis). Histopathologic examination shows moderate to severe morphologic abnormality. This type occurs in 10% of cases.

Nephrotic syndrome is a chronic disease characterized by periods of remission (urinary protein excretion and serum albumin normalize) and relapses (recurrence of proteinuria and hypoalbuminemia after complete remission). Most children are steroid responders, with remission subsequent to treatment with steroids. Of the remainder, most are steroid resistant and show no response to steroids. A small number of cases are either partial responders with minimal response to steroids or are steroid dependent and require high doses of prednisone with frequent relapses.

Etiology and Incidence

Nephrotic syndrome occurs as a result of immune, systemic, nephrotoxic, allergic, infectious, malignant, vascular, or idiopathic processes. The actual mechanism of nephrotic syndrome has been extensively studied, and the understanding of its histopathology is better than the understanding of its pathogenesis. The primary mechanism is believed to be immunologic rather than renal (Finberg & Kleinman, 2002).

The incidence of nephrotic syndrome is 1.2 to 2.3 per 100,000, with a 15 times greater incidence in children than in adults. Sixty-six percent to 80% of cases are MCNS, with a peak incidence at 2 to 6 years. Eighty-five percent of patients are steroid responders. In early childhood, the male-to-female ratio is 2:1; however, by midadolescence, the rate of occurrence is equal (Varade, 2001).

Clinical Findings

History. The following may be reported:
- Edema, which is a cardinal clinical feature, especially periorbital edema, in dependent areas (tight shoes or underwear) and lax tissues (puffy eyes)
- Low urine production
- Gastrointestinal symptoms: anorexia, paleness, listlessness, diarrhea, vomiting, abdominal pain (right upper quadrant)
- Recent prodromal infection
- Respiratory difficulties secondary to ascites, effusion, pneumonia, if advanced disease

Physical Examination. Findings include
- Edema—periorbital in the morning, dependent in the evening
- Hypertension, normal BP if hypovolemic
- Chronically ill appearing
- Muscle wasting, malnourishment, growth failure if prolonged
- If the disease is progressive, hydrothorax with respiratory difficulty or ascites with labial edema

Laboratory Studies. The following are ordered as indicated:
- UA and microscopic examination, which reveal protein of 2+ or greater, hyaline and fine granular casts, microhematuria in 33%, elevated specific gravity, fat bodies, and casts in urine
- Quantitative urine protein excretion (24-hour collection or protein-creatinine ratio on a random first morning urine)
- CBC; electrolytes, BUN, creatinine (normal); calcium; serum albumin (less than 2 g/dl), total protein; liver enzymes; triglycerides, lipoproteins, cholesterol (elevated); C3 and C4 (normal); ANA
- Consideration of Venereal Disease Research Laboratories (VDRL), hepatitis B surface antigen, HIV, malaria, purified protein derivative (PPD) as indicated by history
- Kidney biopsy is recommended in the following circumstances:
  - If criteria for MCNS are not met
  - If systemic disease is present
  - In the presence of hypertension and hematuria
  - With hypocomplementemia or nonselective proteinemia
  - If the patient is older than 7 years or an adolescent
  - If the patient is nonresponsive to steroids
  - If relapses are frequent

Differential Diagnosis

Infants (newborn to 1 year) usually have congenital renal problems, children 7 years and older are likely to have focal glomerulosclerosis or mesangial proliferative GN, and teens have membranous nephropathy. The differential diagnosis includes hypoproteinemia from starvation, liver disease, and protein-losing enteropathy; none of these conditions has associated proteinuria. GN should also be considered in the differential diagnosis.

Management

Nephrotic syndrome is a complex, often chronic disorder that responds to careful management with a gratifying long-term outcome. The diagnosis is made with 95% certainty on clinical impressions. A major goal is to control edema while awaiting definitive remission. Management involves the following:

- Referral to a nephrologist; initial hospitalization if severe.
- Prednisone (2 mg/kg per day; maximum, 60 mg) to induce remission, which can occur as early as 14 days as evidenced by diuresis. Steroids are continued for at least 4 to 6 weeks. A crushed or quartered pill is economical and often easier to give than liquid. Once remission occurs, steroid therapy is tapered and weaned over several months. Relapses are treated with a short course of steroids and the patient weaned as soon as the proteinuria resolves. Consultation with a nephrologist is important because of the constantly changing strategies for managing these children.
- Activity and diet recommendations. No limitation is placed on activity. During active disease, salt may be restricted. At other times, a diet appropriate for age is recommended. A high-protein, low-salt/no-salt diet with less than 35% fat and less than 300 mg of cholesterol per day is sometimes recommended.
- Diuretics and albumin replacement are sometimes used in the acute phase. Monitoring of BP at home is sometimes recommended.
- Proteinuria testing at home is recommended to monitor the child and identify exacerbations as soon as possible. Relapses begin with persistent proteinuria of greater than 2+ every day for 3 days.
- Routine immunizations, including varicella vaccine, should be given during remissions and at least 3 months after immunosuppressive drugs, especially live vaccines. Pneumococcal and influenza vaccines are recommended for these children.
- Monitoring and prompt treatment of infection are essential. Exposure to varicella zoster requires that varicella zoster immune globulin be given within 72 hours of exposure. Sepsis workup should be done with any fever and broad-spectrum antibiotics given until the organism is identified (Lum, 2003).

Complications

Children with nephrotic syndrome are susceptible to pneumococcal, *Escherichia coli*, *Pseudomonas*, and *Haemophilus influenzae* infection because of stasis of fluid; such infection is seen as peritonitis, pneumonia, cellulitis, or septicemia. Hypertension or hypotension is a possibility. Because the child is in a hypercoagulable state, thromboembolism is possible. Protein losses and compromising edema are also potential complications.

Patient Education/Prognosis

The prognosis is good in steroid responders, with resolution by adolescence without any residual renal dysfunction (Burg et al, 2002). Families must know that relapses are the rule. An understanding of the disease process, side effects of steroids, recognition of infection, and the importance of monitoring proteinuria for relapses is crucial. If chronic steroid treatment is needed, the child and family must understand the side effects of the medication.

Nephritis or Glomerulonephritis

Description

Nephritis is a noninfectious, inflammatory response of the kidneys characterized by varied degrees of hypertension, edema, proteinuria, and hematuria that can be either microscopic or macroscopic with dysmorphic RBCs and casts. Nephritis is classified as acute, intermittent, or chronic. Primary GN occurs when the original and predominant structure impaired is the glomerulus. Secondary GN occurs when renal involvement is secondary to systemic disease (e.g., lupus, HSP, primary vasculitis, Goodpasture syndrome, or drug hypersensitivity reactions). Involvement can be in the glomerulus or the interstitium and either localized in one part of the kidney or generalized throughout. GN refers to inflammation primarily in the glomeruli; interstitial nephritis refers to inflammation in the interstitium primarily caused by drug reactions. Poststreptococcal GN (PSGN) is the classic form of GN.

Acute nephritis most commonly occurs as PSGN, which is characterized by a history of streptococcal infection within the last 2 weeks and an acute onset of edema, oliguria, hypertension, and gross hematuria. Consider an alternative diagnosis if the following findings are present:

- Nephrotic levels of protein
- Lack of evidence for a postinfection mechanism
- Rapidly deteriorating renal function
- Clinical or laboratory findings suggesting other forms of GN, for example, rash, positive ANA

Intermittent gross hematuria and proteinuria syndromes include the following:

- IgA nephropathy, or Berger disease, is the most common chronic GN in children of European-Asian descent and is uncommon in blacks; it has a 2:1 male preponderance (Blowey, 2002). It is an immunologic entity causing recurrent gross and microscopic hematuria and often proteinuria. It is present in about one third of persons biopsied for persistent microscopic hematuria (Blowey, 2002). It is often precipitated by viral infections or strenuous exercise, and each episode lasts less than 72 hours. BP is normal, no edema is present, and C3 is normal. Definitive diagnosis is made by biopsy. The prognosis is good in the absence of elevated serum creatinine or nephrotic-range proteinuria, although progression to chronic renal insufficiency can occur in 10% to 30% (Blowey, 2002). Berger disease and idiopathic hypercalciuria (see the section on hematuria) are responsible for 50% or more cases of isolated hematuria in children.

- Hereditary or familial nephritis involves many disorders, but the best known is Alport syndrome. More common and severe in males, with onset before 15 years of age in 75% of children, this condition is inherited as an X-linked dominant trait. The initial manifestation is isolated, persistent microscopic hematuria with intermittent macrohematuria and variable proteinuria occurring with an upper respiratory infection or exercise. Laboratory abnormalities are variable; biopsy verifies the diagnosis. Extrarenal abnormalities, including neurogenic deafness (hearing loss in 50% with females often spared), ocular abnormalities (30%), and macrothrombocytopenia, are often found (Fouser, 1998). Vision and hearing screening is essential with referral for any abnormalities. Severe forms of the disease can lead to end-stage renal disease, which is often heralded by hypotension.
- Familial or benign recurrent nephritis, now also called thin-basement-membrane disease, is a disorder inherited as an autosomal dominant trait with unknown etiology. Macroscopic and microscopic hematuria and mild proteinuria, often precipitated by upper respiratory tract infection, characterize episodes. Laboratory values other than the UA are normal. The diagnosis is confirmed by biopsy, which may not be needed if the disease is mild and confirmed in relatives. In the absence of notable proteinuria, deafness, ocular defects, and renal failure, and with normal biopsy findings, the prognosis is excellent.
- Chronic nephritis is most commonly known as membranoproliferative GN (MPGN) and is distinguished by four types based on biopsy. Chronic nephritis can be found after acute nephritis or when investigating nonspecific complaints such as anorexia, intermittent vomiting, and malaise. It is manifested by diminished renal function that ultimately has detrimental effects on other organ systems. Types I and II may respond to steroids, but the overall prognosis is guarded.

Pyelonephritis, discussed later in the UTI section, is inflammation of the renal parenchyma, calyces, and pelvis caused by bacteria.

Etiology and Incidence

The inflammatory response of the kidneys results from various causes such as infection, an immunologic response, a drug or toxin, and vascular or systemic disorders. PSGN is an immune response by the host to a Group A β-hemolytic streptococcal infection, whereas acute postinfectious GN (APGN) can be caused by bacterial, fungal, viral, parasitic, or rickettsial agents.

PSGN is the most common form of nephritis in childhood, occurs more often in males (2:1), peaks at 7 years of age, and is unusual in children younger than 3 years or in adults. The incidence of APGN is difficult to determine because of the large number of patients with subclinical cases, most younger than 5 to 10 years (Blowey, 2002; Varade, 2001).

Clinical Findings

History. The following may be reported:

- Streptococcal skin (more likely) or pharyngeal infection within the past 2 to 3 weeks (PSGN). Classically, a latent period of 7 to 10 days elapses between infection and the onset of symptoms; if less than 5 days or more than 14 days, consider other causes.
- Abrupt onset of gross hematuria.
- Reduced urine output.
- Lethargy, anorexia, nausea, vomiting, abdominal pain.
- Chills, fever, backache (pyelonephritis).
- Medication taken in the last few weeks.

Physical Examination. Findings to look for include the following:

- Hypertension that is transient and resolves in 1 to 2 weeks
- Edema, especially periorbital edema, of abrupt onset with weight gain
- Ear malformations
- Flank or abdominal pain or a mass (in polycystic kidney or malignancy, e.g., Wilms' tumor)
- Costovertebral angle tenderness (in pyelonephritis)
- Circulatory congestion—dyspnea, cough, pallor, pulmonary edema if severe
- Oliguria, with diuresis in 5 to 7 days
- Rashes or arthralgias (with SLE, HSP, or impetigo)
- Evidence of trauma or abuse

Laboratory Studies. The following are done as indicated:

- UA with microscopic examination—tea color, elevated specific gravity, macrohematuria and microhematuria, proteinuria not exceeding the amount of hematuria, pyuria in PSGN; granular, hyaline, WBC, or RBC casts and dysmorphic RBCs
- Serum C3/C4 (low early in disease, returning to normal in 6 to 8 weeks), total protein and albumin (elevated)
- CBC, erythrocyte sedimentation rate (ESR), ASO titer (elevated), Streptozyme test (positive), anti-DNA antibody titer
- Electrolytes, BUN, creatinine, and cholesterol
- Fluorescent antinuclear antibody (lupus), hepatitis titers, sickle cell or hemoglobin electrophoresis, tuberculin PPD, and fluorescent treponemal antibody absorption (syphilis)

Differential Diagnosis

Acute nephritis also occurs as part of systemic illnesses such as SLE, HSP, hemolytic-uremic syndrome, vasculitis, or as a reaction to drugs or irradiation.

Management

See Fig. 35-8. Consultation with a nephrologist is recommended in all cases.

- PSGN treatment is supportive because resolution occurs spontaneously 90% of the time within 6 to 24 months. The course does not seem to be affected by corticosteroids, immunosuppression, or other treatment modalities. During the peak of oliguria and hypertension in the first few days of illness, hospitalization may be required with fluid and sodium limitation and diuretic, antihypertensive, and antibiotic treatment if cultures are positive. Resolution occurs once diuresis begins. Gross hematuria persists for 1 to 2 weeks, urine can be abnormal for 6 to 12 weeks, and microscopic hematuria can persist for up to 2 years. Complement levels return to normal in 3 to 6 weeks.
- Acute nephritis—possible hospitalization with treatment as just described.
- IgA nephropathy—annual follow-up with BP, UA, and determination of renal function.
- Benign familial or hereditary nephritis—perform audiometry and review family medical history. Hereditary markers are being developed for this disease.
- Benign recurrent nephritis—monitor UA and renal function every 1 to 2 years.
- Chronic nephritis—a team approach is required to adequately provide care.

Complications

Prolonged oliguria and renal failure can occur if acute nephritis progresses. Hypertensive encephalopathy or congestive heart failure can occur secondary to PSGN. Irreversible parenchymal damage causes hypertension and renal insufficiency.

Prognosis

Patients with PSGN may have macrohematuria or microhematuria for up to 6 to 12 months, but the long-range outcome is excellent. Thin-basement-membrane disease has a good outcome. IgA nephropathy with severe histologic findings has a poor outcome, especially if the child is black.

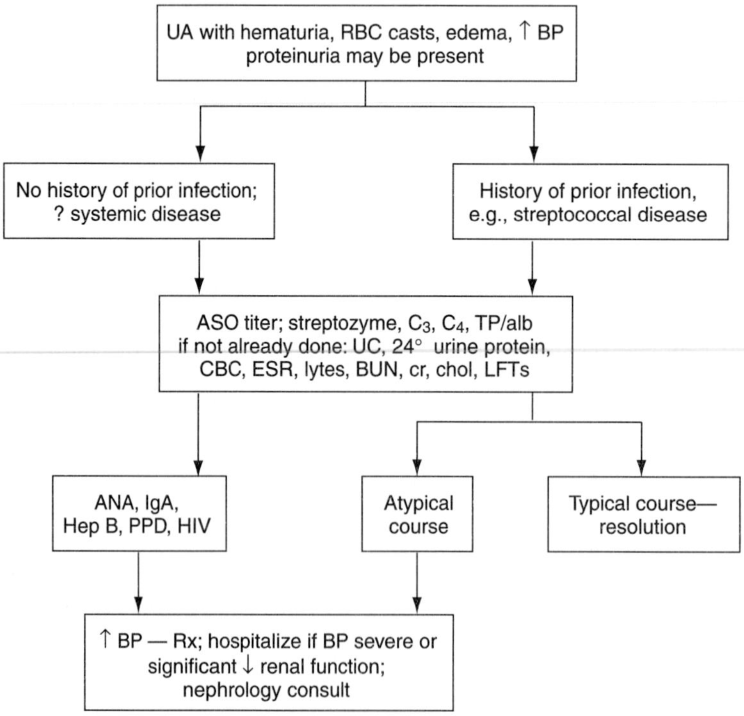

FIGURE 35-8 Evaluation of nephritis. *alb*, Albumin; *ANA*, antinuclear antibody; *ASO*, antistreptolysin O; *BP*, blood pressure; *BUN*, blood urea nitrogen; *C3*, complement 3; *C4*, complement 4; *CBC*, complete blood count; *chol*, cholesterol; *cr*, creatinine; *ESR*, erythrocyte sedimentation rate; *HepB*, hepatitis B; *HIV*, human immunodeficiency virus; *IgA*, immunoglobulin A; *LFT*, liver function test; *PPD*, purified protein derivative; *RBC*, red blood cell; *Rx*, prescribe; *TP*, total protein; *UA*, urinalysis.

Renal Tubular Acidosis

Description

Dysfunction of renal tubule transport capability results in a condition known as renal tubular acidosis (RTA). Three distinct types of RTA have been identified. Type I, classic or distal RTA (dRTA), occurs when the defect is in the distal tubule. When the defect occurs in the proximal tubules, it is known as proximal RTA (pRTA), type II, or bicarbonate-wasting RTA. Type III has been reclassified as a subtype of type I that occurs primarily in preterm infants. Type IV, also known as hyperkalemic RTA, occurs with problems in the functioning of aldosterone most commonly following relief of obstructive uropathy (Chan, Scheinman, & Roth, 2001).

The diagnosis depends on a combination of clinical features, laboratory values, and response to treatment

- RTA is suggested by a serum carbon dioxide level below 20, especially if the anion gap is normal (12 ± 4 mEq/L). Anion gap = $Na^+ - (Cl^- + HCO_3^-)$.
- dRTA (type I) is suggested by hypokalemia, hyperchloremia with a serum CO_2 less than 16, and urine pH greater than 5.5
- pRTA (type II) is suggested by hypokalemia, hyperchloremia with a serum CO_2 less than 16, and urine pH less than 5.5
- Type IV is suggested by hyperkalemia

Fanconi syndrome is an uncommon and more complex form of pRTA (type II) with associated glycosuria, phosphaturia, aminoaciduria, and a defect in vitamin D metabolism manifested as nausea, anorexia, intermittent vomiting, and possibly rickets.

Etiology and Incidence

The dysfunction in the transport capability of the renal tubules affects either the reabsorption of filtered bicarbonate, excretion of hydrogen ion, or both and results in a metabolic acidosis. RTA is often an isolated and primary problem with unknown cause, but diseases or intoxication can cause it. It is seen most typically in children evaluated for growth failure and is often revealed when illness, dehydration, or starvation stresses a child. RTA is more common in males than females, with pRTA being the most common form seen in children.

The proximal tubule, which normally absorbs 85% of bicarbonate, is able to reabsorb only 60% of bicarbonate from filtered urine in patients with pRTA. The distal tubule continues to function and reabsorbs approximately 15% of the bicarbonate, and the urine is acidified (pH less than 5.5). However, a large amount of bicarbonate is wasted. As the body adapts, a new threshold for serum bicarbonate is set, usually around 14 to 16 mEq (Dell & Avner, 2004).

A defect in the ability of the distal renal tubule to excrete hydrogen is the cause of dRTA. This defect causes complete loss of reabsorption of the final 15% of bicarbonate and an inability to acidify urine (pH greater than 5.5). Type IV RTA is characterized by a deficiency in the production or responsiveness of aldosterone and impaired ammonia production. Type IV RTA is often associated with an obstructive uropathy or other transient phenomenon in infancy (Alon, 2002; Friedman, 2002).

Clinical Findings

History. The following information is often reported:

- Failure to gain weight (especially) and height—the most common symptoms
- Polyuria and polydipsia
- Muscle weakness (due to hypokalemia)
- Irritability before eating, satiation after eating, vomiting, diarrhea, or constipation in dRTA
- Preference for liquids over solid foods, poor appetite, or anorexia, especially with type IV

Physical Examination. Findings can include:

- Arrested growth curve toward the end of the first year with consistent growth before that
- Normal physical examination and development

Laboratory Studies. The following studies are recommended:

- Serum electrolytes, including CO_2 (hypokalemia, hyperchloremic metabolic acidosis), renal function tests (BUN, creatinine), calcium, phosphorus, alkaline phosphatase, and UA (first morning void) to test for glucose and pH

If any of the laboratory findings are abnormal, consider the following:

- A 24-hour creatinine clearance to establish the normal GFR, calcium (for calcium-to-creatinine ratio; normal: less than 0.21 mg/dl), citrate, potassium oxalate (Chan, Scheinman, & Roth, 2001)
- Renal ultrasonography to determine the anatomy and rule out nephrocalcinosis (low; normal: greater than 180 mg/g of creatinine), nephrolithiasis, hydronephrosis, obstructive uropathy, and parenchymal damage

Differential Diagnosis

Primary RTA must be differentiated from secondary RTA, which can be due to many disease states or conditions, such as other causes of growth failure (FTT), hypothyroidism, and systemic acidosis.

Management

Goals of management include correcting the acidosis and maintaining normal bicarbonate (greater than 20 mEq/L), thereby restoring growth and minimizing complications.

- Oral alkalizing medications given to achieve these goals include the following:
  - Bicitra (sodium citrate and citric acid or Shohl solution), which equals 1 mEq bicarbonate per milliliter and is relatively pleasant tasting.
  - Polycitra (sodium and potassium citrate and citric acid), which equals 2 mEq bicarbonate per milliliter and is less palatable. Giving it in juice, water, or formula may ease its administration. Polycitra is especially useful if the child is hypokalemic or requires an excess quantity or if compliance is an issue.
  - $NaHCO_3$ tablets are available in 325 mg strength (4 mEq bicarbonate) and 650 mg strength (8 mEq bicarbonate).
  - Eight ounces of baking soda mixed with 2.65 L of distilled water equals 1 mEq/ml of bicarbonate.
  - Dosing is determined by the type of RTA. Distal RTA requires low doses, often between 2 and 5 mEq/kg per day. Proximal RTA requires high doses, often between 5 and 15 mEq/kg per day and sometimes as high as 20 mEq/kg per day. The dose must be titrated to the child's response as determined by weight and laboratory results (CO_2 and electrolytes). Initiate medication at 3 mEq/kg per day and check laboratory results in a few days. Titrate the dose until a serum bicarbonate level of 20 to 22 mEq/L is achieved (Friedman, 2002).
- To maintain as normal a bicarbonate level as possible, doses should be given frequently throughout the day (with meals) and as late as possible at night (at bedtime). A larger dose at bedtime has been advocated to coincide with growth hormone secretion at night in order to maximize growth (Chan, Scheinman, & Roth, 2001).
- The response to medication helps confirm the diagnosis and type of RTA. dRTA has a rapid response to treatment, and normal bicarbonate levels are maintained with little difficulty. pRTA requires higher doses to normalize bicarbonate and is less easily maintained. Type IV RTA requires mineralocorticoid treatment if aldosterone is deficient.
- Maximizing caloric intake to enhance growth can be accomplished as follows:
  - Give solid foods first at meals and snacks and avoid water and noncaloric foods.
  - Provide nutritional supplements.
- Meticulous follow-up is imperative.
  - Weight and laboratory results should be monitored biweekly to monthly until weight gain is established and CO_2 is stabilized. Weighing on the same scale and by the same person is essential.
- Pseudoephedrine should be avoided because it is minimally excreted in alkalinized urine and associated with a risk of intoxication.
- Referral to a pediatric nephrologist is necessary for any child whose laboratory values are not normalizing and who is not growing well with treatment, has unusual laboratory results, has type IV RTA, or has any complication of RTA.

Complications

It is rare to have complications with pRTA. Hypercalciuria leading to nephrocalcinosis, nephrolithiasis, renal parenchymal destruction, and occasionally renal failure can occur with dRTA. Rickets are sometimes found in type IV RTA.

Patient Education, Prevention, and Prognosis

Isolated pRTA responds quickly to treatment, with children showing catch-up growth and obtaining normal maximal height. pRTA resolves spontaneously without recurrence of symptoms, often within 1 to 2 years but at worst over the first decade of life (Constantinescu & Satlin, 2002; Dell & Avner, 2004). dRTA usually lasts a lifetime, and type IV resolves with correction of the underlying problem.

Wilms' Tumor

Description

Wilms' tumor, the most common malignancy of the genitourinary tract, is typically recognized as a firm smooth mass in the abdomen or flank. It is staged according to the National Wilms' Tumor Study as follows:

- Stage I is limited to the kidney and can be completely excised with the capsular surface intact (35%).
- Stage II extends beyond the kidney but can still be completely excised (30%).
- Stage III has postsurgical residual nonhematogenous extension confined to the abdomen (20%).
- Stage IV has hematogenous metastasis, most frequently to the lung (12%).
- Stage V is bilateral kidney involvement (3% to 5%) (Nachman & Abelson, 2002; Steinhurz, 2002).

Etiology and Incidence

This malignancy is manifested as a solitary growth in any part of either or both kidneys. Two forms are recognized: heritable (less than 1%) and nonheritable. An important feature of Wilms' tumor is the occurrence of associated congenital anomalies in 15% of children, including renal abnormalities such as cryptorchidism, hypospadias, duplication of the collecting system, ambiguous genitalia (4.4%), hemihypertrophy (2.9%), aniridia (1.1%), cardiac abnormalities, and Beckwith-Wiedemann, Drash, and Perlman syndromes. Wilms' tumor will develop in 15% to 20% of children with neurofibromatosis. It occurs with equal frequency in both sexes and has a 3:1 black-to-white incidence. Fifty-five percent occur on the left side. The incidence of Wilms' tumor is 1 per 10,000/year in children younger than 15 years, or about 400 to 500 cases annually, with 80% being diagnosed before 5 years of age. The peak incidence and median age at diagnosis fall at 3 years (Ferguson, 2002; Nachman & Abelson, 2002; Steinhurz, 2002).

Clinical Findings

History

- The most frequent finding is increasing abdominal size or an actual palpable mass.
- Pain is reported if the mass has undergone rapid growth or hemorrhage (25% to 50%).
- Fever, dyspnea, diarrhea, vomiting, weight loss, or malaise may be reported.

Physical Examination

- A firm, smooth abdominal or flank mass that does not cross the midline may be noted.
- BP is elevated if renal ischemia is present (rare).
- A left varicocele is found in males if the spermatic vein is obstructed.
- A careful examination is needed to rule out congenital anomalies.

Laboratory Studies

- Chest and abdominal radiography is performed to differentiate neuroblastoma, which is usually calcified.
- Abdominal ultrasonography is used to differentiate a solid from a cystic mass or hydronephrosis and multicystic kidney.
- UA demonstrates hematuria in 25% to 33% of children.
- A CBC, reticulocyte count, and liver and renal chemistry studies are performed.
- A computed tomography (CT) scan of the chest, abdomen, and pelvis to stage the disease and bone marrow is often done by the oncology team.

Differential Diagnosis

Neuroblastoma is the main differential diagnosis (the mass often crosses the midline). Multicystic kidney, hydronephrosis, renal cyst, or other renal malignancies are additional conditions to consider.

Management

Diagnostic workup is the initial urgent priority, with subsequent timely referral to a pediatric cancer center for treatment. Surgery is scheduled to remove the affected kidney and possibly the ureter and adrenal gland; combined chemotherapy and radiotherapy are instituted if the disease is advanced or histologic findings are unfavorable. Close follow-up after the initial treatment should be coordinated with the cancer team.

Complications

The lungs and liver are the most common sites of metastasis. High BP is possible because of renal ischemia and will occasionally lead to cardiac failure. Scoliosis resulting from radiation therapy is uncommon because the radiation is carefully controlled.

Patient Education, Prevention, and Prognosis

The prognosis is determined by the histology of the neoplasm, by the patient's age (the younger the better), the size of the tumor, positive nodes, and, most significantly, the extent or stage of the disease. If the child has favorable histologic parameters, the 4-year survival rate is as follows: 97% if stage I, 92% if stage II, 87% if stage III, and 73% if stage IV. Forty-five percent of relapses occur within 6 months, 28% more within 12 months (D'Angio et al, 1989; Nachman & Abelson, 2002).

LOWER GENITOURINARY TRACT DISORDERS

Urinary Tract Infection/Pyelonephritis

Description

Not only are UTIs frequently seen in primary care, but they are also the most commonly seen serious bacterial infection in young febrile children without an obvious source of infection. Because young children have limited symptoms, a high degree of suspicion must be maintained to diagnose UTI. Inflammation and infection can occur at any point in the urinary tract, so a UTI must be identified according to location. Bacteriuria is bacteria in the urine without other symptoms and is notable as a marker for possible underlying anatomic abnormality. Cystitis is infection of the bladder that produces lower tract symptoms. Pyelonephritis is the most severe type of UTI involving the renal parenchyma or kidneys and must be identified because of its potential for causing renal damage. Clinical signs thought to indicate pyelonephritis are a febrile infant with no other sign of infection or an older child with significant bacteriuria, systemic symptoms, or renal tenderness. UTIs may also be differentiated according to the type of infection. A UTI may be symptomatic or asymptomatic. It may also be complicated or uncomplicated. A *complicated UTI* is defined both as a UTI with fever, toxicity, dehydration, and poor compliance or occurring in a child younger than 3 to 6 months and as a UTI associated with a structural or functional abnormality such as vesicoureteral reflux (VUR), obstruction, voiding dysfunction, instrumentation, or pregnancy. Additionally, a UTI must be identified as a first occurrence, recurrent (within 2 weeks with the same organism or any reinfection with a different organism), or chronic (ongoing, unresolved, often caused by an abnormality or resistant organism). Finally, age at the time of occurrence and gender of the child are important factors in determining the course of treatment. (Pyelonephritis, although an upper tract disorder, is discussed in this section because it can be an infection ascending from the lower tract.)

It should be noted that evaluation and treatment of UTIs have changed dramatically over the last 30 years because of new knowledge regarding the pathogenesis of infection, especially kidney damage, and because of new imaging technologies and treatment. Therefore the practitioner must remain alert to new information as it becomes available (Larcombe, 2002.).

Etiology and Incidence

The organism most commonly associated with UTI is *E. coli* (75% to 95%), although other organisms such as *Enterobacter, Klebsiella, Pseudomonas,* and *Proteus* can be found. Several factors are believed to contribute to the etiology of UTIs. Most UTIs are thought to be ascending—that is, the infection begins with colonization of the urethral area and ascends the urinary tract. If the infection progresses to the kidney, intrarenal reflux deep into the kidneys can lead to scarring. This damage to the kidney occurs in the composite papillae, which have wide and gaping openings allowing intrarenal reflux. Simple papillae have angled, slitlike openings that resist intrarenal reflux (Fig. 35-9). The composite papillae are located in the upper and lower poles of the kidney, which is the usual site of scarring.

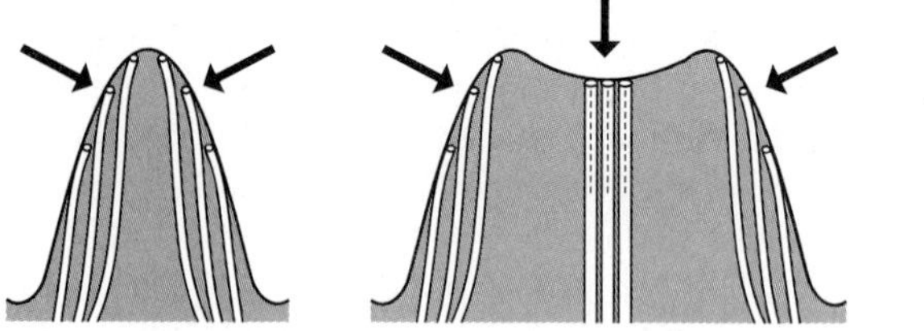

FIGURE 35-9 Most renal papillae are conical, with papillary ducts that open obliquely into the renal pelvis *(left)*. These do not allow intrarenal reflux. But some kidneys have compound papillae, formed by the fusion of conical papillae *(right)*. These have papillary ducts with gaping openings at right angles to urine flow and do permit intrarenal reflux. (From Ransley PG: Intrarenal reflux: anatomical, dynamic and radiological studies—part I, *Urol Res* 5:61-69, 1977.)

Host resistance factors and bacterial virulence factors are also important in the etiology of UTIs. Host resistance factors include the presence of a structural abnormality or dysplasia (such as VUR, obstruction, or any other anatomic defect) or the presence of functional abnormalities (such as dysfunctional voiding or constipation). Other factors affecting resistance include female gender (having a short urethra), poor hygiene, irritation from bubble baths, sexual activity or sexual abuse, and pinworms.

Several bacterial factors are known, but the two most important ones are adherence and virulence of the bacteria. Bacteria that have fimbriae or pili are able to anchor or adhere to the surface of the bladder mucosa. This adherence allows the bacteria to resist the bladder's defensive cleansing flow of urine and causes tissue inflammation and cell damage. Adherence may also play a role in bacteria ascending the urinary tract. Virulence refers to the toxicity of substances released by bacteria. The greater the virulence, the greater the damage to the urinary tract. Both of these factors enhance colonization of the urinary tract and aid in the persistence and impact of the bacteria.

The incidence of UTI in newborns is 1% to 1.4%, with a greater frequency in premature and low-birth-weight infants, as well as a slightly greater frequency in uncircumcised males. One study showed a UTI incidence of 1:47 in uncircumcised males during the first year of life, compared with 1:445 in circumcised males and 1:49 in females (Schöen, Colby, & Ray, 2000). After the first year of life it is also more common to find a UTI in females than in males (1:10). The overall incidence is 3% to 5% in girls and 1% in boys (Elder, 2004). Symptomatic UTI is found in 3% to 8% of females and 1% to 2% of males. By 11 years of age, 3% of girls and 1% of boys will have had a UTI (Finberg & Kleiman, 2002; Larcombe, 2002). The incidence of UTI is often increased in adolescents girls as they become sexually active. Recurrence is common, often within the first year after the initial infection.

Clinical Findings

History

- The following information should be elicited:
- Previous infection? How diagnosed? Workup done? Results?
- Hygiene habits
- Voiding and bowel patterns: frequency, completeness, dribbling, daytime enuresis, and weak stream
- Irritants such as bubble bath, nylon underwear, or clothing (spandex, tight pants or shorts that rub)
- Masturbation, sexual activity, or sexual abuse
- Family history of VUR, recurrent UTI, or kidney problems
- Other infection: pinworms, diaper rash

Physical Examination

- See Table 35-2 for age-related symptoms.
- BP, temperature, and general appearance (toxic appearing?)
- Growth parameters—growth may be decreased with chronic UTI or renal insufficiency
- Flank pain or tenderness in the costovertebral angle
- Abdominal examination—suprapubic tenderness, bladder distention or a flank mass (obstructive signs), mass from fecal impaction
- Genitalia—vaginal erythema, edema, irritation, or discharge; labial adhesions; uncircumcised male, urethral ballooning; weak, dribbling, threadlike stream
- Neurologic examination (if voiding is dysfunction)—perineal sensation, lower extremity reflexes, sacral dimpling, or cutaneous abnormality

Laboratory Studies. The method used to collect urine has an impact on the interpretation of results. Urine collected in a bag, because of the high degree of contaminants, is accurate only if negative. Voided midstream clean-catch specimens are somewhat more accurate, especially if collected as a first morning specimen and kept refrigerated (less than 24 hours) until analysis and can be used on toilet-trained children. Having the female child sit backward on the toilet separates the labia and decreases contamination (Plachter, Schulman, & Canning, 1999). In assessing for infection, suprapubic bladder aspiration is the most accurate method (99%), but sterile catheterization is 95% sensitive (Table 35-3). Either one of these collection methods should be used in very ill children and infants. Refer to the diagnostic studies section in the first part of this chapter to review other pertinent information.

- UA has limited value in diagnosing UTI because it can be negative even with a positive culture. It should be used only to raise or lower suspicion. Suspicious findings include foul odor, cloudiness, nitrites and/or leukocytes, alkaline pH, proteinuria, hematuria, pyuria, and bacteriuria.
  - Nitrite chemical tests are reliable on urine specimens collected after sleeping all night or when gram-negative bacteria are present and when the urine has been in the bladder for 4 hours or longer. False-positive results are rare, whereas false-negative results are common.
  - Leukocyte esterase chemical tests detect pyuria, but pyuria may arise from causes other than UTI.
- Microscopic evaluation of uncentrifuged urine is helpful if bacteria are seen.
- Gram stain is helpful if bacteria are identified.
- Urine culture by standard culture methods or by dipslide is essential to confirm the diagnosis. See Table 35-3 for evaluation of culture results. If culture growth is 10,000, repeat the culture unless the sample was collected by suprapubic aspiration or catheterization.
- Bacterial identification and determination of sensitivities are necessary in patients who appear toxic or could have pyelonephritis, have relapses or recurrent UTI, or are nonresponsive to medication.
- Blood culture should be done if sepsis is suspected or in infants younger than 1 year (see Chapter 24, Fever without a Focus).
- CBC (elevated WBC count), ESR, C-reactive protein, BUN, and creatinine should be done if the child appears ill and pyelonephritis is suspected.

Differential Diagnosis

The differential diagnosis includes a foreign body, urethritis, vaginitis, viral cystitis, sexual abuse, dysfunctional voiding, dysuria-pyuria syndrome, appendicitis, pelvic

TABLE 35-2 ***Clinical Findings of Urinary Tract Infection in Children of Various Ages***

Neonates	Infants	Toddlers and Preschoolers	School-Age Children and Adolescents
Jaundice	Malaise	Altered voiding pattern	"Classic dysuria" with frequency, urgency, and discomfort
Hypothermia	Irritability	Malodor	Malodor
Failure to thrive	Difficulty feeding	Abdominal/flank pain*	Enuresis
Sepsis	Poor weight gain	Enuresis	Abdominal/flank pain*
Vomiting or diarrhea	Fever*	Vomiting or diarrhea*	Fever/chills*
Cyanosis	Vomiting or diarrhea	Malaise	Vomiting or diarrhea*
Abdominal distention	Malodor	Fever*	Malaise
Lethargy	Dribbling	Diaper rash	
	Abdominal pain/colic		

*Findings especially likely with pyelonephritis.

TABLE 35-3 ***Criteria for Diagnosis of Urinary Tract Infections***

Method of Collection	Colony Count (Pure Culture)	Probability of Infection (%)
Suprapubic aspiration	Any organism	>99
Catheterization	$>10^5$	95
	$\geq 10^4$-10^5	Infection likely, especially if obstruction or if frequent voider
	10^3-$<10^4$ single organism	Suspicious, repeat
	$<10^3$	Infection unlikely
Clean voided		
Boy	$>10^4$, single organism	Infection likely
Girl	Three specimens, $>10^5$	95
	Two specimens, $>10^6$	90-95
	One specimen, $>10^6$	80-90
	5×10^4-10^5	Suspicious, infection possible, repeat
	10^4-5×10^4	Suspicious, if symptomatic, repeat
	10^4-5×10^4	Infection unlikely if asymptomatic
	$<10^4$	Infection unlikely

Modified from Feld LG, Greenfield SP, Ogra PL: Urinary tract infections in infants and children, *Pediatr Rev* 11:71-77, 1989; Rushton HG: UTI in children: epidemiology, evaluation and management, *Pediatr Clin North Am* 44:1133-1169, 1997; Hoberman A, Wald ER: UTI in young children: new light on old questions, *Contemp Pediatr* 14(11):140-156, 1997; Heldrich FJ: UTI diagnosis: getting it right the first time, *Contemp Pediatr* 12(2):110-133, 1995; Opas LM: UTI: burning issues (unpublished manuscript), Los Angeles, 1999.

abscess, and pelvic inflammatory disease. Any child who has fever without focus, a fever of unexplained origin, FTT, chronic diarrhea, or recurrent abdominal pain should be evaluated for UTI.

Management

1. Goals of treatment are to quickly identify the extent and level of infection, to treat appropriately to eradicate infection and provide symptomatic relief, to find and correct anatomic or functional abnormalities, and to prevent recurrence and new or progressive renal damage. When deciding on a treatment plan, the child's age, sex, and symptoms and the suspected location of the UTI must be kept in mind.
2. Bacteriuria. Whether asymptomatic bacteriuria should be treated is controversial. Those who advocate treatment do so with the intent of preventing further infection or sequelae and identifying any underlying abnormalities.
3. Afebrile UTI (Fig. 35-10):
   a. Antibiotic treatment for 10 days (Tran, Muchant, & Aronoff, 2001). First-line drugs as recommended by the American Academy of Pediatrics (AAP) practice parameter on UTIs (AAP, 2002) are as follows:

- Trimethoprim-sulfamethoxazole (6 to 12 mg/kg trimethoprim plus 30 to 60 mg/kg per day sulfamethoxazole in two divided doses if older than 2 months).
- Amoxicillin (40 mg/kg per day in two or three divided doses) if no resistance is found in the community.

Also recommended are the following:

- Sulfisoxazole (120 to 150 mg/kg per day in three or four divided doses if older than 2 months).
- Nitrofurantoin (4 to 8 mg/kg per day four times a day if older than 1 month).

If allergic to the drugs just mentioned or a broader spectrum is needed:

- Cefixime (8 mg/kg per day in one or two doses)
- Cephalexin (50 to 100 mg/kg per day in three or four divided doses)
- Cefprozil (30 mg/kg per day in two divided doses)
- Cefpodoxime (10 mg/kg per day in two divided doses)
- Loracarbet (15 to 30 mg/kg per day in two divided doses)

   b. Follow-up urine culture should be done 48 to 72 hours after initiating treatment, especially if symptoms persist or organism resistance is found in the community.

- If the culture is sterile, continue antibiotic therapy.
- If the culture is not sterile or if no clinical improvement is seen, urine should be sent for bacterial identification and sensitivity studies, and an alternative broad-spectrum antibiotic should be used pending those results. Culture should be repeated after 48 to 72 hours and, if sterile, antibiotic therapy continued.

   c. Follow-up cultures should be obtained 3 to 4 days after finishing antibiotic treatment.

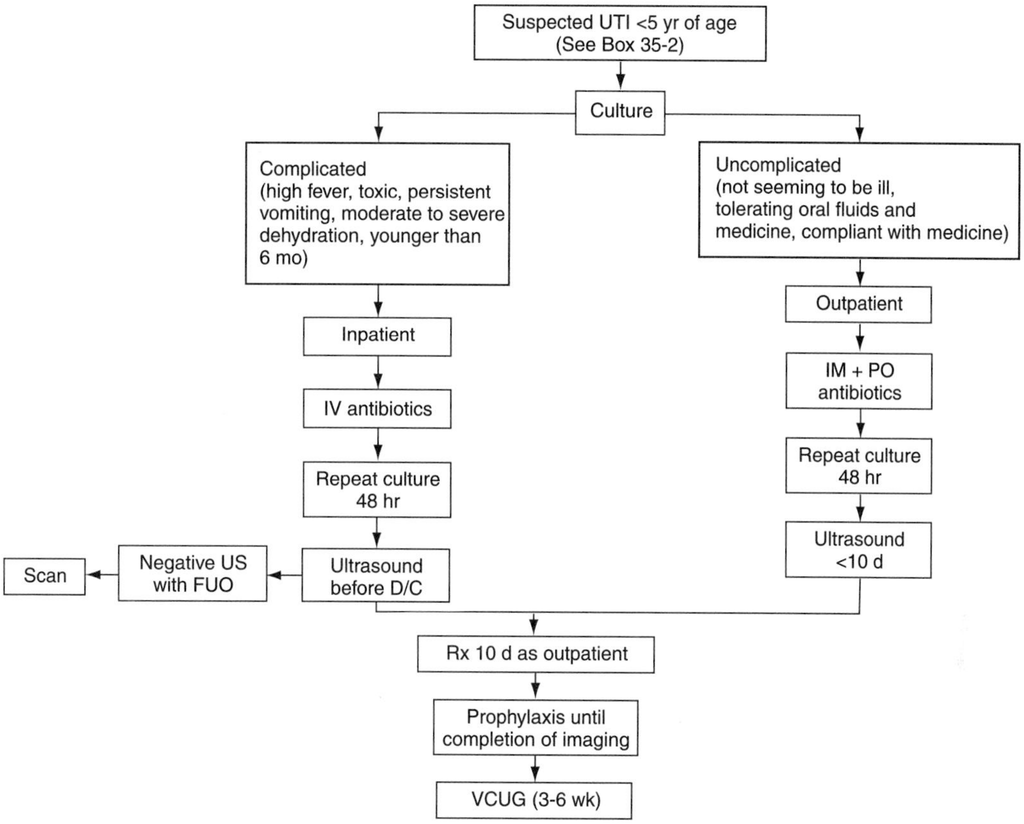

FIGURE 35-10 Evaluation of urinary tract infection (UTI) in a child less than 5 years of age. *D/C*, Discharge; *FUO*, fever of unknown origin; *IM*, intramuscular; *IV*, intravenous; *PO*, oral; *Rx*, prescribe; *US*, ultrasonogram; *VCUG*, voiding cystourethrogram; *VUR*, vesicoureteral reflux. (Adapted with permission from Opas LM: UTI: burning issues [unpublished manuscript], Los Angeles, 1999.)

d. Repeat urine culture should be done with any fever, illness, dysuria, or frequency. Because recurrent UTI is so common, monitoring urine culture at 1, 3, and 6 months is often recommended.

e. If the child is younger than 5 years, once a sterile urine is obtained, low-dose prophylaxis should be continued until radiologic workup is completed (see number 5).

f. Phenazopyridine (Pyridium) may be given at 100 mg for ages 6 to 12 years and 200 mg for those older than 12 years three times per day for dysuria.

4. Febrile UTI. Because fever is often an indicator of pyelonephritis, treatment must be initiated promptly to prevent or minimize sequelae (Newman et al, 2002) (see Fig. 35-10).

a. Uncomplicated (not seeming to be ill, tolerating oral fluids and medicine, mildly dehydrated, with good compliance):

- Parenteral antimicrobials are administered intramuscularly for the first 24 hours or until afebrile with a normal ESR and sterile culture are recommended (AAP, 2002).
  - Ceftriaxone (Rocephin), 75 mg/kg every 24 hours, is often used.
  - Cefotaxime, 150 mg/kg per day divided every 6 hours.
  - Ceftazidime, 150 mg/kg per day divided every 6 hours.
  - Ceftazolin, 50 mg/kg per day divided every 8 hours.
  - Tobramycin, 5 mg/kg per day divided every 6 hours.
  - Ticarcillin, 300 mg/kg per day divided every 6 hours.
  - Ampicillin, 100 mg/kg per day divided every 6 hours.
  - Gentamicin, 7.5 mg/kg per day divided every 8 hours.
- Oral antibiotics (see the section on cystitis) are administered following intramuscular therapy for a total of 10 to 14 days, followed by prophylaxis until the radiologic workup is complete; if pyelonephritis is the final diagnosis, continue prophylactic antibiotics for 6 months.
- Repeat urine culture after 48 hours of antibiotic therapy and 1, 2, 3, and 6 months after infection.
- Ultrasonography should be performed as soon as convenient, VCUG within 6 weeks.

b. Complicated (high fever, toxic, persistent vomiting, moderate to severe dehydration, poor compliance, younger than 3 to 6 months):
- Inpatient treatment consists of intravenous antibiotics (see intramuscular antibiotics earlier) until afebrile for 24 to 36 hours with a normal ESR and sterile culture.
- The remainder of treatment is as presented earlier.

5. Radiologic workup:
   a. Box 35-2 lists the suggested criteria for the radiologic workup of children with UTI; Table 35-4 details radiologic studies that can be done.
   b. In a child older than 10 years with a first uncomplicated UTI and no voiding dysfunction before the UTI, no further workup is needed at this time.
   c. Renal and bladder ultrasonography should be done during hospitalization or within 10 days in any child younger than 10 years (Friedman, 2002; most conservative recommendation, see Box 35-2), any child with a complicated UTI, or any child with a history of dysfunctional voiding.
- If the ultrasonogram is normal in a child older than 5 years but with complicated UTI or in a child with previous dysfunctional voiding, start prophylaxis and perform VCUG.
- If the ultrasonogram is normal in a child younger than 5 years, start prophylaxis and perform VCUG.
- If the ultrasonogram is normal in a child younger than 5 years with complicated UTI, start prophylaxis and perform VCUG and consult with a pediatric nephrologist regarding the need for a dimercaptosuccinic acid (DMSA) nuclear scan.
- If the ultrasonogram is abnormal, start prophylaxis and perform VCUG. Depending on the abnormality, the child may need referral to a urologist.

   d. VCUG should be done after the infection is treated, once the patient is asymptomatic with sterile urine culture. Waiting until 4 to 6 weeks after infection is often recommended to allow any inflammatory changes to subside, although it has been reported that early (less than 7 days) VCUG does not change the incidence of reflux (Mahant, To, & Friedman, 2001).
- Prophylaxis should be continued until the VCUG is complete and results are known.
- If reflux is present, prophylaxis is needed for 1 year, at which time repeat VCUG should be done. If repeat VCUG shows resolved reflux, prophylaxis is discontinued.

   e. Nuclear scans (DMSA or technetium-labeled diethylenetriamine pentaacetic acid [Tc-DTPA]) can be performed to diagnose acute pyelonephritis and to evaluate for scarring. These tests are especially helpful in neonates and in children with fever of unknown origin. However, they are the most expensive test available and should be ordered only as indicated and after consultation with a pediatric nephrologist (Kraus, 2001).
- Any evidence of acquired kidney damage requires antibiotic suppression therapy.

6. Recurrent infection (two or more in 1 year):
   a. Initial treatment is as for urinary tract infection.
   b. Perform a radiologic workup if not previously done.
   c. Once urine is sterile, administer prophylactic antibiotics and monitor urine cultures for 6 to 12 months (see Fig. 35-10 and Box 35-2).

Complications

Recurrent infection, chronic UTI, FTT, and irreversible renal scarring (the most significant complication) can occur. Major risk factors for renal damage include delay in treatment of pyelonephritis, age younger than 1 year, anatomic or neurogenic obstruction, severe reflux, dysplasia, and multiple infections (Patterson & Strife, 2000). The same acute inflammatory process responsible for eradication of bacteria is also responsible for damage to renal tissue and subsequent scarring.

Patient Education and Prevention

- Clear explanation of the etiology, potential complications, and overall treatment plan, including both short- and long-term plans.
- Frequent and complete voiding and increased quantities of fluids, especially water. Sometimes scheduled voiding times or double voiding (voiding and then immediately attempting to void again) can be helpful.
- Proper hygiene and avoidance of irritants such as bubble baths and perfumed soaps. Avoidance of tight pants, especially spandex pants, is recommended along with cotton underwear. Treat perineal inflammation to help avoid UTI.
- Sexually active females should be encouraged to drink water before intercourse and void immediately afterward.
- Home monitoring of urine with nitrite sticks on first morning urine is helpful. If positive or questionable or the child is symptomatic, a culture must follow.
- Decrease intake of bladder irritants such as the "four *C*'s" (caffeine, carbonated beverages, chocolate, citrus) and aspartame (Nutrasweet), alcohol, and spicy foods.
- Avoid constipation. Stool softeners and timed defecation may be helpful.
- Three-day rule. To avoid delay in treatment, no infant or young child with unexplained fever should go longer than 3 days without examination of urine.
- Cranberry juice is considered helpful in preventing the adherence of *E. coli* in the urethra (see Chapter 43).

BOX 35-2 *Radiologic Workup and Prophylaxis for Urinary Tract Infections*

Why Do a Workup?

- To identify any structural or functional abnormality of the urinary tract
- To identify any renal scarring or damage

Who Requires a Workup?

Recommendations vary among experts. Those who recommend the most aggressive workup do so to identify scarring early and prevent further damage.

- All children with the first infection (Chon, Lai, & Dairiki, 2001)
- Infants or any child younger than 5 years old (Opas, 1999)
- All children younger than 6 years old (Elenberg & Travis, 2002)
- Any child with pyelonephritis
- Any child younger than 8 years old with acute symptoms, especially fever or toxicity (at least 50% have reflux or obstructive lesions)
- All children younger than 10 years old and all children 10 years old and older with signs and symptoms of pyelonephritis who respond slowly to therapy and are prepubertal (Friedman, 2002)
- Males with a first infection; females after a second infection if no other criteria are met
- Any child with suspicious factors (e.g., high blood pressure, abnormal urine stream, poor growth) or with a positive family history of UTI or abnormal voiding patterns
- Adolescents with pyelonephritis or after a second UTI with documented culture and no history of recent sexual activity

What Should Be Done?

- Renal and bladder ultrasonography: done initially in all children
- VCUG: done if ultrasound is abnormal, if child is younger than 5 years old, or if voiding dysfunction was present before UTI
- Nuclear imaging scan: done to detect renal scars or parenchymal inflammation
- Intravenous pyelogram: done if further definition of structure or function of the kidney is needed

When Should It Be Done?

- Ultrasonography: during hospitalization or within 10 days in any child younger than 5 years old or with complicated UTI
- VCUG: after urine has become sterile and the patient is asymptomatic; some authorities recommend 4 to 6 weeks after the diagnosis of UTI
- As follow-up for pyelonephritis and vesicoureteral reflux

When Should Prophylaxis Be Used?

- After resolution of UTI and before radiologic workup
- To suppress recurrent UTI after radiologic workup

What Should Be Used for Prophylaxis?

Approximately one third to one half the treatment dosage of antibiotic should be given at bedtime. Although prophylaxis is generally recommended, well-designed, randomized, placebo-controlled trials are still required to determine if long-term, low-dose antibiotic administration prevents urinary tract infection in children (AAP, 2002; Johnson, 1999; Williams, Lee, & Craig, 2001).

- Nitrofurantoin (1 to 2 mg/kg qd if older than 2 months of age); max dose 50 mg; expensive
- TMP (2 mg/kg) and SMX (10 mg/kg) qd if older than 2 months of age; TMP (5 mg/kg) and SMX (25 mg/kg) bid twice per week (max dose 40 mg); a yearly CBC should be done to monitor for neutropenia
- TMP (2 mg/kg, max dose 50 mg) at bedtime if older than 3 months of age
- Sulfisoxazole (10-20 mg/kg divided every 12 hours if older than 2 months of age)
- Penicillin or ampicillin can be used for a newborn or premature infant
- Nalidixic acid (30 mg/kg divided every 12 hours)
- Methenamine mandelate (75 mg/kg divided every 12 hours)

---

bid, Twice daily; *CBC,* complete blood count; *qd,* every day; *SMX,* sulfamethoxazole; *TMP,* trimethoprim; *UTI,* urinary tract infection; *VCUG,* voiding cystourethrography.

TABLE 35-4 *Radiologic Studies Done for Evaluation of Urinary Tract Infection*

Study	Cost	Advantages	Disadvantages	Use
USN	Least expensive	Shows structure, shape, and growth Detects structural abnormality, obstruction, pyelonephritis, large scars Painless, low risk, no radiation, noninvasive, available	Does not detect small scars of VUR Poor visualization of ureters Does not measure renal function or transient injury to kidney	Initial evaluation and follow-up
VCUG, radiographic	Least expensive	Detects and grades VUR—if high or low pressure, high or low bladder volumes, during voiding, during early or late bladder filling Visualize bladder and urethra (especially in males) and diverticula	Does not detect obstruction, pyelonephritis, scars Risk of urethral trauma from catheterization Greater radiation than with scan	Initial evaluation In infants and children younger than 5 yr with abnormal USN or dysfunctional voiding
VCUG, nuclear	More expensive	Visualize bladder and reflux Constantly monitors for transient reflux Less radiation	Discomfort of catheterization No urethral visualization Unable to grade reflux	Follow-up of VUR To evaluate siblings of child with VUR Follow-up of surgery
IVP	Less expensive	Detects obstruction, pyelonephritis, large scars, stones, nephrocalcinosis Details pelvicaliceal system, shows ureters Estimates renal function Readily available	Does not detect small scars or VUR Risk of allergic reaction, acute renal failure, pain of injection, radiation Requires good renal function Only identifies structural damage	Better defines level of obstruction Not used very often
Nuclear scans • DMSA • Tc-DTPA	Most expensive	Detects acute inflammation, scars, and obstruction Earlier detection of parenchymal damage—large or small scars, permanent or focal—than with IVP (1-3 yr) Good in neonates Shows renal outline, estimates renal and tubular function, measures changes Less radiation	Does not detect VUR or measure renal function Does not evaluate calyces, ureters, bladder, or urethra	Follow-up Fever of unknown origin and negative USN in neonates To diagnose APN To detect renal scars
CT scan (contrast)	Expensive	Detects obstruction, pyelonephritis, large scars	Does not detect small scars or VUR Risk of allergic reaction, acute renal failure	Trauma

APN, acute pyelonephritis; *CT*, computed tomography; *DMSA*, dimercaptosuccinic acid; *IVP*, intravenous pyelography; *Tc-DTPA*, technetium-labeled diethylenetriamine pentaacetic acid; *USN*, ultrasound; *VCUG*, voiding cystourethrography; *VUR*, vesicoureteral reflux.

Vesicoureteral Reflux

Description

Regurgitation of urine from the bladder up the ureter to the kidney is called vesicoureteral reflux (VUR). Primary VUR is the most common type and is typified by a congenital, abnormally short ureter and ineffective valve. Secondary VUR is due to bladder outlet obstruction and can be functional or structural. It is graded according to an international classification (Fig. 35-11). Grades I, II, and III (low grade) describe reflux to the renal pelvis with little or no distention. Grades IV and V (high grade) include definite distention of the ureters and renal pelvis and can include hydronephrosis or reflux into the intrarenal collecting system (American Urological Association Practice Parameters, Guidelines and Standards Committee, 1997).

Etiology and Incidence

Reflux occurs because of congenital abnormalities and can persist with recurrent infection. Reflux provides a route for bacteria to ascend to the kidney and cause pyelonephritis. VUR is the most common anatomic abnormality found in children with UTI, with an incidence of 20% to 50% when studied after the first UTI (Decter, 2001; Ingelfinger, 2002). Approximately 30% to 40% of siblings of children with reflux also have reflux, and 50% of children whose mothers have reflux also have reflux (Elder, 2004; Ingelfinger, 2002).

Clinical Findings

History. The history assesses for a previous UTI, voiding pattern or dysfunction, and asymptomatic or UTI symptoms.

Laboratory Studies. The following, if not already done, are ordered as indicated to identify obstructive uropathy and dysplasia:

- Ultrasonography
- VCUG—establishes the presence of reflux, determines the grade, and gives high detail
- Nuclear scan—uses less radiation to identify VUR but gives less detail (no grading) and requires someone skilled in interpretation; most helpful in long-term follow-up and with neonates
- IVP—may be done if the VCUG is positive because it gives more defined structural and functional information
- Ultrasonography and IVP possibly normal even in the presence of reflux

Management

The goal of treatment is the prevention of infection and subsequent scarring. Early identification and appropriate treatment of infection achieve this goal.

Management involves the following (Tables 35-5 and 35-6):

- Grades I, II, and III reflux. Most children outgrow their reflux and should be left to do so. Grades I and II VUR resolve spontaneously in up to 85% of children (Opas, 1999) and 77% of grades III and IV (Smellie et al, 2001). Primary VUR resolves spontaneously in 85%; secondary VUR resolves with correction of the underlying problem (Arant, 2002).
  - Prophylactic antibiotics to prevent UTI (see Box 35-2) should be continued until the child has been infection free for 12 months as documented by urine cultures and a negative VCUG for reflux. If antibiotics are not

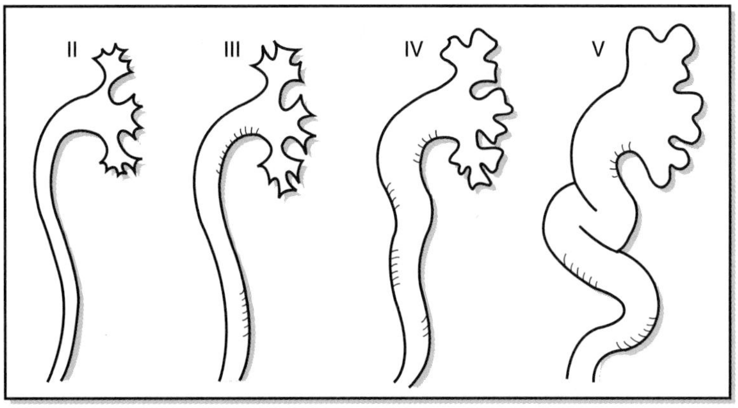

FIGURE 35-11 International reflux grading. Grade I: ureter only. Grade II: ureter, pelvis, and calyces; no dilation, normal calyceal fornices. Grade III: mild or moderate dilation or tortuosity (or both) of ureter, and mild or moderate dilation of renal pelvis but no or slight blunting of the fornices. Grade IV: moderate dilation or tortuosity (or both) of ureter and moderate dilation of renal pelvis and calyces. Complete obliteration of sharp angles of fornices but maintenance of papillary impressions in majority of calyces. Grade V: gross dilation and tortuosity of ureter; gross dilation of renal pelvis and calyces; papillary impressions are no longer visible in majority of calyces. (From Lebowitz RL et al: International system of radiographic grading of vesicoureteral reflux, International Reflux Study in Children, *Pediatr Radiol* 15(2):105, 1985.)

TABLE 35-5 *Treatment Recommendations for Children without Scarring at Diagnosis*

Recommendations were derived from a survey of preferred treatment options for 36 clinical categories of children with reflux.
The recommendations are classified as follows:

Guidelines = treatments selected by 8 or 9 of 9 panel members, given the strongest recommendation language.
Preferred options = treatments selected by 5-7 of 9 panel members.
Reasonable alternatives = treatments selected by 3-4 of 9 panel members.
No consensus = treatments selected by no more than 2 of 9 panel members.

The treatment recommendations apply to both boys and girls with primary vesicoureteral reflux (VUR).

Clinical Presentation (Age at Presentation)		Treatment: Initial (Antibiotic Prophylaxis or Open Surgical Repair)			Treatment: Follow-up* (Continued Antibiotic Prophylaxis, Cystography, or Open Surgical Repair)		
VUR Grade Laterality	**Age (Years)**	**Guideline**	**Preferred Option**	**Reasonable Alternative**	**Guideline**	**Preferred Option**	**No consensus†**
I-II unilateral or bilateral	<1	Antibiotic prophylaxis					Boys and girls
	1-5	Antibiotic prophylaxis					Boys and girls
	6-10	Antibiotic prophylaxis					Boys and girls
III-IV unilateral or bilateral	<1	Antibiotic prophylaxis			Bilateral: surgery if persistent‡	Unilateral: surgery if persistent‡	
	1-5	Unilateral: antibiotic prophylaxis	Bilateral: antibiotic prophylaxis			Surgery if persistent‡	
	6-10		Unilateral: antibiotic prophylaxis Bilateral: surgery	Bilateral: antibiotic prophylaxis		Surgery if persistent‡	
V unilateral or bilateral	<1		Antibiotic prophylaxis		Surgery if persistent‡		
	1-5		Bilateral: surgery Unilateral: antibiotic prophylaxis	Bilateral: antibiotic prophylaxis Unilateral: surgery	Surgery if persistent‡		
	6-10	Surgery					

From American Urological Association Pediatric Vesicoureteral Reflux Clinical Guidelines Panel: *The management of primary vesicoureteral reflux in children: clinical practice guidelines*, Baltimore, 1997, The Association, p 52.
*For patients with persistent uncomplicated reflux after extended treatment with continuous antibiotic therapy.
†No consensus was reached regarding the role of continued antibiotic prophylaxis, cystography, or surgery.
‡The duration of reflux regarding the length of time that clinicians should wait before recommending surgery is dependent on the child's age, whether the disease is unilateral or bilateral, the grade of the reflux at diagnosis, and the percent chance of reflux resolution from diagnosis to 5 years (AUA, 1997, p 23, Table 2).

taken or the child has recurrent infection, surgery may be needed.

- Interval urine cultures are performed as indicated and with symptoms or unexplained illness (see Fig. 35-10).
- Radiologic studies—ultrasonography, VCUG, or renal scan—every 12 months to monitor reflux, renal growth, and scarring.
- CBC, BUN, and creatinine annually to monitor renal function.
- Circumcision may be recommended for the male infant (Cascio, Colhoun, & Puri, 2001).
- In children with reflux who are toilet trained, regular, low volitional low-pressure voiding with complete bladder emptying should be encouraged. If uninhibited

TABLE 35-6 *Treatment Recommendations for Children with Scarring at Diagnosis*

Recommendations were derived from a survey of preferred treatment options for 36 clinical categories of children with reflux. The recommendations are classified as follows.

Guidelines = treatments selected by 8 or 9 of 9 panel members, given the strongest recommendation language.
Preferred options = treatments selected by 5-7 of 9 panel members.
Reasonable alternatives = treatments selected by 3-4 of 9 panel members.
No consensus = treatments selected by no more than 2 of 9 panel members.

The treatment recommendations apply to both boys and girls with primary vesicoureteral reflux (VUR).

Clinical Presentation (Age at Presentation)		Treatment: Initial (Antibiotic Prophylaxis or Open Surgical Repair)			Treatment: Follow-up[*] (Continued Antibiotic Prophylaxis, Cystography, or Open Surgical Repair)		
VUR Grade Laterality	**Age (Years)**	**Guideline**	**Preferred Option**	**Reasonable Alternative**	**Guideline**	**Preferred Option**	**No consensus[†]**
I-II unilateral or bilateral	<1	Antibiotic prophylaxis					Boys and girls
	1-5	Antibiotic prophylaxis					Boys and girls
	6-10	Antibiotic prophylaxis					Boys and girls
III-IV unilateral	<1	Antibiotic prophylaxis			Girls: surgery if persistent[‡]	Boys: surgery if persistent[‡]	
	1-5	Antibiotic prophylaxis			Girls: surgery if persistent[‡]	Boys: surgery if persistent[‡]	
	6-10		Antibiotic prophylaxis		Girls: surgery if persistent[‡]		
II-IV bilateral	<1	Antibiotic prophylaxis			Girls: surgery if persistent[‡]		
	1-5		Antibiotic prophylaxis	Surgery	Girls: surgery if persistent[‡]		
	6-10	Surgery					
V unilateral or bilateral	<1		Antibiotic prophylaxis	Surgery	Girls: surgery if persistent[‡]		
	1-5	Bilateral: surgery	Unilateral: surgery			Surgery if persistent[‡]	
	6-10	Surgery					

From American Urological Association Pediatric Vesicoureteral Reflux Clinical Guidelines Panel: *The management of primary vesicoureteral reflux in children: clinical practice guidelines*, Baltimore, 1997, The Association, p 52.
[*]For patients with persistent uncomplicated reflux after extended treatment with continuous antibiotic therapy.
[†]No consensus was reached regarding the role of continued antibiotic prophylaxis, cystography, or surgery.
[‡]The duration of reflux regarding the length of time that clinicians should wait before recommending surgery is dependent on the child's age, whether the disease is unilateral or bilateral, the grade of the reflux at diagnosis, and the percent chance of reflux resolution from diagnosis to 5 years (AUA, 1997, p 23, Table 2).

bladder contractions are suspected, anticholinergic therapy may be helpful (American Urological Association Practice Parameters, Guidelines and Standards Committee, 1997).

- Grades IV and V reflux are managed medically or surgically by a pediatric urologist and pediatric nephrologist (American Urological Association Practice Parameters, Guidelines and Standards Committee, 1997; Capozza & Caione, 2002; Mevorach et al, 2002).
- Adolescents may need surgery because reflux in this age-group is rarely outgrown.
- Surgery is indicated for progressive renal injury and breakthrough infection (especially acute pyelonephritis) or with associated anatomic abnormalities.
- Nephrology consultation is indicated in the presence of notable scarring, a solitary or atrophic kidney, hypertension, elevated creatinine, or evidence of abnormal kidney function with any grade of reflux.

Complications

Preexisting renal damage may be present, and new renal scarring can occur. Children with grades III or IV reflux have up to 50% reported incidence of scarring at the time of diagnosis (Decter, 2001). These complications can lead to ongoing renal disease, atrophy, growth failure, elevated BP, and decreased renal functioning.

Patient Education and Prevention

- VUR does not cause scarring, infection does—but VUR is a risk factor for pyelonephritis and subsequent scarring.
- Screening ultrasonography should be done on an infant born to parents with VUR, on any young siblings of a child with VUR, and on any older siblings with any history of UTI.
- Management, prevention of UTIs, and compliance must be understood by families. The necessity of routine urine culture should also be emphasized. The potential for untreated, chronic UTI leading to chronic renal disease must be explained. Other points to emphasize include the following:
    - Prompt treatment of UTI should be instituted.
    - Prophylactic medicines are best given at night because of urinary stasis while asleep.
    - BP and growth should be monitored.
    - Measures as discussed in the Patient Education and Prevention section of UTIs should be followed.

COMMON GENITOURINARY CONDITIONS IN MALES

Hypospadias

Description

Hypospadias is a common congenital abnormality in which the urethral opening is on the ventral surface (underside) of the penis. Chordee, a ventral bowing of the penis, occurs when a tight band of fibrous tissue pulls on the penis. Torsion refers to rotation of the penis to the right or left.

Etiology and Incidence

The etiology of hypospadias is unclear. It is believed that the endocrine system probably has an important role, but what that role is remains unclear. The primitive gonad in the eighth week of embryonic development differentiates into male or female. As the genital tubercle enlarges, developmental arrest occurs along the line of urethral fusion and causes hypospadias.

Hypospadias occurs in 1 in 300 infant boys (Ingelfinger, 2002). There was a major increase in incidence in the 1990s, especially in low-birth-weight babies and babies whose mothers had taken fertility drugs or undergone invitro fertilization. The cause of this may be due to genetic factors (e.g., endocrine abnormalities) or environmental factors (e.g., androgen blockers and estrogen or endocrine disruptions), and it probably occurs early in gestation (Bukowski & Zeman, 2001; Hussain et al, 2002; Kurzrock, 2002). Risk is increased if family members have hypospadias: 8% if the father, 14% if a sibling, and 21% if two family members. Hypospadias occurs more commonly in whites than in African Americans, in Italians and Jews, and in winter conceptions. Nine percent of boys with hypospadias also have undescended testicles, inguinal hernia, or hydrocele.

Clinical Findings

History

- A family history of a male relative with genitourinary problems is reported.
- The child sits to void or holds his penis to direct the stream.

Physical Examination. In a newborn, the classic finding is a dorsally hooded foreskin. It is essential to visualize the urethral meatus. Pulling the ventral shaft skin in a downward and outward direction facilitates visualization. Anatomic classification is made by location:

- Anterior (70%), glanular, coronal, or anterior penile
- Middle (10%)
- Posterior (20%), scrotal, penoscrotal, or posterior penile

Other findings include:

- Urinary stream that aims downward rather than straight
- Inguinal hernia or undescended testicles (9%) (Bukowski & Zeman, 2001)
- Chordee

Differential Diagnosis

The differential diagnosis includes intersex abnormalities.

Management

Circumcision must not be done because the foreskin is used in the surgical repair. Referral should be made to a urologist at birth for evaluation. Surgery to correct hypospadias is best done at around 6 to 12 months of age. Considerations in scheduling earlier surgery include the following: it is psychologically less damaging; a caudal block is easily performed; the wound heals more rapidly; and there is more time to repair complications before toilet training begins. Surgery scheduled later minimizes anesthesia risk, the larger anatomy makes surgery easier, and the patient can participate in the decision-making process (Bukowski & Zeman, 2001). Repair is usually accomplished in a one-stage outpatient procedure unless it is a complex defect.

Complications

Peer taunting of boys with unrepaired hypospadias and problems with erections if chordee is not repaired are possible complications. Intersex abnormalities are possible if associated with cryptorchidism. Fistulas and urethral or meatal stenosis are potential complications of surgery.

Patient Education

Hypospadias is usually an isolated anomaly that does not require further workup. Education and reassurance regarding cause, repair, and outcome should be provided.

Undescended Testes—Cryptorchidism

Description

Cryptorchidism describes a testis that does not reside in and cannot be manipulated into the scrotum. A retractile testis is out of the scrotum but can be brought into the scrotum and remains there. A gliding testis can be brought into the scrotum but returns to a high position in the scrotum once released. An ectopic testis lies outside the normal path of descent. An ascended testis is one that has fully descended but has spontaneously reascended and lies outside the scrotum. A trapped testis is one dislocated after herniorrhaphy. Any testis that is not in the scrotum is subject to progressive deterioration. Undescended testes are a common disorder that often causes great anxiety for parents.

Etiology and Incidence

Testes develop in the abdomen and descend in the seventh fetal month to the upper part of the groin, subsequently progressing through the inguinal canal into the scrotum. Failure of the testes to descend can be caused by mechanical lesions or can be secondary to hormonal, chromosomal, enzymatic, or anatomic disorders.

Undescended testis is the most common genitourinary disorder in boys. It is more common in preterm, low-birth-weight, and twin infants (Callaghan, 2000). The incidence of cryptorchidism is 0.2% to 1.8% in young adults, 0.5% to 0.8% in 1-year-olds, 2.5% to 4% in term infants, 20% to 30% in premature infants, over 60% if infant birth weight is under 1500 g, and nearly 100% in 900 g neonates (Ferrer & McKenna, 2000; Reiter & Saenger, 2002). A great majority of undescended testes descend spontaneously by 6 months to 1 year of age. The frequency of bilateral occurrence is 10% to 25%, and unilateral involvement (55% to 66%) is more likely to be right-sided. Retractile testes are bilateral and most common in boys 5 to 6 years of age (Pillai & Besner, 1998).

Clinical Findings

History. The history can include the following:

- Family history of undescended testes or testicular malignancy
- Testes sometimes felt during the infant's bath
- Associated urinary problems
- Prematurity
- Risk factors (Callaghan, 2000): first-born, cesarean section, toxemia, hypospadias, congenital subluxation of the hip, low birth weight, winter conception
- Other congenital, endocrine, chromosomal, or intersex disorders

Physical Examination. Having the child sit cross-legged or frog-legged, squat, or stand can facilitate testicle descent and palpation. Findings include the following:

- Scrotal rugae less full
- Bilateral or unilateral absence of a testicle
- Retractile testes, which move between the scrotum and external ring but can be manipulated to the lower part of the scrotum and remain there; especially common with stimulation or cold between ages 3 months and 7 years
- Gliding testes, which lie between the scrotum and external ring and can be manipulated to the lower part of the scrotum but return to the high position
- Location:
  - Prescrotal (at the external inguinal ring), 25%
  - Canalicular, high or low (between the external and internal rings), the most common type, 40%
  - Ectopic (superficial inguinal, femoral, or perineal), 25%
  - Intraabdominal (above the internal inguinal ring), not palpable, occurring in less than 15% of males with undescended testes
  - Indirect inguinal hernia, 90% (Pillai & Besner, 1998)

Laboratory Studies. None are indicated except in newborns with potential sex abnormalities, hypopituitarism, or congenital adrenal hyperplasia. The risk of intersex abnormality is 27% if hypospadias and unilateral or bilateral cryptorchidism are present.

Differential Diagnosis

Retractile testes, anorchism, and chromosomal abnormalities are the differential diagnoses.

Management

The goals of treating undescended testes are to improve fertility outcome, decrease malignancy potential, and minimize the psychologic stress associated with an empty scrotum. Management has come full circle from an initial recommendation for surgery, to treatment with hormonal therapy, and back to early surgical intervention. Both forms of treatment are still options.

- If the testes are undescended by 6 months of age with the peak of postnatal testosterone, they are unlikely to descend spontaneously. The American Academy of Pediatrics, Action Committee of the Urology Section (1996), issued a statement recommending orchiopexy by 1 year of age if performed by a skilled pediatric urologist or surgeon with an attendant skilled pediatric anesthesiologist. Surgical repair can be done by inguinal incision, laparoscopy, or the intraabdominal route, depending on placement of the testes.
- Hormonal therapy can be used to differentiate a retractile testis from a true cryptorchid one. Human chorionic gonadotropin (hCG) by the intramuscular route is the only approved method in the United States, although intranasal gonadotropin-releasing hormone (GnRH) is used in some countries.
- In a child younger than 1 year, regular examination to assess the position of the testes should be performed at every well-child care visit. If the testes remain undescended, referral to a pediatric urologist or surgeon should occur by 1 year of age. Referral should also occur if a retractile testis retracts following palpation.
- If undescended testes are found after 1 year of age, the child should be immediately referred to a pediatric urologist or surgeon for treatment.

Complications

Reascent, poor development, infertility, malignancy, vulnerability to trauma, testicular torsion, and inguinal hernia are possible complications.

Patient Education

Families and patients should be informed of the following:

- Histologic changes have been shown in an undescended testis as early as 6 months of age, with irreversible changes shown by 2 years of age contributing to infertility and playing a role in malignancy (Ferrer & McKenna, 2000).
- Infertility as a complication of cryptorchidism has been reported in as many as 32% to 40% of men with unilateral undescended testes and in 59% to 70% if bilateral (Ferrer & McKenna, 2000).
- Testicular malignancy in males with cryptorchidism is reported to have an incidence 4 to 10 times higher than the general population. Correction of undescended testes does not diminish the incidence of testicular cancer (Reiter & Saenger, 2002). Malignancy is more common with an intraabdominal testis. A progressive increase in the incidence of testicular tumor as the age at orchiopexy increases has been observed. A testicular neoplasm in one child mandates examination of his male siblings. Testicular self-examination should be taught to all adolescents but to these young men especially. The website for the Testicular Cancer Awareness Week (2002; available at *www.tcaw.org*) has a patient handout sheet on testicular self-examination and also provides the opportunity to sign up to receive monthly reminders to perform testicular self-examination (Fig. 35-12).
- No evidence has indicated that undescended testes resolve with puberty; retractile testes generally settle into the scrotum by puberty.
- Open discussion of the problem, management, and potential complications is essential both initially and over time.

Hydrocele

Description

A common cause of painless scrotal swelling is a *hydrocele*, a collection of serous fluid in the scrotal sac. A noncommunicating hydrocele has a collection of fluid only in the scrotum. If the processus vaginalis remains patent so that fluid moves from the abdomen to the scrotum, it is called a *communicating hydrocele* and is more likely to be associated with a hernia (Fig. 35-13).

Etiology

Incomplete closure of the processus vaginalis through which the testes descend into the scrotum allows a hydrocele to develop. Incidence is 0.5% to 2% of males, appearing primarily under 1 year of age (Adelman & Joffe, 1999; Kaplan, 2000; Schnitzer, 2002).

Clinical Findings

Hydroceles that persist beyond 1 year of age are assumed to be in conjunction with a hernia. In older children, hydroceles appear after trauma or with inflammatory illness or neoplasm.

History. The history includes the following:

- Intermittent or constant bulge or lump in the scrotum, often more distally placed. Scrotal size increases with activity and decreases with rest.
- Overlying skin may be tense.
- The hydrocele has not caused distress or vomiting.

Physical Examination. Findings include the following (Table 35-7):

In the realm of "if it ain't broke, don't fix it," there's been a substantial increase in information about prostate cancer. However, testicular cancer is the most common cancer in men ages 15-40, an age when we don't want to admit the possibility of illness. If detected early, it is among the easiest to cure. For men in this age group it is suggested a once-a-month simple self-examination. This can help catch this cancer at an early stage.

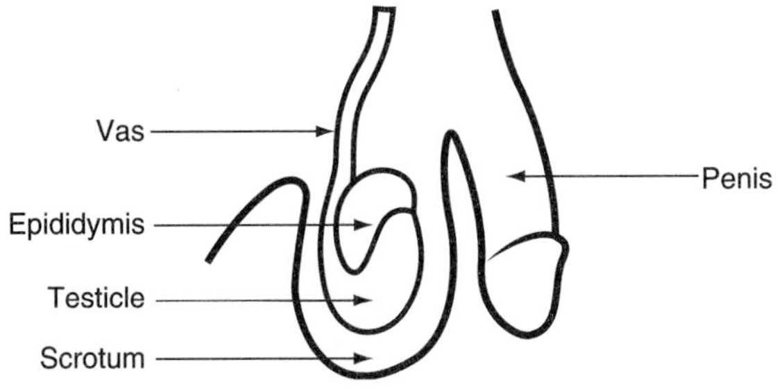

The most convenient time to examine yourself is while taking a shower or bath. The warm water causes the skin to relax, making the examination of the underlying tissues easier.

First:

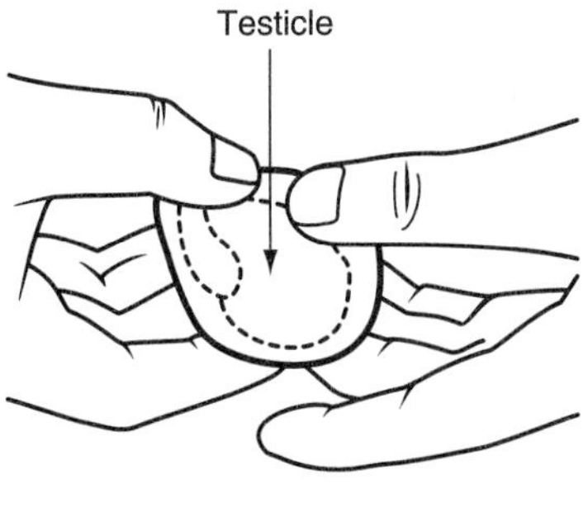

Examine your testicles. Slowly roll each testicle between thumb and forefingers. Try to find any hard, nonsensitive bumps.

Second:

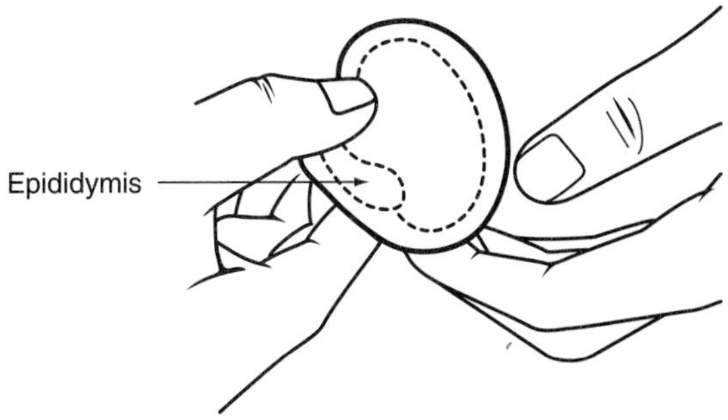

Examine the epididymis for lumps. This crescent-shaped cord is behind each testicle. This area is tender so do not be alarmed.

Third:

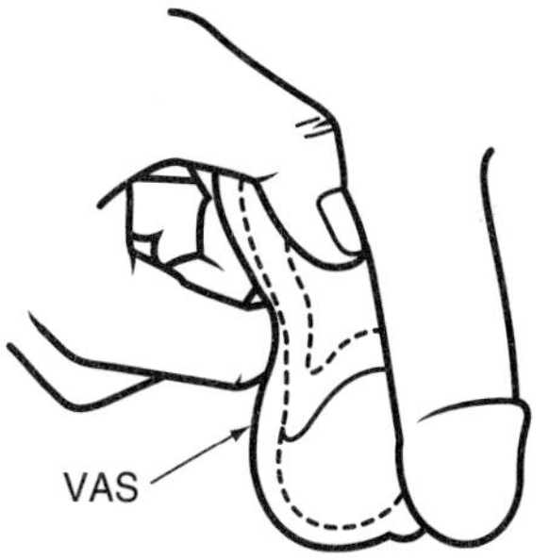

Examine the VAS, the sperm carrying tube that extends from the epididymis of each testicle.

Symptoms:
In early stages, testicular cancer may be symptomless. When symptoms do occur, they include:
- Lump on testicle, epididymis, or vas
- Enlargement of a testicle
- Heavy sensation in groin area or testicles
- Dull ache in groin or abdomen area

If you find a lump or have any of the above symptoms, see your doctor or nurse practitioner immediately for an accurate diagnosis.

FIGURE 35-12 Self-examination for testicular cancer. (From National Men's Resource Center: *Self exam for testicular cancer: "in the shower" guide*, San Anselmo, CA, 1994, The Center.)

- Asymmetry or a scrotal mass present; if swelling is present in the inguinal area, a hernia is probable
- Testes descended
- Usually unilateral swelling
- Translucent on transillumination (pink or red glow)
- Noncommunicating hydrocele—scrotal sac tense, slightly blue tinged, fluctuant, and does not reduce; no swelling in the inguinal region
- Communicating hydrocele—fluid in the scrotal sac comes and goes (probably flat in the morning, swollen later in the day)

Differential Diagnosis

Hernia, undescended testicle, retractile testicle, and inguinal lymphadenopathy are the differential diagnoses.

Management

The following steps are taken:
- Noncommunicating hydrocele—Fluid is generally absorbed spontaneously; no treatment is indicated unless the hydrocele is so large that it is uncomfortable or persists longer than 1 year.

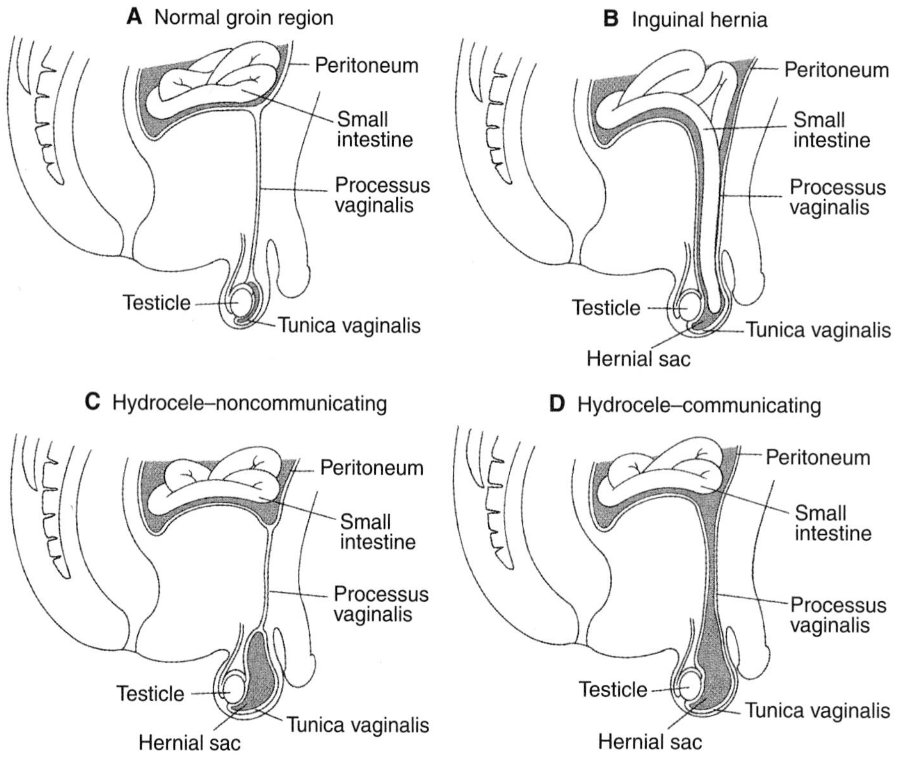

FIGURE 35-13 Hydroceles and hernias. **A**, Groin region of the normal male infant. **B**, An inguinal hernia is the protrusion of bowel into the groin region. **C**, A hydrocele is a collection of fluid within the processus vaginalis. In a noncommunicating hydrocele, the scrotal swelling does not change in size or shape because there is no connection with the abdominal cavity. **D**, In a communicating hydrocele, the processus vaginalis remains open from the scrotum to the abdominal cavity, and scrotal swelling may vary in size during the course of an infant's day. (From Betz CL, Hunsberger M, Wright S: *Family-centered nursing care of infants*, ed 2, Philadelphia, 1994, WB Saunders.)

TABLE 35-7 ***Physical Findings in Scrotal Swellings***

Condition	Tender	Red	Blue	Cremasteric Reflex	Transillumination
Chronic					
Hydrocele	−	−	+	+	+
Tumor	−	−	−	+	−
Varieocele	−	−	−	+	−
Acute					
Torsion					
Newborn	−	−	+	−	−
Other	+	+	−	−	−
Torsion of appendage	+	+	−	+	−
Epididymitis	+	+	−	+	−
Trauma	+	−	+	±	−

From Kaplan GN: Scrotal swelling in children, *Pediatr Rev* 21(9):312, 2000.

- Communicating hydrocele—Can resolve, but more likely to develop a true hernia requiring surgical repair. Refer if persistent after 1 year of age; surgical intervention is suggested.
- Surgery is usually done on an outpatient basis.

Patient Education

Reassurance is needed that the increased size of the scrotal sac will resolve, usually by 1 year of age, and involves no danger. Signs of hernia must be explained, and parents must be alerted to observe and report any abnormal findings.

Spermatocele

Description

A benign, painless scrotal mass or cyst on the head of the epididymis or testicular adnexa containing sperm is called a *spermatocele.*

Etiology and Incidence

A spermatocele is an uncommon finding, much less than 1%, but, when found, is usually in the neonatal period, late childhood, or early adolescence and peaks at 14 years (Adelman & Joffe, 1999).

Clinical Findings

History

- Scrotal swelling but asymptomatic otherwise

Physical Examination

- Painless, mobile cystic nodule usually less than 1 cm in size, superior and posterior to the testicle that transilluminates
- No change in size with the Valsalva maneuver

Differential Diagnosis

A varicocele and an epididymal cyst (identical in appearance, but not containing sperm) are the differential diagnoses.

Management

No treatment is required unless the cyst is large and painful. Refer to a urologist if needed.

Patient Education, Prevention, and Prognosis

Any pain or discomfort should be reported. Testicular self-examination would assist in early detection of this disorder.

Varicocele

Description

A varicocele is a benign enlargement or dilation of testicular veins causing a painless scrotal mass of varying size that may feel like a "bag of worms." It is usually found on the left side.

Etiology and Incidence

The etiology of varicoceles is probably multifactorial, with the physiologic changes associated with puberty playing some role. A varicocele is caused by valvular incompetence of the spermatic vein resulting in dilated or varicose veins. Varicoceles are rare before 10 years of age and may be indicative of malignancy. They occur in 5% of adolescent males and 15% of adult males (Elder, 2004). In males ages 10 to 25 years of age the weighted average is 16% (Adelman & Joffe, 2000) and as many as 20% of adolescents and young adults (Kaplan, 2000). Up to 85% to 95% arise on the left side, and 22% occur bilaterally (Pillai & Besner, 1998).

Clinical Findings

History

- Usually a painless swelling is noted in the left side of the scrotum, occasionally a "dull ache" or "heavy" feeling if large.
- Pain can occur with strenuous physical activity.
- Scrotal swelling with prolonged standing causes pain; swelling and pain resolve on reclining.

Physical Examination

- In the standing position, a "bag of worms" can be felt posterior and superior to the testis that collapses on lying and enlarges with the Valsalva maneuver.
- Measure and compare the size of both testes (length, width, and depth) using a standard orchidometer.
- Grade 3 varicoceles, the classic "bag of worms," are larger than 2 cm and easily visualized; grade 2 varicoceles are 1 to 2 cm in diameter and are easily palpable when the adolescent is standing, but not visualized; grade 1 varicoceles are the most common, very small, and difficult to palpate (the Valsalva maneuver may help).

Laboratory Studies

- Serial ultrasonography to measure testicular size every 6 to 12 months
- Ultrasonography to rule out malignancy in children younger than 10 years

Differential Diagnosis

Varicoceles must be differentiated from other testicular masses such as lipoma, hernia, hydrocele, spermatocele, and tumors.

Management

- Asymptomatic grade 1 varicoceles with normal testicular volumes usually do not require intervention in adolescence. Ultrasonographic monitoring of testicular size can be done every 6 months. Any change in comfort level should be reported.
- Referral to a surgeon or urologist should be made if the varicocele is grade 2 or 3, if the varicocele is painful, if the difference in testicular volume is marked (greater than 2 mm by ultrasound), if the varicocele is right sided or bilateral, or if testicular growth becomes retarded over a 6- to 12-month period (Adelman & Joffe, 1999; Kass, 2001).
- Treatment by spermatic vein embolization or ligation may be attempted in adolescents. Ligation is the usual procedure and has few complications; embolization is a 3-hour procedure with a high complication rate (Pillai & Besner, 1998).

Complications

Atrophy or testicular growth arrest as noted by a discrepancy in testicular size can occur. Lower fertility rates with decreased sperm concentration and motility have been noted and are factors in an aggressive surgical approach for the adolescent male with grade 2 or 3 varicocele. Hydrocele may be an insignificant complication following surgery.

Patient Education, Prevention, and Prognosis

A varicocele is the most common cause of infertility. Because of this, early identification is essential. All patients should be counseled about the long-term risks to fertility. Correction of testicular atrophy and an improved sperm count and fertility have been noted in 80% to 90% of those undergoing surgery early in adolescence. Testicular self-examination would assist in early detection of this disorder (Kass, 2001).

Inguinal Hernia

Description

A scrotal or inguinal swelling (or both) that includes abdominal contents is an inguinal hernia (see Fig. 35-12). In females, inguinal hernias cause swelling in the inguinal area and labia majora.

Etiology and Incidence

Incomplete closure of the processus vaginalis through which the testes descend into the scrotum allows the presence of abdominal contents in the inguinal canal (labia majora) or scrotum and thus the development of a hernia. Males who are obese or weight lifters or have a family history of undescended testes are at high risk for hernias (Sheldon, 2001).

Inguinal hernias are much more common in males than in females, occuring in 1% to 5% of boys (6:1). Premature infants are at increased risk (7% to 30% of males, 2% of females), with an additional 60% risk of incarceration (Schnitzer, 2002). Over 50% of hernias are diagnosed during the first year of life, with the peak incidence in the first 3 months of life. Bilateral hernias are common (10% to 20%). Unilateral hernias are more likely to occur on the right side (50% to 60%) than the left (30%) (Ingelfinger, 2002; Katz, 2001). Indirect hernias are a congenital condition and are the most common type in children younger than 3 years. Direct hernias increase in incidence after 3 years and are usually acquired.

Clinical Findings

History

- Family history of undescended testes
- Swelling in the inguinal area, scrotum, or both that comes and goes and increases with crying or straining
- Weight lifting or obesity
- Prematurity

Physical Examination. Findings include the following:

- Swelling is found in the inguinal area, scrotal area (labia majora in females), or both.
- The hernia is reducible with pressure on the distal end.
- Transillumination does not occur unless the bowel is filled with fluid.
- Direct hernias push outward through the weakest point in the abdominal wall.
- Indirect hernias push downward at an angle into the inguinal canal.
- The child is fussy and has a distended abdomen if the hernia is incarcerated.
- Silk glove sign—a sensation of two surfaces rubbing against each other while one palpates the spermatic cord as it crosses the pubic tubercle.

Laboratory Studies. An abdominal radiograph can be helpful if air is present below the inguinal ligament. Ultrasonography can differentiate a hernia from a hydrocele and is especially helpful if an incarcerated hernia is suspected.

Differential Diagnosis

Hydrocele, undescended testes (coexist in 15%), and inguinal lymphadenopathy are included in the differential diagnosis.

Management

If a child is seen with a hernia, an attempt should be made to reduce it (Katz, 2001) and the child should be referred to a surgeon or urologist for repair within 1 to 2 weeks. Even if no swelling is seen at the visit but is elicited by the history, the child should be referred to a surgeon or urologist. Inguinal hernias do not resolve spontaneously. Premature infants can be deferred until 42 weeks of gestation if the hernia is reducible. If the hernia is not easily reduced, if it is painful, or if a hard, tender, or red mass is present, refer immediately. If reduction has been difficult and ischemia is ongoing, hospitalization and surgical repair within 24 to 48 hours are indicated.

Complications

Incarceration and strangulation of a hernia cause pain, irritability, erythema, vomiting, and abdominal distention. The risk of incarceration is greater than 60% in premature infants, so repair is recommended before discharge (Schnitzer, 2002). Two thirds occur in patients younger than 1 year, and incarceration and strangulation are rare after 5 years of age (Schnitzer, 2002). Either of these conditions should be treated as a surgical emergency.

Patient Education

Because of the 40% to 60% contralateral occurrence of hernias in children, bilateral exploration is usually done at the time of surgery in infants younger than 1 year. If surgery is deferred, parents must be aware of the signs and symptoms of incarceration (tenderness, redness, crying, nausea, vomiting, abdominal distention) and be cautioned to seek immediate evaluation by a medical provider should they occur.

Testicular Masses

Description

A mass located on the testicle is most often a malignancy.

Etiology and Incidence

Testicular tumors are most common between 15 and 35 years of age but can be found anytime after 14 years. Three percent of all cancer deaths in this age-group are due to testicular cancer, affecting 1 in 10,000 teens. Bilateral tumors occur in 2% to 4% of patients (Adelman & Joffe, 1999); however, one third of all tumors are benign (Kaplan, 2000).

Clinical Findings

History

- Sensation of fullness or heaviness
- Possibly no complaints because testicular masses cause little or no pain and are often small
- Cryptorchidism, trauma, and atrophy

Physical Examination

- A hard, painless lump the size of a pea is palpated on the testis. Note the character and extension of the mass.
- The mass does not transilluminate.
- A hydrocele is present in 10% of malignancies; swelling in up to 73% of malignancies (Adelman & Joffe, 1999).
- The abdomen and supraclavicular areas should be assessed for any palpable nodes.

Laboratory Studies

- Levels of α-fetoprotein and the β-unit of hCG
- Scrotal sonography to establish the exact location of the mass and differentiate a cystic from a solid mass
- CT scan to evaluate for metastasis

Differential Diagnosis

Intratesticular masses, which are almost always malignant, must be differentiated from extratesticular masses such as hernia, varicocele, hydrocele, or spermatocele.

Management

Any child or adolescent with a testicular mass must be referred immediately for further evaluation. Treatment is dependent on the stage and type of tumor and can include orchiectomy, irradiation, and chemotherapy.

Complications

Metastasis may have occurred before the initial tumor is noticed. Pay attention to complaints about back or abdominal pain, unexplained weight loss, dypsnea (pulmonary metastases), gynecomastia, supraclavicular adenopathy, urinary obstruction, or a "heavy" or "dragging" sensation (Adelman & Joffe, 1999).

Patient Education, Prevention, and Prognosis

Early detection and therapeutic intervention can lead to a 90% survival rate. Ninety percent of relapses occur in the first 12 months after treatment. Testicular examination must not only be routinely done during physical examinations but must also be taught to adolescent males (see Fig. 35-12).

Phimosis and Paraphimosis

Description

Phimosis refers to a foreskin that is too tight to be retracted over the glans penis. Physiologic or primary phimosis occurs over the first 6 years of life when the glans has not completely separated from the epithelium (Sheldon, 2001). Pathologic or secondary phimosis occurs when the foreskin cannot be retracted after previously being retracted or after puberty. Paraphimosis is the opposite, a retracted foreskin that cannot be reduced to the normal position.

Etiology and Incidence

Phimosis can be congenital or acquired from infection and inflammation under the foreskin. Paraphimosis occurs if the foreskin does not return to its normal position after retraction. Constriction of the penis results in edema of the glans, pain, and possible necrosis. Paraphimosis is most common in adolescents and can follow masturbation, sexual abuse, or forceful retraction.

Clinical Findings

History

- May be a history of infection or inflammation of the penis
- Retraction of the foreskin with an inability to reduce it (paraphimosis)
- Pain and dysuria

Physical Examination

- Phimosis—a tight, pinpoint opening of the foreskin with minimal ability to retract the foreskin; foreskin flat and effaced
- Pathologic phimosis—thickened rolled foreskin
- Paraphimosis—edema and bluish discoloration of the glans and foreskin

Management

Management includes the following:

- Phimosis:
  - Normal cleansing with gentle stretching of the foreskin until resistance. Most foreskins are retractable by 5 years of age. Never forcefully retract the foreskin.

 - Circumcision is indicated if urinary obstruction or infection is present (Langer & Coplen, 1998). Urinary obstruction is evidenced by a ballooning of the foreskin with urination and an abnormal intermittent urinary stream.
 - Topical application of nonsteroidal antiinflammatory ointment is advocated by some (Atilla et al, 1997), a steroid cream by others (Orsola, Caffaratti, & Garat, 2000; Webster & Leonard, 2002), and EMLA cream, which allows for stretching of the prepuce and producing a retractable foreskin (Super, 2001).
- Paraphimosis:
 - A trial of ice may be done to reduce the swelling and allow reduction of the foreskin. Reduction may be accomplished by using the index and third fingers to hold the penis with gauze proximal to the foreskin and by pushing the glans penis back with the thumbs. If this technique is not successful, surgical release of the constricting band must be done to prevent necrosis of the glans.
 - Severe paraphimosis is a surgical emergency.
 - Investigation of events leading to the paraphimosis is needed to rule out sexual abuse.

Complications

Infection, urinary obstruction, and reflux can occur with phimosis. Necrosis of the penis is possible with paraphimosis.

Patient Education

A tight foreskin in uncircumcised males is normal and usually resolves by 6 years of age. It is not an indication for circumcision. The foreskin of infants and children should never be forced back.

Balanitis and Balanoposthitis

Description

Balanitis is an inflammation of the glans; balanoposthitis is an inflammation of the foreskin and glans penis occurring in males with phimosis or in uncircumcised males.

Etiology

Accumulation of debris under the foreskin, probably resulting from poor hygiene, irritates the foreskin and glans and leads to infection. Skin flora are the usual causes of infection, but gram-negative bacteria can be involved. Occasionally, trauma or allergy can be the cause (Langer & Coplen, 1998).

Clinical Findings

History. A fussy infant and pain and dysuria in an older child are reported.

Physical Examination. Edema and inflammation are found.

Management

Antibiotics, both topically and orally, as directed by the cultures along with warm soaks in the bathtub are prescribed. Depending on the swelling, topical steroids might also be prescribed (Super, 2001).

Complications

Paraphimosis can occur.

Patient Education

A review of proper hygiene and the removal of irritants is needed. Occurrence is not an indication for circumcision.

Scrotal Trauma

Description

Trauma to the scrotum most often occurs as a result of sports participation or play.

Etiology and Incidence

Direct blows to the scrotum and straddle injuries are the most common causes of trauma. In a prepubertal child, the testicle is often spared damage because of the small size and mobility of the testes. Damage can occur when the testicle is forcibly compressed against the pubic bones. Significant injury (swelling, discoloration, and tenderness) from minor trauma suggests an underlying tumor.

Clinical Findings

History

- Pain after some type of injury; older children and adolescents usually report a specific mechanism of injury, as well as time and place (Kaplan, 2000).
- Swelling and discoloration occur.

Physical Examination

- Swelling, discoloration, ecchymosis, and tenderness of the scrotum
- Transillumination may be poor if a hematoma is present

Laboratory Studies. A CT scan may be useful to differentiate the degree and type of injury.

Differential Diagnosis

Urethritis, epididymitis, orchitis, and prostatitis should all be included in the differential diagnosis. Degrees of injury include the following:

- Traumatic epididymitis—inflammation, but no infection. Pain and tenderness with scrotal erythema and edema and a tender indurated epididymis develop

within a few days after injury. UA and Doppler ultrasonographic findings are normal. The course is usually acute, but short lived.
- Intratesticular hematoma.
- Hematocele with contusion and ecchymosis of the scrotal wall with severe scrotal injury.
- Testicular torsion.

Management

- NSAIDs, cool compresses, scrotal support or elevation, and bed rest are modalities used to help relieve pain.
- An enlarging scrotum merits immediate surgical exploration, as does hematocele.

Complications

On rare occasion, testicular rupture can occur and be manifested by massive swelling and ecchymosis.

Patient Education, Prevention, and Prognosis

An athletic cup should be worn when participating in any sport in which injury could occur. A testicular hematoma should be considered cancer until proved otherwise.

Testicular Torsion

Description

Testicular torsion, a severely painful condition of acute onset in which interruption of the blood supply to the testis causes subsequent ischemic injury, results in an emergency surgical situation.

Etiology and Incidence

Normal fixation of the testis is absent, so the testis can rotate and block lymphatic and then blood flow. Torsion can occur after physical exertion or trauma or on arising.

Torsion occurs at any age but most commonly in adolescence, with a peak at 15 to 16 years (1 in 4000 males younger than 25 years and a cluster in infancy) (Adleman & Joffe, 2000; Doody & Ryan, 1999). The left side is twice as likely to be involved because of the longer spermatic cord.

Clinical Findings

History. The following may be reported:
- Unilateral pain that starts acutely and gradually and progressively worsens (the cardinal symptom); it can be scrotal or testicular and may worsen if elevated.
- Minor trauma, physical exertion, or onset of acute pain on arising is possible.
- Prior episodes of transient pain are reported in up to 50% of patients (Adelman & Joffe, 2000).
- Nausea, vomiting, or anorexia may occur.
- May be described as abdominal or inguinal pain by the embarrassed child.
- Fever is minimal or absent.

Physical Examination. Findings include the following:
- Ill-appearing and anxious male resisting movement.
- Gradual, progressive swelling of involved scrotum with redness, warmth, and tenderness.
- The ipsilateral scrotum can be edematous, erythematous, and warm.
- Testis swollen larger than opposite side, elevated, lying transversely, exquisitely painful.
- Spermatic cord thickened, twisted, and tender.
- Slight elevation of the testis increases pain (in epididymitis it relieves pain).
- Transillumination can reveal a solid mass.
- The cremasteric reflex is absent on the side with torsion.
- Neonate—hard, painless, nontransilluminating mass with edema or discolored scrotal skin.

Laboratory Studies. Potential studies to consider include
- CBC (possible elevated WBC count); probably not useful
- UA (usually normal)
- Radiographic imaging (color ultrasonography or nuclear scintigraphy) to measure intratesticular blood flow if the diagnosis is in question (Bennett et al, 2002; Kadish, 2001)

Differential Diagnosis

Torsion of the testicular or epididymal appendage, acute epididymitis (mild to moderate pain of gradual onset), orchitis, trauma (pain is better within an hour), hernia, hydrocele, and varicocele are included in the differential diagnosis.

Management

Testicular torsion is a surgical emergency, and identification with prompt surgical referral must occur immediately. If surgery is performed within 3 hours, the testicle salvage rate is 100%, the rate drops to 92% by 6 hours, 62% between 6 and 12 hours, and 38% at 12 to 24 hours (Adelman & Joffe, 2000). Occasionally, manual reduction can be performed, but surgery should follow within 6 to 12 hours to prevent retorsion, preserve fertility, and prevent abscess and atrophy. Contralateral orchiopexy may be done because of a 50% occurrence of torsion in nonfixed testes. Rest and scrotal support do not provide relief.

Complications

Testicular atrophy, abscess, or decreased fertility and loss of the testis as a result of necrosis can occur if the torsion persists more than 24 hours.

Epididymitis

Description

Epididymitis is an inflammation of the epididymis that is painful and acute.

Etiology and Incidence

Epididymitis is commonly caused by *Neisseria gonorrhoeae* or *Chlamydia trachomatis* in the sexually active adolescent, with infection already existing in the urethra or bladder. However, it can also be caused by a viral, coliform bacterial, or tubercular infection; by chemical irritation; by anomalies of the genitourinary tract; or by dysfunctional voiding (Kadish, 2001).

Epididymitis is rare before puberty except with genitourinary tract abnormalities and occurs primarily in sexually active adolescents. In children younger than 2 years, it can be secondary to urogenital anomalies.

Clinical Findings

History. The following may be reported:

- Sexual encounters within 45 days
- Painful scrotal swelling, usually gradual but can be acute in onset
- Dysuria and frequency or obstructive voiding
- Trauma (less than 50%; Kadish, 2001)
- Fever, nausea, vomiting (less than 50%; Kadish, 2001)

Physical Examination. Findings include the following:

- Scrotal edema and erythema are noted.
- The epididymis is hard, indurated, enlarged, and tender; the spermatic cord is tender.
- The testis has normal position and consistency.
- The cremasteric reflex is normal (not present in older adolescents).
- Prehn's sign—elevation of testis relieves pain (in torsion it increases pain)—can be elicited.
- Hydrocele may be present as a reaction to inflammation.
- Urethral discharge may be present, purulent in gonorrhea, and scant and watery in chlamydial infection if associated with urethritis.
- Rectal examination reveals prostate tenderness and can produce a urethral discharge.

Laboratory Studies. The following are done as indicated:

- UA (pyuria and occasional bacteria may be present) and Gram stain and culture for gonococci and chlamydia on first morning urine
- CBC (elevated WBC count)
- Urethral culture and Gram stain (nucleic acid amplification tests may be done for gonococci and chlamydia)
- Testing for other STDs if the epididymitis is due to sexual activity
- Doppler ultrasonography or radionuclide imaging to differentiate torsion of the testis
- Follow-up VCUG, ultrasonography, or both in younger children and those who deny sexual activity to rule out urogenital problems

Differential Diagnosis

The differential diagnosis includes testicular torsion of the spermatic cord or appendix testis, hernia, hydrocele, varicocele, spermatocele, trauma, tumor, or concomitant urethritis. Testicular cancer has been confused with epididymitis.

Management

Management is directed toward symptom relief and treatment of a causative organism if found. The following steps are taken:

- Bed rest, scrotal support, and elevation; apply ice packs as tolerated.
- Sitz baths and analgesics or NSAIDs are administered to relieve pain.
- Antibiotic treatment (Centers for Disease Control and Prevention, 2002):
  - First line: ceftriaxone (250 mg intramuscularly one time) plus doxycycline (100 mg twice a day for 10 days)
  - Alternative treatments: ofloxacin (300 mg twice a day for 10 days) or levofloxacin (500 mg once a day for 10 days)
- Referral to a urologist is indicated if a solitary testicle is involved, if a prompt response to treatment does not occur, or if a question about the diagnosis remains.
- Treatment of sexual partner(s) from the last 60 days is indicated if caused by an STD. Intercourse should be avoided until cured.
- If prepubertal, a sonogram and voiding cystogram are needed to rule out structural problems.
- Follow-up is needed within 3 days if no improvement is seen or if symptoms recur after treatment. Follow-up after antibiotics is recommended to ensure that no palpable mass remains.

Complications

Infertility, abscess formation, testicular infarction, and late atrophy are possible.

Patient Education

Because epididymitis is an STD, partners must be evaluated and treated. Patients must understand the sexually transmitted nature of this disease. Pain and edema usually resolve within 1 week.

RESOURCE BOX

American Association of Kidney Patients
1-800-749-2257
www.aakp.org
Newsletter, informational materials, networking, advocacy, maintain research registry

American Foundation for Urologic Disease
1128 N. Charles St.
Baltimore, MD 21201
1-410-468-1800
1-800-242-2383
Fax: 1-410-468-1808
E-mail: admin@afud.org
www.afud.org
Organization that helps the prevention and cure of urologic diseases with its research, advocacy, and education of health care professionals and the public.

IgA Nephropathy Support Network
1-215-884-9038
www.niddk.nih.gov/health/kidney/summary/iganeph/iganeph.htm
Newsletter, informational materials, networking, referrals to local resources, maintain research registry

National Institute of Diabetes and Digestive and Kidney Disease
1-301-496-3583
www.niddk.nih.gov/index.htm

National Kidney and Urologic Diseases Information Clearinghouse
9000 Rockville Pike
Baltimore, MD 20892
1-301-651-4415
1-800-891-5390
Fax: 1-301-907-8906
www.niddk.nih.gov/health/kidney/nkudic.htm

National Kidney Foundation
1-212-889-2210
1-800-622-9010
www.kidney.org
Newsletter, informational materials, referrals to local resources, local chapters, fund research

REFERENCES

Adelman WP, Joffe A: The adolescent male genital examination: what's normal and what's not, *Contemp Pediatr* 16(7):76-92, 1999.

Adelman WP, Joffe A: The adolescent with a painful scrotum, *Contemp Pediatr* 17(3):111-128, 2000.

Alon US: Renal tubular acidosis. In Finburg L, Kleinman RE, editors: *Saunders manual of pediatric practice*, ed 2, Philadephia, 2002, WB Saunders.

Al-Orifi F et al: Urine culture from bag specimens in young children: are risks too high? *J Pediatr* 137:221-226, 2000.

American Academy of Pediatrics: The diagnosis, treatment, and evaluation of the initial urinary tract infection in febrile infants and young children. In *Pediatric clinical practice guidelines and policies: a compendium of evidence-based research for pediatric practice*, ed 2, Elk Grove Village, IL, 2002, American Academy of Pediatrics.

American Academy of Pediatrics, Action Committee of the Urology Section: Timing of elective surgery of the genitalia of children with particular reference to the risks, benefits and psychological effects of surgery and anesthesia, *Pediatrics* 97:590-594, 1996.

American Academy of Pediatrics, Committee on Practice and Ambulatory Care: Recommendations for preventive pediatric health care, *Pediatrics* 105(3):645-646, 2000.

American Urological Association Practice Parameters, Guidelines and Standards Committee: *Report on the management of primary vesicoureteral reflux in children*, Baltimore, MD, 1997, American Urological Association.

Arant BS: Vesicoureteral reflux and evidence-based management, *J Pediatr* 139(5):620-621, 2002.

Atilla MK et al: A nonsurgical approach to the treatment of phimosis: local nonsteroidal anti-inflammatory ointment application, *Urology* 158:196-197, 1997.

Bender JU, Swinford RD: Hematuria and proteinuria. In Burg FD et al, editors: *Gellis and Kagan's current pediatric therapy*, ed 17, Philadelphia, 2002, WB Saunders.

Bennett S et al: Ultrasound findings as predictors of clinical outcomes in the acute scrotum (abstract 427). Program and abstracts of the American Urological Association 97th Annual Meeting in Orlando, FL, May 25-30, 2002.

Betz CL, Hunsberger M, Wright S: *Family-centered nursing care of children*, Philadelphia, 1994, WB Saunders.

Blake DR, Woods ER: The future is here: noninvasive diagnosis of STDs, *Contemp Pediatr* 18(2):71-87, 2001.

Blowey DL: Acute glomerulonephritis. In Finburg L, Kleinman RE, editors: *Saunders manual of pediatric practice*, ed 2, Philadephia, 2002, WB Saunders.

Boineau FG, Lewy JE: Evaluation of hematuria in children and adolescents, *Pediatr Rev* 11(4):101-107, 1989.

Boschert S: Undescended testis may decrease fertility later, *Pediatr News*, Feb 7, 1998.

Bright Futures: guidelines for health supervision of infants, children and adolescents, ed 2, revised, Arlington, VA, 2000-2002, National Center for Education in Maternal and Child Health.

Bukowski TP, Zeman PA: Hypospadias: of concern but correctable, *Contemp Pediatr* 18(2):89-109, 2001.

Burg FD et al, editors: *Gellis and Kagan's current pediatric therapy*, ed 17, Philadelphia, 2002, WB Saunders.

Callaghan P: Undescended testis, *Pediatr Rev* 21(11):395, 2000.

Capozza N, Caione P: Dextranomer/hyaluronic acid copolymer implantation for vesico-ureteral reflux: a randomized comparison with antibiotic prophylaxis, *J Pediatr* 140(2):230-234, 2002.

Cascio S, Colhoun E, Puri P: Bacterial colonization of the prepuce in boys with vesicoureteral reflux who receive antibiotic prophylaxis, *J Pediatr* 139(1):160-162, 2001.

Centers for Disease Control and Prevention: 2002 guidelines for the treatment of sexually transmitted diseases, *Morb Mortal Wkly Rep* 51(RR-6), May 10, 2002. Available at *www.cdc.gov/std/treatment/default.htm* (accessed Sept 30, 2002).

Chan KM, Scheinman JI, Roth KS: Renal tubular acidosis, *Pediatr Rev* 22(8):277-286, 2001.

Chon CH, Lai FC, Dairiki LM: Pediatric urinary tract infections, *Pediatr Clin North Am* 48(6):1441-1460, 2001.

Constantinescu AR, Satlin LM: Renal tubulopathies. In Burg FD et al, editors: *Gellis and Kagan's current pediatric therapy*, ed 17, Philadelphia, 2002, WB Saunders.

D'Angio GJ et al: Treatment of Wilms' tumor: results of the Third National Wilms' Tumor Study, *Cancer* 64(2):349-360, 1989.

Decter RM: Vesicoureteral reflux, *Pediatr Rev* 22(6):205-209, 2001.

Dell KM, Avner ED: Tubular disorders. In Behrman RE, Kliegman RM, Jensen HB, editors: *Nelson textbook of pediatrics*, ed 17, Philadelphia, 2004, WB Saunders.

Dershewitz RA, editor: *Ambulatory pediatric care*, ed 3, Philadelphia, 1999, JB Lippincott.

Doody EP, Ryan DP: Genital pain. In Dershewitz RA, editor: *Ambulatory pediatric care*, ed 3, Philadelphia, 1999, JB Lippincott.

Elder JS: Urinary tract infections. In Behrman RE, Kliegman RM, Jensen HB, editors: *Nelson textbook of pediatrics*, ed 17, Philadelphia, 2004, WB Saunders.

Elenberg E, Travis LB: Urinary tract infection and perinephric/intranephric abscess. In Burg FD et al, editors: *Gellis and Kagan's current pediatric therapy*, ed 17, Philadelphia, 2002, WB Saunders.

Ferguson WS: Visceral tumors. In Burg FD et al, editors: *Gellis and Kagan's current pediatric therapy*, ed 17, Philadelphia, 2002, WB Saunders.

Ferrer FA, McKenna PH: Current approaches to the undescended testicle, *Contemp Pediatr* 17(1):106-111, 2000.

Finberg L, Kleinman RE: *Saunders manual of pediatric practice*, ed 2, Philadelphia, 2002, WB Saunders.

Fouser L: Familial nephritis/Alport syndrome, *Pediatr Rev* 19(8):265-267, 1998.

Friedman AL: Nephrology: fluids and electrolytes. In Behrman RE, Kliegman RM, editors: *Nelson essentials of pediatrics*, Philadelphia, 2002, WB Saunders.

Gallo AM, Schmeissing K, Langman CB: Think of genetic hypercalciuria when a child has urinary tract findings, *J Pediatr Health Care* 13(1):7-11, 1999.

Graff SL: *A handbook of routine urinalysis*, Philadelphia, 1983, JB Lippincott.

Heldrich FJ: UTI diagnosis: getting it right the first time, *Contemp Pediatr* 12(2):110-133, 1995.

Hogg R et al: Recognizing and treating the nephrotic syndrome: avoid unnecessary delays, *Contemp Pediatr* 17(11):84-93, 2000.

Hussain N et al: Hypospadias and early gestation growth restriction in infants, *Pediatrics* 109(3):473-478, 2002.

Ingelfinger JR: Disorders of the bladder and urethra, ureter and collecting system. In Burg FD et al, editors: *Gellis and Kagan's current pediatric therapy*, ed 17, Philadelphia, 2002, WB Saunders.

Johnson CE: New advances in childhood urinary tract infections, *Pediatr Rev* 20(10):335-342, 1999.

Kadish H: Painful subject: pinpointing the cause of acute scrotal swelling, *Contemp Pediatr* 18(5):95-101, 2001.

Kaplan GW: Scrotal swelling in children, *Pediatr Rev* 21(9):311-314, 2000.

Kass EJ: Adolescent varicocele, *Pediatr Clin North Am* 48(6):1559-1570, 2001.

Katz DA: Evaluation and management of inguinal and umbilical hernias, *Pediatr Ann* 30(12):729-735, 2001.

Kraus SJ: Genitourinary imaging in children, *Pediatr Clin North Am* 48(6):1381-1424, 2001.

Kurzrock EA: Hypospadias. In Behrman RE, Kliegman RM, editors: *Nelson essentials of pediatrics*, Philadelphia, 2002, WB Saunders.

Langer JC, Coplen DE: Circumcision and pediatric disorders of the penis, *Pediatr Clin North Am* 45:801-812, 1998.

Langman CBL: Hematuria and proteinuria. In Dershewitz RA, editor: *Ambulatory pediatric care*, ed 3, Philadelphia, 1999, JB Lippincott.

Larcombe J: Urinary tract infection, *Clinical Evidence*, June 2002, pp 65-67.

Liao JC, Churchill BM: Pediatric urine testing, *Pediatr Clin North Am* 48(6):1425-1440, 2001.

Lum GM: Kidney and urinary tract. In Hay WW et al, editors: *Current pediatric diagnosis and treatment*, New York, 2003, McGraw-Hill.

Mahant S, To T, Friedman J: Timing of voiding cystourethrogram in the investigation of urinary tract infections in children, *Pediatrics* 139(4):568-571, 2001.

Mevorach R et al: Endoscopic treatment of vesicoureteral reflux with copatite: the first 50 patients (abstract 429). Program and abstracts of the American Urological Association 97th Annual Meeting in Orlando, FL, May 25-30, 2002.

Nachman JB, Abelson HT: Wilms tumor. In Behrman RE, Kliegman RM, editors: *Nelson essentials of pediatrics*, ed 4, Philadelphia, 2002, WB Saunders.

Newman TB et al: Urine testing and urinary tract infections in febrile infants seen in office settings, *Arch Pediatr Adolesc Med* 156(1):44-54, 2002.

Opas LM: UTI: burning issues (unpublished manuscript), Los Angeles, 1999.

Orsola A, Caffaratti J, Garat JM: Conservative treatment of phimosis in children using a topical steroid, *Urology* 56(2):307-310, 2000.

Patel HP, Bissler JJ: Hematuria in children, *Pediatr Clin North Am* 48(6):1519-1538, 2001.

Patterson LT, Strife CF: Acquired versus congenital renal scarring after urinary tract infection, *J Pediatr* 136(1):2-4, 2000.

Pillai SB, Besner GE: Pediatric testicular problems, *Pediatr Clin North Am* 45:813-830, 1998.

Plachter NB, Schulman SL, Canning DA: Identification and management of urinary tract infection in the preschool child, *J Pediatr Health Care* 13(6):268-272, 1999.

Ransley R: Intrarenal reflux: anatomical, dynamic and radiological studies—part I, *Urol Res* 5(2):61-69, 1977.

Reiter EO, Saenger PH: Undescended testes. In Finberg L, Kleinman RE: *Saunders manual of pediatric practice*, ed 2, Philadelphia, 2002, WB Saunders.

Ruley EJ: Hematuria. In Hoekelman RA et al, editors: *Pediatric primary care*, ed 4, St Louis, 2001a, Mosby.

Ruley EJ: Proteinuria. In Hoekelman RA et al, editors: *Pediatric primary care*, ed 4, St Louis, 2001b, Mosby.

Schnitzer JJ: Hernias and hydroceles. In Burg FD et al, editors: *Gellis and Kagan's current pediatric therapy*, ed 17, Philadelphia, 2002, WB Saunders.

Schöen EJ, Colby CJ, Ray GT: Newborn circumcision decreases incidence and costs of urinary tract infection during the first year of life, *Pediatrics* 105(4):789-793, 2000.

Sheldon CA: The pediatric genitourinary examination: inguinal, urethral and genital diseases, *Pediatr Clin North Am* 48(6):1339-1380, 2001.

Smellie JM et al: Outcome at 10 years of severe vesicoureteric reflux managed medically: report of the international reflux study in children, *Pediatrics* 139(5):656-663, 2001.

Sparrow MM: Nephrology. In Gunn VL, editor, Johns Hopkins Hospital: *The Harriet Lane handbook*, ed 16, St Louis, 2002, Mosby.

Steinhurz PG: Wilms tumor. In Finburg L, Kleinman RE, editors: *Saunders manual of pediatric practice*, ed 2, Philadephia, 2002, WB Saunders.

Sugunendran H et al: Comparison of urine, first and second endourethral swabs for PCR based detection of genital *Chlamydia trachomatis* infection in male patients, *Sex Transm Infect* 77(6):423-426, 2001.

Super DM: Phimosis. In Hoekelman RA et al, editors: *Pediatric primary care*, ed 4, St Louis, 2001, Mosby.

Testicular Cancer Awareness Week: Available at *www.tcaw.org/issues/getagrip.html* (accessed Sept 30, 2002).

Tran D, Muchant DG, Aronoff SC: Short-course versus conventional length antimicrobial therapy for uncomplicated lower urinary tract infections in children: a meta-analysis of 1279 patients, *J Pediatr* 139(1):93-99, 2001.

US Preventive Health Services Task Force: *Guide to clinical preventive services*, 2002. Available at *www.ahrq.gov/clinic/cps3dix.htm* (accessed Dec 2003).

US Public Health Service: Recommendations. Available at *www.ahrq.gov/clinic/prevenix.htm* (accessed Dec 2003).

Varade WS: Nephrotic syndrome. In Hoekelman RA et al, editors: *Pediatric primary care*, ed 4, St Louis, 2001, Mosby.

Vogt BA: Identifying kidney disease: simple steps can make a difference, *Contemp Pediatr* 14(3):115-127, 1997.

Warshaw BL: Nephrotic syndrome in children, *Pediatr Ann* 23(9):495-504, 1994.

Webster TM, Leonard MP: Topical steroid therapy for phimosis, *Can J Urol* 9(2):1492-1495, 2002.

Williams G, Lee A, Craig J: Antibiotics for the prevention of urinary tract infection in children: a systematic review of randomized controlled trials, *J Pediatr* 138(6):868-874, 2001.

Woodhead JC: Urinary tract infections. In Dershewitz RA, editor: *Ambulatory pediatric care*, ed 3, Philadelphia, 1999, JB Lippincott.

36 Gynecologic Conditions

Linda M. Kollar, Nancy Barber Starr

Gynecologic concerns or problems in the child or adolescent provide the nurse practitioner (NP) varied and interesting challenges regarding health and medical matters, as well as psychosocial interventions. Sensitivity and comfort with these issues aid the NP in working with the child or adolescent and the parent. Educating children and adolescents about their bodies as they mature is essential. Approaching issues that may be considered personal or embarrassing openly and directly allows more comprehensive care and anticipatory guidance. Establishing and maintaining a good relationship with both parents and adolescents helps ease the transition during which adolescents take an increasingly larger role in determining their own care.

Gynecologic issues range from normal transitions that may be perceived as abnormal to serious systemic diseases or abnormalities. The practitioner is required to have a high level of suspicion in all cases in order not to miss any significant signs. At the same time, most conditions are normal and can be easily addressed, reassuring the child or adolescent that all is well and that her body is developing normally.

STANDARDS OF CARE

One of the goals of *Healthy Children 2010: National Health Promotion and Disease Prevention Objectives for the Year 2010* (U.S. Department of Health and Human Services, 2003) (see Appendix D) is "a society where Healthy sexual relationships, free of infection as well as coercion and unintended pregnancy are the norm." The *Guide to Clinical Preventive Services*, third edition (U.S. Preventive Services Task Force, 2003), recommends screening for syphilis in endemic areas (all pregnant women and persons at increased risk of infection) and for asymptomatic infection with *Chlamydia trachomatis* (all sexually active female adolescents, high-risk pregnant women, and other asymptomatic women at high risk of infection). Routine screening for genital herpes simplex virus (HSV) infection is not recommended. Further recommendations include counseling all adolescent patients about risk factors for infection with human immunodeficiency virus (HIV) and other sexually transmitted diseases (STDs) and offering testing for syphilis, gonorrhea, hepatitis B, HIV, and chlamydia infection.

The American Academy of Pediatrics, the American Nurses Association, and the American Medical Association (AMA) *Guidelines for Adolescent Preventive Services (GAPS)* recommends as a routine part of health supervision that adolescents (both male and female) be asked annually about sexual health behavior (Elster & Kuznets, 1994). Sexually active adolescents should have an annual Papanicolaou (Pap) smear and be screened for STDs. Adolescents who have reached 18 years of age, have vaginal symptoms, have been exposed to human papillomavirus (HPV), or engage in high-risk behaviors should also have an annual vaginal examination and Pap smear. Adolescents should receive counseling about responsible sexual behavior, including using contraception and condoms to prevent pregnancy and infection with STDs and HIV, abstention from intercourse as the surest way to prevent STDs and pregnancy, and the benefit of postponing future sexual relationships. Providers should be involved in making these objectives a major priority within community health practice, with a special emphasis in school health settings and school-based clinics (Elster & Kuznets, 1994; U.S. Public Health Service, 2003).

ANATOMY AND PHYSIOLOGY

During the first 8 weeks of gestation, male and female fetuses are sexually undifferentiated, both having one pair of gonads and a pair of ducts. At 8 weeks, the male gonad produces testosterone and antimüllerian hormone (AMH), which causes the gonads to become testes and the tubules to become the vas deferens. In the female, the gonads do not produce testosterone or AMH, so ovaries are formed from the gonads, and the ducts become the uterus and fallopian tubes. External genital structures are also undifferentiated until 8 weeks of gestation, at which time the presence or lack of testosterone causes the external genitalia to develop as either male or female. By 9 months of gestation, all internal and external genital structures are present.

In utero, maternal estrogen thickens and enlarges the genital structures. After birth, maternal hormones are withdrawn resulting in the desquamation of the hypertrophic walls of the uterus. The mucus from the cervix results in the physiologic leukorrhea of the newborn period. As the hormonal influences continue to decrease, the endometrial shedding is often accompanied by bleeding.

Between 8 weeks and 7 years of age, without maternal or endogenous estrogens, the labia majora are flat, the labia minora are thin, and neither offer protection to the genitalia. The absence of fat pads results in open labia whenever the child is in the squatting position. In addition, this thin atrophic genital epithelium is readily traumatized.

Between 6 and 8 years of age, sexual maturation is triggered by the presence of adrenal androgens and then estrogen in females and testosterone in males. In the female, this causes labial thickening and enlargement and sometimes a physiologic leukorrhea. The ovaries contain the lifetime number of immature ova at birth, with the ova maturing generally one per cycle from puberty to menopause. In the male, the production of sperm by the testes begins and continues throughout the life span.

The structure and function of the reproductive system are controlled by the hypothalamic-pituitary-ovarian (HPO) axis (also called the hypothalmic-pituitary-gonadal axis). This complex process begins in the neurologic system (the hypothalamus), involves the endocrine system (the anterior pituitary), and completes its cycle with the gonads (ovaries or testes). The hypothalamus releases gonadotropin-releasing hormone, which stimulates the anterior pituitary to release the gonadotropins, luteinizing hormone (LH), and follicle-stimulating hormone (FSH). These, in turn, stimulate the gonads to release the sex hormones. See Figs. 9-3 and 9-4 and Chapter 9 for a discussion of Tanner staging. Initially, this cycle causes sexual maturation, and, once that is completed, the ongoing release of hormones controls the menstrual cycle, pregnancy, and lactation. The primary female hormones are estrogen and progesterone, with small amounts of androgens (Fig. 36-1).

PATHOPHYSIOLOGY AND DEFENSE MECHANISMS

Pathophysiology

The primary disorders of the gynecologic system can be classified as menstrual cycle disorders, inflammatory reactions, infection, and reproductive problems.

Menstrual Cycle Disorders

Pubertal development is a complex but normal process. Adolescents may be seen with common menstrual problems such as mittelschmerz or dysmenorrhea. Abnormal uterine bleeding, endometriosis, and amenorrhea are three less common disorders that require the NP to differentiate normal growth and developmental variations from systemic disorders or disease (especially neurologic, endocrine, and reproductive problems). The female athlete is especially prone to exercise-related menstrual problems.

Inflammatory Reactions

An inflammatory response can occur in either the external or internal genitalia. Local reactions involve the external genitalia and can be caused by dermatologic disorders or skin irritation from such factors as normal leukorrhea, chemical or allergic reactions, or nonspecific causes. Internal inflammation caused by infection is not always obvious.

Infections

The warm, moist environment of the reproductive tract provides an ideal place for infection. Viral pathogens, such as HSV and HPV, or fungal infection can manifest as a vulvitis or vaginal infection. *Trichomonas*, a protozoan infection, colonizes the vaginal vault. By contrast, bacterial infections caused by chlamydia and gonorrhea ascend into the upper genital tract where pelvic inflammatory disease (PID) or tubal damage can occur.

Reproductive Problems

Reproductive problems occur as a result of structural, hormonal, or endocrine disorders or as sequelae of infection. Refer to an obstetric text for further information.

Defense Mechanisms

The gynecologic system has both anatomic and physiologic defense mechanisms. The labia majora and the pubic hair provide a barrier that serves as the first line of defense. The vagina, serving as an exit for mucosal secretion, menstrual

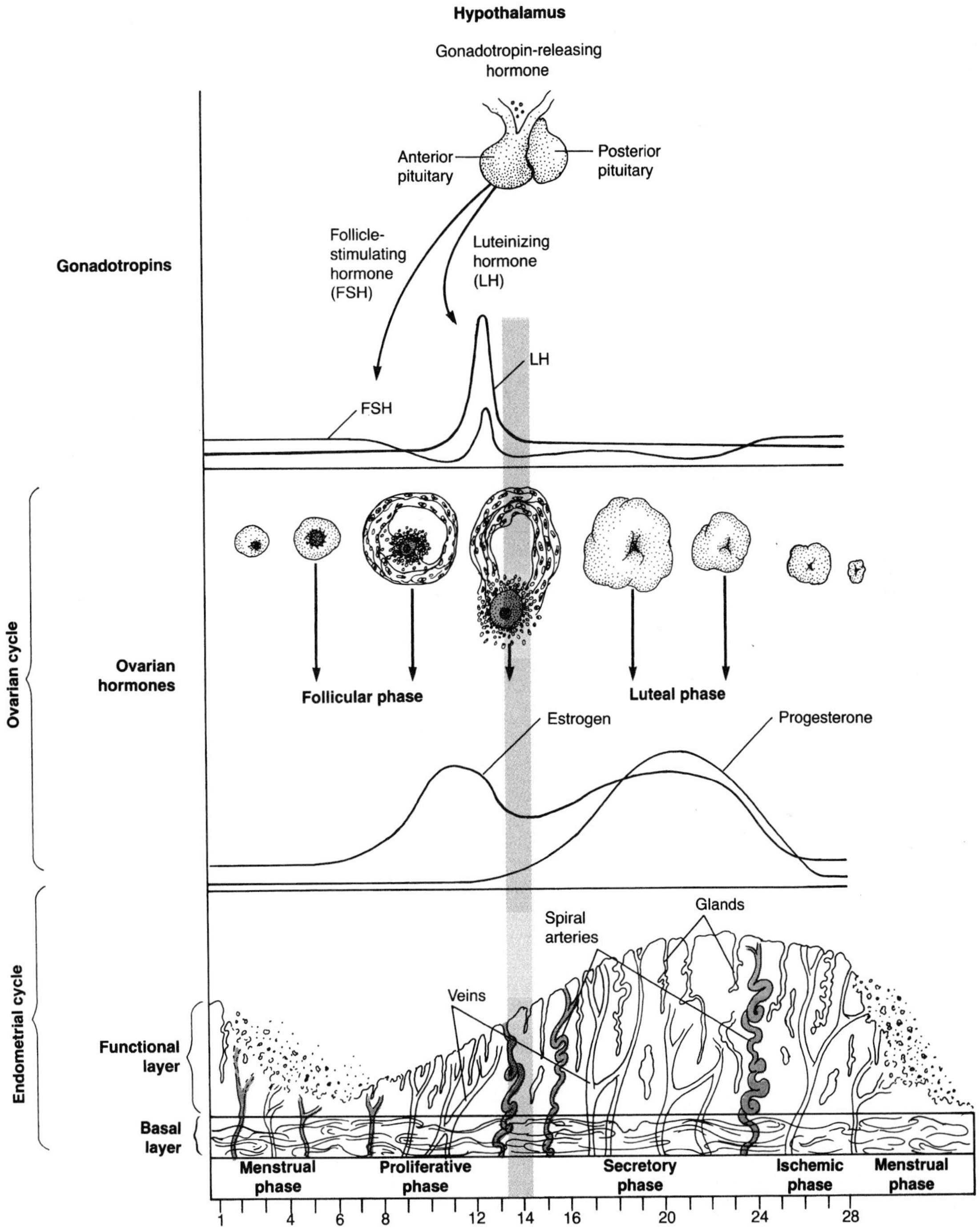

FIGURE 36-1 Female reproductive cycle showing changes in hormone secretion and in the ovary, and the uterine endometrium. (From Gorrie T, McKinney E, Murray S: *Foundations of maternal newborn nursing*, ed 2, Philadelphia, 1998, WB Saunders.)

fluids, and products of conception, also provides a means of defense with its natural downward and outward flow of secretions.

Additionally, with increasing estrogen exposure, the vaginal epithelial tissue thickens and an acid pH develops, discouraging infection. The small external cervical os, a thick mucous plug, and the downward flow of cervical secretions provide barriers to entry to the uterus. A chemical barrier is also established by the cervical enzymes and antibodies.

ASSESSMENT OF THE GYNECOLOGIC SYSTEM

History

The history includes assessment of the following:

- Family history: maternal age at menarche; dysmenorrhea or endometriosis; diabetes mellitus; thyroid, bleeding, and clotting disorders; malignancy; genetic disorders
- Pubertal development: age at breast and pubic hair development; menstrual history: age at menarche, length of cycles, longest and shortest interval between menses, duration of flow, estimated blood loss, last normal menstrual period, dysmenorrhea, knowledge about pubertal development
- Vaginal discharge or bleeding, onset, duration, presence of odor or itching, abdominal pain, urinary symptoms, hygiene habits, use of douche, use of sanitary pads or tampons, bubble bath
- Sexual history: sexual activity (voluntary or forced); type of activity (oral, vaginal, anal, and heterosexual, homosexual, bisexual); age at first intercourse, number of sexual partners in previous 60 days, 12 months, lifetime; exposures to infection; previous infections; previous STDs, last Pap test, history of abnormal Pap test, knowledge about sexuality and discussions with parent/guardian (see Chapter 20)
- Contraceptive history: type, duration, and frequency of use, problems and satisfaction
- Obstetric history, as appropriate
- Review of systems: general health, growth, stressors, medications, substance use, urinary, gastrointestinal, endocrine and dermatologic

All adolescents should be separated from their parent/guardian for the sexual and social history. A discussion of confidentiality with both the guardian and the adolescent should precede the history.

Physical Examination

When a child or adolescent has gynecologic complaints, a complete physical examination is still required. When a gynecologic examination is performed, the child or adolescent should maintain a feeling of being in control. It is important to establish rapport, preserve modesty, and obtain consent to examine. Give the adolescent as many choices as possible in the situation, whether she would like someone else in the room with her, position of the table, use of a hand mirror to observe, and when possible, the timing of the examination. This requires flexibility and time from the care provider but demonstrates respect for the adolescent (Hennigen, Kollar, & Rosenthal, 2000).

Prepubertal Child

There are a variety of positions in which to examine the vulva, vestibule, and lower vagina of a prepubescent girl. Lying on a table, supine, with feet together and knees out ("frog-legged") is generally the most comfortable for patients and provides ease of examination and obtaining of cultures, if necessary. Another alternative is sitting up in the parent's lap with feet and knees frog-legged. Putting the parent on the examination table with feet in the stirrups and the child on his or her lap with feet to the outside of the parent's legs is another alternative. If examination of the entire vagina is necessary, putting the child in knee-chest position on the examination table is the best position for noninvasive, internal examination of the vulva, vagina, and possibly the cervix.

Examine or note the following:

- Breasts, abdomen, and inguinal area
- Presence and distribution of pubic hair
- Presence and distribution of body hair: face, chest, back, abdomen, legs, arms
- Presence of psoriasis or seborrhea
- State of hygiene
- Size of clitoris (approximately 3 × 3 mm prepubertal)
- Signs of estrogenization (pubertal vaginal mucosa—moist, thin, and red; postpubertal vaginal mucosa—moist and dull pink)
- Sexual maturity rating (SMR) or Tanner staging (see Chapters 9 and 20 and Figs. 9-3 and 9-4)
- Anus for cleanliness, excoriation, or erythema

The hymen, normally smooth and continuous, can be described as crescent shaped, annular, or redundant (Fig. 36-2). The significance of the diameter of the hymenal opening as a diagnostic finding is debated. Both transverse and anterior-posterior diameter are dependent on age, relaxation, method of examination, and type of hymen. In general, the older and more relaxed the child, the larger the opening. It is also larger with retraction and in the knee-chest position. In the 3- to 6-year-old, a range of normal findings for the transverse diameter is 1 to 6 mm and for the anterior-posterior diameter 1 to 7 mm. Obesity in young children is associated with hymenal openings larger than average for age (e.g., a 2-year-old with a 4 mm opening when average is 2 mm).

Adolescent

- Inspect the skin for acne.
- Examine the breasts; note Tanner stage.
- Palpate the thyroid.
- Inspect hair distribution on face, chest, back, arms, legs, and abdomen.
- Inspect the external genitalia and determine Tanner stage.

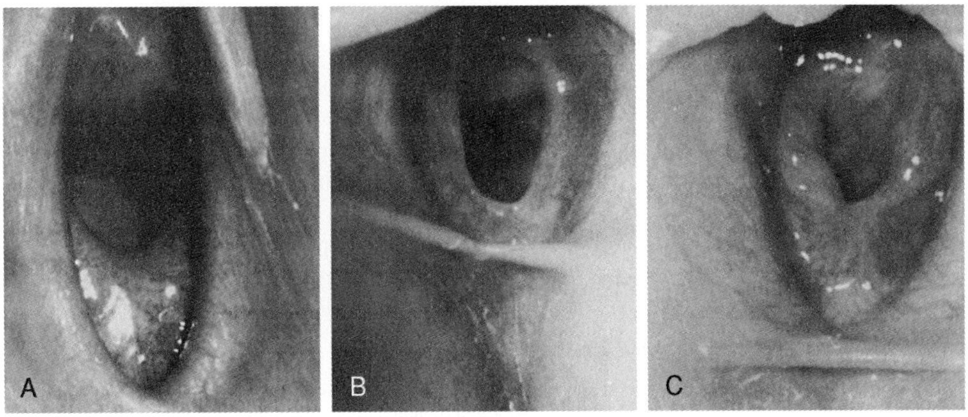

FIGURE 36-2 Types of hymens, photographed through a colposcope. **A**, Crescentic hymen. **B**, Annular hymen. **C**, Redundant hymen with crescent appearance after retraction. (From Emans S, Laufer M, Goldstein D: *Pediatric and adolescent gynecology*, ed 4, Philadelphia, 1998, Lippincott-Raven.)

- Vaginal examination alone may be adequate to assess for irregular bleeding, severe dysmenorrhea, vaginal discharge, and amenorrhea. However, an internal examination and a bimanual examination may be necessary based on symptoms and history.

Diagnostic Studies

Routine care of the child and adolescent without gynecologic complaints does not require any diagnostic studies.

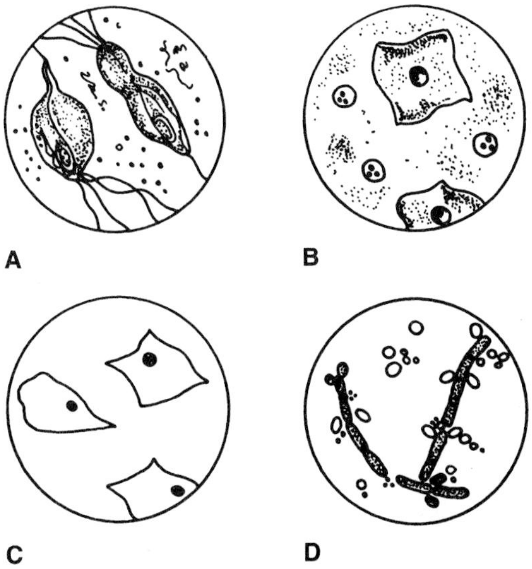

FIGURE 36-3 Fresh vaginal smear showing **A**, *Trichomonas;* **B**, clue cells of bacterial vaginosis; **C**, leukorrhea; **D**, *Candida.* **A, B**, and **C** are saline preparations; **D** is a potassium hydroxide (KOH) preparation. (From Emans S, Laufer M, Goldstein D: *Pediatric and adolescent gynecology*, ed 4, Philadelphia, 1998, Lippincott-Raven.)

Cervical cancer screening with Pap testing should begin approximately 3 years after the young woman has initiated sexual intercourse and no later than 21 years of age (Saslow et al, 2002).

The following studies can be helpful as diagnostic tools. Specific studies and techniques are discussed with each diagnosis. Collection of specimens must be done with care. Techniques that are helpful include using a small amount of saline as a vaginal wash, using a soft plastic eyedropper or feeding tube, or using a moistened cotton swab.

- Web preps. A saline slide of secretions for microscopic examination (Fig. 36-3). Adding potassium hydroxide (KOH) can cause a fishy odor (positive whiff test) in the presence of certain bacteria.
- pH of vaginal mucus (neutral in prepubescent; less than 4.5 once pubertal) and/or Gram's stain
- Rapid detection tests, cultures, serologic blood tests, and Pap smears (sexually transmitted diseases)
- Other tests including pregnancy test by urine or serum, Biggy agar culture (suspected yeast infection), ultrasound

MANAGEMENT STRATEGIES

Anticipatory Guidance

Anticipatory guidance related to gynecologic issues is important to both the child/adolescent and parents. Good genital hygiene can help avoid some potential problems. The transition to puberty and establishment of menses may be eased with appropriate education. With the advent of puberty and the increasing interest in sexuality, much guidance is needed before initiation of sexual activity. Guidance should continue as the teenager contemplates or initiates sexual activity. See Chapters 9 and 20 for further discussion of these topics.

Counseling and Education

Counseling and education related to disorders of the gynecologic system need to be tailored to the child or adolescent and the parents. Confidentiality is a matter to be established with both the parents and the adolescent. Some states have specific laws that allow the NP to treat for obstetric and family planning conditions in adolescents without parental knowledge or consent. Additional team members can be involved, depending on the diagnosis. Coordination, interpretation, and follow-up of these details are important tasks. The resources in the box at the end of the chapter offer the NP additional information.

SPECIFIC GYNECOLOGIC PROBLEMS OF CHILDREN AND ADOLESCENTS

Labial Adhesions

Description

The fusion of tissue between the labia minora that appears to cover the vaginal opening is a common, benign condition in infants and prepubertal girls. It is also called agglutination, synechia vulvae, or vulvar adhesion if only the lower half of the labia minora is involved (Fig. 36-4).

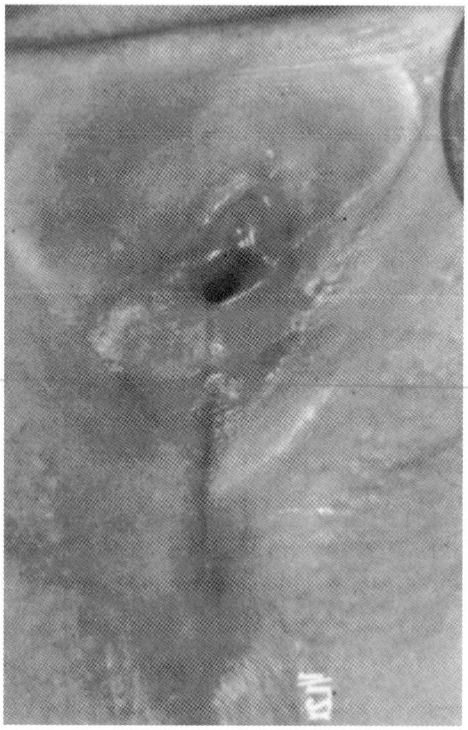

FIGURE 36-4 Labial adhesions that are thinned and almost translucent inferiorly following topical estrogen therapy. (From Craighill MC: Pediatric and adolescent gynecology for primary care pediatricians, *Pediatr Clin North Am* 45:1668, 1998.)

Etiology and Incidence

Before puberty, the vaginal tissues are in a hypoestrogenized state and are prone to inflammation and denudation. As the tissues heal, adhesion of the labia occurs. Mechanisms for the initial insult are irritation, infection, and trauma. The most common precipitant is an asymptomatic, nonspecific vulvovaginitis caused by poor hygiene. There is debate about whether lack of hygiene, masturbation, fondling, and subsequent irritation from sexual abuse are potential causes in older females. Labial adhesions occur primarily in girls 3 months to 6 years of age but can persist until puberty (Emans, Laufer, & Goldstein, 1998).

Clinical Findings

History. The history can include the following:

- Concern about rash in genital area
- Parental concern about vaginal opening
- Dysuria, difficult voiding, or local discomfort

Physical Examination. Physical examination reveals a thin, flat membrane of varying length from the posterior fourchette to the clitoris. The degree of opening near the clitoris varies. The vulva appears flat with a central line of fusion. The urethra may or may not be visualized, and there may be urinary dribbling.

Differential Diagnosis

Scarring, imperforate hymen, clitoral hypertrophy, and intersex problems are the differential diagnosis.

Management

The treatment of labial adhesions is somewhat controversial; Table 36-1 outlines steps that are generally accepted. In asymptomatic labial adhesions, observation is often the best treatment. The presence of symptoms of urinary tract infection, pain with activity, and change in behavior dictates treatment (Bacon, 2002). Forceful separation is always contraindicated because it may result in both trauma to the child and recurrence of adhesions.

Complications

Urinary tract infections and readhesion following mechanical lysis can occur.

Patient Education

Premarin cream can cause breast tenderness and transient enlargement and vulvar pigmentation or erythema, which resolves with discontinuation of the cream. The incidence of recurrence can be decreased with careful attention to perineal hygiene and the daily application of A and D ointment until puberty.

TABLE 36-1 *Treatment of Labial Adhesions*

Degree of Involvement	Treatment	Prognosis
No urinary tract infection, no obstruction, no parental concern.	No treatment. Reassure and observe.	Resolution with puberty and estrogenization of tissue.
Opening ensures urinary and vaginal drainage, but treatment desired.	Apply ointment (e.g., A and D or Vaseline) nightly with cotton-tipped swab with gentle pressure. Following separation, maintain good hygiene and mild ointment (e.g., Vaseline) nightly for 6-12 mo.	Separation within 8 wk. If not, double check technique to ensure gentle pressure is being applied. If persists, see use of estrogen cream below.
Urinary and vaginal drainage impaired.	Apply estrogen-containing 1% cream (e.g., Premarin) qd or bid for 2-3 wk with cotton-tipped swab. Use gentle pressure until separation occurs. Following separation, use Vaseline nightly as outlined above. Alternative treatment is to use transdermal estrogen patch (Climara or FemPatch [change weekly], Alora or Vivelle [change twice a week], or Estraderm [cannot be cut]). Other patches may be cut to alter dosage. Apply near labial adhesions. Continue use for 1 mo following separation (Craighill, 1998).	Separation usually occurs within 8 wk (80%-90%) (Emans, Laufer, & Goldstein, 1998). If not, check technique to ensure pressure is being applied. If unresponsive, may treat with 5% Xylocaine ointment or EMLA cream and gentle teasing of adhesions with a swab. Always avoid forceful separation.

Mittelschmerz

Description

Pelvic pain that occurs at the time of ovulation, midway between menstrual periods, is referred to as *mittelschmerz* (middle pain) (Table 36-2).

Etiology and Incidence

See Table 36-2 for etiology. Incidence is unknown, although some ultrasonographic studies have detected normal follicular fluid in 40% of normal women's midmenstrual cycle that is probably from follicular cyst rupture (Emans, Laufer, & Goldstein, 1998).

Clinical Findings

History

- See Table 36-2
- Recurrent discomfort at same time in each cycle
- Pain occasionally severe and crampy, persisting up to 3 days
- Occasional slight vaginal bleeding

Physical Examination. See Table 36-2.

Differential Diagnosis

Included in the differential diagnosis are appendicitis, torsion or rupture of an ovarian cyst, and ectopic pregnancy.

Management

- The benign nature of the pain must be explained to the adolescent.
- A heating pad may provide some relief.
- Analgesics, especially prostaglandin inhibitors (ibuprofen, naproxen), may be used. Box 36-1 lists dosages.
- Rarely, oral contraceptives may be prescribed for relief (see Chapter 20).

Patient Education

- Provide reassurance and comfort measures as outlined in the management section.
- The adolescent should be encouraged to return if the pain worsens or changes, or if the adolescent is concerned.

Dysmenorrhea

Description

Painful menstruation with cramping in the lower abdomen or pelvis is the most common gynecologic problem seen in adolescence. Primary dysmenorrhea has no pelvic pathology identified, whereas secondary dysmenorrhea is due to a pelvic pathology.

TABLE 36-2 *Evaluation and Treatment of Menstrual Disorders*

	Etiology	History	Physical Examination and Laboratory Tests	Management
Mittelschmerz	Unclear, but pain probably caused by rapid enlargement of dominant follicle before follicular rupture	Pain occurs midway between cycles; dull, achy pain in lower abdomen lasting few minutes to several hours	Pain on palpation in either or both sides of lower abdomen overlying ovaries	Explain benign nature; heating pad; analgesics, especially PG inhibitors; follow up if pain changes
Dysmenorrhea	Primary: caused by exaggerated production of PGs; secondary: caused by infection, or abnormality	Onset 6-24 mo after menarche; pain begins with menses, lasts less than 2 days; mild to severe cramping in lower midabdominal area radiating to back, thighs, labia majora	Normal PE except for pain with examination of lower abdomen	PG inhibitors at onset of menses for duration of pain; follow up by phone or if pain changes; refer for gynecologic care if fails to respond after 6 mo
Endometriosis	Bleeding from ectopic endometrial tissue outside pelvic cavity causes pain, irritation of nerve endings, and uterine contractions	Progressive dysmenorrhea; onset before menses continuing for several days; unresponsive to OC or PG inhibitors in moderate to severe forms; irregular or excessive bleeding	Small papules on labia, vagina clear to red; limited or fixed uterine mobility; pelvic tenderness; uterosacral ligament nodules or tenderness with movement	Refer to gynecologist for management
Dysfunctional uterine bleeding	Defect in the maturation of negative feedback system of estrogen and follicle-stimulating hormone causing disorderly endometrial shedding	Bleeding that may be excessive in quantity or duration, irregular in occurrence	Normal PE except pale if Hgb is low; observe for androgen excess, galactorrhea; rule out pregnancy, STD	*Hgb >12 g*: PG inhibitor or OC; iron supplement; menstrual calendar; reevaluate in 3 mo *Hgb 10-12 g*: as above, OC preferred; folic acid supplement; reevaluate monthly *Hgb <10 g*: hospitalize

Hgb, Hemoglobin; *OC*, oral contraceptive; *PE*, physical examination; *PG*, prostaglandin; *STD*, sexually transmitted disease.

BOX 36-1 *Common Prostaglandin Inhibitors Used to Treat Adolescent Menstrual Disorders*

- Ibuprofen (Advil, Motrin): 400-800 mg 3-4 times a day with a loading dose of 800 mg and a max dose of 3.2 g/day
- Naproxen: 500 mg at onset followed by 250-500 mg every 6-12 hr
- Naproxen sodium (Aleve, Anaprox): 550 mg at onset followed by 275 mg every 6-12 hr; max dose 1375 mg per 24 hr
- Mefenamic acid: 500 mg at onset followed by 250 mg every 6 hr
- Flurbiprofen: 50 mg every 6 hr; 100 mg every 8-12 hr
- Meclofenamate: 100 mg initially; 50-100 mg every 6 hr

Etiology and Incidence

Primary dysmenorrhea is painful menses caused by an exaggerated production of, or response to, prostaglandins, causing uterine hypercontractility, tissue ischemia, and nerve hypersensitivity. The elevations of prostaglandins are brought about by falling progesterone levels during the luteal phase. Secondary dysmenorrhea may be prompted by endometriosis; complications of pregnancy; outflow obstruction; ovarian cysts, fibroids, or other uterine abnormalities; or infection. Dysmenorrhea is present in more than 50% of female adolescents and has been reported in up to 90% of adolescents. It is the leading cause (greater than 10%) of absenteeism from school or work, with increasing incidence in those who describe the pain as severe (Emans, Laufer, & Goldstein, 1998; Schroeder & Sanfilippo, 1999).

Clinical Findings

History. The history should assess the following:

- Primary dysmenorrhea (see Table 36-2)
  - Family history of dysmenorrhea
  - Menstrual history
  - Sexual activity
  - Sexual abuse
  - Number of days of school or activities missed
  - Timing, location, and character of pain
  - Systemic symptoms associated with prostaglandin release such as nausea, vomiting, diarrhea, headache, fatigue, nervousness, dizziness, urinary frequency, lower back or thigh pain
  - Medications or treatments used
  - Cigarette smoking
- Secondary dysmenorrhea
  - Family history of endometriosis
  - History of infection, menorrhagia, intermenstrual bleeding, or abnormal vaginal discharge
  - Onset (with menarche or later than 2 to 3 years after)
  - Pelvic pain at times other than menstruation (worsens over time)
  - Character of pelvic pain (dull and constant rather than crampy)
  - Dyspareunia

Physical Examination. A complete physical examination is recommended. A pelvic examination is deferred only if the adolescent is not sexually active, if the dysmenorrhea does not interfere with daily activities and is mild, or if the dysmenorrhea is responding to treatment. A rectovaginal examination is an integral part of the assessment but will typically fail to identify an abnormality in primary dysmenorrhea.

Laboratory Studies. The following are ordered as indicated:

- Sedimentation rate if PID is suspected
- Pap test and pregnancy test
- Cervical cultures for gonorrhea and chlamydia
- Pelvic ultrasonogram if abnormalities are suspected
- Renal ultrasonogram and intravenous pyelogram if uterine malformation found

Differential Diagnosis

Endometriosis, PID, obstructive malformations or other pathology of the reproductive tract, and psychogenic etiology are included in the differential diagnosis. Nongynecologic causes of pelvic pain such as Crohn's disease and irritable bowel syndrome should be considered.

Management

The following steps are recommended:

- Primary dysmenorrhea:
  - Prostaglandin synthetase inhibitors provide relief in 75% to 90% of patients (Emans, Laufer, & Goldstein, 1998; WebMD Scientific American Medicine, 2002). They should be administered at onset of menses or, if cramping precedes menses, at onset of symptoms. Treat the patient for the duration of the pain, usually 1 to 2 days. The trial period should extend for three cycles; if no relief is experienced, an alternative prostaglandin inhibitor should be tried. See Box 36-1 for specific prostaglandin inhibitors. Ibuprofen and naproxen are widely used in clinical practice (Shroeder & Sanfilippo, 1999). Nonsteroidal antiinflammatory drugs (NSAIDs) are advantageous as first-line therapy because they need to be taken for only 2 to 3 days. Taking NSAIDs with food helps prevent abdominal complaints.
  - Oral contraceptives (OCs) are widely used for dysmenorrhea and are thought to act by suppressing ovulation and reducing endometrial growth and, thus, total prostaglandin production. The efficacy of low-dose combined OC pills, however, has not been demonstrated with randomized controlled trials in adolescents (Davis & Westhoff, 2001). A combination 20 to 35 μg estrogen-progestin pill is used for a 3- to 6-month trial if prostaglandin inhibitors are not successful. OCs can be continued if contraception is needed. OCs offer many noncontraceptive advantages, including protection from endometrial and ovarian cancer, decreased symptoms of PID, decreased iron deficiency, and slowed progress of endometriosis.
  - Application of heat provides short-term relief.
  - Acupuncture and high-frequency transcutaneous electrical nerve stimulation (TENS) have been shown to provide relief.
  - Cyclooxygenase-2 (COX-2) inhibitors such as Celebrex and Vioxx are promising agents under study (WebMD Scientific American Medicine, 2002).
  - Follow up by telephone or visit to adjust dose or change medication as needed. The adolescent should be seen again in 3 to 4 months.
  - If there is failure to respond after 6 months of treatment or if pain worsens over time, the patient should be referred for gynecologic care to rule out endometriosis or other etiology.
- Secondary dysmenorrhea:
  - Requires referral for gynecologic care.
  - Explain that the pain is not "in the patient's head" and can be managed.
  - Assist with stress control to alleviate pain.

Complications

Sexual abuse (26% to 28%) and an increased occurrence of irritable bowel syndrome have been found in association with dysmenorrheal and chronic pelvic pain (Schroeder & Sanfilippo, 1999).

Patient Education and Prevention

- Encourage exercise and stress reduction to help control pain.
- A well-balanced diet with ample amounts of fiber and water, as well as decreasing caffeine and chocolate intake, may be useful to control dysmenorrhea. Supplementation with thiamine, 100 mg daily, has been found to be better than placebo in controlling dysmenorrhea (Gokhale, 1996). Herbal teas, fruits, and vegetables may also help, but there is insufficient evidence to determine the effectiveness (WebMD Scientific American Medicine, 2002).
- Smoking cessation may help decrease dysmenorrhea. A longitudinal study of women found that 41% of smokers compared with 26% of nonsmokers experienced moderate or severe dysmenorrhea (Chen et al, 2000).

Endometriosis

Description

Endometriosis is the proliferation of ectopic endometrial tissue outside the pelvic cavity. It is primarily manifested by dysmenorrhea that progressively worsens. Other symptoms include dyspareunia, noncyclic pelvic pain, and subfertility.

Etiology and Incidence

The cause of endometriosis is unknown. Risk factors include early menarche and late menopause. Several theories have been developed to explain the possible cause of endometriosis, including retrograde menstruation; coelomic metaplasia; lymphatic, vascular, and iatrogenic dissemination; genetic factors; and immunologic or hormonal problems or defects. See also Table 36-2.

The incidence rate in adolescents is difficult to obtain because endometriosis has only recently been studied in this age-group. Estimates of 7% in the population with a first-degree relative with endometriosis, and 1% otherwise, are reported. Average age of onset is 14.7 years, 2.9 years after menarche (Emans, Laufer, & Goldstein, 1998). Approximately 50% of adolescents with untreatable dysmenorrhea or pelvic pain have a diagnosis of endometriosis (Cramer & Missmer, 2002). The incidence of endometriosis in adolescents increases with age, from 12% among 11- to 13-year-olds to 54% among 20- to 21-year-olds (Propst & Laufer, 2000).

Clinical Findings

History. The history can include the following (see Table 36-2):

- First-degree relative with endometriosis
- Deep unilateral or bilateral pain described as sharp or dull
- Chronic pelvic pain that is acyclic and mildly to severely disabling, disrupting routine and causing missed school days or emergency department visits without definitive diagnosis
- Bladder and bowel dysfunction; rectal pain
- Dyspareunia
- Cyclic leg pain

Physical Examination. The following may be seen (see Table 36-2):

- Small papules on labia, vagina, or cervix that are clear to red in color in adolescents (in young women they become bluish to brownish)
- Tender, enlarged, or fixed ovaries
- Adnexal masses, thickening, or tenderness
- Most commonly in adolescents the pelvic examination is unremarkable with mild to moderate pelvic tenderness on palpation

Laboratory Studies. The following are ordered as indicated:

- Complete blood count (CBC), urinary assay, and endocervical cultures for gonorrhea and chlamydia to rule out infectious cause
- Ultrasound (normal in most cases)

Differential Diagnosis

Primary dysmenorrhea, PID, chronic anovulation with cystic ovaries, eating disorders, lactose intolerance, irritable bowel syndrome, chronic constipation, and depression are included in the differential diagnosis.

Management

- The goal in treating endometriosis is to control pain by hormonal alteration of the menstrual cycle to produce a pseudopregnancy, pseudomenopause, or chronic anovulation. Decreasing circulating estrogen decreases the proliferation of endometrial tissue. Young women with endometriosis should be referred to a gynecologist for management.
- Hormonal treatment with danazol, medroxyprogesterone, gestrinone, or gonadotropin-releasing hormone (GnRH) analogs for 6 months have been shown to be effective in pain control for women with endometriosis (American College of Obstetricians and Gynecologists, 2000). The evidence is unclear if surgical treatment (resection/destruction of visible lesions) in addition to medical treatment is more effective (Olive & Pritts, 2001).

- Supportive phone follow-up for side effects of medications and painful flare-ups is essential.
- See at 1- to 3-month intervals to provide support and reevaluate.
- Diet and exercise are important aspects in coping with chronic pain.
- Stress reduction techniques and support groups may also be helpful.
- A website specific to adolescent endometriosis is available (see Resource Box).

Complications

Miscarriage and infertility can occur. Endometriomas are rare in the adolescent age-group. Gastritis that may be treated with histamine-2 blockers is seen frequently.

Prognosis and Prevention

Endometriosis is a chronic disease, and remission and exacerbation are to be expected. Stressful events often cause exacerbation. The goals of treatment are to control pain and prevent infertility.

Dysfunctional Uterine Bleeding

Description

Dysfunctional uterine bleeding (DUB) refers to abnormal menstrual bleeding that is excessive, prolonged, or unpatterned. It can be described as follows:

- *Oligomenorrhea:* more than 35 days between menses or four to nine periods per year
- *Polymenorrhea:* less than 21 days between menses
- *Menorrhagia:* excessive flow or duration of menses
- *Metrorrhagia:* irregular frequency of cycles with bleeding between cycles
- *Menometrorrhagia:* excessive amount of bleeding with irregular frequency
- *Amenorrhea:* absence of bleeding

The bleeding is unrelated to structural or systemic disease and commonly occurs during anovulation. DUB is a diagnosis of exclusion, so any other causes of pathology must first be ruled out. DUB can be classified as mild, moderate, or severe based on hemoglobin level, duration of cycle, and quantity of bleeding.

Etiology and Incidence

The mechanism of DUB appears to be a delay in the maturation of the negative feedback cycle and is not related to structural pathology or medical illness (Emans, Laufer, & Goldstein, 1998). Estrogen production continues without the balancing decrease in FSH, which would suppress estrogen. This results in abnormal endometrial thickening. The abnormal endometrium then sheds in a disorderly manner manifested by heavy, irregular, or prolonged bleeding. There is great variation in what is considered to be a normal menstrual cycle, especially in adolescents. Normal can range from 21 to 45 days between periods, with duration of flow from 3 to 7 days and 30 to 40 ml of blood loss (10 to 15 soaked tampons or pads) per cycle. Periods that last longer than 8 to 10 days and blood loss in excess of 80 ml are considered excessive (Emans, Laufer, & Goldstein, 1998).

Abnormal uterine bleeding is especially common in adolescents (Bravender & Emans, 1999; Rimsza, 2002). Anovulation is the most common cause of DUB and occurs in approximately 50% of females in the first 2 years of their menstrual cycles. However, up to 33% of adolescents can have anovulatory cycles in the fifth year after menarche (Hillard, 1999; Rimsza, 2002). Adolescents with sustained anovulation (e.g., due to eating disorders, weight fluctuations, competitive athletics, chronic illness, or endocrine disease) have an increased incidence of DUB. Anovulation can also be due to stress or illness, thus appearing in adolescents after several years of regular cycles. DUB persists for up to 2 years in 60% of patients, 4 years in 50%, and 10 years in 30% (Emans, Laufer, & Goldstein, 1998).

Clinical Findings

History. The history should assess the following:

- Family history of bleeding disorders or dyscrasias, thyroid dysfunction, diabetes mellitus, or diethylstilbestrol (DES) exposure
- Menstrual history: onset, pattern, duration, quantity, and color; last menstrual period; breakthrough bleeding; dysmenorrhea; passing of clots, number of tampons, pads, or sponges used; longest and shortest intervals between cycles
- Associated menstrual symptoms
- Postcoital bleeding
- Sexual activity and contraception used
- Sexual abuse
- Previous infection or STDs
- Vaginal discharge, pelvic pain
- Galactorrhea, hirsutism (endocrine disease), or other chronic disease
- Bleeding gums, nosebleeds, bruises, hemorrhage (bleeding disorders)
- Hair loss, sleep disorders, cold intolerance, constipation (thyroid symptoms)
- Recent stressors, medications, or substance use
- Exercise patterns
- Weight, eating patterns, weight fluctuations, laxative use, body image

- Genital trauma
- Impact of bleeding on lifestyle

Physical Examination. The physical examination should include the following:

- Height, weight, body mass index (BMI), body type, and fat distribution
- Vital signs (temperature, pulse, respiratory rate, and blood pressure) sitting and standing
- Observation for acne, hirsutism, clitoromegaly (evidence of androgen excess)
- Breast examination for galactorrhea
- Thyroid palpation
- Observation for petechiae, bruising, pale color
- Abdominal examination for mass or tenderness
- Pelvic examination, including digital/speculum examination for foreign bodies, cervical lesions
- Tanner staging
- Bimanual and rectoabdominal examination

Laboratory Studies. The following are ordered as indicated:

- Pregnancy test regardless of sexual history
- CBC with differential, platelet count, reticulocyte count
- Sedimentation rate (if infection or inflammation is suspected)
- Coagulation studies: prothrombin time, partial thromboplastin time, bleeding time (if bleeding disorder is suspected or significant drop in hemoglobin)
- Thyroid function test, blood sugar, prolactin level (if systemic disease is suspected)
- Wet preparations and culture for gonorrhea, chlamydia, *Trichomonas* if patient is sexually active
- Ultrasonogram of pelvis if mass is palpated, anomaly is suspected, bimanual examination cannot be completed, or condition is unresponsive to treatment

Differential Diagnosis

The differential diagnosis includes pregnancy or pregnancy-related complications (postabortion, ectopic pregnancy); stress; excessive participation in athletics; eating disorders, including obesity; drug use; systemic diseases such as blood dyscrasias (20% of patients with coagulation defects have excessive menstrual bleeding); infection (e.g., STDs); trauma, including forceful intercourse or rape; foreign bodies, including intrauterine device; tumors; anomalies; endometriosis; endocrine disorders (e.g., thyroid disorder, diabetes mellitus); debilitating or chronic diseases (especially hepatic or renal diseases); reproductive tract disorders, including malignancy; and medications, including OCs, progesterone implants, and injectables (Bacon, 2000; Hillard, 1999).

Management

The goals in managing DUB include controlling bleeding, preventing endometrial hyperplasia, preventing and treating anemia, restoring quality of life, and preventing recurrence.

- Mild DUB: a shortened cycle or menses longer than normal with flow slightly to moderately increased or unpredictable; hemoglobin greater than 12 g/dl:
  - Observe and reassure.
  - Have patient start and maintain a menstrual calendar.
  - Prescribe iron supplementation and dietary interventions to prevent anemia.
  - Use prostaglandin inhibitors to reduce heavy bleeding (see Box 36-1).
  - Consider OCs for 3 to 4 months to decrease menorrhagia and stabilize menses (see Chapter 20).
  - Reevaluate every 3 months.
- Moderate DUB: shortened (1 to 3 weeks), irregular cycle with moderate to heavy bleeding, hemoglobin between 10 and 12 g/dl:
  - Prescribe OCs, initially 35 to 50 μg monophasic, subsequently monophasic or triphasic for three to six cycles.
  - Alternatively, prescribe a progestin such as medroxyprogesterone acetate (5 to 10 mg every day for 10 to 14 days started on the fourteenth day of cycle for 1 to 2 months). OCs are more effective at stopping active bleeding.
  - Have patient start and maintain a menstrual calendar.
  - Prescribe iron supplementation with 1 mg folic acid per day.
  - Reevaluate at least monthly until condition is stable.
  - Reassess after 6 months.
- Severe DUB: irregular, prolonged, heavy bleeding; hemoglobin less than 10 g/dl:
  - Hospitalize if actively bleeding; treatment may include transfusion, intravenous hormonal therapy, and dilation and curettage.
  - Manage as moderate DUB if not actively bleeding.

Complications

Anemia, profuse bleeding, shock, and side effects of OCs can occur. A long history of anovulation and DUB increases the risk of infertility and endometrial carcinoma.

Patient Education and Prognosis

- Encourage teen to keep a calendar of bleeding days and amounts. This includes keeping track of the number of pads or tampons used in order to increase accuracy.
- Introduce the idea of taking OCs as a treatment. Helping parents and adolescents understand the usefulness of OCs as a medication minimizes stigma they may feel

and helps avoid discontinuation of this method before optimal treatment of symptoms is achieved.
- Discuss decision making about initiation of sexual intercourse and STD prevention.
- Prognosis is excellent if DUB is due to anovulation and immaturity of the HPO axis; these adolescents respond well to treatment, and about half return to regular menstrual patterns within 4 years of menarche (Bravender & Emans, 1999).

Amenorrhea

Description

Amenorrhea is lack of menstruation and is described as either primary or secondary. *Primary amenorrhea* is defined as any one of the following (Apgar, 2002; Emans, Laufer, & Goldstein, 1998; Pletcher & Slap, 1999; Prose, Ford, & Lovely, 1998):
- Absence of menarche by 16 years of age with normal pubertal growth and development
- Absence of any pubertal development (breast budding is initial sign in most females) by 13 years of age (14 years if thin, chronically ill, or athlete)
- Absence of menarche 2 to 3 years after beginning puberty, especially if Tanner stage 4 or 5

Secondary amenorrhea (also called *postmenarchal amenorrhea*) is defined as the absence of menstruation for at least three cycles or more than 6 months in females who have an established menstrual pattern.

Etiology and Incidence

There are multiple etiologies for primary and secondary amenorrhea. When evaluating a young woman for amenorrhea, pregnancy should be ruled out first, regardless of sexual history given. Primary or secondary amenorrhea occurs within three broad categories: generalized pubertal delay, otherwise normal puberty, or specific genital tract abnormalities. Evaluation of the young woman is guided by these three general categories. Constitutional delay without pathology is the most common cause of amenorrhea with pubertal delay (Pletcher & Slap, 1999).

Clinical Findings

History. The history should assess the following:
- Maternal and sibling age of menarche
- Family history of menstrual irregularities
- Family history of eating disorders, diabetes, thyroid disease, or genetic disorders
- Any prenatal exposure to hormones
- Detailed history of growth and pubertal development (sequence and tempo)
- Menstrual calendar (last menses, number and pattern of cycles, age at menarche)
- Chronic systemic disease or illness or previous surgery, radiation, or chemotherapy
- Nutrition, including eating habits, dieting, weight fluctuations
- Exercise patterns, including amount and intensity, level of participation, weigh-ins, or standards for weight that must be kept
- History of stress fractures
- Bowel patterns or abdominal pain
- Headache or visual change
- Galactorrhea, hirsutism, acne
- Medication use (contraceptives, phenothiazides, antihypertensives)
- Sexual activity, contraceptive use
- Stress, recent change in environment, or depression
- Substance use

Physical Examination. The physical examination should include the following:
- Height, weight, BMI, nutritional status, body habitus, blood pressure, pulse
- Sexual maturation rating
- Complete neurologic examination, including cranial nerves, funduscopic examination, and visual fields
- Midline facial defects or other congenital anomalies or stigmata of Turner syndrome
- Palpation of thyroid, dry skin, pitted nails
- Cachexia, lanugo, parotid enlargement, bradycardia, hypotension, hypothermia (anorexia nervosa)
- Breast examination with gentle compression to identify galactorrhea (elevated prolactin)
- Palpation of abdomen and groin for masses, tenderness
- Rectal examination for fissure, fistula, skin tags, or occult blood
- Examination of skin, hair, and genitalia for signs of virilization
- External genital examination for estrogenization of vaginal mucosa (indicates ovarian function), vaginal and hymenal patency, and clitoromegaly (androgen excess)
- Digital vaginal examination and speculum examination if any abnormality is suspected
- Bimanual examination

Laboratory Studies. The following may be indicated:
- Pregnancy test regardless of sexual history
- Smear for vaginal estrogenization
- Thyroid function studies
- Complete blood count
- Erythrocyte sedimentation rate
- Serum prolactin (elevated in pituitary adenoma)
- LH, FSH (elevated in ovarian failure), estradiol

- Chromosome analysis (if stigmata of Turner syndrome present)
- Dehydroepiandrosterone sulfate (DHEA-S), testosterone, and 17-hydroxyprogesterone if there are signs of androgen excess
- Assessment of body fat percentage
- Bone age if no breast development (marked delay equals less than 75% of chronologic age)
- Ultrasound (to determine normal anatomy)
- Magnetic resonance imaging (MRI) or computed tomography (CT) scan (intracranial lesion) if central nervous system lesion suspected

Differential Diagnosis

The differential diagnoses for primary amenorrhea and secondary amenorrhea are essentially identical. The only exceptions are a few genetic conditions that cause primary amenorrhea (e.g., Turner syndrome). Box 36-2 summarizes the differential diagnoses for amenorrhea. An important marker of hypogonadotropic hypogonadism is the female athlete triad of amenorrhea, eating disorder, and osteoporosis (Emans, Laufer, & Goldstein, 1998; Greydanus & Patel, 2002), especially common in gymnasts, figure skaters, ballet dancers, and long-distance runners at elite or highly competitive levels. The pressure for the ideal body for the sport and the intense exercise required may lead to this triad.

BOX 36-2 *Differential Diagnosis of Amenorrhea*

Hypergonadotropic States (Elevated FSH and LH)

Ovarian dysgenesis (Turner syndrome)
Ovarian failure (idiopathic, chemotherapy, infection, trauma, autoimmune)
Androgen insensitivity
Congenital defects in steroid synthesis

Hypogonadotropic States (Low FSH, LH)

Constitutional delay of puberty
Anorexia nervosa
Exercise-induced amenorrhea
Inflammatory bowel disease
Systemic illness
Stress
Deficiency of GnRH
Panhypopituitarism

Normal FSH, LH

Outflow obstruction
Müllerian agenesis
Asherman syndrome
Polycystic ovary syndrome (ratio of LH to FSH may be high)
Partial 21-hydroxylase deficiency

From Mitan LA, Slap GB: Adolescent menstrual disorders, *Med Clin North Am* 84:854, 2000.
FSH, Follicle-stimulating hormone; *GnRH*, gonadotropin-releasing hormone; *LH*, luteinizing hormone.

Management

The treatment of amenorrhea depends on its cause. Restoration of ovulatory cycles leads to the best long-term prognosis. If genital examination is normal, proceed as outlined in Fig. 36-5. When considering whom to evaluate, the following guidelines may be helpful (Emans, Laufer, & Goldstein, 1998):

- Abrupt cessation of menses for 4 months after regular cycles have begun
- Persistent oligomenorrhea after 2 years of regular cycles
- Persistent amenorrhea 6 months after OC use or 12 months after Depo-Provera use
- No obvious cause
- Presence of any signs of estrogen deficiency or androgen excess

For optimal long-term prognosis, management is directed toward restoring ovulatory cycles. This is often accomplished through estrogen-progestin therapy. Anxiety about amenorrhea is common, and frequent reassurance is necessary. Young women should be made aware of the long-term skeletal effects of amenorrhea and instructed on adequate diet, reasonable exercise, and calcium supplementation to avoid osteoporosis.

Vulvovaginitis and Vaginal Discharge

Description

Vulvovaginitis refers to inflammation, often with discharge, from infection or irritation. Vulvitis alone refers to erythema and pruritus; vaginitis refers to discharge with pruritus and irritation that may be secondary to the vulvitis.

Etiology and Incidence

Age is important in differentiating the etiology of vulvovaginitis. In prepubescent children, several factors make vulvovaginitis a common problem. The lack of estrogen stimulation leaves the vulvar skin thin and the vaginal mucosa atrophic, and contributes to minimal vaginal secretions with neutral pH. The lack of pubic hair and labial fat pads diminishes barrier protection, and the proximity of the vaginal opening to the anus predisposes prepubertal females to irritation and infection of the vulva and vagina.

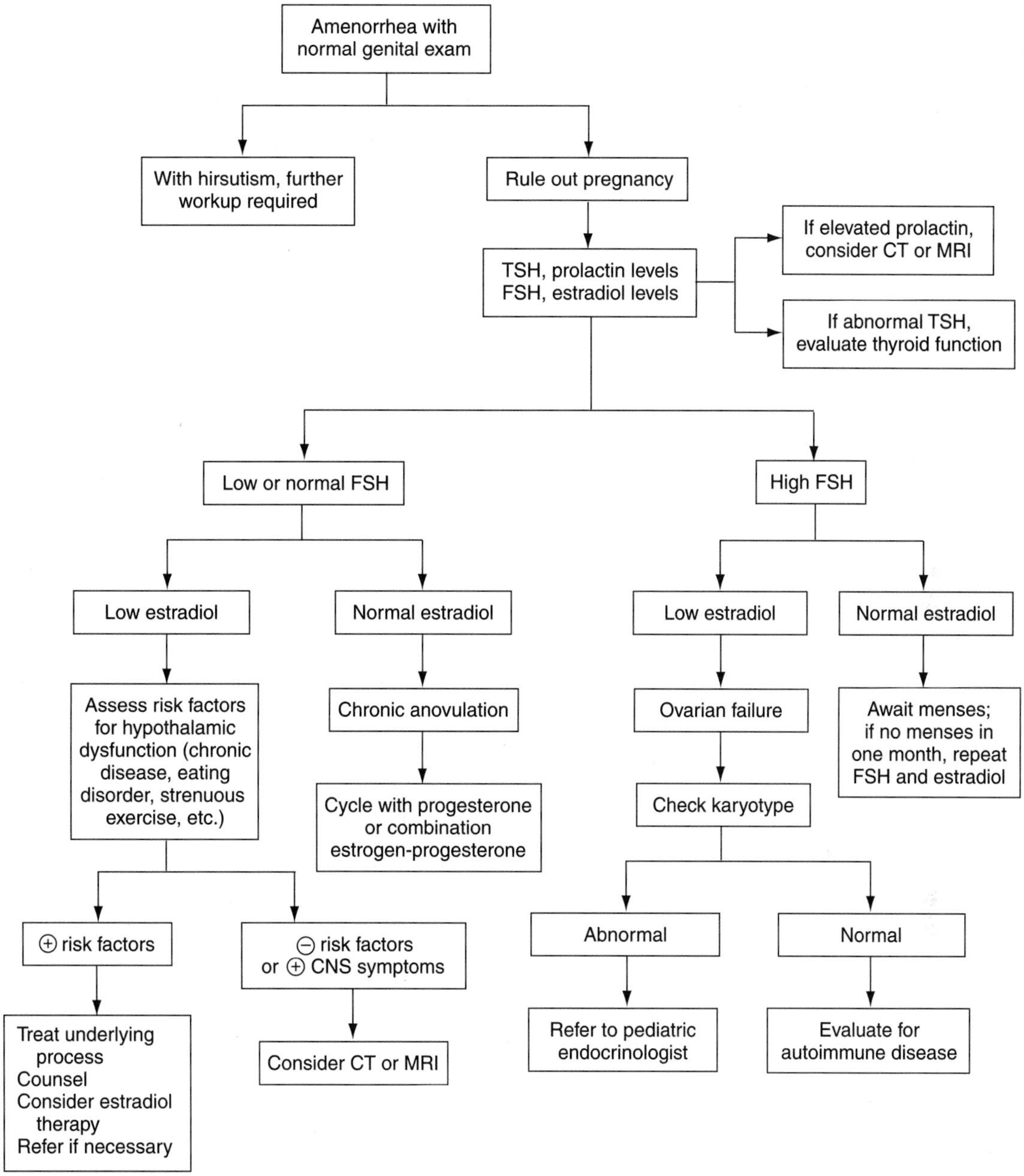

FIGURE 36-5 Evaluation of amenorrhea with a normal genital tract. *CNS*, Central nervous system; *FSH*, follicle-stimulating hormone; *TSH*, thyroid-stimulating hormone. (From Prose C, Ford C, Lovely L: Evaluating amenorrhea: the pediatrician's role, *Contemp Pediatr* 15:106, 1998.)

Poor hygiene, including wiping technique and lack of handwashing, and irritants such as bubble bath, harsh soaps, sand from playtime, or tight-fitting clothing provide additional insults. Prepubescent vulvovaginitis most commonly is nonspecific (up to 80%). Other causes include foreign bodies (most often toilet paper), bacterial infection (often group A β-hemolytic streptococci), or pinworms (Emans, Laufer, & Goldstein, 1998; Smith & Lohr, 1999).

At puberty, the pH changes from 7 to 4.5, vaginal mucosa thickens, acidogenic bacteria predominate, and lactobacillus stabilizes the environment, all offering protection from infection. Adolescent vulvovaginitis is most often due to a specific cause, often secondary to sexual contact. Normal physiologic leukorrhea occurs 6 to 12 months before puberty. *Monilia*, group A β-hemolytic streptococci or other infections, foreign bodies (toilet paper fragments, tampon), and pinworms are possible causes. Bacterial vaginosis, *Trichomonas*, or other STDs (discussed later in this chapter) must also be considered. Up to one half of female gynecologic complaints are related to vulvovaginitis. Bacterial vaginosis, *Monilia*, *Trichomonas*, or mixed-flora infections are the most common infecting agents (Preminger & Pokorny, 1998).

Clinical Findings

The clinical findings pertaining to vaginitis are found in Table 36-3.

History. The history can include the following:

- Prepubertal child and adolescent
  - Previous occurrences and treatment used
  - Genital irritation, itching, pain, and inflammation
  - Vaginal discharge—note onset, quantity, color, type (bloody, mucoid), odor, consistency, and duration
  - Urinary complaints, including dysuria and enuresis
  - Recent medications, especially antibiotics
  - Perineal hygiene or anal pruritus
  - Underlying illnesses (e.g., *Streptococcus* infection, dermatosis, diabetes, immunosuppression)
  - Possible trauma, foreign body, or sexual abuse
  - Use of harsh soaps and bubble bath
- Prepubertal child
  - Superabsorbent diapers
  - Tight-fitting or nylon underwear or clothing
  - Nighttime perianal itching
- Adolescent
  - History of sexual activity or menstrual irregularities
  - Exposures to STDs
  - Use of contraception

Physical Examination. A good light and magnifying glass may aid in the physical examination. Prepubertal examination includes inspection, possible vaginal otoscopy in frog-leg or knee-chest position, and rectal examination. Adolescent examination may also include pelvic and bimanual examination. See Table 36-4 for physical examination findings.

Laboratory Studies. The following should be considered:

- Urinalysis for white blood cells (WBCs), yeast, or trichomonads
- pH of vaginal secretions
- Wet preparation with saline for WBCs; pseudohyphae or yeast buds; motile, pear-shaped, flagellated clue cells or epithelial cells sprinkled with bacteria; bacteria; wet preparation with 10% KOH for whiff test and better visualization of *Monilia* (branching pseudohyphae and spores) (see Fig. 36-3)
- Gram stain
- Rapid antibody tests for *Streptococcus* or *Trichomonas*
- Culture of *Monilia*, *Streptococcus*, or *Trichomonas*
- DNA probes or urine testing for STDs
- Pinworm eggs visualized on tape slide under microscope

Differential Diagnosis

Atopic dermatitis, psoriasis, seborrhea, or other dermatosis; labial adhesions; polyps or tumors; systemic diseases

TABLE 36-3 ***Evaluation and Treatment of Vaginitis***

	Signs and Symptoms	Vaginal Discharge	Etiology	Laboratory Data	Treatment
Nonspecific vaginitis	Itching, burning; dysuria; varied vulvitis	Scant to copious; brown to green; mucoid; foul smelling	Irritation from contact with various substances; poor hygiene	pH variable; no odor on whiff test; micro: leukocytes, bacteria, debris; normal UA	Refractory cases may need topical estrogen or antibiotics
Physiologic leukorrhea	None or minimal itch or burn; minimal vulvitis; 6-12 mo before menarche; possible mild erythema	Scant to moderate; clear to white; odorless; nonirritating	Endogenous hormones 6-12 mo before menarche	pH <4.5; no odor on whiff test; micro: epithelial cells, lactobacilli; normal UA (see Fig. 36-3)	No treatment needed; explain and reassure
Chemical or mechanical	Itch, erythema, vulvar inflammation, dysuria	Scant amount yellow to white	Bubble bath, perfumed soap, lotion; tight-fitting clothes, sand or dirt from playground, obesity	pH <4.5; no odor on whiff test; micro: leukocytes, epithelial cells	Remove irritant; topical steroids

TABLE 36-3 *Evaluation and Treatment of Vaginitis—cont'd*

	Signs and Symptoms	Vaginal Discharge	Etiology	Laboratory Data	Treatment
Foreign body	Dysuria, discomfort, bleeding, minimal vulvar excoriation; history of foreign body in other orifices	Purulent, persistent, dark brown, foul smelling (18%), bloody (82%)	Toilet paper (prepubescent); tampons (adolescent); condoms or object used for masturbation	pH >4.5; odd odor on whiff test; micro: WBCs, epithelial cells with bacteria and debris; UA normal	Remove foreign body with forceps or by irrigating with saline and small feeding tube; knee-chest position may work best
Bacterial	Acute respiratory, enteric, or skin infection	Green color, foul, copious with possible bleeding	*Streptococcus* (most common), *Escherichia coli, Enterococcus, Shigella, Staphylococcus*, or other bacteria	Strep test positive; culture positive	Penicillin, erythromycin, amoxicillin, broad-spectrum cephalosporin or other antibiotic as indicated
Candidiasis	Itching, burning, vulvar inflammation, dysuria, dyspareunia; history of antibiotic or steroid use	Thick, white, curdy cottage cheese adherent, odorless; vulva red, edematous with satellite lesions	Recent antibiotic or steroid use; diabetes or immunodeficiency; *Candida albicans*; pregnancy	pH <4.5; no odor on whiff test; micro: fungal hyphae and buds or spores, culture positive for *Monilia*; UA with WBCs	Imidazoles or triazoles topically or intravaginally; ketoconazole orally
Pinworms	Recent exposure to pinworms; perineal itching especially at night; anal excoriation, erythema, and lesions from scratching	No discharge	*Enterobius vermicularis* spread from anus	Normal UA; tape test reveals eggs	Mebendazole 100 mg once; repeated in 2 wk; treat family members
Bacterial vaginosis	Foul odor, especially after menses or intercourse; often asymptomatic; no inflammation; abdominal pain or irregular prolonged bleeding	Homogeneous, thin milky white discharge adherent* to vaginal walls and pools in posterior fornix; increased amount	*Gardnerella vaginalis* and anerobic bacteria; caused by replacement of normal vaginal flora; may or may not be sexually transmitted	pH >4.5*; fishy odor on whiff test*; micro: clue cells,* few lactobacilli, gram-negative rods, no WBCs (see Fig. 36-3)	May resolve without treatment; treat only if symptomatic with metronidazole for 7 days or clindamycin; increased risk for pelvic inflammatory disease
Trichomonas	Lower abdominal discomfort, dysuria, symptoms worse before and after menses; history of sexual contact; vulvar itching and erythema	White to yellow-grey, frothy, foul odor, profuse, purulent, slightly watery; vaginal mucosa erythematous, cervix friable with petechiae	*Trichomonas vaginalis*, flagellated protozoa, primarily sexually transmitted	pH >4.5, frequently has fishy odor on whiff test; micro: motile, flagellated organisms, WBC >10/hpf on UA (see Fig. 36-3)	Metronidazole for 7-10 days; prepubertal 15 mg/kg in three divided doses or 40 mg/kg in single dose; postpubertal 2 g in single dose

*Need three of these for findings to diagnose bacterial vaginosis.
hpf, High-power field; *micro*, microscopic examination; *UA*, urinalysis; *WBC*, white blood cell.

TABLE 36-4 *Sexually Transmitted Disease: History, Physical Examination, and Initial Treatment*

	History	Physical Examination	Treatment
Gonorrhea (GC)	Often asymptomatic (33%); dysuria; vaginal discharge or bleeding; dyspareunia	Profuse, thick, green discharge, urethritis, cervicitis; Skene's or Bartholin's gland abscess; exudative pharyngitis	Ceftriaxone 125 mg (IM) one time *or* Ciprofloxacin 500 mg one time* *or* Levofloxacin 250 mg one time* *or* Ofloxacin 400 mg PO one time* *If chlamydial infection not ruled out also give* Azithromycin 1 g PO in single dose *or* Doxycycline 100 mg PO bid for 7 days† Report to state health department Do culture and sensitivity 2 weeks after treatment if symptoms persist.
Chlamydia	Often is asymptomatic (30%-70%); spotting, vaginal discharge; dysuria, pyuria; mild abdominal pain or foreign body sensation in eyes possible	Clear to white or yellow discharge, mucopurulent cervicitis with edema, erythema, hypertrophy; Fitz-Hugh–Curtis syndrome (right upper quadrant pain); conjunctivitis	Azithromycin 1 g PO in a single dose *or* Doxycycline 100 mg PO bid for 7 days† Alternative medications: erythromycin ethylsuccinate 800 mg PO qid for 7 days *or* Ofloxacin 300 mg PO bid for 7 days* Levofloxacin 500 mg PO for 7 days* Report to state health department Do follow-up cultures 3 wk after treatment if symptoms persist; rescreen in 3-4 mo after a positive test
Syphilis	*Primary*: vaginal, anal, or oral chancre *Secondary:* copper-penny rash especially on palms and soles, adenopathy, alopecia	Single painless papule with serous discharge, smooth base, raised edges; painless regional lymphadenopathy	Benzathine penicillin G IM 2.4 million U *or* If penicillin allergy and not pregnant: Doxycycline 100 mg PO bid for 14 days† *or* Tetracycline 500 mg PO qid for 14 days† Test for GC, chlamydia, and HIV at time of infection and in 3 mo Follow with RPR or VDRL every 6-12 mo Report to state health department
Herpes simplex virus (HSV)	Painful rash, blisters and ulcers; HSV-1 of mouth and face; burning and irritation 24 hr before; dysuria; other systemic complaints	Clear to white to yellow discharge; vesicles on erythematous base that become ulcers in 1-3 days; extragenital lesions	Acyclovir 400 mg tid for 7-10 days (primary) or 5 days (recurrent) *or* 200 mg five times a day for 7-10 days (primary) or 5 days (recurrent); sitz bath, dry heat, lidocaine jelly 2%; treat *Monilia* vaginitis that often accompanies or follows HSV
Human papillomavirus (HPV)	Asymptomatic or subclinical unrecognized; can be painful	Warts, friable or pruritic (or both); moist, cauliflower-like anogenital and inguinal 4-6 wk after exposure	*Patient applied treatment*: Podofilox or imiquimod *Provider applied treatment:* Cryotherapy, podophyllin resin, trichloroacetic acid or bichloroacetic acid, or surgical removal

bid, Twice a day; *HIV*, human immunodeficiency virus; *IM*, intramuscular; *PO*, by mouth; *qid*, four times daily; *RPR*, rapid plasma reagin; *VDRL*, Venereal Disease Research Laboratories.

*Contraindicated under 18 years of age, in pregnancy, or during lactation.

†Contraindicated under 8 years of age.

such as Kawasaki or Crohn; other STDs; and sexual abuse are included in the differential diagnosis.

Management

General treatment measures for any type of vulvovaginitis are listed in Box 36-3. Specific recommendations include the following:

1. Prepubertal nonspecific etiology:
- If persistent, prescribe antibacterial cream at night (e.g., Bactroban, Sultrin, or clindamycin) for 2 weeks.
- If persistent after 3 weeks, rule out pinworms, and then prescribe a trial of amoxicillin, Augmentin, or one of the cephalosporins.
- If symptoms still persist, prescribe estrogen cream at bedtime for 2 to 3 weeks, then every other night at bedtime for 2 weeks to thicken vulvar epithelium.
- If recurrent vulvovaginitis appears, a 1- to 2-month course of low-dose cephalexin or trimethoprim-sulfamethoxazole (TMP-SMX) at bedtime should be tried.
- If a specific infection is found, treat as outlined herein or refer to appropriate section.
- If therapy fails, refer to a gynecologist.
- If an STD is found in a child, a complete workup for sexual abuse is indicated.

2. Contact dermatitis:
- Topical steroids and hormonal cream can be used to thicken vaginal skin and minimize irritation.

3. Foreign body:
- Prepubertal: Irrigate with warm normal saline with a small feeding tube at the hymenal opening with the child in the frog-leg position.
- Adolescent: Do a pelvic examination followed by irrigation and cultures as indicated.
- A broad-spectrum antibiotic, such as amoxicillin or a cephalosporin, may be indicated if infection is apparent.

4. Bacterial infection:
- Obtain cultures and prescribe appropriate treatment; penicillin or erythromycin is usually used.

5. Monilial infection:
- There are multiple preparations, but the "azole" drugs are recommended as being more effective than nystatin. There are many preparations, some obtainable over the counter (OTC), in single-dose to 7-day dose cream or suppository (Centers for Disease Control and Prevention [CDC], 2002b; Emans, Laufer, & Goldstein, 1998). For sexually active adolescents, many of these preparations are oil based and may weaken latex condoms or diaphragms.
  - Butoconazole 2% cream (5 g, one applicator) intravaginally for 3 days (OTC)
  - Clotrimazole 100 mg vaginal tablet for 7 days or 2 tablets for 3 days or 1% cream (5 g, one applicator) intravaginally for 7 to 14 days (OTC) or 500 mg vaginal tablet in single application
  - Miconazole 200 mg vaginal suppository for 3 days (OTC) or 100 mg vaginal suppository for 7 days (OTC) or 2% cream (5 g, one applicator) intravaginally for 7 days (OTC)
  - Terconazole 80 mg vaginal suppository for 3 days or 0.4% cream for 7 days or 0.8% cream for 3 days
  - Tioconazole 6.5% ointment (5 g, one applicator) intravaginally one time (OTC)
  - Nystatin 100,000 U vaginal tablet for 14 days
  - Fluconazole 150 mg orally one time or 5.5 mg/kg suspension in a single dose
- Treatment failure or recurrence may occur because of increasing resistance of organisms.
- If appropriate, evaluate for STDs.

BOX 36-3 *General Treatment Measures for Vulvovaginitis*

1. Hygiene
   - Wash hands frequently
   - Wipe front to back
   - Change underwear every day
   - Blow dry perineal area with cool to warm air (especially if overweight)
2. Clothing
   - Wear absorbent white underwear, changing once or twice daily; do not wear underwear at night
   - Wear loose clothing—no pantyhose or tight clothes
   - Avoid spandex and sleeper pajamas
   - Change out of swimsuit after swimming
3. Comfort and healing measures
   - Take sitz bath with thorough drying
   - Blow dry for 10-15 min once or twice daily with cool to warm air or pat dry with towel
   - Apply hydrocortisone cream 1% once or twice daily for itching
   - Use oral diphenhydramine or hydroxyzine if itching is severe
4. Protective measures
   - Avoid bubble baths and perfumed lotions or powder
   - Use mild soap (e.g., Dove, Basis, Neutrogena)
   - Avoid shampoo in bath water
   - Use protective ointment twice a day (e.g., Vaseline, A and D, Aquaphor)
   - Avoid bleach or fabric softener in wash, double rinse
   - Urinate with knees spread apart to minimize urinary reflux

- Complicated candidal infections (severe local, recurrent in abnormal host) require documentation by culture, workup for predisposing conditions, longer duration of treatment, and treatment of partners.
- Complementary medicine recommendations include intravaginal garlic for 10 to 12 hours; decreasing foods high in simple carbohydrates; avoiding foods with yeast or mold; increasing fiber, garlic, ginger, cinnamon; live lactobacillus (1 to 2 billion live organisms per day) and acidophilus in diet.

6. Pinworms:
- Mebendazole (100 mg tablet, repeated in 2 weeks).
- Handwashing is important to minimize the spread of infection.
- See Chapter 33 for further discussion.

7. Bacterial vaginosis:
- If asymptomatic, treatment is not recommended.
- If symptomatic, the following drugs are recommended except in pregnancy (CDC, 2002b): metronidazole 500 mg orally two times a day for 7 days or metronidazole gel 0.75% once a day vaginally for 5 days, or clindamycin vaginal cream 2% at bedtime for 7 days. Treatment of partners is not recommended, but evaluation for other STDs may be indicated. Treatment in pregnancy (CDC, 2002b): metronidazole 250 mg three times daily for 7 days or clindamycin 300 mg orally twice daily for 7 days.
- Recurrence is not uncommon.
- Latex in condoms may be weakened by clindamycin vaginal cream. Abstain from consuming alcohol while taking metronidazole.

8. Trichomonas:
- Oral metronidazole 2 g dose once or 500 mg twice a day for 7 days.
- Recurrent disease: 500 mg twice a day for 7 days. If repeated failure: 2 g daily for 3 to 5 days.
- Testing for other STDs is needed; treat sexual partners.
- Abstinence from sexual activity is required until treatment is complete and partners are asymptomatic. Latex in condoms may be weakened by medications.
- Abstain from consuming alcohol while taking medication.
- If prepubertal, workup for sexual abuse is necessary.

9. Gonorrhea or chlamydia in prepubescent children needs to be evaluated and treated as child abuse. See the following section, Chapter 19, and the 2002 CDC guidelines for treatment of sexually transmitted diseases (CDC, 2002b) for more details.

Complications

Labial adhesions can occur. Bacterial vaginosis can contribute to cervical neoplasm, PID, endometritis, postsurgical infection (abortion), abnormal Pap results, and adverse pregnancy outcomes. Trichomonas is associated with adverse pregnancy outcomes, especially premature rupture of membranes and preterm delivery.

Patient Education, Prognosis, and Prevention

- Follow up in 5 days if there is no improvement.
- Recurrence is common, especially with poor hygiene, in obese girls, and during upper respiratory infection.
- Protective measures for the sexually active adolescent include recommending not using diaphragm or condom until 3 days after treatment with topical vaginal cream or tablet.
- Recommend not using tampons or frequent changes of tampons and use of a pad especially at night.

Sexually Transmitted Diseases

Description

Multiple organisms are responsible for STDs in children and adolescents. Gonorrhea (GC), chlamydia, syphilis, HSV, and HPV are the most common STDs affecting the lower female reproductive tract. *Trichomonas* (discussed in previous section), hepatitis B, and HIV infections also are recognized as STDs. See Chapter 24 for discussion of hepatitis B and HIV (systemic STDs). The term *sexually transmitted infection* is sometimes used to refer to asymptomatic infection. Diagnosis can also be made in terms of the location of the infection (e.g., vaginitis, cervicitis, or urethritis).

STDs are a significant public health problem, placing a heavy financial health burden on society, having a tremendous impact on individuals' lives, and playing an important role in the transmission of HIV. The past 40 years have brought progress in treating STDs, with historic low incidence rates for GC and syphilis. However, the highest STD rates in the industrial world still occur in the United States.

Etiology and Incidence

Considered an epidemic, STDs have the highest rates in adolescents, documented as 3 million of the 12 million reported cases per year, or one case in every eight 13- to 19-year-olds. Adolescents at highest risk for acquiring STDs include youths in detention facilities, male homosexuals, and injection drug users. Minorities, especially African Americans, are disproportionally affected. More than 1 million teenage girls with STDs become pregnant, raising concerns about perinatal transmission (CDC, 2002b).

Factors contributing to this epidemic are the increasingly early age and frequency of sexual activity, inconsistent use of contraceptive and protective devices, the physiologic characteristics that predispose adolescents to infection, adolescents' lack of access to and use of health care, and societal influences (Box 36-4). Another factor that may contribute to higher reported numbers of STDs is the increased use and availability of accurate screening tests for diseases, especially chlamydia.

Most STDs must be reported, and the NP must be aware of each state's specific rules. All 50 states allow adolescents to be evaluated and to receive treatment for STDs confidentially. Management of children younger than 13 years old with STDs requires a coordinated effort between the clinician and child protective authorities.

Gonorrhea, caused by *Neisseria gonorrhoeae*, a nonmotile, gram-negative diplococcus, is often found in carriage with *Chlamydia* or other STDs. The gonorrhea rate for 2002 was 125 cases per 100,000, which was slightly lower than 2000 and 2001 but exceeds the 19 cases per 100,000 *Healthy people 2010* objective (CDC, 2003). The highest rate for adolescents occurred in the 15- to 19-year-old group. There are more reported cases of GC in African Americans than Caucasians (40:1). The infection is often asymptomatic, with as many as 80% of young women infected with GC reporting no symptoms (Stamm & McGregor, 2001). GC can progress to PID and persists perinatally for up to 6 months.

BOX 36-4 *Risk Factors for Sexually Transmitted Diseases*

- Adolescent younger than 15 years of age
- Sexually active adolescent, especially with two or more partners in 6 months, high frequency of intercourse, or high rate of new partners
- Use of drugs or alcohol, or other high-risk behaviors
- Pregnancy or abortion
- Homosexual
- Victim of abuse, rape, or incest
- Incarcerated, runaway, homeless, in group shelter or detention home
- Clients in sexually transmitted disease (STD) clinics or with any other STD or previous history of STD
- Lack of family availability; low level of parental support and monitoring
- Beliefs about normative behaviors among peers
- Inappropriate health care behaviors (e.g., not seeking medical care, not adhering to treatment regimen, failure to recognize symptoms, delay in notifying partners, nonuse of barrier contraceptive)

Data from Biro FM, Rosenthal SL: Adolescent STDs: diagnosis, developmental issues, and prevention, *J Pediatr Health Care* 9:256-262, 1995; Bonny AE, Biro FM: Recognizing and treating STDs in adolescent girls, *Contemp Pediatr* 15:119-143, 1998; Emans S, Laufer MR, Goldstein D: *Pediatric and adolescent gynecology*, ed 4, Philadelphia, 1998, Lippincott-Raven.

C. trachomatis infection is the most frequently reported bacterial STD, with a rate of 296.5 cases per 100,000 reported in 2002 (CDC, 2003). *Chlamydia* is present in 8% to 40% of sexually active teenage females. Adolescent patients age 15 to 19 years old have 46% of chlamydial infections, whereas 20- to 24-year-olds represent 33%. *Chlamydia* is reportable in all states and in all prepubescent children. It persists for up to 3 years perinatally and can progress to PID.

Syphilis, caused by *Treponema pallidum*, is a motile spirochete with a rate of 24 cases per 100,000. The majority of the cases occur in the southern United States (CDC, 2003). Coinfection with HIV exists in up to 15% of cases.

There are two identified serotypes of herpes: HSV-1 and HSV-2. Although either type may infect any part of the body, most recurrent genital herpes is a result of HSV-2. Asymptomatic HSV infections are responsible for the transmission of most cases of genital herpes. Type 2 is reportable in prepubescent children in some states.

HPV is a small DNA virus. More than 30 types of HPV can infect the genital tract. Visible warts are usually caused by HPV types 6 or 11. A person may be infected with multiple types of warts. Types 16, 18, 31, 33, and 35 have been strongly associated with cervical cancer, as well as vulvar, penile, and anal squamous intraepithelial neoplasia (CDC, 2002b).

Clinical Findings

History. Many patients are asymptomatic. The history should assess the following:

- Type of sexual activity (including oral, vaginal, anal sex/intercourse) and contraceptive use
- Number of sexual partners over 60 days, 12 months, and lifetime; heterosexual or homosexual (or both) activity
- Known exposure or previous STDs
- Use of drugs or alcohol
- Vaginal discharge (amount, color, odor), pruritus, irregular or painful bleeding, dysmenorrhea, dyspareunia
- Dysuria, urinary urgency or frequency
- Abdominal or pelvic pain
- Skin rashes or lesions, ulcers, warts
- Systemic symptoms such as fever, malaise, headache
- See Box 36-4 for risk factors for STDs and Table 36-4 for history specific to each STD
- See Chapter 20 for further details on obtaining history

Physical Examination

The physical examination should include the following:

- General examination—skin rashes and lesions, lymphadenopathy
- Abdominal examination—hepatic or splenic enlargement or tenderness in right upper quadrant

- Pelvic examination—inspection of external genitalia and vaginal mucosa, vaginal pH and discharge, cervical erythema, friability and mucopus, bimanual examination for motion tenderness, uterine size, adnexal tenderness
- Rectal examination
- Colposcopy of cervix, vagina, and vulva—recommended only for abnormal Pap test results and sexual abuse examination
- See Table 36-4 for physical findings specific to each STD

Laboratory Studies. In deciding the types of studies to order, the NP needs to know the difference in types and accuracy of tests. Methods that are sufficiently accurate for adolescents (presumptive tests) are not adequate for children who are being evaluated for possible abuse.

- Gonorrhea. Gram stain of vaginal discharge that shows gram-negative diplococci in polymorphonuclear leukocytes and culture on selective media with determination of penicillin resistance are definitive tests for gonorrhea. Nucleic acid amplification testing is now commercially available for GC testing. The four tests currently available are polymerase chain reaction (PCR), ligase chain reaction (LCR), strand-displacement amplification (SDA), and transcription-mediated amplification (TMA). Many fewer organisms are needed for detection allowing for reliable urine, vaginal, and cervical swab testing. The availability of urine testing has opened the way for noninvasive specimen collection (Blake & Woods, 2001).
- *Chlamydia.* Culture is the only acceptable method to diagnose possible sexual abuse cases; PCR, LCR, SDA, or TMA probes are acceptable in adolescents, especially in high-prevalence populations. Screening of asymptomatic sexually active young people is essential because about 50% of men and 75% of women with *Chlamydia* will report no symptoms (Grimes, 2000).
- Syphilis. Direct visualization with dark-field microscopy or direct immunofluorescent antibody (DFA) test is definitive. Serologic nontreponemal tests (Venereal Disease Research Laboratories [VDRL], rapid plasma reagin [RPR], or automated reagin test) correlate with disease activity, decline after treatment, and are used to monitor disease progress. Treponemal tests (fluorescent treponemal antibody absorption [FTA-ABS] or microhemagglutination test for *Treponema pallidum* [MHA-TP]) are confirmatory, but once positive, they usually remain so for years.
- Herpes. Culture of scraped vesicle or ulcer is most accurate. Tzanck stain, DFA, and enzyme immunoassay (EIA) are quicker but less sensitive. Blood tests are being studied but are not routinely used because they are not readily available.
- Human papillomavirus. Virapap is the specific test. Pap testing can show koilocytosis; dysplasia, atypia, or cervical intraepithelial neoplasia is suspicious. The use of HPV nucleic acid tests for typing visible genital warts is not recommended. Biopsy for histologic and cytologic microscopic evaluation and typing by DNA hybridization are more specific but rarely needed.

Differential Diagnosis

Chancroid, lymphogranuloma venereum, cytomegalovirus, hepatitis, granuloma inguinale, and molluscum are included in the differential diagnosis.

Management

The guidelines identified in this section are those recommended by the CDC (2002b) for uncomplicated, initial treatment of STDs. Other recommendations and options for children weighing less than 45 kg and for recurrent and complex cases can also be found in this literature or in adolescent gynecology or child abuse literature.

The goals of treatment include making a prompt diagnosis, determining the mode of acquisition, instituting appropriate treatment, preventing complications, contacting appropriate authorities, ensuring appropriate follow-up, and educating the adolescent and partner about risk reduction. All adolescents in the United States can consent to confidential diagnosis and treatment of STDs.

Several options for treatment are given for each disease (see Table 36-4). When determining appropriate treatment, consideration should be given to the site of infection, the resistance patterns in the community, concurrent infections, side effects of the medication, and cost. See Box 36-5 for general treatment measures for STDs.

1. Gonorrhea (uncomplicated, patient greater than 45 kg):
- See Table 36-4.
- Cefixime 400 mg orally in a single dose is recommended as the single-dose treatment. In October 2002, Wyeth Pharmaceutical ceased production of cefixime and it will only be available until the company inventory is depleted (CDC, 2002a).
- Fluoroquinolones should not be used for treatment of GC if the infection was acquired in Asia, the Pacific Islands (including Hawaii), or California because the prevalence of fluoroquinolone-resistant *N. gonorrhoeae* is high in those areas.
- Evaluate and treat all partners exposed in the previous 30 to 60 days, and treat last sexual partner if more than 60 days since last intercourse.

2. *Chlamydia*, uncomplicated genital infection:
- See Table 36-4.
- Treat last partner and any partner exposed within the 60 days before the onset of symptoms.

BOX 36-5 *General Treatment Measures for Sexually Transmitted Diseases*

1. Have patient abstain from sexual intercourse until patient and partner are cured (treatment complete and symptoms resolved). Consequences of untreated sexually transmitted diseases (STDs) should be explained.
2. Test for other STDs, including hepatitis B, human immunodeficiency virus, bacterial vaginosis, and *Trichomonas*.
3. Notify, examine, and treat all partners of patient for any STD identified or suspected.
4. Report STDs to state health department. Reporting to appropriate authorities is important to identify those at risk, recognize new strains, and assess extent of infection in community and the effect of prevention efforts.
5. Provide regular sex health assessment including Papanicolaou testing, vaginal examination, and testing for STDs.
6. Give hepatitis B vaccine if not done already.
7. Discuss safer sex practices, including abstinence and use of condoms.
8. Educate and counsel about complications and transmission of STDs, as well as perinatal consequences.

- Rescreen 3 to 4 months after positive test because a high prevalence of *C. trachomatis* infection is found in women with a chlamydial infection in the preceding several months. Reinfection is usually the cause of infection and elevates the risk for PID.

3. Syphilis, primary or secondary:

- See Table 36-4.
- The same laboratory tests (RPR or VDRL) should be used for follow-up and should decrease fourfold by 6 months and become nonreactive 1 year after treatment in primary cases. If still reactive after 12 months, re-treat and reevaluate for HIV.
- Treat all partners exposed during symptomatic period and for the 3 months before onset of infection.
- An acute febrile reaction (Jarisch-Herxheimer reaction) with myalgia, headache, and other symptoms can occur within 24 hours after treatment.
- Refer if symptoms of secondary or tertiary syphilis are present.

4. Genital herpes: no treatment eradicates the disease. Treatment or prevention of acute outbreaks is the goal of therapy.

- See Table 36-4.
- Famciclovir 250 mg three times a day for 7 to 10 days (primary) or 125 mg twice a day for 5 days (recurrent) [no pediatric data available] *or*
- Valacyclovir 1 g twice a day for 7 to 10 days (primary) or 500 mg twice a day for 3 to 5 days (recurrent) or 1.0 g once a day for 5 days (no pediatric data are available)
- Use daily suppressive treatment if episodes occur six times or more in a year. This reduces the frequency of episodes by more than 70% to 80%. Safety and efficacy is established with patients receiving daily acyclovir for 6 years and with valacyclovir or famciclovir for 1 year.
    - Acyclovir 400 mg orally twice a day *or*
    - Famciclovir 250 mg orally twice a day *or*
    - Valacyclovir 500 mg once a day or 1000 mg once a day
- Test for other STDs as indicated.
- Counsel to abstain from sexual activity when active lesions are present and inform sexual partners.
- Inform that transmission of HSV can occur during asymptomatic periods.
- Stress the risk of perinatal infection and follow pregnancies closely.
- Educate regarding course of disease, self-inoculation, transmission, and asymptomatic viral shedding.
- Suggest dietary modifications including increased intake of vitamin C, B-complex and B_6 vitamins, zinc, and calcium to boost the immune system. A diet high in lysine and low in arginine (e.g., eating fish, chicken, cheese, and most fruits and vegetables and avoiding chocolate, peanuts, and white and wheat flour) may be helpful.

5. Human papillomavirus: no treatment eradicates this disease. The goal should be to remove visible warts and reduce symptoms. The benefit of identification and treatment of subclinical infections has not been established. Patient preference and treatment availability should guide treatment course; spontaneous resolution will occur in most cases. Warts on moist surfaces respond better to topical treatment than do warts on drier surfaces.

- Patient-applied treatment: treat with (1) podofilox 0.5% solution or gel twice a day for 3 days, no treatment for 4 days, for a total of four cycles (safety in pregnancy has not been established) or (2) imiquimod 5% cream applied with finger at bedtime three times a week for up to 16 weeks. Wash treated area with mild soap and water 6 to 10 hours after application. Warts should clear after 8 to 10 weeks. Safety in pregnancy is not determined.
- Provider-applied treatment: treat external visible warts with (1) cryotherapy with liquid nitrogen or cryoprobe every 1 to 2 weeks, or (2) 10% to 25% podophyllin resin in benzoin washed off in 1 to 4 hours to decrease local irritation, repeated weekly (safety in pregnancy not

established), or (3) trichloroacetic acid (TCA) or bichloroacetic acid (BCA) applied in small amounts, dried to frosting consistency, followed by powder or baking soda to remove unreacted acid, repeated weekly, or (4) surgical removal with scissors, shave, curette, or electrosurgery.
- Change treatment if there is no response after three patient-applied treatments or six provider-applied treatments.
- Use only one treatment modality at a time to avoid increased complications.
- Advise patient that an inflammatory reaction is common before resolution.
- After cryotherapy, pain, necrosis, and blistering are common.
- Refer patients with cervical warts, suspected abuse, or extensive lesions in difficult areas for gynecologic treatment. Intralesional interferon or laser surgery may be necessary in severe cases.
- No change in the schedule for Pap testing is necessary with clinical warts.
- Advise patient that recurrence is common, most often in the first 3 months following treatment.
- Remember that latent perinatal transmission of virus can be present for 1 to 3 years.

Complications

In general, perinatal transmission, disseminated infection, and increased risk for chronic hepatitis are possible. PID, ectopic pregnancy, and infertility are possible sequelae to GC and chlamydia. Tertiary disease is a risk with syphilis. An increased incidence of HIV infection occurs with syphilis and HSV infection. HPV infection is linked with cervical dysplasia.

Patient Education and Prevention

- Prevention occurs at a variety of levels and in a variety of ways. The following approaches are recommended (Bonny & Biro, 1998; Stevens-Simon, 1998):
  - Primary prevention seeks to reduce the number of new cases of STDs. This best occurs before sexual debut, focusing on delaying initiation of sexual intercourse, encouraging noncoital sexual behavior, promoting condom negotiating skills, and avoiding exposure to STDs if the intent is to become sexually active. These topics must be addressed specifically, using knowledge, attitudes, and behaviors to guide education. Developmental needs, cultural values, misperceptions, and social skills are areas to be addressed. Peer facilitators are often useful. Hepatitis B and possibly hepatitis A immunizations are recommended.
  - Secondary prevention seeks to reduce the numbers of existing cases by early detection and treatment through well-woman care, annual Pap testing, and STD screening recommended every 6 months for those at risk. Access to health care for treatment and follow-up, monitoring for sequelae, partner notification, and evaluating risk behaviors are important aspects to successful secondary prevention.
  - Tertiary prevention seeks to minimize the psychologic and biologic sequelae of STDs. This includes minimizing perinatal complications and infant morbidity and mortality rates and reducing the frequency of PID and its complications. Identifying coping strategies and means of increasing self-esteem are also important aspects.
- Treatment of any STD in a child should be coordinated with the laboratory, child protective services, and the state authorities.
- Important family factors that reduce risk behaviors include the following:
  - Perceived parental support
  - Degree of family closeness
  - Communication among family members (when parent-child communication is good, adolescents are more likely to postpone sexual intercourse, have fewer partners when sexually active, and increase the use of condoms and contraception [Kollar, 2002])
  - Parenting style
  - Parental supervision and monitoring

Pelvic Inflammatory Disease

Description

Considered an ascending infection, PID refers to infection and inflammation involving the upper genital tract (uterus, fallopian tubes, ovaries, or peritoneal tissue). PID is either acute (less than 3 weeks' duration) or chronic. The classic picture is acute salpingitis that causes lower abdominal pain, vaginal discharge, and fever with an onset after menses. However, PID is difficult to diagnose because symptoms are widely varied (CDC, 2002b).

Etiology and Incidence

PID is often a polymicrobial infection, with GC and chlamydia being the two most common STDs causing PID. Vaginal flora, other aerobic and anaerobic organisms, group B streptococcus, genital mycoplasma, and gram-negative bacteria also are implicated. There are 1 million new cases of PID every year, with the highest incidence occurring in adolescents and young adults (AAP, 2003). The two risk factors considered to be most significant among teenagers are multiple sexual partners and the high prevalence of STDs in this age-group. Other risk factors include increased susceptibility of adolescents to infection, cervical ectopy and thinner cervical mucus, recent instrumentation or intrauterine device use, previous PID, history of lower genital tract infection (including *Chlamydia, Trichomonas*, and bacterial vaginosis), and nonuse of contraceptives of any type. Use of OCs decreases the incidence of PID sevenfold (Pletcher & Slap, 1999).

Clinical Findings

PID in adolescents is often subtle and can go undiagnosed, contributing to the inflammatory sequelae. Criteria for diagnosis of PID have been identified, including a set of minimal, low-threshold criteria prompting early intervention (Box 36-6).

History

- Sexual history, including number of partners and type of activity
- Last menstrual period, contraceptive use, and previous STD or PID

BOX 36-6 *Criteria for Diagnosing Pelvic Inflammatory Disease*

Minimum criteria for treating pelvic inflammatory disease (PID) in sexually active adolescents with no other cause for illness identified:
Uterine/adnexal tenderness *or*
Cervical motion tenderness
Additional criteria that support a diagnosis of PID:
Oral temperature >101° F
Abnormal mucopuruluent cervical or vaginal discharge
Presence of WBCs in saline microscopy of vaginal secretions
Elevated erythrocyte sedimentation rate
Elevated C-reactive protein
Laboratory documentation of cervical infection with gonorrhea or chlamydia
Most specific criteria for diagnosing PID, warranted in selected cases:
Endometrial biopsy with histopathologic evidence of endometritis
Transvaginal sonography or magnetic resonance imaging showing thickened fluid-filled tubes with or without free pelvic fluid or tubo-ovarian complex
Laparoscopic abnormalities consistent with PID

Adapted from Centers for Disease Control and Prevention: Guidelines for treatment of sexually transmitted diseases, *MMWR Morb Mortal Wkly Rep* 51(RR6-80), 2002; American Academy of Pediatrics: *2003 red book: report of the Committee on Infectious Diseases*, ed 26, Elk Grove Village, IL, 2003, American Academy of Pediatrics.

- Lower abdominal pain or tenderness (acute onset with gonorrhea, subtle with chlamydia)
- Intermenstrual bleeding
- Malaise, dysuria, nausea, vomiting, chills, dyspareunia

Physical Examination

- Abdominal examination—bilateral lower quadrant tenderness (most common initial symptom) and possibly right upper quadrant pain (Fitz-Hugh-Curtis syndrome: inflammation of liver capsule); occasional peritoneal signs
- Speculum examination—cervical or vaginal mucopurulent discharge
- Bimanual examination—cervical motion tenderness or adnexal tenderness (may be unilateral)

Laboratory Studies

- CBC (WBCs greater than 10,000), erythrocyte sedimentation rate (greater than 15 mm/hr), C-reactive protein (elevated)
- Microscopic examination of cervical discharge (more than 5 WBCs)
- Gram stain of cervical mucus (gonorrhea)
- Direct immunofluorescence antibody or polyclonal enzyme-linked immunoassay test (chlamydia)
- Serologic test (syphilis)
- Pregnancy test (ectopic)
- Urinalysis and culture if symptoms of pyelonephritis or cystitis
- Pelvic ultrasound (if adnexal enlargement or tubo-ovarian abscess suspected)
- Culdocentesis (pus)

Differential Diagnosis

Acute appendicitis, ectopic pregnancy, twisted ovarian cyst, ruptured corpus luteum cyst, salpingitis, tubo-ovarian abscess, endometriosis, acute pyelonephritis, gastroenteritis, vaginitis, and functional pain are included in the differential diagnosis.

Management

- Goals of treatment include the relief of acute discomfort and prevention of infertility and other sequelae. More than one diagnosis is possible. Empiric treatment should be initiated in sexually active young women if the minimum criteria are met. Treatment should be initiated as soon as possible with broad-spectrum coverage to minimize long-term sequelae.
- Hospitalization is recommended in the following situations: surgical emergency cannot be excluded; pregnancy; lack of response to oral antibiotics; inability to tolerate oral antibiotics; severe illness with nausea, vomiting, or high temperature; or tubo-ovarian abscess (CDC, 2002b).
- Treatment regimens are delineated in Table 36-5.

TABLE 36-5 ***Outpatient Treatment Regimens for Pelvic Inflammatory Disease***

	Regimen A	Regimen B	On Discharge
Oral	Ofloxacin 400 mg orally twice daily for 14 days* *or* Levofloxacin 500 mg orally once daily for 14 days* *with or without* metronidazole 500 mg twice daily for 14 days	Ceftriaxone 250 mg IM in a single dose *or* Cefoxitin 2 g IM in a single dose plus probenecid 1 g orally in a single dose *or* Other parenteral third-generation cephalosporin *Plus* Doxycycline 100 mg twice daily for 14 days *with or without* metronidazole 500 mg orally twice daily for 14 days	
Parental	Cefoxitin 2 g IV every 6 hr *or* cefotetan 2 g IV every 12 hr *plus* Doxycycline 100 mg PO or IV every 12 hr, both continued until 48 hr after improvement; oral treatment with doxycycline preferred even when hospitalized because of pain with infusion	Clindamycin 900 mg IV every 8 hr *plus* Gentamicin 2 mg/kg IV or IM loading dose followed by 1.5 mg/kg every 8 hr, both continued until 48 hr after improvement	Doxycycline 100 mg twice a day for a total of 14 days from time medication was initiated *or* Clindamycin 450 mg orally four times a day for a total of 14 days

IM, Intramuscular; *IV*, intravenous; *PO*, by mouth.
*Contraindicated under 18 years of age, in pregnancy, or during lactation.

RESOURCE BOX

National Resources for Pediatric and Adolescent Gynecology

American College of Obstetricians and Gynecologists (ACOG) (pamphlets)
1-202-638-5577
1-800-762-2264
www.acog.com

American Social Health Association (pamphlets)
1-800-783-9877
www.ashastd.org

Centers for Disease Control and Prevention (CDC) STD Hotline
1-800-227-8922
www.cdc.gov/std

Education Training Resource Associates (pamphlets)
1-800-321-4407
www.etr.org

Endometriosis information
www.youngwomenshealth.org

Focus on the Family
1-800-232-6459
Videos: *No Apologies: The Truth about Life, Love and Sex;* and *Sex, Lies and . . . the Truth*

Medical Institute for Sexual Health (medical data)
1-512-328-6268
www.medinstitute.org

National Abstinence Clearinghouse
1-888-577-2966
www.abstinence.net

National Herpes Hotline
1-919-361-8488
www.ashastd.org/hotlines/herphotline.html

National STD Hotline
1-800-227-8922 or
1-809-765-1010
www.ashastd.org/NSTD/

North American Society for Pediatric and Adolescent Gynecology (NASPAG)
1-215-955-6331
www.naspag.org/index.html

Planned Parenthood Federation of America
1-800-669-0156
www.plannedparenthood.org

RESOURCE BOX

National Resources for Pediatric and Adolescent Gynecology—cont'd

Project Reality, Choosing the Best Abstinence Program
1-847-729-3298
www.projectreality.org

Sex Information and Education Council of the United States (SIECUS)
1-212-819-9770
www.siecus.org

Society for Adolescent Medicine
1-816-224-8010
www.adolescenthealth.org

Teen Aid, Inc. (abstinence curricula)
1-800-357-2868
www.teen-aid.org

- Follow up within 72 hours. If there has been no response, reevaluate diagnosis and treatment. Parenteral therapy should be started and continued until defervescence, evidenced by decreased abdominal tenderness and decreased uterine, adnexal, and cervical motion tenderness.
- Treatment of any sexual partners exposed within 60 days of onset of symptoms is imperative. No intercourse until partners have been treated.
- Follow up 7 to 10 days after treatment.
- Rescreen for *Chlamydia* and GC 4 to 6 weeks after treatment.
- HIV screening should be offered.

Complications

Infertility (15% to 30% attributable to PID, higher with subsequent episodes), tubo-ovarian abscess, ectopic pregnancy (50% of cases), chronic pelvic pain (18% of cases), dyspareunia, repeated PID, tubal scarring, and extrapelvic infection are possible complications (CDC, 2002b).

Prevention

Decrease prevalence and transmission of STDs by promoting abstinence and barrier methods (condoms, diaphragms, cervical caps, spermicidal foams). Screen sexually active adolescents for gonorrhea and chlamydia every 6 months.

REFERENCES

American Academy of Pediatrics: *2003 red book: report of the Committee on Infectious Diseases*, ed 26, Elk Grove Village, IL, 2003, American Academy of Pediatrics.

American College of Obstetricians and Gynecologists: Medical management of endometriosis, *Int J Gyneacol Obstet* 71:183-196, 2000.

Apgar BS: Diagnosis and management of amenorrhea, *Clin Fam Pract* 4:54-60, 2002.

Bacon JL: Dysfunctional uterine bleeding, *Female Patient* 3(suppl):21-28, 2000.

Bacon JL: Prepubertal labial adhesions: evaluation of a referral population, *Am J Obstet Gynecol* 187: 327-332, 2002.

Biro FM, Rosenthal SL: Adolescent STDs: diagnosis, developmental issues, and prevention, *J Pediatr Health Care* 9:256-262, 1995.

Blake DR, Woods ER: The future is here: noninvasive diagnosis of STDs, *Contemp Pediatr* 18:71-87, 2001.

Bonny AE, Biro FM: Recognizing and treating STDs in adolescent girls, *Contemp Pediatr* 15:119-143, 1998.

Bravender T, Emans S: Dysfunctional uterine bleeding, *Pediatr Clin North Am* 46(3):545-553, 1999.

Centers for Disease Control and Prevention: Discontinuation of cefixime tablets in the United States, *MMWR Morb Mortal Wkly Rep* 51:1052, 2002a.

Centers for Disease Control and Prevention: Sexually transmitted diseases: treatment guidelines, *MMWR Morb Mortal Wkly Rep* 51(RR-6):i-80, 2002b.

Centers for Disease Control and Prevention: *Sexually transmitted disease surveillance*, Atlanta, 2002, Centers for Disease Control and Prevention. Available at *www.cdc.gov/std/stats/natoverview.htm* (accessed Dec 2003).

Chen C et al: Prospective study of exposure to environmental tobacco smoke and dysmenorrhea, *Environ Health Perspect* 108:1019-1022, 2000.

Craighill MC: Pediatric and adolescent gynecology for primary care pediatricians, *Pediatr Clin North Am* 45:1659-1688, 1998.

Cramer DW, Missmer SA: The epidemiology of endometriosis, *Ann N Y Acad Sci* 955:11-22, 2002.

Davis AR, Westhoff CL: Primary dysmenorrhea in adolescent girls and treatment with oral contraceptives, *North Am Soc Pediatr Adolesc Gynecol* 14:3-8, 2001.

Elster A, Kuznets N: *AMA guidelines for adolescent preventive services (GAPS)*, Baltimore, 1994, Williams & Wilkins.

Emans S, Laufer MR, Goldstein D: *Pediatric and adolescent gynecology*, ed 4, Philadelphia, 1998, Lippincott-Raven.

Gokhale LB: Curative treatment of primary (spasmodic) dysmenorrhoea, *Indian J Med Res* 103:227-231, 1996.

Greydanus DE, Patel DR: The female athlete: before and beyond puberty, *Pediatr Clin North Am* 49:829-855, 2002.

Grimes DA: STD update: incidence trends and new screening tests, *Contracept Rep* 11:4-10, 2000.

Hennigen L, Kollar LM, Rosenthal SL: Methods for managing pelvic examination anxiety: individual differences and relaxation techniques, *J Pediatr Health Care* 14:9-12, 2000.

Hillard PA: Diagnosing and controlling abnormal uterine bleeding, *Contemp Adolesc Gynecol* 4:4-7, 1999.

Kollar LM: STD update: testing, treatment and the NP's role in prevention. Presentation at 23rd Annual NAPNAP Conference, Reno, NV, 2002.

Mitan LA, Slap GB: Adolescent menstrual disorders, *Med Clin North Am* 84:851-868, 2000.

Olive DL, Pritts EA: Treatment of endometriosis, *N Engl J Med* 345:266-275, 2001.

Pletcher JR, Slap GB: Menstrual disorders: amenorrhea, *Pediatr Clin North Am* 46:505-518, 1999.

Preminger MK, Pokorny SF: Vaginal discharge—a common pediatric complaint, *Contemp Pediatr* 15:115-122, 1998.

Propst AM, Laufer MR: Diagnosing and treating adolescent endometriosis, *Contemp Pediatr* 17:71-78, 2000.

Prose CC, Ford CA, Lovely LP: Evaluating amenorrhea: the pediatrician's role, *Contemp Pediatr* 15:83-110, 1998.

Rimsza ME: Dysfunctional uterine bleeding, *Pediatr Rev* 23(7):227-233, 2002.

Saslow D et al: American Cancer Society guideline for the early detection of cervical neoplasia and cancer, *CA Cancer J Clin* 52:342-362, 2002.

Schroeder B, Sanfilippo JS: Dysmenorrhea and pelvic pain in adolescents, *Pediatr Clin North Am* 46:555-571, 1999.

Smith DE, Lohr JA: Vulvovaginitis. In Dershewitz R, editor: *Ambulatory pediatric care*, ed 3, Philadelphia, 1999, JB Lippincott.

Stamm CA, McGregor JA: Diagnosing and treating STDs in young women, *Contemp Pediatr* 18:53-67, 2001.

Stevens-Simon C: Providing effective reproductive health care and prescribing contraceptives for adolescents, *Pediatr Rev* 19(12):409-417, 1998.

US Department of Health and Human Services: *Healthy People 2010* objectives. Available at *http://web.health.gov/healthypeople* (accessed Nov 26, 2003).

US Preventive Services Task Force: *Guide to clinical preventive services*, 2003. Available at *www.ahrq.gov/clinic/cp3dix.htm* (accessed Dec 2003).

US Public Health Service: Recommendations, 2003. Available at *www.ahrq.gov/clinic/prevenix.htm* (accessed Dec 2003).

WebMD Scientific American Medicine: Treatment steps for primary dysmenorrhea, *Clinical Advisor*, Oct 2002, p 105.

37 Dermatologic Diseases

Peggy Vernon, Nancy Barber Starr

The skin is the body's largest organ and one of its most important. The condition of the skin reflects physical and emotional health, plays a major role in defining identity and supporting survival, and often gives clues to underlying conditions. Skin functions are multiple. Beauty is often defined by the appearance of the skin. Emotions are expressed by blushing and sweating. Skin conveys many impressions through its sensory functions, including reaction to touch, heat, cold, pressure, and pain. Additionally, the skin provides a protective physiologic covering, the first line of defense against injury from chemical, physical, and microorganic invaders. Homeostasis is maintained through fluid regulation and thermoregulation.

Disruptions in the skin account for 20% to 30% of all pediatric office visits (Hurwitz, 1993). The primary care provider plays an essential role in maintaining skin integrity, identifying and minimizing skin disruptions, maximizing healing, and educating parents and children about skin care.

SKIN DEVELOPMENT

Skin development is constant from embryogenesis throughout life. During the embryonic period (the first 2 months of gestation), the skin differentiates into several layers. During the fetal period, appendages (hair, nails, and sebaceous, apocrine, and eccrine glands) develop and all skin layers continue to mature. Neonatal skin continues to change and develop throughout childhood and adolescence, achieving adult skin thickness and characteristics in the late teenage years. Melanin in the skin reaches adult levels by 1 year of age. Vascularization is well developed by the end of the second year of life. Cutaneous nerves develop until puberty and beyond. Sebaceous glands cease production between 6 and 12 months of age but become active again at around 7 years of age. Eccrine sweat function begins between 2 and 18 days of age, although full function is not in place until 2 or 3 years of age. The apocrine glands become active at puberty. Hair goes through three stages: growth (anagen), rest (telogen), and regression (catagen), with approximately 1 cm of growth per month. Nails, formed in the fifth fetal month, are spoon shaped and thin from infancy until 2 to 3 years of age.

ANATOMY AND PHYSIOLOGY

The skin, covering the entire surface of the body, is composed of three layers: the epidermis, the dermis, and the subcutaneous layer (Fig. 37-1). Skin thickness varies from 0.5 mm on the eyelids to 3 to 4 mm on the palms and soles.

The epidermis, the thinner outer layer, comprises five layers of stratified squamous epithelium. The outer horny layer is responsible for much of the barrier protection against microorganisms and irritating chemicals. It also impedes the exchange of fluids and electrolytes with the environment and provides strength of the skin. Melanin serves to protect DNA from damage by ultraviolet (UV) light irradiation. It is produced in the basal layer of the epidermis and contributes to the color of the skin, eyes, and hair. The water content of the environment influences the epidermal barrier, with either excess or inadequate amounts contributing to microscopic and macroscopic breaks.

The thicker middle layer, the dermis, contributes strength, support, and elasticity to the skin. It also regulates heat loss, provides host defenses of the skin, and aids in nutrition and other regulatory functions. The dermis is primarily composed of fibrous connective tissue, with

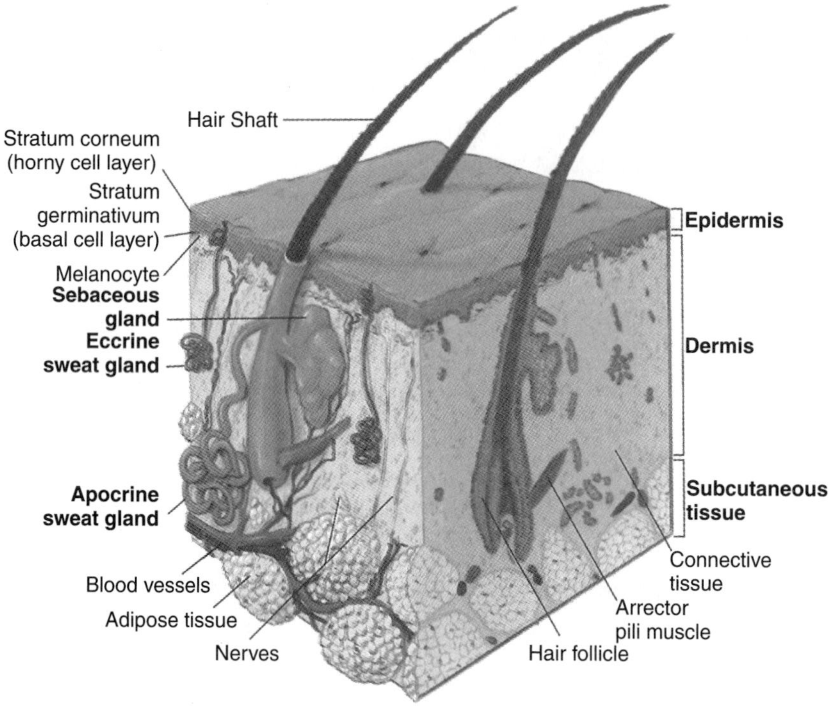

FIGURE 37-1 Structure of the skin. (From Jarvis C: *Physical examination and assessment*, ed 2, Philadelphia, 1996, WB Saunders.)

some elastic fibers and a mucopolysaccharide gel. It includes mast cells, inflammatory cells, and blood and lymph vessels, as well as cutaneous nerves that elicit sensations (touch, pain, itch, warmth, and cold).

Underlying the dermis is subcutaneous tissue primarily composed of adipose tissue. Networks of arteries lie here and branch into the dermis as small arterioles. The subcutaneous tissue is an insulator, a cushion against trauma, and a source of energy and hormone metabolism (see Fig. 37-1).

Skin appendages include the hair, nails, sweat glands, and sebaceous glands. Hair follicles are found over the entire body except for the palms, soles, knuckles, distal and interdigital spaces, lips, glans and prepuce of the penis, and areolae and nipples. Two types of hair can be found on the body. Terminal hair is thick and visible and found on the scalp, axillae, and pubis. Very fine vellus hair is found over the remainder of the body. The visible portion of the hair is the shaft. The root of the hair is embedded in the dermis as a pilosebaceous unit, consisting of a hair follicle and a sebaceous gland. The hair shaft may be straight, wavy, helical, or spiral. Following an acute febrile illness or stress, many hairs convert from anagen to telogen stage, resulting in a noticeably thinned amount of hair for several months.

Nails are epidermal cells converted to keratin that grow continually. The body of the nail (or nail plate) is visible. The nail bed, underneath the nail plate, is composed of layers of epidermis and dermis, which serve as structural support. The root of the nail lies just under the epidermis.

Sweat glands can be grouped into three categories: eccrine, ceruminous, and apocrine. Eccrine glands are numerous and are distributed over the entire body. The coiled bodies of the eccrine glands lie in the dermis and empty onto the surface of the skin, helping maintain fluid and electrolyte balance and body temperature, as well as providing some excretory function. Ceruminous glands, thought to be modified sweat glands, are located in the external ear canal and secrete a waxy pigmented substance, cerumen. Apocrine glands, located primarily in the axillary, genital, and periumbilical areas, are larger coils than eccrine glands. They open into hair follicles, require androgens to stimulate their secretions, and are thought to be responsible for body odor.

Sebaceous glands, found in conjunction with hair follicles, are distributed over the entire body except the soles, palms, and dorsa of the feet. These glands secrete sebum (oil) when stimulated by androgen and function to prevent excessive water evaporation, minimize heat loss, and lubricate hair.

SPECIAL DERMATOLOGIC CONSIDERATIONS IN CHILDREN WITH DARK SKIN OR FROM DIVERSE CULTURAL OR ETHNIC GROUPS

Knowledge of the normal variations in children both with different levels of pigmentation of the skin and from diverse ethnic or cultural groups is important for assessing and treating dermatologic conditions (Dinulos & Graham, 1998; Smith & Burns, 1999). Skin reactions to injury, inflammation, common skin conditions, and cultural practices are varied. A wise clinician listens to parents, because they are often the first to detect subtle changes in color or texture of the skin.

Cutaneous Reaction Patterns

African American children may have an exaggerated cutaneous response to common disorders of the skin. Three identified patterns are pigment lability, follicular response, and mesenchymal response (Dinulos & Graham, 1998). Pigment lability manifested as postinflammatory hypopigmentation or hyperpigmentation is common. If superficial, with changes in the epidermis only, normal pigmentation returns in about 6 months (e.g., in diaper rash, seborrhea, tinea, pityriasis alba). If dermal changes occur, dermal tattooing may occur, causing permanent changes or changes that last for years (e.g., excoriated acne, impetigo, varicella, contact dermatitis). The exaggerated follicular response can be seen in prominent papules and follicles, especially with atopic dermatitis, pityriasis rosea, or tinea versicolor. The mesenchymal response causes hypertrophic scars and keloids (which extend beyond the edge of the scar), often following varicella, ear piercing, burns, or any surgical procedure. Other exaggerated responses include lichenification and vesicular or bullous reaction to bites or staphylococcal infection.

Normal Variations and Common Problems

The following are normal variations or common problems in children with darker skin:

- Variation in color and texture of skin from one part of the body to another
- Pigmentation of gingiva, mucous membrane, sclerae, and nails correlates with degree of cutaneous pigmentation
- Increased areas of melanin in thicker-skinned areas (elbow, knee)
- Futcher's (Voigt's, Ito's) lines—vertical lines separating hyperpigmented extensor surfaces from less pigmented ventral surfaces (upper arms, chest, abdomen)
- Mongolian spots and increased numbers of café au lait spots (see discussion later in chapter)
- Normal exfoliation produces a fine layer of gray scales
- Color alterations (jaundice, anemia, cyanosis)—difficult to assess
- Kinky, wooly, tightly curled hair with closely knit growth that tangles when dry and mats when wet
- Tinea versicolor (see section on fungal disorders), initially papular with hypopigmentation or hyperpigmentation, occurring only on the face
- Atopic dermatitis (see Chapter 25) with prominent follicular pattern with pityriasis alba and postinflammatory hypopigmentation
- Pityriasis rosea (see section on papulosquamous disorders) often confused with tinea, primarily follicular, inverse distribution (face, neck, extremities, and torso)

Conditions occuring more commonly in African American children include tinea capitis, tinea versicolor, papular urticaria, infantile acropustulosis, dermatosis papulosa nigra, lichen nitidus, lichen spinulosis, pseudofolliculitis barbae, transient neonatal pustular melanosis, and acanthosis nigricans. Lichen planus is more severe and keloids are more frequent. Lice are less common in African American children.

Cultural or Ethnic Practices

Grooming, cosmetic, or healing practices of cultural or ethnic groups contribute to various conditions that may be seen. These include the following:

- Hair pomade—acne
- Bleaching creams—discoloration and erythematous nodules
- Chemical or thermal hair straighteners—alopecia, fragile hair shaft, scalp contact dermatitis
- Coining—petechiae and ecchymoses, especially on chest and back
- Cornrowed hair or tight ponytails—traction alopecia
- Cupping—circular ecchymoses on neck, chest, back, and arms
- Henna—orange discoloration of skin, increased bilirubin in infants if applied topically
- Scars or tattoos from decorative practices
- Healing practices used during significant illness that produce burns—circular 1 to 2 cm scars on chest, periumbilicus, wrists, ankles, or back

PATHOPHYSIOLOGY AND DEFENSE MECHANISMS

Disruption of the skin and subcutaneous tissue occurs through a variety of assaults. These include

- Bacterial, fungal, and viral infections
- Allergic and inflammatory reactions

- Infestations
- Vascular reactions
- Papulosquamous and bullous eruptions
- Congenital lesions
- Hair and nail disorders

The skin's outer layers provide the body's first line of defense from chemical, physical, and microorganic injury. The epidermis provides a functional barrier, the dermis provides strength and protection through the cutaneous nerves, and the subcutaneous tissue ensures insulation, cushion from injury, energy source, and hormonal metabolism. These layers, in turn, protect the other body systems. The water content of the skin enhances the protective barrier of the skin. If the skin becomes too dry or too wet, breaks in the barrier occur that elicit an inflammatory response. As a continuously growing system, the skin not only heals itself but controls growth or colonization of microorganisms by continual shedding.

ASSESSMENT OF THE SKIN AND SUBCUTANEOUS TISSUE

History

The history should assess the following:

- History of present illness
  - Onset and length of present or recent illness? Treatment used and effect?
  - Recent travel
  - Most common concerns: pruritus, scaling, and alterations in cosmetic appearance (Weston, Lane, & Morelli, 2002)
  - Three key questions to ask: How long have you had it? Does it itch? What have you used to treat it?
  - Rash, lesions, discharge
  - Associated systemic symptoms: fever, malaise
  - Exposures or allergies: medication, foods, animals, plants? Known allergens? New substances? Persons with similar symptoms or illness? What soaps, shampoos, lotions, and detergents are used?
  - All medication taken over the last few days, including creams, ointments, powders, or lotions (it is often helpful to have patients bring medications they have used to the appointment)
  - Prior incidents of similar rash
- Family history
  - Similar symptoms
  - Skin disorders or allergies
- Review of systems and past medical history
  - Usual state of health and recent illnesses
  - Skin, hair, and nails: skin type, recent and long-term changes, previous incidence of skin disease
  - Eyes, ears, nose, and throat: swelling, itching, crusting, discharge or circles around eyes, nasal mucus discharge, patency or irritation, dry mouth, lesions, or pain
  - Chest: wheezing, coughing, or respiratory difficulty

Physical Examination

A key question is, "Does the patient appear ill?" This clinical impression is important to differentiate the few serious illnesses from the majority of dermatologic conditions. The entire body needs to be examined, not just exposed skin. Attention should be given to the eyes, nose, mouth, lymph nodes, and lungs because a skin disorder may be a cutaneous manifestation of other disease. The dermatologic examination includes a thorough look at the skin, scalp, hair, palms and soles, nails, and anogenital region.

Special techniques for examination of the skin may be required. Good light (daylight is best) is essential to a good examination. A source of direct light, such as a gooseneck lamp, is the best alternative. Other helpful tools include a magnifying glass, a ruler, a glass slide, and a Wood's lamp (UV light). A glass slide gently pressed on the skin (diascopy) allows viewing of the skin with and without capillary filling. A Wood's lamp is used to examine fluorescent-positive fungal infections and depigmenting skin disorders such as vitiligo.

Identification of the type of lesion and correct use of terminology are essential to good dermatologic care. Essential documentation includes the following:

- Location and type of lesion
- Color, color changes, size, and shape
- Arrangement (e.g., isolated, grouped, linear, annular, zosteriform)
- Pattern (e.g., sun-exposed area, symmetry)
- Distribution of lesion (e.g., regional, generalized)
- Border (e.g., indistinct, well circumscribed)
- Consistency (e.g., firm, soft, mobile)

Primary skin lesions (Box 37-1) include changes that arise from previously normal skin. These descriptions should be memorized and used. *Secondary* skin lesions (Box 37-2) result from changes in primary lesions. *Vascular* skin lesions (Box 37-3) involve the blood supply. Other useful descriptive terms are listed in Box 37-4. The presence of vesicles, pustules, scaling, and color changes should be noted as essential for differential diagnosis (Weston, Lane, & Morelli, 2002).

Diagnostic Studies

A few simple laboratory tests are helpful in identifying or excluding dermatologic disorders. Proper procurement of the sample is important. Scraping of lesions can be done with a no. 15 blade or a toothbrush and scales or debris

BOX 37-1 *Primary Skin Changes to Lesions*

Macule—flat, nonpalpable, discolored lesion, 1 cm or smaller
Patch—macule, larger than 1 cm
Papule—solid, raised lesion of varied color with distinct borders, 1 cm or smaller
Plaque—solid, raised, flat-topped lesion with distinct borders, larger than 1 cm
Nodule—raised, firm, movable lesion with indistinct borders and deep palpable portion, 2 cm or smaller
Tumor—large nodule, may be firm or soft
Wheal—fleeting, irregularly shaped, elevated, itchy lesion of varied size, pale at center, slightly red at borders
Vesicle—blister filled with clear fluid
Bulla—vesicle larger than 1 cm
Cyst—palpable lesion with definite borders filled with liquid or semisolid material
Pustule—raised lesion filled with pus, often in hair follicle or sweat pore
Comedo—plugged, dilated pore; open (blackhead), closed (whitehead)

BOX 37-2 *Secondary Skin Changes to Lesions*

Crusts—dried exudate or scab of varied color
Scales—thin, flaking layers of epidermis
Desquamation—peeling sheets of scale
Lichenification—thickening of skin with deep visible furrows
Excoriation—abrasion or removal of epidermis; scratch
Fissure—linear, wedge-shaped cracks extending into dermis
Erosion—oozing or moist, depressed area with loss of superficial epidermis
Ulcer—deeper than erosion; open lesion extending into dermis
Atrophy—thinning skin, may appear translucent
Scar—healed lesion of connective tissue
Keloid—healed lesion of hypertrophied connective tissue
Striae—fine pink or silver lines in areas where skin has been stretched

placed on a glass slide or in culture material. It is important to scrape under any scabs to get the organisms. Moistening the lesion may facilitate this. Scrapings can be obtained from the edges of skin lesions; from plucked hair, including the root; from the nail plate; or from subungual debris. Laboratory tests that can be used include the following:

- Microscopic examination of skin scrapings.
- Potassium hydroxide (KOH) can be used to examine for fungal disorders (hyphae or spores; Fig. 37-2). Add a drop of KOH 20% to dissolve debris and cover with a coverslip. Let sit for 20 to 30 minutes or heat gently (do not boil). Use ×10 magnification to examine.
- Wright, Giemsa, or Gram stains are used to examine for bacteria or herpes simplex or herpes zoster giant cells. Allow scrapings to air-dry, then stain with Wright or Giemsa stain. Use ×40 magnification to examine for bacteria.
- Tzanck's smear for herpes, varicella, or zoster.
- Microbial culture of lesions for bacteria, viruses, or fungi. Simple, inexpensive culture methods for fungal organisms (Dermatophyte Test Medium or InTray CCD [includes *Candida*]—see Resource Box) can be done at room temperature. Skin or nail scrapings or hairs, including the root, are applied so that they break the agar surface. A color change is noted in 1 to 5 days.
- Patch or skin testing for allergic or contact reactions is usually done by dermatologists or allergists.
- Skin biopsy following local anesthesia may be done by punch or shave method for any tumor, palpable purpura, persistent dermatitis, or blister that is not otherwise definitively diagnosed. Such procedures often require referral to a dermatologist.
- Complete blood count (CBC) and erythrocyte sedimentation rate (ESR) may be done to evaluate infection or inflammation.

MANAGEMENT STRATEGIES

Hydration and Lubrication

Maintenance of skin hydration is essential to prevent and treat skin conditions. If the skin is overhydrated, the bonds between cells at the stratum corneum loosen and the barrier is broken. If the skin is too dry, it cracks, again breaking the barrier.

Bathing

Although less frequent bathing is often recommended, especially with dry skin or in dry climates, proper bathing and lubrication will enhance addition and retention of water in the skin. Lukewarm, not hot, water should be used. The bath should not last long enough for skin to become supersaturated. In general, mild soaps such as Dove, Neutrogena, Aveeno, or Purpose should be used. Soap substitutes include Cetaphil and Purpose Gentle Cleansing Wash. Bubble-bath solutions are especially irritating and should be avoided. Soaping and shampooing

BOX 37-3 *Vascular Skin Lesions*

Angioma or hemangioma—papule made of blood vessels
Ecchymosis—bruise, purple to brown in color, macular or papular, varied in size
Hematoma—collection of blood from ruptured blood vessel, larger than 1 cm
Petechiae—pinpoint, pink to purple macular lesions that do not blanch, 1 to 3 mm
Purpura—purple macular lesion, larger than 1 cm
Telangiectasia—collection of macular or raised, dilated capillaries

BOX 37-4 *Descriptive Terms for Dermatologic Lesions*

Acral—involving extremities (hands, feet, ears, etc.)
Annular—ring-shaped
Arcuate—arc-shaped
Circinate—circular
Confluent—running together
Contiguous—touching or adjacent
Discrete—distinct and separate
Diffuse or generalized—scattered, widely distributed
Eczematous—referring to vesicles with oozing crust
Grouped—arranged in sets
Guttate—small, droplike
Herpetiform—referring to grouped vesicles resembling those of herpes
Iris—arranged in concentric circles, one inside the other
Linear—arranged in a line
Localized—in a limited area
Nummular—coin-shaped
Pedunculated—having a stalk
Polycyclic—oval with more than one ring
Reticular—netlike
Serpiginous—snakelike, creeping
Symmetric—balanced on both sides
Telangiectatic—referring to dilated terminal vessels
Umbilicated—depressed or shaped like a navel
Verrucous—wartlike
Zosteriform—resembling shingles, following a nerve root or dermatome

should be done at the end of the bath followed by thorough rinsing. The skin should be gently dried and a lubricating agent applied immediately. See Chapter 25 for further information on lubricating baths. Baths including baking soda or Aveeno colloidal ointment may be helpful

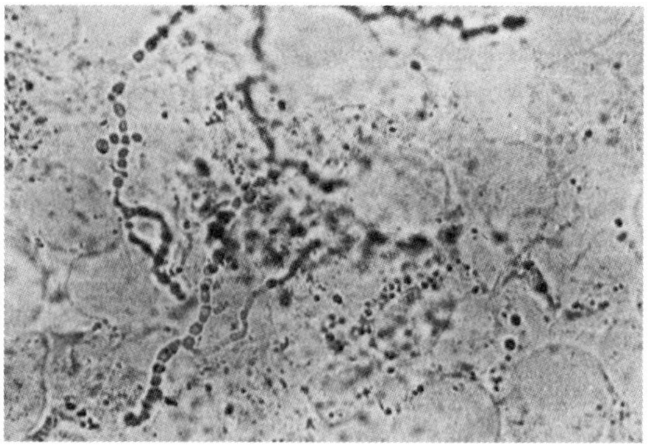

FIGURE 37-2 Fungal elements (hyphae) as seen on microscopic examination of a potassium hydroxide preparation. (From Hurwitz S: *Clinical pediatric dermatology*, ed 2, Philadelphia, 1993, WB Saunders, p 374.)

to relieve pruritus. Tar baths can be used for psoriasis (e.g., Zetar, Polytar, or Balnetar). It is worth noting that bathing and other heat exposures can make a rash seem worse temporarily.

Environmental Considerations

Because water is essential to skin integrity, environmental humidity also plays a role. Excessive humidity (greater than 90%) or deficient humidity (less than 10%) can cause disruption of the skin. Macerated skin, for example, benefits from less humidity (e.g., wet dressings enhance evaporation and relieve symptoms). Itching from excessively dry skin is often relieved by increased humidity provided by humidified heating in winter or by using a vaporizer or humidifier. In hot temperatures, itching can be alleviated by cool air conditioning. Water consumption also plays a role in maintaining proper skin hydration, and children should be encouraged to drink plenty of water.

Skin Care Agents

Soaps, Oils, and Colloids. Mild soaps include Dove, Aveeno, Neutrogena, Basis, Alpha Keri, Oilatum, and Lubriderm. Cetaphil lotion and Purpose Gentle Cleansing Wash are soap substitutes. Bath oils include Alpha Keri and Domol. Colloids include Aveeno.

Moisturizers and Lubricants. Moisturizers and lubricants treat chronic dryness and inflammation of the skin by retaining water in the skin. Composed of petrolatum or a mixture of petrolatum and lanolin, moisturizers and lubricants are most effective when applied to damp skin. Petrolatum-based lubricants include Moisturel, Purpose, Dermasil cream, Vaseline Pure Petrolatum Jelly, and Vaseline Dermatology Formula Lotion. Petrolatum and lanolin combinations include Aquaphor ointment, Eucerin cream and lotion, Lubriderm lotion, and Keri Creme. Glycerin preparations without lanolin or petrolatum include Corn Huskers Lotion, Cetaphil, Keri Light, and Neutrogena.

Sunscreens and Sunblocks. Sunscreens and sunblocks protect the skin from UV light and are graded by their ability to provide sun protection. A fragrance-free sunscreen with a minimum sun protection factor (SPF) of 15 is recommended. Sunscreens that act by absorbing UV light in the B range include para-aminobenzoic acid (PABA) or PABA esters, cinnamates, salicylates, benzophenones, and anthranilates. Only benzophenones protect from UV rays in the longer UVA range. Sunblocks, including titanium dioxide, zinc oxide, and talc, scatter light and are especially useful on the nose, ears, and lips (see Box 37-10).

Wet Dressings

When skin is in an acute stage of oozing, crusting, or itching, wet dressings are useful to help dry the skin, decrease itching, and remove crusts. Thin cloths such as diapers, handkerchiefs, or strips of sheets make the best wet dressings. Dressings should be wet with lukewarm water and applied for 10 to 20 minutes four to six times daily for 48 to 72 hours. During the treatment, dressings must be kept wet either by removing and rewetting or by applying water. Alternative solutions include saline (1 tsp salt with 1 pt of water) or Burow solution (one Domeboro [aluminum acetate; calcium acetate] tablet with 1 pt of water). Creams or ointments applied following wet dressings enhance absorption of the medication in the cream. A slightly more intense technique includes applying a steroid ointment or cream to the skin, followed by a wet dressing and then a dry dressing (e.g., a sleeper, pajamas, or long johns are wetted and put on, and covered with a dry sleeper or long johns) (Weston, Lane, & Morelli, 2002). The dressing is changed every 6 hours for 24 to 72 hours or is used overnight for 5 to 10 nights. Care must be taken to avoid excessive steroidal absorption using this technique by applying steroid only to areas needing it, especially in infants and young children.

Occlusive Dressings

Occlusive dressings decrease evaporation of water from the skin and enhance hydration and absorption of topical medications. Plastic wrap is placed over the affected area after hydrating the skin and applying cream or ointment; these dressings should not be left on longer than 8 hours. Ointments, oils, urea compounds, and propylene glycol used alone are occlusive. Skin folds serve as naturally occurring occlusive areas. Lichen simplex chronicus, dyshidrotic eczema, and psoriasis are skin conditions that benefit from occlusion.

Other Considerations

- Irritants and sensitizing agents such as wool, sweat, and saliva should be avoided.
- Allergens and foods that most commonly cause skin reactions include milk, eggs, wheat, tomato, citrus, chocolate, fish, and nuts.

Medications

Topical therapeutics are most commonly used for dermatologic conditions. Topical therapy can achieve the following goals:

- Restore hydration
- Alleviate symptoms
- Reduce inflammation
- Protect the skin
- Reduce scale and debris
- Cleanse and debride
- Eradicate causative organisms

Thought must be given not only to the medication used in treating skin conditions but also to its preparation (Box 37-5) and vehicle (Fig. 37-3), including stabilizers, preservatives, and perfumes (Orchard & Weston, 2001). Sensitization, and thus aggravation rather than relief of symptoms, is occasionally caused by the medication vehicle or its preparation. Common agents causing sensitization include ethylenediamine, lanolin, parabens, thimerosal, diphenhydramine, "caines," and neomycin. The following guidelines for use of preparations may be helpful:

- Acute inflammation—wet dressings, powders, suspension lotions, alcohol- or water-based lotions, or aerosols
- Chronic inflammation—creams, oil-based lotions or gels, ointments
- Patient's tolerance for and willingness to use certain vehicles
- Patient's environment (dry or humid)

All preparations of topical medication except powders have enhanced absorption if applied to skin immediately after it has been saturated with water. Absorption is also enhanced by occlusion (skin folds or plastic wraps; see previous discussion). Application of the topical medication is best done in one direction, preferably along the hair follicles, without rubbing, applied with a single motion. Use an adequate but not excessive amount.

Antibacterial Agents

Topical antiseptics, soap, and antibacterial soap reduce the number of bacteria on the skin and provide thorough cleansing. Examples of antiseptics include povidone-iodine (Betadine), chlorhexidine gluconate (Hibiclens), and

BOX 37-5 *Preparations of Topical Medications*

Shampoos—liquid soaps or detergents for cleaning the hair (e.g., tar for psoriasis or seborrhea)
Powders—absorb moisture and reduce friction, provide cooling, decrease itching, increase evaporation
Pastes—made of a combination of powder and oil, which makes them somewhat difficult to apply and remove, but effective in providing dryness and protection for skin
Lotions—mixtures of powder and water, useful for drying, cooling, and soothing actions; *emulsion lotions* contain some oil, so are not as drying as lotions; lotions come in suspension or solution
Gels—alcohol based, provide good penetration of skin, but can burn on application; primarily used for acne and in hairy areas
Creams—contain more water than oil and therefore are less occlusive; better used with less-dry skin, in high-humidity areas, in summertime, and on parts of body that naturally cause occlusion (body folds); often accepted better by patient but must be applied every 2 to 3 hours
Ointments—best used with dry skin; composed primarily of oil with little or no water; provide most potent concentration of medication because of their occlusive action on skin; generally need to be used only every 12 hr; tend to leave a greasy feeling and can cause heat retention from decreased evaporation; come as water in oil, absorbent, or water repellent
Oils—fluid fats that hold medication to the skin as barriers or occlusive agents

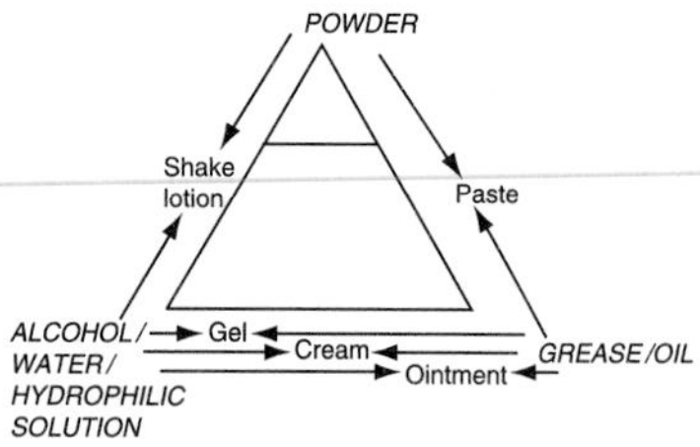

FIGURE 37-3 Vehicles for dermatologic therapy. See Box 37-5 for description.

pHisoDerm. Topical antibiotics such as mupirocin (Bactroban), applied directly to the skin, are used to treat minor skin infections. Neomycin should be avoided because of the high incidence of contact sensitization. Oral antibiotics used to treat more significant bacterial infections include penicillins, erythromycin, cephalosporins, and tetracycline.

Antifungal Agents

Antifungal agents are used to treat *Candida, Malassezia (Pityrosporum)*, and dermatophyte infections. Many topical antifungals are over-the-counter medications. Oral antifungals are used for hair and nail infections or refractory skin infections. They are used with caution in children, not only because of the side effects but also because the newer agents are not Food and Drug Administration (FDA) approved for children, or clinical experience with children is minimal. The traditional drugs are usually the first line of treatment. Antifungal agents are listed in Table 37-4 in the section on fungal infections.

Antiviral Agents

Topical antivirals are used to control cutaneous herpes infections. Oral antivirals, such as acyclovir for herpes infections, are used in more complicated or extensive cases.

Wart therapy agents destroy keratinocytes. These include salicylic acid and lactic acid collodion, salicylic plaster, salicylic solution, liquid nitrogen, cantharidin, podophyllum, and trichloroacetic acid.

Antiacne Agents

Topical keratolytics are used in acne to relieve follicular obstruction by inhibiting bacteria and promoting peeling of the skin. Benzoyl peroxide and retinoic acid are two main agents. Topical antibiotics have few side effects and are most effective in maintaining control of acne. Common ones used include clindamycin, erythromycin, and meclocycline. Systemic antibiotics are effective in inflammatory acne. Tetracycline and erythromycin are the most commonly used. Oral retinoid (isotretinoin), effective in nodulocystic acne not responding to other treatment, is contraindicated in pregnancy because of its teratogenic effects (see Table 37-8).

Antiinflammatory Agents

Topical glucocorticoids are frequently used to reduce inflammation, to decrease itching, and for vasoconstriction without having the widespread systemic effects of oral steroids. They are subdivided into three categories: low-potency, moderate-potency, and high-potency agents (Table 37-1).

High-potency steroids should not be used in children. Only low-potency agents should be used on the face, in the diaper area, and in young children, and only for short periods of time. Steroids are also classified as fluorinated or nonfluorinated. Nonfluorinated steroids are less potent and have fewer side effects; fluorinated steroids are rarely used in pediatrics.

Oral glucocorticoids (prednisone) are used only in acute situations and are limited to short courses. Intralesional

TABLE 37-1 *Topical Steroid Preparations*

Group (Potency)	Drug (Brand Name)	Dosage Form
VI (low)	Alclometasone dipropionate (Aclovate)	0.05% cream, ointment
	Desonide (DesOwen)	0.05% cream, ointment, lotion
	Triamcinolone acetonide (Kenalog)	0.025% cream
	Fluocinolone acetonide (Synalar)	0.01% solution
	Hydrocortisone (Hytone, Nutracort)	0.5%, 1%, 2.5% cream, ointment, lotion, solution
V (medium)	Triamcinolone acetonide (Aristocort A, Kenalog)	0.1% cream, lotion, 0.025% ointment
	Flurandrenolide (Cordran)	0.05% cream, lotion
	Fluticasone propionate (Cutivate)	0.05% cream
	Prednicarbate (Dermatop)	0.1% cream
	Hydrocortisone butyrate (Locoid)	0.1% cream
	Fluocinolone acetonide (Synalar)	0.025% cream
	Hydrocortisone valerate (Westcort)	0.2% cream
IV (medium)	Flurandrenolide (Cordran)	0.025%, 0.05% ointment
	Mometasone furoate (Elocon)	0.1% cream, lotion
	Triamcinolone acetonide (Kenalog)	0.1% cream, ointment
	Betamethasone valerate (Luxiq)	0.12% foam
	Fluocinolone acetonide (Synalar)	0.025% cream, ointment
	Hydrocortisone (Westcort)	0.2% ointment
III (medium)	Clocortolone pivalate (Cloderm)	0.01% cream
	Fluticasone propionate (Cutivate)	0.005% ointment
	Amcinonide (Cyclocort)	0.1% lotion
	Betamethasone dipropionate (Diprosone)	0.05% cream
	Mometasone furoate (Elocon)	0.1% cream, lotion, ointment
	Halcinonide (Halog)	0.025% cream, solution
II (high)	Amcinonide (Cyclocort)	0.1% ointment
	Betmethasone dipropionate (Diprolene)	0.05% cream, ointment, gel, lotion
	Betamethasone dipropionate (Diprosone)	0.05% ointment
	Halcinonide (Halog)	0.025% ointment
	Fluocinonide (Lidex)	0.05% cream, ointment, solution
	Desoximetasone (Topicort A)	0.25% cream, 0.5% gel, solution
I (super)	Clobetasol propionate (Cormax, Temovate, Embeline)	0.05% cream, ointment, gel, solution
	Flurandrenolide (Cordran Tape)	24-inch and 80-inch rolls, patches
	Clobetasol propionate (Olux)	0.05% foam
	Diflorasone diacetate (Psorcon)	0.05% cream, ointment
	Halobetasol propionate (Ultravate)	0.05% cream, ointment

From Taketomo CK, Hodding JH, Kraus DM: *Pediatric dosage handbook*, ed 9, Hudson, OH, 2002, Lexi-Comp; Wynne AL, Woo TM, Millard M: *Pharmacotherapeutics for nurse practitioner prescribers*, Philadelphia, 2002, FA Davis.

steroid injections may be used by the dermatologist to control localized eczema, lichen planus, or psoriasis.

A key to using steroids is to be familiar with a few low-, medium-, and high-level steroids and use them consistently. Use the lowest possible potency that has the desired effect, and with the least possible frequency. Brand name preparations often have a more consistent base and potency. Only low-potency or medium- to low-potency steroids (in severe cases) should be used on the face, groin, and axillae. Remember that ointments are more potent than creams, and lotions are better in hairy areas. Absorption is enhanced in areas that are traumatized or denuded. Side effects are possible when using topical steroids, especially with prolonged use or more potent preparations. Common side effects with long-term use include skin atrophy, striae, increased fragility of the skin, hypopigmentation, secondary infection, acneiform eruption, folliculitis, miliaria, hypertrichosis, telangiectasia, and purpura.

Antipruritic Agents

Antihistamines are used both for sedation and to relieve itching. The most commonly used antihistamines are hydroxyzine and diphenhydramine. Topical antihistamines, especially diphenhydramine HCl (Benadryl) and “caine” medications, should be avoided because of the possibility of contact sensitization. Menthol and pramoxine are topical anesthetics that do not cause sensitization (Paller, 1999). Nonsteroidal antiinflammatory drugs (NSAIDs) are used for relief of pain and in the treatment of sunburn. Ibuprofen and indomethacin are the two mainstays.

Immunodulators

This relatively new class of topical medication is used for short-term or intermittent long-term treatment of atopic dermatitis when conventional therapy is inadvisable, ineffective, or not tolerated. Immunodulators are expensive and cannot be used in children under 2 years old. See Chapter 25 for more information.

Scabicides and Pediculocides

These agents are toxic to mites and lice. Crotamiton (Eurax), permethrin (Elimite, Nix), pyrethrin plus piperonyl butoxide, and lindane (Kwell) are commonly used. Lindane must be used with caution in pregnancy and in young infants.

Hair and Scalp Preparations

Antimicrobial, tar, keratolytic, and detergent shampoos are agents used on the hair and scalp.

Herbal Remedies

Herbal remedies are often used to treat acne, minor wounds, eczema, yeast and fungal infections, herpes simple virus, and poison ivy (Gardiner, Coles, & Kemper, 2001). See Chapter 43 for more information.

Other Medications and Treatments

Other medications and treatments used in dermatologic care include retinoids, topical tars, anthralin, calcipotriene (a vitamin D analog), masking preparations, agents to relieve excessive sweating (aluminum chloride or chlorohydrate), cytotoxic and immunosuppressive agents, and phototherapy.

Counseling and Anticipatory Guidance

Spending adequate time with the patient and parents to discuss the child's skin condition and the family's concerns and needs is essential to the successful management of skin and subcutaneous disorders. Education regarding the disease, plan of treatment, and potential risks and benefits should be provided. Because disorders of the skin are so visible, time must be spent discussing the short- and long-term prognoses, as well as potential plans to prevent complications, recurrence, and spread.

Ideas for preventive care for the dark-skinned patient should be implemented in routine care. The following are initial areas to include:

- Avoid acne or contact dermatitis
- Avoid pomades
- Avoid traction alopecia
- Immunize for varicella to prevent scarring
- Use insect repellents to minimize insect bite reactions
- Treat early signs and symptoms of pruritic or inflammatory conditions (acne, eczema) and infections
- Use moisturizing agents and eliminate soaps for dry, itchy skin
- Use oral antipruritics for dry, itchy skin
- Caution about the use of topical medications, especially high-potency steroids, benzoyl peroxide, and isotretinoin
- Avoid trauma and any procedures that can induce keloids

BACTERIAL INFECTIONS OF THE SKIN AND SUBCUTANEOUS TISSUE

Diagnosis and treatment of common bacterial infections are listed in Table 37-2.

Impetigo

Description

Impetigo is a bacterial infection of the superficial layers of the skin. Nonbullous impetigo usually follows some type of skin trauma (e.g., bites, abrasions, varicella) or other skin disease (most commonly atopic dermatitis). Bullous impetigo develops on intact skin and is caused by *Staphylococcus aureus* toxin production (see Color Fig. 14).

Etiology and Incidence

Impetigo is the primary bacterial infection of the skin in children. Nonbullous impetigo accounts for more than 70% of cases. Bullous impetigo occurs sporadically and is more common in infants and young children. *S. aureus*, the primary pathogen responsible for 70% to 85% of impetigo cases, usually spreads from hands, nasal discharge, or droplets. *Streptococcus pyogenes*, responsible for 30% to 40% of cases, is found most commonly in preschool children and is uncommon under 2 years of age on open skin. Both organisms may be found in an impetiginous lesion. Impetigo occurs more frequently with poor hygiene; during the summer months; in warm, humid climates; and in lower socioeconomic groups (American Academy of Pediatrics [AAP], 2003; Darmstadt & Sidbury, 2004; Weston, Lane, & Morelli, 2002). Streptococcal types that cause pharyngitis rarely cause impetigo and vice versa.

TABLE 37-2 *Diagnosis and Treatment of Common Bacterial Infections*

Infection	Causative Organism	Presentation	Area of Involvement	Treatment	Prevention
Impetigo	*Staphylococcus aureus* or *Streptococcus*	Honey-colored crust on erythematous base, or blisters that rupture, leaving varnish-like coat	Superficial layers of skin (epidermis)	Topical antibiotic if minor, oral antibiotics if more significant infection	Moisturize skin; thorough cleansing of any break in skin
Cellulitis	Most commonly *Streptococcus*	Erythema, swelling, tenderness	Dermis and subcutaneous tissue	Oral antibiotic depending on likely organism; often penicillin or dicloxacillin	Same as above
Folliculitis	*S. aureus*	Pruritus, erythematous papule or pustule at hair follicle	Hair follicle	Warm compresses, topical keratolytics, topical antibiotics, or antistaphylococcal antibiotic if severe	Same as above; good hygiene and antibacterial soap

Clinical Findings

History

- Pruritus, spread of the lesion to surrounding skin, and earlier skin disruption at the site
- Weakness, fever, diarrhea may accompany bullous impetigo

Physical Examination. The following can be found:

- Nonbullous, classic, or common impetigo—begins as macules that progress to vesicles or pustules, which rupture, leaving moist, honey-colored, crusty lesions on mildly erythematous, eroded skin; less than 2 cm in size; little pain but rapid spread
- Bullous impetigo—large, superficial, annular or oval pustular blisters that rupture, leaving thin varnish-like coating or scale
- *S. aureus* lesions—usually on the face, trunk, extremities; superficial blisters that rupture, leaving the skin with a scalded appearance
- *S. pyogenes* lesions—on traumatized skin, lower extremities; punched-out ulcers with crusts
- Lesions most common on face, extremities, or perineum; satellite lesions near the primary site, although they can be found anywhere on the body
- Lymphadenopathy in up to 90% (Darmstadt & Sidbury, 2004)

Laboratory Studies. Gram stain and culture are ordered if identification of the organism is needed.

Differential Diagnosis

Herpes simplex, varicella, nummular eczema, contact dermatitis, tinea, kerion, and scabies are included in the differential diagnosis.

Management

Management involves the following:

- Topical antibiotics may be used if the impetigo is superficial, nonbullous, or localized to one or two lesions. Topical treatment alone provides clinical improvement but may prolong the carrier state (Weston, Lane, & Morelli, 2002). Mupirocin ointment or bacitracin (AAP, 2003) is used three times a day for 7 to 10 days. If there is no improvement in 3 days, oral antibiotics should be started.
- Oral antibiotics. Treatment for *S. aureus* and *S. pyogenes* is usually recommended because coexistence is common.
  - Cephalexin 40 mg/kg per day for 10 days.
  - Dicloxacillin 15 to 50 mg/kg per day for 10 days.
  - Cloxacillin 50 to 100 mg/kg per day for 10 days.
  - Erythromycin 40 mg/kg per day for 10 days; note that there is increasing resistance in some communities, up to 10% to 52% (Weston, Lane, & Morelli, 2002).
  - If streptococcus is cultured, treat with penicillin V 125 to 250 mg twice a day for 10 days.
- For widespread infection with constitutional symptoms and deeper skin involvement, use oral antibiotic active against β-lactamase-producing strains of *S. aureus* such as dicloxacillin, cloxacillin, or cephalexin.
- If an infant has bullous impetigo, use parenteral β-lactamase-resistant antistaphylococcal penicillin such as methicillin, oxacillin, or nafcillin.
- If there is failure to respond in 7 days, swab beneath the crust and do Gram stain, culture, and sensitivities.
- If there is recurrence, evaluate with nasal culture and treat with topical mupirocin to the nares twice a day for 1 to 5 days to eradicate staphylococcus carriage (AAP, 2003).

- Local care of lesions before applying ointment may be helpful. Soak with Burow solution compresses to remove crusts and cleanse with soap.
- Educate regarding cleanliness, handwashing, and spread of disease.
- Exclude from day care or school until treated for 24 hours.
- Schedule a follow-up appointment in 48 to 72 hours if not improved, and in 10 to 14 days.

Complications

- Cellulitis may occur in up to 10% of cases with nonbullous form (Darmstadt & Sidbury, 2004), ecthyma (infection involving entire epidermis), or erysipelas (spreading cellulitis with induration).
- Lymphangitis, suppurative lymphadenitis, guttate psoriasis, erythema multiforme, scarlet fever, acute rheumatic fever, or glomerulonephritis may occur following infection with some strains of streptococcus.
- *Staphylococcal scalded skin syndrome (SSSS)* results from circulating toxin. Unusual over 5 years of age, SSSS manifests abruptly with fever, malaise, and tender erythematous skin, especially in the neck folds and axillae, rapidly becoming crusty around the eyes, nose, and mouth. The Nikolsky sign (peeling of skin with a light rub to reveal a moist red surface) is a key finding. Treatment with oral dicloxacillin, avoidance of steroids, minimal handling, and use of ointments as the skin heals results in quicker healing without scarring over 10 to 14 days (Hurwitz, 1993; Weston, Lane, & Morelli, 2002). Severe cases are dealt with as burn victims.

Patient Education and Prevention

- Thorough cleansing of any breaks in the skin helps prevent impetigo.
- Postinflammatory pigment changes can last weeks to months.

Cellulitis

Description

Cellulitis is a localized bacterial infection often involving the dermis and subcutaneous layers of the skin commonly seen following a disruption of the skin surface from an insect or animal bite, trauma, or a penetrating wound. Periorbital cellulitis is discussed in Chapter 29.

Etiology and Incidence

In children, cellulitis is often facial (one cheek), perivaginal, or perianal, or involves a joint or an extremity. Most cases of cellulitis are caused by streptococci, although *Haemophilus influenzae* (especially in children under 2 years of age) and *S. aureus* (increasing incidence) are also found. Seventy percent of cases of perianal cellulitis are found in males 6 months to 10 years of age. Cellulitis of the cheek is most common in 3-month-olds to 3-year-olds (Weston, Lane, & Morelli, 2002).

Clinical Findings

History

- A previous skin disruption at the site
- Fever, malaise, irritability, anorexia, vomiting, and chills can be reported
- Recent sore throat or upper respiratory infection
- Anal pruritus, blood-streaked stools, and stool retention (perianal cellulitis)

Physical Examination. The following can be seen:

- Erythematous, tender, swollen, warm areas of skin with irregular borders
- Blue to purple tinge to the skin, often produced when the causative organism is *H. influenzae* (in 3-month-olds to 3-year-olds)
- Lymphadenitis proximal to the site
- Bright erythema 2 to 3 cm around anus, superficial, well-marginated, not indurated "ring around the anus" (perianal cellulitis)

Laboratory Studies. CBC and blood culture are done if the child appears ill or toxic or is under 1 year of age. Gram stain and culture of the area can also be done. Blood culture should be done if *H. influenzae* is suspected (Weston, Lane, & Morelli, 2002).

Differential Diagnosis

Early erythema nodosum, subcutaneous fat necrosis, giant urticaria, contact dermatitis, and panniculitis are included in the differential diagnosis. Blood culture should be done if *H. influenzae* is suspected (Weston, Lane, & Morelli, 2002).

Management

Immediate antibiotic therapy is needed.

- Significant infection: An initial intramuscular (IM) dose of antibiotic chosen according to suspected organism (systemic penicillin such as benzathine penicillin 600,000 to 1,200,000 U if *Streptococcus* is suspected) or a third-generation cephalosporin such as ceftriaxone 50 to 75 mg/kg IM every 12 hours. Hospitalization may be required if the child is very young, febrile, and acutely ill or has facial, orbital, or periorbital cellulitis.
- Oral antibiotics:
  - Cephalexin 50 to 75 mg/kg per day for 10 days.
  - Dicloxacillin 50 to 100 mg/kg per day for 10 days if *Staphylococcus* is suspected.

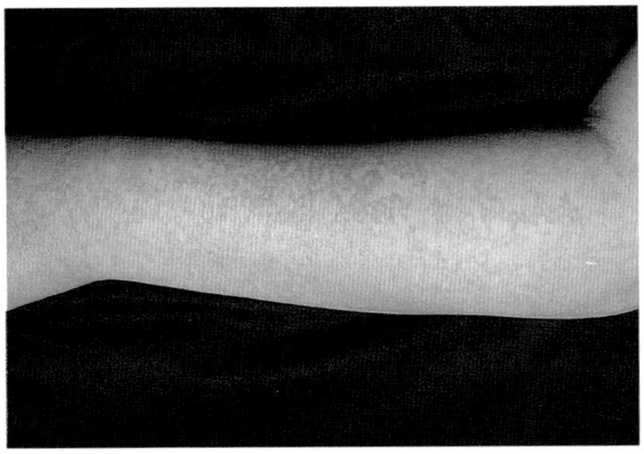

COLOR FIGURE 1 Erythema infectiosum ("fifth disease") with reticulate, lace-like eruption of erythema infectiosum. (From Callen JP, Greer KE, Paller AS: *Color atlas of dermatology*, ed 2, Philadelphia, 2000, WB Saunders, p. 49.)

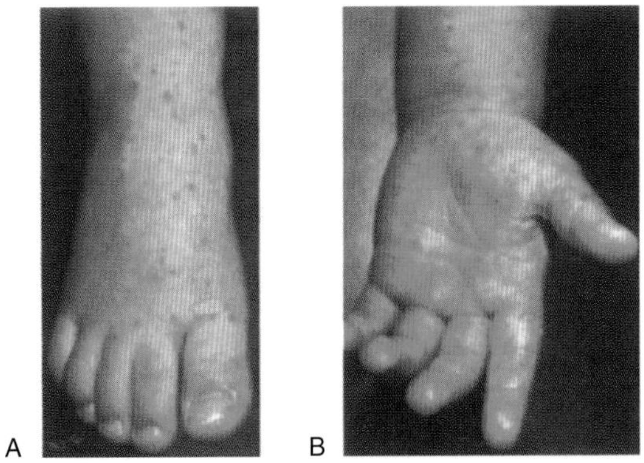

COLOR FIGURE 2 Lesions on the feet **(A)** and hands **(B)** in hand-foot-and-mouth disease. (From Aly R, Maibach H: *Atlas of infections of the skin*, Philadelphia, 1999, WB Saunders, p. 240.)

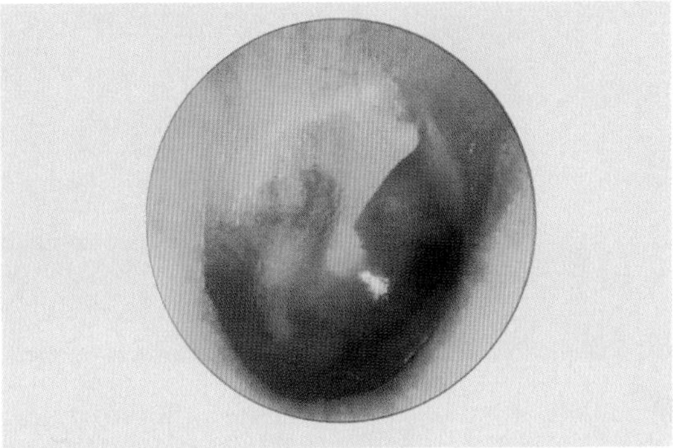

COLOR FIGURE 3 Normal right tympanic membrane. (Photograph courtesy of Sylvan Stool, MD, The Children's Hospital, Denver, CO.)

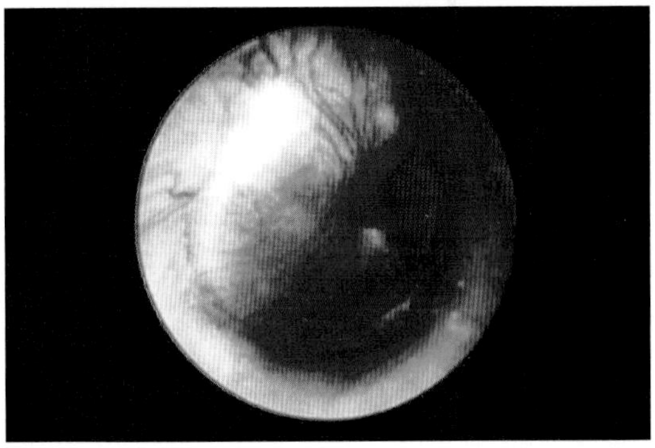

COLOR FIGURE 4 Acute otitis media of the right ear. (From the American Academy of Pediatrics Online Learning in Otitis Media: *www.aap.org/otitismedia/www/*. Developed by the University of Colorado Health Sciences Center, Department of Pediatrics.)

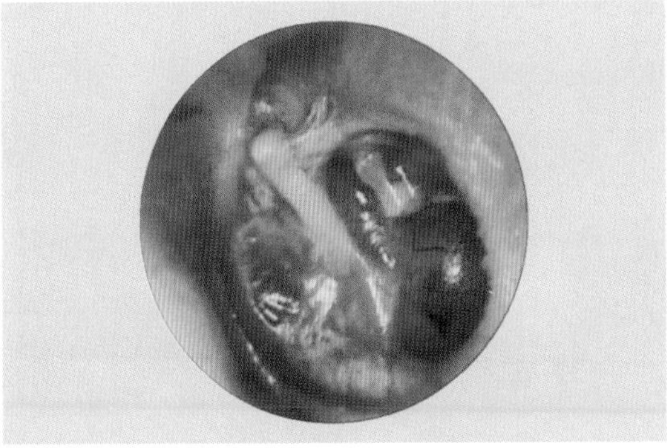

COLOR FIGURE 5 Left ear with posterior retraction. (Photograph courtesy of Sylvan Stool, MD, The Children's Hospital, Denver, CO.)

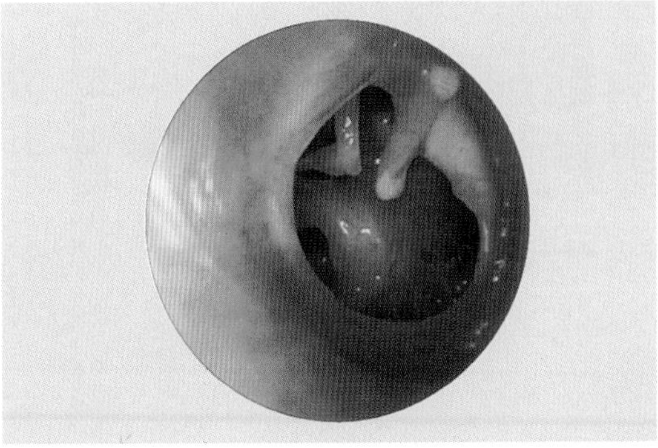

COLOR FIGURE 6 Near total perforation of the right ear. (Photograph courtesy of Sylvan Stool, MD, The Children's Hospital, Denver, CO.)

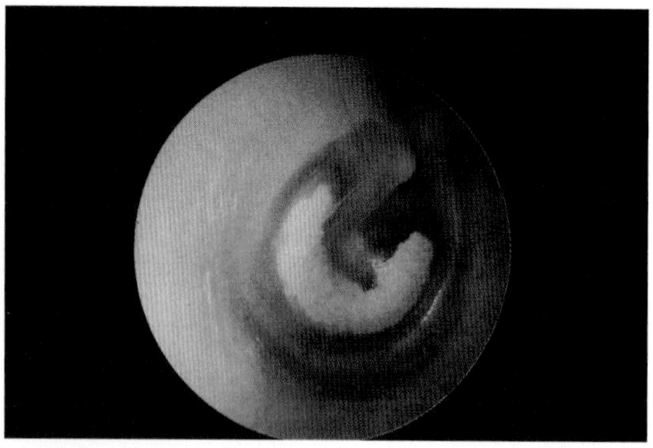

COLOR FIGURE 7 Tympanosclerosis of the right ear. (Photograph courtesy of Sylvan Stool, MD, The Children's Hospital, Denver, CO.)

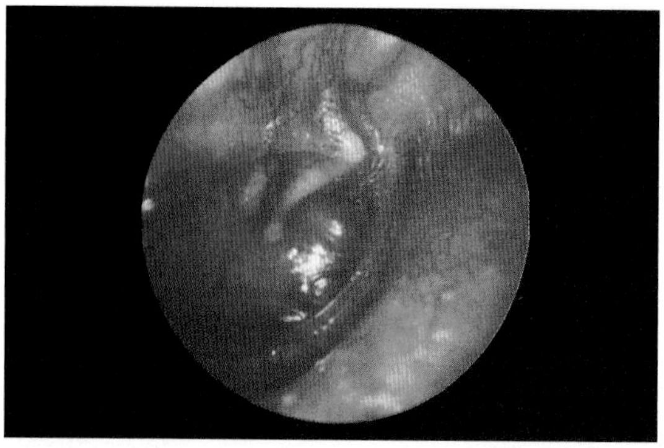

COLOR FIGURE 8 Severely retracted, opaque right tympanic membrane in otitis media with effusion. (From Bluestone CD, Klein JO: *Otitis media in infants and children*, ed 2, Philadelphia, 1995, WB Saunders.)

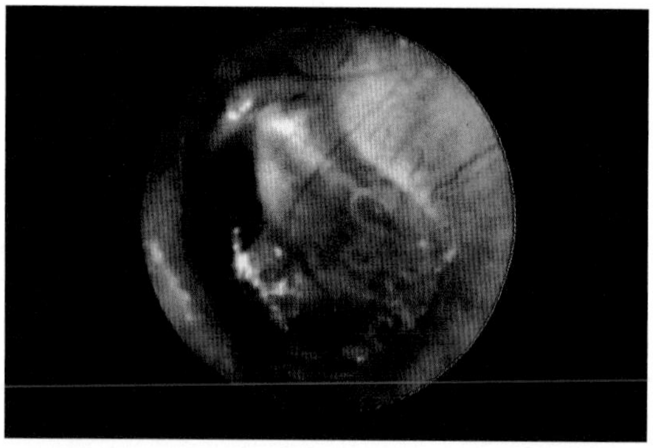

COLOR FIGURE 9 Serous effusion. (From the American Academy of Pediatrics Online Learning in Otitis Media: *www.aap.org/otitismedia/www/*. Developed by the University of Colorado Health Sciences Center, Department of Pediatrics.)

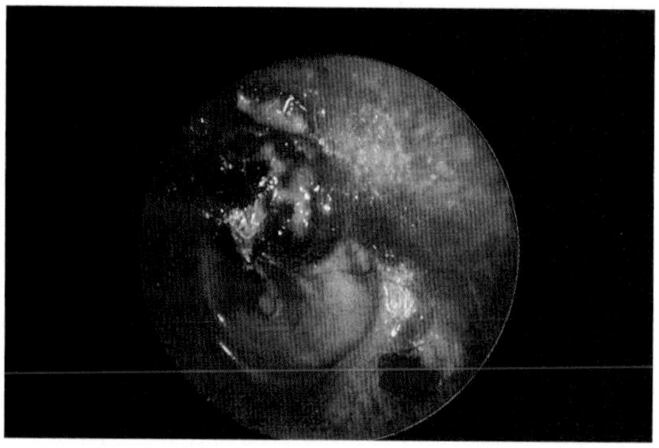

COLOR FIGURE 10 Cholesteatoma of the left ear. (Photograph courtesy of Sylvan Stool, MD, The Children's Hospital, Denver, CO.)

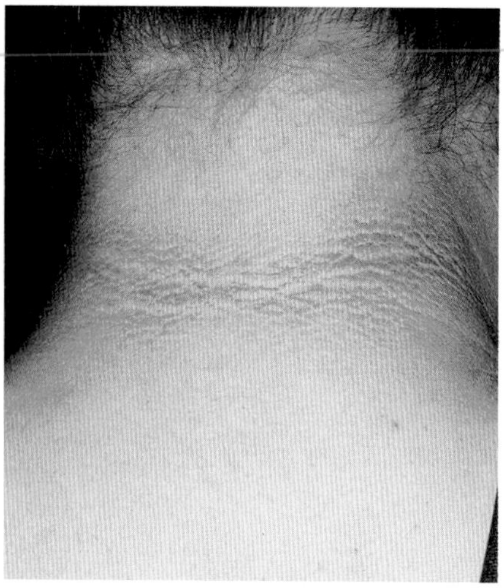

COLOR FIGURE 11 Acanthosis nigricans. Note the thickened, velvety, hyperpigmented skin. (From Habif TP et al: *Skin disease: diagnosis and treatment*, St Louis, 2001, Mosby.)

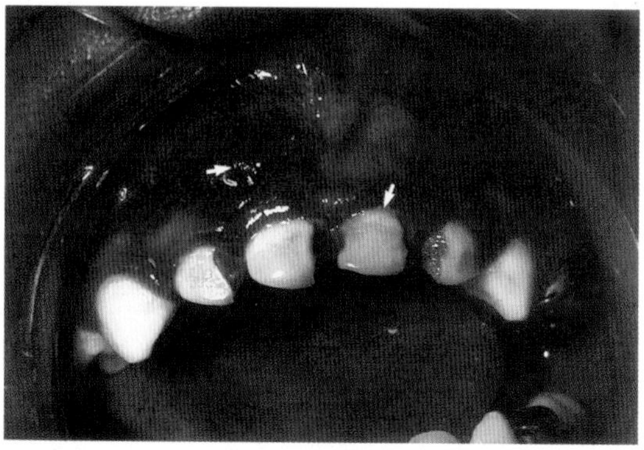

COLOR FIGURE 12 Early childhood caries. Classic appearance of demineralized cervical enamel adjacent to decayed areas. Draining sinus tract (parulis) and edematous red gingival margin (gingivitis) are evident. (Photograph courtesy of Charles Poland, DDS.)

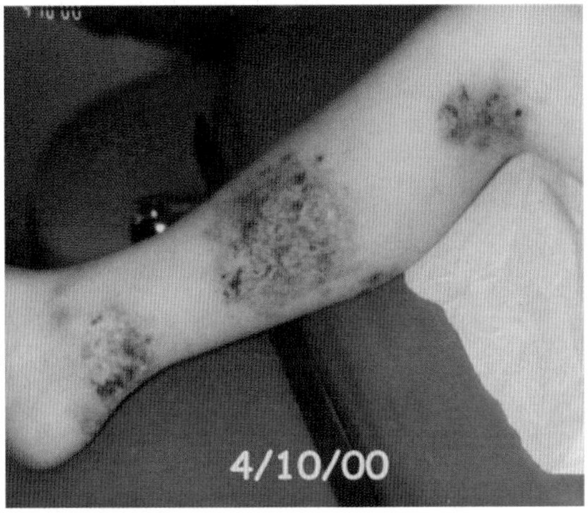

COLOR FIGURE 13 Acute atopic dermatitis. (Photograph courtesy of Peggy Vernon, RN, MA, CPNP, Aurora/Parker Skin Care Center, CO.)

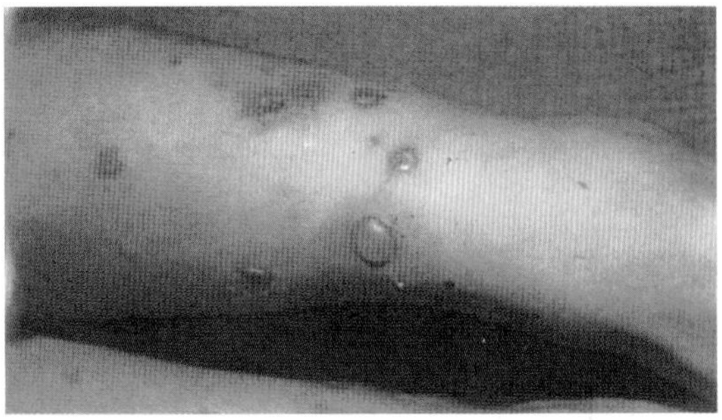

COLOR FIGURE 14 Bullous impetigo on the legs with several lesions in different stages. (From Aly R, Maibach H: *Atlas of infections of the skin*, Philadelphia, 1999, WB Saunders, p. 117.)

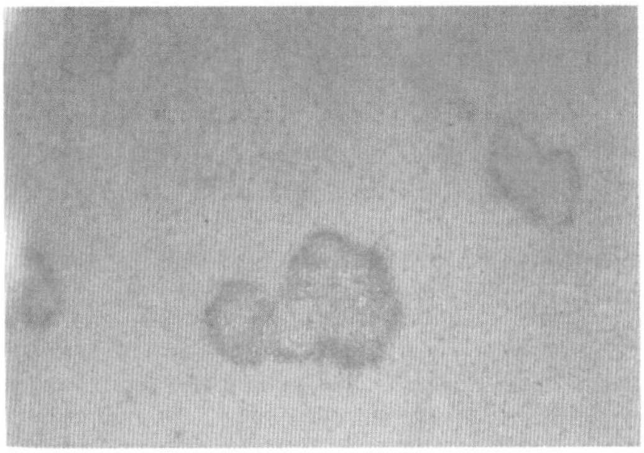

COLOR FIGURE 15 Tinea corporis. Lesions are annular with a raised inflammatory edge and central clearing. (From Aly R, Maibach H: *Atlas of infections of the skin*, Philadelphia, 1999, WB Saunders, p. 23.)

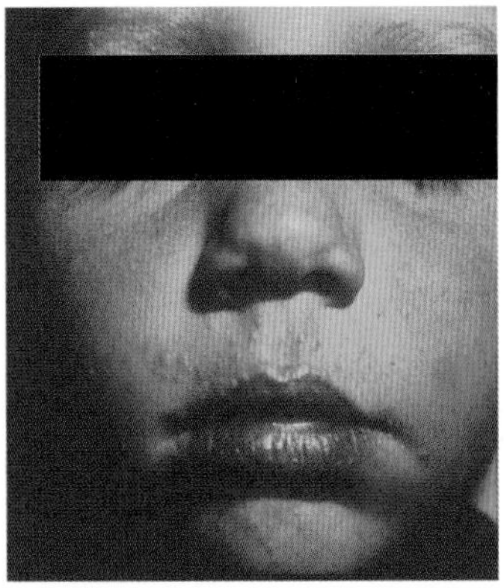

COLOR FIGURE 16 Oral herpes simplex infection in a preschooler. (Photograph courtesy of Peggy Vernon, RN, MA, CPNP, Aurora/Parker Skin Care Center, CO.)

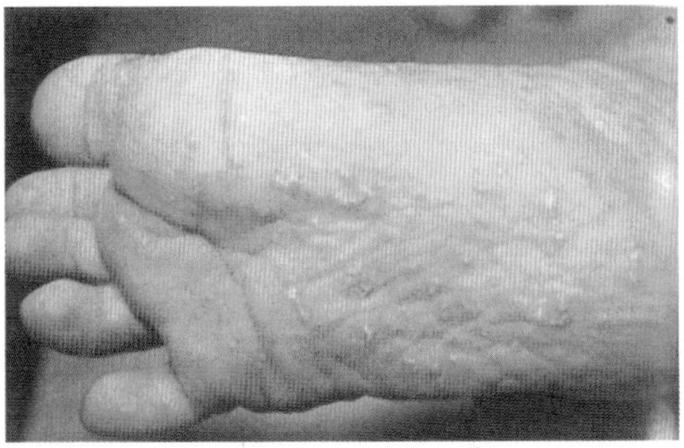

COLOR FIGURE 17 Scabies in an infant with multiple burrows and pustules on soles. (From Aly R, Maibach H: *Atlas of infections of the skin*, Philadelphia, 1999, WB Saunders, p. 176.)

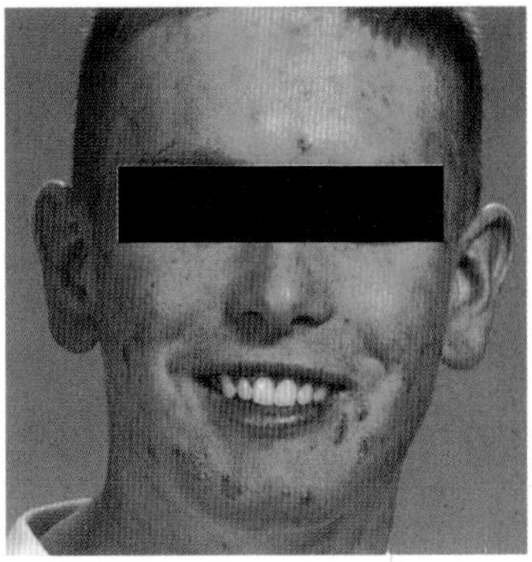

COLOR FIGURE 18 An adolescent with acne vulgaris. (Photograph courtesy of Peggy Vernon, RN, MA, CPNP, Aurora/Parker Skin Care Center, CO.)

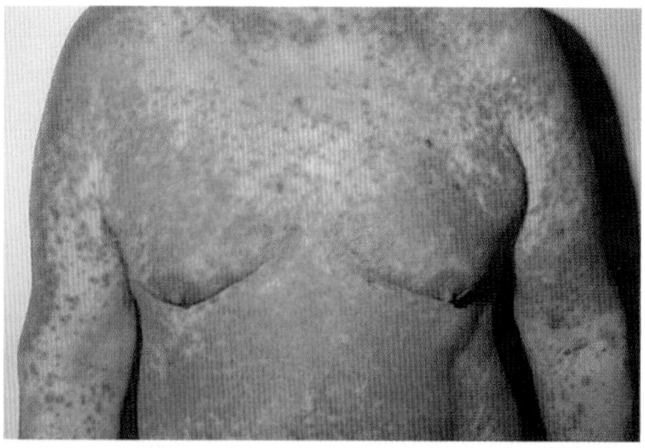

COLOR FIGURE 19 Allergic drug eruption is an erythematous and symmetric rash, usually generalized. (From Lookingbill DP, Marks JG: *Principles of dermatology*, ed 2, Philadelphia, 1993, WB Saunders, p. 218.)

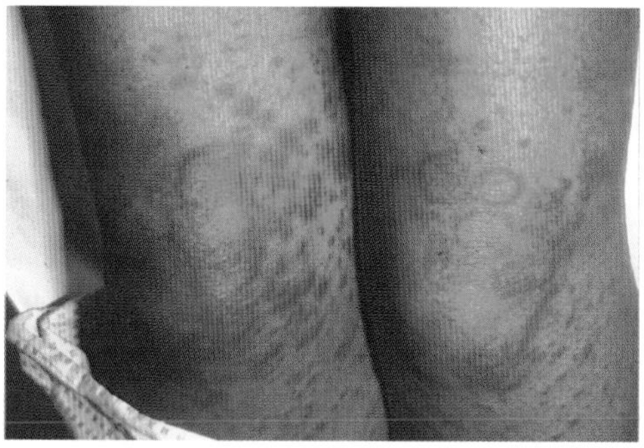

COLOR FIGURE 21 Erythema multiforme secondary to herpes simplex. (From Arndt KA et al: *Primary care dermatology*, Philadelphia, 1997, WB Saunders.)

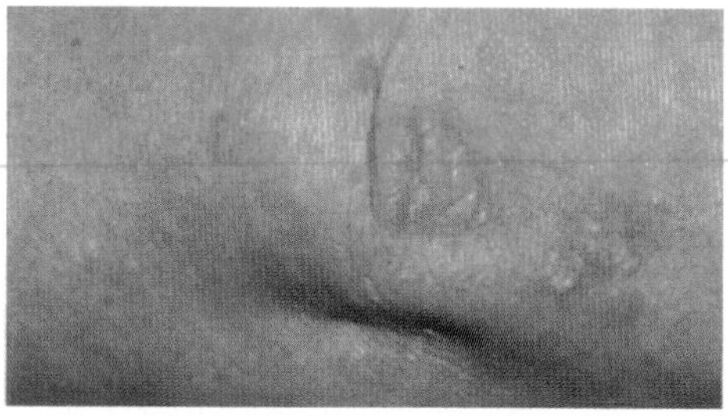

COLOR FIGURE 23 Plaque-like erythematous lesions of psoriasis. (From Aly R, Maibach H: *Atlas of infections of the skin*, Philadelphia, 1999, WB Saunders, p. 239.)

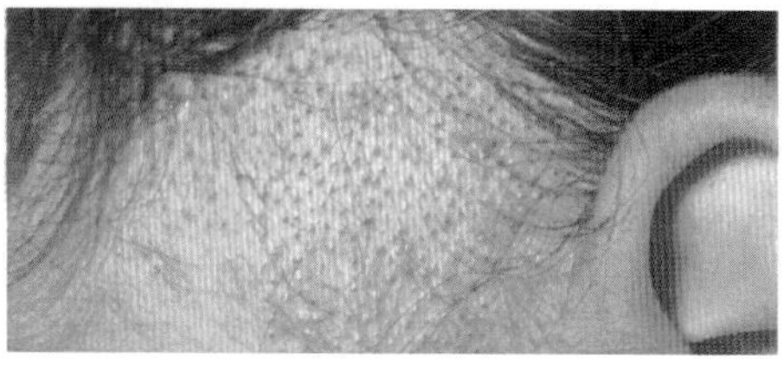

COLOR FIGURE 25 Tinea capitis showing a black dot variety with minimal inflammation. (From Aly R, Maibach H: *Atlas of infections of the skin*, Philadelphia, 1999, WB Saunders, p. 20.)

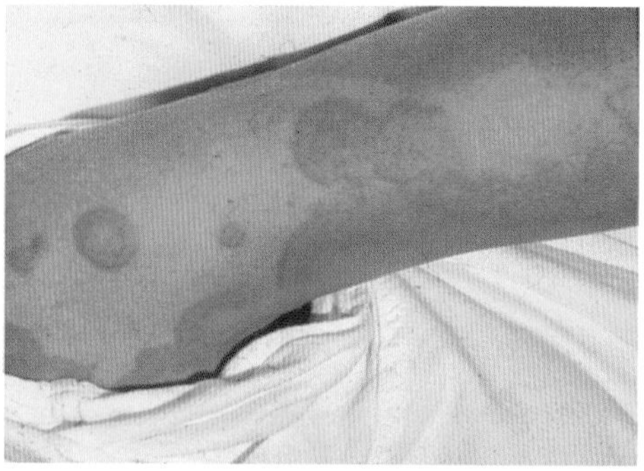

COLOR FIGURE 20 Urticaria. (Photograph courtesy of Frank Parker, MD, Oregon Health Sciences University, Portland, OR.)

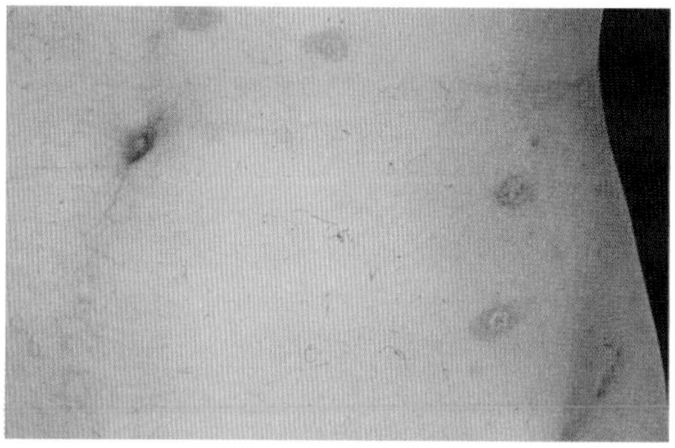

COLOR FIGURE 22 Pityriasis rosea. (Photograph courtesy of Peggy Vernon, RN, MA, CPNP, Aurora/Parker Skin Care Center, CO.)

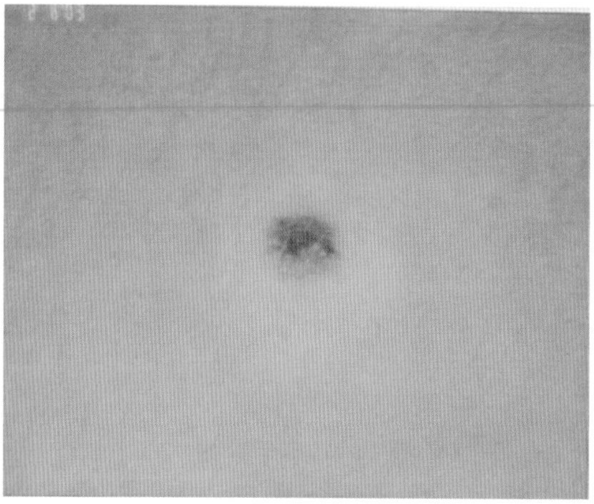

COLOR FIGURE 24 Halo nevus. (Photograph courtesy of Peggy Vernon, RN, MA, CPNP, Aurora/Parker Skin Care Center, CO.)

- Penicillin 30 to 60 mg/kg per day for 10 days if *Streptococcus* is suspected (usually perianal).
- Amoxicillin clavulanate 50 to 80 mg/kg per day for 10 days if *H. influenzae* is suspected; methicillin or a third-generation cephalosporin.

- Follow up in 24 hours to assess response and observe toxicity. Continue daily visits until child is recovering.

Complications

Recurrent perianal streptococcal infection, septicemia, necrotizing fasciitis, and toxic shock syndrome are possible complications.

- *Necrotizing fasciitis*, commonly called *flesh-eating strep*, is an acute, rapidly progressing necrotic invasion of group A streptococcus through the skin and subcutaneous tissue to the fascial compartments. It is found when local resistance is decreased, general debilitation is present, or perforating trauma has occurred. Necrotizing fasciitis occurs most commonly in children as a complication of varicella (AAP, 2003); the peak incidence is in December through March (Working Group on Prevention of Invasive Group A Streptococcal Infections, 1998). Children with diabetes who are in ketoacidosis and immunosuppressed children are most susceptible (Weston, Lane, & Morelli, 2002). Necrotizing fasciitis begins as cellulitis (usually on the leg, or on the abdomen in infants) with severe pain, edema, fever, and bullae on an erythematous surface. It quickly progresses to ulcer, eschar, and gangrene within 2 days. Prompt treatment (surgical debridement, fluid management, and prolonged antibiotic treatment) may be lifesaving, because the overall mortality rate is as high as 15% to 20% (Working Group on Prevention of Invasive Group A Streptococcal Infections, 1998).
- *Toxic shock syndrome (TSS)* is an acute febrile illness that causes significant fever, vomiting and diarrhea, engorged mucous membranes, hypotension, a diffuse macular or sunburn-like rash, and multiple organ system involvement. Either staphylococcal (more common) or streptococcal (more severe disease) organisms can cause TSS. Initially recognized in menstruating adolescents, TSS is also found in males and younger children. When streptococcus is the causative organism, it is usually associated with bacteremia or focal tissue invasion that is rapidly progressive and characterized (85%) by sudden, severe, localized pain out of proportion to physical findings. Treatment is intensive, requires hospitalization, and consists of fluid management, antibiotics, and other supportive measures. Mortality rates of up to 10% have been reported (AAP, 2003; Weston, Lane, & Morelli, 2002). See Chapter 24 and Box 24-4 for the Centers for Disease Control and Prevention (CDC) case definition of streptococcal TSS.

Prevention

- Thorough cleansing of any break in the skin helps prevent cellulitis.
- Perianal spread can occur through shared bath water.

Folliculitis and Furuncle

Description

A superficial bacterial inflammation of the hair follicle is called *folliculitis*; a deeper infection with involvement of the base of the follicle and deep dermis is called a *furuncle* (boil) (Fig. 37-4).

Etiology and Incidence

Obstruction of the follicular orifice is the most important factor contributing to the development of folliculitis, but a moist environment, maceration, poor hygiene, occlusive emollients, and prolonged submersion in contaminated water are also factors. *S. aureus* is the most common causative organism, except for *Pseudomonas aeruginosa*, which causes hot-tub folliculitis. These infections are more common in males than in females.

Clinical Findings

History. The following can be reported:

- Pruritus with folliculitis; tenderness with furuncle
- Hot-tub exposure
- Irritating surface agent
- Occasional fever, malaise, or lymphadenopathy

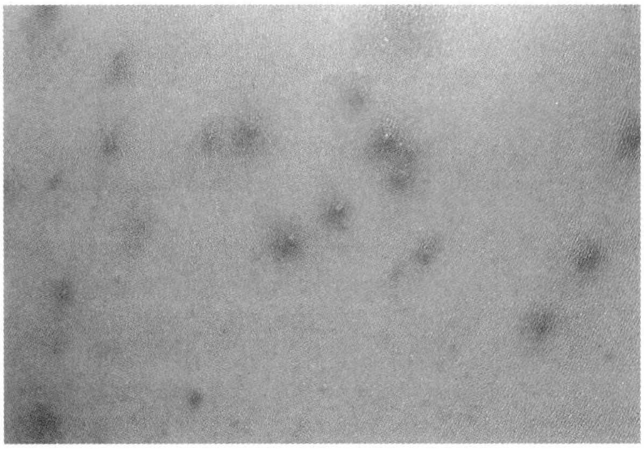

FIGURE 37-4 Staphylococcal superficial folliculitis. Multiple pustules on a red base. (From Weston WL, Lane AT, Morelli JG: *Color textbook of pediatric dermatology*, ed 3, St Louis, 2002, Mosby, p 51.)

Physical Examination. The child often is asymptomatic, but the following can be seen:

- Discrete, erythematous 1 to 2 mm papules or pustules centered around a hair follicle
- Involvement of face, scalp, extremities, buttocks, and back
- Nodules with larger areas of erythema and tenderness (furuncle)
- Pruritic papules, pustules, or nodules deep red to purple in color, most dense in areas covered by swimsuit 8 to 48 hours after exposure (hot-tub folliculitis)

Laboratory Studies. Gram stain and culture are occasionally ordered.

Differential Diagnosis

Candida infection, tinea, acne pustules, and chemical folliculitis constitute the differential diagnosis.

Management

The following steps are taken:

1. Warm compresses after washing with soap and water several times a day
2. Topical keratolytics such as benzoyl peroxide 5% to 10% (twice a day for 5 days), especially if chronic or recurrent
3. Superficial folliculitis: apply topical antibiotic such as erythromycin or clindamycin in cream, gel, solution, or ointment (twice a day for 10 to 14 days)
4. Antistaphylococcal β-lactamase–resistant antibiotics such as dicloxacillin 15 to 50 mg/kg per day for 7 to 10 days or cephalexin 40 to 50 mg/kg per day for 7 to 10 days in severe or widespread cases
5. Review of good personal hygiene habits
6. Follow-up treatment in 1 week for folliculitis, in 1 day for furuncle or abscess, which may need incision and drainage
7. Identify and eliminate predisposing factors
8. If recurrent, look for nasal or skin carrier state

Complications

Deep abscess formation or carbuncles can occur. Sycosis barbae occurs on the chin, upper lip, and jaw, especially in adolescent black males.

Patient Education and Prevention

Good personal hygiene and an antibacterial soap minimize spread to other household members. Hot-tub folliculitis resolves in 5 to 14 days but can recur up to 3 months after exposure.

FUNGAL INFECTIONS OF THE SKIN

Diagnosis and treatment of common fungal infections are listed in Table 37-3.

Candidiasis

Description

Candidiasis is a fungal infection of the skin or mucous membranes commonly called a *yeast infection* or *thrush.* See Chapters 34 and 36 for discussion of oral and vaginal candidiasis.

Etiology and Incidence

Candida albicans is commonly found on skin and oral, vaginal, and intestinal mucosal tissue. Although *Candida* is part of the normal flora, overgrowth and penetration of inflamed skin can occur on the skin or mucous membranes. Candidiasis is more common in infants, obese children, adolescents, and chronically ill or immunocompromised children. It also is often seen as a secondary infection in persistent diaper rashes or with antibiotic, oral steroid, or oral contraceptive use.

Clinical Findings

History. The history often includes antibiotic or steroid use over the previous weeks and occurrence of a rash in a moist, warm area.

Physical Examination. The following can be seen:

- Mouth—white plaques on an erythematous base that adhere to mucous membranes tightly and bleed when scraped; outer lips cracked (cheilitis)
- Corners of mouth—fissured and inflamed (perlèche or angular cheilitis)
- Intertriginous areas (neck, axillae, or groin)—bright erythema in flexural folds
- Diaper area—moist, beefy-red macules and papules with sharply marked borders and satellite lesions; erosions may also be present
- Vulvovaginal area—thick, cheesy, yellow discharge; erythema; edema; and itching

Laboratory Studies. If treatment failure or questionable diagnosis occurs, KOH-treated scrapings of satellite lesions or mucosa reveal yeast cells and pseudohyphae (see Fig. 37-2).

Differential Diagnosis

The differential diagnosis includes erythema toxicum, miliaria, staphylococcal pustulosis, transient neonatal pustulosis, neonatal herpes simplex, and congenital syphilis.

Management

The following steps are taken:

- Skin infection: Topical antifungals (Table 37-4) such as nystatin, miconazole, clotrimazole, ketoconazole, ciclopirox, or econazole applied to skin result in improvement within 3 to 5 days. These may be used at every diaper change for 2 to 3 days until improvement begins.

TABLE 37-3 ***Diagnosis and Treatment of Common Fungal Infections***

Infection	Causative Organism	Clinical Findings	Management	Complications
Candidiasis	*Candida albicans*	Moist, bright-red diaper rash with sharp borders, satellite lesions; associated white spots in mouth, mucous membranes, or corner of mouth	Topical or oral antifungal, generally nystatin; diaper area hygiene	Paronychia or onychomycosis
Tinea corporis	*Trichophyton tonsurans, Microsporum canis, Epidermophyton floccosum*	Pruritic, slightly erythematous circular lesion with a slightly raised border and central clearing; well demarcated	Topical antifungals; identify and treat source; exclude from day care until treated; use oral medications for resistant cases	Tinea incognita from steroid treatment
Tinea cruris	Same as for tinea corporis	Raised-border, scaly lesion on upper thighs and groin; penis and scrotum spared; symmetric	Same as for tinea corporis; loose clothes, absorbent powder	Possible secondary infection
Tinea pedis	Same as for tinea corporis	Vesicles and erosions on instep; fissure between toes with scaling and erythema; diffuse scaling on weight-bearing surfaces with exaggerated scaling in creases; pruritus	Same as for tinea corporis; absorbent powder; cotton socks; open-toed shoes; moisturize	Reinfection common
Tinea versicolor	*Malassezia furfur* or *Malassezia ovalis*	Multiple scaly, discrete oval macules on neck, shoulders, upper back, and chest; hypopigmented to hyperpigmented areas; fail to tan in summer	Selenium shampoo; ketoconazole shampoo; topical imidazoles	50% recurrence rate

- Oral infection: Administer nystatin oral solution four times a day swabbed onto mucous membranes for 5 to 14 days, or gentian violet 1% to 2% aqueous solution applied twice a day, or clotrimazole troches 10 mg tablet dissolved slowly in the mouth five times a day for 14 days in children over 3 years of age. If breastfeeding, the mother should put the solution on her nipples to eliminate reinfection. A second course is sometimes needed to clear the infection.
- If inflammation is present, alternate nystatin cream and 1% hydrocortisone for 1 or 2 days.
- If recalcitrant infection or nail involvement occurs, oral fluconazole or itraconazole 5 mg/kg per day for 21 days may be recommended if over 6 months of age.
- Keep area dry and cool. Minimize skin irritation:
  - Frequent diaper changes.
  - Leave diaper area open to air.
  - Blow-dry with warm air for 3 to 5 minutes at diaper change (especially helpful in intertriginous areas in infants and obese children).
  - Avoid rubber pants.
  - Use mild soap and water; rinse well; avoid diaper wipes.
  - Avoid other powders and medications, especially antibiotics and steroids.
  - Discontinue oral antibiotics and steroids when possible.
  - Discard or sterilize pacifiers.
- Cold milk compresses (if child is not allergic to milk): Mix equal parts skim milk and water with ice cubes in a bowl; saturate cloth and apply repeatedly until warm for 5 to 10 minutes three times a day in conjunction with hydrocortisone and antifungal creams (Weinberg, 1998).

Complications

Chronic mucocutaneous candidiasis resulting from immunologic deficit can occur and is heralded by widespread involvement (oral, skin, nails). Paronychia may occur with thumb-sucking.

Patient Education

Treatment failure is usually due to lack of compliance.

Tinea Capitis

See later section on alopecia.

TABLE 37-4 *Antifungal Medications*

Drug (Trade Name)	Strength and Formulation	Application	Indications/Side Effects
Topical Medications			
Imidazoles			
Clotrimazole (Lotrimin)	1% C, L, S, Su	bid	Erythema, stinging, blistering, peeling, edema, pruritus, hives, burning; fungistatic
Econazole nitrate (Spectazole)	1% C	qd/bid	Burning, pruritus, stinging, erythema; may have antibacterial effects; fungistatic
Ketoconazole (Nizoral)	2% C, Sh	qd/bid	Irritation, pruritus, stinging; fungistatic
Miconazole nitrate (Micatin, Monistat)	2% C, P, S, Su	qd/bid	Irritation, dermatitis, pruritus; economical; fungistatic
Oxiconazole nitrate (Oxistat)	1% C, L	qd/bid	Pruritus, burning, irritation, erythema, folliculitis; fungistatic
Sulconazole nitrate (Exelderm)	1% C, S	qd/bid	Pruritus, burning, stinging; fungistatic
Allylamines			
Butenafine HCl (Mentax)		qd	Irritation; fungicidal
Naftifine HCl (Naftin)	1% C, G	qd/bid	Burning, stinging, erythema, pruritus, irritation; fungicidal
Terbinafine HCl (Lamisil)	1% C	qd/bid	Pruritus, irritation, burning; fungicidal
Ethanolamine			
Cyclopirox olamine (Loprox)	1% C, L	bid	Irritation, erythema, burning; fungicidal
Others			
Calcium undecylenate (Caldesene, Cruex)	10%-20% P, C, O, L	bid	Irritation
Gentian violet	1%-2% S	bid	Staining
Nystatin (Mycolog-II,* Mycostatin, Nilstat, Mytrex*)	100,000 U/g C, L, P, O, Su	bid/tid	Rare adverse reactions; effective against yeast only; fungistatic
Selenium sulfide (Excel; Head & Shoulders Intensive Treatment Dandruff Shampoo; Selsun Blue)	1% Sh, 2.5% L, Sh	qd	For tinea capitis (reduces transmission), tinea versicolor, and seborrheic dermatitis (shampoo may be used as lotion)
Sodium thiosulfate; salicylic acid (Tinver)	25% L	qd/bid	For tinea versicolor
Tolnaftate (Desenex, Tinactin)	1% C, P, S	bid	Rare adverse reactions; fungistatic
Oral Medications			
Clotrimazole	10 mg tab	1 tab five times a day dissolved slowly in mouth	Treatment of oral candidiasis; gastrointestinal symptoms; hepatotoxicity
Fluconazole	10-40 mg/ml; 50, 100, 150, 200 mg capsules	3-6 mg/kg/day in single dose	Approved for pediatric use for oropharyngeal, esophageal, or disseminated candidiasis; possible drug interactions
Griseofulvin	Ultramicrosized	5-10 mg/kg in single dose; maximum dose 750 mg/kg	Mainstay of therapy; fungistatic; excellent safety profile and extensive use; monitor CBC, LFTs, renal function at 4-6 wk and every 4-6 wk while on treatment; possible drug interactions
	Microsized	10-20 mg/kg/day given qd or bid; maximum dose 1000 mg/kg	
Itraconazole	Liquid Su not recommended; 100 or 200 mg capsules	5-10 mg/kg/day as single dose or given in 2 doses; 3- to 16-year-olds treated with 100 mg/day or 3-5 mg/kg/day	Not approved for pediatric use; used in treatment failures or for onychomycosis by some; monitor CBC, LFTs; pulse doses often used at 4-6 wk and every 4-6 wk while on treatment; broadest spectrum; possible drug interactions
Ketoconazole	100 mg/tsp Su 200 mg tab	3.3-6.6 mg/kg/day in single dose	Less effective than griseofulvin and higher risk of hepatotoxicity

TABLE 37-4 Antifungal Medications—cont'd

Drug (Trade Name)	Strength and Formulation	Application	Indications/Side Effects
Nystatin	100,000 U/ml	Infants: 2 ml qid after meals Children/adolescents: 400,000-600,000 U tid pc	Treatment of oral candidiasis
Terbinafine	250 mg tab	<20 kg, 1/4 tab; 20-40 kg, 1/2 tab; >40 kg, 1 tab	Not approved for pediatric use; few studies in children; costly; possible drug interactions Duration of the treatment; tinea capitus 4 wk, tinea corporis 2 wk, tinea pedis 2 wk, finger onychomycosis 6 wk, toenail onychomycosis 12 wk

Data from American Academy of Pediatrics: Recommended doses of parenteral and oral antifungal drugs. In *2003 red book: report of the Committee on Infectious Diseases*, ed 26, Elk Grove Village, IL, 2003, American Academy of Pediatrics, pp 722-724; Baranowitz SA: Personal communication, 2002.
bid, Twice a day; *C*, cream; *CBC*, complete blood count; *G*, gel; *L*, lotion; *LFTs*, liver function tests; *O*, ointment; *P*, powder; *qd*, every day; *S*, solution; *Sh*, shampoo; *Su*, suspension; *tid*, three times daily.
*Nystatin; triamcinolone acetonide.

Tinea Corporis

Description

Tinea corporis, commonly called *ringworm*, is a superficial fungal skin infection found on the face or body. It is also identified by the part of the body affected, for example, tinea manuum (hand), tinea faciei (face) (see Color Fig. 15).

Etiology and Incidence

Tinea corporis is caused by the dermatophytes *Microsporum canis, Trichophyton tonsurans*, and *Epidermophyton floccosum*. Transmission comes as the stratum corneum is invaded following direct contact with infected humans, animals, or fomites. The exact mechanism is unknown but is probably due to a toxin causing an inflammatory response. Infection is common, and it increases with age, hot and humid climates, and crowded living conditions (Weston, Lane, & Morelli, 2002).

Clinical Findings

History. Contact with a person or animal with ringworm is sometimes reported.

Physical Examination

- One or more flat, scaling, mildly erythematous circular patches with raised borders
- Spread peripherally and clear centrally or may be inflammatory throughout with superficial pustules
- Often prominent over hair follicles

Laboratory Studies. If treatment failure or questionable diagnosis occurs:

- KOH-treated scrapings of border of lesion reveal hyphae and spores (see Fig. 37-2).
- Fungal culture.
- Wood's lamp is helpful but does not fluoresce all tinea infections.

Differential Diagnosis

Pityriasis rosea, nummular eczema, psoriasis, seborrhea, contact dermatitis, tinea versicolor, granuloma annulare, and Lyme disease are in the differential diagnosis.

Management

Management involves the following:

- Topical antifungals (see Table 37-4) such as miconazole or clotrimazole are applied three times a day until 1 to 2 weeks after tinea is resolved, usually a minimum of 4 weeks (AAP, 2003). Prescriptive antifungals (e.g., econazole, ciclopirox) penetrate the skin more effectively but are more expensive.
- Extensive infection, or tinea unresponsive to topical treatment, may be treated orally with griseofulvin (see Table 37-4) for 4 to 8 weeks; it must be taken with fatty foods and can cause headache, nausea, diarrhea, or crampy abdominal pain. Monitor CBC, liver function tests (LFTs), and possibly renal function tests if treatment

duration is longer than 3 months; obtain initial laboratory panel at 4 to 6 weeks, repeat every 4 to 6 weeks.
- Identify and treat contacts.
- Educate about communicability of lesions and length of treatment.
- Exclude from day care or school until treatment has begun.
- Follow up in 2 weeks or sooner if lesions are not responding. If unresponsive, diagnosis is incorrect or resistance is possible. Culture to confirm diagnosis and change class of antifungal used.

Complications

Tinea incognito occurs when tinea has been treated with hydrocortisone; signs and symptoms of infection are minimized, but the infection persists.

Patient Education

Find the source of infection and treat or eliminate it to prevent recurrence. Treat skin and 1 cm area beyond the border. Keep skin dry following application of antifungal

Tinea Cruris

Description

Tinea cruris, commonly called *jock itch*, is a superficial fungal skin infection found on the groin, thighs, and intertriginous folds.

Etiology and Incidence

Caused by the dermatophyte *E. floccosum* or, occasionally, *Trichophyton rubrum* or *Trichophyton mentagrophytes*, tinea cruris rarely occurs before adolescence and is more common in males, obese individuals, or those experiencing chafing from tight clothes or moisture. It is extremely common and often occurs with tinea pedis (AAP, 2003).

Clinical Findings

History
- Hot, humid weather, tight clothing, or contact sport such as wrestling
- Often associated with tinea pedis

Physical Examination
- Bilateral, symmetric, scaly, erythematous to slightly brown, sharply marginated lesions with a raised border
- Occurs on inner thighs and inguinal creases; penis and scrotum spared

Laboratory Studies. If treatment failure or questionable diagnosis occurs:
- KOH scraping reveals hyphae and spores
- Fungal culture

Differential Diagnosis

Psoriasis, candidiasis, contact dermatitis, seborrhea, intertrigo, and erythrasma are in the differential diagnosis.

Management

Management is the same as for tinea corporis. Duration of treatment is usually 4 to 6 weeks. If griseofulvin is required, a treatment course of 2 to 6 weeks is usually indicated (see Table 37-4). Additionally:
- Advise the patient to wear cotton underwear and loose clothing and to use absorbent powder.
- Maintain good hygiene following a wrestling event (e.g., bathing, sole use of towel).
- Do not use steroids because of risk of atrophy and striae.

Tinea Pedis

Description

Tinea pedis is a superficial fungal skin infection found on the feet, commonly called *athlete's foot.* There are three clinical forms: (1) vesicles and erosions on the instep of one or both feet; (2) an occasional fissure between the toes with surrounding scale and erythema; and (3) rare diffuse scaling on the weight-bearing surface of the foot with exaggerated scaling in creases (moccasin foot).

Etiology and Incidence

Caused by the dermatophytes *T. rubrum* and *E. floccosum* or *T. mentagrophytes*, tinea pedis rarely occurs before adolescence and is more common in males (AAP, 2003; Weston, Lane, & Morelli, 2002). It often occurs with tinea cruris.

Clinical Findings

History. The following are sometimes reported:
- Sweaty feet
- Use of nylon socks or nonbreathable shoes
- Exposure in family or at school
- Itching, stinging, foul odor
- Microtrauma to feet—cracks, abrasions, nicks, cuts
- Contact with damp areas (e.g., swimming pools, locker room, showers)

Physical Examination. Findings include the following:
- Red, scaly, cracked rash on soles or interdigital spaces and instep, especially between the third, fourth, and fifth toes
- Infection initially white, peeling lesions becoming erythematous, vesicular, macerated, or fissured, and scaly
- Dorsum of foot remains clear
- Chronic infection manifested by a moccasin pattern with diffuse scaling and erythema

Laboratory Studies. Laboratory studies are the same as those for tinea corporis.

Differential Diagnosis

Contact dermatitis, atopic dermatitis, dyshidrotic eczema, psoriasis, and juvenile plantar dermatosis (red, dry fissures of weight-bearing surface) are in the differential diagnosis.

Management

Management is the same as that for tinea corporis. Antifungal medication should be applied 1 cm beyond the borders of the rash for 7 days after clearing. Usual treatment is 3 to 6 weeks. If griseofulvin is required, treatment for 6 to 8 weeks is usually recommended. Additionally:

- Advise patient to keep feet dry, use absorbent powder and cotton socks, avoid scratching, and wear shoes that allow the feet to breathe or go barefoot when home.
- Rinse feet with plain water or water and vinegar; dry carefully, especially between the toes. Moisturize and protect feet to prevent splitting and cracking.
- Aluminum chloride (Drysol) may be used for hyperhidrosis.
- Tennis shoes may be washed in the machine with soap and bleach.
- Physical education or sports may be continued, because tinea pedis is not so common.
- Follow up in 2 to 3 weeks or sooner if lesions are not responding.

Complications

A secondary bacterial infection, indicated by foul odor, can occur. An allergic reaction to fungus, called an *id response*, is manifested by a vesicular eruption on the palms and sides of fingers and occasionally on the trunk and extremities.

Tinea Versicolor

Description

Tinea versicolor is a superficial fungal infection, also called *pityriasis versicolor*, that tends to be persistent and occurs predominantly on the trunk. The lesions do not tan in the summer and become relatively darker in winter months.

Etiology and Incidence

This infection is caused by a yeastlike organism, *Malassezia furfur*, and occurs more commonly in adolescents than in younger children, in chronically ill and immunocompromised children, and in warmer seasons and humid climates (AAP, 2003; Weston, Lane, & Morelli, 2002).

Clinical Findings

History. The infection is associated with warm, humid weather. Occasional mild itching may occur.

Physical Examination. Multiple, annular, scaling, discrete macules ranging from hypopigmented to hyperpigmented (salmon-colored to brown) are seen on the neck, shoulders, upper back and arms, chest midline, and face (especially in children).

Laboratory Studies. KOH scrapings, though not necessary, reveal short curved hyphae and circular spores ("spaghetti and meatballs"). Scrapings fluoresce yellow-orange under Wood's lamp if not cleansed recently.

Differential Diagnosis

Pityriasis alba, pityriasis rosea, vitiligo, postinflammatory hypopigmentation or hyperpigmentation, seborrhea, and secondary syphilis are included in the differential diagnosis.

Management

The following steps are taken:

- Selenium 2.5% lotion or 1% shampoo and ketoconazole 2% shampoo are considered the treatments of choice, applied from face to knees for 30 minutes every day for 7 days; follow with monthly application for 3 months (Weston, Lane, & Morelli, 2002). Sodium hyposulfite or thiosulfate can also be used.
- Topical imidazoles (clotrimazole, miconazole, ciclopirox, or terbinafine solution) or topical azoles (ketoconazole or oxiconazole) applied twice daily for 2 to 4 weeks can be used instead of selenium (see Table 37-4).
- Resistant cases or tropical climates are sometimes an indication for oral antifungal treatment such as with ketoconazole or fluconazole or itraconazole given in a single daily dose for 2 weeks.
- Follow up in 1 month.

Patient Education

- Fifty percent have recurrences within 1 to 10 years.
- Sun exposure makes lesions appear hypopigmented as the surrounding skin tans.
- Repigmentation takes several months.
- If the patient is taking oral antifungal medication, encourage exercise to induce sweating because this may enhance concentration of medication in the skin.
- Skin irritation occurs with overnight application.
- Absence of flaking when skin is scraped is a sign of effective treatment.

VIRAL INFECTIONS OF THE SKIN

Herpes Simplex

Description

In the active state, herpes simplex virus (HSV) causes contagious infections of the skin and mucous membranes ranging from mild to life threatening. Primary infection with HSV type 1 (HSV-1) usually occurs as acute gingivostomatitis (see Chapter 34). The virus then becomes dormant in certain nerve cells until reactivated by triggering factors such as stress, menses, illness, sunburn and windburn, and fatigue. HSV-1 causes recurrent herpes labialis infection, commonly called *cold sores* or *fever blisters* (see Color Fig. 16). HSV-2 infection commonly occurs as a neonatal infection (see Chapter 39) or herpetic vulvovaginitis (see Chapter 36) or progenitalis. Type 1 can also be found in the genital area; type 2 is found on the lips and mouth. Herpetic keratoconjunctivitis is discussed in Chapter 29; other information may be found in Chapter 24.

Etiology and Incidence

HSV-1 is transmitted by close contact with skin, mucous membranes, and body fluids, often through a break in the skin or by autoinoculation. Lesions occur in children of all ages, are contagious as long as they are present, and have an incubation period of 2 to 12 days. Primary lesions usually occur before 5 years of age, are more painful and extensive, and last longer. HSV-1 is responsible for gingivostomatitis, herpes labialis, and hand and finger infections. HSV-2 infection occurs most commonly in adolescents as a sexually transmitted disease and in infants from transmittal during delivery; in children, the possibility of sexual abuse must be considered.

Clinical Findings

History. In primary herpes, fever, malaise, sore throat, and decreased fluid intake can occur. In recurrent HSV infection, there is often a painful prodrome of burning, tingling, and itching at the involved site. Recent acute febrile illness or sun exposure may also be reported.

Physical Examination. The following are seen on physical examination:

- HSV-1
  - Gingivostomatitis—pharyngitis with grouped erythematous-based vesicles that ulcerate and form white plaques on mucosa, gingiva, tongue, palate, lips, chin, and nasolabial folds; lymphadenopathy and halitosis are present
  - Herpes labialis—cluster of small, clear, tense vesicles with an erythematous base that become weepy and ulcerated, progressing to crustiness, usually only on one side of the mouth
  - Hand or fingers—deep-appearing vesicles
  - Common sites of involvement: lips, hand, fingers, nose, cheek, forehead, and eyes; can also occur in the genital area
- HSV-2
  - Grouped vesicopustules and ulceration with edema
  - Primary lesions on vaginal mucosa, labia, or perineum in females and on the penile shaft or perineum in males; oral lesions are possible
  - Recurrent lesions on labia, vulva, clitoris, or cervix in females and on the prepuce, glans, or sulcus in males
  - Regional lymphadenopathy

Laboratory Studies. A Tzanck smear can be done on fluid from the lesions to identify epidermal giant cells. Viral cultures are the gold standard for definitive diagnosis. Direct fluorescent antibody (DFA) tests, enzyme-linked immunosorbent assay (ELISA) serology, and polymerase chain reaction (PCR) tests can be done but are usually only used with severe forms of HSV infection.

Differential Diagnosis

The differential diagnosis includes aphthous stomatitis, hand-foot-and-mouth disease, varicella, impetigo, folliculitis, and erythema multiforme.

Management

Management can be guided by considering the host (e.g., age, area and extent of involvement, and immune status), the organism (is it definitely HSV?), and the drug needed (Table 37-5).

1. Burow solution compresses three times a day to alleviate discomfort
2. Acyclovir 20 to 40 mg/kg per day orally five times a day for 5 days or 200 mg every 4 hours five times a day for 7 to 10 days may be indicated to help shorten the course and alleviate symptoms for children over 2 years of age with the following conditions:
   - Any underlying skin disorder (e.g., eczema)
   - A severe case
   - An immunocompromised disease
   - Systemic symptoms with primary genital infection
   - Occasionally for initial severe gingivostomatitis
3. Antibiotics for secondary bacterial (usually staphylococcal) infection:
   - Mupirocin topically three times a day for 5 days
   - Erythromycin 40 mg/kg per day for 10 days
   - Dicloxacillin 12.5 to 50 mg/kg per day for 10 days
4. Oral anesthetics for comfort; use with caution in children (children should be able to rinse and spit)
   - Viscous lidocaine (xylocaine) 2% topical
   - Liquid diphenhydramine alone or combined with Maalox (aluminum hydroxide; magnesium hydroxide) as a 1:1 rinse (maximum of 5 mg/kg per day diphenhydramine in case it is swallowed); can also be applied with Q-Tips to the lesions
5. Newborn infant, immunosuppressed child, child with infected atopic dermatitis, or child with a lesion in the

TABLE 37-5 ***Diagnosis and Treatment of Herpes Simplex (HS) and Herpes Zoster (HZ)***

	Presentation	Clinical Findings	Treatment	Education
HS	Gingivostomatitis as primary infection; herpes labialis or herpes facialis as recurrent infection	Pharyngitis with erythematous vesicles on/in mouth; small, clear vesicles on erythematous base progressing to crusting	Burow solution; acyclovir in primary case or underlying disorder; antibiotics if secondary infection; oral anesthetics; supportive care	Degree and duration of contagion; triggers to infection
HZ	Reactivation of latent varicella virus, especially after mild cases or in infants <1 yr of age or immunocompromised host	Two to three clustered groups of vesicles on erythematous base, especially over thoracic or lumbosacral dermatomes; pain, itch, tingle is minimal in children	Burow solution; antihistamine; drying lotions; possible acyclovir; silver sulfadiazine (Silvadene cream); antibiotics if secondary infection	New vesicles occur for up to 1 wk; take 2-3 wk to resolve; contagious for varicella; varicella vaccine to prevent

eye or on the eyelid margin: consult with or refer to an appropriate provider

6. Offer supportive care such as antipyretics, analgesics, hydration, and good oral hygiene
7. Exclude from day care only during the initial course (gingivostomatitis) and if the child cannot control secretions
8. Recurrent, frequent, and severe HSV infection may be treated with acyclovir prophylaxis for 6 months

Complications

Herpetic whitlow, occurring on a finger or thumb, is a swollen, painful lesion with an erythematous base and ulceration resembling a paronychia. It occurs on fingers of thumb-sucking children with gingivostomatitis or adolescents with genital HSV infection. Therapy with oral acyclovir 200 mg five times a day for 5 to 10 days may speed healing. *Eczema herpeticum* or *Kaposi's varicelliform eruption* is discussed in Chapter 24. HSV has also been implicated as a possible cause of erythema multiforme and Stevens-Johnson syndrome.

Patient Education, Prognosis, and Prevention

Recurrence of infection, possible triggering factors, and avoidance measures should be discussed. Triggers can include physical and psychologic stress, trauma, fever, exposure to UV light, illness, menses, and extreme weather. Contagiousness of lesions and oral secretions must be understood. Explanation of the course of primary disease, with fever lasting up to 4 days and lesions taking at least 2 weeks to heal, is important. Famciclovir and perciclovir are in clinical trials for use in children. Vaccines are under development to decrease transmission and minimize recurrence.

Herpes Zoster

Description

Herpes zoster (HZ) is a recurrent varicella infection commonly called *shingles* (Fig. 37-5).

Etiology and Incidence

Caused by reactivation of the latent varicella infection, HZ occurs in 10% to 20% of all persons, is rare in childhood, and occurs more frequently with increasing age (three times

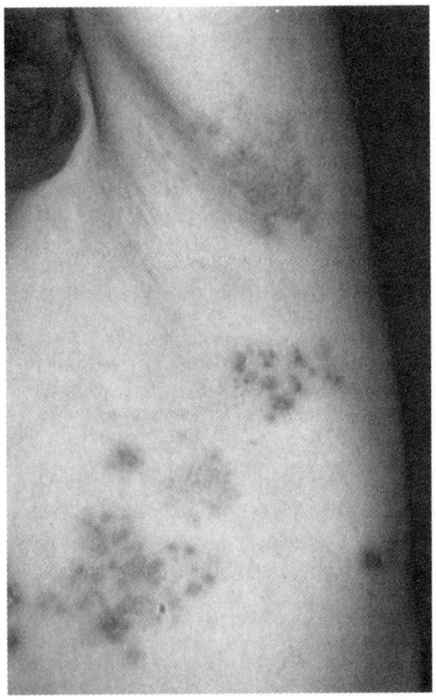

FIGURE 37-5 Herpes zoster. Typical segmented papulovesicular eruptions on an inflammatory base occur in an interrupted band with dermatomal distribution. (From Hurwitz S: *Clinical pediatric dermatology*, ed 2, Philadelphia, 1993, WB Saunders, p 325.)

more common in adolescents than preschoolers). HZ is more common following mild cases of varicella, following varicella before 1 year of age (threefold to twentyfold increased risk), and in immunocompromised children. Reoccurrence of HZ is about 4% (Myers, Stanberry, & Seward, 2004).

Clinical Findings

History. Burning, stinging, or tingling precedes eruption by about 1 week, though this is less common in children. The lesions can be extremely itchy and painful.

Physical Examination. Findings include the following:
- Two or three clustered groups of macules and papules progress to vesicles on an erythematous base. These vesicles become pustular, rupture, ulcerate, and crust.
- Lesions develop over 3 to 5 days and last 7 to 10 days.
- Lesions are commonly seen on thoracic (50% to 70%), lumbosacral (20%), and fifth cranial nerve (10%) dermatomes with scattered lesions outside borders (Weston, Lane, & Morelli, 2002).
- Lesions do not cross midline (key to diagnosis).
- Lymphadenopathy may occur.

Laboratory Studies. The Tzanck smear or viral culture can be done to distinguish from HSV infection. Bacterial culture or Gram stain can be used to distinguish from impetigo.

Differential Diagnosis

Local cutaneous HSV infection and impetigo are in the differential diagnosis.

Management

Management steps include the following:
1. Apply Burow solution compresses three times a day to alleviate discomfort.
2. Administer antihistamines for itching, analgesics for discomfort.
3. Lotions such as calamine help dry lesions and decrease itching.
4. Antiviral medications:
   - Acyclovir 800 mg orally every 4 hours five times a day for 7 to 10 days helps shorten the course and alleviate symptoms in immunocompromised or significantly ill children. Acyclovir has not been fully studied in children under 2 years of age.
   - Famciclovir 500 mg every 8 hours for 7 days at the earliest sign of HZ or within 48 to 72 hours of onset, or valacyclovir 1 g orally three times a day for 7 days at the earliest sign of HZ or within 48 hours of onset, has been approved for adults but not for children with HZ (AAP, 2003).
5. Silver sulfadiazine (Silvadene) cream may provide comfort and speed healing of lesions (Kurtz, 2002).
6. Antibiotics for secondary bacterial (usually staphylococcal) infection:
   - Mupirocin topically twice a day
   - Dicloxacillin 12.5 to 25 mg/kg per day for 7 to 10 days
7. Refer for immediate ophthalmologic examination if eyes, forehead, or nose is involved.

Complications

Complications are rare except in immunocompromised children. Occasionally, HZ is the initial finding in acquired immunodeficiency syndrome (AIDS), especially if more than one dermatome is involved (Weston, Lane, & Morelli, 2002).

Patient Education, Prevention, and Prognosis

- New vesicles appear for up to 1 week and take 2 to 3 weeks to resolve. Illness is usually mild.
- The child is contagious for varicella until lesions are crusted and should be excluded from day care until this occurs. However, if the lesions can be covered, the child may return to child care (AAP, 2003).

Molluscum Contagiosum

Description

A benign, common childhood viral skin infection with little health risk, molluscum contagiosum often disappears on its own in a few weeks to months and is not easily treated (Fig. 37-6).

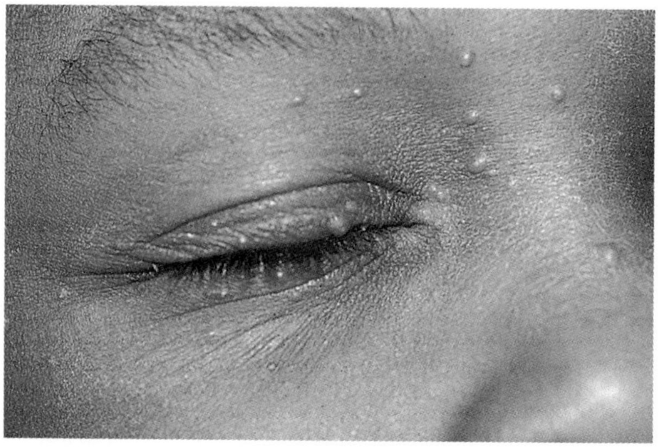

FIGURE 37-6 Multiple molluscum papules on an infant's face. (From Weston WL, Lane AT, Morelli JG: *Color textbook of pediatric dermatology*, ed 3, St Louis, 2002, Mosby, p 51.)

Etiology and Incidence

This highly contagious poxvirus that attacks skin and mucous membranes is spread by direct contact, by fomites, or by autoinoculation. It is commonly found in children and adolescents (AAP, 2003). Three types are identified. Lesions found on the extremities, neck, and head are usually type 1; genital lesions are usually type 2 or 3. The incubation period is about 2 months; the child is contagious as long as lesions are present.

Clinical Findings

History

- Itching at the site
- Possible exposure to molluscum contagiosum

Physical Examination. Findings include the following:

- Very small, firm, pink to flesh-colored discrete papules 1 to 6 mm in size (occasionally up to 15 mm), progressing to become umbilicated papules with a cheesy core; keratinous contents may extrude from the umbilication.
- Face, axillae, antecubital area, trunk, crural area, and extremities are the most commonly involved areas; palms, soles, and scalp are spared.
- Papules are few in number, usually 2 to 20.
- Sexually active or abused children can have genitally grouped lesions.
- Children with eczema or immunosuppression can have severe cases; those with human immunodeficiency virus (HIV) infection or AIDS can have hundreds of lesions.

Differential Diagnosis

Warts, closed comedones, small epidermal cysts, blisters, folliculitis, and condyloma acuminatum are included in the differential diagnosis.

Management

- Untreated lesions take 1 to 5 years to resolve. Mechanical removal of the central core is often done to prevent spread and autoinoculation. Using eutectic mixture of local anesthetics (EMLA) cream (lidocaine; prilocaine) 30 to 45 minutes before the procedure reduces discomfort.
- Curettage is done with a sharp blade to remove the papule. Piercing the papule and expressing the plug can also be done, but this procedure is painful.
- Nightly application of surgical tape (Scotch or adhesive tape can be used) for 1 month followed by removal of lesions.
- Topical medications may prove beneficial. Recheck the patient in 1 to 2 weeks to determine need for re-treatment.
  - Liquid nitrogen may be applied for 2 to 3 seconds (easiest but also painful).
  - Trichloroacetic acid 25% to 50% applied by dropper to the center of the lesion, followed by alcohol (use with caution).
  - Cantharidin 0.7% in collodion applied by dropper to the center of the lesion, followed by alcohol. Salicylic or lactic acid or potassium hydroxide or podophyllin.
  - Podofilox (Condylox) 0.5% topical solution or gel, or imiquimod 5% (Aldara) applied daily with a toothpick or Q-Tip.
  - Tretinoin cream applied to lesion nightly.
  - Silver nitrate, iodine 7% to 9%, or phenol 1% applied for 2 to 3 seconds.
  - Cimetidine 30 to 40 mg/kg per day in two divided doses orally.
- Sexual abuse of children with genitally grouped lesions should be suspected and evaluated.
- Evaluate for HIV infection if hundreds of lesions are found.

Complications

Molluscum dermatitis, a scaly, erythematous, hypersensitive reaction, can occur and will respond to moisturizer; avoid hydrocortisone because it will cause molluscum to flare. Inflammation of the eyes or conjunctiva and scarring can occur.

Patient Education and Prevention

Patients are contagious, but there is no need to exclude them from day care or school. Children with impaired immunity, atopic dermatitis, or traumatized skin are at greater risk for broader spread. Severe inflammation is possible several hours after application of cantharidin. Scarring is unusual.

Warts

Description

A common childhood skin infection characterized by a proliferation of the epidermis, warts are rarely a serious health concern but present cosmetic problems for children and their families.

Etiology and Incidence

Warts are viral-induced epithelial tumors caused by human papillomavirus (HPV). Warts occur in approximately 5% of children by 11 years of age (Weston, Lane, & Morelli, 2002). They are among the most common skin disorders in children. The transmission of warts from person to person is dependent on viral and host factors, such as quantity of virus, location of warts, preexisting skin injury, and cell-mediated immunity. Although 65% of all warts resolve spontaneously within 2 years, there is a high recurrence rate.

Clinical Findings

History. The history can include exposure to someone with warts. Trauma promotes inoculation of the virus (Koebner phenomenon); therefore warts are commonly seen on the extremities. However, they can occur anywhere on the body, including the face, scalp, and genitalia.

Physical Examination

- *Common* warts (verruca vulgaris) are usually elevated, flesh-colored single papules with scaly, irregular surfaces and occasionally black pinpoints, which are thrombosed blood vessels. They are usually asymptomatic and multiple in number and are found anywhere on the body, although most commonly on the hands, nails, and feet (Fig. 37-7).
- *Periungual* warts are common warts occurring around the cuticles of the fingers or toes.
- *Plantar* warts (mosaic) are common warts found on weight-bearing surfaces of the feet. Found alone or grouped, plantar warts grow inward and disrupt skin markings.
- *Filiform* warts project from the skin on a narrow stalk and are usually seen on the face, lips, nose, eyelids, or neck.
- *Flat* warts (verruca plana or juvenile warts) are seen most commonly on the face, neck, and extremities. They are small, slightly elevated papules and number from few to several hundred.
- *Condylomata acuminata* on genital mucosa and adjacent skin are multiple, confluent warts with irregular surfaces, light in color, and cauliflower-like in appearance. See Chapter 36 for more detail.

Differential Diagnosis

The differential diagnosis is calluses, corns, foreign bodies, moles, and comedones.

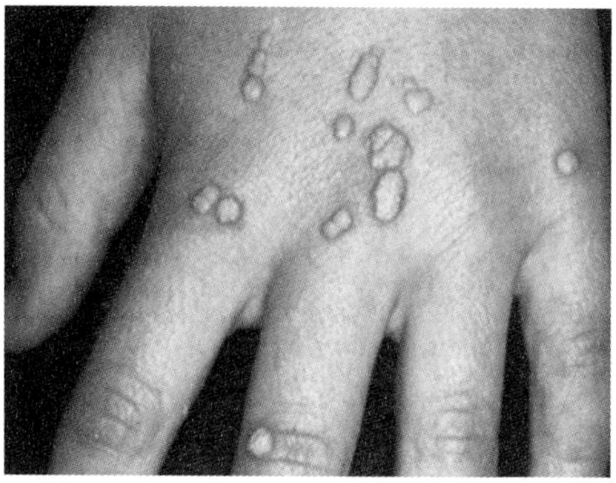

FIGURE 37-7 Multiple common warts (verruca vulgaris). (From Hurwitz S: *Clinical pediatric dermatology*, ed 2, Philadelphia, 1993, WB Saunders, p 329.)

Management

There is no single effective treatment for warts. The recurrence rate for warts is high, and it is unlikely that the wart will resolve with a single treatment. No treatment is necessary if the warts are asymptomatic. The decision to treat should be based on location, number and size of lesions, discomfort, and whether the warts are cosmetically objectionable. Treatment should not be harmful, and scarring should be avoided. Genital warts found in young children or in adolescents who are not sexually active should create suspicion of sexual abuse. Specific treatment options are outlined in Box 37-6. Follow up in 2 to 3 weeks to evaluate response.

Complications

Scarring from removal can occur. A ring of satellite warts may develop at the edge of the blister following cantharidin. Immunocompromised hosts can have extensive involvement.

Patient Education

A blister, sometimes hemorrhagic, may form 1 to 2 days after freezing. Redness and itching may herald regression of a wart. Parents and patients must be warned that multiple or prolonged treatment is often necessary.

INFESTATIONS OF THE SKIN

Diagnosis and treatment of pediculosis and scabies are listed in Table 37-6.

Pediculosis

Description

Pediculosis (lice infestation) affects the head, body, or pubic area. Pediculosis capitis (head) is most common, pediculosis corporis (body) is uncommon, and pediculosis pubis (pubic area) is considered a sexually transmitted disease. Infestation is defined by some as presence of either nits or lice, and by others as presence of lice alone. The gold standard for diagnosis of pediculosis is finding live lice on the head (AAP, 2003; Bloomfield, 2002; Pollack, Kiszewski, & Spielman, 2000; Williams et al, 2001).

Etiology and Incidence

Lice infestation is caused by two subspecies of *Pediculus humanus* (head and body) or by *Phthirus pubis* (pubic). The adult female louse, which survives by sucking human blood, deposits 6 to 10 eggs per day at the base of the hair shaft within a waterproof, gluelike substance. The eggs

BOX 37-6 *Treatment Options for Warts*

Keratolytics eliminate the wart by causing topical peeling and an inflammatory response. They are often available over the counter, cause little pain, and are low in cost and risk, but are slow to work.

- Salicylic acid paints with a concentration of greater than 20% are applied with a toothpick once or twice a day for 4 to 6 weeks. On thick skin, a combination of 16.7% salicylic acid and 16.7% collodion is more effective. This method is useful for common or periungual warts, but it is not effective with warts larger than 5 mm in diameter.
- Salicylic acid plasters with 40% concentration (e.g., Occlusal, Duofilm, Mediplast) are cut to size and taped in place for 3 to 5 days. After the plaster is taken off, the area should be soaked for 45 minutes and the dead epidermis removed. A new plaster is then applied. Treatment can last 3 to 6 weeks. This method is useful for plantar warts.
- Retinotic acid gel 0.025% to 0.05% applied once or twice daily brings resolution in 4 to 6 weeks. This method is useful for flat warts, but it does not work for common, plantar, or peringual warts.
- Occlusion with duct tape for 6½ day, off for ½ day, followed by soaking and scraping of epidermis is easy, painless, and inexpensive.

Destructive agents eliminate the wart by causing necrosis and blister formation. Most techniques are painful and require patient cooperation.

- Cryotherapy. Liquid nitrogen is applied for 2 to 10 seconds after an area 1 to 3 mm beyond the wart turns white or patient complains of pain to induce blister formation above the dermal-epidermal junction. Care must be taken not to freeze the wart too vigorously. Caution should be used when freezing warts over joints and the lateral aspects of digits. This method is uncomfortable and often not tolerated by children. Re-treatment is often necessary.
- Cantharidin 0.7% is applied directly to the wart with a toothpick and covered with tape for 24 hours. This is a potent blistering agent that creates a blister in 2 to 3 days that is sloughed after 7 to 14 days. This method is useful for periungual and some plantar warts. Do not use on other body surfaces.
- Podophyllum 25% solution is alcohol applied to the wart with a toothpick; it should be washed off in 4 hours; may be repeated in 1 week. Podofilox, available over the counter for home use, is applied twice a day for 3 days. After a 4-day rest period, the 3-day cycle may be repeated as necessary. This technique is useful for common or genital warts.
- Surgical excision of warts can lead to scarring that can be more painful than the wart itself, but can be highly effective for large individual warts. Surgery by snipping with scissors, not scalpel, is useful for filiform warts.
- Laser treatments are often as effective as cryosurgery but can be painful and require several treatments for complete resolution.

Immunotherapy modalities stimulate an immune response to HPV. These newer treatment modalities do not have controlled studies evaluating their effectiveness.

- Oral cimetidine, a histamine$_2$ receptor blocking agent, may improve immunity to HPV. It is used in conjunction with other modalities at a dose of 20 to 30 mg/kg divided twice a day for 3 to 4 months.
- Imiquimod cream applied daily creates cell-mediated immunity in surrounding areas and is often effective as a home treatment. It is applied for 1 to 2 months.
- Contact sensitization and interferon injection are methods used by dermatologists, usually in adult patients.

HPV, Human papillomavirus.

mature in 7 to 10 days and begin laying eggs in another 7 to 10 days. Typically, no more than 12 to 24 head lice infest a child at a time (AAP, 2002), though in a 30-day life span, one louse can lay 150 to 300 eggs. Transmission of pediculosis occurs by direct or indirect contact, often by sharing hairbrushes, caps, clothing, or linen or through close living quarters, poor hygiene, or sexual activity (pubic lice).

Pediculosis capitis is considered an epidemic in the United States, with estimates ranging from 6 to 12 million cases per year (AAP, 2002; CDC, 2002). However, head lice are not considered a health hazard because they do not spread disease (AAP, 2002). All socioeconomic groups are affected, but lice are most common in school-age white females, with the peak season occurring from August to November. Lice are uncommon in blacks, with a ratio of 1:34 relative to whites (Weston, Lane, & Morelli, 2002). Pediculosis corporis is uncommon in childhood. If pediculosis pubis is found in a child, sexual abuse must be considered.

As with other medications, lice appear to have a growing resistance to available treatment options mainly in children who have been treated multiple times. European,

TABLE 37-6 ***Diagnosis and Treatment of Pediculosis and Scabies***

	Clinical Findings	Treatment
Pediculosis (head lice)	History of infestation; itchy scalp, scratches; postoccipital nodes; occasional visualization of mites or nits (small white oval cases), commonly on back of head, nape of neck, behind ears, possibly eyelashes	*Key* to treatment is proper technique! *First step* is pediculocide (permethrin or pyrethrin) *Second step* is removal of nits by combing hair with fine-toothed comb in 1-inch sections with special attention to nape of neck and behind ears *Third step* is to cleanse the environment: check family, friends, day care/school contacts; clean sheets, towels, clothing, headgear; store other items in plastic for 2 wk; vacuum; soak brushes and combs; follow up in 2 wk with daily recheck at home; return to school after treatment
Scabies	*Key finding*: itching, worse at night, and complaints more significant than findings; fitful sleep, crankiness; curving burrows, especially in webs of fingers, sides of hands, folds of wrist, armpits, forearms, elbows, belt line, buttocks, proximal half of foot and heel; may be <10 lesions total; secondary excoriation; infants may have lesions on palms, soles, scalp, face, posterior auricle and axilla, folds, red-brown in color, dozens in number	Pharmacologic treatment with permethrin 5%, repeated in 1 wk; antihistamine, hydrocortisone, nonsteroidal antiinflammatory drugs for itching; simultaneously treat family members (even if asymptomatic), friends, school/day care contacts; cleanse environment: linens and clothing, vacuum, store anything else in plastic bags for 1 wk; rash and itch persist for up to 3 wk after treatment; return to school 24 hr after treatment

South American, and Israeli scientists have documented this resistance, and it is being studied in the United States. This has led to the trial of many alternative treatment options.

Clinical Findings

History. The following may be elicited:

- A history of infestation in a family, friend, or day care contact
- Dandruff-like substance in the hair
- Itching of the scalp, scratching, and irritability if infestation has been present for a few weeks

Physical Examination. Findings include the following:

- Head lice:
  - Mites can be visualized; the nits or eggs can be seen as small, white oval cases attached tightly to a hair shaft (Fig. 37-8).
  - Care must be taken to differentiate hair casts, epithelial cells, and other debris from nits.
  - Common sites are the back of the head, nape of the neck, and behind the ears; eyelashes can be involved.
  - Scalp excoriations and occipital or cervical adenopathy can be present.
- Body lice:
  - Excoriated macules or papules may be present.
  - Belt line, collar, and underwear areas are common sites.

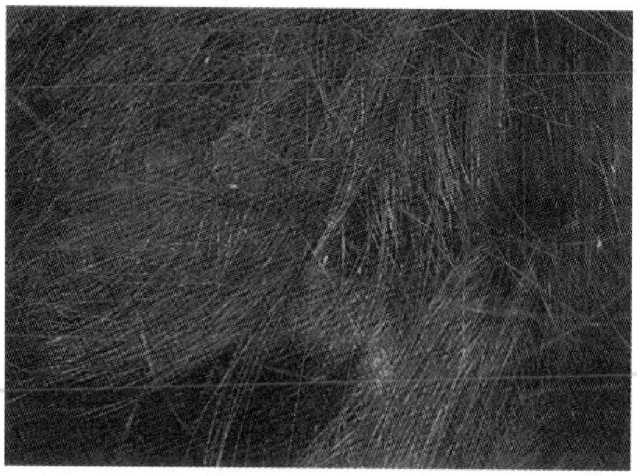

FIGURE 37-8 Pediculosis capitis. Oval, grayish to yellowish white nits are present in the hair of the scalp. (From Hurwitz S: *Clinical pediatric dermatology*, ed 2, Philadelphia, 1993, WB Saunders, p 418.)

  - A hemorrhagic pinpoint macule is seen where the louse extracted blood.
  - Axillary, inguinal, or regional lymphadenopathy can be present.
- Pubic lice:
  - Excoriation and small bluish macules and papules may be present.
  - Eyelashes can be involved; spread to other short-haired areas (thighs, trunk, axillae, beard) may occur.
  - Rule out sexual abuse.

Laboratory Studies. The following can be helpful:

- Nits fluoresce under a Wood's lamp.
- Microscopic examination of a hair shaft can more clearly identify nits.
- Test for other sexually transmitted diseases, especially gonorrhea and syphilis, with pubic lice.

Differential Diagnosis

Scabies (see Table 37-6), dermatitis herpetiformis, and necrotic excoriations are in the differential diagnosis.

Management

Treatment options are varied and controversial, ranging from standard over-the-counter pharmaceutical products, to prescriptive drugs, to many alternatives, to actually dangerous substances. Correct diagnosis is imperative in determining accurate management. One study (Williams et al, 2001) found that only 31% of children with nits had live lice, and only 18% of children with nits developed lice over the next 14 days. Children with five or more nits within 0.25 inch of the scalp were more likely to develop lice, but even in this group, only 32% became infested. This study argues that most children with nits will not become infested and therefore should not be excluded from school or treated with a pediculocide. Rather, they should have regular follow-up with a thorough 5- to 10-minute examination to exclude the presence of lice over the next 14 days. If live lice are found, treatment should then be undertaken.

Pediculocides are toxic substances and should be used only as directed, and with care. If a child is younger than 2 years of age, do not use pediculocides, only manual removal (CDC, 2002). The National Pediculosis Association (NPA) also advises caution in children with chronic illness, undergoing chemotherapy, using medications, or already overexposed to pediculocides, as well as pregnant or nursing mothers who apply the pediculocide (NPA, 2002a). Treatment failure is common, and it is debated whether failure is due to poor technique or actual medication resistance (Pollack, Kiszewski, & Spielman, 2000). The FDA has mandated a change in labeling of over-the-counter lice products in hopes of improving treatment success while minimzing potential harm. A meta-analysis review of controlled clinical trials for treatment of pediculosis showed no evidence that one pediculocide had greater effect than another (Dodd, 2002). This analysis also showed that combing alone was not a curative treatment. Recommendations were to follow local resistance patterns when determining treatment.

1. The *first step* is application of a pediculocide. Proper technique is key to success. If the hair is to be shampooed, do not use a shampoo containing conditioner or cream rinse. Shampoo the child's hair over a sink, not in the tub or shower. Keep the pediculocide out of the eyes. If applying solution to damp hair, make sure it is damp, not wet (dilutes the pediculocide). Do not rewash the hair for 1 or 2 days following treatment. Re-treatment is recommended in 7 to 10 days.
   - Permethrin 1% cream rinse (Nix), also called pyrethrum, is the current treatment of choice for head lice because of its safety, efficacy, and 10-day residual. Hair should be shampooed and towel-dried, permethrin applied and left on for 10 minutes, and then rinsed. Hair should not be rewashed for at least 24 to 48 hours. Re-treatment is advised in 7 to 10 days.
   - Lindane is an organochloride that kills mites, nits, and ova effectively, but safety is a concern because of potential central nervous system effects on the child and potential environmental effects through ineffective removal from wastewater. It is contraindicated for pregnant women and infants. Lindane has been banned in California for the treatment of lice and scabies. The NPA, *Consumer Reports,* the Cancer Prevention Coalition, and the Public Citizen Health Research Group have all issued statements calling for a ban on lindane (*Consumer Reports,* 1998; NPA, 2002b). Eighteen countries outside of the United States have banned it. The CDC (2002) has stated that it "is probably safe when used as directed, but overuse, misuse, or accidentally swallowing can be toxic to the brain and nervous system." For head lice, a 1% lindane shampoo is used for no more than 10 minutes, rinsed, and repeated 1 week later; for body lice, cream or lotion may be applied for 8 to 12 hours and then rinsed off; for pubic lice, a 1% shampoo is used for 10 minutes, then rinsed off and repeated in 1 week (Weston, Lane, & Morelli, 2002).
   - Pyrethrin is a natural extract from the chrysanthemum plant. It is effective as a pediculocide but not as an ovicide. Commonly found as RID, A-200, Pronto, or Triplex, it is usually a 10-minute shampoo applied to dry hair, with repeat application in 7 to 10 days. It is contraindicated in children with allergy to ragweed.
   - Malathion lotion 0.5% is an organophosphate with a pine needle oil base. It is a potent lice killer that binds to the hair shaft for 4 weeks. It has been repeatedly withdrawn from the U.S. market but is once again available. The drug is flammable, and if ingested causes severe respiratory distress. It must be used with extreme caution. The CDC states that "when used as directed it is very effective in treating lice" (CDC, 2002). No safety studies are available for children under 6 years of age.

- Ivermectin in topical 0.8% solution (not available in the United States) or orally as a 200 μg/kg single-dose tablet (available, but not approved as a pediculocide nor for use in children younger than 5 years of age) is sometimes used to treat apparently resistant lice (Bell, 1998).

2. The *second step* is ensuring removal of nits, although this is not an absolutely necessary step (AAP, 2002, 2003; Pollack, Kiszewski, & Spielman, 2000). Again, proper technique is the key to success. Covering hair with a warm, damp towel for 30 minutes before nit removal may help loosen nits. Hair should be wet when combed. A good light, a magnifying glass, and tweezers are useful. A wide-toothed comb may be used initially to straighten the hair.
   - A proper comb has fine teeth. Most pediculocides include a nit-removal comb. The LiceMeister comb from the NPA (see Resource Box) has been developed to efficiently remove nits. The correct technique in combing the hair is also essential. A minimum of 20 to 30 minutes should be spent combing damp hair. Working from the top of the scalp down, 1-inch sections should be divided out and combed. Special attention should be paid to the nape of the neck and behind the ears.
   - Some products claim to dissolve the substance (cement) that attaches the nit to the hair to facilitate removal. A 1:1 vinegar-to-water solution applied to the scalp for 30 minutes, covered with a warm, moist towel, may also help.
   - If eyelashes are involved, coat with petroleum jelly (Vaseline) two to three times a day for 8 to 14 days with manual removal of nits.
   - Comb-outs and inspection should be repeated every night for 2 to 3 weeks to ensure cure.
3. The *third step* is thorough cleansing of the environment.
   - Examination of family members, friends, school, and day care contacts is essential. Treatment of family members, even if nothing is found, is sometimes recommended to prevent recurrent infection, although this practice is now being discouraged because of the emergence of resistant lice and toxicity of pediculocides.
   - Cleansing of sheets, towels, clothing, and headgear by hot-water washing and machine-drying on hot cycle for 20 minutes, ironing, or dry-cleaning is essential.
   - Any item that cannot be washed or dry-cleaned should be stored in a plastic bag for 2 weeks.
   - Hot ironing or vacuuming of play areas, floors, rugs, and furniture is an important step in cleansing.
   - Brushes, combs, and hair accessories should be soaked in pediculocide, alcohol, or Lysol for 1 hour, followed by hot-water rinse.
   - Spraying or fumigating the house is not recommended.
4. *Alternative treatments* are often herbal or essential oils such as olive oil, pine oil, tea-tree oil, margarine, mayonnaise, dog shampoo, and petroleum jelly, all of which are said to suffocate and thereby kill the lice. Certain recommendations are definitely to be avoided, including wrapping the hair in plastic and putting the child under a hair dryer or washing the hair with gasoline or kerosene.
5. *Treatment failure* is not unusual. Common mistakes include the following:
   - Misdiagnosis
   - Improper use of pediculocide
   - Dilution of pediculocide by applying to wet hair, not damp hair
   - Use of a shampoo with conditioner or cream rinse (decreases adherence of the pediculocide to the hair shaft)
   - Inadequate combing techniques
   - Not cleansing personal care items
   - Not screening and treating family members and close contacts
6. Recommendations for dealing with potential *resistance* are varied. Neither formal recommendations nor FDA approval regarding any of these methods has yet been made. Some methods for treating resistant lice that are currently being discussed include the following:
   - Use Nix creme rinse for 4 to 8 hours instead of 10 minutes.
   - Use Nix creme rinse under a shower cap overnight.
   - Use Elimite cream (five times stronger than Nix) overnight.
   - Use crotamiton 10% (Eurax) lotion applied to the scalp and left for 24 hours before rinsing. (One study showed no difference in resistance [Pollack, Kiszewski, & Spielman, 2000].)
   - Use trimethoprim-sulfamethoxazole to kill symbiotic bacteria on which lice survive.
   - Use oral ivermectin 200 μg/kg as a single dose, repeated in 10 days if the child weighs more than 15 kg (AAP, 2003).
7. Nix creme rinse has received FDA approval for *prophylaxis* for institutional use when 20% of the population is infested or for use in immediate household members (PDR, 2002).
8. Body lice may be treated with improved hygiene and cleaning clothes. Infested clothing should be washed and dried at hot temperatures. No pediculocides are required (AAP, 2003).
9. Pubic lice are treated as pediculosis capitis.

Patient Education and Prevention

Items for discussion include the following:

- Follow-up visits in 10 to 14 days are helpful in individual cases to ensure complete resolution of infestation. However, daily to weekly checks for lice or nits should be carried out at home.
- Educate family members about the expected course and that lice infestation is not a social disease.
- Educate family members about the need to avoid excessive or unnecessary re-treatment because of the toxic hazard of medications. Do not use extra amounts; do not treat more than three times with the same medication without being seen by a care provider; do not mix pediculocides.
- The child can return to school following initial treatment. The "no nits" policy is controversial and has no documented effectiveness in controlling pediculosis outbreaks. However, close contacts in the neighborhood or at school, camp, or child care should be informed and checked regularly for infestation.

See Resource Box for education materials and information.

Complications

Secondary bacterial infection can occur, and school absenteeism can result from the strict enforcement of the "no nit" policy.

Scabies

Description

Scabies is caused by the itch mite, *Sarcoptes scabiei*, which burrows under the skin and causes intense itching. There are many different forms of presentation (see Color Fig. 17).

Etiology and Incidence

Scabies is a highly contagious infestation spread through close contact and shared clothing or linen. The female mite burrows into the skin, laying up to three eggs a day as she travels. The eggs hatch in about 2 weeks, and the new mites repeat the process. Sensitization, which causes intense itching, occurs approximately 3 weeks after infestation. Incubation is 1 to 2 months following contact. Scabies occurs in all socioeconomic groups and in all age-groups. However, infestation of African Americans is rare.

Clinical Findings

History. The following can be reported:

- *Key finding*: Itching, worse at night, initially mild but progressively more intense
- Fitful sleep, crankiness, or rubbing of hands and feet (infants)

Physical Examination. Findings include the following:

- Complaints are significantly greater than examination findings.
- Characteristic lesions include curving burrows, especially on webs of fingers and sides of hands, folds of wrists and armpits, forearms, elbows, belt line, buttocks, genitalia, or proximal half of foot and heel.
- Secondary lesions include itchy papules that can be excoriated, urticarial papules with excoriation, nodules from inflammatory response, and crusting and excoriation (signs of secondary infection).
- Infants classically have vesicular lesions on palms, soles, scalp, face, posterior auriculae, and axillae, concentrated in the folds; head and neck lesions typically are red-brown vesiculopustules or nodules. However, any child younger than 2 years of age can have an unusual manifestation.
- Infants classically have dozens of lesions; older children may have fewer than 10.

Laboratory Studies. The following are done as indicated:

- Microscopic examination of scrapings from an unscratched burrow in saline or mineral oil can reveal an eight-legged mite, eggs, or feces. Do not use KOH because it dissolves the mites, eggs, and feces.
- Burrow ink test: Apply a drop of ink or rub a washable felt-tipped pen across suspected burrow. Wipe off excess ink, and examine with magnifying glass for an ink-stained burrow.

Differential Diagnosis

Papular urticaria, atopic dermatitis, contact dermatitis, insect bites, folliculitis, lichen planus, and dermatitis herpetiformis are included in the differential diagnosis.

Management

Management involves the following:

1. Pharmacologic treatment begins with applying a thin layer of scabicide to the entire body, excluding the eyes. Areas of special importance are under the fingernails, the scalp, behind the ears, all folds and creases, and the feet and hands. In general, the scabicide should be reapplied in 7 days on all symptomatic patients.
   - Permethrin 5% lotion (Elimite) is the drug of choice for treating scabies because of its safety and efficacy (less than 2% absorbed; cure rate 89% to 92% [Morgan-Glenn, 2001]). It can be used on infants as young as 2 months of age. Apply for 8 to 14 hours, then rinse off. Re-treat in 1 week. In infants, special application is needed to head, postauricular area, and hands and feet.

- Lindane 1% cream is effective but has potential central nervous system effects (absorption up to 10% [Morgan-Glenn, 2001]). It is contraindicated in children less than 6 months (some say under 2 years) of age, in pregnancy or breastfeeding, and in children who have seizures. (See discussion of lindane under Pediculosis.) When lindane is used, it is applied and left on for 8 to 12 hours before washing off. Repeat application is recommended in 1 week. The CDC (2002) recommends an alternative scabicide (usually permethrin) in children under 10 years of age.
- Crotamiton 10% cream (Eurax) applied to the whole body has been used in infants, but it is not as effective as permethrin or lindane. It must be applied daily for 5 days or to the whole body for 48 hours, rinsed, and repeated. Re-treatment in 2 weeks is suggested.
- Sulfur cream or ointment 5% to 10% in petrolatum is an old treatment that is not highly effective, is smelly, and stains. However, it may be used in pregnant or lactating women, infants, and young children; it is applied nightly for 3 nights and washed off 24 hours after the final application.
- Ivermectin 200 μg orally in a single dose is effective for crusted (Norwegian) scabies or refractory infection (AAP, 2003). Ivermectin is not FDA approved for this, nor is it recommended under 5 years of age (Weston, Lane, & Morelli, 2002).

2. Antihistamines (hydroxyzine or diphenhydramine) or topical 1% hydrocortisone can be helpful for itching.
3. Simultaneous treatment of family members, friends, and school and day care contacts, even if asymptomatic, is essential.
4. At time of treatment, linens and any clothing worn over the last 48 hours should be washed with hot water, put in a hot dryer for 20 minutes, or dry-cleaned. The house should be vacuumed.
5. Nonwashable items should be stored in sealed plastic bags for 1 week.
6. A follow-up visit in 2 weeks can be scheduled to determine success of treatment.
7. Reasons for treatment failure include wrong diagnosis, medication not applied to the whole body, not treating all members of the household, or use of crotamiton. In addition, the child may develop postscabetic eczema that is not indicative of treatment failure. Evaluate and treat with topical corticosteroids.
8. Although resistance has been reported, it is not common and is usually due to treatment failure rather than resistance (Schwade, 1999).

Complications

A secondary bacterial infection is possible. Postscabetic syndrome is common, with visible lesions and pruritus persisting for days to weeks following treatment and nodular lesions persisting for weeks to months. Norwegian scabies is a nonpruritic crusted, scaling infestation with thousands to millions of mites occurring in immunosuppressed or institutionalized patients.

Patient Education, Prognosis, and Prevention

- Educate the family about the course of disease. Rash and itching persist for up to 3 weeks following treatment. Avoid overbathing and further irritation of the skin.
- The child should not be infectious 24 hours after treatment and may return to school or day care.

ALLERGIC AND INFLAMMATORY REACTIONS OF THE SKIN

Acne

Description

Acne is a disorder of the sebaceous follicle in which excess sebum, keratinous debris, and bacteria accumulate, producing microcomedones. The microcomedones may be noninflamed or inflamed lesions. Although rarely a serious medical disorder, acne occasionally heralds underlying disease. It is often of significant concern to the adolescent, having a serious effect on social development (see Color Fig. 18).

Etiology and Incidence

Four mechanisms contribute to the sebaceous follicle disorder: (1) follicular plugging with keratinous material; (2) bacterial colonization with overgrowth of anaerobic organisms deep in the follicle, primarily *Propionibacterium acnes*; (3) sebum overproduction and increased androgen production with an expansion of the follicle; and (4) inflammation due to trapping of *P. acnes* and sebum (Kristal & Silverberg, 1998). Acne is a common skin disease, occurring in up to 80% to 85% of all persons 12 to 24 years of age and appearing as early as 8 to 10 years of age in the form of a microcomedo (Mancini, 2000). It is more common in females than in males but appears earlier in males. Acne tends to improve in the summer and worsen with menses and stress (Weston, Lane, & Morelli, 2002).

Clinical Findings

History. Information to obtain includes the following:

- Family history of acne
- Stage of pubertal development and menstrual history
- Facial products used, especially occlusive products or pomades

- Oral and prescription medication, especially oral contraceptives, antibiotics, or steroids
- Any current or previous acne treatment and results
- Sports participation, especially if wearing football pads or other protective devices
- Jobs such as cooking at a fast-food grill or working at a gas station
- Other medical conditions

Physical Examination. Lesions most commonly are found on the face, back, and chest.

- Noninflammatory lesions:
  - Open comedo (blackhead)—a noninflammatory lesion or papule, firm in consistency, caused by blockage at the mouth of the follicle and occurring on the face, upper back, shoulders, and chest. The black color comes from oxidized melanin. This is the main lesion in early adolescence.
  - Closed comedo (whitehead or microcomedo)—a noninflammatory lesion, semisoft in consistency, caused by blockage at the neck of the follicle. This is a precursor to inflammatory acne.
- Inflammatory lesions occur secondary to rupture of noninflamed lesions into the dermis.
  - Papule—a "bump" in the follicle caused by bacterial overgrowth and rupture of the follicle wall
  - Pustule—raised, superficial, exudate-filled lesion
  - Excoriation and crusting of lesions—caused by manipulation
  - Nodule—firm, erythematous, and deeper in location, caused by rupture of a plug
  - Cyst—raised, large lesion, soft in consistency without erythema, formed from multiple ruptures and reencapsulations
  - Scar—red or purple hue initially, depressed or close to the skin
  - Sinus tracts—confluent nodules likely to cause scarring

The severity of acne is determined by the quantity, type, and spread of lesions (Table 37-7). It is helpful to use a diagram of the face or a grading graph to identify the number and type of lesions present. This allows more precise follow-up of the patient. If only open and closed comedones are found, the disorder is called *comedonal acne.* Most adolescents have a combination of comedones, red papules, and pustules called *papulopustular acne,* which can be mild or severe. *Nodulocystic acne* is the most severe form and requires more intensive intervention. Specific types of acne include *frictional,* occurring from rubbing of bras, tight clothes, or headbands; *pomadal,* along the temple and forehead, due to pomades or oil-based cosmetics; *athletic,* on forehead, chin, or shoulders, due to helmets and pads; and *hormonal,* with a beard distribution.

TABLE 37-7 ***Grading Scale for Acne Severity***

Scale	Definition
0	None: skin is clear
1	Few comedones
2	Mild comedones, few papules, minimal erythema
3	Comedones, papules, pustules, erythema
4	Moderate comedones, greater number of papules, pustules extending over wider area of face, chest, shoulders, back, increasing erythema
5	Comedones, increasing number of papules, pustules, nodules with erythema
6	Comedones, papules, pustules, nodules, cysts; scarring may or may not be present with hyperpigmentation

Differential Diagnosis

Cosmetic, mechanical, environmental, or drug-induced acne; rosacea; flat wart; milia; periorial dermatitis; and folliculitis are included in the differential diagnosis.

Management

The goals of acne management are (1) to counteract the excess production of sebum, (2) to counteract the abnormal desquamation of epithelial cells, (3) to decrease the proliferation of *P. acnes,* and (4) to decrease scarring. Choice of treatment depends on the extent, severity, and duration of disease; type of lesions; and psychologic effects the adolescent is experiencing (Table 37-8 and Box 37-7).

1. *Education* is the first priority. The adolescent must have realistic expectations and an understanding of the pathophysiology and the process of treatment, including the fact that the acne often worsens before improving.
   - Wash face twice a day with a mild soap such as Dove, Neutrogena, or Aveeno Cleansing bar. Scrubbing, rubbing, picking, and squeezing should be avoided. Medication should be applied lightly; do not rub in.
   - Use of a comedo extractor can cause scarring and should be discouraged. Hot soaks applied to pustules may help their resolution.
   - If makeup is used, a nonacnegenic makeup is best.
   - Identify aggravating substances such as oil-based cosmetics, pomades, hair spray, mousse, and face creams.
   - Identify possible aggravating factors such as menses; stress; hot, humid weather; and jobs involving frying oil or grease.

TABLE 37-8 *Treatment of Acne*

Type of Acne	Lesions	Initial Treatment	If Not Improving
Comedonal	Open or closed comedones	Benzoyl peroxide 5% gel qd (if mild) *or* Tretinoin (Retin A) 0.025% cream qd (if moderate) *or* Adapalene 0.1% gel	Combine benzoyl peroxide with tretinoin *or* Increase strength to 0.05%
Mild papulopustular	Red papules, few pustules	Benzoyl peroxide 5%-10% qd *or* Adapalene 0.1% gel *or* Azelaic acid bid (if mild) *or* Topical antibiotic bid *or* Erythromycin 3% with 5% benzoyl peroxide qd-bid (if moderate) *or* Clindamycin 1% with 5% benzoyl peroxide qd-bid	Increase benzoyl peroxide to bid *or* Combine benzoyl peroxide with tretinoin (for comedones) Substitute topical antibiotic bid (for inflammatory)
Moderate to severe papulopustular	Red papules, many pustules	Benzoyl peroxide 5% *and* tretinoin 0.025% *or* Adapalene 0.1% gel *or* Azelaic acid (if comedonal) *or* Topical antibiotic bid (if no comedones) *and* oral antibiotic bid	Increase strength of treatment *or* Refer to dermatologist
Nodulocystic, scarring, or unresponsive	Red papules, pustules, cysts, and nodules	Oral antibiotics bid *and* tretinoin 0.05% qd *or* Adapalene 0.1% gel *and* benzoyl peroxide 10% gel bid (if comedonal)	Refer to dermatologist for oral isotretinoin

bid, Twice a day; *qd*, every day.

BOX 37-7 *Medications Commonly Used in Treating Acne*

Topical Keratolytic or Comedolytic Agents

Retinoids
- Tretinoin (Retin A, Avita) 0.01% to 0.025% gel; 0.025% to 0.1% cream; 0.1% microgel
- Adapalene (Differin) 0.1% gel or cream

Benzoyl peroxide 2.5% to 20% gel, 5% and 10% cream, 5% to 20% lotion or wash
Azelaic acid (Azelex) 20% cream (Finevin)

Topical Antibiotics

Clindamycin 1% solution, lotion, gel, pledget
Erythromycin 1% to 2% solution, 3% gel or swabs
Erythromycin 3% with benzoyl peroxide 5% gel (Benzamycin)
Clindamycin 1% with 5% benzoyl peroxide (Benzaclin or Duac)

Oral Antibiotics

Tetracycline 500 to 1000 mg given in one to four divided doses
Erythromycin 500 to 2000 mg given in one to four divided doses
Minocycline 50 to 200 mg given in one or two divided doses
Doxycycline 50 to 200 mg given in one or two divided doses
Trimethoprim with sulfamethoxazole is used but is not approved by the Food and Drug Administration

- Reassure the patient that no scientific evidence indicates that any particular foods adversely affect acne; however, a well-balanced diet is important to maintaining healthy skin.
- Discuss psychosocial concerns and provide support.
- Remind the patient that results take months and that adherence to treatment is essential to improvement.
- Sun exposure helps clear acne for some adolescents but may worsen it for others. Use of sunscreen is recommended, and caution about sun exposure should be given if using medication that increases photosensitivity.

2. *Topical keratolytic* or *comedolytic agents* are used to minimize follicular obstruction and break up microcomedones. A minimum of 4 to 6 weeks of treatment is required before improvement, but these agents control 80% of acne (Weston, Lane, & Morelli, 2002). Many strengths and forms are available, the strongest being the gels, if tolerated. A general rule is to start low (in strength) and slowly (in frequency), and advance as tolerated or needed. There are two classes: retinoids (tretinoin and adapalene), and agents that possess both antibacterial and keratolytic propetics (benzoyl peroxide and azelaic acid). Each works by a different mechanism; therefore they can be used together, as well as interchangeably. Dryness, erythema, irritation, and scaling can occur with these products, and the strength and frequency of use must be adjusted for this.
   - Tretinoin (Retin-A, Avita) is a keratolytic that causes sun sensitivity. A pea-sized application should be made 20 minutes after washing the face. Initially it is used every other night, advancing to every night. If the skin is very sensitive, applications of 15 to 30 minutes just before bedtime may be used, with the duration gradually advanced.
   - Adapalene (Differin) is a newer formulation with less irritation, more activity, and less photosensitivity.
   - Azelaic acid (Azelex, Finevin) is antibacterial and keratolytic. Used twice a day, it is a newer agent that is useful in individuals with sensitive or dark skin.
   - Benzoyl peroxide is used once or twice a day, depending on the severity of acne and dryness of skin; it is also considered antibacterial by some.
3. *Topical antibiotics* are used to control the inflammatory process, usually most helpful in moderate inflammatory acne. Additionally, they are used as maintenance to control acne after initial treatment with oral antibiotics. Topical antibiotics are applied to the entire skin surface, not just to problem areas. The solution should not be applied until 30 minutes after shaving. Erythromycin can have up to a 50% resistance rate (Morelli, 2002).
   - Topical clindamycin is used twice a day.
   - Topical erythromycin is used twice a day.
   - Topical sulfacetamide is used twice a day.
   - Topical erythromycin with benzoyl peroxide (Benzamycin gel) and clindamycin with benzoyl peroxide (Benzaclin or Duac) are combination products that are more effective than either drug alone and have less resistance from *P. acnes*. This combination is especially effective in mild to moderate inflammatory acne or as an adjunct to oral therapy.
4. *Oral antibiotics* are used in addition to topical keratolytics and topical antibiotics to decrease the concentration of *P. acnes* and to decrease the degree of inflammation if there is no response to topical agents. Antibiotics are taken for 1 to 6 months and often require 3 to 4 weeks to see improvement. Once improvement is noted, dose should be tapered to daily dose and then discontinued. Tetracycline and erythromycin are the antibiotics most commonly used, but minocycline, doxycycline, and trimethoprim with sulfamethoxazole are also used.
   - Tetracycline should be taken 1 hour before or 2 hours after eating with 8 oz of water. Tetracycline should not be used by pregnant or breastfeeding adolescents or in children under 9 years of age. Photosensitivity reactions can occur, but it has been used for over 40 years and is a favorite of many clinicians.
   - Erythromycin can be taken with food.
   - Minocycline can be taken with food and achieves a higher concentration in the follicles. However, side effects include blue-black discoloration in scars and photosensitivity and hypersensitivity reactions.
   - Doxycycline also can be taken with food but has the highest rate of photosensitivity reactions.
   - Trimethoprim with sulfamethoxazole has not been approved for this use but is sometimes tried before isotretinoin.
5. *Oral retinoids* are used for severe, resistant nodulocystic acne. Isotretinoin (Accutane) Amnesteem is contraindicated in pregnancy and usually requires evaluation by a dermatologist before use. The usual course is 20 weeks, there are many side effects, and CBC, LFTs, and urinalysis must be monitored every month while the patient is on the medication. Roche Pharmaceutical Company, the maker of Accutane, provides at no cost an educational packet for patients, *Pregnancy Prevention Program for Women on Accutane.*
6. *Oral contraceptives* (Ortho Tri-Cyclen is the only one approved by the FDA for treatment for acne), antiandrogens (spironolactone), and intralesional steroid therapy are sometimes used in unresponsive cases. Erythromycin-zinc combination is used in Europe and

Russia with success but has not been approved in the United States.
7. Noncomedogenic moisturizers (Moisturel, Purpose lotion, Neutrogena Moisture) can be used for dryness, which is common with treatment. Noncomedogenic makeup is also available and helpful in treating these patients.
8. Follow-up visits should occur at least every 4 to 6 weeks until control is established. Control is indicated by clearing of lesions or the appearance of only a few new lesions every 2 weeks. Referral to a dermatologist should be made for nonresponsive or severe cases.

Complications

Failure can be due to lack of patient motivation, lack of education, inappropriate treatments, initial treatment that was too strong, or expectations of a quick fix. Psychologic effects are real and include decreased self-esteem and poor body image, problems with interpersonal relationships, self-consciousness, embarrassment, depression, and decreased athletic participation, especially in gymnastics, swimming, and wrestling. Resistance of *P. acnes* to tetracycline, erythromycin, and minocycline is increasing.

Atopic Dermatitis

See Chapter 25.

Contact Dermatitis

Description

Contact dermatitis is an acute or chronic inflammation resulting from a hypersensitivity reaction to a substance. The causative agents are either irritants or allergens. Common types of contact dermatitis are the following:

- *Dry skin dermatitis* caused by extremely low humidity (less than 30%) or use of excess soaping or cleansing creams
- *Nickel dermatitis* from contact with jewelry, belts, snaps, or eyeglasses
- *Lip-licker dermatitis* due to constant lip-licking, most often in dry, cold weather
- *Phytophotodermatitis* occurs with sun exposure following contact with plants or juices such as limes, lemons, carrots, celery, figs, parsnips, or dill; manifests as a blistered lesion on an erythematous base and may be confused with a burn
- *Plant oleoresins* such as poison ivy, oak, or sumac
- *Juvenile plantar dermatosis*, manifested as dryness, cracking, and erythema of weight-bearing surfaces of the feet, initially the big toes, mimicking tinea pedis, often found in children with atopic dermatitis (see Chapter 25)
- *Latex dermatitis*

Etiology and Incidence

Irritant dermatitis, the most common form, occurs when a substance has a toxic effect on the skin. The severity of the rash depends on the length of exposure and the concentration of the irritant. Substances such as saliva, urine, and feces; baby wipes; bubble bath; overbathing; and adhesives often cause irritation. Diaper dermatitis is the most common form (see following section). Allergic reactions occur as an immunologic response to an antigen penetrating the skin. Common causes are contact with shoes, nickel, clothes with woolen or rough textures, topical medications (e.g., neomycin and lanolin), perfumed soaps or cosmetics, preservatives, or poison ivy, oak, or sumac. Sometimes the cause is obvious; often no specific cause can be identified. Occurring at any age, contact dermatitis (mostly irritant) is extremely common in children, with an incidence of 5% to 20% of all cases of dermatitis (Weston, Lane, & Morelli, 2002).

Clinical Findings

History. The following information should be sought:

- Contact with any new or unusual substances
- Repeated exposure to any substance or item
- Diarrhea or infrequently changed diapers
- Rash localized to specific area(s)

Physical Examination. The area of involvement offers clues to the causative agent. Often the rash is localized to one area and has sharp borders. Common examples include a linear-type rash secondary to wearing a necklace or bracelet, circular areas from snaps on clothing, or involvement of the earlobes from jewelry or the toes and dorsum of the foot from shoes. The duration and concentration of exposure also affect the intensity of the rash. Minimal contact may produce only mild erythema, whereas prolonged or concentrated contact may produce significant erythema, edema, and blistering with possible crusting and secondary infection. Irritant reactions tend to be immediate, whereas allergic ones are delayed.

- A chafed appearance with shiny, mild to severely erythematous, peeling, or dry, fissured skin may be seen if the reaction is due to an irritant.
- In the diaper area around the anus, the rash is often due to diarrhea; if the skin is affected but the folds are spared, urine is often responsible.
- Erythema, vesicles, and weeping may be present in the acute stage of allergic contact dermatitis.
- Hyperpigmentation and lichenification are seen in chronic conditions.

Differential Diagnosis

The differential diagnosis includes atopic dermatitis, impetigo, herpes simplex, psoriasis, and seborrhea.

Management

Appropriate skin care, recognizing and eliminating offending agents, and treatment of inflammation are the keys to managing contact dermatitis successfully.

- Identify and avoid the substance causing dermatitis.
- For dermatitis in the diaper area, change diapers frequently, keep the area dry and cool (use air-drying as much as possible), and avoid rubber pants. Hydrocortisone 1% may be used cautiously for a period of no more than 5 days. Secondary infection with *Candida* is often present and must be treated with an antifungal agent such as nystatin.
- Burow solution soaks or oatmeal baths and cool compresses applied for 20 minutes every 4 to 6 hours soothe vesicular rashes.
- Apply water and either petrolatum-based or lanolin-and-petrolatum-based emollients to the skin to restore moisture to areas of dryness and chafing.
  - Petrolatum-based emollients include dimethicone (Moisturel), white petrolatum, and Vaseline Dermatology Formula.
  - Lanolin-and-petrolatum–based emollients include Aquaphor, Eucerin, Lubriderm, and Alpha Keri. Do not use if there is inflammation.
- Topical corticosteroids used two to three times daily give relief in 2 or 3 days, although it may take 2 or 3 weeks for complete healing. Occasionally, oral corticosteroids are used for short periods of time (10 to 14 days, tapered the last 7 days) if the area of involvement exceeds 10% of the skin surface.
- Oral antihistamines are helpful if itching and scratching are problems.
- Resolution may take 2 to 3 weeks. Referral to a dermatologist or an allergist for patch testing may be indicated if the dermatitis worsens, fails to respond, or recurs.

Diaper Dermatitis

Description

Diaper dermatitis is most commonly an inflammatory disorder of the skin due to irritation causing breakdown of the skin's natural barrier (Table 37-9).

Etiology and Incidence

Factors contributing to diaper dermatitis include the following:

- Improper hygiene and cleansing methods
- Chemical irritation caused by prolonged contact with skin products, urine, feces, or breakdown products
- Mechanical irritation from diapers, rubber pants, or skin folds
- Other skin dermatoses aggravated by wearing diapers (e.g., seborrhea, atopic dermatitis, or psoriasis)

Diaper rash is most commonly due to irritation from the wetness of urine, combined with friction and occlusion from diapers, and the by-products of feces. The initial rash is termed *irritant contact diaper dermatitis.* A variation of this is called *tidewater* or *tidemark dermatitis* and is found at the diaper edges from either chafing or irritation from talcum powder. *Jacquet's dermatitis,* a severe form manifested by punched-out lesions or erosions primarily on the labia and buttocks, is especially prone to secondary infection.

Approximately 50% of infants develop diaper rashes, less than 2% of which are serious, usually between 9 and 12 months of age (Hansen et al, 1998; Weston, Lane, & Morelli, 2002).

Clinical Findings

History. The following should be assessed:

- Type of diapers and diaper covering used; any recent change in brand
- Frequency of diaper changes and methods of cleansing used
- Any new baby care products used
- Frequency of wet diapers and stools
- Medication taken or used on rash
- Present or recent use of antibiotics

Physical Examination. Findings can include the following:

- Chemical causes
  - Shiny, peeling, erythematous macular or papular rash confluent in the diaper area, sparing folds
  - Head of penis erythematous and dry
  - Erythema primarily on buttocks and around anus (fecal irritation)
- Mechanical causes
  - Erythematous, macerated (acute) or dry (chronic), hyperpigmented area prominent along edges of diaper or plastic pants
  - Erythematous, macerated folds caused by overlapping skin
- Hygiene problems
  - Any finding listed previously
  - Poor hygiene in general

Differential Diagnosis

Differential diagnosis includes contact dermatitis; bacterial, viral, or monilial infection; atopic dermatitis; psoriasis; seborrhea; scabies; and congenital syphilis.

TABLE 37-9 *Diagnosis and Treatment of Diaper Dermatitis*

Type	Cause	Presentation and Location	Other Characteristics	Treatment
Irritant contact dermatitis	Related to wearing diapers; contact with urine and feces	Chapped, shiny, erythematous, parchment-like skin with possible erosions on convex surfaces; creases spared	Peak at 9-12 mo; may progress to involve creases; skin may be dry	Frequent diaper changes, gentle cleansing; greasy lubricant; sitz bath, air-dry; hydrocortisone for inflammation
Candidiasis	Related to wearing diapers; a superinfection with *Candida*	Shallow pustules, fiery-red scaly plaques on convex surfaces, inguinal folds, labia, and scrotum	Satellite lesions, oral thrush; recent antibiotic or diarrhea; occurs at any age	Antifungal cream plus same measures as for contact dermatitis
Miliaria or intertrigo	Related to wearing diapers; due to heat and occlusion	Discrete vesicles or papules (miliaria); erythematous, scaly, maceration in folds of skin	Sweat retention or friction associated	Self-limited (miliaria); avoid precipitating factors; care as for contact dermatitis
Seborrhea	Exaggerated by wearing diapers; overgrowth of *Malassezia* yeast in areas of sebaceous gland activity	Greasy, erythematous scales, well circumscribed in creases of skin, groin; spared convex surfaces	Onset at 3-4 wk of age; also occurs on face or body; often superinfected with *Candida*	Ketoconazole is treatment of choice, or hydrocortisone
Atopic dermatitis (AD)	Exaggerated by wearing diapers; exact cause unknown	Increased number of lines in skin; areas of excoriation in folds and convex surfaces and buttocks; less widespread	AD in other areas; usually begins in first year of life; scratches skin with diaper change; hyperlinear skin folds with diffuse borders	Skin care as for contact dermatitis and as indicated for AD (see Chapter 25); antibiotics for bacterial infection
Psoriasis	Exaggerated by wearing diapers; psoriasis evolves as response to chronic trauma	Erythematous, well-defined sharp, scaly plaques on convex surfaces and inguinal folds; less widespread	Psoriasis affects other places; rare occurrence, if found, usually at 6-18 mo	Treatment often required for weeks or until toilet trained; steroids; ketoconazole if *Candida* present
Bacterial dermatitis	Usually due to staphylococcal or streptococcal infection	Red, denuded areas or fragile blisters; crusting and pustules in suprapubic area and periumbilicus	Usually in newborn, can occur anywhere	Econazole or ketoconazole cream if yeast present as well; mupirocin if minimal; cephalexin, amoxicillin, or erythromycin if extensive

Management

The best treatment is prevention!

1. Keep diaper area dry, clean, and aerated:
   - Frequent diaper changes are essential; every 1 to 2 hours is recommended with one change at night and a minimum of eight changes in a 24-hour period. Cleanse the area well with water at every diaper change and use mild soap, rinsing well following a stool. Avoid vigorous cleansing because this can worsen matters. Avoid using wipes.
   - Use a greasy lubricant if skin is dry.
   - Use a protective barrier ointment or cream such as Desitin (cod liver oil with zinc oxide), A and D ointment, Aquaphor, petrolatum, or zinc oxide at first sign of irritation.
2. Proper use of diapers:
   - Frequent changes are essential.
   - Use thick or absorbent diapers to pull wetness away from skin.
   - Avoid use of rubber or plastic pants.

   - Cloth diapers should be soaked, prerinsed, washed in a mild soap, double-rinsed with 1/4 cup of vinegar, and dried in the sun if possible.
   - Disposable diapers must be large enough not to bind and should never be worn with rubber pants.
3. Treatment of diaper rash:
   - Sitz baths in warm water for 10 to 15 minutes four times a day.
   - Expose diaper area to air by leaving diaper off or by blow-drying with low heat three or four times a day.
   - Burrow solution soaks or compresses four times a day if skin is weepy.
   - Undecylenic acid (Desenex) or calcium undecylenate (Caldescene) powder to decrease the friction and moisture in tidewater dermatitis.
   - Hydrocortisone 0.5% or 1% three times a day for no more than 5 days, especially if skin is dry, for moderate to severe diaper dermatitis. Do not use fluorinated steroids.
   - Increase intake of fluids to dilute urine. In older infants, 2 to 3 oz of cranberry juice acidifies the urine.
   - If the rash has been present for more than 3 days, or if there is no response to the aforementioned measures, add a topical antifungal cream such as clotrimazole or miconazole. If there is still no response, a trial of oral antifungal is indicated (see section on monilial dermatitis).
   - Any recalcitrant rash should be referred to a dermatologist.
   - Follow up by phone in 1 to 2 days. If not improved, reassess within 1 week.

Complications

Secondary infection with bacteria, viruses, or fungi can occur (see previous sections). *Red flags*: severe erosions or ulcers; bullae or pustules; large papules or nodules, purpura, or petechiae; and redness or scaliness over entire body.

Seborrhea

Description

Seborrhea is a chronic inflammatory dermatitis commonly called *cradle cap* in infants or *dandruff* in adolescents.

Etiology and Incidence

The condition is thought to be related to overproduction of sebum, because it commonly occurs in areas with large numbers of sebaceous glands. It may be an overgrowth of *Malassezia ovalis (Pityrosporum ovale)* (a saprophytic yeast), which is present on everyone's body. Seborrhea occurs most often in early infancy and adolescence, is associated with blepharitis, and is more common in spring and summer.

Clinical Findings

History. Note age of onset (infancy or adolescence).

Physical Examination. In infants, erythematous, flaky to thick crusts of yellow, greasy scales occur predominantly on the scalp but also on the face, behind the ears, on the neck and trunk, and in the diaper area.

In adolescents, there are mild flakes with some erythema and yellow, greasy scales on the scalp, forehead, and eyebrows; behind the ears; on the face and flexural surfaces; and in intertriginous areas.

Differential Diagnosis

Atopic dermatitis, psoriasis, *Candida* infection, contact dermatitis, tinea, scabies, and pityriasis rosea are included in the differential diagnosis.

Management

Seborrhea in infants may be self-limited. However, in adolescents, it is usually chronic and recurring. The following measures are helpful in either age-group:

- Shampoo or wash areas daily with a mild soap. In more resistant cases, use antiseborrheic shampoos (e.g., Nizoral, Sebulex, Selsun, Head & Shoulders) every other day for infants or daily for adolescents. Tar shampoos can be used for adolescents if needed. Shampoo should be left on the scalp for 5 to 10 minutes before scrubbing crusts and then rinsing.
- Mineral oil, baby oil, or petroleum jelly placed on thick crusts 10 to 15 minutes before washing softens them, followed by gentle brushing during shampooing to remove crusts.
- If inflammation is marked, low-potency steroid creams can be applied twice a day to the face or three times a day to other body areas for several days and then weaned. A low- to moderate-strength steroid solution can be applied to the scalp if inflammation is present.
- Oral biotin can sometimes improve the condition.
- Educate parents about the etiology, control measures, and the need to continue treatment for a few days after resolution.
- Follow up in 1 to 2 weeks.

Complications

Secondary infection with bacteria or *Candida* can occur. Severe, generalized seborrhea is found in up to 83% of persons infected with HIV.

Sunburn

Description

Sunburn is an injury to the skin occurring from overexposure of the skin to the UV rays of the sun. The incidence of skin cancer is increasing as a result of overexposure to the sun and the use of tanning beds.

Etiology and Incidence

Excessive sun exposure causes a change in the skin's blood flow, cell kinetics, and pigment products. Damage to the skin by sun (primarily ultraviolet B [UVB]) includes erythema, pigmentary or texture changes, and potential carcinogenesis. Injury to the skin begins as quickly as 30 minutes after exposure, peaks at 24 hours, and may last for 72 hours. Other factors that contribute to sun sensitivity are medications (especially griseofulvin, NSAIDs, oral contraceptives, tetracycline, topical diphenhydramine, and tretinoin) and some illnesses.

Children are at increased risk for sunburn because of the greater amount of time they spend outdoors. Most people receive 80% of their lifetime exposure to sun by the time they are 18 to 21 years of age (Chamlin, 2002; Weston, Lane, & Morelli, 2002). Blistering sunburns before 20 years of age more than double the chance of skin cancer. Factors contributing to the degree of burn include the coloring of skin and hair (Box 37-8) and amount of previous sun exposure. Burns are less common in children with darker hair and skin because of their increased amount of melanin. Timing of sun exposure, latitude, and altitude affect skin sensitivity, because UV rays are strongest between 10 AM and 2 PM, at higher altitudes, and nearer the equator. Sunburn can occur on cloudy days, and reflection from sand, water, snow, and concrete increases the risk. One study showed that sunscreen use in children and adolescents was 34.4%, with 83% of respondents reporting at least one sunburn during the previous summer and 36% reporting three or more. Tanning beds were used by nearly 10% (Geller et al, 2002). Of this 10%, 40% were girls 17 to 18 years of age, 26% were youths 15 to 18 years of age, 30% were youths whose caregiver used tanning devices, and 16% were females (Cokkinides et al, 2002).

BOX 37-8 *Skin Types and Protection Needs*

I: Fair (Celtic)—always burns, never tans; sun protection factor (SPF) 15 or greater
II: Fair (white)—easily burns, minimally tans; SPF 15
III: Lightly pigmented (dark white)—sometimes burns, gradually tans; SPF 8 to 10
IV: Pigmented (Mediterranean, Asian, Hispanic)—minimally burns, always tans; SPF 6 to 8
V: Moderately pigmented (American Indian, Hispanic, Mideastern)—rarely burns, profusely tans; SPF 4
VI: Heavily pigmented (American and African black)—rarely burns, tans deeply; no or low SPF needed

Clinical Findings

History

- Length and time of sun exposure
- Previous sunburns, especially blistering ones
- Any medications currently taken
- Chills, headache, and fatigue with moderate to severe burn
- Family history of melanoma or other skin cancer

Physical Examination. Findings include the following:

- Mild or first-degree burns are evidenced by erythema, tenderness, and mild pain.
- Moderate or second-degree burns involve a greater degree of erythema, increased pain, edema, and blisters.
- Severe or third-degree burns involve greater areas of skin and include systemic symptoms of headache, fever, and fatigue.
- Erythema and tenderness are evident from 30 minutes to 4 hours after exposure; 2 to 7 days later, affected layers of the epidermis are shed.

Differential Diagnosis

The differential diagnosis includes photosensitization from medication, xeroderma pigmentosum, lupus erythematosus, viral exanthem, dermatomyositis, and porphyrias.

Management

The degree of burn helps determine which of the following strategies is most appropriate. Prevention is the best intervention (see Patient Education and Prevention).

- Use cool water, saline compresses, or ice packs at least four times a day to ease pain and reduce swelling. Baking soda or cornstarch baths help cool skin. White vinegar or milk compresses help initiate healing.
- Administer prostaglandin inhibitors such as ibuprofen 5 to 10 mg/kg per dose given as soon as possible and every 6 to 8 hours for the next 2 to 3 days or acetaminophen for fever and pain relief.
- Low-dose cortisone creams 0.5% or 1% two to three times a day, used with caution because of the increased absorption through damaged skin, help reduce inflammation and pain.
- Local anesthetic sprays or first-aid creams with benzocaine are contraindicated because of the risk of sensitization.

- Skin emollients such as aloe vera gel or moisturizer are helpful if skin is dry. Jojoba oil and vitamin E creams are sometimes helpful. Avoid petrolatum, butter, or any occlusive ointment because their occlusive properties intensify the burn.
- Extra fluid intake prevents dehydration and restores natural moisture balance.
- If blisters break, dead skin needs to be trimmed and an antibiotic ointment such as polymyxin B sulfate and bacitracin zinc (Polysporin) applied.

Complications

Photoaging, including telangiectasia and actinic keratosis, cataracts, retinal damage, heat stroke, and a change in immune response are possible complications of sunburn (Kim, Ghali, & Tunnessen, 1997).

The incidence of skin cancer (basal cell carcinoma, squamous cell carcinoma, and malignant melanoma) is increasing rapidly, with 1 million cases diagnosed annually; 2% occur in children (Chamlin, 2002; Kim, Ghali, & Tunnessen, 1997). Risk factors include fair skin, history of multiple blistering sunburns, presence of multiple atypical moles, development of new nevi, and family history of melanoma. Basal and squamous cell carcinomas are slow-spreading cancers, directly linked with chronic exposure to UV light. Basal cell carcinomas occur in varied forms, as nodular, pearly, pigmented lesions often on the hand, neck, or head. Squamous cell carcinomas are quickly growing, firm indurated nodules with or without ulceration on sun-exposed areas, especially the rim of the ear, face, lips, and mouth. Malignant melanomas account for 5% of skin cancers but 75% of deaths (Kim, Ghali, & Tunnessen, 1997). Melanomas manifest as new lesions or as changes in existing moles. In preadolescents, melanoma often is nodular, grows rapidly, and itches or bleeds. In adolescents, melanoma manifests as enlarging or changing lesions with irregular color or borders (Chamlin, 2002). There is a link to multiple severe, blistering sunburns, but family history is a more important factor. Any change in a mole, especially with rapid asymmetric growth, crusting, ulceration, or color variation, needs immediate evaluation. Treatment consists of surgical removal and histologic evaluation. All school-age children and adolescents should be taught to do a monthly skin examination (Box 37-9).

Patient Education and Prevention

- Remember that a tan is not a sign of good health, but of skin injury. There is no such thing as a healthy tan. Never seek a tan; seek the shade. Avoid tanning devices or parlors.
- Know your skin type and protection needs (see Box 37-8).

BOX 37-9 *Monthly Skin Examination*

The **ABCDE**s of skin examination:
- **A**symmetry
- **B**order irregularity or notching
- **C**olor variation, especially if multicolored
- **D**iameter greater than 6 mm
- **E**levation, especially if asymmetric

Note any new growths, itchy patches, nonhealing sores, changes in size, irritability, or different sensation in any moles

Process of Skin Examination

Use a full-length mirror, a hand mirror, and a brightly lit room

Examine the following areas:
- Front and back, right and left sides with arms raised
- With elbows bent, forearms, back of arms and palms
- Back of legs and feet, toes and soles
- Back of neck and scalp
- Back and buttocks

From Starr NB: Skin smarts: the essentials of skin protection, *J Pediatr Health Care* 13(3):136-138, 1998.

- Avoid the sun between 10 AM and 2 PM. Learn the "shadow rule"—seek shade if your shadow is shorter than you are tall. Most newspapers print in the weather section the predicted index of UV exposure (1 to 10) as prepared by the National Weather Service.
- Cover up with hats, sunglasses, and clothing.
  - Hats with a wide (3-inch) brim are recommended.
  - Sunglasses should be worn beginning in infancy. Large-framed, wraparound lenses provide the best protection. UV protection is provided by a chemical added to the lenses and is indicated by one of the following labels: UV absorption to 400 nm, special purpose, meets American National Standards Institute (ANSI) UV requirements.
  - Tight-weave, long-sleeved, long-pants clothing with sunscreen applied to the skin underneath provides maximum protection. Color, weight, stretch, wetness, and quality of material all affect the amount of protection offered. *Solumbra* and *SunSkins* offer clothes that provide an SPF of 30 and block 97% of UV rays. *Shades* offers clothes that provide 81% UV protection. *Stingray* offers swimwear that blocks 99% of the sun's rays (see Resource Box).
- Use a sunscreen that is broad spectrum and provides protection from both UVB and UVA light (Box 37-10).

BOX 37-10 *Sunscreen Recommendations*

Sunscreens block the rays of the sun to help prevent sunburn. Sun protection factor (SPF) is the length of time an individual can be exposed to sun without burning if sunscreen is used appropriately. The substantivity of a sunscreen describes its adherence. Sweat resistant (effective for up to 30 minutes of heavy, continuous perspiration), water resistant (effective for up to 40 minutes of swimming), and waterproof (effective for up to 80 minutes of immersion) are different types of substantivity. Specific recommendations include the following:

Use SPF 15 or greater, nonalcohol base, without lanolin, paraben, or fragrance. Use a waterproof product when in water but reapply every 80 minutes with continuous water exposure.

Apply at least 30 minutes before exposure to sun; reapply at least every 2 hours while in the sun, and after swimming, toweling, or heavy perspiration.

Apply liberally (1 oz for an adult) and, for better coverage, use cream instead of lotion.

Pay special attention to eyelids, nose, cheeks, ears, neck, scalp, shoulders, hands, and feet. Use a lip balm with SPF 15 or greater.

Do not use sunscreen on infants younger than 6 months of age, but keep baby out of the sun completely, using shade, brimmed hat, and protective clothing.

Use sunscreen daily in summer or in warm climates. Use even on overcast or cloudy days.

Extra protection is needed with increasing altitude, closer location to the equator, and sand, snow, concrete, or water reflection.

Set an example by using sunscreen.

Sunscreens are available in various chemical combinations (e.g., para-aminobenzoic acid [PABA], PABA esters, cinnamates, benzophenes, salicylates, octocrylene, dibenzoylmethane) and vehicles (e.g., emollient for dry skin, gel or lotion for oily skin, noncomedogenic for acne-prone skin). If a child is sensitive to one, try a sunscreen with different ingredients.

A PABA-free sunscreen is recommended for children. Dibenzoylmethane provides the most protection from ultraviolet A.

Sunblocks scatter and reflect light. Zinc oxide, titanium oxide, or a combination product such as Sportz Bloc is useful for especially sensitive areas such as the nose or previously burned areas.

From Starr NB: Skin smarts: the essentials of skin protection, *J Pediatr Health Care* 13(3):136-138, 1998.

- Teach sun protection early on, by example, as well as words. "Block the Sun, Not the Fun" is a program with curricula, family support materials, and educational posters sponsored by the American Academy of Dermatology (AAD) and Coppertone to educate elementary school–age children to reduce sun exposure and increase protective behavior. See AAD in Resource Box.
- "Choose Your Cover" is a CDC program to increase awareness and change social norms related to skin protection and tanned skin.
- Guidelines for school programs to prevent skin cancer were released by the CDC in 2002 (Glanz, Saraiya, & Wechsler, 2002).
- Do monthly skin checks (see Box 37-9).

Drug Eruptions

Description

Drugs taken systemically can result in a variety of skin reactions or rashes. The three most common types found in children are (1) morbilliform (measles-like) rash, (2) urticaria, and (3) erythema multiforme rash (Table 37-10). Urticaria and erythema multiforme are discussed in the section on vascular reactions later in this chapter. Other reactions not discussed here include acute generalized exanthematous pustulosis, erythema nodosum, leukocytoclastic vasculitis, fixed drug eruption, allergic contact dermatitis, photosensitivity, acneiform eruptions, and pigmentary changes.

Etiology and Incidence

The morbilliform rash, also called an exanthematous rash, is the most common allergic skin reaction to a drug. The rash may be an immunologic or nonimmunologic reaction to the drug. The most common drugs causing reactions are the penicillins; sulfonamides; cephalosporins, especially cefaclor; erythromycin; NSAIDs; barbiturates; isoniazid; carbamazepine; phenytoin; and fluconazole, ketaconazole, and itraconazole (Richards, 1999; Weston, Lane, & Morelli, 2002). Onset of a rash often is within 1 week of starting the medication but can be as late as 2 weeks or more and can occur after the medication has been stopped. Incidence is between 8% and 11% for all courses

TABLE 37-10 ***Differentiating Drug Eruptions, Urticaria, and Erythema Multiforme***

	Etiology	Clinical Findings	Treatment
Drug eruption	Reaction to medication, especially penicillin, cephalexin, erythromycin, sulfa drugs, NSAIDs, barbiturates, isoniazid, carbamazepine, phenytoin	Symmetric, macular, erythematous to papular, confluent morbilliform rash; intense itching; patches of normal skin throughout; begins on trunk, extends distally, including palms and soles; face with confluent erythema	Stop drug and label as allergen to the child; antihistamine, antipruritics, lubricate skin; prednisone if severe; rash can last 7-14 days; medical alert bracelet
Urticaria	Hypersensitive reaction; immunologic antigen-antibody response to release of histamines; often unknown cause; possible reaction to food, drug, insect bite/sting, pollen; possible reaction to infection, especially streptococcal, sinus, mononucleosis, hepatitis	Family history of hives; rapid onset; possible atopy; intense itching; mild erythema, annular, raised wheals with pale centers; lesions scattered or coalesced; *key finding*: appear suddenly, fade from 20 min to 24 hr; blanch with pressure; associated edema of eyelids, lips, tongue, hands, feet	Quick resolution; identify and remove or treat offending agent if possible; stop antibiotic; give oral antihistamines; topical antipruritics; epinephrine or prednisone if anaphylactic, angioedema, or refractory; refer if >6 wk duration
Erythema multiforme (minor)	Immune-mediated hypersensitivity reaction often to infection, especially HSV, also to many other agents	History of infection, especially herpes labialis; variety of lesions on skin and mucous membranes—macules, papules, vesicles, early lesions such as urticaria; *key finding*: target or iris lesions; *key finding*: lesions fixed, symmetric, typical distribution on hands, feet, elbows, knees, also face, neck, trunk; possible oral mucous membrane involvement	Identify, treat, discontinue trigger if possible; treat infection; supportive measures for hydration, prevention of secondary infection, relief of pain; oral antihistamines, cool compresses; oral lesions—mouthwash, topical anesthetics; lesions last 5-7 days, recur in batches over 2-4 wk, resolve without scarring or sequelae

HSV, Herpes simplex virus; *NSAIDs*, nonsteroidal antiinflammatory drugs.

of antibiotics (Richards, 1999). Repeated exposure can progress to anaphylaxis (Weston, Lane, & Morelli, 2002).

Clinical Findings

History. The following can be reported:

- Medication taken within the last 3 weeks
- Intense itching
- Rash worsens even after medicine is discontinued for up to 5 days
- Possible systemic symptoms—fever, arthralgia, arthritis, lymphadenopathy, edema

Physical Examination. Findings include the following (see Color Fig. 19):

- Often begins as a fairly symmetric, macular erythematous rash that becomes papular and confluent.
- Patches of normal skin scattered throughout areas of involvement.
- Rash begins on the trunk, where it is brighter red, more confluent, and extends distally to the extremities, including the palms and soles.
- The face often has confluent areas of erythema.

Laboratory Studies. The following are ordered if necessary for differential diagnosis:

- CBC, monospot test, C-reactive protein (CRP), antinuclear antibodies, antistreptolysin O (ASO), cold agglutinins
- Chest radiograph

Differential Diagnosis

Viral exanthem; measles; toxic erythema such as in scarlet fever, staphylococcal scarlatina, or Kawasaki's disease; morbilliform rash (if the patient has mononucleosis and is taking amoxicillin); toxic shock syndrome; roseola; and erythema infectiosum are included in the differential diagnosis.

Management

Decisions about whether a drug is to be implicated depend on the patient's previous history of taking the drug, the experience of the general population with the drug, the morphology and timing of the rash, and other possible explanations for the rash (e.g., viral illness). The following steps are taken:

1. Discontinue the suspected drug.
2. Label the patient's medical record with the potential allergen.
3. Prescribe antihistamines if itching is present; recommend a lubricant and antipruritics as adjuncts.
4. Prescribe prednisone 1 to 2 mg/kg per day for 5 to 7 days if significant reaction.
5. Schedule follow-up visit as determined by severity of reaction and other illness.
6. Refer to allergist for skin testing to confirm allergy if there are limited or no alternative medications, for desensitization, to clarify drug allergy, for severe parental anxiety, or if symptoms were severe and life threatening.

Complications

Body heat and water loss can occur if the rash is severe. Progression of the rash if medicine is continued can lead to toxic epidermal necrolysis or Stevens-Johnson syndrome (see section on erythema multiforme), or allergic interstitial nephritis.

Patient Education and Prevention

- The rash can last 7 to 14 days with itching present and worsening before getting better.
- There is potential risk from further exposure to that drug or related ones; alternative therapies should be explained.
- Identification and communication of the child's allergy are imperative. In life-threatening allergies, wearing a medical alert bracelet or necklace is essential.

VASCULAR REACTIONS OF THE SKIN

Urticaria

Description

Urticaria is a hypersensitivity reaction commonly called *hives* (see Color Fig. 20). Transient or acute urticaria lasts less than 8 weeks; chronic, recurrent, or persistent urticaria lasts more than 8 weeks. Papular urticaria occurs in reaction to mosquito or flea bites. Physical causes of urticaria include dermatographism, cholinergic reactions (e.g., response to heat, exercise, hot baths), pressure, water, and cold.

Etiology and Incidence

Urticaria is caused by a complex interplay of immunologically mediated antigen-antibody responses to the release of histamine from mast cells. Vasodilation and increased vascular permeability cause erythema and the characteristic wheal. Onset is usually rapid, and resolution occurs within a few days of onset. The cause often remains a mystery (idiopathic). Possible causative factors include the following:

- Reactions to foods (e.g., nuts, eggs, shellfish, strawberries, tomatoes), drugs (salicylates and penicillins are the two most common), animal stings (e.g., bees, wasps, scorpion, spider, jellyfish), or pollen
- Response to bacterial, viral, or fungal infections, especially streptococcal or sinus infection, mononucleosis, hepatitis, adenoviruses and enteroviruses, or parasites
- Response to physical stimuli (e.g., heat or cold, sun or water, tight clothing, vibrations) or stress
- Genetic origin
- Concurrent with inflammatory systemic diseases (e.g., collagen-vascular or inflammatory bowel disease)

Urticaria may be seen in 3% of preschoolers and 2% of older children (Weston, Lane, & Morelli, 2002). Of all cases of urticaria, only 5% are immunoglobulin E (IgE) or allergy mediated. Fifteen percent are physical urticarias, and the remainder are idiopathic (Leickly, 2000; Weston & Badgett, 1998). Portals of entry include infection (most common), ingestion, injection, inhalation, immunologic (rare), and idiopathic.

Clinical Findings

History. The following should be assessed:

- Family or previous history of hives, angioedema, connective tissue disease, juvenile arthritis
- Possibility of atopy
- Intense itching
- Ingestion (within 4 hours) of nuts, shellfish, chocolate, berries, spices, egg white, milk, fish, sesame
- Ingestion or injection of medicines (penicillin, sulfa drugs, sedatives, diuretics, analgesics, acetylsalicylic acid), additives, or preservatives
- Injection of diagnostic agents, vaccine, insect venom, blood, medicine
- Infection with upper respiratory infectious agent, virus, streptococcus, mononucleosis; hepatitis; parasites
- Inhalation of animal danders, pollen, dust, smoke, or aerosols
- Cold, heat, exercise, sun, water, pressure, or vibration

Physical Examination. Location of lesions may help determine the cause (e.g., a lesion around the mouth or tongue is likely due to an ingested agent). Findings can include the following:

- Mildly erythematous, annular, raised wheals or welts with pale centers from 2 mm to 20 cm in diameter
- Lesions scattered or coalesced but generalized
- Lesions appear suddenly and fade in anywhere from 20 minutes to less than 24 hours, reappearing in other areas later; if fixed more than 48 hours, it is not urticaria
- Lesions blanch with pressure
- Heat seems to intensify the lesions
- Associated edema of eyelids, lips, tongue, hands, feet, and genitalia
- Wheals after rubbing or stroking the skin (dermatographism)
- Papulovesicular lesions with central punctate lesion and wheals most common in toddlers (papular urticaria)
- Large, blotchy erythematous lesions with 1 to 3 mm central wheals (cholinergic urticaria)

Laboratory Studies. If urticaria with possible anaphylaxis from an insect bite is suspected, referral to an allergist for testing and hyposensitization is needed. If fever is present, evaluation for underlying disease can be useful.

Differential Diagnosis

Contact dermatitis, atopic dermatitis, scabies, erythema multiforme (lesions are fixed with dusky centers and appear within 72 hours), mastocytosis, reactive erythemas, vasculitis, psoriasis, and juvenile arthritis are also included in the differential diagnosis (see Table 37-10).

Management

The following steps are taken:

1. Identify and remove the offending substance if possible. Stop all antibiotics. Avoid any possible food or environmental trigger.
2. Test for dermatographism by stroking the skin, for cholinergic urticaria by applying heat or observing immediately after exercising, for cold urticaria by applying cold packs, for pressure urticaria by applying weighted bands for several minutes, and for water urticaria by applying wet compresses.
3. Administer medications as indicated:
   - Oral antihistamines such as diphenhydramine 5 mg/kg per day or hydroxyzine 2 to 4 mg/kg per day every 4 to 6 hours until itching and urticaria are resolved. Nonsedating antihistamines are less effective, but if needed, astemizole, cetirizine, or loratadine is best. Urticaria is less likely to recur if the antihistamine is continued for 1 to 2 weeks after resolution.
   - Topical antipruritics may be helpful.
   - Aqueous epinephrine 1:1000 (subcutaneously 0.01 ml/kg up to 0.3 ml) may be needed if anaphylaxis or significant angioedema with swelling of mucous membranes and airway is present.
   - Prednisone 1 to 2 mg/kg per day for 1 week with rapid taper only if refractory to other measures or if angioedema is present with swelling of lips and face.
4. Follow-up visit if not improved within 48 hours.
5. Chronic urticaria persisting longer than 6 weeks needs evaluation for infection or systemic causes or referral for further evaluation.

Complications

Angioedema or anaphylaxis occurs by the same mechanism as urticaria.

- Anaphylactic symptoms require emergency intervention.
- Angioedema is an extension of the reaction into the subcutaneous tissue. It occurs in 50% of children with urticaria at some time during the episode and involves the face (especially the eyes), the hands, and feet 85% of the time (Weston & Badgett, 1998). Angioedema is gradual in onset and often involves reaction to medication (Wolf, 1999). Pseudoephedrine as an adjunct to antihistamine may be helpful. Hereditary angioedema is rare (0.4%) (Weston & Badgett, 1998); however, it is life threatening and usually manifests in adolescence, often following trauma (e.g., dental work, surgery, accident). It is manifested by repeated episodes of swelling of the extremities (75%), face, and throat (30%), accompanied by abdominal pain (52%) that becomes progressively more severe (Weston & Badgett, 1998). Severe airway edema, if untreated, is often the cause of death.
- Serum sickness begins with hives but has other systemic symptoms, for example, fever, arthralgias, malaise, lymphadenopathy, proteinuria.
- If urticaria is from a drug reaction, rechallenge with the drug is more likely to cause anaphylaxis.

Patient Education and Prevention

The following are needed:

- Explanation of causes, course, and treatment. The cause often cannot be found, and control of symptoms is the main goal of treatment. The entire episode usually resolves in 24 to 48 hours, rarely extending beyond 3 to 4 weeks. Further evaluation is needed only if urticaria lasts longer than 8 weeks. (See Leickly [2000] for details.)
- Papular urticaria hypersensitivity often declines within 6 to 12 months.
- Physical urticarias last 2 to 4 years in most cases, but occasionally persist into adulthood.

- Occasionally macular blue-brown lesions are found on resolution of urticaria.
- Avoid allergen if known; wear a medical alert bracelet in case severe reaction occurs; refer for hyposensitization if life-threatening symptoms occur.
- Carry an anaphylactic kit if indicated.

Erythema Multiforme

Description

Erythema multiforme (EM) minor is a self-limited, immune complex hypersensitivity reaction characterized by skin and mucous membrane involvement in response to a variety of agents (see Color Fig. 21). EM major is a separate entity with two variants, Stevens-Johnson syndrome (SJS) and toxic epidermal necrolysis (TEN). Four main types of EM major have been identified (Weston, Lane, & Morelli, 2002):

- Typical SJS with macules and blisters, and mucous membrane involvement on less than 10% of the body surface
- An overlap of SJS and TEN with 10% to 30% of the body surface involved
- A TEN with large confluent areas of the face and trunk involving more than 30% of the body surface
- TEN with "spots," or many red macules with blisters involving more than 10% of the body

Etiology and Incidence

Although not clearly understood, EM minor is thought to be an immune-mediated hypersensitive reaction with lesions similar to a graft-versus-host reaction. Infection is the primary precipitating event in EM minor in children and adolescents, most notably due to HSV, with Epstein-Barr virus (EBV), cytomegalovirus (CMV), or other human herpes viruses being the other implicated viruses (Weston, Lane, & Morelli, 2002). EM major is more commonly related to medications (specifically anticonvulsants, sulfa drugs, penicillins, NSAIDs, and salicylates). Infection, immunizations, foods, and systemic disease also have been implicated. Early recognition and immediate discontinuation of any drug involved shortens the course and prevents serious complications (Weston, Lane, & Morelli, 2002).

Erythema multiforme occurs in healthy individuals of any age, but the highest incidence is in 20- to 40-year-olds. However, 20% to 50% of all cases are seen in children, most commonly in adolescents. EM is more common in males and in the winter months. Recurrence occurs in approximately 33% of cases (Weston, Lane, & Morelli, 2002). TEN occurs most commonly after 10 years of age as a complication of a drug, most commonly a sulfonamide, penicillin, NSAID, anticonvulsant, or barbiturate (Paller, 1999).

Clinical Findings

History. The following are sometimes reported:

- Recent or current infection with a viral (HSV, EBV), bacterial (mycoplasma), fungal, or protozoal agent; 50% of cases have a history of herpes labialis within 7 to 10 days before onset of rash (Weston, Lane, & Morelli, 2002)
- Recurrence, especially with herpes simplex (EM minor) or mycoplasmal pneumonia (EM major)
- Use of sulfa drugs, penicillin, salicylates, anticonvulsants, or barbiturates
- Prodrome to EM major includes a distinct prodrome lasting 1 to 14 days with fever, malaise, sore throat, cough, headache, vomiting, diarrhea, chest pain, myalgia, and arthralgia
- Exposure to UV light or trauma to area

Physical Examination. Lesions vary from patient to patient, within a single episode, and with recurrence.

- EM minor:
  - A variety of lesions on skin and mucous membranes, including macules, papules, vesicles of varying size; early lesions often mistaken for urticaria; lesions may fuse to form large annular plaques.
  - A diagnostic clue is the presence of target lesions (a distinct dark central area with possible blistering or necrosis and an outer ring of erythema) or iris lesions (with a central blister or whitish area, a middle dusky zone, and an outer erythematous ring).
  - Lesions are fixed (another diagnostic clue), tend to be symmetric, and have a typical distribution predominantly on the hands, feet, elbows, and knees, but also on the face, neck, and trunk.
  - Mucous membranes are usually spared, but a single surface, usually lips and mouth, may be involved, including blisters, crusted and swollen lips, and tongue lesions.
- EM major (SJS or TEN):
  - Onset is sudden and widespread, with high fever and weakness; child or adolescent appears ill.
  - At least two mucous membranes are involved, including the oral mucosa and bulbar conjunctiva, genitalia, rectum, nasopharynx, esophagus, respiratory mucosa, or gastrointestinal mucosa.
  - Extensive blisters, bullae, crusts, erosions, and ulcerations are present; rash begins on trunk and disseminates to extremities; often no target lesions are present, and there are areas of skin that are spared.

- The TEN rash has rapidly coalescing target lesions and widespread bullae that become full-thickness epidermal peeling within 24 hours.

Laboratory Studies. The following are ordered as indicated by the clinical condition of the child:

- Chest radiograph to screen for mycoplasmal pneumonia if respiratory symptoms are present
- Tzanck's preparation to screen for herpes
- CBC and urinalysis to screen for leukocytosis and renal involvement

Other studies may be indicated if EM major is suspected.

Differential Diagnosis

Urticaria can be differentiated by lack of itching, lability of lesions, and shorter-lasting hives that are pale centrally, not target or iris lesions. Viral exanthems are more centrally located, confluent, and less erythematous. Purpura is present in vasculitis. In staphylococcal scalded skin syndrome, the skin peels superficially (not full-thickness) and is significantly red. Also included in the differential diagnosis are Kawasaki disease and lupus erythematosus (see Table 37-10).

Management

Care for EM minor is generally supportive, because the condition is self-limited. Children with EM major require hospitalization and intensive support and intervention.

- EM minor:

1. Identify, discontinue, or treat the stimulus, if possible.
2. Treat precipitating infection as appropriate.
   - If HSV, a 5-day course of oral acyclovir 400 mg/day at the onset of each episode, or if recurrent, a 6-month course.
3. Supportive measures to maintain hydration, prevent secondary infection, and relieve pain.
   - Mild analgesics, cool compresses, and oral antihistamines such as diphenhydramine.
   - Soothing mouthwashes or topical anesthetics such as Kaopectate or Maalox mixed in equal parts with diphenhydramine.
   - Topical intraoral anesthetics, such as dyclonine liquid or viscous lidocaine, are sometimes used with caution in older children and adolescents.
   - Debridement of oral lesions with half-strength hydrogen peroxide.
   - Intravenous fluids if oral hydration is not adequate.
4. The role of steroids in treating EM is controversial. Some believe they may be helpful in recurrent cases or early in the course of the disease to moderate symptoms. In evolving SJS or TEN, however, steroids may increase the risk of secondary infection and delay wound healing.

- EM major:
  - EM major can be life threatening and requires hospitalization, burn care, and daily ophthalmologic care.

Complications

Dehydration from reduced oral intake is the most common complication. With EM major there is a mortality rate of 5% to 70%, with morbidity including pneumonitis, renal disease, keratitis, and other ophthalmologic disorders.

Patient Education and Prevention

EM minor lesions last 5 to 7 days, recur in batches over 2 to 4 weeks, but resolve without scarring or sequelae, except for transient desquamation, scaling, or hyperpigmentation. Recurrence of EM minor is common, often once or twice a year.

PAPULOSQUAMOUS ERUPTIONS OF THE SKIN

Pityriasis Rosea

Description

Pityriasis rosea (PR), meaning rose-colored flaking, is a common, mild, self-limited papulosquamous disease (see Color Fig. 22).

Etiology and Incidence

It is debated whether PR is caused by human herpesvirus (HHV) 7. It is minimally contagious and occurs most commonly in the fall, early winter, and spring months in temperate climates. Fifty percent of all cases occur before 20 years of age, most commonly in adolescence (Hartley, 1999).

Clinical Findings

History. Although there is usually no prodrome, mild symptoms of malaise and fever before onset of rash are sometimes reported.

Physical Examination. Findings include the following:

- Herald spot—1 to 10 cm solitary, ovoid, slightly erythematous lesion that enlarges quickly with central clearing, usually occurring 1 to 30 days before the onset of rash *(key finding)*
- Generalized, symmetric, small macular to papular, thin, round to oval lesions, thin scale centrally with thicker scale peripherally, pale pink in color, more common on trunk and proximal extremities from neck to knees, sparing the palms and soles, but also found on face and neck 7 to 15 days after the herald spot

- Christmas tree pattern—rash, especially on back, follows skin lines with oval lesions running parallel
- Oral lesions have punctate hemorrhages, erosions or ulcerations, erythematous macules, or annular plaques
- In blacks, 2 to 3 mm papular lesions are more common on the neck, proximal extremities, inguinal and axillary areas, less common on trunk
- Atypical disease occurs in 25% (Hartley, 1999), most typically young children, girls, and blacks, as inverse PR with involvement of usually spared areas (face, axilla, groin)

Laboratory Studies. If needed, a KOH preparation of a skin scraping is done to rule out tinea; a Venereal Disease Research Laboratories (VDRL) test is done to rule out secondary syphilis.

Differential Diagnosis

Psoriasis, guttate psoriasis, nummular eczema, scabies, tinea (especially the herald patch), secondary syphilis, drug eruptions, or viral exanthems should be ruled out in the differential diagnosis.

Management

The following steps are taken:

- Application of calamine, tepid baths with Aveeno, antihistamines, emollients, or mild topical steroids is done as needed for itching.
- Minimal sun exposure can help lesions resolve more quickly. Avoid sunburn.
- For oral lesions, triamcinolone acetonide (Kenalog in Orabase) in dental paste may be applied, or in patients over 8 years of age, mouthwash with tetracycline and diphenhydramine.

Patient Education and Prevention

PR is a benign, self-limited, and noncontagious disease that has three cycles (emerging, persisting, and fading) with resolution spontaneously in 4 to 12 weeks. Transient pigmentary changes can occur, especially in blacks.

Psoriasis

Description

Psoriasis, a chronic skin disorder with spontaneous remissions and exacerbations, is characterized by thick silvery scales, its distribution pattern, and an isomorphic (Koebner's phenomenon) response (see Color Fig. 23). Types of psoriasis include guttate psoriasis (following a streptococcal infection), psoriasis vulgaris, napkin psoriasis (occurring in the diaper area), inverse psoriasis (limited to areas that are normally spared), localized pustular psoriasis, generalized pustular or psoriatic erythroderma, and psoriatic arthritis.

Etiology and Incidence

Though the cause is unknown, there is a familial predisposition (35%) and probable polygenic inheritance pattern. An accelerated epidermal proliferation of keratinocytes and dermal vascular abnormalities contribute to the characteristic look of the lesions. Trigger factors including infection, local trauma, stress, and certain drugs (corticosteroids, lithium, NSAIDs) play a role in psoriasis.

Psoriasis occurs in 1% to 3% of the population, with 25% to 45% of cases appearing before 10 to 16 years of age. It is diagnosed in infancy (2%), childhood (10%), and adolescence (25%). It is more common in whites than in blacks and in males than in females. Guttate psoriasis is the first sign of psoriasis in 15% to 34% of children (Chen and Cunningham, 2001; Paller, 1999; Weston, Lane, & Morelli, 2002).

Clinical Findings

History. The following may be reported:

- Family history in approximately one third of cases
- Streptococcal pharyngitis before onset
- Trauma before onset
- Itching (variable)

Physical Examination. Findings include the following:

- The scalp (encircling the hairline and external ears), elbows, knees, and buttocks (especially the diaper area in infants) are the most common sites of involvement. In children, the face may also be involved. Lesions are often found around areas of trauma (e.g., genitalia, palms, soles).
- *Plaque psoriasis.* Discrete, initially erythematous, symmetric, well-marginated rash becoming papular with silver scales that may be trivial to widespread.
- *Acute guttate (teardrop) psoriasis.* Widespread, symmetric, round, or oval 0.5 to 2 cm lesions occurring primarily on the trunk and proximal extremities, occasionally on the face, and rarely on the palms or soles. There is less scaling than in psoriasis vulgaris.
- *Psoriasis vulgaris.* Well-circumscribed, erythematous plaques with silvery-white scales concentrated on elbows, knees, scalp, and hairline, but also seen on eyebrows, around ears, and in intergluteal fold and genital area.
- *Koebner's phenomenon (isomorphic response).* The occurrence of psoriasis 1 to 3 weeks after trauma (e.g., bites, scratch, abrasion, sunburn, pressure) (45% of cases; Weston, Lane, & Morelli, 2002).
- *Auspitz's sign.* Bleeding occurs when a scale is removed.

- *Nail signs.* Nails have "ice pick" pits and ridges, are thick and discolored, and can have splinter hemorrhages and be separated from the nail bed; present in 15% of cases (Weston, Lane, & Morelli, 2002).
- *Napkin psoriasis.* Appears eczematous, affecting inguinal and gluteal folds.

Laboratory Studies. The following are to be considered:

- ASO if guttate pattern
- KOH and culture to rule out fungal infection
- VDRL to rule out secondary syphilis

Differential Diagnosis

Pityriasis rosea, seborrhea, *Candida* infection, contact or irritant dermatitis, atopic dermatitis, tinea, dyshidrosis, secondary syphilis, and other nail-pitting conditions are included in the differential diagnosis.

Management

In children, treatment should be as conservative as possible. Medications and treatments should be rotated for best effectiveness. The following are options for management:

- Sun exposure in moderate amounts alleviates lesions. Avoid sunburn.
- Emollient cream such as petrolatum, Eucerin, Aquaphor, or Cetaphil for dry skin can minimize trauma and subsequent psoriasis and may improve psoriasis.
- Apply topical steroids, moderate or strong and sometimes fluorinated, two to three times a day for 2 to 3 weeks. They should be used intermittently but not discontinued spontaneously, because worsening can occur. Monitoring of the patient during use is important. Small localized lesions can be treated with topical, fluorinated steroids. A moderate-potency steroid can be used on thick plaques and larger areas. Severe plaques on the elbows and knees may need a higher-potency steroid (see Table 37-1). Systemic steroids are not indicated and may worsen the condition, causing pustular flare. Consultation with a dermatologist is often indicated.
- Tar or keratolytic shampoos (ketoconazole [Nizoral], anthralin, salicylic acid [P & S]) can be used on the scalp. Tar preparations can also be used on the skin alone or in combination with UV light treatment.
- Mineral or olive oil and warm towels to soak and remove thick plaques.
- Keratolytic agents such as sulfur 3% or salicylic acid 3% to 6% to reduce thick, unresponsive plaques. Salicylic acid blocks UVB and should not be used in combination with phototherapy.
- Anthralin ointment for plaques that are resistant to steroids and tar. In high strengths (1% and higher), apply ointment for 10 to 30 minutes once a day and then wash off. In lower strengths, leave ointment on for 8 hours. Strength used is determined by tolerance. Anthralin stains skin and clothing and can irritate skin.
- Vitamin D analog (Calcitrol) produces improvement in 60% of patients (Paller, 1999) but is approved for use only in children over 12 years of age.
- Tazorotene (Tazorac) is a retinoid that may be effective in management of plaque psoriasis.
- Balneo phototherapy combines magnesium-rich Dead Sea salt baths with ultraviolet light treatments for 4 to 6 weeks or 15 to 25 treatments. This natural treatment may bring 80% to 85% clearance of skin lesions or remission (Mikula, 2003).
- Follow up every 2 weeks until psoriasis is controlled and during exacerbations, and then as needed.
- Refer to a dermatologist if psoriasis is not responsive. Other treatment options include UV light treatment, psoralens, intralesional steroids, retinoids, cyclosporine, and immunotherapy.

Complications

The following complications are possible:

- *Candida* infection as a secondary infection in the diaper area.
- *Pustular psoriasis.* Unusual in childhood. Generalized or local multiple 1 to 2 mm pustules with erythema and scaling also involving palms and soles. Accompanied by malaise, fever, and leukocytosis. Should be referred to a dermatologist.
- *Exfoliative erythroderma.* Rare manifestation, including desquamation and loss of hair and nails with previous history of psoriasis. Should be referred to a dermatologist.
- *Psoriatic arthritis.* An inflammatory arthritis that is rare (1%) but increasing in frequency, most common in females age 9 to 12 years (Paller, 1999; Weston, Lane, & Morelli, 2002). Rheumatoid factor is negative, cutaneous symptoms mild or absent. Prognosis is good.

Patient Education and Prevention

Emotional support and education are the most important aspects in dealing with psoriasis. Areas for discussion include the following:

- Psoriasis is chronic and involves spontaneous remissions and exacerbations. Control and relief are sought, but cure is not available at this time. Treatment may require up to 1 month to determine effectiveness.
- Guttate psoriasis often resolves with antibiotic treatment for streptococcal infection. Psoriasis vulgaris may persist for months to years.
- Lifestyle changes help prevent recurrence. These include avoidance of cutaneous injury, streptococcal infection,

sunburn, stress, itching, bites, tight clothes and shoes, some medications (e.g., oral steroids, NSAIDs), and occlusive dressings. Good skin care, including regular use of emollients, may improve psoriasis and minimize recurrences.
- Psoriasis tends to improve during summer and with pregnancy.
- Psoriasis is considered stable if there are either no new plaques or if existing plaques are not enlarging.

Lichen Striatus

Description

Lichen striatus is peculiar to childhood, characterized by unilateral shiny papules along embryonic lines, or lines of Blaschko.

Etiology and Incidence

Although the etiology is unknown, it is most common in females between 2 and 12 years of age. Lesions spontaneously disappear after 1 week to 3 years. Short relapses have occurred on occasion.

Clinical Findings

History. Lesions appear spontaneously without prodrome.

Physical Examination. Findings include the following:
- Linear, shiny hypopigmented or flesh-colored, flat-topped papules with adherent scale
- Limited to one extremity, initially lesions coalesce in a linear distribution down an extremity
- Lesions involving a nail bed will result in nail deformity
- Rarely are lesions noted on the face
- May be asymptomatic or may be intensely pruritic
- May resolve with hyperpigmentation that lasts several months

Laboratory Studies. A skin biopsy is diagnostic when in doubt.

Differential Diagnosis

The unilateral linear lesions are characteristic. However, differential diagnosis includes lichen planus, lichen nitidus, psoriasis, epidermal birthmarks, and linear Darier's disease.

Management

Lesions are resistant to treatment, and treatment is unnecessary for asymptomatic cases. However, pruritis may be relieved with the use of group I or group II topical steroids, or intralesional steroid injections.

Patient Education and Prevention

Lichen striatus is a benign, self-limited, noncontagious disorder that results in complete resolution.

Keratosis Pilaris

Description

Keratosis pilaris is a common finding on the extensor aspects of the extremities, buttocks, and occasionally the cheeks.

Etiology and Incidence

The etiology is unknown. Some believe it to be a disorder of abnormal keratinization; others believe it to be a response to drying of the skin surface. Keratosis pilaris is more common in children with atopic disorders; in those living in cold, dry climates; and in winter months.

Clinical Findings

History. Keratosis pilaris appears spontaneously, without prodrome. It is usually asymptomatic, although most patients are bothered by the appearance and seek treatment.

Physical Examination. Findings include the following:
- Rough dry skin on the posterior upper arms, anterior thighs, buttocks, and cheeks
- Small papules with follicular plugs of stratum corneum
- Occasional diffuse eruption with small sterile pustules

Laboratory Studies. Skin biopsy reveals inflammation outside the hair follicle.

Differential Diagnosis

Microcomedones of acne, molluscum contagiosum, warts, milia, and folliculitis are often confused with keratosis pilaris.

Management

It is important to recognize keratosis pilaris as a benign disorder to avoid detrimental treatment. Management includes the following:
- In mild cases, the use of lubricants and emollients to moisturize skin is sufficient for improvement.
- Topical keratolytics combined with lactic acid 12%, urea creams, and lubricants are applied several times daily.
- Antibiotics active against *S. aureus* are useful for folliculitis.

Treatment takes weeks to months for improvement, and recurrence is common when treatment is stopped.

Patient Education and Prevention

The chronic but benign nature of keratosis pilaris should be stressed. Treatment takes weeks to months, and recurrence is common.

CONGENITAL LESIONS OF THE SKIN

Vascular and Pigmented Nevi

Description

Nevi are a common finding in children. The two most common types are vascular nevi (vascular malformations and hemangiomas) and pigmented nevi (mongolian spots, café au lait spots, acquired melanocytic nevi, acanthosis nigricans, and lentigines).

Etiology and Incidence

Vascular nevi are caused by a structural abnormality (malformations) or by an overgrowth of blood vessels (hemangiomas) and are flat, raised, or cavernous. Flat lesions or vascular malformations include salmon patches (also called macular stains), an innocent malformation occurring in 30% to 70% of newborns, and port-wine stains, occurring in 3 per 1000 newborns. Raised or cavernous lesions, also called hemangiomas, are present in up to 10% of newborns. Hemangiomas occur more commonly in females (75%) and in 22% to 30% of premature infants weighing less than 1500 g (Achauer and Vanderkam, 2000; Paller, 1999; Weston, Lane, & Morelli, 2002).

Pigmented nevi are caused by an overgrowth of pigment cells. Pigmented nevi most commonly seen are mongolian spots (up to 90% in blacks, 81% in Asians, 70% in Hispanics, and in East Indians; less than 10% in whites), café au lait spots (12% to 22% in blacks, 0.3% to 19% in whites), and acquired nevi, the most common tumor of childhood, 2% of which are atypical (Dinulos & Graham, 1998; Paller, 1999; Tekin, Bodurtha, & Riccardi, 2001; Weston, Lane, & Morelli, 2002).

Clinical Findings

History. The following should be noted:

- Presence from birth, or age first noted
- Progression of lesion
- Familial tendencies for similar nevi, especially for history of melanoma

Physical Examination. Findings include the following (Box 37-11):

- Vascular malformations or flat vascular nevi are present at birth and grow commensurate with the child's growth.
- Hemangiomas are classified as superficial, deep, or mixed. They are not present at birth, but usually emerge by 1 month of age. They may manifest as a pale macule, a telangiectatic lesion, or a bright-red nodular papule. Involution occurs slowly but spontaneously, often between 12 and 24 months of age, heralded by gray areas in the lesion followed by flattening from the center outward. Most are flat by 5 to 7 years of age, the remainder by puberty. Most hemangiomas appear as normal skin after involution, but others may have residual changes such as telangiectasias, atrophy, fibrofatty residue, and scarring (Lebwohl et al, 2002). During the proliferative phase, hemangiomas grow rapidly and form nodular compressible masses, ranging in size from a few millimeters to several centimeters. Occasionally, they may cover an entire limb, resulting in asymmetric limb growth. Rapidly growing lesions may ulcerate.
- Pigmented nevi may be present at birth or may be acquired during childhood.
- Atypical nevi are larger than acquired nevi; have irregular, poorly defined borders; and have variable pigmentation.

Differential Diagnosis

Hematomas or ecchymoses of child abuse are occasionally confused with some nevi. Non–insulin-dependent diabetes mellitus (NIDDM) often causes acanthosis nigricans.

Management

1. Flat vascular nevi:
- Salmon patches.
  - Fade with time, usually by 5 or 6 years of age.
- Port-wine stains.
  - A permanent defect that grows with the child, so cosmetic covering is often used.
  - Refer to a dermatologist for possible laser treatment or corrective cosmesis.
  - If forehead and eyelids are involved, there is potential for multiple syndromes, including Sturge-Weber, Klippel-Trenaunay-Weber, and Parkes-Weber. Neurodevelopmental and ophthalmologic follow-up is needed.
  - Angiomatous papules and underlying soft tissue hypertrophy develop over years.
2. Hemangiomas:
- Reassure and educate the family about the nature and course of this nevus. A word that there is no relationship to anything the mother did during pregnancy is often appreciated.
- Frequent follow-up, especially during the growing phase. Sequential photographs are helpful.
- If the lesions are strategically placed (eye, lip, oral cavity, ear, airway, diaper area), very large, or grow very quickly, prompt referral to a dermatologist is indicated because early treatment is most effective.
- If treatment is required during the proliferative stage, steroids (intralesional and oral) are prescribed until growth is stabilized, then tapered over 4 to 6 weeks, with a 30% to 90% success rate. Indications for steroid treatment are interference with physiologic functions (e.g., breathing, hearing, eating, vision), recurrent bleeding or

BOX 37-11 *Common Vascular and Pigmented Lesions*

I. Vascular malformations or flat vascular nevi
   A. Salmon patch or nevus flammeus
      1. Light-pink macule of varying size and configuration
      2. Commonly seen on the glabella, back of neck, forehead, or upper eyelids
   B. Port-wine stain or nevus flammeus
      1. Purple-red macules that occur unilaterally, tend to be large
      2. Usually occur on face, occiput, or neck, although they may be on extremities
II. Hemangiomas
   A. Superficial (strawberry) hemangiomas are found in the upper dermis of the skin and account for the majority of hemangiomas
   B. Deep cavernous hemangiomas are found in the subcutaneous and hypodermal layers of the skin; although similar to superficial hemangiomas, there is a blue tinge to their appearance
      1. With pressure, there is blanching and a feeling of a soft, compressible tumor
      2. Variable in size, they can occur in places other than skin
   C. Mixed hemangiomas have attributes of both superficial and deep hemangiomas
III. Pigmented nevi
   A. Mongolian spots
      1. Blue or slate-gray, irregular, variably sized macules
      2. Common in the presacral or lumbosacral area of dark-skinned infants; also on the upper back, shoulders, and extremities
      3. The majority of the pigment fades as the child gets older and the skin darkens
      4. Solitary or multiple, often covering a large area
   B. Café-au-lait spots
      1. Tan to light-brown macules found anywhere on the skin; oval or irregular in shape; increase in number with age
   C. Acquired melanocytic nevi are benign, light brown, to dark brown, to black, flat, or slightly raised, occurring anywhere on the body, especially on sun-exposed areas, above the waist
      1. *Junctional nevi* represent the initial stage, with tiny, hairless, light brown to black macules
      2. *Compound nevi*—a few junctional nevi progress to these more elevated, warty, or smooth lesions with hair
      3. *Dermal nevi* are the adult form, dome shaped with coarse hair
      4. *Atypical nevi* usually appear at puberty, have irregular borders, variegated pigmentation, are larger than normal nevi (6-15 mm); usually found on trunk, feet, scalp, and buttocks
      5. *Halo nevi* appear in late childhood with an area of depigmentation around a pigmented nevus, usually on trunk (see Color Fig. 24)
   D. Acanthosis nigricans is velvety brown rows of hyperpigmentation in irregular folds of skin, usually the neck and axilla; tags may also be present
   E. Lentigines are small brown to black macules 1-2 mm in size appearing anywhere on the body in school-age children
   F. Freckles: 1-5 mm light brown pigmented macules in sun-exposed areas

ulceration, high-ouput congestive heart failure, Kasabach-Merritt syndrome, rapid growth that distorts facial features, or presence in the diaper area. Interferon may also be used (Achauer & Vanderkam, 2000).

- Treatment by surgery, cryotherapy, radiation, or injecting sclerosing agents often leads to scarring.
- Danger of cardiovascular complications, disseminated intravascular coagulation, or compression of internal organs with large, deep lesions.
- Regression occurs in 25% of cases by 2 years of age, in 40% to 50% by 4 years of age, in 60% to 75% by school age, and in 95% by adolescence. Scarring may be present if ulceration has occurred; loose skin and telangiectasis follow in 30% to 50% of cases (Paller, 1999). Laser therapy is effective management for residual telangiectasias (Lebwohl et al, 2002).

3. Pigmented nevi. Educate family about the nature of these lesions:

- *Mongolian spots*: Document to distinguish from bruise; fade with time, usually no traces by adulthood.
- *Blue nevus*: Heavily pigmented melanocytes in papule or nodule that can develop melanoma.

- *Café au lait spots*: If six or more lesions larger than 0.5 cm in diameter are present (or more than three in Caucasians [Tekin, Bodurtha, & Riccardi, 2001]) or if axillary freckling or tumors are also present, refer child to rule out neurofibromatosis or other genetic disorder.
- *Acquired melanocytic nevi*: Giant nevi (e.g., bathing trunk nevus) are at increased risk of developing melanoma (Bittencourt et al, 2000) and need referral to a dermatologist. If more than 15 acquired nevi are present, monitor for atypical nevi (Chamlin, 2002).
- *Atypical nevi* appear most commonly in adolescents and require regular follow-up because of increased risk for melanoma. However, melanoma often manifests with new lesions rather than from transformation of current ones. (See section on sunburn complications.)
- *Halo nevus*: A depigmented ring around a pigmented nevi.
- *Spitz nevus*: A smooth, pink to brown, dome-shaped papule often occurring on head and neck.
- *Fried-egg mole*: A compound nevi with flat border and raised darker center.
- *Acanthosis nigricans* is characterized by hyperpigmentation and a velvety thickening of irregular folds of the neck and axilla. It is more common in Native American, African American, and Hispanic adolescents. A decrease in weight sometimes results in resolution of lesions. It can also be a manifestation of NIDDM in children.
- *Lentigines*: May fade or disappear with time but are also associated with various syndromes.
- *Nevus spilus* is a light-brown speckled lentiginous nevi with darker papules within it; it can be congential or acquired and has potential to develop melanoma.
- Refer to dermatologist (Box 37-12).

Complications

Ulceration, infection, platelet trapping, airway or visual obstruction, or cardiac decompensation can occur with large vascular nevi. Kasabach-Merritt syndrome occurs when thrombocytopenic hemorrhage occurs in a large, deep hemangioma. Melanoma in congenital nevi (see discussion in complications of sunburn) is possible, and monitoring of these lesions is important. Changes of particular concern are development of an off-center nodule or papule, color change, bleeding, persistent irritation, erosion, ulceration, and rapid growth.

An autosomal dominant, familial, atypical mole and melanoma syndrome has been identified genetically. Children with multiple atypical nevi and family members with melanoma are at risk for childhood melanoma (Chamlin, 2002; Morelli & Weston, 1999).

BOX 37-12 *When to Refer to a Dermatologist*

- Suspicious nevus (as identified by ABCDE signs [see Box 37-9])
- Rapidly growing or changing nevus
- More than 50 nevi
- One or more atypical nevi
- One or more first-degree relatives with melanoma
- Giant or large congenital nevus
- Signs of excessive sun exposure (increased nevi and freckles in exposed areas)
- History of immunosuppression and multiple nevi on examination

Adapted from Chamlin SL, Williams ML: Pigmented lesions in adolescents, *Adolesc Med* 12(2):v, 195-212, 2001, with permission from Hanley & Belfus, Inc.

Patient Education and Prevention

Monitoring those nevi that are at risk for developing melanoma is important. Teaching the family to watch nevi for any changes is also important. See sunburn complications section for more information.

Vitiligo and Hypopigmentation

Description

Lack of pigment in the skin causing white or light-colored areas can be either hypopigmentation or vitiligo. Two types of vitiligo have been identified: Type A has a generalized, acral symmetric distribution; type B has a segmental, dermatome distribution.

Etiology and Incidence

Vitiligo, presumed to be an immune disorder, occurs in 1% to 2% of the U.S. population, with 50% of cases beginning before 20 years of age. It appears more commonly in children with various systemic or immune disorders (Hurwitz, 1993; Weston, Lane, & Morelli, 2002). Hypopigmentation follows inflammation or injury to the melanocytes in the skin resulting from diseases such as atopic dermatitis, psoriasis, or pityriasis rosea, or from abrasions, burns, injury from liquid nitrogen, or severe sunburn.

Clinical Findings

History. The following should be elicited:

- Family history of vitiligo, halo nevi, traumatic depigmentation of skin, or markedly premature graying of the hair (30% of cases) (Hurwitz, 1993)

- Onset of depigmentation (birth or more recent)
- Presence of any systemic or skin diseases
- Any recent trauma to the skin

Physical Examination. Findings include the following:

- Vitiligo
  - Flat, milk-white macules or papules with scalloped, distinct borders of varied size
  - Symmetric or asymmetric, possibly following a nerve segment
  - Few to multiple, seen most commonly on face and trunk
- Hypopigmentation
  - Macules and patches with irregular mottling and borders
  - Linear or patterned
  - Possibly associated hyperpigmented areas

Laboratory Studies. For vitiligo, a skin biopsy and CBC, fasting glucose, thyroid function and antithyroid antibodies, early-morning serum cortisol, and VDRL are sometimes indicated.

Differential Diagnosis

Pityriasis rosea, pityriasis alba, tinea versicolor, and albinism (eye color affected and onset at birth) are included in the differential diagnosis.

Management

The following steps are taken:

- Vitiligo:
  - Broad-spectrum sunscreens are used to decrease the tanning of normal skin.
  - Cover-up agents such as skin dyes and walnut oil may be used.
  - Mild to moderate steroids may show success in some patients.
  - Refer for treatment with psoralens. May be used in combination with UVA radiation (best used in children under 9 years of age). UVB may also be used.
  - Family should be encouraged to be in a support group because this is a highly disfiguring condition, especially for those with dark complexion.
- Hypopigmentation:
  - Reassure family that repigmentation will occur. Hypopigmentation is self-limited and lasts only a few months.

Complications

With vitiligo, complications include thyroid disease, diabetes mellitus, pernicious anemia, Addison's disease, uveitis, alopecia areata, and severe sunburn.

HAIR AND NAIL DISORDERS

Alopecia, hair loss from areas of skin normally producing hair, can be limited to one area or scattered over the scalp, and can be complete or leave residual hairs of differing lengths. The three main causes of hair loss are tinea capitis, traumatic alopecia, and alopecia areata (Table 37-11).

Tinea Capitis

Description

Ringworm of the scalp and hair may be seen in four different manifestations: (1) diffuse fine scaling without obvious hair breaks and with subtle to significant hair loss; (2) discrete areas of hair loss with stubs of broken hairs (black-dot ringworm) (see Color Fig. 25); (3) "classic" patchy hair loss and scaly lesions with raised borders; and (4) scaly, pustular lesions, or kerions. Tinea capitis occurs in a noninflammatory stage for 2 to 8 weeks, then becomes inflammatory.

Etiology and Incidence

The fungus invades the scalp and hair shaft, causing an inflammatory response and fragile hair shaft. *T. tonsurans* is the causative organism 90% to 95% of the time, and the infection is near epidemic in the United States, but *M. canis* or other species can be responsible (AAP, 2003; Weston, Lane, & Morelli, 2002). Tinea capitis is transmitted by humans sharing hats, combs, and brushes, or by cats, dogs, or rodents. Tinea capitis is the most common dermatophyte infection, occurring primarily in children 3 to 9 years of age (AAP, 2003; Weston, Lane, & Morelli, 2002). It is more common in boys than in girls and in blacks.

Clinical Findings

History. Hair loss, itching, and contact with another person or pet with ringworm are sometimes reported.

Physical Examination. Findings include the following:

- Scaling, erythema, or crusting usually occurs.
- Bald patches or areas of broken hairs are noted.
- Occipital or posterior cervical adenopathy may be significant.
- *Microsporum* species leaves the hair broken and lusterless with a fine gray scale on the scalp.
- *T. tonsurans* manifests as black-dot tinea, with tiny black dots that are the remainder of hair that has broken off at the shaft; no scalp scale is present (most common).
- A boggy, inflamed mass filled with pustules (kerion) is a delayed allergy reaction; cervical lymphadenopathy, fever, and leukocytosis may be present.
- The inflammatory stage is noted by widespread pustules, suppuration, and kerion formation.

TABLE 37-11 Diagnosis and Treatment of Alopecia

	Etiology	Clinical Findings	Treatment
Tinea capitis	*Trichophyton tonsurans* 90%-95%; *Microsporum canis*; others	Fine diffuse scaling without obvious hair breaks and subtle to significant hair loss; hair loss discrete with stubs of broken hair; patchy hair loss with scaling and raised borders to lesions; scaly, pustular lesions or kerions	Griseofulvin taken with fatty food until 2 wk after negative culture; monitor CBC, LFTs, renal function at 4 wk and every 4-8 wk; prednisone if kerion present; culture family members; sporicidal shampoo; keep from school 1 wk; follow-up in 2 wk; launder sheets, clothes, vacuum house
Traumatic alopecia	Chemical, thermal, traction (hairstyling), friction (trichotillomania)	*Traumatic*: incomplete hair loss with varying lengths *Traction*: erythema and pustules, thins and breaks in certain areas, especially linear *Trichotillomania*: circumscribed hair loss with irregular borders and broken hair of varied lengths, no erythema or scarring, especially frontal, parietal, or temporal	*Traction*: avoid hairstyles that precipitate; mild shampoo, gentle brushing; short course of antibiotics if pustules *Trichotillomania*: discussion with parents, oil at night, counseling if entrenched, other interventions if significant
Alopecia areata	Autoimmune mechanism	Family history; single or multiple round or oval patches of complete or near-complete hair loss; no erythema or scaling, scalp smooth with fine new hair growth, usually frontal or parietal; "exclamation hairs" present; nail ridging or pitting; occasional loss of body or pubic hair	Discussion and support; often self-limited course; if extensive, refer to dermatologist for alternative treatments; supportive care—prescription for wig, refer to National Alopecia Foundation

CBC, Complete blood count; *LFTs*, liver function tests.

Laboratory Studies. Examine hair scrapings as follows:

- Wood's light fluoresces yellow-green (positive with *M. canis*, negative with *T. tonsurans*).
- KOH examination of scraped hair: Wait 20 to 40 minutes after application of KOH to examine. If Wood's light was positive, under microscopy the KOH-prepared outer surface of hair is coated with tiny mats of spores; if Wood's light was negative, hyphae and spores are present in hair shaft.
- Fungal culture of a completely plucked hair (use a Kelly clamp) is most reliable.

Differential Diagnosis

Traumatic alopecia, alopecia areata, hypothyroid and hyperthyroid hair loss, seborrhea, atopic dermatitis, psoriasis, impetigo, and folliculitis are included in the differential diagnosis.

Management

The following steps are taken:

- Griseofulvin microsize 15 to 20 mg/kg per day, occasionally up to 25 mg/kg per day (maximum dose 1 g); if no response, once daily after a meal with fatty food such as ice cream to enhance absorption. Treatment should be continued until 2 weeks after resolution, a minimum of 4 to 12 weeks (AAP, 2003). Topical antifungals are ineffective.
- Terbinafine (Lamisil) is not approved by the FDA for this indication. However, some studies have been done in children showing it to be effective for resistant cases. See Table 37-4 for dosing.
- If a long-standing kerion with severe inflammation is present, prednisone 1 to 2 mg/kg per day for 5 to 14 days. Antibiotic treatment is not indicated.
- Family members and pets should be checked for infection by fungal culture and treated if positive. More than

50% are positive (Weston, Lane, & Morelli, 2002), so do not rely on lack of symptoms. Asymptomatic carriers are common.

- Shampooing with selenium sulfide 2.5% or econazole or ketoconazole 2% (two times per week for 4 weeks) decreases spore viability and keeps other household members from being infected.
- Child should be kept out of school for 1 week.
- A follow-up visit should be scheduled after 2 weeks to evaluate response to treatment. Medication should be continued until 2 weeks after culture is negative. Follow-up should be continued every 2 to 4 weeks until new hair growth is evident.
- Monitoring of CBC, LFTs, and possibly renal function tests is recommended at 4 weeks and every 4 to 8 weeks thereafter if griseofulvin is continued for more than 3 months.
- If resistance to griseofulvin is encountered, oral itraconazole, terbinafine, fluconazole, and ketoconazole have been used but are not all approved for use in children under 18 years old.

Complications

An "id" reaction is a hypersensitivity reaction to the fungus, not to the medication with which it is being treated. It manifests either as a red, superficial edema or as scaly, red plaques and papules and is treated with 1 to 2 weeks of topical or systemic steroids. Permanent hair loss and scarring can occur with an untreated kerion.

Patient Education and Prevention

- Sites and modes of transmission are identified (*M. canis*, animal source; *T. tonsurans*, human source) and treated.
- Side effects of medication should be explained and monitored.
- Hair regrowth is slow (3 to 12 months), and, if a kerion was present, hair loss can be permanent.
- Laundering sheets and clothes in a hot-water wash or hot dryer cycle and vacuuming may decrease spread in the family.
- Grooming practices (e.g., hair traction, greasy pomades, infrequent shampooing) may be predisposing factors.
- There is a high rate of asymptomatic carriers; culture is the only definitive means of identification.

Traumatic Alopecia

Description

Traumatic hair loss can be due to chemical or thermal traction or friction. The most common forms are traction alopecia and trichotillomania. Trichotillomania is considered a behavior disorder.

Etiology and Incidence

Traction alopecia, commonly seen in black females, is due to hair styling. Common causes are cornrows, ponytails, or braids; tight curlers; or excessive brushing.

Trichotillomania (TTM) occurs in 0.6% to 4% of the population, with up to 10% having had the habit at some point in time. The mean age of onset is 8 years in males and 12 years in females (Messinger, 1999). Current research indicates etiology is multifactorial, looking at genetic predisposition along with environmental and behavioral variables working together to result in TTM. It is often seen in children with other obsessive-compulsive habits such as thumb-sucking or nail-biting. TTM is classified as an impulse control disorder in the *Diagnostic and Statistical Manual of Mental Disorders*, Fourth Edition (DSM-IV) (Whitaker, Wolf, & Keuthen, 2003).

Clinical Findings

History. The history can include the following:

- Various methods of hair styling with tight pull on hair
- Habits such as nail-biting, finger-sucking, or hair-twirling
- Any recent life changes or stressors
- Medications (anticonvulsants, antithyroids, beta blockers, isotretinoin, lithium, oral contraceptives, vitamin A supplements, warfarin)
- Excess time spent lying in supine position

Physical Examination. The following findings are present:

- Traumatic alopecia
  - Incomplete hair loss with hair of varying lengths
- Traction alopecia
  - Possible erythema and pustules
  - Thinning and breaking in certain areas, tending to occur in a linear pattern related to hairstyle
- Trichotillomania
  - Circumscribed hair loss with irregular borders and broken hairs of varied length
  - No erythema or scaling of the scalp
  - Commonly found on frontal eyelashes, parietal, and temporal areas with peripheral sparing, but also eyebrows

Differential Diagnosis

The differential diagnosis includes tinea capitis, alopecia areata, neonatal occipital alopecia, rub alopecias in atopic dermatitis, and child abuse (make sure no one but the child is pulling out the hair).

Management

The following steps are taken:

1. Traction alopecia:

- Avoid any hairstyle or device that causes traction on the hair, including cornrows, ponytails, braids, and curlers.

- Use only mild shampoo, shampoo infrequently, use wide-toothed combs with rounded ends, and brush gently.
- A short course of antibiotics is prescribed if pustules are present.

2. Trichotillomania:

- A straightforward discussion and ongoing support of the child and parents are essential. In very young children, trichotillomania is usually benign and resolves spontaneously. Older children and adolescents, however, may require individual and family therapy. Attempt to find means to relieve stress and cope with any traumatic events. The following strategies may be helpful (Thomson, 2002):
  - Helping hands—using the hands "together to solve the problem you used to have"; as one hand lifts, the other gives it a pat for not pulling.
  - Mirroring—the child imagines seeing himself or herself as he or she would like to, noting feelings of pride at the image, enforcing determination to control habit.
- Applying oil to the hair at night makes it slippery and harder to pull.
- Medication, behavior therapy, habit reversal, relaxation, and hypnosis are modalities sometimes used.

Complications

Trichobezoars (hairballs) in the child with trichotillomania can cause gastrointestinal symptoms. Some children with trichotillomania have extensive psychopathology.

Patient Education and Prevention

The cause of the hair loss must be discussed and support offered to resolve issues. New hair growth can take 3 to 6 months.

Alopecia Areata

Description

Alopecia areata is an asymptomatic, complete hair loss occurring primarily in frontal or parietal areas (Fig. 37-9).

Etiology and Incidence

The cause of alopecia areata is unknown, but is thought to be an autoimmune mechanism. It is unusual under 2 years of age but can be seen anytime throughout childhood. There is a 10% to 42% familial occurrence (Weston, Lane, & Morelli, 2002).

Clinical Findings

History. The history can include other family members with alopecia areata.

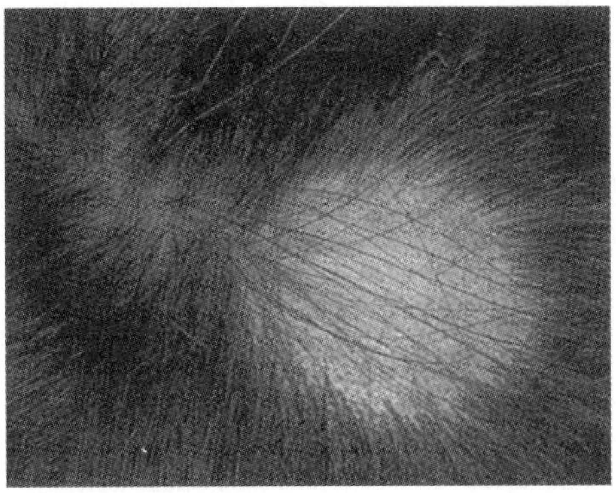

FIGURE 37-9 Alopecia areata with sharply defined oval patches of hair loss. (From Hurwitz S: *Clinical pediatric dermatology*, ed 2, Philadelphia, 1993, WB Saunders, p 486.)

Physical Examination

Findings include the following:

- Single or multiple (up to three) round or oval patches of complete or nearly complete hair loss without erythema or scaling. Scalp is smooth with fine new hair growth.
- The frontal and parietal areas are involved 90% of the time.
- "Exclamation hairs" are narrower at the base, short, and broken off.
- Nail ridging or pitting (a helpful distinguishing factor).
- Occasional loss of body or pubic hair, or eyelashes or eyebrows.
- Possible atopic dermatitis or vitiligo.

Laboratory Studies. The following are sometimes performed:

- KOH examination or fungal culture to rule out tinea
- Skin biopsy

Differential Diagnosis

Tinea capitis versus traumatic alopecia is the differential diagnosis.

Management

No pharmacologic intervention for this condition has proved helpful. The following steps should be taken:

- Open discussion and support of the child and parents. If only one or two patches are present, reassure that regrowth will occur.
- If extensive involvement, refer to a dermatologist for potential treatment options. These include potent topical steroids, intralesional steroids, minoxidil, anthralin, or contact sensitization.

- Recommend wearing a wig, depending on the severity of involvement; prescribing the wig as a medical treatment helps defray the cost.

Complications

Self-esteem issues are common. *Ophiasis* is a form of alopecia areata that begins in the frontal or occipital hairline and spreads along the hair margins. *Alopecia totalis* is a loss of all the hair on the scalp. *Alopecia universalis* is a loss of all the hair on the body.

Patient Education, Prognosis, and Prevention

All families should be put in touch with the National Alopecia Areata Foundation (see Resource Box). The condition is self-limited in most (95%) school-age children and adolescents (Weston, Lane, & Morelli, 2002). Full recovery, often within 1 year, is more likely if three or fewer areas are involved and if onset is in late childhood. However, the greater the hair loss, the longer it takes for regrowth. Prognosis is guarded in infants and toddlers. Approximately one third of patients will have a recurrence within months to years, with a worsening prognosis with each episode.

Onychomycosis

Description

Onychomycosis is a fungal infection of the nail(s) with tinea or *Candida* (Fig. 37-10). One or two nails are often involved. The infection may be superficial, hypertrophic (onychauxic), or cause separation of the nail plate from the tissue (onycholytic).

Etiology and Incidence

The infecting organism invades the nail, proliferates, and destroys the nail integrity, causing separation of the nail plate from the nail bed. The infection originates at the distal edge of the nail. It is uncommon during the first two decades of life, with a worldwide prevalence of 0% to 2.6%, limited almost exclusively to adolescents and adults. Often there is concurrent tinea pedis or tinea manuum. There may be a relation to the use of occlusive shoes. The causative organisms include *Trichophyton rubrum, Trichophyton mentagrophytes, E. floccosum,* and *Candida albicans.* However, 50% of the time another condition is responsible for dystrophic nail.

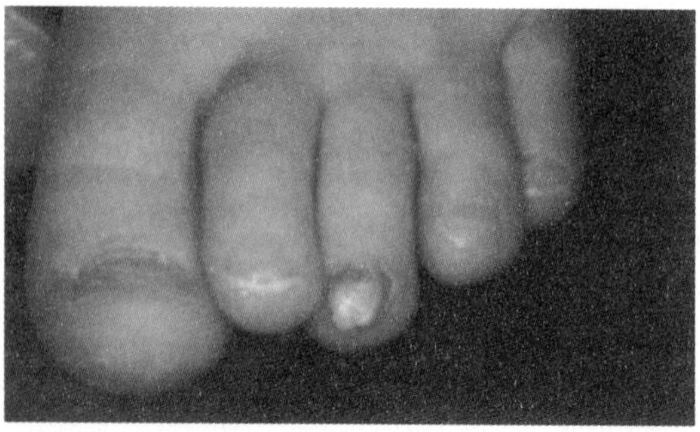

FIGURE 37-10 Onychomycosis (tinea unguium). Thickening and discoloration on the toe of a 4½-year-old child caused by tinea infection. (From Hurwitz S: *Clinical pediatric dermatology*, ed 2, Philadelphia, 1993, WB Saunders, p 386.)

Clinical Findings

History. The adolescent may report a thickened, discolored nail.

Physical Examination

- Opaque white or silvery nail that becomes thick, yellow, with subungal debris
- Toenails are involved more often than fingernails with tinea
- Fingernails are involved more often than toenails with *Candida*
- Seldom symmetric; it may be one to three nails on one extremity

Laboratory Studies. KOH preparations and fungal cultures of the material under the nail are helpful in confirming the diagnosis.

Differential Diagnosis

Psoriasis (involves all nails and includes pitting), hereditary nail defects, dystrophy secondary to eczema or chronic paronychia, lichen planus, and trauma are the differential diagnoses.

Management

1. Itraconazole pulse therapy—5 mg/kg per day orally for 1 week each month for 3 to 5 months is the recommended threatment (Weston, Lane, & Morelli, 2002). Itraconazole capsules are recommended over suspension to minimize effects (Spray and Siegfried, 2001).
2. Successful treatment is difficult and requires oral medication. Griseofulvin can be used, but side effects, length of treatment, and the high recurrence rate following treatment make successful management uncommon. Only 17.5% of cases respond to 6 to 12 months of griseofulvin therapy (Weston, Lane, & Morelli, 2002).
3. Oral terbinafine, ketoconazole, and itraconazole on a daily basis for 4 to 8 weeks have a better short-term success rate than griseofulvin, but relapse rates are not known.

- The FDA-approved drugs and doses for young adults over 18 years of age are as follows:
  - Itraconazole 100 mg two times a day for 12 weeks for toenails.
  - Terbinafine 250 mg/day for 12 weeks for toenails.
- Suggested pediatric dosages are as follows:
  - Itraconazole 3 mg/kg per day, although pulse dosing (see no. 1) is the recommended method.
  - Terbinafine (greater than 40 kg: 250 mg/day; 20 to 40 kg: 125 mg/day; less than 20 kg: 62.5 mg/day) used for 6 to 8 weeks for fingernails or 12 weeks for toenails.
  - Fluconazole 3 to 6 mg/kg once weekly for 6 to 8 weeks for fingernails or 12 weeks for toenails (Rostan & Fitzpatrick, 2002).

4. Ciclopirox in nail lacquer (Penlac) used daily is a new agent that has high cure rates in adults but has not been studied in children (Rostan & Fitzpatrick, 2002; Weston, Lane, & Morelli, 2002).
5. If triazoles are used, a careful review of current medications must be taken because there are many interactions. Monitoring of CBC and hepatic function is recommended at onset of therapy and every 4 to 6 weeks.
6. *Candida* infection is treated with topical application of ketoconazole (Nizoral) under occlusion (plastic glove covered by a cotton sock at bedtime) for 3 to 4 weeks.
7. Follow-up visits at 1-month intervals to monitor laboratory values are recommended; long-term follow-up every 6 months is suggested.

Patient Education, Prognosis, and Prevention

The unfortunate truth to communicate is that cure is difficult to obtain and relapse is common.

Paronychia

Description

Chronic or acute inflammation and infection around a fingernail or toenail is called *paronychia.*

Etiology and Incidence

Infection of a nail with bacteria (often *S. aureus,* occasionally *Streptococcus* or *Pseudomonas*), *Candida* (in infants with thrush or thumb-sucking or when hands are immersed in water a lot), or herpes is common in school-age children and adolescents. It is more common with tight shoes or when nails are malaligned, cut with rounded edges, or too short.

Clinical Findings

History. Tenderness and drainage are reported, as well as discomfort, especially with walking.

Physical Examination. Findings include the following:

- Proximal nail fold erythematous, swollen, and tender; if chronic, may not be tender
- Purulent exudate expressed
- Cuticle broken or absent
- Nontender erythema and edema with thickened, disrupted nail (*Candida* infection, often with secondary bacterial infection)

Laboratory Studies. A culture of the exudate is occasionally done.

Differential Diagnosis

Herpetic whitlow (grouped vesicules on an erythematous base) and eczematous inflammation should be ruled out.

Management

Management includes the following:

- Systemic oral antibiotic if acute infection.
- If *Candida* is suspected, nystatin cream under occlusion (a plastic glove covered by a cotton stocking) every night for 3 to 4 weeks.
- If purulent area is full, loosen cuticle from nail with a no. 11 blade to allow exudate to escape.
- Frequent warm soaks, after which cotton pledgets are inserted beneath the nail to lift it up.
- Instruction on proper trimming of nails and care of toenails:
  - Wear wide-toed shoes.
  - Trim nails straight across and not too short.
  - If condition is recurrent, refer for surgical removal of lateral portion of nail.
- Follow-up visit in 1 month.

Complications

Recurrent infection is possible.

BODY ART

Tattoos and Body Piercing

Description

A tattoo is an indelible mark fixed on the body by insertion of pigment under the skin. Body piercing is the creation of a hole anywhere in the body (typically the ear, eyebrow, lip, naris, tongue, navel, nipple, or genitalia) to insert jewelry. Both tattoos and piercing are considered forms of *body art,* or embellishment of one's appearance, that have been practiced throughout the ages in many cultures as rites of passage, as means of showing status or membership in a particular group, or as proof of virility.

Etiology and Incidence

A tattoo is accomplished by injection of an insoluble ink via a uniform series of punctures into the dermal layer of the skin. Piercing is accomplished by inserting a sharp implement through the skin. Most tattoos or piercings are done in unregulated, unlicensed tattoo parlors, although some adolescents may tattoo or pierce themselves or their peers. Some states have legislation preventing tattooing of minors in tattoo parlors or requiring parental consent.

Questioned as to why they obtained tattoos, 81% of adolescents in one study related it to "personal identity, be myself; I don't need to impress people any more" (Armstrong & Murphy, 1998). Four reasons given by adolescents for body piercing are as follows: "it is a form of body art," "it is fashionable," "it makes a personal statement," and "it is daring" (Armstrong, 1996). Piercing is considered less permanent than a tattoo. Adults and parents may see piercing or tattooing as a deviant behavior, a strange new trend, a fetish, a fad, or a fashion (Muldoon, 1997).

Both tattooing and piercing have an increased incidence in the United States, especially in the adolescent population. Ten percent to 13% of adolescents 12 to 18 years of age have tattoos (Carroll et al, 2002). The average age at first tattoo is 14 years; the average age at first piercing is 15 years (Armstrong & Murphy, 1998; Armstrong & Pace Murphy, 1997).

A study by Carroll and colleagues (2002) surveying 484 teenagers found that teens who participate in piercing, tattooing, and branding are also more likely to engage in other risk-taking behaviors such as eating disorders, drug use, increased sexual activity, and suicide. Of note, as the number of body piercings increased, the use of drugs increased.

Clinical Findings

History. Questions to discuss include the following:

- When and where was the body art obtained?
- Where is it located and what care is being given?
- Were there any complications?

Physical Examination. Any symptoms of infection—erythema, crusting, or scabs?

Differential Diagnosis

Branding, the burning of the skin aimed at creating a permanent scar in a desired design via blowtorch or wire coat hanger in hot oil, is one differential diagnosis. *Self-mutilation*, a self-directed violence that ranges from altering physical appearance (e.g., ear piercing) to extreme forms (e.g., amputation), is another consideration. Some forms are considered normal, but deviant forms are physically damaging, done in response to crisis, and demonstrate disconnectedness and alienation from others (Dallam, 1997).

Management

1. Aftercare for tattoos:
- Perform basic wound care, including not touching for 24 hours.
- A moderate amount of oozing and local swelling is normal for 48 hours.
- Scab should be left alone except for the application of ointment.
- Protect from rough surfaces that can traumatize; protect from sunburn.
- Review signs and symptoms of infection.

2. Aftercare for body piercings (Table 37-12):
- Wash hands before touching; wash area with soap twice daily.
- A moderate amount of oozing and swelling is normal; if crusts appear, remove with wet swab.
- Tongue:
  - Use ice to minimize swelling.
  - Rinse mouth 10 to 12 times a day with half-strength Listerine, twice a day with carbamide peroxide (Gly-Oxide).
  - No deep kissing for 48 hours; once healed, use dental dams for dental work and avoid smoking.

TABLE 37-12 *Healing Time for Body Piercings*

Type of Piercing	Time to Heal
Cheek	2-4 mo
Clitoris	4-10 wk
Ear cartilage	2 mo-1 yr
Ear lobe	6-8 wk
Eyebrow	6-8 wk
Frenum (underneath tongue)	2-6 mo
Inner labia	4-8 wk
Lip	2-3 mo
Male genitalia	4 wk-6 mo
Nasal septum	6-8 mo
Nasal bridge	8-10 wk
Navel	2 mo-1 yr
Nipple	2-6 mo
Nostril	2 mo-1 yr
Outer labia	2-4 mo
Tongue	4-6 wk

Data from Martel S, Anderson JE: Decorating the "human canvas": body art and your patient, *Contemp Pediatr* 19(8):86-102, 2002; Schnare SM: Tattooing, branding, and body piercing, *Womens Health Care* 1(4), 2002.

- Navel:
  - Slowest to heal, most likely area to reject jewelry.
  - Cleanse twice a day with antibacterial soap.
  - Avoid handling; avoid clothing that rubs for up to 1 year.
- Nipples and genitalia:
  - Cleanse twice a day with antibacterial soap twice a day.
  - Avoid manipulation and tight garments; cotton clothes are ideal.
  - Latex barriers must be used with sexual activity.

3. Healing times are variable and should be considered. A tattoo may take 2 to 3 weeks to heal. Body piercing, depending on the site, can take from 4 to 8 weeks for ears, to 6 to 12 months for navel and genital piercings.
4. Infection can be treated with dicloxacillin 500 mg four times a day for 10 days. Whether or not to remove jewelry should be decided by whether it will provide a source of chronic drainage, become an obstacle to healing, or be an ongoing source of infection.
5. Screen for high-risk behaviors.

Complications

The most common complications of tattooing or body piercing include infections, allergic reactions to the dyes or jewelry, and the transmission of blood-borne diseases, primarily hepatitis B and C, and, potentially, HIV. Other reported complications of tattoos include skin neoplasms, syphilis, leprosy, cutaneous tuberculosis, tetanus, hyperplasia, and granuloma annulare. Complications of piercings also include excessive bleeding, nerve damage, keloids, dental fracture, soft tissue damage, and speech impediments.

Patient Education, Prognosis, and Prevention

Providing information and encouraging teenagers to thoroughly research and consider the idea of getting a tattoo or body piercing is an important area of education. Removal of tattoos is expensive, not necessarily completely successful, and fraught with complication (scarring, rashes). Box 37-13 is a helpful handout that covers much of the important information to be discussed. Maintaining an

BOX 37-13 *So You're Thinking about Getting a Tattoo or Body Piercing*

Know the Facts: Make an Informed Decision

Unsterile tattooing and piercing equipment and needles can spread serious infections, hepatitis, or possibly even human immunodeficiency virus (HIV).

The law in many states prohibits the tattooing of minors.

Asking a friend to apply a tattoo may ruin a friendship if the tattoo doesn't look like you thought it would.

Tattoos and permanent makeup are not easily removed and in some cases may cause permanent discoloration. Think carefully before getting a tattoo.

Tattoo removal is very expensive. A tattoo that costs $50 to apply may cost over $1,000 to remove.

Blood donations cannot be made for 1 year after getting a tattoo, body piercing, or permanent makeup.

Before You Get a Tattoo or Body Piercing

First: Talk to your friends or others who have been tattooed or pierced.
Ask them about their experience, the cost, pain, healing time, and so on.
Ask them what they would do if they had a chance to do it over again.

Second: Understand that you do not have to tattoo or pierce your body to belong.
Remember that you are directly involved in decisions that affect your health and body.
You can always change your mind or wait if you are not sure.

Third: Because of potential complications, if you decide to get a tattoo or body piercing, never tattoo or pierce your own body or let a friend do it.

Health Risks to Consider Before You Act

Both tattooing and piercing involve puncturing the skin to introduce a foreign material, jewelry, or ink, and the procedures carry similar risks. The primary health concern is introducing blood-borne germs or viruses into your body.

Blood-borne illnesses such as hepatitis B and C, tetanus, tuberculosis, and HIV infection can lead to serious health problems or death.

Localized infections such as *Staphylococcus* or *Pseudomonas* infection can lead to illness, deformity, and scarring.

Continued

BOX 37-13 *So You're Thinking about Getting a Tattoo or Body Piercing—cont'd*

Tattoo troubles: Tattoos are open wounds that may become infected. The new tattoo must be kept clean. It must also be kept moist with an ointment to prevent a scab from forming. If you are allergic to the inks in the tattoo, the site will not heal properly and scarring may occur.

Piercing problems: Complications depend on where the body has been pierced. Navel infections are the most common; it takes approximately 1 year for navel piercings to heal. Ear cartilage heals slowly. Tongue piercings may lead to tooth damage from biting on the jewelry, partial paralysis if the jewelry pierces a nerve, and extreme inflammation during the first few days.

Selecting a Tattoo Artist or Piercer

Visit several piercers or tattooists. The work area should be kept clean and have good lighting. If they refuse to discuss cleanliness and infection control with you, go somewhere else.

Consent forms (which the customer must fill out) should be handled before tattooing. Reputable piercing and tattoo studios will not serve a minor without signed consent from parents. Check the laws in your state about tattooing of minors if you are under 18.

The tattooist or piercer should have an *autoclave*—a heat sterilization machine used to sterilize equipment between customers.

Packaged, sterilized needles should be used only once and then disposed of in a biohazard container.

Immediately before tattooing or piercing, the tattooist or piercer should wash and dry his or her hands and wear latex gloves. These gloves should be worn at all times during the tattoo or piercing procedure. If the tattoo artist or piercer leaves the procedure or touches other objects, such as the telephone, new gloves should be put on before the procedure continues.

A piercing gun should not be used because it cannot be sterilized properly. Only jewelry made of a noncorrosive metal, such as surgical stainless steel, niobium, or solid 14-karat gold, is safe for a new piercing.

Leftover tattoo ink should be disposed of after each procedure. Ink should never be poured back into the bottle and reused.

By Barbara Freyenberger in Armstrong ML, Murphy KP: Adolescent tattooing, *Prev Researcher* 5(3):1-4, 1998.

RESOURCE BOX

Dermatologic Conditions

American Academy of Dermatology
1-800-462-DERM
1-312-856-8888
www.aad.org
www.coppertone.com
"Block the Sun, Not the Fun" program available

Association of Professional Piercers
519 Castro Street, Box 120
San Francisco, CA 94114
www.safepiercing.com

Cancer Research Foundation of America
1-703-836-4412
www.preventcancer.org/kids

Cancer Research Institute or Cancer Care, Inc. (Melanoma Initiative)
1-800-813-HOPE
www.preventcancer.org/index.cfm

Dermatology Links
www.slider.com/Health/Medicine/Medical_Specialties/Dermatology_2e.htm

Dermatology Online Atlas/Erlangen University
www.derma.med.uni-erlangen.de/bilddb/
Extensive online image database with more than 500 diagnoses; search engine for diagnosis

Dermatology Online Journal
www.dermatology.cdlib.org
Printed journal format with editorials, articles, case reports, and original articles

Electronic Textbook of Dermatology
www.telemedicine.org/stamford.htm
From the Internet Dermatology Society

RESOURCE BOX

Dermatologic Conditions—cont'd

FIRST: Foundation for Ichthyosis and Related Skin Types
1-800-545-3286
1-610-789-3995
www.scalyskin.org
Newsletter, informational materials (including Spanish), networking, referrals to local resources, advocacy, funds research, maintains research registry

Hemangioma Hope
c/o Cindy Dougan
1-814-898-1054
www.hemangiomahope.org
Newsletter, informational materials, networking

National Alopecia Areata Foundation
1-415-456-4644
www.alopeciaareata.com
Newsletter, informational materials (including Spanish), networking, local chapters, advocacy, funds research

National Organization for Albinism and Hypopigmentation (NOAH)
1-800-473-2310
www.albinism.org
Newsletter, informational materials, chapters, advocacy, research

National Pediculosis Association (NPA)
1-718-449-NITS (1-718-449-6487)
www.headlice.org

National Psoriasis Foundation
1-503-244-7404
www.psoriasis.org
Newsletter, informational materials, networking, referrals to local resources, advocacy, funds research, maintains research registry

National Vitiligo Foundation
1-903-534-2925
www.nvfi.org

Nevus Network
1-703-492-0253
www.nevusnetwork.org
Newsletter, informational materials (including Spanish, French), networking, funds research, maintains research registry

OC (Obsessive-Compulsive) Foundation (information on trichotillomania)
1-203-878-5669
www.trich.org/home/default.asp
Newsletter, informational materials, networking, referrals to local resources, advocacy, local chapters, funds research

Skin Cancer Foundation
1-212-725-5176
www.skincancer.org

Trichotillomania Learning Center
www.trich.org

Trichotillomania: A Guide
www.miminc.org

open, nonjudgmental attitude in discussing the options and in caring for adolescents who have body art is also essential. Alternatives to discuss include temporary stick-on tattoos and use of henna or other body paints (Montgomery & Parks, 2001).

REFERENCES

Achauer BM, VanderKam VM: Treating vascular birth marks with laser surgery, *Contemp Pediatr* 17(3):91-109, 2000.

American Academy of Pediatrics: *2003 red book: report of the Committee on Infectious Diseases*, ed 26, Elk Grove Village, IL, 2003, American Academy of Pediatrics.

American Academy of Pediatrics: Clinical report: head lice, *Pediatrics* 110(3):638-643, 2002.

Armstrong ML: You pierced what? *Pediatr Nurs* 22(3):236-238, 1996.

Armstrong ML, Murphy KP: Adolescent tattooing, *Prev Researcher* 5(3):1-4, 1998.

Armstrong ML, Pace Murphy KP: Tattooing and other adolescent risk behavior warranting health education, *Appl Nurs Res* 10:181-189, 1997.

Bell TA: Ivermectin and the LiceMeister Comb in the treatment of resistant pediculosis, *Pediatr Infect Dis J* 17:923, 1998.

Bittencourt FV et al: Large congenital melanocytic nevi and the risk for development of malignant melanoma and neurocutaneous melanocytosis, *Pediatrics* 106(4):736-741, 2000.

Bloomfield D: Head lice, *Pediatr Rev* 23(1):34-35, 2002.

Carroll ST et al: Tattoos and body piercings as indicators of adolescent risk-taking behaviors, *Pediatrics* 109(6):1021-1027, 2002.

Centers for Disease Control and Prevention: Treating head lice, 2002. Available at *www.dpd.cdc.gov/dpdx/html/headline.htm* (accessed Nov 6, 2002).

Chamlin SL: Shedding light on moles, melanoma, and the sun, *Contemp Pediatr* 19(6):102-114, 2002.

Chen N, Cunningham BB: Psoriasis: finding the right approach for your patients, *Contemp Pediatr* 18(8):86-93, 2001.

Cokkinides VE et al: Use of indoor tanning sunlamps by US youth, ages 11-18 years, and by their parent or guardian caregivers: prevalance and correlates, *Pediatrics* 109(6):1124-1130, 2002.

Dallam SJ: The identification and management of self-mutilating patients in primary care, *Nurse Pract* 22(5):151-164, 1997.

Darmstadt GL, Sidbury R: The skin. In Behrman RE, Kliegman RM, Jenson HB, editors: *Nelson textbook of pediatrics*, ed 17, Philadelphia, 2004, WB Saunders.

Dinulos JG, Graham EA: Influence of culture and pigment on skin conditions in children, *Pediatr Rev* 19(8):268-275, 1998.

Dodd CS: Interventions for treating head lice. Cochran Library, Oxford: Update Software, 2002. Available at *www.medscape.com/newarticle/435115* (accessed Nov 6, 2002).

Gardiner P, Coles D, Kemper KJ: The skinny on herbal remedies for dermatologic disease, *Contemp Pediatr* 18(7):103-114, 2001.

Geller AC et al: Use of sunscreen, sunburning rates, and tanning bed use among more than 10,000 US children and adolescents, *Pediatrics* 109(6):1009-1014, 2002.

Glanz K, Saraiya M, Wechsler H: Guidelines for school programs to prevent skin cancer, *MMWR Morb Mortal Wkly Rep* 51(RR04):1-16, 2002.

Hansen RC et al: Dealing with diaper dermatitis, *Contemp Pediatr* May supplement:5-10, 1998.

Hartley AA: Pityriasis rosea, *Pediatr Rev* 20(8):266-269, 1999.

Hurwitz S: *Clinical pediatric dermatology*, ed 2, Philadelphia, 1993, WB Saunders.

Jarvis C: *Physical examination and assessment*, ed 2, Philadelphia, 1996, WB Saunders.

Kim HJ, Ghali FE, Tunnessen WW: Here comes the sun, *Contemp Pediatr* 14(7):41-69, 1997.

Kristal L, Silverberg N: Acne: simplifying a complex disorder, *Contemp Pediatr* (suppl):3-10, 1998.

Kurtz ML: Treatment of herpes zoster. Personal communication, Nov 2002.

Lebwohl M et al: *Treatment of skin disease*, St Louis, 2002, Mosby.

Leickly FE: When the road gets bumpy: managing chronic urticaria, *Contemp Pediatr* 17(5):58-73, 2000.

Mancini AJ: Acne vulgaris: a treatment update, *Contemp Pediatr* 17(12):122-133, 2000.

Martel S, Anderson JE: Decorating the "human canvas": body art and your patient, *Contemp Pediatr* 19(8):86-102, 2002.

Messinger ML: Trichotillomania, *Pediatr Rev* 20(7):249-250, 1999.

Mikula C: Balneo phototherapy for psoriasis: modern application of an age-old treatment, *Adv Nurse Pract* 11(1):53-56, 2003.

Montgomery DF, Parks D: Tattoos: Counseling the adolescent, *J Pediatr Health Care* 15(1):14-19, 2001.

Morelli JG: Resistance to enythromycin in acne. Personal communication, Nov 2002.

Morelli JG, Weston WL: Sun, kids, moles, and melanoma, *Contemp Pediatr* 16(6):61-76, 1999.

Morgan-Glenn PD: Scabies, *Pediatr Rev* 22(9):322-323, 2001.

Muldoon KA: Body piercing in adolescents, *J Pediatr Health Care* 11:298-301, 1997.

Myers MG, Stanberry LR, Seward JF: Varicella-zoster virus. In Behrman RG, Kliegman RM, Jenson HB, editors: *Nelson textbook of pediatrics*, ed 17, Philadelphia, 2004, WB Saunders.

National Pediculosis Association: AAP issues guidelines allowing children in school with lice and nits, 2002a. Available at *www.headlice.org/news/aapresponse.htm* (accessed Oct 30, 2002).

National Pediculosis Association: Lindane educational research network, 2002b. Available at *www.headlice.org/lindane/index.htm* (accessed Oct 30, 2002).

Orchard D, Weston WL: The importance of vehicle in pediatric topical therapy, *Pediatr Ann* 30(4):208-210, 2001.

Paller A: Dermatologic problems. In Dershewitz RA, editor: *Ambulatory pediatric care*, ed 3, Philadelphia, 1999, Lippincott-Raven.

Physician's desk reference for nonprescription drugs and dietary supplements, ed 23, Montvale, NJ, 2002, Thomson Medical Economics.

Pollack RJ, Kiszewski A, Spielman A: Overdiagnosis and consequent mismanagement of head louse infestations in North America, *Pediatr Infect Dis J* 19:689-693, 2000.

Richards CA: Some antibiotics are commonly associated with skin rashes, *Infect Dis Child* 12(2):24-25, 1999.

Rostan EF, Fitzpatrick RE: Fungal infections of the skin. In Burg FD et al, editors: *Gellis and Kagan's current pediatric therapy*, ed 17, Philadelphia, 2002, WB Saunders.

Schnare SM: Tattooing, branding, and body piercing, *Womens Health Care* 1(4), 2002.

Schwade S: Reports of resistant scabies out of proportion, *Pediatr News* 33:21, 1999.

Smith W, Burns C: Managing the hair and skin of African American pediatric patients, *J Pediatr Health Care* 13(2):72-78, 1999.

Spray A, Siegfried E: Dermatologic toxicology in children, *Pediatr Ann* 30(4):197-202, 2001.

Taketomo CK, Hodding JH, Kraus DM: *Pediatric dosage handbook*, ed 9, Hudson, OH, 2002, Lexi-Comp.

Tekin M, Bodurtha JN, Riccardi VM: Café-au-lait spots: pediatrician's perspective, *Pediatr Rev* 22(3):82-89, 2001.

Thomson L: Hypnosis for habit disorders, *Adv Nurse Pract* 10(7):59-62, 2002.

Weinberg S: Secondary infection often occurs with diaper dermatitis, *Infect Dis J* 11:42-43, 1998.

Weston WL, Badgett JT: Urticaria, *Pediatr Rev* 19:240-244, 1998.

Weston WL, Lane AT, Morelli JG: *Color textbook of pediatric dermatology*, ed 3, St Louis, 2002, Mosby.

Whitaker H, Wolf KA, Keuthen N: Chronic hair pulling: recognizing trichotillomania, *Clin Rev* 13(3):37-44, 2003.

Williams LK, Reichart A, Mackenzie WR, et al: Lice, nits, and school policy, *Pediatrics* 107(5):1011-1015, 2001.

Wolf RL: Urticaria, angioedema, anaphylaxis, and serum sickness. In Dershewitz RA, editor: *Ambulatory pediatric care*, ed 3, Philadelphia, 1999, Lippincott-Raven.

Working Group on Prevention of Invasive Group A Streptococcal Infections: Prevention of invasive group A streptococcal disease among household contacts of case-patients, *JAMA* 279:1206-1210, 1998.

Wynne AL, Woo TM, Millard M: P*harmacotherapeutics for nurse practitioner prescribers*, Philadelphia, 2002, FA Davis.

38

Musculoskeletal Disorders

Margaret A. Brady, Catherine E. Burns

Orthopedic conditions in children are disruptions to the major structural system of the body. A variety of conditions can cause orthopedic findings, including child abuse. There also can be iatrogenic deformities that result from cultural practices such as using a cradleboard. Disorders of the musculoskeletal system present unique problems, because growth and development of this system contribute to the evolution of pathology over time. For example, untreated developmental dysplasia of the hip results in derangement of the hip socket with limping and eventual wearing away of the femoral head. Limited mobility, pain, and deformity interfere with the lifestyle of the child. Children with functional disability may not be able to fully participate in all activities with peers and family or have access to various occupations. They may also face challenges related to self-esteem. Nurse practitioners (NPs) must be vigilant and seek to help children and their families avoid these problems.

NPs play a significant role in the management of children with orthopedic problems, although, in many cases, specialists manage specific conditions. The NP assesses development of the musculoskeletal system, identifies problems for early intervention, focuses on lifestyle and injury prevention, monitors the long-term outcomes of orthopedic care, and helps the family to integrate orthopedic care with the daily living activities at home and school. Assisting the family to cope with the issues of disability, deformity, and long-term care is another important role that must be addressed in the care of these children.

ANATOMY AND PHYSIOLOGY

Ossification of the fetal skeleton begins during the fifth month of gestation. The clavicles and skull bones are the first to ossify, followed by the long bones and spine. Bone age, measured by radiographs of the wrists, can be used to quantitatively determine somatic maturation and serves as a mirror that reflects the tempo of growth. In adolescents, the skeletal growth spurt begins at about Tanner stage 2 in girls and Tanner stage 3 in boys. It is at its peak around stage 4 and then ends with stage 5. The growth spurt lasts longer in boys than in girls. The pelvis widens early in pubescent girls. In both sexes, the legs usually lengthen before the thighs broaden. Next, the shoulders widen and the trunk completes its linear growth. Bone growth ends when the epiphyses close.

Long bones have a growth plate, or physis, at each end, which separates the epiphysis from the diaphysis or shaft. Openings through this plate allow blood vessels to penetrate from the epiphysis. In the growth plate, chrondrocytes produce cartilage cells, dead cells are absorbed, and the calcified cartilage matrix is converted into bone. The entire growth plate area is weaker than the remaining bone, because it is less calcified. Because the blood supply to the growth plate comes primarily through the epiphysis, damage to epiphyseal circulation can jeopardize the survival of the chondrocytes. If chondrocytes stop producing, growth of the bone in that area stops (Fig. 38-1).

The length of long bones comes from growth at the epiphyseal plates. The diameter of long bones increases as a result of deposition of new bone on the periosteal surface and resorption on the surface of the medullary cavity. Growth of the small bones, hip, and spine comes from one or more primary ossification centers in each bone. Apophyses are the sites for connection of tendons to bone. In children, these sites, similar to epiphyses, allow for growth and are weaker than bone. These sites can become inflamed with stress.

The development of bones and muscles is influenced by use. Thus, in infants and toddlers, the legs straighten and

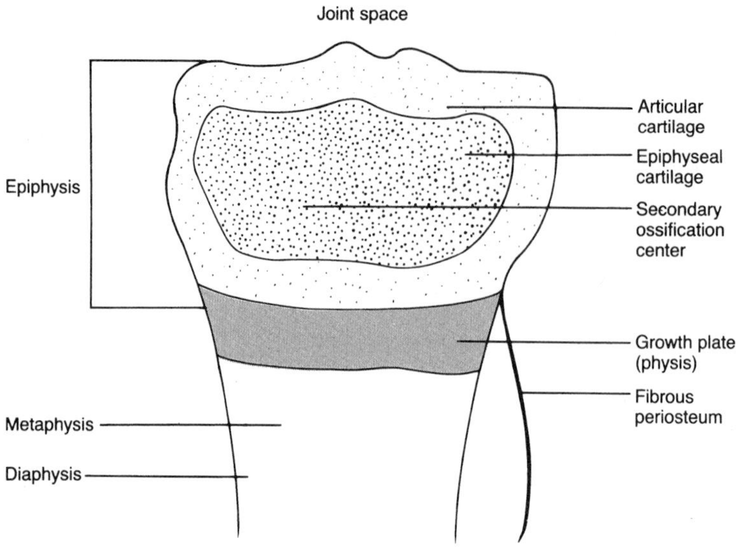

FIGURE 38-1 Anatomy of long bones. (Modified from Shapiro F: Epiphyseal disorders, *N Engl J Med* 317:1702-1710, 1987.)

lengthen with the stimulus of weight bearing and independent walking. The infant is born with the full complement of muscle fibers. Growth in muscle length results from lengthening of the fibers, and growth in bulk comes from hypertrophy. Length of muscles is related to growth in length of the underlying bone. If a limb is not used, it grows minimally. Furthermore, if muscles and bones are not used in their intended normal manner, such as occurs with spastic diplegia, the forces for development tend to stimulate growth in abnormal patterns. Thus scoliosis can develop or bowlegs may increase in severity. Muscle contractures occur if muscles are not used regularly and put through their full range of motion. The growth of fibrous tissue, tendons, and ligaments is also dependent on mechanical demands.

PATHOPHYSIOLOGY AND DEFENSE MECHANISMS

Pathophysiology

Muscles and bones can be affected by localized or systemic problems. Thus the initial orthopedic problem can be symptomatic of a larger problem.

Systemic Problems

Systemic problems can include chronic conditions, such as hemophilia, sickle cell disease, and arthritic diseases; neurologic problems, such as cerebral palsy; and various cancers, including osteosarcomas and leukemias. Children with metabolic problems such as vitamin D–resistant rickets have bony deformities. Acute systemic problems can also affect the musculoskeletal system. For example, viruses and bacteria can infect joints and bones. In developing countries, tubercular infections of bones are common and devastating. Thus the NP must assess patients from a broad perspective, asking questions about other body systems and ordering appropriate laboratory studies that might identify systemic problems.

Genetic Problems

Many genetic problems have an orthopedic component. For example, osteogenesis imperfecta is a genetically based orthopedic condition known for multiple fractures. Children with Down syndrome are more likely to have hip problems. Children with Marfan syndrome have defective connective tissue, have disproportionately long limbs, and may develop scoliosis or dislocate a patella. Severe scoliosis may develop in children with neurofibromatosis. Mucopolysaccharidosis disorders and other syndromes, such as Turner and Noonan, can result in affected children having short stature.

Many orthopedic problems have a multifactorial inheritance pattern. Thus, if one child in a family has a dislocated hip or scoliosis, the risks increase for other children and offspring. The NP needs to understand the genetic disorder in order to monitor related orthopedic problems, consider the genetic implications, and provide families with appropriate genetic information or refer them for genetic counseling (see Chapter 41).

Uterine Packing Deformations

The developing fetus moves its body parts frequently, and this movement influences musculoskeletal development. When the baby fills the uterine space, movements are restricted and body parts begin to assume the shape in which they are fixed. Because much of the bony structure is cartilaginous, molding occurs with relative ease. Thus the tibia are normally bowed. Occasionally, a foot is turned awkwardly, the legs might be fixed straight up with the feet near the ears, or the neck may be tipped to one side. The outcomes are deformities in various degrees. The longer the position is maintained, the more severe the problems are. In general, there is a tendency for bowing and late deformations to straighten. More severe deformities need to be referred to orthopedists for treatment as soon as they are found because a softer skeleton is easier to realign in a positive direction.

Injuries

Ligamentous injuries can produce joint instability. Unstable joints should always be referred to an orthopedist. The most common injuries to muscles produce bleeding in the muscle, at the muscle-tendon junctions, or at tendon insertion points. Muscle hematomas generally heal in 3 weeks, but significant muscle bleeding can lead to scarring. Injuries sufficient to produce significant soft tissue damage also can damage the underlying bone.

Trauma to the bone can cause a fracture, dislocation of the epiphysis (an orthopedic emergency), or damage to the periosteum covering the bone, with bleeding in the space between the two tissues. The effects of fractures through the growth plates of long bones is discussed later in this chapter. Fractures that are misaligned generally have related soft tissue damage. Damage to the nerves and vascular supply must be carefully assessed. Management of traumatic injuries is discussed in Chapter 40.

The possibility of child abuse should always be considered when orthopedic injuries, especially fractures, are present. The rule of thumb is that the injury history should match the appearance of the problem and be consistent with the child's developmental capabilities. Certain injuries, such as spiral fractures of the long bones, are especially suspect, because few independent activities of the child can produce these injuries. They occur with wrenching motions such as when a child's arm or leg has been jerked. Multiple fractures in various stages of healing must be considered evidence of child abuse until proved otherwise. In contrast to intentionally inflicted injuries associated with fracturing, toddler fractures are typically accidental spiral fractures of the distal one third of the tibia and are often the result of a simple fall associated with running or playing or stepping on an object on the floor. This type of accidental injury occurs in the 2- to 4-year-old child, occasionally up to 6 years of age (Behrman, Kliegman, & Jenson, 2004).

Defense Mechanisms

Fracture Healing

Fractures heal by the creation of a callus at the fracture site. The process is the same in children as in adults. However, children produce callus more quickly than adults do. Likewise, young children heal faster because of their growth potential and thicker, more metabolically active periostium. When the fracture occurs, there is damage to the blood vessels, destruction of bone matrix, and death of bone cells adjoining the fracture site. The body reabsorbs the clot and dead cells, while the periostium responds by producing new fibroblasts that invade the fracture site. Immature bone is formed with irregular trabeculae, creating the callus. Normal stresses then cause the bone to remodel into the optimal shape, and the callus bone is gradually replaced by lamellar bone.

Growth Plate Fractures. Fractures of the long bones can produce permanent deformities in children if the fracture occurs through the growth plate. The outcomes depend on the fracture location and type, the age of the child, the status of the blood supply to the physis, and the treatment. The Salter-Harris classification is used to describe epiphyseal fractures, which are divided into five types (Fig. 38-2). The number is a guide to the frequency of that type of fracture, as well as an indicator of the prognosis for further epiphyseal growth. Thus type I is the most frequent type of epiphyseal injury and has a good prognosis; type V is the rarest type of epiphyseal fracture and has the worst prognosis because it results in premature closure of the growth plate.

Type I fractures involve a separation through the physis; type II fractures occur when there is a shearing force applied that fractures a portion of the physis with extension through the metaphyses. For both types, part of the perichondrium is preserved, and the blood supply to the growth plate is maintained. With no disruption to the growth plate, there will be no permanent, worsening deformity as the child grows. Type I and II fractures do not require perfect anatomic alignment to heal with a good functional prognosis. Closed reduction is generally the treatment for type I and II fractures; a type II fracture of the distal femur, however, requires anatomic alignment by either open or closed reduction.

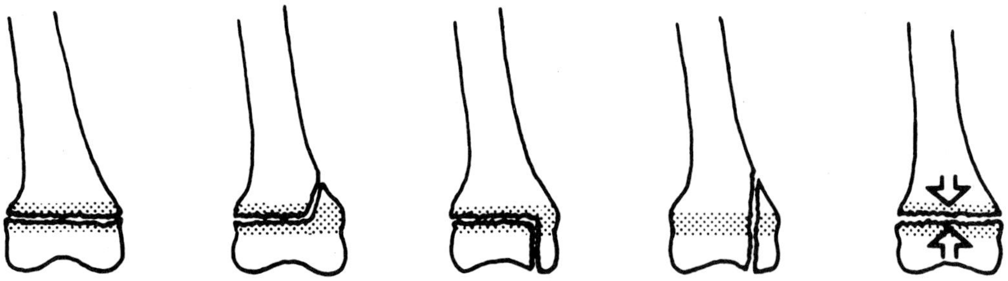

FIGURE 38-2 Salter fracture types. Salter-Harris classification of epiphyseal fractures. Type I: The epiphysis separates from the metaphysis. The germinal cells remain with the epiphysis, usually uninjured. Healing is rapid and growth is seldom arrested. Type II: Similar to type I, except that a small piece of metaphysis breaks free to remain with the epiphysis. Healing is rapid, and growth is usually normal. Types I and II are the most common. Type III: Separation passes a variable distance along the growth plate and then enters the joint. Accurate reduction of the intraarticular fracture is necessary to prevent lateral traumatic arthritis. Open reduction may be needed. Growth disturbances are not usually a problem. Type IV: The fracture extends from the joint across the growth plate and into the metaphysis. This usually requires open reduction to prevent unilateral growth arrest and traumatic arthritis from malposition. Type V: This is a crushing injury that leads to death of the germinal cells of the epiphyseal cartilage and arrest of growth. This type is rare. (From Behrman R, editor: *Nelson textbook of pediatrics*, ed 14, Philadelphia, 1992, WB Saunders.)

Type III involves fracture through a portion of the physis with extension to the epiphysis and into the joint. Type IV fractures involve the metaphysis, physis, and epiphysis. Types III and IV are more serious fractures that must be promptly realigned, usually with open reduction, to prevent growth arrest. The prognosis for types III and IV is fair and depends on the severity of the injury and the accuracy in achieving anatomic alignment through open reduction. Growth arrest and progressive deformities can result from these fractures.

Type V fractures are rare but have serious effects when they occur. This fracture results from a crush injury to the physis, often from a fall from a height, and the growth plate cells are crushed. No further growth occurs at that growth plate unless the epiphyseal blood supply was preserved. Sometimes this fracture is missed on radiographic study because no fracture line can be discerned (Behrman, Kliegman, & Jenson, 2004).

Shaft Fractures. There is a tendency for the long bones to remold into the most normal position possible when they are fractured in places along the shaft. Young children may not fracture bones all the way across (the greenstick fracture). As with adults, young children can experience complete fractures or stress fractures. Complete fractures are common in children and occur when both sides of the bones are fractured. Their classification depends on the direction of the line of fracturing with a spiral, transverse, oblique, or comminuted pattern of fracture (Behrman, Kliegman, & Jenson, 2004).

ASSESSMENT OF THE ORTHOPEDIC SYSTEM

See Table 38-1 for orthopedic terminology.

History

- History of present illness
  - Onset: appearance of first symptoms; insidious or sudden; association with injury or strain; accompanied by any constitutional symptoms or signs (e.g., fever, malaise, swelling, ecchymosis)
  - Pain: location and character, course of radiation, severity, extent of disability produced, effect of various activities including weight bearing, relief measures, changes from day to night or from day to day, child's refusing to move the painful part or assuming a pain-relieving position, effects of previous treatment, presence of pain or discomfort in other parts of the body
  - Deformity: character (swelling, inflammation, contracture, joint stiffness, unusual positioning, appearance); first appearance and who noted it; association with injury or disease; rate of change; extent of disability; a cosmetic problem or a cause of embarrassment
  - Injury: how, when (time and date), why, and where; mechanism or manner in which injury was produced

TABLE 38-1 ***Orthopedic Terminology***

Descriptive Terms for Positions

Term	Definition
Abduction	Movement away from midline
Adduction	Movement toward midline
Dorsiflexion	Movement of toes/foot or fingers/hand toward dorsal surface (up)
Eversion	Same as pronation: palmar surface turned away from midline
External rotation	Turning anterior surface of limb outward or away from midline
Internal rotation	Turning anterior surface of limb inward or toward midline
Inversion	Same as supination: palmar surface turned toward midline
Luxation	Dislocation
Plantar flexion	Movement of toes/foot or fingers/hand toward plantar surface (down or toes pointed)
Pronation	Palmar surface turned downward or toward posterior surface of body
Subluxation	Partial dislocation
Supination	Palmar surface turned upward or toward anterior surface of body
Valgus	Deviation away from midline, a >< shape of the two legs, for instance
Varus	Deviation toward midline, a <> shape of the two legs, for instance

Descriptive Positions for Parts of Long Bone

Term	Definition
Apophysis	Insertion point of tendon on long bone
Diaphysis	Shaft or middle part of long bone
Epiphysis	Distal side of growth plate, a secondary ossification center separated from parent bone
Metaphysis	Proximal side of growth plate, on edge of parent bone
Perichondrium	Membrane of fibrous connective tissue surrounding cartilage
Physis	Growth plate

Descriptive Terms for Feet

Term	Definition
Calcaneus	Ankle fixed in position of dorsiflexion (foot up)
Malleolus	Medial or lateral bony prominence of ankle
Pes cavus	Foot with a high arch
Pes planus	Flatfoot
Pronation	Foot where center of weight lies over medial side of foot rather than being centered—foot sags toward center; often associated with flatfoot
Talipes equinovarus	Clubfoot

  - Altered function: weakness, limp, decreased range of motion
  - Altered gait patterns: toe-walking, in-toeing or out-toeing
  - Other factors or constraints: type of shoe worn (e.g., platform shoes); use of backpack and amount of weight in backpack, amount of time spent at repetitive tasks or at computer station
- Family history
  - Any family members with musculoskeletal problems; many orthopedic problems have a genetic component
- Medical history
  - Pregnancy history and birth history: breech delivery, shoulder presentation, multiple births, oligohydramnios, asphyxia at birth
  - Development history: milestones met at appropriate age such as first walking and sitting
  - Illnesses, accidents or surgeries: trauma, meningitis, juvenile arthritis
- Review of systems
  - Any infections, constitutional diseases, or congenital problems that might have an orthopedic component

Physical Examination

Special orthopedic examination techniques are described in the following paragraphs.

Range-of-Motion Examination

Passive range of motion, in which the examiner moves the joint, provides information about joint mobility and stability. It can also provide information about the limits of tendons and muscles that are contracted. It is necessary to find the bony limits of movement. An excessive range of motion can indicate an unstable joint. Active range of motion, in which the child moves the joint, provides information about both muscle and bony structures working together for functional movement. To assess such problems as developmental dysplasia of the hip, passive range of motion must be used. Note pain, stiffness, limitations or deviations, and rigidity. The normal values of joint motion are age related, which must be kept in mind (e.g., external hip rotation is greatest in early infancy).

Gait Examination

Observe the child walking without shoes and with only minimal covering. Inspect from the front, side, and back as the child walks normally, on his or her toes, and then on heels. The gait should be smooth, rhythmic, and efficient. The gait cycle includes the heel-strike, foot-flat, toe-off, and swing phases. Ankle, knee, and hip movements should be symmetric and full with little side-to-side movement of the trunk.

The smaller child has a faster gait than the larger child, but less distance is covered with each stride. This is related to the smaller child's poorer balance. With a short, quick stride, each leg is off the ground for less time. The feet are spread wider and, in the toddler, the arms may be held up to increase balance. The mature pattern develops by about age 3 years.

Antalgic gaits serve to reduce stress or pain at the affected area. For example, the toe-off phase is restricted if the toe is sore. A Trendelenburg gait in which the trunk tips over the affected hip indicates hip disease and might or might not be painful, because it also involves muscle weakness around the hip joint.

Posture

To assess posture adequately, the child should be examined undressed to his or her underwear. The examiner needs to look at the child from the front, side, and back.

- Pelvis and hips should be level. Place hands on the iliac crest to test for a pelvic tilt caused by limb length discrepancy.
- Legs should be symmetric in shape and size. The patellae should be straight ahead.
- The feet should point straight ahead, with an imaginary line from the center of the heel through the second toe. There should be an arch (except in babies, in whom a fat pad obscures the arch) and straight heel cords.
- The spine should be straight, and the back should look symmetric, with shoulder and scapula heights and waist angles equal. There should be slight lordotic curves at the cervical and lumbar areas.

SPECIAL EXAMINATIONS

Hip Examinations

Galeazzi Maneuver

The Galeazzi maneuver includes flexing the hips and knees while the infant or child lies supine, placing the soles of the feet on the table near the buttocks, and then looking at the knee heights for equality (Fig. 38-3). The Galeazzi sign is positive if the knee heights are unequal.

Barlow Maneuver

The Barlow maneuver dislocates a dislocatable hip posteriorly. The hip is flexed, and the thigh is brought into an adducted position. From that position, the femoral head drops out of the acetabulum or can be gently pushed out of the socket. The dislocation should be palpable as it occurs. The maneuver needs to be done gently in a noncrying neonate in order to keep from damaging the femoral head. The hips should be examined one at a time. The hip generally spontaneously relocates after release of the posterior force.

Ortolani Maneuver

The Ortolani maneuver can be done after the Barlow maneuver or separately. The Ortolani maneuver reduces a posteriorly dislocated hip. It is done to reduce a recently dislocated hip and is not done forcefully. The thigh is flexed and then abducted while pushing up with the fingers located over the trochanter posteriorly. The femoral head is lifted anteriorly into the acetabulum. A clunk and a palpable jerk are obtained as the femoral head is relocated. A mild clicking sound is not a positive Ortolani sign. These are common and normal sounds that are fine, of short duration, and high pitched. Of note, the hip may be dislocated easily only during the first month or two of life. The Ortolani maneuver is most likely to be positive in infants 1 to 2 months of age. The examiner should not still be charting "no hip click" on examinations at 6 months of age. Dislocation can occur late in infancy. However, if this occurs, the NP will note limited abduction on the side of the dislocation (Fig. 38-4).

Trendelenburg Sign

The Trendelenburg sign is elicited by having the child stand and then raise one leg off the ground. If the pelvis drops on the raised leg side, the sign is positive and indicates weak hip abductor muscles on the side that is bearing the weight. Normally, the muscles around a stable hip are strong enough to maintain a level pelvis if one leg is raised (see Fig. 38-3). With bilaterally dislocated hips, a wide-based Trendelenburg limp is noted.

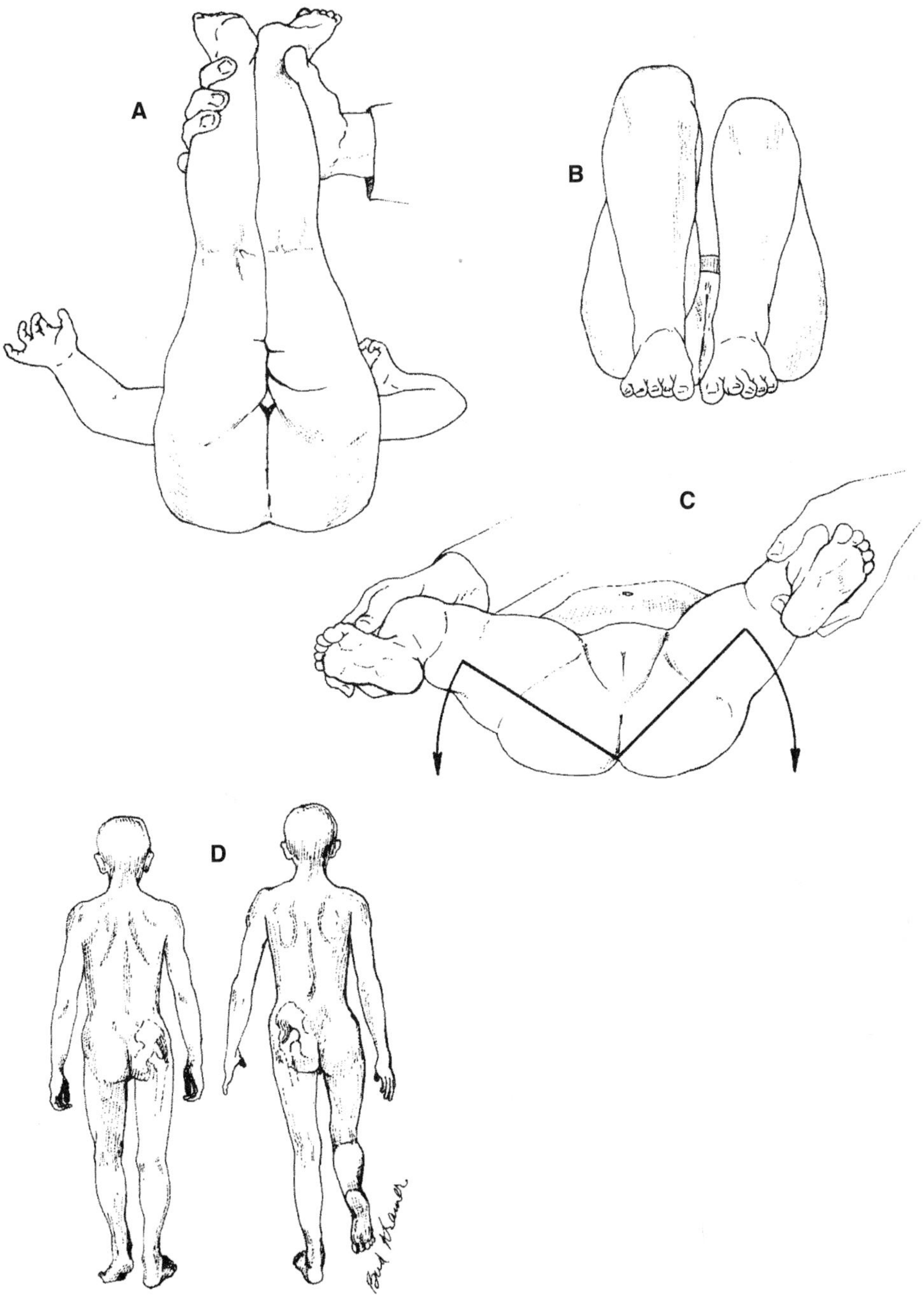

FIGURE 38-3 Physical findings in congenital hip dislocation. **A**, Thigh-fold asymmetry is often present in infants with unilateral hip dislocation. An extra fold can be seen on the abnormal side. The finding is not diagnostic, however. It may be found in normal infants and may be absent in children with hip dislocation or dislocatability. **B**, Leg length inequality is a sign of unilateral hip dislocation (Galeazzi sign). It is not reliable in children with dislocatable but not dislocated hips or in children with bilateral dislocation. **C**, Limitation of hip abduction is often present in older infants with hip dislocation. Abduction of greater than 60 degrees is usually possible in infants. Restriction or asymmetry indicates the need for careful radiologic examination. **D**, Trendelenburg sign. In single-leg stance, the abductor muscles of the normal hip support th pelvis. Dislocation of the hip functionally shortens and weakens these muscles. When the child attempts to stand on the dislocated hip, opposite side of the pelvis drops. When bilateral dislocation is present, a wide-based Trendelenburg limp will result. (From Scoles P: *Pedi orthopedics in clinical practice*, ed 2, St Louis, 1988, Mosby.)

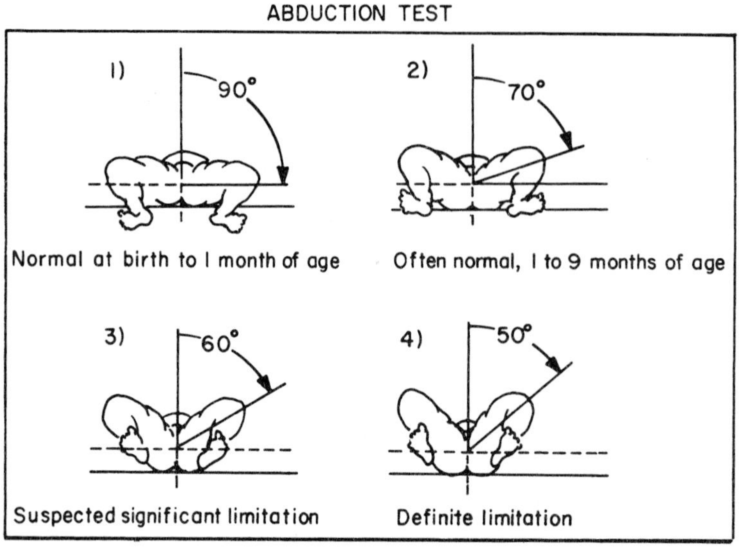

FIGURE 38-4 Hip abduction test. The child is placed supine, and the hips are flexed 90 degrees and fully abducted. Although the normal abduction range is quite broad, one can suspect hip disease in any patient who lacks more than 35 to 45 degrees of abduction. (From Chung SMK: *Hip disorders in infants and children*, Philadelphia, 1981, Lea & Febiger.)

Medial Rotation (Internal Rotation)

The child is placed prone, and the knees are flexed 90 degrees. Medial rotation is measured as the legs are allowed to fall apart as far as possible, using gravity alone or with light pressure. The angle between vertical (0 degree) and the leg position is the medial rotation. It is measured for each leg (Fig. 38-5). Asymmetric hip rotation is abnormal.

Lateral Rotation (External Rotation)

Lateral rotation is measured by allowing the legs to cross while the child is still prone. The angle between vertical and the leg position is measured for each leg (see Fig. 38-5). Again, asymmetric hip rotation is abnormal.

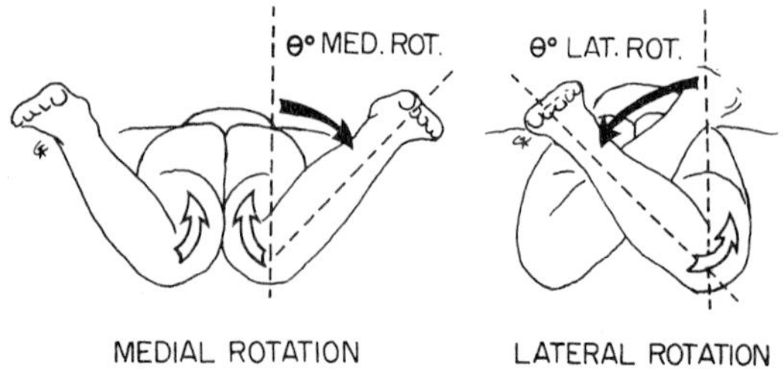

FIGURE 38-5 Medial and lateral rotation measurement. With the patient lying prone and the knees flexed 90 degrees, the femurs are examined for their range of motion at the hips in extension. (From Behrman R, editor: *Nelson textbook of pediatrics*, ed 14, Philadelphia, 1992, WB Saunders.)

Back Examination

Adam Position or the Adam Forward Bend Position

Adam's test looks for asymmetry of the posterior chest wall on forward bending. This position allows for evaluation of structural scoliosis. The child bends at the waist to a position of 90 degrees back flexion with straight legs, ankles together, and arms hanging freely or with palms together but not touching the toes or floor (Fig. 38-6). The back is inspected for asymmetry of the height of the curves on the two sides. The examiner should be seated in front of the child to best visually scan each level of the spine. If a rib hump is present, a scoliometer, if available, can be used to measure the angular tilt of the trunk. Other characteristics of scoliosis to look for include unequal scapula heights, unequal waist angles, asymmetry of the elbow to flank distance, and some deviation of the spine from a straight head-to-toe line. Looking primarily at the straightness of the spine, however, can be misleading, because scoliosis involves both rotation and misalignment of the vertebrae. Adam's position accentuates the rotational deformity of scoliosis.

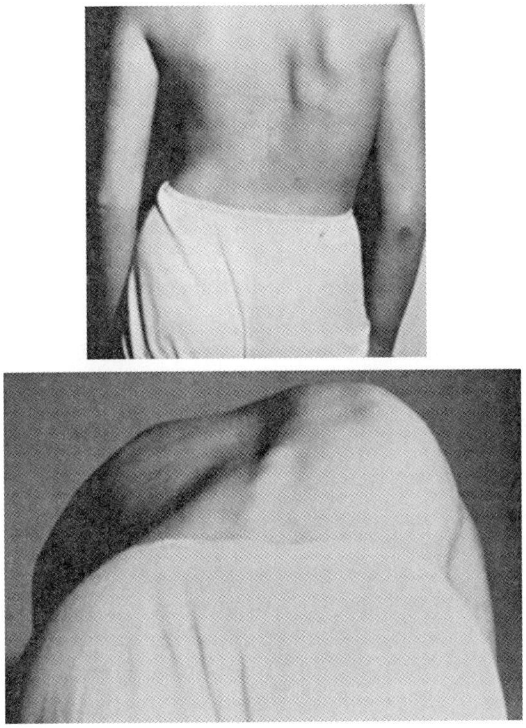

FIGURE 38-6 Adam's position with rib hump of structural scoliosis. Lateral curvature of thoracic and lumbar segments of the spine, usually with some rotation of involved vertebral bodies. Functional scoliosis is flexible; it is apparent with standing and disappears with forward bending. It may be compensatory for other abnormalities such as leg length discrepancy. Structural scoliosis is fixed; the curvature is visible both on standing and on bending forward. Note rib hump with forward flexion. At greatest risk are females age 10 through adolescence. (From Delp MH, Manning RT: Major's physical diagnosis: an introduction to the clinical process, ed 9, Philadelphia, 1981, WB Saunders.)

DIAGNOSTIC STUDIES

Radiographs are an important diagnostic tool for the musculoskeletal system. Anteroposterior and lateral views of the affected area, bone, or joint are typically ordered to analyze the anatomic structures. Views of both extremities may be ordered so that comparisons can be made. Computed tomography (CT) scans augment radiographs to detail specific areas of the body, especially in identification of soft tissue lesions. CT is useful in detailing the relationship of bones to their contiguous structures. Magnetic resonance imaging (MRI) can provide additional information, such as the degree of bone demineralization before the tissue loss is radiographically apparent, whereas 30% to 50% of bone density must be reduced to show a change on conventional radiography. MRI is particularly useful in assessment of soft tissue lesions and allows distinction among different muscles or muscle groups, as well as among different cartilage structures. It also can distinguish among various physiologic changes that occur in bone marrow related to age and disease process. Ultrasonography also provides information about cartilaginous areas or tissues not visible on radiograph. Bone scans (scintigraphy) demonstrate abnormal uptake earlier than conventional radiographs and are useful in detecting causes of obscure skeletal pain because this study is more sensitive than radiographs (Behrman, Kliegman, & Jenson, 2004).

It is important to remember that false-negative imaging studies can occur in early stages of disease (e.g., osteomyelitis) or conditions (e.g., developmental hip dysplasia of the newborn). Also, in those circumstances in which a child will most likely be referred to a specialist, it may be more prudent to defer to the specialist to order imaging studies rather than expose the child to unnecessary radiation.

Various laboratory studies can indicate systemic disease, infection, or inflammation. They also can provide an understanding of muscle metabolism (e.g., lactic acid, pyruvates, carnitine).

Some bony lesions may need to be biopsied for diagnosis, and muscle tissue frequently needs to be sampled to determine specific disease pathology.

MANAGEMENT STRATEGIES

Counseling

Counseling for orthopedic problems involves several components. The family should understand and have time to ask questions about all of the following issues:

- The pathology, including possible etiologies
- The treatment plan
- The prognosis with and without treatment
- Any genetic implications of the diagnosis
- Long-term care issues

Counseling also helps families cope with the diagnosis and its short-term and long-term implications. Congenital problems are often identified at birth or shortly thereafter. Families need to be given the diagnosis truthfully, humanely, and as soon as possible. Issues of etiology need to be discussed to address parents' feelings of guilt for causing the problem and to discuss genetic implications, if any. A plan of care that is mutually agreed on by the family and care provider must be developed before the infant is discharged from the hospital or clinic.

Exercise

All children need exercise to promote their growth and development. Even children with disabling conditions can exercise in some way. Exercise for children should be fun and perceived as play, not work. Often, physical therapists or the child's orthopedist can provide ideas for safe, therapeutic play or sports activities. At school, children with orthopedic problems should engage in physical activities that are as much a part of the regular physical education class as possible.

Anticipatory Guidance: Musculoskeletal Development

Families are sometimes concerned about problems that providers believe are within normal limits and do not require an orthopedic referral. The NP should provide the child's family with a description of the child's predicted musculoskeletal development. Timelines and markers that parents can use to monitor their child's development are particularly helpful in allowing families to understand their child's pattern of growth. Misperceptions about the implications of minor variations need to be clarified, and the family should always be given the opportunity to return for further assessment or discussion if concerns remain. Examples of common concerns are flat feet in infants and toddlers, "bowing" of legs in toddlers, and "knock-knees" in preschool children.

Shoes

The use of therapeutic shoes to correct orthopedic problems is controversial. Studies confirm that therapeutic shoes do little to correct deformities. Shoes for the average child should keep the feet warm and protected from injury. Shoes should be selected to fit properly and comfortably with room for growth. High-top shoes for toddlers may have the advantage of staying on pudgy little feet better, but they do not provide additional support. Toddler feet do not need extra support. Staheli (2003b) identifies five features (the "five *F*'s") of a good shoe:

- Flexible—to allow as much free motion as possible; for young children, test to see if the shoe can be flexed in the parent's hand
- Flat—do not allow high heels
- Foot shaped—avoid pointed toes or other shapes that are not the normal configuration of the foot
- Fitted generously—better to be too large than too small
- Friction similar to skin—the soles should have the same friction as skin so that they are not slippery

Shoe modifications may be needed in certain conditions. Shoe lifts are needed if limb length differences exceed 2.5 cm. Orthotics also can be used in certain orthopedic situations to more evenly distribute pressure on the sole of the foot and facilitate function.

Care of Children in Casts

Children in casts need special attention, and their parents need instructions for care and monitoring for problems. If a plaster cast is used, the major concern is wetness—urine, feces, or environmental substances. The cast absorbs it all. Therefore attention needs to be given to protecting the cast (including a fiberglass cast) from moisture at all times. If the cast becomes wet, a hair dryer can be used for drying small areas; for larger casts, drying may affect only the surface. Good pediatric nursing texts can provide ideas for caring for infants in spica casts—the most difficult to manage. For all casts, openings should be inspected and smelled to help identify pressure sores inside the casted areas. The heel is particularly vulnerable to pressure sores.

The child's cast should be kept cool, clean, and dry. Cover the cast with plastic wrap or a plastic bag when the child bathes or is in a situation in which the cast may get wet.

A child in a cast needs to have developmental stimulation, physical contact, changes in environment, and opportunities to make choices and control his or her care within limits, just as any other child does. Parents need to be instructed to use extra care when picking up a child with a cast—the weight can cause trauma if not supported. Depending on cast material used and how quickly they dry, special care must be taken until the cast is completely dry to prevent compression of the cast material.

Splints and Braces

Splints and braces need to be monitored for good fit and correct use. Splints are useful to provide temporary immobilization.

Genetics Counseling

See Chapter 41.

Physical Therapy

Physical therapists can help restore or maintain function or teach new motor skills. The physical therapist should be accustomed to dealing with children. Physical therapy is especially important to prevent deformities, teach new motor skills, and rehabilitate injuries.

SPECIFIC ORTHOPEDIC PROBLEMS OF CHILDREN

Brachial Plexus Injuries

Description

Brachial plexus injuries are stretch or traction injuries, in which innervation to the arm is disrupted, resulting in paralysis. They are typically classified using Narakas criteria as types I through IV (Table 38-2). Narakas type I involves C5 and C6, affecting the shoulder and bicep muscles. Narakas type II involves shoulder, biceps, and forearm extensors with C5 through C7 nerve root injuries. Recovery is usually complete for types I and II. Narakas type III has variable recovery with complete paralysis of the limb caused by C5 through T1 nerve root injury. Narakas type IV also involves C5 through T1 with complete paralysis of the limb, as well as Horner syndrome. Recovery of function in the shoulder and biceps is fair to poor with hand recovery variable in types III and IV. Brachial plexy injuries can also be classified as type I (Erb's palsy), type II (Erb-Duchenne-Klumke palsy), or type III (lower palsy). Erb's palsy designates C4 through C6 involvement; Erb-Duchenne-Klumpke palsy involves the entire brachial plexus; and lower plexus injury involves C8 and T1 nerve roots (Drendel, Esterhai, & Sawyer, 2002; Hansen & Bateman, 2002).

Etiology

Brachial palsies generally occur through traumatic stretching of the neck and shoulder during birth, producing damage to the brachial plexus. Shoulder dystocia, fetal macrosomia, prolonged and difficult labor and delivery, the use of forceps or vacuum, and vaginal breech deliveries are linked with this type of birth injury. However, there may be no predisposing risk factor, and there is some evidence that the injury may also occur in utero. The incidence ranges from 0.38 to 2.6 per 1000 full-term births (Hansen & Bateman, 2002).

TABLE 38-2 *Brachial Plexus Injury Using Narakas Classification*

Name	Nerve and Muscle Involved	Prognosis
Narakas type I	C5 and C6; shoulder and biceps	Recovery usually complete
Narakas type II	C5-C7; shoulder, biceps, and forearm extensors	Recovery usually complete
Narakas type III	C5-T1	Variable with complete paralysis of limb; shoulder and biceps recovery is fair to poor with hand recovery variable
Narakas type IV	C5-T1	Complete paralysis of the limb as well as Horner syndrome; shoulder and biceps recovery is fair to poor with hand recovery variable

Clinical Findings

History. There may be a history of a traumatic delivery, often of a large baby.

Physical Examination. Findings depend on the type (I through IV) and include the following (Drendel, Esterhai, & Sawyer, 2002; Hansen & Bateman, 2002):

- Neonate cannot abduct the arm from the shoulder or rotate the arm externally and cannot supinate the forearm; infant keeps the shoulder in adduction and internal rotation and cannot flex the elbow (Erb's palsy)
- Absent bicep reflex with absent Moro reflex on the affected side
- Limp wrist and hand with absent grasp reflex (lower plexus involvement)
- Moro reflex absent or incomplete on affected side
- Horner syndrome (ipsilateral ptosis, miosis, enophthalmos, anhidrosis) if the sympathetic fibers of the T1 nerve root are involved
- Occasionally, hand paralysis with normal shoulder movement, which is a rare occurrence of an isolated C8 through T1 injury

Traumatic delivery causing brachial plexus injury also can cause the following associated injuries:

- Rupture of intraabdominal structures, especially liver and spleen
- Fracture of the skull, clavicle, or humerus
- Damage to the sternocleidomastoid muscle with resulting limitation of neck movement (a "sternocleidomastoid tumor" indicates the injury, which results in torticollis if prompt and vigorous physical therapy is not initiated)
- Impaired respiratory effort

Diagnostic Studies. Chest radiograph is needed to rule out fractures of the clavicle or humerus or humeral-epiphyseal separation. Electromyographic studies and radiographs of the clavicle and cervical spine are ordered as indicated.

Differential Diagnosis

Consider dislocation, fracture of the arm or clavicle, cerebral lesions, and cervical column lesions.

Management

The following steps are taken:

- Refer to an orthopedist for immobilization for the first 2 weeks, followed by physical therapy and splints to prevent contractures.

- Physical therapy may be necessary to maintain a full range of motion.
- Recovery of nerve function needs to be monitored using a standardized tool such as the British Muscle Movement Scale. If there is little to no recovery of biceps function by 4 months of age, surgical exploration of the brachial plexus with possible nerve grafting or transfer may be necessary.
- Counsel the family, including explanation of the injury, its prognosis, and its management. The child should be held and cared for as any other baby.

Complications

Paralysis can be permanent. Contractures can occur if regular physical therapy is not started and continued for as long as the paralysis lasts. Physical findings are important to rule out concurrent injuries from traumatic delivery. Brachial plexus injury may be associated with phrenic nerve palsy.

Prognosis

Recovery may or may not be complete and requires time, 18 months in mild cases. Improvement is generally seen in the first few days to weeks, with 75% to 95% resolving spontaneously during the first year of life (Hanson & Bateman, 2002). If there has been no improvement by 2 to 3 months of age, the infant needs evaluation for nerve root avulsion and, depending on the results, possibly surgery. The prognosis for complete recovery of upper brachial plexus injury is excellent, with a more guarded prognosis for lower brachial plexus injury (types III and IV).

Clavicle Fracture

Etiology and Incidence

In neonates, this fracture occurs often during the birth process. Most clavicle fractures occur during normal labor and delivery. However, risk factors include shoulder dystocia, a large neonate, and increased gestational age. Because the clavicle is the first bone to ossify, it is the bone most frequently fractured at birth, with the right fractured more often than the left. It may be a complete or greenstick fracture and typically involves the middle third of the clavicle. The incidence of neonatal clavicle fractures is 4.7 per 1000 live births (Hansen & Bateman, 2002). Childhood fractures of the clavicle are related to trauma.

Clinical Findings

History. In the neonate, assess the following:

- History of difficult delivery—large baby and shoulder dystocia—or a normal labor and delivery
- Irritability when infant is moved or lifted
- In the older child, assess the following:
  - History of fall or trauma

Physical Examination. In all children, look for the following:

- Pain occurring with shoulder movement
- Decreased arm movement on affected side (asymmetric spontaneous arm movements) or absent Moro reflex
- Palpable swelling and crepitus elicited over fracture site
- Callus felt over fracture site within a few days
- Spasm of sternocleidomastoid muscle on affected side
- An associated Erb's palsy

Diagnostic Studies. In the neonate, radiographs should be used to confirm the diagnosis. Clavicle shaft fractures can be difficult to see radiographically in children but are clinically identifiable. Radiographs can be helpful in identifying a fracture near the shoulder joint.

Differential Diagnosis

Brachial palsy, shoulder dislocation, or other bony problem should be considered.

Management

Management involves the following:

- Neonate:
  - Incomplete fractures that do not cause pain need no treatment.
  - Immobilization of the shoulder is an option when movement results in a painful arm (usually with a complete fracture). Pin the sleeve of the infant's arm to the front of the shirt for 1 to 2 weeks.
  - Generally, the neonate is just moved gently without undue stress to the arm and shoulder until a callus forms.
- Older child:
  - Sling immobilization for comfort is often sufficient.
  - A figure-eight clavicle brace can be used if displacement results in a decreased shaft length. However, it is uncomfortable to wear and its effectiveness is questionable.
  - Protection for 4 to 5 weeks is generally sufficient in that union requires about 4 weeks of healing.
  - An older child may need analgesics or a nonsteroidal antiinflammatory drug (NSAID) for pain.
  - The rare open fractures or those with severe tenting need to be surgically corrected.

Prognosis

The prognosis is excellent. Often the injury in neonates is identified only at later primary care visits, when the callus lump is palpated. The child may be irritable until the fracture is stable. Parents need information and emotional support. The infant is usually asymptomatic within 7 to 10 days. In older children with fractures, healing is almost always universal with reduction seldom necessary. Bone remodeling is generally complete. A large callus often appears at the healing site; however, the callus typically resolves in 6 to 12 months, making cosmetic surgery unnecessary (Copley, 2002).

Rib Problems—Costochondritis

Description

Costochondral disease (costochondritis) is a benign disorder marked by pain that is localized at the costosternal or costochondral junction where the sternum, ribs, and costal cartilages connect. It involves musculoskeletal discomfort and is a common complaint.

Etiology

Trauma to the area and unaccustomed physical effort (lifting heavy objects or coughing) are factors known to cause costochondritis.

Clinical Findings

History. Pain localized to the costosternal or costochondral junction is the major symptom. Characteristics of the pain include the following (Schaller, 1996):

- Acute or gradual onset
- Sharp, darting, or dull quality
- Short duration of hours or lasting days
- Occasional complaints of a feeling of tightness caused by muscle spasm
- No exacerbation of pain with respiratory or mild movements

Physical Examination. The major clinical finding on examination is localized tenderness of one or more costochrondral joints with palpation of the costal cartilage. The presence of pain, swelling with or without redness, and tenderness at the costal cartilage is referred to as Tietze syndrome.

Diagnostic Studies. No diagnostic studies are needed because history and physical findings are the key to the diagnosis.

Differential Diagnosis

Rib fractures are the key differential diagnosis if pain is associated with an injury. Childhood rheumatic diseases also can have complaints similar to costochondritis but generally have other characteristic physical findings. Costochondritis is one of the differential diagnoses of pediatric chest pain (see Chapter 31).

Management

Treatment consists of the use of mild analgesia to relieve discomfort and avoidance of strenuous activity. Parents and children need to be reassured that this is a benign, self-limited condition and is not related to cardiac disease.

Back Problems

Back Pain

Description. Children do not commonly complain of severe back pain. Younger children who have such complaints should be carefully evaluated for occult pathology. Complaints of back pain in adolescents deserve attention but have a lesser index of suspicion of occult pathology but, again, deserve cautious evaluation. The older the child is the more likely the etiology of back pain is similar to that of adults (Sussman & Turker, 2002). Back pain can result from sprains of the ligaments or muscles (or both) of the back caused by injury. However, the etiology of this pain is obvious from the history, which usually points to athletic or other types of injury such as a fall or automobile accident (Eilert, 2001).

Clinical Findings. The following findings should alert the NP to possible pathology:

- Night pain
- Pain that prohibits play or activities
- History of trauma (vertebral fracture)
- Positive neurologic or musculoskeletal signs on examination

In school-age children and adolescents, back pain can be associated with a history of the following:

- Carrying heavy backpacks
- Wearing high heels or platform shoes (females)

Questions about the onset, duration, location, frequency, and intensity of the pain are key questions to ask to form an initial impression (Richards, 2003).

Diagnostic Studies. A complete blood count with differential, erythrocyte sedimentation rate, and C-reactive protein are useful screening tests, particularly in young children with constitutional symptoms or those complaining of night pain (Richards, 2003).

Differential Diagnosis. Occult pathology should be ruled out. Diskitis, vertebral osteomyelitis, vertebral fracture, or tumor can cause significant back pain in toddlers. Older children can experience these same problems, as well as intervertebral disk herniation or vertebral end-plate fractures.

Management. Treatment is determined by the findings on history and physical examination and can include referral for radiographs (anteroposterior and lateral views) and imaging studies or referral to a subspecialist physician or pediatrician. If the back pain is due to injury, pain management and physical therapy may be part of the treatment plan.

Scoliosis

Description. Scoliosis is a structural lateral curvature of the spine greater than 10 degrees in the coronal plane of the spine. It also involves significant transverse and sagittal plane rotations. There are seven classifications of scoliosis:

- Idiopathic: thought to be caused by equilibrium dysfunction, familial tendency, or asymmetric growth; within this classification there are three types divided by age at manifestation:
  - Infantile (0 to 3 years)
  - Juvenile (3 to 10 years)
  - Adolescent (puberty to maturity)
- Paralytic: secondary to muscle imbalance in the growing spine caused by primary neuromuscular problems (e.g., cerebral palsy or muscular dystrophy)
- Congenital: associated with a structural anomaly present at birth (e.g., hemivertebrae)
- Mesenchymal: associated with connective tissue problems (e.g., Marfan syndrome)
- Posttraumatic: following injury, thoracoplasty, or irradiation
- Tumors: secondary to bone tumors or other lesions constricting the spine
- Other causes/miscellaneous: examples include metabolic disturbances or dystrophies

Structural scoliosis is the general term used to indicate a true deformity of the vertebrae rather than a postural problem (*secondary* or *functional scoliosis*). Approximately 10% of the population has mild truncal asymmetry. However, curves greater than 10 degrees in children are abnormal and can progress to significant curves in the growing child (Bennett, 2002a; Staheli, 1998).

Etiology. The etiology of scoliosis varies by its classification. Secondary or functional scoliosis, when there is the appearance of a lateral curvature but no structural change in the vertebral column, is due to such secondary problems as leg length inequality, poor posture, or muscle spasm. Congenital scoliosis is due to bony deformity caused by failure in formation or segmentation of vertebrae during fetal development (e.g., neural tube disorders). Paralytic or neuromuscular scoliosis is caused by myopathies and upper or lower neuron diseases (e.g., muscular dystrophy, cerebral palsy, and polio). Mesenchymal or constitutional scoliosis is associated with syndromes (e.g., Marfan syndrome or diastrophic dwarfism). Miscellaneous scoliosis has numerous etiologies that do not fit one of the other classifications. Idiopathic is the most common type of scoliosis. Its etiology is unknown but often has a familial or genetic pattern. Hormonal changes play a role in the disease process, and a rapid growth period is believed to be a significant factor in the progress of curvature associated with idiopathic scoliosis (Sussman & Turker, 2002). Females with this type of scoliosis are more likely than males to have lateral curvatures that progress. The most common type of idiopathic scoliosis is found in adolescents and is the major focus of the remaining discussion.

Small to moderate scoliotic curves do not increase significantly after skeletal growth is complete (i.e., skeletal maturity is reached). Double "S" curves and more severe curves are more likely to progress during the growth years. For a given child, however, the ability to predict progression is difficult because even small curves can progress to severe deformity. Thus regular monitoring of the curve is important (Table 38-3).

Incidence. Idiopathic scoliosis is found in children from around the world. Small curves (less than 10 degrees) of the spine occur in 2% to 4% of the adolescent population, and only 0.1% to 0.3% of these adolescents progress to have significant curves (greater than 20 degrees). The female-to-male ratio is equal but jumps to 5:1 for curves greater than 21 degrees. The majority of adolescents with idiopathic scoliosis have a right thoracic curve. Juvenile manifestation is uncommon, and infantile scoliosis is rare in the United States (Bennett, 2002a).

Clinical Findings

History. It is generally painless, and insidious onset is typical. Generally there is no significant history. The NP should assess the following:

- Family history of scoliosis
- Etiologic factors related to the various causes of structural scoliosis

The presence of pain with a lateral curvature of the spine suggests an inflammatory or neoplastic lesion as the cause of the scoliosis.

Physical Examination. The predominant features in the child who is standing with weight equally on both feet, legs straight, and arms hanging loosely at the sides include the following, although the location of the curve affects the findings:

- Painless lateral curvature of the spine with greater than 10 degrees of rotation.
- The curve can have one turn ("C curve") or may include two compensating curves ("S curve").
- Lateral deviation and rotation of each vertebra is accentuated by looking at the ribs, as well as the spinal column itself.

TABLE 38-3 *Scoliosis, Kyphosis, and Lordosis*

	Curve	Etiology	Clinical Findings	Radiographs	Management	Prognosis
Scoliosis	Lateral	Classifications: idiopathic (most common); neuromuscular; constitutional; secondary; congenital; miscellaneous; functional (leg length discrepancy—not scoliosis)	Hx: positive family hx; related to etiologies (classifications); painless curvature	PA and lateral standing views to identify degree of curve; >15 degrees abnormal; may have one curve (C) or two curves (S); vertebrae show lateral deviation and rotation	Referral to orthopedic surgeon; brace or surgery; need to monitor progression of curve	Most curves do not increase after growth complete; females with idiopathic scoliosis more likely to have curve progress
Kyphosis	AP curve of thoracic spine	Familial (Scheuermann's disease); secondary to tumor, trauma, etc., congenital; postural, not true kyphosis	Postural round back	Narrow disk space and loss of normal anterior height of vertebrae	Postural: PT, dancing, and swimming can be helpful; if structural: refer to an orthopedic surgeon for observation, bracing, or surgery	
Lordosis	AP curve of lumbar spine	Due to hip contractures; physiologic; family and racial groups, before puberty	Abdomen and buttock protuberant; if due to hip contractures, lordosis disappears when sitting	Standing lateral views	Lumbar spine flattens and lordosis disappears when child bends forward, it is physiologic and no treatment; if fixed, refer to an orthopedist	

AP, Anteroposterior; *Hx*, history; *PA*, posteroanterior; *PE*, physical examination; *PT*, physical therapy.

- Unequal shoulder heights.
- Congenital scoliosis may be visible in the infant lying prone; it is sometimes more prominent if the infant is suspended prone. Inspect for skin abnormalities, sacral dimple, and hairy patches.
- Unequal scapula prominences and heights. Note that the muscle masses may be somewhat unequal, especially if the child uses one shoulder more than the other as in carrying books. Look for bony, not muscular, prominence.
- Unequal waist angles—the hip touches arm and the contralateral arm hangs free.
- Unequal rib prominences and chest asymmetry.
- Unequal rib heights when the child stands in the Adam forward bend position (see Fig. 38-6).
- The presence of a left-sided curve should be viewed with caution and is suggestive of neuropathology.

The physical examination should also include the following:

- Observation for equal leg lengths
- Examination of the skin for hairy patches, nevi, café au lait spots, lipomas, dimples
- Neurologic examination
- Cardiac examination for Marfan syndrome

Diagnostic Studies. The clinical diagnosis is always confirmed by radiograph, although some newer techniques of curve measurement are being studied. If a scoliometer is used to measure the tilt of the rib hump, readings of greater than 5 degrees indicate the need for radiographs. The anteroposterior (AP) and lateral standing views on trifold, full-length films are recommended with shielding. The radiograph identifies the degrees of curvature and is the only way to assess the status of the back accurately.

In infants, the rib vertebral angle difference is an important measurement for orthopedists.

The radiograph is an important baseline study, in that the rate of change of the curve determines the severity of the problem and appropriate treatment. The curves of idiopathic adolescent scoliosis are classified radiographically as thoracic, double major, thoracolumbar, double thoracic, and lumbar. The Risser sign is an iliac apophysis maturation index of bone growth and is useful in determining the likelihood of curvature progression. MRI should be ordered if intraspinal anomalies are suspected; bone scans are useful if osteoid osteoma is a differential diagnosis (Bennett, 2002a).

Differential Diagnosis. Structural scoliosis must be differentiated from functional scoliosis. The latter disappears when the child is placed in Adam's position, whereas the former is enhanced in this position. Persistent functional scoliosis to one side in a child with a neuromotor problem can eventually become structural and must be managed with physical therapy or other means to prevent progression.

Consider systemic problems such as neurofibromatosis, cerebral palsy, multiple sclerosis, Rett syndrome, rickets, tuberculosis, and tumor.

Management. The goal of treatment is not full correction of the deformity but to prevent increasing deformity (Bennett, 2002a; Staheli, 1998; Sussman & Turker, 2002).

- Refer to an orthopedic surgeon. Because most treatment relies on growth to assist in correcting the problem, referrals need to be made as early as possible. Most curves require only observation; however, bracing and surgical correction of large curves may be necessary. Bracing is only effective to control a curve and not to decrease its magnitude. It is effective with skeletally immature spines and is considered when curvatures reach 20 to 25 degrees.
- For congenital, constitutional, neuromuscular, or miscellaneous scoliosis, treatment depends on the etiology and severity of the curve and the rate of its progression. Bracing may be tried, is controversial, and is generally not effective. Bracing may help reduce compensatory curves in congenital scoliosis. Rapidly increasing curves need early operative treatment (e.g., spinal fusion and instrumentation). Supervision needs to be maintained until growth is complete. Exercises are not helpful. Paralytic scoliosis is treated with surgery.
- For idiopathic scoliosis, treatment varies depending on age at manifestation. Infantile scoliosis often involves a left thoracic curvature in males and resolves spontaneously in 90% of children. Nonresolving and progressive infantile curves are treated with bracing. Juvenile scoliosis occurs more often in females, is generally progressive, and commonly is a right thoracic curvature that requires treatment with bracing. Adolescent scoliosis has a 3:2 female-to-male ratio and can resolve, remain static, or increase. Mild curves need observation and reassurance only; curves greater than 25 degrees and less than 45 degrees need brace management and observation; curves greater than 45 degrees or curves expected to progress to that range in children who are not candidates for bracing need surgical intervention—instrumentation and fusion. Bracing and casting after surgery may be necessary.
- Monitoring or treatment (or both) is necessary until growth is complete.
- Physical therapy and chiropractic manipulation have not been shown to alter the progression of curvature.
- Support must be given to the child and family through the diagnostic and treatment phases, considering school and peer factors. Assist the child with psychologic adjustment issues that arise if casting, bracing, or surgery is recommended and instituted. Some specific concerns of the child can include self-esteem problems, managing hostility and anger, learning about the disease and its care, wondering about the long-term prognosis, and concerns about clothing and participation in sports and other activities.

Parents often worry about the long-term prognosis and finances to cover care, experience guilt for possibly causing the problem (if it is thought to be genetic) or not identifying the problem earlier, and feel concern about the possible pain and treatment that the child will experience.

Complications. Progressive scoliosis can result in a severe deformity of the spinal column. Severe deformities can result in impairment of respiratory and cardiovascular function, as well as limitation of physical activities and decreased comfort. The psychologic consequences of an untreated scoliosis deformity can be severe.

Prevention. Prevention is not possible; however, early identification of children with scoliosis can help them avoid more expensive, invasive care and prevent the long-term consequences of the disorder. School screening clinics, recommended by the American Academy of Orthopedic Surgeons and the Scoliosis Research Society, have been instituted in many parts of the country to help identify affected children as early as possible. Several studies conducted in the 1960s and 1970s demonstrated that, when children had been screened at school, a trend toward fewer curves requiring surgery and an overall decrease in the magnitude of curves being treated were seen. Screening is effective, however, only if identified children are referred for care. Their parents must be notified, a referral arranged, and follow-up ensured.

Kyphosis

Description. Kyphosis is an AP curve of the thoracic spine with the apex posterior (i.e., the back is prominent). Normally, the thoracic spine is kyphotic (20 to 40 degrees). The most common clinical type of kyphosis is usually postural (postural round back). The curvature of the spinal column points backward, and when viewed from the side, gives the appearance of being humpbacked. In postural kyphosis, the Adam's test demonstrates normalization of the lateral spine profile when viewed from the side (see Table 38-3).

Scheuermann's disease is a common pathologic form of kyphosis that is most commonly seen in adolescent males. It causes low back pain. In Scheuermann's kyphosis, radiographs demonstrate wedging of three adjacent thoracic vertebrae and the presence of end-plate intrusions, known as Schmorl's nodes. Kyphosis in children can be secondary to congenital deformity, tumor, trauma, infection, or such problems as achondroplasia. A radiograph can be useful to identify nonpostural causes. The radiograph shows narrowed disk space, loss of normal anterior height of the involved vertebrae, and other findings. In Scheuermann's kyphosis, the Adam's test demonstrates more or less acute angulation of the back when observed from the side (Neyt & Weinstein, 2003).

Management. Postural kyphosis needs to be managed by referral to a physical therapist. Activities such as dancing or swimming, which require a full range of motion of the shoulders, back, and arms, can be helpful. If the problem is structural and not functional, a referral to an orthopedic surgeon is warranted. If pain is a problem, immobilization of the back in a brace is an option. For mild curves, observation and bracing are the usual options for skeletally immature spines. This is the usual therapy for Scheuermann's kyphosis. For severe and congenital kyphosis (greater than 65 degree curves), anterior and posterior spinal surgery with instrumentation and fusion is the appropriate management strategy (Bennett, 2002a).

Lumbar Lordosis

Description. Lumbar lordosis, or hyperlordosis, is an AP curve of the lumbar area of the spine (i.e., the child stands with the abdomen and buttocks protuberant). It sometimes occurs with kyphosis. Lordosis can be a secondary result of a hip problem in which full extension is limited by hip flexion contractures or from lumbosacral deformities. Physiologic lordosis is commonly seen in families, certain racial groups, and just before onset of puberty. Physiologic lordosis is not a fixed deformity. In lordosis the curvature points forward; the apex of the curve is anterior (Neyt & Weinstein, 2003).

Management. If the NP suspects lumbar lordosis, have the child bend forward. If the lumbar spine flattens and the lordosis disappears in the forward bending position, it indicates that the spine is flexible and the lordosis is only physiologic. This child should be seen for follow-up in 6 to 12 months. If the lordosis persists in the forward bending position, this indicates a fixed structural deformity and needs referral to an orthopedist. Lordosis resulting from hip flexion contractures is absent while sitting and commonly seen in children with cerebral palsy, spina bifida, and developmental dysplasia of the hip (see Table 38-3).

Hip Problems

Developmental Dysplasia of the Hip

Description. *Developmental dysplasia of the hip* (DDH), formerly *congenital dislocated hip*, is the term used to describe a variety of disorders resulting in abnormal development of the hip joint. These disorders include dysplasia, subluxation, or complete dislocation of the femoral head out of the pelvic acetabulum. Dysplasia is characterized by a shallow acetabulum with an immature hip/acetabulum. In subluxation, the hip is unstable, and the head of the femur can slide in and out of the acetabulum. DDH may have occurred congenitally or developed in infancy or childhood.

Etiology. The etiology of DDH is multifactorial, with mechanical, environmental, and physiologic factors and a genetic predisposition for the condition. Physiologic factors include the hormonal effect of maternal estrogen and relaxin on joint laxity that can contribute to DDH in the neonatal period. Mechanical factors include uterine packing stresses (e.g., breech position), especially during the last trimester if the fetal pelvis becomes locked in the maternal pelvis. Sometimes the condition is found at birth, but frequently the actual dislocation occurs postnatally, even after some months. In cultures that swaddle infants in an extended position or place them on cradleboards, the incidence of DDH is greater than normal because of such neonatal positioning.

The mechanism for dislocation is considered to be related to distention of the joint capsule, which allows the femoral head to disengage from the acetabulum. If the head is relocated soon after birth, the soft tissues tighten around the joint within a few weeks. All newborns have normal laxity of their joints. However, if the hip is persistently dislocated, soft tissue and bony parts become deformed.

The hip can dislocate noncongenitally in children with certain muscular or neurologic disorders that affect the use of the lower extremities, such as cerebral palsy, arthrogryposis, or myelomeningocele. Dislocation results from the abnormal use of the extremity over time.

Incidence. The incidence of DDH is estimated to be 10 per 1000 live births and is more common in females (80%). It is found more commonly with breech births. A positive family history (genetic risk factors) increases the risk for having a child with this problem. Other risk factors seen in infants that are associated with DDH include oligohydramnios, torticollis, metatarsus adductus, and lower limb deformities such as clubfoot and dislocated knee (Bennett, 2002b; Shah, 2002).

Clinical Findings

History. The history may include a positive family history; associated neck, knee, and foot deformities noted at or shortly after birth; and breech delivery. The left hip is more commonly involved.

Physical Examination. A hip examination should be performed on children as part of their well-child supervision until they are 2 years of age. Findings of DDH include the following (Bennett, 2002b):

- The early phase, or loose phase, can extend for the first 6 months and is characterized by positive Ortolani or Barlow sign (or both). These signs are seen in infants typically for the first 2 to 3 months of age.
- The late phase occurs after the early phase and by 6 months and is characterized by the following:
  - Limited abduction of the affected hip and shortening of the thigh, which becomes well established and must be relied on as the primary sign in the older infant (see Fig. 38-4).
  - Normal abduction with comfort is 70 to 80 degrees bilaterally. Limited abduction includes those cases with less than 60 degrees of abduction or unequal abduction from one side to the other (see Fig. 38-4).
  - Unequal knee heights (Galeazzi sign [see Fig. 38-3]).
- Other findings include asymmetry of inguinal or gluteal folds (thigh-fold asymmetry is not related to the disorder [see Fig. 38-3]) and unequal leg lengths, shorter on the affected side.

In the ambulatory child who was not diagnosed earlier or was not corrected, the following might also be noted:

- Short leg with toe-walking on the affected side
- Positive Trendelenburg sign (see Fig. 38-3)
- Marked lordosis
- Painless limping or waddling gait with child leaning to the affected side

If the hips are dislocated bilaterally, asymmetries are not observed. Limited abduction is the primary indicator in this situation (see Fig. 38-4). Also, in the subluxed hip (not frankly dislocated), limited abduction again is the primary indicator.

Diagnostic Studies. Radiologic evaluation of the newborn to detect DDH is unreliable, because so much of the hip joint is cartilaginous in young infants. Also, the dislocation may be so recent that pathologic changes in addition to the loose capsule may not yet have developed. Ultrasound study provides useful information, especially in neonates with suspicious findings or when hip risk factors are present. If an infant's hip is unstable by examination, the diagnosis is made. By 2 to 3 months of age, radiography is reliable. A single AP view is adequate.

Differential Diagnosis. The condition is relatively unique.

Management. The goal of management is to restore the articulation of the femur within the acetabulum.

- Refer to an orthopedist promptly while the infant is still in the newborn nursery, if possible. Any child with subluxed, dislocatable, and dislocated hips needs to be referred. The earlier treatment is begun, the better the prognosis is for functional development of the acetabulum. The treatment of choice for subluxation and reducible dislocations identified in the early phase is a Pavlik harness. If the hip is irreducible in the early phase, a Pavlik harness may be tried. However, if it is not successful, a closed reduction followed by Pavlik harness or spica cast is the preferred treatment. A Pavlik harness is fitted to hold the hip in flexion and abduction until stable, permitting flexion motion. If the diagnosis is delayed past about 6 months of age, traction with closed reduction is often first tried. However, traction with open reduction is often necessary to bring the femoral head into place. A femoral and pelvic osteotomy is the treatment of choice in children 18 months of age or older with DDH. Surgery is done to bring the acetabulum down over the femoral head when the possibility of further positive development of the joint ceases.
- Triple diapering is not helpful, because the musculoskeletal forces far outweigh the force that can be exerted by the diaper material.
- Continue long-term monitoring of hip development if neonatal hip instability was noted at birth. A small percentage of infants are noted to have hip instability at birth, versus the 1% of infants with classic DDH. The majority of neonatal hip instability resolves spontaneously. Close observation of these children is recommended.
- The child with a Pavlik harness should be seen weekly to ensure that it fits properly. It is worn 24 hours a day except for bathing until a normal pelvic radiograph is obtained.
- The earlier treatment is started with the Pavlik harness, the better the prognosis for a successful outcome. Generally the harness is worn full-time for 2 months and then

worn during waking hours for decreasing periods of time.
- Support the child and family through the treatment phases. Explain management goals clearly. Caring for a child in a Pavlik harness or spica cast requires special knowledge. Cast care, skin care, and car safety when the child cannot easily be placed in a car seat are all issues to be addressed (One way to provide for child safety restraints is to cut out the sides of the car seat to accommodate the frog position.) Also see Chapter 11 for reference to safety restraints for children with special conditions. Furthermore, the child needs special attention to maintain developmental stimulation while immobilized.

Complications. The long-term outcomes depend on the age at diagnosis, the severity of the joint deformity, and the effectiveness of therapy. Untreated cases may result in a permanent dislocation of the femoral head so that it lies just under the iliac crest posteriorly. Clinically, the child has limited mobility of this artificial joint and related short leg. Forceful reduction can result in avascular necrosis of the femoral head with permanent hip deformity. Redislocation or persistent dysplasia can occur. Adult degenerative arthritis is associated with acetabular dysplasia.

Prevention. The condition cannot be prevented, but early identification resulting in early treatment significantly reduces the long-term consequences of the problem. Screening of all neonates and infants should include full hip abduction, examination for unequal folds and unequal leg lengths, and Barlow, Ortolani, and Galeazzi maneuvers at every examination. The hip can dislocate at any point in early development, even up to the point of first ambulation. In older children, limited abduction, gait, and standing position, including the Trendelenburg position, add important information. Charting should always include notation about hip findings because these can change at subsequent visits.

Legg-Calvé-Perthes Disease

Description. Legg-Calvé-Perthes disease (LCPD) is idiopathic, juvenile avascular necrosis of the femoral head.

Etiology. There is an initial ischemic episode of unknown etiology that interrupts vascular circulation to the capital femoral epiphysis. The articular cartilage hypertrophies, and the epiphyseal marrow becomes necrotic. The area revascularizes, and the necrotic bone is replaced by new bone. This process can take 18 to 24 months. There is a critical point in these dual processes when the subchondral area becomes weak enough that fracture of the epiphysis occurs. At this time, the child becomes symptomatic. With fracturing, further reabsorption and replacement by fibrous bone occurs, and the shape of the femoral head is altered. Articulation of the head in the hip joint is interrupted. The bone reossifies with or without treatment, but the femoral head flattens and enlarges, causing joint deformity (Shah, 2002).

Incidence. The disorder is five times more common in boys and most commonly occurs between 4 and 8 years of age. It occurs bilaterally in approximately 10% to 12% of cases. Children with bilateral LCPD typically are treated at a younger age and have more associated anomalies. Genetics do not appear to be a major predisposing factor. Approximately 10% of children with LCPD have a history of breech delivery, low birth weight, or abnormal birth presentations; 17% have a history of preceding trauma. LCPD in girls tends to be a more serious problem with a poor prognosis (Warren, 2002b).

Clinical Findings

History. There can be an acute or chronic onset with or without a history of trauma to the hip such as jumping from a high place.
- Acute onset (Warren, 2002b)
  - Sudden onset of pain in the groin or knee often occurring at night with pain on weight bearing or stiffness
  - Some children may have little restriction in motion of the hip
- Chronic
  - Recurring pain (mild or aching) at the hip or referred to the knee, anterior thigh, or groin for days to weeks and limp
  - Insidious limping generally in the morning and after activities
  - Stiffness in the morning or after rest

Physical Examination. Findings may include the following:
- Antalgic gait (usually the first sign) with a component of shortening and positive Trendelenburg sign
- Muscle spasm
- Decreased abduction, internal rotation, and extension of the hip
- Pain on rolling the leg internally
- Short stature if bone age is delayed

Diagnostic Studies. Routine AP pelvis and frog-leg lateral views are used to confirm the diagnosis. Alterations seen can include smaller epiphysis, increased epiphyseal density, subchondral fracture line, lateralization of the femoral head, and other features. Changes in the epiphysis margin are discerned by the orthopedist and radiologist (Fig. 38-7). However, there may be no radiographic findings early in the disease. Bone scans and MRI are helpful in recognizing early disease but are of limited value in assessing the extent of involvement or following disease progression. Radiographic changes are helpful in predicting poorer outcomes and the need for aggressive management (Warren, 2002b).

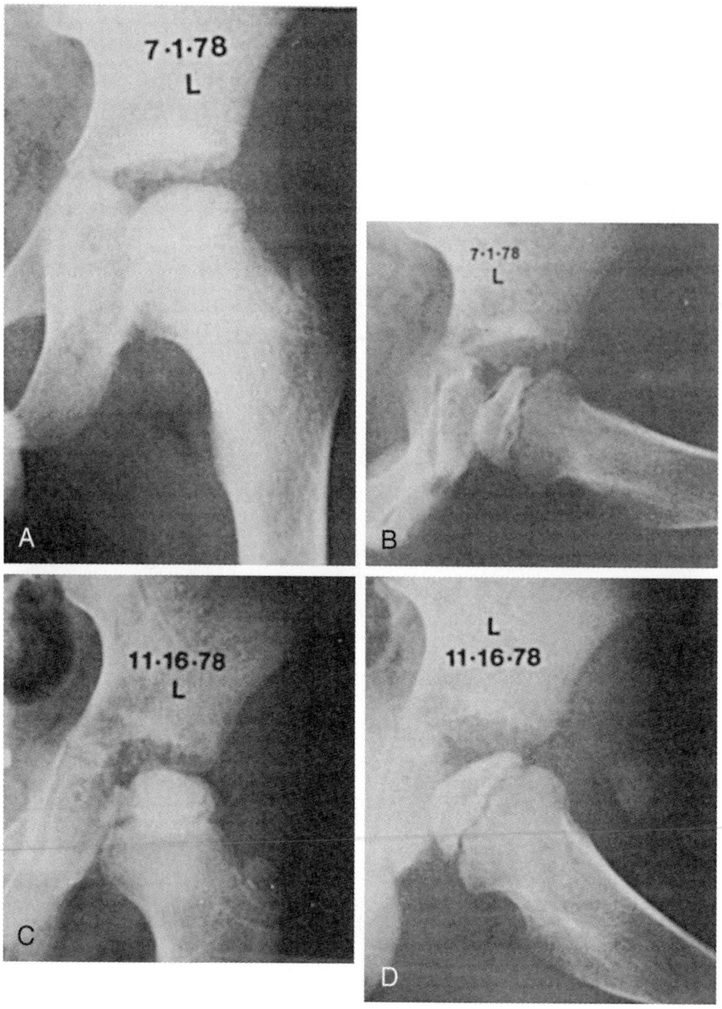

FIGURE 38-7 Radiologic evolution of Legg-Calvé-Perthes disease. **A**, Anteroposterior view of left hip in a 7-year-old boy with hip pain of 4 weeks' duration. No abnormality is obvious. **B**, Frog-leg lateral view demonstrates area of microfracture and compaction of the anterolateral portion of the secondary ossification center of the proximal femur. Treatment with an abduction brace was started. **C**, Four months later, increased radiodensity is noted in the infarcted segment. **D**, Slight collapse of the infarcted area has occurred but no further extension into the remainder of the epiphysis has taken place.

Differential Diagnosis. Acute and chronic infections, sickle cell disease, toxic synovitis, Gaucher's disease, slipped capital femoral epiphysis, and other hip dysplasia problems may occur with similar features. Generally, slipped capital femoral epiphysis occurs in obese preadolescent and adolescent boys.

Management. The following steps are taken (Shah, 2002; Warren, 2002b):

- Refer to an orthopedist immediately and ensure access to care for the child and family. Most cases of LCPD are mild and need no treatment because they are self-limited. However, all children with LCPD require frequent follow-up and monitoring by the orthopedist. Initial bed rest and possibly femoral abduction traction may be used to reduce hip irritability (1 to 2 weeks). Physical therapy may then be needed to reduce residual stiffness. The orthopedist works to prevent extrusion and collapse of the femoral head and attain or maintain a round shape using nonoperative or operative procedures, or both. Containment of the femoral head within the acetabulum is important. For moderate to severe cases, bracing and surgical intervention are the treatment options. Bracing is continued 24 hours a day for 6 to 18 months. Operative treatment is generally used in older children, for those who are not satisfactory candidates for bracing, or for those with extensive necrosis of the femoral head.

- Educate the family regarding the condition and its management and the risk for development of the condition on the other side.
- Support and monitor the child throughout treatment and recovery, including during interruption of school or other activities. The management of LCPD often involves several years of treatment and monitoring.

Complications. Osteoarthritis related to femoral head deformity and decreased use of the hip joint may occur, depending on the femoral head remodeling status. Older children have a poorer prognosis owing to the decreased opportunity for femoral head remodeling in the remaining growth period. Females with LCPD also have a poor prognosis.

Prevention. The condition is not preventable, but early identification and treatment reduce the long-term complications of the disorder such as premature degenerative arthritis in early adult life.

Slipped Capital Femoral Epiphysis

Description. Slipped capital femoral epiphysis (SCFE) is a condition in which the upper femoral epiphysis gradually slips from its functional position in the hip joint, and the femoral neck assumes a more varus angle. During the process, the physis of the femur (the growth plate area) becomes less competent, resulting in a weakening of the perichondrial ring. This weakening allows the epiphysis to slip posteriorly and medially, while the femoral neck moves anteriorly and proximally. The displacement involves a gradual slippage. Because the blood supply to the epiphysis crosses the weakened area, the epiphysis is at risk for avascular necrosis. The condition resolves when the growth plate closes with whatever position the epiphysis has taken in relation to the femoral shaft (Shah, 2002).

Etiology and Incidence. The etiology is unknown and thought to be multifactorial. Possible causes include mechanical susceptibility or vulnerability of the hip, endocrinopathies or systemic disease (e.g., hypothyroidism, hypopituitarism, hypogonadism, and chronic renal failure), trauma resulting from repetitive shear stress, inflammatory changes, and familial association in 5% of cases (Warren, 2002c). Obesity increases the shear forces across the femoral head and growth plate. Obese children develop SCFE at an earlier age.

SCFE is the most common hip disorder in adolescents and is associated with genetic, racial, and geographic risk factors. The problem occurs more commonly in males (2:1 to 3:1), especially those who are skeletally immature and obese. Affected males are generally between 10 and 12 years of age and females are between 11 and 12 years of age (before menarche), but the condition can occur anywhere from 9 to 15 years of age. African American males and females have a higher incidence, and about 5% have a positive family history. Polynesian populations are also at risk. Bilateral involvement occurs in 20% to 25% of cases. The majority of children are above the 90th percentile for weight. Incident rates vary in the United States, from 0.71 per 100,000 in New Mexico to 3.41 per 100,000 in Connecticut (Warren, 2002c).

Clinical Findings. The findings are similar to those of younger children with LCPD.

History. The following may be reported:

- Acute (symptoms within 3 weeks) or chronic (more than 3 weeks) thigh or knee pain
- Acute-on-chronic slip can also be reported (acute episode of further slippage in a child with previous slippage)
- Sometimes a history of mild trauma to the hip area

Physical Findings. Findings include the following:

- Pain in the groin or diffusely over the knee or anterior thigh
- Pain and decreased internal rotation
- Antalgic limp with short leg component (50% are up to 1 inch shorter on affected side)
- External rotation of the leg when walking
- External rotation of the thigh when the hip is flexed
- Thigh atrophy
- Limited abduction and extension

Diagnostic Studies. AP pelvis, frog-leg lateral, and true lateral views of the pelvis are obtained. Radiographic findings include flattening of the epiphyseal prominence, widening or irregularity of the growth plate, and narrowing of the area if the epiphysis has slipped posteriorly. The varus angle between the femoral head and the shaft is also assessed (Fig. 38-8). Computed tomography is used for preoperative planning because it provides measurements of the percentage of epiphysial slip, as well as the head-shaft and head-neck angles. SCFE is classified by grade and severity of the slip.

Differential Diagnosis. LCPD, sepsis of the hip joint, and osteoarthritis should be considered.

Management. The following steps are taken:

- Refer immediately to an orthopedic surgeon because there is risk of an acute and more devastating slip, which can occur at any time. Assist the family to attain prompt intervention. Immediate hospitalization is needed once the diagnosis is made.
- Place the patient on non–weight-bearing crutches until admitted to the hospital. Wheelchair sitting is not advised, because acute flexion can cause further slippage. Adequate instruction should be given so that the child will not fall on the crutches, another risk factor for an acute slip.

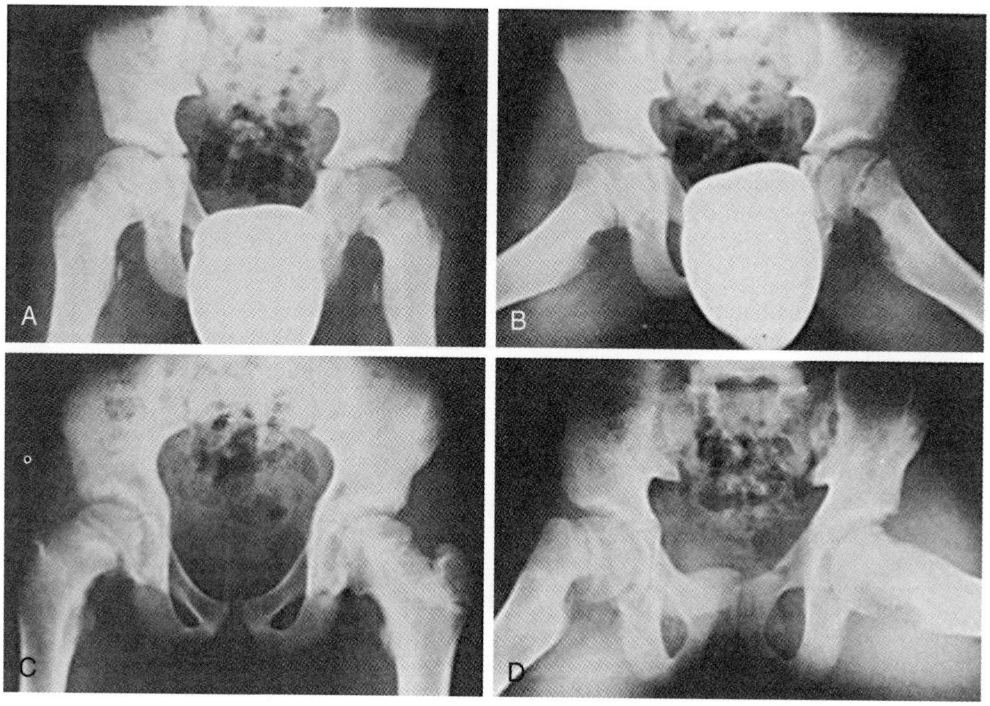

FIGURE 38-8 Acute slipped capital femoral epiphysis in a 10-year-old boy with acute left hip and thigh pain. **A**, Anteroposterior views of both hips. A line drawn along the superior surface of the femoral head, as seen on the right side, should intersect a corner of the femoral head. The left femoral head has slipped inferiorly. **B**, Frog-leg lateral roentgenograms of both hips demonstrate the mild displacement of the left femoral head more clearly. There is no evidence of remodeling in this acute slip. **C**, The left hip was treated by open epiphysiodesis; the bone graft placed across the growth plate is evident and the left growth plate has closed. At this time, 2 years after the onset of left hip pain, the patient had slight right hip pain of 3 months' duration. **D**, Lateral roentgenograms demonstrate moderate to severe slip of the right femoral head.

- For mild to moderate slips, in situ fixation of the epiphysis to the femur with a metallic screw or pins is the accepted treatment of choice. The screw or pins are removed after the growth plate closes. For very severe slippage, osteotomy is sometimes required. Spica cast immobilization is sometimes used for acute slips but has disadvantages. Traction can be used to gently reduce an acute-on-chronic slip.
- Inform the family about the condition and its management and the risk for slippage on the other side if only one side is treated.
- Support and monitor the child throughout the treatment phase, which includes interruption of school and activities during the recovery period. Contact sports are usually restricted by the orthopedist until growth is complete.

Complications. Avascular necrosis of the femoral head or, more commonly, chondrolysis of the cartilage lining the hip joint with narrowing of the hip joint is possible. A bilateral slip may have occurred on the other side at the time of diagnosis or can occur at a later time (Warren, 2002c).

Prevention. SCFE is not a preventable condition. However, identification of the condition during the preslip period, when complaints of hip or referred knee pain, loss of motion, or weakness in the hip are present, allows early intervention that can prevent deformity and long-term sequelae such as premature degenerative arthritis in early adult life. If the child is overweight, advise about the need for weight reduction.

Femoral Anteversion

Description. Everyone has some degree of femoral anteversion. By age 10 to 12 years, the normal angle of anteversion is 10 to 15 degrees. Younger children have a somewhat wider angle. Increased femoral anteversion (more than 2 standard deviations [SD] from the mean) is called femoral torsion and can be either medial or lateral. Medial femoral torsion or medial antetorsion generally occurs around 2 to 3 years of age and lasts until about 5 years of age. It is a condition in which the head and neck of the femur are rotated at an increased angle anteriorly in relation to the femoral shaft. Femoral anteversion is also called *internal femoral torsion.*

Etiology. A family history is often identified, and it occurs more commonly in girls. "W" sitting can increase the deformity. Physiologically, the condition produces an in-toeing gait because the anteriorly directed femoral neck internally rotates to a more neutral position and the head of the femur fits neatly into the acetabulum. This results in internal rotation of the lower femur and leg with the feet in-toeing. Increased femoral anteversion generally is more severe between ages 4 and 6 years but resolves as the child grows and the tibia rotate laterally.

Clinical Findings

History. The following may be reported:

- In-toeing gait, perhaps more severe with fatigue
- Runs awkwardly (looks like an "egg beater")
- Possible family history
- Usually a history of "W" sitting (TV squat)

Physical Examination. Findings include the following:

- In-toeing gait with patellae medial
- Internal (medial) rotation normally less than 70 degrees (mild deformity—70 to 80 degrees; moderate—between 80 and 90 degrees; severe—greater than 90 degrees [Staheli, 1998, 2003a] [see Fig. 38-5])
- External (lateral) rotation decreased (limited to 0-10 degrees)
- Knees medially rotated ("kissing patella") when standing

Diagnostic Studies. Radiographs are not merited unless surgery is contemplated.

Differential Diagnosis. Consider other rotational deformities such as internal tibial torsion or metatarsus adductus. Cerebral palsy with a "scissoring gait" might be mistaken for severe femoral anteversion.

Management. Management includes observation of the child and referral to an orthopedist if medial rotations are significant (no external rotation of the hip in extension) or the child or family has significant concerns. Nonoperative management strategies such as shoe modifications, twister cables, and night splints have all been found to be ineffective. Operative correction is successful but carries the risk of complications. Osteotomy is rarely performed and is done only in the child older than 8 years with significant cosmetic and functional deformity. The natural history of the condition is for the medial, or internal, rotation to decrease, giving some improvement (Eilert, 2001; Staheli, 2003a).

Complications. Studies have shown that the condition does not cause flatfoot, bunions, knee problems, back difficulties, difficulties in running, or degenerative arthritis of the hip in adults (Staheli, 2003a). It is primarily a cosmetic problem unless severe enough to interfere with activities. Self-esteem can be affected.

Prevention. The condition cannot be prevented, but its aggravation can be minimized by discouraging "W" sitting, which places the weight of the upper body directly on the femoral neck, thus increasing the molding in the abnormal direction. Ballet lessons or activities such as skating, bicycle riding, or skiing can help mildly affected children learn to point their feet straight ahead, but such activities do not modify the bony structures (Eilert, 2001).

Knee Problems

Genu Varum

Description. Genu varum, or bowing of the legs, can be a physiologic or developmental variation of normal or a pathologic condition, which involves a rotational deformity. The term *bowlegs* is used to describe physiologic variations of the normal knee angle resulting in bowing of the legs that is typically seen in children up to 2 years old but can be considered normal until age 3 years. Most bowing resolves spontaneously but can progress to persistent or pathologic varus (Warren, 2002a). The angle between the tibia and femur is in pronounced varus (up to 15 degrees) in normal children before 1 year of age. This is considered a uterine packing effect. The angle approaches neutral by 18 months and then proceeds to a valgus angle, with an average angle of 12 degrees from 2 to 3 years of age. The angle then gradually decreases to 8 degrees in females and 7 degrees in males by adulthood. Varus that continues after 30 months of age is considered persistent and needs to be differentiated from pathologic tibia vara such as seen in Blount disease. If the varus angle is greater than 15 degrees in infants, does not begin to decrease in the second year, is asymmetric, is associated with short stature, or is rapidly progressing, the condition is considered pathologic. Knee angle variations that fall 2 SD beyond the mean are outside the normal range of varus and are considered pathologic. The typical pattern of normal bowing seen in children is a symmetric lateral bowing of both tibia in the first year followed by bowlegs in the second year.

Etiology. If the varus does not resolve or increases it may represent Blount disease, rickets, tumor, neurologic problems, infection, or other conditions. A Salter fracture through the tibial growth plate can result in later genu varum as growth across the plate progresses unevenly.

Blount disease (tibia vara) is rare and represents 1% of all cases of genu varum. It is seen more frequently in the African American, Hispanic, and Scandinavian populations, is associated with obesity and early walkers, and commonly has a positive family history. Blount disease can occur in infancy (18 months to 3 years), school years (4 to 10 years), and during adolescence (11 years and older) and affects the proximal tibia (Drendel, Esterhai, & Sawyer, 2002).

Clinical Findings

History. When considering a diagnosis of pathologic genu varum, the NP should assess the following:

- Progression since birth; increasing deformation is problematic
- Risk factors such as metabolic disease

Older children may complain of stiffness or aching after activities (Warren, 2002a).

Physical Examination. Findings include the following:

- Tibial-femoral angle greater than 15 degrees
- Associated internal tibial torsion, common
- Intercondylar (knees) distance with the ankles together—measurement greater than 4 to 5 inches suggestive of the need for additional evaluation
- Joint laxity of the lateral collateral ligaments in older children

Diagnostic Studies. Radiographs are not necessary for physiologic bowlegs. Irregularity in the proximal medial tibia metaphysis with medial slipping of the physis and lateralization of the tibia are characteristic radiographic findings seen in infantile Blount disease. The radiographic findings in adolescent Blount disease differ in that the typical finding is narrowing of the medial physis only, with epiphysis not affected (Warren, 2002a).

Differential Diagnosis. Physiologic, persistent, and pathologic genu varum must be differentiated. Metabolic (rickets) or neurologic problems, Blount disease, infections, tumor, osteochondrodysplasias, and internal tibial torsion should be ruled out.

Management

- In physiologic genu varum (no increasing deformity):
  - No active treatment and resolves spontaneously. Denis Browne sleeping splints, corrective shoes, and passive exercises have not proved useful.
  - Reassure parents; provide information about the natural progression of the problem.
  - Observe the child's condition over time (in 3 to 6 months) to be sure the problem is resolving, especially during the second year of life. Photographs of the legs for the chart can be helpful.
- In pathologic genu varum (increasing deformity):
  - Refer to an orthopedist. Blount disease may be treated with a Blount brace in the early stages of the disease because the bowing is reversible. In later stages of the disease, in older children, or if the disease is progressing, osteotomy is the treatment of choice. Other conditions need to be treated according to the etiology.
  - Monitor to be sure braces are used consistently with good fit.
  - Observe to be sure the problem is not worsening.

Complications. Knee degeneration and deformity result if pathologic genu varum is not treated.

Prevention. Early identification and referral reduce the complexity and expense of treatment, as well as the residual deformities.

Genu Valgum

Description. Genu valgum is commonly referred to as *knock-knees.* Females tend to have a somewhat higher degree of valgus knee posture than males, leveling off by age 7 at 5 to 9 degrees compared with 4 to 7 degrees for boys. Physiologic genu valgum tends to peak at around 24 to 36 months and lasts until about 7 to 8 years of age.

Etiology. The condition can be considered developmental or physiologic in children starting anywhere from 2 to 4 years of age. It can be pathologic in the following situations: found in child older than 6 to 7 years; tibial-femoral angle greater than 15 degrees valgus; increasing in severity; and found in the presence of asymmetry, short stature, or obesity (Warren, 2002a). Causes of pathologic genu valgum include osteochondrodysplasias, physeal injury, tumor, myelodysplasia, and cerebral palsy.

Clinical Findings

History. The NP should assess the following:

- Progression of the deformity
- Risk factors as listed under etiology
- Joint pains or stiff gait caused by adduction of the thighs and abrasions

Physical Examination. Findings include the following (Warren, 2002a):

- Bilateral tibial-femoral angle less than 15 degrees of valgus in the child up to 7 years of age is considered normal and can be safely ignored; a valgus angle greater than 15 degrees is outside the range of normal.
- Unilateral deformity.
- Awkwardness of gait.
- Subluxing patella.
- Intermalleolar (ankles) distance with the knees together—measurement greater than 4 to 5 inches suggests the need for additional evaluation (Mankin & Zimbler, 1997).
- Genu valgum associated with short stature should be referred (Eilert, 2001).

Diagnostic Studies. No radiographic studies are needed unless a pathologic condition is suspected.

Differential Diagnosis. Rule out pathologic conditions of genu valgum.

Management. Management is the same as for physiologic and pathologic genu varum. However, for pathologic genu valgum, the types of braces prescribed are different, as are the surgical procedures. Bracing, usually at night, is used with deformities greater than 15 to 20 degrees, especially if there is a family history. Epiphyseal stapling or osteotomy may be needed if the deformity persists after age 10 years or if ligamentous or patellofemoral instability is present (Warren, 2002a). For most children with genu valgum before age 6 years, the condition resolves spontaneously.

Prevention. Preventive measures are the same as those for genu varum.

Osgood-Schlatter Disease

Description. Osgood-Schlatter disease (OSD) is caused by inflammation of the tibial tubercle, an apophysis site.

Etiology and Incidence. OSD is caused by repetitive microtrauma to the tibial tubercle apophysis, which results in inflammation, microfractures, and new bone formation at the tibial tubercle apophysis. Overuse of the muscles that attach to the apophysis is a factor. Tight muscles resulting from the slow rate of muscle growth relative to bone growth also are believed to be a factor. With the end of growth, the apophysis fuses to the shaft of the tibia and pain diminishes. Thus the incidence declines in older adolescents and in adults (Drendel, Esterhai, & Sawyer, 2002).

OSD is the most common cause of knee pain in adolescents who engage in active sports that typically entail sprinting and jumping. It is most often unilateral and occurs in boys between ages 10 and 15 years and in girls between ages 8 and 14 years (Weimer, 2002).

Clinical Findings

History. The following may be reported:

- Recent physical activity such as playing track, soccer, or football; surfboarding commonly produces the condition.
- Pain increases during and immediately after the activity and decreases when the activity is stopped for a while.

Physical Examination. Characteristic findings include the following:

- Point tenderness, pain, prominence over the tibial tubercle
- Pain with knee extension against passive resistence or with full passive knee flexion
- Possibly reduced knee range of motion
- Bilateral findings (frequent)

Differential Diagnosis. Other knee derangements, tumors (osteosarcoma), and hip problems with referred pain should be considered. The referred pain of hip problems is diffuse across the distal femur without point tenderness at the tibial tubercle.

Management. The following steps are taken:

- Avoid or modify activities that cause pain until the inflammation subsides; symptoms can last for 12 to 18 months.
- Applying ice to the site after activity may help.
- Try hamstring and quadriceps stretching exercises before sports.
- Use of NSAIDs is recommended by some but thought ineffective by others. Because this condition may last up to 12 to 18 months, chronic use of NSAIDs may be problematic.
- A neoprene sleeve over the knee may help stabilize the patella.
- Apply a knee immobilizer if pain is severe and persistent.
- Casting may be suggested for the noncompliant adolescent.

Complications. In the postpubertal child, a residual ossicle in the tendon next to the bone may cause persistent pain. Surgical removal is indicated and will relieve the pain.

Prevention. The condition cannot be prevented, but earlier management may decrease the length of disability and the discomfort associated with it. Avoid overuse and encourage balanced training and adequate warm-up before exercise or sports participation.

Tibial Torsion

Description. Tibial torsion is a common problem in children that involves the twisting of the long bone along its long axis. *Tibial version* is the term used to describe the normal variation in tibial rotation. At birth, the tibias have a mean lateral rotation of 2.2 degrees and rotate laterally over time, with an adult mean lateral tibial rotation of about 23 degrees. Tibial torsion describes those rotations that are outside the range of normal. Medial tibial torsion (MTT) consists of abnormal medial rotation or twisting, resulting in in-toeing of the feet; lateral tibial torsion (LTT) consists of abnormal lateral rotation resulting in out-toeing (Dise, 2002).

Etiology. Tibial torsion may be congenital, developmental, or acquired.

Incidence. MTT is the most common cause of in-toeing during the second year of life and is often noted around 6 to 12 months of life. Lateral tibial torsion is a cause of out-toeing in late childhood and is usually an acquired deformity. Contracture of the iliotibial band is the underlying problem.

Clinical Findings

Physical Examination. Observe the child's gait for in-toeing. The thigh-foot angle (TFA) is used to assess tibial rotation. With the child prone and the knees flexed 90 degrees, the foot and thigh are viewed from directly above (looking downward at the angle of the thigh and foot). The foot should be relaxed. MTT exists if the TFA is negative by more than 10 to 20 degrees (minus 10 to minus 20 degrees) bearing in mind the child's age. In-toeing is expressed in negative values (Fig. 38-9). The normal range at 13 years of age is −5 to +30 degrees. Abnormal lateral torsion is

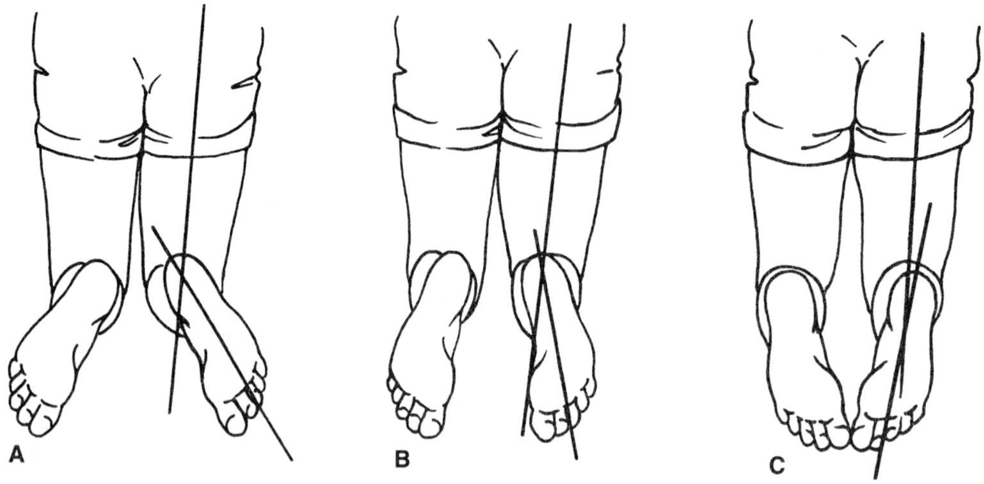

FIGURE 38-9 Thigh-foot angle. With the child in the prone position and the knees flexed and approximated, the long axis of the foot can be compared with the long axis of the thigh. The long axis of the foot bisects the heel and the second toe or lies between the second and third toes. External tibial torsion, **A**, produces excessive outward rotation. Normal alignment, **B**, is characterized by slight external rotation. Internal tibial torsion produces inward rotation of the foot and is a negative angle, **C**. (From Thompson GH: Gait disturbances. In Kliegman RM, Nieder ML, Super DM, editors: *Practical strategies in pediatric diagnosis and therapy*, Philadelphia, 1996, WB Saunders.)

associated with forward-pointing patellae and outward-pointing feet. A TFA measurement of greater than +30 degrees indicates abnormal lateral tibial torsion (Dise, 2002).

Diagnostic Studies. Radiographs are usually not necessary.

Differential Diagnosis. Genu varum in which the problem originates at the knee with a tibial-femoral angle, femoral torsion (femoral anteversion), adducted great toe, and metatarsus adductus also produce in-toeing gaits. Adducted great toe (the searching toe) is a benign condition that resolves spontaneously. Lateral femoral torsion also causes an out-toeing gait.

Management

- Treatment of tibial version (the normal variation in tibial rotation) is observation and monitoring of the child.
- MTT should be referred to an orthopedist if the problem is significant (greater than +20 by age 3 years). Stretching exercises or external rotational splints may be recommended. Surgical intervention may be needed for severe cases that persist into late childhood and cause significant functional problems.
- Shoes have been shown to be ineffective for the treatment of MTT. The avoidance of certain postures (e.g., sleeping in the knee-chest position and sitting with the feet tucked under the buttocks) thought to exacerbate MTT is controversial.
- LTT with TFA greater than +30 degrees should be referred to an orthopedist. It usually worsens with growth and does not correct spontaneously. Medial femoral torsion with pain also should be referred (Dise, 2002).

Complications. There are no complications with normal tibial versions and no interference with activities. Tibial torsion (the TFA is outside the acceptable range of normal) can lead to significant functional problems in severe cases.

Popliteal Cysts

Description. Popliteal cysts, or Baker cysts, are synovial lesions that result from herniation of the synovium of the knee joint into the popliteal space. In children, they are benign cysts and are not associated with intraarticular defects.

Clinical Findings. The major findings are swelling behind the knee with or without mild discomfort.

Diagnostic Studies. Ultrasonography, transillumination of cyst, and diagnostic aspiration of synovial fluid are the usual diagnostic studies.

Management. Observation is the treatment of choice because the majority of these cysts resolve on their own in 1 to 2 years (Eilert, 2001). The rare, large, painful, and persistent cyst should be referred to an orthopedic surgeon.

KNEE INJURIES AND FOOT PROBLEMS

Knee Injuries

Chapters 40 and 15 discuss issues related to the musculoskeletal examination and common sports injuries. Table 38-4 outlines the etiology, assessment, management, and differential diagnosis of common knee injuries that are seen in children and young adults.

TABLE 38-4 *Characteristics of Various Types of Knee Injuries and Conditions*

Condition	History/Mechanism of Injury	Clinical Findings	Management	Differential Diagnosis/ Prognosis/Comments
Quadriceps contusion	Typically a sports injury that results in bruising/contusion of the quadriceps muscle Injury can sometime result from minor trauma	Pain, swelling, and restriction of passive knee flexion	Rest, ice, compression wrap, and elevation (RICE) Flexion of the knee is the last function to return to normal so is a good indicator for return to sport	In teens, rule out rhabdomyosarcoma of the quadriceps, Ewing sarcoma, and osteosarcoma if there is swelling and pain in thigh without clear history of trauma
Meniscal tear (torn cartilage)	Associated with a significant injury in a youth Tear of a normal meniscus is rarely seen in children <12 yr old Congenital abnormal cartilage (discoid) can tear at any age	Pain, swelling and limping Joint line tenderness and positive McMurray sign Can be isolated or occur in combination with ACL or MCL injuries	RICE initially MRI if suspected tear; arthrography with MRI to rule out nerve injury with a prior tear Meniscectomy generally relieves symptoms	75% of patients develop degenerative articular changes on x-ray by age 30 yr A small percentage of youths develop degenerative changes 3 to 5 yr after injury Chrondral fractures or injuries to articular cartilage have similar history and physical findings
Sprain of the anterior cruciate ligament (ACL)	Acute injury; typically there is a twisting or hyperextension while the foot is planted and knee extended Report of a "popping" feeling and knee shifting or pulling apart	Swelling/effusion and pain Instability with lateral movement Positive Lachman's test	Following the injury, a knee brace or immobilizer is used until swelling and pain subside ACL reconstruction	Associated with MCL and meniscal tears
Sprains of the medial collateral ligament (MCL)	Valgus stress to an extended knee Reports tearing sensation with medial pain, swelling, stiffness	Instability with lateral movement Tenderness over the MCL If tenderness extends along the distal femoral physis, suspect physeal fracture	Ice, elevation, compression, splint or hinged knee brace Plain radiographs to look for physeal and epiphyseal fractures in skeletally immature children Surgical repair on an isolated collateral ligament is not beneficial	Combined ACL and MCL injuries are common Physeal fractures are more common than MCL sprains in youths
Osteochondritis dissecans	Juvenile and adolescent types Common 10-15 yr of age; boys more common than girls Etiology—may be trauma or may involve metabolic or genetic factors Pain increased with activity and diminished with rest plus intermittent effusions Locking and catching are unusual findings but may be present if bone fragments detached	Activity-related pain and swelling	Plain radiographs or MRI; 4-6 wk on immobilization and non-weight bearing if <12 yr of age Youths >12 yr, arthroscopic surgery	Mimics symptoms of a torn meniscus Articular cartilage transplantation for selected patients

Continued

TABLE 38-4 Characteristics of Various Types of Knee Injuries and Conditions—cont'd

Condition	History/Mechanism of Injury	Clinical Findings	Management	Differential Diagnosis/ Prognosis/Comments
Dislocation of the patella	Associated with patellar malalignment Pain and swelling Most occur in youths <20 yr old Family history in 20%-30%	Most cases involve lateral dislocation Massive and tense effusion Tenderness at the medial border of the patella and medial retinaculum Guarding with gentle pressure on the medial patella with lateral displacement	Nonoperative management: 1-2 wk of joint rest with splint or knee immobilizer, then intensive rehabilitation Isometric exercises Surgical correction for recurrent dislocations or chronic instability	Outcomes with nonoperative therapy vs. acute surgery are similar Patellar dislocation tends to recur (recurrence is more frequent in younger child) but decreases over time Degenerative arthritis is common with or without surgery with recurrent dislocations

Data from Anderson SJ: Lower extremity injuries in youth sports, *Pediatr Clin North Am* 49:627-641, 2002; Staheli LT, editor: *Pediatric orthopedic secrets*, ed 2, Philadelphia, 2003, Hanley & Blefus; Drendel AL, Esterhai JL, Sawyer JR: Orthopedic problems of the extremities. In Burg FD et al, editors: *Gellis and Kagan's current pediatric therapy*, ed 17, Philadelphia, 2002, WB Saunders.
MRI, Magnetic resonance imaging.

Foot Problems

Pes Planus

Description. Physiologic pes planus (flatfoot) is commonly seen in neonates and toddlers and is due to a fat pad in the arch that makes the appearance of the arch seem flat. This generally resolves by 2 to 3 years of age but in a small percentage of cases can persist into adulthood. Flexible flatfoot is often familial, common, and benign. The arch is seen when the foot is suspended but flattens with weight bearing. Rigid flatfoot is pathologic.

Etiology. Flatfoot is the result of soft tissue laxity, muscular weakness, or a tight Achilles tendon. There is often a familial tendency toward the problem. Flatfoot also is associated with certain syndromes (Marfan and Down syndromes), myelodysplasia, cerebral palsy, and obesity. Flatfoot may be secondary to muscle imbalance or weakness, a bony abnormality, or shortened heel cords (Dise, 2001).

Clinical Findings

History. Onset is noticed with weight bearing. The flexible flatfoot is painless and asymptomatic.

Physical Examination. The NP should assess the following:
- Is there an arch in the suspended foot or when the child toe-stands?
- Can an arch be molded with pressure by the examiner's fingers?
- Is the Achilles tendon tight?
- Is there abnormal shoe wear on the inner side?

Differential Diagnosis. Congenital vertical talus should be considered if the foot is rigid and no arch can be molded or if the foot has a rocker-bottom appearance. Calcaneovalgus foot might be considered also.

Management. Management involves the following:
- Only symptomatic feet and rigid flatfoot should be treated; refer to an orthopedist.
- For painful, flexible flatfoot, a removable, longitudinal arch support may be recommended by the orthopedist.
- If the Achilles tendon is tight, passive stretching may be helpful.
- Routine radiographs are not indicated unless pathologic flatfoot is suspected.

Complications. Flatfoot should be considered a variation of normal unless there is pain or rigidity. Congenital vertical talus is difficult to treat and should not be missed. Some cases of flatfoot are symptomatic in adulthood, and, in severe cases, the bones of the feet adapt to abnormal position with pronation and possible development of bunions.

Patient Education. Parents need to understand that special shoes do not cure the problem and arch supports do not help the foot to "grow" an arch. The so-called Thomas heel is considered ineffective as a treatment.

Metatarsus Adductus

Description. Metatarsus adductus (MA) is a condition in which the hindfoot is straight but the forefoot is adducted, giving the foot a curved, in-toeing shape. It is often bilateral.

Etiology and Incidence. When the foot is flexible, the condition is usually considered a result of uterine packing, with some tightness of the soft tissues in the area of the arch. A nonflexible foot, especially with heel valgus, or persistence may indicate a more serious problem.

Flexible MA is common (1 in 1000 births) and is seen more often in girls than boys. In 10% of cases, it is associated with DDH (Drendel, Esterhai, & Sawyer, 2002).

Clinical Findings

History. There can be a family history.

Physical Examination. Findings include the following:

- The lateral border of the foot has a convex shape. Normally, this border should look straight. Sometimes spreading of the toes is noted with a wider space between the first and second toes.
- The foot should normally be straight. If one draws a line from the middle of the heel it should pass through the second toe or between the second and third toes (Mankin & Zimbler, 1997). In MA, the forefoot has an increased angle (greater than 15 degrees) or resists stretching (Fig. 38-10).
- To determine whether the foot is flexible or rigid, the heel is grasped with one hand while the forefoot is abducted with the other hand. In flexible MA, the forefoot can be abducted past midline.

Diagnostic Studies. Radiographic studies need to be ordered if the foot is not flexible or MA persists beyond 6 months of age.

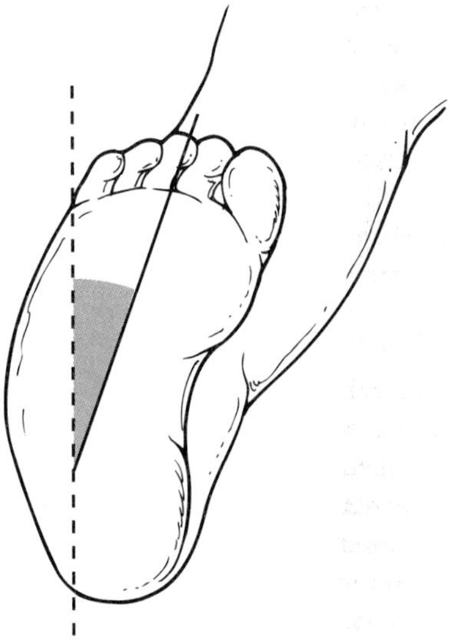

FIGURE 38-10 Metatarsus adductus angle. An angle created by the intersecting lines that is greater than 15 degrees indicates metatarsus adductus.

Differential Diagnosis. Consider congenital vertical talus, which will be rigid, or clubfoot, in which the foot is inverted and in the pointed-toe position.

Management. Management involves the following:

- For the flexible foot that can be brought past midline, the soft tissues can be stretched by the parents with each diaper change. Stretching is done as described under physical examination when the examiner determines whether the foot is flexible. Instruct the parents to hold the stretch to the count of five and repeat five times. The soft tissues should blanch with each stretch. Be sure that the parent is not just pushing on the great toe. If no improvement is evident by 6 months of age, a short course of serial stretching and casting is appropriate. However, most cases resolve spontaneously (Drendel, Esterhai, & Sawyer, 2002).
- For the nonflexible foot:
  - Refer to an orthopedist when the problem is identified.
  - Educate the family that the treatment for infants may include serial short-leg casts or braces to stretch the foot (two or three casts for 2 weeks per cast) or other management if the bones of the foot are more severely affected. If the child is older than 2 to 3 years of age, surgery may be needed to correct the problem.
- Corrective shoes, having the child wear shoes on the opposite foot, or night splints are not helpful for flexible MA.

Complications. Early intervention can prevent more intensive therapeutic measures to correct the deformity.

Talipes Equinovarus

Description. Talipes equinovarus (clubfoot) has three elements: the ankle is in equinus (the foot is in a pointed-toe position), the sole of the foot is inverted as a result of hindfoot varus or inversion deformity of the heel, and the forefoot has the convex shape of metatarsus adductus (forefoot adduction). The foot cannot be manually corrected to a neutral position with the heel down.

Etiology. The etiology of clubfoot may be idiopathic (which tends to be hereditary), neurogenic as seen with myelomeningocele, or associated with certain syndromes such as arthrogryposis and Larsen syndrome. It varies in severity, with uterine positioning a factor in mild clubfoot. The incidence is 1:1000 live births, with approximately 50% of cases being bilateral. The problem is congenital and can be identified in neonates. It is more common in boys (Drendel, Esterhai, & Sawyer, 2002; Eilert, 2001).

Clinical Findings

History. Clubfoot is present at birth.

Physical Examination. The foot appears as described previously.

Diagnostic Studies. AP and dorsiflexion lateral views of the foot are done.

Management. The following steps are taken:

- Refer to an orthopedist as early as possible, ideally in the newborn nursery, because the joints are most flexible in the first hours and days of life. The foot can become rigid in a matter of days. The orthopedist may begin with serial manipulation and casting for 6 weeks. Surgical correction may be required for severe cases that do not respond to serial casting and is usually performed between ages 9 and 12 months.
- Monitor throughout childhood, because the condition can recur. Postcorrection night splinting may be needed. Older children with rigid bony deformities often require osteotomy, tendon transfers, and fusions.

Complications. With growth, the abnormality can become increasingly distorted, making correction more difficult. Calf hypoplasia and a shorter than normal foot can occur even with correction.

Overriding Toes

Overriding toes are generally identified at birth. Efforts to tape them into a correct position or otherwise modify their position are usually futile. Overriding of the second, third, and fourth toes generally resolves with time. Occasionally, if severe, they can be surgically improved. Shoe fit can be a problem.

In-toeing and Out-toeing Rotational Problems

When a child has an in-toeing or out-toeing gait, the degree of rotation and source of the rotational deformity must be assessed. These include internal femoral torsion (femoral anteversion), internal tibial torsion, and metatarsus adductus. The causes of in-toeing usually are physiologic, are related to age, and resolve as the child grows (Table 38-5). In addition, in-toeing in children can vary with activities and from step to step.

Clinical Findings

History. The NP assesses the following:

- Onset of problem
- Increasing or decreasing deformity
- Treatments used to date
- Degree of interference with activities
- Effects on self-image for older children
- Neurologic history

Physical Examination. The physical examination involves the following:

- Observe the gait. Note that the slightly older child may consciously or unconsciously improve or worsen the gait for the examiner. Asking the child to run may also be helpful.
- Lay the child prone on the examining table.
- Examine for femoral anteversion (medial and lateral rotations).
- Examine for internal or external tibial torsion (TFA).
- Examine for MA or other deformity.

The child may have a combination of any or all of the aforementioned problems.

Management. See the individual diagnoses for management strategies.

OTHER COMMON MUSCULOSKELETAL SYSTEM FINDINGS NEEDING ATTENTION

Toe-Walking

Description

Most young children walk on their toes until they establish the heel-toe pattern, usually within the first 6 months of

TABLE 38-5 ***Typical Cause of In-toeing and Out-toeing Rotational Problems***

	Cause	Typical Finding	Age at Manifestation
In-toeing	Equinovarus	Plantar foot flexion, forefoot adduction, and hindfoot varus	At birth
	Metatarsus adductus	Curved foot—refer if not flexible	Birth-6 mo
	Abducted great toe	Searching toe—resolves spontaneously	Toddler period
	Medial tibial torsion	Refer if thigh-foot angle (TFA) >-10 to -20 degrees	12-18 mo
	Internal femoral torsion	Refer if >70 degrees medial and <10 degrees lateral hip rotation	2-5 yr
Out-toeing	Physiologic infantile out-toeing	Feet may turn out when infant is positioned upright—resolves spontaneously	Early infancy
	Lateral tibial torsion	Refer if TFA $>+30$ degrees	Late childhood
	Lateral femoral torsion	Refer if >2 SD of the mean	Late childhood

$>$, Greater than; $<$, less than.

walking. Consistent toe-walking is frequently associated with neurologic problems such as cerebral palsy. Autistic children or those with early muscular dystrophy may toe-walk. Children with tight heel cords may toe-walk. Unilateral toe-walking can be associated with a short leg, as found with a dislocated hip. Toe-walking also can be a habit, especially in children who used walkers. In these children, toe-walking generally resolves before age 3 years and is not associated with any musculoskeletal deformity. It is important to differentiate between the idiopathic toe-walker and the child who toe-walks because of a neuromusculoskeletal condition associated with tight heel cords and contractures.

Clinical Findings

History. The NP should assess

- Onset
- Severity
- Neurologic history
- Use of walker

Physical Examination. The NP should

- Look at shoe wear to assess extent of toe-walking. For example, is the heel worn?
- Assess for tight heel cords. The foot should be brought beyond a 90-degree angle.
- Conduct a neurologic assessment.
- Measure leg lengths and examine hips.

Management

Management depends on the etiology. Orthopedic management is needed for tight heel cords, unequal leg lengths, and hip problems.

Ganglions of the Hands

Description

Ganglions are the most common benign lesions of soft tissue in children (see discussion of popliteal cysts). A ganglionic cyst is an acquired, mucinous, fluid-filled, painless lesion that originates from the synovial-lined space.

Clinical Findings

Ganglions of the hand are hard, fixed masses commonly found on the wrist (commonly dorsal) and flexor aspects of the finger. Transillumination of the cyst with an otoscope or examination by ultrasonography plus findings on physical examination are keys to the diagnosis.

Management

Ganglionic cysts in children are rarely symptomatic and usually regress spontaneously. The likelihood of recurrence with any form of treatment is higher in children than the recurrence rate in adults with ganglionic lesions (Ezake & Hollier, 2003). Conservative care with rest and splinting can be tried. Refer for needle aspiration or surgical excision (the most reliable method to eliminate a ganglion) if conservative care fails to result in partial or complete resolution. Steroid injections are not advised.

Leg Aches of Childhood

Description

Transient aches are common complaints during childhood that have been reported to occur in 13% of boys and 18% of girls, usually involving the lower extremities. The term *growing pains* has been used to describe this discomfort but not without controversy, because musculoskeletal growth has never been proved to be the cause of these aches or pains. *Leg aches* is the term now most commonly used. Their cause is unknown or idiopathic; a common theory is that thigh and calf muscle fatigue is responsible. Differentiating benign leg aches of childhood from more serious pathology is important. Onset is common at about 4 years of age, and they can affect children up to 12 years of age (McCarthy, 2003).

Clinical Findings

History. Pain or leg aches are typically described as

- Occurring characteristically in the evening or late in the day; may wake child up from sleep
- Pain gone in the morning with no limitation of activity
- Poorly localized and bilateral
- Occurring commonly in the front of the thighs, in the calves, and behind the knees
- Transient and occurring over a period of time as long as several years
- Not associated with a limp or disability (McCarthy, 2003)

Physical Examination. Normal physical examination with no tenderness, guarding, or reduced range of joint motion. Have the child stand on tiptoes and heels. Measurement of leg lengths should be taken if leg length inequality is suspected.

Diagnostic Studies. Radiographs and blood work are not necessary if a classic history is given and there are no physical findings.

Differential Diagnosis

Neoplastic lesions, leukemia, sickle cell anemia, and subacute osteomyelitis must be ruled out.

Management

Reassure the parents that these are common complaints that are benign and generally resolve spontaneously. Symptomatic treatment with heat and analgesic may be of benefit. Stress the need for parents to bring the child in for reevaluation if there is a change in symptoms or other signs emerge. Refer a child if the pain is localized to one region, is associated with swelling or other constitutional symptoms, is increasing in severity, or alters gait.

Limps

Description

Children limp for reasons including pain, deformity, or weakness. Limps must always be carefully assessed and managed. Limps may be of several types.

- *Antalgic.* This is a gait caused by pain that increases with the normal stresses of walking. The child tries to get weight off the affected side quickly; thus the normal walking cadence is off, with a shortened stance phase. Examples of antalgic gaits: The child with a sore knee walks with a fixed knee, whereas the child with a sore toe tries not to roll off the toe at the toe-off phase of the stride. A child with appendicitis may also have an antalgic gait, with a slight slumping posture and a shortened stride on the right resulting from psoas muscle irritation.
- *Trendelenburg gait* or *abductor lurch.* This gait is caused by a hip problem such as hip dysplasia. The child tilts over the affected hip with each stride to decrease the mechanical stresses while the opposite side is off the ground during the swing-through phase of the gait.
- *Equinus* or *toe-to-heel gait.* This is caused by lack of neurologic coordination, creating an unsteady, wide-based gait. For example, children with cerebral palsy often exhibit this characteristic toe-to-heel sequence during the stance phase of their gait because of heel-cord contractures.
- *Circumduction.* This gait allows a functionally longer leg to progress forward using a circular swing motion. Children with leg length inequality and painful foot or ankle conditions use this gait.

Clinical Findings

History. A careful history is needed, including

- Onset
- Location of pain
- Changes in limp or pain during the day or since onset
- Interference with activities
- Past medical history, including injury or illness
- Review of systems

Physical Examination. The NP should do the following:

- Identify the type of limp from the gait.
- Examine the hips, legs, feet, and back for range of motion, asymmetry, changes in tissues, and signs of infection.
- Complete a neurologic examination, including strength, reflexes, balance, and coordination.
- Assess Trendelenburg sign for hip stability.

Diagnostic Studies. Studies are ordered appropriate to the findings and history. Knee pain and limp may be referred from the hip.

Differential Diagnosis

Age is an important factor in diagnosing the many causes of limping. Fracture, developmental dysplasia of the hip, Legg-Calvé-Perthes disease, slipped capital femoral epiphysis, tumor, infection, juvenile arthritis, and others should be considered (Table 38-6).

Management

Refer the patient to an orthopedist immediately unless the etiology is a mild strain or a local lesion that can be managed conservatively by the primary care provider.

Overuse Syndromes of Childhood and Adolescence

Description

Overuse syndrome is caused by repetitive movement injury that causes microtrauma. Osgood-Schlatter disease, discussed earlier, is a classic example of an overuse injury commonly seen in children age 10 to 14 years. Other typical overuse injuries of childhood are varus overload of the elbow ("Little League elbow"), proximal humeral epiphysiolysis ("Little League shoulder"), patellofemoral pain syndrome, shin splints, and stress fractures (Table 38-7).

Management

Treatment often involves resting and icing the extremity or joint, doing retraining and strengthening exercises, gradually reintroducing activities, and using analgesics. NSAIDs help reduce the inflammatory component of the trauma. Patient and parent education is important to prevent further injury and disability and to allow the child to return to safe sport participation.

Muscle Diseases

Description

Muscle diseases in children are rare. However, there are many types of problems that can affect muscle metabolism or function. It can be difficult to discern whether the lack of good muscular function is due to problems of enervation or an inability of the muscle to contract efficiently.

TABLE 38-6 ***Differential Diagnosis of Limping***

Condition	Age	Pain ±	Historical Findings	Clinical Findings	Causative Factors	Management
Developmental dysplasia of the hip	T, C, A	−	Breech delivery; metatarsus adductus; torticollis; poor treatment outcomes if not diagnosed at birth or shortly afterward	Limited abduction; Trendelenburg; radiography at 2-3 mo; shortening of leg; acetabular dysplasia	Familial; joint laxity, positioning, maternal hormones	Newborn: no triple diapers; Pavlik harness to hold hips in flexion—see weekly; after 6 mo, traction or open reduction; after 18 mo, osteotomy
Leg length inequality	T, C, A	−	None	Circumduction gait; joint contracture; >1 cm discrepancy in leg lengths	Congenital; neurogenic; vascular; tumor; trauma; infection	Shoe lifts; epiphysiodesis (fusion of growth plate to arrest growth of the opposite side), if discrepancy 2-6 cm
Neuromuscular (NM) disease	T, C, A	−	Depends on cause	Depends on cause; equinus or abductor gait	Cerebral palsy, muscular dystrophy, and other NM diseases	Referral to appropriate specialists
Discitis	T, C, A	+	Varied: fever, malaise, unwilling to walk, backache	Stiff back, ↑ ESR; x-ray 2-3 wk; early bone scan	Bacterial infection in disk space *(Staphylococcus aureus)* or inflammatory response	Immobilization and antistaphylococcal antibiotic therapy
Septic arthritis	T, C, A	++	Moderate to high fever, malaise, arthralgias; irritability; progressive course	Redness, warmth and swelling of joint—knee or hip; limited hip motion; ESR >25 mm/hr	*S. aureus* likely organism	Appropriate antibiotic coverage (7 days, IV; 3-4 wk total)
Osteomyelitis	T, C, A	+	Fever	Refusal to walk or move limb; point tenderness; 7-10 days to see radiographic bony changes	*S. aureus* likely organism	Appropriate antibiotic coverage (generally 7 days, IV; 4-6 wk total or until ESR normal)
Neoplastic	T, C, A	+	Depends on type of neoplasm	Varied	Neoplasm—benign or malignant	Referral to oncologist
Trauma	T, C, A	+	Depends on type (fractures, strains, sprains)	Varied	Varied	Rule out physical abuse if discrepancy related to developmental capabilities, injury history, and type of injury
Occult trauma: toddler fracture	T	+	Well child	Commonly spiral fracture of tibia; refusal to walk, mild soft tissue swelling; radiograph	Trauma	See trauma above

Continued

TABLE 38-6 *Differential Diagnosis of Limping—cont'd*

Condition	Age	Pain ±	Historical Findings	Clinical Findings	Causative Factors	Management
Transient synovitis	3-8 yr	+	Mild to moderate fever, mild irritability; resolves within 1 wk	Limited hip motion; ESR <25 mm/hr	Inflammatory reaction; unknown etiology; often URI (50%) prior	Rest
Juvenile arthritis (JA)	Childhood until 16 yr	+	Fever, rashes, ↑ WBC count; some iritis; joint stiffness and swelling; S & S >3 mo	Mono/polyarticular arthropathy; + ANA (25%-88%); ↑ ESR in moderate/severe JA	Unknown; genetic (HLA) or environmental	Treat with nonsteroidal antinflammatory agents initially; may need sulfasalazine, methotrexate; corticosteroids; joint replacements when older
Slipped capital femoral epiphysis	9-15 yr	+	>90 percentile weight; African American; male	Limited abduction and extension; external rotation of thigh if hip flexed	Multifactorial: mechanical; endocrine; trauma; familial	Needs immediate surgery; non–weight-bearing crutches until admitted (sitting not advised); bilateral involvement does occur
Legg-Calvé-Perthes disease	4-8 yr	+	Acute/chronic onset; pain in hip, groin, knee; stiffness; male	+ Trendelenburg, shortening; ↓ abduction, internal rotation, hip extension; + radiographs but not early	Familial; breech birth; prior trauma (17%)	In female, tends to be more serious problem; bed rest, traction, then PT; bracing and surgery may be needed; bilateral involvement does occur

Adapted from Behrman R, Kliegman RM, Arvin AM, editors: *Nelson textbook of pediatrics*, ed 15, Philadelphia, 1996, WB Saunders; Staheli L: *Fundamentals of pediatric orthopedics*, ed 2, Philadelphia, 1998, Lippincott-Raven.

A, Adolescent (≥11 yr); *ANA*, antinuclear antibody; *C*, child (4-10 yr); *ESR*, erythrocyte sedimentation rate; *HLA*, human leukocyte antigen; *PT*, physical therapy; *S & S*, signs and symptoms; *T*, toddler (1-3 yr); *URI*, upper respiratory infection; *WBC*, white blood cell.

TABLE 38-7 ***Overuse Injuries of Childhood: Characteristic Features and Their Treatment***

Condition	Clinical Findings	Treatment	Comments
Osgood-Schlatter disease	Swelling and tenderness/pain over tibial tubercle	Nonsteroidal antiinflammatory drugs (NSAIDs), knee pad, knee immobilizer if severe pain for 1-2 wk	Most resolve with time (12-18 mo), x-ray only if pain persists (soft tissue swelling and ossicle); if pain persists, consider surgical incision of ossicle
Patellofemoral pain syndrome	Anterior knee pain	Rest, NSAIDs, retraining, and strengthening of quadriceps muscles	Arthroscopic surgery only if recurring problems
Proximal humeral epiphysiolysis ("Little League shoulder")	Shoulder pain—gradual onset; pain ↑ with throwing, especially curve ball	Modify activity; gradual restart but limit intensity and frequency of throwing with retraining	Seen in skeletally immature children; radiographs—widening proximal humeral physis
Shin splints	Pain along medial border of tibia; child does prolonged running	NSAIDs; ice after running; retraining and muscle strengthening after inflammation ↓; gradual return to running	Associated with poor running technique, hard running surface, muscle weakness; inadequate running shoes; sudden increase in running; is an inflammatory response
Stress fractures	Tenderness and swelling at site	Reduce or eliminate activity that caused injury for 10-14 days; may need to cast	Due to microtrauma; most commonly seen in active teens but can occur during childhood; proximal tibia most common site
Varus overload of the elbow ("Little League elbow")	Elbow pain with activity; locking and ↓ extension of elbow; medial humeral epicondyle tenderness	Rest; NSAIDs; ice; when pain free, gradual return to activity with retraining; surgery if elbow instability	Leads to osteochondral lesions and stress fractures if severe; radiographs—widening proximal physis; also seen in gymnasts

Clinical Findings

History. The following may be reported:

- Failure to achieve motor milestones
- Loss of motor skills such as the ability to climb stairs easily
- Easy fatigue with physical activity
- A history of good days and bad days with relation to ability to accomplish physical activities
- Increasing difficulties with motor activities

Physical Examination. Findings include the following:

- Fibrotic or "doughy" feel to the muscles
- Muscle hypertrophy, especially of the calf muscles
- Muscle wasting
- Fibrillations or fasciculations
- Muscle contractures
- Weakness
- Positive Gowers' sign

Gowers' sign is obtained by asking the child to get up off the floor without help. The sign is positive if the child uses his or her arms to push off from the legs, gradually standing in a segmented fashion.

Management

Referral is necessary. These conditions may need to be handled by an interdisciplinary team with orthopedic, metabolic, and physical therapy, social service, and nursing care. Genetics counseling may be necessary, depending on the diagnosis. The muscular dystrophies, for instance, are autosomal dominant and can appear in several children in a family.

Patient and family support is needed. Muscle diseases are chronic, debilitating, and sometimes fatal conditions. Helping the child to lead as normal a life as possible while coping with his or her condition is a major task. The family may need help maintaining caregiving and coping with the implications of the diagnosis.

RESOURCE BOX

National Organizations for Musculoskeletal Disorders

Orthopedic Conditions

Brachial Plexus–Erb's Palsy Support and Information Network
1-414-836-9955
www.ubpn.org

Cherub Association of Families and Friends of Children with Limb Disorders
1-716-773-2769
www.steps-charity.org.uk

Scoliosis and Kyphosis
www.srs.org
A pamphlet with information and advice for parents; order from Scoliosis Research Society

The Spinal Connection
1-800-673-6922
1-781-341-6333
E-mail: scoliosis@aol.com
A newsletter published by the National Scoliosis Foundation, Inc.

Muscle Diseases

Muscular Dystrophy Association
1-800-572-1717
www.mdausa.org

REFERENCES

Behrman RE, Kliegman RM, Jenson HB, editors: *Nelson textbook of pediatrics*, ed 17, Philadelphia, 2004, WB Saunders.

Bennett J: Scoliosis and kyphosis. In Finberg L, editor: *Saunders manual of pediatric practice*, ed 2, Philadelphia, 2002a, WB Saunders.

Bennett J: Dysplasia of the hip. In Finberg L, Kleinman RE, editors: *Saunders manual of pediatric practice*, ed 2, Philadelphia, 2002b, WB Saunders.

Copley AB: Orthopedic trauma. In Burg FD et al, editors: *Gellis and Kagan's current pediatric therapy*, ed 17, Philadelphia, 2002, WB Saunders.

Dise TL: Flatfleet and tibial torsion. In Finberg L, Kleinman RE, editors: *Saunders manual of pediatric practice*, ed 2, Philadelphia, 2002, WB Saunders.

Drendel A, Esterhai JL, Sawyer JR: Orthopedic problems of the extremities. In Burg FD et al, editors: *Gellis and Kagan's current pediatric therapy*, ed 17, Philadelphia, 2002, WB Saunders.

Eilert RE: Orthopedics. In Hay WW et al, editors: *Current pediatric diagnosis and treatment*, ed 15, New York, 2001, McGraw-Hill.

Ezake M, Hollier LH: Acquired hand problems. In Staheli LT, editor: *Pediatric orthopedic secrets*, ed 2, Philadephia, 2003, Hanley & Belfus.

Hansen CA, Bateman DA: Birth injuries. In Burg FD et al, editors: *Gellis and Kagan's current pediatric therapy*, ed 17, Philadelphia, 2002, WB Saunders.

Mankin KP, Zimbler S: Gait and leg alignment: what's normal and what's not, *Contemp Pediatr* 14:41-70, 1997.

McCarthy RE: Leg aches. In Staheli LT, editor: *Pediatric orthopedic secrets*, ed 2, Philadephia, 2003, Hanley & Belfus.

Neyt JG, Weinstein SL: Kyphosis and lordosis. In Staheli LT, editor: *Pediatric orthopedic secrets*, ed 2, Philadephia, 2003, Hanley & Belfus.

Richards BS: Back pain. In Staheli LT, editor: *Pediatric orthopedic secrets*, ed 2, Philadephia, 2003, Hanley & Belfus.

Schaller JG: Nonrheumatic conditions mimicking rheumatic diseases of childhood. In Behrman R, Kliegman RM, Arvin AM, editors: *Nelson textbook of pediatrics*, ed 15, Philadelphia, 1996, WB Saunders.

Scoles P: *Pediatric orthopedics in clinical practice*, ed 2, St Louis, 1988, Mosby.

Shah SA: The hip. In Burg FD et al, editors: *Gellis and Kagan's current pediatric therapy*, ed 17, Philadelphia, 2002, WB Saunders.

Staheli LT: *Fundamentals of pediatric orthopedics*, ed 2, Philadelphia, 1998, Lippincott-Raven.

Staheli LT: In-toeing and out-toeing. In Staheli LT, editor: *Pediatric orthopedic secrets*, ed 2, Philadephia, 2003a, Hanley & Belfus.

Staheli LT: Shoes for children. In Staheli LT, editor: *Pediatric orthopedic secrets*, ed 2, Philadephia, 2003b, Hanley & Belfus.

Sussman M, Turker RJ: Disorders of the shoulder girdle and spine. In Burg FD, Ingelfinger JR, Wald ER, et al, editors: *Gellis and Kagan's current pediatric therapy*, ed 17, Philadelphia, 2002, WB Saunders.

Warren FH: Genu varum and genu valgum. In Finberg L, Kleinman RE, editors: *Saunders manual of pediatric practice*, ed 2, Philadelphia, 2002a, WB Saunders.

Warren FH: Legg-Calvé-Perthes disease. In Finberg L, Kleinman RE, editors: *Saunders manual of pediatric practice*, ed 2, Philadelphia, 2002b, WB Saunders.

Warren FH: Slipped capital femoral epiphysis. In Finberg L, Kleinman RE, editors: *Saunders manual of pediatric practice*, ed 2, Philadelphia, 2002c, WB Saunders.

Weimer SM: Osgood-Schlatter disease and other apophysitides. In Finberg L, Kleinman RE, editors: *Saunders manual of pediatric practice*, ed 2, Philadelphia, 2002, WB Saunders.

39 Perinatal Conditions

Deborah K. Parks, Robert J. Yetman

The neonatal period is a highly vulnerable time for the infant. In the United States, about two thirds of all deaths in the first year of life occur among infants less than 28 days of age (Behrman, Kliegman, & Jensen, 2004). Mortality risk is highest during the first 24 hours of life. Because serious health problems can arise for the infant in the hours after the initial transition to extrauterine life, the nurse practitioner (NP) must be prepared to manage these problems while providing psychosocial support and education for the families. An understanding of the physiology of fetal development, risk factors for potential problems, and pertinent physical findings prepares the NP to effectively assist the newborn's transition to extrauterine life.

STANDARDS OF CARE

The *Healthy People 2010* objectives (U.S. Department of Health and Human Services, 2003) related to maternal, infant, and child care are included in Appendix D. The overall goal of these objectives is to improve maternal health and pregnancy outcomes and reduce rates of disability in infants, thereby improving the health and well-being of women, infants, children, and families in the United States. The health of a population is reflected in the health of its most vulnerable members. A major focus of many public health efforts, therefore, is improving the health of pregnant women and their infants, including reductions in rate of birth defects, risk factors for infant death, and death of infants and their mothers.

The *Guide to Clinical Preventive Services* (U.S. Preventive Services Task Force, 2002) recommends the following preventive services for neonates:

- Prenatal screening for D (Rh) incompatibility, Down syndrome, and neural tube defects (including provision of appropriate folic acid prophylaxis).
- Neonatal screening for sickle hemoglobinopathies to identify infants who may benefit from antibiotic prophylaxis to prevent sepsis. All screening efforts must be accompanied by comprehensive counseling and treatment services.
- Screening for congenital hypothyroidism with thyroid function tests on dried blood spot specimens for all newborns during the first week of life.
- Screening for phenylketonuria (PKU) with a phenylalanine level on a dried blood spot for all newborns before discharge from the nursery. Infants who are tested before 24 hours of age should receive a repeat screening test by 2 weeks of age.
- Ocular antibiotic prophylaxis of all newborn infants to prevent gonococcal ophthalmia neonatorum.
- Routine newborn hearing screening is less clear. A review of the literature did not contribute to the group reaching consensus. The group concluded that newborn hearing screening led to earlier identification of hearing loss, but few data supported long-term benefit.

Put Prevention into Practice: The Clinician's Handbook of Preventive Services (U.S. Public Health Services, 2003) outlines recommendations from major authorities. These authorities recommend that newborn screening be performed according to each state's regulations. Specific recommendations regarding screening for hypothyroidism, PKU, and hemoglobinopathies are detailed in this handbook.

Bright Futures: Guidelines for Health Supervision of Infants, Children, and Adolescents (Green, 2002) has detailed anticipatory guidelines for the newborn, first-week, and 1-month health supervision visits. *Guidelines for Perinatal Care*, 5th edition, from the AAP and the American College of Obstetricians and Gynecologists (Gilstrap & Oh, 2002) is another thorough compendium of standards of caring for the newborn.

ANATOMY AND PHYSIOLOGY

Intrauterine-to-Extrauterine Transition

The infant's intrauterine-to-extrauterine transition requires many biochemical and physiologic changes. In utero, the placenta provides metabolic functions for the fetus. Oxygenated blood from the placenta arrives to the fetus through the umbilical vein. Because of high pulmonary vascular pressure, this blood is shunted from the right to the left side of the heart through the foramen ovale, or to the systemic circulation through the ductus arteriosus. At birth, the umbilical cord is severed. Simultaneously, the infant begins to breathe and the high pulmonary vascular pressure drops, allowing blood flow to the lungs for oxygenation. The foramen ovale and ductus arteriosus are no longer necessary and close after birth. The newborn becomes dependent on gastrointestinal tract function to absorb nutrients, renal function to excrete wastes and maintain chemical balance, liver function to metabolize and excrete toxins, and the functions of the immunologic system to protect against infection. Many newborn problems are related to poor transition to extrauterine life due to asphyxia, premature birth, congenital anomalies, or adverse effects of delivery.

A predictable series of changes or reactivities in vital signs and clinical appearance take place after the delivery of most normal infants (Fig. 39-1). The first period of reactivity includes sympathetic system changes such as tachycardia, rapid respirations, transient rales, grunting, flaring and retractions, a falling body temperature, hypertonus, and alerting exploratory behavior. Parasympathetic system changes during the first period of reactivity include the initiation of bowel sounds and the production of oral mucus.

After an interval of sleep, the infant enters the second period of reactivity. During this time the oral mucus again becomes evident, the heart rate become labile, the infant becomes more responsive to endogenous and exogenous stimuli, and meconium is often passed.

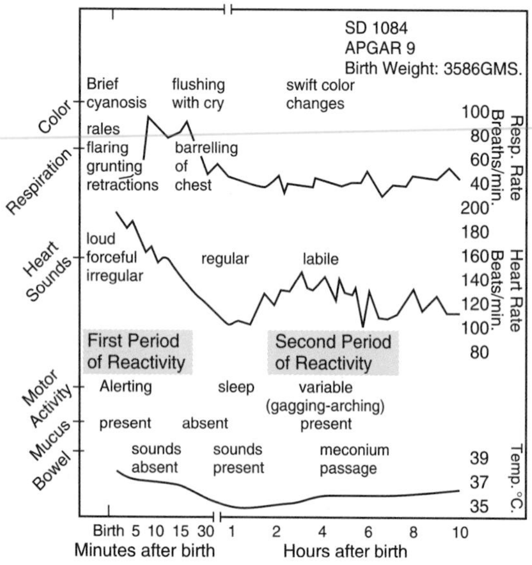

FIGURE 39-1 Summary of normal transition. (From Desmond MM, Rudolph AJ, Phitaksphraiwan P: The transitional care nursery, *Pediatr Clin North Am* 13:651-668, 1966.)

PATHOPHYSIOLOGY
High-Risk Pregnancy

High-risk pregnancies are defined as those in which factors exist that increase the chances of abortion, fetal death, premature delivery, intrauterine growth retardation, fetal or neonatal disease, congenital malformations, mental retardation, and other handicaps. Identification of high-risk pregnancies is the first step toward prevention of neonatal problems (Box 39-1). Comprehensive and frequent prenatal visits for high-risk pregnancies are aimed at preventing complications in the newborn.

Acquired Health Problems

In utero exposure to poor nutrition, alcohol, drugs, viruses or bacteria, and maternal conditions such as hypertension and diabetes can result in prematurity and abnormalities at birth. The risk of neonatal problems increases with maternal age younger than 16 years and older than 40 years.

Genetic Problems

The presence of chromosomal abnormalities, congenital anomalies, inborn errors of metabolism, mental retardation, and familial diseases increases the risk of the same condition in the infant. Because many conditions are not easily identifiable on physical examination, exploring family histories to determine if a newborn is at risk for any inheritable diseases is important. Anticipation of various inherited conditions leads to their early identification and management of potential problems.

Perinatal Complications and Injuries

Perinatal complications occur immediately before or during birth. Prolonged or dysfunctional labor increases the risk of fetal distress. Prolonged rupture of the membranes and chorioamnionitis increase the risk of infant infection, and ruptured placenta previa increases the risk of infant blood loss. Cesarean deliveries, the use of forceps or vacuum extraction, and the type of maternal anesthesia used also pose risks. The term *birth injury* includes mechanical and anoxic trauma incurred by an infant during labor and delivery. The incidence of birth injuries has been estimated at 2 to 7 per 1000 live births; these injuries represent 2% to 3% of infant deaths. Predisposing risk factors include macrosomia, prematurity, cephalopelvic disproportion,

BOX 39-1 *High-Risk Infants*

Demographic Social Factors

Maternal age less than 16 years or greater than 40 years
Developmentally delayed mother
Illicit drug, alcohol, cigarette use
Poverty
Unmarried
Emotional or physical stress

Medical History

Diabetes mellitus
Hypertension
Asymptomatic bacteriuria
Rheumatologic illness (SLE)
Chronic medication
PKU, CHD, or other genetic factors

Prior Pregnancy

Intrauterine fetal demise
Neonatal death
Prematurity
Intrauterine growth retardation
Congenital malformation
Incompetent cervix
Blood group sensitization, neonatal jaundice
Neonatal thrombocytopenia
Hydrops
Inborn errors of metabolism

Present Pregnancy

Vaginal bleeding (abruptio placentae, placenta previa)
Sexually transmitted diseases (colonization: herpes simplex, group B streptococcus, HIV)
In vitro fertilization or chemically enhanced pregnancy
Multiple gestation
Preeclampsia
Premature rupture of membranes
Short interpregnancy time
Polyhydramnios or oligohydramnios
Acute medical or surgical illness
Inadequate prenatal care

Labor and Delivery

Premature labor (less than 37 weeks)
Postdates (greater than 42 weeks)
Fetal distress
Immature L/S ratio: absent phosphatidylglycerol
Breech presentation
Meconium-stained fluid
Nuchal cord
Cesarean delivery
Forceps delivery
Apgar score less than 4 at 1 minute

Neonate

Birth weight less than 2500 g or greater than 4000 g
Birth before 37 or after 42 weeks of gestation
SGA, LGA growth status
Tachypnea, cyanosis
Congenital malformation
Pallor, plethora, petechiae

Adapted from Behrman RE, Kliegman RM, Jensen HM, editors: *Nelson textbook of pediatrics*, ed 15, Philadelphia, 2004, WB Saunders, p 574.
CHD, Congenital heart disease; *HIV*, human immunodeficiency virus; *LGA*, large for gestational age; *L/S*, lecithin-sphingomyelin ratio; *PKU*, phenylketonuria; *SGA*, small for gestational age; *SLE*, systemic lupus erythematosus.

dystocia, prolonged labor, and breech presentation (Behrman, Kliegman, & Jensen, 2004). Birth injuries include caput succedaneum, cephalhematoma, subcutaneous fat necrosis of the face or scalp, fractures of the skull, subconjunctival and retinal hemorrhages, intracranial hemorrhage, peripheral nerve palsies (brachial, phrenic, facial), fractured clavicle or humerus, ruptured liver or spleen, and hypoxic-ischemic insults. Proper steps to monitor and treat an infant with perinatal complications and injuries must be undertaken immediately after birth. The NP must be familiar with perinatal conditions that subject the newborn to a higher risk and be prepared to intervene quickly based on the available perinatal information.

ASSESSMENT OF THE NEONATE

History

The history includes the following:

- Past maternal history
- Past obstetric history
  - Number of previous pregnancies, number of infants born alive
  - Number of elective or spontaneous abortions; number of preterm and term deliveries
  - Cesarian deliveries and indications for them
  - Health status of living children; if deceased, age and cause of death

- Family history
  - Genetically acquired conditions, birth defects, mental retardation, or other diseases
  - Hypertension, hyperlipidemias, heart disease, or familial cancers
  - Age and health status of living relatives
  - Causes of death of family members
- Current obstetric history
  - Medical history
  - Age of mother
  - Prenatal care
  - Infections, illnesses, medications during pregnancy
  - Hypertension or glucose intolerance
  - Duration of labor, duration of ruptured membranes, and presentation and route of delivery
  - Polyhydramnios (excessive fluid) or oligohydramnios (little to no fluid)
  - Infant meconium stained or amniotic fluid foul smelling
  - Forceps used
  - Fever
- Social history
  - Emotional stressors during pregnancy
  - Unplanned or unwanted pregnancy
  - Financial and emotional support
  - Dietary considerations (e.g., strict vegan diet)
  - Alcohol, cigarettes, or drugs used during pregnancy
  - Educational background of parents
  - Father's anticipated involvement in raising infant

Physical Examination

Immediately after Birth

Apgar Score. Immediate evaluation of the newborn infant at 1 and 5 minutes of age can be a valuable routine procedure. An Apgar score is assigned to the baby based on the criteria in Table 39-1.

- Apgar score 8 to 10
  - Vigorous, pink, and crying
  - Requires only warming, drying, gentle stimulation
  - Occasionally requires oxygen for a short period of time
- Apgar score 5 to 7
  - Cyanotic
  - Slow, irregular respirations
  - Good muscle tone and reflexes
  - Responds to bag-and-mask ventilation
- Apgar score 4 or less
  - Limp, pale, or blue
  - Apneic, slow heart rate
  - Maximal resuscitative efforts with bag and mask, chest compressions, intravenous volume expansion, and drug therapy

The 5-minute Apgar score is an indication of how well the resuscitation efforts have succeeded. Caution must be exercised when using the Apgar score to predict long-term outcomes of mortality and developmental delay. Only when combined with other factors such as fetal status, umbilical cord or scalp blood pH, evidence of organ injury, or seizures can the Apgar score be useful in determining long-term outcome (AAP, 1996b; Van de Riet et al, 1999). In actual practice, the decision to resuscitate an infant is based on the heart rate, color, and respiratory rate rather than the 1-minute Apgar score (Fig. 39-2).

Gestational Age. Assessment of an infant's gestational age is based on the physical examination. The assessment is

- Done promptly after birth to confirm maternal factors (Fig. 39-3)
- Based on the mother's menstrual history, obstetric milestones achieved during pregnancy, and prenatal ultrasonograms

An infant's length, weight, and fronto-occipital head circumference are measured and plotted on growth curves

TABLE 39-1 ***Apgar Scores***

Sign	Score 0	Score 1	Score 2
Heart rate (beats/min)	Absent	Slow (<100)	>100
Respiratory effort	Absent	Weak cry; hypoventilation	Good; strong cry
Muscle tone	Limp	Some flexion of extremities	Well flexed
Reflex irritability (response of skin stimulation to feet)	No response	Some motion	Cry
Color	Blue; pale	Body pink; extremities blue	Completely pink

From Apgar V: Evaluation of the newborn infant. Second report, *JAMA* 168:1985, 1958.

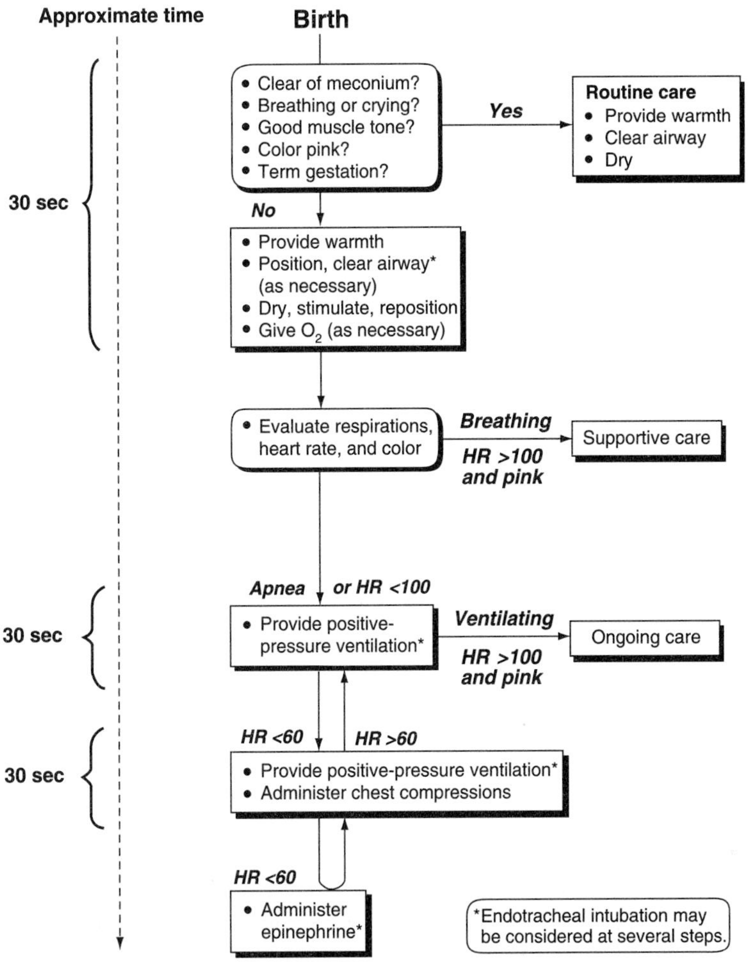

FIGURE 39-2 Resuscitation in the delivery room. (From Niermeyer S, Kattwinkel J, Van Reempts P: International guidelines for neonatal resuscitation: an excerpt from the guidelines 2000 for cardiopulmonary resuscitation and emergency cardiovascular care: international consensus on science, *Pediatrics* 106(3):29, 2000.)

based on gestational age (Fig. 39-4). Infants whose weights fall above the 90th percentile for age are classified as large for gestational age (LGA); those whose measurements fall below the 10th percentile for age are classified as small for gestational age (SGA). Those whose measurements fall between the 10th and 90th percentiles are classified as appropriate for gestational age (AGA).

Temperature. Body surface area of the newborn infant relative to its weight is approximately three times that of the adult. Estimated rate of heat loss in the newborn is four times that of an adult (Behrman, Kliegman, & Jensen, 2000). Body temperature falls precipitously in a cool environment unless adequate precautions are taken.

- Towel-dry infant after birth to prevent evaporative heat loss
- Use radiant warmer
- Wrap infant in warm blankets and cover head to reduce heat loss when baby is to be held by parents

Lungs. During a vaginal delivery, the squeezing action on an infant's chest as it passes through the pelvis and vagina results in expulsion of amniotic fluid from the lungs. Further expulsion of amniotic fluid from the lungs and reversal of high pulmonary vascular resistance ensue with an infant's first large breaths. Careful bulb suctioning assists in clearing the amniotic fluid from the oropharynx. An infant born by cesarean delivery does not experience the squeezing action of a vaginal birth and is dependent on respiratory efforts and appropriate bulb suctioning to adequately clear the amniotic fluid. Auscultation of the newborn's lungs reveals bronchovesicular or bronchial breath sounds. Fine crackles can be present during the first few hours of life.

MATURATIONAL ASSESSMENT OF GESTATIONAL AGE (New Ballard Score)

NAME ____________________ SEX ____________________

HOSPITAL NO. ____________________ BIRTH WEIGHT ____________________

RACE ____________________ LENGTH ____________________

DATE/TIME OF BIRTH ____________________ HEAD CIRC. ____________________

DATE/TIME OF EXAM ____________________ EXAMINER ____________________

AGE WHEN EXAMINED ____________________

APGAR SCORE: 1 MINUTE ____________ 5 MINUTES ____________ 10 MINUTES ____________

NEUROMUSCULAR MATURITY

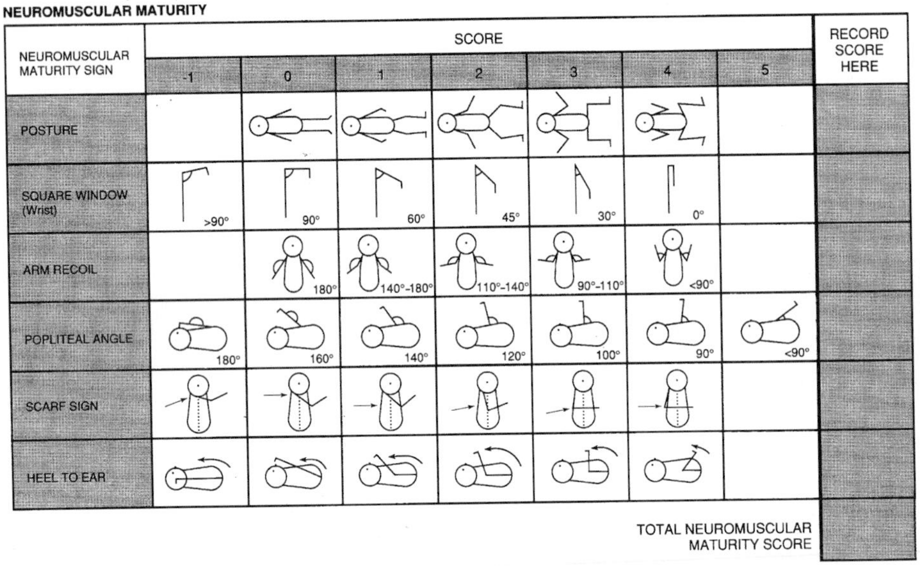

NEUROMUSCULAR MATURITY SIGN	SCORE -1	0	1	2	3	4	5	RECORD SCORE HERE
POSTURE								
SQUARE WINDOW (Wrist)	>90°	90°	60°	45°	30°	0°		
ARM RECOIL		180°	140°-180°	110°-140°	90°-110°	<90°		
POPLITEAL ANGLE	180°	160°	140°	120°	100°	90°	<90°	
SCARF SIGN								
HEEL TO EAR								

TOTAL NEUROMUSCULAR MATURITY SCORE

SCORE

Neuromuscular ____________

Physical ____________

Total ____________

MATURITY RATING

score	weeks
-10	20
-5	22
0	24
5	26
10	28
15	30
20	32
25	34
30	36
35	38
40	40
45	42
50	44

PHYSICAL MATURITY

PHYSICAL MATURITY SIGN	SCORE -1	0	1	2	3	4	5	RECORD SCORE HERE
SKIN	sticky friable transparent	gelatinous red translucent	smooth pink visible veins	superficial peeling &/or rash, few veins	cracking pale areas rare veins	parchment deep cracking no vessels	leathery cracked wrinkled	
LANUGO	none	sparse	abundant	thinning	bald areas	mostly bald		
PLANTAR SURFACE	heel-toe 40-50 mm:-1 <40 mm:-2	>50 mm no crease	faint red marks	anterior transverse crease only	creases ant. 2/3	creases over entire sole		
BREAST	imperceptible	barely perceptible	flat areola no bud	stippled areola 1-2 mm bud	raised areola 3-4 mm bud	full areola 5-10 mm bud		
EYE/EAR	lids fused loosely: -1 tightly: -2	lids open pinna flat stays folded	sl. curved pinna; soft; slow recoil	well-curved pinna; soft but ready recoil	formed & firm instant recoil	thick cartilage ear stiff		
GENITALS (Male)	scrotum flat, smooth	scrotum empty faint rugae	testes in upper canal rare rugae	testes descending few rugae	testes down good rugae	testes pendulous deep rugae		
GENITALS (Female)	clitoris prominent & labia flat	prominent clitoris & small labia minora	prominent clitoris & enlarging minora	majora & minora equally prominent	majora large minora small	majora cover clitoris & minora		

TOTAL PHYSICAL MATURITY SCORE

GESTATIONAL AGE (weeks)

By dates ____________

By ultrasound ____________

By exam ____________

Reference
Ballard JL, Khoury JC, Wedig K, et al: New Ballard Score, expanded to include extremely premature infants. *J Pediatr* 1991; 119:417-423. Reprinted by permission of Dr Ballard and Mosby-Year Book, Inc.

FIGURE 39-3 Classification of newborns by intrauterine growth and gestational age. (From Ballard JL, Khoury JC, Wedig K, et al: New Ballard score, expanded to include extremely premature infants, *J Pediatr* 119:417-423, 1991.)

CLASSIFICATION OF NEWBORNS (BOTH SEXES) BY INTRAUTERINE GROWTH AND GESTATIONAL AGE [1,2]

NAME ______ DATE OF EXAM ______ LENGTH ______

HOSPITAL NO. ______ SEX ______ HEAD CIRC. ______

RACE ______ BIRTH WEIGHT ______ GESTATIONAL AGE ______

DATE OF BIRTH ______

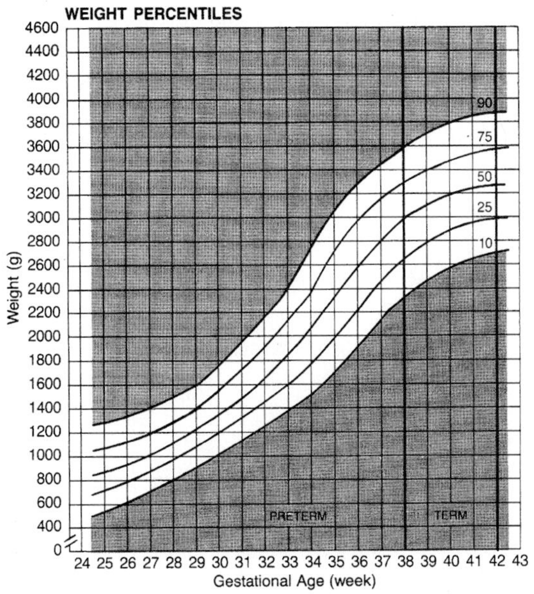

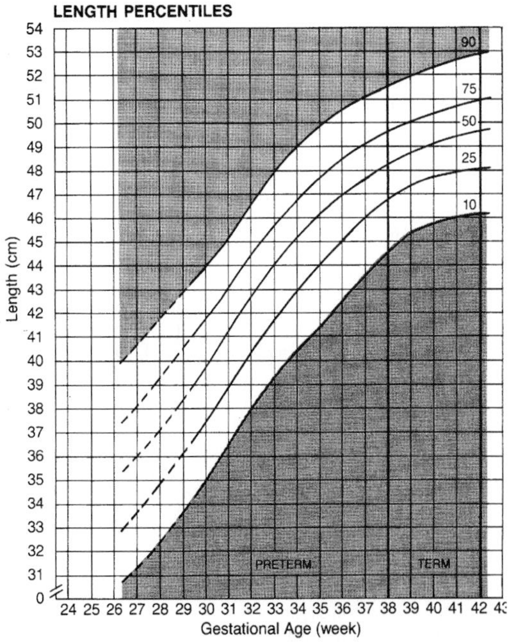

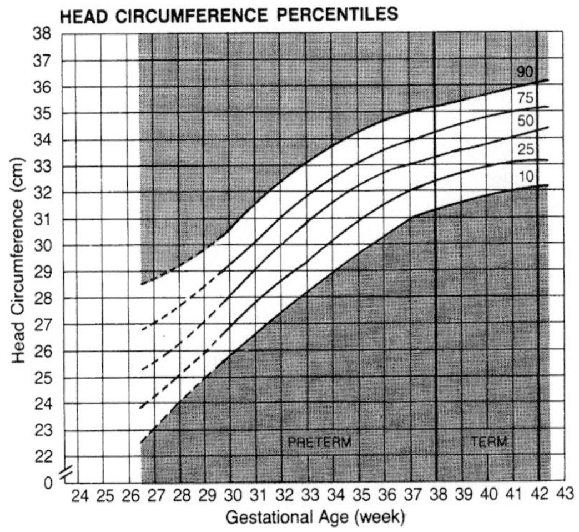

CLASSIFICATION OF INFANT*	Weight	Length	Head Circ.
Large for Gestational Age (LGA) (>90th percentile)			
Appropriate for Gestational Age (AGA) (10th to 90th percentile)			
Small for Gestational Age (SGA) (<10th percentile)			

*Place an "X" in the appropriate box (LGA, AGA or SGA) for weight, for length and for head circumference.

References

1. Battaglia FC, Lubchenco LO: A practical classification of newborn infants by weight and gestational age. *J Pediatr* 1967; 71:159-163.
2. Lubchenco LO, Hansman C, Boyd E: Intrauterine growth in length and head circumference as estimated from live births at gestational ages from 26 to 42 weeks. *Pediatrics* 1966; 37:403-408.

Reprinted by permission from Dr Battaglia, Dr Lubchenco, *Journal of Pediatrics* and *Pediatrics*.

A service of **SIMILAC® WITH IRON** Infant Formula

The Ross Hospital Formula System

A5860(0.05)/JULY 1993

ROSS PRODUCTS DIVISION
ABBOTT LABORATORIES
COLUMBUS, OHIO 43215-1724

LITHO IN USA

FIGURE 39-4 Newborn maturity rating and classification. (From Ross Hospital Formula System, Ross Products Division, Abbott Laboratories, Columbus, Ohio; adapted from Battaglia FC, Lubchenco LO: A practical classification of newborn infants by weight and gestational age, *J Pediatr* 71:159-163, 1967; Lubchenco LO, Hansman C, Boyd E: Intrauterine growth in length and head circumference as estimated from live births at gestational ages from 26 to 42 weeks, *Pediatrics* 37:403-408, 1966.)

Umbilical Cord. The normal umbilical cord contains two thick-walled arteries and a single thin-walled vein. Vessel numbers other than this are abnormal and can be associated with congenital anomalies. The umbilical cord is clamped using sterile technique to avoid infection and bleeding.

After Stabilization

A more complete physical examination is done after stabilization (Table 39-2, Fig. 39-5). When performing the physical, the infant's gestational age, age in hours, and stage of transition must be considered.

Diagnostic Studies

Newborn Screening

All states require screening of infants for a variety of congenital abnormalities, although the tests performed vary from state to state. Screening panels may include PKU, congenital hypothyroidism, galactosemia, hemoglobin type, homocystinuria, tyrosinemia, maple syrup urine disease, sickle cell trait, and congenital adrenal hyperplasia. Testing for cystic fibrosis and the organic acidemias is less widely performed. The ideal timing of these tests is usually after the infant is older than 24 hours of age to ensure the baby's feeding and production of metabolites. Early discharge

TABLE 39-2 ***Physical Examination Findings***

System	Findings
Vital signs and measurements	Check vital signs frequently in the first hours after birth, then every 6-8 hr when stable. Evaluate ability to maintain temperature above 97° F after transition to extrauterine environment. *Failure to maintain temperature* requires evaluation for other problems, particularly sepsis. Respirations should remain between 30 and 60 breaths/min. Heart rate should remain between 120 and 160 beats/min. Significant molding of the head requires repeated measurements to verify size. Daily weight losses of up to 10% or so in the first 2-3 days of life are not abnormal, because normal infants excrete a large amount of water in the first days of life. *Weight loss of greater than 10%* is abnormal and often due to poor intake or excessive losses
Skin	Lanugo and vernix. Lanugo is fine dark hair, prominent over the trunk and shoulders. It is seen in infants born prematurely, becoming less prominent as the gestation approaches term. Thick, greasy, white vernix is more common on prematurely born infants' skin. Dry and cracked skin. This is normal over the first several days of life. If associated with thin subcutaneous fat (parchment-like), it is suggestive of a postmature infant, fetal growth retardation, or both. *Cyanosis.* Acrocyanosis, bluish changes in the color of the hands and feet, and generalized mottling of the skin are frequently noted in the first several days of life when an infant loses body heat. *Central cyanosis* beyond the first few moments of life is abnormal and can represent a significant problem with oxygenation. *Pallor.* Many perinatal events can result in pallor, indicating a significant disruption of the infant's circulatory system. Specific causes include anemia, sepsis, cold stress, hypoglycemia, and seizures. Plethora. An excessively reddish discoloration to the skin can be caused by polycythemia or hyperthermia. Infants born to diabetic mothers can be plethoric. *Meconium staining.* Stress before birth can cause the first stool to pass in utero. If this greenish-black meconium remains in the amniotic fluid for a prolonged period, staining of the infant's skin and fingernails results. *Jaundice.* See the discussion of jaundice in the text under Hematologic Conditions.
Head	Sutures and molding. Vaginally delivered infants demonstrate some degree of molding, usually elongation of the anteroposterior diameter of the skull; if delivered by cesarean method, there are minimal alterations to the shape of the head. Fontanels. The anterior fontanel is usually about 2-3 cm in diameter; the posterior fontanel is about 1 cm in diameter. Both are usually slightly depressed (see Fig. 39-5).
Face	Symmetric structures of the face should be apparent, although unilateral facial edema as a result of delivery conditions can occur normally. Overall view of the face may reveal maxillary or mandibular hypoplasia, distortion, or hemifacial hypoplasia.
Eyes	Size, shape, and position of eyes. Too small or large, too widely spaced, or abnormal upward or downward slanting of palpebral fissures should alert the practitioner to potential congenital problems.

TABLE 39-2 *Physical Examination Findings—cont'd*

System	Findings
	Uncoordinated eye movements. Intermittent uncoordinated eye movements (disconjugate gaze) during the first weeks after birth are common, improving by 2-4 mo of age and resolving by 6 mo of age. *Fixed disconjugate gaze* is abnormal, even in the neonate Conjunctivae. Reddening in the first 24-48 hr of life due to chemical irritation of the eyes from silver nitrate drops or erythromycin ointment is normal. *Purulent discharge* in the first days or weeks of life can be associated with gonococcus, chlamydia, or herpes. Conjunctival hemorrhages secondary to delivery resolve spontaneously over the first weeks of life. Sclerae. Yellowing is associated with hyperbilirubinemia. Small hemorrhages secondary to delivery resolve spontaneously over the first weeks of life. Thinning of the sclera, common in blacks, is manifested by dark blue or black patches. Blue sclerae are associated with osteogenesis imperfecta. Red reflex. Shining an ophthalmoscope white light through the pupil reveals the "red reflex," a disc ranging from pearly gray to orange in color. *Absence of a red reflex* may indicate the presence of lens opacities secondary to cataracts, congenital infection (rubella), or calcium metabolism abnormality. A *white reflex* can indicate retinoblastoma. Absence of the expected red reflex indicates the need for an immediate ophthalmologic evaluation.
Ears	Identify normalcy in the size, rotation, shape, position, and patency of the external auditory canal. Presence of low-set ears should prompt careful examination for other dysmorphic features. Abnormalities in shape require thorough physical examination, especially of the genitourinary system. Assessment of hearing is done by noting a startle response to a loud noise, avoiding any tactile sensations such as a wind current on the face due to clapping near the ear. Auditory brain response testing should be ordered for any infant in whom a question of hearing exists. Screening for universal detection of infants with hearing loss is recommended and is especially important for high-risk infants (e.g., family history, in utero infection, craniofacial anomalies). Preauricular skin tags or significant pits should be noted (can be a genetic red flag). See text section on skin dimpling.
Nose	Patency of the nasal passages can be tested by closing the mouth and one nostril at a time or by passing a small catheter into the nasopharynx to see if the passage is clear. Nasal flaring is a sign of respiratory distress that can be caused by any number of abnormalities, including mechanical obstruction, parenchymal lung disease, or acidosis.
Mouth	Size and symmetry of the lips: • Thin lips with a smooth philtrum (the area between lips and nose) are associated with fetal alcohol syndrome. • *Asymmetric movements* while crying can be due to nerve palsies or absence of perioral muscles. Cleft lip and palate can be associated with midline central nervous system abnormalities. Incomplete cleft palates are recognized by digital examination of the mouth for bony defects of the hard palate in the presence of normal palatal mucosa. Excessive salivation can be related to reflux of gastric contents or esophageal atresia. Epstein pearls are small, white epithelial inclusion cysts on the palate and gums. An excessively large tongue can be associated with genetic or metabolic abnormalities such as hypothyroidism or Down syndrome. Natal teeth are sometimes seen at birth (approximately 1 in 3000 live births). If they are extremely loose, aspiration is a concern. Consultation with a pediatric dentist is indicated.
Neck	Webbing. Redundant skin is seen in trisomy 21, Turner syndrome, and Noonan syndrome. Short neck indicates the possibility of Klippel-Feil syndrome or other vertebral problems. Masses: • Thyroglossal duct cysts (midline) or branchial cleft cyst (along the edge of the sternocleidomastoid muscles) can be found. • Other masses that can be seen include a hematoma in the sternocleidomastoid muscle, cystic hygromas, and, rarely, goiters. • Torticollis. Asymmetric shortening of the sternocleidomastoid muscle results in preferential turning of the head to one side, not to be confused with irritability on neck movement associated with meningitis or subarachnoid hemorrhage. Hematoma of the sternocleidomastoid muscle can result in the development of torticollis and requires early management.

Continued

TABLE 39-2 *Physical Examination Findings—cont'd*

System	Findings
Thorax	Shape, symmetry. Rounded appearance measuring about 2 cm less than the fronto-occipital head circumference (approximately 33 cm): • *Minimization of rounding* occurs with respiratory distress syndrome, atelectasis, and other diseases of decreased expansion of the chest. • Accentuation is seen in meconium aspiration. Wide-spaced nipples and a shieldlike appearance are characteristic of Turner syndrome. Chest movement on inspiration should be symmetric and unlabored. Movement of the abdomen with respirations is normal. *Asymmetric movement* occurs with unilateral pneumothorax. *Intercostal, subcostal, or supracostal retractions* indicate respiratory distress. Clavicles. Vaginally delivered large for gestational age babies are especially prone to fractures of the clavicle (see perinatal injury section in text). Breast bones. Pectus excavatum (concave chest) and pectus carinatum (pigeon chest) are occasionally seen. If severe, both can lead to restrictive lung disease later in life. Nipples: • Fullness and sometimes secretion of a white milky substance are normal and are secondary to maternal hormonal stimulation. • Redness surrounding the nipple, especially with purulent drainage, occurs in neonatal mastitis.
Lungs	General. Coughing, retractions, and an intermittently increased respiratory rate occur immediately after birth, resolving by about 12 hr of age to smooth and unlabored respirations at a rate of 30 to 60 breaths/min. Respiratory distress. *Tachypnea, apnea* (pauses in respiration longer than about 15 sec), *grunting* (an infant's attempt to increase functional residual capacity, thereby improving gas exchange), *interclavicular, subclavicular, or supraclavicular retractions, nasal flaring,* and *central cyanosis* all indicate distress. Auscultation: • Rales or crackles are commonly heard immediately after birth as lung fluid is resorbed. Beyond the immediate postpartum period, *rales* can indicate pneumonia, delayed resorption of lung fluid, meconium aspiration, or pulmonary edema. • *Unilateral absence of breath sounds* occurs in pneumothorax, atelectasis, and pleural effusion. • *Bowel sounds over the chest,* especially with a scaphoid abdomen and significant respiratory distress, indicate a diaphragmatic hernia with displacement of abdominal contents into the chest.
Heart	Inspection. Observe neonate for adequacy of perfusion. Respiratory distress is common with cardiac abnormalities. Edema as a result of cardiac failure is rarely seen in the newborn. Palpation: • *Point of maximal impulse is displaced* from the fourth left intercostal space with pneumothorax, situs inversus, or dextrocardia. • *Thrills or heaves* are associated with murmurs and cardiac abnormalities. Auscultation. Heart rate is normally 120 to 160 beats/min. Detection of skipped beats warrants electrocardiogram. *Heart sounds may be muffled or displaced* in the infant with a pneumothorax. Murmurs. Common in the newborn period, many murmurs disappear after a few hours or a few days. Significant murmurs need to be investigated whenever heard. Pulses. Brachial or radial pulses are compared with femoral or dorsalis pedis pulses for symmetry of impulse and strength in pulse. Delay or relative weakness of lower extremity pulses occurs in coarctation of the aorta. Blood pressure. By Doppler device using a 2.5-4.0 cm wide and 5.0-9.0 cm long cuff, compare with normals for age and gestation. Systolic blood pressures greater than 96 mm Hg are considered significant hypertension in the newborn, and systolic blood pressures exceeding 106 mm Hg are considered severe hypertension (National High Blood Pressure Education Program Working Group, 1996).
Abdomen	General: • Normal abdomen is slightly protuberant, is soft, moves smoothly with respirations, and has fine bowel sounds scattered throughout. *Absent bowel sounds* can indicate ileus. • The liver is usually palpated 1-2 cm below the right costal margin; the spleen tip is sometimes felt at the left costal margin; kidneys, deep within lateral aspects of the abdomen measuring 3-4 cm in size, are usually palpable. • Pain is indicated by crying, grimacing, or forceful resistance with palpation. Umbilical hernias. Midline outpouching from the sternum to the umbilicus is seen with weak abdominal musculature (diastasis recti); a large and protuberant umbilicus occurs with an umbilical hernia.

TABLE 39-2 *Physical Examination Findings—cont'd*

System	Findings
	Umbilical vessels. The normal cord contains two arteries and a single vein. Absence of the second artery can be associated with congenital abnormalities. Vomiting and abdominal distention. Regurgitation of large volumes of feeding is not expected. *Bilious vomiting* is always abnormal and usually a sign of obstruction. *Abdominal distention* with enlargement of any of the organs of the abdomen or failure to pass stool is abnormal. Meconium ileus with failure to pass stool in the first 24-48 hr of life is associated with cystic fibrosis.
Genitalia	Male: • The penis should have the urethral opening at the tip of the phallus with completely developed foreskin. Chordee means that the distal end of the penis is bent. • Testes not located in the scrotal sac or inguinal canal but retrievable to the scrotum are normal. Testes not located in or relocated in the scrotal sac from the canal are considered to be undescended. • Hydrocele is identified by transilluminating fluid collection around the testis and is regarded as normal unless associated with inguinal hernia or lasts more than 12 mo. • Inguinal hernia with displacement of intestines into the scrotal sac is frequently nontransilluminating and is associated with bowel sounds. Inguinal hernias are sometimes apparent and reduced at other times. A surgical consultation is indicated. Female: • Labia majora are large and completely surround the labia minora. • Labia and vagina should be open, often with a white discharge. • Blood-tinged fluid in small amounts by day 2-3 is normal. *Ambiguous genitalia* are genitalia that do not appear to be completely masculinized or feminized. An endocrine referral is important. Anus and rectum. Patency of the rectum and placement of the anus should be noted. A small amount of blood streaking in the diaper, especially with a small anal fissure, is common.
Extremities, back, hips	Molding. Intrauterine constraint and resultant molding cause mild curvatures of the forefeet (metatarsus adductus vs. varus [in-toeing or out-toeing]) or the tibia (genu varum [bowleg], genu valgum [knock-knee]), or both. See Chapter 38 for more information. Contractures of the joints and molding of the bones occur if amniotic fluid was decreased and is abnormal. Fractures: • Skull fractures can occur as a result of extensive molding of a large head. • Femora and humeri can fracture with difficult deliveries and use of instrumentation. • *Multiple fractures* can indicate osteogenesis imperfecta. Spine. Dimples, hemangiomas, tufts of hair, or other lesions along the spine may be associated with spinal abnormalities such as spina bifida occulta. Hips. See Chapter 38 for information about eliciting Ortolani and Barlow signs. Both are indicators of dislocated or dislocatable hips.
Neurologic examination	Muscle tone. Observe tone, movement, and symmetry of the extremities while the infant is awake. Reflexes. Elicit the following: • Rooting • Sucking • Palmar grasp • Moro reflex • Ankle clonus (3-4 beats of clonus at ankle is normal) • Stepping and placing response • Galant reflex • Asymmetric tonic neck reflex Cranial nerves. Cranial nerve I (olfactory) is rarely tested. Vision (cranial nerve II) is tested by an infant's response to a bright light. Cranial nerves III, IV, and VI are tested by noting an infant's ability to gaze in all directions, although intermittent disconjugate gaze is normal through 6 mo of age. Adequate sucking and swallowing confirm presence of cranial nerves V, IX, X, and XII. Symmetric movement of the face with crying confirms presence of cranial nerve VII. Hearing (cranial nerve VIII) is assessed by startle to loud noise.

Italicized findings indicate "red flags."

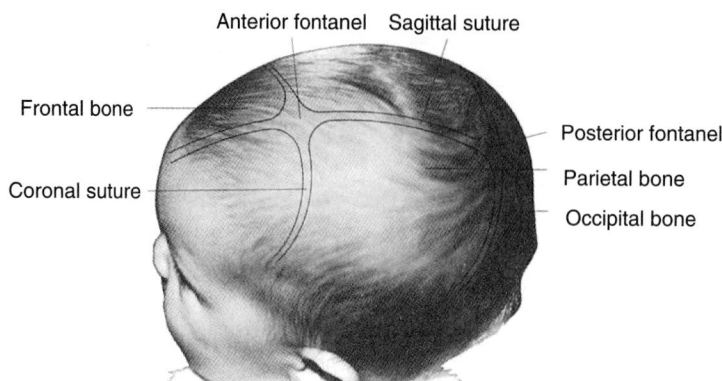

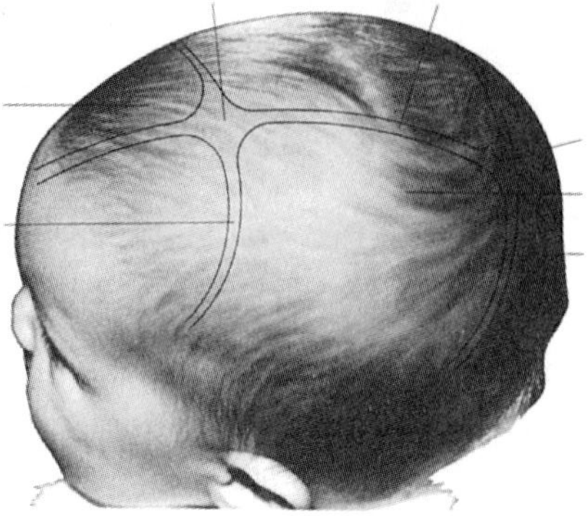

FIGURE 39-5 Fontanels and sutures. (From Betz CL, Hunsberger M, Wright S: *Family-centered nursing care of children*, ed 2, Philadelphia, 1994, WB Saunders, p 124.)

often necessitates repeating some tests (Box 39-2). Two screenings approximately 2 weeks apart are required in some states.

Special Screening

Although most infants require no special screening tests, some are at risk for complications in the newborn period. Infants born to mothers with poorly controlled diabetes and LGA or SGA infants are at higher risk for hypoglycemia and are screened for serum glucose levels. Similarly, infants demonstrating Coombs' test positivity because of maternal-child blood incompatibility are screened for hemolysis. Some nurseries screen both mothers and infants for syphilis; mothers should be screened for hepatitis B unless done prenatally. Universal hearing screening is recommended by some experts (AAP, 1999a), and special attention is paid to any newborn at higher risk for hearing loss due to low birth weight, rubella or other infection, malformation, trauma, asphyxia, prematurity, intensive care unit stay, or antibiotics.

BOX 39-2 *Newborn Screening for Metabolic Disorders*

- All infants should be screened before discharge.
- All infants screened before 24 hours of age should be rescreened before 14 days of age.
- All infants should be tested before the seventh day of life.

1. For some diseases, such as phenylketonuria, the infant needs to be fed so that the intake or production of amino acids exceeds the infant's capacity to metabolize or excrete them.
2. Rescreening is now recommended in many states. Nurse practitioners need to be aware of the need for retesting, especially when infants are discharged early.
3. Cord blood is not acceptable for newborn screening because most metabolites accumulate after birth.
4. Filter papers should be used, preferably with 1 drop of blood filling the entire circle. Blood should not be added from the other side of the paper. If a capillary tube is used, it should not touch the paper. For sick infants, venous blood may be used, but care must be taken that no heparin or hyperalimentation components are included. To prevent hemolysis, the needle should not touch the paper.
5. The filter paper must not be contaminated in any way. The specimen should be dried while lying flat and not exposed to heat or sunlight. Remember that mailboxes may be hot in the summer!
6. Demographic data must be clearly written to ensure follow-up of abnormal results.
7. Specimens should be mailed within 24 hours of collection via first-class mail to avoid delays in reaching the laboratory.
8. Premature or sick infants should be screened by the seventh day of life.
9. Transfusions may temporarily affect results, so specimens should be collected before plasma or blood products are administered.

Adapted from Buist N, Tuerck J: The practitioner's role in newborn screening, *Pediatr Clin North Am* 39:199-211, 1992.

MANAGEMENT STRATEGIES

Initial Care

Following birth, newborns require special care and observation as they master the transition to the extrauterine environment. Additional components of care at this period include prophylaxis for eye infection with silver nitrate or antibiotic ointment and vitamin K injection for hemorrhagic disease.

Establishing Feeding

Whether breastfeeding or bottle-feeding, infant and parents must be well established in initiating feeding before discharge. Follow-up care must be scheduled to ensure adequate nutrition. See Chapters 12 and 13 for more detailed information on breastfeeding and formulas.

Anticipatory Guidance before Discharge

Physical Care

Umbilical Cord. Applying alcohol to the base of the cord traditionally has been recommended to aid in cord separation. Recent recommendations question the utility of this practice and suggest that air-drying by tucking the diaper below the cord is preferable (Mendenhall & Eichenfield, 2000). After cord separation, which usually occurs at 10 to 14 days of life, a slight bloody discharge for 1 to 2 days can be seen. Bellybands or coins to cover the navel are avoided, because these increase the chance of infection. If a foul-smelling discharge or erythema appears around the umbilicus, the infant should be evaluated immediately for sepsis. A granuloma sometimes appears after the cord falls off. An application of silver nitrate helps heal the granuloma.

Circumcision. Circumcision is the removal of the foreskin that normally covers the glans penis. Much controversy surrounds this procedure's medical necessity and the use of anesthesia during the procedure (AAP, 1999b). The decision to circumcise is the parents' responsibility. Proponents of circumcision claim that it keeps the glans cleaner; the chance for developing urinary tract infections is reduced (although the chance of urinary tract infections in uncircumcised males is only 1%); it prevents penile cancer, phimosis, balanitis, adhesions, and occlusion of the urethral meatus; and the boy may look more like his peers. The opponents of circumcision claim that it does not prevent sexually transmitted disease; that good hygiene prevents penile cancer; that circumcision leaves the glans open to the chance of cautery burns and meatal stenosis; and that because fewer boys are being circumcised, these boys will not be different from many of their peers.

Contraindications to circumcision include epispadias or hypospadias, ambiguous genitalia, exstrophy of the bladder, familial bleeding disorders, and illness. Complications of circumcisions include infections, bleeding, gangrene, scarring, meatal stenosis, cautery burns, urethral fistula, amputation or trauma to the glans, and pain. For infants who undergo circumcision, procedural anesthesia is recommended. For the circumcision procedure a variety of anesthesia techniques are available, including application of topical anesthetics (EMLA cream), dorsal penile nerve block, and subcutaneous ring block. Postoperative pain relief measures in the form of sucrose on a pacifier, acetaminophen, soft music, and physiologic positioning of the infant in a padded environment are helpful (AAP, 1999b; Joyce, Keck, & Gerkensmeyer, 2001).

Care of the uncircumcised baby includes gentle cleaning. The skin normally adheres to the penis and is not retractable at birth but loosens as the baby grows. The parents should be counseled not to force the foreskin back. If the baby is circumcised, the penis should be cleansed daily with cotton balls dipped in tap water followed by the application of a small amount of petroleum jelly to the tip of the penis with each diaper change. The petroleum jelly is needed only for the first 2 to 3 days after the circumcision.

Bathing, Oils, and Powders. Counsel parents to test the temperature of the water before bathing the infant. The infant should not be immersed in a tub of water and should be sponge-bathed until the umbilical cord separates and the navel appears healed. Mild cleansing agents such as Dove, Caress, Neutrogena, and Basis are gentle enough for infants' skin. Encourage parents to hold the baby to make him or her feel secure in the water and to never leave the baby alone in the tub.

Oils and powders are not recommended for infants' skin. Oils and greasy substances tend to clog the skin's pores and can cause acne or rashes. Powders should be avoided, because inhaling the talc could lead to respiratory problems. For dry skin, Keri, Eucerin, Aveeno, or Cetaphil lotion is recommended.

Diapers. There is much controversy about whether disposable or cloth diapers are the better choice for infants. The need for frequent changing and proper cleansing is the important message to deliver.

Sleep Position

In 1992 the preponderance of available evidence suggested that the prone sleeping position was associated with an increased incidence of sudden infant death syndrome (SIDS). The AAP issued a statement in that year suggesting that healthy infants, when being put down for sleep, be positioned on their side or back (AAP, 1992). These statements were updated by the AAP in 1996 and 2000, suggesting that *healthy* infants continue to be placed in a nonprone position (wholly on the back preferred), that soft surfaces and gas-trapping objects should be avoided in an infant's sleeping environment, that co-sleeping can be hazardous, that overheating should be avoided, and that "tummy time" during the awake period is recommended for developmental reasons and to help prevent flat spots on the occiput (AAP, 1996a, 2000a). Encourage parents to ensure that their child care center and other caregivers (e.g., grandparents) are following these guidelines (Moon, 2000). SIDS is discussed later in this chapter.

Injury Prevention

Counsel parents on the appropriate use and installation of a crash-tested safety seat when driving with their infant. They should take the infant home from the hospital in a safety seat. At the first visit, the NP should check for appropriate positioning and belt use because 80% of car seats are used inappropriately (American Academy of Pediatrics & Oregon Department of Transportation, 2000) (Fig. 39-6).The house should be childproofed before the infant is taken home. Falls and burns are the most common injuries to neonates. Parents should be counseled to avoid shaking their baby for any reason. Refer to Chapter 11 for more information.

Parenting

The parenting role is stressful, even if all goes well. Fatigue and maternal depression resulting from hormonal shifts are common. Encourage parents to identify and make use of supportive people, arrange time for rest and time alone, and keep their expectations reasonable. When a mother seems to be having significant symptoms, it is imperative the NP also keep in mind the possibility of severe postpartum depression and be ready to intervene on the behalf of the infant, the mother, and the family.

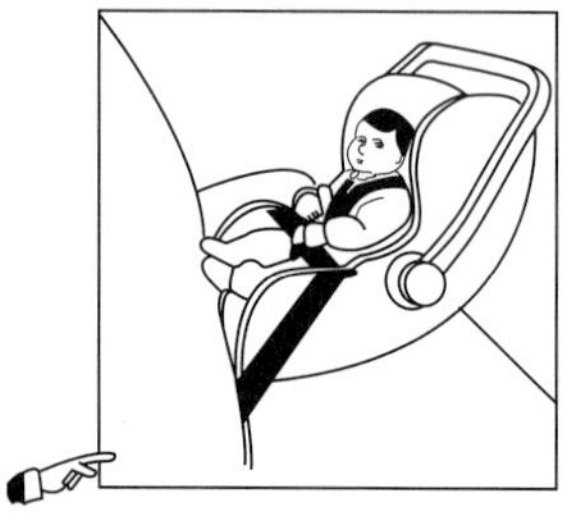

FIGURE 39-6 Proper placement of infant car seat. (Adapted from American Academy of Pediatrics, Oregon Department of Transportation: *One-minute safety checkup*, Elk Grove Village, IL, 2000, American Academy of Pediatrics.)

Early Discharge and Follow-up

Newborns are often discharged after a minimal time of observation. Although this is a common practice, infants can experience difficulty with breastfeeding, poor weight gain, jaundice, and dehydration (Kiely, Drum, & Kessel, 1998). Guidelines for early discharge of normal, healthy newborns are listed in Box 39-3. Plans for follow-up care

BOX 39-3 *Guidelines for Early Discharge of Normal, Healthy Newborns*

Antepartum, intrapartum, and postpartum course for baby and mother must be normal
Vaginal delivery
Single, appropriate for gestational age, term (38 to 42 weeks) baby
Stable vital signs for at least 12 hours before discharge:
- Axillary temperature of 36.1° to 37° C in open crib
- Heart rate 100 to 160 beats per minute
- Respiratory rate less than 60 breaths per minute

Passage of urine and stool
Two successful feedings have been accomplished
Normal physical examination
No excessive bleeding at circumcision site for at least 2 hours
No significant jaundice in first 24 hours
Mother knowledgeable in the care of the infant, including the following:
- Feeding
- Normal stool and urine frequency
- Skin, genital, and cord care
- Ability to identify illness (especially jaundice)
- Proper safety (car seat, sleeping position)
- Smoke alarms in the home

Social support and continuing health care identified
Infant laboratory data, including maternal syphilis and hepatitis B and infant blood type and Coombs' testing completed
Appropriately timed neonatal screening completed
Social situation adequate: include such areas as drug abuse, previous child abuse, mental illness, lack of social support, lack of permanent home, history of domestic violence, or teenage mother
Appropriate early follow-up care within 48 hours of discharge identified

Adapted from American Academy of Pediatrics: Hospital stay for healthy term newborns, *Pediatrics* 96:788-790, 1995; National Association of Pediatric Nurse Associates and Practitioners: Newborn discharge and follow-up care, *J Pediatr Health Care* 11:147-148, 1997.

within 48 to 72 hours, as well as for ongoing health maintenance, should be confirmed before discharge. Box 39-4 gives guidelines for the 48- to 72-hour follow-up visit of the healthy, normal newborn. Even newborns who are hospitalized longer need follow-up care within the first few days of life. All parents leaving the hospital with a newborn should have a confirmed time and place for follow-up, as well as contacts in case of an emergency or questions.

Premature Infants and Newborns with Special Needs

Premature infants have special needs that must be arranged before discharge. Guidelines for discharge and follow-up of the premature infant are detailed in Box 39-5. Newborns with special needs caused by anomalies, disease states, social situation, or other variables also need arrangements made before discharge to provide support, education, and follow-up.

COMMON NEONATAL CONDITIONS

Skin Conditions

Milia

Description, Etiology, and Incidence. Milia are multiple, firm, pearly, opalescent white papules scattered over the forehead, nose, and cheeks. Their intraoral counterparts are called Epstein pearls. Histologically, milia represent superficial epidermal inclusion cysts filled with keratinous material associated with the developing pilosebaceous follicle. They are found in about 40% of newborns (McMillan, 1999).

Management. No treatment is necessary because milia exfoliate spontaneously in most infants over the first few weeks of life.

Sebaceous Hyperplasia

Description and Etiology. Sebaceous hyperplasia is characterized by prominent yellow-white papules at the opening of each pilosebaceous follicle, predominantly over the nose, forehead, upper lip, and cheeks. The overgrowth of sebaceous glands in response to the same androgenic stimulation that occurs in adolescence causes sebaceous hyperplasia.

Management. No treatment is required. These tiny papules diminish in size and disappear entirely within the first few weeks of life.

Erythema Toxicum

Description, Etiology, and Incidence. Firm, yellow-white 1 to 2 mm papules or pustules with a surrounding erythematous flare characterize erythema toxicum. Lesions are clustered in several sites. These lesions usually develop at 24 to 48 hours of age. The cause is unknown, although examination of a Wright-stained smear of the lesion reveals numerous eosinophils. Up to 50% of infants develop erythema toxicum, with the incidence higher in term than in premature infants.

Differential Diagnosis. Pyoderma, candidiasis, herpes simplex, transient neonatal pustular melanosis, and miliaria should be considered (Table 39-3).

Management. No treatment is required because the course is brief and transient.

Transient Neonatal Pustular Melanosis

Description, Etiology, and Incidence. Transient neonatal pustular melanosis is characterized by superficial vesiculopustules that rupture easily and leave a halo of white scales around a central pinhead-sized macule of hyperpigmentation. Pustular melanosis is caused by increased melanization

BOX 39-4 *Guidelines for 48- to 72-Hour Follow-up Visit of the Normal, Healthy Newborn*

1. Assess the infant's general health, hydration, and jaundice; identify any new problems; review feeding
2. Assess quality of bonding
3. Reinforce maternal and family education
4. Review outstanding laboratory data
5. Perform neonatal screen if indicated
6. Develop plan for health care maintenance, including emergency care, preventive care, and periodic screenings
7. Ensure mother has postpartal examination scheduled
8. Ask if mother has immediate birth control needs
9. Assess family support resources (especially if teen, immigrant family, or single parent)

Adapted from American Academy of Pediatrics: Hospital stay for healthy term newborns, *Pediatrics* 96:788-790, 1995.

BOX 39-5 *Guidelines for Discharge and Follow-up of the High-Risk Neonate*

Discharge Planning

Identify all active medical or social problems through a review of the medical record and physical examination of infant
Ensure adequacy of immunizations based on infant's chronologic age
Screen for anemia and begin iron or vitamins if necessary
Review with family member medications, feeding schedules, signs of illness, and appropriate response for infants with active medical conditions
Identify family and community resources if infant is to be discharged on home oxygen therapy
Ensure adequate training of family members in cardiopulmonary resuscitation and, if applicable, on home apnea monitor use
Counsel family in car seat adaptations for the premature infant
Consider need for visiting nurse, social service, respite care, support groups, early intervention services, or referral to the Women, Infants, and Children (WIC) Program
Ensure appropriate hearing screen has been completed

Follow-up Planning

Schedule follow-up hearing screen (if necessary) for infants with:
- Craniofacial abnormalities
- In utero infections
- Birth weight less than 1500 g
- Meningitis
- Exchange transfusion for hyperbilirubinemia
- Use of ototoxic medications
- Apgar score of 0 to 4 at 1 minute or 0 to 6 at 5 minutes
- Mechanical ventilation for 5 days or longer
- Stigmata of syndrome associated with hearing loss
- Family history of deafness

At 4 to 6 weeks of chronologic age, schedule a dilated indirect ophthalmoscopic examination for neonates with a birth weight of 1500 g or less or with a gestational age of 28 weeks or less, as well as those infants greater than 1500 g with an unstable clinical course thought to be at high risk for retinopathy of prematurity by their attending physician (American Academy of Pediatrics, American Association for Pediatric Ophthalmology and Strabismus, American Academy of Ophthalmology, 1997)
Follow-up visits every 1 to 2 weeks, especially if infant is on oxygen therapy
Growth and development should be of prime interest at each routine outpatient visit with referral for formal developmental assessment if any concerns are identified

of the epidermal cells, with sites of predilection being the trunk, limbs, palms, and soles. It is more common in black than in white infants.

Differential Diagnosis. Pyoderma and erythema toxicum are the differential diagnoses.

Management. No treatment is required. The pustular phase rarely lasts more than 2 to 3 days; hyperpigmented macules can persist for as long as 3 months.

Sucking Blisters

Description and Etiology. Sucking blisters are solitary or scattered superficial bullae on the upper limbs and lips of infants at birth, commonly found on the radial aspect of the forearm, the thumb, and the index finger. These blisters result from vigorous sucking on the affected part in utero.

Management. No treatment is required. These bullae resolve rapidly without sequelae.

Cutis Marmorata

Description and Etiology. Cutis marmorata is a lacy, reticulated red or blue cutaneous vascular pattern appearing over most of the body surface. The vascular change is a response to exposure to low environmental temperatures. It

TABLE 39-3 Comparison of Erythema Toxicum and Herpes Simplex Virus

Erythema Toxicum	Herpes Simplex Virus
Benign, self-limited	Pathologic, progressive
No specific maternal history	Frequently a history of maternal disease
Usually seen only in term infants	Can occur in infants of any gestational age
Begins on the second or third day of life, lasting as long as 1 wk	Often begins late in the first week of life or early in the second week of life
Rash is evanescent, often involving the face, trunk, and extremities	Can be superficial and localized only to the presenting part (vertex or buttocks) or widespread and disseminated without cutaneous involvement
1-2 mm white papules or pustules on an erythematous base that occasionally may become vesicular	May manifest similar to sepsis without cutaneous findings, or as grouped vesicles on an erythematous base on the presenting part about days 9-11 of life
Wright or Giemsa stain of lesion scraping demonstrates large numbers of eosinophils and no organisms; cultures are sterile	Direct fluorescent antibody staining or enzyme-linked immunoassay detection of herpes simplex virus antigens of vesicle scrapings, or growth of the organism from vesicle fluid, is diagnostic
No specific therapy necessary	Acyclovir and other antiviral agents

represents an accentuated physiologic vasomotor response that disappears with increasing age. Persistent and pronounced cutis marmorata occurs in Down and trisomy 18 syndromes.

Management. Cutis marmorata usually resolves with warming of the infant.

Harlequin Color Change

Description and Etiology. Harlequin color change is a division of the body skin coloring from forehead to pubis into red and pale halves. The cause is unknown.

Management. No treatment is indicated, because this is a transient and benign condition.

Mongolian Spots, Café au Lait Spots, Salmon Patch (Nevus Simplex), and Port-Wine Stain (Nevus Flammeus, Port-Wine Nevus)

See Chapter 37 for a discussion of these skin conditions.

Nevus Sebaceus

Description and Etiology. Nevus sebaceus is a yellowish, hairless, sharply demarcated smooth plaque on the head and neck. Histologically, these nevi contain an abundance of sebaceous glands. With maturity, usually during adolescence, the lesions become verrucous with large rubbery nodules. During adulthood, the lesions are complicated by secondary malignancies, most commonly basal cell carcinoma.

Management. Total excision before the onset of adolescence is recommended. Refer to a pediatric dermatologist.

Skin Dimpling

Description and Etiology. Skin dimpling is the presence of deep skin dimples over bony prominences and in the sacral area. Skin dimples, as well as pits and creases, occur in normal infants and in those with dysmorphologic syndromes such as congenital rubella, deletion of the long arm of chromosome 18, and the cerebrohepatorenal syndromes.

Management. No treatment is indicated.

Preauricular Sinus Tracts and Pits

Description and Etiology. Sinus tracts and pits occur anterior to the pinna. Resulting from imperfect fusion of the tubercles of the first and second branchial arches during gestational development, tracts and pits can be unilateral or bilateral; they are familial, more common in females and blacks, and occasionally associated with other anomalies of the ears and face.

Management. Excision is required if tracts and pits are chronically infected and draining.

Amniotic Constriction Bands

Description and Etiology. Fibrous strands that encircle fetal parts can cause permanent depression of the underlying tissue, producing defects in the extremities and digits. Found in otherwise normal infants, bands are thought to result from intrauterine rupture of the amnion with formation of fibrous strands. Sometimes there are associated abnormalities, including craniofacial anomalies and thoracic or abdominal wall defects.

Management. Treatment depends on the severity of deformities produced. Constriction bands on the limbs can be managed in consultation with plastic surgery.

Supernumerary Nipples

Description and Etiology. Solitary or multiple accessory nipples and sometimes areolae occur in unilateral or bilateral distribution along a line from the midaxilla to the inguinal area. The cause is unknown. Urinary tract anomalies rarely can occur in children with this finding.

Management. Usually no treatment is necessary unless the accessory nipple becomes symptomatic.

Branchial Cleft and Thyroglossal Cysts and Sinuses

Description and Etiology. Cysts and sinuses in the neck can be unilateral or bilateral and open onto the cutaneous surface or drain into the pharynx. Thyroglossal cysts and fistulas are similar defects located in or near the midline of the neck, extending to the base of the tongue. Thyroglossal cysts occasionally contain aberrant thyroid tissue, as well as mucinous material. Cysts and sinuses in the neck can be formed along the course of the first and second branchial clefts as a result of improper closure during embryonic life. These anomalies can be inherited as autosomal dominant traits.

Management. Antibiotic therapy is indicated for infections of the cysts or sinuses, which rarely occurs in the neonatal period. Surgical excision is recommended for thyroglossal cysts.

Head, Face, and Eye Conditions

Caput Succedaneum

Description and Etiology. Caput succedaneum is a diffuse swelling of the soft tissue of the scalp with possible bruising; the swelling usually crosses the suture lines (Fig. 39-7). Caput succedaneum originates from trauma as the baby descends through the birth canal.

Clinical Findings

History. Primigravida and traumatic delivery may be part of the history.

Physical Examination. Findings include the following:
- Obvious swelling and bruising in the parietal regions of the scalp
- Swelling that crosses suture lines
- Frequently associated with molding

Differential Diagnosis. Cephalhematoma is the differential diagnosis.

Management. No treatment is necessary, because swelling resolves spontaneously over a few days. If the lesion is large, observe the baby for the development of jaundice as the blood from bruising is resorbed.

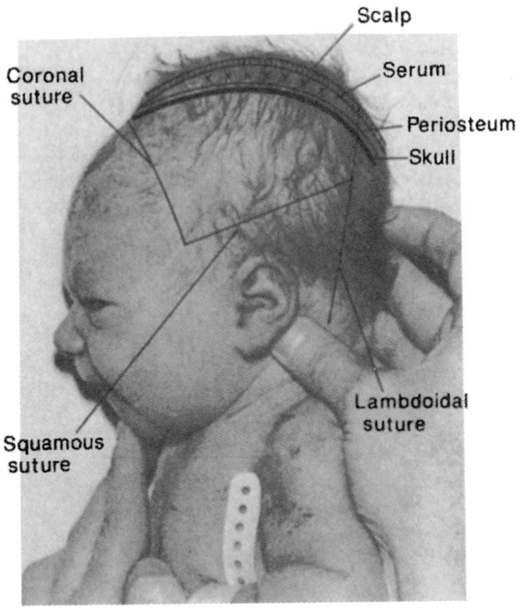

FIGURE 39-7 Caput succedaneum. (From Betz CL, Hunsberger M, Wright S: *Family-centered nursing care of children*, ed 2, Philadelphia, 1994, WB Saunders, p 124.)

Cephalhematoma

Description and Etiology. Cephalhematoma is a collection of blood in the subperiosteal area of the scalp that does not cross the suture lines. Frequently, no noticeable bruising of the area is seen (Fig. 39-8). Cephalhematoma

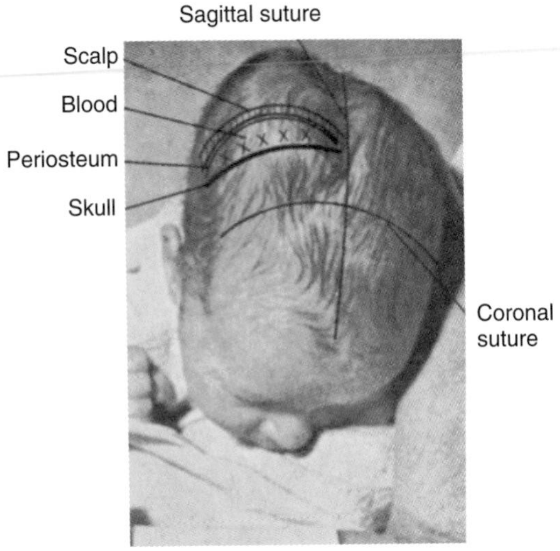

FIGURE 39-8 Cephalhematoma. (From Betz CL, Hunsberger M, Wright S: *Family-centered nursing care of children*, ed 2, Philadelphia, 1994, WB Saunders, p 124.)

results from trauma occurring during a difficult delivery. The swelling appears hours to days after delivery.

Clinical Findings

History. Primigravida and traumatic delivery may be part of the history.

Physical Examination. Findings include the following:

- Swelling in the parietal area that does not cross suture lines
- Rarely associated with a skull fracture, coagulopathy, or intracranial hemorrhage

Differential Diagnosis. Caput succedaneum and cranial meningocele should be considered.

Management. No treatment is indicated because the condition resolves in a few weeks to months. Calcification of the hematoma occurs, which can be felt as bony prominences. Observe for hyperbilirubinemia.

Craniotabes

Description and Etiology. Craniotabes is thinning of the bone of the scalp. This is a normal variation of the parietal bone, usually near the sagittal suture line.

Clinical Findings

History. Prematurity can be part of the history.

Physical Examination. Findings include a "ping-pong ball" effect when pressing on the parietal bone.

Management. No treatment is necessary because craniotabes resolves spontaneously. If persistent, pathologic causes such as rickets should be investigated.

Cleft Lip and Palate

Description, Etiology, and Incidence. Cleft lip is failure of embryonic structures surrounding the oral cavity to join. Cleft palate appears when the palatal shelves fail to fuse. There are various degrees of clefts. Genetic factors influence the development of cleft lip more than cleft palate; however, both occur sporadically. A combination of cleft lip and cleft palate is more common than one without the other. Cleft lip with or without cleft palate occurs in about 1 in 1000 births. Cleft palate alone occurs in 1 in 2500 births (Behrman, Kliegman, & Jensen, 2004). Clefts are more common in males than in females.

Clinical Findings

Physical Examination. Findings include the following:

- A varying degree of cleft, from a small notch to a complete separation
- Unilateral or bilateral cleft
- Involvement of the soft palate, hard palate, or both
- A bifid uvula, which may indicate a submucosal cleft palate

Management and Complications. Surgical repair is indicated, and the timing is individualized. Special nipples and feeding techniques are used until surgery can be performed. Breastfeeding and bottle-feeding may be successful depending on the severity of the cleft. Speech evaluation and perhaps therapy are necessary in later years. Dental restoration is often needed. Team management is often beneficial. Middle ear, nasopharyngeal, sinus infections, and associated hearing loss can occur.

Congenital Cataracts, Glaucoma, and Retinopathy of Prematurity

See Chapter 29.

Cardiac Conditions

See Chapter 31.

Respiratory Conditions

Respiratory Distress Syndrome

Description, Etiology, and Incidence. Respiratory distress syndrome (RDS), formerly called hyaline membrane disease, occurs secondary to atelectasis of the lungs. This is the most common pulmonary disease in the newborn (Table 39-4). Surfactant deficiency is the underlying cause of the disease, resulting in alveolar atelectasis and decreased lung compliance. The incidence is 1% of all live births but only 0.5% of term births. The incidence rises rapidly below 33 to 34 weeks of gestational age. An estimated 50% of all neonatal deaths result from RDS or its complications (Behrman, Kliegman, & Jensen, 2004). The incidence increases with decreasing gestational age and/or weight.

Clinical Findings

History. The history can include the following:

- Diabetic mother
- Preterm delivery
- Multiple prior pregnancies
- Cesarean delivery
- Precipitous delivery
- Asphyxia
- Cold stress
- Previous affected siblings

Physical Examination. Findings include the following:

- Tachypnea
- Grunting
- Intercostal retractions
- Nasal flaring
- Duskiness, cyanosis
- Breath sounds normal or diminished with harsh tubular quality
- Fine rales on deep inspiration

Radiologic and Laboratory Findings. A radiograph of the chest shows a fine reticular granularity of the parenchyma

TABLE 39-4 ***Clinical Comparison of Transient Tachypnea of the Newborn and Respiratory Distress Syndrome***

Transient Tachypnea of the Newborn	Respiratory Distress Syndrome
Seen only in infants delivered at or near term, often in infants born by cesarean section	Found only in premature infants, with the greatest incidence in infants weighing <1500 g
Increased respiratory rate is invariably present; grunting and intercostal retractions are not common	Usually, respiratory rate is increased, infants grunt at expiration, nasal flaring is noted, and sternal and intercostal retractions are commonly seen
Cyanosis is not a prominent feature	Cyanosis in room air is a prominent feature
Air exchange is good; rales and rhonchi are usually absent	Auscultation reveals diminished air entry
Begins at birth, usually resolving in the first 24-48 hr of life	Progressive respiratory distress in the first hours of life
Chest radiograph shows central perihilar streaking with slightly enlarged heart	Chest radiograph demonstrates reticulogranular, ground-glass appearance and air bronchograms
Typical course involves gradual decrease in respiratory rate with resolution in the first 5 days of life	Course variable depending on infant's gestational weight and age; classically, respiratory distress syndrome begins to improve after about 72 hr of symptoms
No specific therapy other than maintaining oxygenation is usually necessary	Artificial surfactant, as well as administration of steroids to the mother, can reduce the severity of this disease; mechanical ventilation is commonly needed

and air bronchograms. Blood gas results indicate hypoxemia, hypercarbia, and metabolic acidosis.

Management, Prognosis, and Prevention. Supportive care and mechanical ventilation are used as indicated. The immediate use of exogenous surfactant has been found to reduce mortality rates and improve short-term respiratory status in preterm infants (AAP, 1999c). The prognosis depends on the severity of the disease and the birth weight of the infant. The only effective preventive measure is prevention of prematurity. Administration of synthetic corticosteroids to selected women 48 to 72 hours before delivery is also used to reduce the severity of the problem.

Transient Tachypnea of the Newborn

Description and Etiology. Transient tachypnea of the newborn (TTN) is a respiratory condition that results from incomplete evacuation of fetal lung fluid in full-term infants. TTN results from decreased pulmonary compliance and tidal volume and increased dead space secondary to slow absorption of fetal lung fluid. It is more common in cesarean deliveries.

Clinical Findings

History. TTN usually disappears within 24 to 48 hours.

Physical Examination. Findings include the following:

- Tachypnea
- Expiratory grunting
- Paucity of auscultation findings
- Intercostal retractions
- Cyanosis that responds to minimal oxygen

Radiologic Findings. A chest radiograph shows prominent pulmonary vascular markings, fluid lines along fissures, overaeration, flat diaphragms, and occasionally pleural fluid.

Differential Diagnosis. The differential diagnosis is RDS (see Table 39-4).

Management and Prognosis. If the infant is not in significant respiratory distress, close observation and transcutaneous oxygen saturation monitoring can be sufficient until the tachypnea resolves. The need for supplemental oxygen therapy provided in a hood should be based on close oxygen monitoring. The use of mechanical ventilation in TTN is rare. Infants usually recover rapidly within 24 to 48 hours with no treatment.

Meconium Aspiration Syndrome

Description, Etiology, and Incidence. Meconium aspiration syndrome occurs in term or postterm infants. This syndrome is a serious pulmonary disorder characterized by small airway obstruction, chemical pneumonitis, and secondary respiratory distress. Fetal distress and anoxia increase intestinal peristalsis and relax the anal sphincter to release meconium into the amniotic fluid. Thick meconium is aspirated either in utero or with the first breath. Approximately 5% to 15% of all newborns are meconium stained, but only a fraction of these infants develop respiratory problems.

Clinical Findings

History. The history includes meconium in the amniotic fluid and below the vocal cords on resuscitation.

Physical Examination. Findings include the following:
- Tachypnea
- Intercostal retractions
- Grunting
- Cyanosis within hours of delivery

Radiologic Findings. A chest radiograph shows patchy infiltrates, coarse streaking of both lung fields, and flattening of the diaphragm.

Management, Prognosis, and Prevention. An infant born with meconium present in the amniotic fluid should undergo suctioning of the mouth and hypopharynx immediately after delivery of the head. Depressed infants and those delivered through thick meconium should undergo visualization of the larynx with removal of any meconium noted. Infants with meconium in the larynx or those who remain depressed should receive endotracheal intubation, with suction applied directly to the endotracheal tube to remove meconium from the airway. Treatment includes supportive care and standard management of respiratory distress. Severe meconium aspiration cases are managed by extracorporeal membrane oxygenation (ECMO). The mortality rate of meconium-stained infants is higher than that of nonstained infants. Meconium aspiration accounts for a significant proportion of neonatal deaths. Residual lung problems are possible. Ultimate prognosis depends on the extent of central nervous system (CNS) injury from asphyxia. DeLee suctioning after the infant's head is delivered is used by some to reduce the risk of meconium aspiration, especially if the baby has not yet breathed deeply.

Gastrointestinal and Abdominal Conditions

Esophageal Atresia and Tracheoesophageal Fistula

Description and Incidence. In esophageal atresia, a blind pouch occurs in the esophagus with or without an associated fistula. Most infants have a proximal pouch, with the associated fistula connecting the distal esophagus and the trachea (Fig. 39-9). This defect occurs in 1 in 4000 births. Approximately one third of affected infants are born prematurely (Behrman, Kliegman, & Jensen, 2004).

Clinical Findings

History. The history includes maternal polyhydramnios and inability to pass a nasogastric tube during resuscitation at birth or afterward in the nursery.

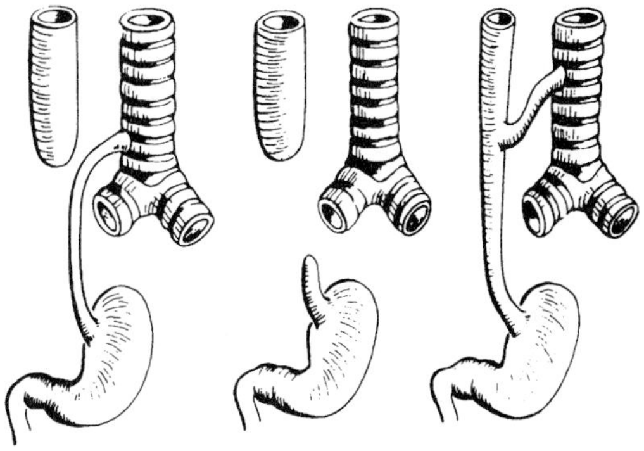

FIGURE 39-9 The three most common types of esophageal atresia and tracheoesophageal fistula (TEF). (From Ein SH: Congenital malformations of the esophagus. In Wyllie R, Hyams JS, editors: *Pediatric gastrointestinal disease*, Philadelphia, 1999, WB Saunders.)

Physical Examination. Findings include the following:
- Excessive oral secretions that require frequent suctioning
- Choking, coughing, and cyanosis, particularly during feedings
- Spitting or vomiting

Radiologic Findings. Chest and abdominal radiographs show the nasogastric tube coiled in the thoracic region. Carefully performed water-soluble x-ray evaluation of the upper esophagus demonstrates the exact location of the atresia and rules out tracheoesophageal fistula.

Differential Diagnosis. RDS, meconium aspiration, and congenital heart disease should be considered.

Management, Complications, and Prognosis. This is a surgical emergency requiring immediate intervention. Preoperatively, the infant should be placed in a prone position and suctioned frequently. A nasogastric tube can be inserted into the blind pouch to prevent aspiration until surgical repair can be accomplished. Pneumonia, atelectasis, aspiration, strictures, and repeated surgery are possible complications. The survival rate postoperatively is almost 100% unless other congenital anomalies are present. Approximately 30% of affected infants have other congenital anomalies, most commonly cardiovascular defects.

Duodenal Atresia

Description and Incidence. Duodenal atresia is a complete obstruction of the duodenum, ending blindly just distal to the ampulla of Vater. Duodenal atresia occurs in 1 in 10,000 births. It is associated with other anomalies in 30% of cases, Down syndrome in 20% to 30% of cases, and prematurity in 50% of cases (Behrman, Kliegman, & Jensen, 2000).

Clinical Findings

History. The history may include the following:

- Maternal polyhydramnios
- Down syndrome
- Premature birth

Physical Examination. Findings include the following:

- Bile-stained vomitus
- Abdominal distention
- Jaundice

Radiologic Findings. Abdominal radiographs show a "double-bubble" pattern in the upright position secondary to air in the stomach and a distended duodenum.

Differential Diagnosis. Malrotation, duodenal obstruction, and annular pancreas should be considered.

Management, Prognosis, and Complications. Surgical intervention is indicated. Feedings should be discontinued and gastric suctioning applied. The prognosis depends on early identification and treatment and other associated anomalies. Aspiration of gastric contents can occur as a complication of this condition.

Volvulus

Description. Volvulus is the twisting of a loop of bowel, causing intermittent or acute pain and obstruction.

Clinical Findings

Physical Examination. Findings include abdominal distention and bilious vomiting.

Radiologic Findings. Intestinal obstruction is demonstrated on abdominal radiograph.

Differential Diagnosis. Duodenal obstruction or atresia and annular pancreas are in the differential diagnosis.

Management, Prognosis, and Complications. Surgical repair and fluid replacement are indicated. The prognosis depends on identification and the urgency of surgery. Perforation, necrosis of the bowel, sepsis, and peritonitis are possible complications.

Pyloric Stenosis

Description and Incidence. Pyloric stenosis is characterized by hypertrophied pyloric muscle, causing a narrowing of the pyloric sphincter. Pyloric stenosis occurs in 3 per 1000 live births, with a fourfold increase in males as compared with females (Behrman, Kliegman, & Jensen, 2004). It tends to be familial and is seen more commonly in white first-born males.

Clinical Findings

History. The history may include the following:

- Regurgitation and nonprojectile vomiting during the first few weeks of life
- Projectile vomiting beginning at 2 to 3 weeks of age
- Insatiable appetite with weight loss, dehydration, and constipation

Investigation of an association between pyloric stenosis and the administration of erythromycin has been suggested.

Physical Examination. Findings include the following:

- Weight loss
- Vomitus that is nonbilious and can contain blood
- A distinct "olive" mass that is often palpated in the epigastrium to the right of midline
- Reverse peristalsis visualized across the abdomen

Radiologic Findings. An upper gastrointestinal series demonstrates a "string sign," indicating a fine, elongated pyloric canal. Ultrasound, with measurement of the pyloric muscle thickness, is used in many centers.

Management and Prognosis. Surgical intervention (pyloromyotomy) is indicated after correction of fluid and electrolyte imbalance. Vomiting can continue for a few days after surgery, so feedings should be introduced gradually. The prognosis is excellent.

Hirschsprung Disease (Congenital Aganglionic Megacolon)

Description and Incidence. Hirschsprung disease is an absence of ganglion cells in the bowel wall, most often in the rectosigmoid region, resulting in a portion of the colon having no motility. This disorder occurs in 1 in 5000 births. It is the most common cause of neonatal obstruction of the colon and accounts for approximately 33% of all neonatal obstructions (Behrman, Kliegman, & Jensen, 2004). The disease is familial, affects males four times more commonly than females, and is common in children with trisomy 21. Additional anomalies are sometimes present.

Clinical Findings

History. The history may include the following:

- Failure to pass meconium within the first 48 hours of life
- Failure to thrive
- Poor feeding
- Chronic constipation
- Down syndrome

Physical Examination. Findings include the following:

- Vomiting
- Abdominal obstruction
- Failure to pass stools
- Diarrhea, explosive bowel movements, or flatus

Radiologic and Laboratory Findings. Radiographs indicate dilated loops of bowel (Fig. 39-10). A biopsy determines the absence of ganglion cells.

Differential Diagnosis. The differential diagnosis includes acquired functional megacolon, colonic inertia, chronic idiopathic constipation, obstipation, small left colon syndrome, meconium plug syndrome, and ileal atresia with microcolon.

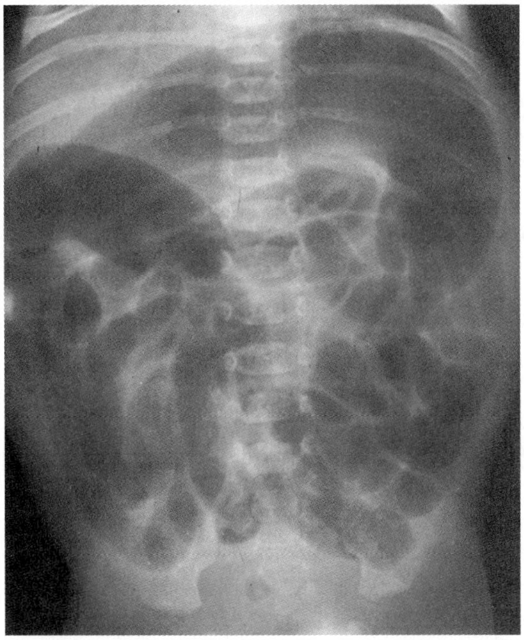

FIGURE 39-10 Dramatic dilation of bowel consistent with Hirschsprung disease. (Photo courtesy of Lawrence H. Robinson, Professor of Radiology and Pediatrics, University of Texas Medical School, Houston, Texas.)

Management. Surgical resection of the affected bowel is indicated, with or without a colostomy.

Imperforate Anus

Description and Incidence. Imperforate anus is the lack of a rectal opening. This condition occurs in about 1 in 5000 births, about half associated with another anomaly (often the VACTERL association consisting of vertebral dysgenesis, anal atresia [imperforate anus], cardiac anomalies, tracheoesophageal fistula, renal anomalies, and limb anomalies).

Clinical Findings

History. The history includes no passage of meconium.

Physical Examination. Findings include no obvious opening in the rectal area.

Radiologic Findings. Endoscopic examination and ultrasound indicate the degree of malformation.

Associated Conditions. Congenital heart disease, esophageal atresia, intestinal atresia, annular pancreas, intestinal malrotation or duplication, bicornuate absence of the musculus rectus abdominis, trisomy 21, finger and hand anomalies, omphalocele, bladder exstrophy, and exstrophy of the ileocecal area are associated conditions (McMillan et al, 1999).

Management. Immediate surgical repair with or without performing a colostomy is indicated. Long-term management related to bowel functioning may be needed because some children will have trouble with bowel emptying or incontinence.

Omphalocele and Gastroschisis

Description and Incidence. An omphalocele is a protrusion of the sac of intestines covered by the peritoneum without overlying skin into the base of the umbilical cord occurring in 1 in 5000 to 10,000 births (Behrman, Kliegman, & Jensen, 2004). Gastroschisis is similar in appearance with intestinal contents protruding through the abdomen with no protective peritoneal covering. Gastroschisis occurs in about 1 in 10,000 to 20,000 live births when there is failure to close the lateral ventral folds of the developing abdominal wall.

Clinical Findings

Physical Examination. Examination reveals a saclike protrusion covered by the peritoneum without overlying skin at the midabdomen.

Associated Conditions. With omphalocele, associated conditions include chromosomal abnormalities, congenital diaphragmatic hernia, and a variety of cardiac problems. Concomitant hypoglycemia and macroglossia suggest Beckwith syndrome. Associated congenital anomalies are rare with gastroschisis.

Management and Complications. Maintain body temperature. Apply protective gauze and wrap abdomen with cellophane to avoid heat and fluid loss. When the infant is stable, surgical repair is indicated. Ileus is a common complication.

Necrotizing Enterocolitis

Description, Etiology, and Incidence. Necrotizing enterocolitis is characterized by varying degrees of mucosal or transmural necrosis of the intestine. The usual onset is in the first 2 weeks of life but can be later in very low birth weight infants. The cause is unknown, but high-risk infants are found to have immature colons that become necrosed from trauma or injury. It occurs in 1% to 5% of neonates, with the vast majority of these cases occurring in premature infants (Behrman, Kliegman, & Jensen, 2004).

Clinical Findings

History. The history can include the following:

- Prematurity, SGA
- Maternal hemorrhage, preeclampsia
- Cocaine exposure in utero
- Exchange transfusions, umbilical catheters
- Asphyxia
- Polycythemia

Physical Examination. Findings include the following:

- Abdominal distention
- Vomiting

- Bloody stools
- Lethargy
- Apnea
- Disseminated intravascular coagulation
- Rapid progression of shock

Laboratory and Radiologic Findings

- Sepsis workup should be done.
- An abdominal radiograph shows pneumatosis intestinalis, a specific air pattern.

Differential Diagnosis. The differential diagnosis includes sepsis, intestinal obstruction, volvulus, Hirschsprung disease, anal fissures, and neonatal appendicitis.

Management, Prognosis, and Complications. Take the following steps:

1. Prescribe systemic antibiotics following sepsis workup as indicated by laboratory results.
2. Stop feedings, initiate gastric suctioning, maintain electrolyte balance, give oxygen as needed, and initiate surgical consultation.
3. Obtain serial abdominal radiographs to follow course of disease.
4. Delay oral feedings in very low birth weight infants for at least 1 week.

The mortality rate is 9% to 25%; 10% develop strictures at the necrotizing site (Behrman, Kliegman, & Jensen, 2004). Malabsorption with short-gut syndrome may complicate management (Finberg & Kleinman, 2002). Ileus and perforation are early complications; strictures and malabsorption are late complications.

Meconium Ileus

Description, Etiology, and Incidence. Meconium ileus is an impaction of the bowel with meconium, causing intestinal obstruction. Meconium ileus is associated with cystic fibrosis and maternal polyhydramnios. About 80% to 90% of patients with meconium ileus have cystic fibrosis; about 10% to 20% of patients with cystic fibrosis have meconium ileus (Behrman, Kliegman, & Jensen, 2000).

Clinical Findings

History. There is a failure to pass meconium within 48 hours of life.

Physical Examination. Findings include abdominal distention and persistent vomiting.

Radiologic Findings. A radiograph shows bowel loops of varying width. There is a grainy appearance at the points of heaviest meconium concentration.

Associated Conditions. Approximately 50% of affected infants have associated intestinal disorders, including atresia, stenosis, volvulus, or perforations (McMillan et al, 1999).

Management and Prognosis. Treatment is individualized; high enemas (with water-soluble contrast material) or laparotomy can be used. The survival rate is good. Referral to a gastrointestinal specialist may be considered.

Diaphragmatic Hernia

Description, Etiology, and Incidence. In diaphragmatic hernia, abdominal contents herniate into the thoracic cavity. Diaphragmatic hernia is caused by failure of the pleuroperitoneal canal to close completely during embryologic development. It occurs with a frequency of about 1 in 5000 live births (Behrman, Kliegman, & Jensen, 2004).

Clinical Findings

History. After birth, immediate respiratory failure occurs secondary to pulmonary hypertension or pulmonary hypoplasia.

Physical Examination. Findings include the following:

- Respiratory distress with tachypnea
- Cyanosis
- Scaphoid abdomen
- Rarely, bowel sounds heard in the chest
- Absence of breath sounds
- Heart tones best heard in the contralateral chest

The amount of respiratory distress depends on the amount of lung capacity. Any child with respiratory distress should be evaluated for diaphragmatic hernia.

Radiologic Findings. A chest radiograph shows fluid and air-filled loops of intestine in the chest. The mediastinum is displaced toward the unaffected side, usually to the right.

Management. Treatment involves the following:

- As soon as the diagnosis is suspected, the infant should be positioned with the head and chest higher than the abdomen.
- Intensive respiratory support, which often includes ECMO
- Surgery
- After surgery, intensive respiratory and metabolic support

Prognosis. The mortality rate is 50% to 60%, depending on the degree of hypoplastic lung.

Hydrocele and Inguinal Hernia

See Chapter 35.

Umbilical Hernia

Definition. Umbilical hernia is a weakness or imperfect closure of the umbilical ring.

Clinical Findings

Physical Examination. Findings include a soft swelling in the umbilical area that can be reduced, often associated with diastasis recti.

Management, Prognosis, and Education. Surgery is not required unless the hernia persists after 5 years of age, strangulates, is nonreducible, or dramatically enlarges. Most umbilical hernias resolve spontaneously by 1 year but can take up to 4 to 5 years; those with fascial defects greater than 1.5 cm in diameter have a lower rate of spontaneous closure. Strangulation is extremely rare (Katz, 2001). Counsel parents to avoid taping coins or placing belly-bands over the umbilicus, because these efforts do not help and can contribute to infection.

Renal Conditions

Acute Renal Failure

Description, Etiology, and Incidence. The newborn normally produces 1 to 3 ml/kg per hour of urine and urinates within the first 48 hours of life.

A stressed neonate may develop decreased renal function. Urine output less than 0.5 ml/kg per 24 hours can indicate acute renal failure and puts the child at risk for disrupted body fluid homeostasis. Multiple causes of renal failure can be identified, including stress during the prenatal period, dehydration, sepsis, anoxia, shock, administration of nephrotoxic drugs, renal dysgenesis, obstructive uropathy, congenital heart disease, hemorrhage, and renal vein thrombosis. Approximately 3% of neonates have some form of renal failure.

Clinical Findings

History. Maternal oligohydramnios may be noted.

Physical Examination. Findings include the following:

- Decreased or no urinary output
- Abdominal mass
- Pallor, edema, lethargy, vomiting, seizures, coma
- High blood pressure
- Pulmonary edema, congestive heart failure, or arrhythmias
- Meningomyelocele
- Prune-belly syndrome

Laboratory Findings. Order the following, as indicated:

- Bladder tap or catheterization to confirm inadequate urinary output
- Urinalysis to rule out hematuria or pyuria
- Urine osmolarity, sodium, and potassium values to indicate kidney filtration ability
- Serum blood urea nitrogen, creatinine, sodium, and potassium values to indicate poor filtration
- Complete blood count including differential and platelets to rule out thrombocytopenia, sepsis, or renal vein thrombosis

Management and Prognosis

- Replace fluid loss (approximately 30 ml/kg per 24 hours), then restrict fluid and diet.
- Maintain strict intake, output, and fluid and electrolyte balance.
- Monitor blood pressure.
- Peritoneal dialysis is sometimes indicated.

The prognosis depends on the degree of renal failure and the cause.

Hydronephrosis

Description and Incidence. Hydronephrosis is a dilation of one or both kidneys frequently caused by an obstruction of the ureteropelvic junction, posterior urethral valves, ectopic ureterocele, prune-belly syndrome, or ureteral or ureterovesical obstructions. Obstructive uropathy occurs in 1 in 1000 births and is slightly more common in males (McMillan et al, 1999).

Clinical Findings

History. The history can include the following:

- Decreased urinary output
- Occasionally found on prenatal ultrasonogram
- Asymptomatic in early stages

Physical Examination. Findings include an abdominal mass.

Management and Prognosis. Surgical repair may be necessary depending on the cause of the hydronephrosis and if spontaneous resolution does not occur by 6 to 12 months of age. The longer the obstruction lasts, the less likely renal function will return to normal.

Cystic Kidney

Description and Incidence. The presence of multiple cysts of various sizes and shapes in the kidney can be either an autosomal dominant or autosomal recessive disease. The autosomal dominant form usually appears in the fourth or fifth decade of life and can be associated with hepatic cysts or cerebral aneurysms. In the autosomal recessive form, which also usually has hepatic cysts, the infant has abdominal masses at birth. The adult form (autosomal dominant) occurs in about 1 in 1000 persons; the juvenile form (autosomal recessive) occurs in about 1 or 2 per 10,000 live births (Blowey, 2002).

Clinical Findings

History. Maternal oligohydramnios may be noted in the juvenile form.

Physical Examination. Findings include the following:

- Abdominal lobular mass
- Hematuria
- Hypertension

Radiologic Findings. A renal scan is done to document the disorder.

Differential Diagnosis. Multicystic dysplasia, hydronephrosis, Wilms' tumor, and renal vein thrombosis are included in the differential diagnosis.

Management and Prognosis. Monitor kidney function and check for enlargement of cysts (with a renal ultrasound) or infection. Nephrectomy is necessary if no regression is seen or a complication occurs. Dialysis or transplantation is sometimes considered. With severe involvement, the neonate dies from pulmonary or renal insufficiency. Hypertension may be difficult to control.

Renal Artery or Vein Thrombosis

Description. Decreased blood flow to the kidney because of thrombus formation is seen.

Clinical Findings

History. In the newborn this condition is often associated with asphyxia, dehydration, shock, and sepsis. Maternal diabetes is a rare cause. Sudden onset of gross hematuria may be noted.

Physical Examination. Findings include a firm flank mass.

Radiologic and Laboratory Findings. Ultrasonography shows marked enlargement of the kidney. The hematocrit is low. The urine contains protein and often blood.

Differential Diagnosis. Other causes of hematuria, such as hydronephrosis, cystic disease, Wilms' tumor, hemolytic-uremic syndrome, and renal abscess, are included in the differential diagnosis.

Management

- Maintain fluid and electrolyte balance.
- Monitor blood pressure.
- Prophylactic anticoagulation therapy is occasionally given to prevent thrombosis in the other kidney.
- Nephrectomy is not necessary unless chronic infection or uncontrollable hypertension occurs.

Neuroblastoma

Description, Etiology, and Incidence. A neuroblastoma is a solid tumor that originates from neural crest tissue along the craniospinal axis. The majority of neuroblastomas develop in the abdomen, usually in the adrenal gland. The cause is unknown. It occurs in 1 in 7000 births and is slightly more common in males (Behrman, Kliegman, & Jensen, 2000).

Clinical Findings

History. An unexplained fever, mass, and symptoms related to the site of the tumor are part of the history.

Physical Examination. Findings include the following:

- Firm, irregular, nontender mass in abdomen
- Pallor
- Hypotension
- Ascites
- Irritability
- Possible external tumors in newborn

Radiologic and Laboratory Findings. These include attempts to stage the disease, including the following:

- Renal radiographs to detect calcifications
- Computed tomography (CT) or magnetic resonance imaging of abdomen
- Radiograph or CT scan of chest
- Bone scan
- Urine catecholamines and vanillylmandelic acid (VMA)
- Bone marrow aspirate

Differential Diagnosis. Wilms' tumor, hydronephrosis, renal vein thrombosis, and lymphoma are included in the differential diagnosis.

Management and Prognosis. Although some neuroblastomas regress without therapy, treatment is surgical removal followed by radiation therapy or chemotherapy. The prognosis depends on the age of the patient and the stage of the tumor. The prognosis is better if complete resection of the tumor is performed or if the patient is younger than 1 year of age.

Renal Agenesis

Description and Incidence. Renal agenesis is failure of the kidney to form normally. Bilateral agenesis is incompatible with life. Bilateral renal agenesis occurs in 1 in 3000 births (Behrman, Kliegman, & Jensen, 2004).

Clinical Findings

History. Maternal oligohydramnios is noted in bilateral agenesis. Unilateral renal agenesis is usually not detected until the child is evaluated for urinary tract infection later in infancy.

Physical Examination. Findings include the following:

- Single umbilical artery associated with unilateral agenesis
- Associated anomalies involving the gastrointestinal or urinary tract and skeleton, especially with Potter syndrome (bilateral agenesis)
- Low-set ears, senile appearance, broad nose, and receding chin consistent with Potter syndrome

Management and Prognosis. Monitor for proteinuria and hypertension. Patients with bilateral disease die within a few months of life. Those with unilateral disease are usually detected with evaluation of the urinary conditions.

Endocrine Conditions

Congenital Hypothyroidism, Congenital Adrenal Hyperplasia

See Chapter 26.

Metabolic Conditions

Hypoglycemia

Description and Etiology. In the term infant serum glucose levels rarely fall below 35 mg/dl in the first 3 hours of life, below 40 mg/dl between 3 and 24 hours of life, or below 45 mg/dl thereafter (Behrman, Kliegman, & Jensen, 2004). Infants at higher risk of developing hypoglycemia include SGA infants and those with diabetic mothers, asphyxia at birth, sepsis, erythroblastosis fetalis, glycogen storage disease, or galactosemia (Table 39-5).

Clinical Findings

History. The history can include the following:

- Risk factors for sepsis or asphyxia
- Infant of a diabetic mother
- SGA

Physical Examination. Findings include the following:

- Lethargy
- Poor feeding and regurgitation
- Apnea
- Jitteriness
- Pallor, sweating, cool extremities
- Seizures

Management and Prognosis. See Management in Table 39-5.

Infants with symptomatic hypoglycemia, particularly low-birth-weight infants and infants of diabetic mothers, are less likely to have normal intellectual development than are asymptomatic infants. Prognosis for normal intellectual

TABLE 39-5 ***Identification and Management of Hypoglycemia, Infant of Diabetic Mother, and Polycythemia in the Newborn***

Condition	Clinical Findings	Workup	Management
Hypoglycemia	Blood glucose <30 mg/dl Infant with history of SGA; poorly controlled diabetic mother (IDDM); at risk for sepsis; asphyxia; erythroblastosis fetalis Lethargy Poor feeding and regurgitation Apnea Jitteriness Pallor, sweating, cool extremities Seizures	Serum glucose—measure within 1 hr of birth, every 2 hr until 6-8 hr of life, then every 4-6 hr until 24 hr of life	Give normoglycemic high-risk infants oral or gavage feedings with breast milk or formula at 1-3 hr of life and continue every 2-3 hr for 24-48 hr Intravenous glucose at 8 mg/kg/min if serum glucose less than 30-35 mg/dl and oral feedings poorly tolerated
Infant of diabetic mother (IDM)	IDDM: large, plump infant with large viscera; puffy facies; plethora; hyperactivity first 3 days; ± hypotonicity, lethargy, poor suck; ± cardiomegaly and murmurs	Intensive observation and care Serum glucose—measure within 1 hr of birth, then every 1 hr for the next 6-8 hr	If clinically well and normoglycemic, initially give oral or gavage feedings with infant formula or breast milk started within 2-3 hr of age and continued at 3 hr intervals If infant is unable to tolerate oral feeding, discontinue feeding and give 10% glucose by peripheral intravenous infusion at a rate of 4-8 mg/kg/hr Treat hypoglycemia, even in asymptomatic infants, with intravenous infusions of glucose
Polycythemia	Cyanosis, tachypnea, respiratory distress Hyperbilirubinemia Infant with history of diabetic mother, IUGR, exposed to chronic hypoxia; recipient of twin-twin transfusion; delayed clamping of umbilical cord; postmaturity; SGA Plethora Feeding disturbance	Hematocrit ≥65%	Phlebotomy and replacement with saline or albumin, or partial exchange transfusion to reduce hematocrit to 50%

Adapted from Burns CE et al: *Pocket reference for pediatric primary care*, Philadelphia, 2001, WB Saunders, pp 430-431.
IDDM, Insulin-dependent diabetes mellitus; *IUGR*, intrauterine growth restriction; *SGA*, small for gestational age.

function is guarded in infants with prolonged and severe hypoglycemia.

Infant of Diabetic Mother

Description and Etiology. An infant of a mother with poorly controlled gestational or insulin-dependent diabetes mellitus is referred to as an infant of a diabetic mother (IDM). Maternal hyperglycemia causes fetal hyperglycemia and hyperinsulinemia, leading to increased hepatic glucose uptake and glycogen synthesis, accelerated lipogenesis, and augmented protein synthesis (Behrman, Kliegman, & Jensen, 2004). See Table 39-5.

Clinical Findings

History. The history includes a mother with poorly controlled diabetes.

Physical Examination. Findings include the following:

- Large and plump neonate with large viscera
- Puffy facies
- Plethora
- Hyperexcitability during the first 3 days of life, although hypotonia, lethargy, and poor sucking also occur

Management, Complications, and Prevention. See Table 39-5.

Cardiomegaly is common (30%), and heart failure occurs in 5% to 10% of infants. Congenital anomalies are increased threefold; cardiac malformations and lumbosacral agenesis are most common. There is a predisposition to obesity in childhood that can extend into adult life. Symptomatic hypoglycemia increases the risk of impaired intellectual development.

Strict management of blood glucose levels in mothers with diabetes decreases the risk of severe problems in the infant.

Orthopedic Conditions

Fractured Clavicle; Brachial Palsy

See Chapter 38.

Polydactyly and Syndactyly

Description and Incidence. Polydactyly is a condition that varies from a skin tag to a formed finger with a nail that extends from the postaxial side. Polydactyly occurs in 1 in 300 in the black population and in 1 in 3000 in the white population. In contrast, syndactyly can be identified by finding fingers or toes fused by skin and sometimes bone. Syndactyly occurs in about 1 in 2000 births and can be seen as part of a variety of syndromes.

Clinical Findings

Physical Examination. In polydactyly a floppy digit is seen on the foot or hand. It varies in degree of formation. Syndactyly is webbing of two digits, partially or to the tip of the digit.

Management. For polydactyly surgical removal of the floppy extra digit is indicated. If the digit is stabilized by bone, surgical removal is deferred until the patient is older, when function can be assessed. For patients with syndactyly treatment is not indicated in the neonate. Surgical separation is recommended at age 2 to 3 years.

Central Nervous System Conditions

Congenital Hydrocephalus

Description, Etiology, and Incidence. Congenital hydrocephalus is an accumulation of cerebrospinal fluid (CSF) in the brain's ventricles at birth. Malformations, infections, intraventricular hemorrhage, and disorders in brain development can lead to congenital hydrocephalus. The incidence varies depending on which of these conditions is causative.

Clinical Findings

History. The history can include vomiting, lethargy, irritability, and poor feeding.

Physical Examination. Findings include the following:

- Head circumference greater than 90% of the standardized growth curve
- Cranial sutures separated by large, tense fontanels

Radiologic Findings. Cranial ultrasonography shows dilated ventricles.

Management. Medications that decrease CSF production (e.g., acetazolamide), a ventriculoperitoneal shunt, or both are used. Referral should be prompt.

Intraventricular Hemorrhage

Description, Etiology, and Incidence. Intraventricular hemorrhage (IVH) occurs within the ventricles of the brain. Risk factors include prematurity, RDS, hypoxemic-ischemic or hypotensive injury, increased or decreased cerebral blood flow, hypertension, hypervolemia, and reduced vascular integrity. There is a 10% to 20% occurrence rate in infants weighing 1500 g or less (Behrman, Kliegman, & Jensen, 2004). The incidence of IVH decreases with increasing gestational age.

Clinical Findings

History. Risk factors for IVH include SGA, prematurity, and others mentioned previously.

Physical Examination. Findings include the following:

- Diminished or absent Moro reflex
- Poor muscle tone, lethargy, somnolence
- Apnea
- Periods of pallor or cyanosis
- Failure to suck well
- High-pitched, shrill cry, seizures

Radiologic Findings. Ultrasonography is used to classify IVH into grades I to IV based on the presence and quantity of blood in the ventricles or brain tissue. Screening cranial ultrasounds should be performed on all infants with a gestational age of less than 30 weeks at 7 to 14 days of age, and optimally should be repeated at 36 to 40 weeks of postmenstrual age (American Academy of Neurology, 2002).

Management and Prognosis. Treatment may involve the following:

- Supportive management and minimal stimulation
- Acetazolamide to decrease CSF production
- Repeated lumbar punctures
- Ventriculoperitoneal shunt or external ventriculostomy

Grade III and IV hemorrhages, periventricular cystic lesions, and moderate to severe ventriculomegaly are all associated with adverse outcome (American Academy of Neurology, 2002).

Hypoxic-Ischemic Insults

Description, Etiology, and Incidence. Three levels of injury (grades I, II, and III, or mild, moderate, and severe) are described (Table 39-6). Brain damage results from fetal hypoxia or ischemia for an extended period of time. The initial hypoxemic or ischemic insult is followed by metabolic and respiratory acidosis. Compensatory mechanisms, such as shunting blood through the ductus to maintain perfusion of the brain, heart, adrenals, kidneys, liver, and intestines, ultimately fail if the insult is severe enough. Depending on the organ most damaged, a variety of signs and symptoms can be seen. Fifteen percent to 20% of infants with hypoxic-ischemic encephalopathy die in the neonatal period; up to 30% develop permanent disabilities. Causes of the initial hypoxic or ischemic insult include abruptio placentae, hemorrhage, cord compression, mechanical injury, severe hypertension or diabetes, and inadequate resuscitation (Behrman, Kliegman, & Jensen, 2004).

Clinical Findings

Physical Examination. Findings include the following:

- Seizure activity
- Pallor
- Cyanosis, apnea
- Bradycardia and unresponsiveness to stimulation

Management and Prognosis. Seizure and symptom management is needed. The prognosis depends on whether the underlying cause can be treated effectively. Severe encephalopathy, characterized by flaccid coma, apnea, and seizures, is associated with a poor prognosis (Behrman, Kliegman, & Jensen, 2000). An infant who remains neurologically abnormal after the initial recovery phase (2 weeks) likely has suffered permanent neurologic impairment. A low Apgar score at 20 minutes, absence of spontaneous respirations, and persistence of abnormal neurologic signs at 2 weeks of age predict death or severe cognitive and motor deficits.

Myelomeningocele

Description, Etiology, and Incidence. A myelomeningocele is the result of failure to close the posterior neural tube and the vertebral column. This is the most severe form of

TABLE 39-6 ***Hypoxic Ischemic Encephalopathy in Term Infants***

Signs	Stage 1	Stage 2	Stage 3
Level of consciousness	Hyperalert	Lethargic	Stuporous, coma
Muscle tone	Normal	Hypotonic	Flaccid
Posture	Normal	Flexion	Decerebrate
Tendon reflexes/clonus	Hyperactive	Hyperactive	Absent
Myoclonus	Present	Present	Absent
Moro reflex	Strong	Weak	Absent
Pupils	Mydriasis	Miosis	Unequal, poor light reflex
Seizures	None	Common	Decerebration
Electroencephalograph	Normal	Low-voltage changing to seizure activity	Burst suppression to isoelectric
Duration	<24 hr if progresses, otherwise may remain normal	24 hr to 24 days	Days to weeks
Outcome	Good	Variable	Death, severe deficits

Modified from Sarnat H, Sarnat M: Neonatal encephalopathy following fetal distress: a clinical and electroencephalopathic study, *Arch Neurol* 33:696, 1976.

neural tube defect. Genetic and environmental factors are both believed to play a causative role. See Chapter 28 for more information.

Clinical Findings

History. Poor intake of folic acid and exposure to hyperthermia or valproic acid are risk factors.

Physical Examination. Findings include the following:

- Saclike cyst containing meninges and spinal fluid covered by thin layer of partially epithelialized skin
- Flaccid paralysis of lower extremities
- Absence of deep tendon reflexes
- Lack of response to touch and pain
- Constant urinary dribbling

Seventy-five percent of cases are found in the lumbosacral area.

Management, Prognosis, and Prevention. Surgical repair and multidisciplinary supportive management are indicated. The mortality rate is 10% to 15% in aggressively treated children (Behrman, Kliegman, & Jensen, 2004). At least 70% have normal intelligence, but seizure disorders, hydrocephalus, and learning disabilities, as well as neurogenic bowel and bladder, are more common than in the general population. Prenatal vitamins and folic acid supplementation (0.4 mg/day) are helpful in preventing neural tube defects and should be taken by any female of childbearing age (AAP, 1999d).

Hematologic Conditions

Polycythemia

Description, Etiology, and Incidence. Polycythemia is characterized by a central hematocrit of 65% or higher. Polycythemia can occur in a variety of conditions, including IDM, cyanotic congenital heart disease, and infants with growth retardation who were exposed to chronic fetal hypoxia that stimulated erythropoietin production and increased red blood cell production. Polycythemia occurs in 1 to 5 per 100 births, depending on the etiology. See Table 39-5.

Clinical Findings

History. The history includes the following:

- Diabetic mother
- Recipient of a twin-twin transfusion
- Delayed clamping of umbilical cord
- Postmature infant
- SGA

Physical Examination. Fifteen percent to 25% of infants with polycythemia are asymptomatic. Findings include the following:

- Plethora
- Feeding disturbances
- Hypoglycemia
- Cyanosis (persistent fetal circulation), tachypnea, respiratory distress
- Hyperbilirubinemia

Management and Prognosis. See Table 39-5. Long-term problems include speech deficits, abnormal fine motor control, reduced IQ, and other neurologic abnormalities.

Hemorrhagic Disease in the Newborn

Description and Etiology. Severe transient deficiencies of vitamin K–dependent clotting factors lead to bleeding. Hemorrhagic disease is caused by a lack of free vitamin K in the mother and absence of bacterial intestinal flora normally responsible for synthesis of vitamin K in the infant. Vitamin K–dependent clotting factors (factors II, VII, IX, X) are normal at birth but decrease within 2 to 3 days. Breast milk is a poor source of vitamin K; late-onset bleeding (occurring 1 to 3 months after birth) rarely may be seen in exclusively breastfed infants. A particularly severe form of deficiency of vitamin K–dependent coagulation factors occurring in the first day of life has been reported in women receiving the anticonvulsants phenytoin and/or phenobarbital.

Clinical Findings

History. The history may include the following:

- Anticonvulsant use by the mother
- Prematurity
- Exclusive breastfeeding without vitamin K supplementation
- Failure to administer parenteral vitamin K at birth
- Neonatal hepatitis or biliary atresia

Physical Examination. Findings include gastrointestinal, nasal, subgaleal, or intracranial bleeding or bleeding at the site of an injection or circumcision.

Laboratory Findings. Prothrombin time, blood coagulation time, and partial thromboplastin time are prolonged.

Differential Diagnosis. This disorder may be the result of disseminated intravascular coagulation or congenital bleeding disorders unrelated to vitamin K.

Management, Prevention, and Prognosis

- Intravenous infusion of 1 to 5 mg of vitamin K is needed. Improvement of coagulation defects and cessation of bleeding should occur within a few hours.
- If a newborn is delivered at home, confirm if vitamin K was given.
- Prevention is achieved by routinely giving 1 mg of natural oil-soluble vitamin K intramuscularly within 1 hour of birth. Prognosis depends on the site and extent of bleeding.

Anemia

Description and Etiology. Anemia is characterized by less than the normal range of hemoglobin for birth weight and postnatal age. Anemia occurs secondary to acute blood loss before or during delivery. Acute blood loss after delivery can be external (gastrointestinal, circumcision site, umbilical stump), internal (fracture site, cephalhematoma, pulmonary hemorrhage, injured internal organ), or secondary to hemolysis or congenital aplastic or hypoplastic anemia.

Clinical Findings

History. The history can include the following:

- Twin-twin transfusion
- Unexpected tearing or delayed clamping of umbilical cord resulting in neonate blood loss
- Internal hemorrhage (due to fracture, cephalhematoma, or internal organ trauma)
- Umbilical stump or circumcision bleeding

Physical Examination. Pallor, congestive heart failure, and shock are possible findings.

Management and Prognosis. Treatment depends on the cause. An asymptomatic full-term infant with a hemoglobin level of 10 g/dl can be observed, whereas a symptomatic neonate born after abruptio placentae or with severe hemolytic disease of the newborn warrants transfusion. Treatment with blood should be balanced by concern about transfusion-acquired infection with cytomegalovirus, human immunodeficiency virus (HIV), and hepatitis B and C viruses. Prognosis depends on the cause and severity of the anemia.

Blood in Vomitus or Stool

Description and Etiology. Bright-red or dark-red blood in the vomitus or stool can be seen without clinical evidence of blood loss. This problem is caused by ingestion of maternal blood during delivery.

Clinical Findings

Physical Examination. Bright-red or dark-red blood is seen in vomitus or stool.

Laboratory Findings. Blood of maternal origin can be differentiated from infant blood by testing for fetal hemoglobin using the Apt test.

Differential Diagnosis. The differential diagnosis includes gastrointestinal bleeding caused by trauma, duplication of bowel, intussusception, volvulus, hemangioma or telangiectasia of bowel, rectal prolapse, vitamin K deficiency, or anal fissure.

Management. No treatment is necessary if blood is of maternal origin.

Jaundice

Description, Etiology, and Incidence. Jaundice, a clinically apparent accumulation of bilirubin in the skin, causes a yellowish orange or sometimes green hue to the skin. Jaundice becomes apparent when serum bilirubin levels exceed 5 to 7 mg/dl and usually advances in a pattern from the infant's head to the toes. Physiologic jaundice is the most common type of jaundice in the newborn period; it appears after the first 24 hours of life, increases at a rate less than 5 mg/dl, and peaks at a total bilirubin usually not exceeding 13 mg/dl with the direct bilirubin not exceeding 2 mg/dl. Physiologic jaundice does not persist beyond 1 week, and the infant shows no signs of illness. Nonphysiologic (pathologic) jaundice appears at less than 24 hours of age and may last longer than 8 days. The rate of increase in total bilirubin is rapid at greater than 0.5 mg/dl per hour. Total bilirubin levels are frequently greater than 12.5 mg/dl before 48 hours of age, or the direct bilirubin exceeds 1.5 to 2 mg/dl. Breast milk jaundice can be divided into early-onset and late-onset types. Early-onset breast milk jaundice develops within 2 to 4 days of birth and is believed to occur as a result of infrequent breastfeeding and insufficient intake leading to decreased intestinal motility. Late-onset breast milk jaundice develops 4 to 7 days after birth, peaks at 10 to 15 days of life, and frequently persists. See Chapter 13 on breastfeeding for more information. Kernicterus or bilirubin encephalopathy involves toxicity of the nervous system resulting from very high levels of bilirubin (Behrman, Kliegman, & Jensen, 2004; Wood, 2001).

Jaundice is observed during the first week of life in approximately 60% of infants. Causes include an increased rate of hemolysis, a decreased rate of conjugation, and abnormalities of liver function (Table 39-7).

- Increased rate of hemolysis: ABO incompatibility, Rh incompatibility, abnormal red blood cell shapes (spherocytosis, elliptocytosis, pyknocytosis, and stomatocytosis), red blood cell enzyme abnormalities (glucose-6-phosphate dehydrogenase deficiency, pyruvate kinase deficiency).
- Decreased rate of conjugation: immaturity of bilirubin conjugation (physiologic jaundice), congenital familial nonhemolytic jaundice (inborn errors of metabolism affecting glucuronyl transferase system and bilirubin transport), breast milk jaundice.
- Abnormalities of excretion or absorption: sepsis, hepatitis (viral, parasitic, bacterial, toxic), metabolic abnormalities (galactosemia, glycogen storage disease, IDM, cystic fibrosis), biliary atresia, choledochal cyst, obstruction of ampulla of Vater (annular pancreas), drugs.

TABLE 39-7 Diagnostic Features of the Various Types of Neonatal Jaundice

Diagnosis	Nature of Van Den Bergh Reaction	Jaundice: Appears	Jaundice: Disappears	Peak Bilirubin Concentration: mg/dl	Peak Bilirubin Concentration: Age (days)	Bilirubin Rate of Accumulation (mg/dl/day)	Remarks
Physiologic jaundice							Usually relates to degree of maturity
Full-term	Indirect	2-3 days	4-5 days	10-12	2-3	<5	
Premature	Indirect	3-4 days	7-9 days	15	6-8	<5	
Hyperbilirubinemia due to metabolic factors							Metabolic factors: hypoxia, respiratory distress, lack of carbohydrate
Full-term	Indirect	2-3 days	Variable	>12	First wk	<5	Hormonal influences: cretinism, hormones
Premature	Indirect	3-4 days	Variable	>15	First wk	<5	Genetic factors: Crigler-Najjar syndrome, transient familial hyperbilirubinemia Drugs: vitamin K, novobiocin
Hemolytic states and hematoma	Indirect	May appear in first 24 hr	Variable	Unlimited	Variable	Usually >5	Erythroblastosis: Rh, ABO Congenital hemolytic states: spherocytic, nonspherocytic Infantile pyknocytosis Drugs: vitamin K; enclosed hemorrhage—hematoma
Mixed hemolytic and hepatotoxic factors	Indirect and direct	May appear in first 24 hr	Variable	Unlimited	Variable	Usually >5	Infection: bacterial sepsis, pyelonephritis, hepatitis, toxoplasmosis, cytomegalic inclusion disease, rubella Drugs: vitamin K
Hepatocellular damage	Indirect and direct	Usually 2-3 days	Variable	Unlimited	Variable	Variable; can be >5	Biliary atresia; galactosemia; hepatitis, infection

From Brown AK: Diagnostic features of the various types of neonatal jaundice, *Pediatr Clin North Am* 9:589, 1962.

Classic physiologic jaundice is characterized by a rise in bilirubin from 1.5 mg/dl in cord blood to 5 to 6 mg/dl on the third day of life, declining to a normal adult level (less than 1.3 to 1.5 mg/dl) by 10 to 12 days in white and black infants. Asian infants reach 8 to 12 mg/dl on day 4 to 5 and decline more slowly. Two percent of Asian newborns and 1% of whites and blacks have serum bilirubin higher than 20 mg/dl in the first week of life. The current estimated minimal level of risk for kernicterus is at 25 to 30 mg/dl in healthy term infants (Robertson, 1998).

Clinical Findings

Family History. The family history may include the following:

- Significant hemolytic disease, anemia
- Inborn errors of metabolism
- Early or severe jaundice

- Ethnic or geographic origin associated with hemolytic anemia
- Hepatobiliary disease

History

- ABO or Rh incompatibilities in previous pregnancies
- Sepsis risk for the infant, such as prolonged rupture of maternal membranes

Physical Examination. Findings include the following:

- Jaundice at birth or at any time during the neonatal period, depending on the underlying condition, with face affected first, followed by the shoulders, chest, and abdomen. Jaundice from deposition of indirect bilirubin in the skin tends to appear bright yellow or orange; jaundice of the obstructive type (direct bilirubin) appears greenish or muddy yellow, with the difference apparent only in severe jaundice. There is no dependable relationship between the intensity of jaundice and the degree of hyperbilirubinemia.
- A crude estimate of the level of jaundice can be based on the dermal zone in which the jaundice is noticed. This estimate should not be used to determine management, but it can help the nurse determine whether drawing a bilirubin is warranted.
  - Head and neck—a mean bilirubin of 6 mg/dl
  - Trunk and umbilicus—a mean bilirubin of 9 mg/dl
  - Groin including the upper thighs—a mean bilirubin of 12 mg/dl
  - Knees and elbows (including the ankles and wrists) or to the feet and hands (including the palms and soles)—a mean bilirubin of 15 mg/dl
- Petechiae, bruising, hepatosplenomegaly, or signs of infection.
- Lethargy, poor feeding, and loss of the Moro reflex are common initial signs of bilirubin toxicity to the brain (kernicterus). These symptoms are subtle and indistinguishable from those of sepsis, asphyxia, hypoglycemia, intracranial hemorrhage, and other acute illnesses in the neonate.
- Diminished tendon reflexes, respiratory distress, failure to suck, opisthotonos, bulging fontanel, twitching of face or limbs, seizures, and a shrill, high-pitched cry are later signs of kernicterus.

Laboratory Findings. Order the following as indicated:

- Total serum bilirubin level (indirect and direct)
- Order the following if the total bilirubin level indicates that further evaluation is necessary. Many times if the nurse suspects that the total bilirubin is going to be in a range significantly elevated for the age of the infant, extra blood can be drawn at the initial blood draw and held for further testing. This eliminates another return visit, stick, and/or unnecessary expense if all of the tests are not later indicated:
  - ABO, Rh, blood type, isoimmune antibodies on mother (should be available at prenatal/delivering hospital)
  - ABO, Rh, blood type, Coombs' test on infant (many times this is done at delivery and held in the hospital's laboratory)
  - Hemoglobin, hematocrit, reticulocyte count

Elevated indirect serum bilirubin with a normal reticulocyte count and negative Coombs' test indicates physiologic jaundice, breast milk jaundice, or congenital familial nonhemolytic jaundice.

Elevated indirect (unconjugated) serum bilirubin with an increased reticulocyte count indicates increased hemolysis secondary to isoimmunization (positive Coombs' test such as caused by ABO or Rh incompatibility), abnormal red blood cell shape, or red blood cell enzyme abnormalities.

Elevated indirect and direct serum bilirubin with a negative Coombs' test and a normal reticulocyte count indicates hepatitis, metabolic abnormalities, biliary atresia, choledochal cyst (in the bile duct), gastrointestinal or pancreatic obstruction, sepsis, or drugs.

Management and Prevention

- The infant's history, course, and physical findings determine the treatment course (Fig. 39-11). Pathologic jaundice requires a more in-depth workup. Risk factors include the following:
  - Appearance of jaundice in first 24 hours of life
  - Rise of bilirubin greater than 0.5 mg/dl per hour
  - Conjugated bilirubin greater than 2 mg/dl
- Treatment level depends on age of infant and total bilirubin level (Table 39-8).
- Phototherapy is used to treat elevated indirect hyperbilirubinemia; it is contraindicated with elevated direct bilirubin. The infant should be dressed only in a diaper and should have eye shields on. Three types of phototherapy are used:
  - Phototherapy via banks of overhead lights placed close to the infant requires eye patches removed at regular intervals, taking care to avoid corneal abrasions; monitoring of temperature; increased fluid intake in response to evaporative water losses; and avoidance of oral drugs because of decreased absorption.
  - Phototherapy via biliblanket (fiberoptic pad) allows ongoing interaction between mother and infant.
  - Phototherapy via bilibed.
- If the infant is breastfeeding and the total bilirubin is greater than 20 mg/dl, the following options exist if physiologic jaundice is assumed (AAP, 1994):
  - Observe.
  - Continue breastfeeding and deliver phototherapy.
  - Supplement breastfeeding with formula with or without phototherapy.

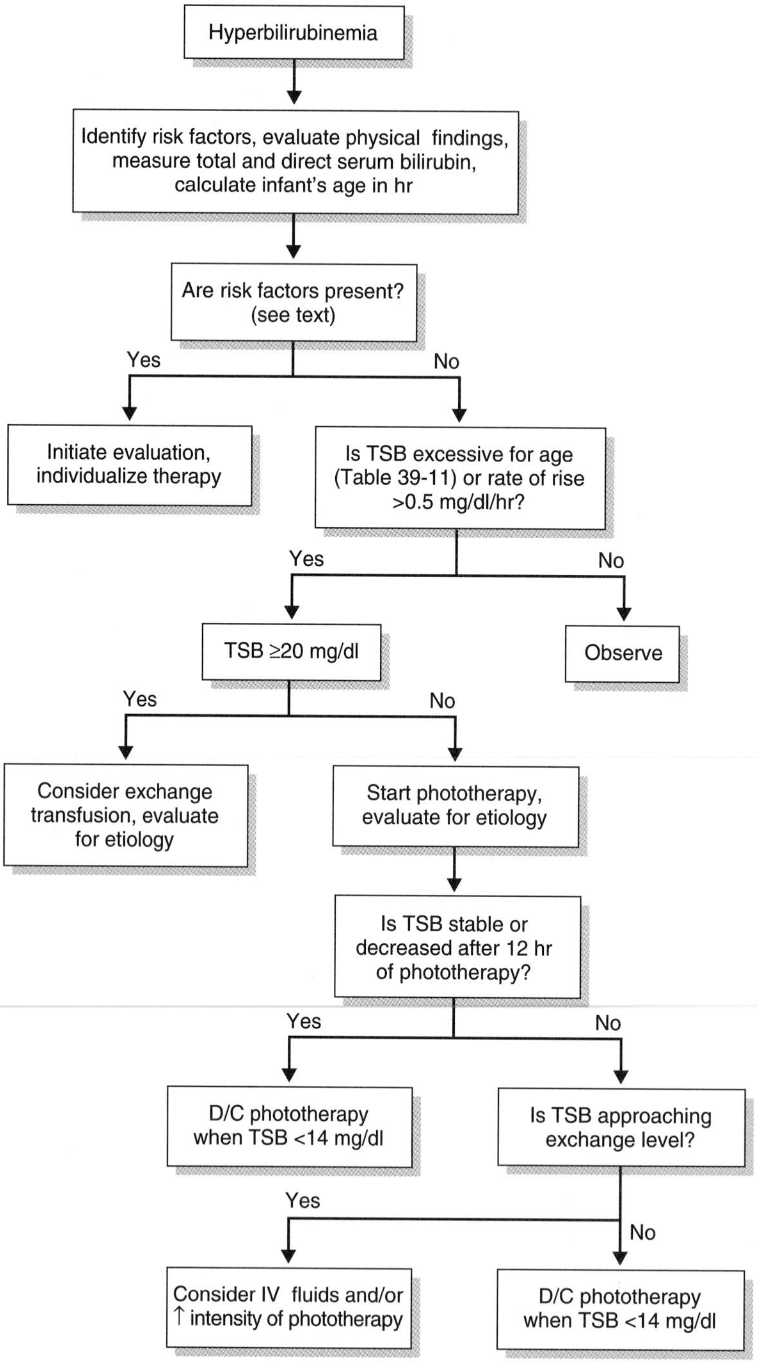

FIGURE 39-11 Management of the full-term newborn with hyperbilirubinemia. *D/C*, Discharge; *IV*, intravenous; *TSB*, total serum bilirubin. (From Banks J, Montgomery D, Coody D, et al: Hyperbilirubinemia in the term newborn, *J Pediatr Health Care* 10:228-230, 1996.)

TABLE 39-8 ***Management of Hyperbilirubinemia in the Healthy Term Newborn***

	Total Serum Bilirubin (TSB) Level, mg/dl (mmol/l)			
Age (hr)	**Consider Phototherapy***	**Phototherapy**	**Exchange Transfusion if Intensive Phototherapy Fails†**	**Exchange Transfusion and Intensive Phototherapy**
≤24‡				
25-48	≥12 (205)	≥15 (260)	≥20 (340)	≥25 (430)
49-72	≥15 (260)	≥18 (310)	≥25 (430)	≥30 (510)
>72	≥17 (290)	≥20 (340)	≥25 (430)	≥30 (510)

Adapted from American Academy of Pediatrics: Practice parameter: management of hyperbilirubinemia in the healthy term newborn, *Pediatrics* 94(4 pt 1):560, 1994.

*Phototherapy at these TSB levels is a clinical option, meaning that the intervention is available and may be used on the basis of individual clinical judgment.

†Intensive phototherapy should produce a decline of TSB of 1-2 mg/dl within 4-6 hr, and the TSB level should continue to fall and remain below the threshold level for exchange transfusion. If this does not occur, it is considered a failure of phototherapy.

‡Term infants who are clinically jaundiced at 24 hr are not considered healthy and require further evaluation.

  - Substitute formula for breastfeeding for 24 hours, having mother continue to pump to maintain supply.
  - Substitute formula for breastfeeding for 24 hours and deliver phototherapy.
- Rebound bilirubin testing (measurement of bilirubin after phototherapy is discontinued) is not required in full-term newborns (Yetman et al, 1998).
- Prevention requires early, frequent feeding. Breastfeeding should begin in the delivery room, occur 10 to 12 times per 24 hours, and include no supplementation.

Infections of the Newborn

Three mechanisms for acquiring neonatal infections exist:

- Transplacental, when the mother acquires an organism that invades her bloodstream and passes through the placenta
- Vertical, when organisms in the vagina invade the amniotic fluid within the uterus
- Horizontal, when the newborn is exposed to environmental agents after birth

Syphilis is transplacentally acquired; herpes, gonorrhea, group B streptococci, *Listeria, Escherichia coli,* and *Chlamydia trachomatis* are typically vertically acquired (Fanaroff & Martin, 2001; Remington & Klein, 2001). Staphylococcal infection is the most common horizontal infection. The most common means for horizontal transmission are the unwashed hands of health care providers.

Risk factors for sepsis (systemic infection) in the newborn include early rupture of amniotic membranes followed by preterm labor, prolonged rupture of membranes, maternal fever, maternal diagnosis of chorioamnionitis, maternal tachycardia, fetal tachycardia, and malodorous amniotic fluid. The neonate with sepsis can be asymptomatic or have nonspecific symptoms (Fanaroff & Martin, 2001; Remington & Klein, 2001). This is in part caused by a delayed immune response to local infection, allowing the neonate to bypass the typical signs and symptoms of infection (e.g., fever). Organisms quickly invade the systemic circulation, and significant deterioration occurs before it can be clinically recognized. Because of the serious nature of neonatal sepsis, significant risk factors or a clinically unstable neonate without perinatal risk factors warrants investigation and initiation of appropriate antibiotics. See Box 39-6 for an overview of neonatal sepsis.

Toxoplasmosis

Organism, Etiology, and Incidence. Toxoplasmosis is an infection caused by *Toxoplasma gondii,* an obligate intracellular protozoan. *T. gondii* infects most species of warm-blooded animals, particularly cats. Cats excrete oocysts in their stools; intermediate hosts include cattle, pigs, and sheep. Humans become infected by consumption of poorly cooked meat or by accidental ingestion of oocysts from soil or in contaminated food. Depending on the timing of the infection, 17% to 65% of untreated women who acquire toxoplasmosis during gestation transmit the parasite to their fetuses (Behrman, Kliegman, & Jensen, 2004). Occurrence is 1 in 1000 to 8000 live births in the United States.

Clinical Findings

History. Prematurity and low Apgar scores are included in the history.

BOX 39-6 *Neonatal Sepsis*

History

"Not doing well"
Temperature instability
Jitteriness
Poor feeding, vomiting
Irritability or lethargy
Apnea
Respiratory distress
Seizures

Physical Examination

Jaundice
Pallor
Petechiae or purpura
Rash
Hepatosplenomegaly
Poor tone and perfusion
Tachycardia or bradycardia
Tachypnea
Cyanosis, grunting, flaring, retractions

Laboratory Evaluation

Blood for CBC with differential, platelet count, and culture—anemia; increase or decrease in WBC count with left shift; thrombocytopenia

Urine—urine culture usually not done in the first 72 hours of life because of low yield

CSF for protein, glucose, cell count, and culture—elevated protein and WBC count; depressed glucose often found in neonatal infections

Management

Combination broad-spectrum antibiotic coverage for gram-positive cocci, gram-negative bacilli, and *Listeria* is recommended. Consider adding coverage for herpes infection if this is a possibility. *Listeria* is treated with ampicillin; group B streptococci can be treated with the penicillins and the cephalosporins; gram-negative organisms are well covered by aminoglycosides and some cephalosporins.

CBC, Complete blood count; *CSF*, cerebrospinal fluid; *WBC*, white blood cell.

Physical Examination. Infants with congenital infection are asymptomatic at birth in 70% to 90% of the cases (AAP, 2003). Findings include the following:

- Jaundice
- Anemia
- Hepatosplenomegaly
- Chorioretinitis
- Microcephaly

Radiologic and Laboratory Findings. Computed tomography of the brain shows calcifications or hydrocephalus. The CSF shows high protein, low glucose, and evidence of *T. gondii.* Serum immunoglobulin G (IgG) and IgM antibodies against toxoplasmosis are seen.

Differential Diagnosis. Sepsis, syphilis, and hemolytic disease are considered in the differential diagnosis.

Management, Prognosis, and Prevention. Oral pyrimethamine, sulfadiazine or triple sulfonamides, spiramycin, and calcium leucovorin are given for 1 year. Treatment usually cures the manifestations of toxoplasmosis such as active chorioretinitis, meningitis, encephalitis, hepatitis, splenomegaly, and thrombocytopenia. Infants with extensive involvement at birth have mild to severe impairment of vision, hearing, cognitive function, and other neurologic functions. No protective vaccine is available. Pregnant women should be informed not to handle raw meat or contaminated cat litter and to wash fruits and vegetables before consumption. Cook meat and eggs well and drink pasteurized milk.

Congenital Rubella

Organism, Etiology, and Incidence. Rubella is an RNA virus. Rubella is transmitted by person-to-person contact; the virus infects the placenta and is transmitted to the fetus. It occurs more frequently in the winter and spring.

Clinical Findings

History. The history can include the following:

- Maternal infection before 16 weeks of gestation
- Negative rubella titers in mother

As many as 50% of infected women are asymptomatic (Behrman, Kliegman, & Jensen, 2004).

Physical Examination. Many infected infants may be asymptomatic in the newborn period. Findings include the following:

- Hearing loss
- Congenital heart disease
- Mental retardation
- Cataract or glaucoma and microphthalmia
- "Blueberry muffin" skin lesions

Laboratory Findings. The rubella virus can be isolated from nasopharyngeal secretions, conjunctivae, urine, stool, and CSF.

Management and Prevention. No specific drug therapy is available. Monitoring and intervention for developmental, auditory, visual, and medical needs improve the quality of life for these children. Congenital rubella is now a rare occurrence because of widespread administration of an effective vaccine (AAP, 2003). All women of childbearing age should have rubella serology titers, and vaccine should be given to IgG-seronegative women who are not pregnant.

Cytomegalovirus

Organism, Etiology, and Incidence. Cytomegalovirus (CMV) is the largest member of the herpesvirus family. CMV is transmitted via intimate and household contact with virus-containing secretions and blood products. When CMV is introduced into a household, it is likely that all members will acquire the infection. CMV is transmitted to the infant via the placenta. Infections are distributed worldwide, and most humans have become infected by the time they reach adulthood. CMV causes congenital infection in 1% to 2% of all live births in the United States. When pregnant women acquire the virus, there is a 30% to 40% transmission rate to the fetus (AAP, 2003; Fanaroff & Martin, 2001; Remington & Klein, 2001).

Clinical Findings

History. Maternal infection and intrauterine growth retardation can be part of the history.

Physical Examination. As many as 90% of infected newborns are asymptomatic. Findings include the following:

- SGA
- Hepatosplenomegaly
- Jaundice
- Petechial rash
- Chorioretinitis
- Cerebral calcifications
- Microcephaly

Laboratory Findings. CMV is isolated in cell cultures from urine, saliva, or other body fluids. Techniques for detection of viral DNA by polymerase chain reaction (PCR) are available from selected laboratories. Proof of congenital infection requires obtaining specimens within 3 weeks of birth. Viral isolation or a strongly positive test for serum IgM anti-CMV antibody is considered diagnostic.

Management, Prognosis, and Prevention. No specific treatment is available for minimally symptomatic immunocompetent neonates (AAP, 2003). Monitor urine for CMV for 18 to 24 months. Serious infections in nonimmunocompromised neonates can be treated with antiviral agents. The outcome of symptomatic congenital CMV infection is poor; there is a 20% to 30% mortality rate and a 90% to 95% morbidity rate, characterized by psychomotor retardation, microcephaly, hearing loss, seizures, and learning disabilities (Behrman, Kliegman, & Jensen, 2004). At greatest risk are susceptible pregnant women exposed to the urine and saliva of CMV-infected children who attend day care centers (AAP, 2003). Handwashing and simple hygienic measures should be reinforced in this population.

Group B Streptococcus

Organism and Etiology. Group B streptococcus (GBS) is a gram-positive diplococcus that is the leading cause of sepsis in infants from birth to 3 months of age resulting in significant perinatal morbidity and mortality rates. Early-onset disease usually occurs within the first 24 hours of life; late-onset disease occurs during the second week of life.

The organism forms colonies in the maternal genitourinary and gastrointestinal tracts. Pregnant women are usually asymptomatic but can manifest chorioamnionitis, endometritis, or urinary tract infection. Infants born of women who are highly colonized are more likely to become colonized. GBS is acquired by newborns following vertical transmission (e.g, ascending infection through ruptured amniotic membranes or contamination following passage through the colonized birth canal). As many as 50% of infants with early-onset disease are symptomatic at birth, indicating an intrauterine infection. The highest attack rate of early-onset GBS is in high-risk deliveries, premature SGA infants, very low birth weight infants, or those with prolonged ruptured membranes; yet full-term infants account for 50% of cases. Colonization of pregnant women and newborns ranges from 5% to 35%. Incidence of GBS is 0.2 to 3.7 cases per 1000 live births (and is decreasing as the use of chemoprophylaxis increases). In untreated, colonized women it occurs in 1 case per 100 to 200 live births (AAP, 2003; Behrman, Kliegman, & Jensen, 2004).

Clinical Findings

History. Risk factors include the following:

- Infants who are less than 37 weeks of gestation
- Rupture of membranes (ROM) of 18 hours or greater
- Maternal fever during labor of 100.4° F oral
- Previous delivery of a sibling with invasive GBS disease
- Maternal chorioamnionitis to include ROM and maternal fever with at least two of the following:
    - Maternal tachycardia (heart rate greater than 90 beats per minute)
    - Fetal tachycardia (heart rate greater than 170 beats per minute)
    - Maternal leukocytosis (white blood cell count greater than 15,000)
    - Uterine tenderness
    - Foul-smelling amniotic fluid

Physical Examination. Findings include the following:

- Poor feeding
- Temperature instability
- Cyanosis, apnea, tachypnea, grunting, flaring, and retracting
- Seizures, lethargy, bulging fontanel
- Rapid onset and deterioration

Laboratory Findings. Cultures of blood, CSF, or both are definitive; antigen identification tests are available but have a false-positive rate of up to 8%.

Differential Diagnosis. RDS, amniotic fluid aspiration syndrome, persistent fetal circulation, meningitis, osteomyelitis, septic arthritis, sepsis from other infections, and metabolic problems are included in the differential diagnosis.

Management, Prognosis, and Prevention. Penicillin G is the treatment of choice for GBS infection. Initiate antibiotic therapy with a penicillin (usually ampicillin) and an aminoglycoside, usually gentamicin, until GBS has been differentiated from *E. coli* or *Listeria* sepsis or meningitis (AAP, 2003).

- Penicillin G intravenous:
  - Infant less than 7 days of age, give 250,000 to 400,000 U/kg per day in three divided doses
  - Infant older than 7 days of age, give 400,000 U/kg per day in four divided doses
- Ampicillin intravenous:
  - Infant less than 7 days of age, give 200 to 300 mg/kg per day in three divided doses
  - Infant older than 7 days of age, give 300 mg/kg per day in four to six divided doses
- Gentamicin doses are as follows (*Harriet Lane Handbook*, 2000):

Gestational Age (weeks)	Age (days)	Dose
≤29 or asphyxia	0-28	2.5 mg/kg q24hr
	>28	3 mg/kg q24hr
30-36	0-14	3 mg/kg q24hr
	>14	2.5 mg/kg q12hr
≥37	0-7	2.5 mg/kg q12hr
	>7	2.5 mg/kg q8hr

Screening of all pregnant women at 35 to 37 weeks of gestation is recommended. Antepartum treatment of asymptomatic mothers carrying GBS is not recommended. Mothers identified antepartum or intrapartum as GBS carriers or with specific risk factors are treated with intravenous ampicillin or penicillin throughout labor until delivery. Treatment given to high-risk patients during labor has decreased transmission of GBS (AAP, 2003).

The mortality rate of early-onset disease ranges from 10% to 40%; mortality rate is highest in very low birth weight infants and in those with low neutrophil count (less than 1500), low Apgar scores, hypotension, apnea, and a delay in starting antimicrobial therapy. Chemoprophylaxis of high-risk, colonized women is an effective method of preventing early-onset GBS infection. Consensus guidelines developed by the Centers for Disease Control and Prevention (CDC) outline steps for a screening-based and risk-factor strategy to prevent GBS (AAP, 2003; CDC, 1996). Treatment consists of intravenous penicillin or ampicillin given to high-risk women at the onset of labor, repeated every 4 hours until the infant is born.

Listeriosis

Organism and Etiology. *Listeria monocytogenes* is a small, gram-positive rod isolated from soil, streams, sewage, certain foods, silage, dust, and slaughterhouses. The food-borne transmission of disease is related to Mexican (soft ripened) cheese, whole and 2% milk, uncooked hot dogs, undercooked chicken, raw vegetables, and shellfish. The newborn infant acquires the organism transplacentally or by aspiration or ingestion at the time of delivery.

Clinical Findings

History. Brown-stained amniotic fluid is seen.

Physical Examination. Findings include the following:

- Generalized symptoms of sepsis
- Whitish posterior pharyngeal and cutaneous granulomas
- Disseminated erythematous papules on skin

Laboratory Findings. Cultures of the blood, CSF, meconium, and urine are done. The CSF shows elevated protein, depressed glucose, and a high leukocyte count. Cultures of the placenta and amniotic fluid also may be helpful.

Management and Prognosis

- Administer intravenous ampicillin and an aminoglycoside (gentamicin) as initial therapy for severe infections.
- After clinical response occurs or for less severe infections in normal hosts, administer ampicillin or penicillin alone.
- The duration of therapy is 10 to 14 days for infections without meningitis and 14 to 21 days for infections with meningitis (AAP, 2003).

Transplacentally acquired listeriosis often results in spontaneous abortion. The death rate of infants with *Listeria* pneumonia noted within 12 hours of birth approaches 100%. Mortality rate varies from 20% to 50% if disease develops between 5 and 30 days of birth, and is especially high in premature infants. Mental retardation, paralysis, and hydrocephalus have been noted in survivors of *Listeria* meningitis (Behrman, Kliegman, & Jensen, 2004; Fanaroff & Martin, 2001; Remington & Klein, 2001).

Congenital Varicella

Organism, Etiology and Incidence. Varicella-zoster virus (VZV) is a herpesvirus. Humans are the only source of infection for this highly contagious virus. The attack rate for congenital varicella syndrome in infants born to mothers with chickenpox during the first trimester is 0.4%; it is 2% when infection occurs between 13 and 20 weeks of gestation.

Clinical Findings

History. There is a history of maternal chickenpox infection.

Physical Examination. Findings may include the following:

- Limb atrophy
- Scarring of the skin of the affected extremity
- Eye manifestations

Laboratory Findings. Diagnosis of VZV is made by immunofluorescent staining of vesicular scrapings.

Management, Prognosis, and Prevention. Some experts recommend acyclovir for pregnant women with varicella, especially in the third trimester (AAP, 2003). Varicella-zoster immune globulin (VZIG) is recommended for the term newborn infant whose mother had an onset of chickenpox within 5 days before delivery or within 48 hours after delivery (and for all preterm infants even if lesions develop more than 1 week before delivery). VZIG is not indicated if the mother has varicella zoster (shingles) only. Airborne and contact precautions are recommended for neonates born to mothers with varicella and, if still hospitalized, are continued until 21 days of age, or 28 days if they received VZIG.

Severe varicella of the newborn infant with fatality rates as high as 30% can result when an infant's mother develops varicella from 5 days before to 2 days after delivery (AAP, 2003). Prevention efforts are targeted to potential mothers. The CDC recommends varicella vaccinations for nonpregnant women of childbearing age with no history of varicella infection (CDC, 1999).

Sexually Transmitted Diseases

Gonorrhea

Organism and Etiology. *Neisseria gonorrhoeae* is a gram-negative diplococcus. *N. gonorrhoeae* infection occurs only in humans. The source of the organism is exudate and secretions of infected mucous membranes. The organism is transmitted primarily through sexual acts and parturition. Gonococcal infections in the newborn are acquired primarily during delivery.

Clinical Findings

History. There is a history of maternal gonococcal infection.

Physical Examination. Findings include conjunctivitis.

Laboratory Findings. Culture of eye exudate is positive for *N. gonorrhoeae.*

Management and Prevention. Administer a single dose of intramuscular ceftriaxone 25 to 50 mg/kg (not to exceed 125 mg) for prophylaxis of infants born to mothers with active gonorrhea (CDC, 2002). Because gonorrheal conjunctivitis can rapidly lead to blindness, all infants are given eye prophylaxis at birth with 1% silver nitrate, 1% tetracycline ophthalmic ointment, or erythromycin 0.5% ophthalmic ointment (AAP, 2003; CDC, 2002).

Chlamydia

Organism, Etiology, and Incidence. Chlamydial infection is caused by an obligate intracellular parasite. *Chlamydia trachomatis* infection is the most common sexually transmitted disease in the United States. Acquisition occurs in approximately 50% of infants born vaginally to infected mothers and in some infants delivered by cesarean section with intact membranes. Of infants acquiring *C. trachomatis* infection, the risk of developing conjunctivitis is 25% to 50% and of pneumonia is 5% to 20% (AAP, 2003).

Clinical Findings

History. There is a history of maternal chlamydial infection.

Physical Examination. Assess for the following:

- Conjunctivitis 1 to 3 weeks after birth (18% to 50%)
- Infant commonly afebrile and with normal activity level
- Pneumonia 2 to 19 weeks after birth (5% to 20%)

Laboratory Findings

- Tests for detection of *C. trachomatis* without cell culture include DNA probe, direct fluorescent antibody (DFA) staining, enzyme immunoassay (EIA), and nucleic acid amplification (PCR, ligase chain reaction [LCR]).
- Routine bacterial cultures are not helpful.
- Gram stain and culture of discharge from the eye (must include epithelial cells from the palpebral conjunctival sac because chlamydia is an obligate parasite) are necessary for diagnosis.

Management and Prevention. Oral erythromycin suspension (50 mg/kg per day in four divided doses for 10 to 14 days) is given for both conjunctivitis and pneumonia (CDC, 2002). Appropriate treatment of the pregnant woman before delivery prevents disease in the newborn. Prophylaxis with oral erythromycin of the asymptomatic infant born to an untreated but chlamydia-positive woman is avoided due to the increased risk of developing hypertrophic pyloric stenosis in the infant.

Syphilis

Organism, Etiology, and Incidence. Syphilis is caused by the spirochete *Treponema pallidum. T. pallidum* crosses the placenta in an infected mother. Routine maternal serologic testing is legally required during prenatal care in all states.

Clinical Findings

History. A history of maternal infection and positive serologic testing in the mother is found.

Physical Examination. The majority of neonates are asymptomatic at birth. Findings include the following:

- Hepatosplenomegaly
- Persistent rhinorrhea
- Maculopapular or bullous dermal lesions
- Failure to thrive, restlessness, fever

Radiologic and Laboratory Findings. Periostitis or osteochondritis is verified by long bone radiography, although the presence of these findings does not affect the management of congenital syphilis (Moyer, 1998). CSF shows high protein, low glucose, high white blood cell count, and positivity on Venereal Disease Research Laboratories (VDRL) test; serum liver enzymes are elevated with liver involvement; and serum rapid plasma reagin (RPR) test is positive.

Management and Prognosis. For proven or highly probably congenital syphilis, the CDC (2002) recommends 10 consecutive days of either crystalline penicillin G 100,000 to 150,000 U/kg per day, given as 50,000 U/kg intravenously every 12 hours during the first 7 days of life and every 8 hours thereafter. Procaine penicillin G 50,000 U/kg intramuscularly daily in a single dose is the only acceptable treatment regimen for congenital syphilis and for all infants born to seropositive mothers without a documented history of adequate treatment. If more than 1 day is missed, the entire course must be restarted. For infants with less certain evidence of syphilis, alternative regimens are available; referral to the latest CDC guidelines is recommended (CDC, 2002). Untreated congenital syphilis can lead to severe multiorgan involvement. Infants who are appropriately treated have a good prognosis.

Herpes Simplex Virus

Description, Etiology, and Incidence. Three clinically distinguishable categories of herpes simplex virus (HSV) infection exist: (1) disseminated disease, (2) CNS disease, and (3) disease restricted to the skin, eyes, and mouth (AAP, 2003) (see Table 39-3). HSV is transmitted by direct contact with infected maternal genitalia during the birth process. Transplacental transmission occurs but has been reported in only a few cases. The risk of neonatal infection is highest with primary genital infection (see Chapter 24 for further discussion).

Clinical Findings

History. The mother has active lesions at vaginal delivery.

Physical Examination. Vesicles in the skin, eye, and mouth are found. Signs or symptoms of encephalitis, pneumonia, or sepsis can also be present.

Laboratory Findings. The virus is isolated in tissue cultures obtained from vesicles, nasopharyngeal or conjunctival swabs, urine, stool, and tracheal secretions and can be tested with culture or rapid diagnostic tests.

Management, Prognosis, and Prevention. Acyclovir 60 mg/kg per day intravenously every 8 to 12 hours is given for 10 to 21 days (CDC, 2002). Treatment with ophthalmic drugs (1% or 2% trifluridine, 0.1% iododeoxyuridine, or 3% vidarabine) is used for infants with ocular involvement (AAP, 2003). Despite effective antiviral therapy, disseminated neonatal HSV infections and localized encephalitis have a considerable morbidity and mortality rate. The risk of acquiring this serious infection is lowered by performing cesarean delivery before rupture of membranes in any pregnancy in which signs or symptoms of HSV infection occur.

Human Immunodeficiency Virus

Etiology and Incidence. Human immunodeficiency virus (HIV), a retrovirus, is transmitted to the newborn via the placenta or at birth secondary to exposure to maternal blood. It is estimated that an infant born to an untreated mother who is HIV positive has a 15% to 30% chance of becoming HIV positive. Half of these infected infants (if untreated) develop acquired immunodeficiency syndrome (AIDS) in the first months of life and die soon thereafter. The other half remain relatively well during infancy but gradually become chronically ill during childhood. Perinatally acquired HIV infections are increasing rapidly in the United States. In approximately 80% of all infected children, transmission occurred from mothers with AIDS. See Chapter 24 for further discussion.

Clinical Findings

History. The history includes an HIV-positive mother. It can also include the following:

- Maternal intravenous drug abuse
- Maternal intercourse with a high-risk male
- Maternal receipt of blood products before April 1985

Physical Examination. Most infants are asymptomatic. Findings *may* include the following:

- Low birth weight
- Microcephaly
- Failure to thrive

Laboratory Findings. HIV DNA PCR is the preferred virologic method for diagnosing HIV infection during infancy. Because of concerns regarding potential contamination with maternal blood, blood samples from the umbilical cord should not be used for diagnostic evaluations. HIV infection can be reasonably excluded among children with two or more negative virologic tests, two of which are performed at age 1 month or older, and one of those being performed at age 4 months or older. Infection with HIV can be reasonably excluded when two HIV DNA PCR assays performed at or beyond 1 month of age and a third performed at 4 months of age or older are negative. See Chapter 24 for the screening schedule for the HIV-exposed infant.

Management, Prognosis, and Prevention. The principal antiretroviral agent used in newborns is zidovudine. The pharmacokinetics, safety, dosing, and uses of nevirapine and several protease inhibitors are under constant review and update, and are available at the HIV/AIDS Treatment Information Service website *(www.hivatis.org)*. Ideally, antiretroviral therapy should be initiated in all HIV-infected infants less than 12 months old as soon as a confirmed diagnosis is established. Other therapy, such as trimethoprim-sulfamethoxazole, is designed to prevent or manage complications. See Chapter 24 for more detail.

Breastfeeding is contraindicated in HIV-positive mothers because of documented transmission via breast milk (CDC, 2002).

Improving the outcomes for HIV-infected infants depends on identifying infants at risk early so that prompt prophylactic strategies and therapeutic interventions can be initiated. Early identification of maternal HIV infection during the antenatal period enables provision of antiretroviral chemoprophylaxis during pregnancy, during labor, and to newborns immediately after birth to reduce the risk of HIV transmission from mother to infant. The use of zidovudine and elective cesarean section can reduce the perinatal transmission to as little as 2% (AAP, 2003). Although research is continuing, vaccines are not yet available. Prevention efforts are targeted at potential mothers, including the reduction of risk factors through behavioral changes.

Drug-Exposed Infants

Cocaine (Crack) Exposure

Description. Cocaine is a local anesthetic and CNS stimulant that is believed to be a teratogen that crosses the placenta.

Clinical Findings

History. Maternal exposure to cocaine or crack and positive urine drug screen for cocaine are found.

Physical Examination. Many infants will show no adverse affects from maternal use of cocaine. Findings may include the following:

- Low birth weight or prematurity
- Fetal distress and meconium staining
- Microcephaly
- Anomalies of the urinary or gastrointestinal tract
- Feeding difficulties, including voracious appetite, poorly coordinated sucking and swallowing, and vomiting
- CNS symptoms of transient irritability, abnormal sleeping patterns, tremors, hypertonia, and lability of mood

There is no clinically documented neonatal withdrawal syndrome for cocaine (AAP, 1998b; Behrman, Kliegman, & Jensen, 2004).

Management, Complications, and Prevention. Take the following steps:

- Offer pacification techniques such as swaddling and decreasing environmental stimuli.
- If symptoms suggest that further treatment is indicated, see following section (Heroin and Methadone Exposure).
- Because cocaine is detectable in breast milk, mothers who use cocaine should not breastfeed.

Prenatal cocaine exposure has been associated in some studies with long-term changes in behavior, including neurobehavioral dysfunction, hyperactivity, aggression, and short attention span; further research is underway (Behrman, Kliegman, & Jensen, 2004; Blatt, Meguid, & Church, 2000). Elimination of in utero exposure to cocaine can occur only if there is identification of a potential problem in a high-risk mother and referral to a substance abuse prevention program.

Heroin and Methadone Exposure

Description. Heroin and methadone are narcotics that cross the placenta.

Clinical Findings

History

- Maternal exposure to heroin or methadone
- Urine drug screen positive for opiates
- Increased incidence of stillbirths and SGA infants, but probably not congenital anomalies

Physical Examination. Findings include the following:

- Tremors and hyperirritability
- Skin abrasions secondary to hyperactivity
- Tachypnea
- Poor feeding
- Diarrhea
- Vomiting
- High-pitched cry
- Fist-sucking
- Low birth weight in 50%

Symptoms of withdrawal occur in up to 75% of infants, usually beginning in the first 48 hours of life, depending on the daily maternal dose, duration of addiction, and time of last maternal dose. A higher incidence of symptomatology is seen if the last dose was taken within 24 hours of birth. Overall, the withdrawal syndrome is more severe and more prolonged with methadone than with heroin (Behrman, Kliegman, & Jensen, 2004).

Differential Diagnosis. The differential diagnosis includes hypoglycemia and hypocalcemia.

Management and Prevention. Supportive management such as swaddling, frequent feedings, and protection from external stimuli is needed. Medications such as phenobarbital, paregoric, and methadone can be used if symptoms such as severe irritability, vomiting and diarrhea, seizures, temperature instability, or severe tachypnea are noted (AAP, 1998b; Behrman, Kliegman, & Jensen, 2000). Pregnant women who are addicted to heroin should be encouraged to enter a treatment program.

Fetal Alcohol Syndrome

See Chapter 41.

SUDDEN INFANT DEATH SYNDROME AND APPARENT LIFE-THREATENING EVENTS

Description, Etiology, and Incidence

The accepted definition of *sudden infant death syndrome* (SIDS) is "the sudden death of an infant under 1 year of age which remains unexplained after a thorough case investigation, including performance of a complete autopsy, examination of the death scene, and review of the clinical history" (Willinger, James, & Catz, 1991). SIDS rarely occurs in the first month of life, with the majority of deaths occurring between 1 and 6 months, peaking at 12 weeks (85% occur between 2 and 4 months of age). It is a diagnosis of exclusion.

An *apparent life-threatening event* (ALTE) is defined as an episode that is frightening to the observer and that is characterized by some combination of apnea (central or occasionally obstructive), color change, marked change in muscle tone, choking, or gagging. In some cases, the observer fears that the infant has died.

The specific cause of SIDS remains unknown; it cannot be predicted or prevented, although placing the infant in a supine position has been shown to decrease the incidence of SIDS and is now the recommended sleep position for infants. Experts have considered as possible causes respiratory obstruction, restrictive clothing, and hyperthermia. Factors associated with SIDS include low birth weight, preterm birth, low maternal age, high parity, maternal smoking and drug use, and poverty.

SIDS is the most common cause of death in infants under 6 months of age, with 85% occurring between 2 and 4 months of age and 95% occurring under 6 months (Behrman, Kliegman, & Jensen, 2004). Approximately 3000 infants per year die of the syndrome. The incidence in the United States is 0.74 per 1000 live births. There is a higher frequency of SIDS in male infants and in the winter months (Behrman, Kliegman, & Jensen, 2004). The National Institutes of Health has monitored sleep position since 1992, and prone sleeping has decreased from 70% to 24%. At the same time the SIDS death rate has fallen by 38% in the United States (AAP, 1996a, 2000a).

Clinical Findings

History

The history can include the following:
- Maternal: cigarette smoking, drug or alcohol abuse during pregnancy; no or poor prenatal care; bottle-feeding; poor education; unmarried; multiparity; maternal age less than 20 years; short intervals between pregnancies; anemia
- Infant: prematurity (less than 37 weeks); low birth weight (less than 250 g) or SGA; twins or other multiple births; Apgar score less than 6 at 5 minutes; apnea; poor weight gain; anemia; intensive care unit stay; neonatal respiratory abnormality, bronchopulmonary dysplasia, previous apparent life-threatening event; many have had cold symptoms a week to a few days before the incident (Behrman, Kliegman, & Jensen, 2004; McMillan et al, 1999)
- Socioeconomic/other: low-income family; crowded living conditions; poor housing conditions; prior SIDS in family; prone sleeping position, soft bedding; race, ethnicity, culture

Physical Examination

Findings include the following:
- No sign of injury
- Frothy blood-tinged secretions in mouth and nares
- Intrathoracic petechiae on autopsy
- Retention of periadrenal brown fat on autopsy

Differential Diagnosis

Aspiration; suffocation; infant botulism or poisoning; cardiac or respiratory disease; hypoxemia; infection; metabolic disorders; child abuse, Munchausen syndrome, or shaken baby syndrome; and CNS abnormalities should be ruled out. Bedsharing, especially if the parent is large, appears to be associated with an increased likelihood of some SIDS-like deaths (Carroll-Pankhurst & Mortimer, 2001).

Some have suggested that a cardiac defect (prolonged QT interval) is strongly associated with SIDS and that routine screening with electrocardiograms may identify infants at risk (Schwartz et al, 1998). The conclusions drawn by these authors have not been met with widespread pediatric acceptance (Lucey, 1999); their recommendations for screening and treatment have not been endorsed by pediatric groups such as the American Academy of Pediatrics.

Management and Prevention

Management is aimed at assisting the family to cope with the loss of the child. The first response of the family is disbelief and shock.
1. Obtain a thorough history from the caretaker within a short period of time after the death. Do not accuse the family of any wrongdoing. Focus the questioning on the cause of death to better understand the circumstances.
2. Reassure caretaker and family that it was not their fault and could not have been prevented.
3. Offer support and counsel to families as soon as possible after death.
4. Supply names of different support groups to help the family overcome grief. Agencies to contact are listed in the Resource Box at the end of the chapter.

5. Provide follow-up for 1 year.
6. Assist surviving siblings. Observe their reaction to the death and refer for counseling if necessary. Help them to understand that it was not their fault and alleviate their feelings of guilt. Allow children to verbalize their feelings. Assist parents to deal with the other children; suggest that parents give extra love, attention, and reassurance to their other children.
7. Evaluate need for home monitoring. Because the rate of SIDS in succeeding children is low (less than 2%) and because monitoring a child cannot prevent a SIDS episode from occurring, the controversy remains about whether to monitor succeeding children (AAP, 2000a; Farrell, Weiner, & Lemons, 2002). Monitors are recommended by some when more than one child in a family has died from SIDS.

See Box 39-7 for measures that aid in the prevention of SIDS.

BOX 39-7 *Measures That Aid in the Prevention of Sudden Infant Death Syndrome*

- Place infants on their backs to sleep until at least 6 months of age. The National Institutes of Health has a "Back to Sleep" program with parent information, stickers, and video (see Resource Box).
- Use a firm mattress. Do not use soft bedding or have stuffed animals in bed. Infants should not sleep in a water bed or in bed with adult.
- Avoid overheating; room temperature should be 68° to 72° F.
- Avoid alcohol and drugs while pregnant and breastfeeding.
- Do not allow cigarette smoking within the house or car.
- For at-risk infants, educate parents and caregivers regarding monitor use and cardiopulmonary resuscitation.

RESOURCE BOX

National Perinatal Resources

Association of Birth Defect Children
1-800-313-2232 (24-hour registry line)
1-407-895-0802
www.birthdefects.org

Association for SIDS and Infant Mortality Professionals
1-612-813-6285
www.asipl.org

Back to Sleep
1-800-505-CRIB
www.nichd.nih.gov/sids/sleep risk.htm

Centers for Disease Control and Prevention
www.cdc.gov/ncidod/diseases
Guidelines for diseases management such as group B streptococcus, varicella, sexually transmitted diseases

Cleft Palate Foundation
1-800-242-5338
1-919-933-9044
www.cleftline.org
Informational materials (including Spanish), networking, referrals to local resources, advocacy, funds research

Compassionate Friends
www.compassionatefriends.org

Family Empowerment Network: Families Affected by Fetal Alcohol Syndrome/Fetal Alcohol Effects
1-800-462-5254
1-608-262-6590
Informational materials (including Spanish), networking, referrals to local resources

Group B Strep Association
www.groupbstrep.org
Newsletter, informational materials, networking, referrals to local resources, advocacy, funds research, maintains research registry

National SIDS Resource Center
1-703-821-8955
www.sidscenter.org

Sudden Infant Death Syndrome Alliance
1-800-221-7437 (SIDS)
www.sidsalliance.org

TEF/VATER International Support Network
1-301-952-6837
www.tefvater.org

REFERENCES

American Academy of Neurology: Practice parameter: neuroimaging of the neonate: report of the Quality Standards Subcommittee of the American Academy of Neurology and the Practice Committee of the Child Neurology Society, *Neurology* 58:1726-1738, 2002.

American Academy of Pediatrics: Positioning and SIDS, *Pediatrics* 89:1120-1126, 1992.

American Academy of Pediatrics: Practice parameter: management of hyperbilirubinemia in the healthy term newborn, *Pediatrics* 94:558-565, 1994.

American Academy of Pediatrics: Hospital stay for healthy term newborns, *Pediatrics* 96:788-790, 1995.

American Academy of Pediatrics: Positioning and sudden infant death syndrome (SIDS): update, *Pediatrics* 98:1216-1218, 1996a.

American Academy of Pediatrics: Use and abuse of the Apgar score, *Pediatrics* 98:141-142, 1996b.

American Academy of Pediatrics: Hospital discharge of high-risk neonate—proposed guidelines, *Pediatrics* 102:411-417, 1998a.

American Academy of Pediatrics: Neonatal drug withdrawal, *Pediatrics* 101:1079-1088, 1998b.

American Academy of Pediatrics: Newborn and infant hearing loss: detection and intervention, *Pediatrics* 103:527-530, 1999a.

American Academy of Pediatrics: Circumcision policy statement, *Pediatrics* 103:686-693, 1999b.

American Academy of Pediatrics: Surfactant replacement therapy for respiratory distress, *Pediatrics* 103:684-685, 1999c.

American Academy of Pediatrics: Folic acid for the prevention of neural tube defects, *Pediatrics* 104:325-327, 1999d.

American Academy of Pediatrics: Changing concepts of sudden infant death syndrome: implications for infant sleeping environment and sleep position, *Pediatrics* 105:650-656, 2000.

American Academy of Pediatrics: *2003 red book: report of the Committee on Infectious Diseases*, ed 26, Elk Grove Village, IL, 2003, American Academy of Pediatrics.

American Academy of Pediatrics, American Association for Pediatric Ophthalmology and Strabismus, American Academy of Ophthalmology: Screening examination of premature infants for retinopathy of prematurity, *Pediatrics* 100:273, 1997.

American Academy of Pediatrics, Oregon Department of Transportation: *One-minute safety checkup*, Elk Grove Village, IL, 2000, American Academy of Pediatrics.

Apgar V: Evaluation of the newborn infant. Second report, *JAMA* 168:1985, 1958.

Ballard JL et al: New Ballard score, expanded to include extremely premature infants, *J Pediatr* 119:417-423, 1991.

Banks J et al: Hyperbilirubinemia in the term newborn, *J Pediatr Health Care* 10(5):228-230, 1996.

Battaglia FC, Lubchenco LO: A practical classification of newborn infants by weight and gestational age, *J Pediatr* 71:159-163, 1967.

Behrman RE, Kliegman RM, Jensen HB, editors: *Nelson textbook of pediatrics*, ed 17, Philadelphia, 2004, WB Saunders.

Betz CL, Hunsberger M, Wright S: *Family-centered nursing care of children*, ed 2, Philadelphia, 1994, WB Saunders.

Blatt SD, Meguid V, Church CC: Prenatal cocaine: what's known about outcomes? *Contemp Pediatr* 17:43-57, 2000.

Blowey DL: Polycystic kidney disease in childhood. In Finberg L, Kleinman R: *Saunders manual of pediatric practice*, ed 2, Philadelphia, 2002, WB Saunders.

Brown AK: Diagnostic features of the various types of neonatal jaundice, *Pediatr Clin North* Am 9:589, 1962.

Buist N, Tuerck J: The practitioner's role in newborn screening, *Pediatr Clin North Am* 39:199-211, 1992.

Carroll-Pankhurst C, Mortimer EA: Sudden infant death syndrome, bedsharing, parental weight, and age at death, *Pediatrics* 107:530-536, 2001.

Centers for Disease Control and Prevention: Prevention of perinatal group B streptococcal disease: a public health perspective, *MMWR Morb Mortal Wkly Rep* 45(RR-7):1-24, 1996.

Centers for Disease Control and Prevention: Prevention of varicella: updated recommendations of the Advisory Committee on Immunization Practices (ACIP), *MMWR Morb Mortal Wkly Rep* 48(RR-06):1-5, 1999.

Centers for Disease Control and Prevention: Sexually transmitted diseases: treatment guidelines, *MMWR Morb Mortal Wkly Rep* 51(RR-6):1-77, 2002.

Desmond MM, Rudolph AJ, Phitaksphraiwan P: The transitional care nursery, *Pediatr Clin North Am* 13:651-668, 1966.

Ein SH: Congenital malformations of the esophagus. In Wyllie R, Hyams JS, editors: *Pediatric gastrointestinal disease*, Philadelphia, 1999, WB Saunders.

Fanaroff AA, Martin RJ: *Neonatal-perinatal medicine: diseases of the fetus and infant*, ed 7, St Louis, 2001, Mosby.

Farrell PA, Weiner GM, Lemons JA: SIDS, ALTE, apnea, and the use of home monitors, *Pediatr Rev* 1:1-9, 2002.

Finberg L, Kleinman R: *Saunders manual of pediatric practice*, ed 2, Philadelphia, 2002, WB Saunders.

Gilstrap LC, Oh W, editors: *Guidelines for perinatal care*, ed 5, Elk Grove Village, IL, 2002, American Academy of Pediatrics and American College of Obstetricians and Gynecologists.

Green M, editor: *Bright Futures: guidelines for health supervision of infants, children, and adolescents*, rev ed 2, Arlington, VA, 2002, National Center for Education in Maternal and Child Health.

Harriet Lane handbook: a manual for pediatric house officers, Baltimore, 2000, Johns Hopkins Hospital.

Joyce BA, Keck JF, Gerkensmeyer J: Evaluation of pain management interventions for neonatal circumcision pain, *J Pediatr Health Care* 15:105-114, 2001.

Katz DA: Evaluation and management of inguinal and umbilical hernias, *Pediatr Ann* 30:729-735, 2001.

Kiely M, Drum MA, Kessel W: Early discharge: risks, benefits, and who decides, *Clin Perinatol* 25:539-553, 1998.

Lubchenco LO, Hansman C, Boyd E: Intrauterine growth in length and head circumference as estimated from live births at gestational ages from 26 to 42 weeks, *Pediatrics* 37:403-408, 1966.

Lucey JF: Comments on a sudden infant death article in another journal, *Pediatrics* 103:812, 1999.

McMillan JA et al: *Oski's pediatrics: principles and practice*, ed 3, Philadelphia, 1999, Lippincott Williams & Wilkins.

Mendenhall A, Eichenfield L: Back to basics: caring for the newborn's skin, *Contemp Pediatr* 17:98-114, 2000.

Moon RY: Infant sleep position policies in licensed child care centers after Back to Sleep campaign, *Pediatrics* 106:576-580, 2000.

Moyer VA et al: Contribution of long bone radiographs to the management of congenital syphilis in the newborn infant, *Arch Pediatr Adolesc Med* 152:353-357, 1998.

National Association of Pediatric Nurse Associates and Practitioners: Newborn discharge and follow-up care, *J Pediatr Health Care* 11(3):147-148, 1997.

National High Blood Pressure Education Program Working Group on Hypertension Control in Children and Adolescents: Update on the 1987 Task Force Report on High Blood Pressure in Children and Adolescents: a working group report from the National High Blood Pressure Education Program, *Pediatrics* 98(4 pt 1):649-658, 1996.

Remington JS, Klein JO: *Infectious diseases of the fetus and newborn infant*, ed 5, Philadelphia, 2001, WB Saunders.

Robertson WO: Personal reflections on the AAP practice parameter on management of hyperbilirubinemia in the healthy term newborn, *Pediatr Rev* 19:75-77, 1998.

Schwartz PJ et al: Prolongation of the QT interval and the sudden infant death syndrome, *N Engl J Med* 338:1709-1714, 1998.

US Department of Health and Human Services: *Healthy People 2010 objectives*, Washington, DC, 2003. Available at *www.health.gov/healthypeople* (accessed Nov 19, 2003).

US Preventive Services Task Force: *Guide to clinical preventive services*, 2002. Available at *www.ahrq.gov/clinic/cps3dix.htm* (accessed Sept 2002).

US Public Health Services: Recommendations. Available at *www.ahrq.gov/clinic/preventix.htm* (accessed Dec 2003).

Van de Riet JE et al: Newborn assessment and long-term adverse outcome: a systematic review, *Am J Obstet Gynecol* 180:1024-1029, 1999.

Willinger M, James LS, Catz D: Defining the sudden infant death syndrome (SIDS): deliberations of an expert panel convened by the National Institute of Child Health and Human Development, *Pediatr Pathol* 11:677-684, 1991.

Wood AJJ: Neonatal hyperbilirubinemia, *N Engl J Med* 344:581-588, 2001.

Yetman RJ et al: Rebound bilirubin levels in infants receiving phototherapy, *J Pediatr* 133:705-707, 1998.

40 Common Injuries

Constance Blair Brehm

Injuries are major pediatric health problems that are best managed with both treatment and prevention strategies. A child with an injury might respond best to (1) a simple home treatment by the parent, caregiver, or supervising adult; (2) intervention by the provider in the primary care setting; (3) referral to a medical specialist or inpatient facility; or (4) a combination of these. Nurse practitioners (NPs) also have a responsibility to assist families to prevent injuries from occurring. Chapter 11 discusses strategies for prevention as part of ongoing health maintenance.

The term *accident prevention* has been replaced by *injury control*, to avoid the connotation that "accidents will happen," implying that nothing can be done to prevent them. Most injuries occur under fairly predictable circumstances to high-risk children and families (Rivara & Grossman, 2000). This chapter focuses on the identification and management of common unintentional pediatric injuries frequently seen in primary care settings. Prevention of nonintentional injuries involves anticipatory guidance to help parents provide a safe environment for their children.

Beyond the first few months of life, injuries are the most common cause of death during childhood and are likewise an important cause of preventable pediatric morbidity and mortality in other age-groups. Injuries cause almost 40% of the deaths among children ages 1 to 4 years and three times more deaths than the next leading cause, congenital anomalies. For the rest of childhood and adolescence up to age 19 years, nearly 70% of deaths are due to trauma, more than all other causes combined (Rivara & Grossman, 2004). Strategies to prevent injuries in children now focus on understanding and modifying risk factors, developing community-wide program approaches, and promoting health policy legislative agendas that focus on injury prevention.

PRINCIPLES OF INJURY CONTROL

In the past, there was an underlying assumption that children were simply "accident prone" because of their highly active and impulsive nature. Earlier prevention efforts often focused on these childhood characteristics. Emphasizing accident proneness is now considered a counterproductive strategy. Injury control plans now focus on education or persuasion of parents and caregivers, changes in product design, and modification of the environment. Those involved in parent safety education agree that it is more advantageous to speak with parents specifically about using child car seat restraints and bike helmets than giving advice that is too general, such as recommendations to closely supervise children and "childproofing" the home. Anticipatory guidance provided by NPs at well-child visits should be geared to the developmental stage of the child. Written materials, audiovisual presentations, peer counseling, and one-to-one interaction with a health professional are all effective teaching and learning strategies. However, safety information should be provided in moderate doses, with reinforcement or repetition at subsequent visits.

Passive injury prevention includes modification of everyday items in the child's environment. Examples include household products, such as the use of child-resistant caps on medicines and cleaning products, and caution in the design of toys so that they do not contain small parts, which are a choking hazard. Other effective strategies for environmental modification include use of smoke detectors, safe roadway design, reduction in traffic volume and speed in residential neighborhoods, and elimination of guns from the child's environment. NPs can advocate for local and national prevention strategies and support such programs as the national SAFE KIDS Campaign. They also can play a key role by supporting injury prevention legislation or initiatives. Public and consumer awareness is crucial for successful prevention programs.

Although most children with serious injuries are seen first in emergency departments (EDs), the NP has a professional obligation to remain current in basic life support techniques. The NP must demonstrate competence in performing emergency cardiopulmonary resuscitation and emergency intervention for choking whether it be for infants, children, or adults. Likewise, all parents and caregivers should be encouraged to enroll in a basic pediatric life support program, especially parents and caregivers of infants and children at risk for cardiopulmonary arrest.

COMMON PEDIATRIC INJURIES

Approach to Trauma

Any child sustaining more than trivial injury must be considered at risk of dying. The NP needs to make an immediate decision about the severity of the trauma. The approach includes primary assessment, evaluation of vital signs, and a quick review of essential functions for all organs. Resuscitation must be initiated if indicated. This takes place in the first 5 to 10 minutes of the assessment process. Secondary assessment follows and includes additional physical examination and radiographs and laboratory tests, if indicated. Physical examination should be repeated serially and compared throughout treatment. Definitive care includes stabilization of the specific local injuries and possible preparation of the patient for transport to an ED if the injury is moderate to severe (Table 40-1).

Trauma to the Skin and Soft Tissue

Abrasions

Description. A simple abrasion represents the loss of mucous membrane or the superficial layer (epidermis) of the skin without loss of dermal integrity. Abrasions are the equivalent of second-degree burns.

Etiology. Abrasions often result from falls or friction accidents. Mechanical means such as dermabrasion can remove the superficial layer of the skin.

Clinical Assessment

History. Seek information about the cause and type of injury and the presence of a foreign object or dirt at the accident scene.

Physical Examination. The extent of the abrasion and the presence of dirt, grime, or other foreign body (e.g., tar) should be determined. Findings include an area of skin that appears scraped off with oozing of serum and blood. Be sure to note redness, heat, and swelling of the area, which may indicate presence of infection. Also assess any punctured body part (most commonly the foot) for circulation, sensation, and function.

Differential Diagnosis. The history of an injury and physical findings are the key to diagnosis. Any other skin condition that can cause loss of epidermis, such as a burn, is included in the differential diagnosis.

Management. Appropriate first aid care is important to prevent infection. Most abrasions can be managed at home unless the abrasion is deep, involves a large area, is associated with severe pain, or has significant dirt, grime, tar, or a foreign body in the wound. The immunocompromised patient may need to be seen. Corneal abrasions are discussed in Chapter 29.

Management of an abrasion includes the following points:

- Thoroughly cleanse the wound. The area can be scrubbed with an antibacterial cleanser using a wet gauze or soft surgical nail brush. Harsh agents such as betadine, alcohol, or peroxide should not be used on open wounds. If dirt or dark-colored matter is not adequately removed, new skin may grow over the particles, resulting in a permanent tattoo. Gentle irrigation with copious amounts of normal saline or water (300 to 1000 ml) is the preferred method to thoroughly cleanse a wound and prevent infection.
- Debride pieces of loose skin with a sterile scissors and remove foreign particles with a tweezers. If tar particles

TABLE 40-1 ***Classification and Disposition of Trauma by Severity***

		Physical Examination			
Category	**History**	**Vital Signs**	**Local Findings**	**Laboratory/Radiographic Studies**	**Probable Disposition**
Mild	Minimal force	Normal	Superficial only	Few	Discharge
Moderate	Significant force	Normal	Suspicious for internal injury	Intermediate	Evaluate
Severe	Critical force	Abnormal	Indicative of internal injury	Many	Immediate therapy; admit

From Ruddy RM, Fleischer GR: Trauma—an approach to the injured child. In Fleischer GR, Ludwig S, Silverman B, editors: *Synopsis of pediatric emergency medicine*, Philadelphia, 2002, Williams & Wilkins, p 462.

are present, the area can be rubbed with petrolatum and then irrigated again.

- Leave small abrasions open to the air or bandage if desired.
- Cover larger abrasions with a nonadherent dressing. Change the dressing in 12 hours, and expose the wound to air within 24 hours.
- Protect abrasions of the hands, feet, or areas overlying joints from friction and dirt until a protective dry scab is formed. Dressings should be changed daily.
- Antibiotic ointment, such as Bacitracin, may be applied to abrasions of the elbows or knees to prevent cracking or reopening of the wound due to constant movement and stretching of the joints. Instruct the parent to wash the area at least daily and reapply ointment and dressing.

Puncture Wounds

Description. Puncture wounds result from penetration of varying levels of the skin and its underlying tissue or structures. These wounds are typically classified as superficial or deep. Because of the potential for serious infection, puncture wounds must be carefully evaluated and treated if indicated. The location and depth of the wound, plus retention of a foreign object, are key risk factors for the subsequent development of infection. For example, deep penetrating wounds and injuries to the forefoot, especially if they involve the plantar fascia, have a higher risk of infection than wounds to the arch or heel area. The forefoot has less overlying soft tissue than other plantar surfaces and is the major weight-bearing area of the foot; therefore cartilage and bone can be involved. In contrast, puncture wounds to muscle, if clean, can be quite deep and still have a relatively low risk of infection.

Etiology and Incidence. Puncture wounds are common pediatric injuries, generally first seen in children at around 2 years of age. A nail, often rusty, is the classic cause of an injury that requires health care intervention. Glass, wood splinters and toothpicks, needles, metal and wire, staples, and thumbtacks are other sources of injury.

Although the majority of puncture wounds heal without problems, a sizable minority of these injuries are complicated by infections that may lead to cellulitis or soft tissue abscesses. The most common causative organisms are *Pseudomonas aeruginosa* and *Staphylococcus aureus. Psuedomonas* osteomyelitis can occur if the puncture wound has penetrated a bone or joint. A classic history is puncture to the foot through a sneaker, as *P. aeruginosa* colonizes on the foam-rubber sole of the sneaker and enters the wound when a nail or other object punctures the foot (Lampe, 2004).

Clinical Assessment. In assessing a child with a minor wound, the NP should exclude more serious, sometimes occult injuries that take precedence in management. Always consider nonaccidental trauma, especially when the history and the injury are inconsistent (Lipton, 2002). Sometimes parents and children will seek care only after symptoms of secondary infection develop.

History. Important information to elicit after a report or suspicion of a puncture wound includes the following:

- Date of injury and wound care provided at the time of initial injury.
- Identification of the agent of injury. If it is not known what object penetrated the skin, the likelihood of an imbedded foreign body is high.
- Condition of the penetrating object. Was the object clean or rusty, jagged or smooth?
- Whether all or part of the foreign object was removed.
- Whether the child was barefoot or what type and condition of footwear was being worn (pertinent to injuries to the foot).
- Immunization status for tetanus coverage.
- Presence of any medical condition that increases the risk for infectious complications.

Physical Examination. Physical examination of the wound must include an assessment of the length and depth of the injury, circulatory status, motor and sensory function, the presence of foreign bodies and contaminants, and the involvement of underlying structures (nerves, tendons, muscles, ligaments, vessels, bones, joints, and ducts) (Lipton, 2002). To examine the foot area (most likely site of puncture wounds) have the patient lie prone and backward on a gurney (or an examination table) so that the head of the table or bed flexes the knee and brings the sole of the foot into clear view. Clean the surrounding skin (irrigate with saline), provide good lighting, and take time to carefully inspect the wound.

The following findings indicate cellulitis:

- Localized pain or tenderness, swelling, and erythema at the puncture site, but may be more obvious on the dorsum of the foot
- Possible fever
- Pain with flexion or extension of the extremity involved
- Decreased ability to bear weight
- Pain along the plantar aspect of the foot during extension or flexion of the toes (can indicate deep tissue injury)

Findings indicative of osteomyelitis-osteochondritis are as noted for cellulitis, with extension of pain and swelling around the puncture wound and to adjacent bony structures. In pyarthrosis (septic arthritis), there are findings of pain, swelling, and decreased range of motion of the affected joint and decreased weight-bearing ability. In the foot, the metatarsophalangeal joint of the great toe is most frequently involved.

Diagnostic Studies. The following are ordered as indicated (Brady, 2002; Staheli, 1998):

- Plain film radiograph should be ordered if a retained foreign body is suspected; if the object is still embedded; if there was penetration of a joint space, the bone or growth cartilage, or the plantar fascia of the foot; or if the puncture site is due to a nail injury and has signs of infection.
- If the radiograph is negative but a retained foreign object is still suspected, computed tomography (CT), ultrasound, and magnetic resonance imaging (MRI) are useful tools.
- Bone scan can be positive within 24 hours of the first appearance of symptoms of osteomyelitis.
- Complete blood count (CBC) may be needed.
- Erythrocyte sedimentation rate (ESR) may be mild to moderately elevated in osteomyelitis-osteochondritis.
- Some recommend a baseline culture of the wound if it is infected.

Differential Diagnosis. A history of penetrating injury and the child's symptoms are the keys to whether the injury represents a superficial wound that will heal uneventfully or develop infectious complications.

Management. Buttaravoli and Stair (2000) outline a practical and straightforward approach to management of puncture wounds:

- If the puncture was created by a slender object such as a sewing needle or thumbtack that was positively removed intact, no treatment other than gentle debridement and irrigation (with large amounts of normal saline) is necessary. For debridement, the puncture wound can be gently shaved using a number 10 scalpel blade to remove the cornified epithelium and debris. If debris is found in the wound, gently slide the plastic sheath of an over-the-needle catheter (such as from an angiocatheter) down the wound track and slowly irrigate with physiologic saline solution, moving the catheter sheath in and out until debris no longer flows from the wound. At times, a small amount of local anesthesia will be necessary to accomplish this.
- If there is any question that a portion of a foreign body may have broken off in the tissues, obtain radiographs. Glass and metal may be visualized on plain films; plastic, aluminum, and wood are more radiolucent and may require ultrasound, CT scan, or MRI for visualization. If radiographs demonstrate that an embedded object has invaded bone, growth cartilage, or a joint space, refer the child immediately to an orthopedic surgeon. Retained foreign bodies increase the potential for infection and should be suspected in patients who have infection or are not responding to treatment of infection. Deep, highly contaminated wounds should also be referred, because debridement in the operating room may be necessary to prevent the catastrophic complications of osteomyelitis (Buttaravoli & Stair, 2000).
- If signs of infection or cellulitis are present, the wound should be cultured. Cultures can also be obtained by needle aspiration if necessary.
- All wound management requires tetanus prophylaxis, if it has been more than 5 years since the last tetanus booster or if the date of the last booster is not known. Consider passive immunization (with Hyper-Tet) and initiation of primary tetanus series in all children who may never have been immunized. This is sometimes the case among immigrant children or those whose parents have refused immunizations for reasons of personal belief.
- Once the wound has been adequately cleansed and debrided, coverage with a Band-Aid or gauze dressing is sufficient. For deep wounds, a small sterile wick of iodoform gauze may be placed inside the wound to keep the edges open. This gauze can be removed after 2 to 3 days, and the subsequent granulation tissue will aid healing. If signs of infection (minor redness or swelling) have appeared, or if the wound was particularly deep and contained debris, prescribe antibiotic coverage with oral dicloxacillin, cephalexin, or erythromycin (best choice if allergic to penicillin) for 10 to 14 days. Change antibiotic coverage only if needed after culture results are known. Schedule return visit to recheck within 48 hours. If pain, erythema, and swelling do not improve within 48 hours of beginning oral antibiotics, consider intravenous antibiotics. For *Pseudomnonas* osteochrondritis, therapy with antipseudomonal antibiotics may be necessary if debridement was not complete or not undertaken (Brady, 2002).

Patient and Parent Education. Instruct parents to allow no weight bearing for 3 to 4 days for a foot injury. Patient education should include observation for signs and symptoms of infection, with the importance of prompt medical attention if there is persistent aching or discomfort.

Ingrown Toenails and Nail Hematoma

Description. Two problems commonly seen in pediatrics are ingrown toenails and nail hematomas from trauma to the nail. Ingrown toenails are caused by any of the following: anatomic predisposition, improper nail trimming, trauma, or constrictive shoes or stockings. Nail hematomas are due to injury and the formation of a subungual hematoma. Nail injuries that involve lacerations or fracture of the distal phalanx should be referred to an orthopedist; uncomplicated nail hematomas can be drained (nail trephination) by primary care providers, typically without local anesthesia.

Management. The treatment for these problems is as follows:

- For ingrown toenail:
  - Pack cotton under the nail edge to elevate the nail from inflamed nailbed.
  - Recommend elevation and soaking of the foot. Cleaning and promotion of drainage may be needed for more severe inflammation.
  - Instruct about wearing properly fitting shoes and correctly trimming the nails. Toenails should be trimmed so that a concave end is left to extend the nail edge beyond the skin.
- For nail hematoma:
  - Determine whether a digital or regional nerve block is needed (the NP may or may not be skilled in this procedure).
  - Attempt to lift the nail to examine for the presence of significant nailbed injuries.
  - Irrigate nail surface with saline solution.
  - Make one or more holes in the area of the nail hematoma with either a portable heat cautery device or a heated paperclip. (Untwist a paperclip and use the rounded tip.)
  - A number 11 scalpel blade is an alternative instrument. Create a small hole or holes in the nail by applying downward pressure with a rotary motion of the scalpel.
  - One or more holes will need to be made to permit continued drainage.
  - Antibiotics generally are not needed.

Lacerations

Description. Lacerations are cuts through the skin; after contusions, they are the most common type of soft tissue injury seen in EDs. The face, scalp, and hands are the most common sites of injury in children. Lacerations often require more complicated treatment than other minor wounds, because they can be associated with occult injuries to the deeper tissues and therefore require careful exploration. Prevention of infection is another major consideration. There are three main classes of lacerations: shear, tension, and compression injuries (Lipton, 2002).

Shear injuries are caused by sharp objects and usually cause little damage to surrounding tissues but can cause nerve, tendon, and vascular damage. They usually heal the fastest and have the lowest incidence of wound infection. The biggest danger of shear injuries is the potential damage to nerve, tendon, and vascular structures. Such injuries require repair of these delicate structures, which should only be attempted in EDs or in the operating room by a skilled surgeon.

Tension lacerations occur when stresses cause the skin to tear. These are accompanied by damage to surrounding tissues. A classic example is when a child falls and bumps his or her head on a dull edge of a piece of furniture, causing the skin to break open in the appearance of a laceration. These lacerations are irregularly shaped.

Compression lacerations occur during a crush injury and have irregular, often stellate wound edges. They can happen from a direct blow by a large blunt object. Because of their association with significant injury to the adjacent skin, they have the highest incidence of wound infection compared with other types of lacerations.

Etiology and Incidence. Lacerations are caused by various forms of trauma. They are common reasons for pediatric health care visits.

Clinical Assessment

History. Important questions to ask include the following:

- How did the injury happen? Determining the mechanism of injury is essential in identifying the presence of contaminants or possible presence of a foreign body, such as dirt, debris, glass, and splinters.
- How long ago (number of hours) did the injury occur? Length of time since injury is a critical factor to consider.
- Does the child have allergies to antibiotics or anesthetics?
- What is the child's tetanus immunization status? Is there a need for further immunization?

Physical Examination. Important points in the examination of the injury are as follows:

- Cleanse the wound (see Management) and cover with saline-soaked gauze until a thorough examination can be made.
- Perform a neurovascular examination of pulses, motor function, and sensation distal to the laceration, and then search for foreign bodies and nerve or tendon injury. Evaluation of range of motion is especially important with wounds involving the distal forearm, wrist, and hand.
- Prepare the wound for exploration and repair (see Management).

Differential Diagnosis. The history and physical examination provide the diagnosis.

Management. Depending on their preparation and experience in the treatment of minor wounds that require suturing, NPs may suture wounds and provide follow-up care. Significant wounds to the face, hands, or genital areas should be referred to specialists, such as an orthopedic surgeon, who specialize in hand repair, or a plastic surgeon for plastic and reconstructive surgery (particularly for the face). Minor lacerations to the scalp or the arms and legs are commonly managed by NPs who have been trained in these techniques.

The steps in wound management are summarized as follows (Selbst & Attia, 2002):

1. *Decision to close the wound.* Compared to adults, children are less likely to get wound infections. In children, the infection rate is about 2% for all sutured wounds. Thus most wounds may be closed *primarily* (i.e., bringing the edges of the skin together, known as "approximation") as soon after the injury as possible to speed healing, prevent infection, and improve the cosmetic result. Delayed closure increases the risk of infection. Some researchers suggest a "golden period" for wound closure of 6 hours. However, wounds considered low risk for infection, such as a clean knife wound to an extremity, can be closed even 12 to 24 hours after the injury. Other guidelines to consider in wound closure include the following:
   - Most wounds to the face are best closed primarily even up to 24 hours after the injury to achieve an optimal cosmetic effect. If the wound is extensive or has high potential for infection (such as a dog bite), the operating room may be the best place for closure.
   - The risk of a laceration becoming infected is greater in areas with lower blood flow. For example, a hand or foot laceration is far more likely to become infected than a scalp laceration, because the extremities of the body have lower blood perfusion than the head and scalp. Contaminated or crush wounds and those involving immunocompromised individuals should be closed promptly, within 6 hours of injury, because they are at high risk of infection.
   - Some contaminated wounds (animal or human bites or those occurring in a barnyard or in an immunocompromised individual) should be left open for healing by *secondary intention,* a process of healing by granulation and reepithelialization, although the scar formation may be more unsatisfactory with this method.
   - If a wound is not closed initially, *delayed primary closure (tertiary closure)* should be considered after the risk of infection decreases (about 3 to 5 days later). This is recommended for selected heavily contaminated wounds and those associated with extensive damage, such as high-velocity missile injuries, crush injuries, and explosion injuries. The wound should be cleaned and debrided and covered at the time of initial treatment and then reassessed in a few days for infection (Selbst & Attia, 2002).
2. *Anesthesia.* Appropriate use of conscious sedation and local anesthetics is essential for successful repair of lacerations in children. Proper wound care includes wound exploration and careful cleansing, which, when added to fear and anxiety, may be extremely painful. Infiltration of the wound with local anesthetic (such as lidocaine) can also help control bleeding. Discussion of anesthesia administration and the details of wound closure techniques are beyond the scope of this text. However, published texts are available that address procedures in primary/ambulatory care that include excellent information on local anesthesia and wound closure. Attendance at workshops that focus on wound management is also helpful.
3. *Hair.* Hair near the wound usually creates minimal difficulty during repair and generally does not need to be removed. In any case hair should not be shaved because to do so can damage hair follicles and increase the risk of infection. Instead, the hair should be clipped with scissors when necessary. Alternatively, petroleum jelly can be used to keep unwanted scalp hair away from the wound while suturing. Eyebrow hair should not be removed because this may lead to abnormal or slow regrowth.
4. *Wound cleansing.* Use of chlorhexidine or povidone-iodine surgical scrub preparations, hydrogen peroxide, or alcohol in the wound itself is not recommended. These agents may be irritating to tissues and may increase infection by damaging white blood cells. The preferred method of wound cleansing is *irrigation* to reduce bacterial contamination and prevent subsequent infection. Normal saline remains the safest and most cost-effective choice for irrigation. The wound should be irrigated with at least 100 to 200 ml for the average 2 cm laceration. More solution may be needed if the wound is unusually large or contaminated. A large irrigating syringe (20 to 50 ml) with an attached splash guard can be used to reduce splatter during irrigation. *Scrubbing* the wound should be reserved for particularly "dirty" wounds in which contaminants are not effectively removed with irrigation alone. It may be necessary to extract some foreign material with fine forceps if it remains adherent after copious irrigation. This will avoid tattooing of the skin and reduce the risk of infection.
5. *Exploration of the wound.* The wound must be explored for presence of foreign bodies, deep tissue layer damage, injury to nerve or blood vessel, or joint involvement. It is imperative that the depth of the wound be determined. Wound probing is done with a Q-Tip, a hemostat, or a needle holder. Deep lacerations should be referred to an ED for layered closure. If tendon injury is suspected or if bone is exposed, referral to an orthopedist is the standard of care.
6. *Wound debridement.* Gentle removal of unattached loose tissues may be done with sterile instruments.

Debridement is advantageous because it creates well-defined wound edges that can be more easily opposed. Although it is helpful to excise necrotic skin, excessive trimming of irregular lacerations should not be attempted. Existing wound irregularity (such as a zigzag wound) is actually helpful in approximation of the edges, and it allows for a more natural appearance in the scar. Excessive removal of tissue can create a defect that is difficult to close or that may increase tension at the wound margin, making scarring more likely.

7. *Wound closure.* Simple, uncomplicated lacerations to the scalp, trunk, arms, or legs may be closed *primarily.* Sutures have been the most commonly used method to close lacerations, with absorbable suture material used for closure of structures deeper than the epidermis and nonabsorbable sutures used to close the outermost layer of a laceration. Deep sutures relieve skin tension, decrease dead space, and probably improve cosmetic outcome. Staples are gaining in popularity for wound closure, particularly in EDs. Staples can be applied rapidly and are associated with a lower infection rate but can be more painful to remove. Surgical tape (Steri-Strips) is rarely used for primary closure because of inadequate strength in areas subject to tension. Tissue adhesives can be applied rapidly and painlessly and will slough off in 7 to 10 days. The adhesive is painted on while manually approximating the skin edges. Adhesive in the wound or between wound margins should be avoided. Table 40-2 compares wound closure techniques.
8. *Dressing.* Dress the wound using a nonadherent gauze for the first layer followed by a second layer of plain gauze if needed. Elasticized gauze (tubular net bandage) can be used to secure dressings.
9. *Immunization.* Give tetanus booster or human tetanus immunoglobulin as indicated.
10. *Antibiotic controversy.* Antibiotic prophylaxis of clean wounds is not indicated. Its use in contaminated wounds may be helpful, but careful wound cleaning is the most effective safeguard in preventing infection.
11. *Suture and staple removal.* Remove sutures or staples depending on their location. See Table 40-3 for a useful guide.

TABLE 40-2 ***Advantages and Disadvantages of Common Wound Closure Techniques***

Technique	Advantages	Disadvantages
Suture	Time honored Meticulous closure Greatest tensile strength Lowest dehiscence rate	Requires removal Requires anesthesia Greatest tissue reactivity Highest cost Slowest application Highest risk of needle stick
Staples	Rapid application Low tissue reactivity Low cost Low risk of needle stick	Less meticulous closure May interfere with imaging techniques
Tissue adhesive	Rapid application Patient comfort Resistant to bacterial growth No need for removal Low cost Low or no risk of needle stick	Lower tensile strength than sutures Dehiscence over high-tension areas Not useful on hands Cannot bathe or swim
Surgical tape	Least reactive Lowest infection rate Rapid application Patient comfort Low cost No risk of needle stick	Frequently falls off Lower tensile strength than sutures Highest rate of dehiscence Requires use of toxic adjuncts Cannot be used in areas with hair Cannot get wet

From Lipton JD: Soft tissue injury and wound repair. In Strange GR et al, editors: *Pediatric emergency medicine: a comprehensive study guide*, ed 2, New York, 2002, McGraw-Hill.

TABLE 40-3 Suture and Staple Removal Guide

Location of Sutures	Length of Time Before Removal
Facial	3-5 days
Upper extremity	7-10 days
Trunk	10 days
Lower extremity	14 days
Over a joint	10-14 days

12. *Bandage.* A nonocclusive bandage can be used to cover the sutured wound.

Patient and Parent Education. Instructions for wound care at home are best given in writing and should include the following information:

- The patient can briefly shower 48 hours after sutures are in place without worrying about the risk of possible infection. However, dry the area well and keep it dry at all other times.
- Note signs and symptoms of infection that warrant an early recheck (redness, swelling, discharge, increasing pain).
- Give instructions about cleansing and bandaging the wound.
- List any restrictions on activities.
- Identify a date for a return appointment.

Burns

Description. A burn injury to one or more layers of the skin and underlying tissues can cause varying degrees of damage. Burns are classified by depth of injury. The traditional classification of burns as first, second, third, or fourth degree is being replaced by the designations of superficial, superficial partial thickness, deep partial thickness, and full thickness (Morgan, Bledsoe, & Barker, 2000).

- Superficial burns (formerly first degree) involve only the epidermis. The skin is erythematous, but there are no blisters. Sensation is preserved. A common example is sunburn. Superficial burns usually heal within 1 week and require only symptomatic treatment.
- Superficial partial-thickness burns (formerly second degree) involve the dermis to a variable degree. The dermal appendages are always preserved and provide a source for regeneration. They are characterized by the presence of marked edema, erythema, blistering, and weeping from the wound. The most common causes are exposure to hot liquids and flames. Healing requires 2 to 3 weeks.
- Deep partial-thickness burns (formerly third degree) are full-thickness injuries. The dermis and dermal appendages are destroyed. The skin appears whitish or leathery. The surface is dry and nontender to palpation. These result from prolonged exposure to fire or hot liquids.
- Full-thickness burns (formerly fourth degree) extend into deep tissues, such as muscle, fascia, nerves, tendons, vessels, and bone.

Burns involving large surfaces of the body generally vary as to their degree of depth. Because burn wounds are dynamic and the effect of dermal ischemia (affected by infection, exposure, and dehydration) may not be readily apparent at first, their depth can change from day to day. The percentage of body surface area (BSA) and the part(s) of the body affected are also key factors to determine treatment, disposition, and prognosis (Table 40-4). Multiple methods have been devised to estimate the BSA affected. For example, the palm of the patient's hand is considered to represent 1% of total BSA. This may be helpful for estimating the extent of small or patchy burns (Morgan, Bledsoe, & Barker, 2000).

Children with burn injuries who meet the following criteria should be admitted to a children's hospital or burn center.

- Superficial and superficial partial-thickness burns involving 10% or more of BSA (considered serious)
- Partial-thickness burns greater than 20% of BSA (require specialized burn care)
- Full-thickness burns greater than 2% of BSA

Burns in certain body locations are high risk for disability. These include greater than 1% burns to the face, perineum, hands, or feet; circumferential burns; or burns overlying joints.

Children with inhalation injury or associated trauma may also require hospital admission (Joffe, 2002).

Etiology and Incidence. Thermal injuries are the second most common cause of death in children in the United States, second only to motor vehicle accidents. These injuries account for approximately 30,000 hospitalizations and more than 3000 deaths annually. Modern technology has increased the exposure of children to potentially injurious thermal energy in their environment. Common modes of injury include scalding, flash injuries from ignition of volatile substances, and contact of clothing with a flame, resulting in ignition of fabrics. However, the house fire is by far the most lethal cause of burns in children and accounts for 45% of burn-related deaths. Much has been done to reduce these injuries through the use of smoke detectors and fire safety instruction programs, yet house fires continue to take the lives of far too many children every year (Strange & Pawel, 2002).

TABLE 40-4 *Estimation of Surface Area Burned Based on Age**

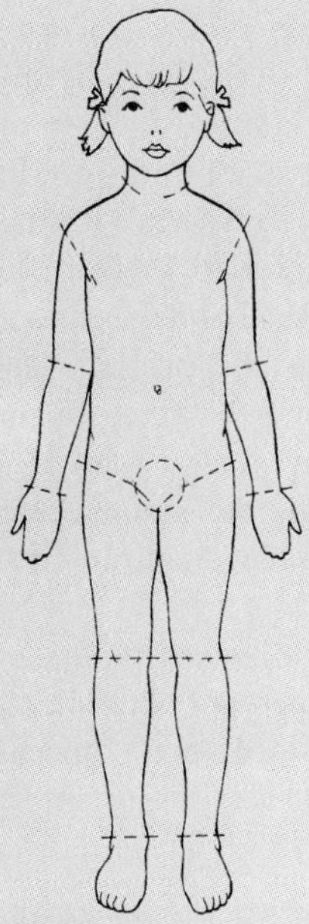

Area	Age (yr) Birth to 1	1-4	5-9	10-14	15	Adult
Head	19	17	13	11	9	7
Neck	2	2	2	2	2	2
Anterior trunk	13	13	13	13	13	13
Posterior trunk	13	13	13	13	13	13
Right buttock	2.5	2.5	2.5	2.5	2.5	2.5
Left buttock	2.5	2.5	2.5	2.5	2.5	2.5
Genitalia	1	1	1	1	1	1
Right upper arm	4	4	4	4	4	4
Left upper arm	4	4	4	4	4	4
Right lower arm	3	3	3	3	3	3
Left lower arm	3	3	3	3	3	3
Right hand	2.5	2.5	2.5	2.5	2.5	2.5
Left hand	2.5	2.5	2.5	2.5	2.5	2.5
Right thigh	5.5	6.5	8	8.5	9	9.5
Left thigh	5.5	6.5	8	8.5	9	9.5
Right leg	5	5	5.5	6	6.5	7
Left leg	5	5	5.5	6	6.5	7
Right foot	3.5	3.5	3.5	3.5	3.5	3.5
Left foot	3.5	3.5	3.5	3.5	3.5	3.5

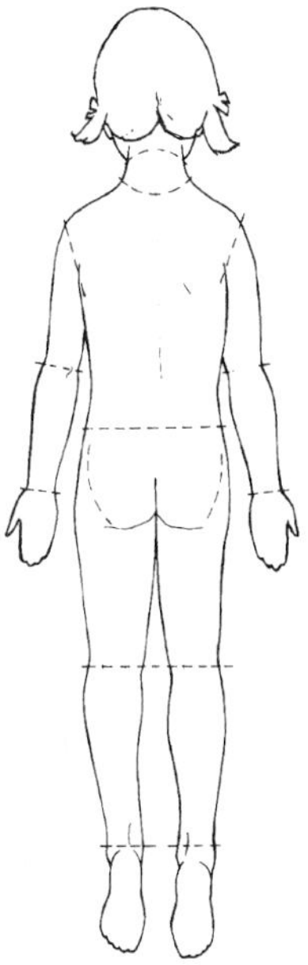

From Joffee M: Burns. In Fleisher GR, Ludwig S, Silverman B, editors: *Synopsis of pediatric emergency medicine*, Philadelphia, 2002, Lippincott Williams & Wilkins, p 529.

*This modification by O'Neill of the Brooke Army Burn Center Diagram shows the change in surface area of the head from 19% in an infant to 7% in an adult. Proper use of this chart provides an accurate basis for subsequent management of the burned child.

The intentional inflicting of burns to a child is, unfortunately, a common form of abuse. Every burn injury in a child should be evaluated for the potential for abuse or neglect. Intentionally inflicted burn injuries often leave a characteristic pattern (see Chapter 19).

Clinical Assessment

History. The following information should be obtained:

- Description of how the burn occurred, including agent of injury and length of time agent was in contact with skin, circumstances surrounding the injury, when it occurred, and likelihood of other injuries such as trauma or smoke inhalation
- Initial and subsequent treatment of burn
- Previous history of burn injuries
- Other current medical problems, medications, allergies, and tetanus status

Physical Examination. The physical examination should begin by doing a primary assessment of the airways. The most common cause of death during the first hour after a burn injury is respiratory impairment (Strange & Pawel, 2002). Inhalation injury produces upper airway edema that can proceed with alarming speed to complete airway obstruction. Inhalation injury should be suspected if there is hoarseness, wheezing, rales, singed nasal hairs, carbonized sputum, cyanosis, or altered mental status. In such cases, immediate emergency intervention (paramedics and immediate transport to the ED) is warranted. Once the patient is stable, a thorough physical examination requires the following determinations:

- Percentage of BSA affected (see Table 40-4)
- Distribution and pattern of the burn with particular concern for circumferential burns to the thorax that may cause poor chest expansion and declining oxygen saturation
- Depth of the burn, classified as superficial, partial thickness, or full thickness
- Assessment of the vascular status of extremities

Diagnostic Studies

- A CBC is indicated to establish baseline levels. The hematocrit will often be elevated secondary to fluid loss. White cell count may also be elevated as an acute phase reaction, but later may be an indicator of infection.

- Serum electrolytes may reveal elevated potassium due to cell breakdown.
- Renal function tests (blood urea nitrogen and creatinine) are used to assess renal and tissue perfusion. A urinalysis, particularly the specific gravity, helps determine hydration status, and presence of myoglobin may suggest acute tubular necrosis.
- Baseline clotting studies and typing and crossmatching may be indicated if there is associated trauma or if surgical intervention, such as grafting, is considered.
- Pulse oximetry, arterial blood gases, and chest radiograph are indicated if there is airway involvement or vascular instability.
- Culturing of critical burn wounds may need to be done weekly or more frequently if infection develops.

Differential Diagnosis. Chapter 19 discusses intentional burn injuries resulting from child abuse. Scalded skin syndrome caused by staphylococcal infection can cause skin exfoliation, but its clinical presentation clearly differentiates it from accidental burn injury. Management is similar to that used for burn management.

Management. Most children with major or serious burns require treatment in the hospital setting and referral to a burn surgeon. Electric and chemical burns also require hospitalization for observation. Children with a burn injury associated with inhalation injury, fractures, suspicion of abuse, uncertainty of follow-up by the parent, or severe pain should also be admitted. The outpatient treatment of minor burns is an option only for superficial burns (first degree) or superficial partial-thickness burns (second degree) to less than 10% of BSA or a burn of less than 1% of BSA to the hands, feet, face, ears, and genitalia. Box 40-1 outlines the primary care management of superficial and partial-thickness burns. Deep partial-thickness burns covering greater than 10% of BSA or full-thickness burns covering more than 2% of BSA should be referred for hospital management by burn specialists.

Patient and Parent Education. The following points are important components of patient and parent education:

- Emphasize use of sunscreen protection to prevent sunburn (see Chapter 37). This is also very important for

BOX 40-1 *Primary Care Setting Management of Superficial and Partial-Thickness Burns*

1. Maintain proper nutrition and hydration to enhance healing.
2. Management of superficial burns:
   - Apply cool compresses.
   - Apply moisturizers to the skin.
   - Administer analgesics, such as acetaminophen or ibuprofen or topical benzocaine spray (over the counter), but be alert for potential hypersensitivity to the product.
3. Management of superficial partial-thickness burns:
   - Monitor the burn daily for the first few days to ensure proper healing and assess for infection.
   - Cleanse the wound by generous irrigation with normal saline solution.
   - Treat very small areas, especially facial wounds, with bacitracin ointment only and leave area open to air.
   - If bullae or blisters are present, do not open or "pop" them. They act as a natural bandage to keep bacteria out. Most will open eventually on their own, but while left intact they protect the underlying skin from infection and allow time for internal healing.
   - Gently debride open blisters to remove devitalized tissue, and residue from prior dressing changes.
   - If the burn is less than or equal to 3% of the body surface area, Vaseline gauze (or fine gauze with Bacitracin ointment) in strips may be applied to the clean debrided area, followed by a dry gauze outer dressing.
   - For burn wounds greater than 3% of the total body surface area, apply silver sulfadiazene (SSD or Silvadene) after the wound is cleansed unless the child has a known sulfa allergy. SSD is an antimicrobial as well as a soothing agent.
   - Apply strips of fine-mesh gauze over the wound. Do not wrap the wound with gauze because wrapped gauze can impair circulation if swelling occurs. Apply additional SSD to gauze strips.
   - Apply a dry outer gauze dressing that can be held in place by a tubular net bandage.
   - Administer adequate analgesic medication. Acetaminophen with codeine may be needed before the wound care is performed and during the day. Switch to over-the-counter acetaminophen or ibuprofen as the pain subsides.
   - Use mittens for young children to prevent scratching if itching occurs as the burn heals; if needed, administer an antihistamine such as diphenhydramine.
   - If a partial-thickness burn involves an extremity, keep it elevated to reduce edema and compromise of blood flow to the burned area. Persons with circumferential burns of an extremity may need to be admitted to the hospital for observation so that compartment syndrome does not develop.

skin that is recovering from a burn, because the skin will be prone to hyperpigmentation from sunlight for up to a year following the burn injury.
- Discuss home and environmental safety issues related to burn prevention at health maintenance visits.
- Reinforce safety issues after a burn injury has occurred (e.g., scald prevention, use of smoke detectors, safekeeping of matches and cigarette lighters, safe use of electric cords and outlets).
- Teach first aid measures for burns (e.g., submerge minor burned area in cold water; rinse chemical burns in cold water, flushing skin thoroughly for at least 20 minutes).
- Inform parents of serious or long-term consequences of burns (e.g., frequent and significant sunburns during early childhood can predispose an individual to skin cancers in later life; electric burns cause thermal injury to skin [contact burn], but, if an arc is created and there is passage of electrical current through the body, there is a potential for cardiac dysrhythmias and neurologic impairment).
- Inform parents that the extent of scarring is difficult to predict with certainty; that scarring depends on depth of burn, length of time needed for healing, whether grafting was done, and the child's age and skin color; and that scars remain immature for the first 12 to 18 months and go through color and texture changes as the child grows. Most scald injuries from hot liquids heal quickly with little or no scarring.
- All skin that has been burned should be protected from sun for at least 12 months. Healed burns remain sensitive to the sun and sunburn more severely than nonburned skin. Encourage parents to avoid sun exposure as much as possible and to use a sunscreen with a sun protection factor (SPF) of 30 (or higher) if sun exposure is unavoidable.

Contusions and Hematomas

Description. A contusion, or bruise, is an injury in which the skin is not broken but trauma has caused effusion into muscle and subcutaneous tissue with injury to the vessels and possibly the nerves. In children, contusions are most often seen on the extremities but can also be found on the face or head.

Etiology and Incidence. Contusions are common in children and are caused by blunt trauma, most often as a result of falling or bumping into objects during play. Participation in contact sports puts children at increased risk for contusions. Bruises to the trunk, face, or head should raise a red flag for possible child abuse. A careful history must be taken to determine whether the explanation of the injury is consistent with the child's condition and his or her independent report of what happened.

Hematomas are localized collections of extravasated blood that are relatively or completely confined within a space or potential space. Hematomas can be associated with most types of minor and major wounds; they must be observed closely for signs of infection and, in some instances, drained.

Clinical Assessment

History. The following should be assessed:
- Cause of bruise
- Treatment given
- History of easy bleeding or bruising, slow healing

Physical Examination. The following should be determined:
- Circulatory status and discoloration
- Motor and sensory function: reduced mobility or range of motion
- Involvement of underlying structures
- Presence of swelling
- Pain or point tenderness
- Limited mobility

Differential Diagnosis. Hemophilia, von Willebrand disease, and purpura should be considered. Myositis ossificans, a complication of contusions rarely seen in children, can be confused with osteogenic sarcoma.

Management.

1. Acute phase, first 24 hours (Buttaravoli & Stair, 2000):
- Prescribe rest, ice, compression, and elevation (RICE):
  - Rest and immobilize the affected part (the ultimate in rest is best achieved with a splint).
  - Ice (or cold compress with an ice bag wrapped in a towel) is applied to the injury for 10 to 20 minutes per hour for the first 24 hours.
  - Compression: application of a pressure bandage helps prevent swelling.
  - Elevation of the affected part (ideally, above the level of the heart) helps prevent swelling.
- Provide appropriate analgesia. A nonsteroidal anti-inflammatory medication, such as ibuprofen, is a good choice.

2. Twenty-four to 48 hours after the acute phase of tenderness and swelling:
- Apply warm compresses or soaks.
- Stretch.
- Do range of motion and strengthening exercises.

3. For 5 to 7 days, avoid exercise that involves the contused area.
4. Reserve radiographs for suspected foreign bodies and bony injuries.
5. Refer severe injuries for orthopedic management.

Complications. Most contusions heal quickly without sequelae, but severe trauma to the quadriceps muscle can lead to myositis ossificans if not treated properly.

Patient and Parent Education. Explain to parents the expected color changes of ecchymosis from the purple discoloration to greenish and that the ecchymosis may also migrate to other surrounding tissues. Arrange for follow-up if there is continuing or increasing discomfort (Buttaravoli & Stair, 2000). Encourage parents to provide their children with a physical environment that minimizes risk of injury.

Sprains and Strains

Description. A sprain is a tear of a ligament joining bone to bone around the joint and is caused most commonly by outside forces, especially contact sports. Strains are tears of the muscle or of fascia joining muscle to bone, often resulting from a dynamic injury and usually not a contact sport.

Sprains and strains may occur concurrently, and both can be graded by severity as a first-degree, second-degree, or third-degree injury. A first-degree sprain involves minimal stretching of a ligament. A second-degree sprain consists of a partial tear (5% to 99% of fibers disrupted) with functional loss and bleeding but still holding. A third-degree sprain is a complete tear with ligamentous instability and often requires casting (Barkin & Rosen, 1999; Buttaravoli & Stair, 2000).

Ankle injuries are the most common acute athletic injury. In pediatrics, 5.5% of ankle injuries are fractures; the others are strains and sprains. Approximately 85% of ankle sprains are due to inversion injuries, 5% are due to eversion injuries, and 10% are combinations of the two (Hergenroeder & Chorley, 2000).

Etiology and Incidence. Sprains are a common athletic injury in children. They most commonly affect the ankle, knee, shoulder, elbow, or wrist and are caused by falls or contact in which the extremity is immobile or moving on one plane and a countervailing force is applied to the joint. In general, the degree of disability immediately after the injury correlates with the severity. For example, if an athlete is injured during a game and cannot walk off the playing field, he or she is more likely to have a serious injury than one who is able to continue playing. Ankle sprains in the child or preadolescent are less common than fractures because the ligaments in this age-group are much stronger than the growth plates or even bone. If a ligamentous injury occurs in a child with an open growth plate, an associated avulsion fracture is almost always present. Once skeletal maturity is reached, however, ankle sprains become the most common of sports injuries (Anderson, 2002).

Assessment

History. The following are assessed:

- Detailed history of the mechanism of injury (e.g., fall, collision, twisting of joint). Some children, especially with more severe sprains, report a "popping" sound or state "my knee gave way."
- Description of symptoms (e.g., onset, location, duration, characteristics, aggravating and relieving factors).
- Type of first aid treatment given.

Physical Examination. The approach to the physical examination depends on the joint involved, the severity of the injury, and the child's ability to cooperate. If the injury is acute, it can be difficult to distinguish the extent of damage. The child may require additional visits for more careful examination as the swelling and pain subside. Always examine the joints and structures located above and below the injury for possible involvement, check function of the injured part, and check circulation and sensation. Any circulatory compromise or marked reduction in sensation (numbness or paralysis) suggests a more serious injury and should be referred to the ED or an orthopedist. During the examination, use the corresponding joint and muscle mass in the other extremity as a control for comparison. Inspect for degree of swelling and ecchymosis over the affected side of the ankle.

Diagnostic Studies. Radiographs are indicated if a fracture or dislocation is suspected. Suspicious findings that suggest the need for radiographs include gross deformity, serious impairment in mobility of the injured area, point tenderness examination, and moderate to severe swelling. Simple radiographs of extremities or other major joint systems are relatively inexpensive and can be useful in distinguishing a sprain or strain from a fracture. Table 40-5 identifies a grading system for ankle injuries. Grades II and III list diagnostic findings suggestive of a patient having a positive extremity radiograph (Mayeda, 1999).

Stiell and colleagues (1995) developed the Ottawa Ankle Rules to guide clinical decision making regarding when radiographs are indicated for certain foot and ankle injuries. Figure 40-1 depicts the Ottawa Ankle Rules. These rules have been applied successfully in adult populations and are shown to save time and money in the health care system without compromising quality of care. Because their appropriateness in pediatric populations is still not confirmed, it is recommended that their use be limited to older children (postpubertal).

The study by Stiell and colleagues (1995) demonstrated that "use of these rules led to a decrease in ankle radiography, waiting time, and costs without an increased rate of missed fractures." The rules state that an ankle radiograph series is required only if there is any pain in the malleolar zone. A foot radiograph is required only if there is any pain in the midfoot zone (see Fig. 40-1). However, their applicability in children has not yet been confirmed.

TABLE 40-5 *Grading of Ankle Injuries*

Severity	Signs and Symptoms	Disability
Grade I (mild)	Minimal swelling (clear definition of Achilles tendon), small area of tenderness, little or no hemorrhage, minimal decreased range of motion	Little or no limp with walking; minimal difficulty hopping
Grade II (moderate)	Moderate swelling (margin of Achilles tendon less defined), more generalized tenderness, some hemorrhage, decreased range of motion	Obvious limping with walking; unable to run, unable to hop, unable to do toe raise
Grade III (severe)	Diffuse swelling (no clear margins of Achilles tendon), widespread tenderness, hemorrhage evident, pronounced decreased range of motion	Unable to bear weight; involuntary guarding with examination

Adapted from Hergenroeder A, Chorley JN: Sports medicine. In Behrman RE, Kliegman RM, Jenson HB, editors: *Nelson textbook of pediatrics*, ed 17, Philadelphia, 2004, WB Saunders, pp 2302-2320.

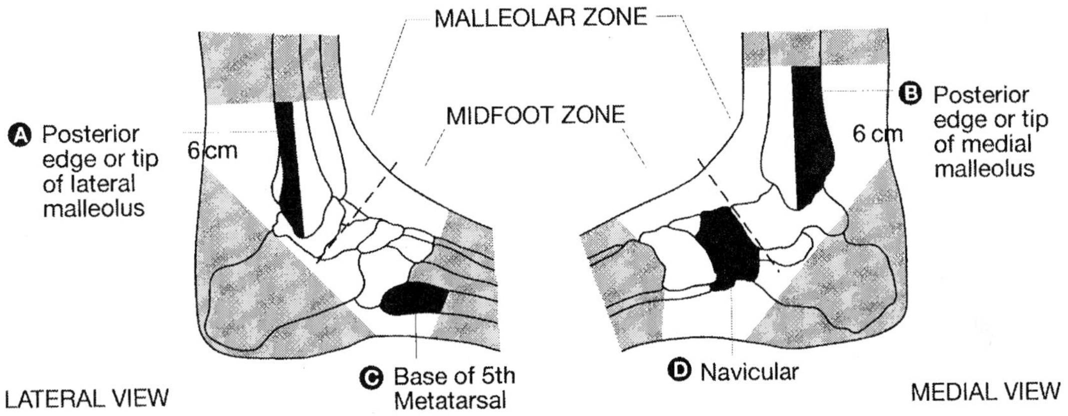

An ankle x-ray series is required only if there is any pain in malleolar zone and any of these findings:
- Bone tenderess at **A**
- Bone tenderness at **B**
- Inability to bear weight both immediately and in emergency department

A foot x-ray series is required only if there is any foot pain in midfoot zone and any of these findings:
- Bone tenderness at **C**
- Bone tenderness at **D**
- Inability to bear weight both immediately and in emergency department

FIGURE 40-1 The use of radiography in acute ankle injuries: Ottawa Ankle Rules. (From Stiell IG et al: A study to develop clinical decision rules for the use of radiography in acute ankle injuries, *Ann Emerg Med* 21:384-390, 1992, with permission from the American Academy of Emergency Physicians.)

The Ottawa Knee Rules (OKR) are also available to use as guides for when to order radiographs in cases of acute knee injury. Studies have demonstrated that relying on the OKR in pediatric populations does not always identify all patients with knee fractures (Khine, Dorfman, Avner, 2001). For this reason liberal referral for radiograph in cases of knee injury is still recommended.

Differential Diagnosis. If there is excessive swelling or discoloration around the joint, suspect a fracture or dislocation, especially of the epiphysis. The degree of pain or pain behavior (i.e., dramatic) does not distinguish a sprain or strain from a fracture. Preverbal children, in particular, may have difficulty localizing pain, may complain of generalized pain, or may experience referred pain in one area caused by injury in an adjacent area. Although trauma is the most common cause of joint pain in children, infectious, rheumatologic, inflammatory, neoplastic, and hematologic abnormalities also should be considered, especially with fever, joint effusion, swelling, or erythema.

Management. Care of sprains and strains differs depending on the grade of injury. Children with severe sprains or strains (third-degree injury) should always be referred to an orthopedic surgeon. Management for lesser injuries is as follows:

1. Acute management for grade I or II sprains and strains:
   - RICE (rest, ice, compression, and elevation of the injured part, as discussed previously). Apply ice immediately for 15 to 20 minutes, and then, depending on the severity of the injury, every 2 to 6 hours for the first 24 to 48 hours. Ice may be applied using massage (a paper cup filled with water and frozen is ideal), ice packs, or immersion of the injured part in an ice water bath. A pressure bandage, such as an Ace wrap, may then be applied with gentle, steady pressure. Take care not to allow impairment of circulation. Elevate the limb. There should be non–weight bearing until pain diminishes.
   - Give nonsteroidal antiinflammatory medication.
   - Heat may be used after 48 hours for mild sprains to facilitate healing.
2. Nonacute/chronic management:
   - May be weight bearing as tolerated.
   - Apply stabilizer or brace for unstable joint. May be needed for 3 to 6 weeks.
   - Recommend rehabilitation exercises, including range of motion and strengthening. Rehabilitation should be gradual, beginning with isometric exercises of muscles and progressing to fuller range of motion and strengthening exercises. There should be no pain or swelling as exercise progresses. A general rule of thumb for return to sport activities for ankle sprains is 1 month for grade I, 2 months for grade II, and up to 3 months for grade III sprains.
   - Apply ice after exercise.
   - Athletes should not return to competition after a sprain until they are pain free and can perform all sports-specific activities.
3. Severe sprains may need casting or surgery (Drendel, Esterhai, & Sawyer, 2002).

Patient and Parent Education. Prevention of injury is key. Teach children and parents the importance of using protective gear (e.g., wrist guards for skaters). Children should also be encouraged to maintain a continuous level of physical activity to maximize muscle strength. See Chapter 15 for a discussion of children's participation in athletic activities.

Prevention of strains can be achieved with consistent stretching, warm-up exercises, and maintenance of muscle strength through regular activity. Strength training may reduce the incidence and severity of overuse injuries. For children who wish to participate in sports activities, advise them to structure a period of conditioning into their schedules.

Fractures and Dislocations

Description. A fracture involves a disruption in the continuity of bone tissue, with bowing or a break, with or without separation. Pediatric patients have unique patterns of fractures due to the immaturity of bone and the dynamic nature of skeletal growth. Fractures are more common than ligamentous injuries or sprains in children due to the relative weakness of the physis or growth plate (Dobiesz & Greenfield, 2002). Fractures that occur in the physis, epiphysis, metaphysis, or diaphysis may be complete, greenstick, buckle, comminuted, avulsed, transverse, oblique, or spiral. Various types of epiphyseal fractures based on the Salter-Harris classification system are discussed in Chapter 38. Stress fractures are discussed later in this chapter.

Dislocations are characterized by displacement of bone ends from their normal position in a joint. There can be wide variation in degree of displacement.

Etiology and Incidence. Fractures are relatively common in children, with Salter II being seen most often (75%). The majority of these injuries occur in children older than 10 years of age. Clavicular fractures may be due to birth trauma and are discussed in Chapter 38. Accidents in which the child tries to break a fall using outstretched arms can result in fractures of the wrist, ulna, radius, or humerus. Direct trauma to bones or joints (e.g., resulting from contact sports, auto accidents, falls) can cause fractures or dislocations.

Clinical Assessment

History. A description of the acute trauma, as well as the signs and symptoms occurring at the time of trauma, provides useful data. An accurate history of the time of the event, mechanism of injury, and direction of forces is important and helps define the type of injury. Often such orthopedic injuries are not witnessed. A child may be too frightened, in too much pain, or too immature to articulate what happened or to give a reliable history. However, children rarely complain about persistent pain unless there is an abnormality. Be sure to question about any history of previous injury and aggravating disease processes, such as preexisting bleeding abnormality. A delay in seeking medical care or a history that is vague or inconsistent with injuries is suggestive of child abuse (see Chapter 19) (Mayeda, 1999).

Physical Examination. Carefully inspect the injured part and the adjacent body parts, keeping in mind that pain and tenderness may be referred from injury in another area. Meticulously check for the following three functions:

1. Motor function, including range of motion, both passive and active. Note any limitations, particularly problems with tendon functioning. This is especially important with hand or finger injuries.
2. Sensory function, especially for any loss of sensation or numbness. Use a body chart to map the location. The existence of point tenderness, produced by palpating over a particular area, is suggestive of possible fracture.
3. Vascular function, especially for evidence of any vascular compromise.

These three functions are easily remembered by using the initials M/S/V.

Significant findings include the following:

- Deformity
- Swelling
- Ecchymosis
- Misalignment of bone or joint
- Loss of function or mobility (especially with dislocation)
- Muscle spasm
- Discoloration (pallor or cyanosis)
- Decrease in vascular function such as capillary refill, diminished or absent pulses

Lacerations with open fractures must be treated promptly in the ED. Dislocations are rare, and when they do occur, they most commonly involve the radial head or patella. Fractures often accompany dislocations because the ligamentous structures are more resistant to trauma (Table 40-6).

Diagnostic Studies. Because of issues such as pain, anxiety, and the possibility of an unreliable or incomplete history, the NP must maintain a high index of suspicion for possible fracture. Radiography must be considered for findings of deformity, marked swelling, pain, ecchymosis, point tenderness, numbness, and loss of function. See Fig. 40-1 for the use of radiography in acute ankle injuries using the Ottawa Ankle Rules. Diagnostic findings suggestive of a patient having a positive extremity radiograph are found in Table 40-7.

Lateral and anteroposterior radiographic views should be obtained. Because of the growth plates, comparison views may be obtained on a selective basis. Early fractures and Salter I fractures do not always appear on radiographs at the time of injury. However, follow-up radiographic studies 7 to 10 days after the trauma may reveal a fracture line. Guidelines for ordering radiography after ankle injuries are discussed earlier in this chapter.

Differential Diagnosis. The cause of a fracture should be determined, because fractures can also be due to pathologic conditions such as osteogenesis imperfecta, sarcoma, hyperparathyroidism, and nutritional deficit (rickets, copper deficiency). Children who are physically abused may have multiple fractures at different stages of healing, repeated fractures, and typically fractures of the skull, ribs, or vertebrae, or spiral, oblique, or transverse fractures in the long bones (especially in children before the age of

TABLE 40-6 ***Assessment and Management of Fractures***

Injury	Clinical Findings	Diagnostic Studies	Management
Fracture/dislocation	Point tenderness over site, generalized pain, deformity, misalignment of bone or joint, loss of function or mobility (especially in dislocation), muscle spasm, discoloration, swelling, lacerations (if open fracture) *Clinical pearl*: tenderness below the lateral malleolus is typically ankle sprain, not fracture; if excessive swelling or discoloration along the joint, suspect fracture or dislocation, especially of epiphysis	Lateral and anteroposterior radiographs; may need to repeat in 10-14 days because early and Salter I fractures may not appear on first films	Referral for casting or other orthopedic interventions
Stress fracture (repeated microtrauma)	Gradual onset of pain with activity that decreases with rest, point tenderness, local swelling; distal atrophy may be noted	Radiograph; if normal, bone scan/ultrasonography	Rest and eliminate activity that caused microtrauma for 10-14 days; casting if complete fracture; retraining

TABLE 40-7 Diagnostic Findings Suggestive of a Patient Having a Positive Extremity Radiograph

Upper Extremity	Lower Extremity
Gross deformity	Gross deformity
Activity restricted	Activity restricted
Bone point tenderness	Bone point tenderness
Pain on motion	Pain on motion
Swelling moderate or severe	Knee injury
Time since injury >6 hr	Foot injury

From Mayeda DV: Management principles. In Barkin RM, Rosen P, editors: *Emergency pediatrics: a guide to ambulatory care*, ed 5, St Louis, 1999, Mosby, p 518.

walking). Chapter 19 discusses findings of child abuse in more detail.

Management. All suspected fractures should be splinted promptly. This stabilizes the fracture to prevent damage to the surrounding soft tissues and also reduces pain, by reducing movement. If the injury is to an extremity, immediate intervention requires application of ice and elevation of the body part to prevent swelling. Uncontrolled swelling can cause neurovascular compromise if confined to a compartment.

Simple fractures can usually be reduced and immobilized easily. They typically heal quickly with no disruption in the child's growth. The potential for impairment to growth plates, joints, tendons, or neurovascular structures following trauma is of serious concern. All children with fractures, other than simple fractures, or dislocations need immediate referral to an orthopedic specialist for management. Open reduction is often necessary with severe fractures.

Because dislocations often involve fractures in addition to the stretching and deforming of the ligaments, it is best to have an orthopedist involved for the dislocation reduction procedure. Analgesia is usually required before the reduction, and radiographic studies should be obtained before and after the reduction. Open dislocations or those associated with neurovascular compromise are true emergencies and must be referred immediately for emergency care. Patients recovering from fractures and dislocations should be provided with appropriate and adequate analgesia, because both fractures and dislocations are painful injuries.

Patient and Parent Education. Patients and parents should be provided with information concerning cast care or application of compression bandages, use of ice to minimize swelling, and keeping the injured part immobilized and elevated as much as possible. They should also be cautioned to carefully observe the injury for signs of worsening pain, circulatory compromise, or delayed healing, and should promptly notify their health care provider if any such signs occur. As with strains and sprains, prevention of injury through use of protective devices, proper conditioning, and attention to the child's physical environment is essential.

Stress Fractures

Description. Stress fractures are classified as overuse injuries and are becoming more common in children. They are caused by repeated muscular action on a bony insertion site or repetitive direct trauma. Bone remodeling cannot keep up with the repeated microtrauma, which leads to bone resorption and fracture.

Etiology. Stress fractures occur in typical locations and are associated with activities and sports. Common sites and causes include the following:
- Metatarsal shaft—running, marching, and ballet
- Tarsal navicular—running, high-impact aerobics
- Distal fibula and proximal tibia—running
- Ribs—coughing and golf
- Neck and shaft of the femur—running, ballet, and gymnastics

Clinical Assessment. Characteristic history includes gradual onset of pain with activity that decreases with rest, point tenderness, and local swelling. Distal atrophy may be noted. The typical history is that of excessive exercising or beginning an aggressive exercise program without preconditioning (see Table 40-6).

Diagnostic Studies. Normal radiographic findings or a zone of radiolucency is the typical finding. Only 10% of stress fractures are initially positive on radiograph. Bone scan may be needed to identify the fracture if radiographs are normal.

Management. Management includes rest and eliminating the repetitive activity that is the source of the microtrauma for 10 to 14 weeks. Noncompliant patients may need to be casted for immobilization. Complete fractures need to be referred to an orthopedic surgeon and most likely will be casted. Retraining is necessary to eliminate the source of the problem, with a gradual return to activity. If symptoms reappear, more rest is needed (Drendel, Esterhai, & Sawyer, 2002; Hergenroeder & Chorley, 2000).

Subluxation of the Radial Head

Description. Subluxation of the radial head, also known as "nursemaid's elbow" or "pulled elbow," occurs frequently in infants and children under age 5 years. Radial head subluxation also can reoccur, with patients age 24 months or younger at greatest risk for recurrence (Chetham, 1999). The injury occurs when abrupt axial traction is applied to the wrist or hand of the extended, pronated forearm of the young child. This action causes the annular ligament to become partially detached from the head of the radius. It then slips into the radiohumeral joint, where it becomes entrapped (Bachman & Santora, 2002).

Etiology. Often subluxation results from an unintentional injury as the parent or caregiver plays with or grabs the child (e.g., when a parent inadvertently yanks the child's arm while crossing a street). It can be a recurrent problem in 30% of cases (not related to child maltreatment). It can also occur if the arm of an infant is trapped beneath the child's trunk as the child is rolled over. The injury is occasionally reported as the result of a fall. However, pulling of the child's arm, especially if this is a recurrent problem, may be the result of inappropriate disciplining or child maltreatment.

Clinical Assessment

History. Often the history is nonspecific as to a report of an injury, and the parent may not have been aware of when the injury occurred. The classic presentation is that of a child who cries with pain and refuses to use an arm after being pulled or lifted by that same arm (Bachman & Santora, 2002).

Physical Examination. Common findings in children include the following:

- The child uniformly holds the arm in pronation with the elbow slightly flexed. The degree of distress may appear minimal, but range of motion of the elbow elicits pain.
- Mild tenderness may be noted with palpation of the radial head.

Diagnostic Studies. Radiographs are not routinely recommended when the history and clinical presentation are classic. However, if obtained, radiography of the elbow is normal.

Differential Diagnosis. Subluxation has a classic history and presentation. However, if the child does not improve after the reduction procedure (see next section), a fracture of the elbow or clavical should be considered, because their clinical presentation may be similar. Consider maltreatment if a recurrent problem or other symptoms or signs are present that lead the NP to suspect child abuse.

Management. Reduction of a subluxed radial head is one of the most gratifying procedures for NPs and parents alike. Two techniques can be used to reduce the radial head: supination and flexion or pronation and flexion. The steps to correct the subluxation involve the following:

- Approach the child in a slow, nonthreatening way and distract the child by talking or other diversionary tactics.
- Use either the supination and flexion technique as illustrated in Fig. 40-2 or the pronation and flexion technique. With the pronation and flexion technique, the examiner hyperpronates the child's forearm by a slight counterclockwise motion and flexes the elbow while applying gentle longitudinal traction (Shah, 2002).
- A palpable or audible "pop" usually signals successful reduction. Typically the patient again reaches for objects with the affected arm within 15 minutes of reduction. No further treatment is necessary.

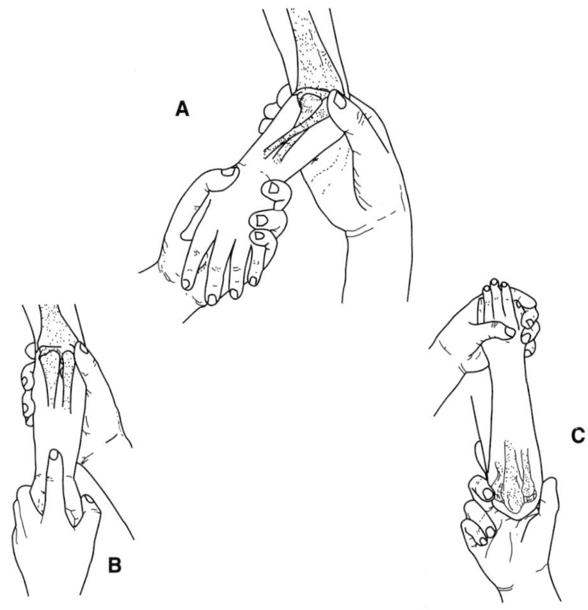

FIGURE 40-2 Reduction of radial head subluxation by supination and flexion technique. **A,** Grasp the palm of the child's hand as if to shake it. Axial traction is applied to the forearm with the wrist adducted to the ulnar side. Pressure is also applied directly over the radial head at the elbow. **B,** The forearm is supinated while axial traction and pressure are maintained over the forearm and radial head, flex the elbow to the shoulder while supination and pressure are maintained over the radial head **(C).** (From Shah B: Reduction of radial head subluxation. In Finberg L, Kleinman RE, editors: *Saunders manual of pediatric practice*, ed 2, Philadelphia, 2002, WB Saunders, p 1162.)

Several attempts (up to three) at reduction may be necessary before the patient resumes normal use of the arm. If normal use does not follow reduction attempts, alternative diagnoses should be considered. In these cases, immobilization with prompt orthopedic follow-up is indicated (Joffe & Loiselle, 2002; Rittenberry & Greenfield, 2002).

Patient and Parent Education. Key points to cover include the following:

- Instruct parents not to lift or pull the child by the hand or elbow.
- The condition tends to recur until the child is approximately 5 years of age in up to 30% of cases.

Compartment Syndrome

Description. Compartment syndrome is a complication of soft tissue injuries (e.g., fractures, crush injuries, and strenuous running). It generally affects the leg and forearm; however, any muscle that is contained by fascia can develop compartment syndrome. Compartment syndrome develops when there is bleeding into a closed fascial space, producing progressive swelling and an increase in intracompartmental pressure. As the pressure increases, venous blood flow is impaired, followed by ischemia, which, if prolonged, results in cell death of the surrounding muscle and nerves (Smith, 2002).

Clinical Assessment. Compartment syndrome is characterized by the "five *P*'s": pain, pallor, paresthesia, pulselessness, and paralysis, with pain being the earliest sign. A child with a splinted fracture should be comfortable with mild analgesia. Acute pain in such a child raises the possibility of compartment syndrome (Smith, 2002).

Chronic compartment syndrome can be seen in runners. It is associated with a history of local pain confined to the muscle (not the bone) with exercise, relief with rest, and rare tenderness and swelling over the muscle compartment.

Management. Prompt recognition of this complication and referral to an orthopedic surgeon are important. The diagnosis is made by direct measurement of compartment pressures. If the syndrome is confirmed, it is treated by immediate fasciotomy. Without treatment, irreversible damage to the compartment structures occurs within 6 to 8 hours after onset and leads to muscle necrosis, fibrosis, and ischemic contracture. With chronic compartment syndrome caused by running, pain prevents resumption of exercise and limits the risk of muscle and nerve damage.

Bites

Animal and Child Bites

Description. Children can be bitten by pets, stray animals, or humans, especially other children. Most bites are to the hand, although pet ferrets may attack a child's face.

Etiology and Incidence. An estimated 1% of ED visits annually in the United States are due to mammalian bites. The vast majority are dog bites (both provoked and unprovoked). Sixty five percent of all dog bites occur in children younger than 11 years of age, with boys being attacked 1.5 times more often than girls. Seventy-five percent of animals who bite children are known to them. The risk of infection from a dog bite, if a child is brought to medical attention within 8 hours, is between 2.5% and 20%. By contrast, the risk of infection of a cat bite (despite early medical attention) is at least 50%. Cat bites cause puncture wounds and tend to be deeper than dog bites, with girls being the more common recipients of the bites. Dog bites can cause abrasions, puncture wounds, and lacerations, with or without an associated avulsion of tissue. Limited data define the incidence of human bite injuries, but it is suspected that human bites are the leading cause of injury in child care centers in the United States. All human bite wounds, regardless of mechanism of injury, should be considered at high risk for infection. Other animal bites, such as rat bites, are not reportable, so there is a paucity of information about their epidemiology (Ginsburg, 2004).

Clinical Assessment. Ask about the circumstances surrounding the bite, including the type of animal, domestic or sylvatic, provoked or unprovoked, and location of the attack. History of drug allergies and immunization status of the child also should be ascertained.

Physical Examination. During physical examination, the wound should be assessed for the type, size, and depth of injury. Explore for the presence of foreign material and the status of underlying structures. If the bite is on an extremity, assess its range of motion. A diagram of the injury should be recorded in the child's chart (Ginsburg, 2004).

Secondary infection is the most common complication of mammalian bites and can lead to cellulitis and lymphangitis, requiring hospitalization. *Streptococcus* and *Staphylococcus* are common organisms associated with infected animal and human bites, with anerobic infection also possible. *Pasteurella multocida* is found in 50% of wound infections from animal bites.

Diagnostic Studies. Obtain wound cultures if indicated to look for aerobic and anerobic microorganisms. A roentgenogram of the affected part should be obtained if it is likely that a bone or joint could have been penetrated or fractured or if retained foreign material is present.

Differential Diagnosis. The differential diagnosis includes lacerations or puncture wounds from other causes.

Management. Management involves both physical and psychologic care of the child and includes the following (Baldwin & Mannheimer, 2002):

- Administer tetanus booster and rabies prophylaxis if indicated (consult with local animal control or public health department).
- Swab the wound with a moistened gauze to remove gross debris. Swab the wound for culture if indicated.
- Anesthetize, clean, and vigorously irrigate the wound with copious amounts of normal saline. Puncture wounds should be thoroughly cleaned and gently irrigated with an angiocatheter, a blunt-tipped needle, or a splash-guard device.
- Debride avulsed or devitalized tissue.
- Superficial wounds that do not involve high-risk structures, such as the fingers, cartilaginous tissue, tendons, bones, and joints, generally do not need to be treated with prophylactic antibiotics.

- Prescribe antibiotics for all human, cat, or rat bites, all but the most trivial of dog bites, and hand puncture wounds, as well as wounds in children who are immunosuppressed or first seen more than 24 hours after injury. These are considered high-risk wounds. Prescribe broad-spectrum antibiotics such as amoxicillin clavulanate or erythromycin until results of cultures are known, and then as indicated by the sensitivity reports. Some sources give prophylactic antibiotics for facial wounds only because of the potential for scarring from infection.
- Some controversy exists over whether bite wounds should be closed primarily with delayed closure (3 to 5 days after injury) or should be allowed to heal by secondary intention (leaving the wound open). Factors to consider are the type, size, and depth of the wound, the anatomic location, the presence of infection, the time interval since the injury, and the potential for cosmetic disfigurement. Surgical consultation should be obtained for all deep or extensive wounds and those involving the bones, joints, or hands. Because of the excellent blood supply to the face, facial lacerations are at less risk for infection. Many plastic surgeons advocate primary closure of facial bite wounds that have been brought to medical attention within 5 hours and have been thoroughly irrigated and debrided. Because of concern about scarring, the NP may refer facial wounds for plastic surgery repair.
- Refer children with severe bites. Hospitalization, reconstructive surgery, and long-term follow-up can also be indicated.
- Discuss the child's fears and management of any behavioral problems that may result.
- Report bites to the appropriate authorities.

Patient and Parent Education. Preventive education and actions should include the following:

- Teach children to avoid stray animals, be cautious around domesticated animals, and not tease or provoke any animal.
- Emphasize the importance of parental supervision of children as they play with pets. Young children, especially, are often unaware of the risks that animals present, and their interactions must be carefully monitored.
- Do not keep typically wild animals as pets in families with very young children.
- Do not allow pets to roam freely.
- Report stray animals promptly to animal control officials.

Hymenoptera

Description. Bees, hornets, yellow jackets, ants, and wasps belong to the Hymenoptera order of insects and have common antigens in their venom. Bees and wasps ordinarily do not sting unless frightened, bothered, or hurt. Yellow jackets are aggressive. Fire ants may cause multiple, painful stings. Reactions to stings by these insects, caused by the Hymenoptera venom, vary from mild, local responses to life-threatening anaphylaxis with wheezing and urticaria. Most children experience only a local reaction, but some children suffer severe systemic reactions, which can progress to medical emergencies unless prompt intervention is initiated.

Etiology. Immunoglobulin E–dependent hypersensitivity is the underlying cause of reactions. Histamines, leukotrienes, prostaglandins, and other inflammatory factors are released, causing local or systemic symptoms. The venom of bees, wasps, and yellow jackets is similar and can cause cross-reactivity (Sorrentino & Monroe, 2002).

Clinical Assessment

History. The child usually reports being bitten or stung. There may be a past history of a local or systemic reaction following an insect bite.

Physical Examination. Findings include the following:

- Mild reaction consists of local redness, pruritus, pain, edema, and possibly generalized urticaria.
- Severe reactions, including anaphylaxis, are characterized by local signs plus any of the following:
  - Difficulty in breathing, wheezing
  - Difficulty swallowing
  - Hoarseness, thickened speech
  - Gastrointestinal disturbances, abdominal pain
  - Dizziness, weakness, confusion
  - Collapse, unconsciousness, even death
- Fire ants bites are characterized by vesicles that develop into sterile pustules.

Diagnostic Studies. Skin testing is not necessary and can be dangerous if there is a history of an allergic response to Hymenoptera sting.

Differential Diagnosis. Other insect bites or dermatologic eruptions that produce similar symptoms are included in the differential diagnosis.

Management. The following steps are taken:

1. For mild local reactions:

- If the stinger is visible, flick it off with the edge of a sharp object (e.g., knife blade or credit card), taking care to not squeeze the attached venom sac.
- Apply ice or cool compresses locally.
- Administer an antihistamine such as diphenhydramine (Benadryl) at 5 mg/kg per day divided every 8 hours for pruritus.
- Calamine lotion or one part meat tenderizer mixed with four parts water may help relieve the discomfort (Taylor, 2002).

2. For moderate to severe allergic reaction:
- Moderate reactions may need to be treated with oral antihistamines, corticosteroids, and inhaled bronchodilators (if wheezing).
- Institute emergency measures for treatment of anaphylactic reactions as follows (Erickson, Herman, & Bowman, 2002):
  - Epinephrine (0.01 mg/kg of 1:1000 aqueous epinephrine at 0.01 ml/kg per dose subcutaneously, repeated at 15- to 20-minute intervals two to three times, not to exceed 0.5 mg total). Administer the dose above the sting site.
  - Antihistamines should be given early but not as a substitute for epinephrine. Diphenhydramine 1 to 2 mg/kg (up to 50 mg) intramuscularly (IM) or intravenously (IV). Ranitidine or cimetidine (an H_2 blocker) may also be added.
  - Glucocorticoids (such as methylprednisolone [Solu-Medrol] at 1 to 2 mg/kg per dose) should be given for their antiinflammatory response, as well as their effect of preventing the late-phase serum sickness response.
  - Bronchodilators are also given if bronchospasm occurs, typically albuterol 0.5% in nebulizer at 0.03 ml/kg per dose in 2 ml of saline.
  - IV fluids should be administered if the child is hypotensive as a result of anaphylactic shock.
  - Administer oxygen.
  - Tracheostomy to be performed if laryngeal edema is life threatening.
  - Hospitalize for anaphylactic shock.

3. Referral to an allergist is indicated for any child who has life-threatening respiratory symptoms (e.g., stridor or wheezing) or hypotension. Venom immunotherapy desensitization is highly effective in preventing further systemic reactions. Children less than 16 years old who have only urticaria or angioedema do not require venom immunotherapy, because only 10% of these children will have systemic reactions with subsequent stings (Erickson, Herman, & Bowman, 2002).

Patient and Parent Education. Key issues to discuss include the following:
- Importance of wearing a medical alert tag or bracelet
- Proper use of an insect sting kit (self-injectable epinephrine pen) and need to have kit always readily available for emergency use
- Prevention of stings by avoiding areas likely to be infested with these insects, not wearing bright-colored clothing, and not using perfumed products

Mosquitoes, Fleas, and Chiggers (Red Bug Mites)

Description. Mosquitoes are the vectors of many important diseases in humans and also cause irritating local skin reactions when they bite. Similarly, flea and chigger bites produce local skin eruptions. The chigger is also known as red bug mite or harvest mite.

Etiology and Incidence. Mosquito bites are the most common insect bites of infants and children. Fleas that commonly attack humans in the United States include the human flea, cat flea, and dog flea. The six-legged larvae of harvest mites are responsible for the skin eruption characteristic of chigger bites. Harvest mites live on grain stems, shrubs, grass, and vines. As humans or animals pass by, the larvae attach themselves to the skin and inject an irritating secretion. The harvest mites then drop to the ground or are scratched off within 1 to 2 days. A seasonal pattern is characteristic of mosquito, flea, and chigger bites.

Clinical Assessment

History. The following may be reported:
- Mosquito or flea bites
  - Known mosquito or flea bite
  - Presence of cat or dog in child's environment
  - Complaints of a brief stinging sensation followed by itching after mosquito bite
- Chigger bites
  - Complaints of itching followed by dermatitis after chigger bite
  - History of playing or walking in grassy areas or other harvest mite habitat near woods and water

Physical Examination. Mosquito bites are characterized by the following:
- Local irritation in unsensitized children
- Urticarial wheals that itch and last several hours to days in sensitized children or firm papules or nodules that last a long period of time
- Central punctum (sometimes noted)
- Secondary impetigo from scratching of skin lesions

Flea bites are characterized by the following:
- Urticarial wheal or papule surrounded by redness in a sensitized person
- Often, central hemorrhagic punctum
- Progression of wheals into bullae in highly sensitized individuals, especially young children
- Grouping of multiple lesions, commonly found on arms, ankles, legs, feet, thighs, waist, and lower abdomen

Chigger bites are characterized by the following:
- Discrete, bright-red papules 1 to 2 mm in diameter that often have hemorrhagic puncta
- Lesions mainly seen on legs (sock area) and belt line but can be widespread
- Wheals, papules, or papulovesicles in sensitized individuals
- Blisters if a secondary hypersensitivity reaction; purpuric lesions or bullae

- Intense pruritus reaching a peak on the second day and decreasing over the next 5 to 6 days, but can persist for months
- Possible secondary impetigo from scratching lesions (Sorrentino & Monroe, 2002)

Diagnostic Studies. The presence of fleas or harvest mites is diagnostic; otherwise, no studies are done.

Differential Diagnosis. The diagnosis is often obvious, but the differential diagnosis can include insect bites that produce similar papular, vesicular lesions, or other skin conditions.

Management. Management consists of controlling pruritus and can include such measures as the following:

- Cool compresses
- Topical corticosteroids (e.g., 1% hydrocortisone cream)
- Oral antihistamines (e.g., diphenhydramine) if topical corticosteroids do not provide relief
- Removal of embedded chiggers (can be withdrawn by covering the insect with alcohol, mineral oil, nail polish, or ointment)
- Treatment of secondary skin lesions as indicated
- Elimination of fleas by treating animals and cleaning carpets, bedding, upholstered furniture; avoid areas that are potentially infested with mosquitoes, fleas, or chiggers
- Insecticides should be used with caution

Patient and Parent Education. Prevention of insect bites is a key component in education. Bites can be prevented by eliminating mosquitoes, fleas, and chiggers from the environment or by preventing their contact with the skin.

- Use insect repellents (generally effective against mosquitoes and harvest mites).
- Wear protective clothing to cover body and tuck pants into shoes or socks.
- Wear neutral-colored clothes (white, green, tan, and khaki do not attract mosquitoes).
- Avoid scented hair sprays, powders, soaps, lotions, creams, and perfumes, because these products can attract all forms of stinging insects.
- Mosquitos are attracted to bright clothing and sweaty skin and are drawn to humans by scent.
- Treat suspected animal carrier for fleas, and spray carpets and other infested areas; spray yards and grassy places for fleas in those environments that the child frequents.
- Vacuum carpets daily if fleas are seen on household pets.
- Avoid playing in areas of harvest mite habitat.

Ticks

Description. Ticks *(Ixodides)* are blood-sucking arachnids. They are vectors of significant diseases such as rickettsial infection (e.g., Rocky Mountain spotted fever and Q fever), relapsing fever, erythema chronicum migrans, and Lyme disease. (See discussion of Lyme disease in Chapter 24).

Etiology and Incidence. Ticks are found in grass, shrubs, vines, and brush and attach themselves to various animals and humans. The female tick sucks blood from the skin and can inject a toxin while sucking blood. Transmission of Lyme disease by the *Ixodes dammini* tick requires a 24-hour tick attachment. Tick bites are most common from early spring to early fall.

Clinical Assessment

History. The practitioner assesses a report of known tick bite and exposure to a tick habitat.

Physical Examination. Findings include the following:

- The initial bite is painless and innocuous; thus the tick is frequently undetected or detected only after several days of attachment.
- An infiltrated lesion with a distinct surrounding erythematous halo develops and can last for 1 to 2 weeks.
- A small pruritic nodule, lasting for months or years, can result if the tick's mouth parts are left in the skin.
- Tick bite pyrexia or tick paralysis, occurring about 6 days after attachment, can result; both disorders are reversible, and symptoms quickly resolve if the tick is removed (Hodge & Tecklenburg, 2002).
- Other signs depend on the tick-related illness that can develop; erythema chronicum migrans can develop around the bite in 2 to 3 weeks and progress to a disseminated rash and Lyme disease.

Diagnostic Studies. Identification of the tick is diagnostic. Diagnostic studies are ordered depending on the disease for which the tick is the vector.

Differential Diagnosis. Many different diseases result from tick bites and their sequelae. The differential diagnosis is variable and depends on the illness for which the tick is the vector. The differential diagnosis of local reactions to simple tick bites includes other insect bites.

Management. Although intervention varies with the specific disease, illnesses resulting from tick bites are best managed with prompt introduction of antibiotics, such as amoxicillin, penicillin, or doxycycline. Recommending antibiotic prophylaxis for asymptomatic deer tick bites remains controversial (Taylor, 2002).

Complete removal of the tick is essential. If fragments of mouth parts or proboscis are left in the skin, local symptoms can continue. To remove ticks, wear gloves and firmly grasp the tick with forceps, tweezers, or gloved fingers as close to the skin as possible (try to grasp its head). Gently pull straight upward with steady, even pressure. Wash the area with soap and water and save the tick for identification (Taylor, 2002). Symptoms of tick bite paralysis can resolve within 24 hours after the tick is removed. Ticks, like chiggers, may also withdraw if they are covered with alcohol, mineral oil, nail polish, or ointment (Richker, 1999).

Patient and Parent Education. The following key points should be made:

- Avoid areas known to be infested with ticks.
- Wear protective clothing—preferably light colored to see ticks better (e.g., long-sleeved shirts tucked into pants and pants tucked into socks).
- Use of insect repellents can help prevent tick bites, but do not apply to face or nonintact skin. Also inform parents that repellents occasionally cause allergic or toxic effects. Use a higher sun protection factor (SPF) of sunscreen if applying insect repellents because the SPF may be decreased. Inspect for ticks after exposure or walking in areas likely to be infested; check for ticks every 2 to 3 hours during a hike; carefully check the scalp, hairline, neck, behind the ears, armpits, legs, back of knees, and groin, because these areas are favorite hiding places of ticks.
- Take a brisk shower after a hike to help remove ticks that are not firmly attached. Wash off tick repellents with soap.

Spiders and Scorpions

Description. Most spider bites are innocuous, causing no reaction or a minor, localized response that can be mistaken for a flea, bedbug, or some other insect bite. There are three spiders common in the North American continent whose bite can cause serious complications: the black widow *(Lactrodectus mactans)*, brown recluse *(Loxosceles reclusa)*, and hobo *(Tegenaria agrestis)* spiders. The black widow spider has a globular body about 1 cm across that is coal black in color with a red or orange hourglass marking on its underside. It is found throughout the United States. The brown recluse spider has an oval light fawn to dark chocolate-brown body; it is approximately 1 cm in length (adults range from 1 to 5 cm in total length), with a dark-brown violin-shaped band extending from its eyes partially down its back. The brown recluse is found in southern and midwestern states. The hobo spider, common to the Pacific Northwest and also found in Montana, Utah, and northern California, measures 1 to 1.5 inches across, including its legs, is brown with gray markings, and has parallel marks on its head and herringbone marks on its rear section. It is often mistaken for the brown recluse.

Scorpions have a stinging apparatus in their tail. They are found in the southwestern and southern United States and live in cool, dark places during the day.

Etiology and Incidence. The black widow spider prefers to live in warm, dark, dry places such as woodpiles, garages, basements, and tool sheds (less frequented outbuildings). It often spins its web on an outdoor privy seat, which explains why many black widow spider bites are received around the genital and buttock areas. The brown recluse spider typically lives in dark, dry places and storage closets among clothes. The brown recluse prefers dark recesses and bites only in self-defense. The hobo spider is found in crawl spaces, wood piles, and other dark areas. Like the brown recluse, the hobo spider bites in self-defense. The venom of the brown recluse and hobo spiders can be hemolytic and necrotizing with extension caused by a spreading factor. Scorpions come out at night and are nonaggressive unless disturbed (Bond, 1999; Taylor, 2002).

Clinical Assessment

History. Assess the known history of a spider bite or activities in, or travel to, an environment that is frequented by these spiders. The characteristic appearance of the spider helps in its identification.

Physical Examination. The characteristic features are identified for each type of spider bite (Taylor, 2002):

- Black widow spider bites:
  - Slight erythema and mild pain. A pinprick sensation is followed by regional lymph node tenderness (30 to 120 minutes later) and a halo lesion at the bite site.
  - Severe, muscle cramping pain starts from 10 minutes to 1 hour after the bite and increases to maximum intensity within 3 hours.
  - Central nervous system symptoms include nausea, vomiting, headache, anxiety, salivation, lacrimation, sweating, hypertension, and tachycardia.
  - Death occurs in 5% of children; most children recover in 2 to 3 days; some experience milder symptoms.
- Brown recluse spider bites:
  - Localized reaction is characterized by mild itching or stinging at time of bite (bite can be painless), with mild to severe pain in about 2 to 8 hours, followed by swelling, itching, and tenderness, a hemorrhagic vesicle (12 to 24 hours later), and finally a gangrenous eschar. Lymphangitis is common if a bite is on an extremity. The lesion takes weeks to months to resolve.
  - Systemic reaction is rare but can occur. It is characterized by nausea, vomiting, chills, fever, malaise, muscle aches and pains, thrombocytopenia, and hemolysis (Bond, 1999).
- Hobo spider bites:
  - Similar to brown recluse spider bites.
- Scorpion bites:
  - Severe local pain and edema occur.
  - Systemic reactions include uncontrolled jerking, muscle fasciculation, facial twitching, hypersalivation, diaphoresis, and respiratory paralysis.

Differential Diagnosis. Other spider bites and conditions that result in similar cutaneous manifestations or systemic findings, or both, are included in the differential diagnosis.

Management. In cases in which venomous spider bites are suspected or confirmed, the patient should be referred to the appropriate medical specialist. Treatment for black widow spider bites includes administration of specific antivenin (in selected cases), intravenous calcium gluconate, muscle relaxants, pain medications, tetanus prophylaxis, and antibiotics if secondary infection develops. Most brown recluse bites tend to heal without incident. Bites with necrotic centers generally require tetanus prophylaxis, pain medication, application of ice or cold compresses, and elevation of the extremity. Scorpion stings may be managed with topical steroids, antihistamines, and cool compresses for local reactions. Children experiencing severe reactions may require the use of antivenin therapy.

Patient and Parent Education. The focus of patient and parent education is prevention. Careful monitoring of environments in which these spiders tend to live and prompt treatment, if bitten, are important points to cover.

Snakebites

Description. Approximately 2500 children per year receive poisonous snakebites in the United States, the majority of which are caused by indigenous pit vipers such as rattlesnakes, cottonmouths, water moccasins, and copperheads. The snake injects venom that contains a variety of toxins into the soft tissue, and the venom can be carried throughout the body via the blood and lymph systems.

Etiology. The snake venom is responsible for the local and systemic reactions that occur. Pit viper venom causes tissue injury, capillary leakage, coagulopathy, and neurotoxicity (Bond, 1999).

Clinical Assessment

History. The NP assesses for a report of a snakebite.

Physical Examination. Characteristic features indicating the presence of venom include the following:

- Severe local reaction soon after the bite, with pain, discoloration, and edema, as well as hemorrhagic effects
- Proximal extension of ecchymosis and swelling during the first few hours after the bite with later fluid-filled or hemorrhagic bullae and necrosis
- Peripheral and central neurologic symptoms
- Evidence of hematologic coagulopathy such as hematemesis, melena, hemoptysis
- Respiratory distress and shock that can lead to death

Diagnostic Studies. Coagulation studies and other laboratory tests are ordered as indicated by the child's condition.

Management. The size of the child, site of the bite, type of snake, and degree of envenomation, plus the effectiveness of treatment, determine whether the snakebite will be fatal. Usually there is a period of 6 to 8 hours between a rattlesnake bite and death in which effective treatment can be instituted to reverse the effects of rattlesnake venom. Treatment includes rapid transportation to a medical center, referral to appropriate medical specialists, antivenin therapy, and treatment for shock and respiratory difficulties. A venous constricting band (not a tourniquet) proximal to the bite can slow the spread of the venom during transit to medical attention.

Patient and Parent Education. Prevention of snakebite is important. Parents and patients who live or vacation in areas where pit vipers are found should be familiar with emergency first aid treatment of snakebites. First aid measures include the following (Bond, 1999):

- Splint the affected extremity and minimize the patient's movements.
- Do not elevate the affected extremity.
- Do not use a tourniquet or ice packs.
- Do not cut the bite area and attempt to suction the venom out.
- Transport immediately to a medical facility.

Head Injuries

Description

The skull of an infant or child is anatomically different from the skull of an adult, a factor that influences how effectively it protects the brain from injury. The brain can better withstand trauma after myelination is complete, the anterior fontanel is closed, and the cranial sutures are fused. Before these events occur, children are particularly vulnerable to cerebral trauma, and this trauma has more severe effects.

In head injuries, irreparable cell damage occurs at the time of the initial trauma, followed by secondary events that can lead to further tissue death. These secondary events are potentially reversible. See Chapter 28 for an in-depth discussion of the brain and its functions.

The discussion of head injury in this chapter is limited to minor closed head injuries and is based on the practice parameter titled "The Management of Minor Closed Head Injury in Children," which was developed by the American Academy of Pediatrics (AAP) and its Committee on Quality Improvement in collaboration with the American Academy of Family Physicians (AAFP) and its Commission on Clinical Policies and Research (AAP, 1999). In addition, indications of impending central nervous system compromise are presented. Head injuries can also be classified as mild, moderate, and severe. Table 40-8 identifies key characteristics that are used in this classification system.

Etiology and Incidence

Head injury is a common cause of trauma in pediatrics, with 2 to 5 million children sustaining head traumas of

TABLE 40-8 ***Classification of Head Injuries Based on Key Characteristics***

Classification	Glasgow Coma Scale*	Neurologic Focal Deficit†	Loss of Consciousness	Other Neurologic Findings
Mild	13-15	No	No or brief loss (<30 min)	May have linear skull fractures
Moderate	9-12	Focal signs	Variable loss	May have depressed skull fracture or intracranial hematoma
Severe	≤8	Focal signs	Prolonged loss	Often have depressed skull fractures and intracranial hematoma

*Either initial or subsequent scores.
†Neurologic focal deficit (e.g., hemiparesis, reflex asymmetry, Babinski sign, abnormal cranial nerve findings).

varying intensities each year in the United States. The level of consciousness is a key determinant of the child's prognosis. Approximately 5000 children die each year from head trauma, and children who survive their injuries have significant long-term disability (Rosman, 2002). Various types of head injuries can result in pathologic conditions: skull fracture, concussion, posttraumatic seizure, cerebral contusion, epidural hematoma, subdural hematoma, cerebral edema, and penetrating injury. A brief description of each is presented in Table 40-9.

Clinical Assessment

History. The following information should be obtained:

- History of how injury occurred; if injury involved a fall, determine height from which the child fell
- Loss of consciousness or memory, confusion, irritability, inappropriate behavior
- Presence of vomiting and frequency
- Presence of headache, description of the headache pain
- Presence of blurred vision, diplopia, or other vision problem

TABLE 40-9 ***Common Types of Head Injuries in Children***

Type of Injury	Characteristics
Skull fracture	Linear, compound, basilar, depressed, and diastatic. Less common in children owing to more elastic skull. Linear is most common type.
Concussion	Transient loss of consciousness with amnesia. Computed topography scan is normal. Child's level of consciousness may be depressed, child may vomit, but neurologic examination becomes normal within hours of treatment.
Posttraumatic seizure	Convulsion resulting from injury that occurs immediately, early (within the first 24 hr), or late (>1 wk after injury). A seizure is the result of a focal injury to the brain.
Cerebral contusion	Bruising of the brain. Injury results form acceleration/deceleration forces. Common features include depressed level of consciousness, headache, and vomiting.
Epidural hematoma	Collection of blood between skull and dura. An overlying fracture is a common association. Classic clinical picture is an initial loss of consciousness, then a lucid interval with subsequent neurologic deterioration.
Subdural hematoma	Collection of blood between dura and brain parenchyma. More common than epidural hematoma. Associated with cerebral contusion following skull fracture or direct trauma or with child abuse. Unconsciousness common with acute subdural hematoma; with chronic subdural hematoma, note growing head in infants or gradual progressive symptoms in older child.
Cerebral edema	Caused by vasogenic, cytotoxic, hydrostatic, or osmotic forces. Significant cause of increased intracranial pressure following injury.
Penetrating injury	Trauma caused by an object such as a bullet entering the brain. In the case of a bullet, the kinetic energy released during its passage through the brain can cause major damage.

- Numbness or loss of sensation, loss of balance, or difficulty walking

A child who is being maltreated may be seen in the ED with head trauma. Reece and Sege (2000) reviewed the histories of a sample of 287 children, ages 1 week to 6 years, who were admitted to a pediatric hospital with head injuries. Eighteen percent of these cases involved suspected child abuse. Based on the findings of this study and others, child abuse should be strongly suspected when such injuries are present in a child without a history of fall or with a history of fall from a relatively low height of less than 4 feet. Reece and Sege (2000) advocate obtaining a skeletal survey for children younger than 3 years when inflicted head injuries are suspected, because younger children are at higher risk. (See Chapter 19 for further discussion of child abuse.)

Physical Examination. Check vital signs (temperature, blood pressure, pulse, and respiration) and compare findings with normal parameters expected for children of varying ages. Perform a thorough physical examination (including a careful oral examination) and a careful neurologic examination. The neurologic examination should include level of consciousness, mental status, motor function (both gross and fine motor), sensory function, cranial nerve functioning, and reflexes. The examiner should be alert to any signs of central nervous system involvement. Evaluation of mental status can be based on the Glasgow Coma Scale (Table 40-10), as discussed in Chapter 28.

TABLE 40-10 ***Glasgow Coma Scale***

Category	Best Response	Score*
Eye opening (E)	Spontaneous	4
	To speech (command)	3
	To pain	2
	None	1
Motor (M)	Obeys (command)	6
	Localizes	5
	Withdraws	4
	Abnormal flexion	3
	Extensor response	2
	None	1
Verbal (V)	Oriented	5
	Confused conversation	4
	Inappropriate words	3
	Incomprehensible sounds	2
	None	1

From Coulter DL: Head trauma. In Finberg LL, editor: *Saunders manual of pediatric practice*, Philadelphia, 1998, WB Saunders, pp 883-885.
*Total score (E + M + V): maximum 15; minimum 3.

Diagnostic Studies. The severity of the head trauma dictates the need for investigative studies. Children with moderate and severe trauma should have a cranial CT scan, as well as routine skull radiographs and other views if there are suspicions or evidence of a neck injury, a suspicious dental trauma, or depressed skull fracture (suspected if there is palpable depression, hemotympanum, or Battle's sign [hemorrhage over the mastoid bone]) (AAP, 1999; Rosman, 2002). Indications for obtaining a CT scan include any of the following:

- History of loss of consciousness (exceeding 1 minute)
- Depressed level of consciousness (lethargy)
- Focal neurologic signs or deficit
- Depressed skull fracture
- Seizures
- Persistent vomiting

CT is the preferred imaging technique because it can be obtained rapidly, and the child can be monitored easily during the study. Skull fractures are better visualized on skull radiographs. Acute hemorrhage is detected more easily by CT than by MRI; however, MRI is the preferred imaging modality for examination of the brain during the recovery period following head trauma and for imagery of the posterior fossa, or to detect hemorrhage when CT is normal but bleeding is suspected (Rosman, 2002). Although CT itself is a safe procedure, some healthy children require sedation or anesthesia (with some risk), so the benefits gained from CT should be carefully weighted against the possible harm of sedating or anesthetizing a child. In addition, CT scans obtained for asymptomatic children may show incidental findings that lead to subsequent unnecessary medical or surgical interventions.

CT scans, MRI, or skull radiographs are not indicated in the following circumstances:

- In instances of minor head trauma with brief (less than 1 minute) loss of consciousness and
  - A normal neurologic examination
  - A Glasgow Coma Scale (GCS) score of 15
  - No complaints of headache, vomiting, memory deficits, or seizures and no history of drug intoxication (Rosman, 2002)
- In instances of minor closed head injury, with no loss of consciousness and no reported or observed neurologic deficits (AAP, 1999)

Differential Diagnosis

History of a head injury is the key to diagnosis. Differentiating minor head trauma that will resolve on its own from more extensive brain injury is problematic at times. Head trauma may cause injuries of the scalp, skull, and intracranial contents. Remember that these injuries may occur alone or in combination (Schutzman, 2002). Children with intracranial lesions after minor closed head injury are not easily distinguishable clinically from the large majority with no intracranial injury. Children with mild nonspecific signs such as headache, vomiting, or lethargy after minor closed head injury may be more likely to have intracranial lesions than children without such signs. However, these clinical signs are of limited predictive value, and most children with headache, lethargy, or vomiting after minor closed head injury do not have demonstrable intracranial injury. In addition, some children with intracranial injury do not have any such signs or symptoms, showing a normal neurologic assessment (AAP, 1999). Because of these findings, some experts recommend a liberal policy on the ordering of cranial CT scans following any head trauma; however, there are drawbacks to routine CT scanning (see discussion in prior section).

Management

Management of the Child with Minor Closed Head Injury and No Loss of Consciousness. Observation in the clinic, office, ED, or home, under the care of a competent caregiver, is recommended for children with minor closed head injury and no loss of consciousness. Observation implies regular monitoring by a competent adult who would be able to recognize abnormalities and seek appropriate assistance.

Management of the Child with Minor Closed Head Injury and Brief Loss of Consciousness. For children with minor closed head injury and brief loss of consciousness (less than 1 minute), and no other neurologic deficits reported or detected on examination, continued observation in the office, clinic, ED, hospital, or home, under the care of a competent caregiver (see definition in preceding paragraph), may be used to evaluate such a child. The use of CT scan, skull radiographs, or MRI in the initial management of children with minor closed head injury and loss of consciousness is not routinely recommended. However, CT scanning along with observation is also accepted.

Management of the Child with Moderate Head Injury. Children with moderate head injuries (GCS score of 9 to 12) may require admission or prolonged observation in the ED until their mental status stabilizes; children with severe head injuries (GCS score of less than 8 or coma and physical findings) need immediate hospital admission. A child with a skull fracture or transient neurologic findings whose level of consciousness is normal may be admitted for overnight observation.

Complications

Complications of head injury can include concussion, posttraumatic seizures, cerebral contusion, epidural hematoma, subdural hematoma, intracerebral hematoma, subarachnoid hemorrhage, acute brain swelling, and penetrating injuries. Intracranial lesions, particularly epidural hematomas, are life threatening and have significant complications. Features indicative of serious injury include loss of consciousness (longer than 1 minute), persistent vomiting, depressed level of consciousness, seizures, unequal pupil size, severe headache, and GCS score of less than 15 (Schutzman, 2002).

Patient and Parent Education

Give all parents or caregivers a "head injury sheet," and make every effort to ensure that they understand the instructions and will comply with them. Salient points to cover in a pediatric head injury information sheet include instructions about when to contact the health care provider or take the child to an ED. Indications are the following:

- Any open head wound
- Increased drowsiness, sleepiness, inability to wake up, unconsciousness
- Vomiting more than one or two times
- Neck pain
- Watery or bloody drainage from ear or nose
- Convulsion, "fit," or fainting
- Unusual irritability, personality change, confusion, or any unusual behavior
- Headache that gets worse or lasts more than a day
- Unequal pupils
- Trouble with vision (blurred), hearing, or speech
- Trouble with walking (e.g., clumsiness or stumbling) or weakness of any muscle of arms, legs, or face

In addition, parents or caregivers should be given the following specific instructions:

- Wake up child every 2 to 4 hours for the first 24 hours after injury; child should wake easily and be able to stay awake for a few minutes.
- Make sure child is moving his or her arms and legs normally.
- Give only acetaminophen, if needed for headache or relief of pain of bumps and bruises.

Parents should also be informed that sometimes symptoms from head trauma occur days, weeks, or months after the initial trauma.

Neurologic sequelae following mild head injury in children often improve or resolve within 9 to 12 months. These sequelae include the following:

- Headache
- Vertigo or dizziness

- Difficulty concentrating or loss of memory
- Depression, fatigue
- Poor school performance and neurobehavioral problems

Heat and Cold Injuries

Frostbite

Description. Frostbite is characterized by ice crystal formation in the tissue and impaired circulation to the affected area, with microvascular changes leading to cellular destruction (Stewart, 1999). Toes, feet, fingers, nose, cheeks, and ears are typical areas of injury.

Etiology. Exposure to temperatures ranging from $-2°$ to $-10°$ C can cause frostbite. Factors such as duration of exposure, increased wind velocity, dependency of the extremity, fatigue, injury, high altitude, immobility, general health, and race can potentiate the effects of cold. Exposure to very cold chemicals (e.g., liquid oxygen) also produces instant frostbite.

Clinical Assessment

History. The NP should assess the following:

- Exposure to cold temperatures
- Complaints of area first feeling a painful cold sensation followed by tingling and numbness
- Complaints of throbbing pain after thawing

Physical Examination. Typical initial findings include the following:

- Frozen area is cold.
- Skin is red at first, then appears pale or waxy white or slightly yellow.

In early stages, tissue blanches; in later stages, it feels doughy or rock hard. On rewarming, the extent of tissue damage becomes apparent. Superficial frostbite is reversible and is often called *frostnip*. These cases are characterized by the following:

- Redness and discomfort
- Skin appearance that returns to normal within a few hours

Deep frostbite occurs when tissues are icy hard and without deep tissue resilience and is characterized by the following signs and symptoms that appear with rewarming:

- Cyanosis or mottling
- Erythema and swelling
- Numbness that evolves into complaints of burning pain
- Vesicles and bullae that appear within 24 to 48 hours
- Gangrene in severe frostbite

Differential Diagnosis. The differential diagnosis includes other conditions that produce similar cutaneous manifestations and injury; a history of exposure to extreme temperatures is the key to the diagnosis.

Management. Severe frostbite should be managed by medical specialists. Treatment includes rapid rewarming procedures, pain management, medical and surgical management of tissue necrosis, prevention of infection, and amputation if needed. Damaged skin should never be massaged or rubbed with snow or ice. Early treatment of mild frostbite includes the following:

- Cover affected area with other body surfaces and warm clothing.
- *Do not use local dry heat*; this practice is dangerous and can cause tissue damage.

Patient and Parent Education. Education of children and parents about the prevention and initial management of frostbite is important. Essential points include advice about the following:

- Use of appropriate clothing when exposed to extreme cold temperatures
- Survival skills for hikers or winter sports participants who are exposed to cold temperatures or who could become lost
- Immediate rewarming of skin that is white by covering with warm clothing or another body surface
- Danger of rubbing affected area with snow or ice or massaging; these practices are contraindicated because they lead to mechanical trauma

Hypothermia

Description. *Hypothermia* is the condition in which body core temperature falls below 35° C. Severe hypothermia is life threatening (Battan & Dart, 2001).

Etiology. Hypothermia can be the result of environmental exposure. Body heat is lost by radiation of heat to nearby objects, evaporation of moisture from the skin and respiratory system, convection of heat from the skin's surface into cooler air, or conduction of heat to objects in direct contact with the body. The effect of cool ambient temperatures is exacerbated by wind, moisture, and lack of appropriate clothing or shelter.

Children are at increased risk of hypothermia because of their relatively larger body surface area, proportionately larger head, smaller body fluid volume, less developed temperature-regulating mechanisms, and less protective body fat. Newborns, particularly low-birth-weight or premature infants, very young children, and children who are ill, fatigued, poorly nourished, or have experienced trauma are at high risk.

Hypothermia, not associated with environmental exposure, may be a sign of other life-threatening illnesses or injuries (e.g., near-drowning in cold water). This secondary hypothermia is not discussed here.

Clinical Assessment

History. The following are assessed:

- Exposure to low ambient temperatures
- Risk factors (e.g., age, physical condition)

Physical Examination. Signs of hypothermia progress from early to late stages and include the following:

- Decreasing body temperature
- Shivering that disappears in late hypothermia
- Pallor or blue lips and skin
- Disorientation, listlessness, sleepiness
- Decreased pulse and respiration
- Coma and death

Diagnostic Studies. No studies are done if hypothermia is mild and responds to basic treatment measures.

Differential Diagnosis. Shock is the differential diagnosis.

Management. For mild hypothermia, in early stages of cooling, remove the child from the cold environment, replace wet clothing, and provide warm liquids. Placing the child in a warm-water bath can be effective. As the body cools further, it can no longer generate adequate heat itself, so external sources of heat must be provided. Again, remove the child from the cold environment, replace wet clothing, and provide heat with warm blankets, heat lamps, hot-water bottles, or, if none of these is available, use the classic technique of placing the child skin-to-skin with a warm person of normal temperature in a sleeping bag or blanket.

Active rewarming by external or core rewarming techniques (e.g., warmed, humidified oxygen and warmed intravenous fluids) is necessary for children with severe hypothermia (Battan & Dart, 2001).

Patient and Parent Education. Instruct parents on the risks of hypothermia in young children. Emphasize the need to monitor children's activities in cold weather and to provide adequate protection from exposure. The higher metabolic rate of normal, healthy children serves to keep them warm, and they may not feel the effects of short-term exposure to the cold. As a result, they may not want a jacket, sweater, hat, or mittens when their parents believe they need them.

Hyperthermia: Common Heat-Related Illness

Description. Hyperthermia is a life-threatening increase in body core temperature. Heat cramps, heat exhaustion, and heat stroke are types of hyperthermia. Heat stroke is a life-threatening condition and is associated with rectal temperatures of over 40° C (Battan & Dart, 2001). Heat cramps and heat exhaustion are discussed in more detail in Chapter 15, because they often occur during sports activities. They are reversible changes; in contrast, heat stroke is a life-threatening condition. This section more specifically discusses heat stroke.

Etiology. Heat-related illness results from an ineffective response of the body's thermoregulatory mechanisms to environmental conditions. Children with some genetic myopathies have malignant hyperthermia, a reaction to anesthesia. All children are at risk for hyperthermia or heat stroke when exposed to high air temperature, especially if the heat is combined with high humidity and if steps are not taken to keep the child cool. Evaporation through sweating is the body's primary cooling mechanism with activity. If air temperature is higher than body temperature, if humidity is high, or if the body is dehydrated, the body's cooling mechanisms and the process of evaporation are compromised and internal body temperature increases. Age, exertion, illness, obesity, and poor nutrition also exacerbate the risk of hyperthermia. Compared with adults, children sweat less, begin to sweat at a higher internal temperature (or set-point), have a higher metabolic rate (thus producing more body heat) and lower cardiac output, and are more susceptible to dehydration (because of proportionately larger body surface area).

Clinical Assessment

History. The practitioner assesses the following (Battan & Dart, 2001):

- Exposure
- Excessive exercise
- Wearing inappropriate clothing
- Inadequate fluid intake or the use of water or other low-sodium fluids during prolonged and strenuous exercise
- Previous episode of heat stroke
- Heat cramps: complaints of intermittent muscle cramping (no rigidity)
- Heat exhaustion: complaints of thirst, headache, fatigue, nausea, and vomiting; core temperature is normal or slightly elevated and the patient still sweats
- Heat stroke: delirium, stupor, or coma—central nervous system dysfunction

Physical Examination. Signs of heat exhaustion include the following:

- Appears anxious and diaphoretic
- Tachycardia with temperature less than 40° C
- Orthostatic hypotension

Signs of heat stroke are progressive and include the following:

- Body temperature above 105° F (40.6° C)
- Hot, dry, red skin
- May or may not sweat
- Initial rapid, strong pulse, progressively becoming weaker
- Initially constricted pupils, progressively dilated
- Initial deep, rapid "snorelike" breathing, progressively becoming weaker

- Tremors, increasing dizziness, and weakness
- Confusion, irritability, anxiety (central nervous system dysfunction)
- Headache
- Loss of appetite, nausea, vomiting
- Decreasing blood pressure
- Seizures, collapse
- Coma and death

Diagnostic Studies. Electrolyte monitoring may be necessary for significant heat cramps and heat exhaustion. Heat stroke requires extensive laboratory studies and monitoring of physiologic parameters.

Differential Diagnosis. Fever differs from hyperthermia in that it is an alteration of the body's hypothalamic set point in response to a pathologic illness or condition.

Management. The management of heat-related illness includes the following:

1. Heat cramps
- Cooling measures
- Oral sodium replacement with electrolyte fluids or liberally salted foods (occasionally IV saline may be needed)

2. Heat exhaustion
- Cool environment
- Intravenous replacement of electrolytes (initial bolus of 10 to 20 ml/kg of normal saline)

3. Heat stroke
- All individuals with heat stroke die without treatment. Heat stroke patients should be transported to a medical facility as quickly as possible. The goal of treatment is to reduce the temperature to less than 100° F or by a total of 4° to 6° F over a 30- to 60-minute period. First aid management includes the following steps:
  - Remove the child from the source of heat.
  - Apply cold packs, wet sheets, or towels. The body responds quickly to cooling of the neck, head, abdomen, and inner thighs.
  - Use a fan to cool and circulate air over child.
  - Be alert for vomiting; prevent aspiration.
- When the body temperature is lowered to the desired level, stop cold packs, monitor, and be prepared to reapply cold packs if temperature increases.
- Other therapies are instituted based on the child's condition (Battan & Dart, 2001).

Patient and Parent Education. Instruct parents on the risks of hyperthermia (e.g., never leave an infant or a child in a closed car or continuously exposed to direct sunlight). Inform parents that children who suffer heat stroke are at higher risk for subsequent heat-related illnesses. Teach ways to prevent hyperthermia, including the following:

- Keep children well hydrated. Offer water often during active play and athletic events or practices. Water is an adequate replacement fluid, although children can also use electrolyte-based sports drinks.
- Make sure children are well rested and have good nutritional intake.
- Provide appropriate clothing (e.g., sunshades, hats, and light-reflective shirts that allow ventilation).
- Regulate children's activity levels to the conditions (e.g., limit active play if it is very hot or humid).
- Acclimatize child gradually to changes in environment.

> RESOURCE BOX
>
> ***National Injury Resources***
>
> **American Burn Association**
> 1-800-548-2876
>
> **Local Poison Control Center**
> The number is listed among emergency numbers in the local telephone book. A call can be made to the local hospital emergency room and advice given according to the local poison control center. One can also call 911 and be transferred to the poison control center; however, not every state or city has a poison control center.

REFERENCES

American Academy of Pediatrics: The management of minor closed head injury in children, *Pediatrics* 104:1407-1415, 1999.

Anderson AC: Injury—ankle. In Fleisher GR, Ludwig S, Silverman BK, editors: *Synopsis of pediatric emergency medicine*, ed 4, Philadelphia, 2002, Lippincott Williams & Wilkins.

Bachman D, Santora S: Orthopedic trauma. In Fleisher GR, Ludwig S, Silverman BK, editors: *Synopsis of pediatric emergency medicine*, ed 4, Philadelphia, 2002, Lippincott Williams & Wilkins.

Baldwin S, Mannheimer A: Animal and human bites and bite-related infections. In Burg FD et al, editors: *Gellis and Kagan's current pediatric therapy*, ed 17, Philadelphia, 2002, WB Saunders.

Barkin RM, Rosen P, editors: *Emergency pediatrics: a guide to ambulatory care*, ed 5, St Louis, 1999, Mosby.

Battan FK, Dart RC: Emergencies, injuries and poisoning. In Hay WW et al, editors: *Current pediatric diagnosis and treatment*, ed 15, Stamford, CT, 2001, Appleton & Lange.

Bond GR: Snake, spider, and scorpion envenomation in North America, *Pediatr Rev* 20:147-151, 1999.

Brady MT: Bone and joint infections. In Burg FD et al, editors: *Gellis and Kagan's current pediatric therapy*, ed 17, Philadelphia, 2002, WB Saunders.

Buttaravoli P, Stair T: *Minor emergencies: splinters to fractures*, St Louis, 2000, Mosby.

Chetham M: Upper extremity injuries. In Barkin RM, Rosen P, editors: *Emergency pediatrics: a guide to ambulatory care*, ed 5, St Louis, 1999, Mosby.

Dobiesz VA, Greenfield RH: Orthopedic injuries. In Strange GR et al, editors: *Pediatric emergency medicine: a comprehensive study guide*, ed 2, New York, 2002, McGraw-Hill.

Drendel AL, Esterhai JL, Sawyer JR: Orthopedic problems of the extremities. In Burg FD et al, editors: *Gellis and Kagan's current pediatric therapy*, ed 17, Philadelphia, 2002, WB Saunders.

Erickson T, Herman BE, Bowman MJ: Spider and arthropod bites. In Strange GR et al, editors: *Pediatric emergency medicine: a comprehensive study guide*, ed 2, New York, 2002, McGraw-Hill.

Ginsburg CM: Animal and human bites. In Behrman RE, Kliegman RM, Jenson HB, editors: *Nelson textbook of pediatrics*, ed 17, Philadelphia, 2004, WB Saunders.

Hergenroeder A, Chorley JN: Sports medicine. In Behrman RE, Kliegman RM, Jenson HB, editors: *Nelson textbook of pediatrics*, ed 16, Philadelphia, 2000, WB Saunders.

Hodge D, Tecklenburg FW: Bites and stings. In Fleisher GR, Ludwig S, Silverman BK, editors: *Synopsis of pediatric emergency medicine*, ed 4, Philadelphia, 2002, Lippincott Williams & Wilkins.

Joffe MD: Burns. In Fleisher GR, Ludwig S, Silverman BK, editors: *Synopsis of pediatric emergency medicine*, ed 4, Philadelphia, 2002, Lippincott Williams & Wilkins.

Joffe MD, Loiselle J: Orthopedic emergencies. In Fleisher GR, Ludwig S, Silverman BK, editors: *Synopsis of pediatric emergency medicine*, ed 4, Philadelphia, 2002, Lippincott Williams & Wilkins.

Khine H, Dorfman DH, Avner JR: Applicability of Ottawa Knee Rule for knee injury in children, *Pediatric Emerg Care* 17(6):401-404, 2001.

Lampe RM: Osteomyelitis and suppurative arthritis. In Behrman RE, Kliegman RM, Jenson HB, editors: *Nelson textbook of pediatrics*, ed 17, Philadelphia, 2004, WB Saunders.

Lipton JD: Soft tissue injury and wound repair. In Strange GR et al, editors: *Pediatric emergency medicine: a comprehensive study guide*, ed 2, New York, 2002, McGraw-Hill.

Mayeda DV: Orthopedic injuries: management principles. In Barkin RM, Rosen P, editors: *Emergency pediatrics: a guide to ambulatory care*, ed 5, St Louis, 1999, Mosby.

Morgan ED, Bledsoe SC, Barker J: Ambulatory management of burns, *Am Fam Physician* 62:2015-2032, 2000.

Reece RM, Sege R: Childhood head injuries. Accidental or inflicted? *Arch Pediatr Adolesc Med* 154:11-15, 2000.

Richker J: Bites. In Barkin RM, Rosen P, editors: *Emergency pediatrics: a guide to ambulatory care*, ed 5, St Louis, 1999, Mosby.

Rittenberry TJ, Greenfield RH: Injuries to the upper extremities. In Strange GR et al, editors: *Pediatric emergency medicine: a comprehensive study guide*, ed 2, New York, 2002, McGraw-Hill.

Rivara FP, Grossman D: Injury control. In Behrman RE, Kliegman RM, Jenson HB, editors: *Nelson textbook of pediatrics*, ed 17, Philadelphia, 2004, WB Saunders.

Rosman NP: Head injury. In Burg FD et al, editors: *Gellis and Kagan's current pediatric therapy*, ed 17, Philadelphia, 2002, WB Saunders.

Schutzman SA: Injury—head. In Fleisher GR, Ludwig S, Silverman BK, editors: *Synopsis of pediatric emergency medicine*, ed 4, Philadelphia, 2002, Lippincott Williams & Wilkins.

Selbst SM, Attia M: Minor trauma—lacerations. In Fleisher GR, Ludwig S, Silverman BK, editors: *Synopsis of pediatric emergency medicine*, ed 4, Philadelphia, 2002, Lippincott Williams & Wilkins.

Shah B: Reduction of radial head subluxation. In Finberg L, Kleinman RE, editors: *Saunders manual of pediatric practice*, ed 2, Philadelphia, 2002, WB Saunders.

Smith JT: Orthopedic problems in children. In Rudolph AM, Kamei RK, Overby KJ, editors: *Rudolph's fundamentals of pediatrics*, ed 3, New York, 2002, McGraw-Hill.

Sorrentino A, Monroe K: Insect stings. In Burg FD et al, editors: *Gellis and Kagan's current pediatric therapy*, ed 17, Philadelphia, 2002, WB Saunders.

Staheli LT: *Fundamentals of pediatric orthopedics*, Philadelphia, 1998, Lippincott-Raven.

Stewart C: Local cold injuries in children: Diagnosis, management, and prevention, *Pediatr Emerg Med Rep* 4(1):1-12, 1999.

Stiell IG et al: Implementation of the Ottawa rules, *JAMA* 271(11):827-832, 1994.

Stiell IG et al: Multicentre trial to introduce the Ottawa rules for use of radiography in acute ankle injuries, *BMJ* 311:594-597, 1995.

Strange GR, Pawel B: Burns and electrical injuries. In Strange GR et al, editors: *Pediatric emergency medicine: a comprehensive study guide*, ed 2, New York, 2002, McGraw-Hill.

Taylor CP: Arthropod bites and stings. In Burg FD et al, editors: *Gellis and Kagan's current pediatric therapy*, ed 17, Philadelphia, 2002, WB Saunders.

41 Genetic Disorders

Pamela J. Hellings, Catherine E. Burns

Genetic disorders occur in approximately 5% of live births. One percent of newborns have a hereditary malformation and 0.5% have an inborn error of metabolism. Up to 50% of spontaneously aborted fetuses have chromosomal defects. A single minor anomaly can occur in up to 13% of newborns (Shapiro, 2000).

The manifestations of genetic diseases can appear immediately after birth or after many years, such as in patients with Huntington chorea. The manifestations can be evidenced in biochemical, reproductive, growth, developmental, or behavioral ways. Therefore the primary health care provider must be constantly vigilant for the possibility of genetic disease. Furthermore, once a genetic condition is suspected, referral to a medical geneticist will not always be required or possible. Primary care providers need to be knowledgeable yet know their own limitations and set personal criteria for referral to specialists.

Caring for children with significant, long-term problems confers enormous responsibilities on the family, community, and society. Prevention of genetic diseases by helping families make decisions about childbearing, screening for early detection to prevent disability, assisting parents to use specialized services, teaching health principles, monitoring and evaluating clients with genetic diseases, and working with families under the stress of caregiving are all roles of the primary care provider. Ethical decision making has a particularly important role in the area of genetics and genetic counseling.

CELLULAR AND MOLECULAR GENETICS

Humans have 46 chromosomes arranged in 23 pairs. Twenty-two pairs are autosomes (the same in males and females) and are homologous because their deoxyribonucleic acid (DNA) is very similar. The remaining pair is the sex chromosomes, with two X chromosomes for females and one X and one Y chromosome for males. They are not homologous. Each chromosome has a long arm (q) and a short arm (p) and is numbered according to its distinct appearance from the largest to the smallest. The gametes (egg and sperm) have half the chromosome complement from the parents (23). During meiosis (formation of the haploid with 23 chromosomes from the egg or sperm) the original paired chromosomes from paternal and maternal sides cross over and exchange genetic material, resulting in extraordinary genetic diversity. The resultant interindividual variation is much greater than intergroup variation. Skin color and hair type have the greatest intergroup variability, unlike the majority of other traits. Fusion at fertilization restores the 46-pair complement, with one of each chromosome pair from each gamete. As a result of genetic variation, a gene may differ from one individual to another in its DNA sequence. These differences in sequencing are called *alleles.* If the two alleles at any given location of a pair of homologous chromosomes are identical, the locus is *homozygous.* If the two alleles are different, the locus is *heterozygous.*

Genes, which carry the information about inherited characteristics from parent to child, are arranged linearly on the chromosomes, each with a specific locus. Thousands of genes are located on each chromosome. Not all genes are active at once; certain mechanisms activate them at various developmental points. In homozygous loci, the genes from a pair of chromosomes carry similar instructions regarding the trait of interest; in heterozygous loci, the instructions are different. In the latter case, one gene may be dominant, with its instructions manifested in the phenotype, as in Huntington chorea, or the genes can be codominant, as in the case of individuals with blood type AB.

The human genome contains 30,000 to 38,000 genes. Genes are composed of deoxyribonucleic acid, commonly referred to as DNA. Each DNA molecule includes pairs of nitrogenous bases—adenine, cytosine, guanine, and thymine (labeled A, C, G, T)—wound around a histone protein core in a double helix. There are more than 3 billion base pairs in the human genome for an individual.

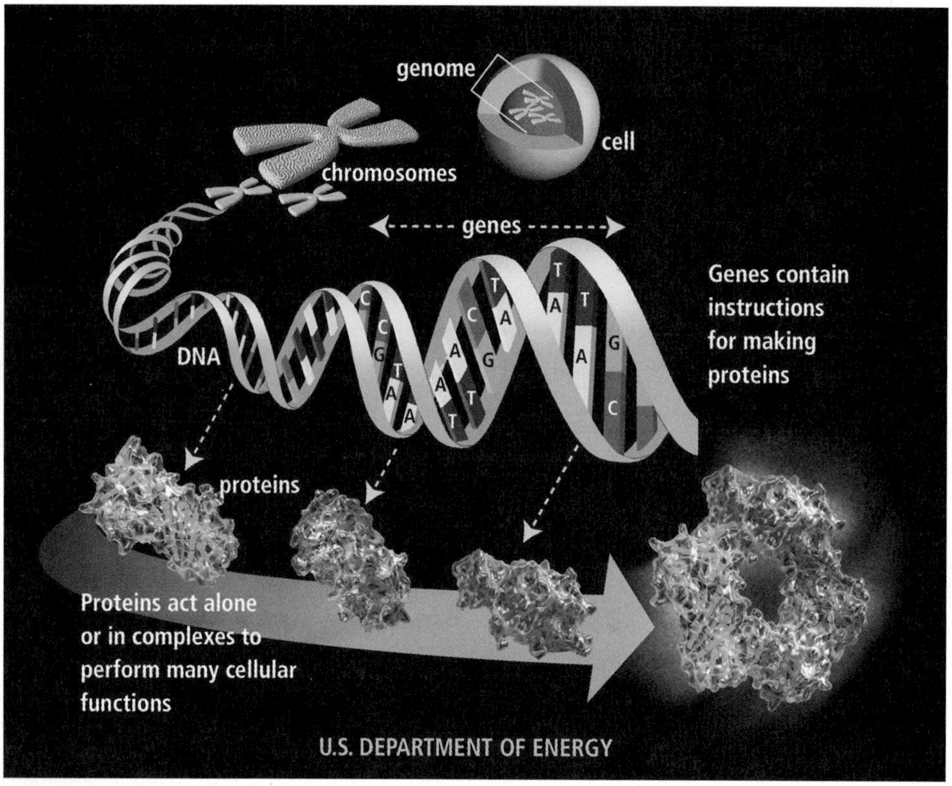

FIGURE 41-1 Genetic diagram.

From the four nitrogenous bases, 64 triple-base combination sequences (codons) of A, C, G, and U (uracil is substituted for thymine in the messenger ribonucleic acid [RNA] at this point) such as GUA, UUG, and CGG are possible (Jorde et al, 2000). Three codons signal the end of a gene (stop codons) and 61 define the 20 amino acids. Thus each amino acid may be specified by more than one codon. The sequence of the amino acids directs the synthesis of proteins in the cell cytoplasm. (Nussbaum, McInnes, & Willard, 2001) (Fig. 41-1).

CAUSES OF GENETIC VARIATION AND GENETIC DISORDERS

Mutations occur when genetic material is permanently changed though alteration, deletion, duplication, or misplacement. Sometimes mutations arise spontaneously, but once the change occurs, it is transmitted to future generations. Mutations are defined as being present in less than 1% of the population. A change in greater than 1% is called a *polymorphism*. Mutations and polymorphisms may be benign, beneficial, or detrimental.

Genetic disorders are classified as *chromosomal disorders*, in which the entire chromosome or large segments of it are duplicated or missing; *single-gene disorders*, in which single genes are altered; and *multifactorial problems*, in which multiple genetic and environmental factors interact. Nontraditional patterns of inheritance are also being described.

Chromosomal Disorders

Chromosomal disorders occur in about 0.4% of live births (Shapiro, 2000). There is also a high frequency of chromosomal disorders in spontaneous abortions and stillbirths. Mental retardation and congenital anomalies commonly occur. The chromosomal disorders include problems of chromosome number (increase or decrease in the number of chromosomes), structure, or both.

Factors related to the occurrence of chromosomal disorders include parental age, nondisjunction (failure of homologous pairs to separate properly during meiosis), and radiation and chemical exposure to the parents. Testing is done through cell culture and chromosome analysis. In addition to the more traditional method of karyotype analysis, in which the total number of each chromosome is identified, staining techniques to identify chromosomal banding assist in the identification of deletions and duplications of chromosomal material. Newer techniques such as fluorescence in situ hybridization (FISH) provide the ability to identify missing, additional, or rearranged chromosomal material for some of the more common abnormalities but must be ordered for the specific location of interest (Jorde et al, 2000).

Single-Gene Disorders

Mendelian theory describes four patterns of inheritance: autosomal dominant, autosomal recessive, X-linked dominant, and X-linked recessive. Dominant problems occur in heterozygotes, where one gene dominates its counterpart from the other parent. Recessive problems occur only when a person is homozygous, with the problem gene appearing on both of the chromosomes of the pair. However, some conditions have reduced *penetrance*, in which a person may have the affected gene (genotype) without expressing the observable characteristics (phenotype), and variable *expressivity*, in which the severity of the disease condition varies greatly. The result is that some children are affected with severe disease whereas others are more mildly affected.

Multifactorial or Multiple Gene Disorders

Multifactorial problems result from the complex interaction of multiple genes in various sites or interaction of genes with the environment. Several terms are used for this group of conditions (e.g., *multifactorial, multiple gene*, and *polygenic*). Cleft lip and palate, spina bifida, hypertension, schizophrenia, pyloric stenosis, diabetes, hypercholesterolemia, Hirschsprung disease, and asthma all fall into this category (Johnson & Robin, 2000).

Multifactorial problems tend to be inherited, and risk for the disease or condition increases if more family members are affected and if the disease has a more severe expression (Jorde et al, 2000).

Nontraditional Inheritance

Three additional patterns of transmission of genetic material from generation to generation have been identified—germline mosaicism, uniparental disomy, and mitochondrial inheritance.

Germline Mosaicism

In this pattern, a mutation occurs in a cell of the developing organism sometime after fertilization. Thus as cells are multiplying, some will begin to reproduce with the mutation while others continue to multiply normally. The outcome is a person with "mosaicism"—some normal and some abnormal cells. Whether the gametes are affected will dictate inheritance to the next generation. Thus the term *germline mosaicism* is used to indicate inheritability of the trait. With germline mosaicism, parents appear normal but have abnormal gametes. The challenge, clinically, is to identify the condition as inheritable. If normal-appearing parents have a first child with a condition such as achondroplasia, which is normally autosomal dominant, the clinician would deduce that the achondroplasia was not inherited in an autosomal dominant manner (in which case one parent would have had the disorder), so it must be a new mutation (usually with normal parents) and germline mosaicism must be considered. The first child may have a new mutation, but the risk of recurrence in a second offspring is not zero, but rather, greater as an inherited condition with a high risk of appearance in subsequent children. It is because of such situations that genetic testing of parents is important to help determine the risk to subsequent children.

Uniparental Disomy

Generally, children receive one chromosome from each parental pair at the time of fertilization. If, by some chance, the child receives two copies of one chromosome of a pair from one parent and none from the other parent, uniparental disomy has occurred. The result is that the child will be homozygous for every gene located on that chromosome, which increases the possibilities of autosomal recessive disorders. The process has been described in some patients with cystic fibrosis. The same process also may result in either Prader-Willi or Angelman syndrome, which involve the same gene loci but differ depending on whether the copies are from the mother or the father (Nicholls, Saitoh, & Horsthemke, 1998).

Mitochondrial DNA Inheritance

Mitochondria in cells also have DNA (mtDNA). Unlike chromosomal DNA, mtDNA is circular and has 13 genes. All inherited mtDNA comes from the ovum—thus it has a maternal transmission pattern. Because each cell has more than one mitochondrion, there are more opportunities for mutations and also for variable expressivity; if many normal mitochondria are present, the effects from the aberrant mtDNA may be minimal. Several biopsies of different tissues will be subjected to both enzymatic and DNA analyses for diagnosis of mtDNA-related diseases. Although rare, mitochondrial diseases do play a role in some more common conditions such as one form of deafness. Hair shaft and pigmented skin lesions have been reported in children with mitochondrial diseases (Bodemer et al, 1999).

Teratogens

Although not strictly genetic in origin, teratogens are often discussed with genetic disorders because the differential diagnosis includes factors that affect the embryo after fertilization, as well as those that affect the DNA of the germ cells or their coming together with fertilization. Fetal alcohol syndrome is an example of a condition in this category. Viral diseases such as rubella, certain drugs, and environmental toxins such as mercury are also considered teratogens.

HUMAN GENOME PROJECT

The Human Genome Project (HGP) is an international effort begun in 1990 with the following goals:

- Sequence the entire genome by 2003 (the sequence is now publicly available)
- Identify genes and their function
- Expand database and data analysis capabilities
- Study the ethical, legal, and social implications of current and anticipated information and technology outcomes of the HGP

Final sequencing of the genome is completed; however, the remaining challenges include identifying all of the genes, understanding their function, and delineating the complex interactions between genes and their environment (Johnson & Robin, 2000). Knowledge about genetics for delivery of primary care clinical services is increasingly important. Nurse practitioners (NPs) must have a firm grasp on genetic principles and, at a minimum, meet the core competencies for all health care professionals developed by a coalition of member organizations representing nursing, medicine, psychology, genetic counseling, and others (National Coalition for Health Professional Education in Genetics [NCHPEG]). The three basic competencies are as follows:

- Appreciate the limitations of one's own genetic expertise
- Understand the social and psychologic implications of genetic services
- Know how and when to make a referral to a genetics professional

In addition, there are detailed recommendations for knowledge, skills, and attitudes that all health professionals need "to prepare for the reality of tomorrow" (NCHPEG, 2000). Finally, the resultant ethical and legal issues will continue to provide formidable challenges for society. NPs must continue to be a part of the societal debate and resolution.

ETHICAL ISSUES

Since 1990, largely due to the work of the HGP, the ability to diagnose a hereditary condition for those who are currently symptomatic or who are presymptomatic, the ability to identify those who are carriers of a genetic condition, and the ability to determine susceptibility to a genetic condition have increased dramatically. However, the availability of this technology raises significant ethical issues. The HGP was concerned about these issues from the beginning and has a branch specifically devoted to oversight of these concerns (the Ethical, Legal, and Social Initiative [ELSI]).

Maintenance of confidentiality is a challenge. The presence of genetic information in the medical record or health insurance diagnostic database and the potential to secure genetic information by accessing DNA databases such as newborn screening specimens mandates policies to maintain the integrity of these records. The potential for discrimination on the basis of genetic diagnosis must be avoided.

During routine testing, it is also possible to discover unanticipated information, for instance regarding the parentage of the child being tested. Situations such as misattribution of paternity and children being raised by nonbiologic parents may be discovered. There is not agreement about whether these findings should be routinely disclosed. Prior agreement in the consent process might assist in the decision about whether to disclose or not.

The availability of presymptomatic testing for conditions that may not become apparent until adulthood such as diabetes, Huntington disease, and breast cancer has raised another set of questions. Should children and adolescents be tested for such conditions? Generally, it is recommended that genetic testing for late-onset conditions be deferred until adulthood when individuals, rather than their parents, can make the decision unless there is evidence that early diagnosis can result in treatment strategies that will alter the progression of the disease (American Academy of Pediatrics [AAP], Committee on Bioethics, 2001).

The ability to screen for a large number of genetic disorders via the newborn screening process has increased the dialogue about which conditions should be included. Because these programs are organized by and paid for through state government, there is large variability in required tests between states. Three principles have been suggested by the Institute of Medicine (IOM) to be used in making decisions about the introduction or continuation of tests:

- Identification of the genetic condition must provide a clear benefit to the child.
- A system must be in place to confirm the diagnosis.

- Treatment and follow-up must be available for affected infants (IOM, 1994).

Mandatory screening for cystic fibrosis and congenital adrenal hyperplasia has been the focus of recent debate.

These are only a few of the ethical issues under current discussion. NPs must be part of the ongoing debate and be aware of the issues, policies, and laws as they work with families who are trying to make decisions.

ASSESSMENT

The NP identifies possible genetic disorders by using the same skills as those used for other pediatric health problems: knowledge of risk factors, collection of a good history, and a complete physical examination augmented with appropriate laboratory or other studies. After the assessment, the NP or other provider determines the operative genetic mechanism and develops and implements a plan of care for the patient and family with consideration of individual, family, and cultural factors. Box 41-1 identifies some common features of children with genetic disorders that should lead the clinician to explore issues of possible genetic problems in the child and family.

Risk Factors

Risk factors include the following:

- Family history of known genetic disorder or recurrent pathologic condition
- Malformations
- Mental retardation
- Metabolic disorders
- Delayed development of secondary sex characteristics
- Sensory deficits
- Progressive disorders
- Neuromuscular disorders
- Affective disorders (e.g., schizophrenia)
- Presence of birth defects
- Mental retardation or learning problems
- Repeated spontaneous abortions or stillbirths
- Maternal factors, including alcohol or drug exposure, medication exposure, age older than 35 years, environmental or occupational toxin exposure
- Family ethnic background (Table 41-1)

BOX 41-1 *Features Suggesting a Genetic Disorder*

Mental retardation/developmental delays
Seizures with mental retardation
Severe hypotonia in infancy
Loss of developmental milestones
Short stature
Failure to thrive/growth retardation
Microcephaly
Dysmorphic features
Two or more physical birth defects
Ambiguous genitalia
Pigmentary skin lesions
Ocular findings or blindness
Deafness

Adapted from Pacific Northwest Regional Genetics Group: *Practical genetics for primary care*, Portland, OR, 1996, Oregon Health Sciences Center, Pacific Northwest Regional Genetics Group.

History

The history of genetic diseases usually includes the following main areas: family history of the disease using a pedigree format, environmental and occupational history, reproductive history, dietary history, medical history of the child, and developmental data. (See Figs. 41-2 and 41-3 for an example of the pedigree notation format.) The pedigree provides a visual map of the occurrence of specific traits and helps identify other family members who might be at risk. Screening questions for genetic disorders that should be asked of all patients are included in Table 41-2. When a genetic disorder is suspected, the history must become more specific, as outlined in Table 41-3. Questions need to address the following:

- A family history is needed to identify family members with conditions that may be genetically transmitted. A pedigree helps display the potential pattern of

TABLE 41-1 *Genetic Risks Associated with Ethnic Background*

Ethnic Background	Genetic Disorder at Higher Risk
Northern European	Cystic fibrosis, phenylketonuria
Jewish (Ashkenazi descent)	Tay-Sachs, Canavan, Gaucher
West African	Sickle cell, sickle cell–hemoglobin C
Mediterranean	ß-thalassemia, sickle cell
French-Canadian	Tay-Sachs, branched-chain ketoaciduria

Instructions:
Key should contain all information relevant to interpretation of pedigree (e.g., define shading)
For clinical (nonpublished) pedigrees, include:
 a) family names/initials, when appropriate
 b) name and title of person recording pedigree
 c) historian (person relaying family history information)
 d) date of intake/update
Recommended order of information placed below symbol (below to lower right, if necessary):
 a) age/date of birth or age at death
 b) evaluation
 c) pedigree number (e.g., I-1, I-2, I-3)

	Male	Female	Sex Unknown	Comments
1. Individual	b. 1925	30 yr	4 mo	Assign gender by phenotype.
2. Affected individual	■	●	◆	Key/legend used to define shading or other fill (e.g., hatches, dots, etc.).
				With ≥2 conditions, the individuals symbol should be partitioned accordingly, each segment shaded with a different fill and defined in legend.
3. Multiple individuals, number known	5	5	5	Number of siblings written inside symbol. (Affected individuals should not be grouped.)
4. Multiple individuals, number unknown	n	n	n	n used in place of ? mark.
5a. Deceased individual	d. 35 yr	d. 4 mo		Use of cross (†) may be confused with symbol for elevated positive (+). If known, write d. with age at death below symbol.
5b. Stillbirth (SB)	SB 28 wk	SB 30 wk	SB 34 wk	Birth of a dead child with gestational age noted.
6. Pregnancy (P)	P b.1925	P 30 yr	P 4 mo	Gestational age and karyotype (if known) below symbol. Light shading can be used for affected and defined in key/legend.
7a. Proband	P↗■	P↗●	P↗◇	First affected family member coming to medical attention.
7b. Consultand	↗□	↗○		Individual(s) seeking genetic couseling/testing.

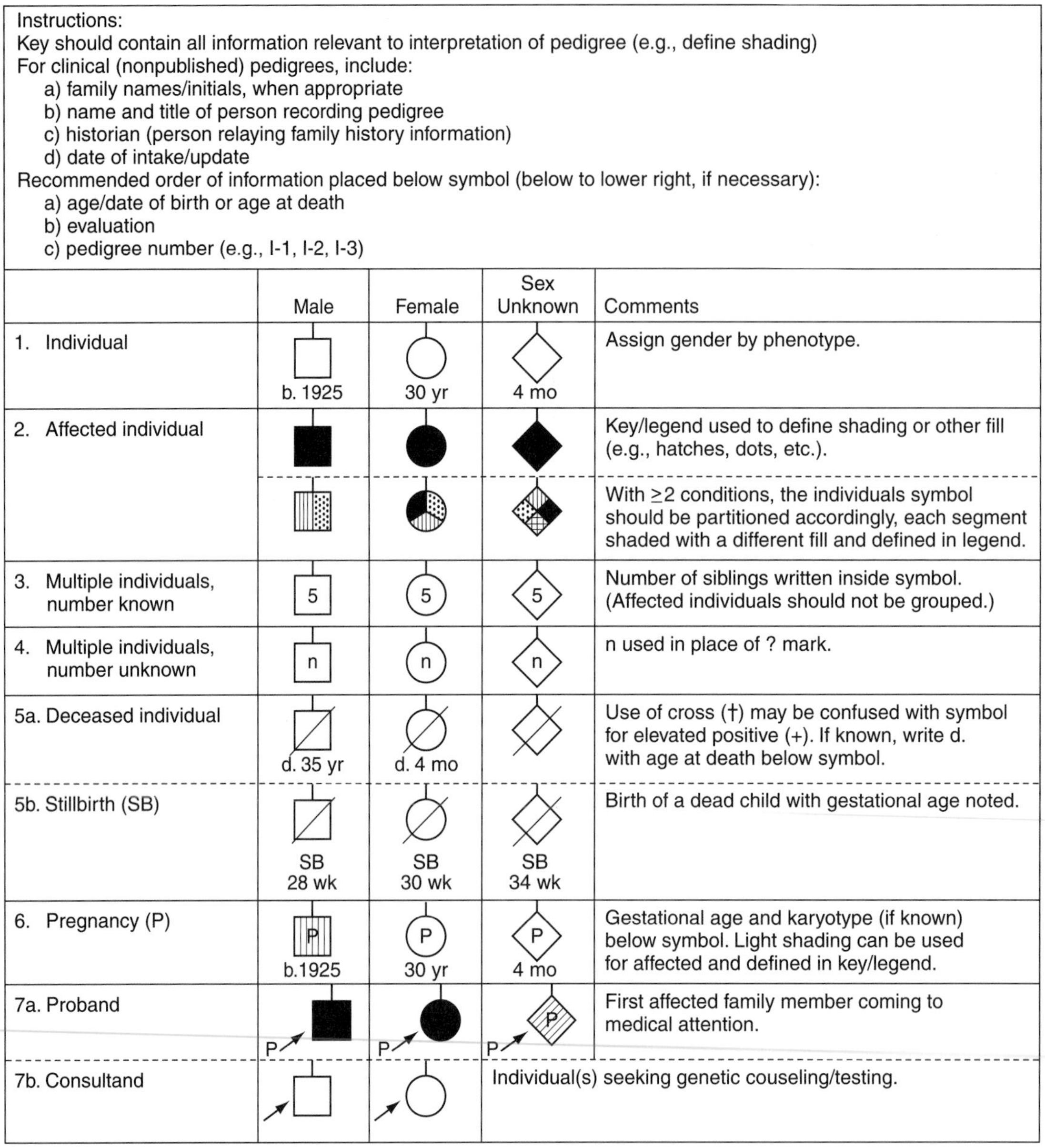

FIGURE 41-2 Pedigree model. Common pedigree symbols, definitions, and abbreviations. (Adapted from Bennett R et al: Recommendations for standardized human pedigree nomenclature, *Am J Hum Genet* 56:745-752, 1995.)

inheritance and visualize the relationships among affected family members. Past and current health of each person in the pedigree, birth histories of other family members, and mental retardation or learning problems of family members are all important areas to explore. Consanguinity should be addressed but is considered less of a risk factor than previously thought.
• The environmental and occupational history is important to know if teratogenic factors might be involved.

• The mother's reproductive history may give information about malformations, genetic conditions, or infectious diseases transmitted to other offspring. Her pregnancy and delivery of the child in question may give other information to determine whether the fetus was affected or whether the condition was a result of trauma, infection, or some other factor occurring during the pregnancy or delivery. If the child was well throughout pregnancy and delivery, one might suspect a postnatal event.

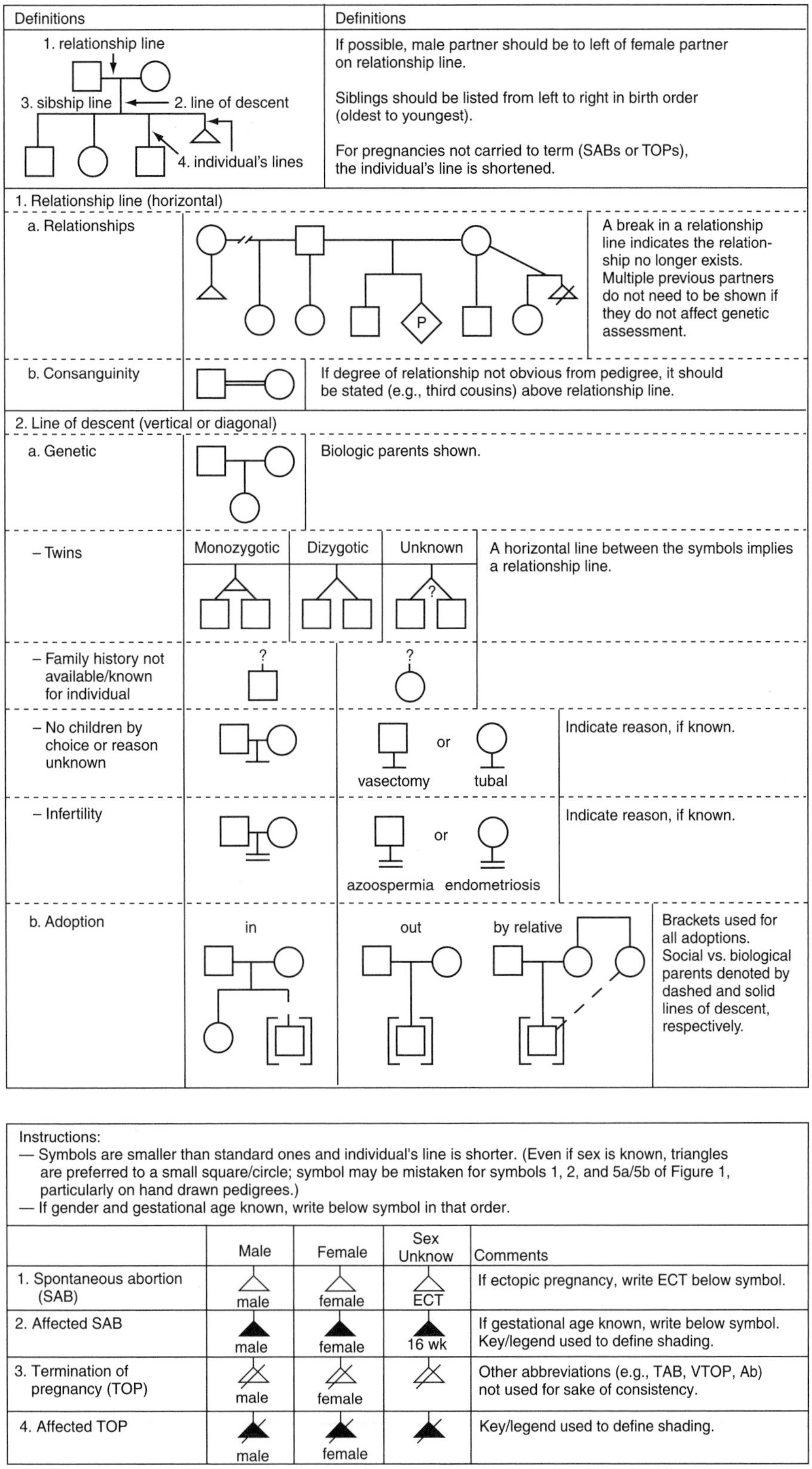

FIGURE 41-3 Pedigree line definitions. (Adapted from Bennett R et al: Recommendations for standardized human pedigree nomenclature, *Am J Hum Genet* 56:745-752, 1995.)

TABLE 41-2 ***General Screening for Genetic Conditions: The History***

Question	Rationale/Comments
Has anyone in the family had a birth defect?	To identify conditions that affect others in the family. If answer is yes, try to get more information about the nature of the defect.
Is there anyone in the family with a stillborn baby or baby who died early in life?	To identify unrecognized genetic disorders. Babies who died very early may have inheritable metabolic disorders. Distinguish from sudden infant death syndrome.
Is there any chance that you and your partner are blood related? Is this pregnancy a product of incest?	Consanguinity of partners closer than first cousins is a risk factor for autosomal recessive disorders. If yes, recommend genetics consultation.
Are there any diseases or traits that run in your family?	Significant if early onset, two or more close relatives affected. Genetic heart disease and genetic cancer risks are important. If yes, recommend genetic consultation and monitoring.
Have you or any of your parents or siblings had three or more miscarriages?	May indicate a chromosome translocation. If yes, order a karyotype of the mother or father (or both).
Does anyone in the family have mental retardation?	Look for multiple members affected and associated with dysmorphic features. If yes, recommend genetic consultation.
What is your ethnic background? Your partner's?	Consider ethnic risk factors and screen if at risk.

Physical Examination

When a genetic disease is being considered, the physical examination focuses on growth, major and minor anomalies, and comparisons with family members. Any major anomaly can have a genetic cause. Three minor anomalies should raise the suspicion of a major anomaly and a genetic disorder.

First, general appearance and familial similarities are assessed. Body size and proportions, measurements and percentiles, and a careful assessment of all systems constitute the remainder of the examination.

Common minor anomalies are identified in Box 41-2. Box 41-3 lists various anomalies by body parts. *Smith's Recognizable Patterns of Human Malformations* (Jones, 1997) includes tables on the size, length, and shape of various body parts that can be used to validate observations presumed to represent pathology.

Dysmorphic features may be recognized and can result from the following:

- *Deformation*—abnormal shape or position of body part caused by external mechanical forces (e.g., clubfoot)
- *Disruption*—defect of organ or large body part caused by external disruption of originally normal process (e.g., amniotic bands)
- *Dysplasia*—abnormal organization of cells into tissues (e.g., polycystic kidneys)
- *Malformation*—abnormal development of an organ or large body part from an intrinsically abnormal process (e.g., cleft palate)

Usually, malformations are genetic in origin with multiple tissues affected. Visual recognition is a major factor in diagnosing genetic diseases. The NP can hone skills by reviewing pictures of patients with various disorders and consulting with experts.

Developmental Assessment

Many genetic disorders cause some degree of mental retardation and central nervous system effects. Developmental assessment is indicated.

Laboratory Studies

Biochemical Studies

Many screening tests are available to check for inborn errors of metabolism. Such tests include those for phenylketonuria (PKU), galactosemia, and others. See Chapter 39 for further discussion.

Molecular Analyses (DNA Studies)

Blood tests to screen for sickle cell disease, the thalassemias, and Tay-Sachs disease are commonly used. Molecular genetic methods are increasingly being used for many disorders, such as cystic fibrosis. Generally, the tests must be ordered with some specificity. Linkage analysis, direct mutation analysis, and molecular cytogenetic analyses are all types of DNA studies. Each has its own advantages and disadvantages (AAP, Committee on Genetics, 2000; Hoyme, 2004).

TABLE 41-3 *Specific Genetic History Questions*

Topic	Specific Items of History
Family history: Helps identify family members with conditions that may be genetically transmitted	1. The pedigree should focus on at least three generations and look for people with similar characteristics. 2. Consanguinity of partners (closer than first cousins) is very important. 3. Note the past and current health of each person listed on the pedigree. 4. Note the age of onset for family members' illnesses. 5. Note multiple miscarriages, stillbirths, and anomalies among families. 6. Family members with learning disabilities or mental retardation are important to document.
Environmental and occupational history	Exposure to environmental toxins, alcohol, cigarette smoke, drugs, or radiation that might affect offspring
Reproductive history: Helps identify malformations, genetic conditions, or infectious diseases transmitted from mother to child 1. Maternal medical history 2. Prenatal history 3. Pregnancy and delivery history	1. Maternal medical history: • Uterine anomalies • Maternal illnesses and diseases (e.g., phenylketonuria, diabetes) • Immunization status 2. Prenatal history. The reproductive history should list every pregnancy, stillbirth, and abortion. Fetuses with significant chromosomal disorders are often aborted, and 5%-7% of stillbirths and perinatal deaths are related to genetic problems: • Recurrent miscarriages • Parity • Advanced maternal or paternal age • Complications of pregnancy • Polyhydramnios or oligohydramnios • Fetal movements • Fetal growth assessments • Prenatal screening results 3. Pregnancy and delivery history: • Breech position • Birth measurements • Gestational age • Results of newborn screening tests • Presence of three or more minor anomalies in neonate • Failure of neonate to adapt to extrauterine life
Dietary history: Helps identify infants with single-gene–related metabolic disorders	1. Infant feeding behavior 2. Formula or food intolerance 3. Temporal relation of symptoms to meals 4. Relation of signs and symptoms to types of food
Medical history of affected child	Use routine past medical history questions—history and current status of illnesses, hospitalizations, surgeries, allergies, injuries, immunizations. List all health care providers involved with the child's care.
Developmental history	1. Achievements of milestones 2. Speech and language development 3. School performance 4. Developmental evaluations 5. Growth

Cytogenetics: Chromosome Studies

Chromosome tests may be needed to identify specific genetic diseases. Fluorescent in situ hybridization (FISH) combines elements of standard cytogenetic technique with molecular technology; probes for specific, extremely small chromosome abnormalities are used. For instance, FISH analysis might identify the deletion of chromosome site 15q11-q13 associated with Prader-Willi.

Imaging Studies

Radiographs and other imaging studies are used to identify skeletal, central nervous system, cardiac, and other anomalies.

BOX 41-2 *Minor Malformations and Variations of Normal*

Large fontanel
Epicanthal folds
Hair whorls
Widow's peak
Low posterior hairline
Preauricular tags or pits
Minor ear anomalies
Protruding ears
Rotated ears
Low-set ears
Darwinian tubercle (blunt point protruding from upper edge of helix)
Digital anomalies
Clinodactyly (curved finger)
Camptodactyly (bent finger)
Syndactyly (webbed finger)
Transverse palmar crease
Shawl scrotum
Redundant umbilicus
Widespread nipples
Supernumerary nipples

From Wardinsky T: Visual clues to diagnosis of birth defects and genetic disease, *J Pediatr Health Care* 8:63-73, 1994.

BOX 41-3 *Malformations of the Body*

Central nervous system (not mental deficiency)
- Hypotonic
- Hypertonic
- Ataxia
- Seizures

Deafness
Brain: major anomalies
- Anencephaly
- Encephalocele
- Hydrocephalus
- Microcephaly
- Macrocephaly
- Meningomyelocele

Cranium
- Craniosynostosis
- Occiput shapes, flat or prominent
- Delayed fontanel closures
- Frontal bossing

Scalp and facial hair patterning
- Multiple hair whorls
- Anterior upsweep
- Posterior midline scalp defects

Facies
- Flat
- Round
- Broad
- Triangular
- Masklike
- Coarse

Ocular region
- Hypotelorism
- Hypertelorism
- Short palpebral fissures
- Inner canthus placement
- Inner epicanthal folds
- Slanted palpebral fissures
- Depth of orbital ridges
- Eye prominence
- Periorbital fullness
- Eyebrow shape and extension
- Ptosis
- Nystagmus
- Strabismus

Eye
- Blue sclera
- Myopia
- Microphthalmos
- Colobomas of iris
- Patterning or color of iris
- Glaucoma
- Keratoconus
- Microcornea
- Corneal opacity
- Lens discolorations/opacities
- Retinal pigmentation

Nose
- Nasal bridge shape
- Short with or without anteverted nostrils
- Hypoplasia of nares
- Prominent nose
- Choanal atresia

Maxilla and mandible
- Malar hypoplasia
- Maxillary hypoplasia often with narrow or high arched palate
- Micrognathia
- Prognathism

BOX 41-3 *Malformations of the Body—cont'd*

Oral region and mouth
- Cleft lip with or without cleft palate
- Abnormal philtrum
- Full lips
- Downturning mouth corners
- Microstomia
- Macrostomia
- Cleft palate or bifid uvula with cleft in lip
- Macroglossia/microglossia
- Hypertrophied alveolar ridges

Teeth
- Adontia
- Hypodontia (including conical teeth)
- Enamel hypoplasia
- Caries
- Early loss
- Irregular placement
- Late eruption
- Other tooth anomalies

External ears
- Low set
- Malformed auricles
- Preauricular tags or pits

Neck, thorax, and vertebrae
- Web neck
- Short neck
- Nipple anomaly
- Clavicle anomalies
- Pectus excavatum or carinatum
- Small thoracic cage
- Rib defects
- Scoliosis
- Other vertebral defects

Limbs
- Arachnodactyly
- Short limbs
- Limb reductions
- Small hands or feet
- Clinodactyly of fifth fingers
- Thumb hypoplasia
- Radius hypoplasia
- Metacarpal hypoplasia
- Polydactyly
- Broad thumb or toe (or both)
- Syndactyly
- Elbow dysplasia
- Patellar dysplasia

Limbs: nails, creases, dermatoglyphics
- Nail hypoplasia or dysplasia
- Single crease (simian)
- Dermal ridge pattern abnormalities

Limbs: joints
- Joint limitations/contractures
- Clubfoot
- Clenched hand
- Joint hypermobility or lax ligaments (or both)
- Joint dislocations

Skin and hair
- Loose/redundant skin
- Pigmentation alterations
- Ichthyotic changes
- Hemangiomas and telangiectasias
- Dimples
- Alopecia
- Hirsutism
- Assorted abnormalities of hair (amount, quality, distribution, color)

Cardiac anomalies

Abdominal
- Hernias
- Hepatosplenomegaly
- Pyloric stenosis
- Incomplete rotation of colon
- Single umbilical artery

Renal
- Kidney malformations
- Renal insufficiency

Genital
- Hypospadias or ambiguous external genitalia
- Micropenis
- Cryptorchidism
- Hypoplasia of labia majora
- Anal defects

Endocrine and metabolic
- Hypothyroidism
- Hypogonadism
- Other endocrine abnormalities
- Hypocalcemia/hypercalcemia
- Hyperlipidemia

Immunoglobulin
- Immunoglobulin deficiency

Hematology-oncology
- Anemia
- Thrombocytopenia
- Lymphoreticular malignancy
- Other malignancies

Unusual growth patterns
- Obesity
- Early macrosomia
- Asymmetry

Adapted from Jones K: *Smith's recognizable patterns of human malformations*, ed 5, Philadelphia, 1997, WB Saunders.

Photography

Photographs provide a visual record of facial and other anatomic variations. They may also be useful in identifying other family members with similar characteristics.

MANAGEMENT STRATEGIES

Primary care management of children with genetic disorders includes a variety of strategies, depending on whether a specific diagnosis has been determined.

Prenatal Screening

Prenatal screening can be done for many diseases if the family history indicates the possibility of a specific disease appearing in offspring. Routine prenatal carrier screening is done for sickle cell disease, Tay-Sachs disease, and the thalassemias. Prenatal carrier screening is done to provide parents with reproductive alternatives. Childbearing women should be referred to obstetric or genetic clinics for prenatal screening and diagnosis. Chorionic villus biopsy sampling for diagnosis of some conditions is done at 8 to 12 weeks of gestation at some specialized centers, and amniocentesis is done at 14 to 20 weeks of gestation. By the fourteenth to sixteenth week of gestation, many imaging studies can also be performed to look for structural anomalies. Maternal serum α-fetoprotein can also be analyzed at 14 weeks. Elevated levels have been associated with neural tube defects, whereas decreased levels have been associated with chromosomal abnormalities. Prenatal diagnosis gives the family information to make decisions, such as possible termination of pregnancies with affected fetuses, artificial insemination or deferral of childbearing, or special preparations at childbirth.

Newborn Genetic Screening

Newborn genetic screening for a variety of metabolic diseases is done routinely (see Box 39-2). The diseases screened for include PKU, hypothyroidism, galactosemia, homocystinuria, maple syrup urine disease, tyrosinemia, sickle cell disease, and others. Different states include slightly different groups of diseases in their panels. The NP should be sure that the routine newborn statewide screening panel blood test is completed correctly.

Screening for other diseases is done if the child falls into a specific target population. Screening of target populations for Tay-Sachs disease and the thalassemias should not be overlooked. Black infants should be screened for sickle cell disease. Screening of newborns is now recommended because prophylactic antibiotics can decrease infections and sickling episodes.

Genetic Disorder Diagnosis

Careful history taking and physical examinations of children should help NPs identify children with genetic diseases. Newborns with obvious defects or dysmorphic features should be evaluated. Children with two major, one major and two minor, or three minor anomalies with other indicators as noted in Box 41-4 should be evaluated for a genetic condition with karyotype analysis. Making the diagnosis may also identify the etiology and the risks for future pregnancies, information that is important for families to have.

In the case of a stillbirth or neonatal death, the infant's features should be documented—preferably photographed. A karyotype on blood and establishment of a fibroblast culture are also important. Head and renal ultrasound should be done if no autopsy is performed.

Children and their families should be referred for diagnosis if genetic disease is suspected. Establishing the correct diagnosis is important for the family and the NP. The recurrence risk, prognosis given the natural history of the condition, guide to appropriate laboratory testing, plan of treatment and management, and facilitation of family coping all require a knowledge of the nature of the disorder.

Telling new parents that their child may have a genetic disorder needs to happen as soon as possible—even if a diagnosis cannot be confirmed. It should be done in a quiet, comfortable place when both parents are present, by

BOX 41-4 *Indications for Karyotype Analysis*

Suspected chromosomal problem
Two major malformations
One major and two minor malformations
Ambiguous genitalia
Congenital heart disease
Hypotonia
Malformed stillborns and normal stillborns when demise is of undetermined etiology
Mental retardation or developmental delay
Growth retardation or short stature
Couple with two or more miscarriages or infertility

Adapted from Pacific Northwest Regional Genetics Group: *Practical genetics for primary care,* Portland, OR, 1996, Oregon Health Sciences Center, Pacific Northwest Regional Genetics Group.

someone with credibility. If possible, the baby should be present and referred to by name. The discussion should include some positive points, as well as the problems to be faced. A follow-up phone call should be planned and additional sources of information identified, including contact with other parents. The parents should have some uninterrupted time with their baby.

Genetic Counseling

Genetic counseling involves open communication with families who have received the diagnosis of a genetic disease. A nondirective approach is desired. Its goals include helping the family to do the following:

- Understand the diagnosis, its course, and its management
- Appreciate the way heredity influences the disorder and the risks of recurrence and carrier status to specific family members
- Understand the alternatives available to reduce the risk of recurrence
- Choose the course of action that is appropriate in view of the risks, family ethics and values, and family goals
- Adjust as well as possible to the disorder, its prognosis, and the risks of recurrence

The process takes time and may require many visits (Hall, 2004; Johnson & Brensinger, 2000). Generally, genetic counseling is provided by specialists. Ethical genetic counseling takes into consideration the principles of beneficence (helping the patient and family) and nonmaleficence (do no harm).

The NP's role in genetic counseling is to perform the following:

- Identify individuals at risk for genetic disorders
- Teach children and families about the genetic counseling process
- Initiate referrals with screening pedigrees, medical records, and appropriate histories and physical examinations
- Evaluate the family's understanding of genetic counseling and provide support as the family makes decisions based on genetic testing information

All families with genetic diseases should receive genetic counseling. The extent of counseling needed determines whether the primary care provider can manage the child and family or whether referral to a genetic clinic would be preferable.

Primary Health Care of Children with Genetic Disorders

Health supervision, screening for complications, and management of the health of the child given the genetic condition at hand are all important. Families with a child with a genetic condition or chronic disease face many challenges and stresses. Stresses can be emotional, social, and financial and demand that families deal with bureaucracies in the health care delivery, education, and health insurance systems (AAP, Committee on Children with Disabilities, 1997).

Primary care and chronic disease management need to be integrated. Monitoring for complications that may emerge is essential. The American Academy of Pediatrics (AAP) has developed an example of health supervision guidelines for children with Down syndrome (AAP, Committee on Genetics, 2001a). It incorporates developmental, psychologic, educational, and medical components. Monitoring for high-risk conditions, including congenital heart disease, thyroid disorders, hearing loss, atlantoaxial subluxation, ophthalmic abnormalities, and growth and development, needs to be integrated into the plan for primary health care. There are similar guidelines for the care of children with neurofibromatosis type 1, Turner syndrome, achondroplasia, sickle cell disease, Marfan syndrome, William syndrome, and fragile X syndrome (AAP, Committee on Bioethics, 2001; AAP, Committee on Genetics, 1995a, 1995b, 1995c, 1996a, 1996b, 2001a, 2001b, 2002). Key features for several genetic disorders are listed in Box 41-5. They illustrate the integration of monitoring for the physiologic, developmental, and psychologic consequences that may occur.

The family's adjustment is a long-term process that requires monitoring and support with new information and resources as the child grows and changes. Some areas to include in planning care are as follows:

- Health education:
  - Educate the family about the condition and its management, including family responsibilities.
  - Answer questions about health care services, and respect the confidentiality of the patient and parents so that information is not shared with insurance companies, employers, or other family members without the client's consent.
  - Provide affected children, within developmental limits, with health education and support to understand and manage their own care.
- Health care services:
  - Provide primary care for health promotion and disease prevention services.
  - Monitor the affected child for growth, development, emergence of new disease manifestations, and complications.
  - Assess the child's developmental age, and recommend appropriate interventions.

BOX 41-5 *Primary Care Monitoring of Children with Common Genetic Disorders*

This box highlights some of the specific monitoring that can be done by primary care providers. It does not serve as a comprehensive guide and assumes the following:

- General health supervision guidelines for all children will be followed as much as possible.
- Genetic counseling will be provided to all families.
- Family support and counseling services will be provided.
- Support groups that might be helpful will be identified for the family.
- Long-term planning will occur.
- Sexual and reproductive issues will be addressed with the child approaching adolescence, including help for both the child directly and the parents.
- School placement and ongoing educational evaluations will occur.
- Care will be coordinated with a clinic specializing in services for children with the specific condition.
- Developmental and behavioral issues will be addressed, with referrals as needed.

Down Syndrome

Cardiac echocardiography: at diagnosis and follow-up as needed if defects identified*
Screen for mitral valve prolapse at adolescence†
Hearing: at 9 mo (or sooner if concerns) and follow-up as needed* (50%-70% will have hearing loss)
Ophthalmologic: at 4 mo (sooner if concerns), 12 mo, 24 mo, then every 2 yr and follow-up as needed*
Thyroid: newborn screen and every 6 mo to age 2 yr, yearly to age 5 yr, then as indicated*
Cervical spine for atlantoaxial instability: at 3 yr, 12 yr, and 18 yr*
Down clinic assessment at 4 mo, 12 mo, then annually to 6 yr, then biannually‡
Early intervention services‡ for developmental delays
Supplemental Security Income referral‡
Use Down syndrome growth charts to evaluate shorter stature and increased weight† and manage obesity
Screen for hip dislocation through age 10 yr†

Neurofibromatosis

To be done at initial evaluation with follow-up as indicated:
Head and spine MRI at diagnosis*
Hearing*§
Blood pressure*§ (renal artery stenosis, aortic stenosis, pheochromocytomas, adrenal tumors, vascular hypertrophic lesions)
Imaging studies of identified affected areas as indicated*§
Vision screening§
Skin evaluations for new neurofibromas and progression of lesions§
Skeletal evaluations for scoliosis, limb abnormalities, localized hypertrophy§

Turner Syndrome

To be done at initial evaluation with follow-up as indicated:††
Cardiac,* echocardiography, or MRI for aortic abnormalities¶
Renal sonogram*¶
Blood pressure because hypertension is common, even without cardiac or renal abnormalities¶
Hearing*¶
Karyotype*¶
Developmental assessment at 3 yr (or sooner if indicated) for mild learning disabilities*
Prepubertal pelvic ultrasonography at time of referral to endocrinology*
Possible referral for growth hormone therapy in mid to late childhood*
Thyroid function at diagnosis and every 1-2 yr because 10%-30% have primary hypothyroidism¶
Vision screening because strabismus, amblyopia, ptosis are common¶
Orthopedic evaluation of developmental dislocated hip, scoliosis¶
Obesity monitoring and management¶
Lymphedema monitoring and management¶

BOX 41-5 *Primary Care Monitoring of Children with Common Genetic Disorders—cont'd*

Short stature management, including growth hormone therapy if the girl drops below the 5th percentile for the normal female growth curve, estrogen therapy for induction of puberty and feminization¶
Fertility counseling and family planning because some women with Turner syndrome can achieve pregnancy without ovarian function via donors¶

Achondroplasia‡‡

MRI of foramen magnum at diagnosis; if small, repeat at 3-6 mo and similarly thereafter; if normal, repeat at 1 yr*
Ultrasonography/CT or MRI of brain at diagnosis; repeat if head growth exceeds achondroplasia growth curves or if symptoms of increased intracranial pressure are present*
Physical therapy to focus on development of gross and fine motor skills*
Monitoring of upper airway restriction, obstructive sleep apnea, and potential for cor pulmonale*
Orthopedic evaluation if bowing of lower extremities progresses because of fibular overgrowth*

Hemophilia and von Willebrand Disease

Developmental screen as follow-up to head trauma**
Adequate protein and calcium intake for bone formation**
Safety: protective helmets, knee pads as needed**
ID bracelet with diagnosis, treatment product, blood type; remember to update annually**
Noncontact sports participation**
Regular dental hygiene care; may need replacement products for dental extractions**
Annual hematocrit**
Annual screen for microscopic hematuria**
Hemophilia management through a hemophilia treatment center

---

*Toomey K: Medical genetics for the practitioner, *Pediatr Rev* 17:163-174, 1996.
†Vessey J: Down syndrome. In Jackson P, Vessey J, editors: *Primary care of the child with a chronic condition*, ed 2, St Louis, 1996, Mosby, pp 371-379.
‡American Academy of Pediatrics, Committee on Genetics: Health supervision for children with Down syndrome, *Pediatrics* 107: 442-449, 2001.
§American Academy of Pediatrics, Committee on Genetics: Health supervision for children with neurofibromatosis, *Pediatrics* 96: 368-372, 1995.
¶Rosenfeld R et al: Recommendations for diagnosis, treatment, and management of individuals with Turner syndrome, *Endocrinologist* 4:351-358, 1994.
**Dragone M, Karp S: Bleeding disorders. In Jackson P, Vessey J, editors: *Primary care of the child with a chronic condition*, ed 2, St Louis, 1996, Mosby, pp 145-170.
††American Academy of Pediatrics, Committee on Genetics: Health supervision for children with Turner syndrome, *Pediatrics* 96:1166-1173, 1995.
‡‡American Academy of Pediatrics, Committee on Genetics: Health supervision for children with achondroplasia, *Pediatrics* 95:443-451, 1995.
CT, Computed tomography; *MRI*, magnetic resonance imaging.

   - Work with the family regarding long-term planning for the child's care, including attention to psychologic, developmental, social, and sexual factors.
   - For conditions without treatment, help families with support for ongoing management, decision making related to experimental treatments that may be offered, and assistance in deciding when residential care or withdrawal of supportive care might be considered.
   - Be an advocate for the family with schools, insurance companies, and others.
   - Support and monitor the care of children with inborn errors of metabolism who need treatment to decrease the offending substrate, increase a deficient substance, provide an enzymatic cofactor, or a combination of these.
- Resources:
   - Know community resources for specific problems that the family may face.
   - Direct the family to financial resources or social services to be sure that necessary care is provided.

  - Direct the family to support groups and local resources.
  - Provide the family with written materials from disease-related organizations.
  - Refer to early intervention and other special educational programs as needed.
  - Direct the family to respite care services as needed.
- Family coping:
  - Evaluate all family members, including siblings and grandparents, for their responses to the child with the diagnosed condition.
  - Support the family through the grief process.
  - Evaluate the parents' coping skills, family dynamics, and psychosocial responses.
  - Assess the adjustment of siblings.

Care needs to be especially vigilant during times of transition. Parents need a support person who will listen to their concerns, joys, and sorrows over time. The NP can be that person.

GENETIC DISORDERS

Various genetic disorders are described in this section. Information is summarized in Tables 41-4 and 41-5.

TABLE 41-4 *Inheritance Patterns with Examples*

Inheritance Pattern	Characteristics	Examples
Chromosomal Abnormalities		
Changes in number of chromosomes	Generally major anomalies and multisystem problems with the trisomies.	Trisomies 21, 18, 13
	Sex chromosome disorders cause sterility and changes in growth patterns. Other changes may be more subtle.	XXY (Klinefelter) XO (Turner)
Changes in structure of chromosomes	Changes may include deletions, duplications.	Cri du chat (46, XY, del [5p]) Cornelia de Lange (duplicated 3q segment), fragile X
Single-Gene Defects		
Autosomal dominant	Affected person from affected parent. Sexes equally affected. Normal offspring will have normal children.	Neurofibromatosis, osteogenesis imperfecta, achondroplasia, Huntington chorea, familial hypercholesterolemia
Autosomal recessive	Both parents heterozygous for trait. High consanguinity risk. Sexes equally affected. Newborn screening may pick up these disorders. Family history usually negative except that siblings may be affected.	Cystic fibrosis, sickle cell, Tay-Sachs, phenylketonuria
X-linked recessive	Males show trait. Female carriers usually do not show trait unless they are homozygous for the abnormal gene.	Hemophilia, Duchenne muscular dystrophy, glucose-6-phosphate dehydrogenase deficiency
Multifactorial	Familial clustering. Sex difference in frequency. No clear biochemical or molecular defect. Considerable variation in expression. Both genetic and environmental components are important.	Cardiac defects, cleft lip/palate, clubfoot, scoliosis, dislocated hip
Germline Mosaicism	Two or more cell lines with differing genotypes in an individual. Gametes of affected adult may be normal or abnormal. Consider if parents seem normal but offspring has an autosomal dominant condition.	Achondroplastic siblings from normal-appearing parents
Uniparental Disomy	Proband has two copies of a chromosome from one parent and none from the other.	Prader-Willi, Angelman
Mitochondrial DNA Disorder	Circular, double-stranded mitochondrial DNA defect, not in nuclear DNA. Variable expression depends on how many mitochondria carry defect.	Leber hereditary optic neuropathy, myoclonic epilepsy, Kearns-Sayre syndrome

TABLE 41-5 *Characteristics of Common Chromosomal Disorders*

Chromosomal Disorder	Principal Clinical Findings of the Diagnosis*
Down syndrome (trisomy 21)	Short stature, brachycephaly, small midface with upturned nose, hypoplastic frontal sinuses, speckled iris, epicanthal folds with palpebral fissures that slant down to midline, small mandible with resulting appearance of large tongue, myopia, small ears, lax joints (including atlantoaxial articulation), short broad hands and feet and digits, single palmar crease, clinodactyly, exaggerated space between great and second toes, developmental delays, hypotonia as infant, congenital heart disease At risk for leukemia, Alzheimer's disease, hypothyroidism
Turner syndrome (XO)	Fetal edema—neonatal carpal or pedal edema (or both) Short stature, sexual infantilism, low hairline, webbed neck, increased carrying angle of arms (cubitus valgus), wide-spaced nipples, horseshoe kidney At risk for bicuspid aortic valve, coarctation of aorta, problems with spatial relationships and visual problem solving, hypertension Difficulties with arithmetic Social development often impaired secondary to not understanding nonverbal communications
Klinefelter syndrome (XXY)	Postpubertal males—infertility, hypogonadism, mild mental retardation, long limbs, gynecomastia
Neurofibromatosis	More than five café au lait spots greater than 5 mm, axillary freckles, Lisch nodules, neurofibromas, optic glioma, megalencephaly At risk for pheochromocytoma, skeletal dysplasia, renovascular hypertension, mental retardation, scoliosis, compromised organs and neurologic system from neurofibroma invasion
Fragile X syndrome	Large ears, macro-orchidism, long narrow face, mental retardation, autistic behavior
Fetal alcohol syndrome	Growth deficiencies, decreased adipose tissue, mental retardation, infant irritability/child hyperactivity, poor coordination/hypotonia, microcephaly, short palpebral fissures, ptosis, retrognathia in infancy, maxillary hypoplasia, hypoplastic long or smooth philtrum, thin vermilion border of upper lip, short upturned nose, micrognathia in adolescence At risk for heart defects, myopia, small teeth with poor enamel, hypospadias, hydronephrosis, hernias

*Not all children will exhibit all findings.

Chromosomal Disorders

As described earlier, chromosomal disorders are problems of chromosome number or structure. Thus with thousands of genes involved for a given chromosome, chromosomal disorders usually result in major, multisystem problems. Only the most common of the many chromosomal disorders are described here.

Changes in Chromosome Number

The trisomies are the most common chromosomal disorders involving a change in chromosome number.

Trisomy 21. *Trisomy 21* (also called *Down syndrome*) occurs in 1 in 600 to 800 live births. More than half of trisomy 21 conceptions are aborted early in pregnancy. Common characteristics include brachycephaly; hypotonia; hyperlaxity; oblique palpebral fissures; protruding tongue; flat nasal bridge; small ears; Brushfield spots on the iris; short, wide hands with palmar simian creases; epicanthal folds; wide gap between the first and second toes; and mental retardation. Complications may include thyroid disease (1% to 6%), leukemia, hip dysplasia, intestinal atresia, and congenital heart disease (30% to 40%). Serous otitis media with hearing loss is common (40% to 60%). Ocular abnormalities occur in about 20% of children with Down syndrome. Prenatal diagnosis from amniocentesis or chorionic villus sampling indicates the condition. Low maternal serum α-fetoprotein concentration, low unconjugated estriol, and elevated human chorionic gonadotropin levels are indicators of Down syndrome.

Health care guidelines have been developed and revised by the AAP (AAP, Committee on Genetics, 2001a) and are summarized in Box 41-5. Early intervention begins in infancy and continues throughout childhood. Education in integrated classrooms in a neighborhood school has been shown to be successful (Van Riper & Cohen, 2001). Most will enter the workforce after high school and may live in group homes as adults. Immunizations are important because these chidren are more susceptible to infections. Cardiac care, hearing screening (as many as 60% have some hearing loss), growth monitoring, and prevention of overweight are important roles for NPs. Thyroid screening;

gastrointestinal care for disorders such as pyloric stenosis, duodenal atresia, Hirschsprung disease, or imperforate anus; atlantoaxial instability screening for those involved in sports; and awareness that leukemia may emerge as a problem are further issues that the NP should monitor (AAP, Committee on Genetics, 2001a; Van Riper & Cohen, 2001).

Trisomy 18. *Trisomy 18*, or a third chromosome 18, occurs in 1 in 6000 live births (Jorde et al, 2003). It is the second most common autosomal chromosomal disorder. These children have mental retardation, failure to thrive, rocker-bottom feet, prominent occiput, small features, short sternum, low-set malformed ears, hypoplasia of the nails, horseshoe kidneys, hernias, flexed and overlapping fingers, micrognathia, and other deformities. Ninety percent have cardiac defects, and only about 5% survive the first year of life. The potential for scoliosis, deafness, and central apnea needs to be monitored.

Trisomy 13. Children with *trisomy 13* have problems so severe that 50% die in the first month of life and 95% die by 3 years of age. Characteristics include mental retardation, failure to thrive, capillary hemangiomas, persistent fetal hemoglobin, microcephaly, cleft lip or cleft palate (or both), microphthalmia, colobomas, apparent deafness, cardiac septal defects, polycystic kidneys, polydactyly, and other features. The incidence is about 1 in 10,000 live births (Jorde et al, 2003).

Other Trisomies. Generally, other trisomies are not compatible with life.

Sex Chromosome Disorders

Sex chromosome disorders involve changes in the number or structure of X or Y chromosomes. Turner syndrome and Klinefelter syndrome are examples of changes in number, and fragile X syndrome involves change in structure.

Turner Syndrome. Turner syndrome (XO) is a disorder of girls in which one X chromosome is present instead of two. The incidence is 1 in 4000 girls. However, about 25% of chromosomally abnormal spontaneous abortions are XO. The girls appear short and have a broad chest, webbed neck, lymphedema of the hands and feet as newborns, cubitus valgus, congenital heart disease (20% to 44%), urinary tract anomalies (45% to 80%), and a low hairline. They will be sterile. Their intelligence is normal. Hormone therapy is important to help with both growth and development of female characteristics. Five percent to 10% have some Y genetic material and are at increased risk for gonadoblastomas.

Klinefelter Syndrome. Klinefelter syndrome (XXY) occurs in 1 in 500 to 1000 boys. Boys with the problem are often not identified until adolescence, when testes fail to enlarge. In addition to prepubertal testes, they can have gynecomastia and decreased body hair. They are usually tall and lanky. They are not feminine in behavior or sexual orientation and usually have normal sexual function. However, they are always sterile.

Other changes in the number of sex chromosomes such as XYY may or may not have clinical implications. Individual counseling is recommended.

Fragile X Syndrome. Fragile X syndrome is the most common inherited cause of mental retardation and is responsible for about 40% of cases of X-linked retardation (Jorde et al, 2003) (Fig. 41-4). Fragile X occurs in both boys (1 in 4000) and girls (1 in 8000) but is more common in males. It is named for the fragile site on the long arm at Xq27.3. The DNA of a normal person contains 10 to 50 copies of the CGG trinucleotide repeat in the region of the FMR-1 gene. A small increase in the number of repeats to between 50 and 200 increases the instability of the area and is called a *premutation.* A man who carries the premutation is a "normal transmitting" male and has normal intelligence but passes the premutation to all of his daughters. If these daughters have sons, there is a great likelihood of further increases in the number of repeats of the CGG/CGG sequence. When the number of repeats exceeds 200, a full mutation (called *symptomatic*) causes moderate to severe mental retardation. The increase in number of CGG repeats is called *allelic expansion.* It may take several generations of expansion in females to finally reach the symptomatic point.

Males with the syndrome have a long face, large ears, prominent forehead and jaw, high-arched palate, macrocephaly, single palmar crease, and hard calluses. Macroorchidism is significant in postpubescent males. They are large individuals in height and weight. Mental retardation is found in essentially all people with the full mutation,

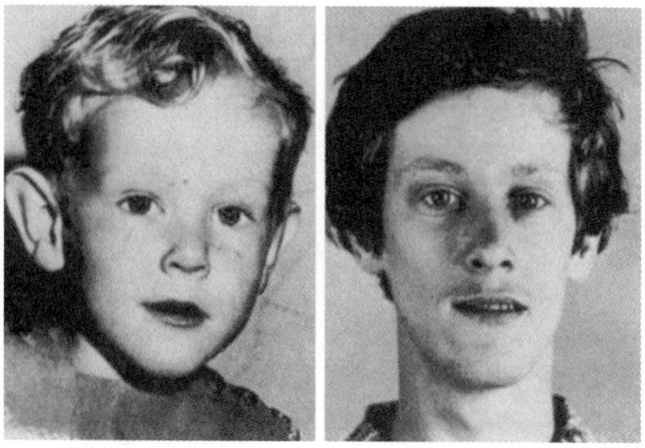

FIGURE 41-4 Children with fragile X syndrome. (From Turner G, Daniel A, Frost M: X-linked mental retardation, macro-orchidism, and the Xq27 fragile site, *J Pediatr* 96:837, 1980.)

although the problem may be milder in females. Behavioral features are important and include hyperactivity, short attention span, perseveration of speech, hand flapping, hand biting, poor eye contact, excessive chewing on clothes, tactile defensiveness, mood instability, shyness, and social anxiety. Seizures occur in approximately 20% of individuals (Hagerman, 1997). Females with the syndrome show varying degrees of mental retardation.

Children with fragile X syndrome and their families need follow-up for connective tissue dysplasias, multidisciplinary team assessment of developmental issues, treatment of behavioral problems and attention-deficit hyperactivity disorder (ADHD), and genetic counseling (Hagerman, 1997).

Other Conditions with Allelic Expansion. Expansions can occur at other sites on autosomes as well, causing problems such as myotonic dystrophy and Huntington disease.

Structural Chromosome Defects

Structural chromosome defects can be of several types. First, *deletions* can occur in which a part of a chromosome is lost. Cri du chat syndrome involves loss of the 5p segment. Some deletions are called *microdeletions* because they can only be identified with high-quality studies. Prader-Willi syndrome is a 15q problem. Children with these syndromes are retarded and obese, with small hands and feet, among other characteristics. If the deletion occurs in chromosome 15 from the father, Prader-Willi syndrome occurs; if the problem stems from chromosome 15 from the mother, Angelman syndrome occurs, with characteristics, including mental retardation and recurrent bouts of laughter, that are very different from those of Prader-Willi syndrome (Nicholls, Saitoh, & Horsthemke, 1998). Prader-Willi and Angelman syndromes may also be caused by uniparental disomy as described previously.

Duchenne muscular dystrophy, Williams syndrome, and DiGeorge syndrome have all been found to include some microdeletions (Shapiro, 2000).

Duplications of sections of chromosomes can occur, such as a duplication of the 3q segment resulting in a Cornelia de Lange–like syndrome. Unbalanced inversions, or the wrong order of genes, are not usually compatible with life. However, children with *translocations* where genetic material is exchanged between nonhomologous pairs may survive. Some children with Down syndrome (1% to 2%) have a translocation rather than a duplication of chromosome 21 (Jorde et al, 2003).

Single-Gene Defects

Single-gene defects follow mendelian rules of inheritance. Because only one gene is involved, the problems may be subtle with few visible anomalies present. The online McKusick catalogue, "Online Mendelian Inheritance in Man" (OMIM), describes more than 9000 single-gene defects or polymorphisms (McKusick, 2002). Inherited biochemical (metabolic) disorders are generally single-gene defects. The reported incidence of inborn errors of metabolism is thought to be 1% to 2% of live births, but this may be underreported because not all are apparent at birth (Lea, 2000).

Autosomal Dominant Disorders

Chromosome pairs 1 to 22 are the autosomes, and pair 23 consists of the sex chromosomes. In autosomal dominant disorders, only one gene of a pair is needed for the problem to appear. The risk for recurrence is 50% if one parent is affected. Unaffected offspring of an affected person have unaffected children; males and females are affected in equal numbers. A Punnett square is used to diagram the inheritance risk for the genotype for each pregnancy and is shown in Fig. 41-5, *A*, for autosomal dominant disorders. Often vertical transmission of the disease phenotype through several generations is identified by a family history, although wide variability in expression can occur. Increased paternal age can have an effect, although fresh gene mutation is frequent. Neurofibromatosis (1 in 4000), tuberous sclerosis (1 in 10,000), achondroplasia (1 in 6000), Huntington disease (1 in 24,000 in the United States), polydactyly (1 in 100 to 300 blacks and 1 in 630 to 3000 whites), osteogenesis imperfecta (1 in 15,000 to 20,000), and familial hypercholesterolemia (1 in 500) are examples of these disorders (Seashore & Wappner, 1996).

Neurofibromatosis is one of the most common genetic disorders seen in children. About 75% of affected individuals have only mild disease manifestations (café au lait spots and cutaneous neurofibromas). Neurofibromatosis I is diagnosed if an individual has at least two of the following seven:

- Five or more café au lait spots greater than 5 mm in diameter in prepubertal individuals or greater than 15 mm in postpubertal individuals (100% of cases)
- Axillary or inguinal freckling (20% to 50% of cases)
- Two or more Lisch nodules on the iris
- Two or more neurofibromas usually appearing in late childhood or with puberty
- A distinctive osseous lesion such as sphenoid dysplasia or scoliosis
- Optic gliomas along the pathway (15% of cases)
- A first-degree relative diagnosed with neurofibromatosis from the previously listed characteristics

Children may have learning disabilities (40%) or ADHD. Speech abnormalities may occur and need to be screened for periodically. Malignancies occur in 6%, and 10% are

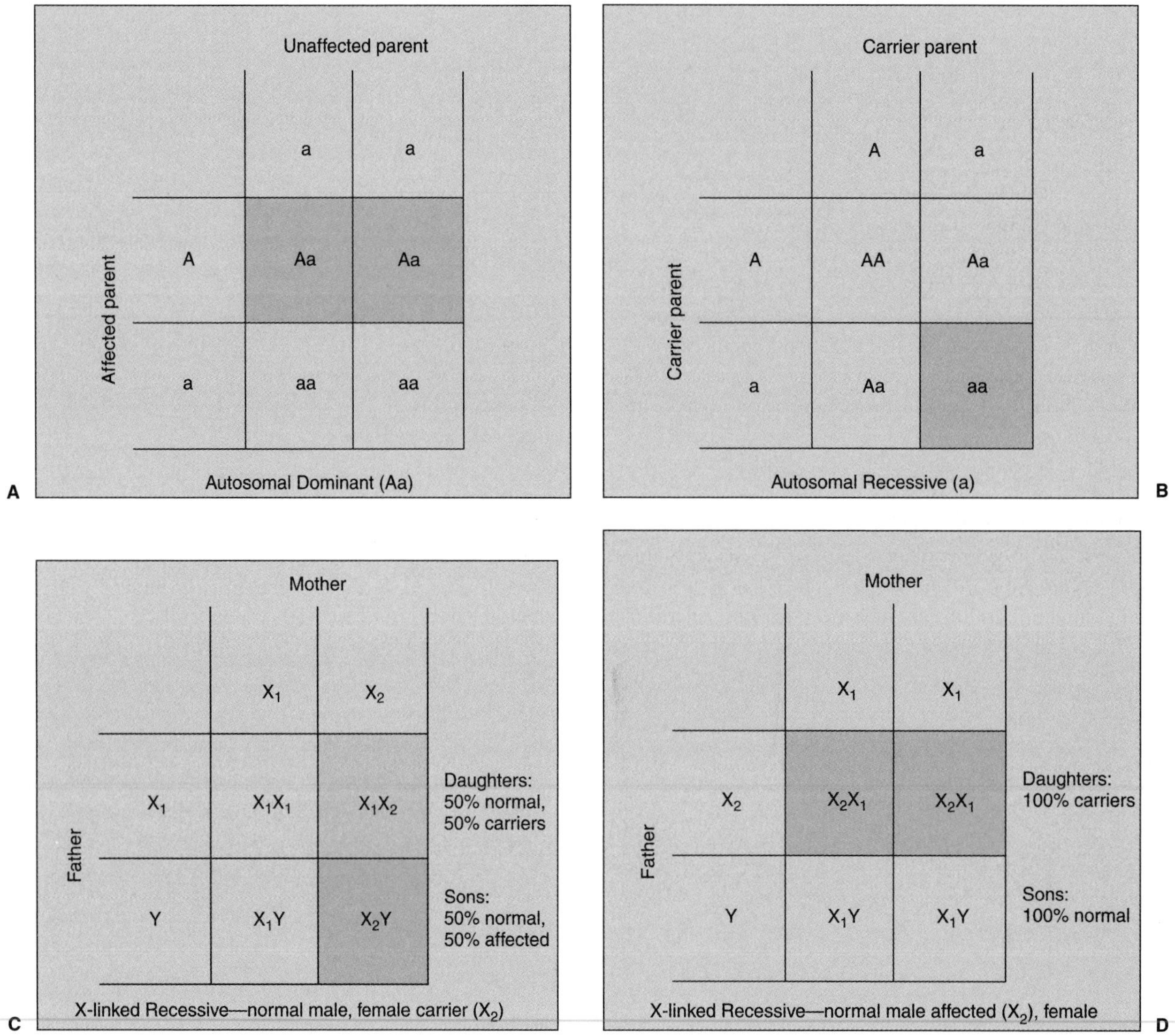

FIGURE 41-5 Punnett squares. (Adapted from Jorde L et al: *Medical genetics*, ed 3, St Louis, 2003, Mosby, pp 63, 65, 94.)

mentally retarded (Shapiro, 2000) (see Box 41-5). Psychologic problems can occur because of the uncertainty of the disease, which is progressive in nature. Care should be multidimensional with attention to neurologic, ophthalmologic, orthopedic, educational, and behavioral issues (Vernon, 2000).

Autosomal Recessive Disorders

These disorders are rare because they require two carriers to mate to produce the condition. Each pregnancy has a 25% chance that the offspring will inherit the condition and a 50% chance that the offspring will be a carrier. Carriers will be heterozygous, but an individual with the condition will be homozygous; that is, both chromosomes of a pair must have the same defect present for expression. The Punnett square for autosomal recessive disorders is shown in Fig. 41-5, *B*. Males and females are affected in equal numbers. The family history is usually negative, although siblings from the same parents may be affected (horizontal transmission). Consanguinity increases the risk for autosomal recessive disorders, and fresh gene mutations are rare. The age of onset of the disease is usually in infancy and often involves an enzyme deficiency or defect; these diseases are usually severe. Prenatal diagnosis and carrier detection are often available. Ethnicity risk factors are most significant for autosomal recessive disorders (see Table 41-1). Uniparental disomy may also result in an autosomal recessive condition (see discussion earlier in this chapter).

Examples of these disorders include some types of congenital hypothyroidism (1 in 4000), PKU (1 in 10,000), galactosemia (1 in 70,000), cystic fibrosis (1 in 1600 whites, the most common lethal inherited disease in the United States), Tay-Sachs disease (1 in 3600 Ashkenazi Jews), sickle cell disease (1 in 600 blacks), and the mucopolysaccharide disorders such as Hurler syndrome (1 in 100,000) (Seashore & Wappner, 1996). Congenital adrenal hyperplasia with ambiguous genitalia is also autosomal recessive.

Newborn blood screening tests are used to identify children with some of these disorders. A metabolic disorder may need to be included in the differential diagnosis in any child with developmental delay or regression, seizures or other neurologic abnormalities, psychosis, failure to thrive, hypoglycemia, unusual odor, abnormal eating patterns, liver disease, or metabolic acidosis.

X-Linked Disorders

In all X-linked disorders, the defective gene lies on the X chromosome. Because men have only one X chromosome, disorders here always yield effects. The Lyon principle explains that one X chromosome in each cell of females is inactivated randomly. If a high number of normal chromosomes are inactivated by chance, the female can exhibit pathology from the aberrant X chromosomes, which then predominate. In other words, females with X-linked disorders may or may not exhibit a given disorder. Prenatal diagnosis is available for many of the X-linked diseases, and the carrier state of the mother can often be determined.

In *X-linked dominant disorders,* affected males transmit the disorder to their daughters, all of whom will be affected, but to none of their sons. There is no carrier state. Fifty percent of the offspring of the daughters have a chance of receiving the affected gene. "X inactivation" lessens the effect in females, and families with the gene often have an excess of female offspring. These disorders are very rare but are characterized by vertical transmission, twice as many affected females as males, and no male-to-male transmission. Vitamin D–resistant rickets (1 in 25,000) is one of the more common examples of an X-linked dominant disorder.

X-linked recessive disorders require two copies of the mutant gene in females or, in males, an affected X chromosome. One in two male children of female carriers may be affected. All daughters of affected males are carriers, and all sons of affected males are normal. The Punnett squares for X-linked recessive disorders in which one parent is a carrier and in which one parent has the disorder are shown in Fig. 41-5, *C,* and Fig. 41-5, *D,* respectively. Generally, females must be homozygous for the abnormal gene before the related disorder is manifested. X-linked recessive disorders are characterized by much greater prevalence in males, lack of male-to-male transmission, and skipped generations representing transmission through carrier females. Some of the X-linked recessive disorders include hemophilia (1 in 8500 males), Duchenne muscular dystrophy (1 in 3300 males), and glucose-6-phosphate dehydrogenase deficiency (1 in 10 black American males).

Teratogens

A variety of drugs and diseases, as well as irradiation, can have significant effects on the developing fetus. Congenital infections include syphilis, rubella, and many others. Maternal PKU and diabetes can also affect fetuses. Fetal alcohol, fetal hydantoin, and fetal warfarin (Coumadin) effects are all described. Alcohol is the most common human teratogen.

Fetal Alcohol Syndrome

Fetal alcohol syndrome (FAS) is severe and occurs in approximately 0.5 to 5 per 1000 children, with fetal alcohol effects occurring more frequently. Characteristics of FAS include growth retardation; facial dysmorphology with an underdeveloped philtrum, thin upper lip, flat midface, short or upturned nose, low nasal bridge, ear anomalies, short palpebral fissures, ptosis, micrognathia, and epicanthal folds; and central nervous system involvement, including microcephaly, structural brain abnormalities, and other neurologic signs such as developmental delays, retardation, poor motor control, attention deficits, hyperactivity, and muscle weakness (Fig. 41-6). Many other anomalies have also been described, including scoliosis, clubfoot, renal and hepatic defects, cardiac defects, cleft lip and palate, ophthalmic abnormalities, hearing loss, and limb reduction.

Other terms used to describe alcohol-related effects not meeting the criteria for FAS include alcohol-related birth defects (ARBDs) and alcohol-related neurodevelopmental disorder (ARND) (AAP, Committee on Substance Abuse and Committee on Children with Disabilities, 2000; Thackray & Tifft, 2001).

Differential diagnoses include Williams syndrome, Noonan syndrome, Dubowitz syndrome, Bloom syndrome, fetal hydantoin syndrome, and maternal phenylketonuria fetal effects. Fragile X syndrome, Turner syndrome, and

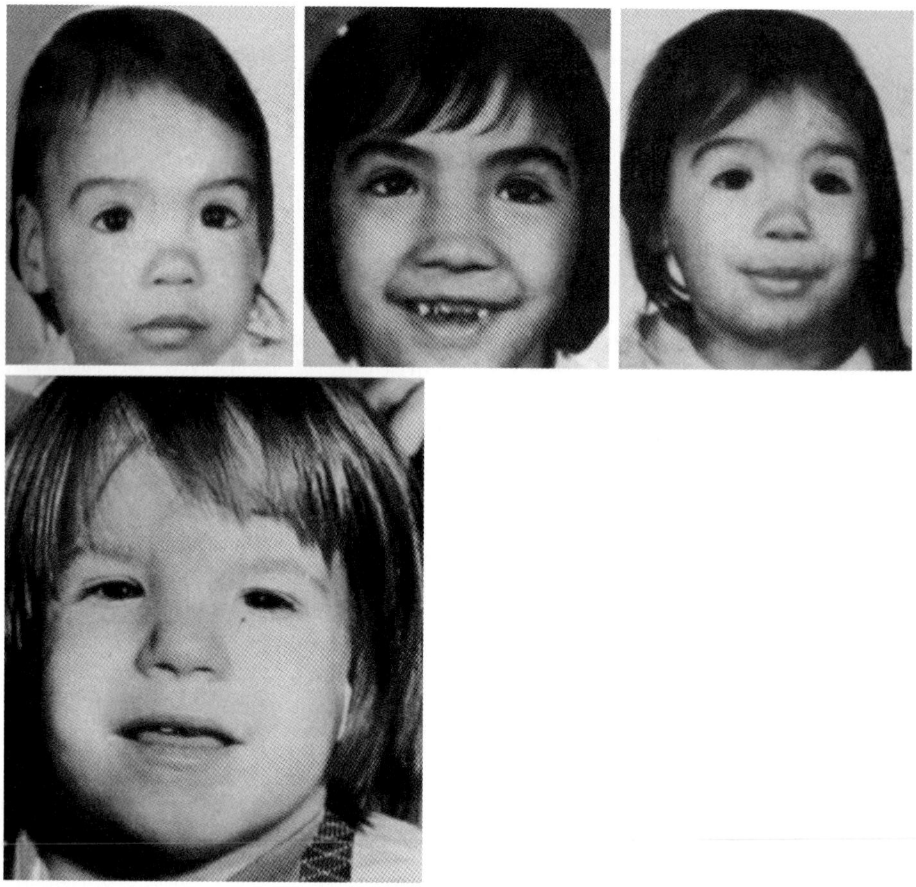

FIGURE 41-6 Children with fetal alcohol syndrome. (From Turner G, Daniel A, Frost M: X-linked mental retardation, macro-orchidism, and the Xq27 fragile site, *J Pediatr* 96:837, 1980.)

others may also have some similar physical, central nervous system, or behavioral features.

Management includes evaluation of growth and nutrition, management of medical problems related to the birth defects, and identification of other medical issues. Educational evaluation and support with community resources will help the child reach his or her potential. Maternal and family help may be useful when children live in impaired homes with continued alcohol use. Other siblings may also be diagnosed with one of the alcohol-related conditions. Abstinence from alcohol during pregnancy is the best prevention for the problem (Thackray & Tifft, 2001).

Genetics and Cancer

"Gene mutations occur in cells of the human body all the time. Cells have the ability to recognize alterations in DNA and, in most instances, correct the change before it is passed on through cell division. Cells' capacity to repair damage from gene mutations may diminish over time, leading to an accumulation of genetic changes that ultimately may cause disease" (Lea, 2000). Cancer must be considered a genetic disease because alterations in the genetic material of cells result in the aberrant cellular growth. Cancer genes are classified into three categories: (1) tumor suppressors—inhibit cellular proliferation; (2) oncogenes—activate cellular proliferation; and (3) defects in DNA repair—increase in number of somatic mutations (Jorde et al, 2003). Errors in any of these areas will result in abnormal cell growth. Chromosomal instability associated with specific conditions also puts the child at risk for certain cancers; for example, Down syndrome is associated with a risk of acute leukemia. Rhabdomyosarcoma, Ewing sarcoma, lymphoma, neuroblastoma, and other cancers are under study. Ultimately, specific gene therapies may be developed to combat these diseases.

RESOURCE BOX

National Resources for Genetic Disorders

GENERAL INFORMATION

Alliance of Genetic Support Groups
www.geneticalliance.org
Referrals to genetic support groups and genetic services via online and toll-free help lines

Association of Birth Defect Children
1-800-313-2232
1-407-245-7035
www.birthdefects.org

Genetic Conditions/Rare Conditions: Support Groups and Information Page
www.kumc.edu/gec/support/groups
Provides information on various genetic conditions and support groups

Human Genome Project Information
www.ornl.gov/hgmis
Information about the Human Genome Project

March of Dimes Birth Defects Foundation
www.modimes.org/index.htm
Resource for health care providers with contact information for genetic clinics and teratology information for all states

National Coalition for Health Professional Education in Genetics
2360 W. Joppa Road, Suite 320
Lutherville, MD 21093
1-410-583-0600
www.nchpeg.org
For health professionals of all types; includes an information center with a collection of links to high-quality genetic education-related websites

National Organization for Rare Disorders (NORD)
55 Kenosia Avenue
PO Box 1968
Danbury, CT 06813-1968
1-800-999-6673 (voicemail only)
1-203-744-0100
www.rarediseases.org
Federation of more than 140 nonprofit volunteer organizations offering information and family support referrals for rare disorders

Office of Genetics and Disease Prevention
Centers for Disease Control and Prevention
www.cdc.gov/genetics

Office of Rare Diseases
National Institutes of Health
www.cancernet.nci.nih.gov/ord/genetics-info
Excellent list of links to genetic resources

Online Mendelian Inheritance in Man (OMIM)
www.ncbi.nom.gov/omim
Database created by V. McKusick, MD; provides a searchable catalogue of virtually all hereditary disorders

ALBINISM AND HYPOPIGMENTATION

National Organization for Albinism and Hypopigmentation (NOAH)
PO Box 959
East Hampstead, NH 03826-0959
1-800-473-2310
www.albinism.org
Newsletter, informational materials, chapters, advocacy, research

DOWN SYNDROME

Association for Children with Down Syndrome, Inc.
4 Fern Place
Plainview, NY 11779
1-516-933-4700 X100
www.acds.org/

National Association for Down Syndrome (Chicago area only)
PO Box 4542
Oak Brook, IL 60522
1-630-325-9112
www.nads.org/

National Down Syndrome Congress
1370 Center Drive, Suite 102
Atlanta, GA 30338
1-800-232-NDSC
www.ndsccenter.org

National Down Syndrome Society
666 Broadway
New York, NY 10012
1-800-221-4602
www.ndss.org

FETAL ALCOHOL SYNDROME

National Organization for Fetal Alcohol Syndrome (NOFAS)
1-800-66-NOFAS
www.nofas.org

Continued

RESOURCE BOX

National Resources for Genetic Disorders—cont'd

Family Empowerment Network: Supporting Families Affected by FAS/FAE
1-800-462-5254
1-608-262-6590
www.fammed.wisc.edu/fen
A national resource, referral, support, and research program serving families affected by fetal alcohol syndrome (FAS) and fetal alcohol effects (FAE) and the providers who work with them; includes information on family retreats, family assessment tools, educational and training programs, resource materials and technical assistance, and a newsletter, the FEN Pen

FRAGILE X SYNDROME

National Fragile X Foundation
1-800-688-8765
1-303-333-6155
www.medhelp.org/www/fragilex
Newsletter, informational materials, networking, local chapters, advocacy, funds research

NEUROFIBROMATOSIS

National Neurofibromatosis Foundation
1-800-323-7938
www.neurofibromatosis.org

NF-2 Sharing Network
10074 Cabachon Ct
Ellicott City, MD 21042-6202
1-410-461-2245 (voice/fax)
Newsletter, informational materials, networking, referrals to local resources, maintains research registry

SHORT STATURE/DWARFISM

Little People of America
www.lpaonline.org
1-888-LPA-2001 (English and Spanish)
Newsletter, informational materials (including Spanish), networking, local chapters

TRISOMIES 13, 18

Support Organization for Trisomy 18, 13, and Related Disorders (SOFT)
1-800-716-7638
www.trisomy.org

TURNER SYNDROME

Turner Syndrome Support Society
www.tss.org.uk

Turner Syndrome Society of the United States
1-800-365-9944
www.turner-syndrome-us.org

REFERENCES

American Academy of Pediatrics, Committee on Bioethics: Ethical issues with genetic testing in pediatrics (RE9924), *Pediatrics* 107:1451-1455, 2001.

American Academy of Pediatrics, Committee on Children with Disabilities: General principles in the care of children and adolescents with genetic disorders and other chronic health conditions (RE9717), *Pediatrics* 99:643-644, 1997.

American Academy of Pediatrics, Committee on Genetics: Health supervision for children with Turner syndrome, *Pediatrics* 96:1166-1173, 1995a.

American Academy of Pediatrics, Committee on Genetics: Health supervision for children with neurofibromatosis, *Pediatrics* 96:368-372, 1995b.

American Academy of Pediatrics, Committee on Genetics: Health supervision for children with achondroplasia, *Pediatrics* 95:443-451, 1995c.

American Academy of Pediatrics, Committee on Genetics: Health supervision for children with fragile X syndrome (RE9626), *Pediatrics* 98:297-300, 1996a.

American Academy of Pediatrics, Committee on Genetics: Health supervision of children with Marfan syndrome (RE9639), *Pediatrics* 98:978-982, 1996b.

American Academy of Pediatrics, Committee on Genetics: Molecular testing in pediatric practice: a subject review (RE0023), *Pediatrics* 106:1494-1497, 2000.

American Academy of Pediatrics, Committee on Genetics: Health supervision for children with Down syndrome (RE0016), *Pediatrics* 107: 442-449, 2001a.

American Academy of Pediatrics, Committee on Genetics: Health care supervision for children with William syndrome (RE0034), *Pediatrics* 107:1192-1204, 2001b.

American Academy of Pediatrics, Committee on Genetics: Health supervision for children with sickle cell disease, *Pediatrics* 109:526-535, 2002.

American Academy of Pediatrics, Committee on Substance Abuse and Committee on Children with Disabilities: Fetal alcohol syndrome and alcohol-related neurodevelopmental disorders (RE 9948), *Pediatrics* 106:358-361, 2000.

Bennett R et al: Recommendations for standardized human pedigree nomenclature, *Am J Hum Genet* 56:745-752, 1995.

Bodemer C et al: Hair and skin disorders as signs of mitochondrial disease, *Pediatrics* 103:428-433, 1999.

Hagerman R: Fragile X syndrome: meeting the challenges of diagnosis and care, *Contemp Pediatr* 14:31-59,1997.

Institute of Medicine: *Assessing genetic risks: implications for health and social policy*, Washington, DC, 1994, National Academy Press.

Johnson K, Brensinger J: Genetic counseling and testing, *Nurs Clin North Am* 35:615-626, 2000.

Johnson M, Robin N: Pediatrics and the Human Genome Project, *Contemp Pediatr* 17:100-112, 2000.

Jones K: *Smith's recognizable patterns of human malformations*, ed 5, Philadelphia, 1997, WB Saunders.

Jorde L et al: *Medical genetics*, ed 2, St Louis, 2000, Mosby.

Lea D: A clinician's primer to human genetics: what nurses need to know, *Nurs Clin North Am* 35:583-614, 2000.

National Coalition for Health Professional Education in Genetics: Core competencies in genetics for all health-care professionals, 2000. Available at *www.nchpeg.org/news-box/corecompetencies000.html* (accessed Dec 1, 2003).

Nussbaum R, McInnes R, Willard H: *Thompson and Thompson genetics in medicine*, ed 6, Philadelphia, 2001, WB Saunders.

Pacific Northwest Regional Genetics Group: *Practical genetics for primary care*, Portland, OR, 1996, Oregon Health Sciences Center, Pacific Northwest Regional Genetics Group.

Seashore M, Wappner R: *Genetics in primary care and clinical medicine*, Stamford, CT, 1996, Appleton & Lange.

Shapiro L: Human genetics. In Behrman R, Kliegman H, Jensen H, editors: *Nelson textbook of pediatrics*, Philadelphia, 2000, WB Saunders.

Thackray H, Tifft C: Fetal alcohol syndrome, *Pediatr Rev* 22:47-55, 2001.

Van Riper M, Cohen W: Caring for children with Down syndrome and their families, *J Pediatr Health Care* 15:123-131, 2001.

Vernon P: Neurofibromatosis: an elephant by another name, *J Pediatr Health Care* 14:244-246, 2000.

Wardinsky T: Visual clues to diagnosis of birth defects and genetic disease, *J Pediatr Health Care* 8:63-73, 1994.

42

Environmental Health Issues

Ardys M. Dunn, Catherine E. Burns

The environment is a basic determinant of human health and illness. Children, because of their developmental immaturity, rapid growth, size, and behavior, are particularly susceptible to environmental threats (Table 42-1). Exposure to toxins or other harmful substances can affect growth and damage organs or body systems during critical periods of development, both prenatally and during childhood. Toxicants that cross the placenta (e.g., carbon monoxide, mercury, lead, cotinine from environmental tobacco smoke) contribute to low-birth-weight babies, spontaneous abortion, intrauterine growth retardation, increased risk of cancer, poor cognitive and behavioral development, and birth defects. Approximately 3% of all babies born in the United States are born with a major birth defect, and the rate of some birth defects is increasing (Kirby, 2002; Waldman & Perlman, 2002).

During childhood, children's rapidly growing tissues more readily absorb environmental toxins; the lungs, skin, and gastrointestinal (GI) tract of newborns are highly permeable and gastric pH is high, facilitating absorption. At the same time, newborns' immature organ systems more slowly metabolize drugs, making it more difficult for infants to detoxify and excrete harmful substances. Children consume more fresh fruit, water, milk, and juice per pound of body weight than adults; many of these products are treated with pesticides or other chemicals. Children engage in more outdoor activities than adults, breathe more pollutants per pound of body weight, and are physically closer to many potentially harmful substances. Crawling on floors, chewing on objects, and running and rolling in grass are behaviors that expose children to environmental toxins and result in respiratory problems, lead poisoning, and pesticide poisoning. Although there is some evidence that the incidence of asthma may be decreasing, nearly 5 million cases have been identified among children, and asthma remains a significant public health problem (Mannino et al, 2002). Adolescents are particularly susceptible to environmental tobacco smoke and occupational hazards.

Children living in poorer communities are at higher risk than others. Poor housing and nutrition, high levels of lead, toxic waste deposits, and limited access to health screening and treatment all contribute to increased risk (Powell & Stewart, 2001).

In addition to the immediate risk during childhood, children have a longer time span for exposure to environmental toxins, and with some conditions children are more likely to suffer health problems than adults exposed to the same substance.

IMPLICATIONS FOR NURSE PRACTITIONERS

Nurse practitioners (NPs) need to be able to give their clients accurate information about environmental health issues. The connection between environment and health is increasingly recognized; a recent study of human exposure to environmental chemicals indicates that most of us may have measurable levels of toxins such as mercury or pesticides in our bodies (Centers for Disease Control and Prevention [CDC], 2001b). The health of children is clearly related to the environment (Woodruff et al, 2003). In many cases, parents or providers may suspect that an illness is associated with environmental conditions, but a direct cause-and-effect relationship is unclear. The NP who is knowledgeable about the potential hazards of environmental exposure will be able to explain the possible

TABLE 42-1 ***Environmental Risk Factors for Children at Different Stages of Development***

Developmental Stage	Developmental Characteristics	Exposure Pathways (Physical Environment)	Biologic Vulnerabilities	Appropriate Responses in the Social Environment
Preconception	Maternal and paternal health status	Maternal/paternal reproductive organs may be compromised Maternal stores of toxicants in bones and fatty tissue can be mobilized during pregnancy	Problems with fertilization, implantation of ovum Damage to ovum or sperm Fetal development	Need for research and education regarding long-term effects of environmental contaminants on reproductive system and subsequent offspring
Prenatal	Fetal development dependent on maternal health status and environmental exposure	Maternal blood supply via placenta Radiation Noise Heat	Tissue differentiation Rapid cell division and growth Organ development Metabolic pathways incomplete	Need for prenatal programs and regulations regarding: Alcohol Cigarettes Drugs Metals
Newborn (0-2 mo)	Nonambulatory Restricted environment High calorie, water intake High air intake Highly permeable skin Alkaline gastric secretions (low gastric acidity)	Food Breast milk Infant formula Dyes in clothing Soaps and shampoos Indoor air Tap/well water in home	Brain Cell migration Neuron myelination Creation of neuron synapses Lungs Developing alveoli Rapid air exchange Narrow airways Bones Rapid growth and hardening Other organs Rapid growth Poor enzyme detoxification	Need for newborn-sensitive programs and regulations regarding: Polychlorinated biphenyls (PCBs) Lead in drinking water Environmental tobacco smoke Need to educate parents and policy makers concerning environmental hazards
Infant/toddler (2 mo-2 yr)	Beginning to walk Oral exploration (mouthing) Restricted environment and near floors Increased time away from parents Minimal variation in diet High intake of fruits, vegetables, and milk products per body weight	Food Baby food Food additives Milk and milk products Air Indoor Layer effects: air near floor contains more toxicants Tap/well water in home and day care Surfaces Rugs Floors Lawns	Brain Creation of synapses Lungs Developing alveoli Rapid air exchange Narrow airways	Need for child-sensitive programs and regulations regarding: Radon in the home Residential pesticide use Lead abatement Environmental tobacco smoke Need to educate parents and policy makers concerning environmental hazards
Preschool child (2-6 yr)	Language acquisition Group and individual play Growing independence Increased intake of fruits and vegetables	Food Fruits, vegetables Milk and milk products Air Day care/preschool Outdoor	Brain Dendritic trimming Neuron myelination Lungs Developing alveoli Increasing lung volume	Need for child-sensitive programs and regulations regarding: Food pesticides Environmental tobacco smoke at home and preschool

TABLE 42-1 *Environmental Risk Factors for Children at Different Stages of Development—cont'd*

Developmental Stage	Developmental Characteristics	Exposure Pathways (Physical Environment)	Biologic Vulnerabilities	Appropriate Responses in the Social Environment
	Day care or preschool attendance	Water Tap/well water and home/day care/ preschool Water fountains Parks and swimming areas		Need to educate parents and policy makers concerning environmental hazards
School-age child (6-12 yr)	Beginning school Playground activities Increased involvement in group activities	Food at home and school Air School Outdoor Water School water fountains Tap/well water Swimming areas Playgrounds Wood preservatives Pesticides and fertilizers Other Arts and crafts supplies	Brain Specific synapse formation Dendritic trimming Lung Volume expansion Metabolic enzymes more active than in younger child	Need for child-sensitive programs and regulations regarding: Asbestos abatement Lead in school drinking water Hazards in arts and crafts material Environmental tobacco smoke Need to educate parents and policy makers concerning environmental hazards
Adolescent (12-18 yr)	Development of abstract thinking Puberty Growth spurt Increased adherence to peer norms	Food Air Water Other Occupation Self-determination: smoking, inhalations	Brain Continued synapse formation Lung Volume expansion Gonad maturation Ova and sperm maturation Breast development Bone growth and calcification Muscle growth	Need for adolescent-sensitive programs and regulations regarding: Child labor and other issues, especially environmental tobacco smoke Need to educate parents and policy makers concerning environmental hazards

Adapted from Gitterman B: Environmental risk factors for children at different stages of development. Personal communication, 1997; Chai S, Bearer CF: A developmental approach to pediatric environmental health. In *Training manual on pediatric environmental health: putting it into practice*, Berkeley, CA, 1999, Children's Environmental Health Network/Public Health Institute.

connections, collect clear assessment data, and work closely with families to make appropriate treatment choices, including referral and consultation with public health authorities. If not personally knowledgeable, the NP should know where to get information. A core competency for all NPs states that the NP "recognizes environmental health problems affecting patients and provides health protection interventions that promote healthy environments for individuals, families, and communities" (U.S. Department of Health and Human Services, 2002).

In addition to direct patient care and education, NPs can collaborate with other health care providers, conduct research to identify environmental problems, and advocate in the public arena (e.g., industry, policy, regulation) for more responsible management of environmental agents that affect health.

RELATIONSHIP BETWEEN ENVIRONMENTAL FACTORS AND HUMAN HEALTH

Although many environmental health hazards have been identified, it is not always possible to determine direct cause and effect. Several difficulties have been noted in making this determination: (1) the extent of exposure may be unclear; (2) there can be a long latency period between exposure and appearance of illness; (3) an individual may have exposure to multiple confounding agents; (4) exposure may need to occur during a "window of vulnerability" (e.g., during the period when a particular body system is forming prenatally) for the agent to have an effect; (5) some individuals may have a genetic susceptibility to an exposure, whereas others do not; and (6) much research in environmental health has been short term, or conducted on animals so results may not translate to human development. Using principles of epidemiologic relationships and toxicology, however, NPs can better understand and explain to their patients the relationship between environment and health.

Epidemiologic Model: Risk Assessment

A first step in an epidemiologic approach (Fig. 42-1) identifies the interactive factors in the environment, including *receptors* (i.e., hosts or living things that are susceptible or exposed to environmental agents); *toxins*, or harmful substances that might cause damage (i.e., the agent); and the environmental *medium*, or route by which exposure could occur (e.g., air, water, food).

A second step of risk assessment using an epidemiologic model is to determine the possibility that harm could occur. A number of questions are asked when making this determination:

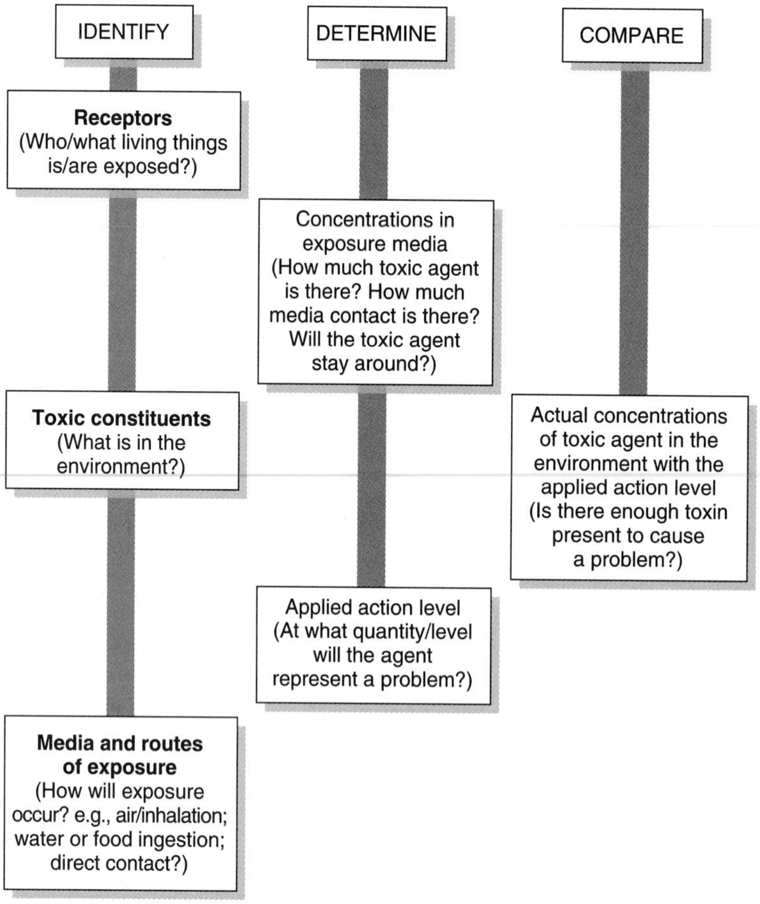

FIGURE 42-1 Risk assessment of environmental hazards. (Adapted from Oregon Poison Center and Health Division, Oregon Department of Human Resources: *Environmental hazards in perspective: seminar syllabus and environmental health resource notebook*, Portland, OR, 1994, Oregon Department of Human Resources.)

- How *susceptible* is the receptor to the agent (e.g., age, sex, genetics, diet, general health)?
- At what quantity (i.e., dose) will the agent present a problem or cause a response in this receptor? This amount is called the *applied action* or dose-response level.
- What is the concentration of the toxic agent? How much is there? How strong is it? How long will it stay around? What is the extent of contact of the toxic agent with the receptor?

A final step in this process compares the actual environmental condition with the applied action level, asking the following question: With the amount of exposure present, is the individual at risk for health problems?

Toxicologic Principles

Toxicologic principles are the same as those the NP has learned related to pharmacologic therapy: exposure, absorption, distribution, metabolism, tissue sensitivity, and effects—therapeutic or toxic. In fact, Paracelsus (1493-1541), considered the "father of toxicology," is reputed to have said, "All substances are poisons; there is none that is not a poison. The right dose differentiates a poison from a remedy."

Exposure

Contact of a biologic, chemical, or physical agent with the outer boundary of an organism (e.g., skin, lungs, GI tract) constitutes exposure. The extent to which exposure creates a problem is an epidemiologic issue (see previous discussion) and depends on factors such as frequency and duration of exposure, concentration of the agent at the point of contact, and the susceptibility of the organism (e.g., an infant's skin burns much more easily than an adult's).

Absorption

Absorption is the process by which an agent is taken into the organism. It occurs in the skin, mucous membranes, lungs, or GI tract (e.g., carbon tetrachloride is absorbed via the skin). Absorption involves active or passive transport (e.g., lipid-soluble chemicals such as polychlorinated biphenyls [PCBs] are passively absorbed through the gut and stored in fat; lead is taken up through active transport in the GI tract and stored in bone or other tissues).

Distribution

Toxic agents are distributed throughout the organism via the blood or lymph systems. The ability of an agent to cross the blood-brain barrier, the amount of blood flow to an organ, and the affinity of tissues to take up a particular agent (e.g., lipid-soluble chemicals are found in fatty tissues) all influence the degree to which a toxicant will be distributed throughout the body.

Metabolism

Metabolic enzymes in the body interact with toxic agents in several ways: (1) oxidation, reduction, and hydrolysis of the agent—the agent can be detoxified, but chemicals can also be activated and made more toxic; and (2) conjugation and breakdown to enhance elimination, usually through the kidney. Metabolism is influenced by the individual's age, sex, nutritional status, genetic makeup, presence of other drugs, and disease or illness.

Tissue Sensitivity

Susceptibility and reaction of tissue to a particular agent can vary.

Toxic Effects

Toxic effects vary by agent, dose, and organ or system affected. They include a wide range of pathologic conditions.

Assessment

Assessment of environmental health hazards should be integrated into regular health appraisals, as well as examinations of ill children. Table 42-2 lists essential questions to ask for an environmental history, including questions related to risk of exposure to lead.

Physical Examination

The physical examination should cover all body systems thoroughly. Evaluate agent-specific findings (e.g., burns caused by chemicals, neurotoxicity caused by mercury), but also look for subtle, nonspecific signs and symptoms (e.g., skin rashes and headaches). The effects of toxicants on the body can be subclinical in many cases, and effects can occur long after exposure.

Laboratory Studies

Laboratory studies can be performed on patients as indicated, based on signs and symptoms. Agent-specific laboratory studies, if available and reliable, can be helpful in determining treatment plans. However, few tests are appropriate for use in the primary care setting because of the following limitations:

- For most toxins, valid and reliable tests have not been developed.
- For those toxins that do have tests, not all laboratories are capable of performing them. The NP should consult with individual laboratories regarding their capabilities.

TABLE 42-2 *Environmental Screening Questions for Pediatric Clients*

1. Has your child had a blood test for lead? _____Yes _____No _____Don't Know
2. Does your child live in or visit regularly (e.g., for day care) a home that was built before 1950? _____Yes _____No _____Don't Know
3. Does your child live in or visit regularly a home built before 1978 that is being or has been recently renovated or remodeled (within the last 6 months)? _____Yes _____No _____Don't Know
4. Does your child have a sibling or playmate who has or did have lead poisoning? _____Yes _____No _____Don't Know
5. Is your child receiving WIC, food stamps, or Medicaid? _____Yes _____No _____Don't Know
6. Does your child or another family member have hobbies that use toxic materials (e.g., model building, stained glass work, cleaning guns)? _____Yes _____No _____Don't Know
7. Is your child exposed to cigarette smoke in his or her environment? _____Yes _____No _____Don't Know
8. If you are breastfeeding your child, are you taking any medications or drugs, do you smoke, or have you been exposed to any toxic substances? (Leave blank if you are not breastfeeding.) _____Yes _____No _____Don't Know
9. Is your child exposed to any of the following substances? _____Yes _____No _____Don't Know
   a. Pesticides or herbicides (e.g., do you use insect or weed killers on your garden or lawn; do you use flea collars or flea baths for your pets? Do you live on a farm or near a farming area, including tree farms)?__________
   b. Asbestos (e.g., does the home or school have exposed insulation, wires, broken tiles or flooring)?__________
   c. Lead or other toxins (e.g., do you use home remedies, or cook with ceramic cookware from Mexico? Are there industries located near the child's home, school, or play areas)?
   d. Radon gas (e.g., in your home basement)?__________
   e. Molds (e.g., wet areas in basements, dry leaves)?__________
   f. Smoke from field burning or wood stoves?_____
10. Are this child's parents working in an environment where they are exposed to toxic substances (e.g., field work, chemical industry, painting)? _____Yes _____No _____Don't Know
11. Does your child's home have safety items in place (e.g., smoke alarms, carbon monoxide detectors, fire extinguishers, electrical outlet covers, fences and gates)? _____Yes _____No _____Don't Know
12. Do you have other questions about your child's possible exposure to environmental toxins?
13. What is your zip code?

Note to providers: Children should be screened for blood lead levels if they

1. Have any signs of lead toxicity, despite answers to environmental questions.
2. Are 1-2 years old and have a "Yes" or "Don't Know" answer to any of questions 1-5.
3. Are 2-6 years old, have never been screened, and have a "Yes" or "Don't Know" answer to any of questions 1-5.
4. Live in a high-risk area. (Contact your state health department for zip code information. CDC has identified areas with ≥27% of housing built before 1950 as high risk.)

From Dunn, Burns, & Settler (2003); CDC (1997).

- Many tests show a wide range of reference levels at which "toxicity" appears.
- There may be little correlation between exposure and levels present in the body at the time the test is done. Levels may have returned to normal, despite damage done to the body; or a one-time sample can reflect recent active exposure, but not measure the total body burden of the contaminant.

Available tests include the following:

- Plasma lead levels
- Gas-liquid chromatography (for PCBs)
- Atomic absorption spectrometry (for mercury)
- Carboxyhemoglobin (for CO poisoning)
- Twenty-four-hour urine (for heavy metals)
- Urinary cotinine assays (for tobacco metabolites)
- Plasma cholinesterase (ChE) levels (for pesticide metabolites, organophosphates)

Management of Environmental Conditions

Management of illness related to environmental factors uses a public health model of primary, secondary, and tertiary prevention. A multidisciplinary approach that includes epidemiology, pediatrics, toxicology, public health, and health economics is necessary in order to treat specific conditions, as well as to prevent exposure to toxins. In addition to providing primary care for acute exposures, NPs can serve to inform patients and families about health risks and the nature of environmental contaminants, advocate for healthy environments in the creation of public policy, and work with other professionals to report, monitor, and control exposures. The regional Pediatric Environmental Health Specialty Units (PEHSUs) and Children's Environmental Health Network are excellent resources for clinical, toxicologic, educational, and policy information and support (see Resource Box).

Primary Prevention

The goal of primary prevention is to keep a condition from occurring and to maintain a level of wellness. Potential environmental hazards can be identified before a health problem has occurred. Health promotion and health education of the individual or public are forms of primary prevention. NPs can find a wealth of information about specific toxins, patient support groups, advocate activities, and safety practices and regulations by accessing sources identified in this chapter (see Resource Box). Primary prevention also includes assessment of communities and populations. Safety inspections in industry and public areas (e.g., school playgrounds); monitoring of lead or radon in buildings; and scientific research to determine connections between environmental agents and disease are all examples of early assessment. It is important to conduct research on children, adapt research methodologies to the unique characteristics of children, and develop biologic markers to better assess the impact of environmental hazards on children (Schwenk et al, 2003).

Primary prevention also takes place at the public policy level. Regulations or legal restrictions can prevent health problems (e.g., through implementation of air and water quality standards, restaurant and food handling regulations, or bans on the use of hydrofluorocarbons). Various U.S. federal agencies function to regulate development and use of hazardous materials (e.g., the Environmental Protection Agency [EPA], the U.S. Consumer Product Safety Commission, and the Occupational Safety and Health Administration [OSHA]). In 1997 the United States joined seven other countries (the G8) in creating the 1997 Declaration of the Environment Leaders of the Eight on Children's Environmental Health, raising the issue of protection of children from environmental threats to an international level (EPA, 2003a).

Secondary Prevention

Secondary prevention involves early detection, treatment, and referral for identified diseases. Testing for serum lead levels is one form of early detection. The general guidelines for management of environmental conditions are found in the next section. Reporting exposures to public health officials helps prevent further contact with the contaminant and can lead to the implementation of abatement procedures. Poisoning due to environmental contaminants is reportable in most states. Check with the county health department and the county agricultural commissioner.

Tertiary Prevention

Tertiary prevention seeks to rehabilitate and restore the environment to a healthful state (e.g., asbestos and lead abatement, "Superfund" and "brownfields" cleanup, restoration of wetlands). Individually, patients can take steps to end exposure to a contaminant (e.g., stop using pesticides in the home, follow directions on pesticide usage exactly) or change other behaviors that exacerbate adverse effects (e.g., radon in combination with tobacco smoke is more harmful). Follow-up is essential, because effects of environmental agents may not appear for months or years.

Prevention and Patient Education

Many health problems are related to environmental factors, but the relationship is not always clear. This uncertainty can be frustrating. NPs may have to tell patients they do not know if there is a connection between a particular environmental factor and illness. It is important to listen to and validate patient concerns; this gives the message that the NP is also concerned and will work with patients to minimize problems. Blanket reassurances are inappropriate, but NPs can provide perspective to patients by explaining the process of environmental effects on health and encouraging patients to actively control their environment. NPs may also serve as liaisons between the family and environmental, community, and specialty health care resources.

COMMON ENVIRONMENTAL AGENTS AND ADVERSE EFFECTS

Growth and development of children, especially cognitive and behavioral, can be significantly limited by environmental agents. This section presents a brief discussion of general pediatric poisoning and some common environmental agents that are particularly hazardous to children.

General Pediatric Poisoning

Description

Poisoning is the process in which a substance that interferes with the body's normal function is taken in by ingestion, inhalation, absorption, or injection. Medications, plants, and chemicals are common causes of poisoning in children.

Etiology and Incidence

Poisoning is a major cause of pediatric injury. It was the third leading cause of injury requiring hospitalization or causing death in a large study of California children, peaking at 1 to 2 years of age and again at 15 to 16 years (Agran et al, 2001). A majority of calls to poison control centers in the United States concern ingestion of toxic and nontoxic substances by young children. The mouthing behavior of infants and normal curiosity of toddlers and preschoolers puts them at high risk for accidental ingestion of toxic materials. Older children may experiment with drugs and household products with the intent of producing hallucinogenic effects.

Assessment

History. The following are assessed:

- Type and amount of substance taken in
- Exact time of intake or exposure
- Route or method of intake
- Reaction or signs and symptoms
- Emergency care given
- Child's health status before poisoning (e.g., any significant chronic illness? Is child taking prescription medication?)

Physical Examination. Findings vary greatly depending on the type and amount of poisonous substance, time since exposure, and susceptibility of the child. Consulting with a poison control center can provide the NP with the information needed to proceed with the physical examination. Information can also be obtained from Material Safety Data Sheets via the Internet (see Resource Box). Reactions can be local or systemic. Questions to consider while conducting the physical examination include the following:

- When did exposure occur?
- Which body system or systems does the poison affect?
- What are specific signs of the poison's effect?
- How quickly does the poison have an effect?
- How susceptible is the child?
- What is the child's age and weight?

Laboratory Studies. Analysis of specimens (e.g., emesis) can be helpful in determining the type of poison, if unknown. Serum levels of the poison can be assessed for some toxicants to determine appropriate treatment of the hospitalized child. In general, however, toxicology screens are not necessary, and diagnosis is made on the basis of history and in consultation with a poison control or pediatric environmental health center.

Differential Diagnosis

A history of exposure distinguishes poisoning or potential poisoning from acute-onset illness. Because there is not always an obvious episode of exposure, the NP should be suspicious of poisoning in otherwise well children who experience sudden seizures, GI distress, or cardiorespiratory collapse.

Management

Management approaches for ingested poisons vary with the type of poison, amount of exposure, time lapse since exposure, and susceptibility of the child. Initial management focuses on airway, breathing, and circulation (the ABCs). No matter what poison was taken in, vital body functions must be maintained.

Subsequent management involves counteracting or neutralizing the effects of the poison (administration of antidotes), decreasing the amount of poison in the system (gastric decontamination), and providing life-support measures while the body detoxifies itself. For some poisons (e.g., warfarin), observation alone may be sufficient (Ingels et al, 2002).

Basic decontamination guidelines for contact contaminants are listed in Box 42-1. The use of gastric decontamination, including lavage, an adsorbent agent (e.g., activated charcoal), catharsis, or whole-bowel irrigation (Bond, 2002), is increasingly coming into question (Ardagh, Flood, & Tait, 2001; Krenzelok, 2002). The American Academy of Clinical Toxicology (AACT) and the European Association of Poisons Centres and Clinical Toxicologists do not recommend gastric decontamination as a routine treatment in poisonings, unless the toxin is life threatening and ingestion has occurred within 60 minutes of treatment (Krenzelok & Vale, 1997). Syrup of ipecac is no longer recommended for use in gastric decontamination.

Prevention and Patient Education

Prevention is the best management for poisonings. Teach parents how to "poison-proof" their home, pointing out connections between the developmental stages of children and sources of poisoning. If a child is exposed to a toxic or potentially toxic substance, instruct parents to call the poison control center *before* instituting treatment.

Lead Poisoning

Description

Lead poisoning is the presence of serum lead levels that cause toxic effects on multiple organ systems. Lead has an

BOX 42-1 *Basic Decontamination Protocol*

Determine the need for decontamination by calling the poison control center in your area.
If clothing has been contaminated, strip the patient and double-bag clothing, then flush the entire body with plain water for 2 to 5 minutes. If contaminated with dust, keep clothing dry; remove carefully to minimize dust becoming airborne; if possible, apply dust mask or respirator to patient before removing clothing (brush dust from face first).
Chemical contamination:
- Scrub or irrigate open wounds for 5 to 10 minutes or longer, using lukewarm water.
- Irrigate eyes with sterile saline, balanced salt solution, or Ringer's lactate for at least 15 to 30 minutes.
- Irrigate face, nose, and ear canals with normal saline, using frequent suction.
- Wash appendages (if that is only body part contaminated) without wetting the whole body, if possible.
- Clean under nails with scrub brush and nail cleaner.

Oily or greasy contamination:
- Cleanse with soap or shampoo, followed by water flushing.

affinity for calcium-binding proteins and may affect any calcium-mediated process. It also affects neurotransmitters and certain enzyme functions (e.g., ferrochelatase in bone marrow). Major toxic effects are caused by disruption of hemoglobin formation and damage to the nervous system, both through direct nerve cell damage and interference with nerve conduction. Over the past 30 years, the definition of the blood lead level considered to be toxic has been revised downward. The current toxic level for clinical assessment is 10 μg/dl or more, but even at lower levels, impairment of cognitive function occurs (Lidsky & Schneider, 2003).

Etiology and Incidence

Although environmental lead sources have decreased in the United States, lead poisoning continues to be a serious environmental health problem for young children. It is estimated that more than 500,000 children age 1 to 5 in the United States have lead levels above 10 μg/dl (Behrman, Kliegman, & Jenson, 2004).

Before 1950, much white house paint was 50% lead and 50% linseed oil. Limits on the lead content of paint began in 1955, and legal restrictions reduced allowable lead to 1% in 1971 and 0.06% by 1977. Homes built before 1960 have been found to have five to eight times the prevalence of lead hazards of homes built between 1960 and 1977 and 14 to 23 times the hazard of homes built between 1978 and 1998 (Jacobs et al, 2002).

Children are at greatest risk in houses where paint is peeling or those where renovation with paint removal is occurring. In some areas, such as coastal towns, many houses are covered with marine paint, designed for boats or other equipment, that still contains lead.

Soil near mines, lead-using industries, and smelters can have high lead levels. Acidic water with low mineral content can leach lead from lead pipes or solder. Hot water may be of more concern than cold. Brass fixtures also contain lead. Food can be a source of lead. Lead from soil can contaminate root vegetables, and cans with soldered seams can leach lead into food. Some other sources of lead are listed in Table 42-3.

Assessment

Screening. Screening for lead poisoning involves two processes: (1) assessing the risk of high-dose exposure using questions developed by the Centers for Disease Control and Prevention (CDC), and (2) blood lead testing. Questions to assess risk of exposure should be asked at every visit between 6 months and 6 years. In addition to the CDC questions, risk assessment questions can include the following:
- Does the child have a parent or guardian with a job or hobby that uses lead?
- Does the child live near a lead smelter, battery recycling plant, or other industry likely to release lead?
- Does the family use ceramic pottery for cooking or food storage?
- Does the family use traditional or folk home remedies?
- Does the child demonstrate pica behavior?
- Does the child have a retained lead bullet internally?
- Has the child recently lived outside the United States? Where?

Routine blood lead testing is not recommended unless children have any sign of lead toxicity or are at risk (see Table 42-2 for risk factors) (CDC, 2002a). There is some evidence that screening after 36 months of age may not be necessary (Karp et al, 2001). If the screening blood lead level is 10 μg/dl or greater, additional assessment and management is recommended (Fig. 42-2).

Physical Examination. Most lead retained by the body is stored in the bones. Although lead affects almost all organ systems, the nervous system, kidneys, and blood are particularly susceptible. Toxicity is a function of both dose and duration of exposure, but clinical signs of toxicity may not

TABLE 42-3 *Common Pediatric Toxicants and Relationship to Disease*

		Health Effects		
Substance	**Source**	**Systems Affected**	**Signs and Symptoms**	**Prevention Strategies**
Lead	Ingestion of particles or inhalation of fumes and particles from: Lead-based paint, caulk Dust, soil, water (lead pipes) Cosmetics Leaded gasoline Solder, ammunition Bearings, fishing weights Folk medicine remedies (e.g., *greta*, *azarcon*, *pay-loo-ah*) Pottery, lead crystal Some dyes used in paper, magazines, plastic wrappers Lead-based insecticides Industries that use/process lead (e.g., smelters, battery manufacturers) Hobbies, stained glass, jewelry	Central nervous system (CNS) Cardiac Gastrointestinal (GI) Renal Some enzymes Thyroid	Anemia Constipation Abdominal pain Anorexia, vomiting Learning disabilities; lower IQ scores Impaired hearing Delayed growth and development Hyperactivity or other behavior problems Agitation or clumsiness Myocardial excitability (with high levels) Headache, increased intracranial pressure Seizures, coma (usually above 70-100 μg/dl), and death	Test blood for lead levels Test soil, water, dust for lead Begin lead abatement as required, using professional experts Repair/replace deteriorating paint (see text) Keep children away from remodeling/demolition projects where lead dust could be released Clean surfaces with cleaning solution; do not dry dust Teach handwashing Keep children from chewing on painted surfaces, eating dirt Use fresh, cold water from taps; when faucet has not been used for 2 hours or more, flush 30-60 seconds until water is noticeably colder Make sure diet has adequate iron, calcium, zinc, and ascorbate, because deficiencies in these enhance lead absorption, retention, and toxicity Use lead-free paints, gasoline, materials for hobbies Do not store or cook food in lead crystal, old or imported pottery Be sure folk remedies are lead free Change work clothes before returning home if job is lead related
Mercury	Food chain; accumulated and concentrated in animals (especially fish), grains, and flour Fungicides Antiseptics Medications Latex paints (added to paints until 1991; older paints still contain Hg) Thermometers and thermostats Fluorescent lights Button/disk batteries Folk medicine remedies or religious practices (e.g., *azogue*)	CNS; GI Respiratory Renal	Five manifestations (see text): Acrodynia: Erythema of palms and soles Pruritis Chronic inorganic mercury intoxication: Tremors Irritability Memory loss Metallic taste in the mouth Gingivostomatitis Renal dysfunction Methyl mercury intoxication: Impaired vision or hearing Numbness or pain in extremities	Do not eat fish or other food sources suspected of being contaminated with mercury; limit intake of fresh water fish caught by family or friends: 6 oz cooked fish per week for pregnant women, women of childbearing years, and nursing mothers; 2 oz for young children (EPA, 2001) Pregnant women should avoid eating swordfish, shark, king mackerel, and tile fish; can eat up to 12 oz of other fish per week (FDA, 2001) Do not allow children to play with glass thermometers, electrical wires, paints, or other materials with mercury Replace mercury thermometers and thermostats

TABLE 42-3 *Common Pediatric Toxicants and Relationship to Disease—cont'd*

		Health Effects		
Substance	**Source**	**Systems Affected**	**Signs and Symptoms**	**Prevention Strategies**
	Burning fossil fuels Mining Smelting Incineration (especially of medical wastes) Industrial discharge Natural seepage from rocks		Birth defects Hypotonia Ataxia Acute inhalation of elemental mercury: Necrotizing bronchitis Pneumonia Fever Acute ingestion of inorganic mercury salts: Nausea and vomiting Intestinal pain Bloody diarrhea Renal necrosis and failure Seizures, coma, and death	NEVER vacuum up mercury spills (this vaporizes and spreads the mercury) Call hazardous materials officials for advice on mercury spills Safely store and dispose of products containing mercury Be sure folk remedies are mercury free Advise families from cultures that use elemental mercury in religious ceremonies of the danger, especially to children
Environmental tobacco smoke (ETS)	Side-stream smoke from tobacco products being used by others (child is inhaling unfiltered smoke) Secondhand smoke exhaled by smoker in child's environment Smoking by child or adolescent	Respiratory Cardiac	Bronchitis Pneumonia Asthma Otitis media Middle ear effusion Premature coronary artery disease (especially white males) Low birth weight (mother exposed to ETS) Sudden infant death syndrome (SIDS)	Adults and siblings in child's environment stop smoking Enroll child in day care that is smoke free Prevent child from starting smoking Recommend smoking cessation programs Health care provider support of decision to stop smoking
Radon	Air Water Is concentrated in basements and low areas	Respiratory	Lung cancer May be some other health effects	Test air in basements and first floor of home for radon levels (see text) Avoid having children play in basements of homes with radon Reduce amount of radon in basements: Seal cracks in foundation of house Cover dirt crawl spaces with impermeable plastic Seal drains Pour concrete floors Provide good ventilation Stop smoking (tobacco smokes acts as a vehicle for radon to enter the body)
Particulate matter	Outdoor: Industrial pollution Gasoline and diesel exhaust Pollens Natural phenomena Forest fires Volcanic activity	Respiratory Cardiovascular	Bronchitis Pneumonia Wheezing Chronic cough Decreased lung function Asthma Cardiovascular conditions Lung cancer	When outdoor air pollution is high, keep children indoors, decrease outdoor playtime Air-condition the home (HEPA systems are most effective) Check heating system to ensure it is clean Cover mattresses, wash bedding frequently

Continued

TABLE 42-3 Common Pediatric Toxicants and Relationship to Disease—cont'd

Substance	Source	Health Effects: Systems Affected	Health Effects: Signs and Symptoms	Prevention Strategies
	Indoor: Wood-burning stoves Dust mites Animal dander Cockroach particles Molds Tobacco smoke			Launder or discard stuffed animals
Molds	Damp areas in the home or school (leaking roofs or plumbing, flooding in basements, backed-up sewers) Humidifiers Steam from shower, bath, or cooking Wet clothes House plants Dry leaves	Respiratory Skin CNS	Allergic reactions: Cough Wheezing or shortness of breath Sinus congestion Watery, itchy, light-sensitive eyes Sore throat Skin rash Headaches, memory loss, mood changes Aches and pains Fever	Maintain dry, clean environment: Clean with hot water and detergent Clean surfaces where mold grows with solution 1 part bleach:4 parts water Dry completely. Allow to dry naturally overnight (EPA, 2003b) Keep humidity low to decrease mold growth If unable to thoroughly clean, discard moldy materials to prevent spores from being released when materials dry
Asbestos	Construction materials: Insulation Ceiling and floor tiles Shingles	Respiratory	Lung irritation Lung disease later in life with repeated exposure	Prevent exposure to asbestos products: If buildings that contain asbestos are in good repair, it may be best to leave asbestos in place; if there is a question, contact a certified asbestos professional to check it Use asbestos abatement measures as appropriate when renovating If parents' workplace is a source of asbestos exposure, remove clothing and bathe before coming in contact with children.
Pesticides	Food Water Direct contact with plants, grass, and other areas treated with pesticides, insecticides, herbicides, or fungicides Direct contact with pesticide through dust, mists, sprays	CNS Immune Endocrine Skin GI	Skin rash Increased risk of cancer Developmental delay Neurotoxicity: Impaired sensation Dizziness Restlessness, confusion, irritability Impaired coordination May disrupt endocrine function May contribute to immune dysfunction Nausea/vomiting Seizures Death by poisoning	Use few or no pesticides in the home; use nonchemical treatments Use only amount recommended, for purpose stated Protect skin from exposure when using; wash thoroughly after use Do not inhale or use on windy day Keep children and pets from treated areas Clean up any spills Keep pesticides from food/dishes Store pesticides safely out of children's reach, in original container Do not mix pesticides Dispose of pesticides at a registered disposal site

TABLE 42-3 *Common Pediatric Toxicants and Relationship to Disease—cont'd*

		Health Effects		
Substance	**Source**	**Systems Affected**	**Signs and Symptoms**	**Prevention Strategies**
				Keep a copy of the label handy Decrease exposure in foods: Vary kinds of fruits and vegetables children eat Grow your own Buy organically grown foods; check USDA labels: "100% organic," "organic" (at least 95% organic content), "made with organic" (70% organic content for up to 3 ingredients), and "organic components" (products with less than 70% organic content) Wash and peel fruits and vegetables (many pesticides are in the product itself; washing and peeling will not remove them) Try to use in-season fruits and vegetables to avoid those sprayed for transport and preservation
Polychlorinated biphenyls (PCBs)	Foods and cooking oil Fish; concentrated in fatty tissues of animals Prenatal exposure via maternal ingestion of contaminated food Breastfeeding Older and deteriorating electrical equipment or wiring; transformers Hydraulic fluids, plasticizers, caulking compounds, paints, adhesives, and flame retardants Pesticides Inks and carbonless paper	CNS Respiratory Hepatic Skin	Prenatal exposure contributes to: Low birth weight Growth delay Developmental delay Decreased IQ scores Neurologic and intellectual impairment Increased respiratory infections Increased behavior problems Smaller male genitalia Chloracne, including cysts (1-10 mm diameter), comedones, papules, hyperpigmentation, conjunctiva, gingiva, and nail changes Childhood exposure leads to: Developmental delays Premature pubertal changes in both boys and girls Acute dermatologic and neurologic problems Chronic liver disease Tooth enamel defects (Jan & Vrbic, 2000)	Avoid PCB-contaminated foods, especially prenatally Avoid environmental exposure from electrical leakage Use professional abatement procedures to dispose of or clean up contaminated materials

Data from AAP (2003); Landrigan (2001); Reigart & Roberts (1999, 2001).
HEPA, High-efficiency particulate air; *USDA*, United States Department of Agriculture.

Child has risk factor from screening criteria		
Yes: Draw venous blood sample and complete laboratory assessment		**No:** Routine screening not recommended; provide caregiver dietary and environmental education

Screening sample: blood lead levels (BLLs)	**Actions to be taken***	**Follow-up BLL monitoring**
<10 μg/dl	Not considered lead poisoning: • Provide caregiver dietary and environmental education • Refer to social services if necessary	If high risk, retest in 6 months If low risk, no further testing needed
10-14 μg/dl	Borderline: Confirmatory venous blood testing within 3 months	Early follow-up within 3 months If follow-up level is 15-19 μg/dl or higher in two tests taken 3 months apart, retest every 1-2 months until results <15 μg/dl for at least 6 months, then retest every 6-9 months
15-19 μg/dl	Confirmatory venous blood testing within 3 months Proceed according to actions for 20-44 μg/dl if: • A follow-up BLL is in this range at least 3 months after initial venous testing or • BLLs increase	Early follow-up within 2 months If levels continue >15 μg/dl, retest every 1-2 months until results <15 μg/dl for at least 6 months, then retest every 3 months until child is 36 months old
20-44 μg/dl	Confirmatory venous blood testing shortly (within 1 week to 1 month; the higher levels in the shorter time) Complete history and physical exam Neurodevelopmental monitoring Lab work: Hgb or Hct and iron status (FEP or ZPP) Abdominal x-ray (if particulate lead ingestion is suspected) with bowel decontamination if indicated	Early follow-up in 1-3 months for BLLs 20-24 μg/dl; in 2 weeks-1 month for BLLs 25-44 μg/dl Retest every 1-2 months until results <15 μg/dl for at least 6 months, then retest every 3 months until child is 36 months old
45-69 μg/dl	Diagnostic venous blood testing within 24-48 hours Complete history and physical examination Complete neurologic exam Lab work: Hgb or Hct and iron status (FEP or ZPP) Abdominal x-ray with bowel decontamination if indicated Chelation therapy	Early follow-up as soon as possible Retest every month until results <15 μg/dl for at least 6 months, then retest every 3 months until child is 36 months old
>70 μg/dl	Medical emergency: Retest immediately as an emergency lab test with venous blood sample Hospitalize for intravenous chelation Proceed according to action for 45-69 μg/dl	Early follow-up as soon as possible Retest every month until results <15 μg/dl for at least 6 months, then retest every 3 months until child is 36 months old

*In all cases of lead toxicity:

- Provide caregiver dietary and environmental education
- Remove child from source of lead if known
- Report to Public Health Department
- Initiate environmental investigation
- Initiate lead hazard control/abatement
- Refer to social services

Adapted from CDC, 1997, pp. 92, 104; CDC, 2002a, pp. 41, 51.

Hgb, Hemoglobin; Hct, hematocrit; FEP, free erythrocytes protoporphyrin; ZPP, zinc protoporphyrin.

FIGURE 42-2 Management recommendations for lead poisoning. (Adapted from Centers for Disease Control and Prevention: *Screening young children for lead poisoning: guidance for state and local public health officials*, Atlanta, 1997, Centers for Disease Control and Prevention; Centers for Disease Control and Prevention: *Managing elevated blood lead levels among young children: recommendations from the Advisory Committee on Childhood Lead Poisoning Prevention*, Atlanta, 2002a, Centers for Disease Control and Prevention.)

accurately reflect the amount of lead in the body. A child can have high blood lead levels (e.g., 45 μg/dl) with no obvious clinical signs. Another child may complain of severe GI problems with a lower lead level (e.g., 15 to 20 μg/dl).

Subclinical Effects. In many cases, changes caused by lead toxicity are subtle enough not to be identified as a clinical problem (see Table 42-3). Findings from early studies related to decreased cognitive function and increased behavior problems continue to be confirmed (Campbell et al, 2000; Needleman et al, 2002).

Clinical Effects. Many children do not demonstrate signs of toxicity until late in the disease. At higher levels, lead affects vitamin D metabolism, nerve conduction velocities, and hemoglobin synthesis. See Table 42-3 for clinical signs and symptoms.

Laboratory Studies. Blood lead testing should be done using venous blood rather than a capillary sample to confirm the diagnosis. Assessment of free erythrocytes protoporphyrin (FEP) and zinc protoporphyrin (ZPP) is helpful because these are elevated due to the biochemical effects of lead. Evaluate iron deficiency, including serum ferritin or low ratio of serum iron to iron binding capacity (Wright et al, 2003).

Differential Diagnosis

GI infections, other causes of anemia, growth retardation, behavior disorders, attention-deficit hyperactivity disorder (ADHD), and central nervous system (CNS) infection are all included in the differential diagnosis.

Management

Management involves preventing the child's exposure to lead in the environment, treating the child for toxicity, monitoring lead levels, correcting dietary deficiencies (if any), and removing lead from the environment (see Table 42-3 and Fig. 42-2). Other children in the same household or environment where exposure could have occurred also should be tested and treated as appropriate.

Prevention and Patient Education

Table 42-3 outlines prevention strategies. Parents need to know that lead abatement is essential; treatments such as chelation therapy and dietary changes are ineffective unless the child is returned to a clean house. Until lead abatement can be implemented, however, parents can work to control lead dust and paint chips in older homes. Conventional vacuums can be used to help control lead dust and high-efficiency particulate air (HEPA) filtering vacuum cleaners can temporarily reduce lead loads, but levels soon rise if the source of lead remains (Yiin et al, 2002). Other strategies parents can use include the following:

- Block access to areas of the room where large peeling paint areas are found.
- Cover smaller peeling areas with sticky-backed paper.
- Damp-mop and damp-dust with household cleaners or lead-specific cleaning products (e.g., Ledizolv) twice weekly to decrease lead dust in the air; do not dry-mop or sweep.
- Pick up and dispose of paint chips with a disposable rag or paper towel soaked in phosphate cleaner.

Inform parents that chelation therapy leads to a rapid fall in blood lead levels, but that most children have a rebound increase within days or weeks of treatment and repeated treatment may be necessary until the lead level is in a safe range.

Mercury

Description

Mercury, like lead, is a heavy metal, and is the second most common cause of heavy metal poisoning. It exists in elemental forms (liquid or vapor), inorganic mercury salts, and organic forms. Organic mercury compounds, such as methyl mercury, are the most toxic and are found in the food chain. CNS tissue is the main target organ for mercury in humans. Once absorbed into the brain, mercury metabolizes to its inorganic form and cannot cross the blood-brain barrier to exit the brain; significant neurologic symptoms can result. The kidney is another major target organ, especially for inorganic mercury poisoning. Mercury may be corrosive to the GI system. The fetus and child are more susceptible to mercury toxicity than are others. Offspring of pregnant females who ingested methyl mercury have been affected by severe, irreversible central and peripheral neurologic conditions (Minamata disease).

Etiology and Incidence

Mercury is pervasive in the environment. Common sources are listed in Table 42-3. Elemental mercury is poorly absorbed in the GI tract, and its use as a dental amalgam is not considered a health risk. However, this volatile metal form of mercury, found in thermometers, can vaporize (e.g., vacuuming up spills can spread the mercury through airborne particles), can be inhaled, and is readily absorbed through the lungs.

Inorganic and organic forms of mercury are also absorbed through inhalation. Inorganic mercury, found in some fungicides, antiseptics, and medications, is poorly absorbed by the gut or through the skin, and does not readily cross the blood-brain barrier. It is excreted in urine. Organic mercury (e.g., methyl mercury) accumulates in the biologic organism, is concentrated in food products (especially fish), and is readily absorbed from the GI tract and through the skin. Organic mercury easily enters the brain, crosses the placenta, and has been found in breast milk.

It is unknown just how prevalent mercury poisoning is, because many signs are common to other conditions. A review of 1999 data from the National Health and Nutrition Examination Survey indicates a low level of toxic impact (CDC, 2001a). This does not, however, minimize the deadly potential of contact with mercury.

Clinical Assessment

History. A thorough history is essential to identify the source of exposure because the signs and symptoms can be very confusing. Questions focus on potential exposure, workplace environment, diet, and whether others in the family are experiencing similar symptoms.

Physical Examination. Five manifestions of mercury poisoning are found clinically (Behrman, Kliegman, & Jenson, 2004, p. 2357):

1. Acrodynia ("pink disease"), most often seen in children:
   - Hypersensitivity reaction with generalized pain, paresthesias
   - Pink, papular, pruritic rash that may involve face, hands, and feet
   - May have morbilliform, vesicular, or hemorrhagic rash
   - Anorexia
   - Weakness, hypotonia, especially of pelvic area
   - Good prognosis when mercury source is removed
2. Chronic inorganic mercury intoxication (signs and symptoms may also be seen with chronic exposure to elemental and organic mercury):
   - Classic triad: tremor, neuropsychiatric disturbance, gingivostomatitis
   - May have sensorimotor neuropathy and visual disturbances
   - Renal dysfunction, nephrotic syndrome
3. Methyl mercury intoxication (Minamata disease):
   - Delayed neurotoxicity, ataxia, paresthesias, tremors, sensory impairment, dementia, death
   - Fetal involvement most severe: low birth weight, profound developmental delays, cerebral palsy, deafness, blindness, seizures
4. Acute inhalation of elemental mercury vapor:
   - Cough, dyspnea, chest pain, fever, headache, GI disturbance
   - Can be self-limited
   - Can progress to necrotizing bronchiolitis; may be fatal
5. Acute ingestion of inorganic mercury salts:
   - Corrosive gastroenteritis within hours, severe GI pain, hematemesis, cardiovascular collapse, renal failure
   - Can be fatal

Laboratory Studies. Blood mercury levels can be used to determine acute mercury exposure, but the blood half-life is short, and levels may not reflect toxicity. A blood level of less than 2 μg/L is considered normal. A 24-hour urine sample in an acid-washed container gives the optimal sample of mercury contamination (less than 10 μg/L is considered normal), but a first morning void may give good information. Hair analysis is not considered reliable.

Differential Diagnosis

The differential diagnosis includes other poisonings, infections of the CNS, and CNS conditions.

Management

Patients should be referred to a center for clinical management. Chelation is the treatment of choice and needs to be conducted at a center where supportive therapy can stabilize the patient during the procedure. Decontamination through gastric lavage may be appropriate to remove ingested inorganic mercury, depending on how recently exposure occurred. Because of mercury's corrosive effect, emesis is not recommended.

Prevention and Patient Education

Stopping exposure is essential (see Table 42-3). Children have been known to innocently play with mercury. Parents need to be reminded of the deadly effect of mercury and encouraged to keep all materials that contain mercury out of children's reach. Mercury spills should be handled by a professional abatement team or cleaned with wet, occlusive materials.

Air Pollution: Indoor and Outdoor

Air quality is an important environmental factor in childhood illness, especially respiratory conditions. Since the 1970s, outdoor air quality has improved in many areas as a result of local, state, and federal regulations, but outdoor air pollution continues to contribute significantly to adverse health effects. Recent relaxation of air quality standards by the U.S. federal government can be expected to again threaten the health of communities. In particular, both children and adults are affected by carbon monoxide, sulfur oxides, hydrocarbons, ozone, particulate matter, and nitrogen oxides. Indoor air quality has declined in the same time period. This is largely attributed to an increase in the use of carpets, wood stove heating, and synthetic and chemically formulated building materials (e.g., pressed wood made with formaldehyde) coupled with more "energy-conserving" construction that makes new homes more "airtight" and reduces ventilation. Because up to 90%

of an individual's time is spent indoors, exposure to airborne toxicants has increased markedly.

As discussed earlier, children are especially susceptible to air quality because they are experiencing rapid lung development; have smaller, narrower airways; breathe more rapidly; are more physically active than adults; and spend more time on the floor. Very young children spend notably more time indoors. This section discusses several of the more common indoor and outdoor airborne toxicants that influence children's health status: environmental tobacco smoke, radon, particulate matter, molds, and asbestos.

Environmental Tobacco Smoke

Description. Environmental tobacco smoke (ETS), the presence of tobacco smoke in the air children breathe, has been associated with chronic and acute respiratory symptoms, recurrent otitis media, middle ear effusions, bronchitis, pneumonia, sudden infant death syndrome (SIDS), asthma, and invasive meningococcal disease (Kriz, Bobak, & Kriz, 2000). Passive smoking has been associated with other health problems such as low birth weight, Legg-Calvé-Perthes disease (Glueck et al, 1998), and appendicitis (Montgomery, Pounder, & Wakefield, 1999). In some conditions tobacco may be a complicating rather than causal factor and other variables such as socioeconomic status and diet must also be considered (Denson, 2001). A meta-analysis noted that the child of a parent who smokes is at approximately twice the risk of having a serious lower respiratory tract infection in infancy or early childhood than the child of a nonsmoker (Li et al, 1999). Pubertal children with a history of long-term exposure to passive cigarette smoke, especially white males, are at increased risk of premature coronary artery disease (Moskowitz, Schwartz, & Schieken, 1999).

Etiology and Incidence. Children, especially very young children, are exposed to tobacco smoke primarily through cigarettes, cigars, or pipes used by parents, other family members, or visitors in the home. Day care providers or teachers also may smoke. Although smoking has decreased in the U.S. adult population, it is estimated that almost 40% of children 5 years of age and younger whose family is low income live with a smoker (Emmons et al, 2001). Many U.S. families, including those with smokers, try to limit their children's exposure to passive smoke; still, a significant number of children are exposed to ETS through visitors, at their grandparents' house, or in other settings (Kegler & Malcoe, 2002; Schuster, Franke, & Pham, 2002). Tobacco smoke is also absorbed into clothing, so even if smokers abstain in the house or around children, their clothes may present a hazard (Noble, 2000).

Active cigarette smoking among high school students peaked between 1997 and 1999, when a high of 36% of students stated that they were current smokers and 17% stated that they were frequent smokers. Since then, high school smoking has decreased, and in 2001 29% of students were current smokers and 14% were frequent smokers, decreasing the amount of smoke in the teenagers' environment (CDC, 2002b).

Assessment. Assessment of the extent to which ETS affects the child's health requires a thorough and accurate history. The physical problems for which children are treated vary, and the NP should suspect tobacco smoke as a factor in children who have recurrent respiratory and ear infections.

History. Collect data about the following:

- The amount of smoke in the child's environment, both in the home and in other locations (e.g., day care, school, home of relatives or friends): How many people smoke, and how much do they smoke? Does the child smoke? The number of smokers in the household is a good indicator of ETS exposure (Kaufman et al, 2002).
- The amount of time the child spends in these environments: How long is the child exposed to ETS? Is the child ever in a car with a smoker?
- Any symptoms related to ETS: Has the child experienced health problems that may be associated with ETS (cough, colds, ear infections, etc.)?

Physical Examination and Laboratory Studies. These will be specific to the physical signs and symptoms of the child (see Table 42-3).

Management. The best treatment for adverse affects of ETS is prevention; every effort should be made to ensure that the child's environment is smoke free (see Table 42-3). Programs such as Keeping Infants Safe from Smoke (KISS) have been shown to have success (Emmons et al, 2001). For those who continue to smoke, smoking outside the home, not smoking in cars, and using adequate ventilation are essential. Alternative day care arrangements should be explored if there is smoking at the child's care center. All children should be informed about the dangers associated with smoking. Nonsmoking children should be praised for their decision to not smoke, and children who smoke should be encouraged and supported in their efforts to quit.

Smoking cessation is a difficult process and depends on a number of biologic, behavioral, and psychosocial factors. In one study, although more than 84% of adolescents had thought seriously about quitting and about 55% had tried to stop in the 6 months before the study survey, only about 15% were able to say they had quit, based on a criterion of "not smoking for the past 30 days" (Zhu et al, 1999). Predictors for success in quitting included (1) being an "occasional" smoker; (2) never having quit or having quit for 14 or more days previously; (3) making a self-prediction that he or she would not be smoking in 1 year; (4) having lower depression scores; and (5) having a mother who does not smoke.

Prevention and Patient Education. Parents are critical in preventing exposure to ETS:

- Parents can create a smoke-free environment by not smoking, stopping, and monitoring the child's exposure.
- Parental disapproval prevents children from becoming smokers (Sargent & Dalton, 2001).
- When parents stop smoking, children do not start, or are more likely to also stop (Chassin et al, 2002).

In the general population, many providers ask their patients about smoking and urge them to stop, but do not provide support and follow-up intervention. Pediatric providers can use the U.S. Agency for Health Care Policy and Research (USAHCPR) guidelines, *Treating Tobacco Use and Dependence: A Clinical Practice Guideline*, to structure their smoking cessation counseling (USAHCPR, 2000). These include the "five *A*'s":

- *Ask about use*: Systematically identify tobacco users and document their status.
- *Advise to quit*: Strongly urge all smokers to quit.
- *Assess willingness to quit*: Identify smokers willing to make an attempt to quit.
- *Assist in quit attempt*: Aid the patient in quitting by offering a plan, providing education and support with nicotine replacement therapy as needed, or referring to a smoking cessation program in the community.
- *Arrange follow-up*: Schedule follow-up contact.

Radon

Description. Radon is a colorless, odorless, radioactive gas that enters homes through soil or water (e.g., basement floors, cracks in concrete foundations, sumps, or drains) (see Table 42-3). As radon decays, some of its products change to an isotope of polonium, which, when inhaled, can cause lung damage leading to cancer. In the atmosphere, radon is diluted and has no health effect. When concentrated in an enclosed area, it represents a risk. Tobacco smoke provides a vehicle for radon to enter the lungs, adding to the risk of radon-induced cancer for smokers and individuals exposed to ETS. Water that has been filtered through the soil can contain radon (e.g., well water), and about 2% to 5% of radon in homes is found in the water supply. Radon in water has been associated with a slightly increased incidence of gastric cancer and leukemia, and there may be some evidence of an effect on chromosomal structure (Bilban & Vaupoti, 2001). The EPA does not yet have standards for safe radon levels in water.

Etiology and Incidence. Radon is generally considered the second leading cause of lung cancer in Americans (EPA, 1994). Because lung cancer typically occurs in older adults and the effect of radon is accentuated by tobacco, the risk of lung cancer in children is very small, and the long-term impact of radon on nonsmokers is unknown (Enflo, 2002). Radon is more prevalent in certain geographic areas. Local health departments can be consulted to determine if radon is a local health risk.

Assessment. In 1988 the Surgeon General recommended that all homes, except residences above the second floor in multilevel buildings, be tested for radon. Radon detector kits can be purchased in hardware, home improvement, or department stores and are available from the National Safety Council (see Resource Box). Measurements are taken using two canisters set side by side in the room, and the device is returned to the manufacturer for analysis. Short-term (2 to 7 days) or long-term (3 to 12 months) testing can be done. The long-term testing gives a more accurate measure of the average radon exposure, because levels fluctuate over time and with changes in seasons. The EPA recommends using the short-term test and suggests the following actions based on findings:

- For levels of 4 to 20 pCi/L, conduct radon remediation within 1 to 2 years.
- For levels of 20 to 200 pCi/L, conduct radon remediation within several months.
- For levels greater than 200 pCi/L, conduct radon remediation within several weeks.

Management. Radon remediation involves decreasing the amount of radon entering the home and removing radon that is present (see Table 42-3). Children should not spend significant amounts of time in high-risk areas of the home.

Particulate Matter

Description. Particulate matter (PM) is one of a cluster of indoor and outdoor air pollutants that have an adverse effect on respiratory and cardiovascular function. Other outdoor air pollutants include ozone, sulfur dioxide (SO_2), nitrogen oxides (NO and NO_2), and carbon monoxide (CO). The diameter of PM is measured in microns, and standards have been set for concentrations of PM_{10} and $PM_{2.5}$. Fine PM (2.5 μm in diameter or smaller) is of growing concern because it can be inhaled and carried deep into lung tissue. Coarse PM (2.5 to 10 μm in diameter) can be filtered by the nasal mucosa or trachea and removed by coughing or sneezing.

Exposure to PM creates an inflammatory response in the body and, in combination with other pollutants, is associated with increased mortality rates and increased hospitalization rates for respiratory or cardiovascular problems (Brook, Brook, & Rajagopalan, 2003). The anatomic structure of the lung may contribute to differential distribution of PM in the pulmonary tree, with subsequent cancer in particular sites (Balashazy, Hofmann, & Heistracher, 2003). Respiratory infections, wheezing, decreased lung function, and asthma hospitalizations have been found to increase with exposure to PM (Brauer et al, 2002); however, studies do not support the contention that PM causes asthma (Hruba et al, 2001).

Etiology and Incidence. PM is a pervasive by-product of industrial production, gasoline and diesel engines, wood-burning stoves, and natural phenomena (e.g., volcanic activity, grass and forest fires, and blowing dust). Residents of urban and industrial areas are exposed to high levels of PM, and concentrations increase in summer months and when there is more combustion present (e.g., rush-hour traffic). The amount of indoor PM, including dust, mites, cockroach particles, and animal dander, varies among households, but many low-income urban residences have high levels of dust, mouse, and cockroach residue.

Assessment. Parents can keep a record of their child's illness episodes to determine if increased air pollution, dust, insects, or pets in the home are associated with illness.

Management. The goal of management is to decease the amount of PM in the environment or limit the child's contact with PM (see Table 42-3).

Molds

Description. Molds are microscopic organisms in the class of bioaerosols, living organisms that release elements into the air. These elements are then inhaled or come into contact with skin or mucous membranes. Although more studies are recommended to confirm a definitive relationship, mold spores are thought to cause allergic reactions (Jacob et al, 2002), and certain fungi can release mycotoxins that elicit irritant and toxic responses (AAP, 2003). Molds thrive in damp spaces, but spores can be found in dust, dry leaves, and storage areas. *Aspergillus* (black mold), *Alternaria, Penicillium,* and *Cladosporium* are common household molds.

Etiology and Incidence. Research on the health effects of molds and the numbers of people affected is limited, but children have an increased risk of cough and wheezing when exposed to damp and mold in the home. Mold in schools has contributed to respiratory problems for children (Meklin et al, 2002). Common sources of mold exposure for children are listed in Table 42-3.

Assessment. Common responses to molds include a spectrum of allergic reactions (see Table 42-3). Assessment questions also are directed at finding the cause of the symptoms:

- Is there a pattern to the symptoms?
- Are they aggravated by any particular environment?
- Are they relieved when the child changes environments?
- What has the family done to remediate the environment?

Differential Diagnosis. The differential diagnosis includes other causes of allergic reactions and upper respiratory infections. Reaction to molds can be confused with pesticide poisoning.

Management. Treatment involves control of allergic symptoms (e.g., antihistamines to control itching or sneezing; see Chapters 25 and 37 for discussion of allergies and their management) and removal of the cause of the problem. Ultimately, the source of moisture must be removed, because maintaining a dry, clean environment minimizes the growth of molds (see Table 42-3). Ozone air cleaners are not effective against molds.

Provide information regarding the connection between exposure to molds, allergic reactions, and respiratory problems. Parents may need support during cleanup, because it may be difficult or nearly impossible to do a thorough job (e.g., mold may have permeated the walls in a rental unit and the family is not able to have them replaced or to move to a more suitable apartment).

Asbestos

Description. Asbestos is the name given to a group of incombustible fibrous magnesium silicate minerals used most often in construction materials. Chrysolite is the only asbestos product still on the market; other forms are found in older buildings. Contamination by asbestos is measured in fibers per cubic centimeter of air. The OSHA workplace standard is 0.1 fibers per cubic centimeter averaged over an 8-hour shift (OSHA, 2002). Levels in schools may range from 0.05 to 0.2 fibers per cubic centimeter, placing schoolchildren at relatively low risk.

Etiology and Incidence. Asbestosis is considered an occupational problem of adults, and smokers are at higher risk of asbestos-induced lung disease than nonsmokers. Childhood exposure to asbestos, however, may contribute to serious illness as an adult. Children can be exposed through direct contact with air in a contaminated building or with material or clothing parents bring home from their work site. An estimated 10,000 schools built between 1946 and 1973 may contain asbestos (American Academy of Pediatrics [AAP], 1994), although it is only considered a hazard if the material is disrupted through deterioration or renovation.

Assessment. Assessment of disease is based on a history of exposure and signs and symptoms of respiratory distress. Any exposure to asbestos fibers is a risk, but repeated inhalation of the fibers is associated with clinical signs of lung disease later in life. There may be a latency period of 20 years or more before conditions such as pleural effusion, lung fibrosis, and mesothelioma in the pleura or peritoneum appear. Controlled studies indicate a significant relationship between cancer and asbestos (Valic, 2002). Exposure to asbestos does not typically produce acute symptoms, although high concentrations of asbestos dust can cause lung irritation, including cough, dyspnea, fatigue, and chest pain.

Management. Preventing unnecessary exposure to asbestos fibers reduces the risk of inhalation and subsequent disease (see Table 42-3). If asbestos is present in the workplace, OSHA standards (not always enforced) require employers to provide workers with full body suits and shoe covers that are left at the work site; parents should be encouraged to work with their employers to minimize the possibility of bringing fibers into the home. The Asbestos Hazard Emergency Response Act (AHERA) sets standards for schools to inspect and manage asbestos contamination (EPA, 2002). The EPA has also adopted OSHA standards and extended protection to the school environment (EPA, 2000). Parents should be informed of the adverse effects of asbestos exposure and reassured that their children are at low risk unless they spend significant amounts of time in older buildings that are in poor repair or undergoing renovation.

Pesticides

Description

Pesticides are chemicals used to kill or control unwanted pests, including plants. Herbicides, fungicides, insecticides, and other products are classified as "general-use" or "restricted-use" pesticides, depending on the toxicity to humans or the environment. Restricted-use pesticides require special handling by certified applicators. Labeling of pesticides varies by toxicity, with a skull and crossbones and the statement "DANGER—POISON" on the most toxic; "WARNING" on less toxic; and "CAUTION" on the labels of the least toxic pesticides. All pesticides are hazardous.

Etiology and Incidence

In 1997 there were over 20,700 registered pesticide products in the United States, with 890 related active ingredients. At that time, an estimated 4.63 billion pounds of all pesticides (including conventional [1 billion pounds], as well as wood preservatives, biocides, and other chemicals) were used in the United States. Usage was in agriculture (806 million pounds) and households (76 million pounds) (EPA, 1999).

Herbicides are the most widely used pesticide, and contaminated food products are a major source of exposure. Because of children's small size and large fruit and vegetable intake per unit of body weight, they ingest pesticides in foods at a disproportionate rate. It is estimated that by age 6 years, the average American child has accumulated 35% of the lifetime allowance of captan, a fungicide used extensively on fruit and a probable human carcinogen (Wiles, 1993). Farmworkers and children who live on or near farms are exposed to agricultural pesticides. Garden and lawn use increases risks to children playing outdoors in these areas. Indoor pesticides are increasingly implicated in childhood illness (Berkowitz et al, 2003).

Assessment

Adverse effects of pesticide exposure can be acute or chronic, and all body systems can be affected, depending on the nature of the toxin and the extent of exposure. Assessment must be comprehensive (see Table 42-3). Much data about pesticide poisoning are based only on studies in adults. There is concern that the effect of pesticides on children differs, and the risk children face for long-term health problems is seriously underestimated. Use of Developmental Neurotoxicity Testing Guidelines is recommended (Tilson, 2000).

A study applying anthropologic methods to community assessment of children's developmental capacity has demonstrated significant developmental differences in native Yaqui children from Mexico exposed to pesticides versus a cohort not exposed (Guillette, 2000). Indoor pesticides are associated with an increased risk of leukemia (Ma et al, 2002). Prenatal exposure to pesticides can affect children as well. In a Southern California study, pesticide exposure, specifically maternal use of flea or tick products during pregnancy, significantly increased the risk of brain tumors in children (Pogoda & Preston-Martin, 1997). Ongoing research in the pediatric population is occurring and should help clarify the relationship between pesticides and health problems (Berkowitz et al, 2003).

Management

Specifics of management depend on the type and amount of pesticide taken in and the route of absorption. Information on treatment is available on product labels. When treating an individual who may have been exposed to pesticides, health care providers, by law, are entitled to access information about the implicated pesticides (see National Pesticide Information Center, Resource Box). The EPA's Worker Protection Standard (WPS) also ensures that providers will be able to access information on general- and restricted-use pesticides. Under the WPS this information can be obtained from employers or manufacturers. Patients may be able to provide the pesticide label. Treatment focuses on supporting life functions:

- ABCs
  - Maintain gas exchange; may need to intubate
  - Prevent aspiration of vomitus
- Consult with a poison control center for direction in management (refer to a center or provider with expertise in this area as soon as possible; see previous discussion for management of general poisonings)
- Seizure control
- Report pesticide exposure to the state health department
- Work with parents, schools, and community agencies to prevent pesticide exposure

Prevention and Patient Education

The risks pesticides present to children are immense. Pesticide exposure occurs in a number of ways and is additive. Regulating the amount of pesticide children take in from any one source is good, but the pattern of multiple contamination must be recognized and a plan to regulate overall exposure developed. Education of parents is the key to prevention of pesticide poisoning in children (see Table 42-3).

Polychlorinated Biphenyls

Description

Polychlorinated biphenyls (PCBs), a family of up to 209 chemicals, are one type of extremely stable organochlorines. Many organochlorines are carcinogens or endocrine disruptors. PCBs used commercially are always mixtures of the various types and are frequently contaminated with furans and dioxins.

PCBs are structurally similar to thyroid hormones. They probably work through changes in hormonal function, altering concentrations of hormones or affecting receptor numbers or affinity. Effects have also been found on the human immune system. Further research is necessary to more definitively connect PCBs with specific neurodevelopmental problems (Ribas-Fito et al, 2001).

Etiology and Incidence

Although banned from production since 1977, PCBs are so stable that they are still commonly found in the environment, even in Arctic mammals (Colborn, Dumanoski, & Myers, 1997). Low levels are found throughout the world, evaporating and returning to earth by rainfall and settling in dust particles. PCBs are not very water soluble, and as a result are not found in high concentrations in drinking water. They dissolve readily in oils, accumulating in the fatty tissues of fish, birds, and mammals. Human exposure comes primarily through ingestion of contaminated foods. The workplace is a major source of exposure to PCBs in the United States. For children, fetal and neonatal exposures are common, usually via maternal ingestion of contaminated food. Schoolchildren can be exposed through deteriorating building materials.

Assessment

History

- History of maternal ingestion of contaminated food
- Skin disorders, including hyperpigmentation, nail changes, and chloracne
- Hepatic dysfunction
- Low birth weight and developmental delays
- Behavioral symptoms
- Frequent respiratory infections

Physical Examination. Clinical effects are listed in Table 42-3.

Laboratory Studies. Increased liver enzymes with severe exposure, although these findings are nonspecific.

Differential Diagnosis

The differential diagnosis includes acne vulgaris, other causes of developmental delay, lead poisoning, and hypothyroidism.

Management

Avoid contact with PCB-contaminated food and environmental sources, especially prenatally. Breastfeeding should not be stopped.

Arsenic

Description

Arsenic is a highly poisonous chemical element that occurs naturally in the environment, in organic and inorganic forms. Arsenic is found in many different compound forms and salts, such as arsenic acid, arsenic trioxide, and arsenate; some compounds (e.g., arsine [AsH_3]) are gaseous, colorless, nonirritating substances with an odor of garlic. Arsenic acts as an enzyme poison in the body and can affect all systems. Long-term, low-level exposure can lead to chronic poisoning and cancer. Acute poisoning is usually paralytic or gastrointestinal in nature. Spontaneous abortion, stillbirth, and preterm birth rates are higher in mothers exposed to arsenic in drinking water (Akhtar Ahmad et al, 2001).

Etiology and Incidence

In addition to its natural occurrence, arsenic is used commercially in pesticides, herbicides, rodenticides, and wood preservatives. Arsenic trioxide is also used in glassmaking and some pigments. Exposure to arsenic occurs in drinking water and contaminated foods. Children can also be exposed through contact with wood used to construct playgrounds that has been treated with chromated copper arsenate (CCA) to prevent decay. Leaching of arsenate into soil and sand of playground areas from treated wood presents a further danger to children (Fields, 2001). Burning treated wood releases arsenic into the air where it can be inhaled.

Assessment

An exposure history is essential in determining whether arsenic poisoning has occurred. Physical signs and symptoms depend on the type of exposure and include the following:

- Cancer, often in the skin with chronic exposure; can appear in any system
- Neurologic: headache, paralysis, delirium, numbness, tremors, decreased reflexes, muscle weakness
- Cardiovascular: decreased circulation to extremities, arrythmias
- GI: nausea, vomiting, diarrhea, pain
- Hematologic: anemia, hemolysis of red blood cells
- Liver damage
- Renal failure

Laboratory Studies. Twenty-four–hour urine sample is the preferred specimen, but serum levels can also be measured.

Management

Prevent exposure by keeping children away from arsenic-containing pesticides. Parents and providers can work with schools and communities to assess for and clean up arsenic contamination of playground areas (Tran et al, 2002). If there is a possibility of arsenic in the water supply, testing is recommended. NPs should also support standards for use and production of arsenic products, such as a 2001 EPA action that lowers the allowable arsenic in drinking water from 50 to 10 μg/L, and the voluntary agreement by the pressure-treated wood industry to phase out use of CCA in wood produced for residential use by December 2003.

Noise

Description

Noise is defined as any sound, but is usually considered loud, harsh, unpleasant, or unwanted. Noise pollution is the presence of irritating, distracting, or physically dangerous noise. Sound has qualities of frequency or pitch (measured in cycles per minute and stated in Hertz [Hz]), intensity or loudness (measured in decibels [dB]), periodicity, and duration (either continuous, short-term, or episodic). The human voice is approximately 50 dB sound pressure levels (AAP, 2003).

The impact of noise on human health is varied. Noise-induced hearing loss (NIHL) and tinnitus are the most obvious effects. Noise also contributes to children's behavior problems and lowered academic performance (Haines et al, 2002; Hygge, Evans, & Bullinger, 2002).

Etiology and Incidence

Hearing loss is a growing problem in the pediatric population, especially among adolescents. Approximately 9.9 per 100,000 individuals suffer NIHL in the total population. Although this number is small, the ratio is significantly higher for children and young adults than other age-groups, with 28 per 100,000 in 6- to 25-year-olds, and 107 per 100,000 in 19-year-old boys (Plontke et al, 2002). As many as 12.5% of 6- to 19-year-olds have evidence of noise-induced hearing threshold shift (Niskar et al, 2001).

Humans are subject to NIHL from exposure to continuous noise or to sudden acoustic trauma that causes damage to the hair cells of the cochlea due to excessive vibration; extreme noise can rupture the tympanic membrane. Noise of more than 85 dB but less than 140 dB leads to temporary hearing loss, most often in the 4000 Hz range. Permanent hearing loss can result from one exposure to a sudden, extreme noise (greater than 140 dB) of short duration, or from ongoing lower levels of noise. Permanent loss is often in the 3000 to 6000 Hz range. Music listened to on headphones and at concerts, firecrackers, electrical tools, airport noise, and even everyday noise of traffic can cause problems (Lercher et al, 2002). Chronic, everyday noise causes sleep disturbance, distraction, decreased concentration, and an increased stress response (e.g., increased heart rate, blood pressure, adrenalin, and cortisol production); these in turn result in personality changes, irritability, poor coping, and lower achievement in children.

Assessment

History. A careful history looks at the following:

- Type of noise in child's environment
- Exposure to chronic noise
- Episodic acoustic trauma
- History of ear disease

Physical Examination. Many states require assessment of newborns for congenital or birth-related hearing loss (see Chapters 17, 30, and 39). This testing establishes a baseline; thereafter children should be assessed for hearing using a pure-tone audiometer at well-child examinations of 4, 5, 10, 12, and 18 years of age. Tympanography and visual examination of the tympanic membrane help rule out otitis media and middle ear effusion.

Management

Noise-induced hearing loss is virtually 100% preventable. The goals of management are to

- Increase awareness of the health hazard noise represents. Parents and children need to understand the relationship between noise and the auditory system. Every well-child visit should include questions related to the child's noise environment, and both children and parents should be given information on the dangers of excessive noise and how to avoid them. NPs can work with parents and schools to offer a hearing loss management curriculum.
- Decrease noise in the environment. Parents and children should be encouraged to minimize noise in their environment, including efforts to
  - Reduce volume on television and radios; turn off "background" TVs and radios.
  - Use headphones cautiously, keeping the volume low enough to hear normal conversation.
  - Avoid loud music, firecrackers, popguns, and other sources of episodic, extreme noise.
  - Avoid loud noises; for example, do not vacuum or use appliances (e.g., blender) with infants nearby.
  - Create a "quiet" place in the home.
- Mitigate exposure to noise. Wear earplugs and earmuffs to protect against "unavoidable" noise. Commercial-quality ear protectors are available for use in the home (e.g., when electrical saws or other loud tools are used). Earplugs can be purchased at any drugstore.
- Implement standards to regulate noise. The Federal Noise Control Act of 1972 provides the mechanism to set standards, rules, and regulations for occupational, industrial, and residential noise (e.g., automobiles, construction). States and municipalities have also established standards for noise control. NPs can be a resource to policy makers by providing information about the health effects of excessive and chronic noise.

RESOURCE BOX

Environmental Health Issues

Agency for Toxic Substances and Disease Registry (ATSDR)
1-404-639-0700
www.atsdr.cdc.gov/

Alliance to End Childhood Lead Poisoning
1-202-543-1147
www.aeclp.org

American Academy of Clinical Toxicology
1-717-558-7750
www.clintox.org/index.html
Position statements on treatment of poisonings

American Council on Science and Health, Inc.
1-212-362-7044
www.acsh.org/

Association of Occupational and Environmental Clinics (AOEC)
http://dmi-www.mc.duke.edu/oem/

Center for Children's Health and the Environment
www.childenvironment.org/
Academic and research policy center on environmental health of children

Centers for Disease Control and Prevention (CDC) National Center for Environmental Health
1-888-232-6789
www.cdc.gov/nceh/

Children's Environmental Health Network
www.cehn.org/

Consumer Product Safety Commission Office of Information
1-800-638-2772
1-301-504-6816
www.cpsc.gov

Environmental Health Perspectives
http://ehp.niehs.nih.gov/children/
Link to Pediatric Environmental Health Specialty Units (PEHSUs)

Environmental Protection Agency (EPA)
www.epa.gov/
The EPA has information on a wide range of environmental toxins. For example:
Molds: www.epa.gov/iaq/molds/moldguide.html
Superfunds: www.epa.gov/superfund/
Brownfields: www.epa.gov/brownfields/
Worker Protection Standard: www.epa.gov/oppfead1/safety/workers/workers.htm

Environmental Working Group (EWG)
www.ewg.org/
Public advocacy and information

Health Care Without Harm
www.noharm.org/
Publication: Going Green: A Resource Kit for Pollution Prevention in Health Care

Continued

RESOURCE BOX

Environmental Health Issues—cont'd

Keeping Infants Safe from Smoke (KISS)
Center for Community-Based Research
Dana-Farber Cancer Institute
www2.dfci.harvard.edu/ccbr/projects_events/past/project_kiss.html
Program to help smokers lower their children's exposure to tobacco smoke

Material Safety Data Sheets
www.ilpi.com/msds/
Information on effects of substances on body

National Environmental Education and Training Foundation
1-202-833-2933
www.neetf.org
Developing initiative to educate health care providers on management of pesticide poisoning (National Pesticide Competency Guidelines)

National Environmental Health Association
1-303-756-9090
www.neha.org/

National Institute of Environmental Health Sciences
www.niehs.nih.gov/
Links to Children's Environmental Health Centers

National Institute for Occupational Safety and Health
www.cdc.gov/niosh/pestsurv/#states
Lists state-based pesticide poisoning surveillance programs

National Institute for Standards and Technology
www.nist.gov/
Laboratory Accreditation Administration: provides list of laboratories that test for asbestos

National Pesticide Information Center (NPIC)
1-800-858-7378
http://npic.orst.edu/

National Safety Council
www.nsc.org/
www.nsc.org/ehc/radon/coupon.htm (form to obtain radon testing kits)

Rocky Mountain Drug Consultation Center
1-800-332-3073
www.rmpdc.org
Pharmaceutical and over-the-counter medication and drug information and consultation services for health care providers; information on poisoning

Scorecard
www.scorecard.org/
Provides information about major pollutants for all zip codes in the United States.

University of Maryland Environmental Health Site for Nurses
www.enviRN.umaryland.edu/

REFERENCES

Agran PF et al: Rates of pediatric and adolescent injuries by year of age, *Pediatrics* 108:e45-e59, 2001.

Akhtar Ahmad S et al: Arsenic in drinking water and pregnancy outcomes, *Environ Health Perspect* 109:629-631, 2001.

American Academy of Pediatrics: *Handbook of common poisonings in children*, Elk Grove Village, IL, 1994, American Academy of Pediatrics.

American Academy of Pediatrics, Committee on Environmental Health: *Handbook of pediatric environmental health*, ed 2, Elk Grove Village, IL, 2003, American Academy of Pediatrics.

Ardagh M, Flood D, Tait C: Limiting the use of gastrointestinal decontamination does not worsen the outcome from deliberate self-poisoning, *N Z Med J* 114:423-425, 2001.

Balashazy I, Hofmann W, Heistracher T: Local particle deposition patterns may play a key role in the development of lung cancer, *J Appl Physiol* 94:1719-1725, 2003.

Behrman R, Kliegman R, Jenson H, editors: *Nelson textbook of pediatrics*, ed 17, Philadelphia, 2004, WB Saunders.

Berkowitz GS et al: Exposure to indoor pesticides during pregnancy in a multiethnic, urban cohort, *Environ Health Perspect* 111:79-84, 2003.

Bilban M, Vaupoti J: Chromosome aberrations study of pupils in high radon level elementary school, *Health Phys* 80:157-163, 2001.

Bond GR: The role of activated charcoal and gastric emptying in gastrointestinal decontamination: a state-of-the-art review, *Ann Emerg Med* 39:273-286, 2002.

Brauer M et al: Air pollution from traffic and the development of respiratory infections and asthmatic and allergic symptoms in children, *Am J Respir Crit Care Med* 166:1092-1098, 2002.

Brook RD, Brook JR, Rajagopalan S: Air pollution: the "heart" of the problem, *Curr Hypertens Rep* 5:32-39, 2003.

Campbell TF et al: Bone lead levels and language processing performance, *Dev Neuropsychol* 18:171-186, 2000.

Centers for Disease Control and Prevention: *Screening young children for lead poisoning: guidance for state and local public health officials*, Atlanta, 1997, Centers for Disease Control and Prevention.

Centers for Disease Control and Prevention: Blood and hair mercury levels in young children and women of childbearing age—United States, 1999, *MMWR Morb Mortal Wkly Rep* 50:140-143, 2001a.

Centers for Disease Control and Prevention: *National report on human exposure to environmental chemicals*, Atlanta, 2001b, Centers for Disease Control and Prevention.

Centers for Disease Control and Prevention: *Managing elevated blood lead levels among young children: recommendations from the Advisory Committee on Childhood Lead Poisoning Prevention*, Atlanta, 2002a, Centers for Disease Control and Prevention.

Centers for Disease Control and Prevention: Trends in cigarette smoking among high school students—United States, *MMWR Morb Mortal Wkly Rep* 51:409-412, 2002b.

Chai S, Bearer CF: A developmental approach to pediatric environmental health. In *Training manual on pediatric environmental health: putting it into practice*, Berkeley, CA, 1999, Children's Environmental Health Network/Public Health Institute.

Chassin L et al: Parental smoking cessation and adolescent smoking, *J Pediatr Psychol* 27:485-496, 2002.

Colborn T, Dumanoski D, Myers JP: *Our stolen future: are we threatening our fertility, intelligence, and survival? A scientific detective story*, New York, 1997, Penguin Group.

Denson KW: Passive smoking in infants, children and adolescents: the effects of diet and socioeconomic factors, *Int Arch Occup Environ Health* 74:525-532, 2001.

Dunn AM, Burns CE, Sattler B: Environmental health of children, *J Pediatr Health Care* 5:223-231, 2003.

Emmons KM et al: A randomized trial to reduce passive smoke exposure in low-income households with young children, *Pediatrics* 108:18-24, 2001.

Enflo A: Lung cancer risks from residential radon among smokers and non-smokers, *J Radiol Prot* 22(3A):A95-A99, 2002.

Environmental Protection Agency: Asbestos worker protection: final rule, *Federal Register* 65(221):69210-69217, 2000.

Environmental Protection Agency: Healthy school environments: asbestos, 2002. Available at *http://cfpub.epa.gov/schools/top_sub.cfm?t_id = 41 & s_id = 42* (accessed 2002).

Environmental Protection Agency: Indoor air: mold, 2003b. Available at *www.epa.gov/iaq/molds/moldguide.html* (accessed 2003).

Environmental Protection Agency: National advice on mercury in freshwater fish for women who are or may become pregnant, nursing mothers, and young children, 2001. Available at *www.epa.gov/ost/fishadvice/advice.html* (accessed 2001).

Environmental Protection Agency: *Pesticides industry sales and usage: 1996 and 1997 market estimates*, Washington, DC, 1999, Office of Prevention, Pesticides, and Toxic Substances, Environmental Protection Agency.

Environmental Protection Agency: *Radon-induced lung cancer*, Washington, DC, 1994, Environmental Protection Agency.

Environmental Protection Agency, Office of Children's Health Protection: 1997 declaration of the environment leaders of the eight on children's environmental health. Available at *http://yosemite.epa.gov/ochp/ochpweb.nsf/content/declara.htm* (accessed 2003a).

Fields S: How dangerous is CCA? *Environ Health Perspect* 109:A263-A269, 2001.

Food and Drug Administration: Consumer advisory: an important message for pregnant women and women of childbearing age who may become pregnant about the risks of mercury in fish, 2001. Available at *www.cfsan.fda.gov/~dms/admehg.html* (accessed 2001).

Gitterman B: Personal communication, 1997.

Glueck CJ et al: Secondhand smoke, hypofibrinolysis, and Legg-Perthes disease, *Clin Orthop* 352:159-167, 1998.

Guillette EA: A broad-based evaluation of pesticide-exposed children, *Cent Eur J Public Health* 8(suppl):58-59, 2000.

Haines MM et al: Multilevel modeling of aircraft noise on performance tests in schools around Heathrow Airport London, *J Epidemiol Community Health* 56:139-144, 2002.

Hruba F et al: Childhood respiratory symptoms, hospital admissions, and long-term exposure to airborne particulate matter, *J Exp Anal Environ Epidemiol* 11:33-40, 2001.

Hygge S, Evans GW, Bullinger M: A prospective study of some effects of aircraft noise on cognitive performance in school children, *Psychol Sci* 13:469-474, 2002.

Ingels M et al: A prospective study of acute, unintentional pediatric superwarfarin ingestions managed without decontamination, *Ann Emerg Med* 40:73-78, 2002.

Jacob B et al: Indoor exposure to molds and allergic sensitization, *Environ Health Perspect* 110:647-653, 2002.

Jacobs DE et al: The prevalence of lead-based paint hazards in US housing, *Environ Health Perspect* 110:A599-A606, 2002.

Jan J, Vrbic V: Polychlorinated biphenyls cause developmental enamel defects in children, *Caries Res* 34:469-473, 2000.

Karp R et al: Should we screen for lead poisoning after 36 months of age? Experience in the inner city, *Ambul Pediatr* 1:256-258, 2001.

Kaufman FL et al: Estimation of environmental tobacco smoke exposure during pregnancy using a single question on household smokers versus serum cotinine, *J Exp Anal Environ Epidemiol* 12:286-295, 2002.

Kegler MC, Malcoe LH: Smoking restrictions in the home and care among rural Native American and white families with young children, *Prev Med* 35:334-342, 2002.

Kirby RS: Chemically induced birth defects, *J Perinatol* 22:687, 2002.

Krenzelok E: New developments in the therapy of intoxications, *Toxicol Lett* 127:299-305, 2002.

Krenzelok E, Vale A: Position statements: gut decontamination. American Academy of Clinical Toxicology; European Association of Poisons Centres and Clinical Toxicologists, *J Toxicol Clin Toxicol* 35:695-786, 1997.

Kriz P, Bobak M, Kriz B: Parental smoking, socioeconomic factors, and risk of invasive meningococcal disease in children: a population based case-control study, *Arch Dis Child* 83:117-121, 2000.

Landrigan PJ: Pesticides and PCBs: does the evidence show that they threaten children's health? *Contemp Pediatr* 18:110-126, 2001.

Lercher P et al: Ambient neighbourhood noise and children's mental health, *Occup Environ Med* 59:380-386, 2002.

Li JS et al: Meta-analysis on the association between environmental tobacco smoke (ETS) exposure and the prevalence of lower respiratory tract infection in early childhood, *Pediatr Pulmonol* 27:5-13, 1999.

Lidsky TI, Schneider JS: Lead neurotoxicity in children: basic mechanisms and clinical correlates, *Brain* 126:5-19, 2003.

Ma X et al: Critical windows of exposure to household pesticides and risk of childhood leukemia, *Environ Health Perspect* 110:955-960, 2002.

Mannino DM et al: Surveillance for asthma—United States, 1980-1999, *MMWR Surveill Summ* 51:1-13, 2002.

Meklin T et al: Indoor air microbes and respiratory symptoms of children in moisture damaged and reference schools, *Indoor Air* 12:175-183, 2002.

Montgomery SM, Pounder RE, Wakefield AJ: Smoking in adults and passive smoking in children are associated with acute appendicitis [letter; comment], *Lancet* 353:379, 1999.

Moskowitz WB, Schwartz PF, Schieken RM: Childhood passive smoking, race, and coronary artery disease risk: the MCV Twin Study, *Arch Pediatr Adolesc Med* 153:446-453, 1999.

Needleman HL et al: Bone lead levels in adjudicated delinquents: a case control study, *Neurotoxicol Teratol* 24:711-717, 2002.

Niskar AS et al: Estimated prevalence of noise-induced hearing threshold shifts among children 6 to 19 years of age: the Third National Health and Nutrition Examination Survey, 1988-1994, United States, *Pediatrics* 108:40-43, 2001.

Noble RE: Environmental tobacco smoke uptake by clothing fabrics, *Sci Total Environ* 262:1-3, 2000.

Occupational Safety and Health Administration: *OSHA fact sheet: asbestos*, Washington, DC, 2002, Department of Labor. Available at *www.osha-slc.gov/SLTC/asbestos/* (accessed 2002).

Oregon Poison Center and Health Division, Oregon Department of Human Resources: *Environmental hazards in perspective: seminar syllabus and environmental health resource notebook*, Portland, OR, 1994, Oregon Department of Human Resources.

Plontke SK et al: The incidence of acoustic trauma due to New Year's firecrackers, *Eur Arch Otorhinolaryngol* 259:247-252, 2002.

Pogoda JM, Preston-Martin S: Household pesticides and risk of pediatric brain tumors, *Environ Health Perspect* 105:1214-1220, 1997.

Powell DL, Stewart V: Children: the unwitting target of environmental injustices, *Pediatr Clin North Am* 48:1291-1305, 2001.

Reigart JR, Roberts JR: Pesticides in children, *Pediatr Clin North Am* 48:1185-1198, 2001.

Reigart JR, Roberts JR: *Recognition and management of pesticide poisonings*, ed 5, Washington, DC, 1999, US Environmental Protection Agency.

Ribas-Fito N et al: Polychlorinated biphenyls (PCBs) and neurological development in children: a systematic review, *J Epidemiol Community Health* 55:537-546, 2001.

Sargent JD, Dalton M: Does parental disapproval of smoking prevent adolescents from becoming established smokers? *Pediatrics* 108:1256-1262, 2001.

Schuster MA, Franke T, Pham CB: Smoking patterns of household members and visitors in homes with children in the United States, *Arch Pediatr Adolesc Med* 156:1094-1100, 2002.

Schwenk M et al: Children as a sensitive subgroup and their role in regulatory toxicology: DGPT workshop report, *Arch Toxicol* 77:2-6, 2003.

Tilson HA: The role of developmental neurotoxicology studies in risk assessment, *Toxicol Pathol* 28:149-156, 2000.

Tran B et al: Arsenic lurks in Canadian playgrounds: is your child safe? 2002, Environmental Defence Canada. Available at *www.edcanada.org/* (accessed 2002).

US Agency for Health Care Policy and Research: Treating tobacco use and dependence: a clinical practice guideline. Available June 2000 at *www.surgeongeneral.gov/tobacco/default.htm* (accessed Jan 16, 2003).

US Department of Health and Human Services: *Nurse practitioner primary care competencies in specialty areas: adult, family, gerontological, pediatric, and women's health*, Rockville, MD, 2002, USDHHS.

Valic F: The asbestos dilemma: I. Assessment of risk, *Arh Hig Rada Toksikol* 53:153-167, 2002.

Waldman HB, Perlman SP: 3,941,553 births in 1998: including tens of thousands with congenital anomalies and abnormal conditions, *ASDC J Dent Child* 69:100-103, 2002.

Wiles R: *Pesticides in children's food*, Washington, DC, 1993, Environmental Working Group.

Woodruff TJ et al: *America's children and the environment: measures of contaminants, body burdens, and illnesses*, ed 2, Washington, DC, 2003, US Environmental Protection Agency.

Wright RO et al: Association between iron deficiency and blood lead level in a longitudinal analysis of children followed in an urban primary care clinic, *J Pediatr* 142:9-14, 2003.

Yiin LM et al: Comparison of techniques to reduce residential lead dust on carpet and upholstery: the New Jersey assessment of cleaning techniques trial, *Environ Health Perspect* 110:1233-1237, 2002.

Zhu SH et al: Predictors of smoking cessation in US adolescents, *Am J Prev Med* 16:202-207, 1999.

43 Complementary Medicine

Catherine G. Blosser

It is estimated that 65% to 80% of the world's population relies on some form of non-Western medicine practice for primary health care (McNeil, 2002). There is an increasing consumer movement toward the use of similar nontraditional medical treatments in the United States. Depending on the region, up to 68% of American adults may have used some type of complementary or alternative medicine (CAM) therapy in their lifetime, and 50% continue to do so (Kessler et al, 2001). Other surveys have placed the use by adults of all CAM therapies over the last 12 months at from 29% to 47% (del Mundo, Shepherd, & Marose, 2002; Ni, Simile, & Hardy, 2002). Rates of CAM use among patients with chronic, recurrent, or incurable conditions tend to be higher (Kemper, 2001). For example, use of specific psychotropic herbal preparations has been reported as high as 67% (Ting, Gross, & Oz, 2002), and a study recently completed in New York revealed that 80% of adolescents reported using CAM therapies for asthma (Reznik et al, 2002). In a 1993 landmark study, patients reported more office visits to practitioners who offered alternative approaches to health and illness than to conventional primary care providers (Eisenberg et al, 1993). In 1990, approximately 40% of these patients told their conventional providers about using nonconventional treatments; surveys in the late 1990s to early 2000s show that this number had increased by only about 10% (Eisenberg et al, 1998; *Landmark Report on Public Perceptions of Alternative Care*, 1998; Winslow & Shapiro, 2002).

Various phrases are used to describe health practices that are not fully embraced by conventional Western medicine practices. These terms include *alternative, complementary, contemporary, holistic, integrative, folk, mind-body medicine, natural, New Age, new medicine, nonconventional, nontraditional, quackery,* and *vernacular medicine.* Dr. Jonas, the first Director of the Office of Alternative Medicine at the National Institutes of Health, observed that these terms represented "practices that aren't part of the politically dominant medical system of a country" (Wysocki, 1997, p. 4). To be acknowledged as a component of the dominant medical system, a particular medical practice must be taught in medical schools, be available in hospitals or conventional health clinics, and be reimbursable by third-party payers (Wysocki, 1997).

Representatives of both dominant and nondominant practices have more routinely used the terms *complementary* and *integrative* instead of *alternative.* The current mainstream view is to regard the CAM movement as a new kind of medicine that will eventually fully integrate modern science while, at the same time, not be limited by it. Advocates of both practices point out that patients benefit when nonconventional and conventional health practices are used collaboratively and when one practice is not an "alternative" to the other. Patients seem to demonstrate this integration, because the 1999 National Health Interview Survey reported that CAM users were also more likely to also use conventional medical services (Ni, Simile, & Hardy, 2002).

Practitioners of complementary therapies view each individual as having unique inner resources for healing, maintaining health, or both. Patients are seen as the primary agents influencing the status of their own health; the practitioner helps mobilize these inherent resources rather than simply administering a "magic bullet." Another practitioner describes the effort as one of augmenting host resistance (enhancing the overall immune response or constitutional state) rather than one of attacking (treating, controlling, and suppressing symptoms) the disease (Schoch, 1999).

This chapter provides an overview of complementary medicine as it is currently practiced and accepted in the United States. Table 43-1 lists many of the complementary therapies in use. Specific applications to pediatric/adolescent diagnoses are discussed in Table 43-5. Nurse practitioners

TABLE 43-1 *Complementary Therapies and Their Applications*

Nonconventional Therapy	Theory Behind Use	Treatment Applications*
Acupressure	Similar principle as acupuncture but uses fingertips instead of needles to apply pressure (see Acupuncture); also incorporates breathing techniques to aid healing by balancing mind-body-spirit; shiatsu, reflexology, jin shin use similar techniques	Muscle tension, targeting a specific organ or glandular systems Usually more acceptable to children than acupuncture
Acupuncture	Hair-thin needles inserted at specific anatomic points alter blockages in energy flow patterns along "meridians" and stimulate body to produce pain-relieving and mood-lifting chemicals or antiinflammatory substances (sterile, disposal needles should always be used) (Acupuncture Scores Points, 1998)	Morning sickness of pregnancy Postoperative dental pain Chronic pain (including headaches) Allergies Asthma Nausea and vomiting (including morning sickness, chemotherapy-induced, and postsurgical) Menstrual cramps Migraine headaches Low back pain Addictions (e.g., smoking) Musculoskeletal pain (e.g., arthritis, fibromyalgia, carpal tunnel syndrome, tendinitis)
Aromatherapy	Uses pure, essential, volatile oils containing oxygenated molecules to transport nutrients to cells of the body; believed to promote immunity and create a cellular environment in which disease-causing bacteria, fungi, and viruses cannot live; aromas of essential oils are either inhaled or absorbed through the skin	Stress and anxiety Fatigue Immune disorders Musculoskeletal pain
Ayurvedic medicine	The traditional form of medicine practiced in Indian cultures; treats imbalances or "dosnas" within body that cause illness by using diet changes, herbal remedies, breath work, physical exercise, hatha yoga, meditation, and rejuvenation or detoxification programs; focuses on preventing disease by enhancing the mind-body connection	For primary health care disorders involving GI systems, GYN, respiratory tract, bones and muscles, circulation (including cardiovascular), emotional/psychological, addictions, ENT
Biofeedback	Empowers the mind to take control of conscious and autonomic processes (Frishberg, 1998); relaxation is focused on one muscle or function rather than on the whole body	Chronic pain Hypertension Insomnia Tension and migraine headaches Incontinence (urine and fecal) Stroke rehabilitation Circulation PTSS and depression Chronic tinnitus Torticollis Chronic facial nerve palsy
Chiropractic (contraindications: malignancies, bone/joint infections, acute fractures, arthropathies)	Regards the spinal column as center of body's well-being; uses manipulation and massage of spinal vertebrae to restore proper flow of nerve impulses necessary for health	Musculoskeletal pain, including chronic low back pain (Abrams, 1997)[†] and headaches Torticollis Whiplash following MVA

TABLE 43-1 *Complementary Therapies and Their Applications—cont'd*

Nonconventional Therapy	Theory Behind Use	Treatment Applications*
Craniosacral mobilization	Manipulates craniosacral mechanisms to free the flow of cerebrospinal fluid pathways that surround brain and spinal cord; flow can be inhibited by injury to the brain, spinal cord, skull, sacrum, and related membranes	TMJ Headaches Skull injuries with resultant chronic pain Poorly fitting dentures Colic, vomiting, hypertonicity, tremor, irritability in infancy Obstetrically complicated delivery for infant Attention-deficit hyperactivity disorder (ADHD)
Herbalism (many phytomedicinals are not recommended for use in children [French, 1996]; see Table 43-4)	Natural herbs are used over pharmaceutical derivatives, practitioners believing them to be as efficacious, gentler, and less toxic; used extensively by naturopathic, homeopathic, and holistic practitioners; appropriate preparation (tea, capsule, topical) of the herb important; the dried or extract form of the plant may be used	Used in place of many pharmaceuticals to treat a myriad of primary health care entities, including PMS, cardiovascular, insomnia, stress, menopause, GI, respiratory, immunity, energy, and memory
Homeopathy	Stimulates a healing response by introducing a substance that is either the same as or similar to the patient's disease; infinitesimal doses of plants, minerals, and animal matter are used; medicinal products are prescribed on the basis of the "law of similars"—the medicine used is "homeopathic" to the symptoms presented	Used by many for wide range of primary care illnesses (e.g., respiratory ailments, headaches, diarrhea, teething, toothaches, arthritis, dermatology problems, GI ailments, depression, and anxiety)
Magnets (contraindications: pacemakers, defibrillators, acute injuries to bone and muscles, first-trimester pregnancy)	Magnets purported to stimulate the blood and draw it more quickly to stressed or injured area, aiding the healing process; may interfere with electric impulses triggering pain or stimulate release of natural body painkillers (endorphins)	Musculoskeletal pain Headaches Nausea
Massage therapy (contraindications: clotting tendencies or communicable skin condition)	Hands-on bodywork techniques that knead and manipulate muscles, soft tissues, and connective tissues of the body; used to promote healing, relaxation, relieve sore and injured muscles, and improve overall sense of well-being and health	Premature infants Cocaine- and HIV-exposed infants Colic in infants Infants with disturbed sleep patterns Autistic children Diabetic children to help normalize glucose levels Asthma Arthritis HIV patients Chronic fatigue syndrome Stress-induced maladies Acute and chronic pain Digestive disorders Circulatory problems Musculoskeletal injuries Headaches
Meditation	A deep relaxation technique that can take many forms, from repeating a mantra to Sufi dancing	Stress-induced maladies Chronic illnesses
Music therapy	Music used to provide rhythmic cues to stimulate brain's motor systems to help build and strengthen connections among nerve cells in the cerebral cortex; boosts immune function in children	Physical rehabilitation of stroke, cerebral palsy, Alzheimer's (O'Brien, 1998), Parkinson's, ADHD, learning disabilities, Downs syndrome Depression and anxiety Hypertension

Continued

TABLE 43-1 ***Complementary Therapies and Their Applications—cont'd***

Nonconventional Therapy	Theory Behind Use	Treatment Applications*
		Pain relief (surgical, during labor) Premature infants (speeds the discharge rate from hospitals; Gideonse, 1998)
Naturopathy	Use natural remedies to help restore health and balance in the body, such as diet, herbal medicine, hydrotherapy, acupuncture, homeopathy, and therapeutic massage; practitioners often use similar diagnostic and testing procedures as Western medicine practitioners	Used by many for most primary health care issues
Nutrition	Stresses wisdom of following healthy, balanced diet to affect diet-related health issues; advocate the food pyramid guidelines	Weight loss Food allergies Vitamin and mineral deficiencies Nonpathological GI conditions (e.g., constipation) Chronic diseases
Osteopathy	Remobilization of joints and tissues to restore them to normal, structural positions and mobility, thus releasing tension in muscles and ligaments	Musculoskeletal pain, including chronic back pain and headaches Torticollis Whiplash following MVA
Pilates	Works on mind-body connection with exercise techniques; relies on exercising with firm support and stretching without straining to improve overall body flexibility and fitness	Restricted body flexibility
Reflexology (use with caution in patients with: deep vein thrombosis, leg ulcers, phlebitis in lower extremities, pregnancy, pacemakers; avoid renal reflexes in patients with suspected renal calculi; avoid kidney/gallbladder reflexes in patients with gallstones)	Massage technique based on the principle that proprioceptive nerve receptors in hands and feet correspond to all parts of the body, including organs and glands; use thumb and fingers to massage reflex areas to detect diseases and to rebalance vital energy; practitioners believe more than 100 medical conditions can be helped	Stress and anxiety Promote circulation Colic, irritability and reflux in infants Headaches Low back pain Some allergic responses Some dermatology conditions GI tract disorders Menstrual problems Arthritis and sciatica
Reiki	A bodywork technique to stimulate healing energy within body	Musculoskeletal maladies Low blood hemoglobin levels Pain control (including from cancer, fractured bones) Stress and grief
Tai chi	Stimulates and balances flow of *chi* or vital energy along acupuncture meridians	Restricted body flexibility, fitness, stamina and energy Stress
Traditional Oriental (Chinese) Medicine	Combines practices and beliefs of acupuncture, acupressure, herbal remedies, massage, dietary changes, and bodywork such as tai chi, breathing, and meditation to stimulate vital body energy to rebalance life force	Used by one fourth of world's population for primary health care disorders involving GI systems, GYN, respiratory tract, bones and muscles, circulation (including cardiovascular), emotional/psychological, addictions, ENT

TABLE 43-1 Complementary Therapies and Their Applications—cont'd

Nonconventional Therapy	Theory Behind Use	Treatment Applications*
Yoga	Works on breathing, body alignment, and posture to improve health; preventitive	Chronic musculoskeletal ailments Stress-related maladies Improving overall body flexibility, fitness, stamina, mental health Asthma Hypertension

*These applications may or may not be supported by scientific research; the listing of these therapies does not imply endorsement of proven efficacy.

†Guidelines for the advocacy of spinal manipulation for acute lower back pain were endorsed in 1994 by the Agency for Health Care Policy and Research of the U.S. Department of Health and Human Services.

ENT, Ears, nose, and throat; *GI*, gastrointestinal; *GYN*, gynecology; *HIV*, human immunodeficiency virus; *MVA*, motor vehicle accident; *PMS*, premenstrual syndrome; *PTSS*, post-traumatic stress syndrome; *TMJ*, temporomandibular joint.

(NPs) and other medical providers need to become familiar with complementary therapies, routinely inquire into their use, and foster open discussion with clients who may be combining conventional and nonconventional treatments. In fact, the most effective treatment may involve using therapeutic applications from several different approaches. Successful practitioners benefit from moving between paradigms without prejudice, gleaning what is of value, and knowing when referral to a complementary medical practitioner is appropriate. As Dr. Jonas so aptly stated, "Alternative medicine is here to stay. It is no longer an option to ignore it or treat it as something outside the normal process of science and medicine" (Jonas, 1998).

HISTORY OF COMPLEMENTARY MEDICAL PRACTICES

Before 1910, many different medical and apprenticeship schools allowed graduates to be licensed and referred to as "doctors." With acceptance of the 1910 Flexner report, all medical training, licensure, and regulation in the United States became standardized; since then, "approved" medical education has been based on science and research. Only training schools that could meet the rigorous Flexner standards were accredited and their graduates recognized as legitimate medical doctors. Although these standards effectively put many charlatans and snake oil medical practitioners out of work, many other nonconventional medical practitioners were also disqualified or their practices severely limited. The philosophies and practices of chiropractic, naturopathy, osteopathy, homeopathy, herbal treatments, and others fell into the unaccredited category. By excluding these disciplines, the medical community failed to consider the efficacy, benefits, and applications of the healing and treatment theories that these other practices had to offer. Rapid advances in immunology and pathology solidly secured the dominance of the rational-empirical approach, which became known as Western or "allopathic" medicine. All ailments were expected to fit within a scientific conceptual framework (Janiger & Goldberg, 1993).

The 1960s brought civil unrest and the questioning of authority in the United States. At the same time, a number of doctors and patients began to express disillusionment with the strict limitations of accepted medical practices. The "holistic" health care movement of the 1970s evolved as patients and disaffected medical practitioners began to refocus health care toward healing, prevention, and the spiritual and environmental factors that affect health. From these contexts the current trend toward combining the best of Western and nontraditional medicine grew.

Certain basic principles are common to all nonconventional treatment modalities (Micozzi, 1997). These principles include the following:

- A focus on wellness—which in turn prevents illness
- Self-healing—focusing external manipulations that stimulate the body's internal healing processes
- Bioenergy—ensuring that the body's energy forces are balanced
- Nutrition, plants, and other natural products—obtaining nutrients from natural food sources to maintain or return to health
- Individuality—recognition and use of the individual's unique constitution, inner resources, and so forth to achieve health

SCIENTIFIC OBSERVATION AND COMPLEMENTARY MEDICINE

Many CAM therapies are effective, yet few have been subjected to the rigorous scientific study that would meet Western criteria. Many mainstream medical practitioners refute claims about the efficacy of CAM treatments and label them quackery or "not scientifically validated." The Office of Technology Assessment points out, in response to this argument, that only about 20% of routine allopathic biomedical therapies have been subjected to the same rigorous, scientific testing standards demanded of complementary medicine treatments (Micozzi, 1997). One only needs to reflect on the recent studies regarding the once-accepted—yet recently disproved—benefit of hormone replacement therapy for cardiovascular health in women (Clinical Evidence Concise, 2003). Also, only 20% of all drugs marketed in the United States have been approved by the Food and Drug Administration (FDA) for use in children or have limited approval for use in children because of the lack of rigorous, scientific clinical trials regarding efficacy of the drugs (Bell, 2002).

Micozzi writes that "one way of studying and understanding alternative medicine is to view it in light of contemporary physics and biology-ecology, and to focus not just on the subtle manipulations of the alternative practitioners but on the physiologic response of the body" (Micozzi, 1996, p. 5). Medical researchers of both disciplines are challenged to apply both Western treatments and successful complementary treatments until advances in physics and biology can explain the mechanisms of their effectiveness.

The National Institutes of Health (NIH) created the Office of Alternative Medicine in 1992 to provide evidence-based research that would move complementary treatments into mainstream medicine, thus enabling greater access and further advancements in the therapies themselves. As of 2002, NIH had increased the budget of the newly renamed National Center for Complementary and Alternative Medicine (NCCAM) by 120%. There are now 12 NCCAM-funded centers that are identifying and studying promising CAM practices using scientific methods to determine effectiveness. The current NCCAM-sponsored portfolio is heavily weighted toward clinical trials; the agency is planning to change this emphasis and fund more studies of the mechanisms underlying CAM practices (NCCAM, 2003). More than 100 research projects are underway.

The goals behind the NCCAM-sponsored research efforts include the following:

- Identifying the role that complementary medical treatments play in clinical outcomes, prevention, and health improvement
- Encouraging independence and collaborative research within the complementary medicine community
- Encouraging the establishment of multidisciplinary research approaches and networking between both conventional and complementary communities
- Basing results on scientifically supported research
- Disseminating data

Examples of some NCCAM-sponsored research projects in pediatrics involve evaluating osteopathic manipulation and echinacea to prevent chronic ear infections; self-hypnosis, acupuncture, and osteopathic manipulation to reduce muscle tension in children with spastic cerebral palsy; and the use of relaxation, guided imagery, and chamomile tea for children with recurrent abdominal pain (Steele Memorial Children's Research Center, 2002). Other studies focus on CAM approaches to arthritis, asthma/allergy, cardiovascular diseases, menopause and "andropause," digestive diseases, immunology, infectious diseases, manual therapies, mental health, mind-body medicine, neurologic diseases, pain, and probiotics.

The greatest body of research into complementary therapies has been done outside the United States; often does not meet U.S. standards of double-blinded, placebo-controlled research models; and is not available in English. European and Indian studies are most closely aligned with our own research designs; the Chinese do not regard double-blind, placebo-controlled human studies as ethical. Many of the large, randomized, controlled studies have been done in Germany, where herbal extracts are regulated and used much the same way as pharmaceutical drugs to treat diseases.

THE USE OF COMPLEMENTARY PRACTICES IN THE UNITED STATES

Recent surveys in the United States and abroad have shown that more than 50% of physicians recommended complementary therapies to patients within the preceding year. Over 50% also had incorporated CAM therapy in their personal health regimens (Kemper, 2001). A small survey of NPs and physician assistants (PAs) in 1997 revealed that 78% of NPs recommended complementary therapies and 75% reported seeing patients benefit from their use (PA and NP Opinions on Alternative Therapies, 1998). This interest in such therapies was also mirrored in another survey conducted of faculty and students employed or enrolled at the University of Minnesota schools of medicine, nursing, and pharmacology. Ninety percent of the combined groups believed that a model that integrated both CAM and allopathic medicine would be most efficacious for clinical care. Eighty-eight percent of the faculty members thought that

CAM should be included in their school's curriculum; the nursing faculty reported the highest interest in practicing such therapies (Kreitzer et al, 2002).

Two thirds of medical schools now offer complementary medicine courses (Knittel, 2002). Columbia, Duke, Harvard, and University of California–San Francisco Medical Centers have also established integrative medicine centers. A Harvard Center for Holistic Pediatric Education and Research survey reported requests for holistic medicine consultations for hospitalized pediatric oncology patients in the areas of nausea, pain, insomnia, and agitation. Specific inquiries were sought about herbs, dietary supplements, nutrition, and mind-body therapies to treat cancer-related symptoms (Kemper & Wornham, 2001). In addition to NCCAM, the American Medical Association, American Academy of Family Practice, American Nurses Association, and other groups (including hospitals) are providing patient and professional education (including hospital staff) in nonconventional treatment options.

Research into complementary practices is increasing and is readily available in the literature and over the Internet. The National Library of Medicine offers a database for MEDLINE searches of more than 82,000 citations under the heading of "alternative medicine." Since 1999, the number of such citations has increased by 63%.

Insurance companies are continuing to study issuing premium coverage for "alternative medical treatments" in response to pressure from policy holders, including employers. Employer-sponsored preferred-provider organization plans are more likely to cover chiropractic and acupuncture services than they were 2 to 4 years ago (Lippman, 2001).

THE ATTRACTION OF COMPLEMENTARY MEDICAL PRACTICES

The CAM therapy literature from 1990 to the present indicates a shift toward a cultural norm of acceptance of complementary therapies rather than a rejection of allopathic medicine. A survey of 1500 adults revealed that the primary reason they chose complementary therapies was their perception of the therapies' effectiveness (Astin, 1998). Negative attitudes toward conventional medical practices or a desire for more control over their health care was not predictive of complementary medicine use. Respondents said they used complementary practices because they believed that they worked, that conventional medical care was not helping them, or that these practices were more reflective of their own values and beliefs about the nature of life and spirituality. Use was not limited to any particular age, race, or gender of the population. However, those more likely to use complementary forms of care were young adult to middle aged, were college educated, and suffered from either anxiety, back problems, urinary tract problems, headaches, muscle sprains/strains, chronic fatigue, addictive problems, or arthritis. Respondents living in the western states were more likely to use CAM therapies. Chiropractic was used most often; herbal/vitamin regimens and body therapy (yoga, massage, relaxation) were used to a slightly lesser extent (Astin, 1998; Elder, Gillcrist, & Minz, 1997). Fifty-eight percent of adult respondents reported using alternative therapy for health promotion or prevention rather than to treat a particular health ailment (Eisenberg et al, 1998). Newer studies (del Mundo, Shepherd, & Marose, 2002) confirm Astin's and Eisenberg's findings.

THE ROLE OF NURSE PRACTITIONERS

NPs are increasingly challenged to offer a more comprehensive management partnership with patients and to form more collaborative and integrative relationships with alternative medicine practitioners. Although NPs may not personally embrace the integration of these therapies in their own practice, they need to have sufficient knowledge, sensitivity, and willingness to support and help the patient make informed decisions about their use.

Sixty-three percent of adults believed that their own medical care would improve if communication between their medical doctor and their alternative care provider increased. The vast majority of patients using alternative methods used them in conjunction with traditional health care. Only 5% to 15% of survey respondents replaced conventional medical care with alternative care (Astin, 1998; *Landmark Report on Public Perceptions of Alternative Care*, 1998).

Landmark Healthcare's (1998) findings that patients want better communication between their conventional and nonconventional practitioners represent an expectation that NPs could readily fulfill. By being broad-minded about the use of alternative therapies, the NP can prevent perceptions similar to the one voiced by one patient: "Why would I bother sharing any kind of information that I might know about how this seemed to help me—they don't want to hear it and I don't want to get yelled at by them" (Elder, Gillcrist, & Minz, 1997, p. 183). This feeling, however, seems to be held by a small minority of patients (del Mundo, Shepherd, & Marose, 2002).

The increasing use of complementary therapies suggests that patients' needs are not being adequately met by allopathic methods. The NP can help identify a better medical approach to illness and prevention for each patient by being more cognizant of that individual's core values, beliefs, and approach to life (Adams et al, 2002).

TALKING WITH PATIENTS

Patients' perceptions of the acceptance they feel from NPs provide an opportunity for open discussion regarding the possible risks and benefits of CAM therapies. NPs are better able to monitor patients when they know the complementary practitioners in their area and establish communication with them, even to the point of sharing the management of patients.

In particular, the patient's health history should be expanded to include the following:

- Alternative products that the patient may be taking, including herbs, "natural products," and homeopathic and nutritional supplements from a health food store
- Other practitioners whom the patient may be seeing
- Other kinds of activities engaged in to address a particular problem
- The perception of any benefit gained from the complementary treatment
- The philosophy and self-care approaches to wellness and illness

The topic must be broached nonjudgmentally to help the family clarify the safety issues and explore how these products or services might fit into the patient management plan. Dr. Jonas states that "the practitioner-patient relationship and the trust that's been developed by looking at mutual goals form the foundation" for ongoing dialogue (Wysocki, 1997). Furthermore, an open, sensitive attitude implies a commitment "to the patients' welfare rather than to the particular system of medicine in which they trained" (Gordon, 1996, p. 2209).

SAFETY AND REGULATORY ISSUES

The NP may find the following risk-benefit issues helpful when recommending, advising against, or proscribing CAM therapies (Adams et al, 2002). These include considering the

- Severity and acuteness of the illness
- Curability of the illness by conventional, allopathic treatment
- Degree of invasiveness of the CAM therapy
- Associated toxicities of the CAM therapy
- Availability and quality of evidence for the CAM therapy
- Patient's knowledge of and willingness to accept the risk and benefits of therapy
- Level of patient's intent to use the CAM therapy
- Concurrent use of any prescribed medications

It is particularly important to ascertain the safety of certain treatment modalities by learning about any alternative product that the patient may be using, including its side effects, possible interactions with other medications, and mechanism of action. Mind-body techniques (e.g., prayer, guided imagery, spiritual healing, relaxation) and acupuncture are unlikely to interact with conventional medications. NPs should be aware of the possible harmful effect of products that are taken at high doses, such as herbal or phytomedicinal products, megadose combination nutritional supplements, colonics, or products taken in unconventional ways. Any treatment must be viewed as hazardous if its use delays the provision of proven conventional care for a serious medical condition.

Contamination and potency are other concerns when patients use herbal or folk remedies. Some traditional folk remedies or herbal preparations manufactured in other countries contain heavy metals, such as lead, zinc, mercury, arsenic, aluminum, and tin. One study, done in 1998, found that imported Asian patent medicines contained undeclared pharmaceuticals or heavy metals 32% of the time. Other problems with herbal products were noted, such as improper labeling of contents and failure to provide adequate amounts of the substance noted on the label (Gardiner & Kemper, 2000; Mortimore & Fischer, 2001). Prior, nonproblematic use of a product by an individual may not be a predictor of a future drug reaction because:

- Consistency of potency between batches of herbal preparations varies
- Herbal products can lack standardization regarding which parts of a plant are used
- Plant ripeness, storage, and regional growth conditions vary

Contamination of plant materials, substitutions, adulterations, incorrect preparations or dosages, and inappropriate labeling and advertising have also contributed to adverse patient reactions. However, few reports of adverse reactions to herbal preparations have been documented, which may be a reflection of either the relatively low risk of these products or underreporting. England and Australia have provided the most complete data to date on documented adverse reactions to herbal preparations. A 2001 survey in the United Kingdom showed a rate of 0.38%; in 2000, Australia reported a 1.16% adverse reaction rate (Ramsay, 2002). The American Association of Poison Control Centers has consistently reported more deaths and adverse reactions due to drugs rather than to vitamins, nutritionals, or herbal preparations. Their 1999 report revealed that 330 nonsuicidal deaths were caused by prescription drugs and over-the-counter preparations (e.g., antidepressants, analgesics, sedatives, and heart drugs) versus 12 deaths due to homeopathic or dietary supplements (Ramsay, 2002). Their latest surveillance report of children under 6 years of age was done in 1998. At that time, no deaths were reported from plants or essential oils, although there were adverse reactions under the plant category (American Association of Poison Control Centers, 1998). Ingestion of toxic ornamental plants rather than herbs accounted for most reports of plant poisonings.

Even though 25% of pharmaceutical drugs are made from herbs, Western medical providers often regard herbal, natural health products (NHPs) as dangerous or ineffective. Since 1993, the Food and Drug Administration (FDA) has had a voluntary system in place, called MedWatch, for reporting adverse reactions to nutritionals and botanicals. Access to MedWatch is available from the FDA's Internet website (see Resource Box). Complaints reported to the FDA have principally involved drugs rather than NHPs (36 drug alerts issued versus 3 alerts for NHPs in 2002) (Food and Drug Administration, 2003). Although many herbs are harmless even in large amounts, others should be prescribed only by a knowledgeable herbalist or botanic professional. *Standardized extracts* are more likely to ensure that a specific amount of an active compound is present, thus avoiding the discrepancies found when different parts of a plant are used or when seasonal or climatic variations occur during cultivation for any given plant or plant part. Western herbalists often use *simples* (the compound is made from one herb), whereas Chinese and Indian (Ayurvedic) medicines often blend together more than one herb (Fugh-Berman, 1997). A general rule is that all herbs need to be respected; they are neither completely safe nor poisonous. Herbs can interact with other herbs or with pharmaceutical drugs. See Table 43-2 for a list of drug categories and herbal product interactions and Table 43-3 for herbs contraindicated in pregnancy and lactation.

The appropriate herb in the appropriate quantity—like pharmaceutical medicines—is necessary to obtain the intended benefits. The medicinal effect of any one herb is thought to be the result of dozens of pharmacologically distinct actions. The herb may be effecting physiologic changes in numerous subtle ways, none of which alone would produce the desired response. This mechanism contrasts with conventional medicines, which generally act by one of a few mechanisms of action and use "physiologically more significant pharmacologic" dosing (Herbal Medicine Taken as a Whole, 1998).

The Dietary Supplement Health and Education Act of 1994 required cautionary labeling for all dietary supplements containing herbs. The American Herbal Products Association has evaluated herbal safety for all botanical ingredients sold in North America (see Resource Box). Each herb has been placed in one of the following classes:

Class 1—herb can be safely consumed when used appropriately
Class 2—the following use restrictions apply:
- Class 2a: for external use only
- Class 2b: not to be used during pregnancy
- Class 2c: not to be used while nursing
- Class 2d: other specific use restrictions as noted

Herbal supplements that carry the United States Pharmacopeia (USP) designation indicate that the manufacturers have voluntarily met USP standards for purity, potency, disintegration, and dissolution. Fact sheets on 28 popular herbal supplements are available from the USP (see Resource Box).

For those who are incorporating CAM therapies into their practices, it is recommended that informed consent be obtained and a reference made to any conventional treatments that may be foregone. One should not refer patients to a CAM practitioner without first having done a complete diagnostic evaluation.

Before expanding their practice, NPs are advised to check the advanced nurse practice act of their state, the policies of their employer, and the relevant standards of practice. NPs may have to pursue a broader interpretation and additional training or certification to ensure compliance with the terms of the nurse practice act.

After a thorough diagnostic evaluation of the patient's complaint, the following steps should be taken by the NP to assist a patient who wishes to try an alternative therapy:

- Assist the patient in identifying a suitable licensed provider.
- Provide the patient with questions to ask the alternative provider during the first consultative visit, including issues of safety and efficacy of any treatment.
- Monitor the patient to review the recommended treatment plan; encourage the patient to keep a symptom diary.
- Monitor the patient's response to treatment at monthly intervals.
- Document all interactions with the patient.

Many states have licensing boards and professional organizations that set standards for nonconventional practitioners, including a requirement to carry malpractice insurance. Further information is available from the Federation of State Medical Boards (see Resource Box). Licensing requirements are subject to change, and patients should be encouraged to review the credentials of any practitioner whom they are considering using. Doctorates in acupuncture or Oriental medicine (OMD degree) are not recognized in the United States.

TABLE 43-2 *Herb-Drug Interactions for Some Drugs Used in Children*

Drug Category	Herbs	Effect of Herb on the Drug's Action
Anesthetics	Kava, valerian	Prolonged sedation—an additive effect
Anticonvulsants	Cis-gamma-linolenic acid–rich herbs (evening primrose oil) Thujone-containing herbs (cedar, tansy, sage)	Decreased therapeutic effect—may decrease seizure threshold, per case reports; mechanism of action unknown
Anticonvulsants	Salicylate-rich herbs (e.g., cramp bark, willow, wintergreen)	Increased therapeutic effect with transcient effects, per case reports; mechanism of action unknown
Anticonvulsant—Phenytoin	Shankapulshpi (an ayurvedic product with many herbs)	Decreases effectiveness of Phenytoin; decreased drug levels in case reports
Antidepressants—bupropion (Wellbutrin)	Cis-gamma-linolenic acid–rich herbs (evening primrose oil)	Lowers seizure threshold and may cause epileptic seizures (Graedon & Graedon, 1999)
Benzodiazepines	St. John's Wort, kava	Decreased drug effect; may increase side effects and sedation; herb binds to GABA receptor sites, per animal and pharmacology studies
Corticosteroids	Laxative herbs (e.g., aloe, cascara, senna, yellow dock), diuretic herbs (e.g., celery seed, corn silk, horsetail, juniper)	Increases side effects; increased potassium loss, per theoretical evidence
Corticosteroids	Licorice	Increased plasma levels due to increase in bioavailability, per case reports and some pharmacological evidence
Corticosteroids	Panax ginseng	CNS stimulation and insomnia, per case reports
General medications	High-fiber herbs (e.g., flax, psyllium, acacia, slippery elm, marshmallow)	Decreased absorption of drugs, per pharmacological studies
General medications	"Hot" remedies (e.g., ginger, garlic, black pepper, red pepper)	Increased absorption by causing vasodilation of intestional wall, per traditional use evidence
Iron	Tannin-rich herbs (e.g., caffeine-containing herbs, cat's claw, tea, uva ursi)	Decreased drug effect because tannin binds with iron to decrease absorption, per theoretic and pharmacologic evidence
Minerals	Fiber-containing herbs (flax, psyllium, acacia, slippery elm, marshmallow)	Decreased bioavailability, especially of Ca, Mg, Cu, Zn with psyllium, per case reports
Monoamine oxidase inhibitors (MAOIs)	Panax ginseng, bioactive amines, licorice	Increased side effects that can lead to toxicity; licorice is reported to be a very strong MAOI, per case reports
Nonsteroidal antiinflammatory drugs (NSAIDs)	Gastric irritant herbs (e.g., caffeine, rue, uva ursi)	Increased side effects and may increase gastric erosion and bleeding, per theoretical evidence
NSAIDs	Nettles	Increased therapeutic effect—increases effect of antiinflammatory activity, per controlled trials
Salicylates	Herbs that alkalinize urine (e.g., uva ursi)	Decreased plasma levels due to increased urine secretion, per pharmacology studies
SSRIs	St. John's Wort	Increased therapeutic effects and side effects
Thyroid hormone	Horseradish	Decreased therapeutic effect by decreasing thyroid function
	Kelp	Increased therapeutic effect because kelp contains iodine, which may lead to hyperthyroidism, per theoretical evidence

Adapted from Hardy M: Herb-drug interactions: an evidence-based table, *Int Med Alert,* Jan 29, 2001, pp. 1-8; Graedon J, Graedon T: *The people's pharmacy: guide to home and herbal remedies,* New York, 1999, Graedon Enterprises, Inc.
CNS, Central nervous system; *GABA,* gamma-aminobutyric acid; *SSRI,* selective serotonin reuptake inhibitor.

TABLE 43-3 *Herbs Contraindicated in Pregnancy and Lactation*

Avoid in Pregnancy	Avoid during Lactation
Aloe	Aloe
Autumn crocus	Buckthorn bark
Black cohosh root	Buckthorn berry
Buckthorn bark and berry	Cascara sagrada bark
Cascara sagrada bark	Coltsfoot leaf
Chaste tree fruit	Senna leaf, peppermint oil, and caraway oil
Cinchona bark	Kava kava
Cinnamon bark	Petasites root
Coltsfoot leaf	Indian snakeroot
Comfrey herb, leaf, and root	Rhubarb root
Echinacea purpurea herb, injectable form	Senna leaf
Fennel oil and seed	Uva ursi
Ginger root	
Indian snakeroot	
Juniper root	
Kava kava	
Licorce root (above 100 mg glycyrrhizin)	
Mayapple root and resin	
Parsley herb and root	
Petasites root	
Rhubarb root	
Sage leaf	
Senna leaf	
Uva ursi leaf	
Herbal Combinations	
Angelica root with gentian root and fennel seed	
Anise oil with fennel oil and caraway oil	
Anise oil with fennel oil, licorice root, and thyme	
Anise oil with fennel seed and caraway seed	
Anise seed with ivy leaf, fennel seed, and licorice root	
Anise seed with marshmallow root, eucalyptus oil, and licorice root >100 mg glycyrrhizin	
Caraway oil and fennel oil	
Caraway oil, fennel oil, chamomile flower	
Caraway seed and fennel seed	
Caraway seed, fennel seed, chamomile flower	
Ivy leaf, licorice root (>100 mg glycyrrhizin), and thyme	
Licorice root, peppermint leaf, German chamomile flower	
Licorice root, primrose root, marshmallow root, and anise seed	
Marshmallow root, fennel seed, Iceland moss, and thyme	
Marshmallow root, primrose root, licorice root (>100 mg glycyrrhizin), and thyme oil	
Peppermint leaf, and fennel seed	
Peppermint leaf, caraway seed, and fennel seed	
Peppermint leaf, caraway seed, fennel seed, chamomile flower	
Peppermint oil and fennel oil	
Peppermint oil, caraway oil, fennel oil	
Peppermint oil, caraway oil, fennel oil, chamomile flower	
Peppermint oil, fennel oil, chamomile flower	
Senna leaf, peppermint oil, caraway oil	

Adapted from Mattison D: Herbal supplements: their safety, a concern for health care providers. March of Dimes website. Available at *www.marchofdimes.com* (accessed Jan 8, 2003).

USING COMPLEMENTARY THERAPIES WITH CHILDREN

Until the late 1990s, the incidence of use of CAM therapies in the pediatric population was unknown. Two studies in 1999 provided data that revealed that approximately 20% to 30% of general pediatric patients had used CAM therapies. Adolescent use was higher, ranging from 50% to 75%. The rates were also high among patients with chronic, recurrent, or incurable diseases (30% to 70%) (Kemper, 2001). These rates are in contrast to the 11% reported in a lone study in Canada in 1997 (Spiegelblatt, 1997).

Reasons cited by parents for choosing alternative medicine for their children include the following (Spigelblatt, 1997; Turow, 1997b):

- Limited access to or dissatisfaction with traditional care
- Ready access to nonconventional practitioners
- Failure of traditional medicine to have an impact on chronic conditions such as degenerative diseases, allergies, asthma, otitis media, musculoskeletal ailments, cancer, rheumatoid arthritis, and cystic fibrosis
- Awareness of complications and side effects produced by pharmaceuticals
- Inadequacy of invasive procedures or diagnostics
- Desire for a more holistic, individualistic form of health care
- Ethnic and cultural beliefs
- Belief that alternative practices are more natural, less harmful, and more effective
- Parents are CAM users
- Belief that by combining conventional and nonconventional treatment a more effective approach to health care is achieved than either practice alone affords
- Awareness of the mind-body connection to affect the immune system response
- Desire for more parental, active participation in their child's treatment

Vitamin or other nutritional supplementation, elimination diets, herbal preparations, aromatherapy, homeopathy, and chiropractics lead the list of the most frequently used CAM therapies in children (Kemper, 2001; Ottolini et al, 2001; Simpson & Roman, 2001). In the study by Ottolini and colleagues (2001), less than half of the families who voiced a desire to discuss the use of CAM options with their physicians had done so. Konefal (2002) observed that physicians were reluctant to respond to patients about CAM modalities because of their traditionally poor communication with CAM practitioners, doubts about CAM practitioner competence, inability to sort out efficacious complementary procedures, and reluctance to participate in offering false hope of obtaining cures.

The rapid shift of interest in CAM therapies has not gone unnoticed by researchers and pediatric care providers. Kemper and colleagues cite studies that show that 50% of physicians (including pediatricians and family medicine residents) use CAM therapies for themselves, and most of these physicians use some CAM therapies in treating their patients or refer them to CAM practitioners (Kemper, 2001; Kemper, Vincent, & Scardapane, 1999; Kemper et al, 2002). The first Pediatric Integrative Medicine Conference in the United States was held in 2000 with more than 300 participants.

There are no guidelines for the use of CAM therapies in children with chronic or disabling conditions. The American Academy of Pediatrics (AAP) has recently issued some advice for physicians counseling families about CAM (AAP, 2001). This policy statement includes advice about the following:

- Seeking information about complementary practices, being prepared to discuss them with patients, and providing information about different approaches to treatment
- Evaluating the scientific evidence for CAM therapies
- Identifying risks or possible deleterious effects
- Educating families about evaluating information
- Avoiding communication of a negative bias or defensiveness about CAM therapies
- Offering to assist in monitoring and evaluating CAM therapies, if chosen by the family

Many of the treatments advocated for children involve the use of herbal preparations. Some of these treatments are discussed in Table 43-5. In children, the most dangerous elements are the pyrrolizidine alkaloids, which can cause liver complications or death. These compounds occur in comfrey, borage, coltsfoot, and species of *Crotalaria* and *Senecio*. These plants are often found in herbal teas, particularly from Jamaica, Africa, and South and Central America. Chaparral, germander, and a Chinese medicine called jin bu huan can also cause liver toxicity. See Table 43-4 for a summary list of these herbs.

Proven research discoveries about CAM therapies in children will help improve the quality of mainstream health care in pediatrics. There are some ongoing, specific research studies that will demonstrate if some CAM therapies are beneficial for certain conditions. The Center for Holistic Pediatric Education based at Harvard University presently has ongoing clinical trials in acupuncture and botanical supplements for cancer treatment. Of the 13 conditions that NCCAM prioritized for 2003 CAM therapy study funding, 9 have potential applicability to children's illnesses (e.g., arthritis, asthma, immunology, probiotics).

The Center for Holistic Pediatric Education and Research, located at Children's Hospital in Boston, is the only academic center devoted to pediatric complementary therapies. It was founded in July 1998. The mission of the center is to advance complementary practices in children into mainstream pediatrics based on scientifically integrated research and to promote collaboration among professionals caring for children. Since its inception, the center has developed a curriculum in holistic pediatrics for medical students and family medicine residents. Research endeavors involve collaboration with other medical schools and research institutes.

THE ROLE OF ALLERGIES AS VIEWED BY COMPLEMENTARY MEDICINE PRACTITIONERS

Complementary practitioners are more likely to identify allergies as being the etiology for many common childhood conditions. Childhood afflictions such as otitis media, upper respiratory infections and other immunologic conditions, atopic dermatitis, asthma, headaches, and hyperactivity/attention-deficit hyperactivity disorder (Box 43-1) are mentioned as being caused by allergies to foods and food additives. These health conditions are believed to result from reactions of the "inner being" to external environmental stimuli, notably foods (Micozzi, 1996). Naturopathic physicians cite genetics, the early introduction of solids, early weaning, genetic reengineering of food components,

TABLE 43-4 ***Herbals: General Precautions about Use in Children***

Herb	Precaution
Ephedra (ma huang)	DO NOT USE
Comfrey (symphytum)	DO NOT USE
Borage *(Borago officinalis)*	DO NOT USE
Coltsfoot *(Tussilago farfara)* and species of *Crotalaria* and *Sececio* in herbal teas	DO NOT USE
Chaparral *(Larrea divaricata)*	DO NOT USE
Germander *(Teucrium chamaedrys)*	DO NOT USE
Jin bu huan	DO NOT USE
Monkshood/wolfbane/aconite	DO NOT USE
Heliotropes	DO NOT USE
Rattlebox *(Leguminosae)*	DO NOT USE
Sassafras	DO NOT USE
Kava kava	DO NOT USE
Goldenseal/roots	Not for infants under 1 month of age
Tea tree oil	Do not prescribe for internal use
Echinacea	Not for children under 2 years of age
Pennyroyal	Do not prescribe for internal use

Data from Eisenberg (1997); Fugh-Berman (1997); Gardiner & Kemper (2000); Mack (1998).

BOX 43-1 ***Elimination and Challenge Diet Regimen***

The elimination diet should last for at least 10 days followed by reintroduction of foods one at a time every 2 days. Symptoms caused by food allergens will usually disappear by the fifth or sixth day of the diet, when the body has thoroughly cleansed itself of the allergen/antibody complexes and the intestines have completely eliminated the allergen-containing food. Should symptoms not disappear, it is recommended that the diet become further restricted. Generally, the fewer known allergens included in the diet, the easier it is to establish a cause. If used for attention-deficit/hyperactivity disorder, severity of hyperactivity is not predictive of outcome on diet (Carter et al, 1994). Behavioral changes may be evidenced by decreased irritability, restlessness, sleep disturbances (Carter et al, 1993; Rowe & Rowe, 1993) and lower scores on Connors' hyperactivity index (Boris & Mandel, 1994).

Eat only these foods before reintroduction of other foods: lamb, chicken, rice, potatoes, bananas, apples, and vegetables in the cabbage family (cabbage, brussels sprouts, broccoli, cauliflower, mustard, radish, turnip, watercress). Do not eat foods that contain artificial colors or preservatives.

If there is a positive response, on reintroduction of eliminated foods more pronounced or acute symptoms will recur. The most common foods that produce symptoms are eggs, wheat, chocolate, nuts, cow's milk, citrus, and cheese. Corn and soy have also been implicated. Avoidance means both eliminating the food in its most identifiable state (e.g., eating a scrambled egg) and identifying it in hidden foods (e.g., breads prepared with eggs). A diary should be kept and wrist pulse recorded, because the pulse may change when an allergen is eaten (Murray & Pizzorno, 1998). Children with atopy are more likely to respond to this diet (Boris & Mandel, 1994). An additive-free diet alone is of little help (Rowe & Rowe, 1993).

and impaired digestion as possible reasons for an increase in food sensitivities (Murray & Pizzorno, 1998).

Holistic medicine practitioners continually stress the importance of breast milk for infants. Newer studies are providing more concrete evidence of the wisdom of this recommendation. One study concluded that allergic disease in childhood was caused by both genetics and exposure to allergens in infancy (Halken & Host, 2001). By breastfeeding (or using a hydrolysed formula) and not introducing solids until after 4 months of age, the incidence of food allergies, atopic dermatitis, recurrent wheezing, and asthma in early childhood were decreased. Those exclusively breastfed for less than 6 months also demonstrated a higher incidence of suspected allergic rhinitis, food allergy–related symptoms, and suspected allergic respiratory symptoms after exposure to pets or pollen during the first 2 years of life (Halken & Host, 2001; Kull et al, 2002). Another study showed that the strongest risk factor for atopic dermatitis (AD) in the first year of life was related to the occurrence of AD in the core family (Schoetzau et al, 2002).

An NP who sees a breastfed infant in whom AD has developed should ask the mother about her use of allergenic foods. Some studies showed that allergens can be transferred through breast milk (Murray & Pizzorno, 1998; Smethurst, 2002), whereas other studies dismissed this association (Halken & Host, 2001). See Table 43-5 (under Colic: Nutritional) for the listing of foods that the mother should avoid if the NP chooses to make this recommendation. The appearance of AD in older or formula-fed infants might lead the NP to suggest eliminating milk, eggs, peanuts, wheat, soybeans, and fish. In those using formula, the use of a hydrolysate formula of pork and soya proteins—or an extensive hydrolysate of casein—has been suggested (Moneret-Vautrin, 2002). Both allopathic and complementary providers agree that early identification of illnesses with allergic etiologies (e.g., AD in infancy) and elimination of allergenic foods from the diet can significantly alter the immunopathogenic mechanisms causing symptoms.

Allergy Testing

Nonallopathic practitioners may advocate laboratory testing for food allergies. Blood testing remains controversial in conventional medical settings, less so with nutritionally oriented practitioners such as naturopaths. It is also of note that a positive skin prick test reaction to egg in infancy was higher in infants with atopic disease (Schoetzau et al, 2002).

SPECIFIC COMPLEMENTARY TREATMENTS FOR CHILDREN AND ADOLESCENTS

Table 43-5 lists some of the complementary treatments that parents of pediatric-age children may be considering or are actually using. NPs may personally want to begin incorporating some complementary approaches into their own practices according to their own comfort level. The families' desires for more integrative health care are more likely to be met when NPs act as advocates, active participants, listeners, and facilitators.

The complementary therapeutics in Table 43-5 were chosen by the specific referenced authors on the basis of evidence-based research as being clinically reasonable or holding clues to promising areas needing further research. Physician authors from both Western medicine and naturopathic professions have been used to compile this table. This information is included for the reader's reference. *Inclusion of a complementary treatment in Table 43-5 does not imply endorsement by this textbook's authors.* Herbal remedies are too numerous to list; it is suggested that the NP use a good reference source that cites research and safety precautions. The Resource Box at the end of this chapter provides several suggestions.

GLOSSARY OF TERMS USED IN THE PREPARATION OF HERBAL TREATMENTS

Knowledge of the following terms will be useful to NPs using Table 43-5 for reference.

Standardized: An herbal product that contains a *specified concentration of one ingredient* of the plant; it may contain other nonstandardized ingredients from the same plant.

Essential oils: Also known as volatile or aromatic oils and found in many plants. These oils are highly concentrated and potent and are not to be taken internally.

Infusion: Preparation similar to tea. The dried herb is steeped in boiling water for 5 to 10 minutes and strained; the preparation can be sweetened to make it more palatable; drink warm or cold.

Tincture: A concentrated extract of an herb made with a mixture of cold water and alcohol (typically 25%, 40%, 60%, or 90% alcohol). The tincture usually is diluted four to five times with water or juice for children; tinctures should not be given internally to children younger than 2 years old.

TABLE 43-5 *Complementary Treatments* for some Common Conditions in Children and Adolescents*

Diagnosis	Treatment Approach	Dosage	Benefit	Possible Side Effects†	Research/Citations
Acne	*Herbal*				
	Goldenseal	Adolescents: use as infusion (wash face)	Antibacterial properties	Nontoxic at recommended dose *Class 2b*	Murray & Pizzorno (1998)
	Tea tree oil	Adolescents: 5% topically, diluted with water once daily (use 15% concentration for severe acne)	Effective against *Proprionibacterium acnes*—antiseptic and antifungal properties	Contact dermatitis	Studies show 5% tea tree oil as effective as 5% benzoyl peroxide (Gardiner, Coles, & Kemper, 2001; Murray & Pizzorno, 1998)
	Salicyclic acid	Adolescents: topically 2-4 times/day (start with 0.5% until tolerated and increase to 2% concentration)	Breaks apart sebum plugs	Redness and irritation	Kemper (1996b)
	Nutritional				
	Vitamin B_6 OR multivitamin with zinc, vitamin B_6, vitamin A, vitamin E, vitamin C, selenium, copper	Adolescents: vitamin B_6, 25 mg bid; one daily multivitamin	Works well for premenstrual aggravation of acne		Kemper (1996b); Murray & Pizzorno (1998)
Anxiety	Yoga		Decreases need for medication, improved self-esteem and ability to cope	Limit some postures in pregnancy, after recent surgery, HTN, glaucoma, acute sciatica, herniated disk, or joint replacement	Ott (2002) (cites studies)
	Aromatherapy				
	Chamomile	Infants/children: put in vaporizer using 2-3 drops of the essential oil	Decreases irritability from illnesses (GI upset, varicella, fevers)	Rare allergic reactions in those hypersensitive to ragweed, aster, chrysanthemums (daisy family of plants) consisting of dermatitis, asthma, dyspnea, anaphylaxis *Class 2b*	Kemper (1996a)
	Music therapy		Listening to music directly influences pulse, BP, electrical activity of muscles; may help nerve cell connections within the cerebral cortex	None	Thaut (1998); Gideonese (1998)

Continued

TABLE 43-5 ***Complementary Treatments* for some Common Conditions in Children and Adolescents—cont'd***

Diagnosis	Treatment Approach	Dosage	Benefit	Possible Side Effects†	Research/Citations
	Massage		Improved behavior, reduced cortisol levels		Field et al (1998)
	Meditation				
	Therapeutic touch				
Aphthous Stomatitis	Herbal				
	Aloe vera	Apply topically several times daily	Accelerates healing; under investigation as antiviral and immunomodulator	Rare allergic reactions if taken internally; rare skin eruptions with topical use *Class 1*	Kemper (1996a); Marcolina (2001) (cites studies)
	Tea tree oil	Apply topically twice daily	Antifungal, antibacterial	Rare allergic reaction DO NOT INGEST	LaValle et al (2000)
	Lactobacillus acidophilus	<12 yr: 2 tablets daily up to 3 times daily >12 yr: 4 tablets up to 3 times daily	Antifungal, antibacterial	None	Graedon & Graedon (1999)
	Vitamins				
	B, B_2, B_6 *Zinc gluconate*	Multivitamin with minerals for age	Nutritional deficiencies in B vitamins occur more frequently in those with canker sores	None	Rini & Bloom (2002); Graedon & Graedon (1999)
Asthma	Nutritional				
	Diet exclusions	Eliminate: milk, chocolate, wheat, citrus, food colorings (tartrazine, sunset yellow, amaranth), food additives (sodium benzoate, 4-hydroxybenzoate esters, sulfites) and tryptophan (amino acid in milk, cheese, turkey, bananas); ensure adequate vitamin C, magnesium, fish in diet		In severe asthma, combined treatment with pharmaceuticals is recommended—nutritionals reduce allergic threshold and can help prevent acute attacks	Many studies cited in Murray & Pizzorno (1998) for these nutritional recommendations Kemper (1996b)

TABLE 43-5 ***Complementary Treatments* for some Common Conditions in Children and Adolescents—cont'd***

Diagnosis	Treatment Approach	Dosage	Benefit	Possible Side Effects†	Research/Citations
	Vegan diet	Vegan diet with exception of cold-water fish for their omega-3 fatty acids—try for 4 months; use onions and garlic liberally PLUS Omega-3 fatty acids (supplement with fish oil)	Alters prostaglandin metabolism, increases intake of antioxidant nutrients and magnesium, eliminates food allergens; onions/garlic inhibit release of inflammatory chemicals; omega-3 fatty acids improve airway responsiveness to allergens		Description of diet in Murray & Pizzorno (1998, p. 265) Kemper (1998) (recommends fish several times a week rather than fish oil supplements)
	Green tea extract OR	Give as watered-down tea, prn	Inhibits histamine release from mast cells by increasing absorption of flavonoids		Murray & Pizzorno (1998);
	Ginkgo biloba extract	<50 lb: 25 mg tid 50-100 lb: 40 mg tid >100 lb: 80 mg tid	Improves respiratory function and reduces bronchial reactivity	Rare side effects (headaches, GI upset) *Class 2d—may potentiate effect of MAO inhibitors*	McGuffin et al (1997); Murray & Pizzorno (1998)
	Vitamin B_6 (effects seen after 1 month)	<50 lb: 8-15 mg/day 50-100 lb: 12-25 mg/day >100 lb: 25-50 mg/day	Reduces side effects in asthmatics being treated with theophylline and reduces number and severity of attacks and other medication use		Murray & Pizzorno (1998); Kemper (1996b, 1998)
	Magnesium	<50 lb: 60-125 mg/day 50-100 lb: 100-200 mg/day >100 lb: 200-400 mg/day	Adequate levels necessary for lung function; affects asthma severity		Murray & Pizzorno (1998); Kemper (1996b)
	Vitamin B_{12}	<50 lb: 300 μg/day 50-100 lb: 500 μg/day >100 lb: 1000 μg/day	Possibly reduces reactions to sulfites		Murray & Pizzorno (1998); Kemper (1996b) (not recommended)
	Vitamin C	10-30 mg/kg/day in divided doses	A major antioxidant in lung lining; asthmatics have higher need for vitamin C; inhibits histamine release		Murray & Pizzorno (1998); Kemper (1996b)
	Acupuncture		Study results mixed; some show modest, temporary effect; ineffective for long-term control		Fugh-Berman (1997); Micozzi (1996) (evidence is mixed)

Continued

TABLE 43-5 ***Complementary Treatments* for some Common Conditions in Children and Adolescents—cont'd***

Diagnosis	Treatment Approach	Dosage	Benefit	Possible Side Effects†	Research/Citations
	Chiropractic				Fugh-Berman (1997) (no evidence of efficacy)
	Homeopathy	Immunotherapy using whatever substance patient is allergic to	Possibly some positive effect	Possible initial exacerbation of symptoms	Fugh-Berman (1997) (one study cited); Kemper (1996b) (no published studies using homeopathic treatments for children)
	Hypnosis	Requires subjects highly susceptible to hypnosis	Reduced symptoms and medication use		Fugh-Berman (1997); Kemper (1996b) (controlled studies cited)
	Biofeedback	Age appropriate	Improved breathing, fewer and less severe asthma attacks		Kemper (1996b) (studies cited)
	Massage		Improves peak air flow, decreases asthma attacks, relieves anxiety, depression	None reported	Green, Moore, & Field (1997) (studies cited); Field et al (1998) (study)
	Yoga		May be helpful in reducing symptoms and reducing medication use; ↑ lung capacity		Fugh-Berman (1997); Kemper (1996b) (cites studies); Ott (2002) (cites studies)
Breastfeeding (Mothers)	Herbal				
	Fish oil (salmon oil is best rather than cod liver oil)	750 mg, 2-3 times daily	Important for hormone, nervous tissue, cellular membrane production	Use with caution in those with diabetes, hypoglycemia, if taking aspirin, NSAIDs, anticoagulants *Do NOT use in those with bleeding disorders* Stop before surgery or dental procedures	LaValle et al (2000)
Burns—First or Second Degree	Herbal				
	Aloe vera	Prepared gel (70% aloe vera) or gel directly from leaves: apply topically several times daily	Antiinflammatory, antibacterial, promotes wound healing	Contact dermatitis *Class 1*	Gardiner & Kemper (2000) (cites studies)

TABLE 43-5 ***Complementary Treatments* for some Common Conditions in Children and Adolescents—cont'd***

Diagnosis	Treatment Approach	Dosage	Benefit	Possible Side Effects†	Research/Citations
	Therapeutic touch		Increased healing	None reported	Kemper (1996b) (cites double-blind study showing statistically significant results)
	Homeopathy				
	Calendula (no other homeopathic remedies recommended)	Popular skin soother, available in skin creams	Some antiinflammatory properties	Rare rash *Class 1*	Kemper (1996b)
Chronic Pain	Combination of acupuncture and hypnosis	Individually tailored program	Significant decrease in pain, per studies	None	Zeltzer et al (2002) (cites study)
Colic	Nutritional				
	12% sucrose solution	Infants: 5½ tsp sugar in 8 oz water: give 2 ml over 30-60 sec for 1-2 days during inconsolable crying	Sucrose analgesia—works by stimulating secretion of endogenous endorphins	None	Markestad (1997) (small double-blind crossover study)
	Herbal				
	Tea with chamomile, mint, fennel, licorice, vervain	Infants: Give in weak tea form (mix ½ to 1 tsp of herb in boiling water; steep 5 min): give ½-4 oz tid-qid	Calming, sedating effects (antispasmodic on smooth muscles of digestive tract)	Rare allergic reaction (dermatitis, asthma, dyspnea, anaphylaxis) in people with hypersensitivity to daisy family (see Anxiety section, chamomile) *Class 2b*	Kemper (1996b)
	Chiropractic	Average of three treatments	Colic relieved	None reported	Kemper (1996b); Fugh-Berman (1997) (noncontrolled study showed 94% resolution but was done in 6-week-old infants over period of 2 wk when spontaneous resolution may have occurred)
	Nutritional				
	Eliminate certain foods in mother's diet if breastfed	Mother should eliminate the following for 1 wk: garlic, cow's milk, fruit, chocolate, coffee, tea, cola, soy, corn, wheat, eggs, cabbage, broccoli, onion, peppers, beans	Colic symptoms improved	None—counsel mother on other appropriate foods of equal nutritional value	Kemper (1996b) (studies equivocal—elimination diet helps in some infants)

Continued

TABLE 43-5 ***Complementary Treatments* for some Common Conditions in Children and Adolescents—cont'd***

Diagnosis	Treatment Approach	Dosage	Benefit	Possible Side Effects†	Research/Citations
	Therapeutic touch		Calming	None reported	Kemper (1996b) (no studies cited)
	Massage	Can be taught to parents; used prn: massage tummy lightly with baby on side, head somewhat down and bottom elevated; give 20-30 min after a meal; can extend massage to include entire body	Calming, relaxes	None if done gently	Kemper (1996b)
Common Cold/Flu	Herbal				
	Echinacea leaves/ stalks/roots	Children >2 yr: tincture 2-5 ml bid—can be diluted in water/juice; use at onset of symptoms only; maximum duration of use 8 wk	Stimulates immune system by boosting macrophages' ability to destroy germs, increases T-cell production, and may have interferon-like effects	Can cause allergic reaction (dermatitis, asthma, dyspnea, anaphylaxis) in people allergic to ragweed and daisy family of plants *Do NOT use in patients with progressive infections (e.g., TB, HIV) or autoimmune diseases*; can interfere with immunosuppressive therapy Preparations not standardized *Class 1*	Kemper (1996a); Bates (1998); Castleman (1995) states "U.S. herb companies market prepackaged echinacea preparations under FDA purity regulations and can be used with confidence" (p. 223); Chamberlain (2002)
	Nutritionals				
	Vitamin C	Children: 250 mg qid or 4-5 glasses of orange juice daily at onset of cold	Reduces symptoms and length of illness by activating neutrophils to oxidize inflammatory mediators and increase extracellular vitamin C	Regarded as safe; diarrhea in high doses	Kemper (1996b); Murray & Pizzorno (1998); Castleman (1995); Turow (1997a)
	Chicken soup; peppers, mustard, horseradish, salsa, other spicy foods	Sip soup slowly throughout the day	Thins nasal secretions, increases nasal and sinus mucous velocity	None reported but use cautiously in children with diarrhea-associated illnesses because of chance of causing hypernatremic dehydration	Kemper (1996b) (proven efficacy incomplete in children but worthwhile to try)

TABLE 43-5 *Complementary Treatments* for some Common Conditions in Children and Adolescents—cont'd*

Diagnosis	Treatment Approach	Dosage	Benefit	Possible Side Effects†	Research/Citations
	Garlic	Raw clove minced in mashed potatoes (1 medium clove = 100,000 U penicillin); do not exceed 2 cloves in 1 day	Kills cold viruses; supports immune function	Safe, occasional GI upset *Class 2c*	Castleman (1995); LaValle et al (2000)
	Zinc lozenges	Children: 15-25 mg sucked every 2 hr for 7 days only	May reduce severity and length of illness by binding rhinoviral docking sites with somatic cells, inhibiting infectivity	Mouth irritation, nausea, vomiting, diarrhea, abdominal pain; can suppress immune system if taken longer than 7 days	Kemper (1996b); Fugh-Berman (1997); Murray & Pizzorno (1998); Turow (1997a); has not been tested or proven effective in children
	Biochemical				
	Saline nose drops/spray	Recipe: $\frac{1}{2}$ tsp salt: 1 cup warm water nasally prn	Helps thin nasal secretions	None reported at recommended dilution	Kemper (1996b)
	Aromatherapy				
	Oils of camphor, eucalyptus, menthol, pine, rosemary, wintergreen, tea tree	Inhaled by vaporizer or steam	Helps relieve congestion; heats nasal passages to a degree that inhibits viral replication	*Class 1*	Kemper (1996b); Turow (1997a)
	Massage				
	Oils of menthol (Vicks Vaporub), Tiger Balm	Infant older than 1 mo: massage face, head, back, lymph glands, chest in gentle downward motion	May cool the nose causing perception of decreased nasal congestion	Safe *Class 1*	Kemper (1996b); Murray & Pizzorno (1998); Turow (1997a)
	Acupuncture		Aids blocked sinuses	Included in 1979 World Health Organization (WHO) list of recognized therapies influenced by acupuncture	Micozzi (1996)
Crohn's Disease (Diarrheal Flare-up)	Nutritional				
	Coconut	Eat 2 coconut macaroon cookies daily (Archway®) or add flaked coconut to cereal (1-2 tsp) or as much as needed for control	Possible antibacterial effect from lauric acid in coconut fat that decreases inflammation	None	Graedon & Graedon (2003) (anecdotal information of efficacy)

Continued

TABLE 43-5 *Complementary Treatments* for some Common Conditions in Children and Adolescents—cont'd*

Diagnosis	Treatment Approach	Dosage	Benefit	Possible Side Effects†	Research/Citations
Diarrhea	Herbal *Berberine-containing plants (goldenseal, barberry, or Chinese remedy "huanglian coptis chinonsis")*	*Goldenseal*: toddlers and older children $1/4$-$1/2$ tsp tincture or $1/8$ tsp fluid extract tid-qid—can be mixed with water or juice *Giardia*: children, 5 mg/kg/day for 6 days	Demonstrated benefits for antimicrobial activity against bacteria (includes *E. coli, Shigella, Salmonella, Klebsiella, F. aerogenes*), fungi, protozoa, including *Giardia* When used with any indicated antibiotics, decreased length of illness	Hypotension or hypertension, nausea, vomiting, diarrhea; *NOT recommended for infants younger than 1 month old* *Class 2b* More effective than Flagyl in treating symptoms but not as effective in clearing from GI tract; best approach to use with standard antibiotic therapy	Kemper (1996b); Murray & Pizzorno (1998) (cite studies) Murray & Pizzorno (1998) (cite studies)
	Lactobicillus acidophilus or *Bifidobacterium bifidum*	5-7 billion organisms/day If using yogurt, make sure it contains these bacteria	Can also be used to decrease incidence of rotovirus diarrhea in infants 5-24 months old; reinforces mucosal wall barrier	Flatulence, constipation *Do NOT use in those with impaired immune systems*	Kemper (1996b) (study cited); Pettit (2002)
	5% carob pod powder	Infants to 1 yr: 1.5 g/kg/day in ORS or formula Children over 1 yr: 1-15 g/kg/day in ORS or milk; stop 24 hr after appearance of formed stools	Acute diarrhea in infants/children; tannins inhibit growth of bacteria and bind bacterial toxins; controlled studies of hospitalized infants showed efficacy of treatment	None Used for centuries in Mediterranean regions *Class 1*	Murray & Pizzorno (1998); Loeb et al (1989)
	Garlic *Best formulations are enteric coated tablets/capsules/dried or powdered garlic, standardized for allilin content*	All ages: 1 clove (or 4 g) chewed, chopped, bruised, or crushed; do not use more than 2 cloves of raw garlic daily	Treats *Entamoeba histolytica*, athlete's foot, vaginal candidiasis; is antimicrobial; organosulfur compounds are believed to interfere with microbial structures/ functions	Garlic breath (try chewing fennel, parsley, fenugreek to counter garlic breath); has anticlotting effect; GI upset, rash, burning mouth, sweating, light-headedness; raw garlic is toxic in high doses	Castleman (1995); Therapeutic Uses of Herbs (1997)

TABLE 43-5 ***Complementary Treatments* for some Common Conditions in Children and Adolescents—cont'd***

Diagnosis	Treatment Approach	Dosage	Benefit	Possible Side Effects†	Research/Citations
	ORS *4 cups water* *½ tsp salt* *1-1½ cups rice cereal for babies* *(2 tbsp sugar can also be added)*	Offer 1 tbsp to 1 oz every 15-30 min; increase as tolerated			WHO (2003)
Eczema/Atopic Dermatitis	Herbal				
	Evening primrose oil	Infants/children: 4 caps/day (300 g) PO Adolescents: 8-12 caps/day Requires 4-12 wk for benefit	Decreased scaling, itching, and general severity; contains high amounts of a fatty acid that children with eczema are thought to have a defect in metabolizing	Very safe; rare, mild GI effects, headache *Class 1*	Fugh-Berman (1996); Gardiner, Coles, & Kemper (2001) (studies cited)
	Echinacea	Apply topically	Promotes healing by stimulating formation of new tissue	Contact dermatitis; use with caution in patients allergic to ragweed and daisy family of plants *Class 1*	Castleman (1995); Kemper (1996b)
	Licorice *(Glycyrrhiza glabra)*	Apply topically as pure glycyrrhetinic acid (commercial product: Simicort from Enzymatic Therapy)	Exerts effect similar to hydrocortisone cream	None *Class 2b*	Murray & Pizzorno (1998) (double-blind, controlled studies cited)
	Chamomile extracts, witch hazel, calendula	Apply topically (commercial product: CamoCare)	May help reduce itching and inflammation; promotes healing	Contact dermatitis; use with caution in patients with allergy to ragweed or daisy family of plants	Murray & Pizzorno (1998); Gardiner & Kemper (2000)
	Nutritional and naturopathic *Diet exclusions*		Improvement in symptoms	Ensure adequate calcium, nutrients	See under Asthma, diet exclusions discussion earlier in chapter
	Breast milk				Refer to Colic, nutritional
	Vitamin C (after diet exclusion and rechallenge)	Infants/children: one 8 oz glass of orange juice daily		None at recommended doses	Kemper (1996b) (cites double-blind, controlled crossover trial of vitamin C with significant improvement of eczema)

Continued

TABLE 43-5 ***Complementary Treatments* for some Common Conditions in Children and Adolescents—cont'd***

Diagnosis	Treatment Approach	Dosage	Benefit	Possible Side Effects[†]	Research/Citations
Elevated Lead Level	Herbal				
	Garlic	Add liberally to foods; see under Common Cold/Flu for dosing information	Helps eliminate lead/heavy metals	*Use with caution in patients with clotting disorders*	Castleman (1995) (based on some European studies)
	Teas from red clover, lemon grass, milk thistle	Tea drinks	Herbalists believe these help detoxify heavy metals	Do not give red clover to children under 2 years old (Castleman, 1995)	Kemper (1996b) (no scientific studies done to date)
Enuresis	Biofeedback	Children >4 yr: program—child voids in front of a uroflow device while being coached; pelvic floor relaxation techniques in front of electromyogram	80%-100% resolution; decreases postresidual void and improves voiding curves	None	Schulman et al (2001) (cite study)
Headaches	*Herbal*				
	Feverfew *(Tanacetum parthenium)*	Children over 2 yr: 25-50 mg bid (start with lower dose and increase as necessary) OR Chew 1-3 leaves daily Change brands if no results seen after a few weeks; try for several months	Prevention of migraines: inhibits release of blood vessel-dilating substances from platelets to decrease production of inflammatory substances and reestablish proper blood vessel tone; benefits are similar to aspirin and NSAIDs, but if NSAIDs do not work, neither will feverfew, because properties are similar	Mouth sores, abdominal pain, allergic reactions usually within first week of use; not to be used during pregnancy or in patients with clotting disorders; sudden cessation may result in rebound headaches *Class 2b*	Murray & Pizzorno (1998) (double-blind studies cited that showed reduction in number and severity of migraines—not for acute attacks); Castleman (1995); Kemper (1996a); McGuffin et al (1997); Therapeutic Use of Herbs (1997)
	Biofeedback	6 yr and up: as needed to master techniques (8-10 wk)	For tension and migraine headaches: patients learn to dilate blood vessels in body to affect blood flow to the head and relax muscles	None	Fugh-Berman (1997) (cites studies showing success rates of 44%-65% for muscle-contraction headaches and 38% for migraines); Kemper (1996b); Murray & Pizzorno (1998); Children Can Take Charge of Migraine (1998); Grazzi et al (2001)

TABLE 43-5 *Complementary Treatments* for some Common Conditions in Children and Adolescents—cont'd*

Diagnosis	Treatment Approach	Dosage	Benefit	Possible Side Effects†	Research/Citations
	Massage	Head, neck, shoulder massage techniques using 1-2 drops peppermint or eucalyptus oil to 1 tsp vegetable oil as massage lotion	Muscle relaxation; oil may help decrease pain sensitivity	None reported	Kemper (1996b) (cites studies showing proven effectiveness)
	Acupuncture	Age when tolerant to needles; nonneedle techniques or Japanese-style acupuncture also available	Use in conjunction with massage and relaxation	None reported	Kemper et al (2000) (cites studies showing effectiveness for migraine prevention and tension headaches)
	Chiropractic	Chiropractors "adjust" all ages: manipulation of cervical/thoracic vertebrae	Pain reduction, acute/chronic	Few complications with cervical manipulation, less with other areas; issues with chiropractics occur when only manipulation is used and more appropriate medical diagnosis and treatment was delayed (e.g., encopresis, ear infections, diabetes, anemia, HTN, tumors)	Fugh-Berman (1997); Nickerson & Silberman (1992)
	Naturopathy and nutritional				
	Elimination diet	Avoid nitrates, nitrites, aspartame, MSG, chocolate, aged cheeses, caffeine, wheat, oranges, eggs, milk, beef, corn, sugar, yeast, shellfish Avoid vitamins A and D and zinc	Benefits children with other allergy symptoms and frequent headaches; vitamin A excess increases intracranial pressure, vitamin D and zinc can cause headaches	None reported	Kemper (1996b, 1998); Murray & Pizzorno (1998) (cites nonrandomized study showing 85% reduction in headaches)

Continued

TABLE 43-5 *Complementary Treatments* for some Common Conditions in Children and Adolescents—cont'd*

Diagnosis	Treatment Approach	Dosage	Benefit	Possible Side Effects†	Research/Citations
	Increase magnesium-rich foods and include ginger and hot peppers, garlic, onion, vegetable oils, fish oils	Adolescents: magnesium 250-400 mg tid plus vitamin B_6 25 mg tid Ginger: daily 1/4 slice fresh or 500 mg qid dried or 100-200 mg tid extract (20% gingerol and shogaol) (for prevention) and 200 mg every 2 hr acute migraine	Low magnesium levels often found in patients with all types of headaches; magnesium maintains blood vessel tone and prevents overexcitability of nerve cells; vitamin B_6 increases intracellular Mg; ginger (contains aspirin-like compounds) exerts antiinflammatory effects and decreases platelet aggregation	Diarrhea, gastric irritation	Kemper (1996b); Murray & Pizzorno (1998) (mixed results on double-blind studies cited)
	Homeopathy	Individualized homeopathic remedies	Reduction in intensity and frequency of attacks	Not recommended for children (Kemper, 1996b)	Fugh-Berman (1997) (cites a double-blind, placebo-controlled study)
Herpes Simplex Labialis	Herbal				
	1% lemon balm extract	Apply topically: 1% dried lemon balm extract cream qid with onset of symptoms or within 72 hr of symptoms for best result	Antiviral compounds; complete healing by eighth day	Use with caution if taking thyroid medication; increases effects of barbiturates	Gardiner, Coles, & Kemper (2001)
	Aloe vera	0.5% aloe vera extract cream applied topically several times daily at onset of symptoms	Speeds healing; antiinflammatory	Contact dermatitis *Class 1*	Same as above
Hyperactivity/ADHD	Music therapy	Have children listen to calm, low-pitched, slow-tempo music	Improved work performance, decrease tension and activity, calming effect on autonomic nervous system	High-pitched music creates tension; low pitch stimulates relaxation; slow tempo is soothing; fast or stimulating music increases anxiety and activity	Kemper (1996b) (cited one study done in Israel showing hyperactive boys doing as well as normal boys when listening to calming music vs no music vs fast-paced music); Klein & Winkelstein (1996); Thaut (1998)

TABLE 43-5 ***Complementary Treatments* for some Common Conditions in Children and Adolescents—cont'd***

Diagnosis	Treatment Approach	Dosage	Benefit	Possible Side Effects†	Research/Citations
	Biofeedback *(Two types: electromyogram and electroencephalogram)*	Takes 6-8 wk (20-40 sessions) to learn techniques, age dependent	More relaxed behavior, improved attention, improved language skills; technique focuses on reducing muscle tension in the forehead and ways to exercise different neurologic pathways to control impulses, ↑ attention, and process information better		Kemper (1996b) (cites studies showing behavioral improvement equal to Ritalin; technique works best if also used with structured scheduling and behavioral rewards)
	Homeopathy				Chan (2002)
	Herbal treatments commonly tried: Valerian, Lemon balm, Kava kava, Melatonin, Pycnogenol, Ginkgo biloba, Blue-green algae	*Cannot be recommended due to lack of studies; kava kava can be toxic (see Table 43-4)*			Chan, Gardiner, & Kemper (2000)
	Evening primrose oil (EPO)	Children: 500-1000 g/daily standardized to contain 8% gamma linolenic acid (GLA)	Improvement on parent and teacher behavioral scales	Safe to try, nausea, diarrhea, headache with high dose or chronic use; flatus, halitosis; increases bleeding time	Chan, Gardiner, & Kemper (2000) (two studies cited)

Continued

TABLE 43-5 *Complementary Treatments* for some Common Conditions in Children and Adolescents—cont'd*

Diagnosis	Treatment Approach	Dosage	Benefit	Possible Side Effects[†]	Research/Citations
	Nutritional/naturopathic				
	Elimination diet	See Box 43-1 Also recommended is the elimination of refined sugars and supplementation with a multivitamin that includes thiamin, niacin, vitamin B_6, magnesium, manganese, potassium, and zinc	Decrease in irritability, insomnia, fidgetiness; improvement seen in up to 73% (Boris & Mandel, 1994) Vitamin deficiencies can result in impaired brain and nervous system function Refined sugars thought to promote reactive hypoglycemia causing increased adrenalin secretion and hyperactivity. (Murray & Pizzorno, 1998)	Elimination diet can put strain on family; dietary management less likely to produce results with discordant marital relationships present (Carter et al, 1993); may need consultation with nutritionist	Studies showed some behavioral changes in hyperactive children (not all studies used subjects meeting DSM III criteria) when challenged by specific food allergens (Carter et al, 1993; Egger, Stolla, & McEwen, 1992; Rowe & Rowe, 1994; Boris & Mandel, 1994; Murray & Pizzorno, 1998); Kemper (1996b) recommends elimination diet after other measures have failed to help (thinks studies fail to prove link between allergies/ sugar and hyperactive behavior in most children; elimination diets possibly more effective in atopic children)
	Nutritional				
	Magnesium	<12 yr: 400 mg daily >12 yr: 400-600 mg daily These doses are > than RDA	Regulates muscles and nerve function, helps with restlessness, irritability, anxiety	Diarrhea, drowsiness, weakness, lethargy if overdose	Starobrat-Hermelin & Kozielec (1997) (cite study)
	Fish oil (omega-3, EPA, DHA)	500-1000 mg/daily or more	Improves visual processing and motor coordination in children with dyslexia and dyspraxia—may help with ADHD	Safe to try	Chan, Gardiner, & Kemper (2000); no studies on ADHD
	Caffeine	Low doses	May boost benefit of Ritalin without increasing side effects	Effects of caffeine (jittery, nervous, anxious, tired with withdrawal)	Kemper (1996b)
	Yoga Meditation Guided therapy		Enhances relaxation	None reported	Kemper (1996b)

TABLE 43-5 ***Complementary Treatments* for some Common Conditions in Children and Adolescents—cont'd***

Diagnosis	Treatment Approach	Dosage	Benefit	Possible Side Effects†	Research/Citations
Jaundice	Therapeutic touch			None reported	Kemper (1996b) (studies done in adults only)
	Prayer therapy		Prayer-healing has been shown to prevent RBCs from breaking down in test tubes; increase in hemoglobin in adults		Kemper (1996b) (studies done in adults only)
Nausea and Vomiting	Herbal				
	Combination tea with chamomile, lemon balm, peppermint	Small, frequent sips	Soothing to stomach upsets	Safe unless existing allergy to ragweed or daisy family of plants *Class 1*	Kemper (1996b)
	Goldenseal or barberry	Tincture: 2-3 drops in 4 oz water, sipped slowly over 1 hr	Especially helpful if child has vomiting and diarrhea	None reported at therapeutic levels; excessive levels can cause GI upset, CNS stimulation *Class 2b*	Kemper (1996b)
	Basil tea	Make with $1/2$ oz dry basil and 1 cup boiling water, steeped 5 min and strained		Not recommended for infants or toddlers *Class 2b*	Kemper (1996b); McGuffin et al (1997)
	Ginger root	$<$ 3 yr: 25 mg qid 3-6 yr: 50-75 mg qid 6-12 yr: 125 mg. qid $>$13 yr: 250 mg qid OR Ginger tea: 1 cup water to 2 slices ginger root (simmer 5 min) OR $1/4$ tsp fresh grated ginger in juice, applesauce, cereal OR Ginger soda (with real ginger)	Helpful to reduce nausea by promoting elimination of intestinal gas and reducing GI spasms	Not for long-term use; use only in recommended doses Large doses can depress CNS, cause cardiac arrthymias, compromise platelet aggregation *Do NOT use in pregnancy* *Class 2b*	Kemper (1996b); Therapeutic Uses of Herbs (1997)

Continued

TABLE 43-5 ***Complementary Treatments* for some Common Conditions in Children and Adolescents—cont'd***

Diagnosis	Treatment Approach	Dosage	Benefit	Possible Side Effects[†]	Research/Citations
	Poultice	Soak cotton flannel cloth in castor oil, lay cloth over abdomen, and cover with towel; have child rest 1 hr, then remove cloth and rinse abdomen with baking soda/water solution	Old folk remedy for nausea		Kemper (1996b)
	Nutritional				
	Vitamin B_6	Motion sickness and nausea of radiation therapy: 10 mg 1 hr before traveling	May help minimize nausea	None reported	Kemper (1996b)
	Hypnosis	Age dependent	Helpful in reducing recurrent vomiting/nausea associated with chemotherapy or motion sickness	None reported	Kemper (1996b)
	Acupressure	Apply pressure 1 inch above wrist crease, between the two tendons leading to the palm; repeat every 2 hr as needed to control nausea	Controls nausea symptoms	None reported	Kemper (1996b) (few studies to date done on children but safe to try, per Kemper)
Onychomycosis	Herbal				
	Tea tree oil *Vicks VapoRub*	Apply topically to affected nails twice daily for 3 mo	Antifungal, antibacterial	Allergic dermatitis in sensitive patients	Gardiner, Coles, & Kemper (2001); Graedon & Graedon (1999)
	Vinegar	Soak affected nails in 50:50 solution white vinegar and water for 30 min daily for several months			
	Vitamin E	Puncture 1 vitamin E capsule; apply oil to affected nail at bedtime (cover with cotton sock) until new nail begins to grow out			

TABLE 43-5 *Complementary Treatments* for some Common Conditions in Children and Adolescents—cont'd*

Diagnosis	Treatment Approach	Dosage	Benefit	Possible Side Effects†	Research/Citations
Otitis Media	Nutritional				
	Elimination diet	Eliminate milk and dairy products, eggs, wheat, corn, oranges, peanut butter, concentrated simple carbohydrates (sugar, honey, dried fruit, concentrated fruit juices, etc.)	Boosts immune system by eliminating allergens known to impede it; decreases congestion of nasal mucous membranes that affect drainage of the eustachian tubes or insults to the integrity of the middle ear	None reported	After elimination diet 86% of food-sensitive patients (71% of subjects) showed significant improvement in serous otitis media recurrence; most subjects allergic to 2-4 foods, most to milk, wheat, egg, peanuts, soy, and corn (Nsouli et al, 1994); tympanostomy tubes deemed inappropriate or of equivocal use in 58% of children (Kleinman et al, 1994)
	Breast milk	All infants			
	Herbal				
	Echinacea	<6 yr: tincture (1:5) 1-2 ml up to tid OR fluid extract (1:1) 1-2 ml up to tid >6 yr: double above doses	Boosts immune system	Safe unless patient has allergy to ragweed or daisy family of plants *Class 1*	Kemper (1996b); Murray & Pizzorno (1998)
Premature Infants	Massage	10-15 min tid	Facilitates growth and development and decreases medical complications	None reported; less duration of massage seems to produce less positive results	Fugh-Berman (1997) (cites several studies supporting massage or stroking)
Presurgery Precautions	STOP THE FOLLOWING: *Vitamin E* *Ginkgo biloba* *Ginseng* *Flax* *NSAIDs, ASA* *Fish oil*		Interfere with platelet function, causing prolonged bleeding		Graedon & Graedon (1999)
PMS	Herbal				
	Black currant seed oil *OR* *Flaxseed oil* *OR* *Evening primrose oil*	As directed on label tid OR 1000 mg tid	Important fatty acids help relieve PMS symptoms and aid glandular function	None Flax needs to be taken with at least 6 oz of water; contraindicated with bowel obstruction	Balch & Balch (1997) (other helpful suggestions offered in this reference); McGuffin et al (1997); Gardiner & Kemper (2000) *Class 1*

Continued

TABLE 43-5 *Complementary Treatments* for some Common Conditions in Children and Adolescents—cont'd*

Diagnosis	Treatment Approach	Dosage	Benefit	Possible Side Effects†	Research/Citations
	Angelica or Dong Quai (Angelica sinensis)	Powered root or tea: 1-2 g tid Tincture (1:5): 4 ml tid Fluid extract: 1 ml tid	Roots contain phytoestrogens, which nourish and tone female glandular and organ system	*Do NOT use if patient is pregnant, is nursing, or has a history of cancer, cardiac disease, or photosensitivity*; occasional light laxative effect *Class 2b*	Murray & Pizzorno (1998) (other helpful preparations offered in this reference; cite supportive studies); Gardiner & Kemper (2000)
	Licorice root (Glycyrriza glabra)	Powered root or tea: 1-2 g tid Fluid extract (1:1): 4 ml tid Dry powdered extract (1:4): 250-500 mg tid	Reduces water retention of PMS; believed to lower estrogen levels and increase progesterone levels	*Do NOT use if patient is pregnant, is breastfeeding, or has glaucoma, diabetes, HTN, or cardiac disease*	McGuffin et al (1997); Therapeutic Uses of Herbs (1998)
	Black cohosh (Cimicifuga racemosa)	1 tablet once or twice daily	Useful for relieving cramps; may help with depression, anxiety, tension, mood swings	Use only with nonpregnant, nonnursing patients; not to be used in patients with cardiac disease or estrogen-dependent cancers Overdose symptoms: nausea, diarrhea, abdominal pain, vomiting, dizziness, headache, tremors, arthalgias *Class 2b*	Gardiner & Kemper (2000); McGuffin et al (1997); Murray & Pizzorno (1998)
	Chasteberry *(Vitex agnus-castus)*	Powdered extract (0.5% agnuside content) 175-225 mg/day Liquid extract: 2 ml/day	Useful with breast tenderness symptoms of PMS; appears to alter GnRH and FSH-RH to normalize secretion of prolactin and estrogen/progesterone ratio	*Do NOT use in pregnant, lactating patients*; occasional minor skin irritations *Class 2b*	McGuffin et al (1997); Murray & Pizzorno (1998)
	Nutritional and naturopathic				
	Calcium	1000 mg/day	Relieves cramping, backache, nervousness		Murray & Pizzorno (1998)
	Magnesium	12 mg/kg/day	Helps with headaches		

TABLE 43-5 ***Complementary Treatments* for some Common Conditions in Children and Adolescents—cont'd***

Diagnosis	Treatment Approach	Dosage	Benefit	Possible Side Effects†	Research/Citations
	Vitamin B complex plus extra vitamin B_6	100 mg tid 50-100 mg/day	B vitamins complement each other Decreases water retention, increases circulation to female organs, helps restore estrogen levels		Balch & Balch (1997); Murray & Pizzorno (1998)
	Vitamin E	400 IU/day	Helps with breast tenderness, depression, irritability; improves oxygen profusion to body		
	Zinc	15-20 mg/day	Promotes hormone balance; controls prolactin secretion		
	Diet	Eat plenty of fresh fruits, vegetables, whole-grain cereals and breads, beans, peas, lentil, nuts and seeds, broiled fowl, fish, high-protein foods as snacks, and soy products; avoid salt, red meats, processed foods, junk/fast foods, caffeine, refined sugar, and dairy products 1 week before menses; increase water intake to 1 quart distilled water/day 1 week before menses and continue 1 week after onset	Red meats and dairy products believed to contribute to hormonal fluctuations; other recommended foods aid in metabolism, maintenance of blood glucose, and absorption of nutrients, and decrease free estrogen in blood; excluding salt decreases bloating and water retention; dairy products and refined sugars also believed to increase excretion of magnesium with resulting impaired estrogen metabolism and moodiness		Micozzi (1996)
	Chiropractic		For cramps: possibly alters prostaglandin levels		Fugh-Berman (1997) (cites studies)
	Acupuncture		For cramps		Fugh-Berman (1997) (cites studies); NIH (1998)
	Yoga				
Skin Irritation/Diaper Rashes	Herbal				
	Aloe vera	All ages: pure gel form, applied topically several times daily	Antibacterial effects; accelerates healing	Contact dermatitis *Class 1*	Kemper (1996a); Murray & Pizzorno (1998); Gardiner, Coles, & Kemper (2001)

Continued

TABLE 43-5 ***Complementary Treatments* for some Common Conditions in Children and Adolescents—cont'd***

Diagnosis	Treatment Approach	Dosage	Benefit	Possible Side Effects†	Research/Citations
	Chamomile	Add essential oil to bath or make as tea and rub affected area	Soothes diaper rash, varicella, contact dermatitis	Contact dermatitis; use in caution in patients with allergy to ragweed or daisy family of plants *Class 1*	Kemper (1996b)
	Nutritional *Zinc*	Formula-fed infants: 10 mg/day for formula-fed infants with history of yeast diaper rashes	May help prevent yeast diaper rashes in formula-fed infants (does not apply to breastfed infants)	None noted	Kemper (1996b) (cites study showing that infants with frequent diaper rashes have lower levels of zinc in their bodies)
	Live Lactobacillus acidophilus bacteria OR Bifidobacterium bifidum	Infants >6 mo: give as yogurt; 1 cup daily 12 mo and over	Thought to help replace the yeast on the skin	None noted	Kemper (1996b)
Teething	Herbal Tea tree oil	Apply topically, diluted with water to gums with Q-Tip *NOT FOR INGESTION*	Antifungal, antibacterial; mouthwash for oral health	Allergic dermatitis in sensitive patients	LaValle et al (2000)
	Clove oil	Apply topically; do not use >48 hr	Antiseptic: good for toothaches, teething; analgesic on mucous membranes; antibacterial and antiviral		
UTI Prevention	Herbal *Cranberry juice, juice extract capsules, or pure cranberry liquid extract mixed with orange juice to decrease tangy taste*	150-600 ml/day children and adolescents; 1-2 capsules once or twice daily for adolescents	Reduces adhesion of gram-negative and gram-positive bacteria to bladder wall cells	Safe: can increase urinary oxalate levels; those with sugar sensitivity should use with caution	Pettit (2002); Gardiner, Conboy, & Kemper (2000) (cites studies)

TABLE 43-5 ***Complementary Treatments* for some Common Conditions in Children and Adolescents—cont'd***

Diagnosis	Treatment Approach	Dosage	Benefit	Possible Side Effects[†]	Research/Citations
Warts (Verruca Vulgaris)	Duct tape occlusive therapy	Cover wart(s) with piece of duct tape for 6 days (if falls off, replace); remove tape: soak wart in warm water and file with emery board; replace tape the next day and repeat regimen for 2 mo or until wart disappears (most resolve in 1 mo)		Allergic reaction to tape	Focht, Spicer, & Fairchok (2002)

*Inclusion of a complementary treatment in this table does not imply endorsement by this textbook's authors; for reference only.

[†]Food supplements and herbal labeling classifications. Class 1—herb can be safely consumed when used appropriately. Class 2—the following use restrictions apply: 2a, for external use only; 2b, not to be used during pregnancy; 2c, not to be used while nursing; 2d, other specific use restrictions as noted.

ADHD, Attention-deficit hyperactivity disorder; *bid*, twice daily; *BP*, blood pressure; *cap*, capsule; *CNS*, central nervous system; *DHA*, docosahexanoic acid; *DSM III*, *Diagnostic and Statistical Manual of Disorders*, third edition; *EPA*, eicosahexaenoic acid; *FDA*, Food and Drug Administration; *FSH-RH*, follicle-stimulating hormone; *GI*, gastrointestinal; *GnRH*, gonadotropin-releasing hormone; *HIV*, human immunodeficiency virus; *HTN*, hypertension; *MAO*, monoamine oxidase; *MSG*, monosodium glutamate; *NIH*, National Institutes of Health; *NSAID*, nonsteroidal antiinflammatory drug; *ORS*, oral rehydration solution; *PMS*, premenstrual syndrome; *PO*, by mouth; *prn*, as needed; *qid*, four times daily; *RBC*, red blood cell; *RDA*, recommended dietary allowance; *TB*, tuberculosis; *tbsp*, tablespoon; *tid*, three times daily; *tsp*, teaspoon; *UTI*, urinary tract infection.

RESOURCE BOX

Complementary Therapies

American Herbal Products Association
1-301-588-1171
www.ahpa.org

Center for Holistic Pediatric Education and Research (CHPER)
1-617-355-2576
www.childrenshospital.org/holistic

Chiropractic and Complementary/Alternative Compilation User's Manual
Palmer Center for Chiropractic Research
www.palmer.edu/carber/manualhome.asp

Cochrane Electronic Library
www.nelh.nhs.uk/cochrane.asp

FDA MedWatch
1-800-FDA-1088
www.fed.gov/medwatch

Federation of State Medical Boards of the United States, Inc.
1-817-868-4000
www.fsmb.org

Herbalgram, American Botanical Council and Herb Research Foundation
1-800-373-7105
www.herbalgram.org

HERBMED
www.herbmed.org

National Center for Complementary and Alternative Medicine (NCCAM)
National Institutes of Health
1-888-644-6226
www.nccam.nih.gov

United States Pharmacopeia (USP)
1-800-227-8772
www.usp.org

Further Reading
Blumenthal M, editor: *Herbal medicine: expanded commission E monographs*, Austin, TX, 2000, American Botanical Council.
Gruenwald J, Brendler T, Jaenicke C, editors: *PDR for herbal medicines*, Montvale, 2000, Medical Economics.
Kemper K: *The holistic pediatrician*, New York, 1996, HarperCollins.

REFERENCES

Abrams G: Chiropractic treatment holds promise for low back pain, *Complement Med Physician* 2(9):66, 1997.

Acupuncture scores points, *University of California Wellness Letter* 14(8):2, 1998.

Adams K et al: Ethical considerations of complementary and alternative medical therapies in conventional medical settings, *Ann Intern Med* 137(8):660-664, 2002.

American Academy of Pediatrics: Policy statement: counseling families who choose complementary and alternative medicine for their child with chronic illness or disability (RE0049), *Pediatrics* 107(3):598-601, 2001.

American Association of Poison Control Centers: 1998 pediatric exposures, American Association of Poison Control Centers, home page, 1998. Available at *www.aapcc.org* (accessed Jan 11, 2003).

Astin J: Why patients use alternative medicine, *JAMA* 279:1548-1553, 1998.

Balch J, Balch P: *Prescription for nutritional healing*, ed 2, Garden City, NY, 1997, Avery.

Bates B: Natural remedies can cause skin reactions, *Pediatr News*, Feb 1998, p 44.

Bell E: Implications of using drugs "off-label," *Infect Dis Child* 15(11):10-11, 2002.

Boris M, Mandel F: Foods and additives are common causes of the attention deficit hyperactive disorder in children, *Ann Allergy* 72:462-468, 1994.

Carter CM et al: Effects of a few food diet in attention deficit disorder, *Arch Dis Child* 69:564-568, 1993.

Castleman M: *The healing herbs: the ultimate guide to the curative power of nature's medicines*, New York, 1995, Bantam.

Chamberlain L: Parents need advice on herbals, *Infect Dis Child* 15(8):74-75, 2002.

Chan E: The role of complementary and alternative medicine in attention-deficit hyperactivity disorder, *J Dev Behav Pediatr* 23(1S):S37-S44, 2002.

Chan E, Gardiner P, Kemper K: "At least it's natural . . .": herbs and dietary supplements in ADHD, *Contemp Pediatr* 17(9):116-130, 2000.

Children can take charge of migraine, *Clin Rev* 8(11):122, 1998.

Clinical Evidence Concise: Secondary prevention of ischaemic cardiac events, *Clinical Evidence Concise*, Issue 9, London, 2003, BMJ Publishing Group.

del Mundo W, Shepherd W, Marose R: Use of alternative medicine by patients in a rural family practice clinic, *Fam Med* 34:206-212, 2002.

Egger J, Stolla A, McEwen L: Controlled trial of hyposensitisation in children with food-induced hyperkinetic syndrome, *Lancet* 339:1150-1153, 1992.

Eisenberg DM: Advising patients who seek alternative therapies, *Ann Intern Med* 127:61-69, 1997.

Eisenberg DM et al: Trends in alternative medicine use in the United States, 1990-1997: results of a follow-up national survey, *JAMA* 280:1569-1575, 1998.

Eisenberg DM et al: Unconventional medicine in the United States: prevalence, costs and patterns of use, *N Engl J Med* 328:246-252, 1993.

Elder NC, Gillcrist A, Minz R: Use of alternative health care by family practice patients, *Arch Fam Med* 6:181-184, 1997.

Field T et al: Children with asthma have improved pulmonary functions with massage therapy, *J Pediatr* 132:854-858, 1998.

Focht D, Spicer C, Fairchok M: The efficacy of duct tape vs cryotherapy in the treatment of verruca vulgaris (the common wart), *Arch Pediatr Adolesc Med* 156(10):971-977, 2002.

Food and Drug Administration: MedWatch home page, 2003. Available at *www.fda.gov/medwatch* (accessed Jan 11, 2003).

French M: The power of plants: an overview of herbal therapies, *Adv Nurse Pract* 4(7):17-21, 1996.

Frishberg M: Alternative medicine gaining wider acceptance, *Common Ground Reflections*, Jan 1998, pp 8-24.

Fugh-Berman A: *Alternative medicine: what works*, Baltimore, 1997, Williams & Wilkins.

Gardiner P, Coles D, Kemper K: The skinny on herbal remedies for dermatologic disorders, *Contemp Pediatr* 18(7):103-113, 2001.

Gardiner P, Conboy L, Kemper K: Herbs and adolescent girls: avoiding the hazards of self-treatment, *Contemp Pediatr* 17(3):133-154, 2000.

Gardiner P, Kemper K: Herbs in pediatric and adolescent medicine, *Pediatr Rev* 21(2):44-57, 2000.

Gideonse T: Music is good medicine, *Newsweek*, Sep 1998, p 103.

Gordon J: Alternative medicine and the family physician, *Am Fam Physician* 54:2205-2212, 1996.

Graedon J, Graedon T: *The people's pharmacy: guide to home and herbal remedies*, New York, 1999, Graedon Enterprises, Inc.

Grazzi L et al: Electromyographic biofeedback-assisted relaxation training in juvenile episodic tension-type headache: clinical outcome at three-year follow-up, *Cephalalgia* 21(8):798-803, 2001.

Green E, Moore B, Field T: Massage therapy: wide-ranging medical applicability and benefit, *Complement Med Physician* 2(9):1, 1997.

Halken S, Host A: Prevention, *Curr Opin Allergy Clin Immunol* 1(3):229-236, 2001.

Hardy M: Herb-drug interactions: an evidence-based table, *Int Med Alert*, Jan 29, pp. 1-8, 2001.

Herbal medicine taken as a whole, *Clin Advisor* 1(11/12):51, 1998.

Janiger O, Goldberg P: *A different kind of healing*, New York, 1993, Putnam.

Jonas W: Alternative medicine—learning from the past, examining the present, advancing to the future, *JAMA* 280:1616-1617, 1998.

Kemper K: Seven herbs every pediatrician should know, *Contemp Pediatr* 13(12):79-91, 1996a.

Kemper K: *The holistic pediatrician*, New York, 1996b, HarperCollins.

Kemper K: Integrated pediatrics: a holistic approach to healing children, *Complement Med Physician* 3(10):1, 1998.

Kemper K: Complementary and alternative medicine for children: does it work? *West J Med* 174:272-276, 2001.

Kemper K et al: Pediatric faculty development in integrative medicine, *Altern Ther Health Med* 8(6):32-33, 2002.

Kemper K et al: On pins and needles? Pediatric pain patients' experience with acupuncture, *Pediatrics* 105(4 pt 2):941-947, 2000.

Kemper K, Vincent E, Scardapane J: Teaching an integrated approach to complementary, alternative, and mainstream therapies for children: a curriculum evaluation, *J Altern Complement Med* 5(3):261-268, 1999.

Kemper K, Wornham W: Consultations for holistic pediatric services for inpatients and outpatient oncology patients at a children's hospital, *Arch Pediatr Adolesc Med* 155(4):449-454, 2001.

Kessler R et al: Long-term trends in the use of complementary and alternative medical therapies in the United States, *Ann Intern Med* 135:262-268, 2001.

Klein S, Winkelstein M: Enhancing pediatric health care with music, *J Pediatr Health Care* 10:74-81, 1996.

Kleinman L et al: The medical appropriateness of tympanostomy tubes proposed for children younger than 16 years in the United States, *JAMA* 271:1250-1255, 1994.

Knittel L: A new medical model: top medical schools are taking an aggressive approach to teaching future doctors about complementary medicine, *Yoga J* 166:35, 2002.

Konefal J: The challenge of educating physicians about complementary and alternative medicine, *Acad Med* 77(9):847-850, 2002.

Kreitzer J et al: Attitudes toward CAM among medical, nursing, and pharmacy faculty and students: a comparative analysis, *Altern Ther Health Med* 8(6):50-53, 2002.

Kull I et al: Breast feeding and allergic diseases in infants—a prospective birth cohort study, *Arch Dis Child* 87(6):478-481, 2002.

Landmark report on public perceptions of alternative care, Sacramento, 1998, Landmark Healthcare.

LaValle J et al: *Natural therapeutics pocket guide 2000-2001*, Hudson, OH, 2000, Lexi-Comp., Inc.

Lippman H: Can complementary and conventional medicine learn to get along? *Business and Health* 9:15, 2001.

Loeb H et al: Tannin-rich carob pod for the treatment of acute-onset diarrhea, *J Pediatr Gastroenterol Nutr* 8:480-485, 1989.

Mack R: "Something wicked this way comes"—herbs even witches should avoid, *Contemp Pediatr* 15(6):49-64, 1998.

Marcolina S: Topical aloe vera for skin and oral wounds, *Altern Med Alert* 1:8-11, 2001.

Markestad T: Use of sucrose as a treatment for infant colic, *Arch Dis Child* 76:356-358, 1997.

Mattison D: Herbal supplements: their safety, a concern for health care providers. March of Dimes website. Available at *www.marchofdimes.com* (accessed Jan 8, 2003).

McGuffin M et al, editors: *American Herbal Products Association's botanical safety handbook*, Boca Raton, FL, 1997, CRC Press.

McNeil D: Health agency embarks on survey of alternative medicine, *Oregonian: International*, Friday, May 17, 2002, p A10.

Micozzi M: *Fundamentals of complementary and alternative medicine*, New York, 1996, Churchill Livingstone.

Micozzi M: The common principles of complementary health care systems: enduring concepts with current clinical relevance, *Complement Med Physician* 2(8):1, 1997.

Moneret-Vautrin D: Optimal management of atopic dermatitis in infancy, *Allerg Immunol (Paris)* 34(9):325-329, 2002.

Mortimore J, Fischer S: Are we ready to give herbal remedies to children? Health Care Agency, County of Orange, California, *Nutrition Times* 3(1):1-3, 2001.

Murray M, Pizzorno J: *Encyclopedia of natural medicine*, ed 2, Rocklin, 1998, Prima Health.

National Center for Complementary and Alternative Medicine: Program FY 2003 research priorities. Available at *www.nccam.nih.gov/research* (accessed Dec 19, 2002).

National Institutes of Health: Consensus conference: acupuncture, *JAMA* 280:1518-1524, 1998.

Ni H, Simile C, Hardy A: Utilization of complementary and alternative medicine by United States adults: results from the 1999 national health interview survey, *Med Care* 40(4):353-387, 2002.

Nickerson J, Silberman T: Chiropractic manipulation in children, *J Pediatr* 12:172, 1992.

Nsouli TM et al: Role of food allergy in serous otitis media, *Ann Allergy* 73:215-219, 1994.

O'Brien M: Integrated geriatrics: optimizing and gentling health care for the elderly, *Complement Med Physician* 3(5):1, 1998.

Ott M: Yoga as a clinical intervention: pain control and stress reduction may be just a breath away, *Adv Nurse Pract* 10(1):81-90, 2002.

Ottolini M et al: Complementary and alternative medicine use among children in the Washington, DC area, *Ambul Pediatr* 1(2):122-125, 2001.

PA and NP opinions on alternative therapies, *Clin News*, Mar/Apr 1998, p 12.

Pettit J: Alternative medicine: cranberry, *Clin Rev* 12(1):43-44, 2002.

Ramsay C: Overkill: The regulation of natural health products in Canada. Fraser Forum, Feb 2002. The Fraser Institute webpage. Available at *www.oldfraser.lexi.net* (accessed Jan 11, 2003).

Reznik M et al: Use of complementary therapy by adolescents with asthma, *Arch Pediatr Adolesc Med* 156(10):1042-1044, 2002.

Rini A, Bloom K: Down in the mouth: update on treatment of oral aphthous ulcers, *Clinical Advisor* 5(2):67-72, 2002.

Rowe K, Rowe K: Synthetic food coloring and behavior: a dose response effect in a double-blind placebo-controlled, repeated-measure study, *J Pediatr* 125:691-697, 1994.

Schoch R: A conversation with Dana Ullman, *Calif Monthly*, Feb 1999, pp 27-30.

Schoetzau A et al: Effect of exclusive breast-feeding and early solid food avoidance on the incidence of atopic dermatitis in high-risk infants at 1 year of age, *Pediatr Allergy Immunol* 13(4):234-242, 2002.

Schulman S et al: Biofeedback methodology: does it matter how we teach children how to relax the pelvic floor during voiding? *J Urol* 166(6):2423-2426, 2001.

Simpson N, Roman K: Complementary medicine use in children: extent and reasons. A population-based study, *Br J Gen Pract* 51(472):914-916, 2001.

Smethurst D: Atopic dermatitis: what are the effects of preventive interventions and treatments? *Clinical Evidence Concise* 7:284-285, 2002.

Spiegelblatt L: Alternative medicine: a pediatric conundrum, *Contemp Pediatr* 14(8):51-64, 1997.

Starobrat-Hermelin B, Kozielec T: The effects of magnesium physiological supplementation on hyperactivity in children with ADHD. Positive response to magnesium oral loading test, *Magnes Res* 10(2):149-156, 1997.

Steele Memorial Children's Research Center in collaboration with the University of Arizona Program for Integrative Medicine: Personal communication, Sept 5, 2002.

Thaut M: Music therapy: the unsung modality, *Complement Med Physician* 3(6):1, 1998.

Therapeutic uses of herbs. Continuing Education #97-005, *Prescriber's Letter*, Fall 1997.

Therapeutic uses of herbs. Continuing Education Booklet, *Prescriber's Letter*, Spring 1998.

Ting W, Gross M, Oz M: The Internet as a research tool in complementary and alternative medicine: a pilot study, *Altern Ther Health Med* 8(3):84-86, 2002.

Turow V: Alternative therapy for colds [letter], *Pediatrics* 100:274-275, 1997a.

Turow V: Chiropractic for children, *Arch Pediatr Adolesc Med* 151:527-528, 1997b.

Winslow C, Shapiro H: Physicians want education about complementary and alternative medicine to enhance communication with their patients, *Arch Intern Med* 162(10):1176-1181, 2002.

World Health Organization: New ORS rehydration formula. Available at *www.who.int* (accessed Feb 23, 2003).

Wysocki S: Unconventional and conventional medicine: searching for common ground, *Contemp Nurse Pract*, Winter 1997, pp 3-15.

Zeltzer L et al: A phase I study on the feasibility and acceptability of an acupuncture/hypnosis intervention for chronic pediatric pain, *J Pain Symptom Manage* 24(4):437-446, 2002.

44

Practice Management Strategies for a Health Care Practice

Denise A. Hall

A successful health care practice requires not only good clinical services, but also sound business planning and efficient day-to-day operations. If the practice has excellent clinical providers but does not pay attention to or does not devote equal resources to its business operation, its future ability to operate will be compromised. This chapter is a primer for setting up and managing a health care practice; it provides a brief overview of key administrative and clinical management strategies necessary for successful practice operations.

Paying attention to business operations in a medical practice can seem like a daunting task at times. Staying current with state and federal regulations, employment laws, and risk management issues requires constant vigilance and attention. Compliance with these legal requirements is only the beginning of ensuring good business operations. Strategic planning; financial management; staff recruiting, training, and retention; efficient administrative operations; marketing; and patient education are all areas that can make or break a practice.

The development of a business plan and an operations plan are two practice management strategies that are instrumental in making a practice successful. Discussion of some of the components of these plans is included in this chapter. For more in-depth information about these and other practice management topics, see the Resource Box at the end of this chapter.

THE BUSINESS PLAN

Developing a business plan is a requisite first step for the development of a new practice and is extremely useful for established practices that may be considering a new project or change in business operations. This plan clearly declares the philosophy and goals of the practice on which an overall strategic plan will be based and how these goals will be reached. Even a simple one- or two-page plan can help provide a formal structure for present and future planning. A vision statement, market analysis, strategic plan, and organizational chart make up a simple business plan for the practice and provide the necessary framework for clinical and administrative operations.

Vision Statement

The vision statement may be one or two simple sentences or one or two paragraphs, but it should summarize the practice's reason for being and the philosophy of the organization. This vision statement is the foundation for all clinical and administrative operations of the practice. A good suggestion is to revisit the vision statement often to ensure that over the years it continues to reflect the mission and values of the practice.

Market Analysis

A market analysis is a primary and critical key task that must be undertaken to better understand the specific demographic makeup of the targeted patient population. This analysis should look at the current and future demand or need for pediatric health care services, as well as the current capacity for providing these services. Factors such as population data, growth projections, primary care competition, and the current economic and business climate are important areas to review. Gathering this information requires time and effort, but is important for good decision making for new business operations and for short- and long-range planning.

Strategic Plan

The vision statement and market analysis are used together to formulate the strategic plan for the practice. A strategic plan is useful for starting a new practice, planning practice growth, or simply developing new projects. It provides both framework and direction for the task at hand and sets the business plan in motion. The strategic plan normally includes the goals and objectives identified by the practice, time elements or a time line, a budget or financial plan, and identification of both physical and human resource requirements.

Organizational Chart

A helpful administrative resource for the strategic plan is the development of an organizational chart. This chart shows titles and reporting responsibilities of the people involved in implementing the business plan of the practice. It not only provides a visual snapshot of the management structure of the practice, but also connects its business plan with the practice's personnel resources. An organizational chart assists the practice in clarifying roles and responsibilities for ownership, management, and staff.

THE OPERATIONS PLAN

Successfully moving the business plan from paper to reality requires additional planning and implementation. The operations plan (OP) provides assistance during this process and helps ensure that key elements for successful practice management are not overlooked. The OP uses the formal business plan for its initial direction but has a different purpose. Its goal is to take a micromanagement view of the business and strategic plan and make them fully functional. Although every practice is individual and distinct, and business plans differ by design and need, the OP establishes systems by which to:

- Identify key practice management areas and practice resources.
- Develop policies and procedures to ensure administrative and clinical quality assurance.
- Monitor, report, and benchmark clinical and administrative results.
- Emphasize quality improvement and customer service.

Operational checklists are included in this chapter for the areas of legal and governance operations, financial, human resources, and clinical operations. The checklists include a basic list of elements and issues that are important in practice operations, regardless of size or strategy.

Legal and Governance Operations

Legal counsel and a certified public accountant (CPA) are valuable resources to have in place when establishing the practice's legal and governance operations. See Table 44-1 for the checklist.

Organizational Structure and Tax Status

Choosing an organizational structure (normally a partnership or corporation) and a tax status are two initial decisions required when starting a practice. Because of the numerous legal and financial implications involved when choosing an organizational structure, it is imperative to have good legal advice during this process. Developing an ongoing relationship with an attorney and accountant with experience in health care organizations is valuable, not only for the start-up phase of a health care practice, but also for ongoing consultation. It is also efficacious to have sound financial and legal advice when drafting the practice's governance documents such as bylaws, articles of

TABLE 44-1 ***Legal and Governance Checklist***

- ☐ Legal counsel
- ☐ Accountant
- ☐ Organizational structure
  - ☐ Partnership, corporation
  - ☐ Tax status
  - ☐ Governance documents
- ☐ Federal tax employer identification number (EIN)
- ☐ Business licenses
- ☐ Provider licenses
- ☐ Insurance requirements
  - ☐ General liability
  - ☐ Professional liability
  - ☐ Workers' compensation
- ☐ Government regulations
  - ☐ Occupational Safety and Health Administration (OSHA)
  - ☐ Health Insurance Portability and Accountability Act (HIPAA)
  - ☐ Clinical Laboratory and Improvement Amendments of 1988 (CLIA)
- ☐ Legal guidelines
  - ☐ Record retention

incorporation, employment agreements, and buy-sell agreements, as well as when reviewing lease documents and contracts.

Federal Tax Identification and Licenses

In addition to appropriate legal documents, the practice will require a federal tax identification number, also called an employer identification number (EIN). A state tax identification number is required for state tax reporting, and most cities require a local business license.

There are also licensing requirements for health care providers. Most states include a state license and a license to dispense drugs (Drug Enforcement Administration [DEA]) as minimum requirements.

Insurance Requirements

The practice should purchase general liability, professional liability, and workers' compensation insurance as part of its required legal and business needs. General liability insurance protects the assets of the business from casualty damage, employee dishonesty, theft, business interruption, and personal injury.

Professional liability policies provide coverage for both the individual providers and the practice in the event of a claim of medical malpractice. Professional liability insurance is written on either a claims-made or an occurrence basis. Because claims-made policies normally require the purchase of a "tail" or extended coverage in the event that the policy is terminated, it is important to understand the differences and which type of coverage is offered under the policy. When purchasing professional liability insurance it is wise to insure the practice, as well as the individual providers. Insuring the practice provides an added layer of protection in the event of a medical malpractice claim, and also includes coverage for clinical and administrative support staff. Limits of $1.5 million to $2 million for each occurrence with an aggregate limit of $3 million to $4 million are now considered a minimum standard of protection.

Workers' compensation insurance protects the practice and its employees against accidents on the job. Examples of accidents that most often happen in a health care practice are needle-stick injuries; injuries caused by lifting or moving patients, equipment, or files; and repetitive motion types of injuries suffered by administrative staff.

Government Regulations

There are numerous and important regulations for health care practices. Special attention must be given to these regulations to ensure awareness, training, and compliance.

Health Insurance Portability and Accountability Act. The newest regulation affecting health care providers is the Health Insurance Portability and Accountability Act (HIPAA) effective April 2003. Although the section of this regulation dealing with the portability of health insurance (Consolidated Omnibus Budget Reconciliation Act [COBRA]) has been in effect since 1996, the newest section regulates how health care providers must protect the privacy of its patients' protected health information (PHI). The primary purpose of the privacy section of HIPAA is to protect the rights of patients by providing them access to their PHI, as well as the ability to control the use and disclosure of their PHI. HIPAA regulations now require health care providers to provide all patients with a "Notice of Privacy Practices." This notice informs patients of their rights under HIPAA and how the practice will use and disclose their PHI for treatment, payment, or health care operations purposes. Other parts of this regulation include requirements for the electronic transfer of PHI and for the development of business associate contracts with organizations with which the practice may share confidential information (outside billing or collection agencies, medical records couriers, transcription companies, answering services, etc.). Other sections of HIPAA contain regulations that require specific security precautions for the safety and confidentiality of health information. Being HIPAA compliant requires the practice to develop policies and procedures that ensure confidentiality of patient information within the practice and to orient and train staff in these areas.

Occupational Safety and Health Administration. The Occupational Safety and Health Administration (OSHA), a division of the Department of Labor, regulates health and safety in the workplace. Medical offices are required to meet safety standards regarding universal precautions, blood-borne pathogens, and tuberculosis and are required to have written policies that enforce these standards. Practices must also provide education and annual training to staff and keep accurate records regarding any injuries and exposures that may have occurred. OSHA standards focus on infection control and contain guidelines for personal protective equipment, frequent handwashing, decontamination, and waste disposal.

Clinical Laboratory and Improvement Amendments of 1988. The Clinical Laboratory and Improvement Amendments of 1988 (CLIA) set performance standards and licensing requirements for hospital and physician-office laboratories based on the complexity of the tests being performed. CLIA standards focus on personnel qualifications of laboratory staff, quality control, quality assurance, and proficiency testing. A procedure manual must be kept up to date that details how to perform every test conducted in the laboratory. Based on the complexity of tests performed, the laboratory will have a CLIA designation of waived, physician-performed microscopy, moderate complexity, or high complexity.

Retention of Records

There are specific guidelines for the retention of all records and business documents in the health care practice. Requirements vary depending on the type of records (medical records, financial records, claims and billing records, staff and employment records). Table 44-2 contains general recommendations for records retention. As the practice gets larger, the retention of records can become an expensive storage problem. New technologies such as optical scanners and electronic file cabinets can help practices meet these requirements in a more efficient manner.

Financial Operations

A financially healthy practice requires the development of an operations budget and constant close attention to its revenues and expenses (Table 44-3). The following steps are recommended:

TABLE 44-2 ***Guidelines for Record Retention***

Document/Records	Months to Keep
Agenda or schedules	24
Bank statements	60
Budgets	60
Cancelled checks	60
Committee meeting minutes	60
Contracts	60 (after expiration)
Employment applications	36
Financial reports	60
Financial statements	Life of organization
Insurance documents	36
Insurance policies	72 (after expiration)
Invoices	72
Policies	Life of organization
Accounts receivable	84
Account reconciliations	24
Reports	60
Tax returns	72
Medical records	Pediatric records should be kept a minimum of 7 yr past age of majority

Developed from recommendations of the American Society of Association Executives and the U.S. Code of Federal Regulations.

- Establish a professional relationship with a bank or other financial institution for the purposes of opening a checking account, a payroll checking account, a savings account, and a line of credit.
- Choose a computerized accounting software package. A packaged accounting software such as Quick Books or Quicken usually meets the needs of a small- to medium-sized practice, whereas larger organizations with multiple locations and many cost centers require a more powerful and sophisticated system. The accountant or bookkeeper should be able to suggest a system that will best meet the needs of the practice. The system should not only be able to manage accounts payables and write checks but should also be able to develop budgets, automate payroll, and provide a standard set of financial reports. The practice's accountant can also help decide whether to operate the accounting system on a cash basis, an accrual basis, or a modified cash basis.
- Establish a chart of accounts. The chart of accounts plays a key role in budgeting and financial reporting. Although any chart of accounts that can break out and report on revenue sources and track expenses by similar types will suffice, the practice may wish to review the chart of accounts recommended by the Medical Group Management Association (MGMA) or a similar consulting group. Setting up the chart of accounts so that financial reports are comparable with those of other similar medical groups can be helpful for the management of revenue and expenses in the practice, as well as for comparison or benchmarking purposes.
- Prepare an operations budget. There are many types of budgets, but an operations budget is a good place to start to be able to (1) plan the operations of the practice based

TABLE 44-3 ***Financial Operations Checklist***

- ☐ Accountant
- ☐ Accounting software
- ☐ Chart of accounts
- ☐ Budgets
  - ☐ Operations
  - ☐ Capital expense
  - ☐ Personnel
- ☐ Bank accounts
- ☐ Financial reports
- ☐ Payroll
- ☐ Revenue cycle

on anticipated revenues and expenses and (2) monitor the revenues and expenses throughout the year. The operations budget should start with a detailed look at the anticipated revenues of the practice (revenues from third-party payers or insurance payers, patient payments, and ancillary services). The fee schedule, insurance reimbursement data, average collection rates, and patient visit data are all important elements used to forecast practice revenues. Revenue projections should not only look back at historical data and current contracts, but should also take into account any anticipated changes that will affect the practice. Potential new sources of revenues, anticipated growth, and changes in contracts can all affect practice revenue and should be included in the budget process.

- Determine salaries and benefits. In most instances, the biggest expense for the health care practice is personnel. Personnel and supporting expenses are listed in the budget as salaries and benefits. Development of this part of the budget will also require projections based on past and projected patient visit data. Determining the number of providers required to support patient visits is necessary, as is determining the number and type of support staff required. A separate personnel budget developed using spreadsheet software such as Excel can help with planning this part of the expense budget. The personnel budget should identify titles, departments, full-time equivalent (FTE) status, hourly rate, salary, and projected annual compensation, including estimated salary increases and overtime. The chart of accounts normally specifies separate line items for budgeted salaries for physicians, nurse practitioners, physician assistants, management, and support staff. In addition, identifying departments or other cost centers in the operations budget can provide valuable information for regular monitoring and reporting of expenses. After the total expenses for salaries are determined, the amount to budget for payroll taxes can be calculated (usually a percentage of the total salary expense). Benefit costs such as health or dental insurance can also be projected using a spreadsheet and then transferred to the operating budget. If practice policies or employment agreements provide additional benefits such as continuing medical education or professional dues, these totals should also be added as a specific line item in the benefits budget category.
- Categorize other expenses in the budget as physical resources, general and administrative expenses, or purchased services. Examples of expenses budgeted as physical resources are rent, janitorial expense, medical supplies (including vaccines), printing of clinical forms, or any expense directly used for the provision of medical services. General and administrative expenses are those that pay for the administrative operations of the practice. Office supplies, administrative printing, telephone (including pagers), insurance, and depreciation expenses are examples of expenses that belong in this category. Expenses that fall under the classification of purchased services are those that are paid to others for specific services provided. Accounting and legal services, answering service, telephone support, computer support, and marketing services are examples.
- Finalize the budget and spread revenue and expense line items over the 12-month period so that they can be tracked, monitored, and reported by month. These expenses can either be spread equally over the 12 months of the year, or they can be adjusted based on known revenue or expense patterns.
- Plan for fixed-asset purchases. If the practice is planning to purchase any furniture or equipment or make significant improvements to the facility that are considered "major" in nature (usually over $500), a capital expense budget and depreciation schedules should also be developed.

Financial Reports

At the minimum, a basic set of monthly financial reports should include a profit and loss (income/expense), an actual profit and loss compared to budget, year-to-date profit and loss compared to budget, and a balance sheet. The practice's accounting software system should have these basic reports, as well as other financial reports that are valuable in tracking the financial performance of the practice and providing the necessary information for financial planning.

Payroll

In a small practice, the accounting software can usually be used to prepare the payroll, calculate withholding taxes, and help ensure that tax deposits are made in a timely manner. Practices with over 25 employees may want to explore using a payroll service for convenience and cost efficiencies. In any case, a method for hourly employees to record and report hours worked will be necessary. There are a variety of ways for employees to track and report time—from manual time sheets to electronic systems that integrate with the payroll or accounting system. If the practice has both exempt (salaried) and nonexempt (hourly) staff, it is usually advisable to have two separate payroll schedules. For example, hourly staff can be paid on a biweekly basis (every 2 weeks), and salaried staff on a semimonthly or monthly basis.

Revenue Cycle

The revenue cycle of the practice is the all-inclusive system that starts with the development of a fee schedule and ends with reimbursement for services performed. Included in the revenue cycle are the following elements:

- Contracts with commercial insurance and Medicare or Medicaid
- Fee schedule
- Charge ticket for coding and billing
- Patient registration form
- Verification of insurance eligibility
- Capture of provided services
- Correct coding of provided services
- Charge entry (manual or electronic)
- Electronic claims submission
- Payment posting (manual or electronic)
- Patient statements
- Accounts receivable management
- Practice management reports

Financial Policies

The development of policies and procedures for financial operations should include guidelines for internal cash controls, making bank deposits, collection of copayments at time of service, insurance verification, methods of payment accepted (check, cash, credit card), timeliness of entry of charges into the practice management system, regular attention to accounts receivable, and collection policies, including potential discharge of patients from the practice. If the practice has decided to outsource any of its accounting, financial, or billing functions, similar policies should be developed and made part of any service contract.

Human Resource Operations

The employees of a practice are instrumental in making a practice successful. They are either an asset to the practice or detrimental to its operations. The staff is not only the largest expense in the practice budget but also functions as the day-to-day marketing and customer service team. Whether by providing clinical or administrative services, the staff represents the practice to current and potential patients every day. Managing staff and the human resource function of a practice is complex and requires a sound knowledge of employment law. Job descriptions are recommended for all employees and can be a valuable tool for use in the hiring, training, and evaluation of practice staff. A basic human resources operations checklist is provided in Table 44-4.

TABLE 44-4 *Human Resources Checklist*

- ☐ State wage and hour laws
- ☐ Federal employment laws
  - ☐ Americans with Disabilities Act (ADA)
  - ☐ Fair Labor Standards Act (FLSA)
  - ☐ Family and Medical Leave Act (FMLA)
  - ☐ Equal Employment Opportunity Commission (EEOC)
  - ☐ Consolidated Omnibus Budget Reconciliation Act (COBRA)
- ☐ Staffing
  - ☐ Exempt and nonexempt
  - ☐ Employment agreements
  - ☐ Personnel forms
- ☐ Salaries and benefits
- ☐ Employee handbook
- ☐ Job descriptions
- ☐ Performance evaluation process
- ☐ Orientation and training
- ☐ Important policies
  - ☐ Confidentiality
  - ☐ Harassment
  - ☐ Nonviolence

Legal Issues for Human Resources

Knowledge of a state's wage and hour laws is necessary. These wage and hour laws help in the development of human resource policies and procedures for the practice. Wage and hour laws will help in the development of the following standards:

- Identify a "work week" for the practice (for example, 12:01 AM Sunday to 12 PM Saturday). This standard is necessary for calculating overtime.
- Identify staff as "nonexempt" or "exempt" from overtime. Nonexempt staff members are normally paid hourly, whereas exempt staff members are paid by salary. The correct classification of staff is critical—misclassification and the failure to pay overtime when required can result in legal recourse, as well as back pay and fines.
- Development of policies for employee rest breaks during the workday
- Payment of wages on involuntary or voluntary termination
- Requirements of the practice for employee's civic obligations such as jury duty or military leave

The practice, depending on its size and its contracts, must be in compliance with the following federal employment laws:

- Americans with Disabilities Act (ADA)
- Family and Medical Leave Act (FMLA)
- Equal Employment Opportunity Commission (EEOC)
- Fair Labor Standards Act (FLSA)
- Consolidated Omnibus Budget Reconciliation Act (COBRA)

Other legal requirements that affect the human resource function include the completion by employees of I-9 (immigration) and W-4 (payroll withholding) forms. These two forms should be completed before the beginning of work. It is generally recommended that the I-9 form be kept separately from the employee's personnel file for confidentiality purposes in the event of an audit.

Compensation and Benefits

Compensation and the use of salary structures or salary ranges are an essential part of human resource management. The marketplace normally plays a large role in establishing these ranges by cities, states, or other specific regions of the country. In addition, the development of job descriptions and a method to evaluate employees' performance are elements that affect salary structure and consequently the personnel costs of the practice. Many human resource consultants suggest linking the performance evaluation to the job description. Various professional organizations and websites provide salary statistics that may be helpful in the development of salary ranges or structures, and at the very least can be used as a method of comparison for the local market.

By offering a good benefits package, the practice can increase its competitiveness in the marketplace and also provide security for employees. A basic benefit package usually includes health and dental insurance, life insurance, vision insurance, 401 K retirement plan, vacation, sick leave, or a combination of vacation and sick leave in a paid time off (PTO) account. More extensive benefits can include tuition allowance, uniform allowance, continuing education, bus passes, parking allowances, long- or short-term disability insurance, or employee assistance programs. A standard benefit package combined with required payroll taxes can add an additional 10% to 20% to the personnel costs of the practice.

Employee Handbook

An employee handbook is an excellent way to communicate personnel policies to staff members. An employee handbook should include the practice's mission statement, confidentiality requirements and agreements, and policies on benefits, vacation, sick leave, time off for bereavement or jury duty, calling in when ill, and leaves of absence. The handbook also communicates the practice's compliance with state and federal regulations. In addition, the practice should develop and include policies on a professional code of conduct, harassment, and nonviolence for inclusion in the handbook. If an employee handbook is developed, an attorney should review it to ensure that it does not contain or imply any language that could be construed as a contract of employment.

Employment Agreements

Health care practices often incorporate employment agreements or a contract of employment for their professional and senior management staff. An employment agreement is a legal contract that specifies the employees' and employers' duties to each other in detail. Counsel from the practice's attorney should be sought when deciding if employment agreements are right for the practice. In any event, an employment agreement should never be construed as a guarantee of employment and should always include a method for termination of the employment by either the employee or the employer during the contract term.

Clinical Operations

An efficient and well-run health care practice often gives the impression that operating or managing a practice is an easy task. Nothing could be further from the truth! A health care practice is a complex business requiring multiple clinical and administrative systems that work well together. Successful day-to-day operations require that both systems operate in conjunction with good customer service. A basic clinical operations checklist is provided in Table 44-5.

Appointment Scheduling

Numerous books and articles have been written on appointment scheduling systems. The practice's scheduling system provides the structure for the clinician's day and either helps to create an office that runs smoothly or contributes to one that is in constant chaos. Important issues in pediatric scheduling require decisions on how to handle well-child visits, ill-child visits, and newborns—how they should be arranged in the schedule and how much time

TABLE 44-5 *Clinical Operations Checklist*

- ☐ Appointment scheduling and phones
  - ☐ Patient flow
  - ☐ Phone system
  - ☐ Phone messages
  - ☐ Telephone triage
  - ☐ Answering service
- ☐ Medical records
  - ☐ Electronic medical record
  - ☐ Charting and documentation
  - ☐ Quality assurance
  - ☐ Medical record forms
- ☐ Practice management information system
- ☐ Standardized procedures
- ☐ Emergency procedures

should be allotted for each type of visit. In a multi-provider practice, probably the most critical element of efficient scheduling is to have a single scheduling philosophy and consistent scheduling rules for the entire practice.

Many practices keep a substantial portion of the daily schedule open for same-day visits. Additionally, the practice may want to consider keeping the first half-hour of the morning open for patients who have been instructed to come in to the office during that time by the provider taking night call. Patients like the fact that they can be assured of being seen first thing in the morning without having to wait until the office opens to phone for an appointment.

Other scheduling concerns that should be addressed in policy statements and standard protocols include how the practice will confirm appointments and how it will deal with late patients, no-show patients, walk-in patients, and urgent or emergency patients.

Practices serving pediatric patients also have found it beneficial to have seasonal schedules. For example, during the winter months it is a good idea to think about reducing the number of well-child appointment slots on Mondays and increasing the number of ill-child slots. Likewise, practices can implement a schedule in the summer months that contains more slots for well-child visits or physical examinations to help meet the demand for school and camp physicals.

Patient Phone Calls

Patient phone calls are a significant factor in the day-to-day operations of any health care practice. Whether calling for prescription refills, for test results, to schedule an appointment, to request a referral, or to ask for advice on home care suggestions during an illness, patients want their concerns handled efficiently and in a timely manner. The practice should have policies and procedures on how these and other types of phone inquiries will be handled and by which staff members. Many of these responsibilities can be handled by clinical support staff such as registered nurses, medical assistants, or referral coordinators. Registered nurses can take patient phone calls, assess the patient, and, depending on the situation and following specific triage protocols, either give medical advice or recommend that an appointment be made. Medical assistants can take messages off a prescription refill line and call in refills. Medical assistants or other support staff can assist the patient in obtaining a referral or an appointment to instigate a referral. Care should be given that staff members functioning in these capacities are neither expected nor allowed to act outside of their clinical competency or scope of practice.

The phone system itself plays a critical role in the scheduling process, practice operations, and good customer service. Does the practice want to have an automated greeting or a live person answer the phone? Both require backup systems to make them work successfully. If the practice uses an automated system, the greeting and subsequent choices for obtaining service should be simple, with only a few choices. If the practice opts for live operators, it should make sure that there are sufficient lines and staff members to handle anticipated volume at various times of the day and week.

Medical Records

Deciding on a medical records system to meet the needs of the practice has traditionally revolved around determining how to organize the medical chart, what type of filing system to use, and development of the policies and procedures required for the medical record functions. With numerous electronic systems available, a new practice should also seriously consider an electronic medical records (EMR) system as a way to not only record the clinical and demographic information on each patient, but also as a way to improve coordination of care. Established practices should also consider an EMR system for all of the aforementioned benefits, realizing, however, that additional planning for incorporating current paper records with the electronic system will be required. Large practices and practices with multiple locations often find that the benefits of the EMR system outweigh the difficulties involved in moving to the electronic system, even if it is a time- and labor-intensive process. There are many types of EMR and electronic medical chart (EMC) systems. Adequately researching how a system works and knowledge of practice styles and outcomes are necessary when deciding on an EMR system.

Practice Management Computer System

A practice management computer system or practice management information system is essential to a modern health care office. The basic system should integrate patient demographic information, the scheduling process, and billing functions. If the practice is interested in adopting an EMR or EMC system immediately or in the future, the software should have an EMR component or be compatible with the desired EMR or EMC system. Many good systems have basic or entry-level systems for small offices that can be upgraded as the practice size and demands of the practice increase. When considering the purchase of a new system, it is a good idea to arrange to visit another practice of similar size that is using the system to see the functions demonstrated in a real-time environment. Scheduling functions, reporting capabilities, and billing functions—inducing the ability to send claims electronically—are key areas to research in a system. In addition, technical support, initial and ongoing training, and system upgrades are important aspects about which to become knowledgeable.

Standardization in the Practice

A medical practice can realize some important benefits by standardizing its practices and procedures. In addition to a standardized appointment schedule, policies and procedures for chart organization and documentation, immunization and well-child schedules, and nursing procedures are areas that lend themselves to conformity. For example, if there are uniform policies and procedures for preparing patients before the clinician's entry into the examination room (vital signs, weighing, measuring, appropriate charting and graphing), support staff can more easily cover for each other and the provider can be confident that all necessary tasks are accomplished.

Emergency Procedures

Practices should develop and implement policies and procedures for handling emergencies in the practice. Emergency protocols should include identification of an emergency, calling 911, definition of levels of emergencies to be handled in the practice, leadership and communication during the emergency, provider and support staff responsibilities, stocking of a "crash cart" to be used in emergencies, having other necessary supplies and equipment, initial and ongoing staff training in cardiopulmonary resuscitation and emergency procedures, documentation and charting of emergencies, and an assessment or critique of all emergencies or training sessions.

Quality Assurance

Developing clinical quality standards for the practice should be a major focus of any clinical checklist for risk management, as well as to improve clinical care. Organizations such as the National Committee for Quality Assurance (NCQA), the American Health Information Management Association (AHIMA), and the Joint Commission on Accreditation of Healthcare Organizations (JCAHO) can provide valuable information and guidance for the development of clinical quality standards. NCQA is a national organization with a primary function of accrediting managed care health plans. Accreditation by NCQA requires health plans to meet standards ranging from access and customer service to preventive medical care; the plans are rated based on their compliance in these areas. Accordingly, NCQA standards are used by health plans when setting quality assurance guidelines for providers in their networks. Many professional liability insurers also use NCQA standards when developing risk management guidelines for their policyholders.

The Medical Record. A review of medical records is a primary focus of accreditation and impromptu site visits by the accrediting bodies mentioned previously. This is because the record serves as legal documentation of all clinical activity. Consequently, the organization, content, and completeness of the medical record can be valuable to ensure quality assurance. The following guidelines for maintaining a clinically and legally sound medical record are suggested by AHIMA and JCAHO:

- Only authorized individuals may make entries in the medical record, and individuals should be trained in documentation practices and documentation standards.
- Every page in the medical record must identify the patient by name and an identifying number.
- Entries made into the medical record should be made as soon as possible after the visit or communication with the patient.
- Every entry in the medical record must be signed or initialed and include a complete date (month, day, year) and time. Entries must be dated at the date and time they are made.
- A signature legend should be maintained by the practice that identifies all signatures and initials appearing in the medical record.
- The medical record should always use factual information. Documentation should clearly identify speculation versus factual information.
- A standard set of abbreviations to be used in the medical record should be developed by the practice.
- All entries in the medical record should be legible.
- If using forms or checklists, all fields should have some entry. If a field is not applicable, an entry such as "N/A" should be made.
- Informed consent should be documented whenever applicable.
- All pertinent communication (and attempts at communication) with the patient or the patient's family should be documented. Messages left on answering machines or voice mail are not considered a valid form of notification.
- When an incident occurs, document the facts of the occurrence in the progress note. Do not chart that an incident report has been completed or refer to the report in charting.
- All entries in the medical record are considered permanent.
- All entries in the medical record should be in blue or black ink. Pencils should never be used.
- If an error is made in an entry, it should be corrected by (1) drawing a thin line through the incorrect entry, ensuring that the inaccurate information is still legible; (2) signing and dating the entry; (3) stating the reason for the error in the margin or above the note; and (4) documenting the correct information.
- If a late entry, addendum, or clarification is added to the medical record, identify it as such and enter the current

date and time. The reason for the late entry should also be noted.

- The medical record should not be removed from the practice site. If it is necessary to transport the medical record, a tracking system and safeguards should be in place to protect confidentiality and protect against loss.
- Policies and procedures should be developed for the destruction of medical records.

Other components of the medical record that ensure both good clinical processes and risk management include:

- A *problem list* that identifies the patient's chronic and significant illnesses. The problem list should appear in a prominent location in the medical record (usually at the front of the medical record).
- *Allergy flags* that indicate known allergies or no known allergies. Allergy flags should be documented on the outside of the medical record and on the problem list. Patients should be questioned about allergies at each visit.
- A *medication list* that contains the patient's acute and chronic medications. This list should be maintained in a prominent location in the medical record. The medication prescribed, the dosage, the date prescribed, and the prescriber should be entered on the medication list. The medication list should also include a record of prescription refills.

Clinical Tracking Systems. Systems that focus on the tracking of necessary medical follow-up appointments, high-risk referrals, and clinical tests ordered are other risk management tools that benefit coordination of care and customer service.

Appointment Tracking. An appointment tracking system helps ensure that patients return to the office as instructed

RESOURCE BOX

Practice Management Strategies for Health Care

ORGANIZATIONS

American Academy of Family Physicians (AAFP)
11400 Tomahawk Creek Parkway
Leawood, KS 66211
1-800-274-2237
www.aafp.org

American Academy of Pediatrics (AAP)
141 Northwest Point Boulevard
Elk Grove Village, IL 60007
1-847-434-4000
www.aap.org

American Health Information Management Association (AHIMA)
233 North Michigan Avenue, #2150
Chicago, IL 60601
1-312-233-1100
www.ahima.org

Medical Group Management Association (MGMA)
104 Inverness Terrace East
Englewood, CO 80112
1-888-608-5601
www.mgma.com

Society of Human Resource Management (SHRM)
1800 Duke Street
Alexandria, VA 22314
1-800-283-SHRM
www.shrm.org

BOOKS (AVAILABLE THROUGH MGMA)

Chart of accounts for healthcare organizations, 1999, MGMA.
Floreen N: *Collections manual for healthcare providers,* Englewood, CO, 1999, MGMA.
Kuehn L: *Health information management: medical record processes in group practice,* 1997, MGMA.
Lucash PD: *Medical practice business plan workbook,* 1999, McGraw-Hill.
Medisphere Health Partners, Inc.: *Managed care contract reference guide,* 1998, MGMA.
Novak A: *Governing policies manual for medical practices,* 1996, MGMA.
Pavlock E: *Financial management for medical groups,* 2000, MGMA.
Physician office safety guide, 1998, MGMA.
Price C, Novak A: *MBA job description manual for medical practices,* 1999, MGMA.
Rowell JC, Green MA: *Understanding health insurance: a guide to professional billing,* 2002, Delmar Thomson Learning.
Schryver D, editor: *An assessment manual for medical groups,* 2002, MGMA.
Warn B, Woodcock E: *Operating policies and procedures manual for medical practices,* 2001, MGMA.

RESOURCE BOX

Practice Management Strategies for Health Care—cont'd

BOOKS (AVAILABLE THROUGH AAP)

A guide to starting a medical office, Elk Grove Village, IL, 1997, American Academy of Pediatrics.

Poole SR: *Developing a telephone triage and advice system for a pediatric office practice*, July 2002, American Academy of Pediatrics.

Schmitt BD: *Pediatric telephone protocols: office version*, ed 9, 2002, American Academy of Pediatrics.

Seidel J, Knapp J: *Childhood emergencies in the office, hospital, and community*, 1992, American Academy of Pediatrics.

OTHER RESOURCES

Annual Business Guide

Reel SJ: Developing a business plan: getting down to specifics, *Adv Nurse Pract* 11(6):53-54, 90, 2003.

Robnett M: Planning your private practice: setting realistic expectations, *Adv Nurse Pract* 11(6):48-49, 2003.

Rollet J: Marketing your practice: strategies that work, *Adv Nurse Pract* 11(6):59-60, 62, 2003.

Zaumeyer C: Financing a private practice: investigating the options, *Adv Nurse Pract* 11(6):56-57, 2003.

Partnerships for Training

Building a Practice in Your Home Community

www.pftweb.org/practice/practice_home_frameset.htm

Site designed to help NPs and others set up and run their own health care practice; a wealth of resources, especially for underserved communities.

Pediatric Coding Alert

1-800-508-2582

2272 Airport Road South

Naples, FL 34112

www.codinginstitute.com

Monthly newsletter for ethically optimizing coding reimbursement and efficiency for pediatric practices.

Pediatric Practice Advisor

1-888-941-4488

15 E. Ridge Pike, Suite 510

Conshohocken, PA 19428

Monthly newsletter containing advice and strategies for pediatric-specific management of offices or clinics.

for any visit that the provider believes is critical. A newborn requiring a repeat bilirubin test is an example of a critical appointment that requires tracking to ensure that the patient complies with the provider's instruction for the repeat testing.

Referral Tracking. If the provider refers the patient to a specialist for a high-risk problem, a tracking system will ensure that the visit was completed and the report from the specialist received and reviewed.

Tests Ordered. A tracking and follow-up system should be implemented to ensure that diagnostic test results are completed and the results are received and reviewed in a timely manner. The system should also include verification that the patient was notified of the test results.

SUMMARY

The above review and checklists can be used for new practices as suggestions for important areas to think about and plan for during the development stages of practice operations. Established practices can use them as a "review of systems" to identify areas that may need improvement. In any case, the topics discussed have been chosen as basic principles for successful practice management.

Appendixes

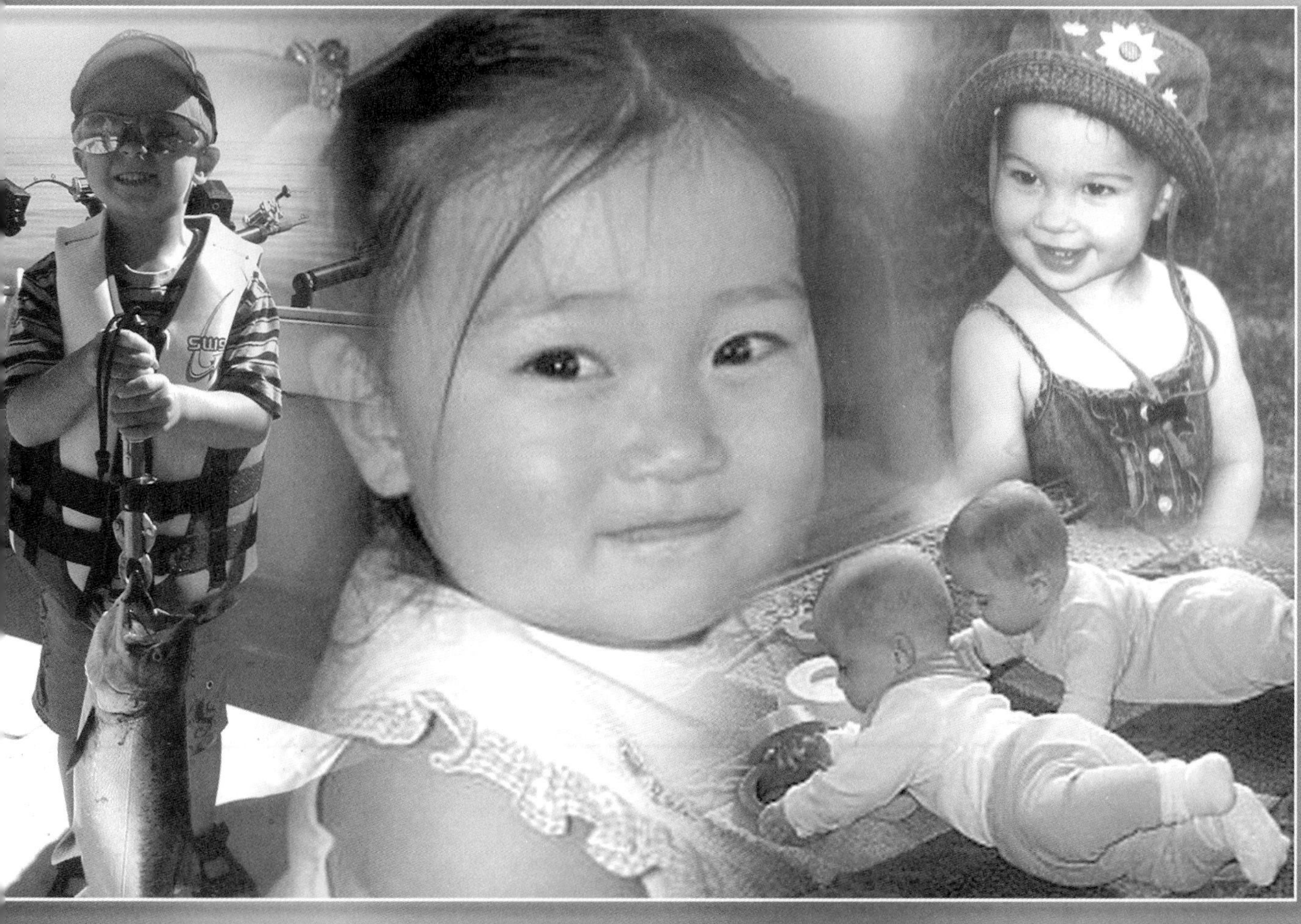

APPENDIX A

Medications

Teri Moser Woo, Catherine G. Blosser

PRESCRIBING MEDICATIONS FOR CHILDREN

Prescribing medications for pediatric patients presents a special challenge. When making treatment decisions, the nurse practitioner (NP) must consider the child's age, the child's developmental level, and any family social and functional issues. Factors that influence compliance such as taste, dosing regimen, and collaborative decision making also need to be considered.

A child's developmental level and age will determine the amount of parental control over the medication administration and assist the NP in determining a successful teaching strategy. For *infants* it is important to take the following into consideration:

- The parent is in total control of administering the medication.
- The parent should be taught how to properly administer medications.
- Determine whether other caregivers will be administering the medication.
- Determine whether a simplified dosing schedule is necessary for a family with children in day care.

Toddlers and *preschoolers* are beginning to exert their independence, and administering medication to this age can be challenging. The key to success with this age is to:

- Discuss medication administration with the parent.
- Choose a medication regimen with the fewest problems with administration.
- Take into account palatability and doses per day to increase compliance.

School-age children developmentally are industrious, and are often the easiest age to which to administer medications. Education should focus on:

- Both the parent *and* the child who will be taking the medication.
- Letting the child choose the formulation, if possible (liquid, chewable, or pills to swallow).
- Avoid dosing during school hours, if possible, to increase compliance.

Adolescent patients often administer their own medication, and compliance rates may vary. The NP needs to more closely collaborate with adolescent patients regarding their medication regimen by:

- Allowing them to have input on dosing schedule and what will work best for them.
- Assisting the family with the transition from parent-controlled to teen-controlled administration.

Medication Administration

Table A-1 lists other measures and strategies that the NP can employ to enhance medication compliance.

Prescribing Drugs "Off-label"

Greater than 80% of drug labeling either has no approval or restricted age approval for pediatric patients (Bell, 2002). Using such drugs "off-label" refers to prescribing the drug outside of the approved indications, dosing recommendations, or age-groups according to the official Food and Drug Administration (FDA)–approved drug's labeling. Using a drug in such a way does not connote unethical use.

Many off-label drugs are used in pediatrics despite lack of pediatric labeling. This has largely resulted from two interrelated factors: (a) pharmaceutical manufacturers did not test the safety and efficacy of drugs in the pediatric age-group, and (b) the preponderance of off-label use in pediatrics has provided little incentive for manufacturers to perform official pediatric clinical trials. Determining the dosage for any pediatric patient using an off-label drug has been a result of proportionately reducing the dose based on weight. However, this does not take into account pediatric metabolism, the drug's pharmacokinetics, adverse

TABLE A-1 ***Factors That Influence Compliance in Prescribing Pediatric Medications***

Factors That Influence Compliance	Interventions That Improve Compliance
Length of treatment. • Poorer compliance for longer length of treatment. • Compliance rates vary with chronic illness.	*Shorten length of treatment if possible.* An example would be to use 5 days of therapy for otitis media rather than 10; this can be accomplished with a number of antibiotics (azithromycin and cefpodoxime at all ages, amoxicillin in children >age 5 yr). *Creative solutions to encourage compliance*: When a child is on medications for a chronic illness, the NP needs to be creative to encourage compliance, because compliance rates vary significantly. Sticker charts or calendars with a small reward for completing a set amount of therapy (e.g., 1 mo) is one strategy (Woo, 2002).
Doses per day: Compliance research in children indicates that the more doses of a medication that need to be administered per day, the poorer the compliance rate. This is particularly significant with working parents and children in school, who often miss midday doses.	*Simplify dosing regimen.* Prescribing medications that require fewer doses per day will increase compliance, with compliance rates of 70%-73% reported in once- or twice-daily dosing regimens, compared with 52% in a three times a day dosing regimen. When the child needs to take the medication at day care or school, dispense two bottles: one for school and one for home. This will ensure fewer missed doses due to forgetting to transport the medication back and forth.
Palatability.	*Choose the best-tasting medication or mask the taste.* If a medication has the same efficacy profile, the best-tasting medication will be easier to administer to young children. There is also the option of using flavoring syrups or crushing tablets such as prednisone and mixing with sweet foods such as chocolate syrup, jam, or pudding (Woo, 2002). Before crushing any tablet or mixing a medication with syrup, the NP should check with a pharmacist to determine if the flavoring is compatible with the medication.
Out-of-pocket costs/family finances.	*Choose the medication that has the lowest out-of-pocket expense for the family.* Asking families about insurance coverage and resources and problem solving with them increases the likelihood that they will fill the prescription.
Family issues: Family issues such as working parents, lack of social support, fatigue, family disruption, and dysfunction all affect the family's ability to comply with the prescribed treatment regimen.	*Assess the family for issues that will affect successful outcome.* If there is poor or less than expected outcome with a treatment regimen, the NP will need to determine if family issues are a factor in compliance and address interventions to assist the family in identifying strategies that will improve success.

effects (e.g., tetracycline and aspirin), and medication delivery form.

The Pediatric Rule of 1994 required that drugs with the potential for use in pediatrics must be evaluated for dosing and efficacy. Further legislation in 1997 (the Modernization Act of 1997) gave 6-month patent extensions to manufacturers that voluntarily conducted clinical trials with pediatric subjects. In 2002 the Pediatric Rule was temporarily suspended, but more recent legislative proposals have called for the reinstatement of the Pediatric Rule, as well as a further proposal to require that pharmaceutical manufacturers test the safety of their drugs in the pediatric population. The new knowledge gained from such clinical trials will provide a higher degree of confidence to providers when prescribing both the older drugs and the almost 200 newer medications presently under study (*Infectious Diseases in Children*, 2002).

MEDICATIONS

Table A-2 is an abbreviated listing of medications used by the NP. It is the responsibility of the reader/prescriber to seek detailed information and thoroughly investigate the drug being prescribed. The textbook's authors take no responsibility for any errors in prescribing. Pharmaceutical references and the FDA often indicate dosages in terms of broad categories of ages, such as "pediatric," "children," and "adult." Wherever possible, specific age or weight-based dosages (or both) are given. The NP will need to use professional judgment when dosing "adolescent" patients; adult dosing is included for that reason.

TABLE A-2 Medications

Generic/Trade Classification	Indications/Dose	Supplied	Remarks
Acetaminophen (Tylenol, Tempra, and others) *Miscellaneous analgesic and antipyretic*	Treatment of mild to moderate pain and fever Children <12 yr: 10-15 mg/kg/dose q 4-6 hr PO (max. 5 doses/day) >12 yr: 325-650 mg q 4-6 hr PO (max. 4 g/day)	80 mg/0.8 ml drops 160 mg/5 ml elixir 80, 160 mg chewable 160, 325, 500 mg tab 80, 120, 325, 650 mg suppository	Drug interactions: barbiturates, carbamazepine, hydantoins, rifampin, sulfinpyrazone. Can cause severe hepatic toxicity with overdose.
Acetaminophen with codeine *Analgesic and antipyretic*	Children: 0.5-1 mg codeine/kg/dose q 4-6 hr PO Adults: 15-60 mg q 4-6 hr PO	Tylenol 120 mg and codeine 12 mg/5 ml elixir #1 tab—Tylenol 300 mg, codeine 7.5 mg #2 tab—Tylenol 300 mg, codeine 15 mg #3 tab—Tylenol 300 mg, codeine 30 mg #4 tab—Tylenol 300 mg, codeine 60 mg	Can cause respiratory depression. Codeine can cause nausea, vomiting, constipation.
Acyclovir (Zovirax) *Antiviral*	*Genital herpes infection*: Adults: 200 mg PO q 4 hr (5 capsules/day) for 10 days; recurrent infection, treat for 5 days; chronic HSV infections: 400 mg PO bid or 200 mg PO 3-5 times a day for 12 mo, then reevaluate; intermittent: 200 mg q 4 hr (5 times a day) for 5 days *Herpes zoster*: Adult dose: 800 mg PO q 4 hr (5 times a day) for 7-10 days *HSV infections in immunocompromised patients, in those with underlying skin disorders, with systemic symptoms, or in severe HSV infections*: Children <12 yr: 10 mg/kg IV over 1 hr q 8 hr for 7 days (5 days for genital herpes) Children >12 yr and adults: 5 mg/kg IV over 1 hr q 8 hr for 7 days (5 days for genital herpes) *Varicella infections*: Children ≥2 yr: 10-20 mg/kg/dose PO qid (max. 800 mg/day) for 5 days Children >40 kg and adults: 800 mg/dose PO qid for 5 days *Mucocutaneous HSV infections*: Children and adolescents: cover all lesions with a thin layer of ointment q 3 hr, 6 times/days for 7 days	200 mg/5 ml suspension 200 mg capsules 400 mg, 800 mg tab 500 mg vial for infection 5% ointment (15, 30 g)	Contraindications: valacyclovir hypersensitivity. Drug interactions: avoid nephrotoxic drugs. Potentiated by probenicid. Therapy should be started at the first sign of infection. Use gloves when applying ointment; apply a thin layer. Adverse effects: renal toxicity (reversible), neurotoxicity, GI disturbances. May have stinging or pain with topical application. Avoid contact with eyes when using ointment.
Adapalene (Differin) *Topical retinoid*	*Treatment of acne vulgaris*: Apply to affected acne areas once daily at bedtime after washing		Adverse effects: erythema, scaling, dryness, pruritis, burning, acne flares. Drug interactions: avoid use until the effects of sulfur or salicylic acid have subsided. Avoid waxed areas.

Continued

TABLE A-2 *Medications—cont'd*

Generic/Trade Classification	Indications/Dose	Supplied	Remarks
			Precautions: avoid use on irritated, eczamatous, or sunburned skin. Avoid contact with eyes, lips, mucous membranes, sun, UV light.
Albuterol sulfate (Proventil, Proventil HFA, Ventolin, Ventolin HFA, Acuneb, Volmax) *Bronchodilator*	*Treatment of bronchospasm*: Children <5 yr: 0.1-0.2 mg/kg/dose PO tid (max. 2 mg tid) Children 6-11 yr: 2 mg PO tid-qid Nebulizer: 0.15 mg/kg/dose q 4 hr prn MDI: children >4yr and adults: 2 inhalations q4-6 hr prn Adults: 2-4 mg PO q4-6 hr or 4-8 mg q12 hr Exercise-induced bronchospasm: >12 yr: 2 inhalations 15 min before exercise	2 mg/5 ml syrup 2, 4 mg tab 4 mg sustained-release tab 5 mg/ml (0.5%) and 0.83% unit-dosed vials (2.5 mg albuterol per vial) inhalation solution 90 μg/metered spray	Common side effects: tachycardia, tremor, palpitations. Do not administer with MAO inhibitors or tricyclic antidepressants. Inhaler use most effective if spacer is used.
Amantadine HCl (Symmetrel) *Antiviral*	Prophylaxis or symptomatic relief of influenza A: Children 1-9 yr: 4.4-8.8 mg/kg/day PO divided bid-tid (max. 150 mg/day) Children 9-12 yr: 100 mg PO bid Children >12 yr and adults <65 yr: 200 mg/d PO; continue 24-48 hr after symptoms disappear	50 mg/5 ml syrup 100 mg capsule	Not recommended for children <age 1 yr. Do not administer with alcohol or stimulants. Reduce dose for renal dysfunction (creatinine clearance <50 ml/min) or hepatic dysfunction. Precautions with seizure disorders, psychiatric disorders, and heart failure.
Ammonium lactate (LAC-Hydrin 12%) *Miscellaneous emollient*	Used in the treatment of moderate to severe xerosis and ichthyosis vulgaris Apply twice daily to affected areas	Lotion (225, 400 g) Cream (280 g, 385 g)	Avoid contact with lips, eyes, mucous membranes. Minimize exposure to sun or UV light. Transient stinging, burning, erythema. Irritation (especially on face), rash, peeling, dryness, hyperpigmentation.
Amoxicillin (Amoxil, Polymax, Trimox, Ultimox) *Penicillin*	Community-acquired pneumonia, sinusitis, skin, otitis, urinary tract, gonorrhea, streptococcal infections Children: <2 yr: high-dose for OM, 80-90 mg/kg/day divided bid or tid ≥2 yr: 40-90 mg/kg/day PO divided bid-tid (do not exceed adult recommended dose) Adults: 250 mg PO bid-tid or 500 mg bid (max. 2-3 g/day) Prophylaxis for otitis media with effusion: 20 mg/kg/day	50 mg/ml drops (15, 30 ml) 125, 200, 250, 400 mg/5 ml suspension 125, 200, 250, 400 mg chewable 250, 500, 875 mg capsule	Can cause a rash if given to a patient with mononucleosis. Usually treat infections for 10 days. Low-risk children >age 5 yr may treat OM for 5-7 days. Drug interactions: cross allergy with cephalosporins or imipenem. Side effects: GI, especially with high-dose (80-90 mg/kg) dosing.
Amoxicillin and clavulanate (Augmentin) *Penicillin, beta-lactamase inhibitor*	Community-acquired pneumonia, otitis media, sinusitis, skin (periorbital cellulitis, human/animal bites) *Dosing based on amoxicillin component*	125, 200, 250, 400 mg/5 ml suspension (75, 150 ml) ES-600: 600 mg/5 ml susp (600 mg amoxicillin and 42.9 mg clavulanic acid)	Drug interactions: cross allergy with cephalosporins or imipenem. Fewer side effects at bid dosing with 45 mg/kg/day. GI side effects—give with food. Peanut butter and cherry yogurt have

TABLE A-2 *Medications—cont'd*

Generic/Trade Classification	Indications/Dose	Supplied	Remarks
	Children ≤40 kg: <12 wk of age 30 mg/kg day divided bid; >12 wk of age 40 mg/kg/day PO tid or 45 mg/kg/day PO bid; ES-600 (≥3 mo) 90 mg/kg/day PO divided bid; do not exceed adult dose Children ≥40 kg and adults: 250-500 mg PO tid (max. 2 g/day) or 875 mg bid	125, 200, 250, 400 mg chewable 250, 500, 875 mg tab (two 250 mg tabs do not equal one 500 mg tab)	been shown to decrease GI side effects. Reduce dose for renal impairment. ES-600 susp NOT interchangable with other strength suspensions. ES-600 susp not recommended for <3 mo of age.
Antipyrine and benzocaine (Auralgan) *Local anesthetic (otic)*	Used for temporary relief of pain associated with otitis media Fill ear canal with drops; may use q 2-4 hr	Otic solution (antipyrine 5.4%, benzocaine 1.4%)	Not for prolonged use. Do not use if TM is perforated.
Atomoxetine HCl (Strattera) *Norephinephrine reuptake inhibitor*	ADHD (nonstimulant) for children, adolescents, adults Children 6-16 yr: Check with current pharmacology reference book	5, 10, 18, 25, 40, 60 mg capsule	Possible drug interactions (use with caution): Paxil, Prozac, quinidine, albuterol. Adverse reactions: abdominal pain, constipation, dyspepsia, nausea/vomiting, decreased weight, anorexia, mood swings, irritability, dry mouth, insomnia. Use with caution in individuals with HTN, tachycardia, cardiovascular disease, asthma.
Azelastine hydrochloride (Astelin) *Antihistamine*	Seasonal allergic rhinitis Children: 5-11 yr: 1 spray each nostril bid; >12 yr: 2 sprays per nostril bid; not recommended <5 yr	Nasal spray (100 sprays/bottle)	Drug interactions: cimetidine, CNS depressants. Caution with other antihistamines. Side effects: bitter taste, fatigue, HA, weight increase, nasal irritation or burning. Children: also conjunctivitis, cough, asthma.
Azithromycin (Zithromax) *Macrolide*	Atypical, community-acquired pneumonia, pharyngitis/tonsillitis (as second-line therapy) Children >6 mo: otitis media 10 mg/kg on day 1, 5 mg/kg on days 2-5; give once daily Children >2 yr: 12 mg/kg/day, days 1-5 Adults: 500 mg on day 1, then 250 mg days 2-5; give once daily Nongonococcal urethritis, cervicitis due to *C. trachomatis*, chanchroid: 1 g as a single dose Pharyngitis, pneumonia, skin and soft tissue disorders, otitis media, sinusitis, pneumonia, streptococcal pharyngitis; nontuberculous mycobacterial infections; nongonococcal urethritis and cervicitis due to *C. trachomatis* (single dose)	250 mg capsules 600 mg tab 100 mg/5 ml, 200 mg/5 ml suspension 1 g single-dose packet	Food decreases bioavailability of capsules. Theophylline effect unknown. Alternative when erythromycin ethylsuccinate not tolerated. Some strains of streptococcus are resistant to azithromycin. Drug interactions: Propulsid, digoxin, theophylline, phenytoin, carbamazepine, triazolam, flucanazole. Side effects: GI upset, abdominal pain. Rare: allergy.

Continued

TABLE A-2 *Medications—cont'd*

Generic/Trade Classification	Indications/Dose	Supplied	Remarks
Bacitracin, neomycin, polymyxin B (Neosporin) *Topical antibiotic*	Used to prevent infection in minor wounds Apply 1-3 times daily	Ointment or cream	High incidence of sensitivity reactions, which can include redness, itching, edema. Do not use in large areas, serious burns, puncture wounds, blisters.
Bacitracin, neomycin, polymyxin B pramoxine (Neosporin Plus) *Topical antibiotic and anesthetic*	Used to prevent infection in minor wounds ≥2 yr: apply 1-3 times daily	Ointment or cream	High incidence of sensitivity reactions, which can include redness, itching, edema. Not recommended for children <2 yr. Do not use in large areas, serious burns, puncture wounds, blisters.
Bacitracin, neomycin, polymyxin B (Neosporin ophthalmic) *Antibiotic (ophthalmic)*	Treatment of external ocular infections Ointment: apply q 3-4 hr for 7-10 days Solution: 3 or 4 times daily	Ophthalmic ointment, solution	Side effects: sensitization, local irritation.
Bacitracin, neomycin, polymyxin B, and hydrocortisone (Cortisporin otic) *Antibiotic, antiinflammatory*	Treatment of topical infections of the external auditory canal Otic suspension: 2-3 drops 3-4 times daily for 7 days	Otic suspension, solution	Otic suspension should be used if tympanic membrane is not intact.
Beclomethasone dipropionate: *Oral inhalation systems* (Beclovent, Vanceril, QVAR) *Glucocorticoid, antiinflammatory*	Maintenance and prophylactic therapy for asthma *NIH asthma guidelines*: Children: Low dose: 84-336 μg/day or 2-8 sprays/day (40-42 μg/spray); 1-4 sprays/day (80-84 μg/spray) Medium dose: 336-672 μg/day or 8-16 sprays/day (40-42 μg/spray); 4-8 sprays/day (80-84 μg/spray) High dose: >672 μg/day or >16 sprays/day (40-42 μg/spray); >8 sprays/day (80-84 μg/spray) Adults: Low dose: 168-504 μg/day or 4-12 sprays/day (40-42 μg/spray); 2-6 sprays/day (80-84 μg/spray) Medium dose: 504-840 μg/day or 12-20 sprays/day (40-42 μg/spray); 6-10 sprays/day (80-84 μg/spray) High dose: >840 μg/day or >20 sprays/day (40-42 μg/spray); >10 sprays/day (80-84 μg/spray)	Beclovent (42 μg/spray); Vanceril (42 μg/spray, 84 μg/spray); QVAR (40 μg/puff, 80 μg/puff MDIs)	Contraindicated in patients with status asthmaticus. Use cautiously in patients with tuberculosis and those on oral steroids. Adverse reactions: hypothalamic-pituitary-adrenal axis suppression during and after the switch from systemic steroids to less systemically available inhaled cortocisteroids, oral candidiasis, headache (oral or nasal delivery systems), nasal irritation (nasal system only). Monitor for linear growth suppression in children if on long-term high-dose therapy. Rinse mouth well following oral inhalation. When changing from oral to inhaled steroids, allow an overlap of at least 2 wk.

TABLE A-2 *Medications—cont'd*

Generic/Trade Classification	Indications/Dose	Supplied	Remarks
Nasal inhalation system (Beconase, Beconase AQ, Vancenase Pocketinhaler, Vancanase AQ) *Glucocorticoid, antiinflammatory*	Used in the treatment of seasonal allergic rhinitis and nasal polyps Nonaqueous sprays: Children 6-12 yr: 1 spray/nostril tid (max. 252 μg/day) Children 12 yr and older: 1 spray/nostril bid-qid (max. 336 μg/day) Aqueous (AQ) sprays: Children 6-12 yr: initially 1 spray/nostril bid increasing to 2 sprays/nostril bid depending on response Children 12 yr and older: 1-2 sprays/nostril bid	Beconase (42 μg/spray), Beconase AQ (0.042%/spray), Vancenase Pocketinhaler (42 μg/spray), Vancenase AQ (84 μg/spray)	
Benzonatate (Tessalon Perles) *Nonnarcotic antitussive*	Used for cough suppression Children >10 yr and older: 100 mg PO tid (max. 6 perles/day)	100 mg perles	Side effects: drowsiness, HA, dizziness, confusion, GI upset, pruritis No respiratory depression. Do not chew perles—can cause oropharyngeal anesthesia.
Benzoyl peroxide (2%, 5%, 10%) (Benzagel, Desquam-E, Desquam-X, Ersa-Gel) *Antibacterial/keratolytic agent*	Used in mild to moderate acne Gel: apply sparingly 1-3 times daily Wash: use on affected area 1-2 times per day; rinse well	2.5%, 5%, 10% gel 5%, 10% wash	Avoid contact with eyes, lips, mucous membranes. Adverse reactions: burning, swelling, peeling, excessive drying. Areas should be cleaned before applying. Can bleach fabrics.
Bethanechol chloride (Duvoid, Urecholine) *Urinary tract and GI tract stimulant*	Used to treat nonobstructive urinary retention, abdominal distention, gastroesophageal reflux Children: 0.6 mg/kg/day PO divided 3 or 4 times daily; for gastroesophageal reflux, 0.1-0.2 mg/kg PO given 30 min-1 hr before meals (max. 4 times daily) Adults: Urecholine 10-50 mg PO bid-qid; 5-10 mg SC q 4 hr for neurogenic bladder; Duvoid 10-15 mg PO bid-qid; 2.5-5 mg SC tid-qid up to 7.5-10 mg q 4 hr for neurogenic bladder	1 mg/ml solution (not available at all pharmacies) 5, 10, 25, 50 mg tab 5 mg/ml injection	Adjunctive therapy for irritable bowel syndrome, colitis, spastic bladder, peptic ulcer disease Contraindicated in patients with hyperthyroidism, hypotension, coronary artery disease, peptic ulcer disease, asthma. Give on empty stomach to prevent nausea and vomiting. Adverse reactions: cramping, nausea, flushing, dizziness, urgency, bronchospasms, fainting. Use in caution in children <8 yr if their urinary retention is due to obstruction.

Continued

TABLE A-2 *Medications—cont'd*

Generic/Trade Classification	Indications/Dose	Supplied	Remarks
Bisacodyl (Dulcolax) *Stimulant laxative*	Used to treat chronic constipation, bowel preparation Children <2 yr: 5 mg rectally Children 3-12 yr: 0.3 mg/kg/day PO or 5-10 mg/day; 5-10 mg rectally Children >12 yr and adults: 10-15 mg PO once daily; 10 mg rectally; up to 30 mg can be used for preparation for bowel procedure	5 mg enteric-coated tab 10 mg rectal suppository	Drug interactions: antacids. Do not crush tablets.
Bitolterol mesylate (Tornalate) *Bronchodilator*	For treatment of acute bronchial asthma, bronchospasms Children >12 yr and adolescents: 2-3 inhalations q 8 hr prn or 1 mg (0.5 ml inhalation solution) via nebulizer q 8 hr (dilute in 2 ml NS); may give nebulizer treatments qid, but no less than 4 hr apart	370 μg/spray MDI 0.2% inhalation solution	Cardiotoxic effects can be increased if used in conjunction with theophylline. Decreases effects of beta-adrenergic blockers (propanolol). Ipratropium may increase duration of bronchodilation. Increased toxicity with MAO inhibitors.
Brompheniramine maleate (Bromphen, Chlorphed, Codimal A, Conjec-B, Cophene-B, Dehist, Dimetone, Nasahist B, Oraminic II, Sinusol-B, Veltane) *Antihistamine*	Children <6 yr: 0.125 mg/kg/dose PO given q 6 hr; max. 6-8 mg/day Children: 6-12 yr, 2-4 mg PO q 6-8 hr; max. 12-16 mg/day Adults: 4-8 mg PO q 4-6 hr, or 8 mg of sustained-release form q 8-12 hr or 12 mg of sustained-release form q 12 hr (max. 24 mg/day) IM/SC/IV: Children <12 yr: 0.5 mg/kg/day divided q 6 hr Children ≥12 yr and adults: 10 mg q 6-12 hr (max. 40 mg/day)	2 mg/5 ml 4 mg tab 8, 12 mg time-released tab 10 mg/ml injection	Adverse effects: drowsiness, sedation, anorexia, dry mouth. Less drowsiness than with other antihistamines. Children <6 yr can experience hyperexcitability. Drug interactions: alcohol and other CNS depressants.
Bropheniramine and pseudoephedrine (Dimetapp Elixir, Dimetapp tablets, Dimetapp Liquigel, Dimetapp Extentabs) *Antihistamine, decongestant*	Children: 6 mo-2 yr: 1/8 to 1/4 tsp q 4 hr (not for use in children under 1 mo of age) 2-6 yr: elixir 2.5 ml (1/2 tsp) q 4 hr 6-12 yr: 1/2 tablet q 4 hr; elixir 5 ml q 4 hr 12 yr and older: 1 liquigel PO q 4 hr; 1 tablet PO q 4 hr; 1 extentab PO q 12 hr; elixir 10 ml q 4 hr	2 mg/12.5 mg (bropheniramе/pseudoephedrine) elixir 4 mg/25 mg tab, liquigel 12 mg/75 mg extentabs	Adverse effects: Drowsiness, excitability; should not be taken by those with HTN, heart disease, diabetes, thyroid disease. Drug interactions: MAO inhibitors, alcohol.
Budesonide (Pulmicort Turbuhaler, Pulmicort Respules) *Corticosteroid*	Maintenance and prophylactic therapy for asthma Turbuhaler: children >6 yr and adults: 1 or 2 inhalations bid	Turbuhaler (200 μg/inhalation) Respules 0.25 mg/2 ml, 0.5 mg/2 ml	Drug interactions: ketoconazole (CYP3A4 inhibitors). Side effects: dry mouth, oral candidiasis, HA, insomnia, GI

TABLE A-2 *Medications—cont'd*

Generic/Trade Classification	Indications/Dose	Supplied	Remarks
	Respules: for use in jet nebulizer; <12 mo not recommended; 12 mo-8 yr previously on bronchodilator alone: 0.5 mg/day once daily or bid; if previously on oral corticosteroids: 1 mg once daily or bid		disturbance. Rinse mouth after use. Rinse face after use if facemask is used with nebulized budesonide.
Budesonide (Rhinocort, Rhinocort Aqua) *Corticosteroid*	Allergic or perennial rhinitis Rhinocort: children ≥6 yr and adults: 2 sprays/nostril bid or 4 sprays/nostril once daily Rhinocort Aqua: not recommended <6 yr; children 6-12 yr: initially 1 spray/nostril once daily, increasing to 2 sprays/nostril once daily (max.); ≥12 yr: 4 sprays/nostril once daily (max.)	32 μg/spray nasal inhaler	Side effects: nasal irritation, epistaxis, pharyngitis, dry mouth. Blow nose before nasal administration.
Calcium (Citracal, Os-Cal, Tums, Caltrate 600, Caltrate Jr, Viactiv, Children's Mylanta) *Antacid, calcium salt*	Adequate intake in terms of elemental calcium (1997 National Academy of Science Recommendations) <6 mo: 210 mg/day PO 6-12 mo: 270 mg/day PO 1-3 yr: 500 mg/day PO 4-8 yr: 800 mg/day PO 9-18 yr: 1300 mg/day PO Antacid use: Children: 2-5 yr, 400 mg up to tid; 6-11 yr, 800 mg up to tid as needed Adults: 1-3 g of elemental calcium chewed every hour, up to 8 g/day	Refer to product listings	Drug interactions: may potentiate digoxin toxicity, may antagonize the effects of calcium channel blockers. Oral calcium administration decreases the absorption of tetracycline, iron, atenolol, quinolone antibiotics, sodium fluoride, and zinc. Adverse reactions: constipation, hypercalcemia.
Carbamazepine (Carbatrol, Epitol, Mazepine, Tegretol) *Miscellaneous anticonvulsant*	Partial, generalized tonic-clonic seizures in children >2 yr <6 yr: initial, 5 mg/kg/day PO: can increase qwk to 10 mg/kg/day divided bid-qid (max. 20 mg/kg/day) 6-12 yr: initially, 100 mg PO bid or 10 mg/kg/day divided bid; can increase by 100 mg/day until therapeutic levels (max. 1000 mg/day) >12 yr: 200 mg PO bid initially; increase by 200 mg/day to therapeutic levels; usual dose: 600-1200 mg/day divided q 6-8 hr Maintenance: 10-20 mg/kg/day PO divided q 6-12 hr	100 mg/5 ml 100 mg chewable 200 mg tab 100, 200, 400 mg XR	Therapeutic range 4-12 μg/ml. Take with food. CBC before therapy (baseline), at 6-12 wk, then annually during long-term therapy. Suspension has to be given 3-4 times daily, tabs 2-4 times daily. XR tabs dosed bid and should not be crushed. Drug interactions: increased plasma levels with CYP3A4 inhibitors (cimetidine, propoxyphene, isoniazid, macrolides, calcium channel blockers, loratadine, fluoxetine, ketoconazole, itraconazole, valproate); decreased plasma levels with CYP3A4 inducers (phenobarbitol, phenytoin, rifampin, theophylline). May increase levels of clomipramine, phenytoin, primidone.

Continued

TABLE A-2 *Medications—cont'd*

Generic/Trade Classification	Indications/Dose	Supplied	Remarks
			May decrease levels of phenytoin, warfarin, doxycycline, theophylline, haloperidol, acetaminophen, alprazolam, clozapine, oral contraceptives, anticonvulsants, and others metabolized by CYP3A4. Cross-sensitivity with tricyclic antidepressants. Adverse reactions: vertigo, diplopia, hyponatremia, drowsiness, hepatotoxicity, aplastic anemia, bone marrow suppression, rash, Stevens-Johnson syndrome, photosensitivity.
Cefadroxil monohydrate (Duricef, Cefadroxil) *First-generation cephalosporin*	Serious skin infections, urinary tract, bone and joint, streptococcal infections Children: <1 yr: 25 mg/kg/day PO bid for 10 days 1-6 yr: 250 mg PO bid for 10 days >6 yr: 500 mg PO bid (up to 2 g/day) >40 kg: 0.5-1 g bid *Skin, soft tissue, UTI*: 1 g daily for 7-10 days	125, 250, 500 mg/5 ml (50, 100 ml) 500 mg capsules 1 g tab	Can dose qd for streptococcal pharyngitis. Use cautiously in patients with serious penicillin hypersensitivity.
Cefdinir (Omnicef) *Cephalosporin antibiotic*	Otitis, sinusitis, pharyngitis, skin infections, community-acquired pneumonia, bronchitis 6 mo-12 yr: 7 mg/kg PO q 12 hr or 14 mg/kg PO qd (max. 600 mg/day) >13 yr: 300 mg PO bid or 600 mg qd Twice-daily dosing for pneumonia and skin infections; once-daily dosing for other infections	300 mg capsules 125 mg/5 ml suspension	Drug interaction: antagonized by magnesium- or aluminum-containing antacids and iron (separate dose by 2 hr). Side effects: GI disturbances, vaginitis.
Cefixime (Suprax) *Third-generation cephalosporin*	Uncomplicated urinary tract infections, bronchitis, pharyngitis, tonsillitis, skin disorders (poor *Staphylococcus aureus* coverage), *Shigella* gastroenteritis, otitis media Children: 8 mg/kg/day PO divided qd-bid (max. dose 400 mg) >50 kg or >12 yr: 200 mg bid or 400 mg qd PO Gonorrhea: 400 mg PO once	100 mg/5 ml (50, 100 ml) 200, 400 mg tab	Can be given as a single dose. Not indicated for infants <6 mo. Treat otitis media with suspension—gives higher therapeutic levels. GI symptoms common, administer with food to decrease GI distress.
Cefotaxime sodium (Claforan) *Third-generation cephalosporin*	Serious infections: skin, septicemia, bone, urinary tract, lower respiratory tract, gynecologic infections, meningitis, and ventriculitis Children 1 mo to 12 yr, <50 kg: 100-150 mg/kg/day divided q 6-8 hr IV/IM	0.5, 1.2 g vial	GI side effects.

TABLE A-2 Medications—cont'd

Generic/Trade Classification	Indications/Dose	Supplied	Remarks
	Children >50 kg or >12 yr with moderate to severe infection: 1-2 g IV/IM q 6-8 hr (max. 12 g/day) Life-threatening infection: 2 g IV q 4 hr (maximum dose 12 g/day)		
Cefpodoxime proxetil (Vantin) *Third-generation cephalosporin*	Children 2 mo-12 yr: *Acute otitis media*: 5 mg/kg PO q 12 hr for 5 days (max. 400 mg/day) *Pharyngitis/tonsillitis and urinary tract infections*: 5 mg/kg PO q 12 hr for 5-10 days (max. 200 mg/day) *Sinusitis*: 5 mg/kg PO q 12 hr for 10 days (max. 400 mg/day) Children ≥13 yr: *Pneumonia*: 200 mg PO q 12 hr for 14 days *Gonorrhea*: 200 mg PO once as a single dose *Skin*: 400 mg PO q 12 hr for 7-14 days *Pharyngitis*: 100 mg PO q 12 hr for 5-10 days *Sinusitis*: 200 mg PO q 12 hr for 10 days *Complicated urinary tract*: 100 mg q 12 hr for 7 days	50, 100 mg/5 ml 100, 200 mg tab	Drug interactions: Antacids, H_2 antagonists, oral anticholinergics may decrease efficacy. Precautions: Penicillin allergy. Impaired renal function. Not indicated for infants <2 mo. Adverse reactions: GI upset
Cefprozil (Cefzil) *Second-generation cephalosporin*	Pharyngitis, skin infections, tonsillitis, acute sinusitis, secondary bacterial infection of acute or chronic bronchitis, urinary tract infection Children 6 mo-12 yr: 15 mg/kg PO q 12 hr for 10 days—otitis media, sinusitis, lower respiratory tract; 7.5 mg/kg PO q 12 hr—pharyngitis, urinary tract; 20 mg/kg PO q 24 hr for 10 days—uncomplicated skin infections ≥13 yr and adults: 500 mg q 24 hr PO—pharyngitis, tonsillitis, acute sinusitis, lower respiratory tract infections, urinary tract; 250 mg q 12 hr (or 500 mg q 24 hr)—uncomplicated skin; 500 mg q 12 hr—skin structure infections	125, 250 mg/5 ml 250, 500 mg tab	Adverse reactions: GI upset, elevated liver enzymes. May be taken without regard to meals. Not indicated for infants <6 mo. Use with caution in penicillin-sensitive patients.
Ceftibuten (Cedax) *Cephalosporin*	Bronchitis, otitis media, pharyngitis, and tonsillitis (limited coverage) Children >6 mo (≤45 kg): 9 mg/kg PO q 24 hr for 10 days (max. 400 mg/day) Children >45 kg or ≥12 yr: 400 mg PO q 24 hr for 10 days	90 mg/5 ml 180 mg/5 ml 400 mg capsule	Reduce dose in patients with renal impairment. Use with caution in patients with penicillin sensitivity. Active against beta-lactamase-producing strains. Give suspension on empty stomach; capsules may be taken with food.
Ceftriaxone (Rocephin) *Third-generation cephalosporin*	Skin, bone and joint, urinary tract, gynecologic, respiratory tract, intraabdominal infections, bacteremia	0.25, 0.5, 1, 5, 10 g vial	Precautions: do not give to hyperbilirubinemic neonates (especially if premature).

Continued

TABLE A-2 *Medications—cont'd*

Generic/Trade Classification	Indications/Dose	Supplied	Remarks
	Children: 50-75 mg/kg/day IV/IM divided 1-2 times daily (max. 2 g/day) Adults: 1-2 g q 12-24 hr IV/IM (max. 4 g/day) *Prophylaxis for high-risk contacts of patients with invasive meningococcal disease*: ≤12 yr: 125 mg IM once; >12 yr: 250 mg IM once *OM*: 50 mg/kg IM once (alternative OM therapy: 50 mg/kg/day for 3 days) max. 1 g/day *Gonorrhea and acute epididymitis*: 250 mg IM once *Meningitis*: 100 mg/kg/day IV/IM (max. 4 g daily)		GI side effects. Mix with lidocaine to prevent pain at IM injection site.
Cefuroxime axetil (Ceftin) *Second-generation cephalosporin*	Pharyngitis, tonsillitis, skin, otitis media, lower respiratory tract, urinary tract, uncomplicated gonorrhea Children: <2 yr: 30 mg/kg/day PO divided bid 2-12 yr: 250 mg PO bid >12 yr and adolescents: 250-500 mg PO bid *Gonorrhea*: 1 g PO as single dose *Lyme disease*: 500 mg PO bid for 20 days	125, 250, 500 mg tab 125 mg/5 ml suspension 250 mg/5 ml suspension	Cefuroxime film-coated tablets and suspension are not bioequivalent and are not to be substituted on a mg/mg basis. Suspension must be administered with food to decrease GI side effects. Tablet may be taken without regard to meals. Swallow tablet whole, do not crush or chew due to bitter taste.
Cephalexin monohydrate (Keflex Pulvules, Cephalexin capsules) *First-generation cephalosporin*	Skin, bone and joint, septicemia, respiratory tract, urinary tract, otitis media, pharyngitis Children: 25-50 mg/kg/day divided tid PO (max. 4 g/day) *OM*: 75-100 mg/kg/day divided tid or qid (max. 4 g/day) for 7-10 days *Pharyngitis, skin and skin structure*: 40 mg/kg/day divided tid or qid for 10 days; may be given bid in those >1 yr *Urinary tract*: 50-100 mg/kg/day divided tid or qid for 7-10 days (max. 4 g/day) Adolescents: 250-500 mg PO tid (max 4 g/day) *Pharyngitis, skin and skin structure infections, uncomplicated cystitis (in those ≥15 yr only)*: 500 mg q 12 hr for 10 days (treat cystitis for 7-14 days)	125, 250 mg/5 ml 250, 500 mg Pulvule capsules	Caution: do not use in patients with immediate-type hypersensitivity to penicillins. Administer on empty stomach. Administer with food if GI upset occurs.
Cetirizine (Zyrtec) *Antihistamine*	Seasonal or perennial rhinitis, chronic idiopathic urticaria Children <2 yr (limited data): 0.25 mg/kg/day PO as a single dose 2-5 yr: 2.5 mg qd to max. of 5 mg PO qd or divided bid	10 mg tab 5 mg/5 ml syrup	Drug interaction: potentiates CNS depression with alcohol or other CNS depressants. Large doses of theophylline may decrease cetirizine clearance with potential increased toxicity.

TABLE A-2 Medications—cont'd

Generic/Trade Classification	Indications/Dose	Supplied	Remarks
	>6 yr, including adolescents: 5-10 mg PO qd as a single dose or divided bid		Contraindications: hydroxyzine sensitivity Warning: doses >10 mg/day may cause significant drowsiness. Side effects: fatigue, dry mouth, somnolence, HA. Children may also have abdominal pain, nausea, vomiting, bronchospasm.
Chloral hydrate (Aquachloral, Chloral Hydrate generic) *Anxiolytic, sedative, hypnotic*	Neonates: 25 mg/kg/dose PO for sedation before procedure Children: sedation, anxiety: 25-50 mg/kg/dose PO q 6-8 hr (max. 500 mg/dose) *Before EEG*: 25-50 mg/kg/dose PO 30-60 min before EEG, may repeat in 30 min to a total maximum of 100 mg/kg or 1 g total for infants and 2 g total for children *Nonpainful procedures requiring sedation*: 50-75 mg/kg PO 30-60 min before procedure; may repeat in 30 min for a total of 120 mg/kg or 1 g total for infants and 2 g total for children Adolescents: 250 mg PO tid for anxiety; 500-1000 mg qhs for insomnia or 30 minutes before procedure for sedation (max. 2 g/day)	500 mg/5 ml 500 mg capsules 324, 500, 648 mg suppositories	Drug interactions: warfarin, furosemide. Prolonged use in newborns can cause hyperbilirubinemia. Administer syrup in one-half glass of water, fruit juice, or ginger ale; may be mixed in infant formula.
Chlorpheniramine maleate (Chlor-Trimeton) *Antihistamine*	Allergic rhinitis, urticaria Children: 2-6 yr: 0.35 mg/kg/day divided q 4-6 hr PO or 1 mg q 4-6 hr, PO (max. 12 mg/day) ≥6-12 yr: 2 mg q 4-6 hr PO ≥12 yr and adolescents: 4 mg q 4-6 hr PO (max. 24 mg/day) or 8-12 mg q 12 hr (time-released)	2 mg/5 ml syrup 2 mg chewable 4, 8, 12 mg tab 8, 12 mg time-released tab, capsule	Adverse effects: CNS sedation, anticholinergic effects.
Ciclopirox olamine (Loprox) *Local antiinfective, antifungal*	Tinea cruris, tinea corporis, tinea pedis, tinea versicolor; also for cutaneous candidiasis Children >10 yr and adolescents: topical—massage into affected area bid for at least 2 wk; treat tinea pedis for 4 wk (safety and efficacy below age 10 not established)	1% cream, lotion, gel	
Cimetidine (Tagamet) *Histamine-receptor antagonist*	Duodenal ulcers, hypersecretory conditions, gastroesophageal reflux Infants: 10-20 mg/kg/day PO divided q 6-12 hr Children: 20-40 mg/kg/day PO divided qid Adults: 300 mg PO qid before meals and qhs	300 mg/5 ml liquid 200, 300, 400, 800 mg tab	Used cautiously in patients with impaired renal or hepatic function. Adverse reactions: dizziness, confusion, headache. Drug interactions: diazepam, theophylline, propranolol, antacids, phenytoin, tricyclic antidepressants, oral contraceptives, warfarin.

Continued

TABLE A-2 *Medications—cont'd*

Generic/Trade Classification	Indications/Dose	Supplied	Remarks
Ciprofloxacin (Cipro, Cipro-IV, Ciloxan Ophthalmic) *Fluoroquinolone*	Lower respiratory tract, sinus, prostate, stomach, skin, bone and joint, urinary tract, infectious diarrhea, gonorrhea, anthrax, tularemia, bacterial conjunctivitis, corneal ulcers Children (oral preparations usually not recommended for children <18 yr): 20-30 mg/kg/day PO divided bid (max. 1.5 g/day) >18 yr: 250-750 mg PO q 12 hr *Gonorrhea*: 250 mg PO once *Postexposure prophylaxis of inhalational anthrax or treatment of cutaneous anthrax*: Children: 15 mg/kg PO q 12 hr for 60 days (max. 1 g/day) Adults: 500 mg PO bid for 60 days *Tularemia*: Children: max. dose 1 g/day PO for 14 days *Conjunctivitis*: Ophthalmic solution: ≥1 yr 1-2 drops each eye q 2 hr while awake for 2 days, then q 4 hr while awake for 5 more days Ophthalmic ointment: ≥2 yr 0.5 inch ribbon in conjunctival sac tid for 2 days then bid for 5 days	250, 500 mg/5 ml suspensions 100, 250, 500, 750 mg tab 0.3% ophthalmic solution and ointment 100 mg/10 ml, 200 mg/20 ml vials for IV use	Oral medication not indicated for children <18 yr. Increases serum theophylline. Antacids decrease absorption. Causes photosensitivity.
Ciprofloxacin hydrochloride and hydrocortisone (Cipro HC Otic) *Antibiotic and steroid*	*Otitis externa*: Children ≥1 yr and adolescents: 3 drops to affected ear bid for 7 days	10 ml bottle	Do not use if TM is perforated. Side effects: HA, pruritus, rash.
Citalopram hydrobromide (Celexa) *Antidepressant*	Treatment of depression: Adults: 20 mg/day PO QAM or qhs; titrated by 20 mg/day in a weekly interval to 40 mg/day	10 mg/5 ml solution 10, 20, 40 mg tab	Do not give if patient is on MAO inhibitors. Drug interactions: MAO inhibitors, tricyclic antidepressants, alcohol, cimetidine, lithium, sumatriptan, metoprolol. Adverse reactions: nausea, dry mouth, insomnia, sweating, sexual dysfunction, tremor, diarrhea, fatigue. Do not abruptly stop drug. Safety and efficacy not established in pediatric patients.
Clarithromycin (Biaxin, Biaxin XL) *Macrolide antibiotic*	Pharyngitis, tonsillitis, sinusitis, lower respiratory tract, upper respiratory tract, skin Children (≥6 mo and to 35 kg): 15 mg/kg/day PO divided q 12 hr for 10 days (max. 500 mg bid) Children >35 kg and adolescents: 250-500 mg PO q 12 hr for 7-14 days Adults: extended-release tabs 1 g qd (sinusitis 14 days; pneumonia and bronchitis 7 days)	250, 500 mg tab 500 mg extended-release tab 125, 250 mg/5 ml granules for suspension	Decrease dose in renal impairment. Drug interactions: theophylline (increased serum levels by 20%), carbamazepine (increased serum levels after only one dose of clarithromycin), terfenadine, digoxin, astemizole, propulsid, and other drugs metabolized by CYP450 isoenzyme CYP3A3/4.

TABLE A-2 *Medications—cont'd*

Generic/Trade Classification	Indications/Dose	Supplied	Remarks
			Rinse mouth following suspension. Do NOT refrigerate suspension because it might gel.
Clemastine fumarate (OTC) (Tavist) *Antihistamine*	Allergic rhinitis, urticaria, allergies Children <6 yr: 0.05 mg/kg/day of clemastine base, 0.335-0.67 mg/day of clemastine fumarate divided bid (max. 1.34 mg daily, 1 mg base) Children 6-12 yr: 0.67-1.34 mg PO bid (max. 4.02 mg/day, 3 mg base) Adults: 1.34-2.68 mg PO bid (max. 8.04 mg/day, 6 mg base)	0.67 mg/5 ml (0.5 mg/5 ml base) syrup 1.34 (1 mg base), 2.68 mg (2 mg base) tab	Treat urticaria at adult doses of 2.68 mg. Administer with food. May cause drowsiness.
Clindamycin (Cleocin T, Clindagel, Cleocin vaginal cream or ovules, Clindets Pledgets) *Topical antibiotic*	Mild to moderate acne, candidiasis vaginitis, vaginal pruritis *Acne*: Children >12 yr: apply thin film to all acne-affected areas twice daily *Bacterial vaginosis*: Nonpregnant: insert 1 full applicator (100 mg cream) intravaginally once daily before bedtime for 3 or 7 days, OR 1 suppository intravaginally at bedtime for 3 days Pregnant (second or third trimester): use cream intravaginally qhs for 7 days	1% topical lotion, gel, solution 2% vaginal cream, 100 mg vaginal suppository	Use if comedones become inflamed; may use alone or with benzoyl peroxide (see below). Solution is flammable—no smoking following application. Discontinue if significant diarrhea occurs. Adverse reactions: dryness, oily skin, irritation; rare: diarrhea, colitis. Avoid eyes and mucous membranes. Discontinue if significant diarrhea occurs. Vaginal cream may weaken latex in condoms for 72 hr after completion of therapy. Wait 30 min after washing face before applying. Can take 6-8 wk to see improvement in acne.
Clindamycin and benzoyl peroxide (Benzaclin) *Topical antibiotic*	Used in mild to moderate acne; use if comedones become inflamed Apply thin film to all acne-affected areas twice daily	1% topical solution	Drug interactions: additive irritation with other topical agents. Avoid erythromycin. Avoid eyes and mucous membranes. Discontinue if significant diarrhea occurs. Wait 30 min after washing before applying. Can take 6-8 wk to see improvement.
Clindamycin hydrochoride (Cleocin HCl) *Miscellaneous antibiotic*	Serious infections involving skin, respiratory tract, sepsis, pelvic and genital tract, intraabdominal areas, bone (staphylococcal and streptococcal organisms) Children: serious infections, 8-16 mg/kg/day divided tid or qid; more serious, 16-20 mg/kg/day PO divided q 6-8 hr for 10 days	75 mg/5 ml 75, 150, 300 mg capsule	Can cause severe colitis. Do not refrigerate suspension; take with a full glass of water.

Continued

TABLE A-2 Medications—cont'd

Generic/Trade Classification	Indications/Dose	Supplied	Remarks
	Adolescents: serious infections, 150-300 mg PO q 6-8 hr (max. 1.8 g/day); more serious, 300-450 mg q 6 hr for 10 days		
Clonidine (Catapress) *Antihypertensive, ADHD treatment*	Hypertension, improves attention in ADHD, tic disorder (including Tourette syndrome) *Hypertension*: Oral: initially 0.005-0.010 mg/kg/day in divided doses q 6-12 hr, increase gradually to achieve desired control (maximum 0.9 mg/day [oral]) *ADHD*: Oral: 0.05 qhs, gradually increasing number of daily doses by 0.05 mg/day q 3-7 days given in 3-4 divided doses (max. 0.3-0.4 mg/day)	0.1, 0.2, 0.3 mg tab 0.1, 0.2, 0.3 mg patch (lasts up to 7 days)	Drug interactions: methlyphenidate may potentially increase ECG effects (ECG abnormalities and 4 cases of sudden death reported); tricyclic antidepressants, beta-blockers, CNS depressants, and alcohol. Do not abruptly discontinue because rapid increase in blood pressure and sympathetic overactivity may occur (increased heart rate, tremors, agitation, anxiety, insomnia, palpitations, sweating). Taper over at least 1 wk. Decrease methlyphenidate dose by 40% if using concurrently with clonidine, consider ECG monitoring.
Clotrimazole (OTC) (Mycelex troches, Lotrimin, Gyne-Lotrimin) *Local antiinfective, antifungal*	*Oral candidiasis*: Children >3 yr and adults: 10 mg troche PO—dissolve slowly, 5 times daily for 2 wk *Vaginal candidiasis*: 1 applicator or 1 vaginal tab qhs for 1-2 wk *Tinea pedis, tinea cruris, tinea corporis, or tinea versicolor*: Topical application of cream bid for 1-8 wk (use for 7 days after rash clears)	10 mg troche 1% cream, solution, lotion 100, 500 mg vaginal tab	Adverse reactions: nausea, vomiting, abnormal liver function tests.
Cloxacillin sodium (Cloxacillin Sodium generic) *Penicillinase-resistant penicillin (antistaphlycoccal)*	Respiratory tract, sinusitis, skin (streptococcal and staphylococcal) Children >1 mo but <20 kg: 50 mg/kg/day PO divided qid (100 mg/day divided qid for very severe infections; max. 4 g/day) Children >1 mo and >20 mg and adolescents: 250 mg PO qid (500 mg qid for very severe infections)	125 mg/5 ml (100, 200 ml bottles) 250, 500 mg capsule	Administer on empty stomach. Not in stock in many pharmacies.
Codeine *Opiate agonist, antitussive, analgesic*	Children: Analgesic: 0.5-1 mg/kg q 4-6 hr PO, IM, SC (max. 60 mg/dose) Antitussive: 2-6 yr: 2.5-5 mg q 4-6 hr PO (max. 30 mg/day); 7-12 yr: 5-10 mg q 4-6 hr PO (max. 60 mg/day) >12 yr and adolescents: Analgesic: 30 mg/dose q 4-6 hr (max. 120 mg/day) Antitussive: 10-20 mg/dose q 4-6 hr (max. 120 mg/day)	15 mg/5 ml solution 15, 30, 60 mg tab 30, 60 mg/ml injection	Respiratory depression, nausea, vomiting, constipation
Cromolyn sodium (Intal, Nasalcrom)	*Prophylaxis in treatment of allergic disorders and asthma*:	Aerosol: 800 μg/metered spray	Not to be used to treat acute asthmatic attacks; may

TABLE A-2 *Medications—cont'd*

Generic/Trade Classification	Indications/Dose	Supplied	Remarks
Mast cell stabilizer	Children >2 yr (oral inhalation): 20 mg via nebulizer qid Children >5 yr and adolescents (oral inhalation): 2 inhalations qid by metered-dose inhaler or 20 mg, oral or nebulizer qid; 1 spray, intranasally, 3 or 4 times daily *Prevention of exercise-induced bronchospasm*: 2 inhalations 10-60 min before exercise	Solution: 10 mg/ml (20 mg) for nebulization Solution, nasal: 5.2 mg/spray	take 3-4 wk for maximum effectiveness in asthma treatment. Adverse reactions: headache, bronchospasm, urticaria, cough, throat irritation. Do not withdraw drug abruptly.
Cromolyn sodium (Opticrom, Crolom, cromolyn sodium generic) *Mast cell stabilizer*	Used for allergic conjunctivitis >4 yr: 1-2 drops q 4-6 hr	4% ophthalmic solution	Side effect: transient ocular burning/stinging
Cyclobenzaprine (Flexeril) *Skeletal muscle relaxant*	Treatment of muscle spasms associated with acute painful musculoskeletal conditions >12 yr: 10 mg 3 times/day (range 20-40 mg/day in 2-4 divided doses, max. 60 mg/day)	10 mg tab	Drug interactions: MAO inhibitors.
Cyproheptadine HCl (Periactin) *Antihistamine*	*Allergic rhinitis, urticaria, allergic conjunctivitis*: Children: 0.25 mg/kg/day PO divided bid-tid or age 2-6 yr: 2 mg PO bid-tid (max. 12 mg/day) 7-14 yr: 4 mg PO bid-tid (max. 16 mg/day) >14 yr: 12-16 mg/day divided tid (max. 0.5 mg/kg/day) *Migraine headaches*: Children: 4 mg bid-tid; adolescents: 4-8 mg 3 times a day	2 mg/ 5 ml syrup 4 mg tab	Experimentally used to stimulate appetite and increase weight gain in children Side effect: weight gain; in some patients, sedative effect disappears within 3-4 days.
Desloratadine (Clarinex) *Antihistamine*	Allergic rhinitis (seasonal or perennial); chronic idiopathic urticaria Children ≥12 yr and adolescents: 5 mg PO once daily; renal or hepatic impairment: 5 mg every other day	5 mg tab	Adverse effects: dry mouth or throat, somnolence, myalgia, dizziness. Safety not established in children <12 yr.
Desmopressin acetate (DDAVP, Stimate) *Posterior pituitary hormone; antidiuretic*	Used in the treatment of diabetes insipidus, temporary polyuria, and some forms of hemophilia *Diabetes insipidus*: Children 3 mo-12 yr: 0.05-0.3 ml/day intranasally divided qd or bid >4 yr: 0.05 mg tab qd, titrate to desired response (0.1-0.8 mg/day) ≥12 yr: 0.05-0.4 ml intranasally daily in 1-3 divided doses; 2-4 μg/day SC or IV divided bid *Nocturnal enuresis*: Children >6 yr: 0.05-0.2 ml intranasally qhs; give 1/2 dose in each nostril; 0.2 mg tab qhs to max. 0.6 mg *Hemophilia A and type I von Willebrand disease*: Children >3 mo and adolescents: 0.3 μg/kg slow IV preoperative	Injection: 4 μg/ml Nasal solution: 0.1 mg/ml 0.1, 0.2 mg tabs, scored	Upper respiratory infections can decrease the absorption of the drug. High incidence of relapse in the treatment of nocturnal enuresis when drug is stopped. Nasal spray may be used intermittently for short periods of time for temporary control of nocturnal enureses. Drug interactions: chlorpropamide, lithium, carbamazepine, epinephrine, fludrocortisone. Observe for signs of water intoxication: headache, drowsiness, listlessness, shortness of breath. Adverse reactions: headache, nausea, nasal congestion, abdominal cramps. When switching to tabs, give first dose 24 hr after last nasal dose.

Continued

TABLE A-2 *Medications—cont'd*

Generic/Trade Classification	Indications/Dose	Supplied	Remarks
Dexamethasone (Decadron) *Glucocorticoid, antiinflammatory*	Used in the treatment of chronic inflammatory disorders, cerebral edema, shock, allergies, croup, hematologic disorders Children (antiinflammatory): 0.03-0.15 mg/kg/day PO, IV, or IM divided bid to qid Adults (antiinflammatory, other uses): 0.5-9 mg/day PO, IV, or IM divided bid-tid *Croup*: 0.6 mg/kg once. Use Decadron IV solution and give PO, mixed in acetaminophen elixir per age to improve compliance over the bitter-tasting suspension.	0.5 mg/5 ml elixir 0.5, 0.75, 4 mg tab 4 mg/ml vial IM injection (5, 25 ml vials) 24 mg/ml vial intravenous (5 ml vial)	Contraindicated in patients with systemic fungal infections. Use cautiously in patients with untreated viral or bacterial infections, renal disease, heart disease, tuberculosis, ulcerative colitis, hypothyroidism, diabetes. Do not give live vaccines to patients on dexamethasone. Can mask signs and symptoms of infection. Drug interactions: oral anticoagulants, oral contraceptives, rifampin, phenytoin, barbiturates, hypoglycemics. Suspension tastes bitter.
Dextroamphetamine saccharate; dextroamphetamine sulfate; amphetamine aspartate; amphetamine sulfate (Adderall, Adderall XR) *Amphetamine, CNS stimulant*	Used in the treatment of ADHD/ADD *Tablets*: 3-5 yr: 2.5 mg qd; increase 2.5 mg/day weekly increments until desired response attained 6 yr and older: 5 mg qd or bid; increase by 5 mg/day weekly increments until desired response attained Give first dose on awakening; additional doses (1 or 2) in 4-6 hr intervals (max. 40 mg/day) *XR capsules*: 6 yr and older: 5-10 mg qd on AM awakening; increase by 5-10 mg/day at weekly intervals (max. 30 mg/day)	5, 7.5, 10, 12.5, 15, 20, 30 mg tab; all tablets are double scored 5, 10, 15, 20, 25, 30 XR capsules	Drug interactions: MAO inhibitors, tricyclic antidepressants, antihypertensives, phenobarbital, meperidine, phenytoin. Abuse potential. Side effects: HTN, insomnia, anorexia, dry mouth, GI disturbance. Can exacerbate tics and Tourette syndrome. Monitor growth in children. XR capsules may be opened and sprinkled on a small amount of applesauce (do not chew).
Dextroamphetamine sulfate (Dexedrine) *Amphetamine, CNS stimulant*	Used in the treatment of ADHD and narcolepsy *Narcolepsy*: Children 6-12 yr: 5 mg PO initially; increase by 5 mg at weekly intervals (max. 60 mg/day) until desired response attained ≥12 yr: 10 mg PO initially; increase by 10 mg at weekly intervals (max. 60 mg/day); give in divided doses or use long-acting forms Spansules: give once daily; if using tablets, give first dose on awakening; additional doses (1-2) at 4-6 hr intervals *ADHD*: Children 3-5 yr: 2.5 mg/day PO initially; increase by 2.5 mg/day in weekly intervals; usual dose 0.1-0.5 mg/kg/day, given in the AM (max. 40 mg/day) Children >6 yr: 5 mg/day PO initially given qd or bid; increase by 5 mg/day in weekly intervals; usual dose 0.1-0.5 mg/kg/day, given in the AM (max. 40 mg/day); additional doses (1-2) at intervals of 4-6 hr	5, 10, 15 mg capsule (spansule), sustained release 5, 10 mg tab 5 mg/5 ml elixir	Contraindicated in patients with hypertension, hyperthyroidism, glaucoma, or cardiovascular disease. Drug interactions: MAO inhibitors, tricyclic antidepressants, phenobarbital, phenytoin; insulin requirements may be altered. Do not give within 6 hr of bedtime. Adverse reactions: GI disturbances, insomnia, dry mouth, anorexia, hypertension, tremor, tachycardia. Avoid caffeine.

TABLE A-2 *Medications—cont'd*

Generic/Trade Classification	Indications/Dose	Supplied	Remarks
Dextromethorphan hydrobromide (Benylin DM, Delsym, Hold, Robitussin DM, Sucrets Cough) *Nonnarcotic antitussive*	Cough suppression Children: 1-3 mo: 0.5-1 mg q 6-8 hr 3-6 mo: 1-2 mg q 6-8 hr 7 mo-1 yr: 2-4 mg q 6-8 hr 2-5 yr: 2.5-5 mg q 4 hr PO (max. 30 mg/day) >6 yr: 5-10 mg q 4 hr PO (max. 60 mg/day) Adolescents: 10-20 mg q 4 hr PO (max. 120 mg/day)	5, 7.5, 10, 15 mg/5 ml syrup 5 mg lozenge 15 mg chewable 30 mg/5 ml extended-release syrup	Anecdotal reports of teenagers abusing dextromethorphan-containing cough medications have increased.
Diazepam (Valium) *Anxiolytic, benzodiazepine, status epilepticus*	*Status epilepticus* (intravenous push): Neonate: 0.25 mg/kg/dose q 15-30 min for 2 or 3 doses (not first-line drug in neonates) Children: >30 days and <5 yr: 0.2-0.5 mg/dose q 2-5 min to a maximum total dose of 5 mg >5 yr: 1 mg/dose q 2-5 min up to a maximum of 10 mg Adults: 5-10 mg; may repeat in 10-15 min intervals to a maximum of 30 mg *Sedation/relaxation*: Children: 0.12-0.8 mg/kg/day PO divided tid-qid >12 yr: 2-10 mg PO bid-qid	5 mg/ml injection 5 mg/ml, 5 mg/5 ml solution 2, 5, 10 mg tab 2.5, 5, 10, 15, 20 mg rectal gel system (pediatric and adult applicator tips)	Controlled substance, schedule IV. Do not use in patients with narrow-angle glaucoma, severe pain. Causes CNS depression. Tablets can be crushed. Complete blood count, liver and kidney function tests should be performed regularly with long-term use.
Dicloxacillin monohydrate (Dynapen) *Penicillinase-resistant penicillin*	Sinusitis, skin, bone and joint, respiratory tract (infections caused by penicillinase-producing staphylococcus) Children <40 kg: 25-50 mg/kg/day PO divided q 6 hr (max. 2 g/day) Children >40 kg and adults: 125-500 mg PO q 6 hr (max. 2 g/day)	62.5 mg/5 ml suspension 250, 500 mg capsule	Drug interactions: warfarin, rifampin, aminoglycosides. Decreases effectiveness of oral contraceptives. Food decreases absorption.
Dicyclomine HCl (Bentyl) *Antimuscarinic, antispasmodic*	Used as adjunctive therapy to treat peptic ulcer disease, functional GI disturbances (acute enterocolitis) Infants >6 mo: 5 mg PO tid-qid Children: 10 mg/dose PO 3-4 times a day Adults: 20 mg PO qid; may increase to 40 mg qid if tolerated and adequate response not obtained at lower dose	10 mg/5 ml syrup 20 mg tab 10 mg capsule	Contraindicated in patients with glaucoma, obstructive GI or GU conditions, myasthenia gravis. Use cautiously in patients with hyperthyroidism, cardiac disease, hypertension. Adverse reactions: hypotonia, dry mouth, blurred vision, palpitations.
Dimenhydrinate (Dramamine) *Antiemetic*	Treat and prevent nausea, vertigo, and vomiting associated with motion sickness Children 2-5 yr: 12.5-25 mg PO q 6-8 hr (max. 75 mg/day) Children 6-12 yr: 25-50 mg PO q 6-8 hr (max. 150 mg/day) Children ≥12 yr and adults: 50-100 mg PO q 4-6 hr (max. 400 mg/day)	12.5 mg/5 ml liquid 50 mg scored tab, chewable tabs	Contraindicated in patients with glaucoma, asthma, seizures. Adverse reactions: drowsiness, dizziness, hypotension, dry mouth, blurred vision.
Diphenhydramine hydrochloride (OTC) (Benadryl) *Antihistamine*	Allergic rhinitis, urticaria, allergic reaction to blood or plasma, motion sickness, vertigo, cough, insomnia, control of dyskinetic movement Children: 5 mg/kg/day divided q 6-8 hr PO/IM/IV (max. 300 mg/day) Adults: 25-50 mg/dose q 4-6 hr PO/IM/IV	12.5 mg/5 ml syrup, elixir 12.5 mg chewable 25, 50 mg tab, capsule 10, 50 mg/ml injection 1%, 2% cream, lotion	Can cause respiratory suppression. Topical diphenhydramine should not be used to treat chicken pox, poison oak, or sunburn or over large areas of the body or on blistered or oozing skin. May cause paradoxic excitation in children.

Continued

TABLE A-2 *Medications—cont'd*

Generic/Trade Classification	Indications/Dose	Supplied	Remarks
Diphenoxylate HCl and atropine sulfate (Lomotil, Lonox) *Antidiarrheal*	Used to treat nonspecific diarrhea Children: <2 yr: not recommended 2-12 yr: 0.3-0.4 mg/kg/day PO divided qid; dose calculated as the diphenoxylate component >12 yr and adolescents: 5 mg PO qid (diphenoxylate)	Solution: diphenoxylate 2.5 mg and atropine 0.025 mg/5 ml Tab: diphenoxylate 2.5 mg and atropine 0.025 mg	Use cautiously in pediatric patients and those with liver disease or ulcerative colitis. Use solution in children ≤12 yr. Drug interactions: MAO inhibitors. Adverse reactions: dizziness, headache, dry mouth, tachycardia, drowsiness. If no response in 48 hr, drug is not likely to be effective.
Docusate sodium (Colace, Correctol, Ducusoft S, DOK, DOS, Liqui-gels, Diocto, Ex-Lax) *Laxative*	Stool softener oral: 5 mg/kg/day in 1-4 divided doses or dose by age <3 yr: 10-40 mg/day divided in 1-4 doses Children 3-6 yr: 20-60 mg/day PO Children 6-12 yr: 40-120 mg/day PO Children >12 yr: 50-360 mg/day PO divided 1-4 times daily	10 mg/ml solution; 16.7 mg/5 ml syrup; 20 mg/5 ml solution 50, 100, 250 mg capsule 100 mg tablet	Drug interactions: mineral oil. Mix liquid with fruit juice or milk to mask taste. Docusate sodium liquid (5-10 ml) instilled into the ear as a ceruminolytic produces ear wax softening within 15 min.
Doxycycline calcium (Doryx, Vibramycin, Vibra-Tabs, Periostat) *Tetracycline*	Used in treatment of infections caused by *Rickettsia, Chlamydia, Mycoplasma*; syphilis, gonorrhea, traveler's diarrhea, postexposure of inhaled or cutaneous anthrax: >8 yr and <45 kg: 4.4 mg/kg/day PO divided bid (max. 200 mg/day) >8 yr and >45 kg: 100 mg/day PO divided bid; 100 mg q 12 hr for severe infections *For postexposure prophylaxis of inhalational anthrax or treatment of cutaneous anthrax*: ≤8 yr: 2.2 mg/kg q 12 hr for 60 days >8 yr (>45 kg) and adolescents: 100 mg q 12 hr for 60 days	50 mg/5 ml suspension 20, 100 mg tab 50, 100 mg capsule	Syrup not available at many pharmacies. Use of outdated product can cause Fanconi-like syndrome. Can cause photosensitivity. Drug interactions: antacids, iron products, zinc, calcium, magnesium reduce absorption. Note: see *MMWR* vol. 50, no. 42 (Oct. 26, 2001) for more information on anthrax dosing.
Econazole nitrate (Spectazole) *Local antiinfective, antifungal*	*For treatment of tinea pedis, tinea cruris, tinea corporis, tinea versicolor*: Children >3 yr and adolescents: apply topically once daily Treat tinea pedis for 4 wk, all others for 2 wk *Cutaneous candidiasis*: Apply topically twice daily for 2 wk (morning and evening)	1% cream	Adverse effects: transient burning/stinging, pruritis, erythema. Instruct patients to use for full length of treatment; do not use around eyes or vaginally
EMLA cream (lidocaine 2.5% and prilocaine 2.5%) *Topical anesthetic*	Used for topical anesthesia before painful procedures 1-3 mo: 1 g with maximum application area of 10 cm^2 4-12 mo: 2 g with maximum application area of 20 cm^2 1-6 yr: 10 g with maximum application area of 100 cm^2 7-12 yr: 20 g with maximum application area of 200 cm^2 These are maximum doses	5, 30 g tubes 1 g disk	Do not use on open wounds. Do not use near eyes. Clean and disinfect area before applying. Apply at least 1 hr before procedure.
Epinephrine HCl (Epinephrine Mist, Primatene Mist, AsthmaHaler,	Bronchodilation; anaphylactic reactions Children: *anaphylaxis or asthma*: 0.01 mg/kg (1:1000) SC repeat q 15 min for 2 doses, then q 4 hr prn (max. 0.5 mg/dose)	1:1000 (1 mg/ml), 1:2000 (0.5 mg/ml), 1:10,000 (0.1 mg/ml) injection	Inhaled $beta_2$-agonist preferred. Rotate injection sites. Adverse effects: ECG changes, restlessness, tremor, nausea, vomiting.

TABLE A-2 *Medications—cont'd*

Generic/Trade Classification	Indications/Dose	Supplied	Remarks
Adrenalin, Ana-Guard, EpiPen, EpiPen Jr; racepinephrine preparations: Breatheasy Inhalant, S-2 Inhalant) *Bronchodilator, vasopressor, cardiac stimulant*	Adults: *anaphylaxis*: 0.1-0.5 mg (1:1000) SC q 5-15 min; *asthma*: 0.3 mg SC q 20 min up to 3 times (max. 1 mg/dose) Inhaler: *Asthma*: children 4 yr and older: 160-250 μg/spray; repeat once if necessary after 1 min, then no sooner than q 3 hr Nebulizer: *Asthma*: children 4 yr and older: 1-3 deep inhalations (depending on response; do not repeat more often than q 3 hr) of racepinephrine or epinephrine solutions	160, 220 μg/metered spray, powder 1% solution (1:100 epinephrine) or 2.25% racepinephrine	
Erythromycin topical (Emgel, Erygel, Akne-Mycin) *Topical antibiotic*	Apply bid to acne-prone areas	2% solution, gel	Cleanse area first, wait 30 min before applying. Wash hands after applying. Additive irritant effects when used with other topical acne products. Contraindicated in patients with known sensitivity to erythromycin.
Erythromycin and benzoyl peroxide topical (Benzamycin Pak) *Topical antibiotic, keratolytic agent*	Used in mild to moderate acne Apply twice daily	3% gel pak (60 per carton) or gel	Should be refrigerated. Expires every 3 mo. Contraindicated in patients with known sensitivity to erythromycin. Should be applied following cleansing. Wash hands after applying.
Erythromycin base, estolate, stearate, ethylsuccinate *Antibiotic*	Upper and lower respiratory tract, otitis media, pharyngitis, syphilis, gonorrhea, skin, gynecologic disorders, and Legionnaires' disease *Erythromycin base* (E-Mycin, ERYC, Ery-Tab, PCE Dispertab, Erythromycin base filmtab) *Erythromycin estolate* (Erythromycin Estolate generic) *Erythromycin stearate* (Erythrocin) *Erythromycin ethylsuccinate* (EES) (E.E.S., EryPed, E.E.E. filmtabs) All four preparations dosed as follows: *Children*: 30-50 mg/kg/day PO divided q 6 hr (do not exceed 2 g/day of base) *Adults*: base: 250-500 mg PO q 6-12 hr; ethylsuccinate: 400-800 mg PO q 6-12 hr; ethylsuccinate delayed release: 333 mg PO q 8 hr *Chlamydia*: base: 500 mg PO qid for 7 days; ethylsuccinate: 800 mg PO qid for 7 days	*Erythromycin base*: 250, 500 mg tablets 250, 333, 500 mg delayed-release tablets or capsules *Erythromycin estolate*: 250 mg capsules 125, 250 mg/5 ml suspension *Erythromycin stearate*: 250, 500 mg tab *Erythromycin ethylsuccinate*: 125 mg pellets in capsule 250 tab, 333 mg delayed-release tab; 250 mg capsule 100 mg/2.5 ml drops 200, 400 mg/5 ml 200 mg chewable tablet; 400 mg tab	Most prescribe tid. GI upset common. Give with food to decrease side effects. Drug interactions: theophylline, carbamazepine, cyclosporine, digoxin, terfenadine, warfarin. Useful in patients allergic to penicillin.
EES and sulfisoxazole combination (Pediazole, Eryzole) *Erythromycin and sulfonamide*	Upper and lower respiratory tract disorders, otitis media Children >2 mo: 40-50 mg/kg/day PO (of EES) divided q 6 hr (max. 2 g erythromycin, 6 g sulfisoxazole/day)	EES 200 mg and sulfisoxazole 600 mg/5 ml	Can be prescribed bid-qid. Drug interactions as with erythromycin.

Continued

TABLE A-2 *Medications—cont'd*

Generic/Trade Classification	Indications/Dose	Supplied	Remarks
Erythromycin ethylsuccinate ophthalmic (Ilotycin, Romycin) *Ocular antibiotic*	Treatment of ocular infections; prophylaxis of ophthalmia neonatorum *Prophylaxis of ophthalmia neonatorum*: instill 0.5-1 cm ribbon of ointment in each conjunctival sac within first hour following birth *Chlamydia infections*: 0.25-inch ribbon twice daily for 2 mo *Other eye infections*: instill 0.25-inch ribbon of ointment in each eye 3 or 4 times daily	Ophthalmic ointment 0.5%	Side effects: ocular irritation or redness after application
Estrogens, conjugated (Premarin cream) *Hormone*	Treatment of vaginal adhesions Apply small amount daily until agglutination resolves	Vaginal cream, 0.625%	Apply small amount of cream to Q-Tip and then gently use Q-Tip to rub cream over labial adhesions. Use for 2 wk, then stop. If excessive amounts used or if prolonged use, estrogen effects may be noted.
Ethosuximide (Zarontin, Ethosuximide Syrup) *Anticonvulsant*	Controls absence seizures 3-6 yr: 10 mg/kg/24 hr to start divided bid; usual maintenance dose 15-40 mg/kg/day (max. 250 mg in 1 dose/day) >6 yr: initially 250 mg bid, increase as needed by 250 mg/day every 4-7 days until seizures controlled; usual maintenance dose 20-40 mg/kg/day (max. 1.5 g/day in 2 divided doses) Dose dependent on drug levels	250 mg capsule 250 mg/5 ml syrup	Therapeutic range: 40-100 μg/ml; toxic: >150 μg/ml. Drug interactions: phenytoin, valproic acid. Side effects: GI disturbances, blood dyscrasias, fatigue, sedation.
Famotidine (Pepcid, Pepcid AC) *GI histamine H_2 agonist*	Duodenal or gastric ulcers, gastroesophageal reflux disease (GERD) Infants and children <16 yr: *Peptic ulcer*: 0.5 mg/kg/day PO qd or divided bid (max. 40 mg/day) *GERD*: 1-2 mg/kg/day PO divided bid (max. 80 mg/day)	40 mg/5 ml suspension 10 mg chewable tab; 10 mg tab (OTC), 20 mg, 40 mg tab	Drug interactions: may give antacids concomitantly. Adverse reactions: HA, constipation, dizziness, diarrhea, somnolence
Felbamate (Felbatol) *Anticonvulsant*	For partial, generalized seizures and Lennox-Gastaut syndrome *Partial and generalized seizures*: Children >14 yr: 1.2-2.4 g/day divided tid-qid (max. 3.6 g/day); **consult with a neurologist before using** *Lennox-Gastaut syndrome*: Children 2 and older: 15-45 mg/kg/day PO tid-qid, but **consult with a neurologist before using**	600 mg/5 ml suspension 400, 600 mg tab	Adverse reactions: drowsiness, lethargy, nausea, vomiting, aplastic anemia, hepatitis, anorexia, ataxia, behavioral changes. LFTs, CBC with differential, platelets, reticulocyte count need to be monitored monthly; blood drug levels are not monitored.
Ferrous sulfate (OTC) (Feosol, Fer-In-Sol, Fer-Gen-Sol, Mol-Iron, Feratab) *Oral iron supplement*	Prevention and treatment of iron deficiency anemia Children to 5 yr: 1-2 mg/kg/day to 15 mg/day for prophylaxis; 3-6 mg/kg/day in divided doses bid-tid for 2-3 mo for treatment of iron deficiency 5-12 yr: prophylaxis: 15-18 mg/day; treatment for iron deficiency anemia: 60 mg elemental iron/day for 2-3 mo	Fer-In-Sol drops: 15 mg/0.6 ml elemental iron Fer-In-Sol syrup: 18 mg/5 ml elemental iron Elixirs (elemental iron): 44 mg/5 ml; 60 mg/5 ml; 25 mg/ml	Concurrent vitamin C (e.g., orange juice) enhances absorption. Contraindicated in patients with enteritis, ulcers, ulcerative colitis, hemochromatosis, hemolytic anemia, hepatitis. Drug interactions: tetracycline, vitamin C, antacids, chloramphenicol. Adverse reactions: GI symptoms, staining of

TABLE A-2 *Medications—cont'd*

Generic/Trade Classification	Indications/Dose	Supplied	Remarks
	Menstruating adolescent females 12-18 yr: prophylaxis: 60-120 mg/day elemental iron 12 and older: prophylaxis: 60 mg elemental iron/day; iron deficiency anemia: 50-100 mg elemental iron tid for 2-3 mo	Tablets: 195 mg (39 mg elemental [ele] iron) 300 mg (60 mg ele iron), 325 mg (65 mg ele iron), 525 mg (105 mg ele iron)	teeth, dark stools. Overdosage can be fatal, at levels between 30-300 mg/kg elemental iron.
Fexofenadine HCl (Allegra, Allegra-D) *Antihistamine*	Treatment of seasonal allergic rhinitis <6 yr: not recommended for Allegra <12 yr: not recommended for Allegra-D 6-11 yr: 30 mg PO bid ≥12 yr: 60 mg bid or 180 mg qd; 60 mg qd if decreased renal function	30 mg, 60 mg, 180 mg capsules Allegra-D: 120 mg pseudoephedrine in each capsule for extended release	Drug interactions: MAO inhibitors, antihypertensives. Side effects: HA, GI upset, insomnia, dry mouth.
Fluconazole (Diflucan) *Antifungal*	For oral, esophageal, systemic candidiasis *Oral candidiasis*: >2 wk of age: 6 mg/kg on day 1, then 3 mg/kg/day for 14 days Adults: 200 mg on day 1, then 100 mg/day for 14 days *Vaginal candidiasis*: Adults: 150 mg PO once	50 mg/5 ml suspension 50, 100, 150, 200 mg tab	Renal and hepatotoxicity have been reported; if abnormal liver or renal function tests occur during therapy, discontinue drug or monitor closely for more severe renal or hepatic injury. Can cause nausea, headache, rash, vomiting, abdominal pain, diarrhea. Decrease dose in renal failure. Drug interactions: warfarin, theophylline, oral hypoglycemics, phenytoin, cyclosporine, rifampin, hydrochlorothiazide, propulsid, astemizole.
Flunisolide (AeroBid, Nasalide, Nasarel) *Glucocorticoid, antiinflammatory*	For treatment of asthma requiring chronic steroid use; nasal solution used to treat seasonal allergic rhinitis *Allergic rhinitis*: Children 6-14 yr: initially, 1 spray each nostril tid or 2 sprays each nostril bid (max. 4 inhalations or sprays daily); titrate dose to lowest effective amount; maintenance, 1 spray each nostril qd Adults: initially, 2 sprays each nostril bid (max. 8 inhalations or sprays daily); titrate dose to lowest effective amount; maintenance, 1 spray each nostril qd *Asthma prophylaxis*: Children 6-15 yr: 2 oral inhalations bid >15 yr: 2 oral inhalations bid (max. 8 inhalations/day) *NIH asthma guidelines*: Children 6-15 yr: low dose, 500-700 μg/day (2-3 sprays); medium dose, 1000-1250 μg/day (4-5 sprays); high dose, >1250 μg/day (>5 sprays/day) Children >15 yr: low dose, 500-1000 μg/day (2-4 sprays); medium dose, 1000-2000 μg/day (4-8 sprays); high dose: >2000 μg/day (>8 sprays/day)	250 μg/metered spray oral inhalant 25 μg/metered spray nasal inhalant	Rinse mouth following oral inhalation. Not recommended for use in children <6 yr. Contraindicated in patients with fungal, untreated bacterial, or viral infections. Not to be used to treat acute asthmatic attacks. Adverse reactions: oral candidal infections, nasal irritation, adrenal suppression, headache. Do not stop drug abruptly. Use caution when transferring from systemic steroids to inhaled steroids.

Continued

TABLE A-2 *Medications—cont'd*

Generic/Trade Classification	Indications/Dose	Supplied	Remarks
Fluoride (many preparations) *Mineral supplement*	Used to prevent dental caries and in treatment of osteoporosis **Caries prevention depends on content of fluoride in child's source of drinking water**: *<0.3 ppm fluoride content of water*: 6 mo-3 yr: 0.25 mg PO daily 3-6 yr: 0.5 mg PO daily 6-16 yr: 1 mg PO daily *0.3-0.6 ppm fluoride content of water*: 6 mo-3 yr: no supplement required 3-6 yr: 0.25 mg PO daily 6-16 yr: 0.5 mg PO daily	Drops calibrated by fluoride ion Luride drops: 0.125 mg/drop Pediaflor drops: 0.5 mg/ml Tri-Vi-Flor drops: 0.25, 0.5 mg/ml Oral solution: 1 mg/ml fluoride ion Chewable tab: 0.25, 0.5, 1 mg fluoride ion Tab: 0.25 mg fluoride ion	**Do not give if fluoride content of drinking water is >0.6 ppm**. Do not give with milk products. Adverse reactions: GI upset; do not swallow rinse or gel. Dental fluorosis can occur if supplements are given unnecessarily. Infants <6 mo should not receive fluoride supplements. This includes those exclusively breastfed.
Fluoxetine (Prozac, Prozac Weekly, Sarafem) *Antidepressant*	*Depression or obsessive-compulsive disorder*: Children <5 yr: no dosing information available Children 7-18 yr: initial dose of 5-10 mg/day or 10 mg given 3 times a week may result in less adverse effects; dose titrated upward weekly (max. 20 mg/day) >18 yr: initially 5 mg/day or 20 mg q 2-3 days; increase dose after several weeks by 20 mg/day increments, titrate dose every few weeks up to maximum dose of 80 mg/day; delayed-release capsules: 90 mg once weekly, starting 7 days after last 20 mg dose *Bulimia*: Adults: 60 mg/day administered in the morning; may need to titrate up or down to this dose, depending on response and side effects *Premenstrual dysphoric disorder*: Adults: 20 mg/day titrated as necessary up to 80 mg/day; start 14 days before expected start of menses and continue through first full day of menses	10, 20, 40, 90 mg capsule; 90 mg delayed-release capsule 20 mg/5 ml solution	Drug interactions: do not use within 14 days of MAO inhibitors. May increase phenytoin, carbamazepine levels. Cautions with antipsychotics, benzodiazepines, and other CNS drugs. Adverse effects: nausea, CNS stimulation, somnolence, HA, tremor, fatigue, mania/hypomania, anorexia, weight loss, GI upset. Slow titration up to effective dose decreases adverse effects. Give last dose of the day before 4 PM to prevent insomnia.
Fluticasone propionate (Flovent, Flonase) *Inhaled Steroid*	Treatment of seasonal or perennial allergic rhinitis and as asthma therapy *Allergic rhinitis (nasal inhalation)*: Children ≥4 yr: 1 spray per nostril/day to max. 2 sprays per nostril/day Adults: 2 sprays each nostril qd Children <4 yr: not recommended *NIH asthma guidelines (oral inhalation)*: Children: low dose, 88-176 μg/day or 2-4 sprays/day (44 μg/spray); medium dose, 176-440 μg/day or 4-10 sprays/day (44 μg/spray) or 2-4 sprays/day (110 μg/spray); high dose, >440 μg/day or >4 sprays/day (110 μg/spray) or >2 sprays/day (220 μg/spray)	50 μg/metered nasal spray 50, 100, 250 μg powder, rotadisk oral inhalation 44 μg, 110 μg, 220 μg/inhalation inhalers	Side effects: nasal irritation, HA, candidiasis, pharyngitis. If exposed to varicella, consider prophylactic therapy to prevent varicella (e.g., varicella zoster immune globulin). Rinse mouth following use.

TABLE A-2 Medications—cont'd

Generic/Trade Classification	Indications/Dose	Supplied	Remarks
	Adults: low dose, 88-264 μg/day or 2-6 sprays/day (44 μg/puff) or 2 sprays/day (110 μg/spray); medium dose, 264-660 μg/day or 2-6 sprays/day (110 μg/spray); high dose, >600 μg/day or >6 sprays/day (110 μg/puff); or >3 sprays/day (220 μg/spray)		
Fluticasone propionate and salmeterol combination (Advair Diskus 100/50, 250/50, 500/50) *Inhaled steroid + long-acting beta agonist*	For long-term asthma control only; prescribe a short-acting inhaled beta-agonist for acute symptoms Children >12 yr and adolescents: *Not previously on an inhaled steroid*: 1 inhalation of 100/50 q 12 hr; if insufficient response after weeks use next higher strength (max. 1 inhalation 500/50 q 12 hr) *Currently using another inhaled steroid*: initial q 12 hr dose depends on dosage of inhaled corticosteroid currently in use (guidelines provided in a pharmacology reference book)	Fluticasone propionate/salmeterol diskus 100 μg/50 μg, 250 μg/50 μg, 500 μg/50 μg	Drug interactions: antagonized by beta-blockers. Avoid other sympathomimetics (except short-acting beta-agonists).
Furazolidone (Furoxone) *Antibacterial, antiprotozoal*	For treatment of bacterial or protozoal diarrhea and enteritis Children (5 mg/kg/day, not to exceed 8.8 mg/kg/day): Infants 1-11 mo: 8-17 mg PO qid for 7 days 1-4 yr: 17-25 mg PO qid for 7 days 5-12 yr: 25-50 mg PO qid for 7 days >12 yr: 100 mg PO qid for 7 days	16.7 mg/5 ml liquid 100 mg tab	Interactions: alcohol, tricyclic antidepressants, tyramine-containing foods, sympathomimetic drugs. Duration of therapy not to exceed 7 days.
Gabapentin (Neurontin) *Anticonvulsant*	For refractory partial-onset seizures (an adjunct drug only) Children ≥3 yr: initially, 10-15 mg/kg/day PO divided bid-tid; maintenance, 30-50 mg/kg/day PO divided bid-tid	250 mg/5 ml solution 100, 300, 400 mg capsule 600, 800 mg tab	Therapeutic blood level: 5-15 μg/ml An adjunct drug only with other convulsants. Adverse reactions: somnolence, dizziness, ataxia, headache, tremor, vomiting, nystagmus, fatigue, behavioral problems in developmentally delayed patients. Other laboratory values that may need monitoring depend on other concurrent anticonvulsants used.
Gentamicin sulfate (Garamycin, Genoptic S.O.P., Gentak, Gentacidin, Ocu-Mycin, Gentafair, Gentasol) *Antibiotic, ophthalmic*	Treatment of ocular infections Solution: 1-2 drops q 4 hr for 5-7 days Ointment: use bid-tid for 5-7 days	0.3% ophthalmic solution, ointment	Transient irritation, burning/stinging, rarely redness and lacrimation. Discontinue if allergic contact dermatitis results.
Griseofulvin (Fulvicin, Grifulvin, Grisactin, Gris-PEG, Griseofulvin Ultra, Fulvicin P/G)	For treatment of tinea corporis, tinea pedis, tinea capitis, tinea unguium, tinea cruris *Tinea pedis, tinea curis, tinea unguium*: Children >2 yr: 7.3 mg/kg/day PO (alternative: 10-15 mg/kg/day PO of	Microsize: 125 mg/5 ml suspension 250 mg capsule 250, 500 mg tab Ultramicrosize:	Give with fatty foods to increase absorption. Use with caution in penicillin-sensitive patients. Adverse reactions: blood dyscrasias, nausea, vomiting,

Continued

TABLE A-2 *Medications—cont'd*

Generic/Trade Classification	Indications/Dose	Supplied	Remarks
Penicillium griseofulvum derivative	ultramicrosize for areas highly resistant) or 10-20 mg/kg/day PO divided bid (microsize); treat tinea pedis for 4-8 wk; treat tinea unguium for 4-6 mo Adults: 660-750 mg/day PO (ultramicrosize) or 1 g/day PO (microsize) *Tinea capitis, tinea corporis*: Children >2 yr (ultramicrosize): 5-10 mg/kg PO once daily (max. 750 mg) for 2-4 wk for tinea corporis; 4-12 wk for tinea capitis Adult: 330-375 mg/day PO (ultramicrosize) or 500 mg/day PO (microsize)	125, 165, 250, 330 mg tab	photosensitivity. Drug interactions: alcohol, barbiturates, warfarin, anticoagulants. Monitor CBC and LFTs after 4-6 wk of treatment and q 4-6 wk of continuing treatment.
Guaifenesin (Breonesin, Hytuss-2X, Humibid Pediatric, Robitussin, many others) *Expectorant*	Controls cough due to minor throat, bronchial irritation <2 yr: 12 mg/kg/day PO divided q 4 hr 2-5 yr: 50-100 mg PO q 4 hr (max. 600 mg/day) 6-11 yr: 100-200 mg PO q 4 hr (max. 1.2 g/day) Children ≥12 yr and adolescents: 200-400 mg PO q 4 hr (max. 2.4 g/day)	67, 100 mg/5 ml syrup 100, 200 mg tab 200 mg capsule 300, 600, 800 mg and 1.2 g sustained release	Side effects: rarely GI upset. Should not be used to treat the chronic coughs of asthma, smoking, or bronchitis.
Guaifenesin and dextromethorphan (Robitussin DM, Tussin DM, many others) *Expectorant and cough suppressant*	Children (dose based on dextromethorphan component): 1-2 mg/kg/day PO divided q 6-8 hr Adults: 60-129 mg/day DM PO divided q 6-8 hr	Syrup: many strengths available; Robitussin DM: guaifenesin 100 mg and dextromethorphan 10 mg/5 ml	See dextromethorphan and guaifenesin listings.
Hydrocodone and acetaminophen (Vicodin) *Opiate agonist, analgesic, antipyretic, antitussive*	Relief of moderate to severe pain; antitussive *Antitussive (based on hydrocodone content)*: Children: 0.6 mg/kg/day PO divided in 3-4 doses; <2 yr: do not exceed 1.25 mg/dose PO; 2-12 yr: do not exceed 5 mg/dose PO; >12 yr: do not exceed 10 mg/dose PO *Analgesic*: Children: dose has not been established Adults: 1-2 tabs PO q 4-6 hr	5 mg hydrocodone and 500 mg acetaminophen tab 2.5 mg hydrocodone and 167 mg acetaminophen/5 ml elixir	Avoid alcohol and other CNS depressants. Elixir is 7% alcohol.
Hydroxyzine hydrochloride (Atarax, Anx, Vistaril) *Miscellaneous anxiolytics, sedative, hypnotic, antihistamine*	*Antiemetic*: Children: 1.1 mg/kg IM; adults: 25-100 mg IM *Anxiety*: Children <6 yr: 50 mg PO divided qid; ≥6 yr: 50-100 mg PO divided qid (max. 600 mg); adults: 50-100 mg PO qid *Preoperative*: Children: 0.6 mg/kg PO or 1.1 mg/kg IM; adults: 50-100 mg PO or 25-100 mg IM *Pruritus*: <6 yr: 50 mg/day PO divided q 6-8 hr; ≥6 yr: 50-100 mg/day PO divided q 6-8 hr; adults: 25 mg PO q 6-8 hr	10 mg/5 ml syrup (Atarax) 25 mg/5 ml suspension (Vistaril) 10, 25, 50, 100 mg tab (Atarax, Anx) 25, 50, 100 mg capsule (Vistaril) 25, 50 mg/ml injection	Interacts with other CNS depressants. Adverse reactions: drowsiness, dry mouth.

TABLE A-2 *Medications—cont'd*

Generic/Trade Classification	Indications/Dose	Supplied	Remarks
Hyoscyamine, atropine, scopolamine, phenobarbital (Donnatal, Antispasmodic, Hyosophen, Bellatal and others) *Antimuscarinic, antispasmodic*	For irritable bowel syndrome: Children: 10 lb: 0.5 ml PO q 4 hr or 0.75 ml q 6 hr 20 lb: 1 ml PO q 4 hr or 1.5 ml q 6 hr 30 lb: 1.5 ml PO q 4 hr or 2 ml q 6 hr 50 lb: 2.5 ml PO q 4 hr or 3.75 ml q 6 hr 75 lb: 3.75 ml PO q 4 hr or 5 ml q 6 hr 100 lb: 5 ml PO q 4 hr or 7.5 ml q 6 hr	Atropine 0.0194 mg, scopolamine 0.0065 mg, hyoscyamine 0.1037 mg, phenobarbital 16.2 mg tab, capsule, or per 5 ml elixir	Contraindicated in patients with glaucoma, GU or GI obstructive disease, tachycardia, myasthenia gravis. Drug interactions: digitalis, griseofulvin, tetracyclines, MAO inhibitors, tricyclic antidepressants, steroids, amantadine, CNS depressants, antihistamines.
Ibuprofen (Advil, Motrin, Nuprin) *Nonsteroidal antiinflammatory, antipyretic*	Management of inflammatory disorders; analgesic for mild/moderate pain; antipyretic; dysmenorrhea Children >6 mo: *Antipyretic*: 5-10 mg/kg/dose q 6-8 hr PO (max. 40 mg/kg/dose) *Juvenile arthritis*: 30-70 mg/kg/day PO divided tid *Analgesic*: 4-10 mg/kg/dose PO divided tid Adults: 200-800 mg/dose tid-qid (maximum 1.2 g/day)	40 mg/ml, 100 mg/5 ml suspension 50 mg,100 mg chewable 100, 200 mg tab (OTC) 300, 400, 600, 800 mg tab (Rx)	Drug interactions: digoxin, methotrexate. Can cause GI upset. Contraindicated in patients with aspirin sensitivities or bleeding disorders.
Imipramine (Tofranil, Tofranil-PM) *Tricyclic antidepressant*	Used in the treatment of childhood enuresis, depression, ADHD *Enuresis*: Children ≥6 yr: 10-25 mg PO initially 1 hr before bedtime; increase by 10-25 mg/dose increments weekly (max. 2.5 mg/kg/day); or 50 mg PO qhs for 6-12 yr; 75 mg PO ≥12 yr Slowly reduce dosage after desired response of several weeks *ADHD*: Children ≥6 yr: 2-5 mg/kg/day PO divided bid-tid *Depression*: Children <12 yr initial 1.5 mg/kg/day PO, increasing as necessary by 1 mg/kg every 3-4 days to maximum of 5 mg/kg/day; >12 yr: initial 30-40 mg/day PO (to 100 mg/day); adults: 50-100 mg/day PO initially divided tid; increase by 25-50 mg to max of 300 mg/day	10, 25, 50 mg tab 75, 100, 125, 150 mg capsule—Tofranil-PM (imipramine pamoate)	Children should have supine and standing blood pressures, ECG, and CBC before therapy and before any increase in dosages ≥3.5 mg/kg/day. Use with caution in patients with cardiac disease, glaucoma, seizure disorders, diabetes. Drug interactions: MAO inhibitors (if given within 14 days), warfarin, CNS depressants, antihypertensive agents. Adverse reactions: drowsiness, dry mouth, GI upset, photosensitivity, arrhythmias. Can take 2-4 wk to see full effects of therapy.
Ipratropium bromide (Atrovent, Combivent, DuoNeb) *Anticholinergic bronchodilator*	Used as adjunctive therapy in asthma with short-acting beta-agonist Children (nebulization): 5-12 yr: 125-250 μg q 4-6 hr (dilute 1/4-1/2 dose vial [2.5 ml] of 0.02% solution to final volume of 3-5 ml with 0.9% sodium chloride inhalation solution) >12 yr (nebulization): 250-500 μg (1/2-1 unit dose [2.5 ml] vial of 0.02% solution) q 6-8 hr; inhaler: 2 inhalations qid Children (oral inhalation) ≥12 yr: initial 2 inhalations (36 μg) q 6 hr (max. 12/day)	18 μg/spray inhaler (Atrovent); 18 μg ipratropium with 90 μg albuterol (Combivent) 0.02% (500 μg ipratropium in 2.5 ml NS [Atrovent]); 0.5 mg ipratropium with 2.5 mg albuterol per 3 ml (DuoNeb) solution for nebulization	Side effects: nervousness, GI disturbances, HA. Albuterol may also be mixed with the nebulized Atrovent solution if used within 1 hr.

Continued

TABLE A-2 *Medications—cont'd*

Generic/Trade Classification	Indications/Dose	Supplied	Remarks
Isoniazid (INH, Laniazid) *Antituberculosis agent*	*Active tuberculosis*: Children: 10-20 mg/kg/day PO divided bid (max. 300-500 mg/day); if compliance in question: 20-40 mg/kg/dose PO biweekly (max. 900 mg), preferably after 1 mo of daily isoniazid treatment Adults: 5-10 mg/kg/day PO qd (usual dose 300 mg/day); 15 mg/kg/dose PO biweekly (max. 900 mg) *Latent tuberculosis or preventive treatment*: Children: 10-15 mg/kg/day PO (max. 300 mg/day) for 9-12 mo Adults: 300 mg/day PO	50 mg/5 ml 100, 300 mg tab	Tablets may be crushed and put into applesauce for children, because the solution is very bitter tasting. Take on empty stomach. Avoid food containing tyramine. Avoid alcohol. Drug interactions: phenytoin, diazepam, carbamazepine. Adverse reactions: peripheral neuritis, seizures, ataxia, stupor, tinnitus, diarrhea. Note: INH is usually used in combination with other antituberculosis agents. Consultation with TB specialist is indicated to prevent development of multidrug-resistant TB.
Isotretinoin (Accutane) *Antiacne agent*	Management of severe recalcitrant cystic acne 0.5-1 mg/kg/day PO divided bid for 15-20 wk (face); 0.5-2 mg/kg/day PO divided bid (chest and back); if relapse occurs, therapy can be reinstated after 8 wk	10, 20, 40 mg capsule	Monitor CBC, platelets, sedimentation rate, triglycerides. Pregnancy category X. Avoid pregnancy during therapy. Two methods of contraception must be used. Acne worsens during first few weeks of therapy. Relapses more likely to occur at the lower doses. No blood donation for at least 1 mo following discontinuation of drug. Avoid other vitamin A products. Adverse reactions: pruritus, photosensitivity, conjunctivitis, cheilitis, epistaxis, bone pain. Depression and suicidal ideation have been reported. Note: Isotretinoin therapy is reserved for use by dermatologists or NPs who have completed special training, due to the serious adverse effects. There is an extensive education and consent program provided by the manufacturer.
Itraconazole *Antifungal*	For onychomycosis; oropharyngeal and esophageal candidiasis in the immunocompromised *Onychomycosis*: ≥18 yr: 100 mg PO bid for 12 wk or pulsed 5 mg/kg/day (up to 400 mg/day) PO divided bid for 1 wk each month for 3-5 mo (recommended regimen) *Oropharyngeal/esophageal candidiasis* (solution): ≥100-200 mg/day swished in mouth for 1-2 wk 100 mg capsule	10 mg/ml solution; 100 mg capsules	Drug interactions: Prolonged effect of benzodiazepines. Adverse reactions: GI, rash, pruritus, urticaria, headache, dizziness, hepatic function abnormalities, hypokalemia, fatigue, fever, myalgia, decreased bone plate activity in animal studies. Drug has been used in children 6 mo-12 yr without unusual adverse effects, but long-term effect of therapy in children is not known. Baseline and monthly CBC and LFTs recommended.

TABLE A-2 Medications—cont'd

Generic/Trade Classification	Indications/Dose	Supplied	Remarks
Kaolin and pectin (OTC) (Kaopectate) *Antidiarrheal*	Used to treat mild diarrhea Children 3-6 yr: 15-30 ml each dose following each loose stool Children 6-12 yr: 30-60 ml each dose Adults: 60-120 ml	Kaolin 975 mg and pectin 22 mg/5 ml suspension	Do not administer for longer than 48 hr. Drug interactions: tetracycline, theophylline, chloroquine, digoxin. Adverse reactions: constipation, fecal impaction. Use cautiously in pediatric patients.
Ketoconazole (Nizoral) *Antifungal*	*Systemic candidiasis, histoplasmosis, blastomycosis, chromomycosis*: Children <2 yr: 3.3-6.6 mg/kg/day PO Children >40 kg and adolescents: initially 200 mg PO qd; may increase to 400 mg qd if no response to lower dose Minimum treatment for candidiasis is 7-14 days; for other systemic fungal infections, use for 6-12 mo *Tinea capitus, tinea pedis, extensive or recalcitrant tinea corporis, tinea cruris, tinea unguium*: Children >40 kg and adolescents: 200-400 mg/day PO for 1-2 mo; for tinea unguium treat for 6-12 mo *Topical treatment of tinea corporis, tinea cruris, tinea versicolor, tinea unguium (onychomycosis)*: Adults and children: apply cream 1 or 2 times daily for 2 wk; for onychomycosis apply once at bedtime and cover with cotton socks; treat for 3-4 wk Shampoo: shampoo twice weekly for 4 wk	200 mg tab (scored) 2% cream 2% shampoo	Adverse reactions: hepatotoxicity, nausea, vomiting. Most effective oral antifungal. Drug interactions: phenytoin, cimetidine, ranitidine, rifampin, terfenadine. Limited experience with this drug in children—need to outweigh risks with benefits. LFTs should be monitored before treatment and during treatment lasting over 4 wk.
Ketorolac tromethamine 0.5% (Acular) *Nonsteroidal antiinflammatory (ophthalmic)*	Used for treatment of ocular itching due to seasonal allergic conjunctivitis Children <3 yr: not recommended Children ≥3 yr and adolescents: 1 drop qid for up to 7 days	Ophthalmic solution 0.5%	Can have transient stinging and burning following instillation. Refrigeration decreases stinging. Contraindicated in patients with soft contact lenses.
Lactulose (Cephulac, Chronulac, Kristalose, and others) *Laxative*	Laxative Children: 0.5-1.0 mg/kg/dose bid PO Adults: 15-30 ml daily PO (max. 3 oz/day) or 10-20 g dissolved in 4 oz water	3.33 g/5 ml solution 10, 20 g packets	Contraindicated in patients with fecal impaction or those with acute abdomen. Use with caution in diabetic patients.
Lamotrigine (Lamictal) *Anticonvulsant*	Partial, absence, atonic, juvenile myclonic seizures; Lennox-Gastaut syndrome (an adjunct drug with valproic acid) *Lennox-Gastaut syndrome* (in combination with valproic acid): Children 2-12 yr: initially, 0.15 mg/kg/day PO divided bid; titrate by 0.15 mg/kg weekly until maintenance dose of 1-5 mg/kg/day is reached (max. 200 mg once or divided bid) *Partial seizures, Lennox-Gastaut* (in combination with valproic acid):	2, 5, 25 mg chewable tab 25, 100, 150, 200 mg tab	Adverse reactions: Stevens-Johnson syndrome, drowsiness, headache, blurred vision, vomiting. Blood levels 2-20 μg/ml. Monitor LFTs, ammonia, prothrombin, partial thromboplastin because of the co-valproic acid therapy.

Continued

TABLE A-2 *Medications—cont'd*

Generic/Trade Classification	Indications/Dose	Supplied	Remarks
	Children ≥16 yr: 25 mg qod for 2 wk, followed by 25 mg once daily for 2 wk; after 4 wk, daily dose may be increased by 25-50 mg every 1-2 wk until effective maintenance dose of 100-400 mg once or twice daily *Monotherapy for partial seizures*: Children ≥16 yr: 50 mg qd for 2 wk, followed by 100 mg/day divided bid for 2 wk; then increase by 100 mg q 1-2 wk until maintenance dose of 500 mg/day divided bid		
Levalbuterol HCl (Xopenex) *Bronchodilator for nebulization*	Prevention and treatment of bronchospasm <6 yr: no clinical trials have been done 6-11 yr: 0.31 mg via nebulization q 6-8 hr, may increase to 1.25 mg q 6-8 hr >12 yr: 0.63 mg q 6-8 hr; may be increased to 1.25 mg q 6-8 hr	0.63 mg/3 ml unit dose, 1.25 mg/3 ml inhalation solution	Drug interactions: beta-blockers, diuretics, digoxin, MAO inhibitors, tricyclic antidepressants. Side effects: tachycardia, elevated heart rate, tremor, nervousness, pain, flu syndrome.
Levetiracetam (Keppra) *Anticonvulsant*	Partial seizures Children <16 yr (consult with a neurologist before using): initially, 10-30 mg/day PO divided bid ≥16 yr: intially, 500 mg PO bid; dose may be increased by 1 g daily at 2 wk intervals (max. 3 g/day)	250, 500, 750 mg tab	Therapeutic level: 20-60 μg/ml. Adverse reactions: somnolence, anxiety, fatigue, behavioral changes, coordination difficulties, dizziness.
Lindane (Kwell, Kwildane, Scabene) *Scabicide, pediculicide*	*Scabies*: Infants: apply thin layer of lotion from head to toe and wash off after 6 hr (this is *not* the first-choice drug in children <2 yr) >2 yr and adolescents: apply thin layer, massage, moving from neck to toes; shower after 8-12 hr; treatment can be repeated in 1 wk *Lice*: Children >2 yr and adolescents: apply to hairy areas and adjacent areas, wash off in 8-12 hr; for scalp, shampoo well for 4-5 min, rinse, and comb hair to remove nits	1% lotion, shampoo	Avoid contact with eyes, mucous membranes, face, and urethral meatus. Use with caution in infants and young children. Body should be clean and dry before application. Do not apply to broken or inflamed skin. Itching may continue for 4-6 wk because of the body's reaction to the infestation rather than to the therapy.
Lodoxamide (Alomide) *Mast cell stabilizer (ophthalmic)*	Used to treat vernal conjunctivitis, vernal keratitis, and vernal keratoconjunctivitis Children >2 yr and adolescents: 1-2 drops qid for up to 3 mo	Ophthalmic solution 0.1%	Contraindicated in patients with contact lenses. Adverse reactions: stinging, blurred vision, transient burning, itching, dry eyes.
Loperamide (OTC) (Imodium, Anti-Diarrheal Formula) *Antidiarrheal*	For the treatment of acute and chronic diarrhea Children 2-5 yr (13-20 kg): initially, 1 mg tid PO 6-8 yr (20-30 kg): initially, 2 mg bid PO 9-12 yr (>30 kg): initially, 2 mg tid PO Second and subsequent doses: 0.1 mg/kg/dose on second and subsequent days of unformed stool Adults: 2 capsules initially, then 1 capsule following each stool (max. 8 capsules/day)	1 mg/5 ml liquid 2 mg capsule, tab	Contraindicated in patients with ulcerative colitis, pseudomembranous colitis, or hepatic disease. Adverse reactions: constipation, abdominal cramping, nausea, vomiting, dizziness. Use cautiously in pediatric patients.

TABLE A-2 *Medications—cont'd*

Generic/Trade Classification	Indications/Dose	Supplied	Remarks
Loracarbef (Lorabid) *Carbacephem*	Upper and lower respiratory tract, otitis, sinusitis, pharyngitis, tonsillitis, uncomplicated cystitis, and pyelonephritis >6 mo: 30 mg/kg/day PO divided bid—otitis media, sinusitis; 15 mg/kg/day PO divided bid—skin, pharyngitis, tonsillitis; 15-30 mg/kg/day PO divided bid—uncomplicated UTI Adults: 200-400 mg PO q 12 hr	100, 200 mg/5 ml 200, 400 mg pulvules	Food limits bioavailability. Strawberry/bubble gum taste. Treat otitis with suspension—better therapeutic outcome. 10% cross-sensitivity in patients with penicillin and cephalosporin allergies.
Loratadine (Claritin, Claritin-D 12 Hour) *Antihistamine*	Nasal and nonnasal symptoms of seasonal allergic rhinitis Children 2-5 yr: 5 mg/day PO (use syrup) ≥6 yr: 10 mg/day PO (do not use Claritin-D combination in children <12 yr) OR <30 kg: 5 mg/day PO; >30 kg: 10 mg/day PO	10 mg tab 10 mg redi-tab 5 mg loratadine/120 mg pseudoephedrine, 10 mg/240 mg extended-release tab 5 mg/5 ml syrup	Give on empty stomach. Possible interaction with macrolide antibiotics, ketoconazole, cimetidine, ranitidine, or theophylline.
Magnesium citrate (Evac-Q-Mag) *Cathartic, laxative*	Children 2-5 yr: 2.7-6.25 g PO once or in divided doses 6-11 yr: 5.5-12.5 g PO once or in divided doses ≥12 yr and adolescents: 11-25 g PO daily or in divided doses	77.5-95 mg/5 ml solution when power mixed	Contraindicated in patients with renal impairment, acute abdominal pain, bowel obstruction, or appendicitis. Drug interactions: tetracycline, digoxin, indomethacin, ketoconazole, iron salts, ciprofloxacin, benzodiazepines, and calcium channel blockers. Chilling magnesium citrate will increase palatability.
Magnesium hydroxide (OTC) (Phillips' Milk of Magnesia) *Laxative*	Used to treat constipation and to induce bowel evacuation Children: 2-5 yr: 5-15 ml PO daily for constipation 6-11 yr: 15-30 ml PO daily for constipation >12 yr and adolescents: 30-60 ml as single dose for constipation	400, 800 mg/5 ml and 1.2 g/5 ml suspension 300, 600 mg tab	Contraindicated in patients with renal failure, intestinal obstruction, fecal impaction. Adverse reactions: abdominal cramps, hypotension, nausea, vomiting. Drug interactions: tetracycline, digoxin, indomethacin, ketoconazole.
Mebendazole (Vermox) *Anthelmintic*	Roundworms, whipworms, hookworms, pinworms *Pinworms*: Adults and children >2 yr: 100 mg PO as single dose; can repeat in 2 wk if infection persists *Roundworm, whipworm, hookworm*: Adults and children >2 yr: 100 mg PO bid for 3 days; can repeat in 3 wk	100 mg tab (chewable)	Few side effects at low doses. Occasional abdominal pain and diarrhea. Can swallow tablets or crush and mix with food. Administer with food.
Medroxyprogesterone acetate (Depo-Provera) *Progestin*	For abnormal uterine bleeding, secondary amenorrhea, or as contraception *Dysfunctional uterine bleeding*: 5-10 mg PO for 5-10 days beginning on day 16 or 21 of cycle *Secondary amenorrhea*: 5-10 mg PO for 5-10 days	2.5, 5, 10 mg tab 150, 400 mg/ml injection	Contraindicated in patients with thromboembolic disease, pregnancy, hepatic disease, breast or genital cancer, cardiovascular disease, undiagnosed vaginal bleeding. Drug interactions: bromocriptine.

Continued

TABLE A-2 *Medications—cont'd*

Generic/Trade Classification	Indications/Dose	Supplied	Remarks
	Contraception: 150 mg IM q 3 mo, first dose given only during first 5 days of normal menstrual period; may give within 5 days postpartum if not breastfeeding or at 6 wk postpartum if breastfeeding		Adverse reactions: depression, weight fluctuations, irregular bleeding, edema, breast tenderness, acne, galactorrhea.
Mefenamic acid (Ponstel) *Nonsteroidal antiinflammatory*	Mild to moderate pain, dysmenorrhea, inflammatory disease >14 yr: 500 mg PO, then 250 mg PO q 6 hr—not to exceed 1 wk	250 mg tab	Adverse reactions: blood dyscrasias. Drug interactions: anticoagulants, phenytoin, sulfonamides, corticosteroids. Take with food.
Metaproterenol sulfate (Alupent) *Bronchodilator*	For reversible airway obstruction due to asthma or chronic obstructive pulmonary disease (COPD) *Oral*: Children: <2 yr: 0.4 mg/kg/dose PO q 8-12 hr 2-6 yr: 1.3-2.6 mg/kg/day PO divided q 6-8 hr 6-9 yr or <27 kg: 10 mg/dose PO q 6-8 hr >9 yr or >27 kg: 20 mg/dose PO q 6-8 hr *Inhaled*: Metered-dose inhaler: children ≥12 yr, 2-3 inhalations q 3-4 hr (max. 12 inhalations/day) q 6-8 hr Nebulizer: children 6-12 yr, 0.1-0.2 ml of 5% solution diluted with NS to volume of 3 ml q 6-8 hr; ≥12 yr, 0.2-0.3 ml of 5% solution diluted with 2.5 ml NS q 6-8 hr	10 mg/5 ml solution 10, 20 mg tab (scored) 0.65 mg/metered spray 0.4%, 0.6%, 5% nebulization solution	Can cause nervousness, restlessness, or tremor. Drug interactions: MAO inhibitors, propranolol. Do not use concurrently with other sympathomimetic bronchodilators. Best results if second inhalation is given 10 min following first.
Methylphenidate (Concerta, Ritalin, Ritalin-SR, Ritalin LA, Methylin, Metadate CD) *CNS stimulant*	Used for the treatment of narcolepsy and ADHD *ADHD*: Children >6 yr: initially, 5 mg PO 1 or 2 times daily with breakfast and lunch; increase by 5-10 mg weekly; usual dose 0.3-0.7 mg/kg/dose given 2 or 3 times daily (max. 60 mg/day) Concerta dosing: if on methylphenidate HCl immediate-release tablet at dose of 5 mg bid-tid or 20 mg of a noncore extended-release tablet, switch to Concerta 18 mg PO qAM; if on methylphenidate HCl tablet of 10 mg bid-tid or 40 mg of a noncore extended-release capsule, switch to Concerta 36 mg PO qAM; to change from methyphenidate HCl tablet of 15 mg bid-tid or noncore sustained-release 60 mg daily, give Concerta 54 mg PO qd; may increase dose in 1 wk intervals (max. 54 mg/day) *Narcolepsy*: Adults: 10 mg PO bid-tid, up to 60 mg/day; give 30-45 min before meals	5, 10, 20 mg immediate-release tablet (Methylin, Ritalin) 10, 20 mg noncore sustained-release tablet (Metadate, Methylin) 20, 30, 40 mg noncore extended-release capsule (Ritalin LA; Metadate CD 20 mg only) 18, 36, 54 mg core, extended-release tablet (Concerta)	Contraindicated in patients with hyperthyroidism, cardiovascular disease, glaucoma, hypertension. Cautious use in patients with tics or Tourette syndrome. Drug interactions: MAO inhibitors, tricyclic antidepressants, anticonvulsants. Adverse reactions: anorexia, insomnia, nausea, weight loss, tachycardia, abdominal pain. May sprinkle Metadate CD 20 mg extended-release capsule contents on applesauce to administer.
Metronidazole (Flagyl, Protostat; MetroGel/Cream/Lotion, Noritate vaginal)	Trichomoniasis, amebiasis, giardiasis, *H. pylori, C. difficile*, anaerobic and mixed aerobic-anaerobic bacterial infections *Amebiasis*:	250, 500 mg tab 375 mg capsule; 750 mg extended-release tab	Adverse reactions: headache, metallic taste, nausea, diarrhea, dizziness, dry mouth. Avoid alcohol (may cause disulfiram-like reaction.)

TABLE A-2 *Medications—cont'd*

Generic/Trade Classification	Indications/Dose	Supplied	Remarks
Antiinfective	Children: 35-50 mg/kg/day PO divided tid; adults 500-750 mg q 8 hr for 5-10 days *Trichomoniasis*: Children: 15-30 mg/kg/day PO divided tid for 7-10 days; adults: 500 mg bid for 7 days; or 2 g single dose; or 2 g divided bid in 1 day *Giardiasis*: Children: 15 mg/kg/day PO tid for 5-7 days; adults 250 mg PO tid for 5-7 days or 2 g as single dose for 3 days *H. pylori*: Adults: 250-500 mg PO tid in combination with at least one other agent effective against *H. pylori* *Anaerobic*: Children: 30 mg/kg/day PO divided q 6 hr; adults: 30 mg/kg/day PO divided q 6 hr *Clostridium difficile* (antibiotic-associated colitis): Children: 30-50 mg/kg/day PO divided q 6-8 hr (max. 2 g/day); adults: 250 mg PO qid or 500 mg tid for 10 days *Pelvic inflammatory disease*: Adults: 500 mg PO bid for 14 days in combination with other antibiotics *Bacterial vaginosis*: Vaginal gel 1 applicator qhs for 5 days or 500 mg PO bid for 7 days	0.75, 1% cream, gel, lotion	Drug interactions: warfarin, phenobarbital, cimetidine. Liquid preparations can be made by a compounding pharmacy.
Miconazole nitrate (Micatin, Desewnex, Lotrimin, Ting, Monistat-Derm, Monistat 1, Monistat 3, Monistat 7, and others) *Local antifungal*	Topical treatment of tinea pedis, tinea cruris, tinea corporis, tinea versicolor: Children >2 yr and adolescents: apply bid for 2-4 wk Vaginal or vulvar candidiasis: 1 applicator or 100 mg vaginal suppository qhs for 7 days or 200 mg suppository qhs for 3 days or one 1200 mg suppository at bedtime	1%, 2% cream, lotion, spray, powder for topical use 100, 200, 1200 mg vaginal suppository	Adverse effects: irritation, burning; vulvovaginal burning, itching, irritation. Rarely HA, pelvic cramps, hives, skin rashes, contact dermatitis
Mineral oil (OTC) (Agoral) *Laxative*	Children: 1-2 ml/kg/dose PO qd or bid Adults: 15-60 ml/day PO as single dose; retention enema, 60-150 ml	Sterile liquid Fleet enema—133 ml	Liquid form contraindicated in children <4 yr due to aspiration potential. Enema form not for use in children <2 yr. Give on empty stomach. Take a multivitamin if on prolonged therapy. Can be mixed with a small amount of ice cream to improve compliance.
Minocycline HCl (Minocin, Dynacin, Vectrin) *Tetracycline*	*Mycoplasma, Chlamydia, Rickettsia, neisserial meningitis carriers (alternative drugs are recommended for prophylaxis when in close contact of individuals with invasive meningococcal disease)*: Children >8 yr: 4 mg/kg/day PO once, followed by 2 mg/kg q 12 hr for 5-7 days Adults: 200 mg initially, then 100 mg bid for 5-7 days	50 mg/5 ml suspension 50, 100 mg capsule	Drug interactions: increases digoxin levels. Avoid penicillins and methoxyflurane. Oral contraceptives may be less effective. Adverse effects: photosensitivity. Nausea, dizziness, blood dyscrasias, pseudotomor cerebri (signs/symptoms include HA and blurred vision), hepatotoxicity. HA at higher doses.

Continued

TABLE A-2 *Medications—cont'd*

Generic/Trade Classification	Indications/Dose	Supplied	Remarks
	Acne resistant to tetracycline or erythromycin: Adolescents: 50-200 mg/day divided bid; decrease dose after improvement		Outdated products can be toxic.
Miralax (see Polyethylene Glycol)			
Mometasone furoate monohydrate (Nasonex) *Corticosteroid*	Treatment of seasonal and perennial allergic rhinitis <3 yr: not recommended ≥3-11 yr: 1 spray each nostril qd >12 yr: 2 sprays per nostril qd	0.05% (50 μg/spray) nasal suspension	Improvement of symptoms should begin in 2 days. If exposed to varicella, consider prophylactic therapy to prevent varicella. Side effects: HA, pharyngitis, epistaxis, cough, URI.
Montelukast sodium (Singulair) *Leukotriene receptor antagonist*	Prophylaxis and chronic treatment of asthma Children: <2 yr: not recommended; 2-5 yr: one 4 mg chewable tab qhs; 6-14 yr: 5 mg qhs; >15 yr: 10 mg qhs	4, 5 mg chewable tab 10 mg tab	Drug interactions: drugs that induce CYP450 (phenobarbital, rifampin). Side effects: asthenia/fatigue, abdominal pain, HA, cough. Not for primary treatment of asthma. Not for monotherapy. Advise patient to take regularly, even during symptom-free periods.
Mupirocin (Bactroban) *Topical antibiotic*	Useful in the treatment of impetigo due to *Staphylococcus, Streptococcus* Apply 3 times daily	2% ointment or cream	Rare reactions: burning/stinging, pain, pruritis, rash, erythema, nausea, abdominal pain, HA, dizziness, stomatitis
Naproxen OTC (Naprosyn, Aleve, Anaprox, Naprelan) *Nonsteroidal*	Antiinflammatory, analgesic Children >2 yr: juvenile arthritis: 2.5-5 mg/kg/day PO q 8-12 hr (max. 15 mg/kg/day); analgesic: 5-7 mg/kg/dose q 8-12 hr Adults: Rheumatoid arthritis: 250-500 mg bid; analgesia: 250 mg PO q 6-8 hr (max. 1250 mg/day) Mild to moderate dysmennorhea: initially 500 mg, then 250 mg PO q 6-8 hr (max. 1250 mg/day)	125 mg/5 ml suspension 250, 375, 500 mg tab 375, 500 mg delayed release	Use cautiously in patients with impaired renal function or burns. Side effects: constipation, heartburn, abdominal pain, nausea. Take with milk, antacids, or food to minimize GI effects. Drug interactions: warfarin, methotrexate.
Nedocromil sodium (Tilade) *Nonsteroidal antiinflammatory*	Used as prophylaxis in treatment of asthma Children <6 yr: not approved Children ≥6 yr (inhalation): 2 inhalations qid; frequency may be reduced to bid-tid, depending on response	1.75 mg/metered spray oral inhalant	Not to be used for acute asthma attacks. Adverse reactions: bad taste, HA.
Neomycin/polymyxin B/hydrocortisone combination (Pediotic, Antibiotic Ear Solution, LazerSporin-C and others) *Otic antibiotic, antiinflammatory*	Used for treatment of superficial bacterial infections of the external ear Children and adults: 1-3 gtts q 6-8 hr for 7-10 days only	0.35%/10,000 U/1% otic suspension or solution	A wick can be used to instill drops—saturate cotton with drops and leave in ear canal. The wick should be replaced daily.

TABLE A-2 Medications—cont'd

Generic/Trade Classification	Indications/Dose	Supplied	Remarks
Nitrofurantoin (Furadantin, Macrobid) *Urinary antiinfective*	Prevention and treatment of urinary tract infections; *Pseudomonas, Serratia,* and *Proteus* are resistant to this drug Children ≥1 mo: 5-7 mg/kg/day PO divided q 6 hr (max. 400 mg/day) for at least 7 days; prophylaxis therapy: 1-2 mg/kg/day PO as a single daily dose (max. 100 mg/day) Adults: 50 mg/dose PO q 6 hr for at least 7 days; prophylaxis: 50-100 mg/dose PO qhs	25 mg/5 ml 25, 50, 100 mg capsule	Drug interactions: avoid magnesium-containing antacids. Can cause discoloration of urine. Do not crush tab. Rinse mouth following administration of suspension to prevent staining of teeth.
Nystatin (Mycostatin, Nilstat, Nystex, O-V Statin) *Antifungal*	Oral *Monilia*: Neonates: 100,000 U (1.0 ml) qid (50,000 U in each cheek) Infants: 200,000 U (2.0 ml) qid (100,000 U in each cheek) Children and adults: troche 200,000-400,000 U qid or 400,000-600,000 U qid *Gastrointestinal infections*: Adults: 500,000-1 million U PO as tab qid *Cutaneous and mucocutaneous candidal infections*: Topical: apply 2 or 3 times daily Vaginal: 1 tab qhs for 2 wk	100,000 U/ml suspension 500,000 U tab 100,000 U vaginal tab 100,000 U/g cream, ointment, powder	Vaginal tabs can be used by pregnant women up to 6 wk before term. Paint oral suspension in infant's mouth to coat lesions. Vaginal tabs can be used orally by immunosuppressed patients to provide prolonged drug contact with oral mucosa.
Ofloxacin otic solution (Floxin Otic, Ocuflox ophthalmic) *Antibiotic, quinolone*	Otitis media with tympanostomy tubes in place, otitis externa, bacterial conjunctivitis, keratitis *Otitis media, otitis externa*: Children 1-12 yr: 5 drops in affected ear bid for 10 days Children >12 yr and adolescents: 10 drops in affected ear bid for 10 days; use for 14 days in chronic suppurative otitis media *Conjunctivitis*: Children ≥1 yr: 1-2 gtts q 2-4 hr while awake for 2 days, then 1-2 gtts qid for 5 days (used more frequently with keratitis)	0.3% otic, ophthalmic solution	Side effects: pruritus, dizziness, vertigo, earache, taste perversion, rash, ocular burning or discomfort. Not recommended for <1 yr of age. Warm bottle in hand 1-2 min before administering otic solution.
Oseltamivir phosphate (Tamiflu) *Antiviral*	Prophylaxis and treatment of symptomatic, uncomplicated acute influenza A or B *Treatment*: ≥1 yr: if <15 kg, 30 mg (2.5 ml oral suspension) bid; >15 to 23 kg, 445 mg (3.8 ml oral suspension) bid; >23 to 40 kg, 60 mg (5 ml) bid; >40 kg, 75 mg (6.2 ml) bid *Prophylaxis*: ≥13 yr: 75 mg once daily for at least 7 days	12 mg/ml suspension 75 mg capsules	Start drug within 24-48 hours of onset of symptoms. Start prophylaxis within 2 days of exposure to an infected person; can be used up to 6 weeks for prophylaxis. Efficacy has not been established in those with underlying pulmonary disease; adjust dose in those with impaired creatinine clearance. Drug is not to be a substitution for influenza vaccination. Adverse effects: vomiting, abdominal pain, epistaxis, otic disorder, conjunctivitis.
Oxcarbazepine (Trileptal) *Anticonvulsant*	Partial seizures (monotherapy or as adjunct therapy)	300 mg/5 ml suspension	Therapeutic blood level: 5-50 μg/ml.

Continued

TABLE A-2 *Medications—cont'd*

Generic/Trade Classification	Indications/Dose	Supplied	Remarks
	Children (monotherapy):intially, 8-10 mg/kg/day PO divided bid; titrate to 30 mg/kg/day PO over 4 wk Children >16 yr (monotherapy): 600 mg/day divided bid, titrated by 300 mg/day weekly to desired response (about 2400 mg/day)	150, 300, 600 mg tab	Side effects: hyponatremia, dizziness, somnolence, diplopia, fatigue, nausea, ataxia; contraindicated if carbamazepine sensitive.
Oxybutynin chloride (Ditropan) *Antispasmodic*	For bladder spasms associated with neurogenic bladder or urinary urgency, leakage, or dysuria Children >5 yr: 5 mg PO bid (max. 15 mg/day) Adults: 5 mg PO 2-3 times daily (max. 20 mg/day)	5 mg/5 ml syrup 5 mg tab; 5, 10, 15 mg extended-release tab	Contraindicated in patients with GI or GU obstruction, myasthenia gravis, glaucoma, ulcerative colitis, unstable cardiac disorders. Drug interactions: CNS depressants. Adverse reactions: GI disturbances, dry mouth, dizziness, decreased sweating, tachycardia. Safety in children <age 5 has not been established.
Palivizumab (Synagis) *Humanized monoclonal antibody*	Prevention of RSV in high-risk pediatric patients Pediatric patients: 15 mg/kg per dose given IM once a month, beginning in the fall before RSV season and continuing monthly through RSV season (November through April in most regions)	50, 100 mg single-use vial	See Chapter 24 for indications for use Side effects: GI disturbances, pain and redness at injection site, URI, rash, SGOT increases.
Penicillin G benzathine (Bicillin LA parenteral) *Penicillin*	*Children*: Streptococcal pharyngitis: <27 kg: 600,000 U IM as a single dose; ≥27 kg: 900,000 U IM as a single dose (AAP recommends 1.2 million units) Prophylaxis of rheumatic fever: 25,000 U/kg IM q 3-4 wk (max. 1.2 million U/dose) Syphilis: 50,000 U/kg IM for 1 dose (max. 2.4 million U) *Adults*: Streptococcal pharyngitis: 1.2 million U IM for 1 dose Prophylaxis of rheumatic fever: 1.2 million U IM q 3-4 wk or 600,000 U bimonthly Syphilis: 2.4 million U IM for 1 dose	300,000, 600,000 U/ml injection	Give deep IM in upper, outer quadrant of buttocks. Give midlateral thigh in infants and small children. Adverse reactions: hypersensitivity, pain at injection site.
Penicillin G benzathine/penicillin G procaine (Bicillin CR parenteral) *Penicillin*	*Children*: Streptococcal pharyngitis: 25,000-50,000 U/kg IM in one dose (max. 1.2 million U); or <14 kg: 600,000 U IM as single dose; 14-27 kg: 900,000 U IM as a single dose; ≥27 kg: 900,000 U IM as a single dose *Adults*: Streptococcal pharyngitis: 2.4 million U IM for 1 dose	150,000/150,000, 300,000/300,000, 450,000/450,000 U/ml injection	Give deep IM in upper, outer quadrant of buttocks. Give midlateral thigh in infants and small children. Adverse reactions: hypersensitivity, pain at injection site. Preferred over Bicillin LA for treatment of streptococcal pharyngitis because Bicillin CR has earlier peak levels of antibiotic.
Penicillin V potassium (Pen-Vee K, Veetids) *Penicillin*	Skin and soft tissue disorders, streptococcal pharyngitis, prophylaxis pneumococcal infection, anthrax *Streptococcal pharyngitis, otitis media, erysipelas, scarlet fever*:	125, 250 mg/5 ml solution 250, 500 mg tab	Food interferes with absorption. May be dosed bid for streptococcal pharyngitis. Drug interactions: tetracycline. Suspension has unpleasant taste.

TABLE A-2 *Medications—cont'd*

Generic/Trade Classification	Indications/Dose	Supplied	Remarks
	Children >1 mo: 15-62.5 mg/kg/day PO divided 3-6 doses; ≥12 yr: 125-250 mg PO q 6-8 hr or 500 mg PO q 12 hr for 10 days *Streptococcus pneumoniae, including otitis media, skin, or skin structure infections*: Children ≥12 yr: 250-500 mg PO q 6 hr (q 6-8 hr for skin-related infections) *Prophylaxis of pneumococcal infection*: Children <5 yr: 125 mg PO bid; >5 yr: 250 mg PO bid *Cutaneous anthrax*: Children ≥2 yr: 25-50 mg/kg/day PO divided bid-qid for 60 days; adults: 200-500 mg/day PO divided qid (children <2 yr should initially be treated with IV rather than oral therapy) *Prophylaxis aerosolized anthrax spores if anthrax found to be penicillin sensitive*: Children <9 yr: 50 mg/kg PO divided qid; >9 yr and adults: 7.5 mg/kg PO qid for 60 days (duration of treatment will also depend on use of anthrax vaccine postexposure)		
Permethrin (Elimite, Nix) *Pediculicide*	Head lice, scabies *Head lice and their eggs*: Adults and children >2 mo: apply cream rinse to hair after shampooing and towel drying, leave on for 10 min, then rinse; can repeat treatment in 7 days if lice are observed *Scabies*: Adults and children >2 mo: apply cream from head to toe; leave on for 8-12 hr before washing off with water; in infants also apply to hairline, neck, scalp, temple, and forehead; may repeat in 1 wk if live mites appear	1% lotion/cream rinse 5% cream	Thorough combing to remove nits from hair is required, as well as cleansing of the equipment. Permethrin 5% cream was shown to be safe and effective when applied to infants <1 mo old for neonatal scabies. Permethrin is a safer alternative than lindane for treating scabies and head lice in young infants.
Phenazopyridine HCl (Azo-Standard, Baridium, Pyridium, and others) *Urinary analgesic*	For pain associated with urinary tract infections or irritation Children 6-12 yr: 4 mg/kg/dose PO tid for 2 days only Children >12 and adolescents: 100-200 mg PO tid	95, 97, 100, 200 mg tab	Contraindicated in patients with liver or kidney disease. Adverse reactions: GI disturbances, headache, vertigo, methemoglobinemia, skin pigmentation. Urine discoloration occurs (orange or red) and stains clothing. May stain soft contact lenses.
Phenobarbital (Luminal) *Barbiturate, anticonvulsant, sedative*	Simple partial, tonic-clonic, febrile seizures; status epilepticus,hyperbilirubinemia, chronic cholestasis *Maintenance for grand mal, partialseizures*: Children: 3-5 mg/kg/day PO divided bid (maintenance 5-10 mg/kg/day)	20 mg/5 ml elixir 15, 16, 30, 32, 60, 65, 100 mg tab 30, 60, 65, 130 mg/ml injection	2-3 wk may be required to achieve full anticonvulsant effect. Therapeutic level 10-45 μg/ml (>50 μg/ml is potentially toxic).

Continued

TABLE A-2 *Medications—cont'd*

Generic/Trade Classification	Indications/Dose	Supplied	Remarks
	Adults: 100-300 mg/day PO qhs (can be divided, but there is no advantage) *Febrile seizures*: 3-4 mg/kg/day PO maintenance *Status epilepticus (not the drug of choice—see diazepam)*: Children: 10-15 mg/kg IV, may repeat q 10-15 min to a total of 20 mg/kg Adults: 10 mg/kg IV, may repeat q 10-15 min to a total of 20 mg/kg		Drug interactions: primidone, valproic acid, warfarin, corticosteroids, oral contraceptives, doxycycline. Do not withdraw drug abruptly. Side effects: sedation, irritability, hyperkinesis, ataxia, slurred speech, nystagmus, Stevens-Johnson syndrome,attention/memory/learning changes.
Phenylephrine HCl (Mydfrin ophthalmic, Neo-Synephrine, Nostril, Vicks Sinex, and others) *Vasoconstrictor, mydriatic, decongestant*	Relief of nasal and nasopharyngeal mucosal congestion; ocular congestion, itching *Nasal congestion*: 0.125% solution: children <6 yr, 1-2 drops q 4 hr for 3 days 0.25% solution: 6-12 yr, 2-3 sprays or drops q 4 hr for 3 days 0.5% solution: ≥12 yr: 2-3 sprays or gtts q 4 hr for 3 days 1% solution: use in adults with severe congestion, 1-2 sprays each nostril no more frequently than q 4 hr *Ocular congestion*: 0.08%-0.25% solution in children >1 yr: 1-2 gtts tid-qid prn	0.125%, 0.25%, 0.5%, 1% nasal solution 0.12%, 2.5%, 10% ophthalmic solution	Available in various combinations, usually 5 mg/ml. Side effects: transient burning, stinging, sneezing, increased nasal discharge, nasal dryness; overuse can cause rebound nasal congestion, which subsides 1 wk or more after discontinuance; rare systemic effects due to absorption. Do not use in those with HTN.
Phenytoin (Dilantin) *Hydantoin derivative, anticonvulsant*	Partial, generalized seizures, status epilepticus,migraines *Seizures*: Neonates: 4-7 mg/kg/day PO divided q 6-8 hr Children: intially, 5 mg/kg/day PO divided q 12 hr; maintenance, 4-8 mg/kg/day (max. 300 mg/day) Adults: initially, 100 mg PO tid, increasing 100 mg q 2-3 wk to reach desired effect; maintenance, 6-7 mg/kg/day divided q 12-24 hr (300-600 mg/day) *Arrhythmias*: Children: 2-5 mg/kg/day PO or IV divided bid Adults: 100 mg bid-qid PO maintenance	125 mg/5 ml suspension (shake well before administering) 50 mg chewable tab 30, 100 mg capsule 100 mg extended capsule 50 mg/ml injection	Therapeutic blood level in neonates: 7.5-15 μg/ml; children and adults: 7.5-20 μg/ml, but clinical response is more meaningful than plasma concentrations. Monitor CBC with differential, and liver enzymes before onset and at regular intervals during first few months of treatment; then blood levels and lab q 6 mo. Phenytoin may alter thyroid hormone demands, requiring monitoring. Drug interactions: alcohol, antihistamines, folic acid, rifampin, antacids. Barbiturates, carbamazepine, theophylline, and calcium can all cause decreased plasma levels of hydantions. Adverse reactions: gingival hyperplasia, blood dyscrasias, rash, hirsutism, anemia, lymphadenopathy, Stevens-Johnson syndrome. Can cause discoloration of urine. Is poorly absorbed in infants and young children.

TABLE A-2 *Medications—cont'd*

Generic/Trade Classification	Indications/Dose	Supplied	Remarks
Polyethylene glycol (Miralax) *Osmotic laxative*	Constipation, encopresis Children: 0.5-1.0 mg/kg/dose PO bid in 4-8 oz water or juice depending on response Adults: 1 heaping tablespoon/day PO (17 g) in 8 oz water, juice, soda, coffee, tea	14 oz, 26 oz, and individual packets	Do not use in patients with known or suspected bowel obstruction. In encopresis, goal is a daily soft, easily passed bowel movement; treatment duration is usually about 6 mo for effective normalization of bowel function.
Prednisolone (Prelone, Pediapred) *Glucocorticoid, antiinflammatory*	For treatment of inflammatory disorders of respiratory and GI tracts, allergic disorders, and rheumatic disease Children: antiinflammatory, 0.1-2 mg/kg/day PO divided 1-4 times daily; asthma, 1-2 mg/kg/day PO divided 1-2 times daily for 3-5 days Adults: 5-60 mg/day PO	5, 15 mg/5 ml solution 5 mg tab	Contraindicated in patients with active, untreated infections, including varicella. Can mask symptoms of infections. Do not abruptly stop drug. Adverse reactions: growth suppression, fractures, GI discomfort, vertigo, acne.
Prednisone (Deltasone, Meticorten, Sterapred) *Glucocorticoid, antiinflammatory*	Used in the treatment of inflammatory disorders, allergic disorders, and hematologic diseases Children: 0.1-2 mg/kg/day PO in 1-4 divided doses Adults: 5-60 mg/day PO divided in 1-4 doses	5 mg/ml (concentrated), 5 mg/5 ml solution 1, 2.5, 5, 10, 20, 50 mg tab	See contraindications and adverse reactions for prednisolone.
Primidone (Mysoline) *Anticonvulsant*	Partial, tonic-clonic, myoclonic seizures Children <8 yr: 50 mg PO qhs for 3 days; 100-125 mg PO bid for days 4-6; 100-125 mg tid for days 7-9; maintenance of 250 mg tid (10-25 mg/kg/day divided tid) Children ≥8 yr: 100-125 mg PO qhs for 3 days; 100-125 mg PO bid for days 4-6; 100-125 mg PO tid for days 7-9; maintenance of 250 mg tid	250 mg/5 ml suspension 50, 250 mg tab	Therapeutic level: 5-12 μg/ml Side effects: drowsiness, ataxia, vertigo, anorexia, nausea/vomiting, rash, aggression.
Promethazine HCl (Phenergan) *Antihistamine, antiemetic, antivertigo, sedative*	Used to treat vertigo,nausea, vomiting *Children*: Antihistamine: 0.1 mg/kg PO q 6 hr during the day and 0.5 mg/kg PO qhs prn (max. 25 mg/dose) Antiemetic: 0.25-0.5 mg/kg q 4-6 hr PO, IM, IV, rectally (max. 25 mg/dose) Motion sickness: 0.5 mg/kg PO 30 min before departure and q 12 hr as needed (max. 25 mg/dose) Sedation: 0.5-1.1 mg/kg/dose q 5 hr as needed PO, IV, IM, rectal *Adults*: Antihistamine: 12.5 mg PO or rectally tid and 25 mg PO or rectally at bedtime; 25 mg IV, IM may be given and repeated in 2 hr; switch to oral route as soon as possible Antiemetic: 12.5-25 mg q 4-6 hr PO, IM, IV, rectally Motion sickness: 25 mg PO 30 min-1 hr before departure, then q 12 hr as needed Sedation: 25-50 mg/kg q 6 hr PO, rectal, IM, IV	6.25, 25 mg/5 ml syrup 12.5, 25, 50 mg tab 12.5, 25, 50 mg suppository 25, 50 mg/ml injection	Drug interactions: MAO inhibitors, CNS depressants. Adverse reactions: confusion, dry mouth, dizziness, drowsiness, blurred vision. IM administration preferred to IV. IV administration can cause hypotension (rapid administration) or hypertension (slow administration). Avoid SC administration—can cause tissue necrosis.

Continued

TABLE A-2 *Medications—cont'd*

Generic/Trade Classification	Indications/Dose	Supplied	Remarks
Pseudoephedrine (OTC) (Sudafed, many others) *Decongestant, sympatomymetic*	Upper respiratory infections *Children*: <2 yr: 4 mg/kg/day PO in divided doses every 6 hr 2-5 yr:15 mg PO q 6 hr (max. 60 mg/day) 6-12 yr: 30 mg PO q 6 hr (max. 120 mg/day) ≥12 yr: 60 mg PO q 6 hr (max. 240 mg/day) OR extended release product: 120 mg PO q 12 hr	Pseudoephedrine hydrochloride: 15, 30 mg/5 ml; 75 mg/0.8 ml oral solutions 30, 60 mg tabs 15 mg chewable tabs 240 mg extended-release tabs 120 mg extended-release film-coated tabs Pseudoephedrine sulfate: 120 mg extended-release tabs	Drug interactions: additive effects with other sympathomymetics. Hypertensive crisis with MAO inhibitors. Adverse effects: tachycardia, palpitations, arrhythmias, CNS excitement.
Pyrantel pamoate (Antiminth, Pin-X, Reese's Pinworm Medicine) *Anthelmintic*	Roundworms, hookworm, pinworms Children >2 yr and adolescents: 11 mg/kg PO as single dose (max. 1 g); for pinworms, repeat in 2 wk	250 mg/5 ml suspension 62.5 mg tab	Suspension can be mixed with milk or juice; can be given with food. Treat all family members. Minimal toxicity. Use with caution in patient who is malnourished, anemic, or has hepatic disease.
Pyrethrins (OTC) (A-200, Licide, Pyrinyl, Pronto, RID, and others) *Pediculicide*	Pediculosis Apply to *dry* hair and affected body areas, leave on 10-20 min (time varies by brand), rinse; repeat in 7-10 days regardless if there is evidence of infestation; do not repeat in <24 hr	Available as gel, shampoo, liquid	Avoid contact with eyes, face.
Ramantadine hydrochloride (Flumadine) *Antiviral*	For prophylaxis or symptomatic treatment of influenza A 1-9 yr: 5 mg/kg daily in 1 or 2 divided doses (max. 150 mg/day); alternative dosing if ≥20 kg: 100 mg/day in 1 or 2 divided doses ≥10 yr: 100 mg bid; alternative dosing if ≥10 yr and ≥40 kg: 200 mg daily in 1 or 2 divided doses: if <40 kg and regardless of age: 5 mg/kg daily in 1-2 divided doses	50 mg/5 ml solution 100 mg coated tablets	Drug should be started within 48 hours of symptom onset; discontinue treatment after 3-5 days or within 24-48 hours after signs and symptoms of illness resolve. For prophylaxis in high-risk individuals, start drug as soon as possible after recognition of the outbreak and continue for at least 2 weeks or until about 1 week after end of outbreak. Children receiving influenza virus vaccine for the first time, may required prophylaxis for up to 6 weeks following the vaccine or until 2 weeks after the second dose of vaccine. For those immunocompromised and unable to take the vaccine, prophylaxis can be used 6-12 weeks during the influenza A outbreak.

TABLE A-2 *Medications—cont'd*

Generic/Trade Classification	Indications/Dose	Supplied	Remarks
			Possible adverse effects: CNS (insomnia, nervousness/ jitteriness, dizziness/ lightheadedness, impaired concentration) and GI (nausea, anorexia, abdominal pain), rash, tinnitus, dyspnea.
Ranitidine HCl (Zantac) *Antiulcer agent*	For treatment of duodenal or gastric ulcers (acute and long-term prophylaxis), GERD, erosive esophagitis *Gastric/duodenal ulcer*: Children 1 mo-16 yr: 2-4 mg/kg/day PO divided q 12 hr (max. 300 mg/day); maintenance: 2-4 mg/kg/day PO divided q 12 hr (max. 150 mg/day) >16 yr: 150 mg bid or 300 mg qhs *GERD and erosive esophagitis*: Children 1 mo-16 yr: 4-10 mg/kg/day PO divided bid (GERD max. 300 mg/day; erosive esophagitis max. 600 mg/day) ≥16 yr: 150 mg bid or 300 mg qhs	25 mg/ml injection 75 mg/5 ml solution 75, 150, 300 mg tab 150 mg capsule 150 mg tab for solution	Use with caution if liver and renal impairment. Adverse reactions: HA, dizziness, sedation, malaise, mental confusion, nausea, vomiting, constipation, rash, arthralgia, bradycardia, or tachycardia.
Rifampin (Rifadin, Rimactane; Rifamate, Rifater [combinations with isoniazid]) *Antituberculosis agent, antibiotic*	*Tuberculosis (should be given in combination with other drugs)*: Infants <1 wk: max. 10 mg/kg/day PO Children: 10-20 mg/kg/day PO divided bid (max. 600 mg/day) Adults: 10 mg/kg/day PO up to 600 mg/day *H. influenzae prophylaxis*: Infants <1 mo: 10 mg/kg/day PO for 4 days; ≥1 mo: 20 mg/kg/day PO for 4 days (max. 600 mg) Adults: 600 mg/day PO for 4 days *Meningococcal prophylaxis, nasal carriers of N. meningitidis*: Children <1 mo: 5 mg/kg/dose PO q 12 hr for 2 days; ≥1 mo: 10 mg/kg PO q 12 hr for 2 days (max. 600 mg/day) Adults: 600 mg PO q 12 hr for 2 days	50 mg/ml 150, 300 mg capsule	Prophylaxis is most effective within 24 hr of exposure and no later than 2 wk. Take on empty stomach. Can discolor body fluids. Drug interactions: verapamil, methadone, digoxin, cyclosporine steroids, oral contraceptives (an alternate form of birth control should be used). Adverse reactions: nausea, vomiting, heartburn, epigastric distress, anorexia, abdominal cramps, flatulence, diarrhea, headache, drowsiness, fatigue, ataxia, confusion. Monitor liver function, CBC, bilirubin during therapy for tuberculosis.
Salicylic acid preparations (DuoFilm; Occlusal-HP; Trans-Ver-Sal, Compound W, Mediplast, Fostex, Clearsil Stri-Dex, Oxy, Noczema, and others) *Keratolytic agent*	For treatment of seborrheic dermatitis, psoriasis, dandruff, warts,and other benign epithelial tumors *Warts*: apply once daily to wart *Seborrhea and dandruff of scalp*: follow package directions *Acne*: use per package directions; usual use is application to all acne-affected areas once or twice daily	Cream, gel, shampoo, bar, lotion, ointment, pledget, solution, plaster	Avoid contact with healthy skin; if used in concentrations >10% protect surrounding area with application of petrolatum to surrounding normal tissue. Contraindicated in diabetics, those with impaired circulation. Not to be used on moles, birthmarks, unusual skin lesions.

Continued

TABLE A-2 *Medications—cont'd*

Generic/Trade Classification	Indications/Dose	Supplied	Remarks
Salmeterol xinafoate (Serevent) *Bronchodilator*	For long-term control therapy in the treatment of asthma Children 4-12 yr: use 1 diskus inhalation q 12 hr Adults and children >12 yr: 2 metered-dose inhalations q 12 hr (max. 4 inhalations/day)	21 μg/inhalation metered-dose inhaler 50 μg/inhalation diskus	Not used as treatment for acute asthma attack. Use cautiously (high incidence of overuse). Patient education is very important. Drug interactions: MAO inhibitors, tricyclic antidepressants. Also available in combination with fluticasone propionate (Advair).
Selenium sulfide (OTC and Rx) (Exsel, Selsun, Selsun Blue) *Local antiseborrheic, antifungal*	For treatment of dandruff, seborrhea, dermatitis of scalp, tinea versicolor *Dandruff, seborrhea, dermatitis of scalp*: Children and adolescents: wash with 1-2 tsp, leave on 2-3 min, rinse well; 2 applications/wk for 2 wk, then q 3-4 wk *Tinea versicolor*: Apply 2.5% lotion or shampoo in thin layer on affected area, leave on for 10-15 min, then rinse; apply once daily for 7 days; may be used prophylactically once a month *Seborrhea (including cradle cap)*: Apply 1% selenium sulfide shampoo in very small amount to scalp, massage in, and rinse well; apply twice weekly for 2 wk; avoid getting in eyes	1% or 2.5% selenium sulfide shampoo—OTC 1%, 2.5% selenium sulfide lotion—Rx	Safety in infants has not been established. Do not use on excoriated or inflamed areas. Avoid getting in eyes.
Sertraline hydrochloride (Zoloft) *Selective serotonin reuptake inhibitor*	Treatment of depression and obsessive-compulsive disorder 6-12 yr: 25 mg PO qd >12 yr: 50-100 mg PO qd; increase at 1 wk intervals (max. 200 mg/day)	25 mg/ml solution 25, 50, 100 mg tab	Drug interactions: cimetidine, diazepam, tricyclic antidepressants, warfarin, tolbutamide. MAOIs may cause hypertensive crisis. Side effects: GI disturbances, sweating, agitation, insomnia, hyperkinesia, malaise, fever.
Simethicone (OTC) (Gas-X, Mylicon, Phazyme, Mylanta, Maalox) *Antiflatulent*	Used to treat flatulence and functional gastric bloating Infants and children <2 yr: 20 mg PO qid 2-12 yr: 40 mg PO qid >12 yr: 40-125 mg PO after meals and qhs	40 mg/0.6 ml; 50 mg/5 ml suspension 80, 125, 150, 166 mg chewable tab 62.5 mg tab; 125, 166 mg capsule	Administer after meals or at bedtime.
Sodium citrate and citric acid (Bicitra, Cytra-2, Shohl's Solution) *Alkalinizing agent*	Used in the management of metabolic acidosis and in conditions requiring alkaline urine Infants and children: 2-3 mEq/kg/day PO divided tid-qid; 15 mEq/kg/day in some conditions Children: 5-15 ml PO diluted, after meals and qhs Adults: 10-30 ml PO diluted in water or juice, after meals and qhs	Solution: sodium citrate 500 mg and citric acid 334 mg/5 ml 1 mEq of sodium and 1 mEq of bicarbonate each in 1 ml of Bicitra	Contraindicated in patients with renal insufficiency and in those with a sodium restriction. Drug interactions: antihypertensives. Adverse reactions: hypernatremia, metabolic alkalosis, diarrhea.
Sodium phosphate (Fleet Enema) *Laxative*	Children >2 yr: 1 oz/20 lb of weight Adolescents and adults: 4 oz (max. 8 oz)	2.25 and 4.5 oz squeeze bottle	Enemas are not recommended for children <2 yr.

TABLE A-2 *Medications—cont'd*

Generic/Trade Classification	Indications/Dose	Supplied	Remarks
Sodium sulfacetamide (Bleph, Isopto, Cetamide, Sulamyd) *Sulfonamide ophthalmic*	For treatment of ocular infections Solution: 1-2 drops 3-4 times daily for 5-10 days; 0.25-inch ribbon of ointment is used 1-4 times daily	10%, 15%, 30% ophthalmic solution 10% ophthalmic ointment	Solution will burn with instillation. Do not use in children <2 mo. Eyes should be cleansed before instillation—inactivated by purulent discharge.
Sorbitol *Laxative*	Children 2-11 yr: 2 ml/kg PO (as 70% solution) Children ≥12 yr and adults: 30-150 ml PO (as 70% solution)	70% oral solution	Use as hyperosmotic laxative as a single dose, at infrequent intervals.
Sulfasalazine (Azulfidine) *Sulfonamide (antibacterial and antiinflammatory)*	For management of ulcerative colitis, Crohn's disease, polyarticular course juvenile arthritis *Ulcerative colitis*: >2 yr: 40-60 mg/kg/day PO divided q 4-8 hr; maintenance: 20-30 mg/kg/day PO divided q 6 hr (max. 2 g/day) Adults: 1-2 g PO q 6-8 hr; maintenance: 2 g/day (max. 4 g/day) *Juvenile arthritis*: Children ≥6 yr: 30-50 mg/kg/day PO divided bid (max. 2 g/day); increase drug slowly in weekly increments to maintenance	500 mg tab; 500 mg delayed-release tablet	Can cause discoloration of urine and skin. GI intolerance is common during first few days. Drug interactions: folic acid, phenytoin, methotrexate, anticoagulants, oral hypoglycemics.
Sulfisoxazole (Gantrisin) *Sulfonamide*	*Urinary tract infections*: >2 mo: 75 mg/kg PO initially, then 25-30 mg/kg PO bid (max. 75 mg/kg/day) Adults: 2 g PO initially, then 1 g bid-tid *Otitis media with effusion prophylaxis*: 50-75 mg/d	500 mg/5 ml 500 mg tab	Not indicated for infants <2 mo. Take on empty stomach.
Sumatriptan (Imitrex) *Selective agonist of vascular serotonin type 1-like receptors*	Acute treatment of migraine HA Children 6-18 yr (limited evidence): 0.6 mg/kg/dose (or 3-6 mg) SC; may repeat once in 2 hr >18 yr: 6 mg SC; repeat in 1 hr to max. 2 doses per 24 hr Oral: 25 mg once; if unsatisfactory response repeat dose at 2 hr intervals to max. 200 mg/day Nasal spray: 5, 20 mg intranasally; can repeat once; max. 40 mg or 4 sprays	0.6 mg/0.5 ml unit dose syringe/vial; 12 mg/ml injection 25, 50, 100 mg tab 5, 20 mg nasal/0.1 ml spray	Drug interactions: MAO inhibitors, SSRIs. Contraindicated in patients with ischemic heart disease or HTN. Side effects: increased blood pressure, flushing, nausea, drowsiness, sweating; local reactions with spray and injection.
Terbinafine HCl (Lamisil) *Antifungal*	For treating tinea pedis, tinea corporis, tinea cruris, tinea versicolor, tinea unguium (onychomycosis) Children ≥12 yr: *Tinea pedis, t. corporis, t. cruris, t. versicolor*: apply cream or solution twice daily for 1-2 wk *Tinea unguium*: <20 kg: 62.5 mg/day PO; 20-40 kg: 125 mg/day PO; >40 kg: 250 mg/day PO; if fingernails affected, treat for 6-8 wk; toenails for 12 wk	1% cream, solution, spray 250 mg tab	Do baseline and monthly CBC, LFTs when treating systemically for onychomycosis. May also concurrently use the cream for onychomycosis (apply once daily to affected nails). Adverse reactions: erythema, pruritis, burning, blistering, swelling, oozing with topical application. Stevens-Johnson syndrome, toxic epidermal necrolysis, hepatic and renal impairment, ocular disturbances, neutropenia with systemic therapy.

Continued

TABLE A-2 *Medications—cont'd*

Generic/Trade Classification	Indications/Dose	Supplied	Remarks
Terbutaline sulfate (Brethine) *Bronchodilator (short-acting beta-adrenergic agonist)*	For asthma exacerbations and COPD Children <12 yr: 0.05 mg/kg/dose PO q 6-8 hr (max. 0.15 mg/kg/dose tid or 5 mg/day); 0.01 mg/kg/dose SC (max. 0.3 mg/dose q 15-20 min for 2 doses only) Children 12-15 yr: 2.5 mg PO tid (max. 7.5 mg/day); SC dose same as above >15 yr: 5 mg PO tid, titrated up as necessary (max. 15 mg/day); SC 0.25 mg, repeated once	2.5, 5 mg tab 1 mg/ml injection	Drug interactions: MAO inhibitors, tricyclic antidepressants, beta-blockers. Can cause tachycardia, tremor, hypertension, headache, palpitations.
Tetracycline (Achromycin, Sumycin) *Tetracycline*	Mycoplasma, *Chlamydia*, rickettsia, acne, exacerbation of bronchitis, *H. pylori* (in combination with other drugs), gonorrhea, tularemia, syphilis (in patients sensitive to penicillin) Children >8 yr: 25-50 mg/kg/day PO divided bid-qid, max. 2 g/day Adults: 250-500 mg PO qid *Acne*: initially, 500 mg bid for 1-2 mo, then lower dose to 500 mg qd for 1-2 mo; maintenance, 125-500 mg/day	125 mg/5 ml suspension 100, 250, 500 mg capsule 250, 500 mg tab	Combination therapy packet (Helidac Therapy) available for treating *H. pylori.* Take on empty stomach. Photosensitivity. Outdated drugs may be toxic. Drug interactions: antacids, milk, zinc, iron, calcium. Pregnancy category D; contraception must be used by sexually active females.
Theophylline (Slo-bid, Slo-Phyllin, Theo-Dur, Theolair, and others) *Respiratory smooth muscle relaxant*	Used as a bronchodilator in the treatment of asthma, COPD; also used for neonatal apnea/bradycardia Infants/newborns for apnea of prematurity: 4 mg/kg/day PO divided q 6 hr 6 wk-6 mo: 10 mg/kg/day PO divided q 6 hr 6 mo-1 yr: 12-18 mg/kg/day PO divided q 6 hr 1-9 yr: 20-24 mg/kg/day PO divided q 6 hr 9-12 yr and adolescent smokers: 15 mg/kg/day PO 12-16 yr (nonsmokers): 13 mg/kg/day PO ≥6 yr (nonsmoking, healthy): 10 mg/kg/day PO	27, 50 mg/5 ml solution 100, 200, 250, 300, 400, 450, 500, 600 mg timed-release tab (8-12 hr) 50, 65, 75, 100, 125, 130, 200, 260, 300 mg sustained-release capsule	Therapeutic levels: 10-15 μg/ml (toxic level >20 μg/ml). After therapeutic level obtained, serum levels should be monitored q 6-12 mo. Factors that affect serum levels: smoking cigarettes or marijuana, charcoal-broiled beef, phenytoin, phenobarbital, carbamazepine, rifampin, IV isoproterenol, fever, illnesses, propranolol, allopurinol, erythromycin, cimetidine, oral contraceptives, ciprofloxacin, troleandomycin. Do not crush Theo-Dur tablets. Use cautiously in patients with hyperthyroidism, hypertension, cardiac disease, or liver disease.
Thiabendazole (Mintezol) *Anthelmintic*	Pinworms, roundworms, whipworms, trichinosis, threadworm, cutaneous larva migrans (dog and cat hookworm) Children and adolescents: 22-25 mg/kg/day PO divided q 12 hr for 2 days (max. 3 g/day); duration of treatment depends on type of helmintic infection	500 mg/5 ml suspension 500 mg chewable tab	Can inhibit metabolism of aminophylline. Side effects: 50% of patients experience nausea, vomiting, dizziness, anorexia. Administer after meals. Chew well before swallowing.
Tiagabine HCl (Gabatril) *Anticonvulsant*	Partial, generalized seizures Children <12 yr: consult with a neurologist for dosing	2, 4, 12, 16, 20 mg tab	Therapeutic level: not determined, but 5-70 μg/ml has been suggested.

TABLE A-2 *Medications—cont'd*

Generic/Trade Classification	Indications/Dose	Supplied	Remarks
	Children 12 yr-18 yr: intially, 4 mg daily for 1 wk, increasing to 4 mg bid on the second week; thereafter, titrate weekly in 4 mg increments until clinical response or maintenance of 32 mg/day is reached divided bid-qid >18 yr: initially, 4 mg/day for 1 wk, increasing by 4-8 mg/day (divided bid-qid) in weekly increments until maintenance (or clinical response) of 32-56 mg/day is reached divided bid-qid		Drug interactions: valproic acid possibly. Adverse reactions: drowsiness, concentration problems, increase of spike and wave of EEG, withdrawal seizures. Titrate doses more slowly in those with renal and hepatic impairment.
Tobramycin sulfate (Tobrex, Aktob, Tobrasol, Tomycine, TobraDex) *Antibiotic (ophthalmic)*	For treating ocular infections of *Chlamydia*, fungi, viruses, most anaerobic bacteria *Mild to moderate infections*: Suspension: 1-2 drops q 4 hr; ointment: 0.5-inch ribbon 2-3 times daily; use for 5-10 days *Severe infections*: Suspension: 2 drops q 30-60 min, decreasing to q 4 hr when improvement occurs; ointment: 0.5-inch ribbon q 3-4 hr until improvement occurs, then q 6-12 h	0.3% ophthalmic suspension, ointment	Adverse reactions: increased lacrimation, itching, eyelid edema, erythema, punctate keratitis.
Tolnaftate (OTC) (Aftate, Breezee Mist, Tinactin) *Antifungal*	Topical treatment of tinea pedis, tinea manuum, tinea cruris, tinea corporis, tinea versicolor Children and adolescents: apply to affected area bid for 2-6 wk	1% cream, powder, solution, spray	
Topiramate (Topomax) *Anticonvulsant*	Partial, generalized seizures Children 2-16 yr: initially, 1-3 mg/kg/day PO given nightly the first week, increasing at 1-2 wk intervals by increments of 1-3 mg/kg/day divided bid to achieve optimal clinical response or 5-9 mg/kg/day divided bid ≥17 yr: initially, 25-50 mg/day PO divided bid, titrating upward by 25-50 mg at weekly intervals to achieve optimal response or maintenance of 400 mg/day divided morning and evening	15, 25 mg sprinkle capsule 25, 100, 200 mg tab	Therapeutic range: 2-25 μg/ml. Adverse reactions: language and coordination difficulties, difficulty concentrating, nervousness, somnolence, fatigue, abnormal vision, anorexia, weight loss, kidney stones. Reevaluate use of this drug during pregnancy.
Tretinoin (Retin-A, Renova, Avita) *Cell stimulant and proliferant*	Used in the treatment of mild to moderate acne Apply a thin layer to acne areas once daily at bedtime; begin with 0.025% cream and increase strength to bid if needed; patients with sensitive skin may need every other night dosing	0.025%, 0.05%, 0.1% cream 0.01%, 0.025%, 0.1% gel 0.05% solution	Do not apply immediately following hydration of skin. Can have exacerbation of acne initially, including hyperpigmentation or hypopigmentation of skin. Avoid contact with abraded skin, eyes, and mucous membranes.

Continued

TABLE A-2 *Medications—cont'd*

Generic/Trade Classification	Indications/Dose	Supplied	Remarks
Triamcinolone acetonide (Azmacort, Nasacort AQ, Aristocort) *Glucocorticoid, antiinflammatory*	Long-term control medication for asthma; seasonal and perennial allergic rhinitis; atopic dermatitis *Topical*: Children and adults: apply thin film 2-3 times daily *Allergic rhinitis (nasal spray)*: Children 6-11 yr: 1-2 sprays/day each nostril Children ≥12 yr and adults: 2 sprays/day each nostril *NIH asthma guidelines (oral inhalation)*: Children 6-12 yr: low dose, 1-2 sprays q 6-8 hr (300-800 μg/day); medium dose, 2-3 sprays q 6-8 hr (800-1200 μg/day); high dose, >3 sprays q 6-8 hr (≥1200 μg/day) Children ≥13 yr: low dose, 1-3 sprays q 6-8 hr (400-1200 μg/day); medium dose, 3-4 sprays q 6-8 hr (1200-1600 μg/day); high dose, >4 sprays q 6-8 hr (≥1600 μg/day)	0.025%, 0.1%, 0.5% cream, ointment 55 μg/nasal spray 100 μg/metered dose, oral inhalation	See contraindications and side effects for flunisolide. Monitor linear growth in children using high-dose inhaled steroids. Rinse mouth with water after using oral inhaled steroids. Reduce oral inhalations from high doses as soon as effective response is achieved.
Trifluridine (Trifluridine Solution, Viroptic) *Antiviral (ophthalmic)*	For treating herpes simplex keratitis (HSV-1 and HSV-2) and keratoconjunctivitis Children <6 yr: not recommended Children ≥6 yr and adults: 1 gtt q 2 hr during day (max. 9 drops/day) for 7 days, decreasing dose to 1 gtt q 4 hr after reepithelialization for 7 days more; do not use for longer than 21 days	1% ophthalmic solution	Adverse effects: transient stinging or burning.
Trimethobenzamide HCl (Tigan, Tebamide) *Antiemetic*	Used for the treatment of nausea and vomiting Children <13.6 kg: 100 mg rectally tid-qid 13.6-45 kg: 100-200 mg PO or rectally tid-qid Alternative dose for children ≤45 kg: 15 mg/kg/day divided tid-qid rectally; 20 mg/kg/day divided tid-qid orally >45 kg: 250 mg PO tid-qid, or 200 mg IM or rectally tid-qid	100, 200 mg capsule 100, 200 mg suppository 100 mg/ml injection	Use cautiously in infants and children and in patients with acute febrile illness. Not effective in the treatment of motion sickness. Can mimic or mask symptoms of Reye syndrome.
Trimethoprim HCl (Primsol, Proloprim, Tripex) *Antibiotic (folic acid inhibitor)*	For treating otitis media, acute uncomplicated UTIs; prophylaxis for UTIs and traveler's diarrhea; *P. carinii* pneumonia (conjunctive therapy) *Otitis media*: Children 6 mo-12 yr: 10 mg/kg/day PO divided q 12 hr for 10 days *UTI*: Children ≥12 yr: 100 mg q 12 hr or 200 mg PO once daily for 10 days	50 mg/5 ml bubblegum-flavored solution 100 mg, 200 mg tab	Adverse effects: rash, diarrhea, rare hematologic effects. May cause folate deficiencies with subsequent bone marrow suppression and blood dyscrasias (avoid large doses or prolonged administration). Use with caution in patients with impaired renal or hepatic function, with known folic acid deficiency, or in children with fragile X chromosome associated with mental retardation.

TABLE A-2 *Medications—cont'd*

Generic/Trade Classification	Indications/Dose	Supplied	Remarks
Trimethoprim (TMP)-sulfamethoxazole (SMX) (Bactrim, Bactrim DS, Septra, Septra DS, Sulfatrim) *Sulfonamide + folic acid inhibitor antibiotic*	Urinary tract infections, bronchitis in adults, otitis media, shigellosis, traveler's diarrhea, *P. carinii* pneumonia Children <2 mo: not recommended Children ≥2 mo: 8 mg TMP/kg/day PO (40 mg/kg SMX/day) PO divided bid or 1 ml/kg/day divided bid (max. 160 mg TMP, 800 mg SMX/day) Adults: 1 DS tablet, 2 regular tabs, or 20 ml of susp PO bid	TMP 40 mg and SMX 200 mg/5 ml suspension TMP 80 mg and SMX 400 mg/tab TMP 160 mg and SMX 800 mg/DS tab	Adverse reactions: Stevens-Johnson syndrome, drug fever, rash. GI side effects minimal. Not effective against streptococcal infections. Drug interactions: warfarin, methotrexate, phenytoin.
Trimethoprim sulfate, polymyxin B sulfate (Polytrim) *Antibiotic ophthalmic*	For ocular infections Children ≥2 mo and adults: 1 gtt q 3 hr for 7-10 days (max. 6 gtts/day)	Ophthalmic solution	Contraindicated in children <2 mo. Less burning than with other preparations.
Valproic acid (Depakene, Depakote) *Carboxylic acid derivative, anticonvulsant*	Generalized seizures if over 10 yr of age, myoclonic, absence seizures Children and adults: initially, 10-15 mg/kg/day PO divided bid-tid; may increase by 5-10 mg/kg/day weekly to max. of 30-60 mg/kg/day; tablet given bid; syrup and sprinkle given tid	250 mg/5 ml syrup 125 mg sprinkle 125, 250, 500 mg delayed-release and extended-release tab	Therapeutic range: 50-120 μg/ml. Take with food. Do not take with carbonated soda. Do not crush or chew tabs. Blood monitoring (baseline, after 1 mo, then q 6-12 mo, and before surgery): LFTs, ammonia, prothrombin, partial thromboplastin, bilirubin. Children <2 yr and those on multiple anticonvulsants are at increased risk of developing hepatotoxicity.
Vancomycin HCl (Vancocin) *Miscellaneous antiinfective*	Methicillin-resistant staphylococcal enterocolitis, *C. difficile*-associated diarrhea/colitis, pseudomembranous colitis Infants and children: 40 mg/kg/day PO divided q 6-8 hr for 7-10 days (max. 2 g/day) Adults: 500 mg-2 g/day PO divided q 6-8 hr for 7-10 days (max. 2 g/day)	250 mg/5 ml, 500 mg/6 ml oral solution 125, 250 mg capsule 1, 10 g solution	Use with caution in neonates and young infants. Unpleasant taste.
Xylitol (OTC) (Carefree, Orbit, Trident) *Natural sweetener*	Used to inhibit dental decay by encouraging remineralization and inhibits plaque formation Children and older (oral): 1 piece of gum chewed for 5 min qid; or 2 mints sucked on for 5 min qid	Gum, mints	Caries-causing bacteria cannot colonize in the presence of Xylitol.
Zafirlukast (Accolate) *Leukotriene receptor antagonist*	Long-term control medication for mild persistent asthma; not for acute asthma attacks Children 7-11 yr: 10 mg PO bid taken 1 hr before or 2 hr after meals ≥12 yr and adolescents: 20 mg PO bid as above	10, 20 mg tab	Not recommended for use in children <7 yr. Drug interactions: potentiates warfarin. Plasma levels reduced by erythromycin, theophylline. Plasma levels increased by aspirin. Caution with drugs metabolized by CYP2C9 (tolbutamide, phenytoin, carbamazepine) or CYP3A4 (dihydropyrinine calcium channel blockers, cyclosporine). Cautious use with calcium channel blockers, cyclosporine, astemizole. Side effects: HA, GI disturbances, dizziness. Rarely hepatic dysfunction.

Continued

TABLE A-2 *Medications—cont'd*

Generic/Trade Classification	Indications/Dose	Supplied	Remarks
Zanamivir (Relenza) *Antiviral*	Treatment of symptomatic, uncomplicated acute influenza A or B; prophylaxis use remains to be established ≥7 years: 2 inhalations (one 5 mg blister per inhalation) twice daily about q 12 hr for 5 days. Two doses should be taken the first day, as long as 2 hours has passed between doses	5 mg powder for inhalation per Rotadisk® foil blister pack used in a Diskhaler®	Drug must be started within 24-48 hours of symptom onset. Consult before using in patients with underlying respiratory disease (asthma, COPD). Patients needing to use an inhaled bronchodilator at the same time as zanamivir should use the bronchodilator first. Adverse effects: possible bronchospasm and decline in pulmonary function tests; diarrhea, nausea, vomiting; nasal symptoms, sinusitis, cough; ENT infections; HA; dizziness; rash. Drug should not be used as a substitute for influenza vaccine.
Zidovudine (AZT) (Retrovir) *Antiviral*	Human immunodeficiency virus (HIV) in combination with other drugs: Children 3 mo-12 yr: 180 mg/m^2 PO q 6 hr (max. 200 mg q 6 hr) >12 yr and adolescents: 600 mg/day PO divided bid-tid	50 mg/5 ml syrup 300 mg tab 100 mg capsule	Dosage is available for neonates and infants <3 mo. Must be taken frequently—around the clock. Adverse effects: GI symptoms, anemia (45%), granulocytopenia, thrombocytopenia. Monitor CBC, platelets. Reduce dose by 30% if hemoglobin <8 g/dl.
Zileutin (Zyflo) *Leukotriene receptor agonist*	Long-term control medication for mild persistent asthma; not for acute asthma attacks Children ≥12 yr and adults: 600 mg PO qid (with meals and at bedtime)	600 mg tab	Drug interactions: propranolol (doubles serum propranolol concentrations), theophylline (doubles serum theophylline levels), warfarin (decreased warfarin clearance, leading to increased prothombin time). Monitor drugs metabolized by CYP3A4. Adverse effects: altered liver function, dyspepsia, headache, headache, myalgia. Monitor liver function before and during every month for the first 3 mo of administration, every 2-3 mo for the first year, and periodically thereafter.
Zonisamide (Zonegran) *Anticonvulsant*	Partial, generalized seizures ≥16 yr: intially, 100 mg PO daily for 2 wk, increasing to 200 mg once daily or divided bid for 2 wk, and then by 100 mg increments q 2 wk thereafter until effective response achieved; usual maintenance, 100-600 mg once daily or divided bid	100 mg capsule	Therapeutic blood levels: 10-40 μg/ml. Plasma clearance is increased with concomitant use of phenytoin or carbamazepine; half-life is decreased with concomitant use of phenytoin, phenobarbital, and carbamazepine. Adverse reactions: behavioral problems, kidney stones, drowsiness, anorexia, abdominal pain, taste perversion, headache, dizziness, ataxia, nystagmus, and others.

Data from American Society of Health-System Pharmacists: *American Hospital Formulary Service (AHFS) drug information 2002*, Bethesda, Md, 2002, American Society of Health-System Pharmacists; Behrman RE, Kliegman RM, Jenson HB: *Nelson textbook of pediatrics*, ed 17, Philadelphia, 2004, WB Saunders; Burg F et al: *Gellis and Kagan's current pediatric therapy*, ed 17, Philadelphia, 2002, WB Saunders; Drug Facts and Comparisons staff: *Drug facts and comparisons*, ed 57, St Louis, 2002, Drug Facts and Comparisons; Takemoto C, Kraus D, Hodding J: *Pediatric dosage handbook*, ed 10, Cleveland, 2003, Lexicomp Inc.

ADD, Attention-deficit disorder; *ADHD*, attention-deficit hyperactivity disorder; *bid*, twice daily; *CBC*, complete blood count; *CNS*, central nervous system; *dl*, deciliter; *ECG*, electrocardiogram; *EEG*, electroencephalogram; *GI*, gastrointestinal; *g*, grams; *GU*, genitourinary; *HA*, headache; *HSV*, herpes simplex virus; *hs*, bedtime; *HTN*, hypertension; *IM*, intramuscular; *IV*, intravenous; *LFTs*, liver function tests; *MAO*, monoamine oxidase; *max.*, maximum; *MDI*, metered-dose inhaler; *μg*, micrograms; *ml*, milliliters; *NIH*, National Institutes of Health; *NS*, normal saline; *OTC*, over the counter; *OM*, otitis media; *PO*, by mouth; *prn*, as needed; *q*, every; *QAM*, every morning; *qd*, every day; *qhs*, bedtime; *qid*, four times daily; *qod*, every other day; *qwk*, every week; *RSV*, respiratory syncytial virus; *Rx*, prescription; *SC*, subcutaneous; *SGOT*, serum glutamic-oxaloacetic transaminase; *SL*, sublingual; *SSRIs*, selective serotonin reuptake inhibitors; *tab(s)*, tablet(s); *tid*, three times daily; *TM*, tympanic membrane; *U*, units; *URI*, upper respiratory infection; *UTI*, urinary tract infection; *UV*, ultraviolet; >, greater than; <, less than; ≥, greater than or equal to; ≤, less than or equal to.

APPENDIX A-1. STEPWISE APPROACH FOR MANAGING ASTHMA

Figure 1. Stepwise Approach for Managing Infants and Young Children (5 Years of Age and Younger) With Acute or Chronic Asthma (Updates EPR-2 Figures 3-4a and 3-6)

Classify Severity: Clinical Features Before Treatment or Adequate Control		Medications Required To Maintain Long-Term Control
	Symptoms/Day / Symptoms/Night	Daily Medications
Step 4 **Severe Persistent**	Continual / Frequent	■ **Preferred treatment:** – **High-dose inhaled corticosteroids** **AND** – **Long-acting inhaled β_2-agonists** **AND**, if needed, – Corticosteroid tablets or syrup long term (2 mg/kg/day, generally do not exceed 60 mg per day). (Make repeat attempts to reduce systemic corticosteroids and maintain control with high-dose inhaled corticosteroids.)
Step 3 **Moderate Persistent**	Daily / >1 night/wk	■ **Preferred treatments:** – **Low-dose inhaled corticosteroids and long-acting inhaled β_2-agonists** **OR** – **Medium-dose inhaled corticosteroids.** ■ Alternative treatment: – Low-dose inhaled corticosteroids and either leukotriene receptor antagonist or theophylline. If needed (particularly in patients with recurring severe exacerbations): ■ **Preferred treatment:** – **Medium-dose inhaled corticosteroids and long-acting β_2-agonists.** ■ Alternative treatment: – Medium-dose inhaled corticosteroids and either leukotriene receptor antagonist or theophylline.
Step 2 **Mild Persistent**	>2/wk but <1x/day / >2 nights/mo	■ **Preferred treatment:** – **Low-dose inhaled corticosteroids (with nebulizer or MDI with holding chamber with or without face mask or DPI).** ■ Alternative treatment (listed alphabetically): – Cromolyn (nebulizer is preferred or MDI with holding chamber) OR leukotriene receptor antagonist.
Step 1 **Mild Intermittent**	≤2 days/wk / ≤2 nights/mo	■ No daily medication needed.

Quick Relief
All Patients

- Bronchodilator as needed for symptoms. Intensity of treatment will depend on severity of exacerbation.
  - Preferred treatment: **Short-acting inhaled β_2-agonists** by nebulizer or face mask and space/holding chamber
  - Alternative treatment: Oral β_2-agonists
- With viral respiratory infection
  - Bronchodilator q4-6hr up to 24 hr (longer with physician consult); in general, repeat no more than once every 6 wk
  - Consider systemic corticosteroid if exacerbation is severe or patient has history of previous severe exacerbations
- Use of short-acting β_2-agonists >2 times a week in intermittent asthma (daily, or increasing use in persistent asthma) may indicate the need to initiate (increase) long-term-control therapy.

Step down
Review treatment every 1 to 6 mo; a gradual stepwise reduction in treatment may be possible.

Step up
If control is not maintained, consider step up. First, review patient medication technique, adherence, and environmental control.

Goals of Therapy: Asthma Control

- Minimal or no chronic symptoms day or night
- Minimal or no exacerbations
- No limitations on activities; no school/parent's work missed
- Minimal use of short-acting inhaled β_2-agonist
- Minimal or no adverse effects from medications

Note

- The stepwise approach is intended to assist, not replace, the clinical decisionmaking required to meet individual patient needs.
- Classify severity: assign patient to most severe step in which any feature occurs.
- There are very few studies on asthma therapy for infants.
- Gain control as quickly as possible (a course of short systemic corticosteroids may be required); then step down to the least medication necessary to maintain control.
- Minimize use of short-acting inhaled β_2-agonists. Over-reliance on short-acting inhaled β_2-agonists (e.g., use of short-acting inhaled β_2-agonist every day, increasing use or lack of expected effect, or use of approximately one canister a month even if not using it every day) indicates inadequate control of asthma and the need to initiate or intensify long-term-control therapy.
- Provide parent education on asthma management and controlling environmental factors that make asthma worse (e.g., allergies and irritants).
- Consultation with an asthma specialist is recommended for patients with moderate or severe persistent asthma. Consider consultation for patients with mild persistent asthma.

APPENDIX A-1. STEPWISE APPROACH FOR MANAGING ASTHMA (continued)

Figure 2. Stepwise Approach for Managing Asthma in Adults and Children Older Than 5 Years of Age: Treatment (Updates EPR-2 Figures 3-4a and 3-6)

Classify Severity: Clinical Features Before Treatment or Adequate Control			Medications Required To Maintain Long-Term Control
	Symptoms/Day **Symptoms/Night**	**PEF or FEV_1** **PEF Variability**	**Daily Medications**
Step 4 **Severe Persistent**	Continual Frequent	≤60% >30%	▪ **Preferred treatment:** – **High-dose inhaled corticosteroids** AND – **Long-acting inhaled β_2-agonists** AND, if needed, – Corticosteroid tablets or syrup long term (2 mg/kg/day, generally do not exceed 60 mg per day). (Make repeat attempts to reduce systemic corticosteroids and maintain control with high-dose inhaled corticosteroids.)
Step 3 **Moderate Persistent**	Daily >1 night/wk	>60%-<80% >30%	▪ **Preferred treatment:** – **Low-to-medium dose inhaled corticosteroids and long-acting inhaled β_2-agonists.** ▪ Alternative treatment (listed alphabetically): – Increase inhaled corticosteroids within medium-dose range OR – Low-to-medium dose inhaled corticosteroids and either leukotriene modifier or theophylline. If needed (particularly in patients with recurring severe exacerbations): ▪ **Preferred treatment:** – **Increase inhaled corticosteroids within medium-dose range and add long-acting inhaled β_2-agonists.** ▪ Alternative treatment: – Increase inhaled corticosteroids within medium-dose range and add either leukotriene modifier or theophylline.
Step 2 **Mild Persistent**	>2/week but <1x/day >2 nights/mo	≥80% 20-30%	▪ **Preferred treatment:** – **Low-dose inhaled corticosteroids.** ▪ Alternative treatment (listed alphabetically): cromolyn, leukotriene modifier, nedocromil, OR sustained release theophylline to serum concentration of 5-15 mcg/mL.
Step 1 **Mild Intermittent**	≤2 days/wk ≤2 nights/mo	≥80% <20%	▪ No daily medication needed. ▪ Severe exacerbations may occur, separated by long periods of normal lung function and no symptoms. A course of systemic corticosteroids is recommended.

Quick Relief
All Patients

- Short-acting bronchodilator: **2-4 puffs short-acting inhaled β_2-agonists** as needed for symptoms.
- Intensity of treatment will depend on severity of exacerbation; up to 3 treatments at 20-minute intervals or a single nebulizer treatment as needed. Course of systemic corticosteroids may be needed.
- Use of short-acting β_2-agonists >2 times a week in intermittent asthma (daily, or increasing use in persistent asthma) may indicate the need to initiate (increase) long-term-control therapy.

Step down
Review treatment every 1 to 6 months; a gradual stepwise reduction in treatment may be possible.

Step up
If control is not maintained, consider step up. First, review patient medication technique, adherence, and environmental control.

Goals of Therapy: Asthma Control

- Minimal or no chronic symptoms day or night
- Minimal or no exacerbations
- No limitations on activities; no school/work missed
- Maintain (near) normal pulmonary function
- Minimal use of short-acting inhaled β_2-agonist
- Minimal or no adverse effects from medications

Note

- The stepwise approach is meant to assist, not replace, the clinical decisionmaking required to meet individual patient needs.
- Classify severity: assign patient to most severe step in which any feature occurs (PEF is % of personal best; FEV_1 is % predicted).
- Gain control as quickly as possible (consider a short course of systemic corticosteroids); then step down to the least medication necessary to maintain control.
- Minimize use of short-acting inhaled β_2-agonists. Over-reliance on short-acting inhaled β_2-agonists (e.g., use of short-acting inhaled β_2-agonist every day, increasing use or lack of expected effect, or use of approximately one canister a month even if not using it every day) indicates inadequate control of asthma and the need to initiate or intensify long-term-control therapy.
- Provide education on self-management and controlling environmental factors that make asthma worse (e.g., allergens and irritants).
- Refer to an asthma specialist if there are difficulties controlling asthma or if step 4 care is required. Referral may be considered if step 3 care is required.

APPENDIX A–2. USUAL DOSAGES FOR ASTHMA MEDICATIONS

Figure 1. Usual Dosages for Long-Term-Control Medications (Updates EPR-2 Figure 3–5a)

Medication	Dosage Form	Adult Dose	Child Dose*	Comments
Inhaled Corticosteroids *(See Estimated Comparative Daily Dosages for Inhaled Corticosteroids.)*				
Systemic Corticosteroids			(Applies to all three corticosteroids)	
Methylprednisolone	2, 4, 8, 16, 32 mg tablets	■ 7.5–60 mg daily in a single dose in AM or qod as needed for control	■ 0.25–2 mg/kg daily in single dose in AM or qod as needed for control	■ For long-term treatment of severe persistent asthma, administer single dose in AM either daily or on alternate days (alternate-day therapy may produce less adrenal suppression). If daily doses are required, one study suggests improved efficiency and no increase in adrenal suppression when administered at 3 PM (Beam et al. 1992).
Prednisolone	5 mg tablets, 5 mg/5 cc, 15 mg/5 cc	■ Short-course "burst": to achieve control 40–60 mg per day as single or 2 divided doses for 3–10 days	■ Short-course "burst": 1–2 mg/kg/day, maximum 60 mg/day for 3–10 days	■ Short courses or "bursts" are effective for establishing control when initiating therapy or during a period of gradual deterioration.
Prednisone	1, 2.5, 5, 10, 20, 50 mg tablets; 5 mg/cc, 5 mg/5 cc			■ The burst should be continued until patient achieves 80% PEF personal best or symptoms resolve. This usually requires 3–10 days but may require longer. There is no evidence that tapering the dose following improvement prevents relapse.
Long-Acting Inhaled Beta$_2$-Agonists				■ Should not be used for symptom relief or exacerbations. Use with corticosteroids.
Salmeterol	MDI 21 mcg/puff	2 puffs q 12 hours	1–2 puffs q 12 hours	■ May use one dose nightly for symptoms.
	DPI 50 mcg/blister	1 blister q 12 hours	1 blister q 12 hours	
Formoterol	DPI 12 mcg/single-use capsule	1 capsule q 12 hours	1 capsule q 12 hours	■ Efficacy and safety have not been studied in children <5 years of age. ■ Each capsule is for single use only; additional doses should not be administered for at least 12 hours. ■ Capsules should be used only with the Aerolizor™ inhaler and should not be taken orally.

Continued

APPENDIX A–2. USUAL DOSAGES FOR ASTHMA MEDICATIONS (continued)

Figure 1. Usual Dosages for Long-Term-Control Medications (Updates EPR-2 Figure 3–5a)

Medication	Dosage Form	Adult Dose	Child Dose*	Comments
Combined Medication				
Fluticasone/Salmeterol	DPI 100 mcg, 250 mcg, or 500 mcg/ 50 mcg	1 inhalation bid; dose depends on severity of asthma	1 inhalation bid; dose depends on severity of asthma	■ Not FDA approved in children <12 years of age. 100/50 for patient not controlled on low-to-medium dose inhaled corticosteroids. 250/50 for patients not controlled on medium-to-high dose inhaled corticosteroids.
Cromolyn and Nedocromil				
Cromolyn	MDI 1 mg/puff Nebulizer 20 mg/ampule	2–4 puffs tid-qid 1 ampule tid-qid	1–2 puffs tid-qid 1 ampule tid-qid	■ One dose prior to exercise or allergen exposure provides effective prophylaxis for 1–2 hours.
Nedocromil	MDI 1.75 mg/puff	2–4 puffs bid-qid	1–2 puffs bid-qid	■ See cromolyn above.
Leukotriene Modifiers				
Montelukast	4 mg or 5 mg chewable tablet 10 mg tablet	10 mg qhs	■ 4 mg qhs (2–5 years of age) 5 mg qhs (6–14 years of age) 10 mg qhs (>14 years of age)	■ Montelukast exhibits a flat dose-response curve. Doses >10 mg will not produce a greater response in adults.
Zafirlukast	10 or 20 mg tablet	40 mg daily (20 mg tablet bid)	■ 20 mg daily (7–11 years of age) (10 mg tablet bid)	■ For zafirlukast, administration with meals decreases bioavailability; take at least 1 hour before or 2 hours after meals.
Zileuton	300 or 600 mg tablet	2400 mg daily (give tablets qid)		■ For zileuton, monitor hepatic enzymes (ALT).
Methylxanthines				
Theophylline	Liquids, sustained-release tablets, and capsules	Starting dose 10 mg/kg/day up to 300 mg max; usual max 800 mg/day	Starting dose 10 mg/kg/day; usual max: ■ <1 year of age: 0.2 (age in weeks) + 5 = mg/kg/day ■ ≥1 year of age: 16 mg/kg/day	■ Adjust dosage to achieve serum concentration of 5–15 mcg/mL at steady-state (at least 48 hours on same dosage). ■ Due to wide interpatient variability in theophylline metabolic clearance, **routine serum theophylline level monitoring is important.** ■ See Figure 3–5a, page 87, EPR-2 for factors that can affect theophylline levels.

* Children ≤12 years of age

APPENDIX A-2. USUAL DOSAGES FOR ASTHMA MEDICATIONS (continued)

Figure 2. Estimated Comparative Daily Dosages for Inhaled Corticosteroids (Updates EPR-2 Figure 3–5b)

	Low Daily Dose		Medium Daily Dose		High Daily Dose	
Drug	**Adult**	**Child***	**Adult**	**Child***	**Adult**	**Child***
Beclomethasone CFC 42 or 84 mcg/puff	168–504 mcg	84–336 mcg	504–840 mcg	336–672 mcg	>840 mcg	>672 mcg
Beclomethasone HFA 40 or 80 mcg/puff	80–240 mcg	80–160 mcg	240–480 mcg	160–320 mcg	>480 mcg	>320 mcg
Budesonide DPI 200 mcg/inhalation	200–600 mcg	200–400 mcg	600–1200 mcg	400–800 mcg	>1200 mcg	>800 mcg
Inhalation suspension for nebulization (child dose)		0.5 mg		1.0 mg		2.0 mg
Flunisolide 250 mcg/puff	500–1000 mcg	500–750 mcg	1000–2000 mcg	1000–1250 mcg	>2000 mcg	>1250 mcg
Fluticasone MDI: 44, 110, or 220 mcg/puff	88–264 mcg	88–176 mcg	264–660 mcg	176–440 mcg	>660 mcg	>440 mcg
DPI: 50, 100, or 250 mcg/inhalation	100–300 mcg	100–200 mcg	300–600 mcg	200–400 mcg	>600 mcg	>400 mcg
Triamcinolone acetonide 100 mcg/puff	400–1000 mcg	400–800 mcg	1000–2000 mcg	800–1200 mcg	>2000 mcg	>1200 mcg

* Children ≤12 years of age.

Note

- **The most important determinant of appropriate closing is the clinician's judgment of the patient's response to therapy.** The clinician must monitor the patient's response on several clinical parameters and adjust the dose accordingly. The stepwise approach to therapy emphasizes that once control of asthma is achieved, the dose of medication should be carefully titrated to the minimum dose required to maintain control, thus reducing the potential for adverse effect.
- Comparative dosages in the EPR-2 were based on a limited number of published comparative clinical trials and extrapolation of differences in topical potency and lung delivery. This updated comparative dosage chart is based on review of recently published clinical trials involving more than 5,000 patients and published reviews (Barnes PJ et al. 1998; Kelly 1998; Pedersen 1997). The key differences from the EPR-2 include a higher dosage of budesonide and recommendations for two newly available medications: beclomethasone HFA and budesonide suspension for nebulization. The rationale for these changes is summarized as follows:
  - The high dose is the dose that appears likely to be the threshold beyond which significant hypothalamic-pituitary-adrenal (HPA) axis suppression is produced, and, by extrapolation, the risk is increased for other clinically significant systemic effects if used for prolonged periods of time (Martin et al. 2002; Szefler et al. 2002).
  - The low and medium dose reflects findings from dose-ranging studies in which incremental efficacy within the low-to-medium dose ranges was established without increased systemic effect as measured by overnight cortisol excretion. The studies demonstrated a relatively flat dose-response curve for efficacy at the medium-dose range; that is, increasing the dose to high-dose range did not significantly increase efficacy but did increase systemic effect (Martin et al. 2002; Szefler et al. 2002).
  - The dose for budesonide dry powder inhaler (DPI) is based on recently available comparative data with other medications, rather than the comparison to budesonide metered-dose inhaler (MDI) that was used in the EPR-2. These new data, including a meta-analysis of seven studies, show that budesonide DPI is comparable to approximately one-half the microgram dose of fluticasone (Barnes NC et al. 1998; Nielsen and Dahl 2000).
  - The dose for beclomethasone HFA is one-half the dose for beclomethasone CFC, based on studies demonstrating that the different pharmaceutical properties of the medications result in enhanced lung delivery for the HFA (a less forceful spray from the HFA propellant and a reengineered nozzle that allows a smaller particle size) (Leach et al. 1998; Busse et al. 1999; Gross et al. 1999; Thompson et al. 1998).
  - The dose for budesonide nebulizer suspension is based on efficacy and safety studies (Baker et al. 1999; Kemp et al. 1999; Shapiro et al. 1998), but no comparative studies with other inhaled corticosteroids are available. It is noted that the efficacy studies did not demonstrate a clear or consistent dose-response, although the high dose of 2.0 mg was effective in a placebo-controlled study in 40 infants with severe asthma (de Blic et al. 1996). In a small open-label long-term safety study, the ACTH stimulated cortisols appeared lower in the 13 infants receiving the high dose of 2.0 mg budesonide compared to infants receiving lower doses, but this was not statistically significant due, perhaps, to the small study size (Scott and Skoner 1999).
- Some doses may be outside package labeling, especially in the high dose range.
- MDI dosages are expressed as the actuater dose (the amount of the drug leaving the actuater and delivered to the patient), which is the labeling required in the United States. This is different from the dosage expressed as the valve dose (the amount of drug leaving the valve, all of which is not available to the patient), which is used in many European countries and in some scientific literature. DPI doses are expressed as the amount of drug in the inhaler following activation.

APPENDIX A–2. USUAL DOSAGES FOR ASTHMA MEDICATIONS (continued)

Figure 3. Usual Dosages for Quick-Relief Medications (Updates EPR-2 Figure 3–5d)

Medication	Dosage Form	Adult Dose	Child Dose*	Comments
Short-Acting Inhaled $Beta_2$-Agonists				
	MDI			
Albuterol Albuterol HFA Pirbuterol	90 mcg/puff, 200 puffs 90 mcg/puff, 200 puffs 200 mcg/puff, 400 puffs	■ 2 puffs 5 minutes prior to exercise ■ 2 puffs tid-qid prn	■ 1–2 puffs 5 minutes prior to exercise ■ 2 puffs tid-qid prn	■ An increasing use or lack of expected effect indicates diminished control of asthma. ■ Not generally recommended for long-term treatment. Regular use on a daily basis indicates the need for additional long-term-control therapy. ■ Differences in potency exist but all products are essentially comparable on a per puff basis. ■ May double usual dose for mild exacerbations. ■ Nonselective agents (i.e., epinephrine, isoproterenol, metaproterenol) are not recommended due to their potential for excessive cardiac stimulation, especially in high doses.
	DPI			
Albuterol Rotahaler	200 mcg/capsule	1–2 capsules q 4–6 hours as needed and prior to exercise	1 capsule q 4–6 hours as needed and prior to exercise	
	Nebulizer solution			
Albuterol	5 mg/mL (0.5%) 2.5 mg/mL 1.25 mg/3 mL 0.63 mg/3 mL	1.25–5 mg in 3 cc of saline q 4–8 hours	0.05 mg/kg (min 1.25 mg, max 2.5 mg) in 3 cc of saline q 4–6 hours	May mix with cromolyn or ipratropium nebulizer solutions. May double dose for severe exacerbations.
	Nebulizer solution			
Bitolterol	2 mg/mL (0.2%)	0.5–3.5 mg (0.25–1 cc) in 2–3 cc of saline q 4–8 hours	Not established	May not mix with other nebulizer solutions.
	Nebulizer solution			
Levalbuterol (R-albuterol)	0.31 mg/3 mL 0.63 mg/3 mL 1.25 mg/3 mL	0.63 mg–2.5 mg q 4–8 hours	0.025 mg/kg (min. 0.63 mg, max. 1.25 mg) q 4–8 hours	0.63 mg of levalbuterol is equivalent in efficacy and side effects to 1.25 mg of racemic albuterol. The product is a sterile-filled preservative-free unit dose vial.

APPENDIX A–2. USUAL DOSAGES FOR ASTHMA MEDICATIONS (continued)

Figure 3. Usual Dosages for Quick-Relief Medications (Updates EPR-2 Figure 3–5d)

Medication	Dosage Form	Adult Dose	Child Dose*	Comments
Anticholinergics				
	MDI			
Ipratropium	18 mcg/puff, 200 puffs	2–3 puffs q 6 hours	1–2 puffs q 6 hours	Evidence is lacking for anticholinergics producing added benefit to $beta_2$-agonists in long-term-control asthma therapy.
	Nebulizer solution			
	0.25 mg/mL (0.025%)	0.25 mg q 6 hours	0.25–0.5 mg q 6 hours	
	MDI			
Ipratropium with albuterol	18 mcg/puff of ipratropium bromide and 90 mcg/puff of albuterol 200 puffs/canister	2–3 puffs q 6 hours	1–2 puffs q 8 hours	
	Nebulizer solution			
	0.5 mg/3 mL ipratropium bromide and 2.5 mg/3 mL albuterol	3 mL q 4–6 hours	1.5–3 mL q 8 hours	Contains EDTA to prevent discoloration of the solution. This additive does not induce bronchospasm.
Systemic Corticosteroids			(Applies to the first three corticosteroids)	
Methylprednisolone	2, 4, 6, 8, 16, 32 mg tablets	■ Short course "burst": 40–60 mg/day as single or 2 divided doses for 3–10 days	■ Short course "burst" 1–2 mg/kg/day, maximum 60 mg/day, for 3–10 days	■ Short courses or "bursts" are effective for establishing control when initiating therapy or during a period of gradual deterioration. ■ The burst should be continued until patient achieves 80% PEF personal best or symptoms resolve. This usually requires 3–10 days but may require longer. There is no evidence that tapering the dose following improvement prevents relapse.
Prednisolone	5 mg tablets, 5 mg/5 cc, 15 mg/5 cc			
Prednisone	1, 2.5, 5, 10, 20, 50 mg tablets; 5 mg/cc, 5 mg/5 cc			
	Repository injection			
(Methylprednisolone acetate)	40 mg/mL 80 mg/mL	240 mg IM once	7.5 mg/kg IM once	May be used in place of a short burst of oral steroids in patients who are vomiting or if adherence is a problem.

*Children ≤12 years of age.

APPENDIX A–2. USUAL DOSAGES FOR ASTHMA MEDICATIONS

Figure 4. Dosages of Drugs for Asthma Exacerbations in Emergency Medical Care or Hospital (Updates EPR-2 Figure 3–10)

	Dosages		
Medication	**Adult Dose**	**Child Dose***	**Comments**
Short-Acting Inhaled $Beta_2$-Agonists			
Albuterol			
Nebulizer solution (5.0 mg/mL, 2.5 mg/3 mL, 1.25 mg/3 mL, 0.63 mg/3 mL)	2.5–5 mg every 20 minutes for 3 doses, then 2.5–10 mg every 1–4 hours as needed, or 10–15 mg/hour continuously	0.15 mg/kg (minimum dose 2.5 mg) every 20 minutes for 3 doses, then 0.15–0.3 mg/kg up to 10 mg every 1–4 hours as needed, or 0.5 mg/kg/hour by continuous nebulization	Only selective $beta_2$-agonists are recommended. For optimal delivery, dilute aerosols to minimum of 3 mL at gas flow of 6–8 L/min.
MDI (90 mcg/puff)	4–8 puffs every 20 minutes up to 4 hours, then every 1–4 hours as needed	4–8 puffs every 20 minutes for 3 doses, then every 1–4 hours inhalation maneuver. Use spacer/holding chamber	As effective as nebulized therapy if patient is able to coordinate.
Bitolterol			
Nebulizer solution (2 mg/mL)	See albuterol dose	See albuterol dose; thought to be half as potent as albuterol on a mg basis	Has not been studied in severe asthma exacerbations. Do not mix with other drugs.
MDI (370 mcg/puff)	See albuterol dose	See albuterol dose	Has not been studied in severe asthma exacerbations.
Levalbuterol (R-albuterol)			
Nebulizer solution (0.63 mg/3 mL, 1.25 mg/3 mL)	1.25–2.5 mg every 20 minutes for 3 doses, then 1.25–5 mg every 1–4 hours as needed, or 5–7.5 mg/hour continuously	0.075 mg/kg (minimum dose 1.25 mg) every 20 minutes for 3 doses, then 0.075–0.15 mg/kg up to 5 mg every 1–4 hours as needed, or 0.25 mg/kg/hour by continuous nebulization	0.63 mg of levalbuterol is equivalent to 1.25 mg of racemic albuterol for both efficacy and side effects.
Pirbuterol			
MDI (200 mcg/puff)	See albuterol dose	See albuterol dose; thought to be half as potent as albuterol on a mg basis	Has not been studied in severe asthma exacerbations.
Systemic (Injected) $Beta_2$-Agonists			
Epinephrine 1:1000 (1 mg/mL)	0.3–0.5 mg every 20 minutes for 3 doses sq	0.01 mg/kg up to 0.3–0.5 mg every 20 minutes for 3 doses sq	No proven advantage of systemic therapy over aerosol.
Terbutaline (1 mg/mL)	0.25 mg every 20 minutes for 3 doses sq	0.01 mg/kg every 20 minutes for 3 doses then every 2–6 hours as needed sq	No proven advantage of systemic therapy over aerosol.

APPENDIX A-2. USUAL DOSAGES FOR ASTHMA MEDICATIONS (continued)

Figure 4. Dosages of Drugs for Asthma Exacerbations in Emergency Medical Care or Hospital (Updates EPR-2 Figure 3-10)

	Dosages		
Medication	**Adult Dose**	**Child Dose***	**Comments**
Anticholinergics			
Ipratropium bromide			
Nebulizer solution (0.25 mg/mL)	0.5 mg every 30 minutes for 3 doses then every 2–4 hours as needed	0.25 mg every 20 minutes for 3 doses, then every 2 to 4 hours	May mix in same nebulizer with albuterol. Should not be used as first-line therapy; should be added to $beta_2$-agonist therapy.
MDI (18 mcg/puff)	4–8 puffs as needed	4–8 puffs as needed	Dose delivered from MDI is low and has not been studied in asthma exacerbations.
Ipratropium with albuterol			
Nebulizer solution (each 3 mL vial contains 0.5 mg ipratropium bromide and 2.5 mg albuterol)	3 mL every 30 minutes for 3 doses, then every 2–4 hours as needed	1.5 mL every 20 minutes for 3 doses, then every 2–4 hours	Contains EDTA to prevent discoloration. This additive does not induce bronchospasm.
MDI (each puff contains 18 mcg ipratropium bromide and 90 mcg of albuterol)	4–8 puffs as needed	4–8 puffs as needed	
Systemic Corticosteroids		(Applies to the first three corticosteroids)	
Prednisone Methylprednisolone Prednisolone	120–180 mg/day in 3 or 4 divided doses for 48 hours, then 60–80 mg/day until PEF reaches 70% of predicted or personal best	1 mg/kg every 6 hours for 48 hours then 1–2 mg/kg/day (maximum = 60 mg/day) in 2 divided doses until PEF 70% of predicted or personal best	For outpatient "burst" use 40–60 mg in single or 2 divided doses for adults (children: 1–2 mg/kg/day, maximum 60 mg/day) for 3–10 days.

*Children ≤12 years of age

Note

No advantage has been found for higher dose corticosteroids in severe asthma exacerbations, nor is there any advantage for intravenous administration over oral therapy provided gastrointestinal transit time or absorption is not impaired. The usual regimen is to continue the frequent multiple daily dose until the patient achieves an FEV_1 or PEF of 50 percent of predicted or personal best and then lower the dose to twice daily. This usually occurs within 48 hours. Therapy following a hospitalization or emergency department visit may last from 3 to 10 days. If patients are then started on inhaled corticosteroids, studies indicate there is no need to taper the systemic corticosteroid dose. If the followup systemic corticosteroid therapy is to be given once daily. One study indicates that it may be more clinically effective to give the dose in the afternoon at 3 PM, with no increase in adrenal suppression (Beam et al. 1992).

REFERENCES (APPENDIX A-2, FIGURES 1 AND 2)

Baker JW, Mellon M, Wald J, Welch M, Cruz-Rivera M, Walton-Bowen K. A multiple-dosing, placebo-controlled study of budesonide inhalation suspension given once or twice daily for treatment of persistent asthma in young children and infants. *Pediatrics* 1999;102(2):414-21.

Barnes NC, Hallett C, Harris TA. Clinical experience with fluticasone propionate in asthma: a meta-analysis of efficacy and systemic activity compared with budesonide and beclomethasone dipropionate at half the microgram dose or less. *Respir Med* 1998;92(1):95-104.

Barnes PJ, Pedersen S, Busse WW. Efficacy and safety of inhaled corticosteroids. New developments. Am J Respir Crit Care Med 1998;157(suppl):S1-S53.

Beam WR, Weiner DE, Martin RJ. Timing of prednisone and alterations or airways inflammation in nocturnal asthma. *Am Rev Respir Dis* 1992; 146(6):1524-30.

Busse WW, Brazinsky S, Jacobson K, Stricker W, Schmitt K, Vanden Burgt J, Donnell D, Hannon S, Colice GL et al. Efficacy response of inhaled beclomethasone dipropionate in asthma is proportional to dose and is improved by formulation with a new propellant. *J Allergy Clin Immunol* 1999;104(6):1215-22

de Blic J, Delacourt C, Le Bourgeois M, Mahut B, Ostinelli J, Caswell C, Scheinmann P. Efficacy of nebulized budesonide in treatment of severe infantile asthma: a double-blind study. *J Allergy Clin Immunol* 1996;98(1):14-20.

Gross G, Thompson PJ, Chervinsky P, Vanden Burgt J. Hydrofluoroalkane-134a beclomethasone dipropionate, 400 μg, is as effective as chlorofluorocarbon beclomethasone dipropionate, 800 μg, for the treatment of moderate asthma. *Chest* 1999;115(2):343-51.

Kelly HW. Comparison of inhaled corticosteroids. *Ann Pharmacother* 1998;32(2):220-32.

Kemp JP, Skoner D, Szefler SJ, Walton-Bowen K, Cruz-Rivera M, Smith JA. Once-daily budesonide inhalation suspension for the treatment of persistent asthma in infants and young children. *Ann Allergy Asthma Immunol* 1999;83(3):231-9.

Leach CL, Davidson PJ, Boudreau RJ. Improved airway targeting with the CFC-free HFA-beclomethasone metered-dose inhaler compared with CFC-beclomethasone. *Eur Respir J* 1998;12(6):1346-53.

Martin RJ, Szefler SJ, Chinchilli VM, Kraft M, Dolovich M, Boushey HA, Cherniack RM, Craig TJ, Drazen JM, Fagan JK et al. Systemic effect comparisons of six inhaled corticosteroid preparations. *Am J Respir Crit Care Med* 2002;165:1377-83.

National Heart, Lung, and Blood Institute, National Asthma Education and Prevention Program. *Guidelines for the diagnosis and management of asthma.* Expert Panel Report 2, Publication No. 97-4051. Bethesda, MD: U.S. Department of Health and Human Services; 1997.

Nielsen LP, Dahl R. Therapeutic ratio of inhaled corticosteroids in adult asthma: A dose-range comparison between fluticasone propionate and budesonide, measuring their effect on bronchial hyperresponsiveness and adrenal cortex function. *Am J Respir Crit Care Med* 2000;162(6): 2053-7.

Pedersen S, OÕByrne PA. comparison of the efficacy and safety of inhaled corticosteroids in asthma. *Allergy* 1997;52(39 suppl):1-34.

Scott MB, Skoner DP. Short-term and long-term safety of budesonide inhalation suspension in infants and young children with persistent asthma. *J Allergy Clin Immunol* 1999;104:(4 Pt 2)200-9.

Shapiro G, Mendelson L, Kraemer MJ, Cruz-Rivera M, Walton-Bowen K, Smith JA. Efficacy and safety of budesonide inhalation suspension (Pulmicort Respules) in young children with inhaled steroid-dependent, persistent asthma. *J Allergy Clin Immunol* 1998;102(5):789-96.

Szefler SJ, Martin RJ, King TS, Boushey HA, Cherniack RM, Chinchilli VM, Craig TJ, Dolovich M, Drazen JM, Fagan JK, et al. Significant variability in response to inhaled corticosteroids for persistent asthma. *J Allergy Clin Immunol* 2002;109(3):410-8.

Thompson PJ, Davies RJ, Young WF, Grossman AB, Donnell D. Safety of hydrofluoroalkane-134a beclomethasone dipropionate extrafine aerosol. *Respir Med* 1998;92(suppl):33-39.

REFERENCES

Bell E: Implications of using drugs "off-label," *Infect Dis Child* 15(11):10, 2002.

Burg F et al: *Gellis and Kagan's current pediatric therapy*, ed 17, Philadelphia, 2002, WB Saunders.

Drug Facts and Comparisons staff: *Drug facts and comparisons*, ed 57, St Louis, 2002, Drug Facts and Comparisons.

Infectious Diseases in Children: Almost 200 new drugs in development for use in children, *Infect Dis Child* 15(10):41, 2002.

Takemoto C, Kraus D, Hodding J: *Pediatric dosage handbook*, ed 10, Cleveland, 2003, Lexicomp Inc.

Woo T: Pediatric patients. In Wynne A, Woo T, Millard M: *Pharmacotherapeutics for nurse practitioner prescribers*, Philadelphia, 2002, FA Davis.

APPENDIX B

Growth Grids

Catherine E. Burns

Growth in height, weight, and head circumference is an important indicator of health for children. However, the health care provider must remember that growth must be assessed accurately to be valid. Growth is modified by a variety of factors including, but not limited to, nutrition, general health, and genetics. The following points may be helpful:

- Measure height of infants and children less than 2 years of age in a recumbent position, holding the infant's or child's head against a headboard and using a footboard against the foot.
- Measure height of children greater than 2 years of age by using a stadiometer or against a wall using a right angle against the head rather than the height measure on a standing scale.
- The body mass index (BMI) is used for assessing the height-weight proportions for all children over 2 years of age. To calculate BMI:
    - ○ Weight (kg) ÷ Stature (cm) ÷ Stature (cm) × 10,000 or
    - ○ Weight (lb) ÷ Stature (in) ÷ Stature (in) × 703
- Measure heights without shoes and infant weights without diapers.
- Chart the height, weight, and head circumference on grids for all visits, not just well-child visits.
- An estimate of adult height in inches can be calculated as follows:
    - ○ Boys: Adult height estimate (in) = (Mother's height [in] + Father's height [in]) + 2.5 ÷ 2
    - ○ Girls: Adult height estimate (in) = (Mother's height [in] + Father's height [in]) − 2.5 ÷ 2

When possible, use growth charts that are specific for children with certain genetic conditions. Down syndrome, Turner syndrome, Williams syndrome, and others have growth charts.

Birth to 36 months: Boys
Length-for-age and Weight-for-age percentiles

NAME ____________________

RECORD# ____________

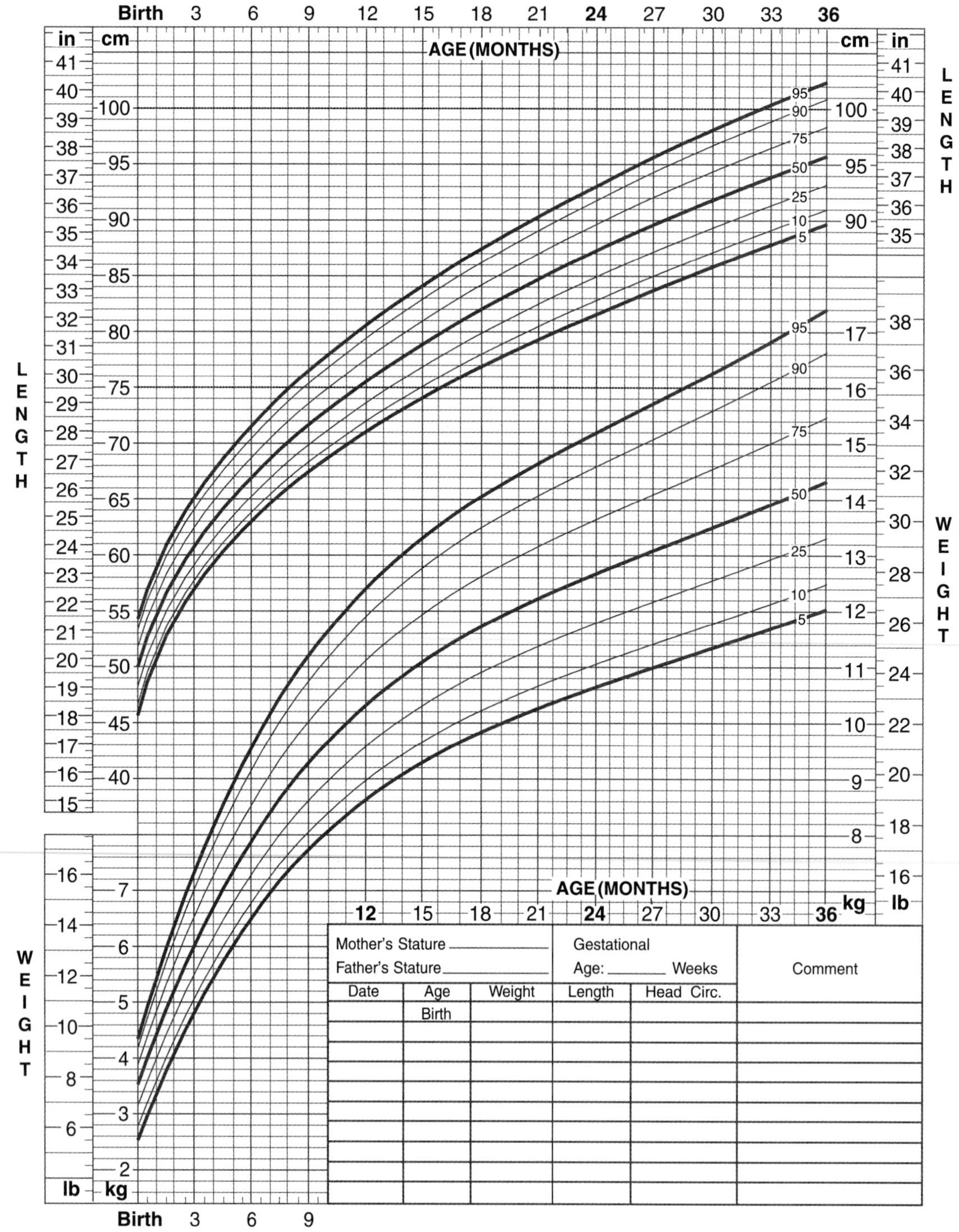

Pubished May 30, 2000 (modified 4/20/01).
SOURCE: Developed by the National Center for Health Statistics in collaboration with the National Center for Chronic Disease Prevention and Health Promotion (2000).
http://www.cdc.gov/growthcharts

CDC
SAFER • HEALTHIER • PEOPLE™

FIGURE B-1 Birth to 36 months: boys' length-for-age and weight-for-age percentiles. (From the National Center for Health Statistics in collaboration with the National Center for Chronic Disease Prevention and Health Promotion, 2000. Available at *www.cdc.gov/growthcharts.*)

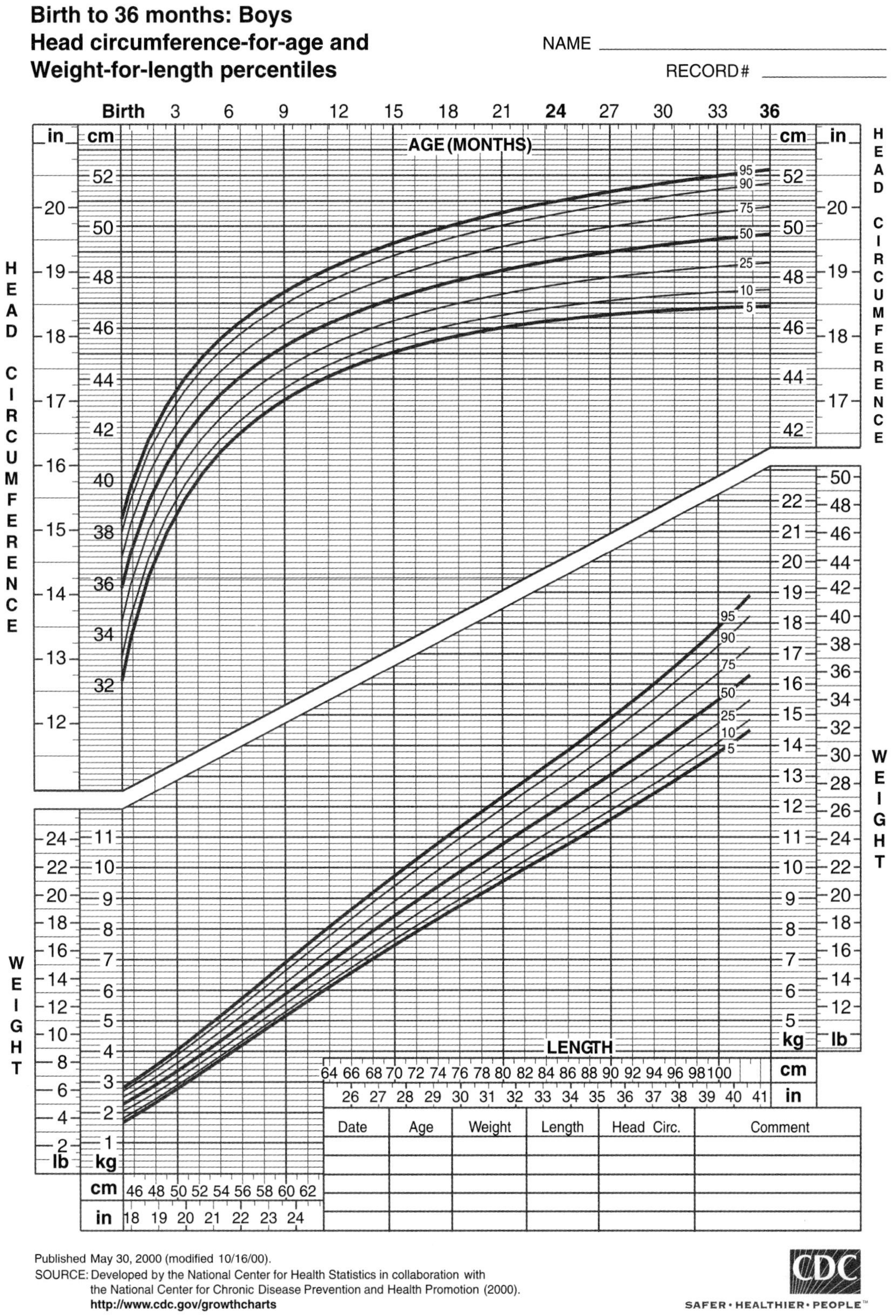

FIGURE B-2 Birth to 36 months: boys' head circumference–for–age and weight-for-length percentiles. (From the National Center for Health Statistics in collaboration with the National Center for Chronic Disease Prevention and Health Promotion, 2000. Available at *www.cdc.gov/growthcharts.*)

Birth to 36 months: Girls
Length-for-age and Weight-for-age percentiles

NAME ____________________

RECORD# ____________

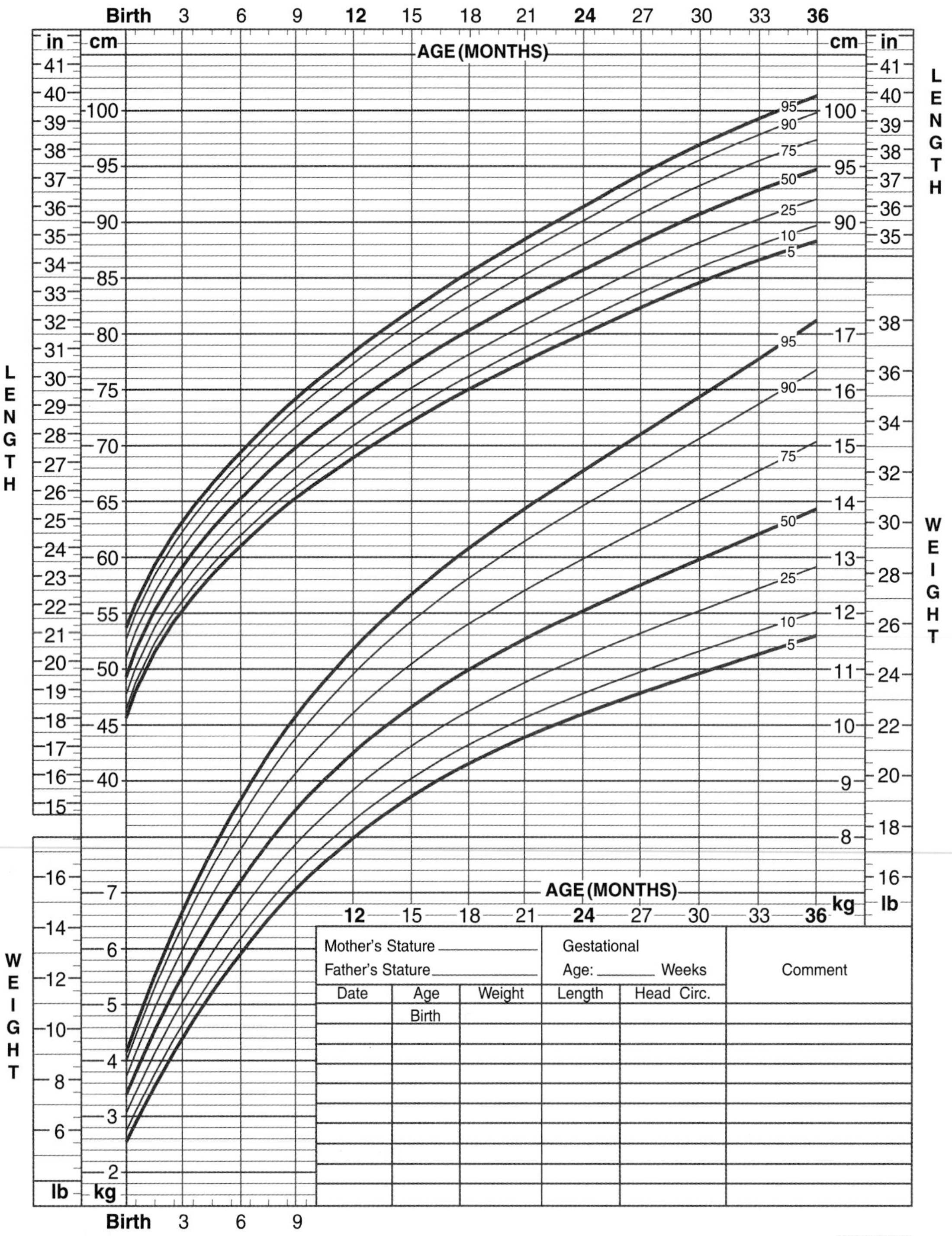

Published May 30, 2000 (modified 4/20/01).
SOURCE: Developed by the National Center for Health Statistics in collaboration with the National Center for Chronic Disease Prevention and Health Promotion (2000).
http://www.cdc.gov/growthcharts

CDC
SAFER • HEALTHIER • PEOPLE™

FIGURE B-3 Birth to 36 months: girls' length-for-age and weight-for-age percentiles. (From the National Center for Health Statistics in collaboration with the National Center for Chronic Disease Prevention and Health Promotion, 2000. Available at *www.cdc.gov/growthcharts*.)

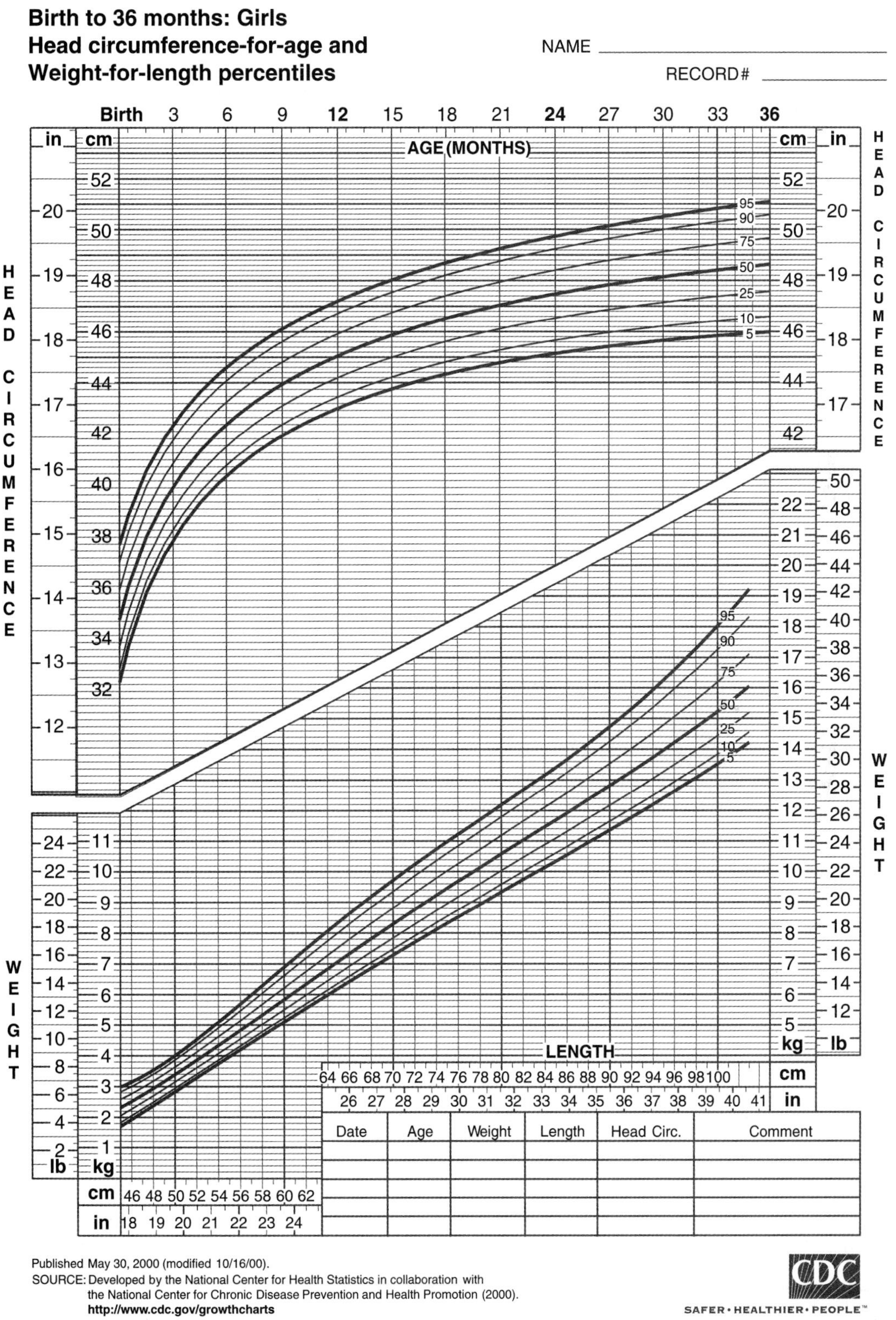

FIGURE B-4 Birth to 36 months: girls' head circumference–for–age and weight-for-length percentiles. (From the National Center for Health Statistics in collaboration with the National Center for Chronic Disease Prevention and Health Promotion, 2000. Available at *www.cdc.gov/growthcharts.*)

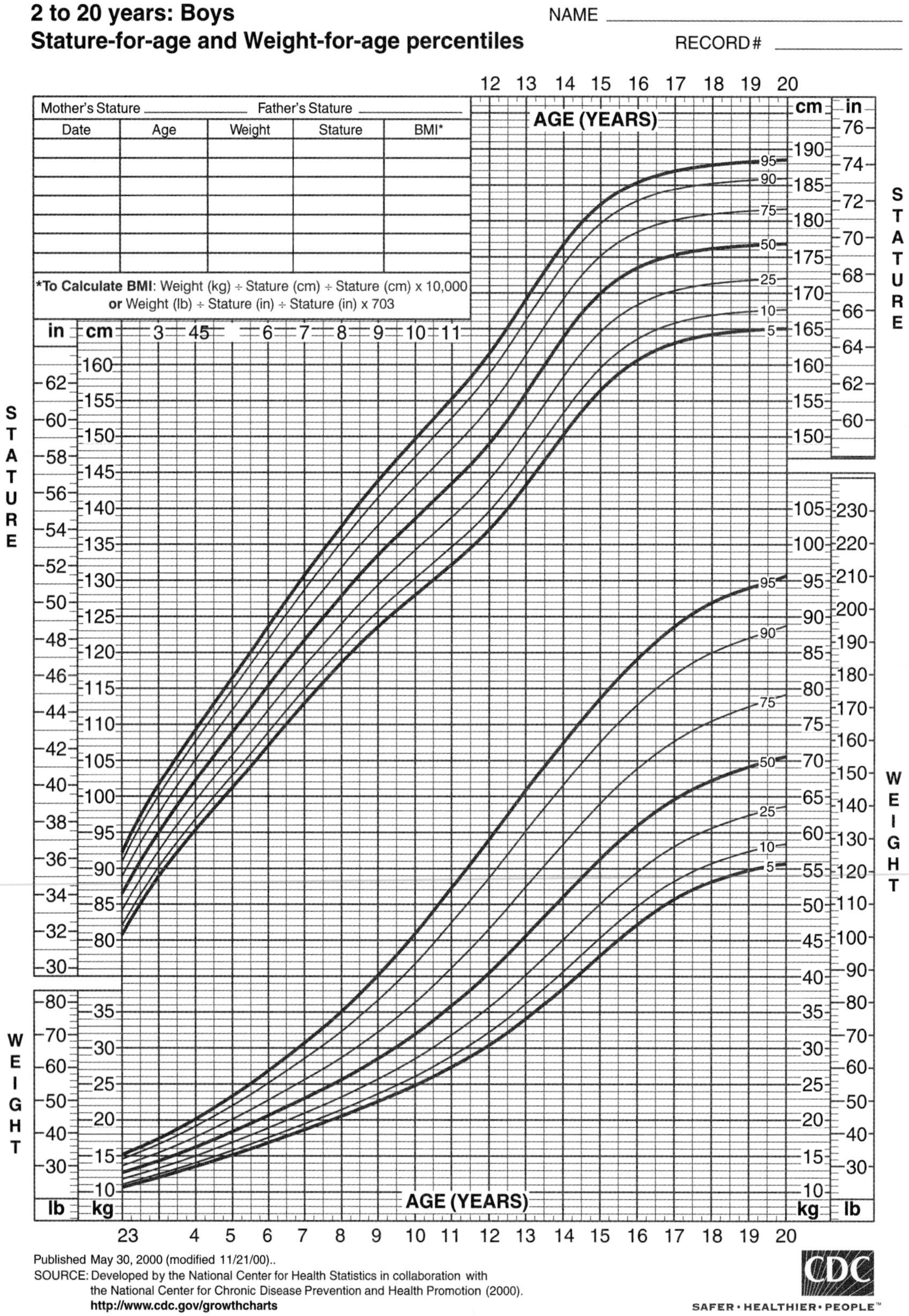

FIGURE B-5 Age 2 to 20 years: boys' weight-for-age and stature-for-age percentiles. (From the National Center for Health Statistics in collaboration with the National Center for Chronic Disease Prevention and Health Promotion, 2000. Available at *www.cdc.gov/growthcharts.*)

2 to 20 years: Boys
Body mass index-for-age percentiles

NAME ______________________

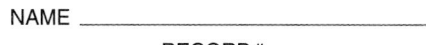

RECORD# __________

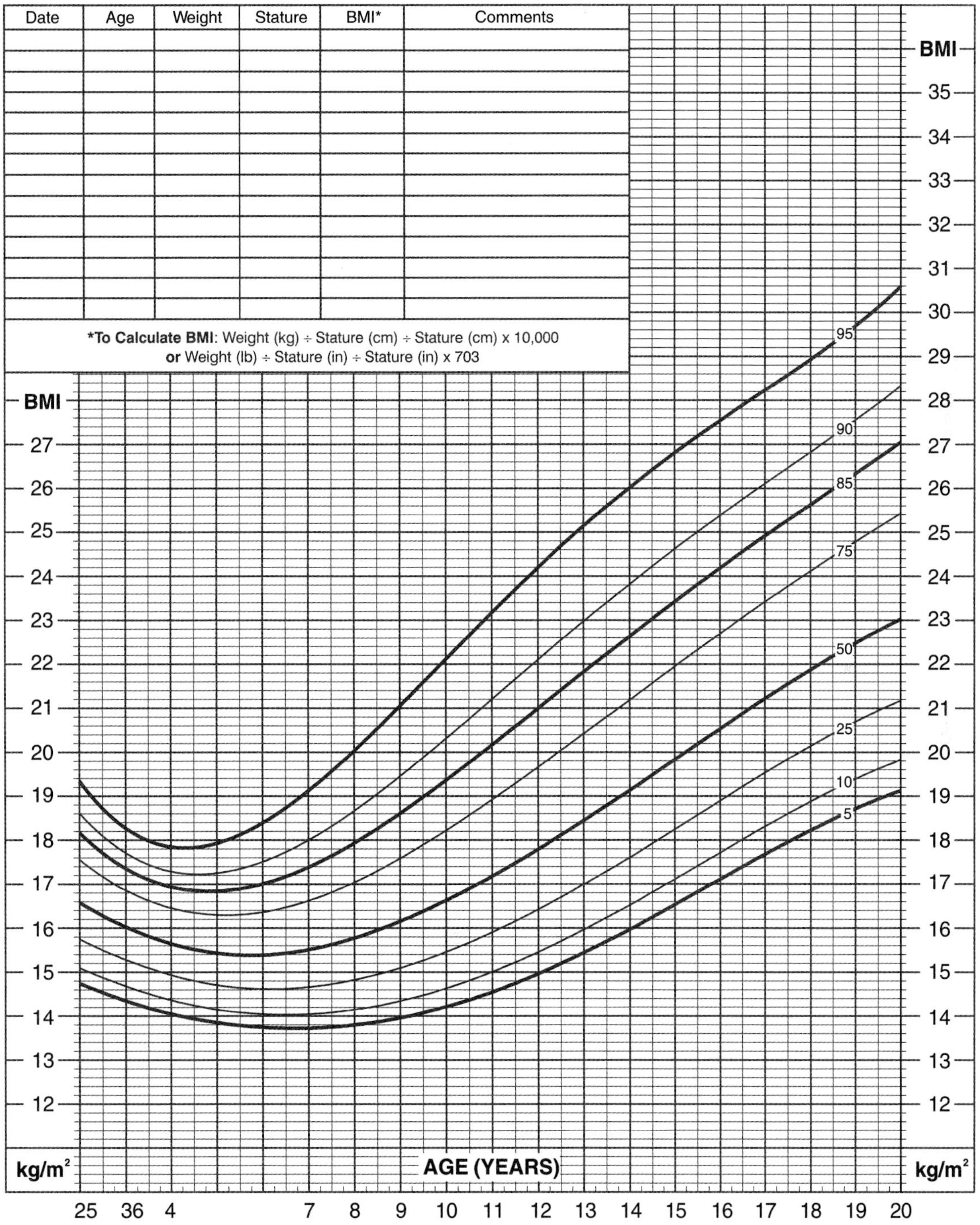

Published May 30, 2000 (modified 10/16/00).
SOURCE: Developed by the National Center for Health Statistics in collaboration with the National Center for Chronic Disease Prevention and Health Promotion (2000).
http://www.cdc.gov/growthcharts

CDC
SAFER • HEALTHIER • PEOPLE™

FIGURE B-6 Age 2 to 20 years: boys' body mass index–for–age percentiles. (From the National Center for Health Statistics in collaboration with the National Center for Chronic Disease Prevention and Health Promotion, 2000. Available at *www.cdc.gov/growthcharts.*)

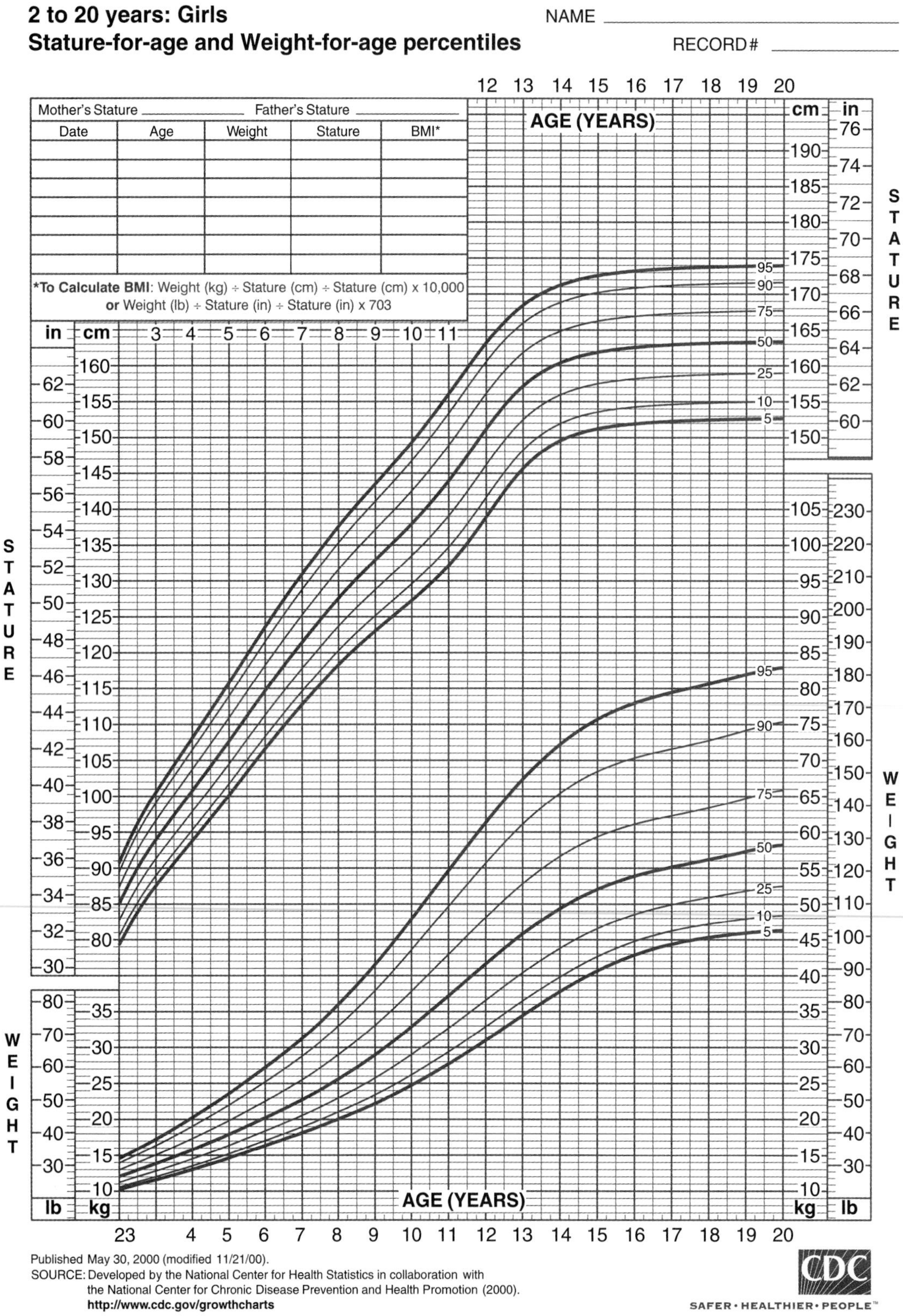

FIGURE B-7 Age 2 to 20 years: girls' weight-for-age and stature-for-age percentiles. (From the National Center for Health Statistics in collaboration with the National Center for Chronic Disease Prevention and Health Promotion, 2000. Available at *www.cdc.gov/growthcharts*.)

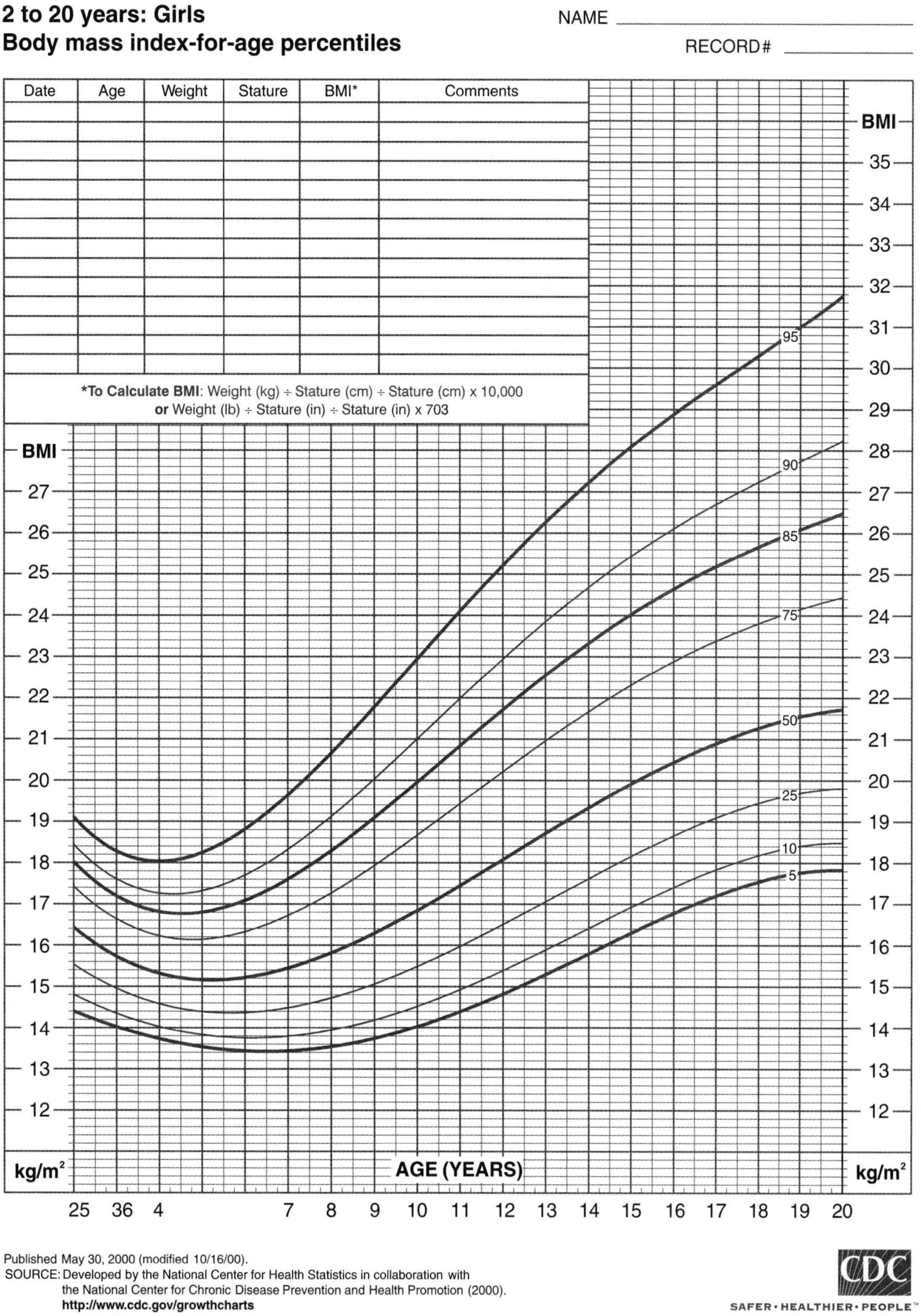

FIGURE B-8 Age 2 to 20 years: girls' body mass index–for–age percentiles. (From the National Center for Health Statistics in collaboration with the National Center for Chronic Disease Prevention and Health Promotion, 2000. Available at *www.cdc.gov/growthcharts.*)

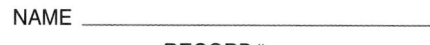

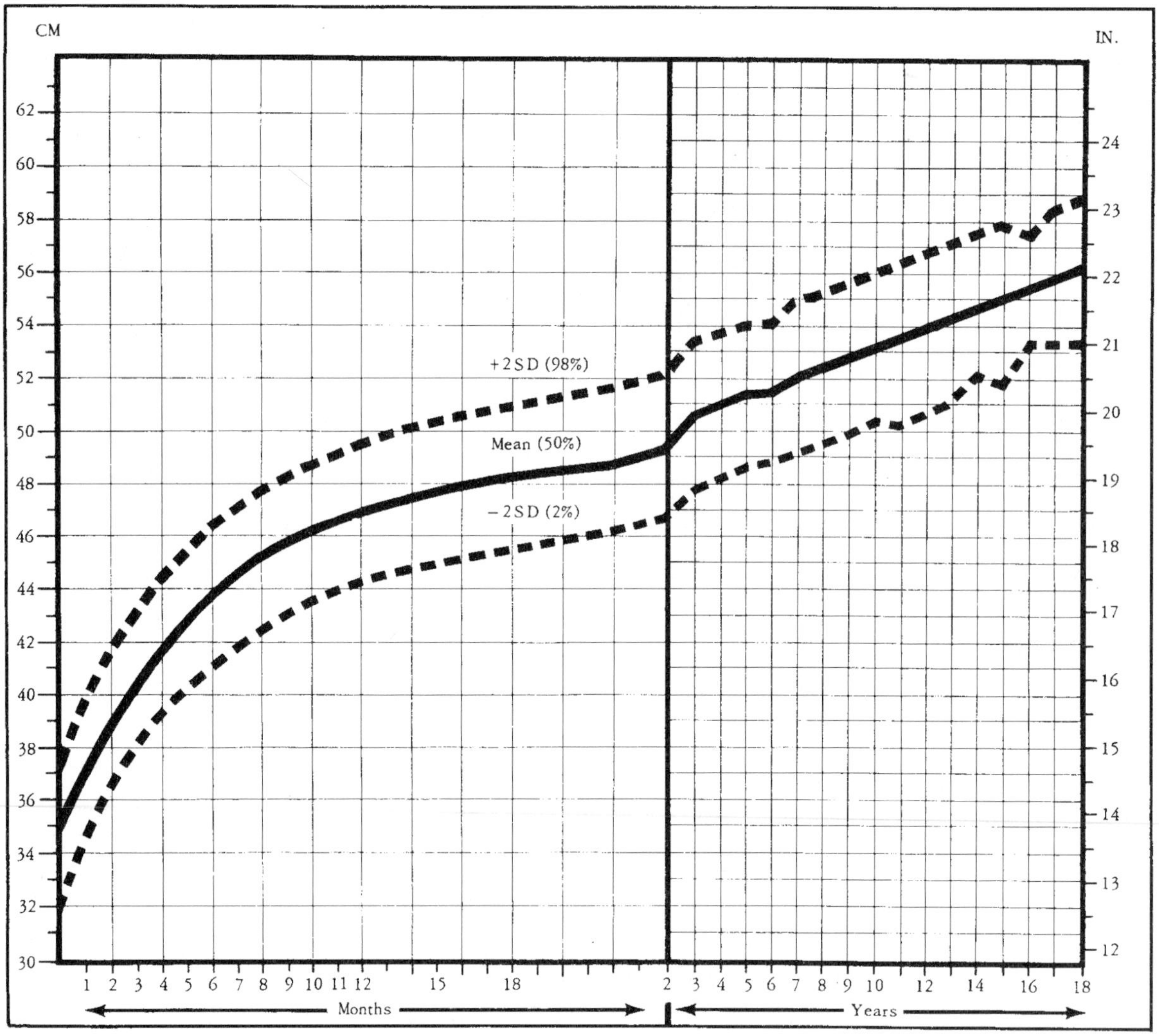

FIGURE B-9 Head circumference chart (boys). (From Nellhaus G: Head circumference from birth to eighteen years. Practical composite international and interracial graphs, *Pediatrics* 41:106-114, 1968.)

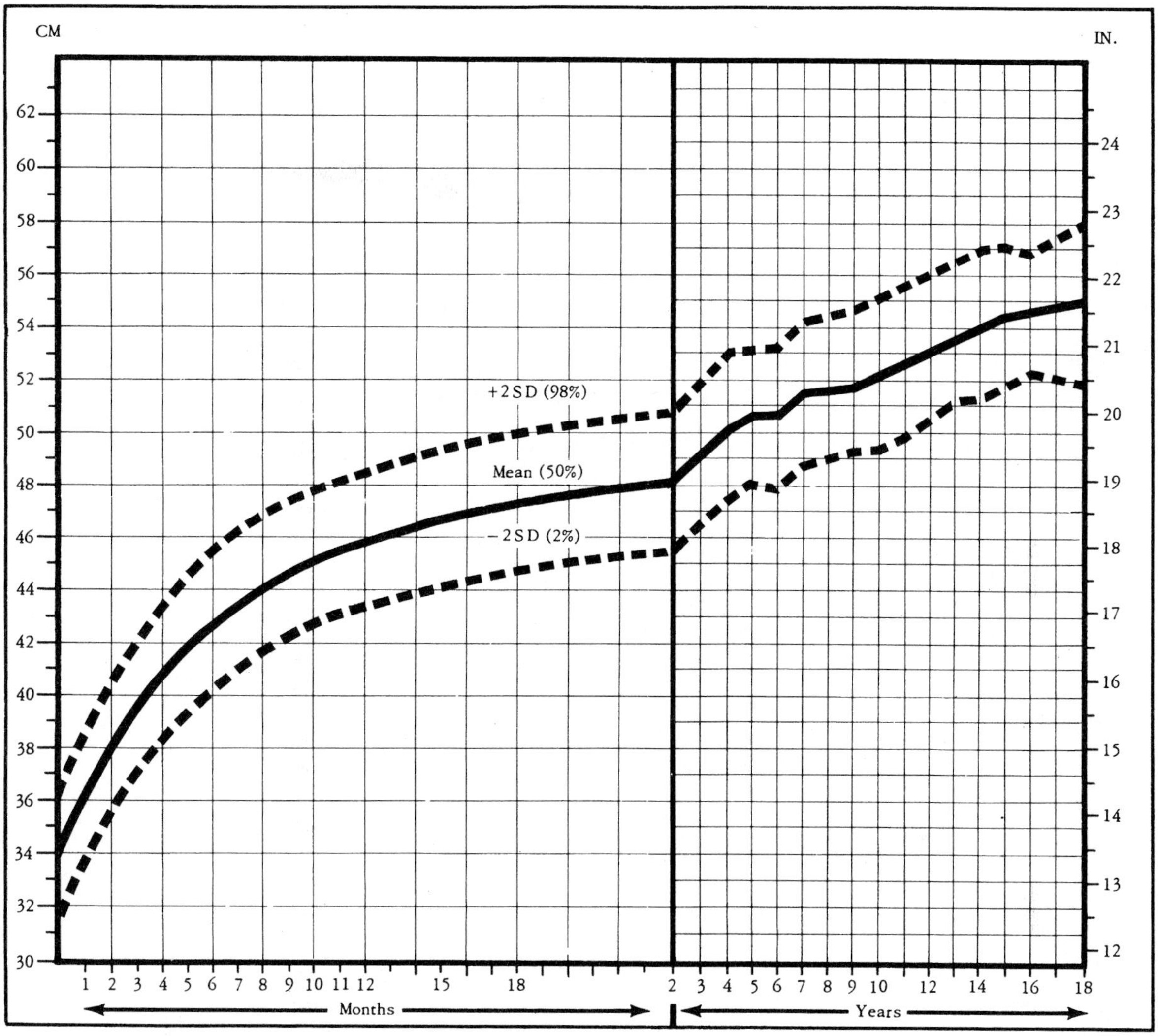

FIGURE B-10 Head circumference chart (girls). (From Nellhaus G: Head circumference from birth to eighteen years. Practical composite international and interracial graphs, *Pediatrics* 41:106-114, 1968.)

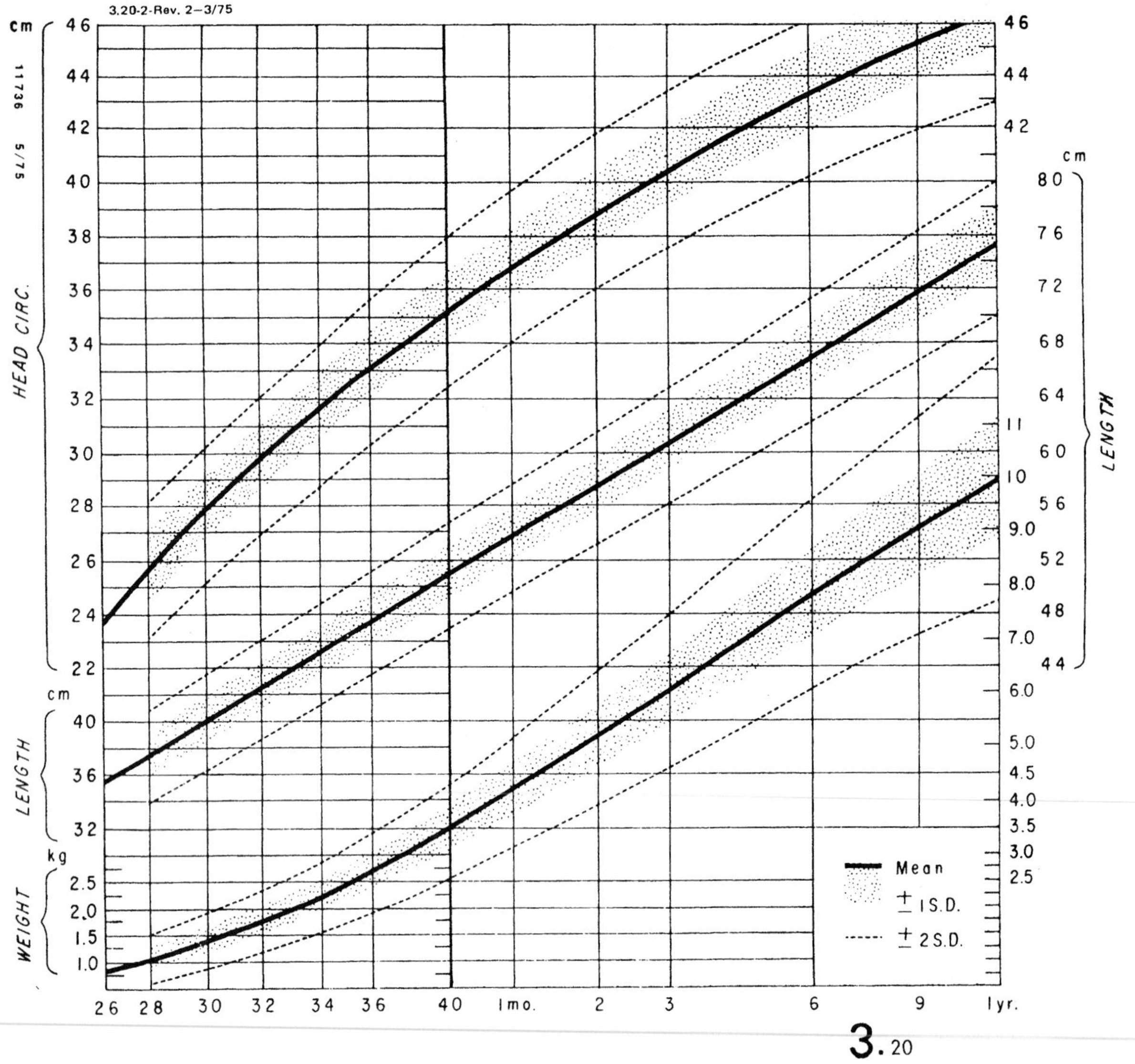

FIGURE B-11 Growth record for premature infants in relation to gestational age and fetal and infant norms. (From Babson S, Benda G: Growth graphs for the clinical assessment of infants of varying gestational age, *J Pediatr* 89:814-820, 1976.)

APPENDIX C

Normal Laboratory Values

Steven Goodstein, Catherine E. Burns

A limited selection of blood chemistry, urine, and hematologic values is presented as the most common laboratory screening tests requested. The authors recognize that the nurse practitioner may have a need for more complex tests, for example, cerebrospinal fluid studies, immunoglobulins, and therapeutic drug levels. The reader is directed to seek the source of these values from the performing laboratory, as well as its respective standards in comparison with control specimens. Some pediatric specimens need to be sent to a special laboratory for appropriate testing.

Laboratories use a variety of analytical methods to determine biochemical and hematologic values. Normal values for laboratory tests vary depending on the procedure used. Normal ranges reflect a combination of the population served, individual biologic differences, specimen collection and handling techniques, and intrinsic laboratory variation. Given this variability, if any questions arise, it is recommended that the reader consult with the reference laboratory for its methods and the established normal range of values for the methods used.

Interpretation of laboratory values can be a complex diagnostic exercise. In Table C-1, the comments in the Interpretation column are intended to offer the reader general ideas about each test and its common use. A skilled clinician uses laboratory data with other clinical data to make decisions, sometimes combining several tests to best understand the physiologic status of the client.

The laboratory values for this appendix have been compiled from tables in Behrman, Kliegman, and Jenson (2000), Burtis and Ashwood (1999), Fishbach (2000), and Free (1996).

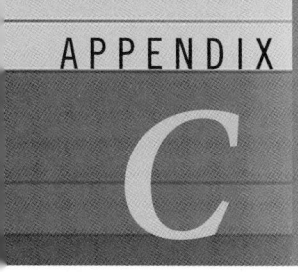

TABLE C-1 *Pediatric Laboratory Values*

Test Name	Reference Range		Interpretation
Blood Chemistry (from Serum)			
Alanine aminotransferase (ALT, SGPT) (U/L)	Newborn/infant	13-45	Liver, heart, and skeletal muscle have significant levels. High levels are associated with hepatic cell damage.
	Adult		
	M	10-40	
	F	7-35	
Amylase (U/L)	Newborn	5-65	Marked rise generally indicates acute pancreatitis.
	Adult	27-131	
Aspartate aminotransferase (AST, SGOT) (U/L)	Newborn	25-75	Elevated levels occur with heart, liver, and muscle disease.
	Infant	15-60	
	Adult	8-20	
Bilirubin, total (mg/dl)	Premature		Elevated levels occur with increased destruction of RBCs or impairment of liver excretory function.
	Cord blood	<2.0	
	0-1 day	<8.0	
	1-2 days	<12.0	
	3-5 days	<16.0	
	Full-term		
	Cord blood	<2.0	
	0-1 day	1.4-8.7	
	1-2 days	3.4-11.5	
	3-5 days	1.5-12.0	
	Adult	0.3-1.2	
Chloride (mmol/L)	Cord blood	96-104	Values increase in metabolic acidosis and other conditions. Decreased values occur with diuresis, GI losses, and other conditions.
	0-30 days	98-113	
	>30 days	98-107	
Cholesterol (5th-95th percentile, mg/dl)	Cord blood		Elevated levels indicate disorders of blood lipids.
	M	44-103	
	F	50-108	
	0-4 yr		
	M	114-203	
	F	112-200	
	5-9 yr		
	M	121-203	
	F	126-205	
	10-14 yr		
	M	119-202	
	F	124-201	
	15-19 yr		
	M	113-197	
	F	119-200	
	20-24 yr		
	M	124-218	
	F	122-216	
Creatinine (mg/dl)	Cord blood	0.6-1.2	Elevated levels indicate impaired renal function, muscle disease, congestive heart failure, shock, dehydration, and other conditions.
	Newborn	0.3-1.0	
	Infant	0.2-0.4	
	Child	0.3-0.7	
	Adolescent	0.5-1.0	
	Adult		
	M	0.7-1.3	
	F	0.6-1.1	
Ferritin (mg/ml)	Newborn	25-200	Ferritin is a more sensitive indicator than iron or TIBC for diagnosing iron deficiency or overload.
	1 mo	200-600	
	2-5 mo	50-200	

TABLE C-1 ***Pediatric Laboratory Values—cont'd***

Test Name	Reference Range		Interpretation
	6 mo-15 y	7-140	
	Adult		
	M	20-250	
	F	10-120	
Glucose (fasting) (mg/dl)	Cord blood	45-96	Fasting low levels may indicate a physiologic response or a disorder in glucose metabolism. Increased fasting levels may indicate diabetes mellitus, pancreatic disorders, endocrine diseases, drugs, and other conditions.
	Premature	20-60	
	Neonate	30-60	
	Newborn		
	1 day	40-60	
	>1 day	50-80	
	Child	60-100	
	Adult	74-106	
Iron (μg/dl)	Newborn	100-250	Decreased levels occur with iron deficiency, blood loss, and other conditions. Elevated levels occur with hemolytic anemias, iron intoxication, hepatitis, and other conditions.
	Infant	40-100	
	Child	50-120	
	Thereafter		
	M	65-175	
	F	50-170	
Lead (whole blood specimen) (μg/dl)	Child	<10	Increased levels indicate lead toxicity.
	Adult	<25	
	Toxic	≥100	
Potassium (mmol/L)	Newborn	3.7-5.9	Decreased levels may indicate shifting of potassium into cells, GI loss, biliary loss, renal loss, and reduced uptake. Increased levels occur with shifts to intracellular fluid, decreased excretion, or increased uptake.
	Infant	4.1-5.3	
	Child	3.4-4.7	
	Thereafter	3.5-5.1	
Sodium (mmol/L)	Newborn	133-146	Decreased levels indicate sodium loss or water excess (caused by numerous conditions). Increased levels may occur with an increase in sodium or an excessive loss of water (caused by numerous conditions).
	Infant	139-146	
	Child	138-145	
	Thereafter	136-145	
Thyrotropin (thyroid-stimulating hormone [TSH]) (μU/L)	Adult	0.4-4.2	Decreased levels are associated with hyperthyroidism. Increased levels are associated with hypothyroidism.
	Birth-4 days	1.0-39.0	
	2-20 wk	1.7-9.1	
	21 wk-20 yr	0.7-6.4	
Thyroxine, free (FT4) (ng/dl)	Newborn	2.6-6.3	Decreased levels are associated with hypothyroidism or overproduction of T3. Increased levels are associated with Graves' disease and thyrotoxicosis from overproduction of T4.
	Adult	0.8-2.7	
Thyroxine, total (T4) (μg/dl)	1-3 days	11.8-22.6	T4 serves as a good index of thyroid function only if binding globulin (TBG) is normal.
	1-2 wk	9.8-16.6	
	1-4 mo	7.2-14.4	
	4-12 mo	7.8-16.5	
	1-5 yr	7.3-15.0	
	5-10 yr	6.4-13.3	
	10-15 yr	5.6-11.7	
	Adult		
	M	4.6-10.5	
	F	5.5-11.0	
Urea nitrogen (BUN) (mg/dl)	Premature (1 wk)	3-25	Measures glomerular function and production/excretion of urea. Decreased with liver failure, malnutrition, and other conditions. Increased with impaired renal function, congestive heart failure, salt/water depletion, shock, and other conditions.
	Newborn	4-12	
	Infant/child	5-18	
	Adult	6-20	

Continued

TABLE C-1 *Pediatric Laboratory Values—cont'd*

Test Name	Reference Range		Interpretation
Hematology (Whole Blood Specimens)			
Erythrocyte count (RBC) (millions of cells/mm^3 [μl])	1-3 days (capillary)	4.0-6.6	Measures total number of RBCs. Decreased with anemia, cell destruction, and decreased production. Increased with increased RBC production, renal disease, tumors, altitude, pulmonary disease, cardiovascular diseases, and other conditions. A relative increase may occur with dehydration.
	1 wk	3.9-6.3	
	2 wk	3.6-6.2	
	1 mo	3.0-5.4	
	2 mo	2.7-4.9	
	3-6 mo	3.1-4.5	
	0.5-2 yr	3.7-5.3	
	2-6 yr	3.9-5.3	
	6-12 yr	4.0-5.2	
	12-18 yr		
	M	4.5-5.3	
	F	4.1-5.1	
	18-49 yr		
	M	4.5-5.9	
	F	4.0-5.2	
Erythrocyte sedimentation rate (ESR, sed rate) (mm/hr)	Westergren, modified		Not diagnostic, but indicates a disease process. Increases occur with collagen diseases, infections, inflammatory conditions, neoplasms, heavy metal poisoning, tissue destruction, and other conditions.
	Child	0-10	
	Adult		
	M <50 y	0-15	
	F <50 y	0-20	
	Wintrobe		
	Child	0-13	
	Adult		
	M	0-9	
	F	0-20	
Hematocrit (HCT, Hct) (% packed erythrocyte volume [erythrocyte volume/whole blood × 100])	1 day	48-69	Low values indicate blood loss or inadequate production or excess destruction of RBCs. High values indicate erythrocytosis, severe dehydration, shock, and other conditions.
	2 days	48-75	
	3 days	44-72	
	2 mo	28-42	
	6-12 yr	35-45	
	12-18 yr		
	M	37-49	
	F	36-46	
	18-49 yr		
	M	41-53	
	F	36-46	
Hemoglobin, total (Hb) (g/dl)	1-3 days	14.5-22.5	Decreased levels are found with anemia, hyperthyroidism, cirrhosis, severe hemorrhage, hemolysis, and systemic diseases. Very low values may lead to heart failure and death.
	2 mo	9.0-14.0	
	6-12 yr	11.5-15.5	
	12-18 yr		
	M	13.0-16.0	
	F	12.0-16.0	
	18-49 yr		
	M	13.5-17.5	
	F	12.0-16.0	
Leukocyte count (white blood cell [WBC] count) (× 1000 cells/mm^3)	Birth	9.0-30.0	Indicates total WBC count circulating in the blood. With some infections, WBCs increase as cells are transported. A low count may occur in overwhelming bacterial infection (sepsis) or with the use of immunosuppressive agents. Elevated levels may occur in response to an underlying disease, a primary cellular disorder (leukemia), pregnancy, corticosteroid treatment, strenuous exercise, and other conditions.
	24 hr	9.4-34.0	
	1 mo	5.0-19.5	
	1-3 yr	6.0-17.5	
	4-7 yr	5.5-15.5	
	8-13 yr	4.5-13.5	
	Adult	4.5-11.0	

TABLE C-1 *Pediatric Laboratory Values—cont'd*

Test Name	Reference Range		Interpretation
Leukocyte differential (%)	Myelocytes	0-0	Describes the proportion of the types of WBCs. Used in conjunction with the total leukocyte count to determine absolute cell counts. Neutrophils: usually increased during bacterial infections. May be decreased in viral infections. Bands are immature; segmented are more mature forms. Eosinophils: increased during allergic responses and parasitic infections. Basophils: increased in allergic reactions, hematologic disorders, and other conditions. Lymphocytes: increased in viral infections. T, B, and natural killer types. Monocytes: increased in severe and recovery stages of infections (phagocytosis). Myelocytes: involved in the early maturation of neutrophils, eosinophils, basophils, and monocytes.
	Neutrophils ("bands")	3-5	
	Neutrophils ("segs")	54-62	
	Lymphocytes	25-33	
	Monocytes	3-7	
	Eosinophils	1-3	
	Basophils	0-0.75	
Platelet count (thrombocyte count)	Newborn	84-478 × $10^3/mm^3$	Decreased platelet counts occur with anemias, some infections, congestive heart failure, bone marrow lesions, and other conditions. Increases occur with malignancies, splenectomy, collagen diseases, some anemias, and other conditions.
	1 wk-adult	150-400 × $10^3/mm^3$	
Reticulocyte count (%)	1 day	<0.4-6.0	Provides an estimate of the rate of RBC production. The percentage may be used to calculate the absolute value. An elevated count with normal hemoglobin indicates RBC loss with bone marrow compensation. A normal reticulocyte count with a low hemoglobin level indicates an inadequate response to anemia. Reticulocyte turns to erythrocyte in 24 hours.
	7 days	<0.1-1.3	
	1-4 wk	<0.1-1.2	
	5-6 wk	<0.1-2.4	
	7-8 wk	<0.1-2.9	
	9-10 wk	<0.1-2.6	
	11-12 wk	<0.1-1.3	
	Adult	<0.5-1.5	
Urine			
Urine, macroscopic	All ages		
Bilirubin		Negative	Increased in hepatocellular disease or intrahepatic/extrahepatic biliary obstruction.
Blood, occult		Negative	RBCs increased in acute glomerulonephritis, acute infections, renal calculi, trauma, and other conditions.
Glucose, qualitative		Negative	Increased when blood glucose level exceeds the reabsorption capacity of the renal tubes (pathologic or benign).
Hemoglobin		Negative	Hemoglobinuria may occur in intravascular hemolysis and other conditions.
Ketones		Negative	Increased with adequate carbohydrate intake or a defect in carbohydrate metabolism. Especially significant with diabetes mellitus.
Leukocyte esterase		Negative	Measures WBCs. Increase indicates inflammation or infection (or both). Associated with certain renal diseases and diseases of the urinary tract or vaginitis.
Nitrite		Negative	Positive associated with urinary tract infection.
pH		4.6-8.0	Indication of acid-base balance.
Protein, qualitative		Negative	Increased in pathologic or physiologic conditions (e.g., fever, stress, strenuous exercises).
Specific gravity		1.001-1.030	Measures the concentrating and diluting ability of the kidney. Associated with tubular damage.
Urobilinogen		0.2-1.0 mg/dl	Increased in liver disease. Decreased in obstruction of bile ducts and other conditions.

Continued

TABLE C-1 *Pediatric Laboratory Values—cont'd*

Test Name	Reference Range		Interpretation
Urine, microscopic			
Casts			
Hyaline		0-1/lpf	Hyaline casts: increased in pathologic or physiologic conditions. Implies damage to the glomerular capillary membrane permitting leakage of proteins through the glomerular filtrate.
Other		None	Other casts: involved in a variety of conditions depending on the type of cast. Involved in tubular epithelial damage (epithelial cell cast), renal infection (WBC cast), vascular disorder (RBC cast), renal disease (granular cast), chronic renal condition (waxy cast), severe renal disease (broad cast), and degenerative tubular disease (fatty cast).
Red blood cells (RBCs)		0-2/hpf	RBCs: denote bleeding into the urinary system.
White blood cells (WBCs)	M	0-3/hpf	WBCs: associated with an inflammatory process.
	F and children	0-5/hpf	
Urine volume (ml/24 hr)	Newborn	50-300	Decreased in dehydration, renal ischemia, renal disease, obstruction, and other conditions. Increased in diabetes insipidus, diabetes mellitus, chronic progressive renal failure, and other conditions.
	Infant	350-550	
	Child	500-1000	
	Adolescent	700-1400	
	Thereafter		
	M	800-1800	
	F	600-1600	

BUN, Blood urea nitrogen; *GI*, gastrointestinal; *hpf*, high-power field; *lpf*, low-power field; *T3*, triiodothyronine; *TBG*, thyroxin-binding globulin; *TIBC*, total iron-binding capacity.

TABLE C-2 *Evaluation of Bleeding Disorders*

Test	Mechanism	Normal Values*	Examples of Disorders
Prothrombin time	Extrinsic to common pathway	Neonate: 12-18 sec Postneonate: <12 sec	Defect in vitamin K–dependent factors, hemorrhagic disease of newborn, malabsorption; liver disease, DIC, oral anticoagulants
Activated partial thromboplastin time (APTT, PTT)	Intrinsic and common pathway	Neonate: 70 sec Postneonate: 25-40 sec	Hemophilia, von Willebrand, heparin, DIC, deficient factors
Thrombin time (TT)	Fibrinogen to fibrin	Neonate: 12-17 sec Postneonate: 10-15 sec	Fibrin split products, DIC, low fibrin level, heparin, uremia
Bleeding time (BT)	Hemostasis, capillary and platelet function	Postneonate: 3-7 min	Platelet dysfunctions, low platelet count, von Willebrand, aspirin
Platelet count (see Table C-1)	—	—	—
Peripheral blood smear	Number and shape of blood cells	—	Platelets: peripheral destruction disorder RBCs: suggest microangiopathic process (e.g., HUS, hemangioma, DIC) WBCs: number and differential suggest infections, leukemias, etc.

*Values will vary from laboratory to laboratory based on the technology used. The values here are typical but should not be considered as absolute normal values. Use the norms recorded on laboratory slips as another guide to decide whether a given value is abnormal or normal. And, of course, use clinical judgment because most disorders are defined by a variety of signs, symptoms, and test values.
DIC, Disseminated intravascular coagulation; *HUS*, hemolytic-uremic syndrome; *RBCs*, red blood cells; *WBCs*, white blood cells.

TABLE C-3 *Red Blood Cell Indices (May Be Used to Differentiate Anemias)*

Index	Definition	Calculation (Usually Done Electronically)
Mean corpuscular volume (MCV)	Average volume of RBC expressed as femtoliters (fl)	Hct (%) × 10/RBC count (×10^{12}/L)
Mean corpuscular hemoglobin (MCH)	Average weight of hemoglobin in an RBC expressed in picograms (pg)	Hb (g/dl) × 10/RBC count (×10^{12}/L)
Mean corpuscular hemoglobin concentration (MCHC)	Average concentration of hemoglobin in the RBC expressed as grams per deciliter (g/dl)	Hb (g/dl) × 100/Hct (%)
Red cell distribution width (RDW)	A measure of anisocytosis; the coefficient of variation of the RBC size determined on automated blood cell counting instruments expressed as a percent	Standard deviation of RBC size/mean corpuscular volume. Normal range: 11.5%-14.5%

NOTE: Normal values will vary depending on the technology used. Generally all of these values are calculated electronically.

Age	MCV (fl)	MCH (pg)	MCHC (g/dl)
0-1 day	95-125	30-42	30-34
2-4 days	98-118	30-42	30-34
5-7 days	100-120	30-42	30-34
8-14 days	95-115	30-42	30-34
15-30 days	93-113	28-40	30-34
1-2 mo	83-107	27-37	31-36
3-5 mo	83-107	25-35	32-36
6-11 mo	78-102	23-31	32-36
1-3 yr	76-92	23-31	32-36
4-7 yr	78-94	23-31	32-36
8 yr-adult	80-94	26-32	32-36

Data from Rodak B: *Hematology clinical principles and applications*, ed 2, Philadelphia, 2002, WB Saunders.

REFERENCES

Behrman R, Kliegman R, Jenson H, editors: *Nelson textbook of pediatrics*, ed 17, Philadelphia, 2004, WB Saunders.

Burtis C, Ashwood E: *Tietz textbook of clinical chemistry*, ed 3, Philadelphia, 1999, WB Saunders.

Fishbach F: *A manual of laboratory and diagnostic tests*, ed 6, Philadelphia, 2000, JB Lippincott.

Free HM, editor: *Modern urine chemistry*, Tarrytown, NY, 1996, Bayer.

APPENDIX D

Healthy People 2010 Objectives Focused on Children and Adolescents

The following goals and objectives are extracted from *Healthy People 2010: Understanding and Improving Health,* second edition (US Department of Health and Human Services, 2000). The objectives included here represent current thinking about the directions that health care should take over the next 10 years and the roles that individuals, schools, communities, and health care providers should assume in creating a more healthy population. Only objectives directly related to the health of infants, children, and adolescents are included in this appendix. Generally, the major child health themes are included. The numbers in parentheses after objectives indicate the objective numbers in the government document.

HEALTHY PEOPLE 2010 GOALS

There are two goals for the nation's health as of 2010: (1) to increase the quality and years of healthy life and (2) to eliminate health disparities. "Healthy People 2010 seeks to increase life expectancy and quality of life over the next 10 years by helping individuals gain the knowledge, motivation, and opportunities they need to make informed decisions about their health. At the same time Healthy People 2010 encourages local and State leaders to develop community wide and statewide efforts that promote healthy behaviors, create healthy environments, and increase access to high-quality health care" (US Department of Health and Human Services, 2000, p. 10). Leading health indicators include the following:

- Physical activity
- Overweight and obesity
- Tobacco use
- Substance abuse
- Responsible sexual behavior
- Mental health
- Injury and violence
- Environmental quality
- Immunization
- Access to health care

HEALTHY PEOPLE 2010 OBJECTIVES

Access to Quality Health Services

Goal: Improve access to comprehensive, high-quality health care across a continuum of care.

1. Increase the proportion of persons with health insurance (1-1).
2. Increase the proportion of insured persons with coverage for clinical preventive services (1-2).
3. Increase the proportion of persons appropriately counseled about health behaviors (1-3).
4. Increase the proportion of persons with a usual primary care provider (1-5).
5. Increase the proportion of physicians, physician assistants, nurses, and other clinicians who receive appropriate training to address important health disparities: disease prevention and health promotion, minority health, women's health, geriatrics (1-7).

Cancer

Goal: Reduce the number of new cancer cases as well as the illness, disability, and death caused by cancer.

1. Increase the proportion of persons who use at least one of the following protective measures that may reduce the risk of skin cancer: avoid the sun between 10 AM and 4 PM, wear sun-protective clothing when exposed to sunlight, use sunscreen with a sun-protective factor (SPF) of 15 or higher, and avoid artificial sources of ultraviolet light (3-9).

Disability and Secondary Conditions

Goal: Promote the health of people with disabilities, prevent secondary conditions, and eliminate disparities between people with and without disabilities in the U.S. population.

1. Reduce the proportion of children and adolescents with disabilities who are reported to be sad, unhappy, or depressed (6-2).
2. Increase the proportion of children and youth with disabilities who spend at least 80% of their time in regular education programs (6-9).
3. Reduce the proportion of people with disabilities reporting environmental barriers to participation in home, school, work, or community activities (6-12).

Education and Community-Based Programs

Goal: Increase the quality, availability, and effectiveness of educational and community-based programs designed to prevent disease and improve the health and quality of life.

1. Increase high school completion (7-1).
2. Increase the proportion of middle, junior high, and senior high schools that provide school health education to prevent health problems in the following areas: unintentional injury; violence; suicide; tobacco use and addiction; alcohol and other drug use; unintended pregnancy, HIV/AIDS, and STD infection; unhealthy dietary patterns; inadequate physical activity; and environmental health (7-2).
3. Increase the proportion of college and university students who receive information from their institution on each of the six priority health-risk areas [injuries, tobacco use, alcohol and illicit drug use, sexual behaviors that cause unintended pregnancy and STDs, dietary patterns that cause disease, and inadequate physical activity] (7-3).
4. Increase the proportion of the Nation's elementary, middle, junior high, and senior high schools that have a nurse-to-student ratio of at least 1:750 (7-4).
5. Increase the proportion of health care organizations that provide patient and family education (7-7).
6. Increase the proportion of patients who report that they are satisfied with the patient education they receive from their health care organization (7-8).
7. Increase the proportion of hospitals and managed care organizations that provide community disease prevention and health promotion activities that address the priority health needs identified by their community (7-9).
8. Increase the proportion of local health service areas/jurisdictions that have established a community health promotion program that addresses multiple *Healthy People 2010* focus areas (7-10).
9. Increase the proportion of local health departments that have established culturally appropriate and linguistically competent community health promotion and disease prevention programs (7-11).

Environmental Health

Goal: Promote health for all through a healthy environment.

1. Reduce the proportion of persons exposed to air that does not meet the U.S. Environmental Protection Agency's health-based standards for harmful pollutants (8-1). [Also 8-2 to 8-4 relate to air quality standards.]
2. [Several objectives relate to healthy water supplies—8-5 to 8-10.]
3. Eliminate elevated blood lead levels in children (8-11).
4. Reduce pesticide exposures that result in visits to a health care facility (8-13).
5. Increase the proportion of the Nation's primary and secondary schools that have official school policies ensuring the safety of students and staff from environmental hazards, such as chemicals in specific classrooms, poor indoor air quality, asbestos, and exposure to pesticides (8-20).

Other standards relate to outdoor air quality, water quality, toxics and waste, healthy homes and healthy communities, infrastructure and surveillance, and global environmental health.

Family Planning

Goal: Improve pregnancy planning and spacing and prevent unintended pregnancy.

1. Increase the proportion of pregnancies that are intended (9-1).
2. Reduce the proportion of births occurring within 24 months of a previous birth (9-2).
3. Increase the proportion of females at risk of unintended pregnancy (and their partners) who use contraception (9-3).
4. Reduce the proportion of females experiencing pregnancy despite use of a reversible contraceptive method (9-4).
5. Increase the proportion of health care providers who provide emergency contraception (9-5).

6. Increase male involvement in pregnancy prevention and family planning efforts (9-6).
7. Reduce pregnancies among adolescent females (9-7).
8. Increase the proportion of adolescents who have never engaged in sexual intercourse before age 15 years (9-8).
9. Increase the proportion of adolescents who have never engaged in sexual intercourse (9-9).
10. Increase the proportion of sexually active, unmarried adolescents age 15 to 17 years who use contraception that both effectively prevents pregnancy and provides barrier protection against disease (9-10).
11. Increase the proportion of young adults who have received formal instruction before turning 18 on reproductive health issues, including the following topics: birth control methods, safer sex to prevent HIV, prevention of sexually transmitted diseases, and abstinence (9-11).

Food Safety

Goal: Reduce the number of food-borne illnesses. (No objectives are specific to children, although all are inclusive of them.)

Human Immunodeficiency Virus Infection

Goal: Prevent HIV transmission and associated morbidity and mortality by (1) ensuring that all persons at risk for HIV infection know their serostatus, (2) ensuring that persons not infected with HIV remain uninfected, (3) ensuring that persons infected with HIV do not transmit HIV to others, and (4) ensuring that those infected with HIV are accessing the most effective therapies possible.

1. Reduce AIDS [and cases of HIV] among adolescents and adults (13-1, 13-5).
2. Reduce the number of new AIDS cases among adolescent and adult men who have sex with men (13-2).
3. Reduce the number of new AIDS cases among females and males who inject drugs (13-3).
4. Increase the proportion of sexually active persons who use condoms (13-6).
5. Increase the percentage of HIV-infected adolescents and adults in care who receive testing, treatment, and prophylaxis consistent with current Public Health Service treatment guidelines (13-13).

Immunization and Infectious Diseases

Goal: Prevent disease, disability, and death from infectious diseases, including vaccine-preventable diseases.

1. Reduce or eliminate indigenous cases of vaccine-preventable diseases (14-1).
2. Reduce chronic hepatitis B infections in infants and young children (perinatal infections) (14-2).
3. Reduce hepatitis B (14-3).
4. Decrease bacterial meningitis in young children (14-4).
5. Reduce invasive pneumococcal infections, hepatitis A, meningococcal disease, Lyme disease, hepatitis C, tuberculosis, invasive early-onset group B streptococcal disease (14-5, 14-6, 14-7, 14-8, 14-9, 14-11, 14-16).
6. Reduce the number of courses of antibiotics for ear infections for young children (14-18).
7. Reduce the number of courses of antibiotics prescribed for the sole diagnosis of the common cold (14-19).
8. Achieve and maintain effective vaccination coverage levels for universally recommended vaccines among young children (14-22).
9. Maintain vaccination coverage levels for children in licensed day care facilities and children in kindergarten through the first grade (14-23).
10. Increase the proportion of young children and adolescents who receive all vaccines that have been recommended for universal administration for at least 5 years (14-24).
11. Increase the proportion of providers who have measured the vaccination coverage levels among children in their practice population within the past 2 years (14-25).
12. Increase the proportion of children who participate in fully functional population-based immunization registries (14-26).
13. Increase the vaccination coverage levels for adolescents (14-27).
14. Increase hepatitis B vaccination coverage among high-risk groups (14-28).
15. Reduce the number of vaccine-associated adverse reactions (14-30).

Injury/Violence Prevention

Goal: Reduce injuries, disabilities, and deaths due to unintentional injuries and violence.

1. Reduce hospitalizations for nonfatal head injuries [also nonfatal spinal cord injuries] (15-1, 15-2).
2. Reduce firearm-related deaths [and injuries]. (15-3, 15-5).
3. Reduce the proportion of persons living in homes with firearms that are loaded and unlocked (15-4).
4. Reduce nonfatal poisonings [and deaths caused by poisonings] (15-7, 15-8).
5. Reduce deaths caused by suffocation [also falls] (15-9, 15-27).
6. Reduce deaths caused by unintentional injuries [also nonfatal unintentional injuries, drownings] (15-13, 15-14, 15-29).

7. Reduce deaths caused by motor vehicle crashes [also pedestrian deaths and injuries, nonfatal motor vehicle injuries] (15-15, 15-16, 15-17, 15-18).
8. Increase the use of safety belts [also child restraints] (15-19, 15-20).
9. Increase the proportion of motorcyclists using helmets [also bicyclists] (15-21, 15-23).
10. Reduce residential fire deaths (15-25).
11. Increase functioning residential smoke alarms (15-26).
12. Reduce hospital emergency department visits for nonfatal dog bite injuries (15-30).
13. Increase the proportion of public and private schools that require use of appropriate head, face, eye, and mouth protection for students participating in school-sponsored physical activities (15-31).
14. Reduce homicides (15-32).
15. Reduce maltreatment and maltreatment fatalities of children (15-33).
16. Reduce the annual rate of rape or attempted rape [also sexual assault] (15-35, 15-36).
17. Reduce physical assaults (15-37).
18. Reduce physical fighting among adolescents (15-38).
19. Reduce weapon carrying by adolescents on school property (15-39).

Maternal, Infant, and Child Care

Goal: Improve the health and well-being of women, infants, children, and families.

1. Reduce fetal and infant deaths (16-1).
2. Reduce the rate of child deaths [also adolescents and young adults] (16-2, 16-3).
3. Reduce maternal deaths (16-4).
4. Increase the proportion of pregnant women who receive early and adequate prenatal care (16-6).
5. Increase the percentage of healthy full-term infants who are put down to sleep on their backs (16-13).
6. Reduce the occurrence of developmental disabilities (16-14).
7. Increase abstinence from alcohol, cigarettes, and illicit drugs among pregnant women (16-17).
8. Reduce the sudden infant death syndrome mortality rate to 0.3 per 1000 live births.
9. Reduce the rate of child mortality to 30 per 100,000 children age 1 to 4 years and 17 per 100,000 children age 5 to 14 years.
10. Increase the proportion of mothers who breastfeed their babies (16-19).
11. Ensure appropriate newborn bloodspot screening, follow-up testing, and referral to services (16-20).
12. Reduce hospitalization for life-threatening sepsis among children 4 years and under with sickling hemoglobinopathies (16-21).

Mental Health and Mental Disorders

Goal: Improve mental health and ensure access to appropriate, quality mental health services.

1. Reduce the suicide rate (18-1).
2. Reduce the rate of suicide attempts by adolescents (18-2).
3. Reduce the relapse rates for persons with eating disorders including anorexia nervosa and bulimia nervosa (18-5).
4. Increase the number of persons seen in primary health care who receive mental health screening and assessment (18-6).
5. Increase the proportion of children with mental health problems who receive treatment (18-7).
6. Increase the proportion of juvenile justice facilities that screen new admissions for mental health problems (18-8).

Nutrition and Overweight

Goal: Promote health and reduce chronic disease associated with diet and weight.

1. Reduce the proportion of children and adolescents who are overweight or obese (19-3).
2. Reduce growth retardation among low-income children under age 5 years (19-4).
3. Increase the proportion of persons age 2 years and older who consume at least two daily servings of fruit (19-5).
4. Increase the proportion of persons age 2 years and older who consume at least three daily servings of vegetables, with at least one third being dark green or orange vegetables (19-6).
5. Increase the proportion of persons age 2 years and older who consume at least six daily servings of grain products, with at least three being whole grains (19-7).
6. Increase the proportion of people age 2 years and older who consume less than 10% of calories from saturated fat (19-8).
7. Increase the proportion of persons age 2 years and older who consume no more than 30% of calories from total fat (19-9).
8. Increase the proportion of persons age 2 years and older who consume 2400 mg or less of sodium daily (19-10).
9. Increase the proportion of persons age 2 years and older who meet dietary recommendations for calcium (19-11).
10. Reduce iron deficiency among young children and females of childbearing age (19-12).

11. Increase the proportion of children and adolescents age 6 to 19 years whose intake of meals and snacks at school contributes to good overall dietary quality (19-15).

Oral Health

Goal: Prevent and control oral and craniofacial diseases, conditions, and injuries and improve access to related services.

1. Reduce the proportion of children and adolescents who have dental caries experience in their primary or permanent teeth (21-1).
2. Reduce the proportion of children, adolescents, and adults with untreated dental decay (21-2).
3. Increase the proportion of children who have received protective sealants on their molar teeth (21-8).
4. Increase the proportion of the U.S. population served by community water systems with optimally fluoridated water (21-9).
5. Increase the proportion of children and adults who use the oral health care system each year (21-10).
6. Increase the proportion of low-income children and adolescents who received any preventive dental health service during the past year (21-12).
7. Increase the proportion of school-based health centers with an oral health component (21-13).
8. Increase the proportion of local health departments and community-based health centers, including community, migrant, and homeless health centers, that have an oral health component. (21-14).

Physical Activity and Fitness

Goal: Improve health, fitness, and quality of life through daily physical activity.

1. Increase the proportion of adolescents who engage in moderate physical activity for at least 30 minutes on 5 or more of the previous 7 days (22-6).
2. Increase the proportion of adolescents who engage in vigorous physical activity that promotes cardiorespiratory fitness 3 or more days per week for 20 or more minutes per occasion (22-7).
3. Increase the proportion of the nation's public and private schools that require daily physical education for all students (22-8).
4. Increase the proportion of adolescents who participate in daily school physical education (22-9).
5. Increase the proportion of adolescents who spend at least 50% of school physical education class time being physically active (22-10).
6. Increase the proportion of adolescents who view television 2 or fewer hours on a school day (22-11).
7. Increase the proportion of trips made by walking [also bicycling] (22-14, 22-15).

Public Health Infrastructure

Goal: Ensure that Federal, Tribal, State, and local health agencies have the infrastructure to provide essential public health services effectively.

These objectives relate to collection and management of national and local data related to health, provision of services by agencies, national performance standards for pubic health services, statutes to support public health, and proportions of agencies that conduct or collaborate on population-based research.

Respiratory Diseases

Goal: Promote respiratory health through better prevention, detection, treatment, and education efforts.

1. Reduce asthma deaths [and hospitalizations and emergency department visits] (24-1, 24-2, 24-3).
2. Reduce activity limitations among persons with asthma (24-4).
3. Reduce the number of school or work days missed by persons with asthma due to asthma (24-5).
4. Increase the proportion of persons with asthma who receive formal patient education, including information about community and self-help resources, as an essential part of the management of their condition (24-6).
5. Increase the proportion of persons with asthma who receive appropriate asthma care according to the NAEPP Guidelines (24-7).
6. Increase the proportion of persons with symptoms of obstructive sleep apnea whose condition is medically managed (24-11).

Sexually Transmitted Diseases

Goal: Promote responsible sexual behaviors, strengthen community capacity, and increase access to quality services to prevent sexually transmitted diseases (STDs) and their complications.

1. Reduce the proportion of adolescents and young adults with Chlamydia trachomatis infections (25-1).
2. Reduce gonorrhea (25-2).
3. Reduce the proportion of persons with genital herpes [and human papillomavirus (HPV)] infection (25-5, 25-6).
4. Reduce the proportion of females who have ever required treatment for pelvic inflammatory disease (PID) (25-6).

5. Reduce HIV infections in adolescent and young adult females age 13 to 24 years that are associated with heterosexual contact (25-8).
6. Reduce neonatal consequences from maternal sexually transmitted diseases, including chlamydial pneumonia, gonococcal and chlamydial ophthalmia neonatorum, laryngeal papillomatosis (from human papillomavirus infection), neonatal herpes, and preterm birth and low birth weight associated with bacterial vaginosis (25-10).
7. Increase the proportion of adolescents who abstain from sexual intercourse or use condoms if currently sexually active (25-11).
8. Increase the number of positive messages related to responsible sexual behavior during weekday and nightly prime-time television programming (25-12).
9. Increase the proportion of youth detention facilities and adult city or county jails that screen for common bacterial sexually transmitted diseases within 24 hours of admission and treat STDs (when necessary) before persons are released (25-14).
10. Increase the proportion of sexually active females age 25 years and under who are screened annually for genital chlamydia infections (25-16).
11. Increase the proportion of primary care providers who treat patients with sexually transmitted diseases and who manage cases according to recognized standards (25-18).

Substance Abuse

Goal: Reduce substance abuse to protect the health, safety, and quality of life of all, especially children.

1. Reduce deaths and injuries caused by alcohol- and drug-related motor vehicle crashes (26-1).
2. Reduce drug-induced deaths [and hospital emergency department visits] (26-3, 26-4).
3. Reduce the proportion of adolescents who report that they rode, during the previous 30 days, with a driver who had been drinking alcohol (26-6).
4. Reduce intentional injuries resulting from alcohol- and illicit drug-related violence (26-7).
5. Increase the proportion of adolescents who remain alcohol and drug free.
6. Reduce past-month use of illicit substances (26-10).
7. Reduce the proportion of persons engaging in binge drinking of alcoholic beverages (26-11).
8. Reduce steroid use among adolescents (26-14).
9. Reduce the proportion of adolescents who use nonprescribed inhalants (26-15).
10. Increase the proportion of adolescents who disapprove of substance abuse (26-16).
11. Increase the proportion of adolescents who perceive great risk associated with substance abuse (26-17).
12. Increase the proportion of persons who are referred for follow-up care for alcohol problems, drug problems, or suicide attempts after diagnosis or treatment for one of these conditions in a hospital emergency department (26-22).

Tobacco Use

Goal: Reduce illness, disability, and death related to tobacco use and exposure to secondhand smoke.

1. Reduce tobacco use by adults (27-1).
2. Reduce tobacco use by adolescents. Increase by at least 1 year the average age of first use of tobacco products by adolescents (27-2).
3. Reduce the initiation of tobacco use among children and adolescents (27-3).
4. Increase the average age of first use of tobacco products by adolescents and young adults (27-4).
5. Increase tobacco use cessation attempts by adolescent smokers (27-7).
6. Reduce the proportion of children who are regularly exposed to tobacco smoke at home (27-9).
7. Reduce the proportion of nonsmokers exposed to environmental tobacco smoke (27-10).
8. Increase tobacco-free environments in schools, including all school facilities, property, vehicles, and school events (27-11).
9. Reduce the illegal sales rate to minors through enforcement of laws prohibiting the sale of tobacco products to minors (27-14).
10. Increase the number of States and the District of Columbia that suspend or revoke State retail licenses for violations of laws prohibiting the sale of tobacco to minors (27-15).
11. Eliminate tobacco advertising and promotions that influence adolescents and young adults (27-16).

Vision and Hearing

Goal: Improve the visual and hearing health of the Nation through prevention, early detection, treatment, and rehabilitation.

1. Increase the proportion of preschool children age 5 years and under who receive vision screening (28-2).
2. Reduce uncorrected visual impairment due to refractive errors (28-3).

3. Reduce blindness and visual impairments in children and adolescents age 17 years and under (28-4).
4. Increase the use of appropriate personal protective eyewear in recreational activities and hazardous situations around the home (28-9).
5. Increase the proportion of newborns who are screened for hearing loss by age 1 month, have audiologic evaluation by age 3 months, and are enrolled in appropriate intervention services by age 6 months.
6. Reduce otitis media in children and adolescents (28-12).
7. Increase the use of appropriate ear protection devices, equipment, and practices (28-16).
8. Reduce noise-induced hearing loss in children and adolescents age 17 years and under (28-17).

REFERENCE

US Department of Health and Human Services: *Healthy people 2010: understanding and improving health*, ed 2, Washington, DC, Nov 2000, US Government Printing Office.

Index

Page numbers followed by "f" denote figures, "t" denote tables, and "b" denote boxes.

B

F

O

DISEASES AND ICD-9-CM CODES

Abdominal mass 789.3
Abdominal pain 789.0
Abrasion (noninfected) 919.0
Abscess 682.9
Acanthosis nigricans 701.2
Acne 706.1
Allergic rhinitis 477.9
Allergy, allergic reaction 995.3
Alopecia 704.00
Amblyopia 368.00
Amenorrhea 626.0
Anaphylaxis 995.0
Anal fissure 565.0
Anemia 285.9
  autoimmune hemolytic 283.0
  iron deficiency 280.9
Anorexia nervosa 307.1
Anxiety 300.00
Apnea, neonatorum 770.81
  with sleep 780.57
Apophysitis 732.9
Appendicitis 540.9
Arthritis, juvenile 714.30
Asthma 493.9
Attention deficit/Hyperactivity disorder 314.01
Autism 299.0
Back pain 724.5
Bacteremia 790.7
Behavior problem 312.9
Behavior disorder V71.02
Bereavement V62.82
Bite/sting 919.4
Birth control counseling/advice V25.09
Birth injuries 767.9
Bleeding 459.0
Breast feeding difficulties 676.8
Bronchiolitis 466.19
Bronchitis 490
Bronchopulmonary dysplasia 770.7
Bulimia 783.6
Burn 949.0
Cafe-au-lait spots 709.09
Candidiasis, unspecified 112.89
Caries, dental 521.00
Celiac disease 579.0
Cellulitis 682.9
Cephalhematoma, newborn 767.1
Cerebral palsy 343.9
Cerumen, impacted 380.4
Cervical adenitis 289.3
Cervicitis 616.0
Checkup, health V70.0
Checkup, newborn V20.2
Child abuse, unspecified 995.50
Child behavior causing concern V61.20
Chlamydial infection, unspecified 079.98
Colic 789.0
Conduct disorder childhood 312.81
Congenital heart disease 746.9
Conjunctivitis 372.30
Constipation 564.00
Constitutional states in development V21
Contraception V25
Contusion 924.9
Convulsions 780.39
Cough 786.2
Counseling V65.40
  counseling on injury prevention V65.43
Croup 464.4
Cryptorchidism 752.51
Cyanosis 782.5
Cystic fibrosis 277.00
Cystitis 595.9
Dacryocystitis 375.30
Deafness 389.9
Deficient diet 269.9
Deformity 738.9
Dehydration 276.5
Depression 311
Dermatitis 692.9
  atopic (eczema) 691.8
  contact 692.9
  diaper 691.10
  seborrheic 691.10
Development delayed 783.40
Development delayed, sexual 259.0
Diabetes mellitus 250.0
Dietary surveillance and counseling V65.3
Diarrhea 787.91
Diminished vision 369.9
Drug reactions, adverse 995.2
Dyslexia, developmental 315.02
Earache 388.70
Eating disorders 307.50
Eczema 692.9
Educational circumstances V62.3
Effusion, joint 719.00
Encephalitis 323.9
Encopresis 787.6
Endocrine, nutritional, metabolic special screening V77
Enuresis 788.30
Epiglottitis 464.30
Epilepsy 345.9
Epistaxis 784.7
Erythema multiforme 695.1
Examination V70.9
  annual V70
  for bacterial and spirochetes, special screening V74
  cervical, Pap V76.2
  child care V20.2
  developmental test V20.2
  ear V72.21
  followup disease V67.59
  general medical V70
  gynecological V72.3
    for contraception V25.40
  health
    infant V20.2
    preschool V70.5
    child V20.2
    school V70.5
  hearing V72.1
Eye deviation 378.87
Failure to thrive 783.4
Family disruption V61.0
Fatigue 780.79
Feeding problem 783.3
  newborn 779.3
Fetal alcohol syndrome 760.71
Fever 780.6
  newborn 778.4
Fifth disease 057.0
Flat feet 734
Floppy infant 781.99
Follow-up examination, unspecified V67.9
Food allergy 693.1
Folliculitis 704.8
Foreign body aspiration 933.1
Fracture 829.0
Fungal infections 117.9
Gait abnormality 781.2
Gastrointestinal reflux 530.81
Gastrointestinal disorders 536.9
Gastroenteritis, viral 558.9
Genu valgum 736.41
Genu varum 736.42
Giardiasis 007.1
Gingivitis 523.1
Glomerulonephritis 583.9
Gonorrhea 098.0
Granuloma 686.1
Group B streptococcal infection 041.02
Group A beta hemolytic infection ______
Gynecomastia 611.1
Hand-foot-mouth disease 074.3
Headache 784.0
Health advice V65.4
  checkup V70.0
  education V65.4
Health problems within family V61.4
  alcoholism within family V61.41
Health supervision of infant or child V20
Hearing loss 389.9
Heart murmur 785.2
Hemangioma 228.0

Source: ICD-9-CM Expert for Physicians, vol 1 and 2. *International Classification of Diseases*, 9th revision, clinical modification 2002, Salt Lake City, UT, 2002, Ingenix.

Continued

Hematuria 599.7
Hemolytic uremic syndrome 283.11
Hemorrhagic disease 287.9
Hepatitis 573.3
Hepatosplenomegaly 571.8
Hernia 553.9
Herpangina 074.0
Herpes simplex virus infection 054.9
High risk sexual behavior V69.2
Hip dysplasia 755.63
Hordeolum (stye) 373.11
Human immunodeficiency virus infection 042
Hydrocele 603.9
Hydrocephalus 331.4
Hypercholesterolemia 272.0
Hypertension 401
Hyperthermia 780.6
Hypogammaglobulinemia, transient of infancy 279.09
Hypoglycemia 251.2
Hypospadias 752.61
Hypothyroidism 244.9
Immunization V05.9
Impetigo 684
Inappropriate diet and eating habits V69.1
Influenza 487.1
Infection 136.9
Infections, congenital 771.89
Ingrown toenail 703.0
Injury 959.9
Intolerance, milk/food 579.8
Irritability (nervous) 799.2
Itch 698.9
Jaundice 782.4
Jaundice, newborn 774.3
Jealousy, sibling 313.3
Kawasaki syndrome 446.1
Keloid 701.4
Kyphosis 737.10
Labial adhesions 752.49
Laceration 998.2
Lack of
- education V62.3
- food 994.2
- housing V60.0

Lactation disorder 676.9
Language disorder – developmental defect 315.31
Laryngitis 464.00
Legal circumstances V62.5
Legg-Calve-Perthes 732.21
Lethargy 780.79
Leukocoria 360.44
Lipid metabolism disorders 272.9
Lice 132.9
Lordosis 737.20
Low birth weight 765.1
Lower respiratory infection 519.8
Lymphadenopathy 785.6
Malaise and fatigue 780.79
Mastoiditis 383.9
Meconium aspiration 770.1
Meningitis 322.9
Menstrual disorders 626.9
Mental and behavioral problems V40
Mental disorders and development, special screening V79
Mental deficiency 319
Metatarsus adductus/valgus 754.60
Microcephaly 742.1
Migraine syndromes 346.0
Misuse of drugs 305.9
Molluscum contagiosum 078.0
Mononucleosis, infectious 075
Movement disorder 339.90
Murmur, functional 785.2
Muscle spasm 728.85
MVA V71.4
Nasal congestion 478.1
Nausea 787.02
Neglect 995.52
Nephrotic syndrome 581.9
Neutrophilic leukocytosis 288.8
Nevus, pigmented (M8720/0) 239.5
Newborn infant, single V30
Noncompliance with treatment V15.81
Nosebleed 784.7
Nystagmus 379.50
Obesity 278.00
Osgood-Schlatter Disease 732.4
Otalgia 388.70
Otitis externa (Swimmer's ear) 380.10
Otitis media 382.9
- serous 381.4
- with rupture 382.01

Parasitic infections 136.9
Parent-child problems V61.2
Pectus excavatum 754.81
Pediculosis 132.9
Pelvic inflammatory disease 614.9
Peptic ulcer disease 533.9
Perforated tympanic membrane 384.81
Pharyngitis 462
Phimosis 605
Pinworms 127.4
Pityriasis rosea 368.13
Physical abuse 995.54
Pica 307.52
Pigmented skin lesions 709.00
Pityriasis rosea 696.3
Platelet disorders (thrombocytopenia) 287.1
Pneumonia 486
- mycoplasma pneumonia 483.0

Pneumothorax 512.8
Polycythemia 238.4
Posttraumatic stress disorder 308.9
Poverty/economic problem V60.2
Puberty V21.1
Puberty, precocious 259.1
Puberty, delayed 259.0
Pregnancy V22.2
Procedure not carried out due to patient decision V64.2
Proteinuria 791.0
Psoriasis 696.1
Psychosocial problem, unspecified V62.9
Pyloric stenosis 537.0
Rales 786.7
Rape V71.5
Rash 782.1
Red eye 379.93
Respiratory distress 786.09
Respiratory distress syndrome 769
Respiratory failure 518.81
Retinopathy of prematurity 362.21
Rett syndrome 330.8
Ringworm 110.9
Rhinitis, allergic 477.9
Roseola 057.8
Rotavirus 008.61
RSV 079.6
Scabies 133.0
Schizophrenia 295.9
Scoliosis 737.30
Seizures 780.30
Sepsis 038.9
Sexual abuse 995.53
Shigella 004.9
Short stature 783.43
Sickle cell disease 282.60
Sinusitis 473.9
Skin infections 686.9
Sleep disorders 780.50
Slipped capital femoral epiphysis 732.9
Small for gestational age 764.0
Social maladjustment V62.4
Speech disorder 784.5
Splenomegaly 789.2
Strep throat 034.0
Stress (emotional) 308.0
Stings 789.9
Suicide risk 300.9
Sunburn 692.71
Syncope 780.2
Tachycardia 785.0
Tachypnea 786.06
Testicular mass 608.89
Thrush 112.0
Tinea capitus 110.0
Tobacco abuse 305.1
Throat pain 784.1
Upper respiratory infection 465.9
Urinary frequency 788.41
Urinary tract infection 599.0
Vaginal discharge 623.5
Vesiculopustular rash 782.1
Viral exanthem 057.9
Viral hepatitis 070.0
Viral syndrome 079.99
Vomiting 787.03
Vulvovaginitis 616.9
Warts, viral 078.14
Weight gain 783.1
Weight loss 783.2
Wheezing 786.07